LIBRARY
University of Glasgow

ALL ITEMS ARE ISSUED SUBJECT TO RECALL

GUL 18-08

Berek & Novak's
Gynecology

Berek & Novak's
Gynecology

Fifteenth Edition

Jonathan S. Berek, MD, MMS

Professor and Chair
Department of Obstetrics and Gynecology
Stanford University School of Medicine
Director, Stanford Women's Cancer Center
Stanford Cancer Institute
Stanford, California

Editorial Assistant & Design
Deborah L. Berek, MA

Illustrations by
Timothy C. Hengst, CMI, FAMI
George Barile

Wolters Kluwer | Lippincott Williams & Wilkins
Health
Philadelphia • Baltimore • New York • London
Buenos Aires • Hong Kong • Sydney • Tokyo

Acquisitions Editor: Sonya Seigafuse
Product Manager: Nicole Walz
Vendor Manager: Alicia Jackson
Senior Manufacturing Manager: Benjamin Rivera
Marketing Manager: Kimberly Schonberger
Design Coordinator: Holly Reid McLaughlin
Production Service: Aptara, Inc.

Printed in the United States of America
Not authorised for Sale in North America or the Caribbean
CIP data available upon request

ISBN-13: 978-1-4511-7556-1
ISBN-10: 1-4511-7556-6

Care has been taken to confirm the accuracy of the information presented and to describe generally accepted practices. However, the authors, editors, and publisher are not responsible for errors or omissions or for any consequences from application of the information in this book and make no warranty, expressed or implied, with respect to the currency, completeness, or accuracy of the contents of the publication. Application of the information in a particular situation remains the professional responsibility of the practitioner.

The authors, editors, and publisher have exerted every effort to ensure that drug selection and dosage set forth in this text are in accordance with current recommendations and practice at the time of publication. However, in view of ongoing research, changes in government regulations, and the constant flow of information relating to drug therapy and drug reactions, the reader is urged to check the package insert for each drug for any change in indications and dosage and for added warnings and precautions. This is particularly important when the recommended agent is a new or infrequently employed drug.

Some drugs and medical devices presented in the publication have Food and Drug Administration (FDA) clearance for limited use in restricted research settings. It is the responsibility of the health care provider to ascertain the FDA status of each drug or device planned for use in their clinical practice.

To purchase additional copies of this book, call our customer service department at (800) 638-3030 or fax orders to (301) 223-2320. International customers should call (301) 223-2300.

Visit Lippincott Williams & Wilkins on the Internet: at LWW.com. Lippincott Williams & Wilkins customer service representatives are available from 8:30 am to 6 pm, EST.

10 9 8 7 6 5 4 3 2 1

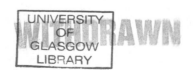

To Deborah—together in life and in print.

Contributors

Lisa N. Abaid, MD, MPH

Gynecologic Oncology Associates
Newport Beach, California

Jean R. Anderson, MD

Professor
Department of Gynecology and Obstetrics
Johns Hopkins University School of Medicine
Baltimore, Maryland

Mira Aubuchon, MD

Assistant Professor
Department of Obstetrics, Gynecology and
    Women's Health
University of Missouri School of Medicine
Columbia, Missouri

Valerie L. Baker, MD

Assistant Professor
Department of Obstetrics and Gynecology
Stanford University School of Medcine
Stanford, California

David A. Baram, MD

Clinical Assistant Professor
Department of Obstetrics and Gynecology
University of Minnesota School of Medicine
Regions Hospital
St. Paul, Minnesota

Rosemary Basson, MD

Clinical Professor
Departments of Psychiatry and Obstetrics & Gynecology
University of British Columbia
University of British Columbia Centre for Sexual Medicine
Vancouver, Canada

Ross S. Berkowitz, MD

William H. Baker Professor of Gynecology
Department of Obstetrics and Gynecology
Harvard Medical School
Director of Gynecology and Gynecologic Oncology
Brigham and Women's Hospital
Dana Farber Cancer Institute
Boston, Massachusetts

Andrew I. Brill, MD

Director of Minimally Invasive Gynecology
Department of Obstetrics and Gynecology
California Pacific Medical Center
San Francisco, California

Lieutenant Colonel Richard O. Burney, MD, MSc

Department of Obstetrics and Gynecology
Madigan Healthcare System
United States Army Medical Command
Tacoma, Washington

Joanna M. Cain, MD

Professor and Vice Chair
Department of Obstetrics and Gynecology
University of Massachusetts Medical School
Worcester, Massachusetts

Daniel L. Clarke-Pearson, MD

Robert A. Ross Distinguished Professor and Chair
Department of Obstetrics and Gynecology
University of North Carolina
Physician and Chief
North Carolina Women's Hospital
University of North Carolina Hospitals
Chapel Hill, North Carolina

Daniel W. Cramer, MD, ScD

Professor
Department of Epidemiology
Harvard Medical School
Boston, Massachusetts

Geoffrey W. Cundiff, MD

Professor and Head
Department of Obstetrics and Gynecology
University of British Columbia
Vancouver Coastal Health
Vancouver, British Columbia

Jessie Dorais, MD

Visiting Instructor
Department of Obstetrics and Gynecology
Division of Reproductive Endocrinology
University of Utah Health Care
Utah Center for Reproductive Medicine
Salt Lake City, Utah

Thomas M. D'Hooghe, MD, PhD

Professor
Department of Reproduction, Regeneration &
    Development
Leuven University
Director, Leuven University Fertility Center
Leuven, Belgium

Oliver Dorigo, MD, PhD

Assistant Professor
Division of Gynecologic Oncology
Department of Obstetrics and Gynecology
David Geffen School of Medicine at UCLA
Los Angeles, California

Sean C. Dowdy, MD,

Associate Professor
Department of Obstetrics and Gynecology
Co-Program Leader, Women's Cancer Program
Mayo Clinic
Rochester, Minnesota

John C. Elkas, MD, JD

Associate Professor
Department of Obstetrics and Gynecology
Virginia Commonwealth University,
  Inova Fairfax Campus
Inova Fairfax Hospital
Falls Church, Virginia

Tommaso Falcone, MD

Professor and Chair
Department of Obstetrics and Gynecology
Cleveland Clinic
Cleveland, Ohio

Carrie E. Frederick, MD

Clinical Instructor
Division of Family Planning
Department of Obstetrics and Gynecology
Stanford University School of Medicine
Sanford, California

Michael L. Friedlander, MBCHB, PhD

Conjoint Professor
University of New South Wales
Prince of Wales Cancer Centre
Sydney, Australia

Joseph C. Gambone, DO, MPH

Professor Emeritus
Department of Obstetrics and Gynecology
David Geffen School of Medicine at UCLA
Los Angeles, California

Francisco Garcia, MD, MPH

Distinguished Outreach Professor
Departments of Public, Health, Obstetrics and Gynecology,
  Clinical Pharmacy, and Nursing
University of Arizona
University Medical Center
Tucson, Arizona

Tracy W. Gaudet, MD

Director
Veteran's Health Administration
Office of Patient-Centered Care and Cultural Transformation
Washington, DC

Armando E. Giuliano, MD

Clinical Professor of Surgery
David Geffen School of Medicine at UCLA
Executive Vice Chair, Surgery
Cedars-Sinai Medical Center
Los Angeles, California

Jonathan L. Gleason, MD

Instructor
Department of Obstetrics and Gynecology
University of Alabama at Birmingham
Birmingham, Alabama

Rene Genadry, MD

Associate Professor
Department of Gynecology and Obstetrics
Johns Hopkins University School of Medicine
Baltimore, Maryland

Donald P. Goldstein, MD

Professor
Department of Obstetrics and Gynecology
Harvard Medical School
Brigham and Women's Hospital
Boston, Massachusetts

Baiba J. Grube, MD

Department of Oncology & General Surgery
Yale School of Medicine
New Haven, Connecticut

Robert E. Gutman, MD

Associate Professor
Department of Obstetrics and Gynecology and
  Urology
Georgetown University
Fellowship Director, Female Pelvic Medicine and
  Reconstructive Surgery
Washington Hospital Center
Washington, DC

Kenneth D. Hatch, MD

Professor
Department of Obstetrics and Gynecology
University of Arizona School of Medicine
Tucson, Arizona

Paula J. Adams Hillard, MD

Professor
Department of Obstetrics and Gynecology
Stanford University School of Medicine
Stanford, California

Christine H. Holschneider, MD

Associate Professor
Department of Obstetrics and Gynecology
David Geffen School of Medicine at UCLA
Los Angeles, California
Chair, Department of Obstetrics and Gynecology
Olive View-UCLA Medical Center
Sylmar, California

John P. Keats, MD

Medical Director, Perinatal Safety
Catholic Healthcare West
San Francisco, Californina

Emily Ko, MD

Clinical Fellow
Division of Gynecologic Oncology
University of North Carolina
Chapel Hill, North Carolina

Oumar Kuzbari, MD

Visiting Instructor
Department of Obstetrics and Gynecology
Division of General Obstetrics and Gynecology
University of Utah Health Care
Utah Center for Reproductive Medicine
Salt Lake City, Utah

Ruth Bunker Lathi, MD

Assistant Professor
Division of Reproductive Endocrinology
Department of Obstetrics and Gynecology
Stanford University School of Medicine
Stanford, California

Camelia A. Lawrence, MD

Breast Surgeon
United Health Services
Wilson Medical Center
Johnson City, New York

Teri A. Longacre, MD

Professor
Department of Pathology
Stanford University School of Medicine
Stanford, California

John R. Lurain, MD

Marcia Stenn Professor of Gynecologic Oncology
Department of Obstetrics and Gynecology
Northwestern University Feinberg School of Medicine
Chicago, Illinois

Javier F. Magrina, MD

Professor
Department of Gynecology
Mayo Clinic Arizona
Director, Gynecologic Oncology
Mayo Clinic Hospital
Phoenix, Arizona

Andrea Mariani, MD

Associate Professor
Department of Obstetrics and Gynecology
Mayo Clinic
Rochester, Minnesota

Otoniel Martínez-Maza, PhD

Professor
Department of Obstetics and Gynecology
David Geffen School of Medicine at UCLA
Los Angeles, California

Howard D. McClamrock, MD

Chief
Division of Reproductive Endocrinology and Infertility
Departments of Obstetrics, Gynecology and Reproductive
 Sciences
University of Maryland
Baltimore, Maryland
Shady Grove Fertility Reproductive Sciences Center
Rockville, MD

Shawn A. Menefee, MD

Associate Clinical Professor
Department of Reproductive Medicine
University of California, San Diego
San Diego, California

Caela R. Miller MD

Assistant Professor
Division of Gynecologic Oncology
Department of Obstetrics and Gynecology
Uniformed Services University of the Health Sciences
Walter Reed National Military Medical Center
Bethesda, Maryland

Malcolm G. Munro, MD

Clinical Professor
Department of Obstetrics & Gynecology
David Geffen School of Medicine at UCLA
Director of Gynecologic Services
Kaiser Permanente, Los Angeles Medical Center
Los Angeles, California

Leena Nathan, MD

Department of Obstetrics and Gynecology
David Geffen School of Medicine at UCLA
Los Angeles, California

Antonia F. Nicosia, MD

Clinical Assistant Professor
Division of Family Planning
Department of Obstetrics and Gynecology
Stanford University School of Medicine
Stanford, California

Thomas E. Nolan, MD, MBA

Professor and Department Head Emeritus
Department of Obstetrics and Gynecology
Louisiana State University Health Science
    Center-New Orleans
New Orleans, Louisiana

Ingrid Nygaard, MD, MS

Professor
Department of Obstetrics and Gynecology
Division of Urogynecology and Pelvic
    Reconstructive Surgery
University of Utah School of Medicine
Salt Lake City, Utah

David L. Olive, MD

Attending Physician
Department of Obstetrics and Gynecology
Meriter Hospital
Wisconsin Fertility Institute
Middleton, Wisconsin

Junko Ozao-Choy, MD

John Wayne Cancer Institute
Santa, Monica, California

Steven F. Palter, MD

Medical Director
Gold Coast IVF
Syosset, New York

William H. Parker, MD

Clinical Professor
Department of Obstetrics and Gynecology
David Geffen School of Medicine at UCLA
Los Angeles, California
Adjunct Faculty
John Wayne Cancer Institute
Santa Monica, California

Arasen A. V. Paupoo, MD, MA

Assistant Professor and Director
Division of Reproductive Endocrinology and Infertlity
Department of Obstetrics and Gynecology
Creighton University School of Medicine
Omaha, Nebraska

C. Matthew Peterson, MD

John A. Dixon Presidential Professor and Chair
Department of Obstetrics and Gynecology
University of Utah School of Medicine
University Hospital
Salt Lake City, Utah

Sharon T. Phelan, MD

Professor
Department of Obstetrics and Gynecology
Health Science Center School of Medicine
University of New Mexico
Albuquerque, New Mexico

Maureen G. Phipps, MD, MPH

Associate Professor
Departments of Obstetrics and Gynecology and
    Community Health
Warren Alpert Medical School of Brown University
Women & Infants Hospital of Rhode Island
Providence, Rhode Island

Andrea J. Rapkin, MD

Professor
Department of Obstetrics and Gynecology
David Geffen School of Medicine at UCLA
Los Angeles, California

Robert W. Rebar, MD

Executive Director
American Society for Reproductive Medicine
Birmingham, Alabama

Holly E. Richter, PhD, MD

Professor and Division Director
Department of Obstetrics and Gynecology
University of Alabama at Birmingham
Birmingham, Alabama

Danielle M. Roncari, MD, MPH

Assistant Professor
Department of Obstetrics and Gynecology
Tufts New England Medical Center
Boston, Massachusetts

Isaac Schiff, MD

Joe Vincent Meigs Professor of Gynecology
Harvard Medical School
Chief, Obstetrics and Gynecology Service
Massachusetts General Hospital
Boston, Massachusetts

Wendy J. Schillings, MD

Department of Obstetrics and Gynecology
Division of Reproductive Endocrinology &
    Infertility/Gynecology
Lehigh Valley Health Network
Allentown, Pennsylvania

Kevin M. Schuler, MD

Fellow
Division of Gynecologic Oncology
Department of Obstetrics and Gynecology
University of North Carolina at Chapel Hill
Chapel Hill, North Carolina

Danny J. Schust, MD

Associate Professor
Department of Obstetrics, Gynecology and Women's Health
University of Missouri
Columbia, Missouri

Jan L. Shifren, MD

Associate Professor
Department of Obstetrics, Gynecology and
   Reproductive Biology
Harvard Medical School
Director, Vincent Menopause Program
Massachusetts General Hospital
Boston, Massachusetts

Eric R. Sokol, MD

Assistant Professor of Obstetrics and Gynecology, and
   Urology (Courtesy)
Co-Chief, Division of Urogynecology and Pelvic
   Reconstructive Surgery
Stanford University School of Medicine
Stanford, California

David E. Soper, MD

Professor and Vice Chair
Department of Obstetrics and Gynecology
Medical University of South Carolina
Charleston, South Carolina

Nada Logan Stotland, MD, MPH

Professor
Department of Psychiatry
Rush Medical College
Chicago, Illinois

Thomas G. Stovall, MD

Clinical Professor
Department of Obstetrics and Gynecology
University of Tennessee, Memphis
Memphis, Tennessee

Phillip Stubblefield, MD

Emeritus Professor
Department of Obstetrics and
   Gynecology
Boston University School of Medicine
Boston Medical Center
Boston, Massachusetts

R. Edward Varner, MD

Professor
Department of Obstetrics and Gynecology
University of Alabama at Birmingham
Birmingham, Alabama

Amy J. Voedisch, MD, MS

Clinical Instructor
Division of Family Planning
Department of Obstetrics and Gynecology
Stanford University School of Medicine
Stanford, California

Mylene W. M. Yao, MD

Chief Executive Officer
UNIVFY
Palo Alto, California

Foreword

Emil Novak of Johns Hopkins University School of Medicine and Hospital edited the ***Textbook of Gynecology***, which was first published in 1941, and remained the standard in the field for many years thereafter. The 14th edition of that landmark text, published in 2007, was given a new title, ***Berek and Novak's Gynecology***, honoring both Dr. Jonathan S. Berek and the late Dr. Novak, whose significant contributions sustained and, where necessary, recalibrated the work through several previous editions, thereby preserving its vitality and relevance for new generations of physicians. The book retains its prominence as one of the major comprehensive textbooks in the discipline, a status it is certain to maintain in the 15th edition.

For this edition, Dr. Berek again assembled an impressive array of contributors—clinicians and researchers, leaders in their respective fields—who bring insightful knowledge and valuable perspectives to their respective areas of expertise. The result is a comprehensive treatment of current practice—but with an eye toward future developments—in the science and practice of gynecology and its related subspecialties. Innovative developments in research and clinical practice are treated in detail. For example, in keeping with the expansion of one gynecologic subspecialty, the chapters on pelvic reconstruction and urogynecology are necessary reading for comprehension of this growing discipline. The substantially expanded field of minimally invasive gynecologic surgery is covered thoroughly in the chapters dealing with endoscopy, hysterectomy, and robotics. Not surprising, given Dr. Berek's reputation as a leader and innovator in gynecologic oncology, this textbook indisputably remains the definitive encyclopedia on that subject. The basic science section is intertwined beautifully with the principles of practice, promoting an understanding of the many changes in clinical medicine in recent years. Compassion and sensitivity are evident throughout the work, especially in the sections dealing with sexuality and related sexual issues.

The traditional areas of gynecology are presented in an exciting format with all the information the practicing gynecologist requires in order to provide excellent patient care. Another attractive feature is that it is published with substantial full-color illustrations and graphics that greatly enhance the readability and accessibility of the material.

Practitioners of the medical specialty of gynecology, both clinicians and researchers, are wholly dedicated to the care and well-being of women. As both a teaching tool and reference, this new edition of ***Berek and Novak's Gynecology*** will prove to be, as previous editions were, an invaluable asset to them as they ply their important work.

Isaac Schiff, MD
Joe Vincent Meigs Professor of Gynecology
Harvard Medical School
Chief, Vincent Obstetrics and Gynecology Service
Massachusetts General Hospital
Boston, Massachusetts

The first edition of *Novak's Textbook of Gynecology*, written by the distinguished Dr. Emil Novak of Johns Hopkins, became a successful and important international reference for the practice of gynecology. This edition is the carefully nurtured descendant of that book and retains the useful format of the prior three editions of the text, enhanced by full-color illustrations and photographic reproductions.

As with the previous editions, the goal is to provide a comprehensive summary of the specialty of gynecology. All chapters were thoroughly revised to provide timely information and references. The illustrations and photographs were updated and made more accessible and informative. Two new chapters are added to the 15th edition—one on uterine fibroids to expand the discussion on this most common of problems for women, and another on robotic surgery to address the increased utilization of this technology in gynecologic operations.

This textbook, originated by the faculty of the Johns Hopkins University School of Medicine, continues to reflect the contributions of that great institution. After the 5th edition and subsequent death of Dr. Novak in 1957, many physicians from Johns Hopkins, and subsequently some members of the Vanderbilt faculty, helped carry the torch—Dr. Edmund R. Novak through the ninth edition in 1979; Drs. Howard W. Jones, Jr. and Georgeanna Seegar Jones through the 10th edition in 1981; and Drs. Howard W. Jones, III, Lonnie S. Burnett, and Anne Colston Wentz through the 11th edition in 1988. These editors, assisted by many contributors from the faculty at Johns Hopkins, especially Drs. J. Donald Woodruff and Conrad G. Julian, helped define the specialty of gynecology during the latter half of the 20th century. These physicians shaped the practice of gynecology as we know it today—its surgical and medical therapies, reproductive endocrinology, assisted reproductive technologies, gynecologic oncology, urogynecology, and infectious diseases. As a graduate of Johns Hopkins University School of Medicine, I am proud to contribute to that rich tradition.

Berek & Novak's Gynecology, 15th edition, is presented in eight sections. The first section, Principles of Practice, includes the initial assessment of the gynecologic patient, the history and physical examination, and communication skills. This section addresses ethical principles of patient care, quality assessment and improvement, and the epidemiology of gynecologic conditions. The second section, Basic Principles, summarizes the scientific basis for the specialty—anatomy and embryology, molecular biology and genetics, and reproductive physiology. The third section, Preventive and Primary Care, emphasizes the importance of primary health care for women, which has evolved to address preventive care, screening, family planning, sexuality, and common psychiatric problems. The fourth section, General Gynecology, reviews benign diseases of the female reproductive tract, the evaluation of pelvic infections, uterine fibroids, pain, intraepithelial diseases, the management of early pregnancy loss and ectopic pregnancy, and the evaluation of benign breast disease. The fifth section, Operative General Gynecology, covers perioperative care and the operative management of benign gynecologic conditions using endoscopy, hysterectomy and robotics. The sixth section is Urogynecology and Pelvic Reconstructive Surgery. The seventh section, Reproductive Endocrinology, summarizes the major disorders affecting the growth, development, and function of women from puberty through menopause. The eighth section, Gynecologic Oncology, covers malignant diseases of the female reproductive tract and breast cancer.

I gratefully acknowledge the many individuals who contributed to this book. I extend my thanks to Tim Hengst, an outstanding medical illustrator, for the excellent illustrations, anatomic drawings, and thematic designs. I am especially grateful to my talented content editor, Deborah Berek, who diligently evaluated and assisted the entire project from the initial manuscripts through page proofs. I appreciate the many people at Lippincott Williams & Wilkins who helped me, especially Charley Mitchell, whom I consider the best editor in medical book publishing and with whom I worked for over a quarter of a century. I extend my gratitude to Sonya Seigafuse and Nicole Walz for their dedication and commitment to enthusiastically and skillfully shepherd the manuscript during the editorial process. I acknowledge the outstanding work of Chris Miller who diligently and expertly worked with me to accomplish the final page layout and formatting of this book. I acknowledge the support of my past mentors—Dean Sherman Mellinkoff, Drs. J. Donald Woodruff, Kenneth J. Ryan, J. George Moore, and William J. Dignam—and I extend my gratitude to my current colleagues Drs. Isaac Schiff, Gautam Chaudhuri, Neville F. Hacker, Beverly Mitchell, and Dean Philip Pizzo. Each of these physicians and scholars graciously provided me with essential guidance and encouragement. My special thanks to Laurie Lacob, Nicole Kidman and Keith Urban, Trisha Yearwood and Garth Brooks for their support of the Stanford Women's Cancer Center—and for their help, encouragement, and friendship that stimulated this project.

The publication of this book marks 6 years of my tenure at the Stanford University School of Medicine. The generosity of spirit and commitment to the cause of women and their health that guides the work of my colleagues at Stanford has been a pleasure and inspiration for me. The local community outside of the university shares this commitment to improving the health and welfare of women, and I am gratified by their efforts to make a difference in the kind of care that is available to women and their families.

I look forward to the specialty's continued positive impact of on the health of women throughout the world. It is my fervent hope that our work will benefit all women and reduce the numbers of those who are afflicted with diseases of the female reproductive tract and the breast. To that end, this book is offered as a resource to assist and encourage all who study the specialty of gynecology.

Jonathan S. Berek

Contents

PRINCIPLES
OF PRACTICE

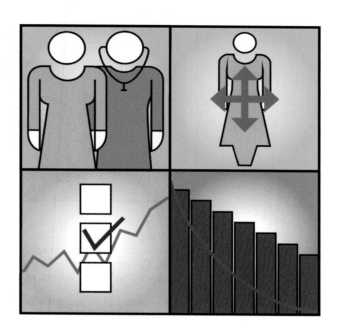

1 Initial Assessment and Communication

Jonathan S. Berek
Paula J. Adams Hillard

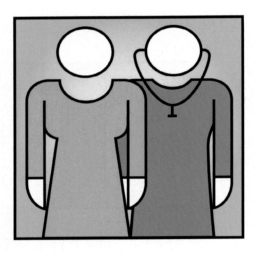

- We are all products of our environment, our background, and our culture. The importance of ascertaining the patient's general, social, and familial situation cannot be overemphasized. The physician should avoid being judgmental, particularly with respect to questions about sexual practices and sexual orientation.

- Good communication is essential to patient assessment and treatment. The foundation of communication is based on key skills: empathy, attentive listening, expert knowledge, and rapport. These skills can be learned and refined.

- The Hippocratic Oath demands that physicians be circumspect with all patient-related information. For physician–patient communication to be effective, the patient must feel that she is able to discuss her problems in depth and in confidence.

- Different styles of communication may affect the physician's ability to perceive the patient's status and to achieve the goal of optimal assessment and successful treatment. The intimate and highly personal nature of many gynecologic conditions requires particular sensitivity to evoke an honest response.

- Some patients lack accurate information about their illnesses. Incomplete or inadequate understanding of an illness can produce dissatisfaction with medical care, increased anxiety, distress, coping difficulties, unsuccessful treatment, and poor treatment response.

- After a dialogue is established, the patient assessment proceeds with obtaining a complete history and performing a physical examination. Both of these aspects of the assessment rely on good patient–physician interchange and attention to details.

- At the completion of the physical examination, the patient should be informed of the findings. When the results of the examination are normal, the patient can be reassured accordingly. When there is a possible abnormality, the patient should be informed immediately; this discussion should take place after the examination, with the patient clothed.

The practice of gynecology requires many skills. In addition to medical knowledge, the gynecologist should develop interpersonal and communication skills that promote patient–physician interaction and trust. The assessment must be of the "whole patient," not only of her general medical status. It should include any apparent medical condition as well as the psychological, social, and family aspects of her situation. **To view the patient in the appropriate context, environmental and cultural issues that affect the patient must be taken into account.** This approach is valuable in routine assessments, and in the assessment of specific medical conditions, providing opportunities for preventive care and counseling on an ongoing basis.

Variables that Affect Patient Status

Many external variables exert an influence on the patient and on the care she receives. Some of these factors include the patient's "significant others"—her family, friends, and personal and intimate relationships (Table 1.1). **These external variables include psychological, genetic, biologic, social, and economic issues.** Factors that affect a patient's perception of disease and pain and the means by which she has been taught to cope with illness include her education, attitudes, understanding of human reproduction and sexuality, and family history of disease (1–3). Cultural factors, socioeconomic status, religion, ethnicity, language, age, and sexual orientation are important considerations in understanding the patient's response to her care.

We are all products of our environment, our background, and our culture. The importance of ascertaining the patient's general, social, and familial situation cannot be overemphasized (4). Cultural sensitivity may be particularly important in providing reproductive health care (5).

The context of the patient's family can and should be ascertained directly. The family history should include a careful analysis of those who had significant illnesses, such as cancer or an illness that the patient perceives to be a potential explanation for her own symptoms. The patient's perspective of her illness can provide important information that informs the physician's judgment; specific questioning to elicit this perspective can improve satisfaction with the interaction (6).

Table 1.1 Variables that Influence the Status of the Patient
Patient
Age
History of illness
Attitudes and perceptions
Sexual orientation
Habits (e.g., use of alcohol, tobacco, and other drugs)
Family
Patient's status (e.g., married, separated, living with a partner, divorced)
Caregiving (e.g., young children, children with disabilities, aging parents)
Siblings (e.g., number, ages, closeness of relationship)
History (e.g., disease)
Environment
Social environment (e.g., community, social connectedness)
Economic status (e.g., poverty, insuredness)
Religion (e.g., religiosity, spirituality)
Culture and ethnic background (e.g., first language, community)
Career (e.g., work environment, satisfaction, responsibilities, stress)

The patient's understanding of key events in the family medical history and how they relate to her is important. The patient's sexual history, relationships, and practices should be understood, and her functional level of satisfaction in these areas should be determined. **The physician should avoid being judgmental, particularly with respect to questions about sexual practices and sexual orientation** (see Chapter 11).

Communication

Good communication is essential to patient assessment and treatment. The patient–physician relationship is based on communication conducted in an open, honest, and careful manner that allows the patient's situation and problems to be accurately understood and effective solutions developed collaboratively. Good communication requires patience, dedication, and practice and involves careful listening and both verbal and nonverbal communication.

The foundation of communication is based on four key skills: empathy, attentive listening, expert knowledge, and the ability to establish rapport. These skills can be learned and refined (4,7,8). When the initial relationship with the patient is established, the physician must vigilantly pursue interviewing techniques that continue to create opportunities to foster an understanding of the patient's concerns (9). Trust is the fundamental element that encourages open communication of the patient's feelings, concerns, and thoughts, rather than withholding information (10).

One very basic element of communication—sharing a common language and culture—may be missing when a clinician interacts with a patient of limited or no English proficiency. Language concordance between physician and patient is assumed in many discussions of communication. More than 18% of Americans speak a language other than English at home, and over 8% have limited English proficiency (11). Language barriers are associated with limited health education, compromised interpersonal care, and lower patient satisfaction in health care encounters (11,12). Medical interpreters can mitigate these effects. The State of California recognized the importance of communication in patient–physician interactions through a provision in the Health and Safety Code that states "where language or communication barriers exist between patients and the staff of any general acute care hospital, arrangements shall be made for interpreters or bilingual professional staff to ensure adequate and speedy communication between patients and staff" (13). Training future physicians to work with interpreters is receiving increasing attention in United States medical schools and will contribute to improved clinical practice and reduce health care disparities (14).

Although there are many styles of interacting with patients, and each physician must determine and develop the best way that she or he can relate to patients, physicians must convey that they are able and willing to listen and that they receive the information with utmost confidentiality (1). **The Hippocratic Oath demands that physicians be circumspect with all patient-related information.** The Health Insurance Portability and Accountability Act (HIPAA), which took effect in 2003, established national standards intended to protect the privacy of personal health information. Initial fears expressed about the impact of HIPAA regulations and the potential for legal liability led to discussions of appropriate communication and physicians' judgments based on the ethical principles of confidentiality in providing good medical care (15,16) (see Chapter 2).

Communication Skills

It is essential for the physician to communicate with a patient in a manner that allows her to continue to seek appropriate medical attention. The words used, the patterns of speech, the manner in which words are delivered, even body language and eye contact, are all important aspects of the patient–physician interaction. The traditional role of the physician was paternalistic, with the physician expected to deliver direct commands or "orders" and specific guidance on all matters (4). Now patients appropriately demand and expect more balanced communication with their physicians. Although they may not have equivalent medical expertise, they do expect to be treated with appropriate deference, respect, and a manner that acknowledges their personhood as equal to that of the physician (17). Doctor–patient communication is receiving more attention in current medical education and is being recognized as a major task of lifelong professional learning and a key element of successful health care delivery (18).

As a result of electronic access to medical information, patients sometimes have more specific medical knowledge of a given medical problem than the physician does. When this is the case, the physician must avoid feeling defensive. The patient often lacks broader knowledge of the context of the problem, awareness of the variable reliability of electronic sources of information, the ability to assess a given study or journal report within an historical context or in comparison with other studies on the topic, knowledge of drug interactions, an ability to maintain objective intellectual distance from the topic, or essential experience in the art and science of medicine. The physician possesses these skills and extensive knowledge, whereas the patient has an intensely focused personal interest in her specific medical condition. Surveys of physicians' perceptions of the impact of Internet-based health information on the doctor–patient relationship found both positive and negative perceptions; physicians express concerns about a hindrance to efficient time management during an office visit, but a positive perception of the potential effects on the quality of care and patient outcomes (19). **A collaborative relationship that allows patients greater interactive involvement in the doctor–patient relationship can lead to better health outcomes** (1,20,21).

Physician–Patient Interaction

The pattern of the physician's speech can influence interactions with the patient. Some important components of effective communication between patients and physicians are presented in Table 1.2. There is evidence that scientifically derived and empirically validated interview skills can be taught and learned, and conscientious use of these skills can result in improved outcomes (8). A list of such skills is found in Table 1.3.

For physician–patient communication to be effective, the patient must feel that she is able to discuss her problems in depth and in confidence. Time constraints imposed by the pressures of office scheduling to meet economic realities make this difficult; both the physician and the patient frequently need to reevaluate their priorities. If the patient perceives that she participates in decision making and that she is given as much information as possible, she will respond to the mutually derived treatment plan with lower levels of anxiety and depression, embracing it as a collaborative plan of action. She should be able to propose alternatives or modifications to the physician's recommendations that reflect her own beliefs and attitudes. There is ample evidence that patient communication, understanding, and treatment outcomes are improved when

Table 1.2 Important Components of Communication between the Patient and Physician: The Physician's Role

The Physician Is:	The Physician Is Not:
A good listener	Confrontational
Empathetic	Combative
Compassionate	Argumentative
Honest	Condescending
Genuine	Overbearing
Respectful	Dogmatic
Fair	Judgmental
Facilitative	Paternalistic

The Physician Uses:
Understandable language
Appropriate body language
A collaborative approach
Open dialogue
Appropriate emotional content
Humor and warmth

Table 1.3 Behaviors Associated with the 14 Structural Elements of the Interview[a]

Preparing the Environment	Negotiating a Priority Problem
Create privacy	Ask patient for priorities
Eliminate noise and distractions	State own priorities
Provide comfortable seating at equal eye level	Establish mutual interests
Provide access	Reach agreement on order of addressing issues

Preparing Oneself	**Developing a Narrative Thread**
Eliminate distractions and interruptions	Develop personal ways of asking patient to tell her story
Focus	Ask when last felt healthy
Self-hypnosis	Ask about entire course of illness
Meditation	Ask about recent episode or typical episode
Constructive imaging	**Establishing the Life Context of the Patient**
Let intrusive thoughts pass through	Use first opportunity to inquire about personal and social details

Observation	Flesh out developmental history
Create a personal list of categories of observation	Learn about patient's support system
Practice in a variety of settings	Learn about home, work, neighborhood, safety
Notice physical signs	**Establishing a Safety Net**
Presentation	Memorize complete review of systems
Affect	Review issues as appropriate to specific problem
What is said and not said	**Presenting Findings and Options**

Greeting	Be succinct
Create a personal stereotypical beginning	Ascertain patient's level of understanding, cognitive style
Introduce oneself	Ask patient to review and state understanding
Check the patient's name and how it is said	Summarize and check
Create a positive social setting	Tape record and give tape to patient

Introduction	Ask patient's perspectives
Explain one's role and purpose	**Negotiating Plans**
Check patient's expectation	Activate patient
Negotiate about differences in perspective	Agree on what is feasible
Be sure expectations are congruent with patient's	Respect patient's choices whenever possible

Detecting and Overcoming Barriers to Communication	**Closing**
Develop personal list of barriers to look for	Ask patient to review plans and arrangements
Include appropriate language	Clarify what to do in the interim
Physical impediments such as deafness, delirium	Schedule next encounter
Include cultural barriers	Say goodbye
Recognize patient's psychological barriers, such as shame, fear, and paranoia	

Surveying Problems	
Develop personal methods of initiation of problem listing	
Ask "What else?" until problems are elicited	

[a]Lipkin M Jr. Physician–patient interaction in reproductive counseling. *Obstet Gynecol* 1996;88:31S–40S.

Derived from **Lipkin M, Frankel RM, Beckman HB, et al.** Performing the interview. In: **Lipkin M, Putnam SM, Lazare A,** eds. *The medical interview: clinical care, education, and research.* New York: Springer-Verlag, 1995:65–82.

discussions with physicians are more dialogue than lecture. In addition, when patients feel they have some room for negotiation, they tend to retain more information regarding health care recommendations. The concept of collaborative planning between patients and physicians is embraced as a more effective alliance than the previous model in which physicians issued orders (22). The patient thus becomes more vested in the process of determining health care choices. For example, decisions about the risks and benefits of menopausal hormone therapy must be discussed in the context of an individual's health and family history as well as her personal beliefs and goals. The woman decides whether the potential benefits outweigh the potential risks, and she is the one to determine whether or not to use such therapy. Whereas most women prefer shared decision making in the face of uncertainty, with an evidence-based discussion of her risks and benefits, others want a more directive approach (23). **The physician's challenge is to be able to personalize the interaction and communication.**

There is evidence that when patients are heard and understood, they become more vocal and inquisitive and their health improves (9). Participation facilitates investment and empowerment. **Good communication is essential to the maintenance of a relationship between the patient and physician that will foster ongoing care.** Health maintenance, therefore, can be linked directly to the influence of positive interactions between the physician and patient. Women who are comfortable with their physician may be more likely to raise issues or concerns and convey information about potential health risks and be more receptive to the physician's recommendations. This degree of rapport may promote the effectiveness of health interventions, including behavior modification. It helps ensure that patients return for regular care because they feel the physician is genuinely interested in their welfare and they have confidence in the quality of the treatment and guidance they receive.

When patients are ill, they feel vulnerable, physically and psychologically exposed, and powerless. The physician, by virtue of his or her knowledge and status, has power that can be intimidating. It is essential that the physician be aware of this disparity so the "balance of power" does not shift too far away from the patient. Shifting it back from the physician to the patient may help improve outcomes (1,20,21). Physicians' behaviors can suggest that they are not respectful of the patient. Such actions as failing to maintain scheduled appointment times, routinely holding substantive discussions when the patient is undressed, or speaking to her from a standing position while she is lying down or in the lithotomy position can emphasize the imbalance of power in the relationship.

In assessing the effects of the patient–physician interaction on the outcome of chronic illness, three characteristics associated with better health care outcomes were identified (21):

1. **An empathetic physician and a high level of patient involvement in the interview.**
2. **Expression of emotion by both patient and physician.**
3. **Provision of information by the physician in response to the patient's inquiries.**

Among patients with diabetes, these characteristics resulted in improved diastolic blood pressure and reduction of hemoglobin A_{1c}. The best responses were achieved when an empathetic physician provided as much information and clarification as possible, responded to the patients' questions openly and honestly, and expressed a full range of emotions, including humor. Responses improved when the relationship was not dominated by the physician (21).

In studies of gender and language, men tend to talk more than women, successfully interrupt women, and control the topics of the conversation (24). As a result, male physicians may tend to take control, and this imbalance of power may be magnified in the field of obstetrics and gynecology, in which all the patients are women. Male physicians may be more assertive than female physicians. Men's speech tends to be characterized by interruptions, command, and lectures, and women's speech is characterized by silence, questions, and proposals (25,26). Some patients may feel more reticent in the presence of a male physician, whereas others may be more forthcoming with a male than a female physician (27). Women's preference for a male or female physician may be based on gender as well as experience, competency, communication styles, and other skills (28,29). Although these generalizations clearly do not apply to all physicians, they can raise awareness about the various styles of communication and how they shape the physician–patient relationship (30,31). These patterns indicate that **all physicians, regardless of their gender, need to be attentive to their style of speech because it may affect their ability to elicit open and candid responses from their patients** (32–34). Women tend to express their feelings in order to validate, share, and establish an understanding of their concerns or establish a shared understanding of their concerns (22,24,25).

Different styles of communication may affect the physician's ability to perceive the patient's status and to achieve the goal of optimal assessment and successful treatment. The intimate and highly personal nature of many gynecologic conditions requires particular sensitivity to evoke an honest patient response.

Style

The art of communication and persuasion is based on mutual respect and fosters the development of the patient's understanding of the circumstances of her health. Insight is best achieved when the patient is encouraged to question her physician and when she is not pressured to make decisions. Patients who feel "backed into a corner" have the lowest compliance with recommended treatments (20).

Following are techniques to help achieve rapport with patients:

1. **Use positive language (e.g., agreement, approval, and humor).**
2. **Build a partnership (e.g., acknowledgment of understanding, asking for opinions, paraphrasing, and interpreting the patient's words).**
3. **Ask rephrased questions.**
4. **Give complete responses to the patient's questions.**

The manner in which a physician guides a discussion with a patient will determine the patient's level of understanding and her ability to successfully complete therapy. The term *compliance* has long been used in medicine; it suggests that the patient will follow the physician's recommendations or "orders." The term is criticized as being overly paternalistic; an alternative term, *adherence* to therapy, was proposed (35–37). This term still implies that the physician will dictate the therapy. A more collaborative approach is suggested by the phrase *successful use* of therapy, which can be credited mutually to the physician and the patient. With this phrase, the ultimate success of the therapy appropriately accrues to the patient (38). If a directive is given to take a prescribed medication without a discussion of the rationale for its use, patients may not comply, particularly if the instructions are confusing or difficult to follow. Barriers to compliance result from practical considerations: Nearly everyone finds a four times daily (qid) regimen more difficult than daily use. A major factor in successful compliance is the simplicity of the regimen (39,40). Practical factors that affect successful use include financial considerations, insurance coverage, and literacy (41). A discussion and comprehension of the rationale for therapy, along with the potential benefits and risks, are necessary components of successful use; but they may not be sufficient in the face of practical barriers. The specifics of when and how to take medication, including what to do when medication is missed, have an impact on successful use. Positive physician–patient communication is correlated with patient adherence to medical advice (42).

The style of the presentation of information is key to its effectiveness. As noted, the physician should establish a balance of power in the relationship, including conducting serious discussions about diagnosis and management strategies when the patient is fully clothed and face-to-face with the physician in a private room. Body language is important during interactions with patients. The physician should avoid an overly casual manner, which can communicate a lack of respect or compassion. The patient should be viewed directly and spoken to with eye contact so that the physician is not perceived as "looking off into the distance" (9).

Laughter and Humor

Humor is an essential component that promotes open communication. It can be either appropriate or inappropriate. Appropriate humor allows the patient to diffuse anxiety and understand that (even in difficult situations) laughter can be healthy (43,44). Inappropriate humor would horrify, disgust, offend, or generally make a patient feel uncomfortable or insulted. Laughter can be used as an appropriate means of relaxing the patient and making her feel better.

Laughter is a "*metaphor for the full range of the positive emotions.*" It is the response of human beings to incongruities and one of the highest manifestations of the cerebral process. It helps to facilitate the full range of positive emotions—love, hope, faith, the will to live, festivity, purpose, and determination (43). Laughter is a physiologic response, a release that helps us feel better and allows us to accommodate the collision of logic and absurdity. Illness, or the prospect of illness, heightens our awareness of the incongruity between our existence and our ability to control the events that shape our lives and our outcomes. We use laughter to combat stress, and stress reduction is an essential mechanism used to cope with illness.

Strategies for Improving Communication

All physicians should appreciate the importance of the art of communication during the medical interview. It is essential that interactions with patients are professional, honorable, and honest. Issues that were reported to be important to physicians regarding patient–physician interactions are presented in Table 1.4. Similarly, patients suggested the importance of many of these same issues in facilitating participatory decision making (45).

Following are some general guidelines that can help to improve communication:

1. **Listen more and talk less.**
2. **Encourage the pursuit of topics introduced by and important to patients.**
3. **Minimize controlling speech habits such as interrupting, issuing commands, and lecturing.**
4. **Seek out questions and provide full and understandable answers.**
5. **Become aware of any discomfort that arises in an interview, recognize when it originates in an attempt by the physician to take control, and redirect that attempt.**

Rank	Physicians' Support Services	Always or Often (%)	Rarely or Never (%)
1	Answering the patient's questions about the disease and its treatment, side effects, and possible outcomes	99	1
2	Making sure that the patient clearly understands the explanation of the medical treatment procedures	99	1
3	Encouraging the patient to develop an attitude of hope and optimism concerning treatment outcome	95	5
4	Adjusting treatment plans to enhance compliance when the patient exhibits noncompliance	88	12
5	Directly counseling family members	87	13
6	Continuing to serve as primary physician when the patient receives supplementary treatment at another facility	85	15
7	Providing referral to social support groups	83	17
8	Providing the patient with educational materials	81	19
9	Helping the patient develop methods to improve the quality of his or her life	74	26
10	Assisting the patient in determining which of his or her coping mechanisms are most productive and helping to activate them	62	38
11	Providing referral to psychological counseling services	57	43

Table 1.4 Importance Attached to the Patient–Physician Relationship[a]

[a]Results of a physician survey of 649 oncologists in regard to patient–physician communication.
Modified from **Cousins N.** *Head first: the biology of hope and the healing power of the human spirit.* New York: Penguin Books, 1989:220, with permission.

6. **Assure patients that they have the opportunity to discuss their problem fully.**

7. **Recognize when patients may be seeking empathy and validation of their feelings rather than a solution. Sometimes all that is necessary is to be there as a compassionate human being.**

In conducting interviews, it is important for the physician to understand the patient's concerns. Given the realities of today's busy office schedules, an additional visit may be required to discuss some issues in sufficient depth. In studies of interviewing techniques it was shown that although clinicians employ many divergent styles, the successful ones tend to look for "windows of opportunity" (i.e., careful, attentive listening with replies or questions at opportune times). This communication skill is particularly effective for exploring psychological and social issues during brief interviews. The chief skill essential to allow the physician to perceive problems is the ability to listen attentively.

An interview that permits maximum transmission of information to the physician is best achieved by the following approach (10):

1. **Begin the interview with an open-ended question.**

2. **As the patient begins to speak, pay attention to her answers, to her emotions, and to her general body language.**

3. **Extend a second question or comment, encouraging the patient to talk.**

4. **Allow the patient to respond without interrupting, perhaps by employing silence, nods, or small facilitative comments, encouraging the patient to talk while the physician is listening.**

5. **The physician should periodically summarize his or her understanding of the history to confirm accuracy.**

6. **Expressions of empathy and understanding at the completion of the interview along with a summary of the planned assessments and recommendations will facilitate the closure of the interview.**

Attentiveness, rapport, and collaboration characterize good medical interviewing techniques. Open-ended questions (*"How are you doing?" "How are things at home?" "How does that make you feel?"*) are generally desirable, particularly when they are coupled with good listening skills (46).

Premature closure of an interview and an inability to get complete information from the patient may occur for several reasons. They may result from failure to recognize the patient's particular concern, from not providing appropriate opportunity for discussion, from the physician's discomfort with sharing the patient's emotion, or perhaps from the physician's lack of confidence that he or she can deal with the patient's concern. One of the principal factors undermining the success of the interview is lack of time. This is a realistic concern perceived by physicians, but skilled physicians can facilitate considerable interaction even in a short time by encouraging open communication (47).

Some patients lack accurate information about their illnesses. Incomplete or inadequate understanding of an illness can produce dissatisfaction with medical care and increased anxiety, distress, and coping difficulties, resulting in unsuccessful treatment and poor treatment response. As patients increasingly request more information about their illnesses and more involvement in decisions about their treatment, and as physicians attempt to provide more open interactive discussions, there is an even greater need to provide clear and effective communication. Although patients vary in their levels of intellectual finesse, medical sophistication, anxiety, denial, and ability to communicate, the unfortunate occurrence of impaired patient comprehension can be the product of poor physician communication techniques, lack of consultation time, and in some cases, the withholding of information considered detrimental to patient welfare (48).

If clinical findings or confirmatory testing strongly suggest a serious condition (e.g., malignancy), the gravity and urgency of this situation must be conveyed in a manner that does not unduly alarm or frighten the individual. Honest answers should be provided to any specific questions the patient may want to discuss (49,50).

Allowing time for questions is important, and scheduling a follow-up visit to discuss treatment options after the patient has an opportunity to consider the options and

recommendations is often valuable. The patient should be encouraged to bring a partner or family member with her to provide moral support, to serve as another listener to absorb and digest the discussion, and to assist with questions. The patient should be encouraged to write down any questions or concerns she may have and bring them with her to a subsequent visit; important issues may not come to mind easily during an office visit. If the patient desires a second opinion, it should always be facilitated. Physicians should not feel threatened by patient attempts to gain information and knowledge.

Valuable information can be provided by interviews with ancillary support staff and by providing pamphlets and other materials produced for patient education. Some studies demonstrated that the use of pamphlets is highly effective in promoting an understanding of the condition and treatment options. Others showed that the use of audiotapes, videotapes, or information on an Internet site has a positive impact on knowledge and can decrease anxiety (51–53).

There are numerous medical Web sites that can be accessed, although the accuracy of the information is variable and must be carefully reviewed by physicians before recommending sites to patients. Physicians should be familiar with Internet sources offering accurate information and be prepared to provide the addresses of these sites if the patient expresses interest (54).

The relationship between the patient and her physician, as with all aspects of social interaction, is subject to constant change. The state of our health is dynamic and it affects our ability to communicate with others, including conversations between patients and physicians. **Open communication between patient and physician can help achieve maximum effectiveness in diagnosis, treatment, and compliance for all patients.**

Talk to the heart, speak to the soul.

Look to the being and embrace the figure's form.
Reach deeply, with hands outstretched.
Talk intently, to the seat of wisdom,
as life resembles grace.

Achieve peace within a fragile countenance.
Seek the comfort of the placid hour
Through joyous and free reflection
know the other side of the flesh's frame.

JSB

History and Physical Examination

After a dialogue is established, the patient assessment proceeds with obtaining a complete history and performing a physical examination. Both of these aspects of the assessment rely on good patient–physician interchange and attention to details. During the history and physical examination, risk factors that may require special attention should be identified. These factors should be reviewed with the patient in developing a plan for her future care (see Chapter 8).

Depending on the setting—ambulatory office, inpatient hospitalization, or outpatient surgical center—record keeping is typically facilitated by forms or templates (either written or electronic), which provide prompts for important elements of the medical, family, and social history. Increasingly, electronic medical records are used in the office and hospital setting. One challenge is that paper and electronic records do not always "mesh," and both paper and electronic records may be periodically unavailable. Efforts to develop patient-held medical records are not yet widely adopted.

History

After the chief complaint and characteristics of the present illness are ascertained, the medical history of the patient should be obtained. It should include her complete medical and surgical history, her reproductive history (including menstrual and obstetric history), her current use of medications (including over-the-counter and complementary and alternative medications), and a thorough family and social history.

A technique for obtaining information about the present illness is presented in Table 1.5. **The physician should consider which other members of the health care team might be helpful in completing the evaluation and providing care. Individuals who interact with the patient in the office—from the receptionists to medical assistants, nurses, advance practice nurses (nurse practitioners or nurse-midwives)—can contribute to the patient's care and may provide additional information or insight or be appropriate clinicians for providing follow-up. In some teaching hospitals, residents or medical students may provide care and participate in an office setting. The role that each of these individuals plays in a given office or health care setting may not be apparent to the patient; care should be taken that each individual introduces her- or himself at the opening of the interaction and explains his or her role on the team. It may be necessary to discuss the roles and functions of each individual member of the team.** In some cases, referral to a nutritionist, physical or occupational therapist, social worker, psychologist, psychiatrist, or sex counselor would be helpful. Referral to or consultations with these clinicians and with physicians in other specialty areas should be addressed as needed. The nature of the relationship between the obstetrician/gynecologist and the patient should be clarified. Some women have a primary clinician whom they rely on for primary care. Other women, particularly healthy women of reproductive age, consider their obstetrician/gynecologist their primary clinician. The individual physician's comfort with this role should be discussed and clarified at the initial visit and revisited periodically as required in the course of care. These issues are covered in Section III, Preventative and Primary Care (see Chapters 8–13). Laboratory testing for routine care and high-risk factors is presented in Chapter 8.

Physical Examination

A thorough gynecologic physical examination is typically performed at the time of the initial visit, on a yearly basis, and as needed throughout the course of treatment (Table 1.6). The extent of the physical examination during the gynecologic visit is often dictated by the patient's primary concerns and symptoms. For example, for healthy teens without symptoms who are requesting oral contraceptives before the initiation of intercourse, a gynecologic examination is not necessarily required. Some aspects of the examination—such as assessment of vital signs and measurement of height, weight, blood pressure, and calculation of a body mass index—should be performed routinely during most office visits. Typically, examination of the breasts and abdomen and a complete examination of the pelvis are considered to be essential parts of the gynecologic examination. It is often helpful to ask the patient if the gynecologic examination was difficult for her in the past; this may be true for women with a history of sexual abuse. For women who are undergoing their first gynecologic examination, it may be useful to ask what they have heard about the gynecologic examination or to state: *"Most women are nervous before their first exam, but afterward, most describe it as 'uncomfortable.'"*

Abdominal Examination

With the patient in the supine position, an attempt should be made to have her relax as much as possible. Her head should be leaned back and supported gently by a pillow so that she does not tense her abdominal muscles. Flexion of the knees may facilitate relaxation.

The abdomen should be inspected for signs of an intra-abdominal mass, organomegaly, or distention that would, for example, suggest ascites or intestinal obstruction. Auscultation of bowel sounds, if deemed necessary to ascertain the nature of the bowel sounds, should precede palpation. The frequency of intestinal sounds and their quality should be noted. In a patient with intestinal obstruction, "rushes," as well as the occasional high-pitched sound, can be heard. Bowel sounds associated with an ileus may occur less frequently but at the same pitch as normal bowel sounds.

The abdomen is palpated to evaluate the size and configuration of the liver, spleen, and other abdominal contents. Evidence of fullness or mass effect should be noted. This is particularly important in evaluating patients who may have a pelvic mass and in determining the extent of omental involvement, for example, with metastatic ovarian cancer. A fullness in the upper abdomen could be consistent with an "omental cake." All four quadrants should be carefully palpated for any evidence of mass, firmness, irregularity, or distention. A systematic approach should be used (e.g., clockwise, starting in the right upper quadrant). Percussion should be used to measure the dimensions of the liver. The patient should be asked to inhale and exhale during palpation of the edge of the liver. Areas of tenderness should be evaluated after the examination of the rest of the abdomen.

Table 1.5 Technique of Taking the History of the Present Illness

1. **The technique used in taking the history of the present illness varies with the patient, the patient's problem, and the physician. Allow the patient to talk about her chief symptom.** Although this symptom may or may not represent the real problem (depending on subsequent evaluation), it is usually uppermost in the patient's mind and most often constitutes the basis for the visit to the physician.

   During the phase of the interview, establish the temporal relation of the chief symptom to the total duration of the illness. Questions such as, *"Then up to the time of this symptom, you felt perfectly well?"* may elicit other symptoms that may antedate the chief one by days, months, or years. In this manner, the patient may recall the date of the first appearance of illness.

   Encourage the patient to talk freely and spontaneously about her illness from the established date of onset. Do not interrupt the patient's account, except for minor promptings such as, *"When did it begin?"* and *"How did it begin?,"* which will help in developing chronologic order in the patient's story.

   After the patient has furnished her spontaneous account (and before the next phase of the interview), it is useful to employ questions such as, *"What other problems have you noticed since you became ill?"* The response to this question may reveal other symptoms not yet brought forth in the interview.

   Thus, in the first phase of the interview, the physician obtains an account of the symptoms as the patient experiences them, without any bias being introduced by the examiner's direct questions. Information about the importance of the symptoms to the patient and the patient's emotional reaction to her symptoms are also revealed.

2. **Because all available data regarding the symptoms are usually not elicited by the aforementioned techniques, the initial phase of the interview should be followed by a series of direct and detailed questions concerning the symptoms described by the patient.** Place each symptom in its proper chronologic order and then evaluate each in accordance with the directions for analyzing a symptom.

   In asking direct questions about the details of a symptom, take care not to suggest the nature of the answer. This particularly refers to questions that may be answered "yes" or "no." If a leading question should be submitted to the patient, the answer must be assessed with great care. Subject the patient to repeated cross-examination until you are completely satisfied that the answer is not given just to oblige you.

   Finally, before dismissing the symptom under study, inquire about other symptoms that might reasonably be expected under the clinical circumstances of the case. Symptoms specifically sought but denied are known as negative symptoms. These negative symptoms may confirm or rule out diagnostic possibilities suggested by the positive symptoms.

3. **The data secured by the techniques described in the first two phases of the interview should now suggest several diagnostic possibilities.** Test these possibilities further by inquiring about other symptoms or events that may form part of the natural history of the suspected disease or group of diseases.

4. **These techniques may still fail to reveal all symptoms of importance to the present illness, especially if they are remote in time and seemingly unrelated to the present problem.** The review of systems may then be of considerable help in bringing forth these data. A positive response from the patient on any item in any of the systems should lead immediately to further detailed questioning.

5. **Throughout that part of the interview concerning the present illness, consider the following factors:**

   a. **The probable cause of each symptom or illness, such as emotional stress, infection, neoplasm.** Do not disregard the patient's statements of causative factors. Consider each statement carefully, and use it as a basis for further investigation. When the symptoms point to a specific infection, direct inquiry to water, milk, and foods eaten; exposure to communicable diseases, animals, or pets; sources of sexually transmitted disease; or residence or travel in the tropics or other regions where infections are known to exist. In each of the above instances, ascertain, if possible, the date of exposure, incubation period, and symptoms of invasion (prodromal symptoms).

   b. **The severity of the patient's illness, as judged either by the presence of systemic symptoms, such as weakness, fatigue, loss of weight, or by a change in personal habits.** The latter includes changes in sleep, eating, fluid intake, bowel movements, social activities, exercise, or work. Note the dates the patient discontinued her work or took to bed. Is she continuously confined to bed?

   c. **Determine the patient's psychological reaction to her illness (anxiety, depression, irritability, fear) by observing how she relates her story as well as her nonverbal behavior.** The response to a question such as, *"Have you any particular theories about or fear of what may be the matter with you?"* may yield important clues relative to the patient's understanding and feeling about her illness. The reply may help in the management of the patient's problem and allow the physician to give advice according to the patient's understanding of her ailment.

Modified from **Hochstein E, Rubin AL.** *Physical diagnosis.* New York: McGraw-Hill, 1964:9–11, with permission.

Table 1.6 Method of the Female Pelvic Examination

The patient is instructed to empty her bladder. She is placed in the lithotomy position (Fig. 1.1) and draped properly. The examiner's right or left hand, depending on his or her preference, is gloved. The pelvic area is illuminated well, and the examiner faces the patient. The following order of procedure is suggested for the pelvic examination:

A. External genitalia

1. Inspect the mons pubis, labia majora, labia minora, perineal body, and anal region for characteristics of the skin, distribution of the hair, contour, and swelling. Palpate any abnormality.

2. Separate the labia majora with the index and middle fingers of the gloved hand and inspect the epidermal and mucosal characteristics and anatomic configuration of the following structures in the order indicated below:

   a. Labia minora

   b. Clitoris

   c. Urethral orifice

   d. Vaginal outlet (introitus)

   e. Hymen

   f. Perineal body

   g. Anus

3. If disease of the Skene glands is suspected, palpate the gland for abnormal excretions by milking the undersurface of the urethra through the anterior vaginal wall. Examine the expressed excretions by microscopy and cultures.

   If there is a history of labial swelling, palpate for a diseased Bartholin gland with the thumb on the posterior part of the labia majora and the index finger in the vaginal orifice. In addition, sebaceous cysts, if present, can be felt in the labia minora.

B. Introitus

With the labia still separated by the middle and index fingers, instruct the patient to bear down. Note the presence of the anterior wall of the vagina when a cystocele is present or bulging of the posterior wall when a rectocele or enterocele is present. Bulging of both may accompany a complete prolapse of the uterus.

The supporting structure of the pelvic outlet is evaluated further when the bimanual pelvic examination is done.

C. Vagina and cervix

Inspection of the vagina and cervix using a speculum should always precede palpation.

The instrument should be warmed with tap water—not lubricated—if vaginal or cervical smears are to be obtained for the test or if cultures are to be performed.

Select the proper size of speculum (Fig. 1.2), warmed and lubricated (unless contraindicated). Introduce the instrument into the vaginal orifice with the blades oblique, closed, and pressed against the perineum. Carry the speculum along the posterior vaginal wall, and after it is fully inserted, rotate the blades into a horizontal position and open them. Maneuver the speculum until the cervix is exposed between the blades. Gently rotate the speculum around its long axis until all surfaces of the vagina and cervix are visualized.

1. Inspect the vagina for the following:

   a. The presence of blood

   b. Discharge. This should be studied to detect trichomoniasis, monilia, and clue cells and to obtain cultures, primarily for gonococci and chlamydia.

   c. Mucosal characteristics (i.e., color, lesions, superficial vascularity, and edema)
   The lesion may be:

      1. Inflammatory—redness, swelling, exudates, ulcers, vesicles

      2. Neoplastic

      3. Vascular

      4. Pigmented—bluish discoloration of pregnancy (Chadwick's sign)

      5. Miscellaneous (e.g., endometriosis, traumatic lesions, and cysts)

   d. Structural abnormalities (congenital and acquired)

Table 1.6 (*Continued*)

2. Inspect the cervix for the same factors listed above for the vagina. Note the following comments relative to the inspection of the cervix:

   a. Unusual bleeding from the cervical canal, except during menstruation, merits an evaluation for cervical or uterine neoplasia.

   b. Inflammatory lesions are characterized by a mucopurulent discharge from the os and redness, swelling, and superficial ulcerations of the surface.

   c. Polyps may arise either from the surface of the cervix projecting into the vagina or from the cervical canal. Polyps may be inflammatory or neoplastic.

   d. Carcinoma of the cervix may not dramatically change the appearance of the cervix or may appear as lesions similar in appearance to an inflammation. Therefore, a biopsy should be performed if there is suspicion of neoplasia.

D. Bimanual palpation

The pelvic organs can be outlined by bimanual palpation; the examiner places one hand on the lower abdominal wall and the finger(s) (one or two) (see Fig. 1.3) of the other hand in the vagina (or vagina and rectum in the rectovaginal examination) (see Fig. 1.4). Either the right or left hand may be used for vaginal palpation. The number of fingers inserted into the vagina should be based on what can comfortably be accommodated, the size and pliability of the vagina, and the weight of the patient. For example, adolescent, slender, and older patients might be best examined with a single finger technique.

1. Introduce the well-lubricated index finger and, in some patients, both the index and the middle finger into the vagina at its posterior aspect near the perineum. Test the strength of the perineum by pressing downward on the perineum and asking the patient to bear down. This procedure may disclose a previously concealed cystocele or rectocele and descensus of the uterus.

   Advance the fingers along the posterior wall until the cervix is encountered. Note any abnormalities of structure or tenderness in the vagina or cervix.

2. Press the abdominal hand, which is resting on the infraumbilical area, very gently downward, sweeping the pelvic structures toward the palpating vaginal fingers.

   Coordinate the activity of the two hands to evaluate the body of the uterus for:

   a. Position

   b. Architecture, size, shape, symmetry, tumor

   c. Consistency

   d. Tenderness

   e. Mobility

   Tumors, if found, are evaluated for location, architecture, consistency, tenderness, mobility, and number.

3. Continue the bimanual palpation, and evaluate the cervix for position, architecture, consistency, and tenderness, especially on mobility of the cervix. Rebound tenderness should be noted at this time. The intravaginal fingers should then explore the anterior, posterior, and lateral fornices.

4. Place the "vaginal" finger(s) in the right lateral fornix and the "abdominal" hand on the right lower quadrant. Manipulate the abdominal hand gently downward toward the vaginal fingers to outline the adnexa.

   A normal tube is not palpable. A normal ovary (about 4 × 2 × 3 cm in size, sensitive, firm, and freely movable) is often not palpable. If an adnexal mass is found, evaluate its location relative to the uterus and cervix, architecture, consistency, tenderness, and mobility.

5. Palpate the left adnexal region, repeating the technique described previously, but place the vaginal fingers in the left fornix and the abdominal hand on the left lower quadrant.

6. Follow the bimanual examination with a rectovaginal–abdominal examination.

   Insert the index finger into the vagina and the middle finger into the rectum very gently. Place the other hand on the infraumbilical region. The use of this technique makes possible higher exploration of the pelvis because the cul-de-sac does not limit the depth of the examining finger.

7. In patients who have an intact hymen, examine the pelvic organs by the rectal–abdominal technique.

Table 1.6 (*Continued*)

E. Rectal examination

1. Inspect the perianal and anal area, the pilonidal (sacrococcygeal) region, and the perineum for the following aspects:

   a. Color of the region (note that the perianal skin is more pigmented than the surrounding skin of the buttocks and is frequently thrown into radiating folds)

   b. Lesions

   1. The perianal and perineal regions are common sites for itching. Pruritus ani is usually indicated by thickening, excoriations, and eczema of the perianal region and adjacent areas.

   2. The anal opening often is the site of fissures, fistulae, and external hemorrhoids.

   3. The pilonidal area may present a dimple, a sinus, or an inflamed pilonidal cyst.

2. Instruct the patient to "strain down" and note whether this technique brings into view previously concealed internal hemorrhoids, polyps, or a prolapsed rectal mucosa.

3. Palpate the pilonidal area, the ischiorectal fossa, the perineum, and the perianal region before inserting the gloved finger into the anal canal.
   Note the presence of any concealed induration or tenderness in any of these areas.

4. Palpate the anal canal and rectum with a well-lubricated, gloved index finger. Lay the pulp of the index finger against the anal orifice and instruct the subject to strain downward. Concomitant with the patient's downward straining (which tends to relax the external sphincter muscle), exert upward pressure until the sphincter is felt to yield. Then, with a slight rotary movement, insinuate the finger past the anal canal into the rectum. Examine the anal canal systematically before exploring the rectum.

5. Evaluate the anal canal for:

   a. Tonus of the external sphincter muscle and the anorectal ring at the anorectal junction

   b. Tenderness (usually caused by a tight sphincter, anal fissure, or painful hemorrhoids)

   c. Tumor or irregularities, especially at the pectinate line

   d. Superior aspect: Reach as far as you can. Mild straining by the patient may cause some lesions, which are out of reach of the finger, to descend sufficiently low to be detected by palpation.

   e. Test for occult blood: Examine the finger after it is withdrawn for evidence of gross blood, pus, or other alterations in color or consistency. Smear the stool to test for occult blood (guaiac).

6. Evaluate the rectum:

   a. Anterior wall

   1. Cervix: size, shape, symmetry, consistency, and tenderness, especially on manipulation

   2. Uterine or adnexal masses

   3. Rectouterine fossa for tenderness or implants
      In patients with an intact hymen, the examination of the anterior wall of the rectum is the usual method of examining the pelvic organs.

   b. Right lateral wall, left lateral wall, posterior wall, superior aspect; test for occult blood

Modified from **Hochstein E, Rubin AL.** *Physical diagnosis.* New York: McGraw-Hill, 1964:342–353, with permission.

Pelvic Examination

The pelvic examination is usually performed with the patient in the dorsal lithotomy position (Fig. 1.1). The patient's feet should rest comfortably in stirrups with the edge of the buttocks at the lower end of the table so that the vulva can be readily inspected and the speculum can be inserted in the vagina without obstruction from the table. Raising the head of the examination table, if possible, may facilitate relaxation. Drapes should be placed to provide a measure of cover for the patient's legs but should be depressed over the abdomen to allow observation of the patient's expression and to facilitate communication.

Before each step of the examination, the patient should be informed of what she will feel next: "*First you'll feel me touch your inner thighs; next I'll touch the area around the outside of your*

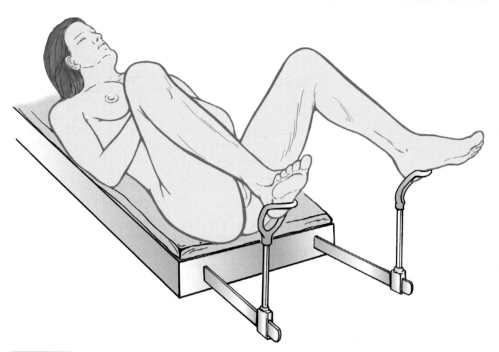

Figure 1.1   The lithotomy position for the pelvic examination.

vagina." The vulva and perineal area should be carefully inspected. Evidence of any lesions, erythema, pigmentation, masses, or irregularity should be noted. The skin quality should be noted as well as any signs of trauma, such as excoriations or ecchymosis. Areas of erythema or tenderness are noted, particularly in women with vulvar burning or pain, as might be seen with vulvar vestibulitis or localized provoked vulvodynia. The presence of any visible lesions should be quantitated and carefully described with regard to their full appearance and characteristics on palpation (i.e., mobility, tenderness, consistency). A drawing of the location of skin lesions is helpful. Ulcerative or purulent lesions of the vulva should be evaluated and cultured as outlined in subsequent chapters, and biopsy should be performed on any lesions. It may be helpful to ask the patient if she is aware of any vulvar lesions and to offer a mirror to demonstrate any lesions.

After thorough visualization and palpation of the external genitalia, including the mons pubis and the perianal area, a speculum is inserted into the vagina. In a healthy adult who is sexually active, a Pederson speculum typically is used. The types of specula that are used in gynecology are presented in Figure 1.2.

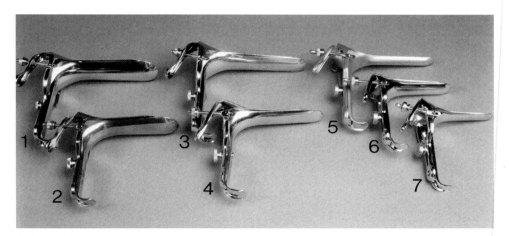

Figure 1.2   Vaginal specula: 1, Graves extra long; 2, Graves regular; 3, Pederson extra long; 4, Pederson regular; 5, Huffman "virginal"; 6, pediatric regular; and 7, pediatric narrow.

The smallest width speculum necessary to produce adequate visualization should be used. The larger Graves speculum may be required in women who have lax vaginal walls, are pregnant, or will be undergoing cervical or endometrial biopsies or procedures. In some women, a longer speculum (either Pederson or Graves) may facilitate visualization of the cervix in a manner that is less uncomfortable to the patient. If any speculum other than the typically sized specula is used, the patient should be informed and encouraged to remind the clinician before her next examination. The speculum should be warmed before it is inserted into the vagina; a heating pad or speculum warmer should be placed under the supply of specula. **If lubrication is required, warm water generally is sufficient or a small amount of lubricant can be used without interfering with cervical cytology testing.** The patient should be asked to relax the muscles of her distal vagina before the insertion of the speculum to facilitate the placement and to avoid startling her by this portion of the examination. After insertion, the cervix and all aspects of the vagina should be carefully inspected. Particular attention should be paid to the vaginal fornices, because lesions (e.g., warts) may be present in those areas and may not be readily visualized.

The appropriate technique and frequency for cervical cytology testing is presented in Chapter 19. **Biopsy should be performed on any obvious lesions on the cervix or in the vagina.** An endometrial biopsy usually is performed with a flexible cannula or a Novak curette (see Chapter 14). Any purulence in the vagina or cervix should be cultured (see Chapter 18). **Testing for sexually transmitted diseases should be performed routinely in adolescents and young adults as recommended by the Centers for Disease Control and Prevention.**

After the speculum is removed and the pelvis palpated, lubrication is applied to the examination glove, and **one or two (the index or index and middle) fingers are inserted gently into the vagina.** In general, in right-handed physicians, the fingers from the right hand are inserted into the vagina and the left hand is placed on the abdomen to provide counter-pressure as the pelvic viscera are moved (Fig. 1.3). In patients with pelvic pain, a stepwise "functional pelvic

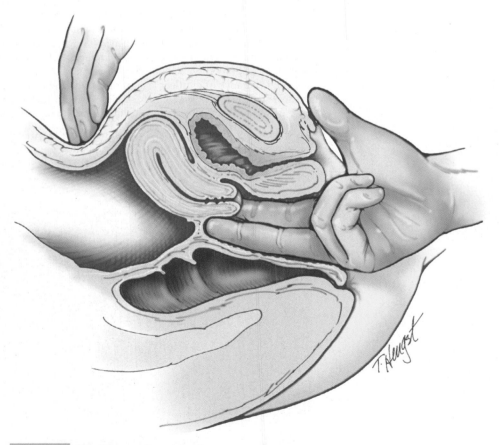

Figure 1.3   **The bimanual examination.**

examination" involves the sequential palpation of anatomic structures, including the pelvic floor muscles, bladder, rectum, cervix, and cul-de-sac. These areas are assessed for tenderness and a specific source of pain. Pelvic floor muscle spasm is a common concomitant of pelvic pain. The vagina, its fornices, and the cervix are palpated carefully for any masses or irregularities. One or two fingers are placed gently into the posterior fornix so the uterus can be moved. With the abdominal hand in place, the uterus usually can be palpated just above the surface pubis. In this manner, the size, shape, mobility, contour, consistency, and position of the uterus are determined. The patient is asked to provide feedback about any areas of tenderness, and her facial expressions are observed during the examination.

The adnexa are palpated gently on both sides, paying particular attention to any enlargements. Again, the size, shape, mobility, and consistency of any adnexal structures should be carefully noted.

When indicated, a rectovaginal examination should be performed to evaluate the rectovaginal septum, the posterior uterine surface, the adnexal structures, the uterosacral ligaments, and the posterior cul-de-sac. Uterosacral nodularity or posterior uterine tenderness associated with pelvic endometriosis or cul-de-sac implants of ovarian cancer can be assessed in this manner. Hemorrhoids, anal fissures, sphincter tone, rectal polyps, or carcinoma may be detected. A single stool sample for fecal occult blood testing obtained in this manner is not adequate for the detection of colorectal cancer and is not recommended (55) (Fig. 1.4).

At the completion of the physical examination, the patient should be informed of the findings. When the results of the examination are normal, the patient can be reassured accordingly. When there is a possible abnormality, the patient should be informed immediately; this discussion should take place after the examination with the patient clothed. A plan to evaluate the findings should be outlined briefly and in clear, understandable language.

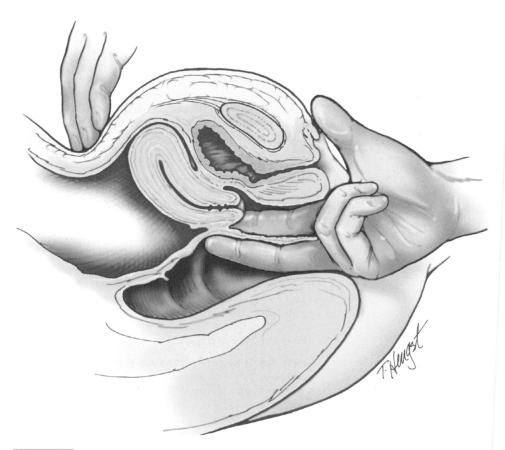

Figure 1.4 The rectovaginal examination.

The implications and timing of any proposed procedure (e.g., biopsy) should be discussed, and the patient should be informed when the results of any tests will be available.

Pediatric Patients

A careful examination is indicated when a child presents with genital symptoms such as itching, discharge, burning with urination, or bleeding. The examiner should be familiar with the normal appearance of the prepubertal genitalia. The normal unestrogenized hymenal ring and vestibule can appear mildly erythematous. The technique of examination is different from that used for examining an adult and may need to be tailored to the individual child based on her age, size, and comfort with the examiner.

A speculum examination should not be performed in a prepubertal child in the office. A young child usually can be examined best in a "frog leg" or "butterfly leg" position on the examining table. Some very young girls (toddlers or infants) do best when held in their mother's arms. Sometimes, the mother can be positioned, clothed, on the examination table (feet in stirrups, head of table elevated) with the child on her lap, the child's legs straddling her mother's legs. The knee-chest position may be helpful for the examination (56). The child who is relaxed and warned about touching will usually tolerate the examination satisfactorily. An otoscope can be used to examine the distal vagina if indicated. Two percent *lidocaine* jelly may be used as a topical anesthetic to facilitate the examination if needed.

Some children who were abused, who had particularly traumatic previous examinations, or who are unable to allow an examination may need to be examined under anesthesia, although a gentle office examination should almost always be attempted first. If the child had bleeding and no obvious cause of bleeding is visible externally or within the distal vagina, an examination under anesthesia is indicated to visualize the vagina and cervix completely. A hysteroscope, cytoscope, or other endoscopic instrument can be used to provide magnification and as a light source for vaginoscopy, which should be performed under anesthesia.

Adolescent Patients

A pelvic examination may be less revealing in an adolescent than in an older woman, particularly if it is the patient's first examination or if it takes place on an emergency basis. **An adolescent who presents with excessive bleeding should have a pelvic examination if she had intercourse, if the results of a pregnancy test are positive, if she has abdominal pain, if she is markedly anemic, or if she is bleeding heavily enough to compromise hemodynamic stability.** The pelvic examination occasionally may be deferred in young teenagers who have a classic history of irregular cycles soon after menarche, who have normal hematocrit levels, who deny sexual activity, and who will reliably return for follow-up. A pelvic examination may be deferred in adolescents who present to the office requesting oral contraceptives before the initiation of intercourse or at the patient's request, even if she has had intercourse. Newer testing methods using DNA amplification techniques allow noninvasive urine testing for gonorrhea and chlamydia (57). Current guidelines recommend that cervical cytology testing in most adolescents be initiated at age 21 (58).

Other diagnostic techniques (such as pelvic ultrasound) can substitute for or supplement an inadequate examination. An examination usually is required when there is a question of pelvic pain, genital anomaly, pregnancy-related condition, or possibility of pelvic infection. **The keys to a successful examination in an adolescent lie in earning the patient's trust, explaining the components of her examination, performing only the essential components, and using a very careful and gentle technique.** It is helpful to ascertain whether the patient had a previous pelvic examination, how she perceived the experience, and what she heard about a pelvic examination from her mother or friends.

Before a first pelvic examination is performed, a brief explanation of the planned examination (which may or may not need to include a speculum), instruction in relaxation techniques, and the use of *lidocaine* jelly as a lubricant can be helpful. The patient should be encouraged to participate in the examination by voluntary relaxation of the introital muscles or by using a mirror if she wishes. If significant trauma is suspected or the patient finds the examination too painful and is truly unable to cooperate, an examination under anesthesia may be necessary. The risks of general anesthesia must be weighed against the value of information that would be obtained by the examination.

Confidentiality is an important issue in adolescent health care. A number of medical organizations, including the American Medical Association, the American Academy of Pediatrics, and the American College of Obstetrics and Gynecologists, endorsed adolescents' rights to confidential medical care. Particularly with regard to issues as sensitive as sexual activity, it is critical that the adolescent be interviewed alone, without a parent in the room. The patient should be asked whether she engaged in sexual intercourse, whether she used any method of contraception, used condoms to minimize the risks of sexually transmitted diseases, or she feels there is any possibility of pregnancy.

Follow-Up

Arrangements should be made for the ongoing care of patients, regardless of their health status. Patients with no evidence of disease should be counseled regarding health behaviors and the need for routine care. For those with signs and symptoms of a medical disorder, further assessments and a treatment plan should be discussed. The physician must determine whether she or he is equipped to treat a particular problem or whether the patient should be directed to another health professional, either in obstetrics and gynecology or another specialty, and how that care should be coordinated. If the physician believes it is necessary to refer the patient elsewhere for care, the patient should be reassured that this measure is being undertaken in her best interests and that continuity of care will be ensured. Patients deserve a summary of the findings of the visit, recommendations for preventive care and screening, an opportunity to ask any additional questions, and a recommendation for the frequency of any follow-up or ongoing care visits.

Summary

The management of patients' gynecologic symptoms, and abnormal findings and signs detected during examination, requires the full use of a physician's skills and knowledge. Physicians are challenged to practice the art of medicine in a manner that leads to effective alliances with their patients. The value of skilled medical history taking cannot be overemphasized. **Physicians should listen carefully to what patients are saying about the nature and severity of their symptoms.** They should listen to what patients may not be expressing: their fears, anxieties, and personal experiences that lead them to react in a certain manner when faced with what is often, to them, a crisis (such as the diagnosis of an abnormality on examination, laboratory testing, or pelvic imaging).

Physicians should supplement their formal education and clinical experience by constantly seeking valid new information and honing their communication skills. To meet the challenges posed by the complexities of patient care, physicians must learn to practice evidence-based medicine, derived from the very latest data of highest quality. Computers make the world of information management accessible to both physicians and patients. Physicians need to search the medical literature to acquire knowledge that can be applied, using the art of medicine, to patient care that maintains health, prevents disease, alleviates suffering, and manages and cures illness.

References

1. **Simpson M, Buckman R, Stewart M, et al.** Doctor-patient communication: the Toronto consensus statement. *BMJ* 1991;303:1385–1387.
2. **Ley P.** *Communicating with patients.* London: Croom Helm, 1988.
3. **Butt HR.** A method for better physician-patient communication. *Ann Intern Med* 1977;86:478–480.
4. **Lipkin M.** The medical interview and related skills. In: **Branch W,** ed. *Office practice of medicine.* Philadelphia: Saunders, 1987:1287–1306.
5. **Omar H, Richard J.** Cultural sensitivity in providing reproductive care to adolescents. *Curr Opin Obstet Gynecol* 2004;16:367–370.
6. **Lang F, Floyd MR, Beine KL, et al.** Sequenced questioning to elicit the patient's perspective on illness: effects on information disclosure, patient satisfaction, and time expenditure. *Fam Med* 2002;34:325.
7. **Beck RS, Daughtridge R, Sloane PD.** Physician-patient communication in the primary care office: a systematic review. *J Am Board Fam Pract* 2002;15:25–38.
8. **Lipkin M Jr.** Physician-patient interaction in reproductive counseling. *Obstet Gynecol* 1996;88:31S–40S.
9. **Branch WT, Malik TK.** Using "windows of opportunities" in brief interviews to understand patients' concerns. *JAMA* 1993;269:1667–1668.
10. **Shenolikar RA, Balkrishnan R, Hall MA.** How patient-physician encounters in critical medical situations affect trust: results of a national survey. *BMC Health Serv Res* 2004;4:24.
11. **Flores G.** Language barriers to health care in the United States. *N Engl J Med* 2006;355:229–231.
12. **Ngo-Metzger Q, Sorkin DH, Phillips RS, et al.** Providing high-quality care for limited English proficient patients: the importance of language concordance and interpreter use. *J Gen Intern Med* 2007;22(Suppl 2):324–330.
13. **California State Legislature.** California Health and Safety Code, in Section 1259. Available at ONECLE: http://law.onecle.com/california/health/1259.html
14. **Lie D, Bereknyei S, Braddock CH 3rd, et al.** Assessing medical students' skills in working with interpreters during patient encounters: a validation study of the Interpreter Scale. *Acad Med* 2009;84:643–650.

15. **Lo B, Dornbrand L, Dubler NN.** HIPAA and patient care: the role for professional judgment. *JAMA* 2005;293:1766–1771.

16. **Angelos P.** Compliance with HIPAA regulations: ethics and excesses. *Thorac Surg Clin* 2005;15:513–518.

17. **Mishler EG, Clark JA, Ingelfinger J, et al.** The language of attentive patient care: a comparison of two medical interviews. *J Gen Intern Med* 1989;4:325–335.

18. **Conti AA, Gensini GF.** Doctor-patient communication: a historical overview. *Minerva Med* 2008;99:411–415.

19. **Kim J, Kim S.** Physicians' perception of the effects of Internet health information on the doctor-patient relationship. *Inform Health Soc Care* 2009;34:136–148.

20. **The Headache Study Group of The University of Western Ontario.** Predictors of outcome in headache patients presenting to family physicians—a one year prospective study. *Headache* 1986;26:285–294.

21. **Kaplan SH, Greenfield S, Ware JE Jr.** Assessing the effects of physician-patient interactions on the outcomes of chronic disease. *Med Care* 1989;27(Suppl):S110–127.

22. **Fallowfield L, Hall A, Maguire GP, et al.** Psychological outcomes in women with early breast cancer. *BMJ* 1990;301:1394.

23. **Walter FM, Emery JD, Rogers M, et al.** Women's views of optimal risk communication and decision making in general practice consultations about the menopause and hormone replacement therapy. *Patient Educ Couns* 2004;53:121–128.

24. **Spender D.** *Man made language.* New York: Routledge & Kegan Paul, 1985.

25. **Tannen D.** *You just don't understand: women and men in conversation.* New York: Ballantine, 1990.

26. **West C.** Reconceptualizing gender in physician-patient relationships. *Soc Sci Med* 1993;36:57–66.

27. **Todd A, Fisher S.** *The social organization of doctor-patient communication,* 2nd ed. Norwood, NJ: Ablex, 1993.

28. **Adams KE.** Patient choice of provider gender. *J Am Med Womens Assoc* 2003;58:117–119.

29. **Plunkett BA, Kohli P, Milad MP.** The importance of physician gender in the selection of an obstetrician or a gynecologist. *Am J Obstet Gynecol* 2002;186:926–928.

30. **Roter D, Lipkin M, Korsgaard A.** Sex differences in patients' and physicians' communication during primary care medical visits. *Med Care* 1991;29:1083–1093.

31. **Roter DL, Hall JA.** Why physician gender matters in shaping the physician-patient relationship. *J Womens Health* 1998;7:1093–1097.

32. **Lurie N, Slater J, McGovern P, et al.** Preventive care for women. Does the sex of the physician matter? *N Engl J Med* 1993;329:478–482.

33. **Sandhu H, Adams A, Singleton L, et al.** The impact of gender dyads on doctor-patient communication: a systematic review. *Patient Educ Couns* 2009;76:348–355.

34. **Bertakis KD.** The influence of gender on the doctor-patient interaction. *Patient Educ Couns* 2009;76:356–360.

35. **Donovan JL.** Patient decision making. The missing ingredient in compliance research. *Int J Technol Assess Health Care* 1995;11:443–455.

36. **Haynes RB, Taylor DW, Sackett DL.** Compliance in health care. Baltimore: Johns Hopkins University Press, 1979.

37. **Osterberg L, Blaschke T.** Adherence to medication. *N Engl J Med* 2005;353:487–497.

38. **Association of Reproductive Health Professionals.** Helping women make choices that facilitate successful contraceptive use. Clinical proceedings: periodic well-woman visit 2004 April. Available online at: http://www.arhp.org/healthcareproviders/cme/onlinecme/wellwoman/helpingwomen.cfm

39. **Erhardt LR.** The essence of effective treatment and compliance is simplicity. *Am J Hypertens* 1999;12(Pt 2):105S–110S.

40. **Krueger KP, Felkey BG, Berger BA.** Improving adherence and persistence: a review and assessment of interventions and description of steps toward a national adherence initiative. *J Am Pharm Assoc* 2003;43:668–678; quiz 678–679.

41. **Parker RM, Williams MV, Baker DW, et al.** Literacy and contraception: exploring the link. *Obstet Gynecol* 1996;88:72S–77S.

42. **Zolnierek KB, Dimatteo MR.** Physician communication and patient adherence to treatment: a meta-analysis. *Med Care* 2009;47:826–834.

43. **Cousins N.** The laughter connection. In: Cousins N, ed. *Head first: the biology of hope and the healing power of the human spirit.* New York: Penguin, 1989:125–153.

44. **Wender RC.** Humor in medicine. *Prim Care* 1996;23:141–154.

45. **Epstein RM, Alper BS, Quill TE.** Communicating evidence for participatory decision making. *JAMA* 2004;291:2359–2366.

46. **Good RS.** The third ear. Interviewing techniques in obstetrics and gynecology. *Obstet Gynecol* 1972;40:760–762.

47. **Levinson W, Chaumeton N.** Communication between surgeons and patients in routine office visits. *Surgery* 1999;125:127–134.

48. **Dunn SM, Butow PN, Tattersall MH, et al.** General information tapes inhibit recall of the cancer consultation. *J Clin Oncol* 1993;11:2279–2285.

49. **Baile WF, Kudelka AP, Beale EA,** et al. Communication skills training in oncology. Description and preliminary outcomes of workshops on breaking bad news and managing patient reactions to illness. *Cancer* 1999;86:887–897.

50. **Maguire P, Faulkner A.** Improve the counselling skills of doctors and nurses in cancer care. *BMJ* 1988;297:847–849.

51. **Dunn RA, Webster LA, Nakashima AK, et al.** Surveillance for geographic and secular trends in congenital syphilis—United States, 1983–1991. *MMWR CDC Surveill Summ* 1993;42:59–71.

52. **Elkjaer M, Burisch J, Avnstrøm S, et al.** Development of a web-based concept for patients with ulcerative colitis and 5-aminosalicylic acid treatment. *Eur J Gastroenterol Hepatol* 2010;22:695–704.

53. **O'Conner-Von S.** Preparation of adolescents for outpatient surgery: using an Internet program. *AORN J* 2008;87:374–398.

54. **Ilic D.** The role of the internet on patient knowledge management, education, and decision-making. *Telemed J E Health* 2010;16:664–669.

55. **ACOG Editorial Committee for Guidelines for Women's Health Care, ed.** *Guidelines for women's health care: a resource manual,* 3rd ed. ACOG: Washington, DC: ACOG, 2007:573.

56. **Emans SJ, Laufer MR, Goldstein DP.** *Pediatric and adolescent gynecology,* 5th ed. Philadelphia: Lippincott Williams & Wilkins, 2005:1076.

57. **Spigarelli MG.** Urine gonococcal/Chlamydia testing in adolescents. *Curr Opin Obstet Gynecol* 2006;18:498–502.

58. **ACOG Committee.** Opinion No. 431: routine pelvic examination and cervical cytology screening. *Obstet Gynecol* 2009;113:1190–1193.

2

Principles of Patient Care

Joanna M. Cain

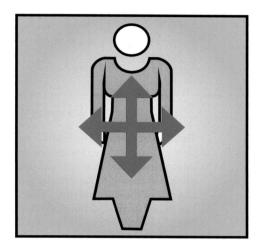

- Professionalism is the foundation of patient care and is as much an ongoing educational endeavor as learning new procedures or techniques.

- The right to privacy prohibits a physician from revealing information regarding the patient unless the patient waives that privilege.

- Informed consent is a process whereby the physician educates the patient about the medical condition, explores her values, and informs her about the risks and benefits of treatment and reasonable medical alternatives.

- The concept of autonomy does not allow a patient's wishes to take precedence over good medical judgment.

- For children, parents are the surrogate decision makers, except in circumstances in which the decision is life threatening and might not be the choice a child would make later, when adult beliefs and values are formed.

- Creating a highly professional environment of safe culture, lack of harassment, high professional behavior standards, and disclosure of unexpected outcomes benefits both patients and health professionals.

The practice of gynecology, as with all branches of medicine, is based on ethical principles that guide patient care. These principles and concepts create a framework for ethical decision making that applies to all aspects of practice:

- **Autonomy:** a person's right to self-rule, to establish personal norms of conduct, and to choose a course of action based on a set of personal values and principles derived from them

- **Confidentiality:** a person's right to decide how and to whom personal medical information will be communicated is part of autonomy

- **Beneficence:** the obligation to promote the well-being of others or, in medicine, to benefit the patient through meeting a goal of medicine by the care offered

- **Covenant:** a binding agreement between two or more parties for the performance of some action

- **Fiduciary Relationship:** a relationship founded on faith and trust and the obligation to act in a trustworthy manner

- **Informed Consent:** the patient's acceptance of a medical intervention after adequate discussion and consideration of the nature of the procedure, its risks and benefits, and alternatives

- **Justice:** the right of individuals or groups to claim what is due to them based on certain personal properties or characteristics

- **Maleficence:** the act of committing harm (*Nonmaleficence* obliges one to avoid doing harm)

Patient and Physician: Professionalism

Health care providers fulfill a basic need—to preserve and advance the health of human beings. Despite the challenges imposed by the commercial aspects of the current medical environment, for most physicians, the practice of medicine remains very much a "calling," a giving of oneself to the greater good. The behavior of health professionals is judged against this list of ethical principles and concepts by other professionals and the public who share the belief in the "calling" of medicine. There are examples of unprofessional behaviors that mar this professional image. They are demonstrably easier to see in others than ourselves, including unprofessionalism in relation to drug companies, shouting at or mistreating others, or inappropriate behaviors with students, patients or colleagues, that abuse professional standing such as boundary violations or learner abuse (1). Lapses do not always represent inherent flaws in professionals, "*most lapses represent deficiencies in judgment and skill. They occur when the physician in question fails to recognize the presence of a challenge to professionalism or lacks the skill to handle a challenge at the time it occurs*" (2). As Lucey and Souba note, the solution to unprofessional behavior is not recrimination but development of a set of skills that allow professionals to recognize and address these professional challenges—and those skills need to be developed and reinforced not just by individuals but by the whole community of practicing physicians throughout their professional careers (2). Professionalism is as much an ongoing educational endeavor as is learning new procedures or techniques, and "*we should assume that our peers want to be professional and that they will welcome interventions from a trusted colleague when circumstances suggest that a lapse is imminent*" (2). Creating an environment where we can help one another in this way improves the quality and safety of the care for our patients by preventing unprofessional behavior. **An environment without fear of recrimination, harassment, or unprofessional behavior promotes speaking up for patients' interests and promotes safer environments for everyone. It is a fundamental principle of excellence in patient care.**

Professionalism has to balance the differences of fiduciary and contractual relationships between physician and patient: "*The kind of minimalism that a contractualist understanding of the professional relationship encourages produces a professional too grudging, too calculating, too lacking in spontaneity, too quickly exhausted to go the second mile with his patients along the road of their distress*" (3). There is a relationship between physician and patient that extends beyond a contract and assumes the elements of a fiduciary relationship—a covenant between parties. **The physician, having knowledge about the elements of health care, assumes a trust relationship with the patient where her interests are held paramount. Both the patient and the physician have rights and responsibilities in this relationship, and both are rewarded when those rights and responsibilities are upheld. Honesty, disclosure, confidentiality, and informed consent are expressions of that trust or covenantal relationship.**

Disclosing Medical Errors and Unanticipated Outcomes

In creating a trustworthy and safe environment, disclosure of unanticipated outcomes can add to the trust patients have in their health care team and ensure that all medical errors or near misses are used to improve the environment of care. If we are obligated as professionals by our trust relationship with our patients, then patients should expect truthfulness, including being made aware of individual or systemic errors, which, as Kohn et al. noted in *To Err Is Human*, are inevitable in the delivery of health care (4). **The climate of no-fault discussion of**

errors creates an environment conducive to restructuring the systems or procedures that make it possible for errors to occur and is critical in development of a safety culture.

Medical errors can create a keen sense of shame, humiliation, and failed responsibility in health professionals, and efforts have begun to identify and develop the skills and methods for disclosing and learning from them (5). Support for individuals facing these feelings and wanting to disclose is critical in this development. **Skills that seem common to disclosure are: telling the medical facts, honesty and truthfulness (responsibility and answering questions), empathy (and apology), stating how future errors will be prevented, and using good communication skills (6). These are skills that require training and development and should not be taken for granted.** Many institutions have risk management groups or other support groups that can be helpful in development of skills and can accompany or lead such a discussion in the absence of those skills. Disclosure and apology cause apprehension for physicians—particularly in the discipline of obstetrics and gynecology where litigation adversely affected practice patterns (defensive medicine) and heightened a reluctance to disclose medical errors for fear of litigation (7). It is interesting to note that **open disclosure overall generated less litigation than failing to disclose, and the growth of compensation with disclosure seems to add to this decrease** (8–12). Apology raises particular anxiety about implying culpability and inciting litigation, so help with framing an apology is always appropriate. **The obligation of trust (fiduciary relationship) that we have with our patients is part of the healing aspects of medicine—and we owe it to our patients and to ourselves to develop the robust curricula and support at all levels of medicine to make disclosure the step toward solution and healing that it can be for both physician and patient.**

Confidentiality

The patient seeking assistance from a health professional has the right to assurance that the information exchanged during that interaction is kept private. **Privacy is essential to the trust relationship between doctor and patient. Discussions are privileged information. The right to privacy prohibits a physician from revealing information regarding the patient unless the patient waives that privilege.** Privileged information belongs to the patient except when it impinges on the legal and ethical rights of institutions and society at large, regardless of the setting. In a court situation, for example, physicians cannot reveal information about their patients unless the patient waives that privilege. If privilege is waived, the physician may not withhold such testimony.

The privilege of privacy must be maintained even when it does not seem intrinsically obvious. A patient's family, friend, or spiritual guide, for example, has no right to medical information regarding the patient unless the patient specifically approves it, except if the patient is unable to provide that guidance because of their medical circumstance. In that circumstance, health providers must exercise their judgment based on their assessment of the involvement of that particular person with the patient's health. This may seem obvious but often can be overlooked, such as when a health care giver receives a call from a concerned relative inquiring about the status of a patient. The response may be a natural attempt to reassure and inform a caring individual about the patient's status. However, for her own reasons, the patient may not want certain individuals informed of her medical condition. Thus, confidentiality has been breached. It is wise to ask patients about who may be involved in decision making and who may be informed about their status. **If a health care giver is unclear of the patient's wishes regarding the person requesting information, the reply should indicate that the patient's permission is necessary before discussing her status. When trying to contact patients for follow-up of medical findings, it is never appropriate to reveal the reason for contact to an individual other than the patient.**

Record Keeping

Health care professionals are part of record-keeping organizations. Those records are used for multiple purposes in medicine and are a valuable tool in patient care. There is an increasing tendency for ancillary organizations to collect, maintain, and disclose information about individuals with whom they have no direct connection (13). Health care professionals must be aware of this practice and its ramifications. Patients sign a document, often without understanding its meaning, upon registering with a health care institution or insurance plan. That document waives the patient's privilege to suppress access and gives insurers, and often other health care providers who request it, access to the medical record. The consequences of such disclosure for patients can be significant in terms of insurance coverage and potential job discrimination (14). Even with health care reform, this continues to be a concern because individuals may have shifts in the pools of insurance available to them and the costs may vary. This concern must be weighed against the need for all health care providers involved with an individual to be informed about past or present diseases or activities that may interfere with or complicate management. The use of illegal drugs, a positive HIV test result, and even a history of cancer or psychiatric illness are all exceptionally important to health care providers in evaluating individual patients. When revealed to outside institutions, these factors may affect the patient's ability to obtain medical care, insurance, or even credit. **Everything that is written in a patient's record should be important to the medical care of that patient, and extrinsic information should be avoided.** It is appropriate for physicians to discuss with patients the nature of medical records and their release to other parties so that patients can make an informed choice about such release.

The Health Insurance Portability and Accountability Act (HIPAA) was enacted in 1996 and the effective compliance of the "privacy rule" was instituted in April 2003, and this rule imposed additional requirements for access to patient records for clinical research and guidelines for protecting electronic medical records. Although the intent of the act was laudable, the extent to which privacy will be improved is unknown, and the potential harm to the public from failure to do critical database research because of its costly requirements may be greater than any benefit. The considerable confusion and misunderstanding of the rules associated with the act are potentially harmful to patients. The exceptions from the requirement to obtain patient authorization to share health information include areas such as patient treatment, payment, operations (quality improvement, quality assurance, and education), disclosure to public health officials and health oversight agencies, and legal requirements (15). **One widely misunderstood feature of the act was whether protected health information could be sent via fax, e-mail or mail to another treating physician (which is allowed)** (16). It is important that researchers understand the influence of these rules in all settings; preplanning for clinical database research to include consent for research database efforts when the patient first enters the office or institution will make this critical research possible (17). **The security of medical records is a concern not just for individual patients and physicians but also for health systems and researchers.**

Legal Issues

The privilege of patients to keep their records or medical information private can be superseded by the needs of society, but only in rare circumstances. The classic legal decision quoted for the needs of others superseding individual patient rights is that of *Tarasoff v. Regents of the University of California* (18). That decision establishes that the special relationship between a patient and doctor may support affirmative duties for the benefit of third persons. It requires disclosure if "*necessary to avert danger to others*" but still in a fashion "*that would preserve the privacy of the patient to the fullest extent compatible with the prevention of the threatened danger.*" This principle is compatible with the various codes of ethics that allow physicians to reveal information to protect the welfare of the individual or the community. In other words, "the protective privilege ends where the public peril begins" (18).

Legislation can override individual privilege. The most frequent example is the recording of births and deaths, which is the responsibility of physicians. Various diseases are required to be reported depending on state law (e.g., HIV status may or may not be reportable in individual states, whereas AIDS is reportable in all states). Reporting any injuries caused by lethal weapons, rapes, and battering (e.g., elder and child abuse) is mandatory in some states and not others. The regulations for the reporting of these conditions are codified by law and can be obtained from the state health department. These laws are designed to protect the individual's privacy as much as possible while still serving the public's interest. **Particularly in the realm of abuse, physicians have a complex ethical role regardless of the law. Victims of abuse must feel supported and assured that the violent act they survived will not have an adverse effect on how they are treated as people.** Their sense of vulnerability and their actual vulnerability may be so great that reporting an incident may increase their risk for medical harm. Despite the laws, physicians have an ethical responsibility to protect the patient's best interest.

Informed Consent

Informed consent is a process that involves an exchange of information directed toward reaching mutual understanding and informed decision making. Ideally, informed consent should be the practical manifestation of respect for patient preferences (autonomy) (19,20). An act of informed consent is often misunderstood to be getting a signature on a document. The intent of the individual involved in the consent process is often the protection of the physician from liability. Nothing could be further from either the legal or ethical meaning of this concept.

Informed consent is a conversation between physician and patient that teaches the patient about the medical condition, explores her values, and informs her about the reasonable medical alternatives. Informed consent is an interactive discussion in which one participant has greater knowledge about medical information and the other participant has greater knowledge about that individual's value system and circumstances affected by the information. This process does not require an arduous lecture on the medical condition or extensive examination of the patient's psyche. It does require adjustment of the information to the educational level of the patient and respectful elicitation of concerns and questions. It also requires acknowledgment of the various fears and concerns of both parties. Fear that the information may frighten patients, fear of hearing the information by the patient, a lack of ability to comprehend technical information, and an inability to express that lack are among the many barriers facing physicians and patients engaging in this conversation. **Communication skills are part of the art of medicine,** and observation of good role models, practices, and positive motivation can help to instill this ability in physicians (21).

Autonomy

Informed consent arises from the concept of autonomy. Pellegrino defines an autonomous person as "*one who, in his thoughts, work, and actions, is able to follow those norms he chooses as his own without external constraints or coercion by others*" (22). This definition contains the essence of what health care providers must consider as informed consent. The choice to receive or refuse medical care must be in concert with the patient's values and be freely chosen, and the options must be considered in light of the patient's values.

Autonomy is not respect for a patient's wishes against good medical judgment. Consider the example of a patient with inoperable, advanced-stage cervical cancer who demands surgery and refuses radiation therapy. **The physician's ethical obligation is to seek the best for the patient's survival (beneficence) and avoid the harm (nonmaleficence) of surgery, even if that is what the patient wishes.** Physicians are not obligated to offer treatment that is of no benefit, and the patient has the right to refuse treatment that does not fit into her values. Thus, this patient could refuse treatment for her cervical cancer, but she does not have the right to be given any treatment she wishes, in this case a treatment that would cause harm and no benefit.

Surrogate Decision Makers

If the ability to make choices is diminished by extreme youth, mental processing difficulties, extreme medical illness, or loss of awareness, surrogate decision making may be required. In all circumstances, the surrogate must make every attempt to act as the patient would have acted (23). The hierarchy of surrogate decision makers is specified by statutory law in each state and differs slightly from state to state. For adults, the first surrogate decision maker in the hierarchy is usually a court-appointed guardian if one exists and second is a durable power of attorney for health care if it exists, followed by relatives by degree of presumed familiarity (e.g., spouse, adult children, parents). For lesbian couples this presents issues in some states and the creation of a durable power of attorney can address this issue proactively. **Physicians should make sure their patients are aware of the need to have clear instructions about who they would want to speak for them if they are not able—in some cases it is not the person specified by the state guidelines.** For example, elderly women may not want their elderly (and slightly senile) spouse making decisions and prefer a friend or children—and should have a durable power of attorney for health care that ensures that will be the case.

For children, parents are the surrogate decision makers, except in circumstances in which the decision is life threatening and might not be the choice a child would make later, when adult beliefs and values are formed. The classic example of this is the Jehovah's Witness parents who refuse life-saving transfusions for their child (24). Although this case is the extreme, it illustrates that the basic principle outlined for surrogate decision making should apply to parents. Bias that influences decision making (in protection of parental social status, income, or systems of beliefs) needs to be considered by physicians because the potential conflict may lead parents to decisions that are not in the best interest of the child. If there is a conflicting bias that does not allow decisions to be made in the best interest of the child or that involves a medical threat to a child, legal action to establish guardianship (normally through a child protective agency by the courts) may be necessary. This action can destroy the patient (child)–physician relationship and the parent–physician relationship. It may affect the long-term health and well-being of the child, who must return to the care of the parents. Such decisions should be made only after all attempts to educate, clarify, and find alternatives are exhausted.

The legal age at which adolescents may make their own decisions regarding their health care varies by state (25). There is a growing trend to increase the participation of adolescents who are capable of decision making for their own health care. Because minors often have developed a value system and the capacity to make informed choices, their ability to be involved in decisions should be assessed individually rather than relying solely on the age criteria of the law and their parents' views.

A unique area for consideration of informed consent is providing care or conducting clinical research in foreign settings or caring for individuals from other countries who have differing viewpoints regarding individual autonomy. For example, if the prevailing standard for decision making by a woman is that her closest male relative makes it for her, how is that standard accommodated within our present autonomy-based system? In international research, these issues presented major concerns when women were assigned to placebo or treatment groups and consent was accepted from male relatives (26). The potential of coercion when no other access to health care is available creates real questions about the validity and freedom of choice for participants in entering clinical research studies in order to access health care in under-resourced areas (27). When caring for patients from certain cultures and foreign countries in daily practice, it is important to recognize that these issues exist in a microcosm. Ensuring that the patient can make the choice herself or freely chooses to have a relative make it for her remains an important element of informed consent.

Beneficence and Nonmaleficence

The principles of beneficence and nonmaleficence are the basis of medical care—the "to do good and no harm" of Hippocrates. These issues can be clouded by other decision makers, consultants, family members, and sometimes financial constraints or conflicts of interest. Of all the principles of good medical care, benefit is the one that continually must be reassessed. Simple questions can help clarify choices. What is the medical indication? How does the proposed therapy address this issue? How much will this treatment benefit the patient? How much will it extend the patient's life? When confronted with multiple medical problems and consultants, physicians should ask how much treatment will be of benefit given all the patient's problems (e.g., failing kidneys, progressive cardiomyopathy, HIV-positive status, and respiratory failure) rather than considering treatment of one problem without acknowledging that the overall benefit is limited by the presence of all the other problems.

An additional area of balancing beneficence and nonmaleficence is ensuring that the medicine we practice is the safest and highest quality relative to medical evidence. The safety and quality agenda in medicine is growing and necessitates consideration of the role of experience (number of procedures, simulation for ongoing maintenance of skills and development of skills, team training) in ensuring that our patients have access to the highest quality of care. When evidence shows improved outcomes for specific interventions—for example, with timing difference in preoperative antibiotics—health care professionals must participate in and embrace efforts to achieve those metrics on behalf of their patients as part of their fiduciary duty and their obligation to seek the benefit of their patients. Steps specific to this in obstetrics and gynecology are listed by the American College of Obstetricians and Gynecologists as developing the commitment to encourage a culture of patient safety, implementing safe medication practices, reducing the likelihood of surgical errors, improving communication with health care providers and patients, and working with patients to improve safety (28).

The benefit or futility of the treatment, along with quality-of-life considerations, should be evaluated for all aspects of patient care. It is best to weigh all of the relevant issues in a systematic fashion. Some systematic approaches depend on a sequential gathering of all the pertinent information in four domains: medical indications (benefit and harm), patient preferences (autonomy), quality of life, and contextual issues (justice) (19). Other approaches identify decision makers, followed by facts, and then ethical principles. It is important for physicians to select an ethical model of analysis under which to practice so that, when faced with troubling and complex decisions, they have sufficient experience with an ethics-based analytic system to help clarify the issues.

Medical Futility

The essence of good medical care is to attempt to be as clear as possible about the outcomes of the proposed interventions. If the proposed intervention (e.g., continued respiratory support or initiating support) has a slight or highly unlikely chance of success, intervention might be considered futile. **Physicians have no obligation to continue or initiate therapies of no benefit** (29). The decision to withdraw or withhold care is one that must be accompanied by an effort to ensure that the patient or her surrogate decision maker is educated about the decision and agrees with it. Other issues, such as family concerns, can and should modify decisions if the overall well-being of the patient and of the family is best served. For example, waiting (within reason) to withdraw life support may be appropriate to allow a family to reach consensus or a distant family member to see the patient for a last time.

Quality of Life

Quality of life is a much used, often unclear term. In the care of patients, quality of life is the effect of therapy on the patient's experience of living based on her perspective. It is perilous and speculative to assume that physicians know what quality of life represents for a particular patient judging from a personal reaction. It is instructive, however, to attempt to guess what it means and then seek the patient's perspective. The results may be surprising. For example, when offered a new drug for ovarian cancer, a patient might prefer to decline the treatment because the side effects may not be acceptable, even when there may be a reasonable chance that her life may be slightly prolonged. Conversely, the physician may not believe that further treatment is justified but the patient finds joy and fulfillment in entering a phase I clinical trial because it adds meaning to her life to give information to others about the possibilities of a new treatment. Informing patients of the experiences of others who had alternative treatments may help in their decision making, but it is never a substitute for the individual patient's decisions.

Professional Relations

Conflict of Interest

All professionals have multiple interests that affect their decisions. Contractual and covenantal relationships between physician and patient are intertwined and complicated by health care payers and colleagues, which create considerable pressure. The conflict with financial considerations directly influences patients' lives, often without their consent. Rennie described that pressure eloquently: "*Instead of receiving more respect (for more responsibility), physicians feel they are being increasingly questioned, challenged, and sued. Looking after a patient seems less and less a compact between two people and more a match in which increasing numbers of spectators claim the right to interfere and referee*" (30). One response to this environment is for the physician to attempt to protect his or her efforts by assuming that the physician–patient relationship is only contractual in nature. This allocation of responsibility and authority to the contract precludes the need for the ethical covenant between the physician and patient. For example, a pre-existing contract, insurance, a relationship with a particular hospital system, or a managed-care plan may discourage referral to a specialist, removing the physician's responsibility. All health care professionals will experience this tension between a covenantal or contractual relationship. A reasonable consideration of that relationship is "*one that allows clients as much freedom as possible to determine how their lives are affected as is reasonably warranted on the basis of their ability to make decisions*" (31).

Health Care Payers

An insurance coverage plan may demand that physicians assume the role of gatekeeper and administrator. Patients can be penalized for a lack of knowledge about their future desires or needs and the lack of alternatives to address the changes in those needs. Patients are equally penalized when they develop costly medical conditions that would not be covered if they moved from plan to plan. These situations often place the physician in the position of being the arbiter of patients' coverage rather than acting as an advocate and adviser. It is an untenable position for physicians because they often cannot change the conditions or structure of the plan but are forced to be the administrators of it.

In an effort to improve physician compliance with and interest in decreasing costs, intense financial conflicts of interest can be brought to bear on physicians by health care plans or health care systems. If a physician's profile on costs or referral is too high, he or she might be excluded from the plan, thus decreasing his or her ability to earn a living or to provide care to certain patients with whom a relationship has developed. Conversely, a physician may receive a greater salary or bonus if the plan makes more money. The ability to earn a living and to see patients in the future is dependent on maintaining relationships with various plans and other physicians. These are compelling loyalties and conflicts that cannot be ignored (32–34).

These conflicts are substantially different from those of fee-for-service plans, although the ultimate effect on the patient can be the same. In fee-for-service plans, financial gain conflicts of interest have the potential to result in failure to refer a patient or to restrict referral to those cases in which the financial gain is derived by return referral of other patients (35). Patients who have poor insurance coverage may be referred differentially from those who have better coverage. Patients may be unaware of these underlying conflicts of interest, a situation that elevates conflict of interest to an ethical problem. A patient has a right to know what her plan covers, to whom she is being referred and why, and the credentials of those to whom she is referred. The reality is that health care providers make many decisions under the pressure of multiple conflicts of interest. Physicians can be caught between self-interest and professional integrity. The outcome for individuals' and society's relationship with health care providers is damaged by failure to recognize and specifically address conflicts of interest that impede decision making (36). **Focusing clearly on the priority of the patient's best interest and responsibly rejecting choices that compromise the patient's needs are ethical requirements.**

Institutions, third-party payers, and legislatures avoid accountability for revealing conflicts of interest to those to whom they offer services. The restrictions of health care plans are never placed in a position as equally prominent as the coverage. The coverage choices can be quite arbitrary, and there is rarely an easily accessible and usable system for challenging them. Whole health systems or options may or may not be covered, but their presence or absence is obscured in the information given to patients. The social and financial conflicts of interest of these payers can directly affect the setting and nature of the relationship between physician and patient. To deal with ambiguous and sometimes capricious decision making, revelation of the conflicts of interest and accountability for choices should be demanded by physicians and patients (37).

Legal Problems

Abuses of the system (e.g., referral for financial gain) led to proposals and legislation, often referred to as Stark I and II, affecting physicians' ability to send patients to local laboratories and facilities in which they have a potential for financial gain. There were clearly documented abuses, but the same legislation would negatively affect rural clinics and laboratories whose sole source of financial support is rural physicians. States vary on the statutory legislation regarding this issue. Regardless of the laws, it is ethically required that financial conflicts of interest are revealed to patients (38,39).

Another abuse of the physician–patient relationship caused by financial conflicts of interest is fraudulent Medicare and Medicaid billings. This activity resulted in the Fraud and Abuse Act of 1987 (42 U.S.C. at 1320a–7b), which prohibits any individual or entity making false claims or soliciting or receiving any remuneration in cash or any kind, directly or indirectly, overtly or covertly, to induce a referral. Indictments under these laws are felonies, with potential fines, jail sentences, and loss of the license to practice medicine. Physicians should be aware of the legal ramifications of their referral and billing practices (40–42).

Harassment

The goal of medicine is excellence in the care of patients and, often, research and education that will advance the practice of medicine. Everyone involved in the process should be able to pursue the common goal on equal footing and without harassment that interferes with employees', learners', or colleagues' ability to work or be promoted equally in that environment. Every office and institution should have an assessment strategy to ensure that the work environment is conducive to focusing on work and learning and not hostile to individuals.

Every office and institution must have written policies on discrimination and sexual harassment that detail inappropriate behavior and state specific steps to be taken to correct an inappropriate situation and make sure they are widely accessible and available. The goal is to ensure appropriate reporting and procedures for taking appropriate action and protecting victims, educating or rehabilitating an offender, and preventing the reoccurrence of the behavior.

The legal sanction for this right is encoded in both statutory law through the Civil Rights Act of 1964 [42 U.S.C.A. at 2000e–2000e–17 (West 1981 and Supp. 1988)] and reinforced with judicial action (case or precedent law) by state and U.S. Supreme Court decisions. Charges of sexual harassment can be raised as a result of unwelcome sexual conduct or a hostile workplace.

Employees are not the only ones to experience sexual or other harassment, learners such as medical students or nursing students can experience it and have a high reported prevalence of it (43). Sexual or other harassment for students can interfere with the educational process and trigger federal discrimination liability, including loss of federal funds encoded in Title IX protections (44).

Stress Management

There is little doubt that the day-to-day stress of practicing medicine is significant. Besides the acknowledged stress of the time pressures and responsibility of medicine, the current health care environment has a detrimental effect on physicians' job security, with concurrent health risks (45). Stress takes a toll on cardiac function and on the practice of medicine and life outside of medicine (46,47).

Responding to stress through drug or alcohol abuse increases overall health and marital problems and decreases effectiveness in practice. In a long-term prospective study of medical students, individuals with high-risk (e.g., volatile, argumentative, aggressive) temperaments were shown to have a high rate of premature death (particularly before 55 years of age) (48). **Adequate sleep, reasonable working hours, exercise, and nutritional balance are directly related to decreases in psychological distress** (49). Simple relaxation training is shown to decrease gastroesophageal reflux in response to stress (50).

The pace that physicians maintain has a seductive quality that can easily mask the need for stress reduction by means of good health practices, exercise, and relaxation training. The answer to increased stress is not to work harder and extract the time for this from the relaxing and enjoyable pursuits that exist outside medicine. The outcome of that strategy (in terms of optimal psychological and physical functioning) is in neither the physician's nor the patient's best interest. Both the welfare of the patient and the welfare of the physician are enhanced by a planned strategy of good health practices and relaxation. This strategy is important to all members of the health care team. By providing such leadership, physicians can contribute to a better work and health care environment for everyone.

Society and Medicine

Justice

Some of the ethical and legal problems in the practice of gynecology relate to the fair and equitable distribution of burdens and benefits. How benefits are distributed is a matter of great debate. There are various methods of proposed distribution:

- **Equal shares** (everyone has the same number of health care dollars per year)

- **Need** (only those people who need health care get the dollars)

- **Queuing** (the first in line for a transplant gets it)

- **Merit** (those with more serious illnesses receive special benefits)

- **Contribution** (those who have paid more into their health care fund get more health care)

Each of these principles could be appropriate as a measure of just allocation of health care dollars, but each will affect individual patients in different ways. Just distribution has become a major issue in health care. The principles of justice apply only when the resource is desired or beneficial and to some extent scarce (51).

The traditional approach to medicine was for practitioners to accept the intense focus on the individual patient. The current changes in medicine will alter the focus from the patient to a population: "*in the emerging medicine, the presenting patient, more than ever before, will be a representative of a class, and the science that makes possible the care of the patient will refer prominently to the population from which that patient comes*" (52). Physicians increasingly are bound by accumulating outcomes data (population statistics) to modify the treatment of an individual in view of the larger population statistics. If, for example, the outcome of radical ovarian cancer debulking is only 20% successful in a patient with a certain set of medical problems, that debulking may be offered instead to someone who has an 85% chance of success. Theoretically, the former individual might have a successful debulking and the procedure might fail in the latter, but population statistics were used to allocate this scarce resource. The benefit was measured by statistics that predict success, not by other forms of justice allocation by need, queuing, merit, or contribution. This approach represents a major change in the traditional dedication of health care solely to the benefits of individual patients. With scarce resources, the overall benefits for all patients are considered in conjunction with the individual benefits for one patient.

There was always an inequity in the distribution of health care access and resources. This inequity is not seen by many health care providers who do not care for those patients who are unable to gain access, such as those who lack transportation or live in rural areas or where limits are imposed by lack of health care providers, time, and financial resources. Social discrimination sometimes leads to inequity of distribution of health care. Minorities are less likely to see private physicians or specialists with clear impacts on outcomes of care, regardless of their income or source of health care funding (53–58). Thus, health care is rationed by default.

Health care providers must shift the paradigm from the absolute *"do everything possible for this patient"* **to the proportionate** *"do everything reasonable for all patients"* (19). To reform the health care system requires judicial, legislative, and business mandates, and attention to the other social components that can pose obstacles to efforts to expand health care beyond a focus on individual patients.

Health Care Reform

The tension between understanding health as an inherently individual matter (in which the receipt of health care is critical to individual well-being) and as a communal resource (in which distribution of well-being throughout society is the goal) underpins much of the political and social debate surrounding health care reform (56). The questions of health care reform are twofold: 1) What is the proper balance between individual and collective good? and 2) Who will pay for basic health care? Because much of health care reform requires balancing competing goals, legislation to achieve reform should specifically address how this balance can be achieved. The role of government should be as follows:

- Regulating access of individuals to health care.

- Regulating potential harms to the public health (e.g., smoking, pollution, drug use).

- Promoting health practices of benefit to large populations (e.g., immunization, fluoridation of water).

Even with the present changes in health care structure in the United States, health care payers, not individual providers, often make decisions regarding both the amount and distribution of resources. The health insurance industry determines what are "reasonable and customary" charges and what will be covered. The government decides (often with intense special-interest pressure) what Medicare and Medicaid will cover (57–60). These decisions directly affect patient care. For that reason, health care providers cannot ethically remain silent when the health and well-being of their individual patients and their communities are adversely affected by health care reform decisions.

Research on the outcomes of care provided by gynecologists or affected adversely by the current system for financing health care (financial aspects, safety, quality-of-life measures, survival, morbidity, and mortality) will allow the discipline to have a voice in determining choices for women's health care. This is an ethically important responsibility for all women's health care providers.

References

1. **Steinman MA, Shlipak MG, McPhee SJ.** Of principles and pens: attitudes and practices of medicine housestaff towards pharmaceutical industry promotions. *Am J Med* 2001;110:551–557.
2. **Lucey C, Souba W.** Perspective: the problem with the problem of professionalism. *Acad Med* 2010;85:1018–1024.
3. **May WF.** Code and covenant or philanthropy and contract. *Hastings Cent Rep* 1975;5:29–38.
4. **Kohn KT, Corrigan JM, Donaldson MS.** *To err is human: building a safer health system.* Washington, DC: National Academy Press, 1999.
5. **Bell SK, Moorman DW, Delbanco T.** Improving the patient, family, and clinician experience after harmful events: the "when things go wrong" curriculum. *Acad Med* 2010;85:1010–1017.
6. **Stroud L, McIlroy J, Levinson W.** Skills of internal medicine residents in disclosing medical errors: a study using standardized patients. *Acad Med* 2009;84:1803–1808.
7. **Lumalcuri J, Hale R.** Medical liability an ongoing nemesis. *Obstet Gynecol* 2010;115:223–228.
8. **Feinmann J.** You can say sorry. *BMJ* 2009;339:b3057.

9. **Kraman SS, Hamm G.** Risk management: extreme honesty may be the best policy. *Ann Intern Med* 1999;131:963–967.
10. **Popp PL.** How will disclosure affect future litigation? *J Heath Risk Manag* 2003;23:5–9.
11. **Boothman RC, Blackwell A, Campbell D Jr, et al.** A better approach to medical malpractice claims? The University of Michigan experience. *J Health Life Sci Law* 2009;2:125–159.
12. **Gallagher T.** A 62 year old woman with skin cancer who experience wrong site surgery. *JAMA* 2009;302:669–677.
13. **Privacy Protection Study Commission.** *Personal privacy in an information society.* Washington, DC: U.S. Government Printing Office, 1977.
14. **Cain J.** Confidentiality. In: APGO Task Force on Medical Ethics. *Exploring medical-legal issues in obstetrics and gynecology.* Washington, DC: APGO, 1994:43–45.
15. **Lo B, Dornbrand L, Dubler N.** HIPAA and patient care: the role for professional judgment. *JAMA* 2005;293;1766–1771.
16. **Centers for Medicare and Medicaid Services.** Is mandatory encryption in the HIPAA Security rule? HIPAA certification compliance. Available online at: http://www.hipaacertification.net/Is-mandatory-encryption-in-HIPAA-Security-Rule.htm
17. **O'Herrin J, Fost N, Kudsk K.** Health insurance portability accountability act (HIPAA) regulations: effect on medical record research. *Ann Surg* 2004;239:772–778.
18. **Tobriner MO.** Majority Opinion, California Supreme Court, 1 July 1976. California Reporter (West Publishing Company) 1976:14–33.
19. **Jonsen AR, Siegler M, Winslade WJ.** *Clinical ethics.* New York: McGraw-Hill, 1992:5–61.
20. **American College of Obstetricians and Gynecologists.** *Ethical dimensions of informed consent.* Committee Opinion No. 108. Washington, DC: ACOG, 1992.
21. **Katz J.** Informed consent: must it remain a fairy tale? *J Contemp Health Law Policy* 1994;10:69–91.
22. **Pellegrino ED.** Patient and physician autonomy: conflicting rights and obligations in the physician-patient relationship. *J Contemp Health Law Policy* 1994;10:47–68.
23. **Buchanan AE, Brock DW.** *Deciding for others: the ethics of surrogate decision making.* New York: Cambridge University Press, 1989.
24. **Ackerman T.** The limits of beneficence: Jehovah's Witnesses and childhood cancer. *Hastings Cent Rep* 1980;10:13–16.
25. **Nocon JJ.** Selected minor consent laws for reproductive health care. In: APGO Task Force on Medical Ethics. *Exploring medical-legal issues in obstetrics and gynecology.* Washington, DC: APGO, 1994:129–136.
26. **Loue S, Okello D.** Research bioethics in the Ugandan context. II. Procedural and substantive reform. *J Law Med Ethics* 2000;28:165–173.
27. **Emanuel E, Wendler D, Grady C.** What makes clinical research ethical? *JAMA* 2000;283:2701–2711.
28. **ACOG Committee.** Opinion 447. Patient safety in obstetrics and gynecology. *Obstet Gynecol* 2009;114:1424–1427.
29. **Jecker NS, Schneiderman LJ.** Medical futility: the duty not to treat. *Camb Q Healthc Ethics* 1993;2:151–159.
30. **Rennie D.** Let us focus your worries! Health care policy: a clinical approach. *JAMA* 1994;272:631–632.
31. **Bayles MD.** The professional-client relationship. In: *Professional ethics: an annotated bibliography of monographs.* Belmont, CA: Wadsworth, 1981.
32. **Ellsbury K.** Can the family physician avoid conflict of interest in the gatekeeper role? An affirmative view. *J Fam Pract* 1989;28:698–701.
33. **Stephens GG.** Can the family physician avoid conflict of interest in the gatekeeper role? An opposing view. *J Fam Pract* 1989;28:701–704.
34. **Miles C.** Resource allocation in the National Health Service. In: Byrne P, ed. *Ethics and the law in health care and research.* New York: Wiley, 1990:117–123.
35. **Cain JM, Jonsen AR.** Specialists and generalists in obstetrics and gynecology: conflicts of interest in referral and an ethical alternative. *Women's Health Issues* 1992;2:137–145.
36. **American College of Obstetricians and Gynecologists.** *Deception.* Committee Opinion No. 87. Washington, DC: ACOG, 1990.
37. **Wrenn K.** No insurance, no admission. *N Engl J Med* 1985;392:373–374.
38. **Hyman D, Williamson JV.** Fraud and abuse: setting the limits on physicians' entrepreneurship. *N Engl J Med* 1989;320:1275.
39. **McDowell TN Jr.** Physician self referral arrangements: legitimate business or unethical entrepreneurialism. *Am J Law Med* 1989;15:61–109.
40. **Stark F.** Ethics in patient referrals. *Acad Med* 1989;64:146–147.
41. **Green RM.** Medical joint-venturing: an ethical perspective. *Hastings Cent Rep* 1990;20:22–26.
42. **Nocon JJ.** Fraud and abuse: employment kickbacks and physician recruitment. In: APGO Task Force on Medical Ethics. *Exploring medical-legal issues in obstetrics and gynecology.* Washington, DC: APGO, 1994:69–74.
43. **Best CL, Smith DW, Raymond, JR Sr, et al.** Preventing and responding to complaints of sexual harassment in an academic health center: a 10-year review from the Medical University of South Carolina. *Acad Med* 2010;85:721–727
44. **Recupero PR, Heru AM, Price M, et al.** Sexual harassment in medical education: liability and protection. *Acad Med* 2004;79:817–824.
45. **Heaney CA, Israel BA, House JS.** Chronic job insecurity among automobile workers: effects on job satisfaction and health. *Soc Sci Med* 1994;38:1431–1437.
46. **Sloan RP, Shapiro PA, Bagiella E, et al.** Effect of mental stress throughout the day on cardiac autonomic control. *Biol Psychol* 1994;37:89–99.
47. **Serry N, Bloch S, Ball R, et al.** Drug and alcohol abuse by doctors. *Med J Aust* 1994;60:402–407.
48. **Graves PL, Mead LA, Wang NY, et al.** Temperament as a potential predictor of mortality: evidence from a 41-year prospective study. *J Behav Med* 1994;17:111–126.
49. **Ezoe S, Morimoto K.** Behavioral lifestyle and mental health status of Japanese workers. *Prev Med* 1994;23:98–105.
50. **McDonald HJ, Bradley LA, Bailey MA, et al.** Relaxation training reduces symptom reports and acid exposure in patients with gastroesophageal reflux disease. *Gastroenterology* 1994;107:61–69.
51. **Daniels N.** Just health care. Cambridge, UK: Cambridge University Press, 1985.
52. **Jonsen AR.** The new medicine and the old ethics. Boston: Harvard University Press, 1990.
53. **Watson SD.** Minority access and health reform: a civil right to health care. *J Law Med Ethics* 1994;22:127–137.
54. **Watson SD.** Health care in the inner city: asking the right question. *North Carolina Law Rev* 1993;71:1661–1663.
55. **Freeman HE, Blendon RJ, Aiken LH, et al.** Americans report on their access to health care. *Health Aff (Millwood)* 1987;6:6–8.
56. **Burris S.** Thoughts on the law and the public's health. *J Law Med Ethics* 1994;22:141–146.
57. **Evans RW.** Health care technology and the inevitability of resource allocation and rationing decisions: part 2. *JAMA* 1983;249:2208–2210.
58. **President's Commission for the Study of Ethical Problems in Medicine and Biomedical and Behavioral Research.** Securing access to health care: the ethical implications of differences in availability of health services. Washington, DC: Government Printing Office, 1983:1–3.
59. **Eddy DM.** What care is essential? *JAMA* 1991;265:786–788.
60. **Committee on Health Care for Underserved Women, ACOG.** The uninsured. *Obstet Gynecol* 2004;104:1471–1473.

3 Safety and Quality

John P. Keats
Joseph C. Gambone

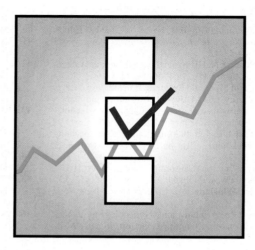

- Quality is the degree to which health services for the individual and populations increase the likelihood of desired health outcomes, consistent with current professional knowledge.

- Each physician assumes a significant responsibility for safety and excellent care in their own practice environment.

- Adverse outcomes and near misses allow the organization to examine its processes of care with an eye to continuous improvement.

- In an assessment of the factors leading up to serious adverse events in hospitals, communication problems were the most frequently identified root cause, occurring in almost three-fourths of cases.

- No one should be hesitant to raise questions and concerns when an unsafe situation is observed.

- Drills and rehearsals for emergency situations improve outcomes and enhance safety.

- Hand washing using appropriate technique before and after every patient encounter should be considered mandatory.

- In the operating room, a preoperative verification process, a marking of the surgical site, and the performance of a time-out should be routine.

- Medication safety is a high priority for quality improvement initiatives. Avoiding abbreviations that may lead to medication error increases patient safety.

- Disruptive behavior in the hospital setting can have adverse effects on patient safety and overall quality of care.

- Professional organizations endorse active disclosure to the patient when adverse events occur, including those caused by error.

- Effective communication with office personnel and with patients is an essential element for creating a culture of safety in the office setting.

What Is Quality Care?

It has been more than a decade since the Institute of Medicine (IOM) published two seminal works in the fields of patient safety and medical care quality: *To Err Is Human* and *Crossing the Quality Chasm* (1,2). Despite the heightened awareness and increased public focus on the crucial issues raised by these publications, there is limited evidence of significant progress toward making this country's health care both safer and better (3). One reason for this absence of momentum may be the very gradual incorporation of an emphasis on the principles of patient safety during medical school and residency. Leaders in the patient safety movement have called for the redesign of education for health care professionals in order to equip these individuals with the essential knowledge, skill, and attitude required to function safely and effectively in the health care delivery environment of the 21st century. Although this imperative affects all health professions, it is particularly compelling in medical education because physicians' actions and decisions indicate parameters for the care that most other health care professionals provide (4).

The IOM defined quality as "the degree to which health services for the individual and populations increase the likelihood of desired health outcomes . . . consistent with current professional knowledge" (5). Of note in this assertion is the recognition that health care quality is important and applicable to entire groups of people, as well as to every single patient. Implicit is the obligation to be sensitive to the flexible meaning of "desired health outcomes," because desired outcomes may differ from the perspective of hospitals, physicians, patients, and their families. Adherence to the definition includes rigorous application of accepted standards of information and treatment to any clinical problem, a process now referred to as evidence-based medical practice (6).

Another construct to define and achieve higher quality health care can be derived from the "Five Rights" of medication administration: right patient, right drug, right dose, right time, and right route (7). The Five Rights of medical quality could be thought of as doing the right thing for the right patient at the right time; doing it right the first time; and doing it right for every patient (8).

The concepts embodied in these two statements are elegantly incorporated into the IOM's six "Aims for Improvement" that are articulated in *Crossing the Quality Chasm* and listed in Table 3.1 (The Six Aims) (2). It is notable that "Safe" is listed first. **Safety has always been considered "first among equals" in the hierarchy of physicians' responsibilities.** This was initially understood as an admonition to individual medical practitioners. However, it is now recognized that fulfilling this promise of safety requires conscientious evaluation and careful renovation of the systems that deliver medical care.

Clinical Variation

Each patient receiving an identical diagnosis might not be given the same treatment. This is known as clinical variation, and can be broadly categorized as falling into two types. One is necessary clinical variation, an alteration in medical practice that is required by the differing needs of individual patients. This modification may be in response to differences in the patients themselves, because of age, overall health status, or other clinical characteristics; or it may be caused by differing desired outcomes as part of a patient-centered approach to care (8). This kind of variation is expected in any system of care. The other type is unexplained clinical variation, which comprises differences in medical care and patient management that are not accounted for by differences in patient symptoms, objective findings, or patients' goals for care. **These treatment discrepancies could account for wide variations in the cost of care without any demonstrable difference in outcomes as measured by morbidity or mortality**

Table 3.1 Six Aims for Quality Health Care	
Care should be:	
Safe (First among equals)	Timely
Effective	Efficient
Patient-centered	Equitable

(9–11). Often this unexplained variation is the result of management choices made by physicians in cases that fall into so-called clinical gray areas, where no single course is clearly correct. Sometimes this variation is both unexplained and unintended. It is this unexplained or unintended variation that is considered one of the greatest barriers to the delivery of consistently high-quality care (12). The specialty of gynecology is subject to this treatment inconsistency. Significant geographic variations in hysterectomy rates, largely unexplained by the clinical characteristics of those local populations, were reported (11,13). Further study and reduction of unnecessary variation in these rates could contribute to making medical care more efficient and equitable.

Role of Organizational Leadership

Creating a safe environment for the delivery of medical care requires the active participation of organizational leadership. Each physician assumes a significant responsibility for safety and excellent care in his or her own practice environment. In the hospital, oversight for issues of safety and quality is shared by the hospital board, executive leadership, and physicians who serve as chief medical officer, vice president of medical affairs, or department chairs. A new position being adopted by many hospitals is the patient safety officer (14). This individual takes direct responsibility for overseeing all aspects of the hospital patient safety program and reports to the hospital chief executive officer or board of directors. It is an emerging role for physicians who want to make patient safety the focus of their professional lives.

An integral part of promoting patient safety is the creation of an organizational culture where patient safety is recognized as everyone's responsibility. Culture in an organization is "the way we do things around here" mindset, and it reflects the attitude of the members of the organization toward what is important and how that fits into the structure of their activities (15). The first step in creating a culture of safety is to measure a starting point for both nursing and physician staff regarding the attitudes and perceptions around patient safety. This can be accomplished using any of several validated tools such as a safety attitude questionnaire or hospital survey on patient safety culture (14). Once areas of deficiency are identified, steps can be taken to improve culture by direct interaction with frontline clinicians to ascertain appropriate changes to the clinical environment to promote safety. This can be done through regular safety meetings or direct observation of the workplace with Executive Walkrounds™ (16).

Another method for improving the safety climate in a hospital is the adoption of the tenets of "Just Culture" (17). **Just Culture recognizes that human error cannot be eliminated from any complex system such as health care.** People sometimes make mistakes. They can be held accountable for following procedural rules to reduce harm to patients resulting from human error. **Adverse outcomes and near misses allow the organization to examine its processes of care with an eye to continuous improvement. With such a system in place, the reporting of safety problems and concerns will often increase dramatically.** This in turn allows the hospital or other health care organization to initiate programs to address these issues and to make "first, do no harm" a reality.

Communication

In an assessment of the factors leading up to serious adverse events in hospitals, communication problems were the most frequently identified root cause, occurring in almost three-fourths of cases (18). Assuring clear and timely communication between all caregivers is perhaps the single most important measure to improve the safety and quality of medical care. In the health care setting, structured communication techniques are referred to under the title "team resource management." The basic principle of team resource management is to foster an atmosphere where individuals with different roles are brought together to achieve a successful outcome to a complex operation (19). Despite differing roles, training, and ranking within a perceived hierarchy, and the fact that some individuals may not have worked together as a team before, it is understood that each participant has an overarching responsibility. That responsibility is to communicate with all team members whenever they see anything that is potentially unsafe or when other team members are not acting appropriately in a given situation. This concept is particularly applicable in the operating room, by nature a highly complex environment. **Everyone present—physicians, nurses, house staff, and technicians—must keep patient safety foremost in their minds. No one should be hesitant to raise questions and concerns when an unsafe situation is observed.**

There are excellent formalized systems to train health care providers in this important skill (19). One of the most comprehensive and well-recognized systems is Team Strategies and Tools to

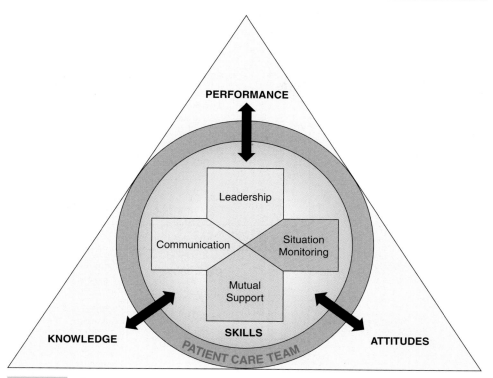

Figure 3.1   The TeamSTEPPS program logo. (From Team STEPPS Program of the U.S. Agency for Healthcare Research and Quality [AHRQ]).

Enhance Performance and Patient Safety (TeamSTEPPS), a joint project of the Agency for Health Care Research and Quality and the Department of Defense (20). The TeamSTEPPS logo (Fig. 3.1) is a visual model representing the four basic teamwork skills of leadership, communication, situational monitoring, and mutual support. The program teaches how the interaction of these skills produces the three desired team outcomes for knowledge, attitudes, and performance, and how these outcomes further reinforce those skills in a reciprocal manner. TeamSTEPPS includes the principles of team resource management, as well as many specific techniques for effective communication. One of the most useful is represented with the acronym SBAR: *S*ituation, *B*ackground, *A*ssessment, and *R*ecommendation (or *R*equest) (21). It is a structured method for relaying information about a changing clinical situation. The initiator of the exchange gives a brief description of the clinical change or concern that is prompting the communication. This is followed by the clinically relevant background information about the patient. The initiator then gives his or her assessment of what he or she thinks is happening with the patient and makes a recommendation or request for action by the other party. It is frequently used by nurses to update on-call physicians about a patient's clinical status, but can also be used between residents and attending physicians or any other pair of providers where concise, clear communication is required.

Certain situations in health care are particularly prone to miscommunication. One example is during the stress of emergency situations, when a physician may be rapidly giving orders for medications, blood transfusions, or procedures to be initiated. A technique referred to as "call-outs" helps ensure that critical orders are received correctly. The person to whom the verbal order is directed repeats the order verbatim to acknowledge he or she has received it and will be responsible for carrying it out. Hearing this call-out assures the ordering physician that the order was received, who will be performing it, and allows an opportunity to correct the order if it was misheard. Similarly, telephone orders are well known to be sources of misinterpretation of physicians' treatment intentions (22). Check-back is a technique to minimize errors in this medium. In a typical situation, a doctor calls a nurse to order a medication for a patient. Check-back has three components. First, the physician gives the medication order to the nurse. Second, the nurse repeats the order back to the physician, specifying medication name, dose, route, and timing of administration. Lastly, the physician confirms back to the nurse that the order was

I	Introduction	Introduce yourself and your role/job (include patient)
P	Patient	Name, identifiers, age, sex, location
A	Assessment	Present chief complaint, vital signs, symptoms, and diagnosis
S	Situation	Current status/circumstances, including code status, level of (un)certainty, recent changes, and response to treatment
S	SAFETY Concerns	Critical lab values/reports, socio-economic factors, allergies, and alerts (falls, isolation, etc.)
THE		
B	Background	Co-morbidities, previous episodes, current medications, and family history
A	Actions	What actions were taken or are required? Provide brief rationale
T	Timing	Level of urgency and explicit timing and prioritization of actions
O	Ownership	Who is responsible (person/team) including patient/family?
N	Next	What will happen next? Anticipated changes? What is the plan? Are there contingency plans?

Figure 3.2 I PASS the BATON. (From Team STEPPS Program of the U.S. Agency for Healthcare Research and Quality [AHRQ]).

correctly received. A handoff of a patient from one physician to another is a third opportunity for miscommunication. This relay team approach to care is occurring more frequently in medical education as a result of residency work-hour restrictions (23). To minimize errors in this setting, it is wise to use a structured script for communicating critical clinical information. One such script from the TeamSTEPPS program is the mnemonic I PASS the BATON, which is essentially a checklist of clinical items to be related to the person assuming the care of the patient (Fig. 3.2) (19). The key point is that management handoffs should be a formal process that does not rely on memory to convey crucial information.

An important feature of team resource management is the ability of any team member to "stop the line"; that is to halt the process or procedure when they feel a risk to patient safety is present. One recommended technique is the "CUS" method. This acronym represents three possible sets of "code words" that any team member may articulate to indicate that the procedure must stop until the safety concern is addressed. The letters in the acronym stand for "I'm *C*oncerned"; I'm *U*ncomfortable"; and "I have a *S*afety concern." Another method is the "Two-Challenge Rule." This indicates that when a team member has a safety concern he or she should bring it to the attention of the physician in charge of the procedure in question. If the concern is not acknowledged or adequately addressed, the team member should address it a second time. If the concern is still unanswered or uncorrected, the team member is then obligated to go up the chain of command to a supervisor or higher-ranking physician to have his or her concerns satisfied.

All of these techniques can contribute to a safer environment for patient care in the operating room, emergency department, and on patient floors. However, none of them can be very effective without practice. The use of drills and simulations to rehearse these techniques in mock emergency situations is well established in anesthesia training programs (24,25). The use of simulators to teach basic surgical techniques including laparoscopy and robotic surgery are becoming more common (26–28). **Drills and rehearsals for emergency situations improve outcomes and enhance safety** (29–31).

Infection Control

Hospital-acquired infections are one of the most common causes of morbidity in hospitalized patients (32). **Reducing the incidence of these infections, and preventing their spread to other patients, should be a top priority for all health care providers.**

Surgical site infections result in an increased length of stay for surgical patients, with all the attendant associated risks and increased costs (33). While not preventable 100% of the time, their incidence can be significantly reduced. There are many operating room techniques available to accomplish this, and they should be used consistently (34). These include avoidance of shaving of the operative site, appropriate antimicrobial skin preparation, preoperative hand antisepsis, use and correct timing of administration of antibiotic prophylaxis, and observance of sterile technique.

In addition to preventing the occurrence of infection, it is equally important to prevent transmission of infection from one patient to another. **One of the most effective, but widely underutilized techniques is simple hand washing.** The effectiveness of hand washing in the prevention of disease transmission was first demonstrated by Ignac Semmelweis in the obstetrical wards of Vienna in the 1840s (35). Despite having this knowledge for over 150 years, compliance with hand-hygiene techniques in the hospital setting remains poor (36). **Hand washing using appropriate technique before and after every patient encounter should be considered mandatory.** Beyond this basic technique, certain infections require special precautions to prevent transmission, known as isolation techniques (37). These involve combinations of masks, gowns, and gloves to prevent contact with infected skin, body fluids, or airborne particles. It includes special handling of trash, linens, and environmental surfaces. The level of precautions to be taken will be determined by the hospital's infection control personnel. The key point is to adhere rigorously to the isolation instructions posted outside the patient's room.

Operating Room Safety

The operating room is by its nature a highly complex health care environment. It is a potential site for adverse events, which can be catastrophic. These include wrong patient surgeries, wrong site surgeries, and retained foreign objects. All of these occur in hospitals, despite recognition that these events should never take place (38,39). The Joint Commission, a national accrediting body for hospitals, has developed the Universal Protocol™ that all surgeons and operating rooms should follow (40). There are three major components of the Universal Protocol. **First is to conduct a preprocedure verification process** that confirms the identity of the patient and his or her understanding of what procedure is to be performed. **Second is marking of the operative site** by the surgeon, which is especially critical in cases involving bilateral structures. This is to be done in the preoperative area with the patient awake as a confirmation of accuracy. **Third is the performance of a surgical "time out"** in the operating room prior to the start of the surgery to confirm the correct patient identity and correct planned procedure. **Failure to perform any of these steps increases the risk of performing the wrong operation on the wrong patient.**

The traditional use of checklists resulted in dramatic increases in the safety of aviation (41). Their use in medicine is recent but is demonstrated to decrease complications significantly when used consistently to verify that procedural steps are not overlooked. A simple five-step checklist for central-line placement in the intensive care unit was shown to reduce the incidence of catheter-related sepsis almost to zero (42,43). Similarly, checklists are advocated for use in the surgical suite to ensure that critical steps for error prevention and patient safety are not overlooked. The World Health Organization (WHO) released a surgical checklist in 2009 under their "Safe Surgery Saves Lives" program (44). It involves items to be reviewed and documented before the induction of anesthesia, before the skin incision, and before the patient leaves the operating room. Use of the WHO checklist was shown to reduce major complications of surgery from 11% to 7% and the inpatient death rate from major surgery from 1.5% to 0.8% (45). The use of checklists such as this to improve patient safety in the operating room should become more widespread.

The inadvertent retention of foreign bodies such as sponges, instruments, or other objects at the conclusion of surgery is a continuing source of patient harm. Risk factors associated with retained foreign bodies are emergency surgery, an unexpected change in surgical procedure, high patient body mass index, and failure to perform sponge and instrument counts (46). Systems must be established to prevent these occurrences, and surgeons need to aware of the contributing risk factors listed above (47). **The most commonly retained item is a surgical sponge. Strict adherence to guidelines for tracking surgical sponges is necessary to reduce the incidence of this serious complication.** One comprehensive program to assist in this adherence is called "Sponge Accounting" (48). It involves standardized counting and recording of sponges at the start of the case and as additional sponges are added to the surgical field. At the conclusion of the surgery, all sponges are placed in special transparent holders to allow visual confirmation that all sponges were taken out of the patient. Other systems employ radiofrequency tagging of all sponges so that retained sponges can be detected easily before the surgical wound is closed (49).

Application of Safety Technology

Computerized physician (prescriber) order entry system (CPOE) is a prescription ordering system where the prescriber enters ordering information directly into a computer. Some of the more sophisticated systems can check for errors and make suggestions based on preprogrammed guidelines and protocols. CPOE is known to reduce serious medical errors and prevent otherwise undetected adverse drug events (ADEs) (50). When CPOE systems are properly designed and implemented, they can improve workflow efficiency by supplying real-time dosing information and other decision support protocols and guidelines. Poorly designed or improperly implemented CPOE systems, however, have the potential to decrease efficiency and increase medication error.

Medication safety is a high priority for quality improvement initiatives. Avoiding abbreviations that may lead to medication error increases patient safety (51). Table 3.2 lists examples of dangerous abbreviations and dose expressions that should be avoided. **Avoiding abbreviations that can be misread is an important and effective improvement, especially when orders are handwritten.** One easily remembered and important rule about the written medication order is "always lead and never follow" a decimal point when using zeros. An order that is written as .1 mg should be written as 0.1 mg—an example of leading with a zero. It can be very dangerous for the written period to be missed, resulting in 1 mg being given to a patient rather than 0.1 mg. The leading zero should alert to the correct dosage. An order that is written as 1.0 mg should be written as 1 mg—never following with a zero, so that a patient is not mistakenly given 10 mg of a drug if the period is missing or not seen. Exclusive use of properly designed and implemented CPOE systems can eliminate misread written orders.

Bar coding of medications improves error occurrence by reducing the rate of wrong medication by nearly 75%. Other types of medication error improvements attributed to bar coding include incorrect dose, wrong patient errors, and wrong time errors, which were reduced substantially through the use of bar coding (52).

The Leapfrog Group, comprised of Fortune 500 companies and other large health care purchasers, has made CPOE one of its top priorities for improving patient safety along with appropriate staffing of intensive care units (ICUs) and appropriate referral of high-risk patients to "centers of excellence." CPOE and bar coding are two safety technologies that are proven to lower the risk of medical errors.

Disruptive Provider Behavior

In 2009, as part of its accreditation standards, the Joint Commission proposed that all health care organizations with professional staffs develop and implement a Code of Conduct Policy along with an education program that addresses disruptive behavior.

Disruptive physician (provider) behaviors include inappropriate conduct in the hospital setting, resulting in conflict or confrontation. These behaviors can range from verbal and even physical abuse to sexual harassment. In recent years disruptive behavior in the hospital setting has become more evident, if not more common. One study showed that the vast majority of surveyed physicians, nurses, and administrators had witnessed disruptive behavior by physicians (53). Nurses and other hospital employees also commit disruptive behavior, but it is far less common than

Table 3.2 Examples of Dangerous Abbreviations and Dose Expressions

Abbreviation/Dose Expression	Intended Meaning	Misinterpretation
AU	Aurio uterque (each ear)	Mistaken for OU (oculo uterque-each eye).
D/C	Discharge, discontinue	Premature discontinuation of medications when D/C (intended to mean "discharge") has been misinterpreted as "discontinued" when followed by a list of drugs.
μg	Microgram	Mistaken for "mg" when handwritten
o.d. or OD	Once daily	Misinterpreted as "right eye" (OD-oculus dexter) and administration of oral medications in the eye
TIW or tiw	Three times a week	Mistaken as "three times a day"
per os	orally	The "os" can be mistaken for "left eye"
q.d. or QD	every day	Mistaken as q.i.d., aspecially if the period after the "q" or the tail of the "q" is misunderstood as an "i"
qn	Nightly or at bedtime	Misinterpreted as "qh" (every hour)
qhs	Nightly at bedtime	Misread as every hour
q6PM, etc.	Every evening at 6PM	Misread as every 6 hours
q.o.d. or QOD	Every other day	Misinterpreted as "q.d." (daily) or "q.i.d." (four times daily) if the "o" is poorly written
sub q	Subcutaneous	The "q" has been mistaken for "every" (e.q., one heparin dose ordered "sub q 2 hours before surgery" misunderstood as every 2 hours before surgery)
SC	Subcutaneous	Mistaken for SL (sublingual)
U or u	Unit	Read as a zero (0) or a four (4), causing a 10-fold overdose or greater (4U seen as "40" or 4u seen as 44")
IU	International unit	Misread as IV (intravenous)
cc	Cubic centimeters	Misread as "U" (units)
×3d	For 3 days	Mistaken for "three doses"
BT	Bedtime	Mistaken for "BID" (twice daily)
ss	Sliding scale (insulin) or (apothecary)	Mistaken for "55"
> or <	Greater than or less than	Mistakenly used opposite of intended
/ (slash mark)	Separates two doses or indicates "per"	Misunderstood as the number 1 ("25 unit/10 units") read as "110" units
Name letters and dose numbers run together (e.g., Inderal 40 mg)	Inderal 40 mg	Misread as Inderal 140 mg.
Zero after decimal point (1.0)	1 mg	Misread as 10 mg if the decimal point is not seen
No zero before decimal dose (.5 mg)	0.5 mg	Misread as 5 mg

Modified from **Reiter RC, Yielding L, Gluck PA.** Clinical performance improvement: assessing the quality and safety of women health care. In: **Hacker NF, Moore JG, Gambone JC, eds.** *Essentials of obstetrics and gynecology,* 4th ed., Philadelphia: Elsevier/Saunders, 2004:52, with permission.

disruptive physician behavior. **Disruptive behavior in the hospital setting can have adverse effects on patient safety and overall quality of care.**

One recommendation for mitigating disruptive behavior among health care professionals when concise and clear communication is needed is the SBAR method, mentioned above. Having an accepted and agreed-upon verbal process to question or suggest changes in patient management improves communication. **Team building that encourages collegial interaction and a sense that all members of the health care team are important and have something to offer can promote a culture that makes disruptive behavior less likely.**

Patient and Family Involvement in Quality and Safety

One of the better definitions of quality is "meeting a customer's (patient's and their families) expectations." Clear and frequent communication between the team of health care professionals and the patient and the patient's family is the most effective way to determine and meet appropriate expectations. The Joint Commission, in collaboration with the Centers for Medicare and Medicaid Services, introduced an initiative they called "Speak Up." The program features brochures, posters, and buttons on a variety of patient safety topics. The program goal is designed to urge patients to take an active role in preventing health care errors by becoming involved and informed participants as members of the health care team. In 2008 a survey conducted by the Joint Commission indicated that campaigns like Speak Up add significant value to the accreditation process (54). Eighty percent of the more than1,900 organizations that responded rated the program as good or excellent.

Another initiative developed at Rand and the University of California–Los Angeles is the PREPARED checklist for informed, collaborative choice (Table 3.3) . Studies show that greater patient (and family) involvement in health care decision making results in improved satisfaction and better outcomes (55). The PREPARED checklist, using each letter in the word and a mnemonic, consists of a structured conversation that includes the *P*lan, *R*eason for the plan, *E*xpectation of benefit, *P*references (e.g., prefer or avoid surgery), *A*lternatives, *R*isks, and *E*xpenses, followed by an informed collaborative *D*ecision to accept or reject the plan.

The use of either or both of these programs should improve overall safety by informing the patient and his or her family about what will happen, what is expected along with the known risks (complications and side effects), so that they can alert the health care team of any expected or unexpected adverse events. Patients and their families traditionally have low self-efficacy or confidence that they can understand and actively participate during their health care. Programs such as Speak Up and PREPARED are shown to increase patient and family member self-efficacy.

Disclosure and Apology for Adverse Events

Organized medicine is increasing its focus on the prevention of medical error. A controversial issue involving medical error is the need to promptly disclose and apologize for any medical errors that occur. In the past many, if not most, health care organizations focused on managing the medical legal risk of medical error. The conventional wisdom was that any disclosure and apology for error would lead to litigation and bigger payouts. **The Joint Commission and other professional organizations require or endorse active disclosure to the patient when adverse events occur, including those caused by error** (56).

Three programs are worth noting in any discussion of disclosure and apology for medical error. First is the University of Michigan's patient safety program, which addresses the need to disclose medical error in several publications (57). Important points are made about a patient's rights concerning disclosure of medical error and that an apology for errors can be a productive benevolent gesture rather than an admission of fault. The authors point out several fallacies about disclosure, including that disclosing medical error always leads to litigation and that error always means negligence.

Lucian Leape, one of the fathers of the modern patient safety movement, pointed out that a patient has an ethical right to full disclosure of medical error (58). Although an apology is not

Table 3.3 PREPARED Checklist Process for Informed Communication	
P lan:	Course of action being considered
R eason:	Indication or rationale
E xpectation:	Chances of benefit and failure
P references:	Patient-centered priorities
A lternatives:	Other reasonable options/plans
R isks:	Potential harms from considered plans
E xpenses:	Direct and indirect costs
D ecision:	Fully informed collaborative choice

an ethical right, it is a therapeutic necessity, according to Leape. Several programs are under way to test the assertion that disclosure and apology can decrease the likelihood of litigation. COPIC, a Colorado medical insurance company, found that full disclosure results in small early settlements and dramatically reduced law suits and payouts (59).

The Sorry Works Coalition, which is a coalition of doctors, insurers, and patient advocates, urges the use of full disclosure and apology for medical errors (60). They point out that the current tort system has failed, resulting in higher and higher malpractice premiums without decreasing the rate of medical error. Demands for caps on malpractice awards and greater disciplinary measures for providers are largely ineffective. The Sorry Works Coalition advocates early disclosure with apology and financial settlements without litigation as the way forward in dealing with medical error.

Safety in the Office Setting

Thus far, most efforts to improve safety involved activities that occur in the inpatient setting. This is a logical initial approach because most risky procedures and tests are performed in the hospital setting. There is a trend to adapt some invasive procedures and tests and offer them in the office setting. Gynecologic procedures such as hysteroscopy and loop excision of the cervix are examples of this. It is anticipated that there will be increasing numbers of "risky" invasive procedures performed in the office setting. The American College of Obstetricians and Gynecologists (ACOG) established a Task Force on Patient Safety in the Office Setting. In addition to the task force and its report, the college developed a patient safety assessment tool and a certification process (61).

The charge to the task force was to "assist, inform and enable Fellows of the College to design and implement processes that will facilitate a safe and effective environment for the more invasive technologies currently being introduced into the office setting." The task force produced a monograph and a publication containing an executive summary of the work and recommendations (62). The task force addressed issues of leadership in the office setting; competency and assessment; teamwork and communication; anesthesia safety; measurement (of processes and outcomes); and tools such as checklists, time-outs, and drills.

In the hospital setting, leadership for safety is provided at multiple levels, starting with the department chair, with assistance from designated personnel in risk management and quality assurance. In the office setting, this responsibility must be assumed by one individual in a solo practice and one or several in a group practice. One individual should be designated as medical director and his or her responsibilities are outlined in Table 3.4.

The process of competency and assessment should be similar to the credentialing and privileging systems that hospitals use. The determination that a provider is qualified (credentialed) and competent to perform specific procedures (privileged) is equally important in the office setting. Procedures initially performed solely in an inpatient setting should be converted to the office setting only after the provider has demonstrated competency in an accredited operating room setting.

Effective communication with office personnel and with patients was identified by the task force as an essential element for creating a culture of safety in the office setting. Regular meetings should be held with all office staff to establish and implement patient safety and quality improvement protocols.

Anesthesia safety is critical for avoiding adverse outcomes in the office setting. As office-based procedures become more invasive, many practices have incorporated certified anesthesia personnel into the office team. The level of anesthesia achieved, not the agents used, should

Table 3.4 Medical Director Responsibilities in an Office Setting
• Motivation of staff to create a "safety culture"
• Credentialing and privileging for office procedures
• Developing/updating/enforcing office policies
• Conducting regular mock safety drills
• Tracking and reporting adverse events
• Establishing a nonpunitive quality improvement process

be the primary issue regarding anesthesia safety. When nonanesthesia certified providers are managing the patient, appropriate credentialing and privileging should be documented.

The task force strongly recommends the use of checklists, drills, and time-outs to verify the appropriate progress of office-based procedures. Checklists improve safety and effectiveness in other industries as well as health care (41–43). Verifying that the correct procedure is being performed on the correct patient during a time-out for confirmation is useful in the office setting, and drills and simulations are essential activities in high-reliability organizations. Advances in technology are expected to move many more invasive procedures into the office setting, and patients and providers will expect that these are performed with high-reliability and safety.

Through the Presidential Task Force Report, ACOG provided a blueprint for improving patient safety in the office setting (61). In parallel with this effort, ACOG convened another ad hoc committee to design a Web-based tool for outpatient practices to perform a self-assessment and gauge the degree to which they have implemented important safety measures. The work of this committee resulted in the Office Patient Safety Assessment (OPSA) tool. ACOG members can utilize this tool online to evaluate the safety environment in their office practices in four major domains. The first is Office Safety Culture, which includes questions about patient identification, team training, and communication. The second is Practice Management, which looks at utilization of electronic health records or other systems to track patient appointments and inquiries, and reporting normal and abnormal diagnostic tests. Third is Medication Safety, which asks about practices related to accuracy of medication lists, medication prescribing, and the dispensing of drug samples. The last domain is Procedures, which evaluates the appropriateness of patient selection for office procedures, equipment availability and maintenance, and safe anesthesia practices. The various elements in these domains provide a roadmap for improvement in those office practices where physicians find they have not yet instituted some of these recommended features (61).

The Business Case for Quality and Safety

Given the evidence that supports efforts to improve the quality and safety of medical care, why is there still much work to do in this crucial area? One explanation is that the misaligned financial incentives inherent in the reimbursement systems for physicians and hospitals are not designed to offer a "business case" for quality in providing medical care (63). This means that there is no monetary reward for improving quality in medicine, and pursuing that goal will result in higher costs. However, Donald Berwick, head of the Centers for Medicare and Medicaid Services (CMS), and others, maintain that it is possible to improve care and dramatically lower costs (64).

How can the application of the quality and safety principles outlined above result in cost savings in the delivery of health care? The business case for quality and safety is built on the concept of the elimination of waste in medical care. Brent James, executive director for the Institute for Healthcare Delivery Research at Intermountain Healthcare in Salt Lake City, identifies two main types of waste in health care (65). The first is *quality waste*, which can be thought of as rework or scrap. This is the failure to achieve the desired outcome of medical care the first time around. This would include such diverse events as medication errors that result in patient harm, hospital-acquired infections, wrong site surgeries, and retained foreign objects at surgery. The second type is *inefficiency waste*. This refers to excessive resource consumption to achieve an outcome when a different alternative is available to more efficiently achieve a similar outcome. An example would be performing an inpatient hysterectomy for menorrhagia that could be treated equally well with outpatient medication or endometrial ablation. James estimated that together these two sources account for as much as 50% of the expenditures on health care in this country (65). Combating these sources of wasted health-care dollars will require a widespread adoption of the principles discussed: the use of evidence-based medical treatments and safety technology; the elimination of unexplained clinical variation in our processes of care; improved teamwork and communication between providers in different disciplines; the direct involvement of patients and their families in monitoring their own care; and all of these under the guidance of committed health care leadership able to rally support for these efforts.

More evidence is emerging to validate these concepts. The Dartmouth Institute found a strong correlation between higher health care quality and cost savings in multispecialty groups (66). In 2010, the Rand Corporation produced a technical report showing that improved patient safety, as measured by a reduction in adverse events at hospitals in California, resulted in a significant reduction in malpractice claims (67). This represents a large potential cost savings and is an attractive alternative solution to the problem of substantial malpractice costs in our current health care system. The twin aims of improving the safety and quality of the medical care are goals that all physicians should actively pursue.

References

1. **Kohn LT, Corrigan JM, Donaldson MS, eds.** Institute of Medicine. *To err is human: building a safer health system.* Washington, DC: National Academies Press, 2000.
2. **Richardson WC, Berwick DM, Bisgard JC, et al.** *Crossing the quality chasm: a new health system for the 21st century.* Washington, DC: National Academies Press, 2001.
3. **Leape LL, Berwick DM.** Five years after to err is human. What have we learned? *JAMA* 2005;293:2384–2390.
4. **Leape LL, Berwick DM, Clancy CM, et al.** *Unmet needs: teaching physicians to provide safe patient care.* Report of the Lucian Leape Institute Roundtable on Reforming Medical Education. National Patient Safety Foundation, 2010.
5. **Lohr KN, ed.** *Medicare: a strategy for quality assurance,* vol. I. Washington, DC: National Academy Press, 1990:21.
6. **Sackett DL.** Evidence based medicine: what it is and what it isn't. *BMJ* 1996;312:71–72.
7. **The "Five Rights";** ISMP Medication Safety Alert! Acute Care; electronic publication April 7, 1999. http://www.ismp.org/Newsletters/acutecare/articles/19990407.asp
8. **Florence Nightingale: measuring hospital care outcomes.** Oakbrook Terrace, IL: Joint Commission on Accreditation of Healthcare Organizations, 1999.
9. **Gawande A.** The cost conundrum: what a Texas town can teach us about health care. *New Yorker Magazine,* June 1, 2009.
10. **Fisher ES, Bynum JP, Skinner JS.** Slowing the growth of health care costs—lessons from regional variation. *N Engl J Med* 2009;360:849–852.
11. **The Dartmouth Atlas of Health Care in Virginia;** The Center for the Evaluative Clinical Sciences, Dartmouth Medical School; The Maine Medical Assessment Foundation AHA Press 2000. http://www.dartmouthatlas.org/downloads/atlases/virginia_atlas.pdf
12. **Berwick D.** Controlling variation in health care: a consultation with Walter Shewart. *Med Care* 1991;29:12.
13. **Women's Reproductive Health:** Hysterectomy Fact Sheet; Centers for Disease Control and Prevention electronic publication on CDC website http://www.cdc.gov/reproductivehealth/womensrh/00-04-FS_Hysterectomy.htm
14. **Frankel A, Leonard M, Simmonds T, Haraden C, eds.** *The essential guide for patient safety officers.* Joint Commission Resources and the Institute for Healthcare Improvement, Oakbrook Terrace, IL, 2009.
15. **Reason J.** Human errors: models and management. *BMJ* 2000;320:768–770.
16. **Frankel A, Graydon-Baker E, Neppl C, et al.** Patient safety leadership WalkRounds™. *Jt Comm J Qual Saf* 2003;29:16–26.
17. **Marx D.** *Patient safety and the "just culture": a primer for health care executives.* New York: Columbia University Press, 2001.
18. **Sentinel Event Alert 30.** *Preventing infant death and injury during delivery.* The Joint Commission, July 21, 2004. http://www.jointcommission.org/assets/1/18/SEA_30.PDF
19. **Helmreich RL, Merritt AC, Wilhelm JA.** The evolution of crew resource management training in commercial aviation. *Int J Aviation Psychol* 1999;9:19–32.
20. **Haig K, Sutton S, Whittington J.** SBAR: a shared mental model for improving communication between clinicians. *Jt Comm J Qual Patient Saf* 2006;32:167–175.
21. **CAPSLINK.** U.S. Pharmacopeia, Center for the Advancement of Patient Safety, December 2003. http://www.usp.org/pdf/EN/patientSafety/capsLink2003-12-01.pdf
22. **Ulmer C, Wolman DW, Johns MME, eds.** *Resident duty hours: enhancing sleep, supervision and safety institute of medicine.* Washington, DC: The National Academies Press, 2009.
23. **Moorthy K.** Simulation based training. *BMJ* 2005;330:493–494.
24. **Holzman RS, Cooper JB, Gaba DM, et al.** Anesthesia crisis resource management: real-life simulation training in operating room crises. *J Clin Anesth* 1995;7:675–687.
25. **Bower J.** Using patient simulators to train surgical team members. *AORN J* 1997;65:805–808.
26. **Larsen C, Soerensen JL, Grantcharov TP, et al.** Effect of virtual reality training on laparoscopic surgery: randomized control trial. *BMJ* 2009;338:b1802.
27. **Lendvay TS, Casale P, Sweet R, et al.** VR robotic surgery: randomized blinded study of the dV-trainer robotic simulator. *Stud Health Technol Inform* 2008;132:242–244.
28. **Thompson S.** Clinical risk management in obstetrics: eclampsia drills. *BMJ* 2004;328:269–271.
29. **Crofts JF, Bartlett C, Ellis D, et al.** Management of shoulder dystocia: skill retention 6 and 12 months after training. *Obstet Gynecol* 2007;110:1069–1074.
30. **Institute for Healthcare Improvement.** http://www.ihi.org/IHI/Topics/PatientSafety/MedicationSystems/Changes/Individual Changes/Conduct+Adverse+Drug+Event+%28ADE%29+Drills.htm
31. **World Health Organization.** *Prevention of hospital acquired infections: a practical guide.* Geneva, Switzerland: World Health Organization Department of Communicable Disease, Surveillance and Response, 2002.
32. **Coella R, Glenister H, Fereres J, et al.** The cost of infection in surgical patients: a case study. *J Hosp Infect* 1993;25:239–250.
33. **Mangram AJ, Horan TC, Pearson ML, et al.** *Guideline for prevention of surgical site infection, 1999.* Centers for Disease Control and Prevention; U.S. Public Health Service, Atlanta, GA, 1999.
34. **Nuland S.** *The doctors' plague: germs, childbed fever, and the strange story of Ignac Semmelweis.* New York: Norton, 2004.
35. **Centers for Disease Control and Prevention.** Guideline for hand hygiene in the health care settings. *MMWR Morb Mortal Wkly Rep* 2002;51:RR-16.
36. **Siegel JD, Rhinehart E, Jackson M, et al.** *2007 Guideline for isolation precautions: preventing transmission of infectious agents in healthcare settings.* Centers for Disease Control and Prevention, Atlanta, GA, 2007.
37. **Serious reportable events.** National Quality Forum Fact Sheet. October 2008. http://qualityforum.org/Publications/2008/10/Serious_Reportable_Events.aspx
38. **Statement on ensuring correct patient, correct site, and correct procedure surgery.** *Bull Am Coll Surg* 2002;87:12.
39. **The Joint Commission.** *Universal protocol.* Available online at: http://www.jointcommission.org/standards_information/up.aspx
40. **Gawande A.** *The checklist manifesto: how to get things right.* New York: Metropolitan Books, 2009.
41. **Pronovost P, Needham D, Berenholtz S, et al.** An intervention to decrease catheter-related bloodstream infections in the ICU. *N Engl J Med* 2006;355:2725–2732.
42. **Gawande A.** The checklist. *New Yorker,* December 10, 2007.
43. **World Health Organization.** Guidelines for safe surgery. 2009. http://whqlibdoc.who.int/publications/2009/9789241598552_eng.pdf
44. **Haynes AB, Weiser TG, Berry WR, et al.** Surgical safety checklist to reduce morbidity and mortality in a global population. *N Engl J Med* 2009;360:491–499.
45. **Gawande AA, Studdert DM, Orav EJ, et al.** Risk factors for retained instruments and sponges after surgery. *N Engl J Med* 2003;348:229–235.
46. **Statement on the prevention of retained foreign bodies after surgery.** *Bull Am Coll Surg* 2005;90:10. http://www.facs.org/fellows_info/statements/st-51.html
47. **Gibbs VC, Auerbach AD.** The retained surgical sponge. In: **Shojania KG, Duncan BW, McDonald KM, Wachter RM, eds.** Making health care safer: a critical analysis of patient safety practices.

Evidence Report/Technology Assessment No. 43. AHRQ Publication No. 01-E058. 2001. Washington, DC. http://archive.ahrq.gov/clinic/ptsafety/summary.htm

48. **No Thing Left Behind®**. A national surgical patient-safety project to prevent retained surgical items. Available online at: www.nothingleftbehind.org.

49. **Rogers A.** Radio frequency identification (RFID) applied to surgical sponges. *Surg Endosc* 2007;21:1235–1237.

50. **King WJ, Paice N, Jagadish R, et al.** The effect of computerized physician order entry on medication errors and adverse drug events in pediatric patients. *Pediatrics* 2003;112:506–509.

51. **Paparella S.** Avoiding dangerous abbreviations and dose expressions. *J Emerg Nurs* 2004;30:54–58.

52. **Reiter RC, Yielding L, Gluck PA.** Clinical performance improvement: assessing the quality and safety of women's health care. In: **Hacker NF, Moore JG, Gambone JC, eds.** *Essentials of obstetrics and gynecology*, 4th ed. Philadelphia: Elsevier/Saunders, 2004:50–51.

53. **Gluck PA.** Physician leadership: essential in creating a culture of safety. *Clin Obstet Gynecol* 2010;53:473–481.

54. **The Joint Commission.** Speak-up program. 2010. Available online at: http://www.JointCommission.org/generalpublic/speak+up/about_speakup.htm

55. **DiMatteo RM, Reiter RC, Gambone JC.** Enhancing medication adherence through communication and informed collaborative choice. *Health Commun* 1994;6:253–255.

56. **LeGros N, Pindall JD.** Active disclosure of unanticipated adverse events. *Health Law* 2002;35:189–210.

57. **Kachalia A, Kaufman SR, Boothman R, et al.** Liability costs before and after implementation of a medical error disclosure program. *Ann Intern Med* 2010;153:213–221.

58. **Leape LL.** Full disclosure and apology—an idea whose time has come. *Physician Exec* 2006;32:16–18.

59. **Liebman CB, Hyman CS.** A mediation skills model to manage disclosure of errors and adverse events to patients. *Health Affairs* 2004;23:22–32.

60. **The Sorry Works Coalition.** Available online at: www.sorryworks.net

61. **American College of Obstetricians and Gynecologists.** Report of the Presidential Task Force on Patient Safety in the office setting. Washington, DC: ACOG, 2010.

62. **Erickson, TB, Kirkpatrick DH, DeFrancesco MS, et al.** Executive summary of the American College of Obstetricians and Gynecologists Presidential Task Force on Patient Safety in the office setting. *Obstet Gynecol* 2010;115:147–151.

63. **Casalino L.** Markets and medicine: barriers to creating a "business case for quality." *Perspect Biol Med* 2003;46:38–55.

64. **Berwick DM, Nolan TW.** Physicians as leaders in improving health care: a new series in Annals of Internal Medicine. *Ann Intern Med* 1998;128(4):289–292.

65. **James B.** Cost of poor quality or waste in integrated delivery system settings. Appendix A: quality and inefficiency waste in the peer-reviewed medical literature. 2010. U.S. Department of Health and Human Services. Agency for Healthcare Research and Quality. Available online at: http://www.ahrq.gov/research/costpqids/cpqidsappa.htm

66. **Weeks WB.** Higher health care quality and bigger savings found at large multispecialty medical groups. *Health Aff* 2010;29:991–997.

67. **Greenberg, Michael D, Amelia M. Haviland, J. Scott Ashwood and Regan Main.** Is Better Patient Safety Associated with Less Malpractice Activity? Evidence from California. Santa Monica, CA: RAND Corporation, 2010. http://www.rand.org/pubs/technical_reports/TR824.

4

Clinical Research

Maureen G. Phipps
Daniel W. Cramer

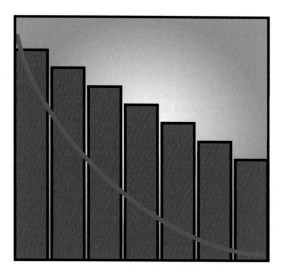

- *Clinical research* includes a range of research disciplines and approaches, including patient-oriented research, clinical trials, epidemiology, and outcomes research.

- *Patient-oriented research* centers on understanding mechanisms of human disease, studies of therapies, or interventions for disease.

- *Clinical trials* use a controlled experimental design to assess the effectiveness of an intervention on an outcome.

- *Epidemiology* is the study of the distribution and determinants of health and disease in specific populations.

- *Outcomes research* and *health services research* include studies that seek to identify the most effective and efficient intervention, treatments, and services for patient care.

- Study designs include *experimental studies* (clinical trials), *observational studies* (cohort studies, case-control studies, and cross-sectional studies), and *descriptive studies* (case reports and case series).

- *Scientific validity* of a research study is evaluated by understanding the study question, how the study was designed, and whether chance, bias, or confounding could have accounted for the findings.

Study Designs

Medical practice is evolving to include complex options for patient treatment and preventive care, in part because clinical research methods and techniques to guide patient care have advanced. To evaluate whether new treatments and diagnostic approaches should be integrated into clinical practice or decide whether observational data reported in the literature is relevant, clinicians should understand the fundamental strengths and limitations of clinical research methods and the level of evidence different types of studies provide.

As outlined by the National Institute of Child Health and Human Development, **clinical research includes patient-oriented research involving understanding mechanisms of human disease, studies of therapies or interventions for disease, clinical trials, and technology development.**

Epidemiologic methods and behavioral research are used in clinical research to examine the distribution of disease and the factors that affect health and how people make health-related decisions. Outcomes research and health services research include studies that seek to identify the most effective and efficient intervention, treatments, and services for patient care (1).

The purpose of a research study is to test a hypothesis about and to measure an association between *exposure (or treatment)* and *disease occurrence (or prevention)*. The type of study design influences the way the study results should be interpreted.

Analytic studies are often subdivided into experimental studies (clinical trials) and observational studies (cohort studies, case-control studies, and cross-sectional studies).

Descriptive studies (case reports and case series) often provide useful information for informing future analytic studies.

The common types of clinical research study methods, considerations for the strength of evidence for the specific study design, and interpretation of the results are presented. Although there is debate about which system should be used for evaluating the strength of evidence from an individual study, **a well-designed and executed clinical trial presents the highest level of evidence** (2). Other types of studies should be designed to best approach the strengths of a clinical trial.

Clinical Trials

Clinical trials include intervention studies where the assignment to the treatment or control condition is controlled by the investigator and the outcomes to be measured are clearly defined at the time the trial is designed. **Features of *randomized clinical trials* include randomization (in which participants are randomly assigned to exposures), unbiased assessment of outcome, and analysis of all participants based on the assigned exposure (an "intention to treat" analysis).**

There are many different types of clinical trials, including studies designed to evaluate treatments, prevention techniques, community interventions, quality-of-life improvements, and diagnostic or screening approaches (3). Since 2007, investigators conducting randomized clinical trials are expected to register the trial to comply with mandatory registration and results reporting requirements (4).

Clinical Trial Phases

New investigational drugs or treatments are usually evaluated by clinical trials in phases with more people being involved as the purpose of the study becomes more inclusive (3).

Phase I Trials   In these trials, researchers test an experimental drug or treatment for the first time in a small group of people (20–80) to evaluate its safety, determine a safe dosage range, and identify side effects.

Phase II Trials   In these, the experimental study drug or treatment is given to a larger group of people (100–300) to see whether it is effective and to further evaluate its safety.

Phase III Trials   In phase III trials, the experimental study drug or treatment is given to large groups of people (1,000–3,000) to confirm its effectiveness, monitor side effects, compare it to commonly used treatments, and collect information that will allow the experimental drug or treatment to be used safely.

Phase IV Trials   These are postmarketing studies that delineate additional information, including the drug's risks, benefits, and optimal use.

Randomized Controlled Double-Blinded Clinical Trial

The *randomized controlled double-blinded clinical trial* is considered the gold standard for evaluating interventions because randomizing treatment assignment and *blinding* both the participant and the investigator are the cornerstones for minimizing *bias*. When studies are not randomized or blinded, bias may result from preferential assignment of treatment based on patient characteristics or an unintentional imbalance in baseline characteristics between treatment groups, leading to *confounding*.

Although not all studies can be designed with blinding, the efforts used in the trial to minimize bias from nonblinding should be explained. Investigators are expected to provide evidence that the factors that might influence outcome, such as age, stage of disease, medical history, and symptoms, are similar in patients assigned to the study protocol compared with patients assigned to placebo or traditional treatment. Published reports from the clinical trial are expected to include a table showing a comparison of the treatment groups with respect to potential confounders and to demonstrate that the groups did not differ in any important ways before the study began.

CONSORT Checklist

Clearly defining the outcome or criteria for successful treatment helps ensure unbiased assessment of the outcome. A well-designed clinical trial has a sufficient number of subjects enrolled to ensure that a "negative" study (one that does not show an effect of the treatment) has enough statistical power to evaluate the predetermined (a priori), expected treatment effect. **The Consolidated Standards of Reporting Trials (CONSORT) Statement is an evidence-based, minimum set of recommendations for reporting on randomized controlled trials developed by the CONSORT Group to alleviate the problems arising from inadequate reporting of randomized controlled trials.** The 25-item CONSORT checklist (Table. 4.1) and flow diagram

Table 4.1 CONSORT Checklist

Section/Topic	Item No.	Checklist Item	Reported on Page No.
Title and abstract			
	1a	Identification as a randomized trial in the title	_____
	1b	Structured summary of trial design, methods, results, and conclusions (for specific guidance see CONSORT for abstracts)*	_____
Introduction			_____
Background and objectives	2a	Scientific background and explanation of rationale	_____
	2b	Specific objectives or hypotheses	_____
Methods			_____
Trial design	3a	Description of trial design (such as parallel, factorial) including allocation ratio	_____
	3b	Important changes to methods after trial commencement (such as eligibility criteria), with reasons	_____
Participants	4a	Eligibility criteria for participants	_____
	4b	Settings and locations where the data were collected	_____
Interventions	5	The interventions for each group with sufficient details to allow replication, including how and when they were actually administered	_____
Outcomes	6a	Completely defined prespecified primary and secondary outcome measures, including how and when they were assessed	_____
	6b	Any changes to trial outcomes after the trial commenced, with reasons	_____
Sample size	7a	How sample size was determined	_____
	7b	When applicable, explanation of any interim analyses and stopping guidelines	_____
Randomization: sequence generation	8a	Method used to generate the random allocation sequence	_____
	8b	Type of randomization; details of any restriction (such as blocking and block size)	_____
Allocation concealment mechanism	9	Mechanism used to implement the random allocation sequence (such as sequentially numbered containers), describing any steps taken to conceal the sequence until interventions were assigned	_____
Implementation	10	Who generated the random allocation sequence, who enrolled participants, and who assigned participants to interventions	_____
Blinding	11a	If done, who was blinded after assignment to interventions (for example, participants, care providers, those assessing outcomes) and how	_____
	11b	If relevant, description of the similarity of interventions	_____
Statistical methods	12a	Statistical methods used to compare groups for primary and secondary outcomes	_____
	12b	Methods for additional analyses, such as subgroup analyses and adjusted analyses	_____

Table 4.1 CONSORT Checklist (*Continued*).

Section/Topic	Item No.	Checklist Item	Reported on Page No.
Results			_____
Participant flow (a diagram is strongly recommended)	13a	For each group, the numbers of participants who were randomly assigned, received intended treatment, and were analyzed for the primary outcome	_____
	13b	For each group, losses and exclusions after randomization, together with reasons	_____
Recruitment	14a	Dates defining the periods of recruitment and follow-up	_____
	14b	Why the trial ended or was stopped	_____
Baseline data	15	A table showing baseline demographic and clinical characteristics for each group	_____
Numbers analyzed	16	For each group, number of participants (denominator) included in each analysis and whether the analysis was by original assigned groups	_____
Outcomes and estimation	17a	For each primary and secondary outcome, results for each group, and the estimated effect size and its precision (such as: 95% confidence interval)	_____
	17b	For binary outcomes, presentation of both absolute and relative effect sizes is recommended	_____
Ancillary analyses	18	Results of any other analyses performed, including subgroup analyses and adjusted analyses, distinguishing prespecified from exploratory	_____
Harms	19	All important harms or unintended effects in each group (for specific guidance see CONSORT for harms)*	_____
Discussions			_____
Limitations	20	Trial limitations, addressing sources of potential bias, imprecision, and, if relevant, multiplicity of analyses	_____
Generalizability	21	Generalizability (external validity, applicability) of the trial findings	_____
Interpretation	22	Interpretation consistent with results, balancing benefits and harms, and considering other relevant evidence	_____
Other Information			_____
Registration	23	Registration number and name of trial registry	_____
Protocol	24	Where the full trial protocol can be accessed, if available	_____
Funding	25	Sources of f funding and other support (such as supply of drugs), role of funders	_____

*We strongly reconmiend reading this statement in conjunction with the CONSORT 2010 Explanation and Elaboration for important clarifications on all the items. If relevant, we also recommend reading CONSORT extensions for cluster randomized trials, nonlnferiority and equivalence trials, nonpharmacological treatments, herbal interventions, and pragmatic trials. Additional extensions are forthcoming: for those and for up-to-date references relevant to this checklist, see www.consort-statement.org.

(Fig. 4.1) offer a standard way for authors to prepare reports of trial findings, facilitating their complete and transparent reporting and aiding their critical appraisal and interpretation (5).

Clinical Trial Design Considerations

Clinical trials are considered a gold standard, because when done well they provide information about both relative and absolute risks and minimize concerns about bias and confounding (see the section on Presenting and Understanding the Results of Analytic Studies). Many clinical research questions are not amenable to clinical trials because of cost restraints, length of time required to complete the study, and feasibility of recruitment and implementation.

When evaluating the results from a clinical trial, consider how restrictive inclusion and exclusion criteria may narrow the participant population to such a degree that there may be concerns about external validity or generalizing the results. Other concerns include blinding, loss to follow-up, and clearly defining the outcome of interest. When the results of a randomized controlled trial do not show a significant effect of the treatment or intervention, the methods should be evaluated to understand what assumptions (expected power and effect size) were made to determine the necessary sample size for the study.

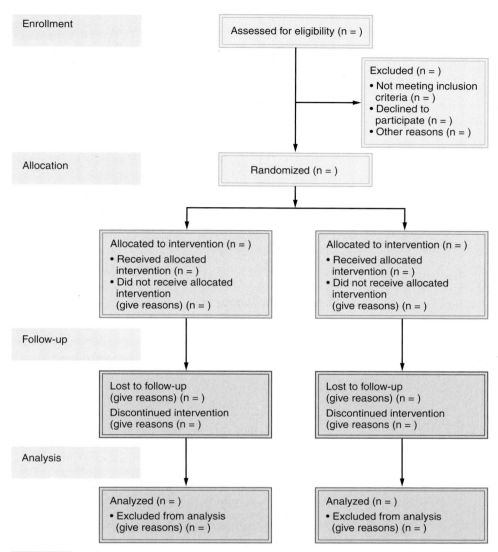

Enrollment

Assessed for eligibility (n =)

Excluded (n =)
• Not meeting inclusion
  criteria (n =)
• Declined to
  participate (n =)
• Other reasons (n =)

Allocation

Randomized (n =)

Allocated to intervention (n =)
• Received allocated
  intervention (n =)
• Did not receive allocated
  intervention
  (give reasons) (n =)

Allocated to intervention (n =)
• Received allocated
  intervention (n =)
• Did not receive allocated
  intervention
  (give reasons) (n =)

Follow-up

Lost to follow-up
(give reasons) (n =)
Discontinued intervention
(give reasons (n =)

Lost to follow-up
(give reasons) (n =)
Discontinued intervention
(give reasons (n =)

Analysis

Analyzed (n =)
• Excluded from analysis
  (give reasons) (n =)

Analyzed (n =)
• Excluded from analysis
  (give reasons) (n =)

Figure 4.1   **CONSORT flow diagram.**

Intention-to-Treat Analysis

Randomized controlled trials should be evaluated with an intention-to-treat analysis, which means that all of the people randomized at the initiation of the trial should be accounted for in the analysis with the group to which they were assigned. Unless part of the overall study design, even if a participant stopped participating in the assigned treatment or "crossed over" to another treatment during the study, they should be analyzed with the group to which they were initially assigned. All of these considerations help to minimize bias in the design, implementation, and interpretation of a clinical trial (6).

Observational Studies

In cases where the exposure and outcome are not amenable to an experimental design, because the exposure is known or suspected to have harmful effects, observational studies may be used to assess association. **Observational studies, including cohort, case-control, and cross-sectional studies, are analytic studies that take advantage of "natural experiments" in which exposure is not assigned by the investigator; rather, the individuals are assessed by the investigator for a potential exposure of interest (present or absent) and outcomes (present or absent).** The timing of the evaluation of the exposure and outcome defines the study type.

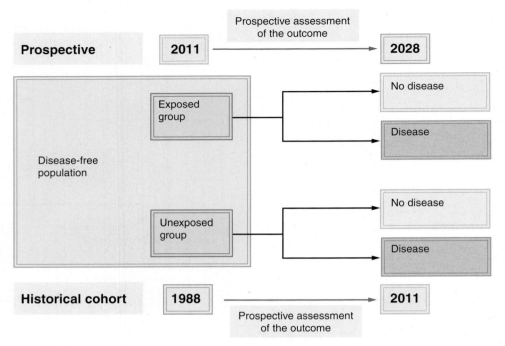

Figure 4.2 Schematic of prospective and retrospective cohort study designs.

Cohort Studies

Cohort studies often are referred to as longitudinal studies. Cohort studies involve identifying a group of exposed individuals and unexposed individuals and following both groups over time to compare the rate of disease (or outcome) in the groups. Cohort studies may be prospective, meaning that the exposure is identified before outcome, or retrospective, in which the exposure and outcome have already occurred when the study is initiated. **Even in a retrospective cohort study, the study is defined by the fact that the cohorts were identified based on the exposure (not the outcome), and individuals should be free of disease (outcome) at the beginning time point for the cohort study** (Fig. 4.2).

In a study that includes a survival analysis, the two cohort groups (exposed and nonexposed) begin with a population that is 100% well (or alive) at the beginning of the study. The groups are followed over time to calculate the percentage of the cohort still well (or alive) at different time points during the study and at the end of the study. Although a survival analysis typically describes mortality after disease (i.e., cancer patients who died within 5 years), it can be adapted to other events and outcomes (e.g., the percentage of women who become pregnant while using long-acting contraceptives).

Cohort Study Design

Strengths of cohort studies include the ability to obtain both attributable and relative risks because the occurrence of the outcome is being compared in two groups (see the section on Presenting and Understanding the Results of Analytic Studies). However, only associations can be established, not causality. Because randomization is not part of the study design, the investigator must consider that a factor associated with the exposure may lead to the outcome rather than the exposure itself. Misclassifying the exposure or the outcome and confounding variables are potential sources of bias in cohort studies.

Given that truly prospective cohort studies can be expensive and take a long time for completion, there should be compelling evidence for the public health importance of the exposure(s) and association(s) being addressed. Issues related to sample size and participant retention in the study protocol are as important in cohort studies as they are in randomized controlled trials.

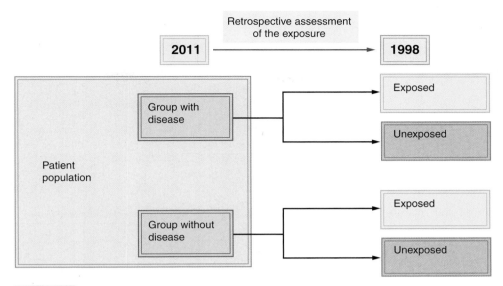

Figure 4.3 Schematic of case control study design.

Case-Control Studies

A case-control study starts with the identification of individuals with a disease or outcome of interest and a suitable control population without the disease or outcome of interest. The controls should represent a sample of the population from which the cases arose and who were at risk for the disease or outcome but did not develop it. The relationship between a particular attribute or exposure to the disease is retrospectively studied by comparing how the cases and controls differed in that exposure (Fig. 4.3).

Odds Ratio

The measure of association for a case-control study is the odds ratio, which is the ratio of exposed cases to unexposed cases, divided by the ratio of exposed to unexposed controls (see the section on Presenting and Understanding the Results of Analytic Studies). **If an entire population could be characterized by its exposure and disease status, the exposure odds ratio would be identical to the relative risk obtainable from a cohort study of the same population.** Although the relative risk (RR) cannot be calculated directly from a case control study, it can be used as an estimate of the relative risk when the sample of cases and controls are representative of all people with or without the disease and when the disease being studied is uncommon. Attributable risk is not directly obtainable in a case-control study.

Case-Control Study Considerations

The advantages of case-control studies are that they are generally lower in cost and easier to conduct than other analytic studies. Case-control studies are most feasible for examining the association between a relatively common exposure and a relatively rare disease. Disadvantages include greater potential for selection bias, recall bias, and misclassification bias.

Case-control studies may be especially prone to selection bias and recall bias. Investigators need to understand sampling issues around which cases and controls were selected for their study and how these may have affected exposure rates. Subtle issues, such as interviewer technique, may affect the likelihood that cases may recall or report exposures more readily than controls.

Cross-Sectional Studies

Cross-sectional studies assess both the exposure and the outcome at the same point in time. Individuals are surveyed to provide a "snapshot" of health events in the population at a particular time. Cross-sectional studies are often called prevalence studies because the disease exists at the time of the study, and the longitudinal follow-up and disease duration are not known. **Prevalence is the existing number of cases at a specific point in time.**

Cross-sectional studies are often done to evaluate a diagnostic test. The value of the test (predictor) is compared with the outcome (disease). The results of these evaluations are often

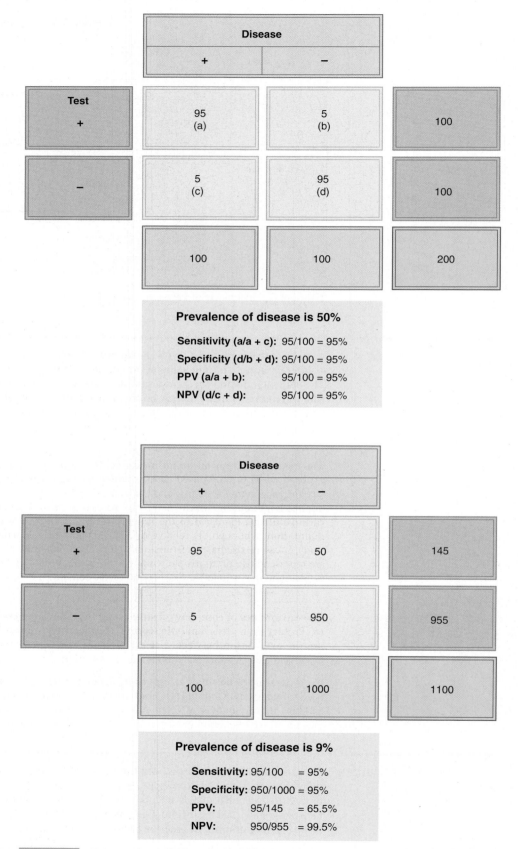

Figure 4.4 Comparison of sensitivity, specificity and predictive values when the prevalence of the disease varies.

presented as *sensitivity* and *specificity*. The sensitivity and specificity represent the characteristics of a given diagnostic test and do not vary by population characteristics. In contrast the negative and positive predictive values of a test do vary with the baseline characteristics of a population such as prevalence of a disease (Fig. 4.4).

Cross-Sectional Study Considerations

Although cross-sectional studies are primarily descriptive, they may contribute information about suggested risk factors for disease by showing how that disease varies by age, sex, race, or geography. In *ecologic studies*, disease rates in various populations are correlated with other population characteristics (e.g., endometrial cancer rates worldwide are positively correlated with per capita fat consumption and negatively correlated with cereal and grain consumption) (7).

Caution must be used in interpreting findings from a cross-sectional study because there is no temporal relationship between the exposure and the outcome; therefore, causality cannot be established. However, cross-sectional data can be valuable in informing analytic study designs or used as supporting data for documenting the consistency of an association.

Descriptive Studies

Descriptive studies, case reports and case series, do not include comparison groups.

Case Reports and Case Series

In a case report or case series, the characteristics of individuals who have a particular disease are described. A case report usually describes an unusual clinical scenario or procedure in a single patient, whereas a case series usually includes a larger group of patients with similar exposures or outcomes. **Just because members of a case series share a particular characteristic, it cannot be assumed that there is a cause-and-effect relationship.**

Hypotheses about exposures and disease may be developed from descriptive studies that should then be explored in analytic studies. Because a case series has no comparison group, statistical tests of association between the exposure and outcome cannot be performed. A case series usually does not yield any measure of association other than estimates of the frequency of a particular characteristic among members included in the case series.

Presenting and Understanding the Results of Analytic Studies

To present the results of clinical trials or observational studies, a variety of rates and measures may be derived, as summarized below. **To judge the scientific validity of the results of clinical studies, an investigator needs to consider whether the finding could have occurred simply by chance, by performing appropriate statistical testing, or if there are other possible explanations for the reported association, including bias or confounding.** Besides statistical significance and freedom from bias or confounding, there are several additional criteria that can be applied to judge whether the treatment truly did affect disease outcome or whether an exposure truly caused the disease, as outlined below.

Rates and Measures

The terminology associated with rates and measures include (Fig. 4.5):

- *Incidence (IR)*—**frequency of newly identified disease or event (outcome).**

- *Prevalence (PR)*—**frequency of an existing disease or outcome during a specified period or point in time.**

- *Odds Ratios (OR)*—**ratio of the probability of an exposure in one group (cases) compared with probability of the exposure in another group (controls).**

- *Relative Risk (RR)*—**ratio of risk in the exposed group compared with the risk in the unexposed group.** If the RR = 1 (or not significantly different from 1) then the risk in the exposed group is equal to the risk in the nonexposed group. RR >1 may suggest a positive association with the exposed group having greater risk than the nonexposed group, whereas a RR <1 implies a negative association with the exposed group having less risk than the nonexposed group.

- *Absolute Risk Reduction (ARR)*—**the difference in risk between the unexposed (control) group and the exposed (treatment) group.**

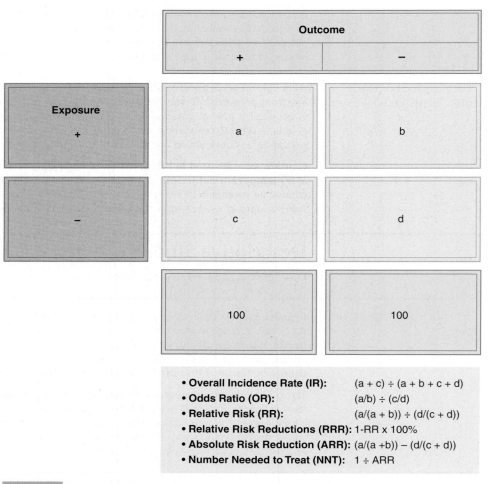

	Outcome	
	+	**−**
Exposure +	a	b
−	c	d
	100	100

- **Overall Incidence Rate (IR):** $(a + c) \div (a + b + c + d)$
- **Odds Ratio (OR):** $(a/b) \div (c/d)$
- **Relative Risk (RR):** $(a/(a + b)) \div (d/(c + d))$
- **Relative Risk Reductions (RRR):** $1\text{-}RR \times 100\%$
- **Absolute Risk Reduction (ARR):** $(a/(a + b)) - (d/(c + d))$
- **Number Needed to Treat (NNT):** $1 \div ARR$

Figure 4.5 Calculating rates and measures.

- *Relative Risk Reduction (RRR)*—the percentage of reduction in the risk comparing the unexposed (control) group to the exposed (treatment) group.

- *Number Needed to Treat (NNT)*—represents the number of people who would need treatment (or the intervention) to prevent one additional outcome (to calculate the NNT, take the inverse of the ARR, i.e., $1 \div ARR$).

- *Sensitivity*—among the people who have the outcome, this is the proportion who have a positive test.

- *Specificity*—among the people who do not have the outcome, this is the proportion who have a negative test.

- *Negative Predictive Value (NPV)*—among the people who have a negative test, this is the proportion who do not have the outcome.

- *Positive Predictive Value (PPV)*—among the people who have a positive test, this is the proportion who have the outcome.

Statistical Testing

Statistical testing is used in clinical research for hypothesis testing in which the investigator is evaluating the study results against the null hypothesis (that there is no difference between the groups). Results from statistical testing allow the investigator to evaluate how likely it is that the study result is caused by chance rather than an intervention or exposure (p value). In the case where a study failed to find a significant difference, it is equally important to describe the likelihood that the study conclusion was wrong and that a difference truly exists. Finally, it is important to provide as precise a measure of the treatment effect or association as possible and convey to the reader the plausible range that the "true" effect resides (or confidence interval).

P Value and Statistical Significance

The *p* value is a reflection of the probability of a *type I error (alpha)*. This reflects the probability that a difference between study groups could have arisen by chance alone. In other words, it is the probability that there is a difference between therapies, interventions, or observed groups when a true difference does not exist.

Historically in the medical literature, a *p* value of less than or equal to 0.05 was used to determine statistical significance. This reflects a probability of 1 in 20 that the null hypothesis was rejected based on the results from the study sample. This *p* value may be adjusted downward if multiple associations are being tested and the chances of false discovery are high. In genome-wide association studies, in which hundreds of thousands of genetic variants are tested between groups, *p* values are frequently set at 10^{-7} (0.0000001).

Beta Error and Power

***Type II (or beta) error* reflects the probability of failing to reject the null hypothesis when in reality it is incorrect (i.e., there truly was a treatment effect or a difference between the observed groups).** In clinical trials it is important for the investigator to address the beta error, even in the design stage of the study. Study planners should calculate the *power* (or 1–the *beta error*) that their study would have to detect an association, given assumptions made about the differences expected between treatments, and design the study size accordingly. Be aware that small clinical trials cited as evidence for "no effect of therapy," may not have an adequate sample size to address the study question; in essence, the study is not powered to detect the difference.

Confidence Intervals

***Confidence intervals* (CI) provide the investigator an estimated range in which the true statistical measure (e.g., mean, proportion, and relative risk) is expected to occur. A 95% confidence interval implies that if the study were to be repeated within the same sample population numerous times, the confidence interval estimates would contain the true population parameter 95% of the time. In other words, the probability of observing the true value outside of this range is less than 0.05.** When evaluating measures of association, such as odds ratio or relative risk with 95% CI, values that include 1 (no difference) are not considered statistically significant.

Meta-analysis

One way of improving precision of the effect measure and narrowing the confidence interval is to perform a meta-analysis in which treatment effects from several clinical trials are aggregated to provide a summary measure. Meta-analysis is a favorite tool of the Cochrane database, with which clinicians should be familiar (8). However, there are important considerations in interpreting the meta-analysis, including whether studies were similar enough in their design to be aggregated. Guides for systematic reviews and meta-analysis that involve randomized controlled trials (i.e., the Preferred Reporting Items for Systematic Reviews and Meta-Analyses [PRISMA] statement) and observational studies (i.e., the Meta-analysis Of Observational Studies in Epidemiology [MOOSE] guidelines) are excellent resources for both the investigator and the reviewer (9,10).

Bias

***Bias* is a systematic error in the design, conduct, or analysis of a study that can result in invalid conclusions.** It is important for an investigator to anticipate the types of bias that might occur in a study and correct them during the design of the study, because it may be difficult or impossible to correct for them in the analysis.

- *Information bias* **occurs when participants are classified incorrectly with respect to exposure or disease.** This may occur if records are incomplete or if the criteria for exposure or outcome were poorly defined, leading to misclassification.

- *Recall bias* **is a specific type of information bias that may occur if cases are more likely than controls to remember or to reveal past exposures.** In addition to establishing well-defined study criteria and accessing complete records, information bias may be reduced by blinding interviewers to a participant's study group.

- *Selection bias* **may occur when choosing cases or controls in a case-control study and when choosing exposed or unexposed subjects in a cohort study. A systematic error in selecting participants may influence the outcome by distorting the**

measure of association between the exposure and the outcome. Including an adequately large study sample and obtaining information about nonparticipants may reduce bias or provide information to evaluate potential selection bias.

Confounding

A *confounder* is a known risk factor for the disease and is associated with the exposure. The confounder may account for the apparent effect of the exposure on the disease or mask a true association. Confounders have unequal distributions between the study groups.

- Age, race, and socioeconomic status are potential confounders in many studies. Results may be adjusted for these variables by using statistical techniques such as stratification or multivariable analysis. Adjusting for confounding variables aids in understanding the association between the outcome and exposure if the confounding variable were constant.

- Multivariable analysis is a statistical technique commonly used in epidemiologic studies that simultaneously controls a number of confounding variables. The results from an adjusted analysis include the adjusted odds ratio or relative risk that reflects an association between the exposure and the outcome and accounts for the specific known confounders that were included in the analysis.

Causality and Generalizability

The criteria needed to establish a causal relationship between two factors, especially exposure and disease, are defined (11). Although there are nine separate criteria for judging whether an association is likely to be causal, several of these criteria are most relevant for clinical studies.

- ***Biologic gradient*** *or* ***dose response*** refers to a relationship between exposure and outcome such that a change in the duration, amount, or intensity of the exposure is associated with a corresponding increase or decrease in disease risk.

- ***Plausibility*** refers to knowledge of the pathologic process of the disease or biologic effects of the exposure that would reasonably support an association. Plausibility overlaps with another concept, *coherence*, which also refers to compatibility with the known biology of the disease.

- ***Experiment*** refers to the evidence that the disease or outcome can be prevented or improved by an experiment that eliminates, reduces, or otherwise counters the exposure.

- ***Consistency*** refers to whether the association was repeatedly observed by different investigators, in different locations and circumstances.

- ***Temporality*** refers to the concept that cause must precede effect. For example, is it possible in a case-control study that symptoms of preclinical disease could lead to the exposure? Investigators must demonstrate that the exposure was present before the disease developed.

- ***Strength*** refers to the strength of association. The further the deviation of the relative risk or odds ratio from 1, the stronger the association and the easier it is to accept that the study results are real. For example, studies have shown that the possession of a BRCA mutation may increase the lifetime risk for ovarian or breast cancer some 30-fold. Although strength is a very important criterion, large-scale genetic studies suggest that other factors are equally important. For example, multiple studies reported several variants at the 8q24 chromosomal region associated with prostate and other cancers (12). Even though possession of one allele may change risk by only about 15% (i.e., OR = 1.15), the consistency and high statistical significance suggest the association cannot be caused by chance and this is considered a true association.

Summary

Reviewing the medical literature is part of the ongoing education for those who provide clinical care. Incorporating research findings into clinical care is enhanced by understanding different study designs, their strengths and weaknesses, and the measures of association they are able to provide. Evaluating whether there is enough evidence available to support changing a specific medication, procedure, or protocol used to care for patients is the

cornerstone to improving clinical practice. In a field that is rapidly progressing, understanding clinical research helps physicians provide optimal care for the women they treat everyday.

References

1. **National Institutes of Health.** Eunice Kennedy Shriver, National Institute of Child Health & Human Development. Clinical research and clinical trials: what is clinical research? 2009. Available online at: http://www.nichd.nih.gov/health/clinicalresearch

2. **Atkins D, Eccles M, Flottorp S, et al.** Systems for grading the quality of evidence and the strength of recommendations I: critical appraisal of existing approaches. The GRADE Working Group. *BMC Health Serv Res* 2004;4:38.

3. **ClinicalTrials.gov** A service of the U.S. National Institutes of Health. 2010. http://www.clinicaltrials.gov/

4. **U.S. Food and Drug Administration.** Regulatory information: Food and Drug Administration Amendments Act (FDAAA) of 2007. Available online at: http://www.fda.gov/RegulatoryInformation/Legislation/FederalFoodDrugandCosmeticActFDCAct/Significant AmendmentstotheFDCAct/FoodandDrugAdministrationAmendments Actof2007/default.htm

5. **Schulz KF, Altman DG, Moher D.** CONSORT Group. CONSORT 2010 Statement: updated guidelines for reporting parallel group randomized trials. *BMJ* 2010;340:c332.

6. **Hulley SB, Cummings SR, Browner WS, et al.** *Designing clinical research.* 3rd ed. Philadelphia: Lippincott Williams & Wilkins, 2007.

7. **Armstrong B, Doll R.** Environmental factors and cancer incidence and mortality in different countries, with special reference to dietary practices. *Int J Cancer* 1975;15:617–631.

8. **The Cochrane Library.** About the Cochrane library. Available online at: http://www.thecochranelibrary.com/view/0/AboutThe CochraneLibrary.html

9. **Liberati A, Altman DG, Tetzlaff J, et al.** The PRISMA statement for reporting systematic reviews and meta-analyses of studies that evaluate health care interventions: explanation and elaboration. *J Clin Epidemiol* 2009;62:e1–34.

10. **Stroup DF, Berlin JA, Morton SC, et al.** Meta-analysis of observational studies in epidemiology: a proposal for reporting. Meta-analysis Of Observational Studies in Epidemiology (MOOSE) group. *JAMA* 2000;283:2008–2012.

11. **Hill AB.** The environment and disease: association or causation? *Proc R Soc Med* 1965;58:295–300.

12. **Yeager M, Chatterjee N, Ciampa J, et al.** Identification of a new prostate cancer susceptibility locus on chromosome 8q24. *Nat Genet* 2009;41:1055–1057.

BASIC PRINCIPLES

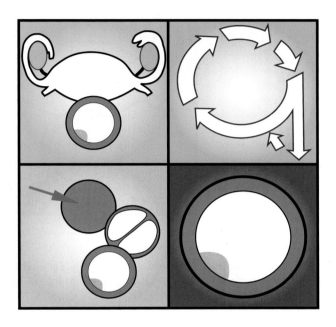

5 Anatomy and Embryology

Eric R. Sokol
Rene Genadry
Jean R. Anderson

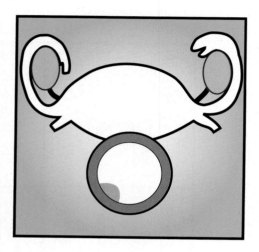

- **Although the basic facts of anatomy do not change, our understanding of specific anatomic relationships and the development of new clinical and surgical correlations continue to evolve.**

- **There is significant variation in the branching pattern of pelvic blood vessels between individuals, and patterns of blood flow may be asymmetric from side to side in the same individual. The pelvic surgeon should be prepared for deviations from "textbook" vascular patterns.**

- **An understanding of the development of pelvic floor disorders and their safe and effective management requires a comprehensive knowledge of the interrelationships between the bony pelvis and its ligaments, pelvic muscles and fasciae, nerves and blood vessels, and pelvic viscera.**

- **Approximately 10% of infants are born with some abnormality of the genitourinary system, and anomalies in one system are often mirrored by anomalies in another system that provide special implications in pelvic surgery.**

- **About 75% of all iatrogenic injuries to the ureter result from gynecologic procedures, most commonly abdominal hysterectomy; risk is increased with distortions of pelvic anatomy, including adnexal masses, endometriosis, other pelvic adhesive disease, or fibroids.**

An understanding of the anatomy of the female pelvis is fundamental to the knowledge base of a practicing gynecologist. Although the basic facts of anatomy and their relevance to gynecologic practice do not change with time, our understanding of specific anatomic relationships and the development of new clinical and surgical correlations continue to evolve.

The anatomy of the fundamental supporting structures of the pelvis, including the genital, urinary, and gastrointestinal viscera, are presented in this chapter. Because significant variation has developed in the names of many common anatomic structures, the terms used here reflect current nomenclature according to the *Nomina Anatomica*; other commonly accepted terms are included in parentheses (1).

Pelvic Structure

Bony Pelvis

The skeleton of the pelvis is formed by the sacrum and coccyx and the paired hipbones (coxal, innominate), which fuse anteriorly to form the symphysis pubis. Figure 5.1 illustrates the bony pelvis as well as its ligaments and foramina.

Sacrum and Coccyx

The sacrum and coccyx are an extension of the vertebral column resulting from the five fused sacral vertebrae and the four fused coccygeal vertebrae. They are joined by a symphyseal articulation (sacrococcygeal joint), which allows some movement.

The essential features of the sacrum and coccyx are as follows:

1. **Sacral promontory**—the most prominent and anterior projection of the sacrum, this is an important landmark for insertion of a laparoscope and for sacrocolpopexy. It is located just below the level of bifurcation of the common iliac arteries.

2. **Four paired anterior and posterior sacral foramina**—exit sites for the anterior and posterior rami of the corresponding sacral nerves; the lateral sacral vessels also traverse the anterior foramina.

3. **Sacral hiatus**—results from incomplete fusion of the posterior lamina of the fifth sacral vertebra, offering access to the sacral canal, which is clinically important for caudal anesthesia.

Laterally, the alae ("wings") of the sacrum offer auricular surfaces that articulate with the hipbones to form synovial sacroiliac joints.

Os Coxae

The paired *os coxae*, or hipbones, have three components: the ilium, the ischium, and the pubis. These components meet to form the acetabulum, a cup-shaped cavity that accommodates the femoral head.

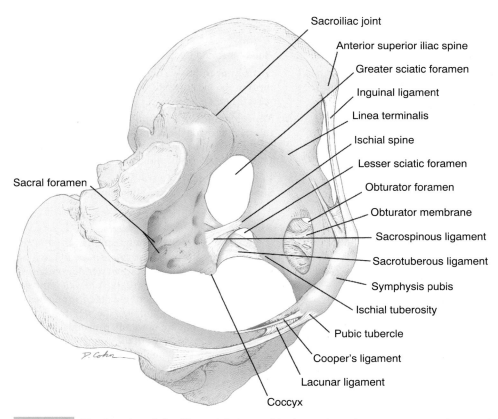

Figure 5.1   The female pelvis. The pelvic bones (the innominate bone, sacrum, and coccyx) and their joints, ligaments, and foramina.

Ilium

1. **Iliac crest**—provides attachments to the iliac fascia, abdominal muscles, and fascia lata.

2. **Anterior superior and inferior spine**—superior spine provides the point of fixation of the inguinal ligament and is clinically important as a lateral landmark for laparoscopic entry.

3. **Posterior superior and inferior spine**—superior spine is the point of attachment for the sacrotuberous ligament and the posterior sacral iliac ligament.

4. **Arcuate line**—marks the pelvic brim and lies between the first two segments of the sacrum.

5. **Iliopectineal eminence (linea terminalis)**—the junction line of the ilium and the pubis.

6. **Iliac fossa**—the smooth anterior concavity of the ilium, covered by the iliacus muscle.

Ischium

1. **Ischial spine**—delineates the greater and lesser sciatic notch above and below it. It is the point of fixation for the sacrospinous ligament and the arcus tendineus fascia pelvis (white line); the ischial spine represents an important landmark in the performance of pudendal nerve block and sacrospinous ligament vaginal suspension; vaginal palpation during labor allows detection of progressive fetal descent.

2. **Ischial ramus**—joins the pubic rami to encircle the obturator foramen; provides the attachment for the inferior fascia of the urogenital diaphragm and the perineal musculo-fascial attachments.

3. **Ischial tuberosity**—the rounded bony prominence upon which the body rests in the sitting position; a clinical landmark for the passage of the inferior arm of anterior vaginal mesh kit systems.

Pubis

1. **Body**—formed by the midline fusion of the superior and inferior pubic rami.

2. **Symphysis pubis**—a fibrocartilaginous symphyseal joint where the bodies of the pubis meet in the midline, allows for some resilience and flexibility, which is critical during parturition.

3. **Superior and inferior pubic rami**—join the ischial rami to encircle the obturator foramen; provide the origin for the muscles of the thigh and leg; provide the attachment for the inferior layer of the urogenital diaphragm; the inferior rami is a clinical landmark for transobturator incontinence sling passage.

4. **Pubic tubercle**—a lateral projection from the superior pubic ramus, to which the inguinal ligament, rectus abdominis, and pyramidalis attach.

Clinical Considerations

Studies using magnetic resonance imaging (MRI) or computed tomography (CT) pelvimetry found an association between the architecture of the bony pelvis, specifically a wider transverse inlet (distance between the most superior aspects of the iliopectineal line) and a shorter obstetric conjugate (shortest distance between the sacral promontory and the pubic symphysis), and the occurrence of pelvic floor disorders (2,3). A loss of lumbar lordosis and a pelvic inlet that is less vertically oriented is more common in women who develop genital prolapse than in those who do not (4,5). A less vertical orientation of the pelvic inlet is thought to result in an alteration of the intra-abdominal forces that are normally directed anteriorly to the pubic symphysis such that a greater proportion is directed toward the pelvic viscera and their connective tissue and muscular supports. It is theorized that women with a wide pelvic inlet are more likely to develop pelvic organ prolapse (2,3). It is speculated that women with these characteristics may be more likely to suffer neuromuscular and connective tissue injuries during labor and delivery, predisposing them to the development of pelvic neuropathy, pelvic organ prolapse, or both. One MRI study, in which only white women were enrolled to remove race as a potential confounder, found that bony pelvis dimensions were similar at the level of the muscular pelvic floor with and without pelvic organ prolapse (6).

Pelvic Bone Articulations

The pelvic bones are joined by four articulations (two pairs):

1. **Two cartilaginous symphyseal joints—the sacrococcygeal joint and the symphysis pubis**—these joints are surrounded by strong ligaments anteriorly and posteriorly, which are responsive to the effect of relaxin and facilitate parturition.

2. **Two synovial joints—the sacroiliac joints**—these joints are stabilized by the sacroiliac ligaments, the iliolumbar ligament, the lateral lumbosacral ligament, the sacrotuberous ligament, and the sacrospinous ligament.

The pelvis is divided into the *greater* and *lesser pelvis* by an oblique plane passing through the sacral promontory, the *linea terminalis (arcuate line of the ilium)*, the pectineal line of the pubis, the pubic crest, and the upper margin of the symphysis pubis. This plane lies at the level of the superior pelvic aperture (*pelvic inlet*) or pelvic brim. The inferior pelvic aperture or *pelvic outlet* is irregularly bound by the tip of the coccyx, the symphysis pubis, and the ischial tuberosities. The dimensions of the superior and inferior pelvic apertures have important obstetric implications.

Ligaments

Four ligaments—inguinal, Cooper's, sacrospinous, and sacrotuberous—of the bony pelvis are of special importance to the gynecologic surgeon.

Inguinal Ligament

The inguinal ligament is important surgically in the repair of inguinal hernia. The inguinal ligament:

1. Is formed by the lower border of the aponeurosis of the external oblique muscle folded back upon itself.
2. Is fused laterally to the iliacus fascia and inferiorly to the fascia lata.
3. Flattens medially into the lacunar ligament, which forms the medial border of the femoral ring.

Cooper's Ligament

Cooper's ligament is used frequently in bladder suspension procedures. Cooper's ligament:

1. **Is a strong ridge of fibrous tissue extending along the pectineal line—also known as the pectineal ligament.**
2. **Merges laterally with the iliopectineal ligament and medially with the lacunar ligament.**

Sacrospinous Ligament

The sacrospinous ligament is often used for vaginal suspension. This ligament offers the advantage of a vaginal surgical route. The sacrospinous ligament:

1. **Extends from the ischial spine to the lateral aspect of the sacrum.**
2. **Is separated from the rectovaginal space by the rectal pillars.**
3. **Lies anterior to the pudendal nerve and the internal pudendal vessels at its attachment to the ischial spine.**

The inferior gluteal artery, with extensive collateral circulation, is found between the sacrospinous and sacrotuberous ligaments and may be injured during sacrospinous suspension (Fig. 5.2) (7). Injury to the inferior gluteal artery, and to the pudendal nerve and internal pudendal vessels, during sacrospinous ligament suspension may be minimized by careful and controlled retraction and suture placement at least two fingerbreadths medial to the ischial spine.

Sacrotuberous Ligament

The sacrotuberous ligament is sometimes used as a point of fixation for vaginal vault suspension. The sacrotuberous ligament:

1. **Extends from the ischial tuberosity to the lateral aspect of the sacrum.**
2. **Merges medially with the sacrospinous ligament.**
3. **Lies posterior to the pudendal nerve and the internal pudendal vessels.**

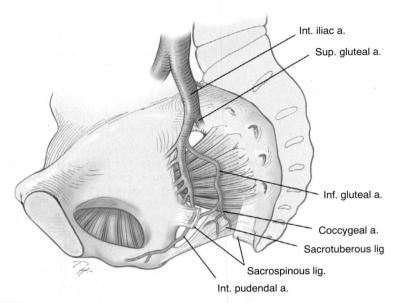

Int. iliac a.

Sup. gluteal a.

Inf. gluteal a.

Coccygeal a.

Sacrotuberous lig

Sacrospinous lig.

Int. pudendal a.

Figure 5.2 Tone drawing of left hemipelvis with sacrospinous ligament reflected. a., artery; Inf., inferior; lig., ligament; n., nerve; Sacrosp., sacrospinous; Sacrotub., sacrotuberous. (Redrawn from **Thompson JR, Gibbs JS, Genadry R, et al.** Anatomy of pelvic arteries adjacent to the sacrospinous ligament: importance of the coccygeal branch of the inferior gluteal artery. *Obstet Gynecol* 1999;94:973–977, with permission.)

Foramina

The bony pelvis and its ligaments delineate three important foramina that allow the passage of the various muscles, nerves, and vessels to the lower extremity.

Greater Sciatic Foramen

The greater sciatic foramen transmits the following structures: the piriformis muscle, the superior gluteal nerves and vessels, the sciatic nerve along with the nerves of the quadratus femoris, the inferior gluteal nerves and vessels, the posterior cutaneous nerve of the thigh, the nerves of the obturator internus, and the internal pudendal nerves and vessels.

Lesser Sciatic Foramen

The lesser sciatic foramen transmits the tendon of the obturator internus to its insertion on the greater trochanter of the femur. The nerve of the obturator internus and the pudendal vessels and nerves reenter the pelvis through the lesser sciatic foramen.

Obturator Foramen

The obturator foramen transmits the obturator nerves and vessels. The obturator neurovascular bundle can be injured during transobturator tape placement, a procedure for treatment of urinary incontinence. Trocar-based mesh kits for anterior and apical vaginal prolapse are often passed through the obturator membrane, just lateral to the descending ischiopubic ramus but medial to the obturator foramen. Injury to the obturator nerves and vessels can be prevented during these procedures by careful identification of anatomic landmarks and placement away from the obturator foramen.

Muscles

The muscles of the pelvis include those of the lateral wall and those of the pelvic floor (Fig. 5.3; Table 5.1).

Lateral Wall

The muscles of the lateral pelvic wall pass into the gluteal region to assist in thigh rotation and adduction. They include the piriformis, the obturator internus, and the iliopsoas.

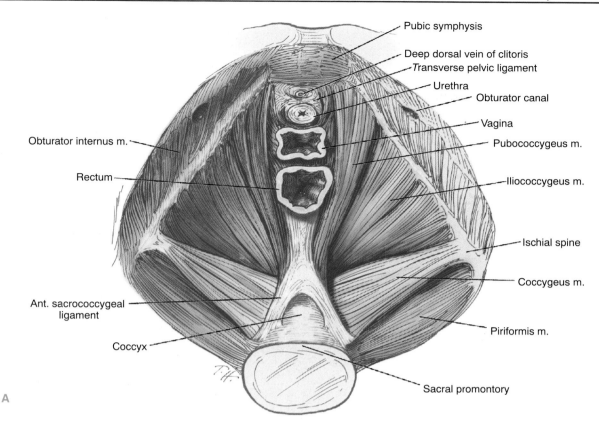

A

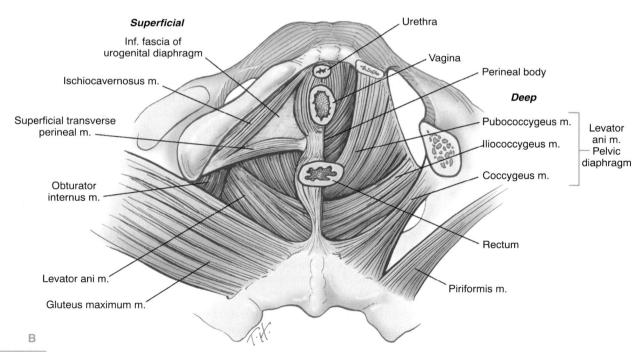

B

Figure 5.3 **The pelvic diaphragm.** A: A view into the pelvic floor that illustrates the muscles of the pelvic diaphragm and their attachments to the bony pelvis. B: A view from outside the pelvic diaphragm illustrating the divisions of the levator ani muscles (superficial plane removed on the right). (*continued*)

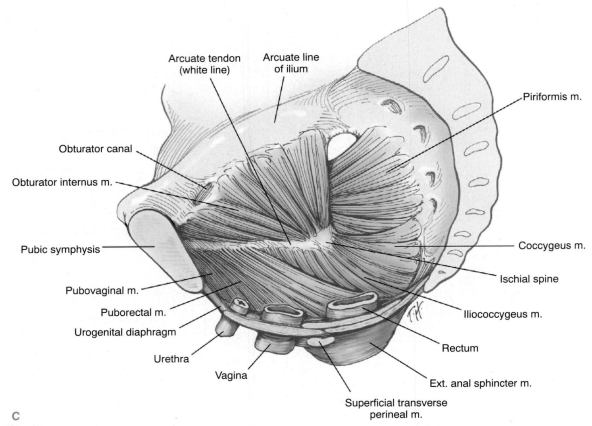

Arcuate tendon
(white line)

Arcuate line
of ilium

Piriformis m.

Obturator canal

Obturator internus m.

Pubic symphysis

Coccygeus m.

Pubovaginal m.

Ischial spine

Puborectal m.

Iliococcygeus m.

Urogenital diaphragm

Urethra

Rectum

Vagina

Ext. anal sphincter m.

Superficial transverse
perineal m.

C

Figure 5.3   (***Continued***) C: A lateral, sagittal view of the pelvic diaphragm and superior fascia of the urogenital diaphragm. The muscles include the deep transverse perineal and sphincter urethrae.

Pelvic Floor

Pelvic Diaphragm

The pelvic diaphragm is a funnel-shaped fibromuscular partition that forms the primary supporting structure for the pelvic contents (Fig. 5.4). It is composed of the levator ani (pubococcygeus, puborectalis, iliococcygeus) and the coccygeus muscles, along with their superior and inferior fasciae (Table 5.1). It forms the ceiling of the ischiorectal fossa.

Levator Ani

The levator ani muscles are composed of the pubococcygeus (including the pubovaginalis and pubourethralis, puborectalis, and the iliococcygeus). The levator ani is a broad, curved sheet of muscle stretching anteriorly from the pubis and posteriorly from the coccyx and from one side of the pelvis to the other. It is perforated by the urethra, vagina, and anal canal. Its origin is from the tendinous arch extending from the body of the pubis to the ischial spine. **This tendineus arch, called the *arcus tendineus levator ani*, is formed by a thickening of the obturator fascia and serves as a lateral landmark and point of attachment for some vaginal suspension procedures.** The levator ani is inserted into the central tendon of the perineum, the wall of the anal canal, the anococcygeal ligament, the coccyx, and the vaginal wall.

The levator ani assists the anterior abdominal wall muscles in containing the abdominal and pelvic contents. It supports the vagina, facilitates defecation, and aids in maintaining fecal continence. During parturition, the levator ani supports the fetal head while the cervix dilates. The anterior portion of the levator ani complex serves to close the urogenital hiatus and pull the urethra, vagina, perineum, and anorectum toward the pubic bone, whereas the horizontally oriented posterior portion (levator plate) serves as a supportive diaphragm or "backstop" behind the pelvic viscera. Loss of normal levator ani tone, through denervation or direct muscle trauma, results in laxity of the urogenital hiatus, loss of the horizontal orientation of the levator plate, and a more bowl-like configuration. These changes can be bilateral or asymmetric (8). Such

	Origin	Insertion	Action	Innervation
Table 5.1 Muscles of the Pelvic Floor				
Lateral Pelvic Wall				
Piriformis	Anterior aspect of S2–S4 and sacrotuberous ligament	Greater trochanter of the femur	Lateral rotation, abduction of thigh in flexion; holds head of femur in acetabulum	S1–S2; forms a muscular bed for the sacral plexus
Obturator internus	Superior and inferior pubic rami	Greater trochanter of the femur	Lateral rotation of thigh in flexion; assists in holding head of femur in acetabulum	(L5, S1) Obturator internus nerve
Iliopsoas	Psoas from the lateral margin of the lumbar vertebrae; iliacus from the iliac fossa	Lesser trochanter of the femur	Flexes thigh and stabilizes trunk on thigh; flexes vertebral column or bends it unilaterally	(L1–L3) Psoas-ventral rami of lumbar nerve (L2–L3) Iliacus-femoral nerve contains the lumbar plexus within its muscle body
Pelvic Floor				
Pelvic Diaphragm				
Levator Ani Pubococcygeus Pubovaginalis Puborectalis	From the tendinous arch, extending from the body of the pubis to the ischial spine	Central tendon of the perineum; wall of the anal canal; anococcygeal ligament; coccyx; vaginal wall	Assists the anterior abdominal wall muscles in containing the abdominal and pelvic contents; supports the posterior wall of the vagina; facilitates defecation; aids in fecal continence; during parturition, supports the fetal head during cervical dilation	S3–S4; the inferior rectal nerve
Coccygeus	Ischial spine and sacrospinous ligament	Lateral margin of the fifth sacral vertebra and coccyx	Supports the coccyx and pulls it anteriorly	S4–5
Urogenital Diaphragm				
Deep transverse perineal	Medial aspect of the ischiopubic rami	Lower part of the vaginal wall; anterior fibers blend with those of the sphincter urethrae	Steadies the central perineal tendon	S2–S4; perineal nerve
Sphincter urethrae	Medial aspect of the ischiopubic rami	Urethra and vagina	Compresses the urethra	S2–S4; perineal nerve

configurations are seen more often in women with pelvic organ prolapse than in those with normal pelvic organ support (9).

Traditional teaching is that the levator ani muscles are innervated by the pudendal nerve on the perineal surface and direct branches of the sacral nerves on the pelvic surface. Evidence indicates that the levator ani muscles are innervated solely by a nerve traveling on the superior (intrapelvic) surface of the muscles without the contribution of the pudendal nerve (10–15). This nerve, referred to as the *levator ani nerve*, originates from S3, S4, and/or S5 and innervates both the coccygeus and the levator ani muscle complex (10). After exiting the sacral foramina, it travels 2 to 3 cm medial to the ischial spine and arcus tendineus levator ani across the coccygeus,

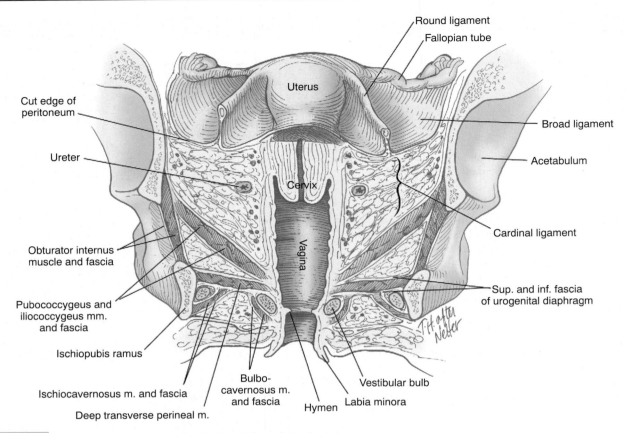

Figure 5.4   **The ligaments and fascial support of the pelvic viscera.**

iliococcygeus, pubococcygeus, and puborectalis. Occasionally, a separate nerve comes directly from S5 to innervate the puborectalis muscle independently. Given its location, the levator ani nerve is susceptible to injury through parturition and pelvic surgery, such as during sacrospinous or iliococcygeus vaginal vault suspensions.

Urogenital Diaphragm

The muscles of the urogenital diaphragm anteriorly reinforce the pelvic diaphragm and are intimately related to the vagina and the urethra. They are enclosed between the inferior and superior fascia of the urogenital diaphragm. The muscles include the deep transverse perineal and sphincter urethrae (Table 5.1).

Blood Vessels

The pelvic blood vessels supply genital structures as well as the following:

- Urinary and gastrointestinal tracts
- Muscles of the abdominal wall, pelvic floor and perineum, buttocks, and upper thighs
- Fasciae, other connective tissue, and bones
- Skin and other superficial structures

Classically, vessels supplying organs are known as *visceral vessels* and those supplying supporting structures are called *parietal vessels*.

Major Blood Vessels

The course of the major vessels supplying the pelvis is illustrated in Figure 5.5; their origin, course, branches, and venous drainage are presented in Table 5.2. In general, the venous system draining the pelvis closely follows the arterial supply and is named accordingly. Not infrequently, a vein draining a particular area may form a plexus with multiple channels. Venous systems, which are paired, mirror each other in their drainage patterns, with the notable exception of the ovarian veins. Unusual features of venous drainage are also listed in Table 5.2.

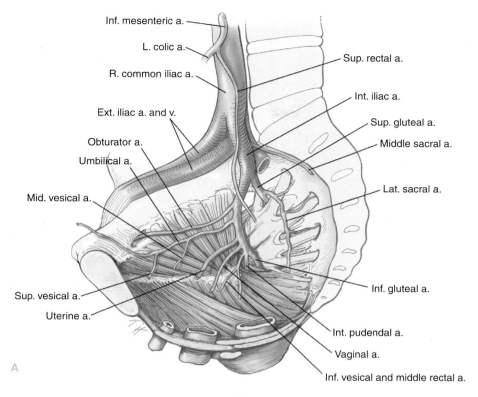

- Inf. mesenteric a.
- L. colic a.
- R. common iliac a.
- Ext. iliac a. and v.
- Obturator a.
- Umbilical a.
- Mid. vesical a.
- Sup. vesical a.
- Uterine a.
- Sup. rectal a.
- Int. iliac a.
- Sup. gluteal a.
- Middle sacral a.
- Lat. sacral a.
- Inf. gluteal a.
- Int. pudendal a.
- Vaginal a.
- Inf. vesical and middle rectal a.

A

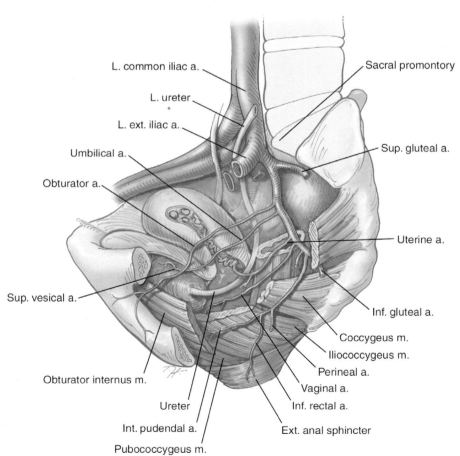

- L. common iliac a.
- L. ureter
- L. ext. iliac a.
- Umbilical a.
- Obturator a.
- Sup. vesical a.
- Obturator internus m.
- Ureter
- Int. pudendal a.
- Pubococcygeus m.
- Sacral promontory
- Sup. gluteal a.
- Uterine a.
- Inf. gluteal a.
- Coccygeus m.
- Iliococcygeus m.
- Perineal a.
- Vaginal a.
- Inf. rectal a.
- Ext. anal sphincter

B

Figure 5.5 **The blood supply to the pelvis.** A: The sagittal view of the pelvis without the viscera. B: The blood supply to one pelvic viscera.

Table 5.2 The Major Blood Vessels of the Pelvis

Artery	Origin	Course	Branches	Venous Drainage
Ovarian	Arises from ventral surface of aorta just below the origin of the renal vessels	Crosses over common iliac vessels; in proximity to ureter over much of its course, crosses over ureter while superficial to the psoas muscle and runs just lateral to the ureter when entering the pelvis as part of the infundibulopelvic ligament	To ovaries, fallopian tubes, broad ligament; often small branches to ureter	Right side drains into the inferior vena cava; left drains into the left renal vein
Inferior mesenteric artery (IMA)	Unpaired left-sided retroperitoneal artery arising from the aorta 2–5 cm proximal to its bifurcation	IMA and its branches pass over the left psoas muscle and common iliac vessels; IMA courses anterior to the ureter and ovarian vessels above the pelvic brim	1. *Left colic*—originates above pelvic brim; supplies left transverse colon, splenic flexure, descending colon 2. *Sigmoid*—several branches; supply sigmoid colon 3. *Superior rectal (hemorrhoidal)*—divides into two terminal branches to supply rectum	Inferior mesenteric vein empties into the splenic vein
Common iliac artery	Terminal division of the aorta at fourth lumbar vertebra	Oblique and lateral course, about 5 cm in length	1. *External iliac* 2. *Internal iliac*	Lie posterior and slightly medial to arteries; drain into inferior vena cava
External iliac femoral artery	Lateral bifurcation of common iliac, begins opposite the lumbosacral joint	Along the medial border of the psoas muscle and lateral pelvic side wall; becomes femoral artery after passing under the inguinal ligament to supply lower extremity	1. *Superficial epigastric*—supplies skin and subcutaneous tissue of lower anterior abdominal wall 2. *External pudendal*—supplies skin and subcutaneous tissue of mons pubis and anterior vulva 3. *Superficial circumflex iliac*—supplies skin/subcutaneous tissues of the flank 4. *Inferior epigastric*—supplies musculofascial layer of lower anterior abdominal wall 5. *Deep circumflex iliac*—supplies musculofascial layer of lower abdominal wall	Lie posterior and then medial to the artery as it enters the anterior thigh; drain into common iliac veins
Internal iliac (hypogastric) artery	Medial bifurcation of common iliac artery, begins opposite the lumbosacral joint; is major blood supply to the pelvis	Descends sharply into the pelvis; divides into an anterior and posterior division 3–4 cm after origin	*Posterior division* 1. *Iliolumbar*—anastomoses with lumbar and deep circumflex iliac arteries; helps supply lower abdominal wall, iliac fossa 2. *Lateral sacral*—supplies contents of sacral canal, piriformis muscle 3. *Superior gluteal*—supplies gluteal muscles	Deep to arteries, from complex plexus; drain into common iliac veins

Vessel	Origin	Course	Distribution	Venous drainage
			Anterior division: 1. *Obturator*—supplies iliac fossa, posterior pubis, obturator internus muscle 2. *Internal pudendal* 3. *Umbilical*—remnant of fetal umbilical artery; after giving off branches, as the medial umbilical ligament 4. *Superior, middle, inferior vesical*—supply bladder and one or more branches to the ureter 5. *Middle rectal (hemorrhoidal)*—supplies rectum, branches to midvagina 6. *Uterine*—supplies uterine corpus and cervix, with branches to upper vagina, tube, round ligament, and ovary 7. *Vaginal*—supplies vagina 8. *Inferior gluteal*—supplies gluteal muscles, muscles of posterior thigh		1. *Inferior rectal (hemorrhoidal)*—supplies anal canal, external anal sphincter, perianal skin, with branches to levator ani 2. *Perineal*—supplies perineal skin, muscles of superficial perineal compartment (bulbocavernosus, ischiocavernosus, superficial transverse perineal) 3. *Clitoral*—supplies clitoris, vestibular bulb, Bartholin gland, and urethra	Drain into internal iliac veins
Internal pudendal artery	Internal iliac artery; provides the major blood supply to the perineum	Leaves the pelvis through the greater sciatic foramen, courses around the ischial spine, and enters the ischiorectal fossa through the lesser sciatic foramen. In its path to the perineum, lies with the pudendal nerve within Alcock's canal, a fascial tunnel over the obturator internus muscle		
Middle sacral artery	Midline unpaired vessel arising from posterior terminal aorta	Courses over lower lumbar vertebrae, sacrum, and coccyx	Supplies bony and muscular structures of posterior pelvic wall	Paired middle sacral veins usually drain into left common iliac vein
Lumbar arteries	Segmental branches arising at each lumbar level from posterior aorta	Pass around the side of the 4 superior lumbar vertebrae, divide into anterior and posterior branches	Supplies abdominal wall musculature (external/internal oblique, transversus abdominis)	Veins into inferior vena cava

General Principles

"Control blood supply" and "maintain meticulous hemostasis" are two of the most common exhortations to young surgeons. In developing familiarity with the pattern of blood flow in the pelvis, several unique characteristics of this vasculature should be understood because of their potential implications to surgical practice:

1. **The pelvic vessels play an important role in pelvic support.** They provide condensations of endopelvic fascia that act to reinforce the normal position of pelvic organs (16).

2. **There is significant anatomic variation between individuals in the branching pattern of the internal iliac vessels.** There is no constant order in which branches divide from the parent vessel; some branches may arise as common trunks or may spring from other branches rather than from the internal iliac. Occasionally, a branch may arise from another vessel entirely (e.g., the obturator artery may arise from the external iliac or inferior epigastric artery). This variation may be found in the branches of other major vessels; the ovarian arteries are reported to arise from the renal arteries or as a common trunk from the front of the aorta on occasion. The inferior gluteal artery may originate from the posterior or the anterior branch of the internal iliac (hypogastric) artery. Patterns of blood flow may be asymmetric from side to side, and structures supplied by anastomoses of different vessels may show variation from person to person in the proportion of vascular support provided by the vessels involved (16). The pelvic surgeon must be prepared for deviations from "textbook" vascular patterns.

3. **The pelvic vasculature is a high-volume, high-flow system with enormous expansive capabilities throughout reproductive life.** Blood flow through the uterine arteries increases to about 500 mL per min in late pregnancy. In nonpregnant women, certain conditions, such as uterine fibroids or malignant neoplasms, may be associated with neovascularization and hypertrophy of existing vessels and a corresponding increase in pelvic blood flow. Understanding the volume and flow characteristics of the pelvic vasculature in different clinical situations will enable the surgeon to anticipate problems and take appropriate preoperative and intraoperative measures (including blood and blood product availability) to prevent or manage hemorrhage.

4. **The pelvic vasculature is supplied with an extensive network of collateral connections that provides a rich anastomotic communication between different major vessel systems** (Fig. 5.6). This degree of redundancy is important to ensure adequate supply of oxygen and nutrients in the event of major trauma or other vascular compromise. Hypogastric artery ligation continues to be used as a strategy for management of massive pelvic hemorrhage when other measures have failed. Bilateral hypogastric artery ligation, particularly when combined with ovarian artery ligation, dramatically reduces pulse pressure in the pelvis, converting flow characteristics from that of an arterial system to a venous system and allowing use of collateral channels of circulation to continue blood supply to pelvic structures. The significance of collateral blood flow is demonstrated by reports of successful pregnancies occurring after bilateral ligation of both hypogastric and ovarian arteries (17). Table 5.3 lists the collateral channels of circulation in the pelvis.

Special Vascular Considerations

To avoid injury to vascular structures and resultant hemorrhage while inserting a trocar into the anterior abdominal wall during laparoscopy, the surgeon should keep in mind certain anatomic relationships. The inferior epigastric artery is a branch of the external iliac artery, arising from the parent vessel at the medial border of the inguinal ligament and coursing cephalad lateral to and posterior to the rectus sheath at the level of the arcuate line. It lies about 1.5 cm lateral to the medial umbilical fold, which marks the site of the obliterated umbilical artery. **During laparoscopy the inferior epigastric artery almost always can be visualized between the obliterated umbilical artery medially and the insertion of the round ligament through the inguinal canal laterally.** This artery can be traced visually cephalad, allowing for safe insertion of lateral port site. The aortic bifurcation occurs at the level of L4 to L5, just above the sacral promontory. Palpation of the sacral promontory to guide trocar insertion allows the surgeon to avoid the major vascular structures in this area (see Fig. 23.4 in Chapter 23). **The left common iliac vein lies medial to the artery and is at risk of injury during umbilical laparoscopic trocar insertion and during dissection for sacrocolpopexy.**

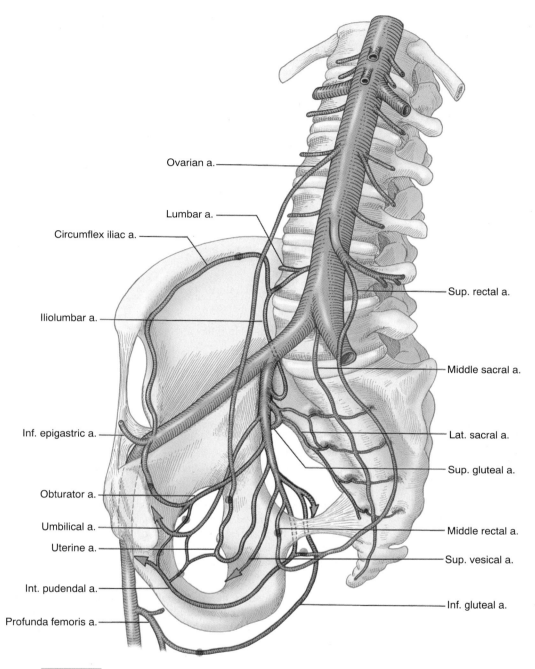

Figure 5.6 **The collateral blood vessels of the pelvis.** (Modified from **Kamina P.** *Anatomie gynécologique et obstétricale.* Paris, France: Maloine Sa Éditeur, 1984:125, with permission.)

Lymphatics

The pelvic lymph nodes are generally arranged in groups or chains and follow the course of the larger pelvic vessels, for which they are usually named. Smaller nodes that lie close to the visceral structures are usually named for those organs. Lymph nodes in the pelvis receive afferent lymphatic vessels from pelvic and perineal visceral and parietal structures and send efferent lymphatics to more proximal nodal groups. The number of lymph nodes and their exact location is variable; however, certain nodes tend to be relatively constant:

1. Obturator node in the obturator foramen, close to the obturator vessels and nerve
2. Nodes at the junction of the internal and external iliac veins

Table 5.3 Collateral Arterial Circulation of the Pelvis	
Primary Artery	*Collateral Arteries*
Aorta	
Ovarian artery	Uterine artery
Superior rectal artery (inferior mesenteric artery)	Middle rectal artery
	Inferior rectal artery (internal pudendal)
Lumbar arteries	Iliolumbar artery
Vertebral arteries	Iliolumbar artery
Middle sacral artery	Lateral sacral artery
External Iliac	
Deep iliac circumflex artery	Iliolumbar artery
	Superior gluteal artery
Inferior epigastric artery	Obturator artery
Femoral	
Medial femoral circumflex artery	Obturator artery
	Inferior gluteal artery
Lateral femoral circumflex artery	Superior gluteal artery
	Iliolumbar artery

3. Ureteral node in the broad ligament near the cervix, where the uterine artery crosses over the ureter
4. The *Cloquet* or Rosenmüller node—the highest of the deep inguinal nodes that lies within the opening of the femoral canal

Figure 5.7 illustrates the pelvic lymphatic system. Table 5.4 outlines the major lymphatic chains of relevance to the pelvis and their primary afferent connections from major pelvic and perineal structures. There are extensive interconnections between lymph vessels and nodes; usually more than one lymphatic pathway is available for drainage of each pelvic site. Bilateral and crossed extension of lymphatic flow may occur, and entire groups of nodes may be bypassed to reach more proximal chains.

The natural history of most genital tract malignancies directly reflects the lymphatic drainage of those structures, although the various interconnections, different lymphatic paths, and individual variability make the spread of malignancy somewhat unpredictable. Regional lymph node metastasis is one of the most important factors in formulation of treatment plans for gynecologic malignancies and prediction of eventual outcome.

Nerves

The pelvis is innervated by both the autonomic and somatic nervous systems. The autonomic nerves include both *sympathetic* (adrenergic) and *parasympathetic* (cholinergic) fibers and provide the primary innervation for genital, urinary, and gastrointestinal visceral structures and blood vessels.

Somatic Innervation

The *lumbosacral plexus* and its branches provide motor and sensory somatic innervation to the lower abdominal wall, the pelvic and urogenital diaphragms, the perineum, and the hip and lower extremity (Fig. 5.8). The nerves originating from the muscles, the lumbosacral trunk, the anterior divisions of the upper four sacral nerves (*sacral plexus*), and the anterior division of the coccygeal nerve and fibers from the fourth and fifth sacral nerves (*coccygeal plexus*) are found on the anterior surface of the piriformis muscle and lateral to the coccyx, respectively, deep in the posterior pelvis. In Table 5.5 each major branch is listed by spinal segment and structures innervated. In addition to these branches, the lumbosacral plexus includes nerves that innervate

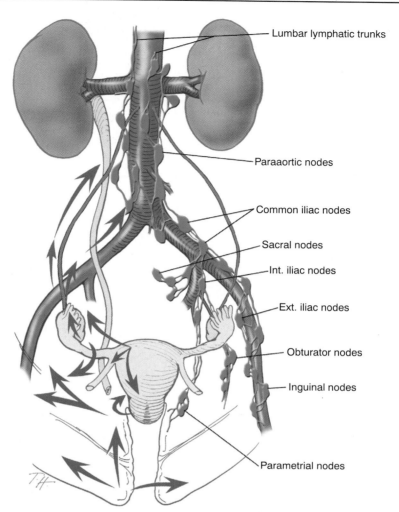

Lumbar lymphatic trunks

Paraaortic nodes

Common iliac nodes

Sacral nodes

Int. iliac nodes

Ext. iliac nodes

Obturator nodes

Inguinal nodes

Parametrial nodes

Figure 5.7   The lymphatic drainage of the female pelvis. The vulva and lower vagina drain to the superficial and deep inguinal nodes, sometimes directly to the iliac nodes (along the dorsal vein of the clitoris) and to the other side. The cervix and upper vagina drain laterally to the parametrial, obturator, and external iliac nodes and posteriorly along the uterosacral ligaments to the sacral nodes. Drainage from these primary lymph node groups is upward along the infundibulopelvic ligament, similar to drainage of the ovary and fallopian tubes to the para-aortic nodes. The lower uterine body drains in the same manner as the cervix. Rarely, drainage occurs along the round ligament to the inguinal nodes.

muscles of the lateral pelvic wall (obturator internus, piriformis), posterior hip muscles, and the pelvic diaphragm. A visceral component, the pelvic splanchnic nerve, is included.

Nerves supplying the cutaneous aspects of the anterior, medial, and lateral lower extremities, and the deep muscles of the anterior thigh, primarily leave the pelvis by passing beneath the inguinal ligament. Nerves supporting the posterior cutaneous and deep structures of the hip, thigh, and leg lie deep in the pelvis and should not be vulnerable to injury during pelvic surgery. **The obturator nerve travels along the lateral pelvic wall to pass through the obturator foramen into the upper thigh, and it may be encountered in more radical dissections involving the lateral pelvic wall, in paravaginal repairs, or in trocar-based incontinence and prolapse procedures.**

The pudendal nerve innervates the striated urethral and anal sphincters and the deep and superficial perineal muscles and provides sensory innervation to the external genitalia. This nerve originates from S2–S4, crosses over the piriformis to travel with the internal pudendal vessels into the ischiorectal fossa through the lesser sciatic foramen, and travels through the pudendal canal (Alcock's canal) on the medial aspect of the obturator internus muscles, where

Table 5.4 Primary Lymph Node Groups Providing Drainage to Genital Structures	
Nodes	**Primary Afferent Connections**
Aortic/para-aortic	Ovary, fallopian tube, uterine corpus (upper); drainage from common iliac nodes
Common iliac	Drainage from external and internal iliac nodes
External iliac	Upper vagina, cervix, uterine corpus (upper); drainage from inguinal
Internal iliac	Upper vagina, cervix, uterine corpus (lower)
Lateral sacral	
Superior gluteal	
Inferior gluteal	
Obturator	
Vesical	
Rectal	
Parauterine	
Inguinal	Vulva, lower vagina; (rare: uterus, tube, ovary)
Superficial	
Deep	

it divides into its three terminal branches to provide the primary innervation to the perineum. Other nerves contribute to the cutaneous innervation of the perineum:

1. **The anterior labial nerve branches of the ilioinguinal nerve**—these nerves emerge from within the inguinal canal and through the superficial inguinal ring to the mons and upper labia majora.

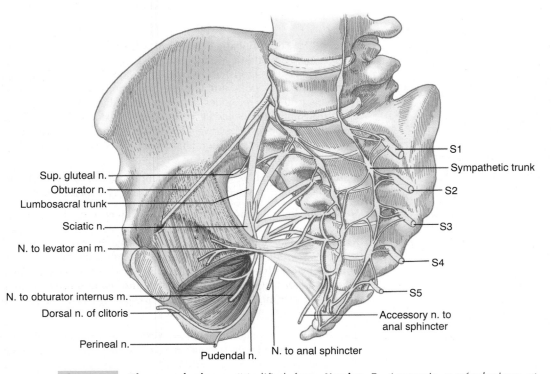

Figure 5.8 The sacral plexus. (Modified from **Kamina P.** *Anatomie gynécologique et obstétricale.* Paris, France: Maloine Sa Éditeur, 1984:90, with permission.)

Table 5.5 Lumbosacral Plexus		
Nerve	*Spinal Segment*	*Innervation*
Iliohypogastric	T12, L1	Sensory—skin near iliac crest, just above symphysis pubis
Ilioinguinal	L1	Sensory—upper medial thigh, mons, labia majora
Lateral femoral cutaneous	L2, L3	Sensory—lateral thigh to level of knee
Femoral	L2, L3, L4	Sensory—anterior and medial thigh, medial leg and foot, hip and knee joints Motor—iliacus, anterior thigh muscles
Genitofemoral	L1, L2	Sensory—anterior vulva (genital branch), middle/upper anterior thigh (femoral branch)
Obturator	L2, L3, L4	Sensory—medial thigh and leg, hip and knee joints Motor—adductor muscles of thigh
Superior gluteal	L4, L5, S1	Motor—gluteal muscles
Inferior gluteal	L4, L5, S1, S2	Motor—gluteal muscles
Posterior femoral cutaneous	S1, S2, S3	Sensory—vulva, perineum, posterior thigh
Sciatic	L4, L5, S1, S2, S3	Sensory—much of leg, foot, lower-extremity joints Motor—posterior thigh muscle, leg and foot muscles
Pudendal	S2, S3, S4	Sensory—perianal skin, vulva and perineum, clitoris, urethra, vaginal vestibule Motor—external anal sphincter, perineal muscles, urogenital diaphragm

2. **The genital branch of the genitofemoral nerve**—this branch enters the inguinal canal with the round ligament and passes through the superficial inguinal ring to the anterior vulva.

3. **The perineal branches of the posterior femoral cutaneous nerve**—after leaving the pelvis through the greater sciatic foramen, these branches run in front of the ischial tuberosity to the lateral perineum and labia majora.

4. **Perforating cutaneous branches of the second and third sacral nerves**—these branches perforate the sacrotuberous ligament to supply the buttocks and contiguous perineum.

5. **The anococcygeal nerves**—these nerves arise from S4 to S5 and also perforate the sacrotuberous ligament to supply the skin overlying the coccyx.

Autonomic Innervation

Functionally, the innervation of the pelvic viscera may be divided into an *efferent* component and an *afferent*, or sensory, component. In reality, afferent and efferent fibers are closely associated in a complex interlacing network and cannot be separated anatomically.

Efferent Innervation

Efferent fibers of the autonomic nervous system, unlike motor fibers in the somatic system, involve one synapse outside the central nervous system, with two neurons required to carry each impulse. In the *sympathetic (thoracolumbar) division*, this synapse is generally at some distance from the organ being innervated; conversely, the synapse is on or near the organ of innervation in the *parasympathetic (craniosacral) division*.

Axons from preganglionic neurons emerge from the spinal cord to make contact with peripheral neurons arranged in aggregates known as *autonomic ganglia*. Some of these ganglia, along with interconnecting nerve fibers, form a pair of longitudinal cords called the *sympathetic trunks*. Located lateral to the spinal column from the base of the cranium to the coccyx, the sympathetic

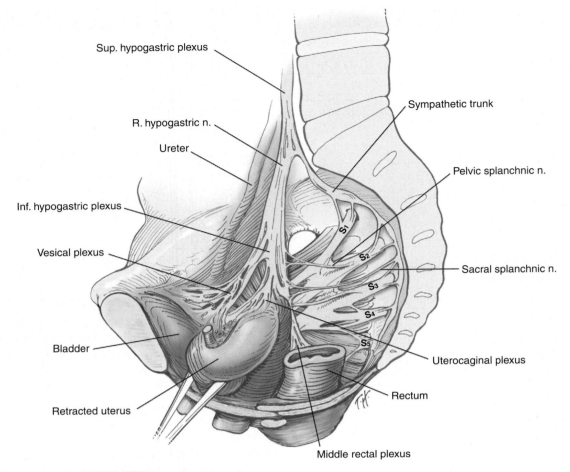

Sup. hypogastric plexus

Sympathetic trunk

R. hypogastric n.

Ureter

Pelvic splanchnic n.

Inf. hypogastric plexus

S1

S2

Vesical plexus

Sacral splanchnic n.

S3

S4

Bladder

S5

Uterocaginal plexus

Rectum

Retracted uterus

Middle rectal plexus

Figure 5.9   The presacral nerves.

trunks lie along the medial border of the psoas muscle from T12 to the sacral prominence and then pass behind the common iliac vessels to continue into the pelvis on the anterior surface of the sacrum. On the anterolateral surface of the aorta, the *aortic plexus* forms a lacy network of nerve fibers with interspersed ganglia. Rami arising from or traversing the sympathetic trunks join this plexus and its subsidiaries.

The ovaries, part of the fallopian tubes, and broad ligament are innervated by the *ovarian plexus*, a network of nerve fibers accompanying the ovarian vessels and derived from the aortic and renal plexuses. The *inferior mesenteric plexus* is a subsidiary of the *celiac plexus* and *aortic plexus* and is located along the inferior mesenteric artery and its branches, providing innervation to the left colon, sigmoid, and rectum.

The *superior hypogastric plexus* (*presacral nerve*) is the continuation of the aortic plexus beneath the peritoneum in front of the terminal aorta, the fifth lumbar vertebra, and the sacral promontory, medial to the ureters (Fig. 5.9). Embedded in loose areolar tissue, the plexus overlies the middle sacral vessels and is usually composed of two or three incompletely fused trunks. It contains preganglionic fibers from lumbar nerves, postganglionic fibers from higher sympathetic ganglia and the sacral sympathetic trunks, and visceral afferent fibers. Just below the sacral promontory, the superior hypogastric plexus divides into two loosely arranged nerve trunks, the *hypogastric nerves*. These nerves course inferiorly and laterally to connect with the inferior *hypogastric plexuses* (*pelvic plexuses*), which are a dense network of nerves and ganglia that lie along the lateral pelvic sidewall overlying branches of the internal iliac vessels (Fig. 5.9).

The inferior hypogastric plexus includes efferent sympathetic fibers, afferent (sensory) fibers, and parasympathetic fibers arising from the pelvic splanchnic nerves (S2 to S4, nervi erigentes).

This paired plexus is the final common pathway of the pelvic visceral nervous system and is divided into three portions, representing distribution of innervation to the viscera:

1. **Vesical plexus**
   - Innervation: bladder and urethra
   - Course: along vesical vessels
2. **Middle rectal plexus (hemorrhoidal)**
   - Innervation: rectum
   - Course: along middle rectal vessels
3. **Uterovaginal plexus (Frankenhäuser ganglion)**
   - Innervation: uterus, vagina, clitoris, vestibular bulbs
   - Course: along uterine vessels and through cardinal and uterosacral ligaments; sympathetic and sensory fibers derive from T10, L1; parasympathetic fibers derive from S2 to S4.

Afferent Innervation

Afferent **fibers from the pelvic viscera and blood vessels traverse the same pathways to provide sensory input to the central nervous system.** They are involved in reflex arcs needed for bladder, bowel, and genital tract function. The afferent fibers reach the central nervous system to have their first synapse within the posterior spinal nerve ganglia.

Presacral neurectomy, in which a segment of the superior hypogastric plexus is divided and resected in order to interrupt sensory fibers from the uterus and cervix, is associated with relief of dysmenorrhea secondary to endometriosis in about 50% to 75% of cases in which it was used (18,19). Efferent fibers from the adnexa travel with the ovarian plexus; thus, pain originating from the ovary or tube is not relieved by resection of the presacral nerve. Because this plexus contains efferent sympathetic and parasympathetic nerve fibers intermixed with afferent fibers, disturbance in bowel or bladder function may result. An alternative surgical procedure is resection of a portion of the uterosacral ligaments; because they contain numerous nerve fibers with more specific innervation to the uterus, it is postulated that bladder and rectal function is less vulnerable to compromise (20).

An anesthetic block of the pudendal nerve is performed most often for pain relief with uncomplicated vaginal deliveries but may provide useful anesthesia for minor perineal surgical procedures. This nerve block may be accomplished transvaginally or through the perineum. A needle is inserted toward the ischial spine with the tip directed slightly posteriorly and through the sacrospinous ligament. As the anesthetic agent is injected, frequent aspiration is required to avoid injection into the pudendal vessels, which travel with the nerve.

Pelvic Viscera

Embryonic Development

The female urinary and genital tracts are closely related, anatomically and embryologically. Both are derived largely from primitive mesoderm and endoderm, and there is evidence that the embryologic urinary system has an important inductive influence on the developing genital system. **About 10% of infants are born with some abnormality of the genitourinary system, and anomalies in one system are often mirrored by anomalies in another system** (19).

Developmental defects may play a significant role in the differential diagnosis of certain clinical signs and symptoms and have special implications in pelvic surgery (21–26). **Thus it is important for gynecologists to have a basic understanding of embryology.**

Following is a presentation of the urinary system, internal reproductive organs, and external genitalia in order of their initial appearance, although much of this development occurs concurrently. The development of each of these three regions proceeds synchronously at an early embryologic age (Table 5.6).

Urinary System

Kidneys, Renal Collecting System, Ureters

The kidneys, renal collecting system, and ureters derive from the longitudinal mass of mesoderm (known as the nephrogenic cord) found on each side of the primitive aorta.

Table 5.6 Development of Genital and Urinary Tracts by Embryologic Age		
Weeks of Gestation	*Genital Development*	*Urinary Development*
4–6	Urorectal septum	Pronephros
	Formation of cloacal folds, genital tubercle	Mesonephros/mesonephric duct
	Ureteric buds, metanephros	
	Genital ridges	Exstrophy of mesonephric ducts and ureters into bladder wall
6–7	End of indifferent phase of genital development	Major, minor calyces form
	Development of primitive sex cords	Kidneys begin to ascend
	Formation of paramesonephric ducts	
	Labioscrotal swellings	
8–11	Distal paramesonephric ducts begin to fuse	Kidney becomes functional
	Formation of sinuvaginal bulbs	
12	Development of clitoris and vaginal vestibule	
20	Canalization of vaginal plate	
32	Renal collecting duct system complete	

This process gives rise to three successive sets of increasingly advanced urinary structures, each developing more caudal to its predecessor.

The *pronephros*, or "first kidney," is rudimentary and nonfunctional; it is succeeded by the "middle kidney," or *mesonephros*, which is believed to function briefly before regressing. Although the *mesonephros* is transitory as an excretory organ, its duct, the *mesonephric (wolffian) duct*, is of singular importance for the following reasons:

1. It grows caudally in the developing embryo to open, for the first time, an excretory channel into the primitive cloaca and the "outside world."
2. It serves as the starting point for development of the metanephros, which becomes the definitive kidney.
3. It ultimately differentiates into the sexual duct system in the male.
4. Although regressing in female fetuses, there is evidence that the mesonephric duct may have an inductive role in development of the paramesonephric or müllerian duct (22).

The ureteric buds, which sprout from the distal mesonephric ducts, initiate the development of the *metanephros*; these buds extend cranially and penetrate the portion of the nephrogenic cord known as the *metanephric blastema.* The ureteric buds begin to branch sequentially, with each growing tip covered by metanephric blastema. Ultimately the metanephric blastema form the renal functional units (the nephrons), whereas the ureteric buds become the collecting duct system of the kidneys (collecting tubules, minor and major calyces, renal pelvis) and the ureters. Although these primitive tissues differentiate along separate paths, they are interdependent on inductive influences from each other—neither can develop alone.

The kidneys initially lie in the pelvis but subsequently ascend to their permanent location, rotating almost 90 degrees in the process as the more caudal part of the embryo in effect grows away from them. Their blood supply, which first arises as branches of the middle sacral and common iliac arteries, comes from progressively higher branches of the aorta until the definitive renal arteries form; previous vessels then regress. **The definitive kidneys become functional in the late 7th to early 8th weeks of gestation.**

Bladder and Urethra

The cloaca forms as the result of dilation of the opening to the fetal exterior. During the 7th week of gestation, the cloaca is partitioned by the mesenchymal urorectal septum into an anterior urogenital sinus and a posterior rectum. The bladder and urethra form from the most superior portion of the urogenital sinus, with surrounding mesenchyme contributing to their muscular and serosal layers. The remaining inferior urogenital sinus is known as the *phallic* or *definitive urogenital sinus.* Concurrently, the distal mesonephric ducts and attached ureteric buds are incorporated into the posterior bladder wall in the area that will become the bladder trigone. As a result of the absorption process, the mesonephric duct ultimately opens independently into the urogenital sinus below the bladder neck.

The *allantois,* which is a vestigial diverticulum of the hindgut that extends into the umbilicus and is continuous with the bladder, loses its lumen and becomes the fibrous band known as the *urachus* or *median umbilical ligament.* In rare instances, the urachal lumen remains partially patent, with formation of urachal cysts, or completely patent, with the formation of a urinary fistula to the umbilicus (23).

Genital System

Although genetic gender is determined at fertilization, the early genital system is indistinguishable between the two genders in the embryonic stage. This is known as the "indifferent stage" of genital development, during which both male and female fetuses have gonads with prominent cortical and medullary regions, dual sets of genital ducts, and external genitalia that appear similar. Male sexual differentiation is an "active" process, requiring the presence of the SRY gene (gender-determining region), located on the short arm of the Y chromosome. Clinically, **gender is not apparent until about the 12th week of embryonic life and depends on the elaboration of testis-determining factor and, subsequently, androgens by the male gonad.** Female development is called the "basic developmental path of the human embryo," requiring not estrogen but the absence of testosterone.

Internal Reproductive Organs

The *primordial germ cells* migrate from the yolk sac through the mesentery of the hindgut to the posterior body wall mesenchyme at about the 10th thoracic level, which is the initial site of the future ovary (Figs. 5.10 and 5.11). Once the germ cells reach this area, they induce proliferation of cells in the adjacent mesonephros and celomic epithelium to form a pair of *genital ridges* medial to the mesonephros. This occurs during the 5th week of gestation. The development of the gonad is absolutely dependent on this proliferation because these cells form a supporting aggregate of cells (the primitive sex cords) that invest the germ cells and without which the gonad would degenerate.

Müllerian Ducts   **The *paramesonephric or müllerian ducts* form lateral to the mesonephric ducts; they grow caudally and then medially to fuse in the midline.** They contact the urogenital sinus in the region of the posterior urethra at a slight thickening known as the *sinusal tubercle.* Subsequent sexual development is controlled by the presence or absence of testis-determining factor, encoded on the Y chromosome and elaborated by the somatic sex cord cells. Testis-determining factor causes the degeneration of the gonadal cortex and differentiation of the medullary region of the gonad into Sertoli cells.

The Sertoli cells secrete a glycoprotein known as *anti-müllerian hormone* (AMH), which causes regression of the paramesonephric duct system in the male embryo and is the likely signal for differentiation of Leydig cells from the surrounding mesenchyme. The Leydig cells produce testosterone and, with the converting enzyme 5α-reductase, dihydrotestosterone. Testosterone is responsible for evolution of the mesonephric duct system into the vas deferens, epididymis, ejaculatory ducts, and seminal vesicle. At puberty, testosterone leads to spermatogenesis and changes in primary and secondary sex characteristics. Dihydrotestosterone triggers the development of the male external genitalia and the prostate and bulbourethral glands. In the absence of testis-determining factor, the medulla regresses, and the cortical sex cords break up into isolated cell clusters (the primordial follicles).

The germ cells differentiate into oogonia and enter the first meiotic division as primary oocytes, at which point development is arrested until puberty. In the absence of AMH, the mesonephric duct system degenerates, although in at least one-fourth of adult women, remnants may be found in the mesovarium (*epoophoron, paroophoron*) or along the lateral wall of the uterus or vagina (*Gartner duct cyst*) (24).

The paramesonephric duct system subsequently develops. The inferior fused portion becomes the *uterovaginal canal,* which later becomes the epithelium and glands of the uterus and the upper vagina. The endometrial stroma and myometrium differentiate from surrounding mesenchyme.

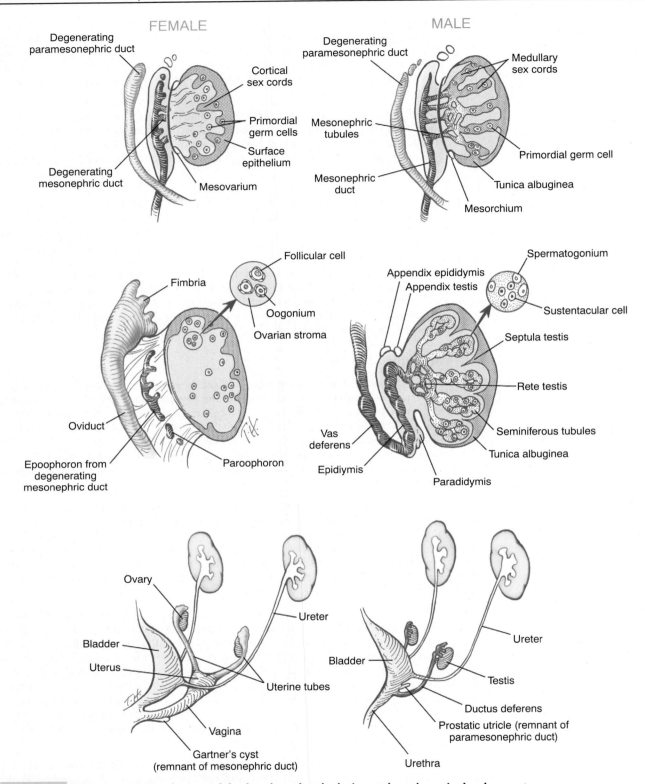

Figure 5.10 The comparative changes of the female and male during early embryonic development.

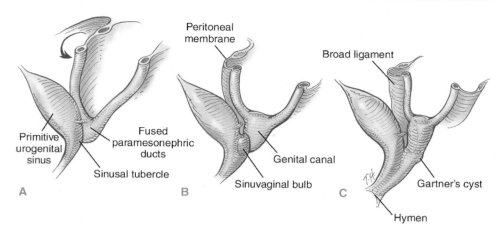

Figure 5.11   **The embryonic development of the female genital tract.** The formation of the uterus and vagina. **A:** The uterus and superior end of the vagina begin to form as the paramesonephric ducts fuse together near their attachment to the posterior wall of the primitive urogenital sinus. **B, C:** The ducts then zipper together in a superior direction between the 3rd and 5th months. As the paramesonephric ducts are pulled away from the posterior body wall, they drag a fold of peritoneal membrane with them, forming the broad ligaments of the uterus. **A–C:** The inferior end of the vagina forms from the sinovaginal bulbs on the posterior wall of the primitive urogenital sinus.

The cranial unfused portions of the paramesonephric ducts open into the celomic (future peritoneal) cavity and become the *fallopian tubes.*

The fusion of the paramesonephric ducts brings together two folds of peritoneum, which become the broad ligament and divide the pelvic cavity into a posterior rectouterine and anterior vesicouterine pouch or cul-de-sac. Between the leaves of the broad ligament, mesenchyme proliferates and differentiates into loose areolar connective tissue and smooth muscle.

Vagina   The *vagina* **forms in the 3rd month of embryonic life.** While the uterovaginal canal is forming, the endodermal tissue of the sinusal tubercle begins to proliferate, forming a pair of *sinovaginal bulbs*, which become the inferior 20% of the vagina. The most inferior portion of the uterovaginal canal becomes occluded by a solid core of tissue (the *vaginal plate*), the origin of which is unclear. Over the subsequent 2 months, this tissue elongates and canalizes by a process of central desquamation, and the peripheral cells become the vaginal epithelium. The fibromuscular wall of the vagina originates from the mesoderm of the uterovaginal canal.

Accessory Genital Glands   **The female accessory genital glands develop as outgrowths from the urethra (*paraurethral* or *Skene*) and the definitive urogenital sinus (*greater vestibular* or *Bartholin*).** Although the ovaries first develop in the thoracic region, they ultimately arrive in the pelvis by a complicated process of descent. This descent by differential growth is under the control of a ligamentous cord called the *gubernaculum*, which is attached to the ovary superiorly and to the fascia in the region of the future labia majora inferiorly. The gubernaculum becomes attached to the paramesonephric ducts at their point of superior fusion so that it becomes divided into two separate structures. As the ovary and its mesentery (the mesovarium) are brought into the superior portion of the broad ligament, the more proximal part of the gubernaculum becomes the *ovarian ligament*, and the distal gubernaculum becomes the *round ligament*.

External Genitalia

Early in the 5th week of embryonic life, folds of tissue form on each side of the cloaca and meet anteriorly in the midline to form the genital tubercle (Fig. 5.12). With the division of the cloaca by the urorectal septum and consequent formation of the perineum, these cloacal folds are known anteriorly as the *urogenital folds* and posteriorly as the *anal folds*. The genital tubercle begins to enlarge. In the female embryo, its growth gradually slows to become the clitoris, and the urogenital folds form the labia minora. In the male embryo, the genital tubercle continues to grow to form the penis, and the urogenital folds are believed to fuse to enclose the penile urethra.

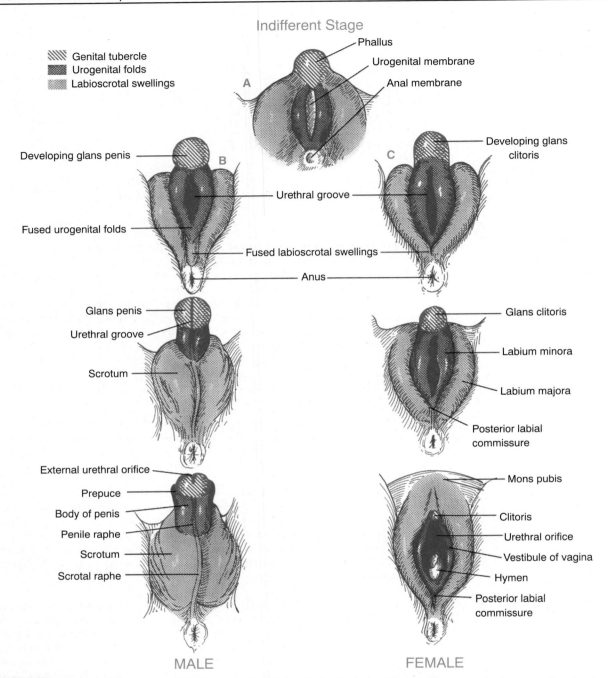

Figure 5.12 **The comparative development of the female and male external genitalia.** **A:** In both sexes, the development follows a uniform pattern through the 7th week and thereafter begins to differentiate. **B:** The male external genitalia. **C:** The female external genitalia.

Lateral to the urogenital folds, another pair of swellings develops, known in the indifferent stage as *labioscrotal swellings*. In the absence of androgens, they remain largely unfused to become the labia majora. The definitive urogenital sinus gives rise to the vaginal vestibule, into which open the urethra, vagina, and greater vestibular glands.

Clinical Correlations   **Developmental abnormalities of the urinary and genital systems can be explained and understood by a consideration of female and male embryologic development. Because of the intertwined development of these two systems, abnormalities in one may be associated with abnormalities in the other** (25).

Urinary System

Urinary-tract anomalies arise from defects in the ureteric bud, the metanephric blastema, or their inductive interaction with each other.

Renal Agenesis   Renal agenesis occurs when one or both ureteric buds fail to form or degenerate, and the metanephric blastema is therefore not induced to differentiate into nephrons. Bilateral renal agenesis is incompatible with postnatal survival, but infants with only one kidney usually survive, and the single kidney undergoes compensatory hypertrophy. Unilateral renal agenesis is often associated with absence or abnormality of fallopian tubes, uterus, or vagina—the paramesonephric duct derivatives.

Abnormalities of Renal Position   Abnormalities of renal position result from disturbance in the normal ascent of the kidneys. A malrotated pelvic kidney is the most common result; a horseshoe kidney, in which the kidneys are fused across the midline, occurs in about 1 in 600 individuals and has a final position lower than usual because its normal ascent is prevented by the root of the inferior mesenteric artery.

Duplication of the Upper Ureter and Renal Pelvis   Duplication of the upper ureter and renal pelvis is relatively common and results from premature bifurcation of the ureteric bud. If two ureteric buds develop, there will be complete duplication of the collecting system. In this situation, one ureteric bud will open normally into the posterior bladder wall, and the second bud will be carried more distally within the mesonephric duct to form an ectopic ureteral orifice into the urethra, vagina, or vaginal vestibule; incontinence is the primary presenting symptom. Most of the aforementioned urinary abnormalities remain asymptomatic unless obstruction or infection supervenes. In that case, anomalous embryologic development must be included in the differential diagnosis.

Genital System

Because the early development of the genital system is similar in both sexes, congenital defects in sexual development, usually arising from a variety of chromosomal abnormalities, tend to present clinically with ambiguous external genitalia. These conditions are known as *intersex conditions* or *hermaphroditism* and are classified according to the histologic appearance of the gonads.

True Hermaphroditism   **Individuals with true hermaphroditism have both ovarian and testicular tissue, most commonly as composite ovotestes but occasionally with an ovary on one side and a testis on the other.** In the latter case, a fallopian tube and single uterine horn may develop on the side with the ovary because of the absence of local AMH. True hermaphroditism is an extremely rare condition associated with chromosomal mosaicism, mutation, or abnormal cleavage involving the X and Y chromosomes.

Pseudohermaphroditism   **In individuals with pseudohermaphroditism, the genetic gender indicates one gender, whereas the external genitalia have characteristics of the other gender.** Males with pseudohermaphroditism are genetic males with feminized external genitalia, most commonly manifesting as hypospadias (urethral opening on the ventral surface of the penis) or incomplete fusion of the urogenital or labioscrotal folds. Females with pseudohermaphroditism are genetic females with virilized external genitalia, including clitoral hypertrophy and some degree of fusion of the urogenital or labioscrotal folds. Both types of pseudohermaphroditism are caused either by abnormal levels of sex hormones or abnormalities in the sex hormone receptors.

Another major category of genital tract abnormalities involves various types of uterovaginal malformations, which occur in 0.16% of women (Fig. 5.13) (26). These malformations are believed to result from one or more of the following situations:

1. Improper fusion of the paramesonephric ducts.
2. Incomplete development of one paramesonephric duct.
3. Failure of part of the paramesonephric duct on one or both sides to develop.
4. Absent or incomplete canalization of the vaginal plate.

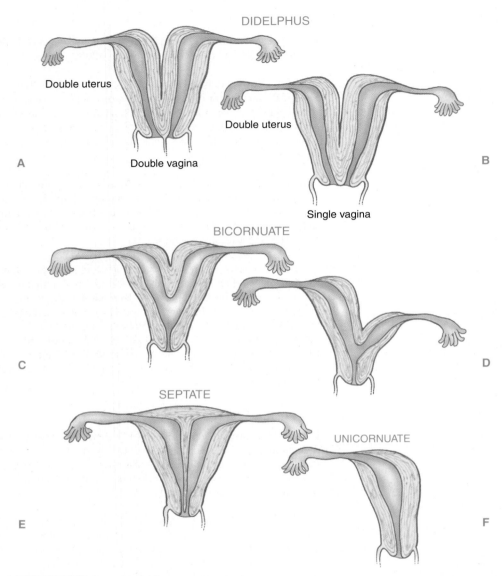

DIDELPHUS

Double uterus

Double uterus

A

Double vagina

B

Single vagina

BICORNUATE

C

D

SEPTATE

UNICORNUATE

E

F

Figure 5.13   **Types of congenital abnormalities.** **A:** Double uterus (uterus didelphys) and double vagina. **B:** Double uterus with single vagina. **C:** Bicornuate uterus. **D:** Bicornuate uterus with a rudimentary left horn. **E:** Septate uterus. **F:** Unicornuate uterus.

Genital Structures

Vagina

A sagittal section of the female pelvis is presented in Fig. 5.14.

The vagina is a hollow fibromuscular tube extending from the vulvar vestibule to the uterus. In the dorsal lithotomy position, the vagina is directed posteriorly toward the sacrum, but its axis is almost horizontal in the upright position. It is attached at its upper end to the uterus just above the cervix. The spaces between the cervix and vagina are known as the *anterior, posterior,* and *lateral vaginal fornices.* **Because the vagina is attached at a higher point posteriorly than anteriorly, the posterior vaginal wall is about 3 cm longer than the anterior wall.**

The posterior vaginal fornix is separated from the posterior cul-de-sac and peritoneal cavity by the vaginal wall and peritoneum. This proximity is clinically useful, both diagnostically and therapeutically. *Culdocentesis,* a technique in which a needle is inserted just posterior to the cervix through the vaginal wall into the peritoneal cavity, is used to evaluate intraperitoneal

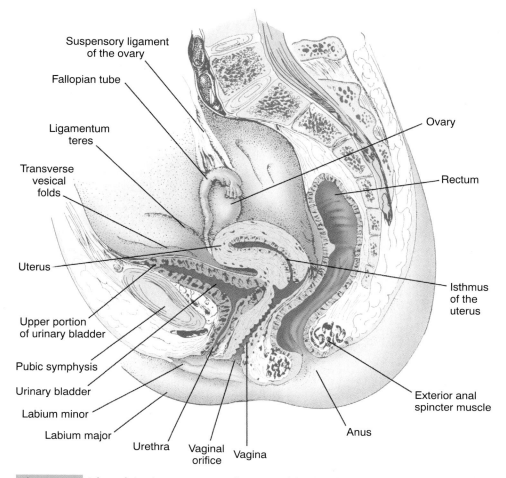

Figure 5.14   **The pelvic viscera.** A sagittal section of the female pelvis with the pelvic viscera and their relationships.

hemorrhage (e.g., ruptured ectopic pregnancy, hemorrhagic corpus luteum, other intraabdominal bleeding), pus (e.g., pelvic inflammatory disease, ruptured intra-abdominal abscess), or other intra-abdominal fluid (e.g., ascites). Incision into the peritoneal cavity from this location in the vagina, known as a *posterior colpotomy*, can be used as an adjunct to laparoscopic excision of adnexal masses, with removal of the mass intact through the posterior vagina.

The vagina is attached to the lateral pelvic wall with endopelvic fascial connections to the *arcus tendineus* (white line), which extends from the pubic bone to the ischial spine. This connection converts the vaginal lumen into a transverse slit with the anterior and posterior walls in apposition; the lateral space where the two walls meet is the *vaginal sulcus*. Lateral detachments of the vagina are recognized in some cystocele formations (lateral cystoceles or paravaginal defects).

The opening of the vagina may be covered by a membrane or surrounded by a fold of connective tissue called the *hymen*. This tissue is usually replaced by irregular tissue tags after sexual activity and childbirth occur. The lower vagina is somewhat constricted as it passes through the urogenital hiatus in the pelvic diaphragm; the upper vagina is more spacious. The entire vagina is characterized by its distensibility, which is most evident during childbirth.

The vagina is closely applied anteriorly to the urethra, bladder neck and trigonal region, and posterior bladder; posteriorly, the vagina lies in association with the perineal body, anal canal, lower rectum, and posterior cul-de-sac. **It is separated from both the lower urinary and gastrointestinal tracts by their investing layers of fibromuscular elements known as the *endopelvic fascia*.**

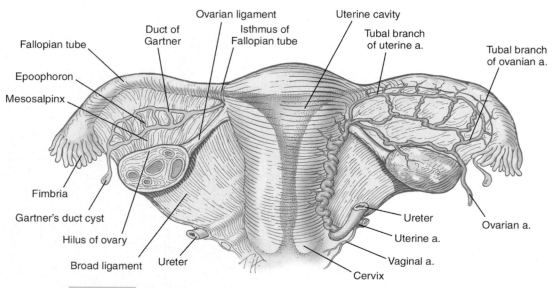

Figure 5.15   **The uterus, fallopian tubes, and ovaries.**

The vagina is composed of three layers:

1. **Mucosa**—nonkeratinized stratified squamous epithelium, without glands. Vaginal lubrication occurs primarily by transudation, with contributions from cervical and Bartholin gland secretions. The mucosa has a characteristic pattern of transverse ridges and furrows known as *rugae*. It is hormonally sensitive, responding to stimulation by estrogen with proliferation and maturation. The mucosa is colonized by mixed bacterial flora with lactobacillus predominant; normal pH is 3.5 to 4.5.

2. **Muscularis**—connective tissue and smooth muscle, loosely arranged in inner circular and outer longitudinal layers.

3. **Adventitia**—endopelvic fascia, adherent to the underlying muscularis.

Blood Supply   The blood supply of the vagina includes the vaginal artery and branches from the uterine, middle rectal, and internal pudendal arteries.

Innervation   The innervation of the vagina is as follows: the upper vagina—uterovaginal plexus; the distal vagina—pudendal nerve.

Uterus

The uterus is a fibromuscular organ usually divided into a lower cervix and an upper corpus or uterine body (Fig. 5.15).

Cervix

The portion of cervix exposed to the vagina is the exocervix or portio vaginalis. It has a convex round surface with a circular or slitlike opening (the external os) into the endocervical canal. **The endocervical canal is about 2 to 3 cm in length and opens proximally into the endometrial cavity at the internal os.**

The cervical mucosa contains both stratified squamous epithelium, characteristic of the exocervix, and mucus-secreting columnar epithelium, characteristic of the endocervical canal. The intersection where these two epithelia meet—the squamocolumnar junction—is geographically variable and dependent on hormonal stimulation. It is this dynamic interface, the transformation zone, which is most vulnerable to the development of squamous neoplasia.

In early childhood, during pregnancy, or with oral contraceptive use, columnar epithelium may extend from the endocervical canal onto the exocervix, a condition known as *eversion* or *ectopy*. After menopause, the transformation zone usually recedes entirely into the endocervical canal.

Production of cervical mucus is under hormonal influence. It varies from profuse, clear, and thin mucus around the time of ovulation to scant and thick mucus in the postovulatory phase of the cycle. Deep in the mucosa and submucosa, the cervix is composed of fibrous connective tissue and a small amount of smooth muscle in a circular arrangement.

Corpus

The body of the uterus varies in size and shape, depending on hormonal and childbearing status. **At birth, the cervix and corpus are about equal in size; in adult women, the corpus has grown to two to three times the size of the cervix.** The position of the uterus in relation to other pelvic structures is variable and is generally described in terms of positioning—anterior, midposition, or posterior; flexion; and version. *Flexion* **is the angle between the long axis of the uterine corpus and the cervix, whereas** *version* **is the angle of the junction of the uterus with the upper vagina.** Occasionally, abnormal positioning may occur secondary to associated pelvic pathology, such as endometriosis or adhesions.

The uterine corpus is divided into several different regions. The area where the endocervical canal opens into the endometrial cavity is known as the *isthmus or lower uterine segment.* **On each side of the upper uterine body, a funnel-shaped area receives the insertion of the fallopian tubes and is called the** *uterine cornu*; **the uterus above this area is the fundus.**

The endometrial cavity is triangular in shape and represents the mucosal surface of the uterine corpus. The epithelium is columnar and gland forming with a specialized stroma. It undergoes cyclic structural and functional change during the reproductive years, with regular shedding of the superficial endometrium and regeneration from the basal layer.

The muscular layer of the uterus, the *myometrium,* **consists of interlacing smooth muscle fibers and ranges in thickness from 1.5 to 2.5 cm.** Some outer fibers are continuous with those of the tube and round ligament.

Peritoneum covers most of the corpus of the uterus and the posterior cervix and is known as the *serosa.* Laterally, the broad ligament, a double layer of peritoneum covering the neurovascular supply to the uterus, inserts into the cervix and corpus. Anteriorly, the bladder lies over the isthmic and cervical region of the uterus.

Blood Supply   The blood supply to the uterus is the uterine artery, which anastomoses with the ovarian and vaginal arteries.

Innervation   The nerve supply to the uterus is the uterovaginal plexus.

Fallopian Tubes

The fallopian tubes and ovaries collectively are referred to as the *adnexa.* The fallopian tubes are paired hollow structures representing the proximal unfused ends of the müllerian duct. They vary in length from 7 to 12 cm, and their function includes ovum pickup, provision of physical environment for conception, and transport and nourishment of the fertilized ovum.

The tubes are divided into several regions:

1. **Interstitial**—narrowest portion of the tube, lies within the uterine wall and forms the tubal ostia at the endometrial cavity.
2. **Isthmus**—narrow segment closest to the uterine wall.
3. **Ampulla**—larger diameter segment lateral to the isthmus.
4. **Fimbria (infundibulum)**—funnel-shaped abdominal ostia of the tubes, opening into the peritoneal cavity; this opening is fringed with numerous fingerlike projections that provide a wide surface for ovum pickup. The fimbria ovarica is a connection between the end of the tube and ovary, bringing the two closer.

The tubal mucosa is ciliated columnar epithelium, which becomes progressively more architecturally complex as the fimbriated end is approached. The muscularis consists of an inner circular and outer longitudinal layer of smooth muscle. The tube is covered by peritoneum and, through its mesentery (mesosalpinx), which is situated dorsal to the round ligament, is connected to the upper margin of the broad ligament.

Blood Supply   The vascular supply to the fallopian tubes is the uterine and ovarian arteries.

Innervation   The innervation to the fallopian tubes is the uterovaginal plexus and the ovarian plexus.

Ovaries

The ovaries are paired gonadal structures that lie suspended between the pelvic wall and the uterus by the infundibulopelvic ligament laterally and the utero-ovarian ligament medially. Inferiorly, the hilar surface of each ovary is attached to the broad ligament by its mesentery (mesovarium), which is dorsal to the mesosalpinx and fallopian tube. Primary neurovascular structures reach the ovary through the infundibulopelvic ligament and enter through the mesovarium. **The normal ovary varies in size, with measurements up to 5 × 3 × 3 cm.** Variation in dimension results from endogenous hormonal production, which varies with age and with each menstrual cycle. Exogenous substances, including oral contraceptives, gonadotropin-releasing hormone agonists, or ovulation-inducing medication, may either stimulate or suppress ovarian activity and, therefore, affect size.

Each ovary consists of a cortex and medulla and is covered by a single layer of flattened cuboidal to low columnar epithelium that is continuous with the peritoneum at the mesovarium. The cortex is composed of a specialized stroma and follicles in various stages of development or attrition. The medulla occupies a small portion of the ovary in its hilar region and is composed primarily of fibromuscular tissue and blood vessels.

Blood Supply   The blood supply to the ovary is the ovarian artery, which anastomoses with the uterine artery.

Innervation   The innervation to the ovary is the ovarian plexus and the uterovaginal plexus.

Urinary Tract

Ureters

The ureter is the urinary conduit leading from the kidney to the bladder; it measures about 25 cm in length and is totally retroperitoneal in location.

The lower half of each ureter traverses the pelvis after crossing the common iliac vessels at their bifurcation, just medial to the ovarian vessels. It descends into the pelvis adherent to the peritoneum of the lateral pelvic wall and the medial leaf of the broad ligament and enters the bladder base anterior to the upper vagina, traveling obliquely through the bladder wall to terminate in the bladder trigone.

The ureteral mucosa is a transitional epithelium. The muscularis consists of an inner longitudinal and outer circular layer of smooth muscle. A protective connective tissue sheath, which is adherent to the peritoneum, encloses the ureter.

Blood Supply   The blood supply is variable, with contributions from the renal, ovarian, common iliac, internal iliac, uterine, and vesical arteries.

Innervation   The innervation is through the ovarian plexus and the vesical plexus.

Bladder and Urethra

Bladder

The bladder is a hollow organ, spherically shaped when full, that stores urine. Its size varies with urine volume, normally reaching a maximum volume of at least 300 mL. The bladder is often divided into two areas, which are of physiologic significance:

1. The **base of the bladder** consists of the urinary trigone posteriorly and a thickened area of detrusor anteriorly. The three corners of the trigone are formed by the two ureteral orifices and the opening of the urethra into the bladder. The bladder base receives α-adrenergic sympathetic innervation and is the area responsible for maintaining continence.
2. The **dome of the bladder** is the remaining bladder area above the bladder base. It has parasympathetic innervation and is responsible for micturition.

The bladder is positioned posterior to the pubis and lower abdominal wall and anterior to the cervix, upper vagina, and part of the cardinal ligament. Laterally, it is bounded by the pelvic diaphragm and obturator internus muscle.

The bladder mucosa is transitional cell epithelium and the muscle wall (detrusor). Rather than being arranged in layers, it is composed of intermeshing muscle fibers.

Blood Supply   The blood supply to the bladder is from the superior, middle, and inferior vesical arteries, with contribution from the uterine and vaginal vessels.

Innervation   The innervation to the bladder is from the vesical plexus, with contribution from the uterovaginal plexus.

Urethra

The vesical neck is the region of the bladder that receives and incorporates the urethral lumen. The female urethra is about 3 to 4 cm in length and extends from the bladder to the vestibule, traveling just anterior to the vagina.

The urethra is lined by nonkeratinized squamous epithelium that is responsive to estrogen stimulation. Within the submucosa on the dorsal surface of the urethra are the paraurethral or Skene glands, which empty through ducts into the urethral lumen. Distally, these glands empty into the vestibule on either side of the external urethral orifice. **Chronic infection of Skene glands, with obstruction of their ducts and cystic dilation, is believed to be an inciting factor in the development of suburethral diverticula.**

The urethra contains an inner longitudinal layer of smooth muscle and outer, circularly oriented smooth muscle fibers. The inferior fascia of the urogenital diaphragm or perineal membrane begins at the junction of the middle and distal thirds of the urethra. Proximal to the middle and distal parts of the urethra, voluntary muscle fibers derived from the urogenital diaphragm intermix with the outer layer of smooth muscle, increasing urethral resistance and contributing to continence. At the level of the urogenital diaphragm, the skeletal muscle fibers leave the wall of the urethra to form the sphincter urethrae and deep transverse perineal muscles. In the coronal plane on MRI studies, the ventral urogenital diaphragm forms an interconnected complex with the compressor urethrae, vestibular bulb, and levator ani. The dorsal part connects the levator ani and vaginal sidewall via a distinct band to the ischiopubic ramus. In the sagittal plane the parallel position of urogenital diaphragm and levator ani can be seen (27).

Blood Supply   The vascular supply to the urethra is from the vesical and vaginal arteries and the internal pudendal branches.

Innervation   The innervation to the urethra is from the vesical plexus and the pudendal nerve.

The lower urinary and genital tracts are intimately connected anatomically and functionally. In the midline, the bladder and proximal urethra can be dissected easily from the underlying lower uterine segment, cervix, and vagina through a loose avascular plane. The distal urethra is essentially inseparable from the vagina. Of surgical significance is the location of the bladder trigone immediately over the middle third of the vagina. Unrecognized injury to the bladder during pelvic surgery may result in development of a vesicovaginal fistula.

Dissection to the level of the trigone is rarely required, and damage to this critical area is unusual.

Lower Gastrointestinal Tract

Sigmoid Colon

The sigmoid colon begins its characteristic S-shaped curve as it enters the pelvis at the left pelvic brim (Fig. 5.16). The columnar mucosa and richly vascularized submucosa are surrounded by an inner circular layer of smooth muscle and three overlying longitudinal bands of muscle called tenia coli. A mesentery of varying length attaches the sigmoid to the posterior abdominal wall.

Blood Supply   The blood supply to the sigmoid colon is from the sigmoid arteries.

Innervation   The nerves to the sigmoid colon are derived from the inferior mesenteric plexus.

Rectum

The sigmoid colon loses its mesentery in the midsacral region and becomes the rectum about 15 to 20 cm above the anal opening. The rectum follows the curve of the lower sacrum and coccyx and becomes entirely retroperitoneal at the level of the rectouterine pouch or posterior cul-de-sac. It continues along the pelvic curve just posterior to the vagina until the level of the anal hiatus of the pelvic diaphragm, at which point it takes a sharp 90-degree turn posteriorly and becomes the anal canal, separated from the vagina by the perineal body.

The rectal mucosa is lined by a columnar epithelium and characterized by three transverse folds that contain mucosa, submucosa, and the inner circular layer of smooth muscle. The tenia of the

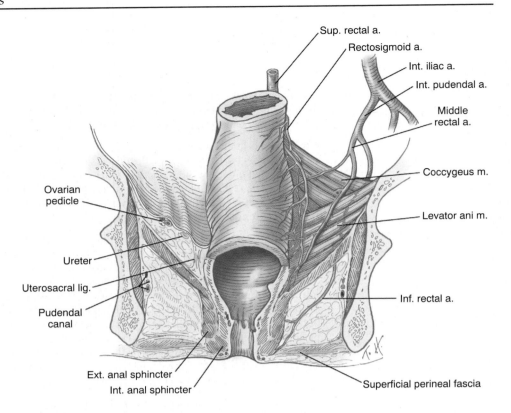

Sup. rectal a.

Rectosigmoid a.

Int. iliac a.

Int. pudendal a.

Middle rectal a.

Coccygeus m.

Levator ani m.

Ovarian pedicle

Ureter

Uterosacral lig.

Pudendal canal

Inf. rectal a.

Ext. anal sphincter

Int. anal sphincter

Superficial perineal fascia

Figure 5.16 **The rectosigmoid colon, its vascular supply, and muscular support.** (Coronal view: peritoneum removed on right.)

sigmoid wall broaden and fuse over the rectum to form a continuous longitudinal external layer of smooth muscle to the level of the anal canal.

Anal Canal

The anal canal begins at the level of the sharp turn in the direction of the distal colon and is 2 to 3 cm in length. At the anorectal junction, the mucosa changes to stratified squamous epithelium (the pectinate line), which continues until the termination of the anus at the anal verge, where there is a transition to perianal skin with typical skin appendages. It is surrounded by a thickened ring of circular muscle fibers that are a continuation of the circular muscle of the rectum, the internal anal sphincter. Its lower part is surrounded by bundles of striated muscle fibers, the external anal sphincter (28).

Fecal continence is provided primarily by the puborectalis muscle and the internal and external anal sphincters. The puborectalis surrounds the anal hiatus in the pelvic diaphragm and interdigitates posterior to the rectum to form a rectal sling. The external anal sphincter surrounds the terminal anal canal below the level of the levator ani. A growing body of literature suggests that both external anal sphincter and levator ani muscles are important for fecal continence and that multiple injuries contribute to pelvic floor dysfunction (29,30) One such MRI study showed that major levator ani muscle injuries were observed in 19.1% women who delivered vaginally with external anal sphincter injuries, 3.5% who delivered vaginally without external anal sphincter injury, and none of the women who delivered by cesarean section before labor. Among women with external anal sphincter injuries, those with major levator ani muscle injuries trended more toward fecal incontinence (29). Further studies suggest that thickening of the internal anal sphincter occurs with aging, and that thinning of the external anal sphincter and a corresponding drop in squeeze pressure correlated with fecal incontinence, but not aging (31).

The anatomic proximity of the lower gastrointestinal tract to the lower genital tract is particularly important during surgery of the vulva and vagina. Lack of attention to this proximity during repair of vaginal lacerations or episiotomies can lead to damage of the rectum and fistula formation or injury to the external anal sphincter, resulting in fecal incontinence. Because of the avascular nature of the rectovaginal space, it is relatively easy to dissect the rectum from the vagina in the midline, which is routinely done in the repair of rectoceles.

Blood Supply   The vascular supply to the rectum and anal canal is from the superior, middle, and inferior rectal arteries. The venous drainage is a complex submucosal plexus of vessels that, under conditions of increased intra-abdominal pressure (pregnancy, pelvic mass, chronic constipation, ascites), may dilate and become symptomatic with rectal bleeding or pain as hemorrhoids.

Innervation   The nerve supply to the anal canal is from the middle rectal plexus, the inferior mesenteric plexus, and the pudendal nerve.

The Genital Tract and Its Relations

The genital tract is situated at the bottom of the intra-abdominal cavity and is related to the intraperitoneal cavity and its contents, the retroperitoneal spaces, and the pelvic floor. Accessing it through the abdominal wall or the perineum requires a thorough knowledge of the anatomy of these areas and their relationships.

The Abdominal Wall

The anterior abdominal wall is bound superiorly by the xiphoid process and the costal cartilage of the 7th to 10th ribs and inferiorly by the iliac crest, anterosuperior iliac spine, inguinal ligament, and pubic bone. It consists of skin, muscle, fascia, and nerves and vessels.

Skin

The lower abdominal skin may exhibit striae, or "stretch marks," and increased pigmentation in the midline in parous women. The subcutaneous tissue contains a variable amount of fat.

Muscles

Five muscles and their aponeuroses contribute to the structure and strength of the anterolateral abdominal wall (Fig. 5.17; Table 5.7).

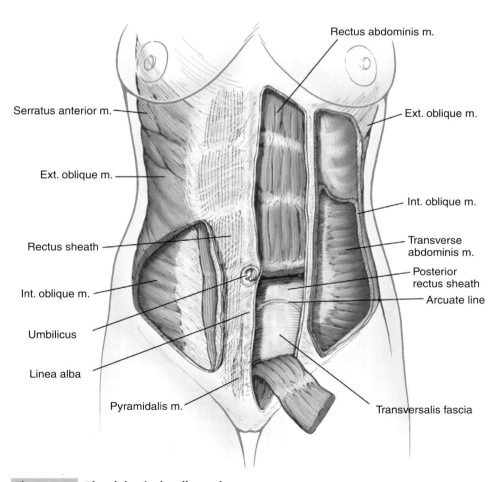

Figure 5.17   The abdominal wall muscles.

95

Table 5.7 Muscles Contributing to the Structure and Strength of the Anterolateral Abdominal Wall			
Muscle	*Origin*	*Insertion*	*Action*
External oblique	Fleshy digitations from the outer surfaces of ribs 5–12	Fibers radiate inferiorly, anteriorly, and medially, in most cases ending in the aponeurosis of the external muscle and inserting into the anterior half of the iliac crest, the pubic tubercle, and the linea alba. The superficial inguinal ring is located above and lateral to the pubic tubercle at the end of a triangular cleft in the external oblique muscle, bordered by strong fibrous bands that transmit the round ligament	Compresses and supports abdominal viscera; flexes and rotates vertebral column
Internal oblique	Posterior layer of the thoracolumbar fascia, the anterior two-thirds of the iliac crest, and the lateral two-thirds of the inguinal ligament	Inferior border of ribs 10–12. The superior fibers of the aponeurosis split to enclose the rectus abdominis muscle and join at the linea alba above the arcuate line. The most inferior fibers join with those of the transverse abdominis muscle to insert into the pubic crest and pecten pubis via the conjoint tendon	Compresses and supports abdominal viscera
Transversus abdominus	Inner aspect of the inferior six costal cartilages, the thoracolumbar fascia, the iliac crest, and the lateral one-third of the inguinal ligament	Linea alba with the aponeurosis of the internal oblique, the pubic crest and the pecten pubis through the conjoint tendon	Compresses and supports abdominal viscera
Rectus abdominis	Superior pubic ramus and the ligaments of the symphysis pubis	Anterior surface of the xiphoid process and the cartilage of ribs 5–7	Tenses anterior abdominal wall and flexes trunk
Pyramidalis	Small triangular muscle contained within the rectus sheath, anterior to the lower part of the rectus muscle	On the linea alba, easily recognizable shape, used to locate the midline, particularly in a patient with previous abdominal surgery and scarring of the abdominal wall	Tenses the linea alba, insignificant in terms of function, and is frequently absent

Fascia

Superficial Fascia

The superficial fascia consists of two layers:

1. **Camper fascia**—the most superficial layer, which contains a variable amount of fat and is continuous with the superficial fatty layer of the perineum.

2. **Scarpa fascia**—a deeper membranous layer continuous in the perineum with Colles fascia (superficial perineal fascia) and with the deep fascia of the thigh (fascia lata).

Rectus Sheath

The aponeuroses of the external and internal oblique and the transversus abdominis combine to form a sheath for the rectus abdominis and pyramidalis, fusing medially in the midline at the linea alba and laterally at the semilunar line (Fig. 5.18). Above the arcuate line, the aponeurosis of the internal oblique muscle splits into anterior and posterior lamella (Fig. 5.18A). Below this line, all three layers are anterior to the body of the rectus muscle

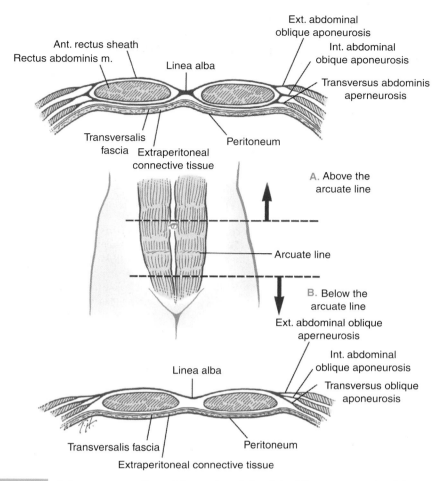

Figure 5.18   **A transverse section of the rectus abdominis.** The aponeurosis of the external and internal oblique and the transversus abdominis from the rectus abdominis. **A:** Above the arcuate line. **B:** Below the arcuate line.

(Fig. 5.18B). The rectus is covered posteriorly by the transversalis fascia, providing access to the muscle for the inferior epigastric vessels.

Transversalis Fascia and Endopelvic Fascia

The transversalis fascia is a firm membranous sheet on the internal surface of the transversus abdominis muscle that extends beyond the muscle and forms a fascia lining the entire abdominopelvic cavity. Like the peritoneum, it is divided into a parietal and a visceral component. It is continuous from side to side across the linea alba and covers the posterior aspect of the rectus abdominis muscle below the arcuate line. Superiorly, it becomes the inferior fascia of the diaphragm. Inferiorly, it is attached to the iliac crest, covers the iliac fascia and the obturator internus fascia, and extends downward and medially to form the superior fascia of the pelvic diaphragm.

Characteristically, the transversalis fascia continues along blood vessels and other structures leaving and entering the abdominopelvic cavity and contributes to the formation of the visceral (*endopelvic*) pelvic fascia (32). The pelvic fascia invests the pelvic organs and attaches them to the pelvic sidewalls, thereby playing a critical role in *pelvic support*. In the inguinal region, the fascial relationships result in the development of the inguinal canal, through which the round ligament exits into the perineum. The fascia is separated from the peritoneum by a layer of preperitoneal fat. Areas of fascial weakness or congenital or posttraumatic and surgical injuries result in herniation of the underlying structures through a defective abdominal wall. The incisions least likely to result in damage to the integrity and innervation of the abdominal wall muscles include a midline incision through the linea alba and a transverse incision through the recti muscle fibers that respects the integrity of its innervation (33).

Nerves and Vessels

The tissues of the abdominal wall are innervated by the continuation of the inferior intercostal nerves T4 to T11 and the subcostal nerve T12. The inferior part of the abdominal wall is supplied by the first lumbar nerve through the iliohypogastric and the ilioinguinal nerves. **Abdominal wall surgical sites below the level of the anterior superior iliac spine have the potential for ilioinguinal or iliohypogastric injury** (34). The primary blood supply to the anterior lateral abdominal wall includes the following:

1. The **inferior epigastric and deep circumflex iliac arteries,** branches of the external iliac artery
2. The **superior epigastric artery,** a terminal branch of the internal thoracic artery

The inferior epigastric artery runs superiorly in the transverse fascia to reach the arcuate line, where it enters the rectus sheath. It is vulnerable to damage by abdominal incisions in which the rectus muscle is completely or partially transected, during placement of lateral laparoscopic ports, or by excessive lateral traction on the rectus. The deep circumflex artery runs on the deep aspect of the anterior abdominal wall parallel to the inguinal ligament and along the iliac crest between the transverse abdominis muscle and the internal oblique muscle. The superior epigastric vessels enter the rectus sheath superiorly just below the seventh costal cartilage.

The venous system drains into the saphenous vein, and the lymphatics drain to the axillary chain above the umbilicus and to the inguinal nodes below it. The subcutaneous tissues drain to the lumbar chain.

Perineum

The perineum is situated at the lower end of the trunk between the buttocks. Its bony boundaries include the lower margin of the pubic symphysis anteriorly, the tip of the coccyx posteriorly, and the ischial tuberosities laterally. These landmarks correspond to the boundaries of the pelvic outlet. The diamond shape of the perineum is customarily divided by an imaginary line joining the ischial tuberosities immediately in front of the anus, at the level of the perineal body, into an anterior urogenital and a posterior anal triangle (Fig. 5.19).

Urogenital Triangle

The urogenital triangle includes the external genital structures and the urethral opening (Fig. 5.19). **These external structures cover the superficial and deep perineal compartments and are known as the** *vulva* (Figs. 5.20 and 5.21).

Vulva

Mons Pubis

The mons pubis is a triangular eminence in front of the pubic bones that consists of adipose tissue covered by hair-bearing skin up to its junction with the abdominal wall.

Labia Majora

The labia majora are a pair of fibroadipose folds of skin that extend from the mons pubis downward and backward to meet in the midline in front of the anus at the posterior fourchette. They include the terminal extension of the round ligament and occasionally a peritoneal diverticulum, the *canal of Nuck*. They are covered by skin with scattered hairs laterally and are rich in sebaceous, apocrine, and eccrine glands.

Labia Minora

The labia minora lie between the labia majora, with which they merge posteriorly, and are separated into two folds anteriorly as they approach the clitoris. The anterior folds unite to form the prepuce or hood of the clitoris. The posterior folds form the frenulum of the clitoris as they attach to its inferior surface. The labia minora are covered by hairless skin overlying a fibroelastic stroma rich in neural and vascular elements. The area between the posterior labia minora forms the vestibule of the vagina.

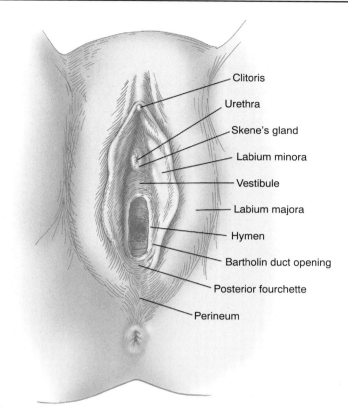

Figure 5.19   **Vulva and perineum.**

Clitoris

Urethra

Skene's gland

Labium minora

Vestibule

Labium majora

Hymen

Bartholin duct opening

Posterior fourchette

Perineum

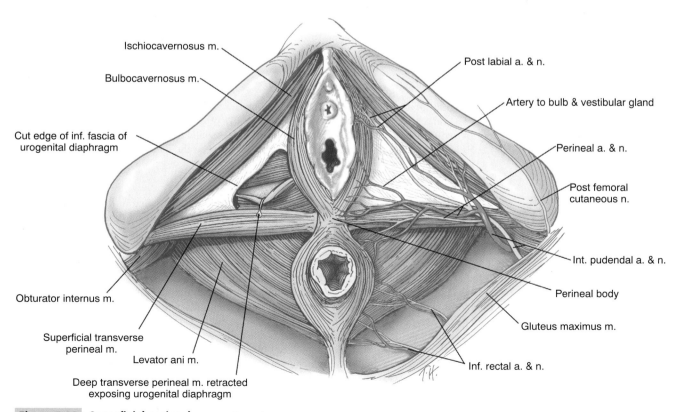

Figure 5.20   **Superficial perineal compartment.**

Ischiocavernosus m.

Bulbocavernosus m.

Cut edge of inf. fascia of urogenital diaphragm

Obturator internus m.

Superficial transverse perineal m.

Levator ani m.

Deep transverse perineal m. retracted exposing urogenital diaphragm

Post labial a. & n.

Artery to bulb & vestibular gland

Perineal a. & n.

Post femoral cutaneous n.

Int. pudendal a. & n.

Perineal body

Gluteus maximus m.

Inf. rectal a. & n.

99

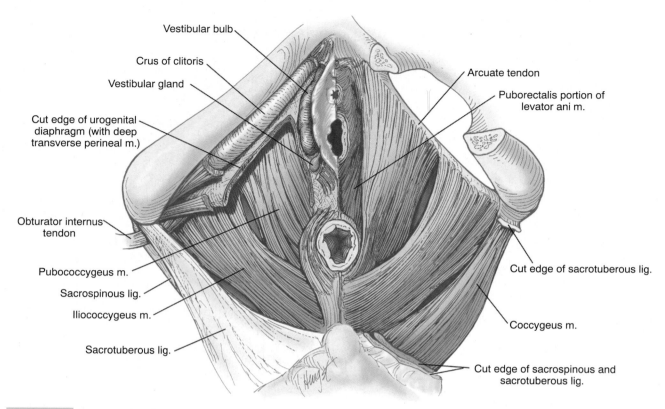

Figure 5.21 **Deep perineal compartment.**

Clitoris

The clitoris is an erectile organ that is 2 to 3 cm in length. It consists of two crura and two corpora cavernosa and is covered by a sensitive rounded tubercle (the glans).

Vaginal Orifice

The vaginal orifice is surrounded by the *hymen*, a variable crescentic mucous membrane that is replaced by rounded caruncles after its rupture. The opening of the duct of the *greater vestibular (Bartholin) glands* is located on each side of the vestibule. Numerous lesser vestibular glands are also scattered posteriorly and between the urethral and vaginal orifices.

Urethral Orifice

The urethral orifice is immediately anterior to the vaginal orifice and about 2 to 3 cm beneath the clitoris. The *Skene (paraurethral) gland* duct presents an opening on its posterior surface.

Superficial Perineal Compartment

The superficial perineal compartment lies between the superficial perineal fascia and the inferior fascia of the urogenital diaphragm (perineal membrane) (Fig. 5.20). The superficial perineal fascia has a superficial and deep component. **The superficial layer is relatively thin and fatty and is continuous superiorly with the superficial fatty layer of the lower abdominal wall (*Camper fascia*).** It continues laterally as the fatty layer of the thighs. The deep layer of the superficial perineal (*Colles*) fascia is continuous superiorly with the deep layer of the superficial abdominal fascia (*Scarpa fascia*), which attaches firmly to the ischiopubic rami and ischial tuberosities. **The superficial perineal compartment is continuous superiorly with the superficial fascial spaces of the anterior abdominal wall, allowing spread of blood or infection along that route.** Such spread is limited laterally by the ischiopubic rami, anteriorly by the transverse ligament of the perineum, and posteriorly by the superficial transverse perineal muscle. The superficial perineal compartment includes the following:

Erectile Bodies

The vestibular bulbs are 3-cm, highly vascular structures surrounding the vestibule and located under the bulbocavernosus muscle. The body of the clitoris is attached by two crura to the internal aspect of the ischiopubic rami. The crura are covered by the ischiocavernosus muscles.

Muscles

The muscles of the vulva are the ischiocavernosus, the bulbocavernosus, and superficial transverse perineal. They are included in the superficial perineal compartment as follows:

Ischiocavernosus

- Origin—ischial tuberosity

- Insertion—ischiopubic bone

- Action—compresses the crura and lowers the clitoris

Bulbocavernosus

- Origin—perineal body

- Insertion—posterior aspect of the clitoris; some fibers pass above the dorsal vein of the clitoris in a slinglike fashion

- Action—compresses the vestibular bulb and dorsal vein of the clitoris

Superficial Transverse Perineal

- Origin—ischial tuberosity

- Insertion—central perineal tendon

- Action—fixes the perineal body

Vestibular Glands

The vestibular glands are situated on either side of the vestibule under the posterior end of the vestibular bulb. They drain between the hymen and the labia minora. Their mucous secretion helps maintain adequate lubrication. Infection in these glands can result in an abscess.

Deep Perineal Compartment

The deep perineal compartment is a fascial space bound inferiorly by the perineal membrane and superiorly by a deep fascial layer that separates the urogenital diaphragm from the anterior recess of the ischiorectal fossa (Fig. 5.21). It is stretched across the anterior half of the pelvic outlet between the ischiopubic rami. The deep compartment may be directly continuous superiorly with the pelvic cavity (35). The posterior pubourethral ligaments, functioning as winglike elevations of the fascia ascending from the pelvic floor to the posterior aspect of the symphysis pubis, provide a point of fixation to the urethra and support the concept of the continuity of the deep perineal compartment with the pelvic cavity.

The anterior pubourethral ligaments represent a similar elevation of the inferior fascia of the urogenital diaphragm and are joined by the intermediate pubourethral ligament, with the junction between the two fascial structures arcing under the pubic symphysis (36). The urogenital diaphragm includes the *sphincter urethrae* (*urogenital sphincter*) and the *deep transverse perineal* (*transversus vaginae*) muscle.

The urogenital diaphragm (perineal membrane) is composed of two regions: one dorsal and one ventral. The dorsal portion consists of bilateral transverse fibrous sheets that attach the lateral wall of the vagina and perineal body to the ischiopubic ramus. This portion is devoid of striated muscle. The ventral portion is part of a solid three-dimensional tissue mass in which several structures are embedded. It is intimately associated with the compressor urethrae and the urethrovaginal sphincter muscle of the distal urethra with the urethra and its surrounding connective tissue. In this region the perineal membrane is continuous with the insertion of the arcus tendineus fascia pelvis. The levator ani muscles are connected with the cranial surface of the perineal membrane. The vestibular bulb and clitoral crus are fused with the membrane's caudal surface (37).

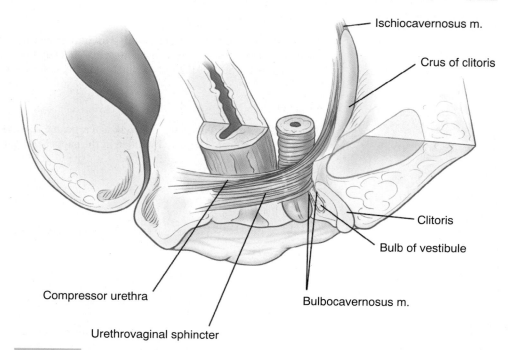

Ischiocavernosus m.

Crus of clitoris

Clitoris

Bulb of vestibule

Compressor urethra

Bulbocavernosus m.

Urethrovaginal sphincter

Figure 5.22 **The complete urogenital sphincter musculature, bladder, and vagina.** (Redrawn from **Haderer JM, Pannu HK, Genadry R, et al.** Controversies in female urethral anatomy and their significance for understanding urinary continence: observations and literature review. *Int Urogynecol J Pelvic Floor Dysfunct* 2002;13:236–252, with permission.)

The sphincter urethrae (Fig. 5.22) is a continuous muscle fanning out as it develops proximally and distally, including the following:

1. **External urethral sphincter**, which surrounds the middle third of the urethra.
2. **Compressor urethrae**, arcing across the ventral side of the urethra.
3. **Urethrovaginal sphincter**, which surrounds the ventral aspect of the urethra and terminates in the lateral vaginal wall.

The deep transverse perineal muscle originates at the internal aspect of the ischial bone, parallels the muscle compressor urethrae, and attaches to the lateral vaginal wall along the perineal membrane. Studies show that a smaller striated urogenital sphincter is associated with stress incontinence and poorer pelvic floor muscle function (38).

The urinary and genital tracts have a common reliance on several interdependent structures for support. **The cardinal and uterosacral ligaments are condensations of endopelvic fascia that support the cervix and upper vagina over the levator plate. Laterally, endopelvic fascial condensations attach the midvagina to the pelvic walls at the arcus tendineus fascia pelvis anteriorly and the arcus tendineus levator ani posteriorly. The distal anterior vagina and urethra are anchored to the urogenital diaphragm and the distal posterior vagina to the perineal body.**

Anteriorly, the pubourethral ligaments and pubovesical fascia and ligaments provide fixation and stabilization for the urethra and bladder. Posteriorly, they rely on the vagina and lower uterus for support. Partial resection or relaxation of the uterosacral ligaments often leads to relaxation of the genitourinary complex, resulting in the formation of a cystocele. Studies indicate that half of the observed variation in anterior compartment support may be explained by apical support (39). Various types and degrees of genital tract prolapse or relaxation are almost always associated with similar findings in the bladder, urethra, or both.

There are three levels of vaginal support as described by DeLancey (Fig. 5.23) (40). Level I support consists of paracolpium that suspends the apical portion of the vagina and is comprised of the cardinal-uterosacral ligament complex. Level II support comprises the

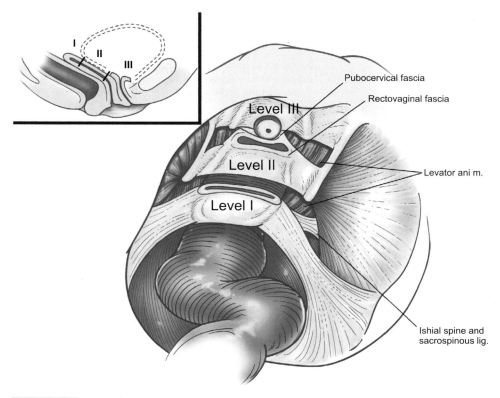

Figure 5.23   DeLancey levels of support. (Modified from DeLancey JOL. Anatomic aspects of vaginal eversion after hysterectomy. *Am J Obstet Gynecol* 1992;166:17–28, with permission.)

paracolpium that is attached to the vagina laterally via the arcus tendineus fasciae pelvis and superior fascia of the levator ani. Level III support consists of the distal vaginal attachments: anteriorly, via fusion of the urethra to the vagina, laterally, to the levators, and posteriorly, with the perineal body.

Clinical Relevance

Disruption of level I support may lead to prolapse of the uterus or vaginal vault, while damage to level II and III supports predispose to anterior and posterior vaginal prolapse. All levels of defective support should be repaired during reconstructive surgery.

Blood Supply   The blood supply to the vulva is as follows:

1. External pudendal artery (from femoral artery), internal pudendal artery
2. Venous drainage—internal pudendal veins

The blood supply to the superficial and deep perineal compartments is as follows:

1. Internal pudendal artery, dorsal artery of the clitoris
2. Venous drainage—internal pudendal veins, which are richly anastomotic
3. Lymphatic drainage—internal iliac chain

Innervation   The innervation to the vulva is from branches of the following nerves:

1. Ilioinguinal nerve
2. Genitofemoral nerve (genital branch)
3. Lateral femoral cutaneous nerve of the thigh (perineal branch)
4. Perineal nerve (branch of pudendal)
5. Superficial and deep perineal compartments, innervated by the perineal nerve

Perineal Body

The perineal body or central perineal tendon is critical to the posterior support of the lower aspect of the anterior vaginal wall. It is a triangle-shaped structure separating the distal portion of the anal and vaginal canals that is formed by the convergence of the tendinous attachments of the bulbocavernosus, the external anal sphincter, and the superficial transverse perinei muscle. Its superior border represents the point of insertion of the *rectovaginal (Denonvilliers) fascia*, which extends to the underside of the peritoneum covering the cul-de-sac of Douglas, separating the anorectal from the urogenital compartment (41). The perineal body plays an important anchoring role in the musculofascial support of the pelvic floor. It represents the central connection between the two layers of support of the pelvic floor—the pelvic and urogenital diaphragm. It also provides a posterior connection to the anococcygeal raphe. Thus, it is central to the definition of the bilevel support of the floor of the pelvis.

Anal Triangle

The anal triangle includes the lower end of the anal canal. The external anal sphincter surrounds the anal triangle, and the ischiorectal fossa is on each side. Posteriorly, the *anococcygeal body* lies between the anus and the tip of the coccyx and consists of thick fibromuscular tissue (of levator ani and external anal sphincter origin) giving support to the lower part of the rectum and the anal canal.

The *external anal sphincter* forms a thick band of muscular fibers arranged in three layers running from the perineal body to the anococcygeal ligament. The subcutaneous fibers are thin and surround the anus and, without bony attachment, decussate in front of it. The superficial fibers sweep forward from the anococcygeal ligament, and the tip of the coccyx around the anus inserts into the perineal body. The deep fibers arise from the perineal body to encircle the lower half of the anal canal to form a true sphincter muscle, which fuses with the puborectalis portion of the levator ani.

The *ischiorectal fossa* is mainly occupied by fat and separates the ischium laterally from the median structures of the anal triangle. It is a fascia-lined space located inferiorly between the perineal skin and the pelvic diaphragm superiorly; it communicates with the contralateral ischiorectal fossa over the anococcygeal ligament. Superiorly, its apex is at the origin of the levator ani muscle from the obturator fascia. It is bound medially by the levator ani and the external sphincter with their fascial covering, laterally by the obturator internus muscle with its fascia, posteriorly by the sacrotuberous ligament and the lower border of the gluteus maximus muscle, and anteriorly by the base of the urogenital diaphragm. It is widest and deepest posteriorly and weakest medially.

An ischiorectal abscess should be drained without delay, or it will extend into the anal canal. The cavity is filled with fat that cushions the anal canal and is traversed by many fibrous bands, vessels, and nerves, including the pudendal and the inferior rectal nerves. The perforating branch of S2 and S3 and the perineal branch of S4 also run through this space.

The *pudendal (Alcock) canal* is a tunnel formed by a splitting of the inferior portion of the obturator fascia running anteromedially from the ischial spine to the posterior edge of the urogenital diaphragm. It contains the pudendal artery, vein, and nerve in their traverse from the *pelvic* cavity to the perineum.

Blood Supply   The blood supply to the anal triangle is from the inferior rectal (hemorrhoidal) artery and vein.

Innervation   The innervation to the anal triangle is from the perineal branch of the fourth sacral nerve and the inferior rectal (hemorrhoidal) nerve.

Retroperitoneum and Retroperitoneal Spaces

The subperitoneal area of the true pelvis is partitioned into potential spaces by the various organs and their respective fascial coverings and by the selective thickenings of the endopelvic fascia into ligaments and septa (Fig. 5.24). It is imperative that surgeons operating in the pelvis be familiar with these spaces, as discussed below.

Prevesical Space

The prevesical (Retzius) space is a fat-filled potential space bound anteriorly by the pubic bone, covered by the transversalis fascia, and extending to the umbilicus between the medial umbilical ligaments (obliterated umbilical arteries); posteriorly, the space extends to the

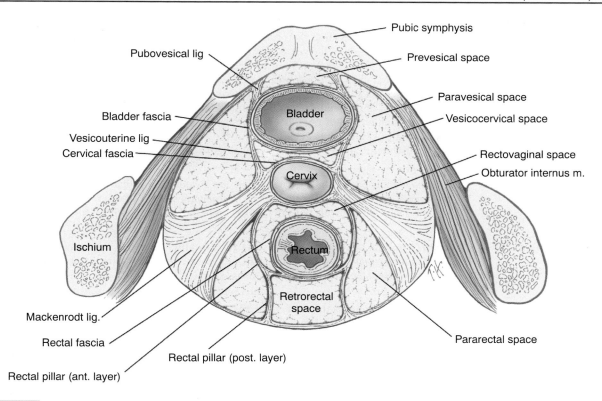

Figure 5.24 **Schematic sectional drawing of the pelvis shows the firm connective tissue covering.** The bladder, cervix, and rectum are surrounded by a connective tissue covering. The Mackenrodt ligament extends from the lateral cervix to the lateral abdominal pelvic wall. The vesicouterine ligament originating from the anterior edge of the Mackenrodt ligament leads to the covering of the bladder on the posterior side. The sagittal rectum column spreads both to the connective tissue of the rectum and the sacral vertebrae closely nestled against the back of the Mackenrodt ligament and lateral pelvic wall. Between the firm connective tissue bundles is loose connective tissue (paraspaces). (From **Von Peham H, Amreich JA.** *Gynaekologische Operationslehre.* Berlin, Germany: S Karger, 1930, with permission.)

anterior wall of the bladder. It is separated from the paravesical space by the ascending bladder septum (bladder pillars).

Upon entering the prevesical space, the pubourethral ligaments may be seen inserting into the posterior aspect of the symphysis pubis as a thickened prolongation of the arcus tendineus fascia. With combined abdominal and vaginal bladder neck suspensory procedures, the point of entry is usually the Retzius space between the arcus tendineus and the pubourethral ligaments.

Paravesical Spaces

The paravesical spaces are fat filled and limited by the fascia of the obturator internus muscle and the pelvic diaphragm laterally, the bladder pillar medially, the endopelvic fascia inferiorly, the lateral umbilical ligament superiorly, the cardinal ligament posteriorly, and the pubic bone anteriorly.

Vesicovaginal Space

The vesicovaginal space is separated from the Retzius space by the endopelvic fascia. This space is limited anteriorly by the bladder wall (from the proximal urethra to the upper vagina), posteriorly by the anterior vaginal wall, and laterally by the bladder septa (selective thickenings of the endopelvic fascia inserting laterally into the arcus tendineus). **A tear in these fascial investments and thickenings medially, transversely, or laterally allows herniation and development of a cystocele.**

Rectovaginal Space

The rectovaginal space extends between the vagina and the rectum from the superior border of the perineal body to the underside of the rectouterine Douglas pouch. It is bound anteriorly by the rectovaginal septum (firmly adherent to the posterior aspect of the vagina), posteriorly by the anterior rectal wall, and laterally by the descending rectal septa separating the rectovaginal space from the pararectal space on each side. The rectovaginal septum represents a firm membranous transverse septum dividing the pelvis into rectal and urogenital compartments, allowing the independent function of the vagina and rectum and providing support for the rectum. It is fixed laterally to the pelvic sidewall by rectovaginal fascia (part of the endopelvic fascia) along a line extending from the posterior fourchette to the arcus tendineus fasciae pelvis, midway between the pubis and the ischial spine (42). An anterior rectocele often results from a defective *septum* or an avulsion of the septum from the perineal body. Reconstruction of the perineum is critical for the restoration of this important compartmental separation and for the support of the anterior vaginal wall (43). **Lateral detachment of the rectovaginal fascia from the pelvic sidewall may constitute a "pararectal" defect analogous to anterior paravaginal defects.**

Pararectal Space

The pararectal space is bound laterally by the levator ani, medially by the rectal pillars, and posteriorly above the ischial spine by the anterolateral aspect of the sacrum. It is separated from the retrorectal space by the posterior extension of the descending rectal septa.

Retrorectal Space

The retrorectal space is limited by the rectum anteriorly and the anterior aspect of the sacrum posteriorly. It communicates with the pararectal spaces laterally above the uterosacral ligaments and extends superiorly into the presacral space.

Presacral Space

The presacral space is the superior extension of the retrorectal space and is limited by the deep parietal peritoneum anteriorly and the anterior aspect of the sacrum posteriorly. It harbors the middle sacral vessels and the hypogastric plexi between the bifurcation of the aorta invested by loose areolar tissue. Presacral neurectomy requires familiarity with and working knowledge of this space. **Abdominal sacrocolpopexy involves dissection in the presacral space down to the anterior longitudinal ligament, which is the point of fixation for the tail of the Y-shaped mesh graft. The surgical space is bound superiorly by the bifurcation of the great vessels and laterally by the ureter on the right and the mesentery of the sigmoid colon and the left common iliac vein on the left. The left iliac vein lies medial to the left iliac artery bounding this space and is more prone to injury during laparoscopic entry or presacral dissection.**

Peritoneal Cavity

The female pelvic organs lie at the bottom of the abdominopelvic cavity covered superiorly and posteriorly by the small and large bowel. Anteriorly, the uterine wall is in contact with the posterosuperior aspect of the bladder. The uterus is held in position by the following structures:

1. The **round ligaments** coursing inferolaterally toward the internal inguinal ring
2. The **uterosacral ligaments**, which provide support to the cervix and upper vagina and interdigitate with fibers from the cardinal ligament near the cervix
3. The **cardinal ligaments**, which provide support to the cervix and upper vagina and contribute to the support of the bladder

Anteriorly, the uterus is separated from the bladder by the vesicouterine pouch and from the rectum posteriorly by the rectouterine pouch or Douglas cul-de-sac. Laterally, the bilateral broad ligaments carry the neurovascular pedicles and their respective fascial coverings, attaching the uterus to the lateral pelvic sidewall.

The broad ligament is in contact inferiorly with the paravesical space, the obturator fossa, and the pelvic extension of the iliac fossa, to which it provides a peritoneal covering, and with the uterosacral ligament. Superiorly, it extends into the infundibulopelvic ligament.

Ureter

In its pelvic path in the retroperitoneum, several relationships are of significance and identify areas of greatest vulnerability to injury of the ureter (Fig. 5.25):

1. **The ovarian vessels cross over the ureter as it approaches the pelvic brim and lie in lateral proximity to the ureter as it enters the pelvis.**
2. **As the ureter descends into the pelvis, it runs within the broad ligament just lateral to the uterosacral ligament, separating the uterosacral ligament from the mesosalpinx, mesovarium, and ovarian fossa.**

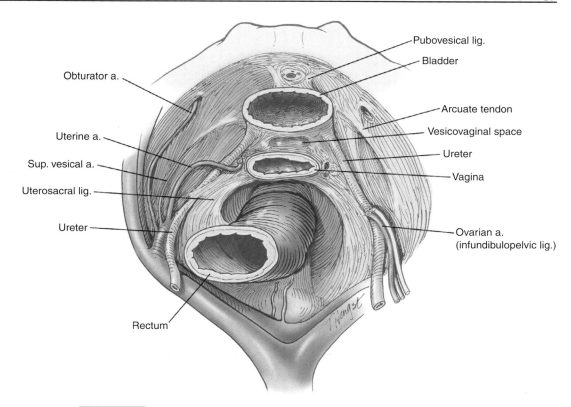

Figure 5.25   The course of the ureter and its relationship to the sites of greatest vulnerability.

3. **At about the level of the ischial spine, the ureter crosses under the uterine artery in its course through the cardinal ligament; the ureter divides this area into the supraureteric parametrium surrounding the uterine vessels and the infraureteric paracervix molded around the vaginal vessels and extending posteriorly into the uterosacral ligament. In this location, the ureter lies 2 to 3 cm lateral to the cervix and in proximity to the insertion of the uterosacral ligament at the cervix. This proximity warrants caution when using the uterosacral ligament for vaginal vault suspension (44,45).**

4. **The ureter then turns medially to cross the anterior upper vagina as it traverses the bladder wall.**

About 75% of all iatrogenic injuries to the ureter result from gynecologic procedures, most commonly abdominal hysterectomy (46). Distortions of pelvic anatomy, including adnexal masses, endometriosis, other pelvic adhesive disease, or fibroids, may increase susceptibility to injury by displacement or alteration of usual anatomy. **Careful identification of the course of the ureter before securing the infundibulopelvic ligament and uterine artery is the best protection against ureteric injury during hysterectomy or adnexectomy. Even with severe intraperitoneal disease, the ureter can always be identified using a retroperitoneal approach and noting fundamental landmarks and relationships.**

Pelvic Floor

The pelvic floor includes all of the structures closing the pelvic outlet from the skin inferiorly to the peritoneum superiorly. It is commonly divided by the pelvic diaphragm into a pelvic and a perineal portion (47). The pelvic diaphragm is spread transversely in a hammocklike fashion across the true pelvis, with a central hiatus for the urethra, vagina, and rectum. Anatomically and physiologically, the pelvic diaphragm can be divided into two components: the internal and external components.

The *external component* originates from the arcus tendineus, extending from the pubic bone to the ischial spine. It gives rise to fibers of differing directions, including the *pubococcygeus*, the *iliococcygeus*, and the *coccygeus*.

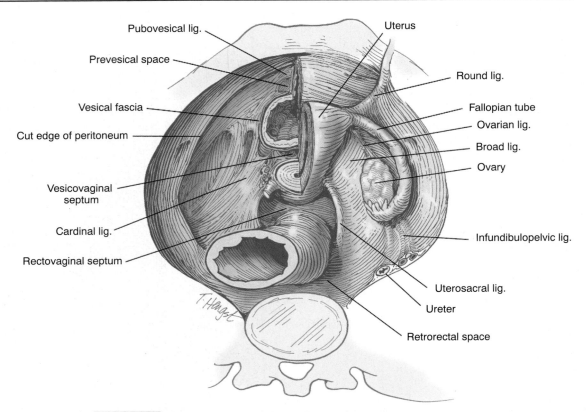

Figure 5.26 The fascial components of the pelvic diaphragm.

The *internal component* **originates from the pubic bone above and medial to the origin of the pubococcygeus and is smaller but thicker and stronger** (47). Its fibers run in a sagittal direction and are divided into the following two portions:

1. *Pubovaginalis* fibers run in a perpendicular direction to the urethra, crossing the lateral vaginal wall at the junction of its lower one-third and upper two-thirds to insert into the perineal body. The intervening anterior interlevator space is covered by the urogenital diaphragm.
2. *Puborectalis* superior fibers sling around the rectum to the symphysis pubis; its inferior fibers insert into the lateral rectal wall between the internal and external sphincter.

The pelvic diaphragm is covered superiorly by fascia, which includes a parietal and a visceral component and is a continuation of the transversalis fascia (Fig. 5.26). The parietal fascia has areas of thickening (ligaments, septae) that provide reinforcement and fixation for the pelvic floor. **The visceral (*endopelvic*) fascia extends medially to invest the pelvic viscera, resulting in a fascial covering to the bladder, vagina, uterus, and rectum. It becomes attenuated where the peritoneal covering is well defined and continues laterally with the pelvic cellular tissue and neurovascular pedicles.**

Musculofascial elements (the hypogastric sheath) extend along the vessels originating from the internal iliac artery. Following these vessels to their respective organs, the hypogastric sheath extends perivascular investments that contribute to the formation of the endopelvic fascia so critical for the support of the pelvic organs.

Thus, the parietal fascia anchors the visceral fascia, which defines the relationship of the various viscera and provides them with significant fixation (uterosacral and cardinal ligaments), septation (vesicovaginal and rectovaginal), and definition of pelvic spaces (prevesical, vesicovaginal, rectovaginal, paravesical, pararectal, and retrorectal).

For its support, the pelvic floor relies on the complementary role of the pelvic diaphragm and its fascia resting on the perineal fibromuscular complex. It is composed of the perineal

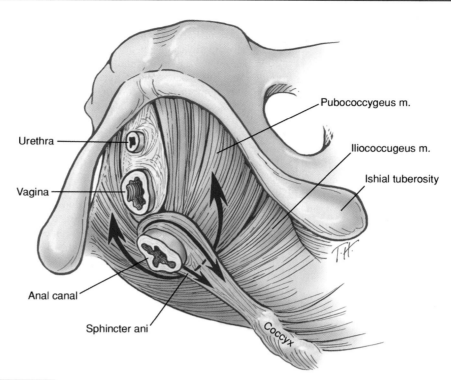

Figure 5.27   **The double-layered muscular support of the pelvic diaphragm.**

Labels: Urethra, Vagina, Anal canal, Sphincter ani, Pubococcygeus m., Iliococcugeus m., Ishial tuberosity, Coccyx

membrane (urogenital diaphragm) anteriorly and the perineal body joined to the anococcygeal raphe by the external anal sphincter posteriorly. This double-layered arrangement, when intact, provides optimal support for the pelvic organs and counterbalances the forces pushing them downward with gravity and with any increase in intra-abdominal pressure (Fig. 5.27). Dynamic imaging techniques, such as MRI, CT, and ultrasonography, increasingly are used to provide additional information in the evaluation of pelvic floor problems by visualizing anatomic landmarks during different functional phases.

Endopelvic Fascia

Controversy exists surrounding the use of the term "fascia" as it applies to the pelvis. Histologic studies reveal that the linings of the levator ani, piriformis, and obturator internus are genuine examples of pelvic fascia. One example in which the term "fascia" is incorrectly used is in reference to the tissue that is plicated in an anterior colporrhaphy. Histologically, it is the muscular lining of the vagina that is plicated. There are no discrete capsules of fascia that separate the bladder and vagina from each other.

The endopelvic fascia is a sheet of fibroareolar tissue following the blood supply to the visceral organs and acts as a retroperitoneal mesentery. The fascia divides the retroperitoneal space into avascular planes. The endopelvic or pubocervical fascia attaches the cervix and vagina to the lateral pelvic sidewall. It is composed of two parts: the parametrium, which is that part connected to the uterus (i.e., the uterosacral and cardinal ligaments), and the paracolpium, which is that part connected to the vagina. The parametrium and cardinal ligaments continue to the vaginal introitus and fuse directly to the supporting tissues associated with the vagina. The uterine and vaginal arteries travel in these structures. The uterosacral ligaments are the posterior components of the cardinal ligaments, extending from the cervix and upper vagina to the lateral sacrum. Lateral pelvic support is provided by linear condensations of obturator and levator ani fascia termed the arcus tendineus fascia pelvis and the arcus tendineus levator ani, respectively. The arcus tendineus levator ani serves as a point of attachment for the pubococcygeus and iliococcygeus muscles and lies on the fascia of the obturator internus muscle. It runs from the posterolateral pubic ramus to the ischial spine. The arcus tendineus fascia pelvis runs from the anterior pubis to the ischial spine as it joins with the arcus tendineus levator ani. It provides lateral (paravaginal) support to the anterior vagina.

Obturator Space

The obturator *membrane* is a fibrous sheath that spans the obturator *foramen* through which the obturator neurovascular bundle penetrates via the obturator *canal*. The obturator internus muscle lies on the superior (intrapelvic) side of the obturator membrane. The origin of the obturator internus is on the inferior margin of the superior pubic ramus and the pelvic surface of the obturator membrane. Its tendon passes through the lesser sciatic foramen to insert onto the greater trochanter of the femur to laterally rotate the thigh. The obturator artery and vein originate as branches of the internal iliac vessels. As they emerge from the cranial side of the obturator membrane via the obturator canal and enter the obturator space, they divide into many small branches, supplying blood to the muscles of the adductor compartment of the thigh. Cadaver work contradicted previous reports that the obturator vessels bifurcate into medial and lateral branches (48). Rather, the vessels are predominantly small (<5 mm in diameter) and splinter into variable courses. The muscles of the medial thigh and adductor compartment are (from superficial to deep) the gracilis, adductor longus, adductor brevis, adductor magnus, obturator externus, and obturator internus. In contrast to the vessels, the obturator nerve emerges from the obturator membrane and bifurcates into anterior and posterior divisions, traveling distally down the thigh to supply the muscles of the adductor compartment. With the patient in the dorsal lithotomy position, the nerves and vessels follow the thigh and course laterally away from the ischiopubic ramus. **Transobturator incontinence slings and anterior trocar-based mesh prolapse kits are often placed beneath the adductor longus tendon and just lateral to the descending ischiopubic ramus in order to avoid the obturator neurovascular bundle, which lies lateral and superior to this relatively safe point of entry through the obturator membrane.**

Summary

New surgical approaches are being developed to solve old problems and often require surgeons to revisit familiar anatomy from an unfamiliar perspective or with a different understanding of complex anatomic relationships. Examples of innovative surgical approaches that require renewed understanding of anatomic relationships include laparoscopic or robotic surgery, midurethral incontinence slings that traverse the obturator or retropubic spaces, and prolapse kits that traverse pararectal and paravesical spaces. Anatomic alterations secondary to disease, congenital variation, or intraoperative complications may make familiar surgical territory suddenly seem foreign. All of these situations require surgeons to be perpetual students of anatomy, regardless of their breadth or depth of experience.

Several strategies for continuing education in anatomy are suggested:

1. **Review relevant anatomy before each surgical procedure.**

2. **Study the gynecologic literature on an ongoing basis—numerous publications document the evolution of newer concepts regarding anatomic issues such as pelvic support.**

3. **Operate with more experienced pelvic surgeons, particularly when incorporating new surgical procedures into practice.**

4. **Periodically dissect fresh or fixed cadaveric specimens; this practice may be arranged through local or regional anatomy boards or medical schools or by special arrangement at the time of autopsy.**

5. **Take advantage of newer computer-generated three-dimensional pelvic models and virtual reality interactive anatomic and surgical simulators, when available, to better understand functional anatomy and to help plan complicated surgical procedures (49,50).**

References

1. **International Anatomical Nomenclature Committee.** *Nomina anatomica.* 6th ed. Edinburgh, Scotland: Churchill Livingstone, 1989.
2. **Sze EH, Kohli N, Miklos JR, et al.** Computed tomography comparison of bony pelvis dimensions between women with and without genital prolapse. *Obstet Gynecol* 1999;93:229–232.
3. **Handa VL, Pannu HK, Siddique S, et al.** Architectural differences in the bony pelvis of women with and without pelvic floor disorders. *Obstet Gynecol* 2003;102:1283–1290.
4. **Mattox TF, Lucente V, McIntyre P, et al.** Abnormal spinal curvature and its relationship to pelvic organ prolapse. *Am J Obstet Gynecol* 2000;183:1381–1384.

5. **Nguyen JK, Lind LR, Choe JY, et al.** Lumbosacral spine and pelvic inlet changes associated with pelvic organ prolapse. *Obstet Gynecol* 2000;95:332–336.
6. **Stein TA, Kaur G, Summers A, et al.** Comparison of bony dimensions at the level of the pelvic floor in women with and without pelvic organ prolapse. *Am J Obstet Gynecol* 2009;200:241.e1–5.
7. **Thompson JR, Gibbs JS, Genadry R, et al.** Anatomy of pelvic arteries adjacent to the sacrospinous ligament: importance of the coccygeal branch of the inferior gluteal artery. *Obstet Gynecol* 1999;94:973–977.
8. **DeLancey JOL, Kearney R, Chou Q, et al.** The appearance of levator ani muscle abnormalities in magnetic resonance imaging after vaginal delivery. *Obstet Gynecol* 2003;101:46–53.
9. **Singh K, Jakub M, Reid WM, et al.** Three dimensional assessment of levator ani morphologic features in different grades of prolapse. *Am J Obstet Gynecol* 2003;189:910–915.
10. **Barber MD, Bremer RE, Thor Kb, et al.** Innervation of the female levator ani muscles. *Am J Obstet Gynecol* 2002;187:64–71.
11. **Snooks SJ, Swash M.** the innervation of the muscles of continence. *Ann R Coll Surg Engl* 1986;68:45–49.
12. **Percy JP, Neill ME, Swash M, et al.** Electrophysiological study of motor nerve supply of pelvic floor. *Lancet* 1981;1:16–17.
13. **Pierce LM, Reyes M, Thor KB, et al.** Innervation of the levator ani muscles in the female squirrel monkey. *Am J Obstet Gynecol* 2003;188:1141–1147.
14. **Bremer RE, Barber MD, Coates KW, et al.** Innervation of the levator ani and coccygeus muscles of the female rat. *Anat Rec* 2003;275:1031–1041.
15. **Vanderhorst VG, Holstege G.** Organization of lumbosacral motoneuronal cell groups innervating hindlimb, pelvic floor, and axial muscles in the cat. *J Comp Neurol* 1997;382:46–47.
16. **Uhlenhuth E, Day EC, Smith RD, et al.** The visceral endopelvic fascia and the hypogastric sheath. *Surg Gynecol Obstet* 1948;86:9–28.
17. **Thompson JD, Rock WA, Wiskind A.** Control of pelvic hemorrhage: blood component therapy and hemorrhagic shock. In: **Thompson JD, Rock JA, eds.** TeLinde's operative gynecology. 7th ed. Philadelphia, PA: Lippincott, 1991:151.
18. **Lee RB, Stone K, Magelssen D, et al.** Presacral neurectomy for chronic pelvic pain. *Obstet Gynecol* 1986;68:517–521.
19. **Polan ML, DeCherney A.** Presacral neurectomy for pelvic pain in infertility. *Fertil Steril* 1980;34:557–560.
20. **Cilento GB, Bauer BS, Retik BA, et al.** Urachal anomalies: defining the best diagnostic modality. *Urology* 1998;52:120–122.
21. **Vaughan ED Jr, Middleton GW.** Pertinent genitourinary embryology: review for the practicing urologist. *Urology* 1975;6:139–149.
22. **Byskov AG, Hoyer PE.** Embryology of mammalian gonads and ducts. In: **Knobil E, Neill JD, eds.** *The physiology of reproduction.* 2nd ed. New York: Raven, 1994:487.
23. **Cilento GB, Bauer BS, Retik BA, et al.** Urachal anomalies: defining the best diagnostic modality. *Urology* 1998;52:120–122.
24. **Arey LB.** The genital system. In: **Arey LB, ed.** *Developmental anatomy.* 7th ed. Philadelphia, PA: Saunders, 1974:315.
25. **Moore KL.** The urogenital system. In: **Moore KL, ed.** The developing human: clinically oriented embryology. 3rd ed. Philadelphia, PA: Saunders, 1982:255.
26. **Semmens JP.** Congenital anomalies of female genital tract: functional classification based on review of 56 personal cases and 500 reported cases. *Obstet Gynecol* 1962;19:328–350.
27. **Brandon CJ, Lewicky-Gaupp C, Larson KA, et al.** Anatomy of the perineal membrane as seen in magnetic resonance images of nulliparous women. *Am J Obstet Gynecol* 2009;200:583.e1–6.
28. **Lawson JO.** Pelvic anatomy. II. Anal canal and associated sphincters. *Ann R Coll Surg Engl* 1974;54:288–300.
29. **Terra MP, Beets-Tan RG, Vervoorn I, et al.** Pelvic floor muscle lesions at endoanal MR imaging in female patients with faecal incontinence. *Eur Radiol* 2008;18:1892–1901.
30. **Heilbrun ME, Nygaard IE, Lockhart ME, et al.** Correlation between levator ani muscle injuries on magnetic resonance imaging and fecal incontinence, pelvic organ prolapse, and urinary incontinence in primiparous women. *Am J Obstet Gynecol* 2010;202:488.e1–6.
31. **Lewicky-Gaupp C, Hamilton Q, Ashton-Miller J, et al.** Anal sphincter structure and function relationships in aging and fecal incontinence. *Am J Obstet Gynecol* 2009;200:559.e1–5.
32. **Curtis AH.** A textbook of gynecology. 4th ed. Philadelphia, PA: Saunders, 1943.
33. **Moore KL.** *Clinically oriented anatomy.* 2nd ed. Baltimore, MD: Williams & Wilkins, 1985.
34. **Whiteside JL, Barber MD, Walters MD, et al.** Anatomy of ilioinguinal and iliohypogastric nerves in relation to trocar placement and low transverse incisions. *Am J Obstet Gynecol* 2003;189:1574–1578.
35. **Oelrich TM.** The striated urogenital sphincter muscle in the female. *Anat Rec* 1983;205:223–232.
36. **Milley PS, Nichols DH.** The relationship between the pubo-urethral ligaments and the urogenital diaphragm in the human female. *Anat Rec* 1971;170:281.
37. **Stein TA, DeLancey JO.** Structure of the perineal membrane in females: gross and microscopic anatomy. *Obstet Gynecol* 2008;111:686–693.
38. **Morgan DM, Umek W, Guire K, et al.** Urethral sphincter morphology and function with and without stress incontinence. *J Urol* 2009;182:203–209.
39. **Summers A, Winkel LA, Hussain HK, et al.** The relationship between anterior and apical compartment support. *Am J Obstet Gynecol* 2006;194:1438–1443.
40. **DeLancey JOL.** Anatomic aspects of vaginal eversion after hysterectomy. *Am J Obstet Gynecol* 1992;166:17–28.
41. **Uhlenhuth E, Wolfe WM, Smith EM, et al.** The rectovaginal septum. *Surg Gynecol Obstet* 1948;86:148–163.
42. **Leffler KS, Thompson JR, Cundiff GW, et al.** Attachment of the rectovaginal septum to the pelvic sidewall. *Am J Obstet Gynecol* 2001;185:41–43.
43. **Nichols DH, Randall CL.** Clinical pelvic anatomy of the living. In: **Nichols DH, Randall CL, eds.** *Vaginal surgery.* Baltimore, MD: Williams & Wilkins, 1976:1.
44. **Barber MD, Visco AG, Weidner AC, et al.** Bilateral uterosacral ligament vaginal vault suspension with site specific endopelvic facial defect repair for treatment of pelvic organs. *Am J Obstet Gynecol* 2000;183:1410–1411.
45. **Buller JL, Thompson JR, Cundiff GW, et al.** Uterosacral ligament: description of anatomic relationships to optimize surgical safety. *Obstet Gynecol* 2001;97:873–879.
46. **Symmonds RE.** Urologic injuries: ureter. In: Schaefer G, Graber EA, eds. Complications in obstetric and gynecologic surgery. Philadelphia, PA: Harper & Row, 1981:412.
47. **Lawson JO.** Pelvic anatomy. I. Pelvic floor muscles. *Ann R Coll Surg Engl* 1974;54:244–252.
48. **Whiteside JL, Walters MD.** Anatomy of the obturator region: relations to a transobturator sling. *Int Urogynecol J* 2004;15:223–226.
49. **Parikh M, Rasmussen M, Brubaker L, et al.** Three dimensional virtual reality model of the normal female pelvic floor. *Ann Biomed Eng* 2004;32:292–296.
50. **Bajka M, Manestar M, Hug J, et al.** Detailed anatomy of the abdomen and pelvis of the visible human female. *Clin Anat* 2004;17:252–260.

6

Molecular Biology and Genetics

Oliver Dorigo
Otoniel Martínez-Maza
Jonathan S. Berek

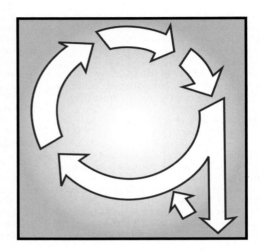

- The regulation and maintenance of normal tissue requires a balance between cell proliferation and programmed cell death, or *apoptosis*.

- The regulation of ovarian function occurs through *autocrine*, *paracrine*, and *endocrine* mechanisms. Disruption of these autocrine and paracrine intraovarian pathways may be the basis of polycystic ovarian disease, disorders of ovulation, and ovarian neoplastic disease.

- Among the genes that participate in control of cell growth and function, *proto-oncogenes* and *tumor suppressor genes* are particularly important.

- Growth factors trigger intracellular biochemical signals by binding to cell membrane receptors. In general, these membrane-bound receptors are *protein kinases* that convert an extracellular signal into an intracellular signal. Many of the proteins that participate in the intracellular signal transduction system are encoded by *proto-oncogenes* that are divided into subgroups based on their cellular location or enzymatic function.

- Oncogenes comprise a family of genes that result from gain of function mutations of their normal counterparts, proto-oncogenes. The normal function of proto-oncogenes is to stimulate proliferation in a controlled context. Activation of oncogenes can lead to stimulation of cell proliferation and development of a malignant phenotype.

- Tumor suppressor genes are involved in the development of most cancers and are usually inactivated in a two-step process in which both copies of the tumor suppressor gene are mutated or inactivated by epigenetic mechanisms like methylation. The most commonly mutated tumor suppressor gene in human cancers is *p53*.

- T lymphocytes have a central role in the generation of immune responses by acting as helper cells in both humoral and cellular immune responses and by acting as effector cells in cellular responses. T cells can be distinguished from other types of

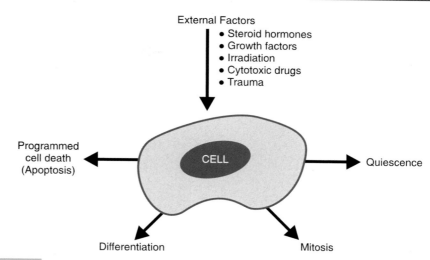

External Factors
- Steroid hormones
- Growth factors
- Irradiation
- Cytotoxic drugs
- Trauma

CELL

Programmed cell death (Apoptosis)

Quiescence

Differentiation

Mitosis

Figure 6.1 **External stimuli affect the cell, which has a specific coordinated response.**

lymphocytes by their cell surface phenotype, based on the pattern of expression of various molecules, as well as by differences in their biologic functions.

- There are two major subsets of mature T cells that are phenotypically and functionally distinct: *T-helper/inducer cells*, which express the CD4 cell surface marker, and the *T-suppressor/cytotoxic cells*, which express the CD8 marker. T_H1 and T_H2 are two helper T-cell subpopulations that control the nature of an immune response by secreting a characteristic and mutually antagonistic set of cytokines: Clones of T_H1 produce interleukin-2 (IL-2) and interferon-γ (IFN-γ), whereas T_H2 clones produce IL-4, IL-5, IL-6, and IL-10.

Advances in molecular biology and genetics have improved our understanding of basic biologic concepts and disease development. The knowledge acquired with the completion of the human genome project, the data available through The Cancer Genome Atlas (TCGA), the development of novel diagnostic modalities, such as the microarray technology for the analysis of DNA and proteins, and the emergence of treatment strategies that target specific disease mechanisms all have an increasing impact on the specialty of obstetrics and gynecology.

Normal cells are characterized by discrete metabolic, biochemical, and physiologic mechanisms. Specific cell types differ with respect to their mainly genetically determined responses to external influences (Fig. 6.1). An external stimulus is converted to an intracellular signal, for example, via a cell membrane receptor. The intracellular signal is transferred to the nucleus and generates certain genetic responses that lead to changes in cellular function, differentiation, and proliferation. Although specific cell types and tissues exhibit unique functions and responses, many basic aspects of cell biology and genetics are common to all eukaryotic cells.

Cell Cycle

Normal Cell Cycle

Adult eukaryotic cells possess a well-balanced system of continuous production of DNA (transcription) and proteins (translation). Proteins are constantly degraded and replaced depending on the specific cellular requirements. Cells proceed through a sequence of phases called the cell cycle, during which the DNA is distributed to two daughter cells (*mitosis*) and subsequently duplicated (*synthesis phase*). This process is controlled at key checkpoints that monitor the status of a cell, for example, the amount of DNA present. The cell cycle is regulated by a small number of heterodimeric protein kinases that consist of a regulatory subunit (cyclin) and a catalytic subunit (cyclin-dependent kinase). Association of a cyclin with a cyclin-dependent kinase (CdkC) determines which proteins will be phosphorylated at a specific point during the cell cycle.

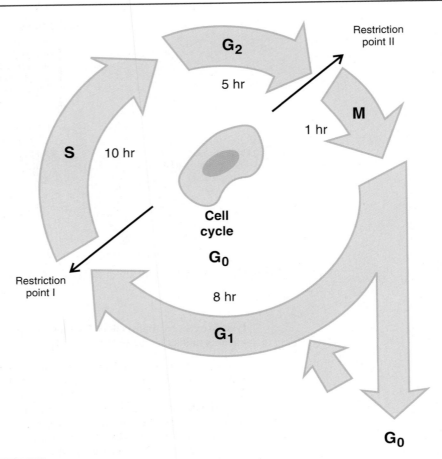

Figure 6.2   The cell cycle.

The cell cycle is divided into four major phases: M phase (mitosis), G_1 phase (period between mitosis and initiation of DNA replication), S phase (DNA synthesis), and G_2 phase (period between completion of DNA synthesis and mitosis) (Fig. 6.2). Postmitotic cells can "exit" the cell cycle into the so-called G_0 phase and remain for days, weeks, or even a lifetime without further proliferation. The duration of the cell cycle may be highly variable, although most human cells complete the cell cycle within approximately 24 hours. During a typical cell cycle, mitosis lasts about 30 to 60 minutes, the G_1 phase 7 to 10 hours, S phase 10 hours, and G_2 phase 5 hours. With respect to the cell cycle, there are three subpopulations of cells:

1. *Terminally differentiated cells* cannot re-enter the cell cycle.
2. *Quiescent (G_0) cells* can enter the cell cycle if appropriately stimulated.
3. *Dividing cells* are currently in the cell cycle.

Red blood cells, striated muscle cells, uterine smooth muscle cells, and nerve cells are terminally differentiated. Other cells, such as fibroblasts, exit from the G_1 phase into the G_0 phase and are considered to be out of the cell cycle. These cells enter the cell cycle following exposure to specific stimuli, such as growth factors and steroid hormones. Dividing cells are found in the gastrointestinal tract, the skin, and the cervix.

G_1 Phase	In response to specific external stimuli, cells enter the cell cycle by moving from the G_0 phase into the G_1 phase. The processes during G_1 phase lead to the synthesis of enzymes and regulatory proteins necessary for DNA synthesis during S phase and are mainly regulated by G_1 cyclin-dependent kinase–cyclin complexes (G_1CdkC). Complexes of G_1CdkC induce degradation of the S phase inhibitors in late G_1. Release of the S phase CdkC complex subsequently stimulates entry into the S phase. **Variations in the duration of the G_1 phase of the cell cycle, ranging**

from less than 8 hours to longer than 100 hours, account for the different generation times exhibited by different types of cells.

S Phase

The nuclear DNA content of the cell is duplicated during the S phase of the cell cycle. The S phase CdkC complex activates proteins of the DNA prereplication complexes that assemble on DNA replication origins during G_1. The prereplication complex activates initiation of DNA replication and inhibits the assembly of new prereplication complexes. This inhibition ascertains that each chromosome is replicated only once during the S phase.

G_2 Phase

RNA and protein synthesis occurs during the G_2 phase of the cell cycle. The burst of biosynthetic activity provides the substrates and enzymes to meet the metabolic requirements of the two daughter cells. Another important event that occurs during the G_2 phase of the cell cycle is the repair of errors of DNA replication that may have occurred during the S phase. Failure to detect and correct these genetic errors can result in a broad spectrum of adverse consequences for the organism and the individual cell (1). Defects in the DNA repair mechanism are associated with an increased incidence of cancer (2). Mitotic CdkC complexes are synthesized during the S and G_2 phases, but are inactive until DNA synthesis is completed.

M Phase

Nuclear–chromosomal division occurs during the mitosis or M phase. During this phase, the cellular DNA is equally distributed to each of the daughter cells. Mitosis provides a diploid (2n) DNA complement to each somatic daughter cell. Following mitosis, eukaryotic mammalian cells contain diploid DNA, reflecting a karyotype that includes 44 somatic chromosomes and an XX or XY sex chromosome complement. Exceptions to the diploid cellular content include hepatocytes (4n) and the functional syncytium of the placenta.

Mitosis is divided into prophase, metaphase, anaphase, and telophase. Mitotic CdkC complexes induce chromosome condensation during the prophase, assembly of the mitotic spindle apparatus, and alignment of the chromosomes during the metaphase. Activation of the anaphase promoting complex (APC) leads to inactivation of the protein complexes that connect sister chromatids during metaphase, permitting the onset of anaphase. During anaphase, sister chromatids segregate to opposite spindle poles. The nuclear envelope breaks down into multiple small vesicles early in mitosis and reforms around the segregated chromosomes as they decondense during telophase. Cytokinesis is the process of division of the cytoplasm that segregates the endoplasmic reticulum and the Golgi apparatus during mitosis. After completion of mitosis, cells enter the G_1 phase and either re-enter the cell cycle or remain in G_0.

Ploidy

After meiosis, germ cells contain a haploid (1n) genetic complement. After fertilization, a 46,XX or 46,XY diploid DNA complement is restored. Restoration of the normal cellular DNA content is crucial to normal function. Abnormalities of cellular DNA content cause distinct phenotypic abnormalities, as exemplified by hydatidiform molar pregnancy (see Chapter 39). **In a complete hydatidiform mole, an oocyte without any nuclear genetic material (e.g., an empty ovum) is fertilized by one sperm. The haploid genetic content of the fertilized ovum is then duplicated, and the diploid cellular DNA content is restored, resulting in a homozygous 46,XX gamete.** Less often, a complete hydatidiform mole results from the fertilization of an empty ovum by two sperm, resulting in a heterozygous 46,XX or 46,XY gamete. In complete molar pregnancies, the nuclear DNA is usually paternally derived, embryonic structures do not develop, and trophoblast hyperplasia occurs. Rarely, complete moles are biparental. This karyotype seems to be found in patients with recurrent hydatidiform moles and is associated with a higher risk of persistent trophoblastic disease.

A partial hydatiform mole follows the fertilization of a haploid ovum by two sperm, resulting in a 69,XXX, 69,XXY, or 69,XYY karyotype. A partial mole contains paternal and maternal DNA, and both embryonic and placental development occur. Both the 69,YYY karyotype and the 46,YY karyotype are incompatible with embryonic and placental development. These observations demonstrate the importance of maternal genetic material, in particular the X chromosome, in normal embryonic and placental development.

In addition to total cellular DNA content, the chromosome number is an important determinant of cellular function. Abnormalities of chromosome number, which often are caused by nondisjunction during meiosis, result in well-characterized clinical syndromes such as trisomy 21 (Down syndrome), trisomy 18, and trisomy 13.

Genetic Control of the Cell Cycle

Cellular proliferation must occur to balance normal cell loss and maintain tissue and organ integrity. This process requires the coordinated expression of many genes at discrete times during the cell cycle (3). In the absence of growth factors, cultured mammalian cells are arrested in the G_0 phase. With the addition of growth factors, these quiescent cells pass through the so-called restriction point 14 to 16 hours later and enter the S phase 6 to 8 hours thereafter. **The restriction point or G_1/S boundary marks the point at which a cell commits to proliferation. A second checkpoint is the G_2/M boundary, which marks the point at which repair of any DNA damage must be completed** (4–7). To successfully complete the cell cycle, a number of cell division cycle (*cdc*) genes are activated.

Cell Division Cycle Genes

Among the factors that regulate the cell cycle checkpoints, proteins encoded by the *cdc2* family of genes and the cyclin proteins appear to play particularly important roles (8,9). Growth factor–stimulated mammalian cells express early-response or delayed-response genes, depending on the chronological sequence of the appearance of specific RNAs. The early- and delayed-response genes act as nuclear transcription factors and stimulate the expression of a cascade of other genes. Early-response genes such as *c-Jun* and *c-Fos* enhance the transcription of delayed-response genes such as *E2Fs*. E2F transcription factors are required for the expression of various cell cycle genes and are functionally regulated by the retinoblastoma (*Rb*) protein. Binding of Rb to E2F converts E2F from a transcriptional activator to a repressor of transcription. Phosphorylation of Rb inhibits its repressing function and permits E2F-mediated activation of genes required for entry into the S phase. Cdk4-cyclin D, Cdk6-cyclin D, and Cdk2-cyclin E complexes cause phosphorylation of Rb, which remains phosphorylated throughout the S, G_2, and M phases of the cell cycle. After completion of mitosis, a decline of the level of Cdk-cyclins leads to dephosphorylation of Rb by phosphatases and, consequently, an inhibition of *E2F* in the early G_1 phase.

Cdks are being evaluated as targets for cancer treatments because they are frequently overactive in cancer disease and Cdk-inhibiting proteins are dysfunctional. The Cdk4 inhibitor P1446A-05, for example, specifically inhibits Cdk4-mediated G_1-S phase transition, arresting cell cycling and inhibiting cancer cell growth (10). SNS-032 selectively binds to Cdk2, -7, and -9, preventing their phosphorylation and activation and subsequently preventing cell proliferation.

As cells approach the G_1-S phase transition, synthesis of cyclin A is initiated. The Cdk2-cyclin A complex can trigger initiation of DNA synthesis by supporting the prereplication complex. The *p34 cdc2* protein and specific cyclins form a complex heterodimer referred to as *mitosis-promoting factor* (MPF), which catalyzes protein phosphorylation and drives the cell into mitosis. Cdk1 assembles with cyclin A and cyclin B in the G_2 phase and promotes the activity of the MPF. **Mitosis is initiated by activation of the *cdc* gene at the G_2-M checkpoint** (11,12). Once the G_2-M checkpoint is passed, the cell undergoes mitosis. In the presence of abnormally replicated chromosomes, progression past the G_2-M checkpoint does not occur.

The *p53* tumor suppressor gene participates in cell cycle control. Cells exposed to radiation therapy exhibit an S-phase arrest that is accompanied by increased expression of p53. This delay permits the repair of radiation-induced DNA damage. In the presence of *p53* mutations, the S-phase arrest that normally follows radiation therapy does not occur (13,14). The wild type *p53* gene can be inactivated by the human papillomavirus E6 protein, preventing S-phase arrest in response to DNA damage (15).

Apoptosis

The regulation and maintenance of normal tissue requires a balance between cell proliferation and programmed cell death, or *apoptosis*. When proliferation exceeds programmed cell death, the result is hyperplasia. When programmed cell death exceeds proliferation, the result is atrophy. Programmed cell death is a crucial concomitant of normal embryologic development. This mechanism accounts for deletion of the interdigital webs, palatal fusion, and development of the intestinal mucosa (16–18). Programmed cell death is also an important phenomenon in normal physiology (19). The reduction in the number of endometrial cells following alterations in steroid hormone levels during the menstrual cycle is, in part, a consequence of programmed cell death (20,21). In response to androgens, granulosa cells undergo programmed cell death (e.g., follicular atresia) (22).

Programmed cell death, or apoptosis, is an energy-dependent, active process that is initiated by the expression of specific genes. This process is distinct from cell necrosis, although both mechanisms result in a reduction in total cell number. In programmed cell death, cells shrink and undergo phagocytosis. Conversely, groups of cells expand and lyse when undergoing cell necrosis. The process is energy independent and results from noxious stimuli. Programmed cell death is triggered by a variety of factors, including intracellular signals and exogenous stimuli such as radiation exposure, chemotherapy, and hormones. Cells undergoing programmed cell death may be identified on the basis of histologic, biochemical, and molecular biologic changes. Histologically, apoptotic cells exhibit cellular condensation and fragmentation of the nucleus. Biochemical correlates of impending programmed cell death include an increase in transglutaminase expression and fluxes in intracellular calcium concentration (23).

Programmed cell death emerged as an important factor in the growth of neoplasms. Historically, neoplastic growth was characterized by uncontrolled cellular proliferation that resulted in a progressive increase in tumor burden. It is recognized that the **increase in tumor burden associated with progressive disease reflects an imbalance between cell proliferation and cell death.** Cancer cells fail to respond to the normal signals to stop proliferating, and they may fail to recognize the physiologic signals that trigger programmed cell death.

Modulation of Cell Growth and Function

The normal cell exhibits an orchestrated response to the changing extracellular environment. The three groups of substances that signal these extracellular changes are steroid hormones, growth factors, and cytokines. The capability to respond to these stimuli requires a cell surface recognition system, intracellular signal transduction, and nuclear responses for the expression of specific genes in a coordinated fashion. **Among the genes that participate in control of cell growth and function,** *proto-oncogenes* and *tumor suppressor genes* **are particularly important.** More than 100 proto-oncogene products that contribute to growth regulation have been identified (24) (Table 6.1). As a group, proto-oncogenes exert positive effects upon cellular proliferation. In contrast, *tumor suppressor genes* exert inhibitory regulatory effects on cellular proliferation (Table 6.2).

Steroid Hormones

Steroid hormones play a crucial role in reproductive biology and in general physiology. Among the various functions, steroid hormones influence pregnancy, cardiovascular function, bone metabolism, and an individual's sense of well-being. The action of steroid hormones is mediated via extracellular signals to the nucleus to affect a physiologic response.

Estrogens exert a variety of effects on growth and development of different tissues. The effects of estrogens are mediated via estrogen receptors (ER), intracellular proteins that function as ligand-activated transcription factors and belong to the nuclear receptor superfamily (25). Two mammalian ERs have been identified: ERα and ERβ. The structure of both receptors is similar and consists of six domains named A through F from the N- to C-terminus, encoded by 8 to 9 exons (26). Domains A and B are located at the N-terminus and contain an agonist-independent transcriptional activation domain (activation function 1, or AF-1). The C domain is a highly conserved central DNA-binding domain composed of two zinc fingers through which ER interacts with the major groove and the phosphate backbone of the DNA helix. The C-terminus of the protein contains domains E and F and functions as ligand-binding domain (LBD–domain E) and AF-2–domain F (Fig. 6.3).

Activation of transcription via the ER is a multistep process. The initial step requires activation of the ER via various mechanisms (Fig. 6.4). For example, estrogens such as 17β-estradiol can diffuse into the cell and bind to the LBD of the ER. Upon ligand binding, the ER undergoes conformational changes followed by a dissociation of various bound proteins, mainly heat shock proteins 90 and 70 (Hsp90 and Hsp70). Activation of the ER also requires phosphorylation by several protein kinases, including casein kinase II, protein kinase A, and components of the Ras/Mapk (mitogen-activated protein kinase) pathway (26). Four phosphorylation sites of the ER are clustered in the NH$_2$ terminus with the AF-1 region.

The activated ER elicits a number of different genomic as well as nongenomic effects on intracellular signaling pathways. The classical steroid signaling pathway involves binding of the activated estrogen receptor to an estrogen responsive element (ERE) on the genome as homodimers and subsequent stimulation of transcription (27,28). The minimal consensus sequence for

Table 6.1 Proto-Oncogenes	
Proto-oncogenes	**Gene Product/Function**
	Growth factors
	Fibroblast growth factor
fgf-5	
Sis	Platelet-derived growth factor beta
hst, int-2	
	Transmembrane receptors
erb-B	Epidermal growth factor (EGF) receptor
HER-2/neu	EGF-related receptor
Fms	Colony-stimulating factor (CSF) receptor
Kit	Stem cell receptor
Trk	Nerve growth factor receptor
	Inner-membrane receptor
bcl-2	
Ha-ras, N-ras, N-ras	
fgr, lck, src, yes	
	Cytoplasmic messengers
Crk	
cot, plm-1, mos, raf/mil	
	Nuclear DNA binding proteins
erb-B1	
jun, ets-1, ets-2, fos, gil 1, rel, ski, vav	
lyl-1, maf, myb, myc, L- myc, N-myc, evi-1	

the ERE is a 13 bp palindromic inverted repeat (IR) and is defined as 5′-GGTCAnnnTGACC-3′. Genes that are regulated by activated ERs include early gene responses such as *c-myc*, *c-fos*, and *d-jun*, and genes encoding for growth factors such as insulin growth factor (IGF-1 and IGF-2), epidermal growth factor (EGF), transforming growth factor-α, and colony-stimulating factor (CSF-1).

Table 6.2 Tumor Suppressor Genes	
p53	Mutated in as many as 50% of solid tumors
Rb	Deletions and mutations predispose to retinoblastoma
PTEN	Dual specificity phosphatase that represses PI3-kinase/Akt pathway activation with negative effect on cell growth
P16^{INK4a}	Binds to cylin-CDK4 complex inhibiting cell cycle progression
FHIT	Fragile histidine triad gene with tumor suppressor function via unknown mechanisms
WT1	Mutations are correlated with Wilms' tumor
NF1	Neurofibromatosis gene
APC	Associated with colon cancer development in patients with familial adenomatous

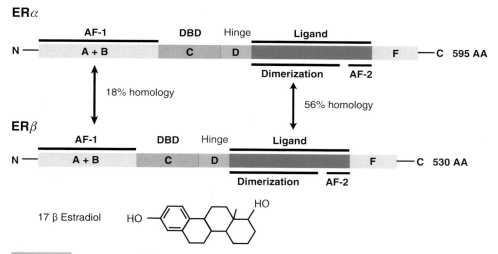

Figure 6.3 **Structure of the two mammalian estrogen receptors.** ERα (595 amino acids) and ERβ (530 amino acids) consist of six domains (A–F from the N- to C-terminus). Domains A and B at the N-terminus contain an agonist-independent transcriptional activation domain (activation function 1, or AF-1). The C domain is the central DNA-binding sequence (DBD). Domains E and F function as ligand binding domain (LBD) and activation function 2 (AF-2). Also shown is the structure of the ER ligand 17β-estradiol.

In addition to the described genomic effects of estrogens, there is growing evidence for nongenomic effects of estrogens on intracellular signal transduction pathways. These effects include rapid activation of the adenylate cyclase, which results in cyclic adenosine monophosphate (cAMP)–dependent activation of protein kinase A (PKA) (29). Estrogens can stimulate the MAPK pathway and rapidly activate the Erk1/Erk2 proteins.

Various ligands with different affinities to the ER were developed and are called *selective estrogen receptor modulators* (*SERMs*). *Tamoxifen*, for example, is a mixed agonist/ antagonist for ERα, but it is a pure antagonist for ERβ. The ERβ receptor is ubiquitously expressed in hormone-responsive tissues, whereas the expression of ERα fluctuates in response to the hormonal milieu. The cellular and tissue effects of an estrogenic compound appear to reflect a dynamic interplay between the actions of these estrogen receptor isoforms. These observations underscore the complexity of estrogen interactions with both normal and neoplastic tissue. Mutations of hormone receptors and their functional consequences illustrate their important contributions to normal physiology. For example, absence of ERα in a male human was reported (30). The clinical sequelae attributed to this mutation include incomplete epiphyseal closure, increased bone turnover, tall stature, and impaired glucose tolerance. The androgen insensitivity syndrome is caused by mutations of the androgen receptor (31). Mutations of the receptors for growth hormone and thyroid-stimulating hormone result in a spectrum of phenotypic alterations. Mutations of hormone receptors may also contribute to the progression of neoplastic disease and resistance to hormone therapy (32,33).

Growth Factors

Growth factors are polypeptides that are produced by a variety of cell types and exhibit a wide range of overlapping biochemical actions. Growth factors bind to high-affinity cell membrane receptors and trigger complex positive and negative signaling pathways that regulate cell proliferation and differentiation (34). **In general, growth factors exert positive or negative effects upon the cell cycle by influencing gene expression related to events that occur at the G_1-S cell cycle boundary (35).**

Because of their short half-life in the extracellular space, growth factors act over limited distances through autocrine or paracrine mechanisms. In the autocrine loop, the growth factor acts on the cell that produced it. The paracrine mechanism of growth control involves the effect of growth factors on another cell in proximity. Growth factors that play an important role in female reproductive physiology are listed in Table 6.3. The biologic response of a cell

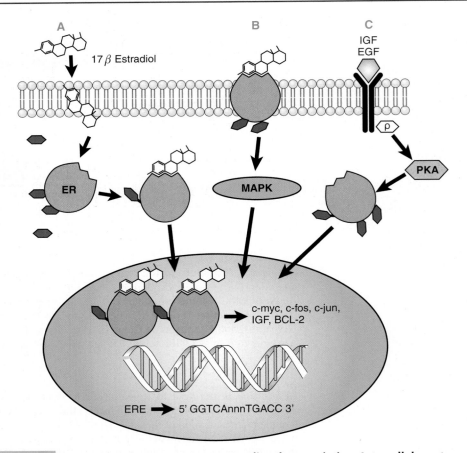

Figure 6.4 **Activation of estrogen receptor mediated transcription. Intracellular estrogen receptor signaling is mediated via different pathways. A:** 17β-estrodiol diffuses through the cell membrane and binds to cytoplasmic ER. The ER is subsequently phosphorylated, undergoes dimerization, and binds to the estrogen response element (ERE) on the promoter of an estrogen responsive gene. **B:** Estrogen ligand binds to membrane-bound ER and activates the mitogen-activated protein kinase (MAPK) pathways that support ER-mediated transcription. **C:** Binding of cytokines such as insulinlike growth factor (IGF) or epidermal growth factor to their membrane receptor can cause activation of protein kinases like PKA, which subsequently activates ER by phosphorylation.

to a specific growth factor depends on a variety of factors, including the cell type, the cellular microenvironment, and the cell cycle status.

The regulation of ovarian function occurs through *autocrine, paracrine,* **and** *endocrine* **mechanisms** (36–42). The growth and differentiation of ovarian cells are particularly influenced by the insulinlike growth factors (IGF) (Fig. 6.5). IGFs amplify the actions of gonadotropin hormones on autocrine and paracrine growth factors found in the ovary. IGF-1 acts on granulosa cells to cause an increase in cAMP, progesterone, oxytocin, proteoglycans, and inhibin. On theca cells, IGF-1 causes an increase in androgen production. Theca cells produce tumor necrosis factor-α (TNF-α) and EGF, which are regulated by follicle-stimulating hormone (FSH). Epidermal growth factor acts on granulosa cells to stimulate mitogenesis. Follicular fluid contains IGF-1, IGF-2, TNF-α, TNF-β, and EGF. **Disruption of these autocrine and paracrine intraovarian pathways may be the basis of polycystic ovarian disease, disorders of ovulation, and ovarian neoplastic disease.**

Transforming growth factor-β (TGF-β) activates intracytoplasmic serine threonine kinases and inhibits cells in the late G_1 phase of the cell cycle (42). It appears to play an important role in embryonic remodeling. Mullerian-inhibiting substance (MIS), which is responsible for regression of the mullerian duct, is structurally and functionally related to TGF-β (43). TGF-α is an EGF homologue that binds to the EGF receptor and acts as an autocrine factor in normal cells.

Table 6.3 Growth Factors that Play Important Roles in Female Reproductive Physiology

Growth Factor	Sources	Targets	Actions
Platelet-derived growth factor (PDGF)	Placenta, platelets, preimplantation embryo, endothelial cells	Endothelial cells Trophoblasts	Mitogen
Epidermal growth factor (EGF)	Submaxillary gland, theca cells Granulosa cells Endometrium	Mitogen	
Transforming growth factor-α (TGF-α)	Embryo, placenta, theca cell, ovarian stromal cell	Placenta Granulosa cells	Mitogen
Transforming growth factor–β (TGF-β)	Embryo, theca cells Endometrium Granulosa cells Theca cells	Mitogen	
Insulinlike growth factor 1 (IGF-1)	Granulosa cells	Theca cells Granulosa cells	Mediates growth hormone activity
Insulinlike growth factor 2 (IGF-2)	Theca cells	Theca cells	Insulinlike
Fibroblast growth factor (FGF)	Granulosa cells	Granulosa cells Angiogenic Mitogen	

As with EGF, TGF-α promotes entry of G_0 cells into the G_1 phase of the cell cycle. The role of growth factors in endometrial growth and function was the subject of several reviews (37–42). Similar to the ovary, autocrine, paracrine, and endocrine mechanisms of control also occur in endometrial tissue.

Intracellular Signal Transduction

Growth factors trigger intracellular biochemical signals by binding to cell membrane receptors. In general, these membrane-bound receptors are *protein kinases* that convert an extracellular signal into an intracellular signal. The interaction between growth factor ligand and its receptor results in receptor dimerization, autophosphorylation, and tyrosine kinase activation. Activated receptors in turn phosphorylate substrates in the cytoplasm and trigger the intracellular signal transduction system (Fig. 6.6). The intracellular signal transduction system relies on serine threonine kinases, *src*-related kinases, and G proteins. Intracellular signals activate nuclear factors that regulate gene expression. **Many of the proteins that participate in the intracellular signal transduction system are encoded by *proto-oncogenes* that are divided into subgroups based on their cellular location or enzymatic function** (44,45) (Fig. 6.7).

The *raf* and *mos* proto-oncogenes encode proteins with serine threonine kinase activity. These kinases integrate signals originating at the cell membrane with those that are forwarded to the nucleus (46,47). Protein kinase C (PKC) is an important component of a second messenger system that exhibits serine threonine kinase activity. This enzyme plays a central role in phosphorylation, which is a general mechanism for activating and deactivating proteins. It also plays an important role in cell metabolism and division (48).

The *Scr* family of tyrosine kinases is related to PKC and includes protein products encoded by the *scr*, *yes*, *fgr*, *hck*, *lyn*, *fyn*, *lck*, *alt*, and *fps/fes* proto-oncogenes. These proteins bind to the inner cell membrane surface.

The *G proteins* are guanyl nucleotide-binding proteins. The heterotrimeric, or large G proteins, link receptor activation with effector proteins such as adenylcyclase, which activates the cAMP-dependent, kinase-signaling cascade (49). The monomeric or small G proteins, encoded by

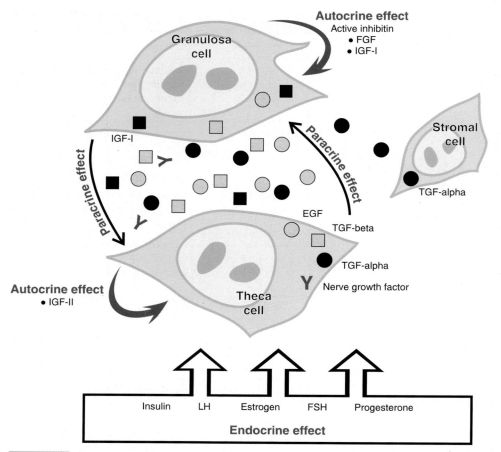

Figure 6.5   **The regulation of ovarian function occurs through autocrine, paracrine, and endocrine mechanisms.**

the *ras* proto-oncogene family, are designated *p21* and are particularly important regulators of mitogenic signals. The *p21 Ras* protein exhibits guanyl triphosphate (GTP) binding and GTPase activity. Hydrolysis of GTP to guanyl diphosphate (GDP) terminates *p21 Ras* activity. The *p21 Ras* protein influences the production of deoxyguanosine (dG) and inositol phosphate (IP) 3, arachidonic acid production, and IP turnover.

The phosphoinositide 3 (PI3) kinase can be activated by various growth factors like platelet-derived growth factor (PDGF) or IGF results. Activation of PI3 kinase results in an increase of intracellular, membrane-bound lipids, phosphatidylinositol-(3,4)-diphosphate (PIP2), and phosphatidylinositol-(3,4,5)-triphosphate (PIP3). The *Akt* protein is subsequently phosphorylated by PIP3-dependent kinases (PDK) for full activation. Activated *Akt* is released from the membrane and elicits downstream effects that lead to an increase in cell proliferation, prevention of apoptosis, invasiveness, drug resistance, and neoangiogenesis (50). The *Pten* (phosphatase and chicken tensin homologue deleted on chromosome 10) protein is an important factor in the PI3 kinase pathway, because it counteracts the activation of *Akt* by dephosphorylating PIP3. Cells with mutated tumor suppressor gene *Pten* and lack of functional *Pten* expression display an increased proliferation rate and decreased apoptosis, possibly supporting the development of a malignant phenotype. *Pten* frequently is mutated in endometrioid adenocarcinoma. Furthermore, lack of functional *Pten* expression was described in endometriosis.

The mammalian target of rapamycin (mTOR) is regulated by the PI3 kinase pathway. mTOR is a serine/threonine protein kinase that regulates a variety of cellular processes, including proliferation, motility, and translation (51). mTOR integrates the input from various upstream pathways, including insulin and growth factors like IGF proteins. The mTOR pathway provides important survival signals for cancer cells and therefore was one focus of targeted drug development (52).

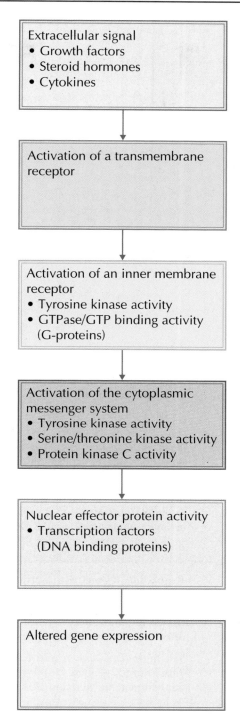

Figure 6.6 **Pathways of intracellular signal transduction.**

For example, *rapamycin* inhibits mTOR by associating with its intracellular receptor FKBP12. Derivates of *rapamycin* like *everolimus* (RAD001) and *temsirolimus* (CCI779) showed promising results in clinical trials (53).

mTOR functions as the catalytic subunit of two different protein complexes. Among the proteins associated with mTOR complex 1 (mTORC1) is mTOR, the regulatory associated protein of mTOR (Raptor), and PRAS40. This complex functions as a nutrient and energy sensor and controls protein synthesis (54). While mTORC1 is activated by insulin, growth factors, amino

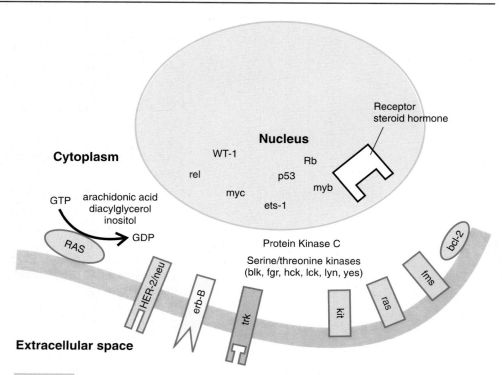

Figure 6.7 **Proto-oncogenes are divided into subgroups based on their cellular location or enzymatic function.**

acids and oxidative stress, low nutrient levels, reductive stress, and growth factor deprivation inhibit its activity.

In contrast, the mTOR complex 2 (mTORC2) contains, among others, mTOR, the rapamycin-insensitive protein Rictor, and mammalian stress-activated protein kinase interacting protein 1 (mSIN1). mTORC2 regulates the cytoskeleton and phosphorylates Akt (55). Its regulation is complex, but involves insulin, growth factors, serum, and nutrient levels.

Expression of Genes and Proteins

Regulation of genetic transcription and replication is crucial to the normal function of the daughter cells, the tissues and ultimately the organism. Transmission of external signals to the nucleus by way of the intracellular signal transduction cascade culminates in the transcription of specific genes and translation of the mRNA into proteins that ultimately affect the structure, function, and proliferation of the cell.

The human genome project resulted in the determination of the sequence of DNA of the entire human genome (56). With the completion of this project, it appears that the human haploid genome contains 23,000 protein coding genes. Sequencing the human genome is a major scientific achievement that opens the door for more detailed studies of structural and functional genomics. **Structural genomics involves the study of three-dimensional structures of proteins based on their amino acid sequences. Functional genomics provides a way to correlate structure and function. Proteomics involves the identification and cataloging of all proteins used by a cell, and cytomics involves the study of cellular dynamics, including intracellular system regulation and response to external stimuli.** The **transcriptome** is the set of all RNA molecules, including mRNA, rRNA, tRNA, and other noncoding RNA produced in one or a population of cells. The transcriptome varies with external environmental conditions and reflects the actively expressed genes. **The *metabolome* describes a set of small-molecule metabolites, including hormones and signaling molecules, that are found in a single organism. Similar to the transcriptome and proteome, the metabolome is subject to rapid changes (57). The *kinome* of an organism describes a set of protein kinases, enzymes that are crucial for phosphorylation reactions.**

Hereditary Cancer   Sporadic Cancer

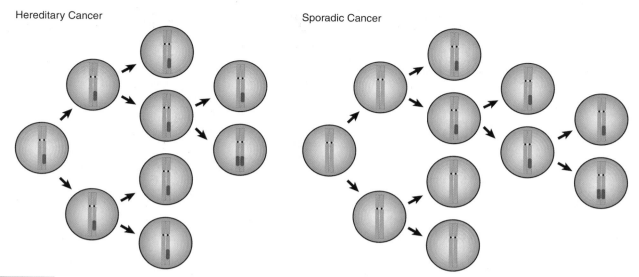

Figure 6.8 **Hereditary and sporadic cancer development based on the Knudson "two-hit" genetic model.** All cells harbor one mutant tumor suppressor gene allele in hereditary cancer. The loss of the second allele results in the malignant phenotype. Sporadic cancers develop in cells with normal genome, therefore requiring both alleles to be inactivated (two hits).

Cancer Genetics

Cancer is a genetic disease that results from a series of mutations in various cancer genes. Uncontrolled cell growth occurs because of accumulation of somatic mutations or the inheritance of one or more mutations through the germline, followed by additional somatic mutations. The mutation in genes that are directly involved in normal cellular growth and proliferation can lead to the development of uncontrolled growth, invasion, and metastasis.

According to the Knudson hypothesis, which was first described in children with hereditary retinoblastoma, two hits or mutations within the genome of a cell are required for a malignant phenotype to develop (58). In hereditary cancers, the first hit is present in the genome of every cell. Only one additional hit is necessary, therefore, to disrupt the correct function of the second cancer gene allele. In contrast, sporadic cancers develop in cells without hereditary mutations in the cancer predisposing alleles. In this case, both hits must occur in a single somatic cell to disrupt both cancer gene alleles (Fig. 6.8).

Most adult solid tumors require 5 to 10 rate-limiting mutations to acquire the malignant phenotype. Among these mutations, some are responsible for causing the cancer phenotype, whereas others might be considered bystander mutations, as with, for example, the amplification of genes that are adjacent to an oncogene. The most compelling evidence for the mutagenic tumor development process is that the age-specific incidence rates for most human epithelial tumors increase at roughly the fourth to eighth power of elapsed time.

Gatekeepers and Caretakers

Cancer susceptibility genes are divided into "gatekeepers" and "caretakers" (59). Gatekeeper genes control cellular proliferation and are divided into oncogenes and tumor suppressor genes. In general, oncogenes stimulate cell growth and proliferation, and tumor suppressor genes reduce the rate of cell proliferation or induce apoptosis. Gatekeepers prevent the development of tumors by inhibiting growth or promoting cell death. Examples of gatekeeper genes include the tumor suppressor gene *p53* and the retinoblastoma gene.

Caretaker genes preserve the integrity of the genome and are involved in DNA repair (stability genes). The inactivation of caretakers increases the likelihood of persistent mutations in gatekeeper genes and other cancer-related genes. The DNA mismatch repair genes, MLH1, MSH2, and MSH6, are examples of caretaker genes.

Hereditary Cancer

Most cancers are caused by spontaneous somatic mutations. However, a small percentage of cancers arise on a heritable genomic background. About 12% of all ovarian cancers and about 5% of endometrial cancers are considered to be hereditary (60,61). Germline mutations require additional mutations at one or more loci for tumorigenesis to occur. These

Table 6.4 Hereditary Cancer Syndromes Associated with Gynecologic Tumors

Hereditary Syndrome	Gene Mutation	Tumor Phenotype
Li-Fraumeni syndrome	TP53, CHEK2	Breast cancer, soft tissues sarcoma, adrenal cortical carcinoma, brain tumors
Cowden syndrome, Bannayan-Zonana syndrome	PTEN	Breast cancer, hamartoma, glioma, endometrial cancer
Hereditary breast and ovarian cancer	BRCA1, BRCA2	Cancer of breast, ovary, fallopian tube
Hereditary nonpolyposis colorectal cancer (HNPCC)	MLH1, MSH2, MSH3, MSH6, PMS2	Cancer of colon, endometrium, ovary, stomach, small bowel, urinary tract
Multiple endocrine neoplasia type I	Menin	Cancer of thyroid, pancreas and pituitary, ovarian carcinoid
Multiple endocrine neoplasia type II	RET	Cancer of thyroid and parathyroid, pheochromocytoma, ovarian carcinoid
Peutz-Jeghers syndrome	STK11	Gastrointestinal hamartomatous polyps, tumors of the stomach, duodenum, colon, ovarian sex cord tumor with annular tubules (SCTAT)

mutations occur via different mechanisms, for example, via environmental factors such as ionizing radiation or mutations of stability genes. **Characteristics of hereditary cancers include diagnosis at a relatively early age and a family history of cancer, usually of a specific cancer syndrome, in two or more relatives.** Hereditary cancer syndromes associated with gynecologic tumors are summarized in Table 6.4.

Various cancer-causing genetic and epigenetic mechanisms are described. On the genomic level, gain of function gene mutations can lead to a conversion of proto-oncogenes into oncogenes, and loss of function gene mutations can inactivate tumor suppressor genes. Epigenetic changes include DNA methylation, which can cause inactivation of tumor suppressor gene expression by preventing the correct function of the associated promoter sequence. Collectively, these genetic and epigenetic changes are responsible for the development of cancer characterized by the ability of cells to invade and metastasize, grow independently of growth factor support, and escape from antitumor immune responses.

Oncogenes

Oncogenes comprise a family of genes that result from gain of function mutations of their normal counterparts, proto-oncogenes. The normal function of proto-oncogenes is to stimulate proliferation in a controlled context. Activation of oncogenes can lead to stimulation of cell proliferation and development of a malignant phenotype. Oncogenes were initially discovered through retroviral tumorigenesis. Viral infection of mammalian cells can result in integration of the viral sequences into the proto-oncogene sequence of the host cell. The integrated viral promoter activates transcription from the surrounding DNA sequences, including the proto-oncogene. Enhanced transcription of the proto-oncogene sequences results in the overexpression of growth factors, growth factor receptors, and signal transduction proteins, which results in stimulation of cell proliferation. One of the most important group of viral oncogenes is the family of *ras* genes, which include *c-H(Harvey)-ras*, *c-K(Kirsten)-ras*, and *N(Neuroblastoma)-ras*.

Tumor Suppressor Genes

Tumor suppressor genes are involved in the development of most cancers and are usually inactivated in a two-step process in which both copies of the tumor suppressor gene are mutated or inactivated by epigenetic mechanisms like methylation (62). The most commonly mutated tumor suppressor gene in human cancers is *p53* (63). The p53 protein regulates transcription of other genes involved in cell cycle arrest such as *p21*. Up-regulation of p53 expression is induced by DNA damage and contributes to cell cycle arrest, allowing DNA repair to occur. p53 also plays an important role in the initiation of apoptosis. The most common mechanism of inactivation of p53 differs from the classic two-hit model. In most cases, missense mutations that change a single amino acid in the DNA binding domain of p53 results in overexpression of nonfunctional p53 protein in the nucleus of the cell.

The identification of tumor suppressor genes was facilitated by positional cloning strategies. The main approaches are cytogenetic studies to identify chromosomal alterations in tumor specimens, DNA linkage techniques to localize genes involved in inherited predisposition to cancer, and examination for loss of heterozygosity or allelic alterations among studies in sporadic tumors. Comparative genomic in situ hybridization (CGH) allows fluorescence identification of chromosome gain and loss in human cancers within a similar experiment.

Stability Genes

The third class of cancer genes is "stability genes," which promotes tumorigenesis in a way different from tumor suppressor genes or amplified oncogenes. The main function of stability genes is the preservation of the correct DNA sequence during DNA replication (caretaker function) (64). Mistakes that are made during normal DNA replication or induced by exposure to mutagens can be repaired by a variety of mechanisms that involve mismatch repair genes, nuclear-type excision repair genes, and base excision repair genes. The inactivation of stability genes potentially leads to a higher mutation rate in all genes. However, only mutations in oncogenes and tumor suppressor genes influence cell proliferation and confer a selective growth advantage to the mutant cell. Similar to tumor suppressor genes, both alleles of stability genes must be activated to cause loss of function.

Genetic Aberrations

Gene replication, transcription, and translation are imperfect processes, and the fidelity is less than 100%. Genetic errors may result in abnormal structure and function of genes and proteins. Genomic alterations such as gene amplification, point mutations, and deletions or rearrangements were identified in premalignant, malignant, and benign neoplasms of the female genital tract (65) (Fig. 6.9).

Amplification

Amplification refers to an increase in the copy number of a gene. Amplification results in enhanced gene expression by increasing the amount of template DNA that is available for transcription. Proto-oncogene amplification is a relatively common event in malignancies of the female genital tract. The *HER2/neu* proto-oncogene, also known as *c-erbB-2* and *HER2*, encodes a 185 *kDa* transmembrane glycoprotein with intrinsic tyrosine kinase activity. It belongs to a family of transmembrane receptor genes that includes the epidermal growth factor receptors (*erbB-1*), *erbB-3*, and *erbB-4*. *HER2/neu* interacts with a variety of different cellular proteins that increase cell proliferation. Overexpression of *HER2/neu* was demonstrated in about 30% of breast cancers, 20% of advanced ovarian cancers, and as many as 50% of endometrial cancers (66). High tissue expression of *HER2/neu* is correlated with a decreased overall survival, particularly in patients with endometrial cancer.

Point Mutations

Point mutations of a gene may remain without any consequence for the expression and function of the protein (gene polymorphism). However, point mutations can alter a codon sequence and subsequently disrupt the normal function of a gene product. The *ras* gene family is an example of oncogene-encoded proteins that disrupt the intracellular signal transduction system following point mutations. Transforming Ras proteins contain point mutations in critical codons (i.e., codons 11, 12, 59, 61) with decrease of GTPase activity and subsequent expression of constitutively active Ras. Point mutations of the *p53* gene are the most common genetic mutations described in solid tumors. These mutations occur at preferential "hot spots" that coincide with the most highly conserved regions of the gene. The *p53* tumor suppressor gene encodes for a phosphoprotein that is detectable in the nucleus of normal cells. When DNA damage occurs, p53 can arrest cell cycle progression to allow the DNA to be repaired or undergo apoptosis. The lack of function of normal *p53* within a cancer cell results in a loss of control of cell proliferation with inefficient DNA repair and genetic instability. Mutations of the *p53* gene occur in approximately 50% of advanced ovarian cancers and 30% to 40% of endometrial cancers but are uncommon in cervical cancer.

Point mutations in the *BRCA1* and *BRCA2* genes can alter the activity of these genes and predispose to the development of breast and ovarian cancer (67). The frequency of *BRCA1* and *BRCA2* mutations in the general population in the United States is estimated at 1:250. Specific

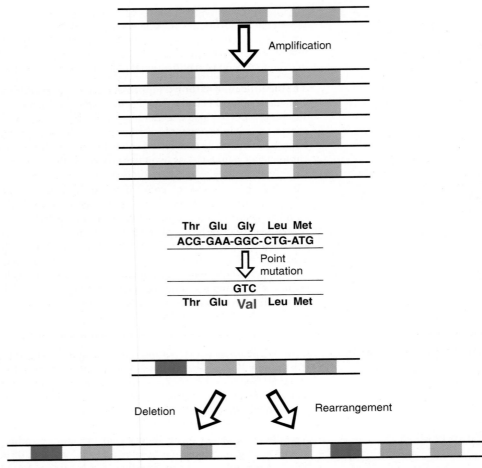

Figure 6.9   Genes can be amplified or undergo mutation, deletion, or rearrangement.

founder mutations were reported for various ethnic groups. For example, two *BRCA1* mutations (185delAG and 5382insC) and one *BRCA2* mutation (6174delT) are found in 2.5% of Ashkenazi Jews of Central and Eastern European descent. Additional founder mutations were described in other ethnic groups, including from the Netherlands (*BRCA1*, 2804delAA and several large deletion mutations), Iceland (*BRCA2*, 995del5), and Sweden (*BRCA1*, 3171ins5).

The BRCA proteins are involved in DNA repair. If DNA is damaged, for example, by ionizing radiation or chemotherapy, the BRCA2 protein binds to the RAD51 protein, which is central for the repair of double-stranded breaks via homologous recombination. BRCA2 regulates the availability and activity of RAD51 in this key reaction. Phosphorylation of the BRCA2/RAD51 complex allows RAD51 to bind to the site of DNA damage and, in conjunction with several other proteins, mediates repair of DNA by homologous recombination. BRCA1 functions within a complex network of protein–protein interactions, mediating DNA repair by homologous recombination and regulating transcription via the BRCA1-associated surveillance complex (BASC).

Deletions and Rearrangements

Deletions and rearrangements reflect gross changes in the DNA template that may result in the synthesis of a markedly altered protein product. Somatic mutations may involve chromosomal translocations that result in chimeric transcripts with juxtaposition of one gene to the regulatory region of another gene. This mutation type is most commonly reported in leukemias, lymphomas, and mesenchymal tumors. The Philadelphia chromosome in chronic myeloid leukemia, for example, is the result of a reciprocal translocation between one chromosome 9 and one chromosome 22. The DNA sequence removed from chromosome 9 contains the proto-oncogene *c-ABL* and inserts into the *BCR* gene sequence on chromosome 22 (Philadelphia chromosome). The resulting chimeric *BCR-ABL* gene product functions as a constitutively active tyrosine kinase and stimulates cellular proliferation by such mechanisms as an increase of growth factors.

Single-nucleotide polymorphism (SNP) describes a variation in the DNA sequence (68). Single nucleotides in the genome differ between paired chromosomes in either one individual or between two individuals. For example, the sequences T**G**ACTA and T**C**ACTA contain one single change in the second nucleotide from guanine (G) to cytosine (C). This results in a G and C allele for this particular gene sequence. SNPs can occur within coding or noncoding sequences of genes or in the intergenic regions. SNPs might not change the amino acid sequence of the protein that is produced (synonymous SNP) or produce a different peptide (nonsynonymous SNPs). If SNPs are located in noncoding regions, various other processes like gene splicing or transcription factor binding might be affected.

The frequency of SNPs in a given population is provided by the minor allele frequency. This frequency differs between ethnic groups and geographic locations. SNPs were associated with various human diseases including cancer disease. They also influence the effect of drug treatment and responses to pathogens and chemicals (69). SNPs are important for the comparison between genomes of different populations for examples providing information about the susceptibility of certain population to develop specific cancers (70).

The Cancer Genome Atlas Project

In 2006 the National Cancer Institute and the National Human Genome Research Institute initiated the Cancer Genome Atlas (TCGA) project. The goal of the project is to provide a comprehensive genomic characterization and sequence analysis of cancer diseases. The initial phase included glioblastoma multiforme, lung, and ovarian cancer (71,72). Many more tumor types will be added to the analysis.

The TCGA is taking advantage of high-throughput genome analysis techniques, including gene expression profiling, SNP genotyping, copy number variation profiling, genome wide methylation profiling, microRNA profiling, and exon sequencing (73). These data are accessible for researchers via the TCGA Web page (74).

Immunology

The immune system plays an essential part in host defense mechanisms, in particular the response to infections and neoplastic transformation. Our increased understanding of immune system regulation provides opportunities for the development of novel immunotherapeutic and immunodiagnostic approaches.

Immunologic Mechanisms

The human immune system has the potential to respond to abnormal or tumor cells in various ways. Some of these immune responses occur in an innate or antigen-nonspecific manner, whereas others are adaptive or antigen specific. Adaptive responses are specific to a given antigen. The establishment of a memory response allows a more rapid and vigorous response to the same antigen in future encounters. Various innate and adaptive immune mechanisms are involved in responses to tumors, including cytotoxicity directed to tumor cells mediated by cytotoxic T cells, natural killer (NK) cells, macrophages, and antibody-dependent cytotoxicity mediated by complementation activation (75).

Adaptive or specific immune responses include humoral and cellular responses. *Humoral immune responses* **refer to the production of antibodies.** Antibodies are bifunctional molecules composed of a variable region with specific antigen-binding sites, combined with a constant region that directs the biologic activities of the antibody, such as binding to phagocytic cells or activation of complement. *Cellular immune responses* **are antigen-specific immune responses mediated directly by activated immune cells rather than by the production of antibodies.** The distinction between humoral and cellular responses is historical and originates from the experimental observation that humoral immune function can be transferred by serum, whereas cellular immune function requires the transfer of cells. Most immune responses include both humoral and cellular components. Several types of cells, including cells from both the myeloid and lymphoid lineages, make up the immune system. Specific humoral and cellular immune responses to foreign antigens involve the coordinated action of populations of lymphocytes operating in concert with one another and with phagocytic cells (macrophages). These cellular interactions include both direct cognate interactions involving cell-to-cell contact and cellular interactions involving the secretion of and response to cytokines or lymphokines. Lymphoid cells are found in lymphoid tissues, such as lymph nodes or spleen, or in the peripheral circulation. The cells that make up the immune system originate from stem cells in the bone marrow.

B Cells, Hormonal Immunity, and Monoclonal Antibodies

B lymphocytes synthesize and secrete antibodies. Mature, antigen-responsive B cells develop from pre-B cells (committed B-cell progenitors) and differentiate to become plasma cells, which produce large quantities of antibodies. Pre-B cells originate from bone marrow stem cells in adults after rearrangement of immunoglobulin genes from their germ cell configuration. Mature B cells express cell surface immunoglobulin molecules that function as receptors for antigen.

Upon interaction with antigen, mature B cells respond to become antibody-producing cells. The process requires the presence of appropriate cell–cell stimulatory signals and cytokines. Monoclonal antibodies are directed against a specific antigenic determinant. In contrast, poly-clonal antibodies detect multiple epitopes that might be presented by just one or a panel of proteins. The in vitro production of monoclonal antibodies, pioneered by Kohler and Milstein in the 1970s, has become an invaluable diagnostic and therapeutic tool, particularly for the management of malignancies (76). The tumor antigen CA125, for example, was detected in a screen of antibodies generated against ovarian cancer cell lines. A radioimmunoassay is widely used to measure CA125 in the serum of patients with ovarian cancer and guide treatment decisions. Therapeutic approaches utilized immunotoxin-conjugated monoclonal antibodies directed to human ovarian adenocarcinoma antigens. These antibodies induce tumor cell killing and can prolong survival in mice implanted with a human ovarian cancer cell line. However, some obstacles limit the clinical use of monoclonal antibodies, including tumor cell antigenic heterogeneity, modulation of tumor-associated antigens, and cross-reactivity of normal host and tumor-associated antigens. No unique tumor-specific antigens were identified. All tumor antigens have to be considered as tumor-related antigens because they are expressed on the malignant as well as the nonmalignant tissues. Because most monoclonal antibodies are murine, the host's immune system can recognize and respond to these foreign mouse proteins. The use of the genetically engineered monoclonal antibodies composed of human-constant regions with specific antigen-reactive murine variable regions can result in reduced antigenicity.

T Lymphocytes and Cellular Immunity

T lymphocytes have a central role in the generation of immune responses by acting as helper cells in both humoral and cellular immune responses and by acting as effector cells in cellular responses. T-cell precursors originate in bone marrow and move to the thymus, where they mature into functional T cells. During their thymic maturation, T cells that can recognize antigen in the context of the *major histocompatibility complex* (MHC) molecules are selected, while self-responding T cells are removed (75).

T cells can be distinguished from other types of lymphocytes by their cell surface phenotype, based on the pattern of expression of various molecules, and by differences in their biologic functions. All mature T cells express certain cell surface molecules, such as the cluster determinant 3 (CD3) molecular complex and the T-cell antigen receptor, which is found in close association with the CD3 complex. **T cells recognize antigen through the cell surface T-cell antigen receptor** (TCR). The structure and organization of this molecule are similar to those of antibody molecules, which are the B-cell receptors for the antigen. During T-cell development, the T-cell receptor gene undergoes gene arrangements similar to those seen in B cells, but there are important differences between the antigen receptors on B cells and T cells. The T-cell receptor is not secreted, and its structure is somewhat different from that of antibody molecules. The way in which the B-cell and T-cell receptors interact with antigens is quite different. T cells can respond to antigens only when these antigens are presented in association with MHC molecules on antigen-presenting cells. Effective antigen presentation involves the processing of antigen into small fragments of peptide within the antigen-presenting cell and the subsequent presentation of these fragments of antigen in association with MHC molecules expressed on the surface of the antigen-presenting cell. T cells can respond to antigens only when presented in this manner, unlike B cells, which can bind antigens directly, without processing and presentation by antigen-presenting cells (75).

There are two major subsets of mature T cells that are phenotypically and functionally distinct: *T-helper/inducer cells,* **which express the CD4 cell surface marker, and the**

T-cytotoxic cells, **which express the CD8 marker.** The expression of these markers is acquired during the passage of T cells through the thymus. CD4 T cells can provide help to B cells, resulting in the production of antibodies by B cells, and interact with antigen presented by antigen-presenting cells in association with MHC class II molecules. CD4 T cells can act as helper cells for other T cells. CD8 T cells include cells that are cytotoxic (cells that can kill target cells bearing appropriate antigens), and they interact with antigen presented on target cells in association with MHC class I molecules. These T cells can inhibit the biologic functions of B cells or other T cells (75). Although the primary biologic role of *cytotoxic T cells* (CTLs) seems to be lysis of virus-infected autologous cells, cytotoxic immune T cells can mediate the lysis of tumor cells directly. Presumably, CTLs recognize antigens associated with MHC class I molecules on tumor cells through their antigen-specific T-cell receptor, setting off a series of events that ultimately results in the lysis of the target cell.

Monocytes and Macrophages

Monocytes and macrophages, which are myeloid cells, have important roles in both innate and adaptive immune responses; macrophages play a key part in the generation of immune responses. T cells do not respond to foreign antigens unless those antigens are processed and presented by antigen-presenting cells. **Macrophages (and B cells and dendritic cells) express MHC class II molecules and are effective antigen-presenting cells for CD4 T cells.** Helper-inducer (CD4) T cells that bear a T-cell receptor of appropriate antigen and self-specificity are activated by this antigen-presenting cell to provide help (various factors—lymphokines—that induce the activation of other lymphocytes). In addition to their role as antigen-presenting cells, macrophages play an important part in innate responses by ingesting and killing microorganisms. Activated macrophages, besides their many other functional capabilities, can act as cytotoxic, antitumor killer cells.

Natural Killer Cells

Natural killer cells are effector cells in an innate type of immune response: the nonspecific killing of tumor cells and virus-infected cells. Therefore, **NK activity represents an innate form of immunity that does not require an adaptive, memory response for optimal biologic function, but the antitumor activity can be increased by exposure to several agents, particularly cytokines such as interleukin-2 (IL-2).** Characteristically, NK cells have a large granular lymphocyte morphology. NK cells display a pattern of cell surface markers that differs from those characteristic of T or B cells. NK cells can express a receptor for the crystallizable fragment (Fc) portion of antibodies, and other NK-associated markers. NK cells appear to be functionally and phenotypically heterogeneous, when compared with T or B cells. The cells that can carry out antibody-dependent cellular cytotoxicity, or antibody-targeted cytotoxicity, are NK-like cells. Antibody-dependent cellular cytotoxicity by NK-like cells resulted in the lysis of tumor cells in vitro. The mechanisms of this tumor cell killing are not clearly understood, although close cellular contact between the effector cell and the target cell seems to be required.

Cytokines, Lymphokines, and Immune Mediators

Many events in the generation of immune responses (as well as during the effector phase of immune responses) require or are enhanced by cytokines, which are soluble mediator molecules (Table 6.5) (77–92). Cytokines are pleiotropic in that they have multiple biologic functions that depend on the type of target cell or its maturational state. Cytokines are heterogeneous in the sense that most cytokines share little structural or amino acid homology. *Cytokines are called monokines if they are derived from monocytes, lymphokines if they are derived from lymphocytes, interleukins if they exert their actions on leukocytes, or interferons (IFNs) if they have antiviral effects.* They are produced by a wide variety of cell types and seem to have important roles in many biologic responses outside the immune response, such as inflammation or hematopoiesis. They may also be involved in the pathophysiology of a wide range of diseases and show great potential as therapeutic agents in immunotherapy for cancer. Although cytokines are a heterogeneous group of proteins, they share some characteristics. For instance, most cytokines are low- to intermediate-molecular weight (10–60 kd) glycosylated-secreted proteins. They are involved in immunity and inflammation, are produced transiently and locally (they act in an autocrine and paracrine rather than an endocrine manner), are extremely potent in small concentrations, and interact with high-affinity cellular receptors that are specific for each cytokine. The cell surface binding of cytokines by specific receptors results in signal transduction followed by changes in gene expression and, ultimately, by changes in cellular proliferation or altered cell behavior, or both. Their biologic actions overlap, and exposure of responsive cells to multiple cytokines can result in synergistic or antagonistic biologic effects.

Table 6.5 Sources, Target Cells, and Biological Activities of Cytokines Involved in Immune Responses

Cytokine	Cellular Source	Target Cells	Biologic Effects
IL-1	Monocytes and macrophages	T cells, B cells Neurons	Costimulator Pyrogen
IL-2	Tumor cells	Endothelial cells	
	T cells	T cells B cells NK cells	Activation and growth Activation and antibody production Activation and growth
IL-3	T cells	Immature hemopoietic stem cells	Growth and differentiation
IL-4	T cells (T_H2)	B cells T cells	Activation and growth; isotype switch to IgE; increased MHCII expression Growth
IL-6	Monocytes and macrophages T cells (T_H17), B cells Ovarian cancer cells Other tumors Tumor cells	B cells T cells Hepatocytes Stem cells Autocrine/paracrine growth and viability-enhancing factor	Differentiation, antibody production Costimulator Induction of acute-phase response Growth and differentiation
IL-10	T cells (Treg, T_H2) Monocytes and macrophages	T cells Monocytes and macrophages B cells	Inhibition of cytokine synthesis Inhibition of Ag presentation and cytokine production Activation
IL-12	Monocytes	NK cells, T cells	Promotes T_H1 cells
IL-13	T cells (T_H2), mast cells, NK cells	B cells, T_H2 cells, macrophages	Regulates IgE secretion by B cell T_H2 development Macrophage activity
IL-15	Dendritic cells, monocytes, placenta, kidney, lung, heart, T cells	Mast cells	NK cell development and function Mast cell proliferation
IL-17	T cells (T_H17)	T cells, fibroblasts	T-cell activation Induces secretion of cytokines by fibroblasts
IL-23	Monocytes, macrophages	CD4+ T cells	Promotes T_H17 cells
IFN-γ	T cells (T_H1)	Monocytes/macrophages	Activation
	NK cells	NK cells, T cells, B cells	Activation Enhances responses
TNF-α	Monocytes and macrophages	Monocytes/macrophages	
	T cells (T_H17) Monokine production Costimulator Pyrogen	T cells, B cells Neurons Endothelial cells Muscle and fat cells	 Activation, inflammation Catabolism/cachexia

IL-1, interleukin-1; T_H1, type 1 T-helper lymphocyte; NK cells, natural killer cells; T_H2, type 2 T-helper lymphocyte; IgE, immunoglobulin E; MHCII, major histocompatibility complex class II; Ag, antigen; IFN, interferon; TNF, tumor necrosis factor.
Modified from **Berek JS**, **Martinez-Maza O.** Immunology and immunotherapy. In: **Lawton FG, Neijt JP, Swenerton KD.** *Epithelial cancer of the ovary.* London, Engl.: BMJ, 1995:224, with permission.

T-cell subsets characterized by the secretion of distinct patterns of cytokines were identified. **T$_H$1 and T$_H$2 are two helper T-cell subpopulations that control the nature of an immune response by secreting a characteristic and mutually antagonistic set of cytokines: Clones of T$_H$1 produce IL-2 and IFN-γ, whereas T$_H$2 clones produce IL-4, IL-5, and IL-10** (86). A similar dichotomy between T$_H$1- and T$_H$2-type responses was reported in humans (87,88). Human IL-10 inhibits the production of IFN-γ and other cytokines by human peripheral blood mononuclear cells and by suppressing the release of cytokines (IL-1, IL-6, IL-8, and TNF-α) by activated monocytes (89–92). IL-10 down-regulates class II MHC expression on monocytes, resulting in a strong reduction in the antigen-presenting capacity of these cells (92). Together, these observations support the concept that IL-10 has an important role as an immune-inhibitory cytokine. Additional T-cell subsets were identified, including Th17 cells and regulatory T cells (Treg). Th17 cells are a distinct, pro-inflammatory T-cell subset, which is functionally characterized by mediating protection against extracellular bacteria and by its pathogenic role in autoimmune disorders (93–98). Th17 cells characteristically produce IL-17, CXCL13 (a B-cell stimulatory chemokine), IL-6, and TNF-α, in contrast to Th2 cells, which characteristically produce IL-4, IL-5, IL-9 and IL-13, or Th1 cells, which produce IFN-γ (Fig. 6.2). Treg cells constitute another subset of CD4-positive T cells that participates in the maintenance of immunologic self-tolerance by actively suppressing the activation and expansion of self-reactive lymphocytes. Treg cells are characterized by the expression of CD25 (the IL-2 receptor chain) and the transcription factor FoxP3 (99,100). Treg cell activity is thought to be important in preventing the development of autoimmune diseases. Removal of Treg may enhance immune responses against infectious agents or cancer. Although much remains to be learned about the role of Treg activity in antitumor immunity, it is clear that such cells may play a role in modulating host responses to cancer.

Because epithelial cancers of the ovary usually remain confined to the peritoneal cavity, even in the advanced stages of the disease, it was suggested that the growth of ovarian cancer intraperitoneally could be related to a local deficiency of antitumor immune effector mechanisms (102,103). Studies showed that ascitic fluid from patients with ovarian cancer contained increased concentrations of IL-10 (102). Various other cytokines are seen in ascitic fluid obtained from women with ovarian cancer, including **IL-6, IL-10, TNF-α,** *granulocyte colony-stimulating factor* (G-CSF), and *granulocyte-macrophage colony-stimulating factor* (GM-CSF) (103). A similar pattern was seen in serum samples from women with ovarian cancer with elevations of IL-6 and IL-10.

TNF-α is a cytokine that can be directly cytotoxic for tumor cells, can increase immune cell–mediated cellular cytotoxicity, and can activate macrophages and induce secretion of monokines. Other biologic activities of TNF-α include the induction of cachexia, inflammation, and fever; it is an important mediator of endotoxic shock.

Cytokines in Cancer Therapy

Cytokines are extraordinarily pleiotropic with a bewildering array of biologic activities, including some outside the immune system (55,56,77,83). Because some cytokines have direct or indirect antitumor and immune-enhancing effects, several of these factors are used in the experimental treatment of cancer.

The precise roles of cytokines in antitumor responses have not been elucidated. Cytokines can exert antitumor effects by many different direct or indirect activities. It is possible that a single cytokine could increase tumor growth directly by acting as a growth factor while at the same time increasing immune responses directed toward the tumor. The potential of cytokines to increase antitumor immune responses was tested in experimental adoptive immunotherapy by exposing the patient's peripheral blood cells or tumor-infiltrating lymphocytes to cytokines such as IL-2 in vitro, thus generating activated cells with antitumor effects that can be given back to the patient (104–106). Some cytokines can exert direct antitumor effects. Tumor necrosis factor can induce cell death in sensitive tumor cells.

The effects of cytokines on patients with cancer might be modulated by soluble receptors or blocking factors. For instance, blocking factors for TNF and for lymphotoxin were found in ascitic fluid from patients with ovarian cancer (106). Such factors could inhibit the cytolytic effects of TNF or lymphotoxin and should be taken into account in the design of clinical trials of intraperitoneal infusion of these cytokines.

Cytokines have growth-increasing effects on tumor cells in addition to inducing antitumor effects. They can act as autocrine or paracrine growth factors for human tumor cells, including those of nonlymphoid origin. For instance, IL-6 (which is produced by various types of human tumor cells) can act as a growth factor for human myeloma, Kaposi's sarcoma, renal carcinoma, and epithelial ovarian cancer cells (77–83).

Cytokines are of great potential value in the treatment of cancer, but because of their multiple—even conflicting—biologic effects, a thorough understanding of cytokine biology is essential for their successful use (104–117).

Factors that Trigger Neoplasia

Cell biology is characterized by considerable redundancy and functional overlap, so a defect in one mechanism does not invariably jeopardize the function of the cell. When a sufficient number of abnormalities in structure and function occur, normal cell activity is jeopardized, and uncontrolled cell growth or cell death results. Either end point may result from accumulated genetic mutations over time. Factors are identified that enhance the likelihood of genetic mutations, jeopardize normal cell biology, and may increase the risk of cancer.

Increased Age

Increasing age is considered the single most important risk factor for the development of cancer (118). Cancer is diagnosed in as much as 50% of the population by 75 years of age (111). It was suggested that the increasing risk of cancer with age reflects the accumulation of critical genetic mutations over time, which ultimately culminates in neoplastic transformation. The basic premise of the multistep somatic mutation theory of carcinogenesis is that genetic or epigenetic alterations of numerous independent genes result in cancer. Factors that are associated with an increased likelihood of cancer include exposure to exogenous mutagens, altered host immune function, and certain inherited genetic syndromes and disorders.

Environmental Factors

A mutagen is a compound that results in a genetic mutation. A number of environmental pollutants act as mutagens when tested *in vitro*. Environmental mutagens usually produce specific types of mutations that can be differentiated from spontaneous mutations. As an example, activated hydrocarbons tend to produce GT transversions (119). A carcinogen is a compound that can produce cancer. It is important to recognize that all carcinogens are not mutagens and that all mutagens are not necessarily carcinogens.

Smoking

Cigarette smoking is perhaps the best known example of mutagen exposure that is associated with the development of lung cancer when the exposure is of sufficient duration and quantity in a susceptible individual. An association between cigarette smoking and cervical cancer has been recognized for decades. **It was determined that the mutagens in cigarette smoke are selectively concentrated in cervical mucus** (59). It was hypothesized that exposure of the proliferating epithelial cells of the transformation zone to cigarette smoke mutagens may increase the likelihood of DNA damage and subsequent cellular transformation.

Others observed that human papillomavirus (HPV) DNA is frequently inserted into the fragile histidine triad (*FHIT*) gene in cervical cancer specimens. The *FHIT* is an important tumor suppressor gene. Cigarette smoking might facilitate the incorporation of HPV DNA into the *FHIT* gene with subsequent disruption of correct tumor suppressor gene function.

Radiation

Radiation exposure can increase the risk of cancer. The overall risk of radiation-induced cancer is approximately 10% greater in women than in men (120). This difference is attributed to gender-specific cancers, including breast cancer. Radiation-induced cancer may be the result of sublethal DNA damage that is not repaired (120). Normally, radiation damage prompts an S-phase arrest so that DNA damage is repaired. This requires normal *p53* gene function. If DNA repair fails, the damaged DNA is propagated to daughter cells following mitosis. If a sufficient number of critical genes are mutated, cellular transformation may result.

Immune Function

Systemic immune dysfunction was recognized as a risk factor for cancer for decades. The immunosuppressed renal transplant patient may have a 40-fold increased risk of cervical cancer (60). Patients infected with HIV who have a depressed CD4 cell count are reported to be at increased risk of cervical dysplasia and invasive disease (116). Individuals who underwent high-dose chemotherapy with stem cell support may be at increased risk of developing a variety of solid neoplasms. These examples illustrate the importance of immune function in host surveillance for transformed cells. Another example of altered immune function that may be related to the development of cervical dysplasia is the alteration in mucosal immune function that occurs in women who smoke cigarettes (60). The Langerhans cell population of the cervix is decreased in women who smoke. Langerhans cells are responsible for antigen processing. It is postulated that a reduction in these cells increases the likelihood of successful HPV infection of the cervix.

Diet

The role of diet in disease prevention and predisposition is widely recognized but poorly understood (116,121). Dietary fat intake is correlated with the risk of colon and breast cancer. Fiber is considered protective against colon cancer. With respect to the female reproductive system, epidemiologic studies provide conflicting results. Deficiencies of folic acid and vitamins A and C were associated with the development of cervical dysplasia and cervical cancer. Considerable research must be performed to clarify the impact of diet on cancer prevention and development.

References

1. **Taylor AM, McConville CM, Byrd PJ.** Cancer and DNA processing disorders. *Br Med Bull* 1994;50:708–717.
2. **Kraemer KH, Levy DD, Parris CN, et al.** Xerodermapigmentosum and related disorders: examining the linkage between defective DNA repair and cancer. *J Invest Dermatol* 1994;103[Suppl 5]:96S–101S.
3. **Jacobs T.** Control of the cell cycle. *Dev Biol* 1992;153:1–15.
4. **Weinert T, Lydall D.** Cell cycle checkpoints, genetic instability and cancer. *Semin Cancer Biol* 1993;4:129–140.
5. **Fridovich-Keil JL, Hansen LJ, Keyomarsi K, et al.** Progression through the cell cycle: an overview. *Am Rev Respir Dis* 1990;142:53–56.
6. **Reddy GP.** Cell cycle: regulatory events in G1-S transition of mammalian cells. *J Cell Biochem* 1994;54:379–386.
7. **Hartwell LH, Weinert TA.** Checkpoints: controls that ensure the order of cell cycle events. *Science* 1989;246:629–634.
8. **Murray AW, Kirschner MW.** Dominoes and clocks: the union of two views of the cell cycle. *Science* 1989;246:614–621.
9. **Lee MG, Norbury CJ, Spurr NK, et al.** Regulated expression and phosphorylation of a possible mammalian cell–cycle control protein. *Nature* 1988;333:257–267.
10. **Vaughn DJ, Flaherty K, Lal P, et al.** Treatment of growing teratoma syndrome. *N Engl J Med* 2009;360:423–424.
11. **Morena S, Nurse P.** Substrates for p34cdc2: in vivo veritas? *Cell* 1990;61:549–551.
12. **Lewin B.** Driving the cell cycle: M-phase kinase, its partners, and substrates. *Cell* 1990;61:743–752.
13. **Kastan MB, Onyekwere O, Sidransky D, et al.** Participation of p53 protein in the cellular response to DNA damage. *Cancer Res* 1991;51:6304–6311.
14. **Kuerbitz SJ, Plunkett BS, Walsh WV, et al.** Wild type p53 is a cell cycle checkpoint determinant following irradiation. *Proc Natl Acad Sci U S A* 1992;89:7491–7495.
15. **Gu Z, Pim D, Labrecque S, et al.** DNA damage–induced p53-mediated transcription inhibited by human papillomavirus type 18 E6. *Oncogene* 1994;9:629–633.
16. **Hammar SP, Mottet NK.** Tetrazolium salt and electron microscopic studies of cellular degeneration and necrosis in the interdigital areas of the developing chick limb. *J Cell Sci* 1971;8:229–251.
17. **Farbman AI.** Electron microscopic study of palate fusion in mouse embryos. *Dev Biol* 1968;18:93–116.
18. **Harmon B, Bell L, Williams L.** An ultrasound study on the meconium corpuscles in rat foetal epithelium with particular reference to apoptosis. *Anat Embryol (Berl)* 1984;169:119–124.
19. **Cotter TG, Lennon SV, Glynn JG, et al.** Cell death via apoptosis and its relationship to growth, development, and differentiation of both tumor and normal cells. *Anticancer Res* 1990;10:1153–1160.
20. **Pollard JW, Pacey J, Cheng SUY, et al.** Estrogens and cell death in murine uterine luminal epithelium. *Cell Tissue Res* 1987;249:533–540.
21. **Nawaz S, Lynch MP, Galand P, et al.** Hormonal regulation of cell death in rabbit uterine epithelium. *Am J Pathol* 1987;127:51–59.
22. **Billig H, Furuta I, Hsueh AJW.** Estrogens inhibit and androgens enhance ovarian granulosa cell apoptosis. *Endocrinology* 1993;33:2204–2212.
23. **Williams GT, Smith CA.** Molecular regulation of apoptosis: genetic controls on cell death. *Cell* 1993;74:777–779.
24. **Baserga R, Porcu P, Sell C.** Oncogenes, growth factors, and control of the cell cycle. *Cancer Surv* 1993;16:201–213.
25. **Hall JM, Couse JF, Korach KS.** The multifaceted mechanisms of estradiol and estrogen receptor signaling. *J Biol Chem* 2001;276:36869–36872.
26. **Katzenellenbogen BS, Choi I, Delage-Mourroux R, et al.** Molecular mechanisms of estrogen action: selective ligands and receptor pharmacology. *J Steroid Biochem Mol Biol* 2000;74:279–285.
27. **Kato S, Endoh H, Masuhiro Y, et al.** Activation of the estrogen receptor through phosphorylation by mitogen-activated protein kinase. *Science* 1995;270:1491–1494.
28. **Klinge CM.** Estrogen receptor interaction with estrogen response elements. *Nucleic Acids Res* 2001;29: 2905–2919.
29. **Lagrange AH, Ronnekleiv OK, Kelly MJ.** Modulation of G protein-coupled receptors by an estrogen receptor that activates protein kinase A. *Mol Pharmacol* 1997;51:605–612.
30. **Smith EP, Boyd J, Frank GR, et al.** Estrogen resistance caused by a mutation of the estrogen receptor gene in a man. *N Engl J Med* 1994;331:1056–1061.
31. **De Bellis A, Quigley CA, Marschke KB, et al.** Characterization of mutant androgen receptors causing partial androgen insensitivity syndrome. *J Clin Endocrinol Metab* 1994;78:513–522.
32. **Fuqua SA.** Estrogen receptor mutagenesis and hormone resistance. *Cancer* 1994;74:1026–1029.
33. **Osborne CK, Fuqua SA.** Mechanisms of tamoxifen resistance. *Breast Cancer Res Treat* 1994;32:49–55.
34. **Pusztal L, Lewis CE, Lorenzen J, et al.** Growth factors: regulation of normal and neoplastic growth. *J Pathol* 1993;169:191–201.
35. **Aaronson SA, Rubin JS, Finch PW, et al.** Growth factor regulated pathways in epithelial cell proliferation. *Am Rev Respir Dis* 1990;142:S7–S10.
36. **Giordano G, Barreca A, Minuto F.** Growth factors in the ovary. *J Endocrinol Invest* 1992;15:689–707.
37. **Baldi E, Bonaccorsi L, Finetti G, et al.** Platelet activating factor in human endometrium. *J Steroid Biochem Mol Biol* 1994;49:359–363.
38. **Gold LI, Saxena B, Mittal KR, et al.** Increased expression of transforming growth factor B isoforms and basic fibroblast growth factor in complex hyperplasia and adenocarcinoma of the endometrium: evidence for paracrine and autocrine action. *Cancer Res* 1994;54:2347–2358.
39. **Leake R, Carr L, Rinaldi F.** Autocrine and paracrine effects in the endometrium. *Ann N Y Acad Sci* 1991;622:145–148.

40. **Giudice LC.** Growth factors and growth modulators in human uterine endometrium: their potential relevance to reproductive medicine. *Fertil Steril* 1994;61:1–17.

41. **Murphy LJ.** Growth factors and steroid hormone action in endometrial cancer. *J Steroid Biochem Mol Biol* 1994;48:419–423.

42. **Laiho M, DeCaprio JA, Ludlow JW, et al.** Growth inhibition by TGF-β linked to suppression of retinoblastoma protein phosphorylation. *Cell* 1990;62:175–185.

43. **Cate RL, Donahoe PK, MacLaughlin DT.** Müllerian-inhibiting substance. In: **Sporn MB, Roberts AB, eds.** *Peptide growth factors and their receptors*, Vol. 2. Berlin: Springer-Verlag, 1990:179–210.

44. **Bates SE, Valverius EM, Ennis BW, et al.** Expression of the transforming growth factor α–epidermal growth factor receptor pathway in normal human breast epithelial cells. *Endocrinology* 1990;126: 596–607.

45. **Hunter T.** Protein kinase classification. *Methods Enzymol* 1991;200: 3–37.

46. **Ralph RK, Darkin-Rattray S, Schofield P.** Growth-related protein kinases. *Bioessays* 1990;12:121–123.

47. **Simon MI, Strathmann MP, Gautam N.** Diversity of G-proteins in signal transduction. *Science* 1991;252:802–808.

48. **Speigel AM.** G-proteins in cellular control. *Curr Opin Cell Biol* 1992;4:203–211.

49. **Hall A.** The cellular function of small GTP-binding proteins. *Science* 1990;249:635–640.

50. **Franke TF, Hornik CP, Segev L, et al.** PI3K/Akt and apoptosis: size matters. *Oncogene* 2003;22:8983–8998.

51. **Hay N, Sonenberg N.** Upstream and downstream of mTOR. *Genes Dev* 2004;18:1926–1945.

52. **Easton JB, Houghton PJ.** mTOR and cancer therapy. *Oncogene* 2006;25:6436–6446.

53. **Motzer RJ, Escudier B, Oudard S, et al.** Phase 3 trial of everolimus for metastatic renal cell carcinoma: final results and analysis of prognostic factors. *Cancer* 2010;116:4256–4265.

54. **Kim D, Sarbassov D, Ali S, et al.** mTOR interacts with raptor to form a nutrient-sensitive complex that signals to the cell growth machinery. *Cell* 2002;110:163–175.

55. **Frias M, Thoreen C, Jaffe J, et al.** mSin1 is necessary for Akt/PKB phosphorylation, and its isoforms define three distinct mTORC2s. *Curr Biol* 2006;16:1865–1870.

56. **Lander ES, Linton LM, Birren B, et al.** International Human Genome Sequencing Consortium. Initial sequencing and analysis of the human genome. *Nature*. 2001;409:860–921. Erratum in: *Nature* 2001;412:565; *Nature* 2001;411:720.

57. **Chan EK, Rowe HC, Hansen BG, et al.** The complex genetic architecture of the metabolome. *PLoS Genet* 2010;6:e1001198.

58. **Knudson AG Jr.** Mutation and cancer: statistical study of retinoblastoma. *Proc Natl Acad Sci U S A* 1971;68:820–823.

59. **Vogelstein B, Kinzler KW.** Cancer genes and the pathways they control. *Nat Med* 2004;10:789–799.

60. **Berends MJ, Wu Y, Sijmons RH, et al.** Toward new strategies to select young endometrial cancer patients for mismatch repair gene mutation analysis. *J Clin Oncol* 2003;21:4364–4370.

61. **King MC, Marks JH, Mandell JB.** Breast and ovarian cancer risks due to inherited mutations in BRCA1 and BRCA2. *Science* 2003;302:643–646.

62. **Sherr CJ.** Principles of tumor suppression. *Cell* 2004;116:235–246.

63. **Kmet LM, Cook LS, Magliocco AM.** A review of p53 expression and mutation in human benign, low malignant potential, and invasive epithelial ovarian tumors. *Cancer* 2003;97:389–404.

64. **Drake AC, Campbell H, Porteous ME, et al.** The contribution of DNA mismatch repair gene defects to the burden of gynecological cancer. *Int J Gynecol Cancer* 2003;13:262–277.

65. **Baker VV.** Update on the molecular carcinogenesis of cervix cancer. *Clin Consult Obstet Gynecol* 1995;7:86–93.

66. **Hogdall EV, Christensen L, Kjaer SK, et al.** Distribution of HER-2 overexpression in ovarian carcinoma tissue and its prognostic value in patients with ovarian carcinoma: from the Danish MALOVA Ovarian Cancer Study. *Cancer* 2003;98:66–73.

67. **Boyd J, Sonoda Y, Federici MG, et al.** Clinicopathologic features of BRCA-linked and sporadic ovarian cancer. *JAMA* 2000;283:2260–2265.

68. **Bacolod MD, Schemmann GS, Giardina SF, et al.** Emerging paradigms in cancer genetics: some important findings from high-density single nucleotide polymorphism array studies. *Cancer Res* 2009;69:723–727.

69. **Goode EL, Maurer MJ, Sellers TA, et al.** Inherited determinants of ovarian cancer survival. *Clin Cancer Res* 2010;16:995–1007.

70. **Notaridou M, Quaye L, Dafou D, et al.** The Australian Ovarian Cancer Study Group/Australian Cancer Study (Ovarian Cancer). Common alleles in candidate susceptibility genes associated with risk and development of epithelial ovarian cancer. *Int J Cancer* 2011;128: 2063–2074.

71. **The Cancer Genome Atlas.** Available at: http://en.wikipedia.org/wiki/The_Cancer_Genome_Atlas. Accessed April 28, 2011.

72. **Cancer Genome Atlas Research Network.** Comprehensive genomic characterization defines human glioblastoma genes and core pathways. *Nature* 2008;455:1061–1068.

73. **Verhaak RG, Hoadley KA, Purdom E, et al.** Integrated genomic analysis identifies clinically relevant subtypes of glioblastoma characterized by abnormalities in PDGFRA, IDH1, EGFR, and NF1. *Cancer Cell* 2010;17:98–110

74. **National Cancer Institute.** The Cancer Genome Atlas. Available at: http://cancergenome.nih.gov./ Accessed April 28, 2011.

75. **Boyer CM, Knapp RC, Bast RC Jr.** Biology and immunology. In: **Berek JS, Hacker NF, eds.** *Practical gynecologic oncology,* 2nd ed. Baltimore, MD: Williams & Wilkins, 1994:75–115.

76. **Kohler G, Milstein C.** Continuous cultures of fused cells secreting antibody of predefined specificity. *Nature* 1978;256:495–497.

77. **Di Giovine FS, Duff GW.** Interleukin 1: the first interleukin. *Immunol Today* 1990;11:13–20.

78. **Hirano T, Akira S, Taga T, et al.** Biological and clinical aspects of interleukin 6. *Immunol Today* 1990;11:443–449.

79. **Watson JM, Sensintaffar JL, Berek JS, et al.** Epithelial ovarian cancer cells constitutively produce interleukin-6 (IL-6). *Cancer Res* 1990;50:6959–6965.

80. **Berek JS, Chang C, Kaldi K, et al.** Serum interleukin-6 levels correlate with disease status in patients with epithelial ovarian cancer. *Am J Obstet Gynecol* 1991;164:1038–1043.

81. **Miki S, Iwano M, Miki Y, et al.** Interleukin-6 (IL-6) functions as an in vitro autocrine growth factor in renal cell carcinomas. *FEBS Lett* 1989;250:607–610.

82. **Wu S, Rodabaugh K, Martínez-Maza O, et al.** Stimulation of ovarian tumor cell proliferation with monocyte products including interleukin-1, interleukin-6 and tumor necrosis factor-α. *Am J Obstet Gynecol* 1992;166:997–1007.

83. **Martínez-Maza O, Berek JS.** Interkeukin-6 and cancer treatment. *In Vivo* 1991;5:583.

84. **Mule JJ, McIntosh JK, Jablons DM, et al.** Antitumor activity of recombinant interleukin-6 in mice. *J Exp Med* 1990;171:629–636.

85. **Fiorentino DF, Bond MW, Mosmann TR.** Two types of mouse helper T cells. IV. $T_H 2$ clones secrete a factor that inhibits cytokine production by $T_H 1$ clones. *J Exp Med* 1989;170:2081–2095.

86. **Mosmann TR, Moore KW.** The role IL-10 in cross regulation of $T_H 1$ and $T_H 2$ responses. *Immunol Today* 1991;12:A49–53.

87. **Del Prete GF, De Carli M, Ricci M, et al.** Helper activity for immunoglobulin synthesis of T helper type 1 ($T_H 1$) and $T_H 2$ human T cell clones: the help of $T_H 1$ clones is limited by their cytolytic capacity. *J Exp Med* 1991;174:809–813.

88. **Romagnani S.** Human $T_H 1$ and $T_H 2$ subsets: doubt no more. *Immunol Today* 1991;12:256–257.

89. **Zlotnik A, Moore KW.** Interleukin-10. *Cytokine* 1991;3:366–371.

90. **Fiorentino DF, Zlotnik A, Mosmann TR, et al.** IL-10 inhibits cytokine production by activated macrophages. *J Immunol* 1991;147: 3815–3822.

91. **Bogdan C, Vodovotz Y, Nathan C.** Macrophage deactivation by IL-10. *J Exp Med* 1991;174:1549–1555.

92. **de Waal Malefyt R, Abrams J, Bennett B, et al.** Interleukin-10 (IL-10) inhibits cytokine synthesis by human monocytes: an autoregulatory role of IL-10 produced by monocytes. *J Exp Med* 1991;174:1209–1220.

93. **Weaver CT, Harrington LE, Mangan PR, et al.** Th17: an effector CD4 T cell lineage with regulatory T cell ties. *Immunity* 2006;24: 677–688.

94. **Katsifis GE, Moutsopoulos NM, Wahl SM.** (2007) T lymphocytes in Sjogren's syndrome: contributors to and regulators of pathophysiology. *Clin Rev Allergy Immunol* 2007;32:252–264.

95. **Korn T, Oukka M, Kuchroo V, et al.** Th17 cells: effector T cells with inflammatory properties. *Semin Immunol* 2007;19:362–371.

96. **Stockinger B, Veldhoen M.** Differentiation and function of Th17 T cells. *Curr Opin Immunol* 2007;19:281–286.

97. **Ouyang M, Garnett AT, Han TM, et al.** A web based resource characterizing the zebrafish developmental profile of over 16,000 transcripts. *Gene Expr Patterns* 2008;8:171–180.

98. **Romagnani S.** Human Th17 cells. *Arthritis Res Ther* 2008;10: 206.

99. **Sakaguchi S, Sakaguchi N, Shimizu J, et al.** Immunologic tolerance maintained by CD25+ CD4+ regulatory T cells: their common role in controlling autoimmunity, tumor immunity, and transplantation tolerance. *Immunol Rev* 2001;182:18–32.

100. **Shevach EM.** CD4+ CD25+ suppressor T cells: more questions than answers. *Nat Rev Immunol* 2002;2:389–400.

101. **Berek JS.** Epithelial ovarian cancer. In: **Berek JS, Hacker NF, eds.** *Practical gynecologic oncology*, 2nd ed. Baltimore, MD: Williams & Wilkins, 1994:327–375.

102. **Gotlieb WH, Abrams JS, Watson JM, et al.** Presence of IL-10 in the ascites of patients with ovarian and other intraabdominal cancers. *Cytokine* 1992;4:385–390.

103. **Watson JM, Gotlieb WH, Abrams JH, et al.** Cytokine profiles in ascitic fluid from patients with ovarian cancer: relationship to levels of acute phase proteins and immunoglobulins, immunosuppression and tumor classification. *J Soc Gynecol Invest* 1993;186:8.

104. **Rosenberg SA.** Immunotherapy of cancer by systemic administration of lymphoid cells plus interleukin-2. *J Biol Response Mod* 1984;3:501–511.

105. **Rosenberg SA, Lotze MT.** Cancer immunotherapy using interleukin-2 and interleukin-2–activated lymphocytes. *Annu Rev Immunol* 1986;4:681–709.

106. **Rosenberg SA, Lotze MT, Muul LM, et al.** Observations on the systemic administration of autologous lymphokine-activated killer cells and recombinant interleukin-2 to patients with metastatic cancer. *N Engl J Med* 1985;313:1485–1492.

107. **Cappuccini F, Yamamoto RS, DiSaia PJ, et al.** Identification of tumor necrosis factor and lymphotoxin blocking factor(s) in the ascites of patients with advanced and recurrent ovarian cancer. *Lymphokine Cytokine Res* 1991;10:225–229.

108. **Rosenberg SA, Lotze MT, Muul LM, et al.** A progress report on the treatment of 157 patients with advanced cancer using lymphokine-activated killer cells and interleukin-2 or high-dose interleukin-2 alone. *N Engl J Med* 1987;316:889–897.

109. **West WH, Tauer KW, Yannelli JR, et al.** Constant-infusion recombinant interleukin-2 in adoptive immunotherapy of advanced cancer. *N Engl J Med* 1987;316:898–905.

110. **Berek JS.** Intraperitoneal adoptive immunotherapy for peritoneal cancer. *J Clin Oncol* 1990;8:1610–1612.

111. **Topalian SL, Solomon D, Avis FP, et al.** Immunotherapy of patients with advanced cancer using tumor-infiltrating lymphocytes and recombinant interleukin-2: a pilot study. *J Clin Oncol* 1988;6:839–853.

112. **Lotzova E.** Role of human circulating and tumor-infiltrating lymphocytes in cancer defense and treatment. *Nat Immunol* 1990;9:253–264.

113. **Garrido MA, Valdayo MJ, Winkler DF, et al.** Targeting human T lymphocytes with bispecific antibodies to react against human ovarian carcinoma cells growing in nu/nu mice. *Cancer Res* 1990;50:4227–4232.

114. **Bookman MA, Berek JS.** Biologic and immunologic therapy of ovarian cancer. *Hematol Oncol Clin North Am* 1992;6:941–965.

115. **Zighelboim J, Nio Y, Berek JS, et al.** Immunologic control of ovarian cancer. *Nat Immunol* 1988;7:216–225.

116. **Berek JS, Martínez-Maza O, Montz FJ.** The immune system and gynecologic cancer. In: **Coppelson M, Tattersall M, Morrow CP, eds.** *Gynecologic oncology.* Edinburgh, Scotland: Churchill Livingstone, 1992:119.

117. **Berek JS, Lichtenstein AK, Knox RM, et al.** Synergistic effects of combination sequential immunotherapies in a murine ovarian cancer model. *Cancer Res* 1985;45:4215–4218.

118. **Newell GR, Spitz MR, Sider JG.** Cancer and age. *Semin Oncol* 1989;16:3–9.

119. **Maher VM, Yang JL, Mah MC, et al.** Comparing the frequency of and spectra of mutations induced when an SV-40–based shuttle vector containing covalently bound residues of structurally-related carcinogens replicates in human cells. *Mutat Res* 1989;220:83–92.

120. **National Research Council.** *Health effects of exposure to low levels of ionizing radiation (BEIR V).* Washington, DC: National Academy Press, 1990.

121. **Yancik R.** *Perspectives on prevention and treatment of cancer in the elderly.* New York: Raven Press, 1983.

7

Reproductive Physiology

David L. Olive
Steven F. Palter

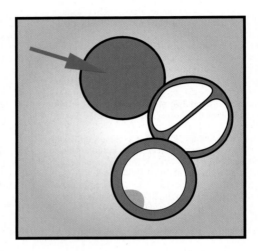

- **The female reproductive process involves the central nervous system (primarily hypothalamus), the pituitary gland, the ovary, and the uterus (endometrium). All must function appropriately for normal reproduction to occur.**

- **Hypothalamic gonadotropin-releasing hormone (GnRH) simultaneously regulates both luteinizing hormone (LH) and follicle-stimulating hormone (FSH) in the pituitary by being secreted in a pulsatile manner. The pulse frequency determines the relative amounts of LH and FSH secretion.**

- **The ovary responds to FSH and LH in a defined, sequential manner to produce follicular growth, ovulation, and corpus luteum formation. The cycle is designed to produce an optimal environment for pregnancy; if pregnancy does not occur, the cycle begins again.**

- **In the early menstrual cycle the ovary produces estrogen, which is responsible for endometrial growth. Following ovulation, progesterone is also produced in significant quantities, which transforms the endometrium into a form ideal for implantation of the embryo. If no pregnancy occurs, the ovary ceases to produce estrogen and progesterone, the endometrium is sloughed, and the cycle begins again.**

The reproductive process in women is a complex and highly evolved interaction of many components. The carefully orchestrated series of events that contributes to a normal ovulatory menstrual cycle requires precise timing and regulation of hormonal input from the central nervous system, the pituitary gland, and the ovary. This delicately balanced process can be disrupted easily and result in reproductive failure, which is a major clinical issue confronting gynecologists. To manage effectively such conditions, it is critical that gynecologists understand the normal physiology of the menstrual cycle. The anatomic structures, hormonal components, and interactions between the two play a vital role in the function of the reproductive system. Fitting together the various pieces of this intricate puzzle will provide "the big picture": an overview of how the reproductive system of women is designed to function.

Neuroendocrinology

Neuroendocrinology represents facets of two traditional fields of medicine: endocrinology, which is the study of hormones (i.e., substances secreted into the bloodstream that have diverse actions at sites remote from the point of secretion), and neuroscience, which is the study of the action of neurons. The discovery of neurons that transmit impulses and secrete their products into the vascular system to function as hormones, a process known as neurosecretion, demonstrates that the two systems are intimately linked. For instance, the menstrual cycle is regulated through the feedback of hormones on the neural tissue of the central nervous system (CNS).

Anatomy

Hypothalamus

The hypothalamus is a small neural structure situated at the base of the brain above the optic chiasm and below the third ventricle (Fig. 7.1). It is connected directly to the pituitary gland and is the part of the brain that is the source of many pituitary secretions. Anatomically, the hypothalamus is divided into three zones: *periventricular* (adjacent to the third ventricle), *medial* (primarily cell bodies), and *lateral* (primarily axonal). Each zone is further subdivided into structures known as nuclei, which represent locations of concentrations of similar types of neuronal cell bodies (Fig. 7.2).

The hypothalamus is not an isolated structure within the CNS; instead, it has multiple interconnections with other regions in the brain. In addition to the well-known pathways of hypothalamic output to the pituitary, there are numerous less well-characterized pathways of output to diverse regions of the brain, including the limbic system (amygdala and hippocampus), the thalamus, and the pons (1). Many of these pathways form feedback loops to areas supplying neural input to the hypothalamus.

Several levels of feedback to the hypothalamus exist and are known as the long, short, and ultrashort feedback loops. The **long feedback loop** is composed of endocrine input from

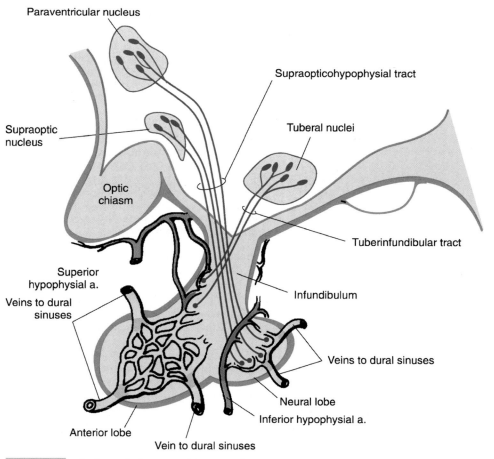

Figure 7.1   The hypothalamus and its neurologic connections to the pituitary.

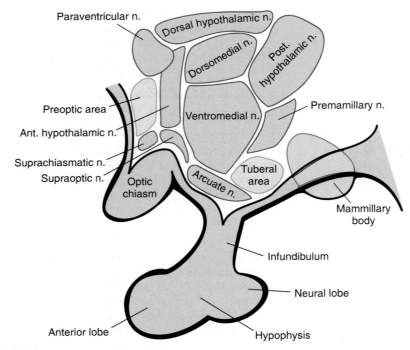

Figure 7.2   **The neuronal cell bodies of the hypothalamus.**

circulating hormones, just as feedback of androgens and estrogens onto steroid receptors is present in the hypothalamus (2,3). Similarly, pituitary hormones may feed back to the hypothalamus and serve important regulatory functions in **short-loop feedback.** Finally, hypothalamic secretions may directly feed back to the hypothalamus itself in an **ultrashort feedback loop.**

The major secretory products of the hypothalamus are the pituitary-releasing factors (Fig. 7.3):

1. *Gonadotropin-releasing hormone (GnRH),* **which controls the secretion of** *luteinizing hormone (LH)* **and** *follicle-stimulating hormone (FSH)*

2. *Corticotropin-releasing hormone (CRH),* **which controls the release of** *adrenocorticotrophic hormone (ACTH)*

3. *Growth hormone–releasing hormone (GHRH),* **which regulates the release of** *growth hormone (GH)*

4. *Thyrotropin-releasing hormone (TRH),* **which regulates the secretion of** *thyroid-stimulating hormone (TSH)*

The hypothalamus is the source of all neurohypophyseal hormone production. The neural posterior pituitary can be viewed as a direct extension of the hypothalamus connected by the fingerlike infundibular stalk. The capillaries in the median eminence differ from those in other regions of the brain. Unlike the usual tight junctions that exist between adjacent capillary endothelial lining cells, the capillaries in this region are fenestrated in the same manner as capillaries outside the CNS. As a result, there is no blood–brain barrier in the median eminence.

Pituitary

The pituitary is divided into three regions or lobes: *anterior, intermediate,* and *posterior.* The *anterior pituitary (adenohypophysis)* is quite different structurally from the *posterior neural pituitary (neurohypophysis),* which is a direct physical extension of the hypothalamus. The adenohypophysis is derived embryologically from epidermal ectoderm from an infolding of Rathke's pouch. Therefore, it is not composed of neural tissue, as is the posterior pituitary, and does not have direct neural connections to the hypothalamus. Instead, a unique anatomic relationship exists that combines elements of neural production and endocrine secretion. The adenohypophysis itself has no direct arterial blood supply. Its major source of blood flow is

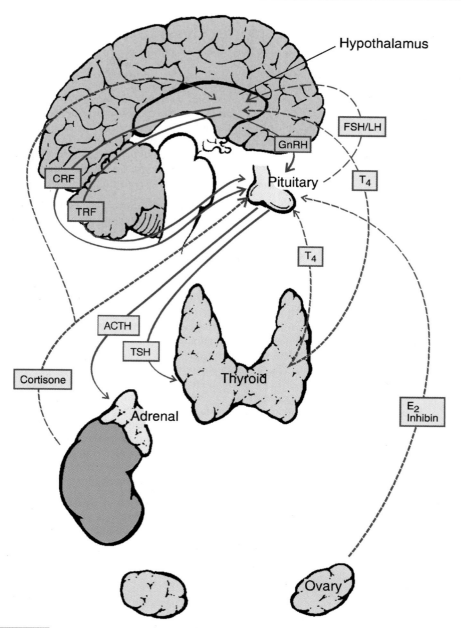

Figure 7.3 The hypothalamic secretory products function as pituitary-releasing factors that control the endocrine function of the ovaries, the thyroid, and the adrenal glands.

also its source of hypothalamic input—the portal vessels. Blood flow in these portal vessels is primarily from the hypothalamus to the pituitary. Blood is supplied to the posterior pituitary via the superior, middle, and inferior hypophyseal arteries. In contrast, the anterior pituitary has no direct arterial blood supply. Instead, it receives blood via a rich capillary plexus of the portal vessels that originates in the median eminence of the hypothalamus and descends along the pituitary stalk. This pattern is not absolute, however, and retrograde blood flow has occurred (4). This blood flow, combined with the location of the median eminence outside the blood–brain barrier, permits bidirectional feedback control between the two structures.

The specific secretory cells of the anterior pituitary are classified based on their hematoxylin- and eosin-staining patterns. Acidophilic-staining cells primarily secrete GH and prolactin and, to a variable degree, ACTH (5). The gonadotropins are secreted by basophilic cells, and TSH is secreted by the neutral-staining chromophobes.

141

Reproductive Hormones

Hypothalamus

Gonadotropin-Releasing Hormone

GnRH (also called luteinizing hormone–releasing hormone, or LHRH) **is the controlling factor for gonadotropin secretion** (6). It is a decapeptide produced by neurons with cell bodies primarily in the arcuate nucleus of the hypothalamus (7–9) (Fig. 7.4). Embryologically, these neurons originate in the olfactory pit and then migrate to their adult locations (10). These GnRH-secreting neurons project axons that terminate on the portal vessels at the median eminence where GnRH is secreted for delivery to the anterior pituitary. Less clear in function are multiple other secondary projections of GnRH neurons to locations within the CNS.

The gene that encodes GnRH produces a 92 amino acid precursor protein, which contains the GnRH decapeptide and a 56 amino acid peptide known as GnRH-associated peptide (GAP). The GAP is a potent inhibitor of prolactin secretion and a stimulator of gonadotropin release.

Pulsatile Secretion

GnRH is unique among releasing hormones in that it simultaneously regulates the secretion of two hormones—FSH and LH. It also is unique among the body's hormones because it must be secreted in a pulsatile fashion to be effective, and the pulsatile release of GnRH influences the release of the two gonadotropins (11–13). Using animals that had undergone electrical destruction of the arcuate nucleus and had no detectable levels of gonadotropins, a series of experiments were performed with varying dosages and intervals of GnRH infusion (13,14). Continual infusions did not result in gonadotropin secretion, whereas a pulsatile pattern led to physiologic secretion patterns and follicular growth. Continual exposure of the pituitary gonadotroph to GnRH results in a phenomenon called *down-regulation*, through which the number of gonadotroph cell surface GnRH receptors is decreased (15). Similarly, intermittent exposure to GnRH will "up-regulate" or "autoprime" the gonadotroph to increase its number of GnRH receptors (16). This allows the cell to have a greater response to subsequent GnRH exposure. Similar to the intrinsic electrical pacemaker cells of the heart, this action most likely represents an intrinsic property of the GnRH-secreting neuron, although it is subject to modulation by various neuronal and hormonal inputs to the hypothalamus.

The continual pulsatile secretion of GnRH is necessary because GnRH has an extremely short half-life (only 2–4 minutes) as a result of rapid proteolytic cleavage. The pulsatile secretion of GnRH varies in both frequency and amplitude throughout the menstrual cycle and is tightly regulated (17,18) (Fig. 7.5). The follicular phase is characterized by frequent, small-amplitude pulses of GnRH secretion. In the late follicular phase, there is an increase in both frequency and amplitude of pulses. During the luteal phase, however, there is a progressive lengthening of the interval between pulses. The amplitude in the luteal phase is higher than that in the follicular phase, but it declines progressively over the 2 weeks. This variation in pulse frequency allows for variation in both LH and FSH throughout the menstrual cycle. For example, decreasing the pulse frequency of GnRH decreases LH secretion but increases FSH, an important aspect of enhancing FSH availability in the late luteal phase. The pulse frequency is not the sole determinant of pituitary response; additional hormonal influences, such as those exerted by ovarian peptides and sex steroids, can modulate the GnRH effect.

Although GnRH is primarily involved in endocrine regulation of gonadotropin secretion from the pituitary, it is apparent that this molecule has autocrine and paracrine functions throughout the body. The decapeptide is found in both neural and nonneural tissues; receptors are present in many extrapituitary structures, including the ovary and placenta. Data suggest that GnRH may be involved in regulating human chorionic gonadotropin (hCG) secretion and implantation, as well as in decreasing cell proliferation and mediating apoptosis in tumor cells (19). The role of GnRH in the extrapituitary sites remains to be fully elucidated.

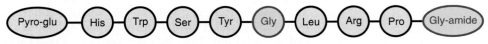

Figure 7.4   Gonadotropin-releasing hormone is a decapeptide.

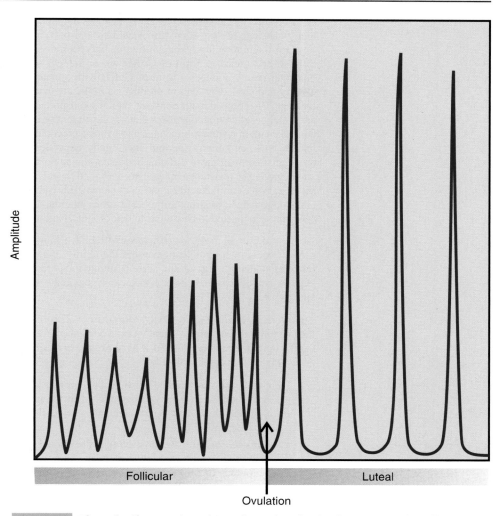

Figure 7.5   The pulsatile secretion of gonadotropin-releasing hormone in the follicular and luteal phases of the cycle.

Gonadotropin-Releasing Hormone Agonists

Mechanism of Action   Used clinically, GnRH agonists are modifications of the native molecule to either increase receptor affinity or decrease degradation (20). Their use leads to a persistent activation of GnRH receptors, as if continuous GnRH exposure existed. As would be predicted by the constant GnRH infusion experiments, this leads to suppression of gonadotropin secretion. An initial release of gonadotropins is followed by a profound suppression of secretion. The initial release of gonadotropins represents the secretion of pituitary stores in response to receptor binding and activation. With continued activation of the gonadotroph GnRH receptor, however, there is a down-regulation effect and a decrease in the concentration of GnRH receptors. As a result, gonadotropin secretion decreases and sex steroid production falls to castrate levels (21).

Additional modification of the GnRH molecule results in an analogue that has no intrinsic activity but competes with GnRH for the same receptor site (22). These GnRH antagonists produce a competitive blockade of GnRH receptors, preventing stimulation by endogenous GnRH and causing an immediate fall in gonadotropin and sex steroid secretion (23). The clinical effect is observed within 24 to 72 hours. Moreover, antagonists may not function solely as competitive inhibitors; evidence suggests they may also produce down-regulation of GnRH receptors, further contributing to the loss of gonadotropin activity (24).

Structure—Agonists and Antagonists   As a peptide hormone, GnRH is degraded by enzymatic cleavage of bonds between its amino acids. Pharmacologic alterations of the structure of GnRH led to the creation of agonists and antagonists (Fig. 7.4). The primary sites of enzymatic cleavage are between amino acids 5 and 6, 6 and 7, and 9 and 10. Substitution of the position-6 amino acid glycine with large bulky amino acid analogues makes degradation more difficult and creates a form of GnRH with a relatively long half-life. Substitution at the carboxyl terminus produces a form of GnRH with increased receptor affinity. The resulting high affinity and slow degradation produces a molecule that mimics continuous exposure to native GnRH (20). Thus, as with constant GnRH exposure, down-regulation occurs. GnRH agonists are widely used to treat disorders that are dependent on ovarian hormones (21). They are used to control ovulation induction cycles and to treat precocious puberty, ovarian hyperandrogenism, leiomyomas, endometriosis, and hormonally dependent cancers. The development of GnRH antagonists proved more difficult because a molecule was needed that maintained the binding and degradation resistance of agonists but failed to activate the receptor. Early attempts involved modification of amino acids 1 and 2, as well as those previously utilized for agonists. Commercial antagonists have structural modifications at amino acids 1, 2, 3, 6, 8, and 10. The treatment spectrum is expected to be similar to that of GnRH agonists, but with more rapid onset of action.

Nonpeptide, small molecule structures with high affinity for the GnRH receptor were developed (25). These compounds demonstrated the ability to suppress the reproductive axis in a dose-related manner via oral administration, unlike the parenteral approach required with traditional peptide analogues (26). Investigation may elucidate an expanded therapeutic role for these antagonists.

Endogenous Opioids and Effects on GnRH   The endogenous opioids are three related families of naturally occurring substances produced in the CNS that represent the natural ligands for the opioid receptors (27–29). **There are three major classes of endogenous opioids**, each derived from precursor molecules:

1. *Endorphins* are named for their endogenous morphinelike activity. These substances are produced in the hypothalamus from the precursor proopiomelanocortin (POMC) and have diverse activities, including regulation of temperature, appetite, mood, and behavior (30).

2. *Enkephalins* are the most widely distributed opioid peptides in the brain, and they function primarily in regulation of the autonomic nervous system. Proenkephalin A is the precursor for the two enkephalins of primary importance: methionine–enkephalin and leucine–enkephalin.

3. *Dynorphins* are endogenous opioids produced from the precursor proenkephalin B that serve a function similar to that of the endorphins, producing behavioral effects and exhibiting a high analgesic potency.

The endogenous opioids play a significant role in the regulation of hypothalamic–pituitary function. Endorphins appear to inhibit GnRH release within the hypothalamus, resulting in inhibition of gonadotropin secretion (31). Ovarian sex steroids can increase the secretion of central endorphins, further depressing gonadotropin levels (32).

Endorphin levels vary significantly throughout the menstrual cycle, with peak levels in the luteal phase and a nadir during menses (33). This inherent variability, although helping to regulate gonadotropin levels, may contribute to cycle-specific symptoms experienced by ovulatory women. For example, the dysphoria experienced by some women in the premenstrual phase of the cycle may be related to a withdrawal of endogenous opiates (34).

Pituitary Hormone Secretion

Anterior Pituitary

The anterior pituitary is responsible for the secretion of the major hormone-releasing factors—FSH, LH, TSH, and ACTH—as well as GH and prolactin. Each hormone is released by a specific pituitary cell type.

Gonadotropins

The gonadotropins FSH and LH are produced by the anterior pituitary gonadotroph cells and are responsible for ovarian follicular stimulation. Structurally, there is great similarity between FSH and LH (Fig. 7.6). They are both glycoproteins that share identical α subunits

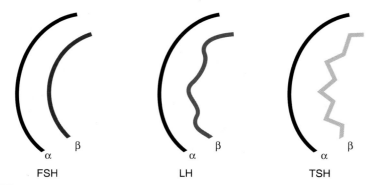

Figure 7.6   **The structural similarity between follicle-stimulating hormone (FSH), luteinizing hormone (LH), and thyroid-stimulating hormone (TSH).** The α subunits are identical, and the β subunits differ.

and differ only in the structure of their β subunits, which confer receptor specificity (35,36). The synthesis of the β subunits is the rate-regulating step in gonadotropin biosynthesis (37). Thyroid-stimulating hormone and placental hCG also share identical α subunits with the gonadotropins. There are several forms of each gonadotropin, which differ in carbohydrate content as a result of posttranslation modification. The degree of modification varies with steroid levels and is an important regulator of gonadotropin bioactivity.

Prolactin

Prolactin, **a 198–amino acid polypeptide secreted by the anterior pituitary lactotroph, is the primary trophic factor responsible for the synthesis of milk by the breast** (38). Several forms of this hormone, which are named according to their size and bioactivity, are normally secreted (39). Prolactin gene transcription is principally stimulated by estrogen; other hormones promoting transcription are TRH and a variety of growth factors.

Prolactin secretion is under tonic inhibitory control by the hypothalamic secretion of dopamine (40). Therefore, disease states characterized by decreased dopamine secretion or any condition that interrupts transport of dopamine down the infundibular stalk to the pituitary gland will result in increased synthesis of prolactin. In this respect, prolactin is unique in comparison with all other pituitary hormones: It is predominantly under tonic inhibition, and release of control produces an increase in secretion. **Clinically, increased prolactin levels are associated with amenorrhea and galactorrhea, and hyperprolactinemia should be suspected in any individual with symptoms of either of these conditions.**

Although prolactin appears to be primarily under inhibitory control, many stimuli can elicit its release, including breast manipulation, drugs, stress, exercise, and certain foods. Hormones that may stimulate prolactin release include TRH, vasopressin, γ-aminobutyric acid (GABA), dopamine, β-endorphin, vasoactive intestinal peptide (VIP), epidermal growth factor, angiotensin II, and possibly GnRH (41–43). The relative contributions of these substances under normal conditions remain to be determined.

Thyroid-Stimulating Hormone, Adrenocorticotropic Hormone, and Growth Hormone

The other hormones produced by the anterior pituitary are TSH, ACTH, and GH. Thyroid-stimulating hormone is secreted by the pituitary thyrotrophs in response to TRH. As with GnRH, TRH is synthesized primarily in the arcuate nucleus of the hypothalamus and is secreted into the portal circulation for transport to the pituitary. In addition to stimulating TSH release, TRH is a major stimulus for the release of prolactin. Thyroid-stimulating hormone stimulates release of T_3 and T_4 from the thyroid gland, which in turn has a negative feedback effect on pituitary TSH secretion. Abnormalities of thyroid secretion (both hyper- and hypothyroidism) are frequently associated with ovulatory dysfunction as a result of diverse actions on the hypothalamic–pituitary–ovarian axis (44).

Adrenocorticotrophic hormone is secreted by the anterior pituitary in response to another hypothalamic-releasing factor, CRH, and stimulates the release of adrenal glucocorticoids.

Unlike the other anterior pituitary products, ACTH secretion has a diurnal variation with an early morning peak and a late evening nadir. As with the other pituitary hormones, ACTH secretion is negatively regulated by feedback from its primary end product, which in this case is cortisol.

The anterior pituitary hormone that is secreted in the greatest absolute amount is GH. It is secreted in response to the hypothalamic-releasing factor, GHRH, and by thyroid hormone and glucocorticoids. This hormone is secreted in a pulsatile fashion but with peak release occurring during sleep. In addition to its vital role in the stimulation of linear growth, GH plays a diverse role in physiologic hemostasis. The hormone plays a role in bone mitogenesis, CNS function (improved memory, cognition, and mood), body composition, breast development, and cardiovascular function. It also affects insulin regulation and acts anabolically. Growth hormone appears to have a role in the regulation of ovarian function, although the degree to which it serves this role in normal physiology is unclear (45).

Posterior Pituitary

Structure and Function

The posterior pituitary (neurohypophysis) is composed exclusively of neural tissue and is a direct extension of the hypothalamus. It lies directly adjacent to the adenohypophysis but is embryologically distinct, derived from an invagination of neuroectodermal tissue in the third ventricle. Axons in the posterior pituitary originate from neurons with cell bodies in two distinct regions of the hypothalamus, the supraoptic and paraventricular nuclei, named for their anatomic relationship to the optic chiasm and the third ventricle. Together these two nuclei compose the hypothalamic magnocellular system. These neurons can secrete their synthetic products directly from axonal boutons into the general circulation to act as hormones. This is the mechanism of secretion of the hormones of the posterior pituitary, oxytocin and arginine vasopressin (AVP). Although this is the primary mode of release for these hormones, numerous other secondary pathways were identified, including secretion into the portal circulation, intrahypothalamic secretion, and secretion into other regions of the CNS (46).

In addition to the established functions of oxytocin and vasopressin, several other diverse roles were suggested in animal models. These functions include modulation of sexual activity and appetite, learning and memory consolidation, temperature regulation, and regulation of maternal behaviors (47). In the human, these neuropeptides were linked to social attachment (48–50). Receptor variants for these two molecules were linked to the spectrum of autistic disorders, suggesting that proper function of these two neuropeptides with their receptors is required for positive group interactive behavior. This relationship is strengthened by a strong association between altruistic behavior and the length of the AVP-1a receptor promoter region (51). It is both surprising and humbling that complex human behaviors may be partially explained by such a relatively simple neuropeptide system. Continuing investigation should help elucidate this physiology and potential therapeutic interventions.

Oxytocin   **Oxytocin is a 9–amino acid peptide primarily produced by the paraventricular nucleus of the hypothalamus** (Fig. 7.7). The primary function of this hormone in humans is the stimulation of two specific types of muscular contractions (Fig. 7.8). The first type, uterine muscular contraction, occurs during parturition. The second type of muscular contraction regulated by oxytocin is breast lactiferous duct myoepithelial contractions, which occur during the milk letdown reflex. Oxytocin release may be stimulated by suckling, triggered by a signal from nipple stimulation transmitted via thoracic nerves to the spinal cord and then to the hypothalamus, where oxytocin is released in an episodic fashion (45). Oxytocin release also may be triggered by olfactory, auditory, and visual clues, and it may play a role in the conditioned reflex in nursing animals. Stimulation of the cervix and vagina can cause significant release of oxytocin, which may trigger reflex ovulation (the Ferguson reflex) in some species.

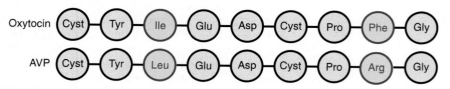

Figure 7.7 **Oxytocin and arginine-vasopressin (AVP) are 9–amino acid peptides produced by the hypothalamus.** They differ in only two amino acids.

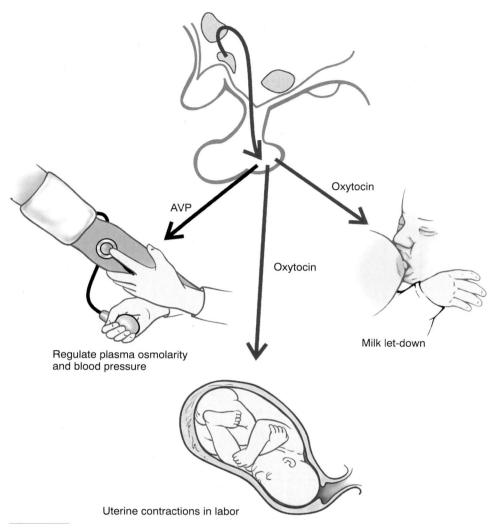

Oxytocin

AVP

Oxytocin

Milk let-down

Regulate plasma osmolarity
and blood pressure

Uterine contractions in labor

Figure 7.8   Oxytocin stimulates muscular contractions of the uterus during parturition and the breast lactiferous duct during the milk letdown reflex. Arginine-vasopressin (AVP) regulates circulating blood volume, pressure, and osmolality.

Arginine Vasopressin   **Also known as antidiuretic hormone (ADH), AVP is the second major secretory product of the posterior pituitary** (Fig. 7.7). It is synthesized primarily by neurons with cell bodies in the supraoptic nuclei (Fig. 7.8). Its major function is the regulation of circulating blood volume, pressure, and osmolality (52). Specific receptors throughout the body can trigger the release of AVP. Osmoreceptors located in the hypothalamus sense changes in blood osmolality from a mean of 285 mOSM/kg. Baroceptors sense changes in blood pressure caused by alterations in blood volume and are peripherally located in the walls of the left atrium, carotid sinus, and aortic arch (53). These receptors can respond to changes in blood volume of more than 10%. In response to decreases in blood pressure or volume, AVP is released and causes arteriolar vasoconstriction and renal free-water conservation. This in turn leads to a decrease in blood osmolality and an increase in blood pressure. Activation of the renal renin–angiotensin system can also activate AVP release.

Menstrual Cycle Physiology

In the normal menstrual cycle, orderly cyclic hormone production and parallel proliferation of the uterine lining prepare for implantation of the embryo. Disorders of the

menstrual cycle and, likewise, disorders of menstrual physiology, may lead to various pathologic states, including infertility, recurrent miscarriage, and malignancy.

Normal Menstrual Cycle

The normal human menstrual cycle can be divided into two segments: the ovarian cycle and the uterine cycle, based on the organ under examination. The ovarian cycle may be further divided into follicular and luteal phases, whereas the uterine cycle is divided into corresponding proliferative and secretory phases (Fig. 7.9). The phases of the ovarian cycle are characterized as follows:

1. **Follicular phase**—hormonal feedback promotes the orderly development of a single dominant follicle, which should be mature at midcycle and prepared for ovulation. The

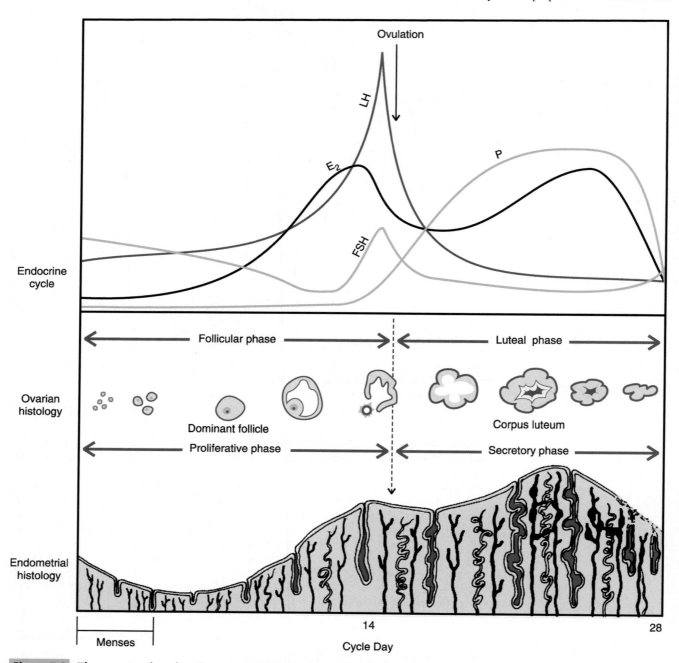

Figure 7.9 **The menstrual cycle.** The *top panel* shows the cyclic changes of follicle-stimulating hormone (FSH), luteinizing hormone (LH), estradiol (E₂), and progesterone (P) relative to the time of ovulation. The *bottom panel* correlates the ovarian cycle in the follicular and luteal phases and the endometrial cycle in the proliferative and secretory phases.

average length of the human follicular phase ranges from 10 to 14 days, and variability in this length is responsible for most variations in total cycle length.

2. **Luteal phase**—the time from ovulation to the onset of menses has an average length of 14 days.

A normal menstrual cycle lasts from 21 to 35 days, with 2 to 6 days of flow and an average blood loss of 20 to 60 mL. However, studies of large numbers of women with normal menstrual cycles showed that only approximately two-thirds of adult women have cycles lasting 21 to 35 days (54). The extremes of reproductive life (after menarche and perimenopause) are characterized by a higher percentage of anovulatory or irregularly timed cycles (55,56).

Hormonal Variations

The relative pattern of ovarian, uterine, and hormonal variation along the normal menstrual cycle is shown in Fig. 7.9.

1. **At the beginning of each monthly menstrual cycle, levels of gonadal steroids are low and have been decreasing since the end of the luteal phase of the previous cycle.**

2. **With the demise of the corpus luteum, FSH levels begin to rise, and a cohort of growing follicles is recruited.** These follicles each secrete increasing levels of estrogen as they grow in the follicular phase. The increase in estrogen, in turn, is the stimulus for uterine endometrial proliferation.

3. **Rising estrogen levels provide negative feedback on pituitary FSH secretion, which begins to wane by the midpoint of the follicular phase.** In addition, the growing follicles produce inhibin-B, which suppresses FSH secretion by the pituitary. Conversely, LH initially decreases in response to rising estradiol levels, but late in the follicular phase the LH level is increased dramatically (biphasic response).

4. **At the end of the follicular phase (just before ovulation), FSH-induced LH receptors are present on granulosa cells and, with LH stimulation, modulate the secretion of progesterone.**

5. **After a sufficient degree of estrogenic stimulation, the pituitary LH surge is triggered, which is the proximate cause of ovulation that occurs 24 to 36 hours later.** Ovulation heralds the transition to the luteal–secretory phase.

6. **The estrogen level decreases through the early luteal phase from just before ovulation until the midluteal phase, when it begins to rise again as a result of corpus luteum secretion.** Similarly, inhibin-A is secreted by the corpus luteum.

7. **Progesterone levels rise precipitously after ovulation and can be used as a presumptive sign that ovulation has occurred.**

8. **Progesterone, estrogen, and inhibin-A act centrally to suppress gonadotropin secretion and new follicular growth.** These hormones remain elevated through the lifespan of the corpus luteum and then wane with its demise, thereby setting the stage for the next cycle.

Uterus

Cyclic Changes of the Endometrium

In 1950, Noyes, Hertig, and Rock described the cyclic histologic changes in the adult human endometrium (57) (Fig. 7.10). These changes proceed in an orderly fashion in response to cyclic hormonal production by the ovaries (Fig. 7.9). Histologic cycling of the endometrium can best be viewed in two parts: the endometrial glands and the surrounding stroma. **The superficial two-thirds of the endometrium is the zone that proliferates and is ultimately shed with each cycle if pregnancy does not occur. This cycling portion of the endometrium is known as the *decidua functionalis* and is composed of a deeply situated intermediate zone (stratum spongiosum) and a superficial compact zone (stratum compactum). The *decidua basalis* is the deepest region of the endometrium. It does not undergo significant monthly proliferation but, instead, is the source of endometrial regeneration after each menses** (58).

The existence of endometrial stem cells was assumed but difficult to document. Researchers found a small population of human epithelial and stromal cells that possess clonogenicity, suggesting that they represent the putative endometrial stem cells (59). Further evidence of the existence of such cells, and their source, was provided by another study that showed endometrial glandular epithelial cells obtained from endometrial biopsies of women undergoing bone marrow

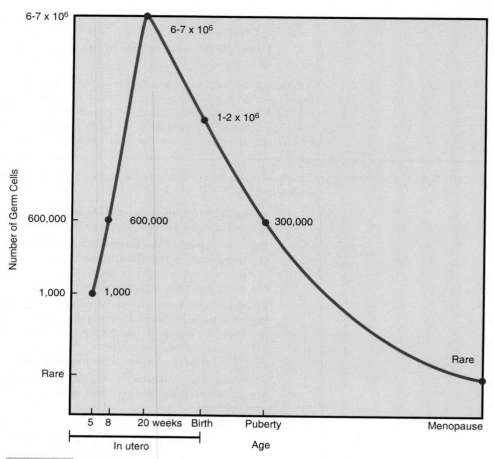

Figure 7.10   The number of oocytes in the ovary before and after birth and through menopause.

transplants, express the HLA type of the donor bone marrow (60). This finding suggests that endometrial stem cells exist, and that they reside in bone marrow and migrate to the basalis of the endometrium. Furthermore, the timing of the appearance of these cells following the transplant was as long as several years. This fact may prove to be of clinical importance in patients with Asherman syndrome who experienced a loss of functional endometrium; repair of the uterine anatomy may eventually result in a functioning endometrial cavity.

Proliferative Phase

By convention, the first day of vaginal bleeding is called day 1 of the menstrual cycle. After menses, the decidua basalis is composed of primordial glands and dense scant stroma in its location adjacent to the myometrium. The proliferative phase is characterized by progressive mitotic growth of the decidua functionalis in preparation for implantation of the embryo in response to rising circulating levels of estrogen (61). At the beginning of the proliferative phase, the endometrium is relatively thin (1–2 mm). The predominant change seen during this time is evolution of the initially straight, narrow, and short endometrial glands into longer, tortuous structures (62). Histologically, these proliferating glands have multiple mitotic cells, and their organization changes from a low columnar pattern in the early proliferative period to a pseudostratified pattern before ovulation. Throughout this time, the stroma is a dense compact layer, and vascular structures are infrequently seen.

Secretory Phase

In the typical 28-day cycle, ovulation occurs on cycle day 14. Within 48 to 72 hours following ovulation, the onset of progesterone secretion produces a shift in histologic appearance of the endometrium to the secretory phase, so named for the clear presence of eosinophilic

protein-rich secretory products in the glandular lumen. In contrast to the proliferative phase, the secretory phase of the menstrual cycle is characterized by the cellular effects of progesterone in addition to estrogen. In general, progesterone's effects are antagonistic to those of estrogen, and there is a progressive decrease in the endometrial cell's estrogen receptor concentration. As a result, during the latter half of the cycle, estrogen-induced DNA synthesis and cellular mitosis are antagonized (61).

During the secretory phase, the endometrial glands form characteristic periodic acid–Schiff positive–staining, glycogen-containing vacuoles. These vacuoles initially appear subnuclearly and then progress toward the glandular lumen (57) (Fig. 7.10). The nuclei can be seen in the midportion of the cells and ultimately undergo apocrine secretion into the glandular lumen, often by cycle day 19 or 20. At postovulatory day 6 or 7, secretory activity of the glands is generally maximal, and the endometrium is optimally prepared for implantation of the blastocyst.

The stroma of the secretory phase remains unchanged histologically until approximately the seventh postovulatory day, when there is a progressive increase in edema. Coincident with maximal stromal edema in the late secretory phase, the spiral arteries become clearly visible and then progressively lengthen and coil during the remainder of the secretory phase. By around day 24, an eosinophilic-staining pattern, known as *cuffing*, is visible in the perivascular stroma. Eosinophilia then progresses to form islands in the stroma followed by areas of confluence. This staining pattern of the edematous stroma is termed *pseudodecidual* because of its similarity to the pattern that occurs in pregnancy. Approximately 2 days before menses, there is a dramatic increase in the number of polymorphonuclear lymphocytes that migrate from the vascular system. This leukocytic infiltration heralds the collapse of the endometrial stroma and the onset of the menstrual flow.

Menses

In the absence of implantation, glandular secretion ceases and an irregular breakdown of the *decidua functionalis* occurs. The resultant shedding of this layer of the endometrium is termed *menses*. The destruction of the corpus luteum and its production of estrogen and progesterone is the presumed cause of the shedding. With withdrawal of sex steroids, there is a profound spiral artery vascular spasm that ultimately leads to endometrial ischemia. Simultaneously, there is a breakdown of lysosomes and a release of proteolytic enzymes, which further promote local tissue destruction. This layer of endometrium is then shed, leaving the decidua basalis as the source of subsequent endometrial growth. Prostaglandins are produced throughout the menstrual cycle and are at their highest concentration during menses (60). Prostaglandin $F_{2\alpha}$ ($PGF_{2\alpha}$) is a potent vasoconstrictor, causing further arteriolar vasospasm and endometrial ischemia. $PGF_{2\alpha}$ produces myometrial contractions that decrease local uterine wall blood flow and may serve to expel physically the sloughing endometrial tissue from the uterus.

Dating the Endometrium

The changes seen in secretory endometrium relative to the LH surge were thought to allow the assessment of the "normalcy" of endometrial development. Since 1950, it was felt that by knowing when a patient ovulated, it was possible to obtain a sample of endometrium by endometrial biopsy and determine whether the state of the endometrium corresponds to the appropriate time of the cycle. Traditional thinking held that any discrepancy of more than 2 days between chronologic and histologic date indicated a pathologic condition termed *luteal phase defect*; this abnormality was linked to both infertility (via implantation failure) and early pregnancy loss (63).

Evidence suggests a lack of utility for the endometrial biopsy as a diagnostic test for either infertility or early pregnancy loss (56). In a randomized, observational study of regularly cycling, fertile women, it was found that endometrial dating is far less accurate and precise than originally claimed and does not provide a valid method for the diagnosis of luteal phase defect (64). Furthermore, a large prospective, multicenter trial sponsored by the National Institutes of Health showed that histologic dating of the endometrium does not discriminate between fertile and infertile women (65). Thus, after half a century of using this test in the evaluation of the subfertile couple, it became clear that the endometrial biopsy has no role in the routine evaluation of infertility or early pregnancy loss.

Ovarian Follicular Development

The number of oocytes peaks in the fetus at 6 to 7 million by 20 weeks of gestation (66) (Fig. 7.10). Simultaneously (and peaking at the 5th month of gestation), atresia of the oogonia occurs, rapidly followed by follicular atresia. At birth, only 1 to 2 million oocytes remain in the ovaries, and **at puberty, only 300,000 of the original 6 to 7 million oocytes are available for ovulation (66,67). Of these, only 400 to 500 will ultimately be released during ovulation.** By the time of menopause, the ovary will be composed primarily of dense stromal tissue with only rare interspersed oocytes remaining.

A central dogma of reproductive biology is that in mammalian females there is no capacity for oocyte production postnatally. Because oocytes enter the diplotene resting stage of meiosis in the fetus and persist in this stage until ovulation, much of the DNA, proteins, and messenger RNA (mRNA) necessary for development of the preimplantation embryo is synthesized by this stage. At the diplotene stage, a single layer of 8 to 10 granulosa cells surround the oogonia to form the primordial follicle. The oogonia that fail to become properly surrounded by granulosa cells undergo atresia (68). The remainder proceeds with follicular development. Thus, most oocytes are lost during fetal development, and the remaining follicles are steadily "used up" throughout the intervening years until menopause.

Evidence has begun to challenge this theory. Studies in the mouse showed that production of oocytes and corresponding folliculogenesis can occur well into adult life (69). The reservoir of germline stem cells responsible for this oocyte development appears to reside in the bone marrow (70). It is not clear whether such stem cells exist in adult humans, and if they do, what clinical function they might provide.

Meiotic Arrest of Oocyte and Resumption

Meiosis (the germ cell process of reduction division) is divided into four phases: prophase, metaphase, anaphase, and telophase. The prophase of meiosis I is further divided into five stages: *leptotene, zygotene, pachytene, diplotene,* and *diakinesis.*

Oogonia differ from spermatogonia in that only one final daughter cell (oocyte) forms from each precursor cell, with the excess genetic material discarded in three polar bodies. When the developing oogonia begin to enter meiotic prophase I, they are known as primary oocytes (71). This process begins at roughly 8 weeks of gestation. Only those oogonia that enter meiosis will survive the wave of atresia that sweeps the fetal ovary before birth. The oocytes arrested in prophase (in the late diplotene or "dictyate" stage) will remain so until the time of ovulation, when the process of meiosis resumes. The mechanism for this mitotic stasis is believed to be an oocyte maturation inhibitor (OMI) produced by granulosa cells (72). This inhibitor gains access to the oocyte via gap junctions connecting the oocyte and its surrounding cumulus of granulosa. With the midcycle LH surge, the gap junctions are disrupted, granulosa cells are no longer connected to the oocyte, and meiosis I is allowed to resume.

Follicular Development

Follicular development is a dynamic process that continues from menarche until menopause. The process is designed to allow the monthly recruitment of a cohort of follicles and, ultimately, to release a single, mature, dominant follicle during ovulation each month.

Primordial Follicles

The initial recruitment and growth of the primordial follicles is gonadotropin independent and affects a cohort over several months (73). The stimuli responsible for the recruitment of a specific cohort of follicles in each cycle are unknown. At the primordial follicle stage, shortly after initial recruitment, FSH assumes control of follicular differentiation and growth and allows a cohort of follicles to continue differentiation. This process signals the shift from gonadotropin-independent to gonadotropin-dependent growth. The first changes seen are growth of the oocyte and expansion of the single layer of follicular granulosa cells into a multilayer of cuboidal cells. The decline in luteal phase estrogen, progesterone, and inhibin-A production by the now-fading corpus luteum from the previous cycle allows the increase in FSH that stimulates this follicular growth (74).

Preantral Follicle

During the several days following the breakdown of the corpus luteum, growth of the cohort of follicles continues, driven by the stimulus of FSH. The enlarging oocyte secretes a glycoprotein-rich substance, the zona pellucida, which separates it from the surrounding granulosa cells (except for the aforementioned gap junction). With transformation from a primordial to a preantral follicle, there is continued mitotic proliferation of the encompassing granulosa cells. Simultaneously, theca cells in the stroma bordering the granulosa cells proliferate. Both cell types function synergistically to produce estrogens that are secreted into the systemic circulation. At this stage of development, each of the seemingly identical cohort members must either be selected for dominance or undergo atresia. It is likely that the follicle destined to ovulate was selected before this point, although the mechanism for selection remains obscure.

Two-Cell, Two-Gonadotropin Theory

The fundamental tenet of follicular development is the two-cell, two-gonadotropin theory (73,75,76) (Fig. 7.11). **This theory states that there is a subdivision and compartmentalization of steroid hormone synthesis activity in the developing follicle.** Most aromatase activity (for estrogen production) is in the granulosa cells (77). Aromatase activity is enhanced by FSH stimulation of specific receptors on these cells (78,79). Granulosa cells lack several enzymes that

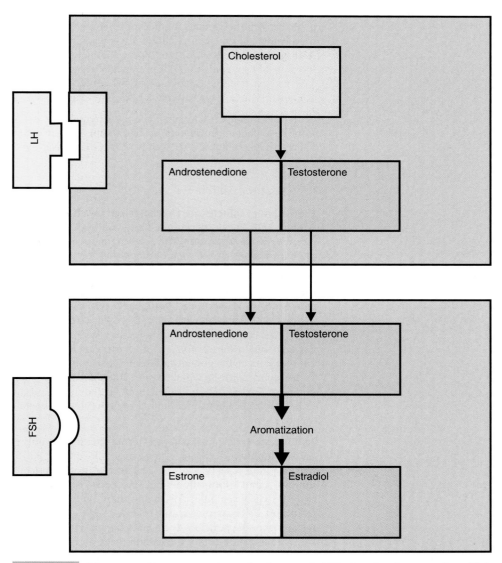

Figure 7.11 **The two-cell, two-gonadotropin theory of follicular development in which there is compartmentalization of steroid hormone synthesis in the developing follicle.** LH, luteinizing hormone; FSH, follicle-stimulating hormone.

occur earlier in the steroidogenic pathway and require androgens as a substrate for aromatization. Androgens, in turn, are synthesized primarily in response to stimulation by LH, and the theca cells possess most of the LH receptors at this stage (78,79). Therefore, a synergistic relationship must exist: LH stimulates the theca cells to produce androgens (primarily androstenedione), which in turn are transferred to the granulosa cells for FSH-stimulated aromatization into estrogens. These locally produced estrogens create a microenvironment within the follicle that is favorable for continued growth and nutrition (80). Both FSH and local estrogens serve to further stimulate estrogen production, FSH receptor synthesis and expression, and granulosa cell proliferation and differentiation.

Androgens have two positive regulatory roles in follicular development. Within the ovary, androgens promote granulose cell proliferation, aromatase activity, and inhibit programmed death of these cells (81).

As the peripheral estrogen level rises, it negatively feeds back on the pituitary and hypothalamus to decrease circulating FSH levels (82). **Increased ovarian production of inhibin-B further decreases FSH production at this point.**

The falling FSH level that occurs with the progression of the follicular phase represents a threat to continued follicular growth. The resulting adverse environment can be withstood only by follicles with a selective advantage for binding the diminishing FSH molecules; that is, those with the greatest number of FSH receptors. The dominant follicle, therefore, can be perceived as the one with a richly estrogenic microenvironment and the most FSH receptors (83). As it grows and develops, the follicle continues to produce estrogen, which results in further lowering of the circulating FSH and creates a more adverse environment for competing follicles. This process continues until all members of the initial cohort, with the exception of the single dominant follicle, have suffered atresia. The stage is then set for ovulation.

Chronic elevation of androgens suppresses hypothalamic–pituitary secretion of FSH, a detriment to the development and maturation of a dominant follicle (81). Clinically, androgen excess results in chronic anovulation, as is seen in polycystic ovarian syndrome.

Preovulatory Follicle

Preovulatory follicles are characterized by a fluid-filled antrum that is composed of plasma with granulosa cell secretions. The granulosa cells at this point have further differentiated into a heterogenous population. The oocyte remains connected to the follicle by a stalk of specialized granulosa known as the *cumulus oophorus.*

Rising estrogen levels have a negative feedback effect on FSH secretion. Conversely, LH undergoes biphasic regulation by circulating estrogens. At lower concentrations, estrogens inhibit LH secretion. At higher levels, estrogen enhances LH release. This stimulation requires a sustained high level of estrogen (200 pg/mL) for more than 48 hours (84). Once the rising estrogen level produces positive feedback, a substantial surge in LH secretion occurs. Concomitant to these events, the local estrogen–FSH interactions in the dominant follicle induce LH receptors on the granulosa cells. Exposure to high levels of LH results in a specific response by the dominant follicle—the result is luteinization of the granulosa cells, production of progesterone, and initiation of ovulation. Ovulation will occur in the single mature, or Graafian, follicle 10 to 12 hours after the LH peak or 34 to 36 hours after the initial rise in midcycle LH (85–87).

As suggested previously, the sex steroids are not the only gonadotropin regulators of follicular development. Two related granulosa cell–derived peptides were identified that play opposing roles in pituitary feedback (88). **The first of these peptides, inhibin, is secreted in two forms: inhibin-A and inhibin-B.** Inhibin-B is secreted primarily in the follicular phase and is stimulated by FSH, whereas inhibin-A is mainly active in the luteal phase (89). **Both forms of inhibin act to inhibit FSH synthesis and release** (90,91). The second peptide, activin, stimulates FSH release from the pituitary gland and potentiates its action in the ovary (92,93). It is likely that there are numerous other intraovarian regulators similar to inhibin and activin, each of which may play a key role in promoting the normal ovulatory process (94). Some of these include follistatin, insulinlike growth factor-1 (ILGF-1), epidermal growth factor (EGF)/transforming growth factor-α (TGF-α), TGF-β1, fibroblast growth factor-β (FGF-β), interleukin-1, tissue necrosis factor-α, OMI, and renin–angiotensin.

Ovulation

The midcycle LH surge is responsible for a dramatic increase in local concentrations of prostaglandins and proteolytic enzymes in the follicular wall (95). These substances progressively weaken the follicular wall and ultimately allow a perforation to form. Ovulation most likely represents a slow extrusion of the oocyte through this opening in the follicle rather than a rupture of the follicular structure (96). Direct measurements of intrafollicular pressures were recorded and failed to demonstrate an explosive event.

Luteal Phase

Structure of Corpus Luteum   **After ovulation, the remaining follicular shell is transformed into the primary regulator of the luteal phase: the corpus luteum.** Membranous granulosa cells remaining in the follicle begin to take up lipids and the characteristic yellow lutein pigment for which the structure is named. These cells are active secretory structures that produce progesterone, which supports the endometrium of the luteal phase. In addition, estrogen and inhibin-A are produced in significant quantities. Unlike the process that occurs in the developing follicle, the basement membrane of the corpus luteum degenerates to allow proliferating blood vessels to invade the granulosa-luteal cells in response to secretion of angiogenic factors such as vascular endothelial growth factor (97). This angiogenic response allows large amounts of luteal hormones to enter the systemic circulation.

Hormonal Function and Regulation   **The hormonal changes of the luteal phase are characterized by a series of negative feedback interactions designed to lead to regression of the corpus luteum if pregnancy does not occur. Corpus luteum steroids (estradiol and progesterone) provide negative central feedback and cause a decrease in FSH and LH secretion. Continued secretion of both steroids will decrease the stimuli for subsequent follicular recruitment. Similarly, luteal secretion of inhibin also potentiates FSH withdrawal. In the ovary, local production of progesterone inhibits the further development and recruitment of additional follicles.**

Continued corpus luteum function depends on continued LH production. In the absence of this stimulation, the corpus luteum will invariably regress after 12 to 16 days and form the scarlike *corpora albicans* (98). The exact mechanism of luteolysis is unclear and most likely involves local paracrine factors. In the absence of pregnancy, the corpus luteum regresses, and estrogen and progesterone levels wane. This, in turn, removes central inhibition on gonadotropin secretion and allows FSH and LH levels to again rise and recruit another cohort of follicles.

If pregnancy does occur, placental hCG will mimic LH action and continually stimulate the corpus luteum to secrete progesterone. Successful implantation results in hormonal support to allow continued maintenance of the corpus luteum and the endometrium. Evidence from patients undergoing oocyte donation cycles demonstrated that continued luteal function is essential to continuation of the pregnancy until approximately 5 weeks of gestation, when sufficient progesterone is produced by the developing placenta (99). This switch in the source of regulatory progesterone production is referred to as the luteal–placental shift.

Summary of Menstrual Cycle Regulation

Following is a summary of the regulation of the menstrual cycle:

1. **GnRH is produced in the arcuate nucleus of the hypothalamus and secreted in a pulsatile fashion into the portal circulation, where it travels to the anterior pituitary.**

2. **Ovarian follicular development moves from a period of gonadotropin independence to a phase of FSH dependence.**

3. **As the corpus luteum of the previous cycle fades, luteal production of progesterone and inhibin-A decreases, allowing FSH levels to rise.**

4. **In response to FSH stimulus, the follicles grow, differentiate, and secrete increasing amounts of estrogen and inhibin-B.**

5. **Estrogen stimulates growth and differentiation of the functional layer of the endometrium, which prepares for implantation. Estrogens work with FSH in stimulating follicular development.**

6. **The two-cell, two-gonadotropin theory dictates that with LH stimulation, the ovarian theca cells will produce androgens that are converted by the granulosa cells into estrogens under the stimulus of FSH.**

7. Rising estrogen and inhibin levels negatively feed back on the pituitary gland and hypothalamus and decrease the secretion of FSH.

8. The one follicle destined to ovulate each cycle is called the dominant follicle. It has relatively more FSH receptors and produces a larger concentration of estrogens than the follicles that will undergo atresia. It is able to continue to grow despite falling FSH levels.

9. Sustained high estrogen levels cause a surge in pituitary LH secretion that triggers ovulation, progesterone production, and the shift to the secretory, or luteal, phase.

10. Luteal function is dependent on the presence of LH. The corpus luteum secretes estrogen, progesterone, and inhibin-A, which serve to maintain gonadotropin suppression. Without continued LH secretion, the corpus luteum will regress after 12 to 16 days. The resulting loss of progesterone secretion results in menstruation.

11. If pregnancy occurs, the embryo secretes hCG, which mimics the action of LH by sustaining the corpus luteum. The corpus luteum continues to secrete progesterone and supports the secretory endometrium, allowing the pregnancy to continue to develop.

References

1. **Bloom FE.** Neuroendocrine mechanisms: cells and systems. In: **Yen SCC, Jaffe RB, eds.** *Reproductive endocrinology.* Philadelphia, PA: Saunders, 1991:2–24.

2. **Simerly RB, Chang C, Muramatsu M, et al.** Distribution of androgen and estrogen receptor mRNA-containing cells in the rat brain: an in situ hybridization study. *J Comp Neurol* 1990;294:76–95.

3. **Brown TJ, Hochberg RB, Naftolin F.** Pubertal development of estrogen receptors in the rat brain. *Mol Cell Neurosci* 1994;5:475–483.

4. **Bergland RM, Page RB.** Can the pituitary secrete directly to the brain? Affirmative anatomic evidence. *Endocrinology* 1978;102:1325–1338.

5. **Duello TM, Halmi NS.** Ultrastructural-immunocytochemical localization of growth hormone and prolactin in human pituitaries. *J Clin Endocrinol Metab* 1979;49:189–196.

6. **Blackwell RE, Amoss M Jr, Vale W, et al.** Concomitant release of FSH and LH induced by native and synthetic LRF. *Am J Physiol* 1973;224:170–175.

7. **Krey LC, Butler WR, Knobil E.** Surgical disconnection of the medial basal hypothalamus and pituitary function in the rhesus monkey. I. Gonadotropin secretion. *Endocrinology* 1975;96:1073–1087.

8. **Plant TM, Krey LC, Moossy J, et al.** The arcuate nucleus and the control of the gonadotropin and prolactin secretion in the female rhesus monkey (Macaca mulatta). *Endocrinology* 1978;102:52–62.

9. **Amoss M, Burgus R, Blackwell RE, et al.** Purification, amino acid composition, and N-terminus of the hypothalamic luteinizing hormone releasing factor (LRF) of ovine origin. *Biochem Biophys Res Commun* 1971;44:205–210.

10. **Schwanzel-Fukuda M, Pfaff DW.** Origin of luteinizing hormone releasing neurons. *Nature* 1989;338:161–164.

11. **Dierschke DJ, Bhattacharya AN, Atkinson LE, et al.** Circhoral oscillations of plasma LH levels in the ovariectomized rhesus monkey. *Endocrinology* 1970;87:850–853.

12. **Knobil E.** Neuroendocrine control of the menstrual cycle. *Recent Prog Horm Res* 1980;36:53–88.

13. **Belchetz PE, Plant TM, Nakai Y, et al.** Hypophyseal responses to continuous and intermittent delivery of hypothalamic gonadotropin-releasing hormone. *Science* 1978;202:631–633.

14. **Nakai Y, Plant TM, Hess DL, et al.** On the sites of the negative and positive feedback actions of estradiol and the control of gonadotropin secretion in the rhesus monkey. *Endocrinology* 1978;102:1008–1014.

15. **Rabin D, McNeil LW.** Pituitary and gonadal desensitization after continuous luteinizing hormone–releasing hormone infusion in normal females. *J Clin Endocrinol Metab* 1980;51:873–876.

16. **Hoff JD, Lasley BL, Yen SSC.** Functional relationship between priming and releasing actions of luteinizing hormone–releasing hormone. *J Clin Endocrinol Metab* 1979;49:8–11.

17. **Soules MR, Steiner RA, Cohen NL, et al.** Nocturnal slowing of pulsatile luteinizing hormone secretion in women during the follicular phase of the menstrual cycle. *J Clin Endocrinol Metab* 1985;61:43–49.

18. **Filicori M, Santoro N, Marriam GR, et al.** Characterization of the physiological pattern of episodic gonadotropin secretion throughout the human menstrual cycle. *J Clin Endocrinol Metab* 1986;62:1136–1144.

19. **Yu B, Ruman J, Christman G.** The role of peripheral gonadotropin-releasing hormone receptors in female reproduction. *Fertil Steril* 2011;95:465–473.

20. **Karten MJ, Rivier JE.** Gonadotropin-releasing hormone analog design. Structure function studies towards the development of agonists and antagonists: rationale and perspective. *Endocr Rev* 1986;7:44–66.

21. **Conn PM, Crowley WF Jr.** Gonadotropin-releasing hormone and its analogs. *Annu Rev Med* 1994;45:391–405.

22. **Loy RA.** The pharmacology and potential applications of GnRH antagonists. *Curr Opin Obstet Gynecol* 1994;6:262–268.

23. **Schally AV.** LH-RH analogues. I. Their impact on reproductive medicine. *Gynecol Endocrinol* 1999;13:401–409.

24. **Halmos G, Schally AV, Pinski J, et al.** Down-regulation of pituitary receptors for luteinizing hormone–releasing hormone (LH-RH) in rats by LH-RH antagonist Cetrorelix. *Proc Natl Acad Sci U S A* 1996;93:2398–2402.

25. **Betz SF, Zhu YF, Chen C, Struthers RS.** Non-peptide gonadotropin-releasing hormone receptor antagonists. *J Med Chem* 2008;51:3331–3348.

26. **Struthers RS, Nicholls AJ, Grundy J, et al.** Suppression of gonadotropins and estradiol in premenopausal women by oral administration of the nonpeptide gonadotropin-releasing hormone antagonist elagolix. *J Clin Endocrinol Metab* 2009;94:545–551.

27. **Hughes J, Smith TW, Kosterlitz LH, et al.** Identification of two related pentapeptides from the brain with potent opiate agonist activity. *Nature* 1975;258:577–580.

28. **Howlett TA, Rees LH.** Endogenous opioid peptide and hypothalamo-pituitary function. *Annu Rev Physiol* 1986;48:527–536.

29. **Facchinetti F, Petraglia F, Genazzani AR.** Localization and expression of the three opioid systems. *Semin Reprod Endocrinol* 1987;5:103.

30. **Goldstein A.** Endorphins: physiology and clinical implications. *Ann N Y Acad Sci* 1978;311:49–58.

31. **Grossman A.** Opioid peptides and reproductive function. *Semin Reprod Endocrinol* 1987;5:115–124.

32. **Reid RI, Hoff JD, Yen SSC, et al.** Effects of exogenous β-endorphin on pituitary hormone secretion and its disappearance rate in normal human subjects. *J Clin Endocrinol Metab* 1981;52:1179–1184.

33. **Gindoff PR, Ferin M.** Brain opioid peptides and menstrual cyclicity. *Semin Reprod Endocrinol* 1987;5:125–133.

34. **Halbreich U, Endicott J.** Possible involvement of endorphin withdrawal or imbalance in specific premenstrual syndromes and postpartum depression. *Med Hypotheses* 1981;7:1045–1058.

35. **Fiddes JC, Talmadge K.** Structure, expression and evolution of the genes for human glycoprotein hormones. *Recent Prog Horm Res* 1984;40:43–78.

36. **Vaitukaitis JL, Ross JT, Bourstein GD, et al.** Gonadotropins and their subunits: basic and clinical studies. *Recent Prog Horm Res* 1976;32:289–331.

37. **Lalloz MRA, Detta A, Clayton RN.** GnRH desensitization preferentially inhibits expression of the LH β-subunit gene in vivo. *Endocrinology* 1988;122:1689–1694.

38. **Brun del Re R, del Pozo E, de Grandi P, et al.** Prolactin inhibition and suppression of puerperal lactation by a Br-ergocriptine (CB 154): a comparison with estrogen. *Obstet Gynecol* 1973;41:884–890.

39. **Suh HK, Frantz AG.** Size heterogeneity of human prolactin in plasma and pituitary extracts. *J Clin Endocrinol Metab* 1974:39:928–935.

40. **MacLeod RM.** Influence of norepinephrine and catecholamine depletion agents synthesis in release of prolactin growth hormone. *Endocrinology* 1969;85:916–923.

41. **Vale W, Blackwell RE, Grant G, et al.** TRF and thyroid hormones on prolactin secretion by rat pituitary cell in vitro. *Endocrinology* 1973;93:26–33.

42. **Matsushita N, Kato Y, Shimatsu A, et al.** Effects of VIP, TRH, GABA and dopamine on prolactin release from superfused rat anterior pituitary cells. *Life Sci* 1983;32:1263–1269.

43. **Dufy-Barbe L, Rodriguez F, Arsaut J, et al.** Angiotensin-II stimulates prolactin release in the rhesus monkey. *Neuroendocrinology* 1982;35:242–247.

44. **Burrow GN.** The thyroid gland and reproduction. In: **Yen SCC, Jaffe RB, eds.** Reproductive endocrinology. Philadelphia, PA: Saunders, 1991:555–575.

45. **Katz E, Ricciarelli E, Adashi EY.** The potential relevance of growth hormone to female reproductive physiology and pathophysiology. *Fertil Steril* 1993;59:8–34.

46. **Yen SCC.** The hypothalamic control of pituitary hormone secretion. In: **Yen SCC, Jaffe RB, eds.** *Reproductive endocrinology.* Philadelphia, PA: Saunders, 1991:65–104.

47. **Insel TR.** Oxytocin and the neuroendocrine basis of affiliation. In: **Schulkin J, ed.** *Hormonally induced changes in mind and brain.* New York: Academic Press, 1993:225–251.

48. **Stein DJ.** Oxytocin and vasopressin: social neuropeptides. *CNS Spectr* 2009;14:602–606.

49. **Donaldson ZR, Young LJ.** Oxytocin, vasopressin, and the neurogenetics of sociality. *Science* 2008;322:900–904.

50. **Yamasue H, Kuwabara H, Kawakubo Y, et al.** Oxytocin, sexually dimorphic features of the social brain, and autism. *Psychiatry Clin Neurosci* 2009;63:129–140.

51. **Israel S, Lerer E, Shalev I, et al.** Molecular genetic studies of the arginine vasopressin 1a receptor (AVPR1a) and the oxytocin receptor (OXTR) in human behaviour: from autism to altruism with some notes in between. *Prog Brain Res* 2008;170:435–449.

52. **McNeilly AS, Robinson IC, Houston MJ, et al.** Release of oxytocin and PRL in response to suckling. *BMJ* 1983;286:257–259.

53. **Dunn FL, Brennan TJ, Nelson AE, et al.** The role of blood osmolality and volume in regulating vasopressin secretion in the rat. *J Clin Invest* 1973;52:3212–3219.

54. **Vollman RF.** The menstrual cycle. In: **Friedman E, ed.** *Major problems in obstetrics and gynecology.* Philadelphia, PA: Saunders, 1977:1–193.

55. **Treloar AE, Boynton RE, Borghild GB, et al.** Variation of the human menstrual cycle through reproductive life. *Int J Fertil* 1967;12:77–126.

56. **Collett ME, Wertenberger GE, Fiske VM.** The effects of age upon the pattern of the menstrual cycle. *Fertil Steril* 1954;5:437–448.

57. **Noyes RW, Hertig AW, Rock J.** Dating the endometrial biopsy. *Fertil Steril* 1950;1:3–25.

58. **Flowers CE Jr, Wilbron WH.** Cellular mechanisms for endometrial conservation during menstrual bleeding. *Semin Reprod Endocrinol* 1984;2:307–341.

59. **Chan RW, Schwab KE, Gargett CE.** Clonogenicity of human endometrial epithelial and stromal cells. *Biol Reprod* 2004;70:1738–1750.

60. **Taylor HS.** Endometrial cells derived from donor stem cells in bone marrow transplant recipients. *JAMA* 2004;292:81–85.

61. **Ferenczy A, Bertrand G, Gelfand MM.** Proliferation kinetics of human endometrium during the normal menstrual cycle. *Am J Obstet Gynecol* 1979;133:859–867.

62. **Schwarz BE.** The production and biologic effects of uterine prostaglandins. *Semin Reprod Endocrinol* 1983;1:189.

63. **Olive DL.** The prevalence and epidemiology of luteal-phase deficiency in normal and infertile women. *Clin Obstet Gynecol* 1991;34:157–166.

64. **Murray MJ, Meyer WR, Zaino RJ, et al.** A critical analysis of the accuracy, reproducibility, and clinical utility of histologic endometrial dating in infertile women. *Fertil Steril* 2004;81:1333–1343.

65. **Coutifaris C, Myers ER, Guzick DS, et al.** Histologic dating of timed endometrial biopsy tissue is not related to fertility status. *Fertil Steril* 2004;82:1264–1272.

66. **Peters H, Byskov AG, Grinsted J.** Follicular growth in fetal and prepubertal ovaries in humans and other primates. *J Clin Endocrinol Metab* 1978;7:469–485.

67. **Himelstein-Braw R, Byskov AG, Peters H, et al.** Follicular atresia in the infant human ovary. *J Reprod Fertil* 1976;46:55–59.

68. **Wassarman PM, Albertini DF.** The mammalian ovum. In: **Knobil E, Neill JD, eds.** *The physiology of reproduction.* New York: Raven Press, 1994:240–244.

69. **Johnson J, Canning J, Kaneko T, et al.** Germline stem cells and follicular renewal in the postnatal mammalian ovary. *Nature* 2004;428:145–150.

70. **Johnson J, Bagley J, Skaznik-Wikiel M, et al.** Oocyte generation in adult mammalian ovaries by putative germ cells in bone marrow and peripheral blood. *Cell* 2005;122:303–315.

71. **Gondos B, Bhiraleus P, Hobel CJ.** Ultrastructural observations on germ cells in human fetal ovaries. *Am J Obstet Gynecol* 1971;110:644–652.

72. **Tsafriri A, Dekel N, Bar-Ami S.** A role of oocyte maturation inhibitor in follicular regulation of oocyte maturation. *J Reprod Fertil* 1982;64:541–551.

73. **Halpin DMG, Jones A, Fink G, et al.** Post-natal ovarian follicle development in hypogonadal (HPG) and normal mice and associated changes in the hypothalamic-pituitary axis. *J Reprod Fertil* 1986;77:287–296.

74. **Vermesh M, Kletzky OA.** Longitudinal evaluation of the luteal phase and its transition into the follicular phase. *J Clin Endocrinol Metab* 1987;65:653–658.

75. **Erickson GF, Magoffin DA, Dyer CA, et al.** Ovarian androgen producing cells: a review of structure/function relationships. *Endocr Rev* 1985;6:371–399.

76. **Erickson GF.** An analysis of follicle development and ovum maturation. *Semin Reprod Endocrinol* 1986;46:55–59.

77. **Ryan KJ, Petro Z.** Steroid biosynthesis of human ovarian granulosa and thecal cells. *J Clin Endocrinol Metab* 1966;26:46–52.

78. **Kobayashi M, Nakano R, Ooshima A.** Immunohistochemical localization of pituitary gonadotropin and gonadal steroids confirms the two cells two gonadotropins hypothesis of steroidogenesis in the human ovary. *J Endocrinol* 1990;126:483–488.

79. **Yamoto M, Shima K, Nakano R.** Gonadotropin receptors in human ovarian follicles and corpora lutea throughout the menstrual cycle. *Horm Res* 1992;37[Suppl 1]:5–11.

80. **Hseuh AJ, Adashi EY, Jones PB, et al.** Hormonal regulation of the differentiation of cultured ovarian granulosa cells. *Endocr Rev* 1984;5:76–127.

81. **Weil SJ, Vendola K, Zhou J, et al.** Androgen receptor gene expression in the primate ovary: cellular localization, regulation, and functional correlations. *J Clin Endocrinol Metab* 1998;83:2479–2485.

82. **Chappel SC, Resko JA, Norman RL, et al.** Studies on rhesus monkeys on the site where estrogen inhibits gonadotropins: delivery of 17 β-estradiol to the hypothalamus and pituitary gland. *J Clin Endocrinol Metab* 1981;52:1–8.

83. **Chabab A, Hedon B, Arnal F, et al.** Follicular steroids in relation to oocyte development in human ovarian stimulation protocols. *Hum Reprod* 1986;1:449–454.

84. **Young SR, Jaffe RB.** Strength-duration characteristics of estrogen effects on gonadotropin response to gonadotropin-releasing hormone in women: II. Effects of varying concentrations of estradiol. *J Clin Endocrinol Metab* 1976;42:432–442.

85. **Pauerstein CJ, Eddy CA, Croxatto HD, et al.** Temporal relationship of estrogen, progesterone, luteinizing hormone levels to ovulation

in women and infra-human primates. *Am J Obstet Gynecol* 1978;130: 876–886.

86. **World Health Organization Task Force Investigators**. Temporal relationship between ovulation and defined changes in the concentration of plasma estradiol-17β luteinizing hormone, follicle stimulating hormone and progesterone. *Am J Obstet Gynecol* 1980;138: 383.

87. **Hoff JD, Quigley NE, Yen SSC**. Hormonal dynamics in mid-cycle: a re-evaluation. *J Clin Endocrinol Metab* 1983;57:792–796.

88. **Demura R, Suzuki T, Tajima S, et al.** Human plasma free activin and inhibin levels during the menstrual cycle. *J Clin Endocrinol Metab* 1993;76:1080–1082.

89. **Groome NP, Illingworth PG, O'Brien M, et al.** Measurement of dimeric inhibin B throughout the human menstrual cycle. *J Clin Endocrinol Metab* 1996;81:1401–1405.

90. **McLachlan RI, Robertson DM, Healy DL, et al.** Circulating immunoreactive inhibin levels during the normal human menstrual cycle. *J Clin Endocrinol Metab* 1987;65:954–961.

91. **Buckler HM, Healy DL, Burger HG.** Purified FSH stimulates inhibin production from the human ovary. *J Endocrinol* 1989;122:279–285.

92. **Ling N, Ying S, Ueno N, et al.** Pituitary FSH is released by het-erodimer of the β-subunits from the two forms of inhibin. *Nature* 1986; 321:779–782.

93. **Braden TD, Conn PM.** Activin-A stimulates the synthesis of gonadotropin-releasing hormone receptors. *Endocrinology* 1992;130: 2101–2105.

94. **Adashi EY.** Putative intraovarian regulators. *Semin Reprod Endocrinol* 1988;7:1–100.

95. **Yoshimura Y, Santulli R, Atlas SJ, et al.** The effects of proteolytic enzymes on in vitro ovulation in the rabbit. *Am J Obstet Gynecol* 1987;157:468–475.

96. **Yoshimura Y, Wallach EE.** Studies on the mechanism(s) of mammalian ovulation. *Fertil Steril* 1987;47:22–34.

97. **Anasti JN, Kalantaridou SN, Kimzey LM, et al.** Human follicle fluid vascular endothelial growth factor concentrations are correlated with luteinization in spontaneously developing follicles. *Hum Reprod* 1998;13:1144–1147.

98. **Lenton EA, Landgren B, Sexton L.** Normal variation in the length of the luteal phase of the menstrual cycle: identification of the short luteal phase. *Br J Obstet Gynaecol* 1994;91:685.

99. **Scott R, Navot D, Hung-Ching L, et al.** A human in vivo model for the luteal placental shift. *Fertil Steril* 1991;56:481–484.

SECTION III

PREVENTIVE AND PRIMARY CARE

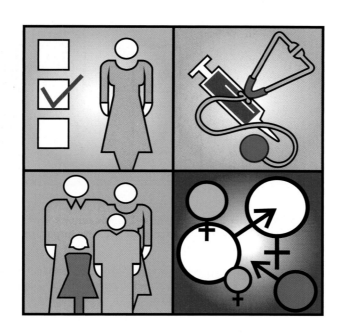

8 Preventive Health Care and Screening

Paula J. Adams Hillard

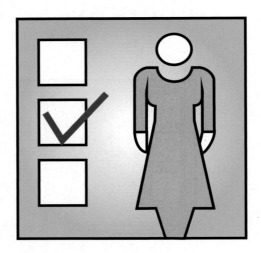

- Preventive health services that encompass screening and counseling for a broad range of health behaviors and risks are important components of general obstetric and gynecologic care.

- Traditional gynecologic care—including cervical cytology testing, pelvic and breast screening examinations, and the provision of contraceptive services—is considered primary preventive care.

- Routine health care assessments for healthy women include a medical history, physical examination, routine and indicated laboratory studies, assessment and counseling regarding healthy behaviors, and relevant interventions, taking into account the leading causes of morbidity and mortality within different age groups.

- Evidence-based guidelines for the provision of periodic health evaluations, screening, and counseling have been developed by the American College of Obstetricians and Gynecologists (ACOG) and other organizations; these guidelines provide the basis for routine preventive health assessment and screening recommendations.

- Preventive services for adolescents should be based on knowledge of the behavioral and medical health risks that place their future health at risk, including substance use and abuse, sexual behaviors that increase the risks of unintended pregnancy and sexually transmitted diseases (STDs), and impaired mental health.

- Obesity, smoking, and alcohol abuse are preventable problems that have a major impact on long-term health; assessment, counseling, and referral for these health risks is a component of periodic health assessment and primary care.

Although obstetricians-gynecologists have focused on the management of abnormal gynecologic conditions, they also have a traditional role of providing primary and preventive care to women, particularly for women of reproductive age. **The obstetrician-gynecologist often serves as a woman's point of entry into the health care system, her primary care clinician, and a source of continuity of care** (1). **Primary care emphasizes health maintenance, preventive services, early detection of disease, and availability and continuity of care. The value of preventive services is apparent in such trends as the reduced mortality rate from cervical cancer that resulted, in large part, from the increased use of cervical cytology testing.** Neonatal screening for phenylketonuria (PKU) and hypothyroidism are examples of effective mechanisms for prevention of mental retardation. Women often regard their gynecologist as their primary care provider; indeed, many women of reproductive age have no other physician. Obstetricians-gynecologists estimated that at least a third of their nonpregnant patients rely on them for primary care (2). As primary care physicians, obstetricians-gynecologists provide ongoing care for women through all stages of their lives—from reproductive age to postmenopause. In this role, some gynecologists include as a routine part of their practices screening for certain medical conditions, such as hypertension, diabetes mellitus, and thyroid disease, and management of those conditions in the absence of complications.

Some traditional aspects of gynecologic practice, such as family planning and preconception counseling, are recognized as effective preventive health measures, although clear and coherent national guidelines and goals for preventing unintended pregnancies have not been a high priority in the United States (3). Preventive medical services encompass screening and counseling for a broad range of health behaviors and risks, including sexual practices; prevention of sexually transmitted diseases (STDs); use of tobacco, alcohol, and other drugs; diet; and exercise.

The Institute of Medicine defined primary care as "*the provision of integrated, accessible health care services by clinicians who are accountable for addressing a large majority of personal health care needs, developing a sustained partnership with patients, and practicing in the context of family and community*" (4). Integrated care is further defined as being comprehensive, coordinated, and continuous. The definition states that primary care clinicians have the appropriate training to manage most problems that afflict patients (including physical, mental, emotional, and social concerns) and to involve other practitioners for further evaluation or treatment when appropriate. Using data from the National Ambulatory Medical Care Surveys, physician specialty groups were analyzed in a study to determine how well these Institute of Medicine primary care definitions applied to the care delivered by each specialty (5). In this analysis, obstetrics and gynecology as a specialty demonstrated some characteristics of primary care that applied to the traditional specialties of internal medicine, family and general physicians, and pediatrics. As a category, however, obstetrics and gynecology was more closely related to medical and surgical subspecialties (5). This analysis would be accepted by many practicing obstetricians and gynecologists who state that the specialty provides both primary and specialty care.

The Institute of Medicine definition includes referral, coordination, and follow-up care, but specifically does not include the function of "gatekeeper" as essential for a primary care clinician. As the US health care system has evolved, health maintenance organizations and insurers have responded to women's resolute support of direct access to obstetricians-gynecologists, a concept also strongly supported by the American Congress of Obstetricians and Gynecologists (6).

There is an increasing emphasis on women's health and gender-specific medicine. Physicians have become more knowledgeable about the differences in pathophysiologic aspects of diseases in women compared with men and thus better equipped to manage them. One example is an increasing emphasis on women's cardiovascular health with preventive care and screening for risk factors.

Gynecologist as Primary Care Provider

The obstetrician-gynecologist frequently serves as a primary medical resource for women and their families, providing information, guidance, and referrals when appropriate. Routine health care assessments for healthy women are based on age groups and risk factors. Health guidance takes into account the leading causes of morbidity and mortality within different age groups. Patient counseling and education require an ability to assess individual needs, to assess stages of readiness for change, and to use good communication skills, including motivational interviewing to encourage behavioral changes and ongoing care (7). A team approach to care is frequently helpful, utilizing the expertise of medical colleagues, such as nurses; advanced practice nurses, including nurse midwives and nurse practitioners; health educators; other allied health professionals, such as dieticians or physical therapists; relevant social services; and other physician specialists. All clinicians, regardless of the extent of their training, have limitations to their knowledge and skills and should seek consultation at appropriate times for the benefit of their patients in providing both reproductive and nonreproductive care.

The National Ambulatory Care Surveys from the Centers for Disease Control and Prevention include obstetrician-gynecologists among primary care specialties as opposed to medical or surgical subspecialties (8). Women's needs for primary care vary across their lifespan. One survey of women's satisfaction with primary care found that women in their early reproductive years (ages 18–34) were more satisfied with care coordination and comprehensiveness when their regular provider was a reproductive health specialist, primarily an obstetrician-gynecologist physician as compared to a generalist, a generalist clinician plus an obstetrician-gynecologist, or no regular provider (9). The scope of services provided by obstetricians-gynecologists varies from one practice or clinician to another and may include more or fewer aspects of well-woman and reproductive health care. It is important to establish with each patient whether she has a primary care clinician and who will be providing primary care and preventive health services (1).

Guidelines for primary and preventive services are issued by a number of medical bodies including the American College of Obstetricians and Gynecologists, the American Academy of Family Physicians, the U.S. Preventive Services Task Force (USPSTF), and the American Medical Association (1,10–14). The guidelines from various organizations differ somewhat in their specific details, and a national guideline clearinghouse for evidence-based clinical practice guidelines, sponsored by the Agency for Healthcare Research and Quality (AHRQ), is available to provide comparisons between guidelines for a given medical condition or intervention (15).

In 2006 in the United States, there were approximately 660 million visits by women to ambulatory medical care providers (16). In the past, approximately eighteen percent of the visits were made to gynecologists (17). Less than a third of ambulatory visits were made by individuals between the ages of 15 and 44 years, and this percentage is declining with an aging population (16). **Normal pregnancy and gynecologic examination were among the most common reasons for care.**

When asked to characterize the nature of an office or clinic visit, obstetricians-gynecologists may or may not identify themselves as primary care providers, depending on a number of variables (18). Those variables may include the patient's age, pregnancy status, whether it is a new versus a return visit, the diagnosis, insurance or referral status, and even geographic practice region. Primary and preventive services clearly within the realm of obstetricians and gynecologists include cervical cytology testing, pelvic examination and breast examination, and family planning services including contraception. **When compared with other physicians, obstetricians-gynecologists are more likely than other physicians to perform cervical cytology testing, pelvic examination, and breast examination.**

Approaches to Preventive Care

In health care, the focus is shifting from disease to prevention. Efforts are under way to promote effective screening measures that can have a beneficial effect on public and individual health. Following is a brief description of programs developed by American College of Obstetricians and Gynecologists (ACOG), the USPSTF, and the American Medical Association to provide guidelines for preventive care.

Guidelines for Primary and Preventive Care

The initial evaluation of a patient involves a complete history, physical examination, routine and indicated laboratory studies, evaluation and counseling, appropriate immunizations, and relevant interventions. Risk factors should be identified and arrangements should be made for continuing care or referral, as needed. **The ACOG recommendations for periodic evaluation, screening, and counseling by age groups, and the leading causes of death and morbidity within different age groups are shown in Tables 8.1 through 8.4 (10). These tables include recommendations for patients who have high-risk factors that require targeted screening or treatment; patients should be made aware of any high-risk conditions that require more specific screening or treatment** (Table 8.5). **Recommendations for immunizations**, indicated according to age group, are available from the U.S. Centers for Disease Control and Prevention (CDC). The CDC recommends HIV screening for pregnant women, adults, and adolescent patients in all health care settings after the patient is notified that testing will be performed, unless the patient declines (opt-out screening) (19). **Subsequent care should follow a specific schedule, yearly or as appropriate, based on the patient's needs and age.**

Table 8.1 Periodic Assessment Ages 13–18 Years

Screening	Evaluation and Counseling
History	**Sexuality**
Reason for visit	Development
Health status: medical, menstrual, surgical, family	High-risk behaviors
Dietary/nutrition assessment	Preventing unwanted/unintended pregnancy
Physical activity	—Postponing sexual involvement
Use of complementary and alternative medicine	—Contraceptive options, including emergency contraception
Tobacco, alcohol, other drug use	Sexually transmitted diseases
Abuse/neglect	—Partner selection
Sexual practices	—Barrier protection
Physical Examination	**Fitness and Nutrition**
Height	Exercise: discussion of program
Weight	Dietary/nutrition assessment (including eating disorders)
Body mass index (BMI)	Folic acid supplementation
Blood pressure	Calcium intake
Secondary sexual characteristics (Tanner staging)	**Psychosocial Evaluation**
Pelvic examination (when indicated by the medical history)	Suicide: depressive symptoms
Skin*	Interpersonal/family relationships
Laboratory Testing	Sexual orientation and gender identity
Periodic	Personal goal development
Chlamydia and gonorrhea testing (if sexually active)[†]	Behavioral/learning disorders
Human immunodeficiency virus (HIV) testing (if sexually active)[‡]	Abuse/neglect
*High-Risk Groups**	Satisfactory school experience
Colorectal cancer screening[§]	Peer relationships
Fasting glucose testing	Date rape prevention
Genetic testing/counseling	**Cardiovascular Risk Factors**
Hemoglobin level assessment	Family history
Hepatitis C virus testing	Hypertension
Lipid profile assessment	Dyslipidemia
Rubella titer assessment	Obesity
Sexually transmitted disease testing	Diabetes mellitus
Tuberculosis skin testing	**Health/Risk Behaviors**
	Hygiene (including dental), fluoride supplementation*
	Injury prevention
	—Exercise and sports involvement
	—Firearms
	—Hearing
	—Occupational hazards
	—Recreational hazards
	—Safe driving practices
	—Helmet use

(Continued)

Table 8.1 (*Continued*)	
Evaluation and Counseling (Continued)	
Skin exposure to ultraviolet rays	***Leading Causes of Death*[¶]**
Tobacco, alcohol, other drug use	1. Accidents (unintentional injuries)
Immunizations	2. Malignant neoplasms
Periodic	3. Intentional self harm (suicide)
Diphtheria and reduced tetanus toxoids and acellular pertussis vaccine booster (once between ages 11–18 years)[‖]	4. Assault (homicide)
Hepatitis B vaccine (one series for those not previously immunized)	5. Diseases of the heart
Human papillomavirus vaccine (one series for those not previously immunized, ages 9–26 years)	6. Congenital malformations, deformations, and chromosomal abnormalities
Influenza vaccine (annually)	7. Chronic lower respiratory diseases
Measles–mumps–rubella vaccine (for those not previously immunized)	8. Cerebrovascular diseases
Meningococcal conjugate vaccine (before entry into high school for those not previously immunized)	9. Influenza and pneumonia
Varicella vaccine (one series for those without evidence of immunity)	10. In situ neoplasms, benign neoplasms, and neoplasms of uncertain or unknown behavior
*High-Risk Groups**	
Hepatitis A vaccine	
Pneumococcal vaccine	

*See Table 8.5.
[†]Urine-based sexually transmitted disease screening is an efficient means for accomplishing such screening without a speculum examination.
[‡]Physicians should be aware of and follow their states' HIV screening requirements. For a more detailed discussion of HIV screening, see Branson BM, Handsfield HH, Lampe MA, Janssen RS, Taylor AW, Lyss SB, et al. Revised recommendations for HIV testing of adults, adolescents, and pregnant women in health-care settings. Centers for Disease Control and Prevention (CDC). *MMWR Recomm Rep* 2006;55(RR-14):1–17; quiz CE1–4. See also Routine human immunodeficiency virus screening. ACOG Committee Opinion No. 411. American College of Obstetricians and Gynecologists. *Obstet Gynecol* 2008;112:401–3.
[§]Only for those with a family history of familial adenomatous polyposis or 8 years after the start of pancolitis. For a more detailed discussion of colorectal cancer screening, see Levin B, Lieberman DA. McFarland B, Smith RA, Brooks D, Andrews KS, et al. Screening and surveillance for the early detection of colorectal cancer and adenomatous polyps, 2008: a joint guideline from the American Cancer Society, the US Multi-Society Task Force on Colorectal Cancer, and the American College of Radiology. American Cancer Society Colorectal Cancer Advisory Group; US Multi-Society Task Force; American College of Radiology Colon Cancer Committee. *CA Cancer J Clin* 2008;58:130–60.
[‖]For more information on the use of Td and Tdap, see Broder KR, Cortese MM, Iskander JK, Kretsinger K, Slade BA, Brown KH, et al. Preventing tetanus, diphtheria, and pertussis among adolescents: use of tetanus toxoid, reduced diphtheria toxoid and acellular pertussis vaccines recommendations of the Advisory Committee on Immunization Practices (ACIP). Advisory Committee on Immunization Practices (ACIP). *MMWR Recomm Rep* 2006;55(RR-3):1–34.
[¶]Leading causes of mortality are provided by the Mortality Statistics Branch at the National Center for Health Statistics. Data are from 2004, the most recent year for which final data are available. The causes are ranked.
From American College of Obstetricians and Gynecologists. Primary and preventive care: periodic assessments. ACOG Committee Opinion No. 452. *Obstet Gynecol* 2009;144:1444–1451.

Guide to Clinical Preventive Services

The USPSTF was commissioned in 1984 as a 20-member nongovernmental panel of experts in primary care medicine, epidemiology, and public health. The USPSTF, comprising primary care providers, now includes nonfederal experts in prevention and evidence-based medicine (such as internists, pediatricians, family physicians, gynecologists-obstetricians, nurses, and health behavior specialists); the task force conducts and publishes scientific evidence reviews on a variety of preventive health services with administrative and research support from the AHRQ. Initial and subsequent reviews and recommendations are being revised and periodically released on the Web site sponsored by the AHRQ (15). The charge to the panel was to develop recommendations for the appropriate use of preventive interventions based on a systematic review of evidence of clinical effectiveness. The panel was asked to rigorously evaluate clinical research to assess the merits of preventive measures, including screening tests, counseling, immunizations, and medications.

Table 8.2 Periodic Assessment Ages 19–39 Years

Screening	Rubella titer assessment
History	Sexually transmitted disease testing
Reason for visit	Thyroid-stimulating hormone testing
Health status: medical, surgical, family	Tuberculosis skin testing
Dietary/nutrition assessment	***Evaluation and Counseling***
Physical activity	***Sexuality and Reproductive Planning***
Use of complementary and alternative medicine	Contraceptive options for prevention of unwanted pregnancy, including emergency contraception
Tobacco, alcohol, other drug use	Discussion of a reproductive health plan§
Abuse/neglect	High-risk behaviors
Sexual practices	Preconception and genetic counseling
Urinary and fecal incontinence	Sexual function
Physical Examination	Sexually transmitted diseases
Height	—Partner selection
Weight	—Barrier protection
Body mass index (BMI)	***Fitness and Nutrition***
Blood pressure	Exercise: discussion of program
Neck: adenopathy, thyroid	Dietary/nutrition assessment
Breasts	Folic acid supplementation
Abdomen	Calcium intake
Pelvic examination: for ages 19–20 years, when indicated by the medical history; age 21 or older, periodic pelvic examination	***Psychosocial Evaluation***
Skin*	Interpersonal/family relationships
Laboratory Testing	Intimate partner violence
Periodic	Date rape prevention
Cervical cytology†:	Work satisfaction
Age 21 years: screen every 2 years	Lifestyle/stress
Age 30 years or older:	Sleep disorders
Option 1: may screen every 3 years after three consecutive negative test results with no history of cervical intraepithelial neoplasia 2 or 3, immunosuppression, human immunodeficiency virus (HIV) infection, or diethylstilbestrol exposure in utero; or	***Cardiovascular Risk Factors***
Option 2: screen every 3 years after negative human papillomavirus DNA test and negative cervical cytology	Family history
Chlamydia and gonorrhea testing (if aged 25 years or younger and sexually active)	Hypertension
Human immunodeficiency virus (HIV) testing‡	Dyslipidemia
*High-Risk Groups**	Obesity
Bone mineral density screening	Diabetes mellitus
Colorectal cancer screening	Lifestyle
Fasting glucose testing	***Health/Risk Behaviors***
Genetic testing/counseling	Breast self-examination‖
Hemoglobin level assessment	Chemoprophylaxis for breast cancer (for high-risk women aged 35 years or older)¶
Hepatitis C virus testing	Hygiene (including dental)
Lipid profile assessment	Injury prevention
Mammography	—Exercise and sports involvement

(Continued)

Table 8.2 *(Continued)*

Evaluation and Counseling *(Continued)*

—Firearms	Influenza vaccine
—Hearing	Measles–mumps–rubella vaccine
—Occupational hazards	Meningococcal vaccine
—Recreational hazards	Pneumococcal vaccine
—Safety belts and helmets	**Leading Causes of Death****
Skin exposure to ultraviolet rays	1. Malignant neoplasms
Suicide: depressive symptoms	2. Accidents (unintentional injuries)
Tobacco, alcohol, other drug use	3. Diseases of the heart
Immunizations	4. Intentional self harm (suicide)
Periodic	5. Human immunodeficiency virus (HIV) disease
Diphtheria and reduced tetanus toxoids and acellular pertussis vaccine (substitute one-time dose of Tdap for Td booster; then boost with Td every 10 years)#	6. Assault (homicide)
Human papillomavirus vaccine (one series for those aged 26 years or less and not previously immunized)	7. Cerebrovascular diseases
Varicella vaccine (one series for those without evidence of immunity)	8. Diabetes mellitus
High-Risk Groups*	9. Chronic liver diseases and cirrhosis
Hepatitis A vaccine (consider combination vaccine for those at risk far hepatitis A and B)	10. Chronic lower respiratory diseases
Hepatitis B vaccine (consider combination vaccine for those at risk for hepatitis A and B)	

*See Table 8.5.

†For a more detailed discussion of cervical cytology screening, including the use of human papillomavirus DNA testing and screening after hysterectomy, see Cervical cytology screening. ACOG Practice Bulletin No. 109. American College of Obstetricians and Gynecologists. *Obstet Gynecol* 2009:114: 1409–20.

‡Physicians should be aware of and follow their states' HIV screening requirements. For a more detailed discussion of HIV screening, see Branson BM, Handsfield HH, Lampe MA, Janssen RS, Taylor AW, Lyss SB, et al. Revised recommendations for HIV testing of adults, adolescents, and pregnant women in health-care settings. Centers for Disease Control and Prevention (CDC). *MMWR Recomm Rep* 2006;55(RR-14):1–17; quiz CE1–4. See also Routine human immunodeficiency virus screening. ACOG Committee Opinion No. 411. American College of Obstetricians and Gynecologists. *Obstet Gynecol* 2008;112:401–3.

§For a more detailed discussion of the reproductive health plain, see The importance of preconception care in the continuum of women's health care. ACOG Committee Opinion No. 313. American College of Obstetricians and Gynecologists. *Obstet Gynecol* 2005;106:665–6.

||Despite a lack of definitive data for or against breast self-examination, breast self-examination has the potential to detect palpable breast cancer and can be recommended.

¶For a more detailed discussion of risk assessment and chemoprevention therapy, see Selective estrogen receptor modulators. ACOG Practice Bulletin No. 39. American College of Obstetricians and Gynecologists. *Obstet Gynecol* 2002;100:835–43.

#For more information on the use of Td and Tdap, see Kretsinger K, Broder KR, Cortese MM, Joyce MP, Ortega-Sanchez I, Lee GM, et al. Preventing tetanus, diphtheria, and pertussis among adults: use of tetanus toxoid, reduced diphtheria toxoid and acellular pertussis vaccine recommendations of the Advisory Committee on Immunization Practices (ACIP) and recommendation of ACIP, supported by the Healthcare Infection Control Practices Advisory Committee (HICPAC), for use of Tdap among health-care personnel. Centers for Disease Control and Prevention; Advisory Committee on Immunization Practices; Healthcare Infection Control Practices Advisory Committee. *MMWR Recomm Rep* 2006;55(RR-17):1–37.

**Leading causes of mortality are provided by the Mortality Statistics Branch at the National Center for Health Statistics. Data are from 2004, the most recent year for which final data are available. The causes are ranked.

From American College of Obstetricians and Gynecologists, Primary and preventive care: periodic assessments. ACOG Committee Opinion No. 452. *Obstet Gynecol* 2009;144:1444–1451.

The task force uses systematic reviews of the evidence on specific topics in clinical prevention that serve as the scientific basis for recommendations. The task force reviews the evidence, estimates the magnitude of benefits and harms, reaches consensus about the net benefit of a given preventive service, and issues a recommendation that is assigned a grade from "A" (strongly recommends), to "B" (recommends), "C" (no recommendations for or against), "D" (recommends against), to "I" (insufficient evidence to recommend for or against) (Table 8.6). The grading system includes suggestions for practice, recommending that the service should be provided, discouraged, or that the uncertainty about the balance of benefits versus harms should be discussed. The levels of certainty regarding net benefit are ranked from high to moderate to low. The task force evaluates services based on age, gender, and risk factors for disease, making recommendations about which preventive services should be included in

Table 8.3 Periodic Assessment Ages 40–64 Years

Screening	Evaluation and Counseling
History	**Sexuality**[||]
Reason for visit	High-risk behaviors
Health status: medical, surgical, family	Contraceptive options for prevention of unwanted pregnancy, including emergency contraception
Dietary/nutrition assessment	Sexual function
Physical activity	Sexually transmitted diseases
Use of complementary and alternative medicine	—Partner selection
Tobacco, alcohol, other drug use	—Barrier protection
Pelvic prolapse	**Fitness and Nutrition**
Menopausal symptoms	Exercise: discussion of program
Abuse/neglect	Dietary/nutrition assessment
Sexual practices	Folic acid supplementation
Urinary and fecal incontinence	Calcium intake
Physical Examination	**Psychosocial Evaluation**
Height	Family relationships
Weight	Intimate partner violence
Body mass index (BMI)	Work satisfaction
Blood pressure	Retirement planning
Oral cavity	Lifestyle/stress
Neck: adenopathy, thyroid	Sleep disorders
Breasts, axillae	**Cardiovascular Risk Factors**
Abdomen	Family history
Pelvic examination	Hypertension
Skin*	Dyslipidemia
Laboratory Testing	Obesity
Periodic	Diabetes mellitus
Cervical cytology (may screen every 3 years after three consecutive negative test results if no history of cervical intraepithelial neoplasia 2 or 3, immunosuppression, human immunodeficiency virus infection (HIV), or diethylstilbestrol exposure in utero, or every 3 years after negative human papillomavirus DNA test and negative cervical cytology[†]	Lifestyle
Colorectal cancer screening (beginning at age 50 years*: colonoscopy every 10 years [preferred])	**Health/Risk Behaviors**
Fasting glucose testing (every 3 years after age 45 years)	Aspirin prophylaxis to reduce the risk of stroke (ages 55–79 years)[¶]
Human immunodeficiency virus (HIV) testing[§]	Breast self-examination[#]
Lipid profile assessment (every 5 years beginning at age 45 years)	Chemoprophylaxis for breast cancer (for high-risk women)**
Mammography (every 1–2 years beginning at age 40 years, yearly beginning at age 50 years)	Hormone therapy
Thyroid-stimulating hormone testing (every 5 years beginning at age 50 years)	Hygiene (including dental)
High-Risk Groups*	Injury prevention
Bone mineral density screening	—Exercise and sports involvement
Colorectal cancer screening	—Firearms
Fasting glucose testing	—Hearing
Hemoglobin level assessment	—Occupational hazards
Hepatitis C virus testing	—Recreational hazards
Lipid profile assessment	—Safety belts and helmets
Sexually transmitted disease testing	Skin exposure to ultraviolet rays
Thyroid-stimulating hormone testing	Suicide: depressive symptoms
Tuberculosis skin testing	Tobacco, alcohol, other drug use

(*Continued*)

Table 8.3 (*Continued*)

Evaluation and Counseling (Continued)

Immunizations	Leading Causes of Death[‡‡]
Periodic	**1.** Malignant neoplasms
Diphtheria and reduced tetanus toxoids and acellular pertussis vaccine booster (substitute one-time dose of Tdap for Td booster; then boost with Td every 10 years)[††]	**2.** Diseases of the heart
Herpes zoster (single dose in adults aged 60 years or older)	**3.** Accidents (unintentional injuries)
Influenza vaccine (annually beginning at age 50 years)	**4.** Chronic lower respiratory diseases
Varicella vaccine (one series for those without evidence of immunity)	**5.** Cerebrovascular diseases
*High-Risk Groups**	**6.** Diabetes mellitus
Hepatitis A vaccine (consider combination vaccine for those at risk for hepatitis A and B)	**7.** Chronic liver disease and cirrhosis
Hepatitis B vaccine (consider combination vaccine for those at risk for hepatitis A and B)	**8.** Septicemia
Influenza vaccine	**9.** Intentional self harm (suicide)
Measles–mumps–rubella vaccine	**10.** Human immunodeficiency virus (HIV) disease
Meningococcal vaccine	
Pneumococcal vaccine	

*See Table 8.5.

[†]For a more detailed discussion of cervical cytology screening, including the use of human papillomavirus DNA testing and screening after hysterectomy, see Cervical cytology screening. ACOG Practice Bulletin No. 109. American College of Obstetricians and Gynecologists. *Obstet Gynecol* 2009;114:1409–20.

[†]Other methods include: 1) fecal occult blood testing or fecal immunochemical test, annual patient-collected (fecal occult blood testing and fecal immunochemical testing require two or three samples of stool collected by the patient at home and returned for analysis. A single stool sample obtained by digital rectal examination is not adequate for the detection of colorectal cancer); 2) flexible sigmoidoscopy every 5 years; 3) double contrast barium enema every 5 years; 4) computed tomography colonography every 5 years; and 5) stool DNA. The American College of Gastroenterology recommends that African Americans begin screening at age 45 years with colonoscopy because of increased incidence and earlier age of onset of colorectal cancer. (Agrawal S, Bhupinderjit A, Bhutani MS, Boardman L, Nguyen C, Romero Y, et al. Colorectal cancer in African Americans. Committee of Minority Affairs and Cultural Diversity, American College of Gastroenterology [published erratum appears in *Am J Gastroenterol* 2005;100:1432]. *Am J Gastroenterol* 2005;100:515, 523; discussion 514.)

[§]Physicians should be aware of and follow their states' HIV screening requirements. For a more detailed discussion of HIV screening, see Branson BM, Handsfield HH, Lampe MA, Janssen RS, Taylor AW, Lyss SB, et al. Revised recommendations for HIV testing of adults, adolescents, and pregnant women in health-care settings. Centers for Disease Control and Prevention (CDC). *MMWR Recomm Rep* 2006;55(RR-14):1–17; quiz CE1–4. See also Routine human immunodeficiency virus screening. ACOG Committee Opinion No. 411. American College of Obstetricians and Gynecologists. *Obstet Gynecol* 2008;112:401–3.

[‖]Preconception and genetic counseling is appropriate for certain women in this age group.

[¶]The recommendation for aspirin prophylaxis must weigh the benefits of stroke prevention against the harm of gastrointestinal bleeding. See Aspirin for the prevention of cardiovascular disease: U.S. Preventive Services Task Force recommendation statement. U.S. Preventive Services Task Force. *Ann Intern Med* 2009;150:396–404.

[#]Despite a lack of definitive data for or against breast self-examination, breast self-examination has the potential to detect palpable breast cancer and can be recommended.

[**]For a more detailed discussion of risk assessment and chemoprevention therapy, see Selective estrogen receptor modulators. ACOG Practice Bulletin No. 39. American College of Obstetricians and Gynecologists. *Obstet Gynecol* 2002;100:835–43.

[††]If Tdap not previously given, give one time, then Td every 10 years thereafter. If Tdap previously given, give Td every 10 years. For more information on the use of Td and Tdap, see Kretsinger K, Broder KR, Cortese MM, Joyce MP, Ortega-Sanchez I, Lee GM, et al. Preventing tetanus, diphtheria, and pertussis among adults: use of tetanus toxoid, reduced diphtheria toxoid and acellular pertussis vaccine recommendations of the Advisory Committee on Immunization Practices (ACIP) and recommendation of ACIP, supported by the Healthcare Infection Control Practices Advisory Committee (HICPAC), for use of Tdap among health-care personnel. Centers for Disease Control and Prevention; Advisory Committee on Immunization Practices; Healthcare Infection Control Practices Advisory Committee. *MMWR Recomm Rep* 2006;55(RR-17):1–37.

[‡‡]Leading causes of mortality are provided by the Mortality Statistics Branch at the National Center for Health Statistics. Data are from 2004, the most recent year for which final data are available. The causes are ranked.

From American College of Obstetricians and Gynecologists, Primary and preventive care: periodic assessments. ACOG Committee Opinion No. 452. *Obstet Gynecol* 2009;144:1444–1451.

routine primary care for which populations. ***Primary preventive measures* are those that involve intervention before the disease develops, for example, quitting smoking, increasing physical activity, eating a healthy diet, quitting alcohol and other drug use, using seat belts, and receiving immunizations. *Secondary preventive measures* are those used to identify and treat asymptomatic persons who have risk factors or preclinical disease but in whom the disease itself has not become clinically apparent.** Examples of secondary preventive measures are well known in gynecology, such as screening mammography and cervical cytology testing.

Table 8.4 Periodic Assessment Ages 65 and Older

Screening	High-Risk Groups[†]
History	Hemoglobin level assessment
Reason for visit	Hepatitis C virus testing
Health status: medical, surgical, family	Human immunodeficiency virus (HIV) testing
Dietary/nutrition assessment	Sexually transmitted disease testing
Physical activity	Thyroid-stimulating hormone testing
Pelvic prolapse	Tuberculosis skin testing
Menopausal symptoms	**Evaluation and Counseling**
Use of complementary and alternative medicine	**Sexuality**
Tobacco, alcohol, other drjg use, and concurrent medication use	Sexual function
Abuse/neglect	Sexual behaviors
Sexual practices	Sexually transmitted diseases
Urinary and fecal incontinence	—Partner selection
Physical examination	—Barrier protection
Height	**Fitness and Nutrition**
Weight	Exercise: discussion of program
Body mass index (BMI)	Dietary/nutrition assessment
Blood pressure	Calcium intake
Oral cavity	**Psychosocial Evaluation**
Neck: adenopathy, thyroid	Neglect/abuse
Breasts, axillae	Lifestyle/stress
Abdomen	Depression/sleep disorders
Pelvic examination*	Family relationships
Skin[†]	Work/retirement satisfaction
Laboratory Testing	**Cardiovascular Risk Factors**
Periodic	Hypertension
Bone mineral density screening (In the absence of new risk factors, screen no more frequently than every 2 years.)	**Dyslipidemia**
Cervical cytology: consider discontinuing at age 65 years or 70 years if patient has had three or more normal results in a row, no abnormal results in 10 years, no history of cervical cancer, no history of diethylstilbestrol exposure in utero, is human immunodeficiency virus (HIV) negative, is not immunosuppressed; if cervical cytology has been discontinued, annual review of risk factors to evaluate need for reinitiation of screening. If cervical cytology is needed: may screen every 3 years after three consecutive negative test results if no history of cervical intraepithelial neoplasia 2 or 3, immunosuppression, HIV infection, or diethylstilbestrol exposure in utero or every 3 years after negative human papillomavirus DNA test and negative cervical cytology.[‡]	Obesity
Colorectal cancer screening[§]: colonoscopy every 10 years (preferred)	Diabetes mellitus
Fasting glucose testing (every 3 years)	Sedentary lifestyle
Lipid profile assessment (every 5 years)	**Health/Risk Behaviors**
Mammography	Aspirin prophylaxis (for women aged 79 years or younger)[‖]
Thyroid-stimulating hormone testing (every 5 years)	Breast self-examination[¶]
Urinalysis	Chemoprophylaxis for breast cancer (for high-risk women)[#]

(Continued)

Table 8.4 (*Continued*)	
Hearing	*High-Risk Groups*[†]
Hormone therapy	Hepatitis A vaccine (consider combination vaccine for those at risk for hepatitis A and B)
Hygiene (including dental)	Hepatitis B vaccine (consider combination vaccine for those at risk for hepatitis A and B)
Injury prevention	Meningococcal vaccine
—Exercise and sports involvement	*Leading Causes of Death*[**]
—Firearms	1. Diseases of the heart
—Occupational hazards	2. Malignant neoplasms
—Prevention of falls	3. Cerebrovascular diseases
—Recreational hazards	4. Chronic lower respiratory diseases
—Safety belts and helmets	5. Alzheimer's disease
Skin exposure to ultraviolet rays	6. Influenza and pneumonia
Suicide: depressive symptoms	7. Diabetes mellitus
Tobacco, alcohol, other drug use	8. Nephritis, nephrotic syndrome, and nephrosis
Visual acuity/glaucoma	9. Accidents (unintentional injuries)
Immunizations	10. Septicemia
Periodic	
Herpes zoster (single dose, if not previously immunized)	
Influenza vaccine (annually)	
Pneumococcal vaccine (once)	
Tetanus-diphtheria booster (every 10 years)	
Varicella vaccine (one series for those without evidence of immunity)	

*When a woman's age or other health issues are such that she would not choose to intervene on conditions detected during the routine examination, it is reasonable to discontinue pelvic exams.
[†]See Table 8.5.
[‡]For a more detailed discussion of cervical cytology screening, including the use of human papillomavirus DNA testing and screening after hysterectomy, see Cervical cytology screening. ACOG Practice Bulletin No. 109. American College of Obstetricians and Gynecologists. *Obstet Gynecol* 2009:114; 1409–20.
[§]Other methods include: 1) fecal occult blood testing or fecal immunochemical test, annual patient-collected (fecal occult blood testing and fecal immunochemical testing require two or three samples of stool collected by the patient at home and returned for analysis. A single stool sample obtained by digital rectal examination is not adequate for the detection of colorectal cancer); 2) flexible sigmoidoscopy every 5 years; 3) double contrast barium enema every 5 years; 4) computed tomography colonography every 5 years; and 5) stool DNA. More frequent testing is recommended for those with other risk factors.
[‖]The recommendation for aspirin prophylaxis must weigh the benefits of stroke prevention against the harm of gastrointestinal bleeding. See Aspirin for the prevention of cardiovascular disease: U.S. Preventive Services Task Force recommendation statement. U.S. Preventive Services Task Force. *Ann Intern Med* 2009;150:396–404.
[¶]Despite a lack of definitive data for or against breast self-examination, breast self-examination has the potential to detect palpable breast cancer and can be recommended.
[#]For a more detailed discussion of risk assessment and chemoprevention therapy, see Selective estrogen receptor modulators. ACOG Practice Bulletin No. 39. American College of Obstetricians and Gynecologists. *Obstet Gynecol* 2002;100:835–43.
[**]Leading causes of mortality are provided by the Mortality Statistics Branch at the National Center for Health Statistics. Data are from 2004, the most recent year for which final data are available. The causes are ranked.
From American College of Obstetricians and Gynecologists, Primary and preventive care: periodic assessments. ACOG Committee Opinion No. 452. *Obstet Gynecol* 2009;144:1444–1451.

The USPSTF is supported by an Evidence-Based Practice Center (EPC), which conducts systematic reviews of the evidence that serve as the scientific basis for USPSTF recommendations. These reviews analyze the effectiveness of various screening measures and tests. Preventive medicine and the discipline of evidence-based medicine have grown and evolved since the release of the first *Guide to Clinical and Preventive Services* in 1989. This document accelerated the trend to replace consensus or expert opinion in clinical recommendations with a more systematic and explicit review of the evidence. The USPSTF has recognized that scientific evidence, including evidence derived from a variety of research designs other than randomized clinical trials, does

Table 8.5 High-Risk Factors

Intervention	High-Risk Factors
Bone mineral density screening*	Postmenopausal women younger than age 65 years: history of prior fracture as an adult; family history of osteoporosis; Caucasian; dementia; poor nutrition; smoking; low weight and BMI; estrogen deficiency caused by early (age younger than 45 years) menopause, bilateral oophorectomy, or prolonged (longer than 1 year) premenopausal amenorrhea; low lifelong calcium intake; alcoholism; impaired eyesight despite adequate correction; history of falls; inadequate physical activity All women: certain diseases or medical conditions and certain drugs associated with an increased risk of osteoporosis
Colorectal cancer screening†	Colorectal cancer or adenomatous polyps in first-degree relative younger than age 60 years or in two or more first-degree relatives of any ages; family history of familial adenomatous polyposis or hereditary non-polyposis colon cancer; history of colorectal cancer, adenomatous polyps, inflammatory bowel disease, chronic ulcerative colitis, or Crohn's disease
Diphtheria and reduced tetanus toxoids and acellular pertussis vaccine‡	Adults who have or who anticipate having close contact with an infant aged less than 12 months and health care providers. When possible, women should receive Tdap before becoming pregnant.
Fasting glucose testing§	Overweight (BMI greater than or equal to 25); first-degree relative with diabetes mellitus; habitual physical inactivity; high-risk race or ethnicity (eg, African American, Latina, Native American, Asian American, Pacific Islander); have given birth to a newborn weighing more than 9 lb or have a history of gestational diabetes mellitus; hypertension; high-density lipoprotein cholesterol level less than 35 mg/dL; triglyceride level greater than 250 mg/dL; history of impaired glucose tolerance or impaired fasting glucose; polycystic ovary syndrome; history of vascular disease; other clinical conditions associated with insulin resistance
Fluoride supplementation	Live in area with inadequate water fluoridation (less than 0.7 ppm)
Genetic testing/counseling	Considering pregnancy and: patient, partner, or family member with history of genetic disorder or birth defect; exposure to teratogens; or African, Cajun, Caucasian, European, Eastern European (Ashkenazi) Jewish, French Canadian, Mediterranean, or Southeast Asian ancestry
Hemoglobin level assessment	Caribbean, Latin American, Asian, Mediterranean, or African ancestry; history of excessive menstrual flow
HAV vaccination	Chronic liver disease, clotting factor disorders, illegal drug user, individuals who work with HAV-infected nonhuman primates or with HAV in a research laboratory setting, individuals traveling to or working in countries that have high or intermediate endemicity of hepatitis A
HBV vaccination	Hemodialysis patients; patients who receive clotting factor concentrates; health care workers and public safety workers who have exposure to blood in the workplace; individuals in training in schools of medicine, dentistry, nursing, laboratory technology, and other allied health professions; injecting drug users; individuals with more than one sexual partner in the previous 6 months; individuals with a recently acquired STD; all clients in STD clinics; household contacts and sexual partners of individuals with chronic HBV infection; clients and staff of institutions for the developmentally disabled; international travelers who will be in countries with high or intermediate prevalence of chronic HBV infection for more than 6 months; inmates of correctional facilities
HCV testing	History of injecting illegal drugs, recipients of clotting factor concentrates before 1987, chronic (long-term) hemodialysis, persistently abnormal alanine aminotransferase levels, recipients of blood from donors who later tested positive for HCV infection, recipients of blood or blood-component transfusion or organ transplant before July 1992, occupational percutaneous or mucosal exposure to HCV-positive blood
HIV testing	More than one sexual partner since most recent HIV test or a sexual partner with more than one sexual partner since most recent HIV test, have received a diagnosis of another STD in the past year, drug use by injection, history of prostitution, past or present sexual partner who is HIV positive or injects drugs, long-term residence or birth in an area with high prevalence of HIV infection, history of transfusion from 1978 to 1985, invasive cervical cancer, sexually active adolescent younger than age 19 years, adolescent entering detention facilities. Recommend to women seeking preconception evaluation.

(Continued)

Table 8.5 (*Continued*)

Intervention	High-Risk Factors
Influenza vaccination	Anyone who wishes to reduce the chance of becoming ill with influenza; anyone who wants to reduce the risk of transmitting it to others; chronic cardiovascular or pulmonary disorders, except hypertension, including asthma; chronic metabolic diseases, including diabetes mellitus, renal dysfunction, hemoglobinopathies, and immunosuppression (including immunosuppression caused by medications or by HIV); hepatic disorders; residents and employees of nursing homes and other long-term care facilities; individuals likely to transmit influenza to high-risk individuals (eg, household members and caregivers of the elderly, children aged from birth to 59 months, and adults with high-risk conditions); those with any condition (eg, cognitive dysfunction, spinal cord injury, seizure or other neuromuscular disorder) that compromises respiratory function or the handling of respiratory secretions, or that increases the risk of aspiration; health care workers; pregnancy during the influenza season; adults older than age 50 years; adolescents who are receiving long-term aspirin therapy who therefore might be at risk for experiencing Reye syndrome after influenza virus infection
Lipid profile assessment	Family history suggestive of familial hyperlipidemia; family history of premature cardiovascular disease (age younger than 50 years for men, age younger than 60 years for women); previous personal history of coronary heart disease or noncoronary atherosclerosis (eg, abdominal aortic aneurysm, peripheral artery disease, carotid artery stenosis); obesity (BMI greater than 30); personal and/or family history of peripheral vascular disease; diabetes mellitus; multiple coronary heart disease risk factors (eg, tobacco use, hypertension)
Mammography	Women who have had breast cancer or who have a first-degree relative (ie, mother, sister, or daughter) or multiple other relatives who have a history of premenopausal breast or breast and ovarian cancers
Meningococcal vaccination	Adults with anatomic or functional asplenia or terminal complement component deficiencies, first-year college students living in dormitories, microbiologists routinely exposed to *Neisseria meningitides* isolates, military recruits, travel to hyperendemic or epidemic areas
MMR vaccination	Adults born in 1957 or later should be offered vaccination (one dose of MMR) if there is no proof of immunity or documentation of a dose given after first birthday; individuals vaccinated in 1963–1967 should be offered revaccination (two doses); health care workers, students entering college, international travelers, and rubella-negative postpartum patients should be offered a second dose.
Pneumococcal vaccination	Chronic illness, such as cardiovascular disease, pulmonary disease, diabetes mellitus, alcoholism, chronic liver disease, cerebrospinal fluid leaks, Hodgkin disease, lymphoma, leukemia, kidney failure, multiple myeloma, nephrotic syndrome, functional asplenia (eg, sickle cell disease) or splenectomy; exposure to an environment where pneumococcal outbreaks have occurred; immunocompromised patients (eg, HIV infection, hematologic or solid malignancies, chemotherapy, steroid therapy); Alaskan Natives and certain Native American populations. Revaccination after 5 years may be appropriate for certain high-risk groups.
Rubella titer assessment	Childbearing age and no evidence of immunity
STD testing	History of multiple sexual partners or a sexual partner with multiple contacts; sexual contact with individuals with culture-proven STD; history of repeated episodes of STDs; attendance at clinics for STDs; women with developmental disabilities; annual screening for chlamydial infection for all sexually active women aged 25 years or younger; other asymptomatic women at high risk for infection and women older than age 25 years with risk factors (new sexual partner or multiple sexual partners); annual screening for gonorrheal infection for all sexually active adolescents and other asymptomatic women at high risk for infection; testing for syphilis for sexually active adolescents who exchange sex for drugs or money, use intravenous drugs, are entering a detention facility, or live in a high prevalence area
Skin examination	Increased recreational or occupational exposure to sunlight; family or personal history of skin cancer; clinical evidence of precursor lesions; fair skin, freckling; light hair; immune suppression; age; xeroderma pigmentosum

(Continued)

Table 8.5 *(Continued)*	
Intervention	*High-Risk Factors*
Thyroid-stimulating hormone testing	Strong family history of thyroid disease; autoimmune disease (evidence of subclinical hypothyroidism may be related to unfavorable lipid profiles)
Tuberculosis skin testing	HIV infection; close contact with individuals known or suspected to have tuberculosis; medical risk factors known to increase risk of disease if infected; born in country with high tuberculosis prevalence; medically underserved; low income; alcoholism; intravenous drug use; resident of long-term care facility (eg, correctional institutions, mental institutions, nursing homes and facilities); health professional working in high-risk health care facilities; recent tuberculin skin test converter (individuals with baseline testing results who have an increase of 10 mm or more in the size of the tuberculin skin test reaction within a 2-year period); radiographic evidence of prior healed tuberculosis
Varicella vaccination	Adults and adolescents aged 13 years or older; all adolescents and adults without evidence of immunity; students in all grade levels, and persons attending college or other postsecondary educational institutions; susceptible persons who have close contact with persons at high risk for serious complications, including health care workers; household contacts of immunocompromised individuals; teachers; daycare workers; residents and staff of institutional settings, colleges, prisons, or military installations; adolescents and adults living in households with children; international travelers; nonpregnant women of childbearing age

Abbreviations: BMI, body mass index; HAV, hepatitis A virus; HBV, hepatitis B virus; HCV, hepatitis C virus; HIV, human immunodeficiency virus; MMR, measles–mumps–rubella; STD, sexually transmitted disease; Tdap, diptheria and reduced tetanus toxoids and acellular pertussis vaccine.

*For a more detailed discussion of bone mineral density screening, see Osteoporosis, ACOG Practice Bulletin No. 50. American College of Obstetricians and Gynecologists. *Obstet Gynecol* 2004;103:203–16.

†For a more detailed discussion of colorectal cancer screening, see Levin B, Lieberman DA, McFarland B, Smith RA, Brooks D, Andrews KS, et al. Screening and surveillance for the early detection of colorectal cancer and adenomatous polyps, 2008: a joint guideline from the American Cancer Society, the US Mutti-Society Task Force on Colorectal Cancer, and the American College of Radiology. American Cancer Society Colorectal Cancer Advisory Group; US Multi-Society Task Force; American College of Radiology Colon Cancer Committee. *CA Cancer J Clin* 2008;58:130–60.

‡For more information, see Broder KR, Cortese MM, Iskander JK, Kretsinger K, Slade BA, Brown KH, et al. Preventing tetanus, diphtheria, and pertussis among adolescents: use of tetanus toxoid, reduced diphtheria toxoid and acellular pertussis vaccines recommendations of the Advisory Committee on Immunization Practices (ACIP). Advisory Committee on Immunization Practices (ACIP). *MMWR Recomm Rep* 2006;55(RR-3):1–34.; Kretsinger K, Broder KR, Cortese MM, Joyce MP, Ortega-Sanchez I, Lee GM, et al. Preventing tetanus, diphtheria, and pertussis among adults: use of tetanus toxoid, reduced diphtheria toxoid and acellular pertussis vaccine recommendations of the Advisory Committee on Immunization Practices (ACIP) and recommendation of ACIP, supported by the Healthcare Infection Control Practices Advisory Committee (HICPAC), for use of Tdap among health-care personnel. Centers for Disease Control and Prevention; Advisory Committee on Immunization Practices; Healthcare Infection Control Practices Advisory Committee. *MMWR Recomm Rep* 2006;55(RR-17):1–37.

§For more information, see Postpartum screening for abnormal glucose tolerance in women who had gestational diabetes mellitus. ACOG Committee Opinion No. 435. American College of Obstetricians and Gynecologists. *Obstet Gynecol* 2009;113:1419–21.

From American College of Obstetricians and Gynecologists, Primary and preventive care: periodic assessments. ACOG Committee Opinion No. 452. *Obstet Gynecol* 2009;144:1444–1451.

not permit "even moderated certainty" about the net benefit of the preventive service. The role of judgment in the domains of the potential preventable burden of suffering from the condition, the potential harm of the intervention, the cost, the context of current practice, and the potential role of other domains are recognized by the task force, with the conclusion that "decision making under conditions of uncertainty is a recurring issue in medicine" (20).

International efforts to categorize the effectiveness of treatments include the Cochrane Library, which produces and disseminates high-quality systematic reviews of health care interventions. These reviews and abstracts are published monthly and are available online and on DVDs by subscription (21). The Cochrane Library provides searchable databases online and through institutional purchase of licenses. Evidence-based guidelines are published in journals available in print and online by discipline (i.e., medicine, mental health, and nursing). Another source of evidence-based information is *Clinical Evidence*, a subscription service published by the *British Medical Journal* in print, via PDA, and online (22). This service describes its content as driven by important clinical questions rather than by the availability of research evidence. The advantages of Web-based sites are the ease of updating and the availability of evidence to clinicians in clinical practice sites throughout the world. Other Web sites that provide tools and information about evidence-based health care include the Oxford Centre for

Table 8.6 U.S. Preventive Services Task Force Ratings

The U.S. Preventive Services Task Force (USPSTF) grades its recommendations according to one of five classifications (A, B, C, D, I) reflecting the strength of evidence and magnitude of net benefit (benefits minus harms). After May 2007, updated definitions of the grades it assigns to recommendations are noted below with "suggestions for practice" with each grade (50).

Grade	Definition	Suggestions for Practice
A	The USPSTF recommends the service. There is high certainty that the net benefit is substantial.	Offer or provide this service
B	The USPSTF recommends the service. There is high certainty that the net benefit is moderate or there is moderate certainty that the net benefit is moderate to substantial.	Offer or provide this service
C	The USPSTF recommends against routinely providing the service. There may be considerations that support providing the service in an individual patient. There is at least moderate certainty that the net benefit is small.	Offer or provide this service only if other considerations support the offering or providing the service in an individual patient
D	The USPSTF recommends against the service. There is moderate or high certainty that the service has no net benefit or that the harms outweigh the benefits.	Discourage the use of this service
I Statement	The USPSTF concludes that the current evidence is insufficient to assess the balance of benefits and harms of the service. Evidence is lacking, of poor quality, or conflicting, and the balance of benefits and harms cannot be determined.	Read the clinical considerations section of USPSTF Recommendation Statement. If the service is offered, patients should understand the uncertainty about the balance of benefits and harms.

Evidence-Based Medicine, the Database of Abstracts of Reviews of Effects (DARE), and the American College of Physicians (ACP) Journal Club (23–25).

Guidelines for Adolescent Preventive Services

Around the same time that clinicians were evaluating the primary health care needs of adults, clinicians who practice adolescent medicine (with backgrounds in pediatrics, internal medicine, family medicine, gynecology, nursing, psychology, nutrition, and other professions) recognized that the guidelines for adult and pediatric health services did not always fit the needs and health risks of adolescence. Neither the ACOG Guidelines for Primary Preventive Care nor the USPSTF recommendations is sufficiently comprehensive or focused on this age group, although both documents include many important aspects of adolescent health care (10,13). The American Medical Association, with the assistance of a national scientific advisory board, developed the Guidelines for Adolescent Preventive Services (GAPS) in response to this perceived need for recommendations for delivering comprehensive adolescent preventive services (13,14,26).

Obstetricians-gynecologists typically see adolescents in crisis to provide care for unintended pregnancies or STDs, including pelvic inflammatory disease. The urgency for preventing these crises is evident. The GAPS report extends the framework of services provided to adolescents. The impetus for developing GAPS was the belief that a fundamental change in the delivery of adolescent health services was necessary. This concept is strongly supported by the Society for Adolescent Medicine, the American Academy of Pediatrics, and the American Academy of Family Physicians (27). Gynecologists could easily provide most, if not all, of the recommended services. The American College of Obstetricians and Gynecologists developed a "Tool Kit" on primary and preventive health care for female adolescents in recognition of the needs of this population, and recommended that the "first visit to the obstetrician-gynecologist for health guidance, screening, and the provision of preventive health care services should take place between the ages of 13 years and 15 years" (28,29). Subsequent annual visits are recommended by ACOG to provide preventive guidance and services including contraception and STD treatment as required. The guidelines and recommendations for adolescent health care address the delivery of health care, focus on the use of health guidance to promote the health and well-being of adolescents and their families, promote the use of screening to identify conditions that occur relatively frequently in adolescents and cause significant suffering either during adolescence or later in life, and provide guidelines for immunizations for the primary prevention of specific infectious diseases. Considerable barriers exist to adolescents' accessing these services, including barriers inherent in the US health care system and legal barriers (30).

The recommendations for adolescent preventive services stem from the conclusion that the current health threats to adolescents are predominantly behavioral rather than biomedical, that more of today's adolescents are involved in behaviors with the potential for serious health consequences, that adolescents are involved in health-risk behaviors at younger ages than previous generations, that many adolescents engage in multiple health-risk behaviors, and that most adolescents engage in at least some type of behavior that threatens their health and well-being (26). **Gynecologists are in a good position to detect high-risk behaviors and to determine whether multiple risk-taking behaviors exist; for example, the early initiation of sexual activity and unsafe sexual practices are associated with substance use** (30,31). Adolescents who are sexually active are much more likely than are adolescents who are not sexually active to have used alcohol (6.3 times greater risk), to have used drugs other than marijuana (four times greater risk), and to have been a passenger in a motor vehicle with a driver who was using drugs (nearly 10 times greater risk) (32). Thus, by being aware of comorbidities, gynecologists can screen for these behaviors and potentially intervene before serious harmful health consequences occur. In recognition of the role that obstetricians-gynecologists could play in providing preventive services for adolescents, ACOG issued guidelines that suggest an initial visit (not necessarily including gynecologic examination) to the obstetrician-gynecologist for health guidance, screening, and the provision of preventive health care service between the ages of 13 and 15 years and subsequent annual preventive health care visits (29).

Counseling for Health Maintenance

During periodic assessments, patients should be counseled about preventive care based on their age and risk factors. **Obesity, smoking, and alcohol abuse are associated with preventable problems that can have major long-term impacts on health.** Patients should be counseled about smoking cessation and moderation in alcohol use and directed to appropriate community resources as necessary. Positive health behaviors, such as eating a healthy diet and engaging in regular exercise, should be reinforced. Adjustments may be necessary based on the presence of risk factors and the woman's current lifestyle and condition. Efforts should focus on weight control, cardiovascular fitness, and reduction of risk factors associated with cardiovascular disease and diabetes (1).

Nutrition

Patients should be given general nutritional information and referred to other professionals if they have special needs (1). **Assessment of the patient's body mass index (BMI; weight [in kilograms] divided by height [in meters] squared [kilograms per square meter]) will give valuable information about the patient's nutritional status.** Tables and methods to calculate BMI are available in print and electronic resources. Patients who are 20% above or below the normal range require evaluation and counseling and should be assessed for systemic disease or an eating disorder. **Of adult women in the United States, 64% are overweight (BMI 25.0–29.9) or obese (BMI ≥30) 36% are obese** (33,34). Overweight and obesity substantially increase the risk of morbidity from hypertension, dyslipidemia, type 2 diabetes, coronary artery disease, stroke, gallbladder disease, osteoarthritis, sleep apnea, and cancers of the endometrium, breast, and colon (35). ACOG has emphasized the role of the obstetrician-gynecologist in the assessment and management of obesity (36).

Central obesity—measured as waist-to-hip ratio—is an independent risk factor for disease. Women with a waist circumference greater than 35 inches are at higher risk of diabetes, dyslipidemia, hypertension, and cardiovascular disease (37). Metabolic syndrome is a complication of obesity that, while somewhat variably defined, includes a clustering of atherogenic dyslipidemia, elevated blood pressure, elevated plasma glucose, and abdominal obesity and confers an increased risk for cardiovascular disease and diabetes (38). One-third to one-half of premenopausal women with polycystic ovarian syndrome (PCOS) meet the criteria for metabolic syndrome (39).

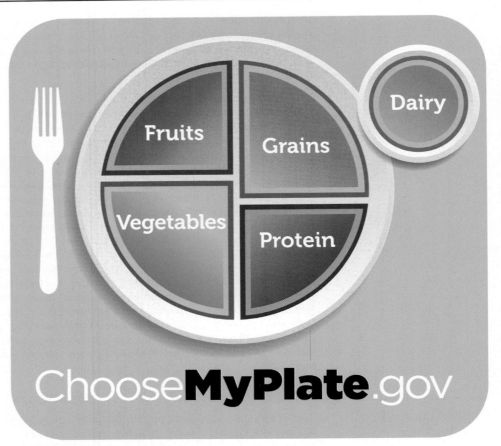

Figure 8.1 *MyPlate Icon.* This is a new communications initiative based on *2010 Dietary Guidelines for Americans,* replacing the Food Pyramid. It is designed to remind Americans to eat healthfully, and illustrates the five food groups using a familiar the familiar mealtime visual of a place setting. (From the United States Department of Agriculture, http://www.ChoseMyPlate.gov)

Key nutritional recommendations were issued by the Dietary Guidelines Advisory Committee to the U.S. Department of Agriculture (40). These recommendations are included in the MyPlate 2010 Guidelines, which has an emphasis on fruits, vegetables, whole grains, and fat-free or low-fat milk and milk products (Fig. 8.1) (41). The guidelines include recommendations to balance food and physical activity and stay within daily calorie requirements.

Fiber content of the diet is being studied for its potential role in the prevention of several disorders, particularly colon cancer. **It is recommended that the average diet for women contain 25 g of fiber per day (40). Whole-grain foods, and vegetables, citrus fruits, and some legumes, are high in fiber and are emphasized in the guidelines for healthy foods.**

Adequate calcium intake is important in the prevention of osteoporosis. A postmenopausal woman should ingest 1,500 mg per day. Adolescents require 1,300 mg per day. Because it may be difficult to ingest an adequate amount of calcium daily in an average diet, supplements may be required.

The U.S. Public Health Service has recommended that women of reproductive age who are capable of becoming pregnant take supplemental folic acid (0.4 mg daily) to help prevent neural tube defects in their infants. Surveys indicate that in 2007, 40% of women of childbearing age consumed a supplement, a percentage that is only half of the *Healthy people 2010* objective of 80% (42). Women who are contemplating pregnancy should be counseled about the risk of fetal neural tube defects and the role of folic acid supplementation prior to conception in their prevention (43).

Alcohol

Alcoholic beverages should be limited to one drink per day for women (40). A simple device called the **T-ACE** questionnaire (**T**olerance; been **A**nnoyed by criticism of drinking; felt need to **C**ut down; need for **E**ye-opener) can be used to elicit information about alcohol use and identify problem drinkers (44). Women should be questioned in a nonjudgmental fashion about their alcohol use and directed to counseling services as required.

Exercise

Exercise can help control or prevent hypertension, diabetes mellitus, hypercholesterolemia, and cardiovascular disease and helps to promote overall good health, psychological well-being, and a healthy body weight. Moderate exercise along with calcium supplementation can help retard bone loss in postmenopausal women. During early menopause, weight-bearing exercise alone is not sufficient to prevent bone loss, although it will slow the rate of bone loss (45). Exercise helps promote weight loss, strength and fitness, and stress reduction. Federal exercise guidelines from the U.S. Department of Health and Human Services note that "regular physical activity reduces the risk of many adverse health outcomes; some physical activity is better than none; for most health outcomes, additional benefits occur as the amount of physical activity increases through higher intensity, greater frequency, and/or longer duration; most health benefits occur with at least 150 minutes (2 hours and 30 minutes) a week of moderate-intensity physical activity, such as brisk walking. Additional benefits occur with more physical activity; both aerobic (endurance) and muscle-strengthening (resistance) physical activity are beneficial; health benefits occur for children and adolescents, young and middle-aged adults, older adults, and those in every studied racial and ethnic group; the health benefits of physical activity occur for people with disabilities; and the benefits of physical activity far outweigh the possibility of adverse outcomes" (46). **To sustain weight loss in adulthood, 60 to 90 minutes of daily moderate-intensity physical activity are recommended.** Cardiovascular conditioning, stretching exercises for flexibility, resistance exercises, or calisthenics for muscle strength and endurance are recommended for most people. Most healthy adults do not need to see a physician before starting a moderate-intensity exercise program, although those with chronic diseases and women over 50 who plan a vigorous program have been advised to do so (40). Women should be counseled about safety guidelines for exercise. Factors that should be considered in establishing an exercise program include medical limitations, such as obesity or arthritis, and careful selection of activities that promote health and enhance compliance (1).

Cardiovascular fitness can be evaluated by measurement of heart rate during exercise. As conditioning improves, the heart rate stabilizes at a fixed level. The heart rate at which conditioning will develop is called the target heart rate (1). The traditional formula for calculating the target heart rate is 220 minus the patient's age times 0.75. A 2010 study examined the definition of a normal heart rate response to exercise stress testing in women and noted that the traditional male-based calculation of target heart rate may not be appropriate for women (47). **The new formula for target heart rate, based on this research, is 206 minus the patient's age times 0.88.**

Smoking Cessation

Smoking is a major cause of preventable illness, and every opportunity should be taken to encourage patients who smoke to quit. Patient education about the benefits of smoking cessation, clear advice to quit smoking, and physician support improve smoking cessation rates, although 95% of smokers who successfully quit do so on their own. Self-help materials are available from the National Cancer Institute, and community-based support groups and local chapters of the American Cancer Society and the American Lung Association. The combination of counseling and medication (nicotine and nonnicotine options) is more effective than either used alone, and Clinical Practice Guidelines on treating tobacco use and dependence from the U.S. Department of Health and Human Services provide recommendations (48).

The "5 As"—*Ask, Advise, Assess, Assist,* and *Arrange*—are designed to be used with smokers who are willing to quit (49). The *Assist* component typically includes first-line pharmacotherapy with *bupropion* or nicotine replacement in the form of gum, inhaler, nasal spray, or patch. In addition, ongoing visits for counseling and support are essential and may include practical counseling and assistance with problem-solving skills and social support during and after treatment. Relapse prevention is important, with congratulations for any successes and encouragement to remain abstinent. Patients who use tobacco but are unwilling to quit at the time of the visit should be treated with the "5 Rs" motivational intervention: *Relevance, Risks, Rewards, Roadblocks,* and *Repetition* (48).

References

1. **ACOG Editorial Committee for Guidelines for Women's Health Care.** Guidelines for women's health care: a resource manual. 3rd ed. Washington, DC: ACOG, 2007:573.

2. **Coleman VH, Laube DW, Hale RW, et al.** Obstetrician-gynecologists and primary care: training during obstetrics-gynecology residency and current practice patterns. *Acad Med* 2007;82:602–607.

3. **Taylor D, Levi A, Simmonds K.** Reframing unintended pregnancy prevention: a public health model. *Contraception* 2010;81:363–366.

4. **Donaldson M, Yordy N, Vanselow N, eds.** *Defining primary care: an interim report.* Institute of Medicine. Washington, DC: National Academy Press, 1994.

5. **Franks P, Clancy CM, Nutting PA.** Defining primary care. Empirical analysis of the National Ambulatory Medical Care Survey. *Med Care* 1997;35:655–668.

6. **American College of Obstetricians and Gynecologists.** *ACOG Legislative Priorities.* ACOG, 2011. Available at http://www.acog.org/departments/dept_web.cfm?recno = 44

7. **ACOG Committee.** ACOG Committee Opinion No. 423: motivational interviewing: a tool for behavioral change. *Obstet Gynecol* 2009; 113:243–246.

8. **Hing E, Burt CW.** *Characteristics of office-based physicians and their practices: United States, 2003–04.* Hyattsville, MD: National Center for Health Statistics, 2007.

9. **Henderson JT, Weisman CS.** Women's patterns of provider use across the lifespan and satisfaction with primary care coordination and comprehensiveness. *Med Care* 2005;43:826–833.

10. **ACOG Committee.** ACOG Committee Opinion No. 452: Primary and preventive care: periodic assessments. *Obstet Gynecol* 2009;114:1444–1451.

11. **American College of Obstetricians and Gynecologists.** Primary and preventive health care for female adolescents. In: *Health care for adolescents.* Washington, DC: American College of Obstetricians and Gynecologists, 2003:1–24.

12. **American Academy of Family Physicians.** *Summary of recommendations for clinical preventive services.* 2010. Available online from: http://www.aafp.org/online/etc/medialib/aafp_org/documents/clinical/CPS/rcps08–2005.Par.0001.File.tmp/February2011CPS03142011.pdf.

13. **U.S. Preventive Services Task Force.** *Recommendations for adults.* 2010. Available online at: http://www.ahrq.gov/clinic/uspstfix.htm

14. **American Medical Association.** *Guidelines for adolescent preventive services (GAPS).* Chicago, IL: American Medical Association, 1997:8.

15. **Agency for Healthcare Research and Quality.** *National guideline clearinghouse.* 2010. Available online at: htp://www.guideline.gov.

16. **Schappert SM, Rechtsteiner EA.** Ambulatory medical care utilization estimates for 2006. *Natl Health Stat Report* 2008;8:1–29.

17. **Brett KM, Burt CW.** *Utilization of ambulatory medical care by women: United States, 1997–98.* Atlanta: U.S. Centers for Disease Control, 2001:1–17.

18. **Scholle SH, Chang J, Harman J, et al.** Characteristics of patients seen and services provided in primary care visits in obstetrics/gynecology: data from NAMCS and NHAMCS. *Am J Obstet Gynecol* 2004;190:1119–1127.

19. **Branson BM, Handsfield HH, Lampe MA, et al.** Revised recommendations for HIV testing of adults, adolescents, and pregnant women in health-care settings. *MMWR Recomm Rep* 2006;55[RR14]:1–17.

20. **Petitti DB, Teutsch SM, Barton MB, et al.** Update on the methods of the U.S. Preventive Services Task Force: insufficient evidence. *Ann Intern Med* 2009;150:199–205.

21. **The Cochrane Collaboration.** *The Cochrane Library.* 2010. Available online at: http://www.thecochranelibrary.com

22. **British Medical Journal.** *Clinical evidence.* 2010. Available online at: http://www.clinicalevidence.bmj.com

23. **University of Oxford.** *Oxford Centre for Evidence Based Medicine.* 2010. [Aim to develop, teach and promote evidence-based health care and provide support and resources ot doctors and health care professionals to help maintain the highest standards of medicine]. Available online at: http://www.cebm.net/

24. **Centre for Reviews and Dissemination.** *Database of abstracts of reviews of effects (DARE).* 2010. [Contains 15,000 abstracts of systematic reviews including over 6000 quality assessed reviews and details of all Cochrane reviews and protocols. The database focuses on the effects of interventions used in health and social care.] Available online at: http://www.crd.york.ac.uk/crdweb/Home.aspx?DB=DARE

25. **American College of Physicians.** *ACP Journal Club.* 2010. [Quality-assessed, clinically rated original studies and reviews from over 130 clinical journals.] Available online at: http://www.acpjc.org/

26. **Elster AB, Kuznets NJ.** *AMA guidelines for adolescent preventive services (GAPS): recommendations and rationale.* Baltimore: Williams & Wilkins, 1994:1–191.

27. **Rosen DS, Elster A, Hedberg V, et al.** Clinical preventive services for adolescents: Position paper of the society for adolescent medicine. *J Adolesc Health* 1997;21:203–214.

28. **American College of Obstetricians and Gynecologists.** *Tool kit for teen care.* Washington, DC: ACOG, 2010.

29. **ACOG Committee on Adolescent Health Care.** *The initial reproductive health visit.* Committee Opinion. Washington, DC: ACOG, 2010.

30. **English A, Ford CA, Santelli JS.** Clinical preventive services for adolescents: position paper of the Society for Adolescent Medicine. *Am J Law Med* 2009;35:351–364.

31. **Zabin LS, Hardy JB, Smith EA, et al.** Substance use and its relation to sexual activity among inner-city adolescents. *J Adolesc Health Care* 1986;7:320–331.

32. **Orr DP, Beiter M, Ingersoll G.** Premature sexual activity as an indicator of psychosocial risk. *Pediatrics* 1991;87:141–147.

33. **Flegal KM, Carroll MD, Ogden CL, et al.** Prevalence and trends in obesity among US adults, 1999–2008. *JAMA* 2010;303:235–241.

34. **Centers for Disease Control and Prevention.** Vital signs: state-specific obesity prevalence among adults—United States, 2009. *MMWR Morb Mortal Wkly Rep* 2010;59:951–955.

35. **Mokdad AH, Ford ES, Bowman BA, et al.** Prevalence of obesity, diabetes, and obesity-related health risk factors, 2001. *JAMA* 2003;289:76–79.

36. **ACOG Committee.** ACOG Committee Opinion No. 319, October 2005. The role of obstetrician-gynecologist in the assessment and management of obesity. *Obstet Gynecol* 2005;106:895–899.

37. **National Heart, Lung, and Blood Institute Obesity Education Initiative.** *The practical guide: identification, evaluation, and treatment of overweight and obesity in adults.* Obesity Education Initiative 2000. Available online at: http://www.nhlbi.nih.gov/guidelines/obesity/practgde.htm

38. **Alberti KG, Eckel RH, Grundy SM, et al.** Harmonizing the metabolic syndrome: a joint interim statement of the International Diabetes Federation Task Force on Epidemiology and Prevention; National Heart, Lung, and Blood Institute; American Heart Association; World Heart Federation; International Atherosclerosis Society; and International Association for the Study of Obesity. *Circulation* 2009;120:1640–1645.

39. **Essah PA, Wickham EP, Nestler JE.** The metabolic syndrome in polycystic ovary syndrome. *Clin Obstet Gynecol* 2007;50:205–225.

40. **U.S. Department of Agriculture.** *Dietary guidelines for Americans.* 2005. Available online at: http://www.health.gov/dietaryguidelines

41. **U.S. Department of Agriculture.** *My pyramid.* 2005. Available online at: http://www.mypyramid.gov

42. **Centers for Disease Control and Prevention.** Use of supplements containing folic acid among women of childbearing age—United States, 2007. *MMWR Morb Mortal Wkly Rep* 2008;57:5–8.

43. **ACOG Committee.** ACOG Committee Opinion No. 313: the importance of preconception care in the continuum of women's health care. *Obstet Gynecol* 2005;106:665–666.

44. **Sokol RJ, Martier SS, Ager JW.** The T-ACE questions: practical prenatal detection of risk-drinking. *Am J Obstet Gynecol* 1989;160:865.

45. **American College of Obstetricians and Gynecologists.** *Osteoporosis.* Washington, DC: American College of Obstetricians and Gynecologists, 2004.

46. **U.S. Department of Health and Human Services.** *2008 physical activity guidelines for Americans.* Washington, DC: U.S. Department of Health and Human Services, 2008:76.

47. **Gulati M, Shaw LJ, Thisted RA, et al.** Heart rate response to exercise stress testing in asymptomatic women: the st. James women take heart project. *Circulation* 2010;122:130–137.

48. **Fiore MC, Jaén CR, Baker TB, et al.** Treating tobacco use and dependence: 2008 update. In: *Clinical practice guideline.* Washington, DC: U.S. Department of Health and Human Services, 2008.

Available online at: http://www.surgeongeneral.gov/tobacco/treating_tobacco_use08.pdf.

49. **Agency for Healthcare Research and Quality.** *Five major steps to intervention (the "5A's").* Available online at: http://www.ahrq.gov/clinic/tobacco/5steps/htm

50. **U.S. Preventive Services Task Force.** *U.S. preventive services task force grade definitions and levels of certainty regarding net benefit.* 2008. Available online at: http://www.uspreventiveservicestaskforce.org/uspstf/grades.htm

9

Primary Care

Sharon T. Phelan
Thomas E. Nolan

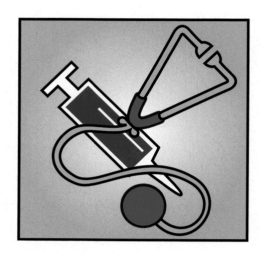

- **Empiric therapy for women with pneumonia should be based on the specific patient profiles and the severity of their pneumonia. All patients with possible community-acquired pneumonia should have a chest radiograph to establish the diagnosis and the presence of complications.**

- **Most patients with hypertension will require two or more antihypertensive medications to achieve optimal blood pressure control less than 140/90 or less than 130/80 mm Hg for patients with diabetes or kidney disease, respectively.**

- **There is an increased use of cholesterol-lowering drugs, including the "statins," a class of drugs that lower cholesterol by blocking a liver enzyme necessary to produce cholesterol, and they are very effective in reducing the risk of heart attacks and deaths.**

- **Type 2 diabetes is frequently not diagnosed until complications appear, and approximately one-third of all people with diabetes may be undiagnosed: individuals at risk should be screened and a comprehensive plan of care initiated for those diagnosed with diabetes.**

- **The sensitive thyroid-stimulating hormone (TSH) assay is the single best screening test for hyperthyroidism and hypothyroidism: in clinical hypothyroidism, the standard treatment is *levothyroxine* replacement, which must be tailored to the individual patient.**

As health care providers for women, gynecologists are responsible for providing care that extends beyond diseases of the reproductive organs to include much of the general medical care of their patients. Broadening the spectrum of care requires adjustments in practice, with less emphasis placed on the surgical aspects of the specialty. Early diagnosis and treatment of medical illnesses can have a major impact on a woman's health. Although timely referral is important for complex and advanced diseases, many conditions can be recognized and treated initially by gynecologists.

Respiratory problems are the most common reasons patients seek care from a physician, so gynecologists should be aware of their pathophysiology. Cardiovascular disease has a significant impact on overall morbidity and is the main cause of death in women. Cardiovascular disease is associated with cigarette smoking, hypertension, hypercholesterolemia, and diabetes mellitus. These conditions are responsive to screening, behavior modification,

and control to lower risk factors. Thyroid disease is a major cause of morbidity for women. Because of the interaction of hormones and the overall effect on the endocrine system, thyroid disease can be of special significance in women. The gynecologist should provide screening and initial therapy for these conditions and assess the need for referral.

Respiratory Infections

Infections of the respiratory system can range from the common cold to life-threatening illness. Those with risk factors should be counseled about preventive measures. Vaccines against flu and pneumonia should be offered as indicated.

Sinusitis

A problem frequently encountered in women is self-diagnosed "sinus problems." Many medical problems—headaches, dental pain, postnasal drainage, halitosis, and dyspepsia—may be related to sinus conditions. The sinuses are not an isolated organ, and diseases of the sinuses are often related to conditions that affect other portions of the respiratory system (i.e., the nose, bronchial tree, and lungs). The entire respiratory system can be infected by one particular virus or pathogen (the sinobronchial or sinopulmonary syndrome); however, the most prominent symptoms are usually produced in one anatomic area. Therefore, during the evaluation of symptoms attributable to sinusitis, the presence of other infections should be investigated.

Multiple infectious and chemical agents or reactions to nervous, physical, emotional, or hormonal stimuli may cause an inflammatory response in the respiratory system (1). Systemic diseases such as connective tissue syndromes and malnutrition may contribute to chronic sinusitis. Environmental factors in the workplace and geographic conditions (e.g., cold and damp weather) may aggravate or accelerate the development of sinusitis. Factors contributing to the development of sinus disease include atmospheric pollutants, allergy, tobacco smoke, skeletal deformities, dental conditions, barotrauma from scuba diving or airline travel, and neoplasms.

Most acute infections (lasting less than 4 weeks) begin with a viral agent in the nose or nasopharynx that causes inflammation, blocking the draining ostia (1). The location of the symptoms varies by anatomic site of infection—maxillary sinus over the cheeks, ethmoid sinus across the nose, frontal sinus in the supraorbital area, and sphenoid sinus to the vertex of the head—and typically last 7 to 10 days, clearing with nothing more than a decongestant. **Viral agents impede the sweeping motion of ciliary function in the sinus and, in combination with edema from inflammation, may occasionally lead to superinfection with bacteria. The most common bacterial agents infecting sinuses are *Streptococcus pneumoniae* and *Haemophilus influenzae*.** Gram-negative organisms are usually limited to compromised hosts in intensive care units. Although less than 2% of acute sinusitis cases transition from viral to bacterial infections requiring antibiotics, more than 85% of patients receive antibiotic prescriptions. Chronic sinusitis (lasting more than 12 weeks) develops from either inadequate drainage or compromised local defense mechanisms. The flora usually is polymicrobial, consisting of aerobic and anaerobic organisms.

Sinus ailments frequently occur in middle-age individuals. Acute infection is usually located in the maxillary and frontal sinuses. Classically, infection in the maxillary sinus results from obstruction of the ostia found in the medial wall of the nose. Fever, malaise, a vague headache, and pain in the maxillary teeth are early symptoms. Reports of "fullness" in the face or exploding pressure behind the eyes often are elicited as well as increasing pain with bending over. Pressure and percussion over the malar areas can cause severe pain. Purulent exudates in the middle meatus of the nose or in the nasopharynx often are present. **Five clinical findings are most useful in diagnosis: (i) maxillary toothache, (ii) poor response to nasal decongestants, (iii) abnormal transillumination, (iv) colored visible purulent nasal secretions, and (v) a history of colored nasal discharge.** When four or more features are present, the likelihood of sinusitis is high, and when none is present, sinusitis is highly unlikely (2). Initial episodes of sinusitis do not require imaging studies; however, when persistent infections occur, studies and referral are indicated. Computed tomography of the sinuses demonstrated that 90% of patients with colds have radiological evidence of sinus disease that usually will resolve in 2 to 3 weeks. Radiographic changes do not reliably identify sinusitis secondary to bacteria. After sinus needle aspiration, about 60% of patients with abnormal radiographic images have positive cultures (3). Unless culture samples are obtained by direct needle drainage, they are contaminated by oropharyngeal flora and are thus of no value. For this reason, therapy usually is empiric.

Systemic decongestants containing *pseudoephedrine* **are useful in shrinking the obstructive ostia and promoting sinus drainage and ventilation.** Topical decongestants should be used for no longer than 3 days because prolonged use may lead to rebound vasodilation and worsening of symptoms. Mucolytics like *guaifenesin* may help thin sinus secretions and promote drainage. Antihistamines should be avoided in acute sinusitis because of their drying effects, which can lead to thickened secretions and poor drainage of the sinuses. Analgesics are recommended for pain relief. Therapies to relieve symptoms include facial hot packs and analgesics. Topical nasal steroids may accelerate the recovery in patients with viral sinusitis and those with a history of chronic rhinitis or recurrent sinusitis who seek treatment of acute rhinosinusitis (4,5). Improvement should be apparent within 48 hours of treatment, but 10 days may be necessary for complete resolution of symptoms. When improvement is not rapid, resistance should be presumed, and other classes of antibiotics should be given (6). In persistent cases, referral to an otolaryngologist for sinus irrigation may be necessary (7).

Broad antibiotic coverage of common aerobes and anaerobes is necessary but should be limited to patients with acute pain, especially unilateral maxillary tooth, facial, or sinus pain, and purulent discharge, particularly if the symptoms initially improved and then worsen. This cluster of symptoms is more suggestive of bacterial rather than viral acute sinusitis. It should be noted that the majority of acute bacterial sinusitis cases resolve in 7 to 10 days without antibiotics, similarly to the viral form. For acute bacterial sinus infections, *amoxicillin* (500 mg three times a day) or *trimethoprim/sulfamethoxazole* (1 tablet twice a day) remains the treatment of choice. *Amoxicillin* is inexpensive, penetrates the sinus tissues well, and can be changed to another antibiotic if symptoms have not improved in 48 to 72 hours. If these give only a minimal or no response after 7 days, consider broader spectrum antibiotics. If beta-lactam resistance is likely, *amoxicillin/clavulanic acid* (875 mg twice daily) or *azithromycin* (5-day course once a day) may be used. Other second-line drugs include *cefuroxime* (250 mg twice daily), *ciprofloxacin* (500 mg twice daily), *clarithromycin* (500 mg twice daily), *levofloxacin* (500 mg once a day), and *loracarbef* (400 mg twice daily). The usual treatment course is 10 to 14 days, and patients should be informed that relapses might occur if the full course of treatment is not completed.

Chronic sinusitis may result from repeated infections with inadequate drainage. The interval between infections becomes increasingly shorter until there are no remissions. Presenting symptoms are recurrent pain in the malar area or chronic postnasal drip. In the preantibiotic era, chronic sinusitis was the result of repeated acute sinusitis with incomplete resolution, whereas allergy is currently a more common cause. Injury of surface ciliated epithelium results in impaired removal of mucus. A vicious cycle ensues of incomplete resolution of infection, followed by reinfection, and ending with the emergence of opportunistic organisms. Allergies have become an important factor in chronic sinusitis. The swelling and edema of the mucosa in conjunction with hypersecretion of mucus leads to ductal obstruction and infection. Chronic sinusitis is associated with chronic cough and laryngitis with intermittent acute infections. Treatment is directed at the underlying etiology: either allergy control or aggressive management of infections. Resistant cases require computed tomography and endoscopic surgery for polyp removal. Nasoantral window formation is a radical surgery that is occasionally necessary.

No clinical criteria can reliably identify those patients who might benefit from treatment with antibiotics. It is reasonable to treat women with presumed bacterial sinusitis if they have high fever, systemic toxicity, immune deficiency, or possible orbital or intracranial involvement (6). Although very rare, untreated sinus infections may have dire consequences, such as orbital cellulitis, leading to orbital abscess, subperiosteal abscess formation of the facial bones, cavernous sinus thrombosis, and acute meningitis. Brain and dural abscesses are rare; when they occur, it usually is the result of direct spread from a sinus. A patient complaining of abnormal vision such as diplopia, changes in mental status, and periorbital edema should prompt a referral to emergency room for evaluation of intracranial or orbital extension. Computed tomography scanning is the most accurate diagnostic tool. The use of aggressive surgical approaches with broad-spectrum antibiotics is necessary for adequate drainage.

Otitis Media

Otitis media remains primarily a disease of children, but may affect adults, often secondary to a concurrent viral infection of the upper respiratory tract. Diagnosis in most cases reveals fluid behind the tympanic membrane. Treatment is directed to symptoms and involves the use of antihistamines and decongestants, despite few data to support their use. Acute otitis media is usually a bacterial infection; *Streptococcus pneumoniae* and *Hemophilus influenza* are the most common pathogens. Symptoms include acute purulent otorrhea, fever, hearing loss, and leukocytosis. Physical examination of the ear reveals a red, bulging, or perforated membrane. Indicated treatment is broad-spectrum antibiotics such as *amoxicillin/clavulanic acid, cefuroxime axetil,* and *trimethoprim-sulfamethoxazole.*

Bronchitis

Acute bronchitis is an inflammatory condition of the tracheobronchial tree. Most often it is viral in origin and occurs in winter. Common cold viruses (rhinovirus and coronavirus), adenovirus, influenza virus, and *Mycoplasma pneumoniae* (a nonviral pathogen) are the most common pathogens involved. Bacterial infections occur less commonly and may be secondary pathogens. Cough, hoarseness, and fever are the usual presenting symptoms. In the initial 3 to 4 days, the symptoms of rhinitis and sore throat are prominent; coughing may last as long as 3 weeks. The prolonged nature of these infections promotes the use of antibiotics to "clear up the infection" (8). Sputum production commonly occurs and may be prolonged in cigarette smokers. Most serious bacterial infections occur in cigarette smokers, who have damage to the lining of the upper respiratory tree and changes in the host flora.

Physical examination discloses a variety of upper airway sounds, usually coarse rhonchi. Rales are usually not present on auscultation, and signs of consolidation and alveolar involvement are absent. **During auscultation of the chest, signs of pneumonia such as fine rales, decreased breath sounds, and euphonia ("E to A changes") should be sought.** If the results of the physical examination are uncertain or the patient's condition appears to be in respiratory distress chest radiography should be performed to detect the presence of parenchymal disease. Paradoxically, as the initial acute syndrome subsides, sputum production may become more purulent. Sputum cultures are of limited value because of the polymicrobial nature of infections. In the absence of complications, treatment is directed to relief of symptoms. The use of antibiotics is reserved for patients in whom chest radiography findings are consistent with pneumonia. Cough is usually the most aggravating symptom and may be treated with antitussive preparations containing either *dextromethorphan* or *codeine.* The efficacy of any expectorant is not proved.

Chronic bronchitis is defined as a productive cough from excessive secretions for at least 3 months in a year for 2 consecutive years. Prevalence is estimated to be between 10% and 25% of the adult population who are smokers. Previously the incidence was lower in women than men, but as the prevalence of cigarette smoking in women increased, so too has the incidence of bronchitis in women. Chronic bronchitis is classified as a form of chronic obstructive pulmonary disease (COPD; e.g., "blue bloaters"). Other causes include chronic infections and environmental pathogens found in dust. The cardinal manifestation of disease is an incessant cough, usually in the morning, with expectoration of sputum. Because of frequent exacerbations, the hospitalizations involved and the complexity of medical management, these patients should be referred to an internist.

Pneumonia

Pneumonia is defined as inflammation of the distal lung that includes terminal airways, alveolar spaces, and the interstitium. Pneumonia may have multiple causes, including viral and bacterial infections or aspiration. Aspiration pneumonia is usually the result of depressed awareness commonly associated with the use of drugs and alcohol or anesthesia. Viral pneumonias are caused by multiple infectious agents, including influenza A or B, parainfluenza virus, or respiratory syncytial virus. Most viral syndromes are spread by aerosolization associated with coughing, sneezing, and even conversation. Incubation is short, requiring only 1 to 3 days before the acute onset of fever, chills, headache, fatigue, and myalgias. Symptom intensity is directly related to intensity of the host febrile reaction. Pneumonia develops in only 1% of patients who have a viral syndrome, but mortality rates may reach 30% in immunocompromised individuals and the elderly. An additional risk is the development of secondary bacterial pneumonias after the initial viral insult. These infections are more common in elderly patients and may explain the high fatality in this group (8). *Staphylococcal* pneumonias, which often arise from a previous viral infection, are extremely lethal regardless of patient age. The best treatment for viral pneumonia is prevention by immunization. Treatment is supportive and consists mostly of administration of antipyretics and fluids.

Bacterial pneumonia is classified as either community acquired or nosocomial, and in many cases the classification determines prognosis and antibiotic therapy. Risk factors that contribute to mortality are chronic cardiopulmonary diseases, alcoholism, diabetes, renal failure, malignancy, and malnutrition. Prognostic features associated with poor outcome include greater than two lobe involvement, respiratory rate greater than 30 breaths per minute on presentation, severe hypoxemia (<60 mm Hg on room air), hypoalbuminemia, and septicemia. Pneumonia is a common cause of adult respiratory distress syndrome (ARDS), with a mortality rate between 50% and 70% (9,10).

Signs and symptoms of pneumonia vary depending on the infecting organism and the patient's immune status. In typical pneumonias, the usual presentation is a patient with high fever, rigors, productive cough, chills, and pleuritic chest pain. Chest radiography often will show infiltrates (11). The following agents, listed in decreasing order, cause two-thirds of all bacterial pneumonias: *Streptococcus pneumoniae, Haemophilus influenza, Klebsiella pneumoniae,* gram-negative organisms, and anaerobic bacteria. Atypical pneumonias are more insidious in onset than typical pneumonias. Patients have moderate fever without the characteristic rigors and chills. Additional symptoms include a nonproductive cough, headache, myalgias, and mild leukocytosis. Chest radiography reveals bronchopneumonia with a diffuse interstitial pattern; characteristically, the patient does not appear to be as ill as the x-ray suggests. Common causes of atypical pneumonia include viruses, *Mycoplasma pneumoniae, Legionella pneumophila, Chlamydia pneumoniae* (also called the TWAR agent), and other rare agents.

A strong index of suspicion is required for diagnosis, especially in elderly and immuno-compromised individuals, who have altered response mechanisms. This is true with "typical agents." Subtle clues in the elderly include changes in mentation, confusion, and exacerbation of other illnesses. The febrile response may be entirely absent, and the results of the physical examination are not predictive of pneumonia. In high-risk groups, an increased respiratory rate of greater than 25 breaths per minute remains the most reliable sign of infection. Mortality in these high-risk groups of patients is strongly correlated with the ability of the host to mount normal defenses to the symptoms of fever, chills, and tachycardia.

All women suspected of having pneumonia should undergo chest radiography to establish the diagnosis and to detect alternate diagnoses such as congestive heart failure and tumors. The chest radiograph can detect complications like pleural effusions and multilobar disease. Laboratory studies helpful in identifying community-acquired pneumonia are sputum Gram stain, sputum culture, and two sets of blood culture. An "adequate sputum" sample (defined as more than 25 neutrophils with less than 10 epithelial cells per low-powered field on microscopic examination) may be difficult to obtain. Respiratory therapists are an excellent resource for inducing sputum. Hospitalized patients undergo assessment of blood–gas exchange by either oximetry or arterial blood–gas analysis. Diagnosis of *Legionella pneumoniae* requires a different laboratory technique: measuring urinary antigen levels. *Mycoplasma pneumoniae* should be suspected when cold agglutinin findings are positive in the presence of the appropriate clinical symptoms.

The American Thoracic Society updated their original guidelines in 2001 (10). These clinical recommendations use an evidence-based approach for the diagnosis and management of community-acquired pneumonia. Therapy should be directed at the responsible or most likely pathogen, but in many cases of pneumonia, the exact cause cannot be determined, and empiric therapy should be initiated. The American Thoracic Society recommends empiric therapy based on four groups of specific patient profiles, the presence of modifying factors, and pneumonia severity (Table 9.1).

- **Group I. Outpatients with no cardiopulmonary disease (congestive heart failure or COPD) and no modifying factors.** These patients are in the lowest-risk group and are usually infected by pathogens such as *Chlamydia pneumoniae, Mycoplasma pneumoniae,* or *Streptococcus pneumoniae.* Patients should be treated with an advanced generation macrolide such as *azithromycin, clarithromycin,* or *doxycycline.*

- **Group II. Outpatients with cardiopulmonary disease or modifying factors.** Patients in this group usually have some comorbidities and are older than 50 years of age. Aerobic gram-negative bacilli, mixed infections with atypical pathogens, and drug-resistant *S. pneumoniae* (DRSP) should be considered in this patient population. Drug recommendations include monotherapy with an antipneumococcal fluoroquinolone, such as *gatifloxacin* or *levofloxacin*; a combination of a macrolide (or *doxycycline*) with a beta-lactam such as *cefpodoxime, cefuroxime,* or *amoxicillin-clavulanate*; or parenteral *ceftriaxone* followed by *cefpodoxime.*

Table 9.1 Modifying Factors that Increase the Risk of Infection with Specific Pathogens

Penicillin-resistant and-drug resistant pneumococci

Age >65 years

| Beta-lactam therapy within the past 3 months |
| Alcoholism |
| Immune-suppressive illness (including therapy with corticosteroids) |
| Multiple medical comorbidities |
| Exposure to a child in a day-care center |

Enteric gram-negatives

| Residence in a nursing home |
| Underlying cardiopulmonary disease |
| Multiple medical comorbidities |
| Recent antibiotic therapy |

Pseudomonas aeruginosa

| Structural lung disease (bronchiectasis) |
| Corticosteroid therapy (>10 mg of prednisone per day) |
| Broad-spectrum antibiotic therapy for >7 days in the past month |
| Malnutrition |

Adapted from **American Thoracic Society.** Guidelines for the management of adults with community-acquired pneumonia. *Am J Respir Crit Care Med* 2001;163:1730–1754.

- **Group III. Inpatients who are not in the intensive care unit and have cardiopulmonary or modifying factors.** Drugs for these patients include intravenous fluoroquinolone monotherapy or a combination of an intravenous beta-lactam agent plus either intravenous or oral administration of an advanced *macrolide* or *doxycycline*. For the small group of inpatients who do not have cardiopulmonary diseases or modifying factors, intravenous *azithromycin* alone can be used. Alternatives include *doxycycline* plus a beta-lactam agent (if *macrolide* allergy or intolerance is present) or monotherapy with an antipneumococcal fluoroquinolone.

- **Group IV. Inpatients in the intensive care unit.** These patients usually have the most severe pneumonia, and all antibiotics are given intravenously. Immediate consultation with an internist, hospitalist, or infectious disease specialist is recommended.

Oxygen therapy and hydration should be initiated in addition to antibiotic therapy. Most patients will have an adequate clinical response within 3 days of treatment. Oral antibiotics may be given when patients meet the following criteria: ability to eat and drink, improvement in cough and dyspnea, afebrile (<100°F) on two occasions 8 hours apart, and a decreasing white blood cell count. If other clinical features are favorable, patients may be switched to oral antibiotics even if febrile. They may be discharged on the same day that oral antibiotics are started if other medical and social factors are favorable.

Vaccination

The *pneumococcal vaccine* should be given to people at high risk for pneumonia, which includes adults 65 years or older and people with special health problems, such as heart or lung disease, alcoholism, kidney failure, diabetes, HIV infection, or certain types of cancer. Repeat vaccination is recommended 5 years after the first dose is given. The vaccine is active against 23 types of pneumococcal strains, and most individuals develop protection within 2 to 3 weeks of inoculations.

The *influenza vaccine* should be given every fall to high-risk groups: individuals 50 years of age or older; anyone with serious long-term health problems such as heart disease, lung disease, kidney disease, diabetes, and weak immune systems as with HIV and AIDS;

Table 9.2 Major Risk Factors for Coronary Artery Disease
Age >55 for men and >65 for women
Family history of cardiovascular disease (men <55 y; women <65 y)
Physical inactivity
Diabetes mellitus
Cigarette smoking
Dyslipidemia
Obesity (body mass index ≥30)
Hypertension
Microalbuminuria or estimated glomerular filtration rate <60 mL/min

Adapted from **Chobanian AV, Bakris GL, Black HR, et al.** The seventh report of the Joint National Committee on Prevention, Detection, Evaluation, and Treatment of High Blood Pressure (JNC VII). *JAMA* 2003;289:2560–2572.

individuals on long-term steroids or receiving cancer treatment; women who are pregnant during the flu season (November through April); and anyone coming in close contact with people at risk of serious influenza like physicians, nurses, and family members. Vaccination is best given from October to mid-November. Antiviral agents should not be used as a substitute for vaccination but may be a useful adjunct. The four agents approved for use in the United States are *amantadine, rimantadine, zanamivir,* and *oseltamivir.* These drugs should be given within 2 days of the onset of symptoms to shorten the duration of uncomplicated illness caused by influenza (11–13).

Cardiovascular Disease

The risk factors for coronary artery disease are presented in Table 9.2. **Central to treating cardiovascular disease is the control of contributing diseases and risk factors through lifestyle modifications** (Table 9.3). Aerobic exercise protects against cardiovascular disease (14). Additional aspects of prevention of myocardial disease, renal disease, and stroke include control of hypertension, identification and control of diabetes and obesity, and control of dietary fats, especially cholesterol, in susceptible individuals (Fig. 9.1). The presence or absence of target organ damage shown in Table 9.4 also determines the risk of coronary artery disease in hypertensive patients.

Hypertension

The relationship between hypertension and cardiovascular events such as stroke, coronary artery disease, congestive heart disease, and renal disease is well known. More than 50 million people in the United States have hypertension. It is found in 15% of the population between the ages of 18 and 74 years; the incidence increases with age and varies with race. The contribution of hypertension to overall cardiovascular morbidity and mortality in women was

Table 9.3 Lifestyle Adjustments to Manage Hypertension
Weight reduction to maintain a body mass index of 18.5–24.9
Limit alcohol use to 2 drinks per day for men (24 oz beer, 10 oz of wine, 3 oz of 80-proof whiskey) and no more than 1 drink per day in women and lighter-weight persons
Regular aerobic exercise (at least 30 minutes per day of brisk walking most days of the week)
Decrease salt intake to less than 2.4 g of sodium or 6 g of sodium chloride per day
Consume a diet rich in fruits, vegetables, and low-fat dairy products with a reduced content of saturated and total fat

Adapted from **Chobanian AV, Bakris GL, Black HR, et al.** The seventh report of the Joint National Committee on Prevention, Detection, Evaluation, and Treatment of High Blood Pressure (JNC VII). *JAMA* 2003;289:2560–2572.

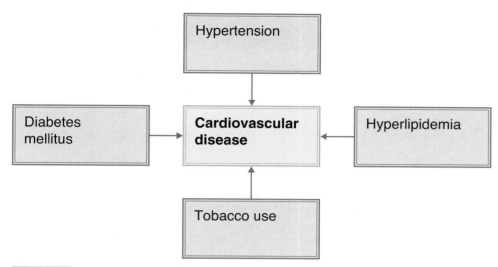

Figure 9.1   Disease and risk factors contributing to cardiovascular disease.

thought to be less important than that in men, but this may reflect the relative absence of research in women (15). After age 50, women have a higher incidence of hypertension than men; this may be a confounding variable related to the overall mortality of men at an earlier age (16). More than 60% of those individuals older than age 60 years can be classified as hypertensive (17). Recognition and treatment of hypertension may decrease the development of renal and cardiac disease.

Epidemiology

The incidence of hypertension is twice as high in African Americans than in whites. Geographic variations exist: the southeastern United States has a higher prevalence of hypertension and stroke, regardless of race (16). One multi-institutional study confirmed an increased incidence of hypertension in African Americans, and that the incidence is increased in individuals with lower levels of education (17). Preventive measures can be most effective in those at highest risk, such as in African American women and individuals from the lowest socioeconomic level (17). The influence of genetic predisposition is poorly understood. Studies of women are limited to those that determine side effects of medication and the impact of certain medications on long-term lipid status (13).

Classically, hypertension is defined as blood pressure levels higher than 140/90 when measured on two separate occasions. Medication may be indicated only for individuals at high risk. Individuals at low risk, such as white women with no other risk factors, may benefit from lifestyle modification alone. Life insurance risk tables indicate that when blood pressure is controlled to lower than 140/90, normal survival occurs over a 10- to 20-year follow-up, regardless of gender. Current recommendations are based on sustained blood pressures higher than 140/90 (18).

Table 9.4 Target Organ Damage
Stroke or transient ischemic attacks
Hypertensive retinopathy
Heart disease
Angina or prior myocardial infarction Congestive heart failure Prior coronary revascularization Left ventricular hypertrophy Chronic kidney disease
Peripheral arterial disease

Adapted from **Chobanian AV, Bakris GL, Black HR, et al.** The seventh report of the Joint National Committee on Prevention, Detection, Evaluation, and Treatment of High Blood Pressure (JNC VII). *JAMA* 2003;289:2560–2572.

Table 9.5 Laboratory Tests and Procedures Recommended in the Evaluation of Uncomplicated Hypertension[a]

Urinalysis
Complete blood count
Potassium
Creatinine or estimated glomerular filtration rate
Calcium
Fasting glucose
Lipid profile that includes HDL, LDL, and triglycerides after a 9- to 12-hour fast
12-lead electrocardiogram

HDL, high-density lipoprotein; LDL, low-density lipoprotein.
[a]If any of the above are abnormal, consultation or referral to an internist is indicated.
Adapted from **Chobanian AV, Bakris GL, Black HR, et al.** The seventh report of the Joint National Committee on Prevention, Detection, Evaluation, and Treatment of High Blood Pressure (JNC VII). *JAMA* 2003;289:2560–2572.

More than 95% of individuals with hypertension have primary or essential hypertension (cause unknown), whereas fewer than 5% have secondary hypertension resulting from another disorder. Key factors to be determined in the history and physical examination include presence of prior elevated readings, previous use of antihypertensive agents, a family history of cardiovascular death before age 55, and excessive intake of alcohol or sodium. Lifestyle modification is considered important in the therapy of hypertension; thus, a detailed history of diet and physical activity should be obtained (14). Baseline laboratory evaluations to rule out reversible causes of hypertension (secondary hypertension) are listed in Table 9.5. Diagnosis and management are based on the classification of blood pressure readings, as presented in Table 9.6.

The Joint National Committee on Prevention, Detection, Evaluation, and Treatment of High Blood Pressure (JNC 7) released their seventh report in 2003. The purpose was to provide an evidence-based approach to the prevention and management of hypertension. **Following are key points of this report:**

- **Systolic blood pressure in those older than 50 years is a more important cardiovascular risk factor than diastolic blood pressure.**

- **Beginning at 115/75 mm Hg, the risk of cardiovascular disease doubles for each increment of 20/10 mm Hg.**

- **Individuals who are normotensive at 55 years of age will have a 90% lifetime risk of developing hypertension.**

- **Patients with prehypertension (systolic blood pressure 120–139 mm Hg or diastolic blood pressure 80–89 mm Hg) require health-promoting lifestyle modifications to prevent the progressive rise in blood pressure and cardiovascular disease.**

- **For uncomplicated hypertension, thiazide diuretic should be used in most cases for medical treatment, either alone or combined with drugs from other classes.**

Table 9.6 Blood Pressure (BP) Classification (Adults 18 Years and Older)

Category	Systolic BP (mm Hg)	Diastolic BP (mm Hg)
Normal	<120	and <80
Prehypertension	120–139	or 80–89
Stage 1 hypertension	140–159	or 90–99
Stage 2 hypertension	>160	or >100

Modified from **Chobanian AV, Bakris GL, Black HR, et al.** The seventh report of the Joint National Committee on Prevention, Detection, Evaluation, and Treatment of High Blood Pressure (JNC VII). *JAMA* 2003;289:2560–2572.

Table 9.7 Drug Choices for Hypertension with Compelling Indications

Compelling Indication	Diuretic	β-Blocker	ACE Inhibitor	ARB	CCB	Aldosterone Antagonist
Heart failure	√	√	√	√		√
Post-MI		√	√			√
High coronary risk	√	√	√		√	
Diabetes	√	√	√	√	√	
Chronic kidney disease	√	√				
Recurrent stroke prevention	√		√			

ACE, angiotensin-converting enzyme; ARB, angiotensin receptor blocker; CCB, calcium channel blocker; MI, myocardial infarction.
Adapted from **Chobanian AV, Bakris GL, Black HR, et al.** The seventh report of the Joint National Committee on Prevention, Detection, Evaluation, and Treatment of High Blood Pressure (JNC VII). *JAMA* 2003;289:2560–2572.

- **Other antihypertensive drug classes (angiotensin-converting enzyme inhibitors, angiotensin-receptor blockers, beta-blockers, calcium channel blockers) should be used in the presence of specific high-risk conditions** (Table 9.7).

- **Two or more antihypertensive medications are required to achieve optimal blood pressure levels (<140/90 mm Hg or <130/80 mm Hg, respectively) for patients with diabetes or chronic kidney disease.**

- **For patients whose blood pressure is more than 20 mm Hg above the systolic blood pressure goal or more than 10 mm Hg above the diastolic blood pressure goal, initiation of therapy using two agents, one of which will be a thiazide diuretic, should be considered.**

Regardless of therapy or care, hypertension will be controlled only if patients are motivated to maintain their treatment plan. If blood pressure control is not easily achieved, if the systolic blood pressure is higher than 180 mm Hg, or if the diastolic reading is higher than 110 mm Hg, referral to an internist is recommended. Referral is indicated if secondary hypertension is suspected or evidence of end-organ damage (renal insufficiency or congestive heart failure) is present.

Measurement of Blood Pressure

An essential variable in evaluation of hypertension is how measurements are obtained and the need to standardize measurements (19). "White coat" or office hypertension (i.e., elevated just by seeing a physician) may occur in up to 30% of patients. For patients who have repeated normal measures outside of the office, it is reasonable to use ambulatory or home monitoring devices. Given the variation of accuracy and patient interpretation, it is advisable for the patient to bring their blood pressure unit into the office to calibrate it against the office-based measurements. In most patients, office readings are sufficient to adequately diagnose and monitor hypertension and eliminate problems of reliability with commercial devices and patient interpretation skills.

Blood pressure protocols for measurement should be standardized. The patient should be allowed to rest for 5 minutes in a seated position and the right arm used for measurements (for unknown reasons, the right arm has higher readings). The cuff should be applied 2 cm above the bend of the elbow and the arm positioned parallel to the floor. The cuff should be inflated to 30 mm Hg above the disappearance of the brachial pulse, or 220 mm Hg. The cuff should be deflated slowly at a rate no more than 2 mm Hg per second.

The cuff size is important, and most cuffs are marked with "normal limits" for the relative size they can accommodate. The most common clinical problem encountered is small cuffs used with obese patients, resulting in "cuff hypertension." Phase IV Korotkoff sounds are described as the point when pulsations are muffled, whereas phase V is complete disappearance. Most experts in hypertension advocate the use of phase V Korotkoff sounds, but phase IV sounds may be used in special circumstances, with the reason documented.

The use of automated devices may help eliminate discrepancies in measurements. Regardless of the method or device used, two measurements should be obtained with less than a 10 mm Hg disparity to be judged adequate. When repeated measures are performed, there should be a 2-minute rest period between readings. Blood pressure has a diurnal pattern, so determinations preferably should be done at the same time. Ambulatory monitoring is not cost-effective in all patients, but may be used to evaluate resistance to therapy, to assess "white coat" hypertension, and to determine whether syncopal episodes are related to hypotension or episodic hypertension (20).

Therapy

Nonpharmacologic interventions or lifestyle modifications should be attempted before initiation of medication unless the systolic blood pressure exceeds 139 mm Hg or the diastolic blood pressure exceeds 89 mm Hg. Drug therapy should be initiated for systolic blood pressure greater than 130 mm Hg or diastolic blood pressure greater than 80 mm Hg in those with diabetes or chronic renal failure. An important element in lifestyle modifications is to modify all contributors to cardiovascular disease. In obese patients, weight loss, especially in individuals with truncal and abdominal obesity, can play a significant role in the prevention of atherosclerosis (14,21). A loss of just 10 pounds was reported to lower blood pressure (22). Inquiries into dietary practices should be made to eliminate excess salt in the diet, specifically certain food groups that are high in sodium, such as canned goods, snack food, pork products, and soy sauce (23). Cholesterol and fat intake in the diet should be limited. Dietary interventions that use calcium, magnesium, and potassium supplementation did not make a clinically significant reduction in pressure (24). **An exercise program, weight loss, and moderating alcohol intake (to no more than two alcoholic beverages per day) contribute to overall cardiovascular health. Aerobic exercise alone may prevent hypertension in 20% to 50% of normotensive individuals** (14).

The goal of therapy is for the patient to lower blood pressure into the "normal range": a systolic reading less than or equal to 120 mm Hg and a diastolic reading less than or equal to 80 mm Hg. If lifestyle modifications are not sufficient to control blood pressure, then pharmacologic intervention is indicated (Fig. 9.2).

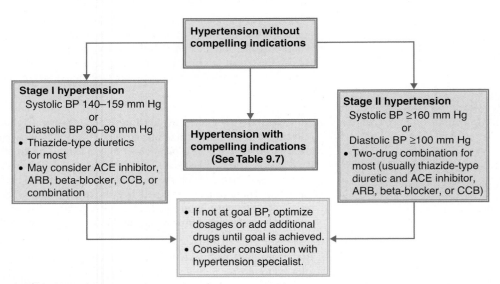

Figure 9.2 **Algorithm for the drug choices for hypertensive patients unresponsive to lifestyle changes.** Goal blood pressure (BP) is <140/90 mm Hg, or <130/80 mm Hg for those with diabetes or chronic kidney disease, respectively. ACE, angiotensin-converting enzyme; ARB, angiotensin-receptor blocker; CCB, calcium channel blocker. (Modified from **Chobanian AV, Bakris GL, Black HR, et al.** The seventh report of the Joint National Committee on Prevention, Detection, Evaluation, and Treatment of High Blood Pressure (JNC VII). *JAMA* 2003;289:2560–2572, with permission.)

Diuretics

The most commonly used medication for initial blood pressure reduction is a thiazide diuretic. The mechanism of action is to reduce plasma and extracellular fluid volume. This lowering of volume is thought to decrease peripheral resistance. Cardiac output initially decreases and then normalizes (25). The important long-term effect is a slight decrease in extracellular fluid volume. The maximum therapeutic dose of thiazides should be lowered to 25 mg, rather than the commonly used 50 mg. The benefit of higher doses is eliminated by the corresponding increase in side effects. Potassium-sparing diuretics (*spironolactone, triamterene,* or *amiloride*) are available in fixed doses and should be prescribed to prevent the development of hypokalemia. Potassium supplementation is less effective than the use of potassium-sparing agents. **Thiazide diuretics are best used in patients with creatinine levels less than 2.5 g/L. Loop diuretics (*furosemide*) work better than thiazide diuretics at lower glomerular filtration rates and higher serum creatinine levels.** Control of hypertension with concurrent renal insufficiency is difficult and is probably best handled by an internist or nephrologist. Thiazides and loop diuretics should not be used concurrently because profound diuresis may occur and lead to renal impairment. Concurrent use of nonsteroidal anti-inflammatory drugs (NSAIDs) limits the effectiveness of this class of drugs. Other side effects that further limit the usefulness of thiazide diuretics include hyperuricemia, which may contribute to acute gout attacks, glucose intolerance, and hyperlipidemias (26). The metabolic side effects of these drugs limit their popularity.

Adrenergic Inhibitors

Beta-blockers were used extensively for years as antihypertensive agents. The mechanism of action is decreasing cardiac output and plasma renin activity, with some increase in total peripheral resistance. As a class, they are an excellent source of first-line therapy, especially for migraine sufferers. The original formulation, *propranolol,* is highly lipid soluble and contributed to bothersome side effects such as depression, sleep disturbances (nightmares in the elderly), and constipation in higher doses. *Propranolol* has a relative lack of beta selectivity, which promotes other undesirable phenomena. Formulations such as *atenolol* are water soluble, are $beta_1$ selective, and have fewer side effects than *propranolol.* At higher doses, $beta_2$ effects emerge. There is no evidence to support speculation that $beta_1$ selective agents may be safe for use in individuals who have asthma. An advantage of water-soluble agents is a longer half-life. Reduced dosing schedules improve compliance. Side effects of beta-blockers include an increase in triglyceride levels and a decrease in high-density lipoprotein (HDL) cholesterol and blunting of adrenergic release in response to hypoglycemia. NSAIDs may decrease the effectiveness of beta-blockers. Contraindications to beta-blockers are asthma, sick sinus syndrome, or bradyarrhythmia. **Beta-blockers are often used for the treatment of angina and after myocardial infarctions. However, if these drugs are acutely withdrawn, a rebound phenomenon of ischemia may occur, leading to acute myocardial infarction.** Despite these potential problems, beta-blockers continue to be useful in counteracting reflex tachycardia, which often occurs with the use of smooth muscle relaxing drugs.

Use of alpha$_1$-adrenergic drugs became popular in men because of their minimal effects on potency and unique relationship to lipids. They may contribute to stress urinary incontinence in women because of altered urethral tone. As single agents, they decrease total cholesterol and low-density lipoprotein (LDL) cholesterol while increasing HDL cholesterol, in contrast to the metabolic effects of beta-blocking agents. Their mode of action is to promote vascular relaxation by blocking postganglionic norepinephrine vasoconstriction in the peripheral vascular smooth muscle. *Prazosin* and *doxazosin* are two preparations available in this class. A serious side effect of these drugs, which is commonly described in the elderly patients, is called the "first-dose effect." In susceptible individuals, severe orthostasis was reported when therapy was initiated but subsided after several days. When alpha$_1$-adrenergic drugs are used in combination with diuretics, hypotension may be further exacerbated. Therapy should begin with small doses taken at bedtime followed by incremental increases. Other side effects that may limit the usefulness of these agents in some patients include tachycardia, weakness, dizziness, and mild fluid retention.

Angiotensin-Converting Enzyme Inhibitors

The angiotensin-converting enzyme (ACE) inhibitors are first-line drugs in the treatment of hypertension. Their rapid rise in popularity results from the introduction of new formulations, which allow dosing once or twice a day with a good therapeutic response. There are relatively few side effects; chronic cough is the most worrisome and is a common reason of discontinuing the use of this group of drugs. Other side effects are occasional first-dose hypotension and blood dyscrasias. Occasionally, patients will suffer from rashes, loss of taste, fatigue, or headaches. Other agents should be considered for patients at risk for pregnancy (a strict contraindication). ACE inhibitors can be used in combination with other agents, including diuretics, calcium channel antagonists, and beta-blocking agents. In contrast to beta-blocking agents, these medications can be used in patients with asthma, depression, and peripheral vascular disease. For unknown reasons, they are less effective in African Americans unless a diuretic is used concomitantly. Use with diuretics increases the effectiveness of both drugs, but hypovolemia may result. If renal failure is present, hyperkalemia may result from potassium supplementation and altered tubular metabolism. Any NSAID, including *aspirin,* may decrease the antihypertensive effectiveness. Use of NSAIDs, volume depletion, and renal artery stenosis may precipitate acute renal failure when administration of an ACE inhibitor is initiated. **Creatinine levels should be measured at the start of therapy and 1 week after initiation of any ACE inhibitor.** An increase of up to 35% of the baseline creatinine value is acceptable, and treatment should be continued unless hyperkalemia develops.

Angiotensin-Receptor Blockers

The angiotensin-receptor blockers such as *losartan* and *valsartan* interfere with the binding of angiotensin II to AT_1 receptors. As with ACE inhibitors, they are effective in lowering blood pressure without causing the side effect of coughing. Angiotensin-receptor blockers have favorable effects on the progression of kidney disease in individuals who have diabetes, and on those without diabetes and congestive heart failure.

Calcium-Channel Blockers

Calcium-channel blockers represent a major therapeutic breakthrough for patients with coronary artery disease. They are effective in patients with hypertension and peripheral vascular disease. The mechanism of action is to block calcium movement across smooth muscle, therefore promoting vessel wall relaxation. Calcium channel blockers are useful in treating concurrent hypertension and ischemic heart disease as an alternative to beta-blockers, if needed. Additionally, these drugs are particularly effective in the elderly and African Americans. Side effects noted include headache, dizziness, constipation, gastroesophageal reflux, and peripheral edema. The addition of long-acting calcium-channel blockers made these preparations more amenable for use in hypertension. A relative contraindication for use of these drugs is the presence of congestive heart failure or conduction disturbances.

Direct Vasodilators

Hydralazine **is a potent vasodilator used for years in obstetrics for severe hypertension associated with preeclampsia and eclampsia.** The mechanism of action is direct relaxation of vascular smooth muscle, primarily arterial. Major side effects include headaches, tachycardia, and fluid (sodium) retention that may result in paradoxical hypertension. Several combinations are used to counter the side effects and enhance antihypertensive effects. Diuretics may be added to reverse fluid retention caused by excess sodium. When used in combination with beta-blockers, tachycardia and headaches may be controlled without compromising the objective of lowering blood pressure. Drug-induced lupus was widely stated as a potential side effect but is rare with normal therapeutic doses of 25 to 50 mg three times daily. *Minoxidil* is another extremely potent drug in this class but is of limited use to the gynecologist because of its side effects in women (beard growth). Because of *minoxidil*'s potency, only experienced practitioners should use it.

Central-Acting Agents

Central-acting agents (*methyldopa* and *clonidine*) have long been used in obstetrics. The mechanism of action is to inhibit the sympathetics in the central nervous system, resulting in peripheral vascular relaxation. Side effects, including taste disorders, dry mouth, drowsiness, and the need for frequent dosing (except for the transdermal form of *clonidine*), limited the popularity of this group of drugs. **Sudden withdrawal of *clonidine* may precipitate a hypertensive crisis and induce angina.** *Clonidine* withdrawal syndrome is more likely to occur with concomitant use of beta-blockers. Compliance is always a major issue, and side-effect profiles contribute significantly to patient nonadherence. With the introduction of new classes of drugs with improved efficacy and reduced side effects, use of medications in this class is expected to decline.

Monitoring Therapy

Blood pressure readings should be monitored frequently by a nurse, the patient, or in the office at 1- to 2-week intervals. If the patient has other diseases (i.e., cardiovascular, renal), therapy should be initiated earlier and directed to the target organ. If lifestyle modification alone is successful, close monitoring is necessary at 3- to 6-month intervals. When lifestyle modification is unsuccessful, a blood pressure medication should be started to decrease target organ disease.

When beginning therapy, concurrent medical conditions treatable with a common agent should be sought. Gender is not an important consideration in choosing an antihypertensive agent. **Concurrent diseases and race are important for patients who:**

- **Have migraine headaches, for which beta-blockers or calcium channel agonists may be the best choice**

- **Are African American and are likely to respond better to a combination of diuretics and calcium channel blockers**

- **Have diabetes, chronic kidney disease, and heart failure, for which ACE inhibitors should be used**

- **Have had myocardial infarctions and should receive beta-blockers because they reduce the risk for sudden death and recurrent myocardial infarctions.**

A summary of the compelling indications for individual drug classes is listed in Table 9.7.

Once antihypertensive medications are initiated, monitoring should be instituted at approximately monthly intervals to determine blood pressures and to assess side effects. Patients with stage II hypertension or with complicated comorbid illnesses may need more frequent monitoring. The serum creatinine and potassium levels should be monitored 1 to 2 times per year. When blood pressure goals are reached, patients may be seen in the office at 3- to 6-month intervals. Patients capable of home blood pressure monitoring should be encouraged to measure blood pressure at the same time twice weekly (20). **If intolerable side effects develop, a different class of medications should be used and the patient's progress monitored.** Patients whose blood pressure is difficult to control with two agents should be considered for referral. Causes of resistance to therapy include diseases missed during the initial evaluation, unrecognized early end-stage disease, and poor compliance. Patients with evidence of target organ disease should be considered for referral to the appropriate specialist for more intensive diagnostic workup and therapy.

Cholesterol

The dietary influence of cholesterol on atherosclerosis and its relationship to hypertension and cardiovascular events (myocardial infarction and stroke) is widely debated in the scientific and lay communities. The controversy centers on the effect of dietary cholesterol in assessing risk and prevention of cardiovascular disease (26,27). Many assume that all cholesterol and fat in the diet have negative health consequences (28). Cholesterol metabolism is complex, and some of our knowledge is extrapolated from animal models. The role of cholesterol testing (who, when, and at what age) is hotly debated among health care professionals, and the test itself is fraught with multiple variables that affect results. Understanding the metabolism of cholesterol will help identify and treat patients at risk of complications from hypercholesterolemia.

Terms and Definitions

Cholesterol is usually found in an esterized form with various proteins and glycerides that characterize the stage of metabolism. The following components are important lipid particles in cholesterol metabolism:

Chylomicrons   **This large lipoprotein particle consists of dietary triglycerides and cholesterol.** Chylomicrons are secreted in the intestinal lumen, absorbed in the lymph, and passed into general circulation. In adipose tissue and skeletal muscle, they adhere to binding sites on the capillary wall and are metabolized for energy production.

Lipoprotein Particle   **Lipoprotein particles are separated into five classes based on physical characteristics.** The various cholesterol metabolites are separated by density. As lipoprotein particles are metabolized and lipids are removed for energy production, they become more dense.

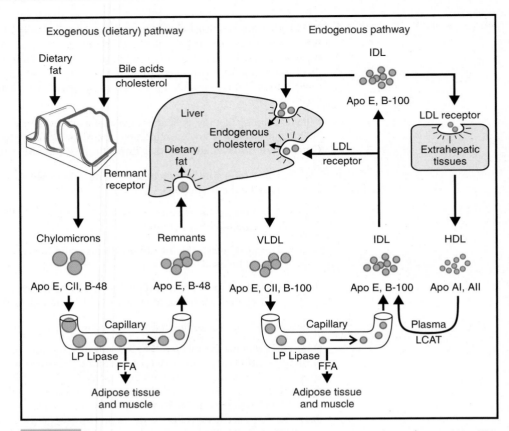

Figure 9.3   **Metabolic pathways of lipid metabolism.** Apo, apoprotein; LP, lipoprotein; FFA, free fatty acid; IDL, intermediate-density lipoprotein; LDL, low-density lipoprotein; VLDL, very-low-density lipoprotein; HDL, high-density lipoprotein; LCAT, lecithin cholesterol acyltransferase.

Attached apoproteins are modified as cholesterol moves from the so-called exogenous pathway (dietary) to the endogenous pathway (postabsorption and metabolization by the liver).

Following are the subdivisions of the lipoprotein classes (Fig. 9.3).

Prehepatic Metabolites

Chylomicrons and remnants are composed of major lipids and apoproteins of the A, B-48, C and E classes. These are large particles made up of dietary cholesterol molecules that are absorbed with triglycerides.

Posthepatic Metabolites

Very low-density lipoproteins (VLDL) are transient remnants found after initial liver metabolism and compose only 10% to 15% of cholesterol particles. They consist of endogenously synthesized triglycerides.

Intermediate density lipoproteins (IDL) consist of cholesterol esters, which are posthepatic remnants derived from dietary sources. Metabolites of IDL are transient lipoproteins measured only in certain pathologic conditions.

Low-density lipoprotein (LDL) is mainly composed of the cholesterol ester and is associated with B-100 apoprotein. LDL cholesterol is approximately 60% to 70% of total cholesterol. Elevated levels of LDL cholesterol are associated with increased myocardial infarction in women older than 65 years of age. There is a structural class called LDL (a′) that is associated with myocardial infarction.

High-density lipoprotein (HDL) is composed of cholesterol esters with apoproteins A-I and A-II. These particles are 20% to 30% of total cholesterol and are the most dense.

Metabolism

Cholesterol metabolism is divided into two pathways: (i) the exogenous pathway derived from dietary sources, and (ii) the endogenous pathway or the lipid transport pathway. Individuals vary in their ability to metabolize cholesterol, with patients classified as normals, hyporesponders, and hyperresponders (29). Hyporesponders may be given cholesterol-loaded diets with no effect on serum cholesterol measurements. Hyperresponders, in contrast, have high serum cholesterol levels, regardless of dietary intake. Explanations for these differences are well described in animal models, but not in humans.

When a meal is eaten, cholesterol is transported as dietary fat. The average daily American diet contains approximately 100 g of triglyceride and approximately 1 g of cholesterol. Triglycerides are found in the core lipoprotein particles and are removed through the capillary endothelium and the chylomicron. Theories suggest that hypo- and hyperresponses to dietary cholesterol may occur secondary to the liver's ability to recognize and metabolize apoprotein E. In the animal model, populations with large numbers of liver receptors for apoprotein E easily metabolize cholesterol and are labeled hyporesponders. Individuals with a reduced number of apoprotein E receptors are unable to metabolize cholesterol as readily, which increases the number of lipid particles. These individuals are considered hyperresponders. Despite dietary cholesterol modification, these individuals continue to have high serum cholesterol levels.

After metabolic degradation of dietary chylomicrons, apoprotein substitution occurs and liver metabolism of cholesterol esters begins. Lipid transport is now in the *endogenous pathway*. Carbohydrates are synthesized to fatty acids and esterified with glycerol to form triglycerides. These newly formed triglycerides are not of dietary origin and are placed in the core of VLDL. These particles are relatively large and carry five to ten times more triglyceride than cholesterol esters with apoprotein B-100. **Hypertriglyceridemia is an independent risk factor for cardiovascular disease.** The relationship between hypertriglyceridemia and cardiovascular disease is well known but poorly defined.

VLDL particles are transported to tissue capillaries, where they are broken down to usable fuels, monoglycerides, and fatty acids. After metabolic enzymatic degradation in the peripheral tissues, IDL remains and is either catabolized in the liver by binding to LDL receptors or modified in the peripheral tissues. As noted previously, they are associated with apoprotein E receptors, the liver recognition receptors. The LDL cholesterol, or the so-called high-risk cholesterol, is found in high circulating levels.

Despite the negative connotation of LDL in cardiovascular disease, it is a very important cellular metabolite and precursor for adrenocortical cells, lymphocytes, and renal cells. The liver uses LDL for synthesis of bile acids and free cholesterol, which is secreted into the bile. In the normal human, 70% to 80% of LDL is removed from the plasma each day and secreted in the bile by utilization of the LDL receptor pathway.

The final metabolic pathway is the transformation of HDL cholesterol in extrahepatic tissue. HDL cholesterol carries the plasma enzyme lecithin cholesterol acyltransferase (LCAT). LCAT allows HDL cholesterol to resynthesize lipids to VLDL cholesterol and recycle the lipid cascade. HDL cholesterol acts as a "scavenger" and therefore reverses the deposit of cholesterol into tissues. There is good evidence that HDL cholesterol is responsible for the reversal of atherosclerotic changes in vessels, hence the term "good cholesterol" (27).

Hyperlipoproteinemia

When cholesterol is measured, various fractions are reported. Plasma cholesterol or total cholesterol consists of cholesterol and unesterified cholesterol fractions. If triglycerides are analyzed in conjunction with cholesterol, then assumptions can be made concerning which metabolic pathway may be abnormal. Elevation of both total cholesterol and triglycerides signifies a problem with chylomicrons and VLDL synthesis. If the triglyceride-to-cholesterol ratio is greater than 5:1, the predominant fractions are chylomicrons and VLDL. A triglycerides-to-cholesterol ratio less than 5:1 signifies a problem in the VLDL and LDL fractions.

Hyperlipoproteinemias are defined by establishing a "normal population" and then setting various limits at the 10th and 90th percentiles. Standards for women set the 80th percentile for cholesterol at 240 mg/dL and the 50th percentile at 200 mg/dL (Table 9.8). A diet low in animal fat and high in vegetable and fiber consumption helps control the level of cholesterol (27–29). Plasma elevations of chylomicrons, LDL, VLDL, various remnants of IDL, and VLDL are classified by the elevated fraction.

Table 9.8 Initial Classification Based on the Total Cholesterol, LDL, HDL, and Triglyceride Levels

Initial Classification

Total cholesterol

<200 mg/dL	Desirable blood cholesterol
200–239 mg/dL	Borderline high blood cholesterol
≥240 mg/dL	High blood cholesterol

LDL cholesterol

<100 mg/dL	Optimal cholesterol
100–129 mg/dL	Near or above optimal
130–159 mg/dL	Borderline high
160–189 mg/dL	High
≥190 mg/dL	Very high

HDL cholesterol

<40 mg/dL	Low HDL cholesterol
≥60 mg/dL	High HDL cholesterol

Triglycerides

<150 mg/dL	Normal
150–199 mg/dL	Borderline high
200–499 mg/dL	High
>500 mg/dL	Very high

LDL, low-density lipoprotein; HDL, high density lipoprotein.
Adapted from **Expert Panel on Detection, Evaluation, and Treatment of High Blood Cholesterol in Adults.** Executive summary of the third report of the National Cholesterol Education Program (NCEP) Expert Panel on the Detection, Evaluation, and Treatment of High Blood Cholesterol in Adults. *JAMA* 2001;285:2486–2497.

Evaluation

There are multiple causes of variation in cholesterol measurements (30,31). **Major sources of variation within individuals include diet, obesity, smoking, ethanol intake, and the effects of exercise.** Other clinical conditions that affect cholesterol measurements include hypothyroidism, diabetes, acute or recent myocardial infarction, and recent weight changes. Measurements can be altered by fasting, position of the patient while the sample is drawn, the use and duration of venous occlusion, various anticoagulants, and the storage and shipping conditions.

Factors Affecting Test Results

Intrapersonal variation is well described. If multiple samples are taken within a given day, weekly and monthly variations can be as high as 6%. **At least two specimens should be taken 1 month apart and should be collected in the same dietary state in order for a lipid value to be considered accurate.**

- **Age and gender contribute to variations in total cholesterol measurements. Before age 50, women have lower lipid values than men, after which age the level in women is higher than in men. This finding may be modified by exogenous oral conjugated estrogens.**

- **Seasonal variation also occurs,** with lipid samples in December or January being found to be approximately 2.5% higher than those measured in June or July.

- **The effect of diet and obesity is well established.** Weight reduction in an obese individual affects the triglyceride level, which may decrease as much as 40%. Total cholesterol and LDL decrease less than 10% with diet; however, HDL increases approximately 10%. Weight gain negates any benefit from prior weight loss. Accuracy of lipid measurements depends on the stability of the patient's weight.

- **Alcohol and cigarette smoking are well-known modifiers of cholesterol. Moderate sustained alcohol intake increases HDL and decreases LDL; there is a complementary increase in triglycerides. Alcohol has a protective effect when taken in moderation (defined as approximately 2 alcoholic drinks [2 ounces of absolute alcohol] per day), but this effect is negated in higher quantities.** The increase in HDL is in the HDL_3 fraction, which is important in the scavenger mechanism of removing LDL. Smoking has the opposite effect, increasing LDL and triglyceride levels and decreasing HDL. HDL_3 decreases with cigarette smoking. The critical number of cigarettes smoked is 15 to 20 per day, regardless of gender, and a variation in the number smoked will affect results. Caffeine has a mixed effect on lipoprotein measurements and should be avoided for 12 hours before blood collection.

- **Exercise is an important variable in the overall risk management of heart disease.** Moderate levels of exercise are as important in overall cardiovascular health as control of hypertension and cessation of cigarette smoking. Strenuous exercise lowers the concentrations of triglycerides and LDL and increases HDL in the serum. Because of these acute blood changes, vigorous exercise should be avoided within 12 hours of drawing the blood for testing.

- **Certain disease states and medications affect cholesterol measurements.** Use of diuretics and *propranolol* increases triglycerides and decreases HDL. Diuretics may increase total cholesterol levels. Diabetes, especially in the presence of poor control, may be associated with very high levels of triglycerides and LDL and decreased levels of HDL. This may explain why these individuals are prone to cardiovascular diseases. Patients with diabetes under tight control have improved lipoprotein profiles.

- **Pregnancy is associated with decreased total cholesterol in the first trimester and continuous increases of all fractions over the second and third trimesters** (32). The LDL and triglyceride concentrations are the lipoproteins most affected by pregnancy.

- **Patients with hypothyroidism have increased levels of total cholesterol and LDL.**

Testing

Because of the diurnal variation of blood triglycerides, blood samples should be collected in the morning after a 12-hour fast. Excessive quantities of water should not be consumed before blood is drawn. After 2 minutes of venous occlusion, serum cholesterol levels can increase 2% to 5%. Therefore, the sample used for cholesterol testing should be collected first if multiple blood samples are required. One of the most important aspects of overall standardization of lipoprotein measurements is the laboratory used. It may be worthwhile to consult a clinical pathologist to determine if the laboratory complies with Centers for Disease Control and Prevention (CDC) standards for cholesterol and lipoprotein measurements.

Management

When hyperlipidemia is confirmed on at least two separate occasions, secondary causes should be diagnosed or excluded by taking a detailed medical and drug history, measuring serum creatinine and fasting glucose levels, and testing thyroid and liver function. Causes of secondary dyslipidemia include diabetes, hypothyroidism, obstructive liver disease, chronic renal failure, and use of medications such as progestins, anabolic steroids, and corticosteroids. **Therapeutic lifestyle changes should be initiated in all patients to reduce their risk of coronary heart disease:**

1. **Reduced intakes of saturated fats (<7% of total calories) and cholesterol (<200 mg per day)**
2. **Therapeutic options for enhancing LDL lowering, such as plant stanols/sterols (2 g per day) and increased viscous (soluble) fiber (10–25 g per day)**
3. **Weight reduction**
4. **Increased physical activity**

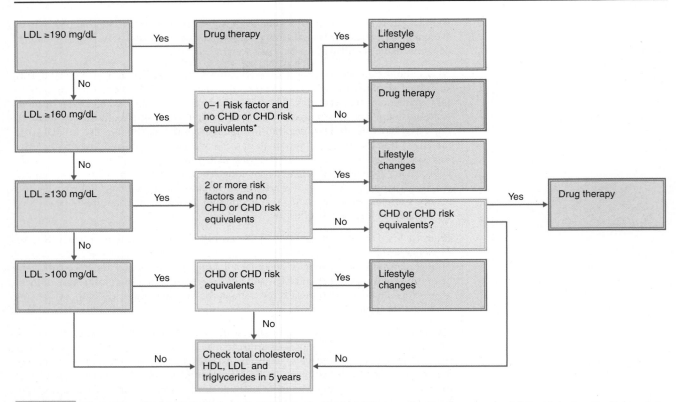

Figure 9.4 **Treatment decisions based on the LDL cholesterol.** LDL, low-density lipoprotein; HDL, high-density lipoprotein. *Coronary heart disease (CHD) risk equivalents: Diabetes or other forms of atherosclerotic disease like peripheral arterial disease, abdominal aortic aneurysm, and symptomatic carotid artery disease. (Adapted from **The Expert Panel on Detection, Evaluation, and Treatment of High Blood Cholesterol in Adults.** Executive summary of the third report of the National Cholesterol Education Program [NCEP] Expert Panel on the Detection, Evaluation, and Treatment of High Blood Cholesterol in Adults. *JAMA* 2001;285:2486–2497.)

Figure 9.4 is a suggested algorithm for cholesterol control based on LDL levels. Cholesterol fat-lowering diet books abound in most bookstores and allow the patient to choose a diet she will best follow. **The role of exercise and cigarette cessation should be stressed to all patients. Patients with a family history of cardiovascular disease (history of premature coronary artery problems and strokes) should be tested and started on conservative programs in their 20s.** After 3 to 6 months, if the LDL remains above 160 mg/dL with zero to one risk factor or above 130 mg/dL with two or more risk factors, then medical therapy should be initiated. Any woman with coronary heart disease or equivalents such as diabetes or other forms of atherosclerotic disease (peripheral arterial disease, abdominal aortic aneurysm, and symptomatic carotid artery disease) should initiate lifestyle changes if her LDL is 100 mg/dL or more and drug therapy if her LDL is 130 mg/dL or more. Anyone with an LDL 190 mg/dL or higher should be considered for drug therapy (33).

The bile acid-binding resins *cholestyramine* and *colestipol* were the mainstay of therapy. Their usefulness is limited by side effects such as constipation, bloating, nausea, and heartburn, and by their tendency to interfere with the absorption of other drugs. *Nicotinic acid* (500 mg three times daily) decreases triglycerides, LDL, and lipoprotein (a') and increases HDL more than any other drug. Flushing, pruritus, gastrointestinal distress, and, rarely, hepatotoxicity are a few of the adverse effects of *nicotinic acid*. Starting at a low dose and pretreating with *aspirin* 325 mg or *ibuprofen* 200 mg can minimize the facial flushing. Fibric acid derivatives like *clofibrate* and *gemfibrozil* are used to lower triglycerides and increase HDL but may increase LDL in some patients. The HMG-CoA (3-hydroxy-3methyl-glutaryl-coenzyme A) reductase inhibitors (statins) include *atorvastatin, fluvastatin, lovastatin, pravastatin,* and *simvastatin.* These medicines inhibit HMG-CoA reductase, the enzyme that catalyzes the rate-limiting step in cholesterol synthesis. **Several clinical trials showed that *pravastatin, simvastatin,* and *lovastatin* have a beneficial effect in cardiovascular disease.** Statins are better tolerated than other lipid-lowering drugs, but reported side effects include severe myalgias, muscle weakness with increases in creatine phosphokinase, and, rarely, rhabdomyolysis, leading to renal failure.

Diabetes Mellitus

Diabetes mellitus (DM) is a chronic disorder of altered carbohydrate, protein, and fat metabolism resulting from a deficiency in the secretion or function of insulin. The disease is defined by the presence of either fasting hyperglycemia or elevated plasma glucose levels based on an oral glucose tolerance testing (OGTT). The major complications of DM are primarily vascular and metabolic. The prevalence of DM is higher in women and certain ethnic groups, although a background rate in the general population is 6.29%, which has increased threefold in 15 years (34). **Risk factors for DM are:**

1. **Age greater than 45 years**
2. **Adiposity or obesity**
3. **A family history of diabetes**
4. **Race/ethnicity**
5. **Hypertension (blood pressure 140/90 mm Hg or greater)**
6. **HDL cholesterol less than or equal to 35 mg/dL and/or a triglyceride level greater than or equal to 250 mg/dL**
7. **History of gestational diabetes or delivery of a baby weighing more than 9 pounds**

Major complications of DM include blindness, renal disease, gangrene of an extremity, heart disease, and stroke. Diabetes is one of the four major risk factors for cardiovascular disease.

Classification

In January 1999, the Expert Committee on the Diagnosis and Classification of Diabetes Mellitus published a report revising the system that was in use since 1979 (35,36). The goal of the revision was to provide guidelines for nomenclature and testing that might reduce diagnostic confusion and improve patient well-being (Table 9.9). The terms *insulin dependent diabetes mellitus* (IDDM) and *noninsulin dependent diabetes mellitus* (NIDDM) were replaced by the terms type 1 and type 2 diabetes mellitus.

Type 1 Diabetes Mellitus

With type 1 diabetes, the major metabolic disturbance is the absence of insulin from the destruction of beta cells in the pancreas. Insulin is necessary for glucose metabolism and cellular respiration. When insulin is absent, ketosis results. The cause of type 1 diabetes is unknown; data suggest an autoimmune association from either a viral infection or toxic components in the environment. Studies in the past decade showed a correlation between many autoimmune diseases and the human leukocyte antigens (HLA).

Insulin-sensitive tissues (muscle, liver, and fat) fail to metabolize glucose efficiently in the absence of insulin. In uncontrolled type 1 diabetes, an excess of counter-regulatory hormones (cortisol, catecholamines, and glucagon) contributes to further metabolic dysfunction. In the absence of adequate amounts of insulin, increasing breakdown products of muscle (amino acid proteolysis), fat (fatty acid lipolysis), and glycogen (glucose glycogenolysis) are recognized. There is an increase in glucose production from noncarbohydrate precursors as a result of gluconeogenesis and ketogenesis in the liver. Without prompt treatment, severe metabolic decompensation (i.e., diabetic ketoacidosis) will occur and may lead to death.

Type 2 Diabetes Mellitus

Type 2 diabetes mellitus is a heterogeneous form of diabetes that commonly occurs in older age groups (>40 years) and more frequently has a familial tendency than type 1 diabetes. This form of diabetes mellitus accounts for approximately 90% to 95% of those with diabetes. The presence of risk factors strongly influences the development of type 2 diabetes in susceptible populations.

Risk factors for type 2 diabetes include ethnicity, obesity, family history of DM, sedentary lifestyle, impaired glucose tolerance, upper-body adiposity, and a history of gestational diabetes and hyperinsulinemia.

In contrast to an absence of insulin that occurs with type 1 diabetes, in type 2 diabetes the altered metabolism of insulin results in insulin resistance. This condition is characterized by

Table 9.9 Classification of Diabetes Mellitus
1. Type 1 diabetes
Characterized by pancreatic destruction leading to insulin deficiency
A. Idiopathic
B. Immune mediated
2. Type 2 diabetes
A combination of insulin resistance and some degree of inadequate insulin secretion
3. Other types of diabetes:
A. Impaired glucose tolerance (IGT)
B. Endocrinopathies (Cushing's, acromegaly, pheochromocytoma, hyperaldosteronism)
C. Drug- or chemical-induced
D. Diseases of the exocrine pancreas (pancreatitis, neoplasia)
E. Infections
F. Genetic defects of beta-cell function and insulin action
G. Gestational diabetes mellitus

Adapted from **The Expert Committee on the Diagnosis and Classification of Diabetes Mellitus.** Report of the Expert Committee on the Diagnosis and Classification of Diabetes Mellitus. *Diabetes Care* 2000;23:S4–S42.

impaired glucose uptake in target tissues. A compensatory increase in insulin secretion results, causing higher-than-normal circulating insulin levels (36). Obesity is present in 85% of affected patients. The cause of type 2 diabetes is unknown, but defects in both the secretion and action of insulin are suspected.

Many patients diagnosed with type 2 diabetes at an early age eventually exhaust endogenous pancreatic insulin and require injected insulin. When under severe stress, such as infection or surgery, they may develop diabetic ketoacidosis or a hyperglycemic hyperosmolar nonketotic state.

Diagnosis

Three methods are available to diagnose diabetes mellitus in nonpregnant women:

1. **A single fasting blood glucose greater than or equal to 126 mg/dL on two separate occasions**
2. **A random blood glucose equal to or above 200 mg/dL in an individual with classic signs and symptoms of diabetes (polydipsia, polyuria, polyphagia, and weight loss)**
3. **A 2-hour OGTT greater than or equal to 200 mg/dL (fasting sample, 60-, and 120-minute samples) after a 75-g load of glucose. A 2-hour OGTT should not be performed if the first two criteria are present.**

Diagnostic criterion for impaired glucose intolerance (IGT) is a fasting glucose greater than or equal to 100 mg/dL but less than 126 mg/dL (36).

A 2-hour OGTT should be performed under the following conditions:

1. A 10-hour fast should precede morning testing.
2. The patient should sit throughout the procedure.

3. No smoking is permitted during the test interval.

4. Caffeinated beverages should not be consumed.

5. More than 150 g of carbohydrates should be ingested for 3 days before the test.

6. No drugs should be taken before the test.

7. The patient should not be bedridden or under stress.

Patients who should be considered for diabetes testing are:

- **All individuals 45 years of age or older (repeat at 3-year intervals)**

- **Persons with classic signs and symptoms of diabetes (i.e., polyuria, polydipsia, polyphagia, and weight loss)**

- **Ethnic groups at high risk (Pacific Islanders, Native Americans, African Americans, Hispanic Americans, and Asian Americans)**

- **Obesity (body mass index >27 kg/m^2)**

- **History of a first-degree relative with diabetes**

- **Women with gestational diabetes or who have delivered a baby weighing more than 9 pounds**

- **Individuals with hypertension (blood pressure >140/90 mm Hg)**

- **An HDL cholesterol level less than or equal to 35 mg/dL or triglyceride level greater than or equal to 250 mg/dL**

- **Presence of impaired glucose tolerance on previous testing**

Assessment of Glycemic Control

The only acceptable method for assessment of glycemic control is determination of blood glucose by direct enzyme analysis, not by measurement of urine values, which do not correlate. Glucometers with memory storage made home glucose monitoring more reliable. Physician treatment guidelines are in Table 9.10 and patient guidelines in Table 9.11. In a 10 multicenters' study, the diabetes control and complication trial (DCCT), performed under the auspices of the National Institutes of Health, showed a marked reduction (40%–50%) in complications of neuropathy, retinopathy, and nephropathy when patients with type 1 diabetes received intensive therapy (accomplished by a team approach) as compared with those who received standard therapy.

Treatment

Type 2 diabetes is treated by a combination of lifestyle adjustments and medications.

Lifestyle

Diet is the most important component of DM management and usually the hardest way to achieve control. **Three major strategies are used: weight loss, low-fat diet (≤30% of calories from fat), and physical exercise.** Obese patients should reduce their weight to ideal body weight. Metabolic advantages of weight reduction are improved lipid profile and improved glucose control secondary to increased insulin sensitivity and decreased insulin resistance. The greater the weight loss, the greater the improvement in lipid disorders. Physical exercise promotes weight loss and improves insulin sensitivity and dyslipidemia in those people who are in high-risk groups for cardiovascular and microvascular diseases (37).

Oral Hypoglycemic Agents

Oral hypoglycemic agents are recommended for many type 2 diabetic patients. The first oral hypoglycemic agents introduced were first- and second-generation sulfonylureas. Other classes of drugs that have different effects in patients with type 2 diabetes—such as biguanides, thiazolidinediones, alpha-glucosidase inhibitors, and *insulin* secretagogues—were introduced. The mode of action of sulfonylureas is based on two different mechanisms: (i) enhanced insulin secretion from the pancreas, and (ii) an extrapancreatic effect that is poorly understood. Endogenous insulin secretion (as measured by C-peptide) is necessary for oral hypoglycemic agents to work. If the fasting blood glucose on an adequate diabetic diet is greater than 250 mg/dL, there is little effect. Frequent evaluation to monitor control (every 3 to 4 months) is important. If glucose levels cannot be controlled with oral hypoglycemic agents (i.e., sulfonylureas) or other

Table 9.10 Physician Guidelines in the Therapy of Diabetes Mellitus

- Establish diagnosis and classify type of diabetes mellitus (DM).

- The oral glucose tolerance test (OGTT) is not recommended for routine clinical use because of its higher cost, time requirement, and limited reproducibility.

- Initiate diabetes education classes to learn blood glucose monitoring and diabetes medications; to learn signs, symptoms, and complications; and to learn how to manage sick days.

- Place patient on ADA diet with appropriate caloric, sodium, and lipid restrictions.

- Establish cardiac risk factors, kidney function (serum creatinine, urine for microalbuminuria).

- If neuropathy is present, refer to a neurologist.

- Establish extent of fundoscopic lesion (refer to ophthalmologist as needed).

- Check feet and toenails at least once a year and refer to a foot specialist.

- Use finger-stick blood glucose for daily diabetic control.

- Follow chronic glycemic control by HgA$_{1c}$ every 2 to 3 months in the office.

- Initial general health evaluation should consist of a complete history and physical examination and the following laboratory tests: CBC with differential, chemistry profile, lipid profile, urinalysis, thyroid function tests, urine for microalbuminuria, and ECG (baseline at age 40 or older, repeat yearly).

- Oral hypoglycemic agents like the sulfonylureas may be considered if fasting blood glucose does not decline or increase and if the patient has diabetes for fewer than 10 years, does not have severe hepatic or renal disease, and is not pregnant or allergic to sulfa drugs.

- While on oral hypoglycemic agents, check the HgA$_{1C}$ every 3 months and at least two times a year if stable.

- If the HgA$_{1C}$ is <7% or the postprandial glucose is <200 mg/dL, omit the oral hypoglycemic agents, place on diet alone, and follow every 3 months.

- If the fasting serum glucose is >200 mg/dL consistently or the HgA$_{1C}$ is more than 10%, consider starting insulin and referring the patient to an internist.

- Administer the flu vaccine every fall and the pneumococcal vaccine every 6 years.

ADA, American Diabetic Association; HgA$_{1c}$, hemoglobin A$_{1C}$; CBC, complete blood count; ECG, electrocardiogram.
Adapted from **The Expert Committee on the Diagnosis and Classification of Diabetes Mellitus.** Report of the Expert Committee on the Diagnosis and Classification of Diabetes Mellitus. *Diabetes Care* 2000;23:S4–S42.

Table 9.11 Patient Guidelines for Treatment of Type 2 Diabetes

- Initiate an ADA reducing diet (50% CHO, 30% fat, 20% protein, high fiber) with three meals a day.

- Maintain ideal body weight or to reduce weight by 5% to 15% in 3 months if obese.

- Modify risk factors (smoking, exercise, fat intake).

- Check fasting blood glucose by finger stick daily for 2 months. If FBS declines, no other therapy is needed. If FBG does not decline or increases, use of an oral hypoglycemic agent may be considered.

ADA, American Diabetic Association; CHO, carbohydrate; FBS, fasting blood glucose.
Adapted from **The Expert Committee on the Diagnosis and Classification of Diabetes Mellitus.** Report of the Expert Committee on the Diagnosis and Classification of Diabetes Mellitus. *Diabetes Care* 2000;23:S4–S42.

medicines (i.e., *metformin*, a biguanide), insulin therapy should be initiated and referral should be considered because of the increased rate of complications.

Thyroid Diseases

Thyroid disorders are more common in women and some families, although the exact rate of inheritance is unknown (38,39). In geriatric populations, the incidence may be as high as 5% (40). The laboratory diagnosis of thyroid disease can be difficult because of altered hormonal states such as pregnancy and exogenous hormones. Thyroid hormones act in target tissues by binding to nuclear receptors, which induce change in gene expression. Extrathyroidal conversion of thyroxine (T_4) to triiodothyronine (T_3) takes place in target tissue. T_3 binds the nuclear receptor with higher affinity than T_4, which makes T_3 more biologically active. Pituitary thyroid stimulating hormone (TSH) and hypothalamic thyrotropin-releasing hormone (TRH) regulate hormone production and thyroid growth by normal feedback physiology. Thyroid-stimulating immunoglobulins (TSI), once known as a long-acting thyroid stimulator (LATS), bind to the TSH receptor, which results in hyperthyroid Graves disease.

More than 99% of circulating T_4 and T_3 concentrations are bound by plasma proteins, predominately to thyroxine-binding globulin (TBG), and the remaining 1% of thyroid hormones are free. Free levels of thyroid hormones remain constant despite physiologic or pharmacologic alterations. Regardless of total serum protein levels, active thyroid hormone remains stable. In healthy women, transitions from puberty to menopause do not alter free thyroid hormone concentrations. Excess endogenous or exogenous sources of estrogen increase TBG plasma concentration by decreasing hepatic clearance. Androgens (especially testosterone) and corticosteroids have the opposite effect by increasing hepatic TBG clearance.

Thyroid function tests may be misleading in women receiving exogenous sources of estrogen because of altered binding characteristics. In euthyroid individuals, elevations of thyroid hormone concentrations arise from three mechanisms: (i) increased protein binding because of altered albumin and estrogen states, (ii) decreased peripheral conversion of T_4 to T_3, or (iii) congenital tissue resistance to thyroid hormones, which is rare. Postmenopausal hormonal therapy and pregnancy alter laboratory findings and complicate interpretation of thyroid function studies. Most laboratories compensate by reporting a free T_4 level that mathematically corrects for physiologic alterations. If questions arise, a clinical pathologist should be consulted.

Hypothyroidism

Overt hypothyroidism occurs in 2% of women, and at least an additional 5% develop subclinical hypothyroidism. This is another disease that disproportionally impacts women five- to eightfold more commonly than men. This is especially true in the elderly, in whom many of the signs and symptoms are subtle. The principal cause of hypothyroidism is autoimmune thyroiditis (Hashimoto's thyroiditis). A familial predisposition is observed in many cases, but the specific genetic or environmental trigger is unknown. The incidence of autoimmune thyroiditis increases with age, affecting up to 15% of women older than 65 years. **Many have subclinical hypothyroidism, which is defined as an elevated serum TSH concentration with a normal serum free T_4 level.** It is uncertain whether treatment will improve quality of life in otherwise healthy patients who have subclinical hypothyroidism (41,42). Chronic autoimmune thyroiditis (Hashimoto's) is the more common cause of hypothyroidism in countries without iodine deficiency. In this process one has both cellular and antibody-mediated destruction of the thyroid, which can result in either a goiter or atrophic thyroid. Autoimmune thyroiditis may be associated with other endocrine (e.g., type 1 diabetes, primary ovarian failure, adrenal insufficiency, and hypoparathyroidism) and nonendocrine (e.g., vitiligo and pernicious anemia) disorders (43). When autoimmune diseases are present, there should be a high degree of suspicion for concurrent thyroid disorders. With postpartum thyroiditis there will be a hyperthyroid phase followed by a hypothyroid phase that can last for months. Iatrogenic causes of hypothyroidism occur after surgical removal or radioactive iodine therapy for hyperthyroidism (Graves) or thyroid cancer. Radiation was used to treat acne and other dermatologic disorders 45 years ago; patients undergoing such treatment have an increased risk of thyroid cancer and require close monitoring. Although worldwide iodine deficiency goiter is the most common form of hypothyroidism, this is uncommon in North America given the iodine supplementation in salt as well as other dietary sources. Hypothyroidism rarely occurs secondary to pituitary or hypothalamic diseases from TSH or TRH deficiency, but this must be considered if symptoms occur after neurosurgical procedures.

Clinical Features

Manifestations of hypothyroidism include a broad range of signs and symptoms: fatigue, lethargy, cold intolerance, nightmares, dry skin, hair loss, constipation, periorbital carotene deposition (causing a yellow discoloration), carpal tunnel syndrome, weight gain (usually less than 5–10 kg), depression, irritability, hyperlipidemia, and impaired memory. Menstrual dysfunction is common, either as menorrhagia or amenorrhea. Infertility may arise from anovulation, but exogenous thyroid hormone is not useful for anovulatory euthyroid women. The finding of hyperlipidemia may be the first indication of hypothyroidism, especially the presence of high triglycerides. Empirical use of thyroid extract should be discouraged.

Hypothyroidism is not a cause of premenstrual syndrome (PMS), but worsening PMS may be a subtle manifestation of hypothyroidism (44). Hypothyroidism may cause precocious or delayed puberty. Hyperprolactinemia and galactorrhea are unusual manifestations of hypothyroidism; however, assessment of thyroid function should be considered. To distinguish primary hypothyroidism from a prolactin-secreting pituitary adenoma, TSH levels should be assessed in women who have amenorrhea, galactorrhea, and hyperprolactinemia.

Diagnosis

Recommendations for screening for thyroid disorders in women range from every 5 years starting at age 35 in women (American Thyroid Association), to age 50 (American College of Physicians), to periodically in older women (American Academy of Family Physicians and American Association of Clinical Endocrinologist), to evidence is insufficient to recommend for or against screening (United States Preventive Services Task Force) (45–49).

Suspected hypothyroidism should always be confirmed with laboratory studies. Primary hypothyroidism is characterized by the combination of an elevated serum TSH with a low serum free T_4 level. Autoimmune thyroiditis can be confirmed by the presence of serum antithyroid peroxidase (formerly referred to as antimicrosomal) antibodies. An elevated TSH with a normal free T_4 level implies subclinical hypothyroidism. Central hypothyroidism, although rare, is distinguished by a low or low-normal serum free T_4 level with either a low or inappropriate normal serum TSH concentration.

Therapy

Synthetic L-thyroxine (T_4) is the treatment of choice for hypothyroidism and is available as generic *levothyroxine*. There is debate about the value of replacing thyroxine in the subclinical hypothyroidism patient. Such replacement did not result in improved survival, decreased cardiovascular morbidity, or improve quality of life (44). The mode of action is by conversion of T_4 to T_3 in peripheral tissues. *Levothyroxine* should be taken on an empty stomach. Absorption may be poor when taken in combination with aluminum hydroxide (common in antacids), *cholestyramine,* ferrous sulfate, or fatty meals. The usual T_4 requirement is weight related (approximately 1.6 μg/kg) but decreases for the elderly. Normal daily dosage is 0.1 to 0.15 mg but should be adjusted to maintain TSH levels within the normal range. TSH levels should be checked in 6 weeks and when dosages or brands are changed.

In the early 1980s, many clinicians thought that increasing the serum T_4 to mildly elevated levels would enhance conversion of T_4 to T_3. Subsequent data proved that even a mild increase of T_4 was associated with cortical bone loss and atrial fibrillation, particularly in older women (44). A low initial T_4 dose (0.025 mg per day) should be initiated in the elderly or patients with known or suspected coronary artery disease. Rapid replacement may worsen angina and in some cases induce myocardial infarction.

Hyperthyroidism

Hyperthyroidism affects 2% of women during their lifetime, most often during their childbearing years and impacts women fivefold more commonly than men. Graves disease represents the most common disorder; it is associated with orbital inflammation, causing the classic exophthalmus associated with the disease and a characteristic dermopathy, pretibial myxedema. It is an autoimmune disorder caused by TSH reception antibodies that stimulate gland growth and hormone synthesis. The etiology of Graves disease in genetically susceptible women is unknown. Autonomously functioning benign thyroid neoplasias are less common causes of hyperthyroidism and are associated with toxic adenomas and toxic multinodular goiter. Transient thyrotoxicosis may be the result of unregulated glandular release of thyroid hormone in postpartum (painless, silent, or lymphocytic) thyroiditis and subacute (painful) thyroiditis. Other rare causes of thyroid overactivity include human chorionic gonadotropin–secreting choriocarcinoma, TSH-secreting pituitary adenoma, and struma ovarii. Factitious ingestion or iatrogenic overprescribing should be considered in patients with eating disorders.

Clinical Features

Symptoms of thyrotoxicosis include fatigue, diarrhea, heat intolerance, palpitations, dyspnea, nervousness, and weight loss. In young patients there may be paradoxical weight gain from an increased appetite. Thyrotoxicosis may cause vomiting in pregnant women, which may be confused with hyperemesis gravidarum (50). Tachycardia, lid lag, tremor, proximal muscle weakness, and warm moist skin are classic physical findings. The most dramatic physical changes are ophthalmologic and include lid retraction, periorbital edema, and proptosis. These eye findings occur in less than one-third of women. In elderly adults, symptoms are often more subtle, with presentations of unexplained weight loss, atrial fibrillation, or new onset angina pectoris. Menstrual abnormalities span from regular menses to light flow to anovulatory menses and associated infertility. Goiter is common in younger women with Graves disease, but may be absent in older women. Toxic nodular goiter is associated with nonhomogeneous glandular enlargement, whereas in subacute thyroiditis the gland is tender, hard, and enlarged.

Diagnosis

Most thyrotoxic patients have elevated total and free T_4 and T_3 concentrations (measured by radioimmune assay). In thyrotoxicosis, serum TSH concentrations are virtually undetectable, even with very sensitive assays (sensitivity measured to 0.1 units). Sensitive serum TSH measurements may aid in the diagnosis of hyperthyroidism. Radioiodine uptake scans are useful in the differential diagnosis of established hyperthyroidism. Scans with homogeneous uptake of radioactive iodine are suggestive of Graves disease, whereas heterogeneous tracer uptake is suggestive of a diagnosis of toxic nodular goiter. Thyroiditis and medication-induced thyrotoxicosis have diminished glandular radioisotope concentration.

Therapy

Antithyroid medications, either *propylthiouracil* (*PTU* 50–300 mg every 6–8 hours) or *methimazole* (10–30 mg per day) are used for initial therapy. After metabolic control is achieved, definitive therapy is obtained by thyroid ablation with radioiodine, which results in permanent hypothyroidism. Both antithyroid drugs block thyroid hormone biosynthesis and may have additional immunosuppressive effects on the gland. The primary difference in oral medications is that *PTU* partially inhibits extrathyroidal T_4-to-T_3 conversion, whereas *methimazole* does not. M*ethimazole* has a longer half-life and permits single daily dosing, which may encourage compliance. Euthyroidism is typically restored in 3 to 10 weeks, and treatment with oral antithyroid agents is continued for 6 to 24 months, unless total ablation with radioiodine or surgical resection is performed. Surgery is less popular because it is invasive and may result in inadvertent parathyroid removal, which commits the patient to lifelong calcium therapy.

The relapse rate with oral antithyroid medications is 50% over a lifetime. Lifelong follow-up is important when medical therapy is used solely because of the high relapse rate. Both medications have infrequent (5%) minor side effects, which include fever, rash, or arthralgias. Major toxicity (e.g., hepatitis, vasculitis, and agranulocytosis) occurs in less than 1%. Agranulocytosis cannot be predicted by periodic complete blood counts; therefore, patients who have a sore throat or fever should stop taking the medication and call their physician immediately.

Therapy with iodine-131 provides a permanent cure of hyperthyroidism in 90% of patients. The principal drawback to radioactive iodine therapy is the high rate of postablative hypothyroidism, which occurs in at least 50% of patients immediately after therapy, with additional cases developing at a rate of 2% to 3% per year. Based on the assumption that hypothyroidism will develop, these patients should be given lifetime thyroid replacement therapy. Beta-adrenergic blocking agents such as *propranolol* or *atenolol* are useful adjunctive therapy for control of sympathomimetic symptoms such as tachycardia (51). An additional benefit of beta-blockers is the blocking of peripheral conversion of T_4 to T_3. In rare cases of thyroid storm, PTU, beta-blockers, glucocorticoids, and high-dose iodine preparations (intravenous sodium iodide) should be administered immediately, and referral to an intensive care unit is advisable.

Thyroid Nodules and Cancer

Thyroid nodules are common and found on physical examination in up to 5% of patients. Nodules may be demonstrated on ultrasound in approximately 50% of 60-year-olds. The vast majority of nodules when discovered are asymptomatic and benign; however, malignancy and hyperthyroidism must be excluded (52). Ultrasound-guided fine-needle aspiration is recommended in the presence of the following factors: history of radiation to the head, neck, or upper chest; family history of thyroid cancer; ultrasound findings suggestive of malignancy; or a nodule larger than 1.5 cm in diameter (53).

Thyroid function tests should be performed before fine-needle aspiration and, if results are abnormal, the underlying disease should be treated. Because most nodules are "cold" on scanning, it is more cost-effective to proceed with tissue sampling rather than scanning. Needle biopsy provides a diagnosis in 95% of cases; in the 5% of patients in whom the diagnosis cannot be established, excisional biopsy is necessary. Only 20% of excisional biopsies of an "indeterminate aspiration" are found to be malignant (54). Lesions that are confirmed malignant on biopsy should be treated with extirpative surgery, and benign nodules should be palpated every 6 to 12 months. *Thyroxine* suppressive therapy for benign nodules is not recommended (53).

Papillary thyroid carcinoma is the most common malignancy, found in 75% of thyroid cancers. For unclear reasons the incidence of papillary cancer increased by almost threefold in the past 30 years, from 2.7 to 7.7 per 100,000 people (55). This may represent the more ready diagnosis of smaller cancers. The majority of cancers are found incidentally during routine examinations. Risk factors include a history of radiation exposure during childhood and family history. Signs include rapid growth of neck mass, new onset hoarseness, or vocal cord paralysis. In the setting of rapid growth, fixed nodule, new onset hoarseness, or the presence of lymphadenopathy, it is important to be sure a fine-needle aspiration is done. Thyroidectomy is the primary treatment with radioactive iodine and TSH suppression with thyroxine. Patients younger than 50 years of age with a primary tumor of less than 4 cm at presentation, even with associated cervical lymph node metastasis, are usually cured. In the elderly, anaplastic tumors have a poor prognosis and progress rapidly despite therapy.

Follicular thyroid cancer is the second most common thyroid cancer, comprising up to 10% of cases. These tend to occur in an older population with peak ages of 40 to 60. It has a threefold greater prevalence in women than men. This form of cancer tends to have vascular invasion, frequently with distant metastases. The prognosis tends to be less favorable with this form of cancer than with papillary cancers, although women do have a better prognosis than men.

Irritable Bowel Syndrome

Irritable bowel syndrome (IBS) is a common problem, affecting about 10% to 15% of the population, with women being twice as likely to have the diagnosis (56). Given that its primary symptom is typically crampy chronic abdominal pain, IBS is often in the differential diagnosis for patients with chronic pelvic pain. Stress and certain foods will often trigger the pain, and defecation often will provide some relief from the pain. Other gastrointestinal symptoms include diarrhea and constipation, gastroesophageal reflux disease, nausea, bloating, and flatulence. What makes this a more difficult diagnosis is the spectrum of additional symptoms, including dysmenorrhea, dyspareunia, fibromyalgia complaints, urinary symptoms of frequency and urgency, and even sexual dysfunction.

This spectrum of symptoms renders diagnosis difficult and led to a consensus group that created the Rome criteria in 1992, revised in 2005 (57). The resulting Rome III criteria are: recurrent abdominal pain or discomfort for at least 3 days per month for 3 months associated with two or more of the following:

- Improvement with defecation

- Onset associated with a change in frequency of stool

- Onset associated with a change in the appearance of the stool

IBS should be a diagnosis of exclusion with consideration initially given to other causes for the dominant symptom. If that is diarrhea, considerations of lactose intolerance, infectious etiology, malabsorption, or celiac disease should be entertained. Symptoms that result in weight loss, rectal bleeding, anemia, or that are noctural or progressive could indicate something other than IBS unless proven otherwise.

A basic workup might include complete blood count and chemistries. Evaluation of diarrhea, if that is the dominant symptom, should potentially include stool cultures if infectious etiology is suspected or 24-hour stool collection (if osmotic) of secretory diarrhea is suspected. Flexible sigmoidoscopy is not done routinely unless needed to rule out inflammatory conditions or malignancy in families with Lynch syndrome. Initiate dietary reviews for lactose intolerance or gluten sensitivity.

Management

General management of IBS can be extremely difficult. Often, the first step is to reassure the patient that this is a functional disease and is not related to cancer or malignancy, assuming those were eliminated by history and examination. Many individuals have some underlying concerns that diagnostic testing needs to be performed or that something is being missed. Constant reassurance is an important aspect of management. The patient needs to be an active participant in her care and understand the chronic nature of the disease. A symptom diary for several weeks may show a link between various foods and stressors that may be modifiable. Some individuals are able to link various stressors in their lives to symptoms while others will not have identifiable causes. **Common triggers include stress, anxiety, medication (antibiotics, antacids), menstrual cycles, abusive relationships, certain foods (lactose, sorbitol), and travel. Patients should be counseled about dietary interventions, including increasing dietary fiber, decreasing total fat intake, and avoiding foods that trigger symptoms.** Stool softeners are recommended for individuals with hard stools, and bulk aiding agents may be helpful for those individuals with constipation. The overuse of laxatives is to be discouraged. Good bowel habits should be discussed. Patients with poor habits should set aside a quiet time every day to attempt defecation. Many individuals get into a habit of ignoring stooling symptoms, leading to further problems with lower gastrointestinal disease.

Antidiarrheal agents, specifically *loperamide* or *diphenoxylate,* are often useful in patients with mild disease. The goal is to reduce the number of bowel movements and help to relieve rectal urgency. Anticholinergics including *hyoscyamine* and *dicyclomine hydrochloride* often are helpful. Powder *opium,* an antidiarrheal, combined with an antispasmodic (*belladonna* alkaloid), is another option for refractory disease. Antispasmodic agents have anticholinergic agents as the primary ingredient, and compliance may be a problem because side effects include dry mouth, visual disturbances, and constipation. These agents can precipitate toxic megacolon, which may result in severe colitis. Toxic megacolon is a medical and potential surgical emergency, in some cases requiring colectomy. **Even though these patients may be extremely difficult to treat, judicious use of symptom-based pharmacologic approaches, reassurance, and patient insight may be helpful. The quality of life for some individuals with IBS is extremely compromised, requiring intense counseling.** It may be difficult to treat them in a busy primary care practice. Those with a concurrent psychiatric disease, such as depression, will often benefit from psychiatric consultation and pharmacologic treatment of the underlying disease in the overall management.

Individuals with chronic, debilitating irritable bowel syndrome should be referred to a gastroenterologist. Any suspicion of organic disease with systemic changes, including weight loss and bloody diarrhea, should be considered for referral.

Studies suggest a relationship between IBS symptoms and an imbalance of central nervous system neurotransmitters related to stress in the environment (58,59). Serotonins (5-hydroxytryptamine or 5-HT) are important in the development of gut disorders. Only 5% of total body serotonin is found in the central nervous system, while 95% is found in the gastrointestinal tract. Other neurotransmitters associated with gastrointestinal disorders include calcitonin, neurotensin, substance P, nitric oxide, vasoactive intestinal peptide, and acetylcholine. These neurotransmitters function at the level of the bowel and the central nervous system.

Several compounds were studied that interact with serotonin receptors in the bowel (5 HT-3 and 5 HT-4). The 5-HT-3 antagonist, *alosetron,* was introduced to treat patients with diarrhea. Patients with other symptoms, including alternating diarrhea and constipation, and individuals with primary constipation received the drug, resulting in severe constipation in approximately one-third of patients. There were reports of ischemic colitis with the use of this drug. Although the drug was withdrawn for a time period, the U.S. Food and Drug Administration allowed its reintroduction. *Tegaserod* is a 5-HT-4 receptor (serotonin receptor) agonist that is approved for short-term use in patients with constipation. It has gastrointestinal stimulatory effects facilitated by intercolonergic transmission as its primary mode of action. There are many 5-HT drugs under development that will be introduced over the next 2 to 5 years.

Gastroesophageal Reflux Disease

The term gastroesophageal reflex disease (GERD) is a commonly used label for many forms of indigestion and heartburn. The American College of Gastroenterology defines it as symptoms or mucosal damage produced by the abnormal reflux of gastric contents into the esophagus (60). The term "abnormal" is key because some reflux is physiologic, usually occurring postprandial and typically being asymptomatic. Given the variation in definition, its prevalence is hard to determine, but it is clear that GERD is more common in the Western world.

Symptoms of GERD include heartburn (burning sensation in the retrosternal area) commonly postprandial, regurgitation gastric contents into mouth, dysphagia from esophageal inflammation, and chest pain that can be confused as angina. **Dysphagia that is progressive is concerning for Barrett's metaplasia or adenocarcinoma and merits an endoscopic evaluation** (61).

Treatment of GERD is multifaceted with lifestyle modification and use of antacids and over-the-counter H_2 receptor antagonists or proton pump inhibitors (PPI). Lifestyle modifications include smoking cessation, avoidance of eating late in the evening, avoidance of being supine after eating, weight loss, avoidance of tight clothing, and restriction of alcohol use. Dietary modifications are helpful but should not be draconian, which will ensure noncompliance. Key foods to try to minimize are fatty foods, chocolate, peppermint, and excessive alcohol. The patient can monitor her own symptoms for the foods that are most problematic for her.

Medications that reduce acid secretions are best and include H_2 blockers or proton pump inhibitors. They do not prevent the reflux but decrease the damage done by the acid when refluxed. Medication needs to be titrated to the severity of the symptoms. H_2 blockers commonly work well for acute pain but in placebo-controlled studies in chronic cases without resolution of heartburn after the common 6-week course, it was found that patients on PPI do better. Maintenance therapy is recommended for patients who have rapid recurrence of symptoms (in less than 2–3 months) after they stop their medication. Otherwise patients can be managed with episodic treatments. **The linkage of *Helicobacter pylori* infections and GERD is poorly understood but seems to be mediated through increased gastric acid secretion.** Treatment can initially worsen GERD and may not improve it (62). Benefits and risks should be discussed with the patient prior to testing and treating for *H. pylori*. The management of GERD during pregnancy is similar to the treatment in the nonpregnant patient.

Carpal Tunnel Syndrome

Carpal tunnel syndrome (CTS) is the cluster of symptoms brought on by compression in the carpal tunnel of the median nerve. These are paresthesia, pain, and weakness. The symptoms are commonly worse at night and may wake the patient from sleep. It is thought women may be more likely to present with complaints of CTS because of their small wrists, repetitive motion injury at work (typing, holding telephone, and reading), and pregnancy with increased edema. The pain and paresthesia can be located in the wrist or hand or can be in the forearm. The weakness may cause a patient to have difficulty opening jars, lifting a plate, turning a doorknob, or holding a glass.

A detailed history is very diagnostic but the use of a couple simple tests can help to confirm it (63). The most common one is the **Phalen maneuver,** in which the patient flexes her palms at the wrist as close to 90 degrees as possible. Then with the dorsal portion of the hands touching and the arms parallel to the floor, the patient presses the flexed hands against each other for approximately 1 minute. This should reproduce her symptoms along the median nerve. The **Tinel test** involves percussion over the top of the carpal tunnel where the median nerve travels. A positive test is when the percussion reproduces the pain and paresthesia. Additional testing such as nerve conduction studies should be reserved for patients who do not respond to conservative management or have significant muscle weakness.

Treatment involves lifestyle modification to decrease repetitive motion injuries or prolonged marked flexion at the wrist. A carpal tunnel brace can be very helpful in maintaining

adequate extension at the wrist, thereby "opening" the tunnel and reducing compression on the medial nerve. Only if these strategies do not work is a surgical intervention indicated.

Mitral Valve Prolapse Syndrome, Dysautonomia, and Postural Orthostatic Tachycardia Syndrome

The terms mitral valve prolapse syndrome (MVPS), dysautonomia, and postural orthostatic tachycardia syndrome (POTS) all refer to a syndrome in which the patient has problems with palpitations, hypotension, syncope, dyspnea, panic/anxiety disorder, numbness, hyperflexible joints, pectus excavatum, and gastric emptying disorders. Initially patients (typically fivefold times more likely to be women) who presented with these symptoms were thought to be somatizing their anxiety disorder. It is now accepted that it is a syndrome that appears to involve the autonomic nervous system (64). This often will present first in early adolescence with gradual worsening of the symptoms. The patients are very slender in build and lose weight to a low body mass index over a number of months as the syndrome evolves. This weight loss is the probable cause of the secondary amenorrhea that prompts these women to seek gynecologic care. The symptoms are not clearly explained by the degree of mitral valve prolapse, so many feel MVPS is a marker for individuals at risk for this complex of symptoms. Increased sympathetic activity is the common pathway for most of the proposed mechanisms for POTS or MVPS. There appears to be a genetic component, with over 10% of patients reporting the diagnosis in family members with orthostatic intolerance (65,66).

A tilt table test is often key to the diagnosis. Treatment focuses on the symptoms and maintaining intravascular volume by encouraging oral intake of water and salts (67). Physical fitness with aerobic exercises to increase muscle mass and reduce dependent pooling of blood; avoidance of smoking, caffeine, and alcohol; and limiting simple carbohydrates will minimize symptoms over time. Additional medications, including adrenoreceptor agonists, acetylcholinesterase inhibitor, mineralocorticoid agonist, beta-blockers, and selective serotonin reuptake inhibitors, may be necessary. Because this is a multifaceted disease, it may be best to refer the patient during the acute phase to a physician who is experienced with this syndrome.

References

1. **Piccirillo JR.** Acute bacterial sinusitis. *N Eng J Med* 2004;351:902–910.
2. **Williams JN, Simel DL.** Does this patient have sinusitis?: Diagnosing acute sinusitis by history and physical examination. *JAMA* 1993;270:1242–1246.
3. **Hirschmann JV.** Antibiotics for common respiratory tract infections. *Arch Intern Med* 2002;162:256–264.
4. **Zalmanovici TA, Yaphe J.** Intranasal steroids for acute sinusitis. *Cochrane Database Syst Rev* 2009;4:CD005149.
5. **Dolor RJ, Witsell DL, Hellkamp AS, et al.** Comparison of cefuroxime with or without intranasal fluticasone for the treatment of rhinosinusitis. *JAMA* 2001;286:3097–3105.
6. **Ahovuo-Saloranta A, Borisenko OV, Kovanen N, et al.** Antibiotics for acute maxillary sinusitis. *Cochrane Database Syst Rev* 2008;2:CD000243.
7. **Kassel JC, King D, Spurling GKP, et al.** Saline nasal irrigation for acute upper respiratory tract infections. *Cochrane Database Syst Rev* 2010;3:CD0068921.
8. **Smith SM, Fahay T, Smucny J, et al.** Antibiotics for acute bronchitis. *Cochrane Database Syst Rev* 2004;4:CD000245.
9. **Nolan TE, Hankins GDV.** Adult respiratory distress. In: **Pastorek J, ed.** *Infectious disease in obstetrics and gynecology.* Rockville, MD: Aspen Publications, 1994:197–206.
10. **Niederman MS, Mandell LA, Bass JB, et al.** American Thoracic Society guidelines for the management of adults with community-acquired pneumonia: diagnosis, assessment of severity, antimicrobial therapy and prevention. *Am J Respir Crit Care Med* 2001;163:1730–1754.
11. **Halm EA, Teirstein AS.** Management of community acquired pneumonia. *N Engl J Med* 2002;347:2039–2045.
12. **Bjerre LM, Verheij TJM, Kochen MM.** Antibiotics for community-acquired pneumonia in adult outpatients. *Cochrane Database Syst Rev* 2009;4:CD002109.
13. **Centers for Disease Control and Prevention.** Prevention and control of influenza: recommendations of the Advisory Committee on Immunization Practices (ACIP). *MMWR Morbid Mortal Wkly Rep* 2000;49[RR3]:1–38.
14. **Chobanian AV, Bakris GL, Black HR, et al.** The seventh report of the Joint National Committee on Prevention, Detection, Evaluation, and Treatment of High Blood Pressure (JNC VII). *JAMA* 2003;289:2560–2572.
15. **Powrie RO.** A 30-year-old woman with chronic hypertension trying to conceive. *JAMA* 2007;298:1548–1559.
16. **Roccella EJ, Lenfant C.** Regional and racial differences among stroke victims in the United States. *Clin Cardiol* 1989;12:IV4–IV8.
17. **Moorman PG, Hames CG, Tyroler HA.** Socioeconomic status and morbidity and mortality in hypertensive blacks. *Cardiovasc Clin* 1991;21(3):179–194.
18. **Arguedas JA, Perez MI, Wright JM.** Treatment blood pressure targets for hypertension. *Cochrane Database Syst Rev* 2009;3:CD004349.
19. **American Society of Hypertension.** Recommendations for routine blood pressure measurement by indirect cuff sphygmomanometry. *Am J Hypertens* 1992;5:207–209.
20. **The National High Blood Pressure Education Program Working Group Report on Ambulatory Blood Pressure Monitoring.** *Arch Intern Med* 1990;150:2270–2280.
21. **Appel IJ, Brands MW, Daniels SR, et al.** Dietary approaches to prevent and treat hypertension: a scientific statement form the American Heart Association. *Hypertension* 2006;47:296.

22. **Selby JV, Friedman GD, Quensenberry CP Jr.** Precursors of essential hypertension: the role of body fat distribution pattern. *Am J Epidemiol* 1989;129:43–53.

23. **Whelton PK, Appel LJ, Espeland, MA, et al.** Sodium reduction and weight loss in the treatment of hypertension in older persons: a randomized controlled trial of nonpharmacologic interventions in the elderly (TONE). *JAMA* 1998;279:839.

24. **Beyer FR, Dickinson HO, Nicolson D, et al.** Combined calcium, magnesium and potassium supplementation for the management of primary hypertension in adults. *Cochrane Database Syst Rev* 2006;3: CD004805.

25. **Wright JM, Musini VM.** First line drugs for hypertension. *Cochrane Database Syst Rev* 2009;3:CD001841.

26. **Freis ED.** Critique of the clinical importance of diuretic-induced hypokalemia and elevated cholesterol level. *Arch Intern Med* 1989; 149:2640–2648.

27. **Brunner E, Rees K, Ward K, et al.** Dietary advice for reducing cardiovascular risk. *Cochrane Database Syst Rev* 2007;4:CD 002128.

28. **Hooper L, Summerbell CD, Higgins JPT, et al.** Reduced or modified dietary fat for preventing cardiovascular disease. *Cochrane Database Syst Rev* 2001;3:CD002137.

29. **Katan MB, Beynen AC.** Characteristics of human hypo- and hyper-responders to dietary cholesterol. *Am J Epidemiol* 1987;125:387–399.

30. **Naughton MJ, Luepker RV, Strickland D.** The accuracy of portable cholesterol analyzers in public screening programs. *JAMA* 1990;263:1213–1217.

31. **Irwig L, Glaszious P, Wilson A, et al.** Estimating an individual's true cholesterol level and response to intervention. *JAMA* 1991;266:1678–1685.

32. **van Stiphout WAHJ, Hofman A, de Bruijn AM.** Serum lipids in young women before, during, and after pregnancy. *Am J Epidemiol* 1987;126:922–928.

33. **Expert Panel on Detection, Evaluation, and Treatment of High Blood Cholesterol in Adults.** Executive summary of the third report of the National Cholesterol Education Program (NCEP) Expert Panel on Detection, Evaluation, and Treatment of High Blood Cholesterol in Adults (Adult Treatment Panel III). *JAMA* 2001;285:2486–2497.

34. **Centers for Disease Control and Prevention.** Diabetes surveillance 2007. Washington DC: U.S. Department of Health and Human Services, Public Health Service, 2007.

35. **The Expert Committee on the Diagnosis and Classification of Diabetes Mellitus.** Report of the Expert Committee on the Diagnosis and Classification of Diabetes Mellitus. *Diabetes Care* 2000;23:S4–S42.

36. **Professional Practice Committee.** American Diabetes Association: clinical practice recommendations 2005. *Diabetes Care* 2005;28:S4–S42.

37. **Wood PD, Stefanick ML, Williams PT, et al.** The effects on plasma lipoproteins of a prudent weight-reducing diet, with or without exercise, in overweight men and women. *N Engl J Med* 1991;325:461–466.

38. **Tunbridge WM, Evered DC, Hall R, et al.** The spectrum of thyroid disease in a community: the Whickham survey. *Clin Endocrinol (Oxf)* 1977;7:481–493.

39. **Vanderpump MP, Tunbridge WM, French JM, et al.** The incidence of thyroid disorders in the community: a twenty-year follow-up of the Whickham survey. *Clin Endocrinol* 1995;43:55–68.

40. **Helfand M, Crapo LM.** Screening for thyroid disease. *Ann Intern Med* 1990;112:840–849.

41. **Helfand M.** Screening for subclincal thyroid dysfunction in nonpregnant adults: a summary of the evidence for the U.S. Preventive Services Task Force. *Ann Intern Med* 2004;140:128–141.

42. **Villar HCCE, Saconato H, Valente O, et al.** Thyroid hormone replacement for subclinical hypothyroidism. *Cochrane Database Syst Rev* 2007;3:CD003419.

43. **Volpé R.** Autoimmunity causing thyroid dysfunction. *Endocrinol Metab Clin North Am* 1991;20:565–587.

44. **Schmidt PJ, Grover GN, Roy-Byrne PP, et al.** Thyroid function in women with premenstrual syndrome. *J Clin Endocrinol Metab* 1993;76:671–674.

45. **Ladenson PW, Singer PA, Ain KB, et al.** American Thyroid Association guidelines for detection of thyroid dysfunction. [erratum appears in Arch Intern Med 2001 Jan 22;161(2):284]. *Arch Intern Med* 2000;160(11):1573–1575.

46. **American College of Physicians.** Clinical guideline, part 1. Screening for thyroid disease. *Ann Intern Med* 1998;129(2):141–143.

47. **American Academy of Family Physicians.** *Summary of Policy Recommendations for Periodic Health Examinations.* Leawood, KS: American Academy of Family Physicians; 2002.

48. **American Association of Clinical Endocrinologists.** 2002 clinical guidelines for the evaluation and treatment of hyperthyroidism and hypothyroidism. *Endocr Pract* 2002;8:457–467.

49. **US Preventative Services Task Force.** Screening for thyroid disease: recommendation statement. *Ann Intern Med* 2004;140: 125–127.

50. **Mori M, Amino N, Tamaki H, et al.** Morning sickness and thyroid function in normal pregnancy. *Obstet Gynecol* 1988;72:355–359.

51. **Zonszein J, Santangelo RP, Mackin JF, et al.** Propranolol therapy in thyrotoxicosis. *Am J Med* 1979;66:411–416.

52. **Hegedus L.** The thyroid nodule. *N Engl J Med* 2004;351:1764–1771.

53. **Tan GH, Gharib H.** Management approaches to nonpalpable nodules discovered incidentally on thyroid imaging. *Ann Intern Med* 1997;126:226–231.

54. **McHenry CR, Walfish PG, Rosen IB.** Non-diagnostic fine needle aspiration biopsy: a dilemma in management of nodular thyroid disease. *Am Surg* 1993;59:415–419.

55. **Howlader N, Noone AM, Krapcho M, et al., eds.** *SEER Cancer Statistics Review, 1975–2008,* National Cancer Institute. Bethesda, MD. Available online at: http://seer.cancer.gov/csr/1975_2008/.

56. **Hungin AP, Whorwell PJ, Tack J, et al.** The prevalence, patterns and impact of irritable bowel syndrome: an international survey of 40,000 subjects. *Aliment Pharmacol Ther* 2003;17:643–650.

57. **Rome Foundation.** Rome III Diagnostic Criteria for Functional Gastrointestinal Disorders. 2010. Available online at: http://www.romecriteria.org/assets/pdf/19_RomeIII_apA_885–898.pdf.

58. **Monnikes H, Schmidt BG, Tache Y.** Psychological stress-induced accelerated colonic transit in rats involves hypothalamic corticotropin-releasing factor. *Gastroenterology* 1993;104;716–723.

59. **Heymann-Monnikes I, Arnold R, Florin I, et al.** The combination of medical treatment plus multicomponent behavioral therapy is superior to medical treatment alone in the therapy of irritable bowel syndrome. *Am J Gastroenterol* 2000;95:981–994.

60. **Devault KR, Castell DO.** Updated guidelines for the diagnosis and treatment of gastroesophageal reflux disease. *Am J Gastroenterol* 2005;100:190.

61. **Kahrilas PJ, Shaheen NJ, Vaezi MF, et al.** American Gastroenterological Association medical position statement on the management of gastroesophageal reflux disease. *Gastroenterology* 2008;135:1383.

62. **Moayyedi P, Soo S, Deeks JJ, et al.** Eradication of *Helicobacter pylori* for non-ulcer dyspepsia. *Cochrane Database Syst Rev* 2006;2:CD002096.

63. **MacDermid JC, Wessel J.** Clinical diagnosis of carpal tunnel syndrome: a systematic review. *J Hand Ther* 2004;17:309.

64. **Freed LA, Levy D, Levine RA, et al.** Prevalence and clinical outcome of mitral valve prolapsed. *N Engl J Med* 1999;341:1.

65. **Jacob G, Biaggioni I.** Idiopathic orthostatic intolerance and postural tachycardia syndromes. *Am J Med Sci* 1999;317:88.

66. **Jacob G, Costa F, Shannon JR, et al.** The neuropathic postural tachycardia syndrome. *N Engl J Med* 2000;343:1008.

67. **Raj SR, Biaggioni I, Yambure PC, et al.** Renin-aldosterone paradox and perturbed blood volume regulation underlying postural tachycardia syndrome. *Circulation* 2005;111:1574.

10 Family Planning

Phillip G. Stubblefield
Danielle M. Roncari

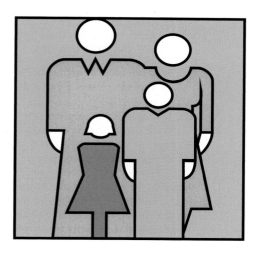

- The most common methods of contraception used in the United States are sterilization, oral contraceptives, and condoms, in that order.

- Latex condoms and other barriers reduce the risk of sexually transmitted diseases (STDs) and cervical cancer.

- The two intrauterine devices (IUDs) available in the United States, the *copper T380A* (*ParaGard*) and the *levonorgestrel T* (*Mirena*), are as effective as tubal sterilization and are associated with a long-term risk of pelvic infection that is no greater than that in the general population.

- The combination estrogen–progestin oral contraceptive, patch, and vaginal ring all provide excellent contraception when used correctly but all increase the risk of venous thrombosis and thromboembolism.

- Present low-dose estrogen–progestin combinations do not increase the risk of heart attack among nonsmokers younger than age 35 years who have no other risks for vascular disease.

- Oral contraceptives do not increase the risk of breast cancer.

- Use of progestin-only injectable and implant hormonal contraceptives results in very low pregnancy rates without the estrogen-associated risk of thrombosis.

- Hormonal contraceptives provide extensive contraceptive and noncontraceptive health benefits, including reduced risk for endometrial and ovarian cancer.

- *Levonorgestrel 1.5 mg* (*Plan B*) and ulipristal acetate are the most effective hormonal means of emergency contraception. Efficacy is greatest within 24 hours of intercourse but remains high at 5 days. The *copper T380A* IUD inserted 5 days after intercourse is even more effective than hormonal methods.

- Long-acting reversible contraceptive (LARC) methods include injectable progestins, subdermal progestin implants, and *copper-* or *levonorgestrel*-releasing intrauterine devices. These offer pregnancy rates comparable to sterilization and are among the safest methods.

- Safe, long-term contraception is provided with laparoscopy and bipolar electrocautery application to three adjacent sites on each tube, the Silastic band, or the *Filshie clip.*

- Hysteroscopic sterilization techniques provide highly effective permanent contraception for women without the use of general anesthesia or abdominal incision.

- Vasectomy provides highly effective, low-cost sterilization for men and is associated with neither heart disease nor prostate cancer.

- Abortion mortality rates fell rapidly with legalization; currently, the overall mortality risk is less than 1 per 100,000, well below the maternal mortality rate of 12.7 per 100,000 live births.

- The risk of abortion mortality increases with gestational age, from 0.1 per 100,000 at 8 weeks or less. Even at 16 to 20 weeks abortion is safer than continuing pregnancy.

The history of contraception is a long one, dating to ancient times. The voluntary control of fertility is especially important in modern society (1). A woman who expects to have no more than one or two children spends most of her reproductive years trying to avoid pregnancy. Effective control of reproduction is essential to a woman's ability to accomplish her individual goals. From a larger perspective, the rapid growth of the human population in this century threatens the survival of all. **At present rates, the population of the world will double in 66 years, and that of the United States will double in 75 years** (2). **For the individual and for the planet, reproductive health requires careful use of effective means to prevent both pregnancy and sexually transmitted disease (STD)** (3).

Table 10.1 Number of Women Aged 15–44 Years, and Percentage Currently Using Contraception Methods According to Age at Interview, United States 2006–2008[a]				
Age	*15–24*	*25–34*	*35–44*	*15–44*
Number of women	20,570,000	19,837,000	21,457,000	61,864,000
Currently using contraception (%)	41.3	67.2	76.5	61.8
Female sterilization (%)	0.7	14.9	33.8	16.7
Male sterilization (%)	0.2	3.9	13.9	6.1
Pill (%)	20.7	20.1	11.5	17.3
Implant, *Lunelle*™ or patch (%)	0.6	1.1	0.4	0.7
Depo-Provera™ (%)	2.7	2.5	0.8	2.0
Contraceptive ring (%)	2.2	1.9	0.5	1.5
Intrauterine device (%)	2.1	4.3	3.8	3.4
Condom (%)	9.9	12.6	7.6	10.0
Periodic abstinence-calendar rhythm (%)	0.2	0.7	0.7	0.5
Periodic abstinence-natural family planning (%)	0	0.3	0.1	0.1
Withdrawal (%)	1.9	4.4	3.3	3.2
Other methods[b] (%)	0.2	0.5	0.2	0.3

[a]Women could list up to four current methods. The method shown above was the most effective method used.
[b]Includes diaphragm (with or without jelly or cream), emergency contraception, female condom, foam, cervical cap, Today™ sponge, suppository or insert, jelly or cream (without diaphragm), and other methods.
From **Vital and Health Statistics.** Use of contraception in the United States 1982–2008. National Survey of Family Growth. Series 23. Number 29. May 2010, Tables 6 and 14.

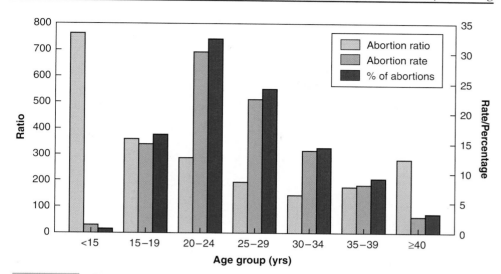

Figure 10.1 **Abortion rate*, ratio+, and percentage of total abortions by age group of women who obtained abortion, United States, 2006§.** *Number of abortions per 1,000 women aged 15–44 years. +Number of abortions per 1,000 live births. §Data from 48 reporting areas, excludes California, Florida, Louisiana, and New Hampshire. (From **Pazol K, Gamble SB, Parker WY, et al.** Abortion surveillance—United States 2005. *MMWR Surveil Sum* 2009;58(SS08):35 [Figure 2].

From puberty until menopause, women are faced with concerns about childbearing or its avoidance: the only options are sexual abstinence, contraception, or pregnancy. The contraceptive choices made by couples in the United States in 2008 are shown in Table 10.1 (4). Oral contraceptives (OCs) were the first choice among women, used by 17.3%. Female sterilization was the second choice, used by 16.7%. With the addition of the 6.1% of couples relying on male sterilization, 22.8% of couples were relying on sterilization, making this the first choice of couples. Condoms were third choice, used by 10%. OC use declines with age, and the rate of sterilization increases. Twenty percent of women under 25 who use contraceptives use OCs and only 0.7% is sterilized. Of women aged 35 to 44 using contraception 17.3% uses OCs and 33.8% is sterilized, as is 13.9% of their consorts (Table 10.1). About 10% of women use more than one method of contraception. **Although use of contraception is high, a significant proportion of sexually active couples (7.4%) does not use contraception, and each year, 2 of every 100 women aged 15 to 44 years have an induced abortion** (4,5). Abortion is an obvious indicator of unplanned pregnancy. Abortion ratios by age group indicate that the use of abortion is greatest for the youngest women and least for women in their late 20s and early 30s who are most likely to continue pregnancies (Fig. 10.1). Use of abortion increases from the late 30s on. **Young women are much more likely to experience unplanned pregnancy because they are more fertile than older women and because they are more likely to have intercourse without contraception.** The effect of age on pregnancy rates with different contraceptive methods is shown in Figure 10.2.

Efficacy

Factors affecting whether pregnancy will occur include the fecundity of both partners, the timing of intercourse in relation to the time of ovulation, the method of contraception used, the intrinsic effectiveness of the contraceptive method, and the correct use of the method. It is impossible to assess the effectiveness of a contraceptive method in isolation from the other factors. The best way to assess effectiveness is long-term evaluation of a group of sexually active women using a particular method for a specified period to observe how frequently pregnancy occurs. **A pregnancy rate per 100 women per year can be calculated using the Pearl formula (dividing the number of pregnancies by the total number of months contributed by all couples, and then multiplying the quotient by 1,200).** With most methods, pregnancy rates decrease with time as the more fertile or less careful couples become pregnant and drop out of the calculations.

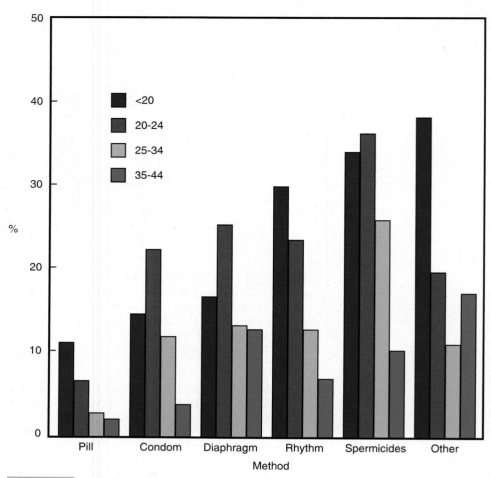

Figure 10.2 **Percentage of women experiencing an accidental pregnancy, in the first 2 years of use, according to method, combined 1988 and 1995 National Survey of Family Growth.** (From Ranjit N, Bankole A, Forrest JD, et al. Contraception failure in the first two years of use: differences across socioeconomic subgroups. *Fam Plann Perspect* 2001;33:25 [Table 6.]).

More accurate information is provided by the life-table method. This method calculates the probability of pregnancy in successive months, which are then added over a given interval. Problems relate to which pregnancies are counted: those occurring among all couples or those in women the investigators deem to have used the method correctly. Because of this complexity, rates of pregnancy with different methods are best calculated by reporting two different rates derived from multiple studies (i.e., the lowest rate and the usual rate), as shown in Table 10.2.

Safety

Some contraceptive methods have associated health risks; areas of concern are listed in Table 10.3. All of the methods are safer than the alternative (pregnancy with birth), with the possible exception of estrogen-containing hormonal contraceptives (pills, patches and ring) used by women older than 35 years of age who smoke (6). **Most methods provide noncontraceptive health benefits in addition to contraception. Oral contraceptives reduce the risk of ovarian and endometrial cancers and ectopic pregnancy. Barrier methods provide some protection against STDs including HIV, cervical cancer, and tubal infertility.**

Medical Eligibility for Contraception

Since 1996 the World Health Organization (WHO) has regularly published Medical Eligibility Criteria for Contraceptive Use (MEC). These recommendations are based on the best evidence available supplemented by expert opinion. **The U.S. Centers for Disease Control undertook a formal process to review and revise the WHO MEC and adapt it to US practice** (7). All

Table 10.2 Percentage of Women Experiencing a Contraceptive Failure During the First Year of Use and the Percentage Continuing Use at the End of the First Year

Method	Women Experiencing Accidental Pregnancy within the First Year of Use (%)		Women Continuing Use at 1 Year (%)
	Typical Use	*Perfect Use*	
No method	85	85	
Spermicides	29	18	42
Periodic abstinence	25		67
Calendar		9	
Ovulation method		3	
Symptothermal		2	
Postovulation		1	
Withdrawal	27	4	43
Cap			
Parous women	32	26	46
Nulliparous women	16	9	57
Sponge			
Parous women	32	20	46
Nulliparous women	16	9	57
Diaphragm	16	6	57
Condom			
Female (Reality)	21	5	49
Male	15	2	53
Combined pill and progestin-only pill	8	0.3	68
Patch (*Evra*™)	8	0.3	68
NuvaRing	8	0.3	68
Intrauterine devices			
ParaGard™ (*Copper T380A*)	0.8	0.6	78
Myrena (*levonorgestrel T*)	0.1	0.1	81
DepoProvera	3	0.3	70
Lunelle	3	0.05	56
Norplant[a] and *Norplant II*	0.05	0.05	84
Implanon™	0.05	0.05	84
Female sterilization	0.5	0.5	100
Male sterilization	0.15	0.10	100

[a]Cumulative 5-year pregnancy rate for pliable tubing, divided by 5.
From **Hatcher RA, Trussell J, Stewart F, et al.** *Contraceptive technology.* 18th ed. New York: Ardent Media, 2004:226, with permission.

present methods of contraception are assigned to one of four categories of suitability of use by women with more than 60 characteristics or conditions. The categories are:

1. A condition for which there is no restriction for the use of the contraceptive method;
2. A condition for which the advantages of using the method generally outweigh the theoretical or proven risks;

Table 10.3 Overview of Contraceptive Methods

Method	Advantages	Disadvantages	Risks	Noncontraceptive Benefits
Coitus interruptus	Available, free	Depends on male control	Pregnancy	Decreased HIV risk
Lactation	Available, free	Unreliable duration of effect	Pregnancy	Decreased breast cancer
Periodic abstinence	Available, free	Complex methodology; motivation is essential	Pregnancy	None
Condoms	Available, no prescription needed	Motivation is essential; must be used each time; depends on man	Pregnancy	Proven to decrease STDs and cervical cancer
Spermicides and sponge	Available, no prescription needed	Must be used each time	Pregnancy	None
Diaphragm/cap	Nonhormonal	Must be used each time; fitting required	Pregnancy, cystitis	Proven to decrease STDs and cervical cancer
ParaGard IUD	Highest efficacy for 12 years, unrelated to coitus	Initial cost; skilled inserter; pain and bleeding	Initial mild risk for PID and septic abortion if pregnancy occurs	None
Mirena IUD	Highest efficacy for 5 years; unrelated to coitus	Initial cost; skilled inserter; amenorrhea for some	Initial mild risk for PID and septic abortion if pregnancy occcurs	Reduced menstrual bleeding; can be used to treat menorrhagia
Oral contraceptives Evra™ patch NuvaRing	High efficacy	Motivation to take daily; cost	Thrombosis; older smokers have increased risk of MI and stroke	Many benefits (see text)
DMPA	High efficacy, convenience	Injection required; bleeding pattern Osteopenia Weight gain	Probably none	Many (see text)
Lunelle™	High efficacy, convenience	Monthly injection	Probably same as orals	Probably same as orals
Implants	Highest efficacy, convenience	Surgical insertion and removal; initial cost; bleeding pattern	Functional cysts	Unknown
Emergency contraception Levonorgestrel Ulipristal	Moderate efficacy	Frequent use disrupts menses	None	Unknown

HIV, human immunodeficiency virus; IUD, intrauterine device; PID, pelvic inflammatory disease; MI, myocardial infarction; *DMPA, depomedroxyprogesterone acetate;* STDs, sexually transmitted diseases.

3. A condition for which the theoretical or proven risks usually outweigh the advantages of using method;

4. A condition that represents an unacceptable health risk if the contraceptive method is used.

Cost

Some methods, such as intrauterine devices (IUDs) and subdermal implants, require an initial high investment but provide prolonged protection for a low annual cost. A complex cost analysis based on the cost of the method plus the cost of pregnancy if the method fails concludes that **sterilization and the long-acting methods are the least expensive over the long term** (8) (Table 10.4).

Table 10.4 Cost per Patient per Year of Contraceptive Methods		
Method	*Cost ($)*	*Cost Multiple ($)*[a]
Vasectomy	55	1.0
Tubal ligation	118	2.14
Intrauterine device	150	2.71
Norplant	202	3.66
Depomedroxyprogesterone acetate	396	7.19
Oral contraceptives	456	8.27
Condoms	776	14.08
Diaphragm	1,147	20.81

[a]For every $1.00 spent on vasectomy, the amount shown would be spent on the method indicated.
From **Ashraf T, Arnold SB, Maxfield M.** Cost effectiveness of levonorgestrel subdermal implants: comparison with other contraceptive methods available in the United States. *J Reprod Med* 1994;39:791–798, with permission.

Long-Acting Reversible Contraceptives

Several contraceptive methods are as effective as sterilization, but are completely reversible. All have the important advantage of being "forgettable," that is, little is required of the user after the method is begun, very much in contrast to methods like the condom that must be used with each act of intercourse, or the OC, which must be taken daily. These forgettable methods have pregnancy rates in typical use of less than 2 per 100 woman-years, are effective for at least 3 months without attention from the user, and are among the safest methods. They include the injectable progestins, *depomedroxyprogesterone acetate* (*DMPA*) and *norethindrone enanthate*, the *etonogestrel* and *levonorgestrel* subdermal implants, copper-bearing intrauterine devices such as the *copper T380A* and the *levonorgestrel*-releasing intrauterine system (9,10).

Nonhormonal Methods

Coitus Interruptus

Coitus interruptus is withdrawal of the penis from the vagina before ejaculation. This method, along with induced abortion and late marriage, is believed to account for most of the decline in fertility of preindustrial Europe (11). Coitus interruptus remains a very important means of fertility control in many countries. Eighty-five million couples are estimated to use the method worldwide, yet it has received little recent formal study. This method has obvious advantages: immediate availability and no cost. The penis must be completely withdrawn both from the vagina and from the external genitalia. Pregnancy has occurred from ejaculation on the female external genitalia without penetration. Coitus interruptus reduces transmission of human immunodeficiency virus (HIV) in mutually monogamous couples (12). Theoretically, some reduction of risk from other STDs would be expected, but this phenomenon apparently was not studied. Efficacy is estimated to range from 4 pregnancies per 100 women in the first year with perfect use to 27 per 100 with typical use (Table 10.2). Jones and colleagues offer a modern review of this practice and conclude that it likely is as effective as the condom (13).

Breastfeeding

Breastfeeding can be used as a form of contraception and can be effective depending on individual variables. The use of contraception during lactation should take into consideration the women's needs and the need to maintain lactation.

Ovulation is suppressed during lactation. The suckling of the infant elevates prolactin levels and reduces gonadotropin-releasing hormone (GnRH) from the hypothalamus, reducing luteinizing hormone (LH) release and thus inhibiting follicular maturation (14). Even with continued nursing, ovulation eventually returns but is unlikely before 6 months, especially if the woman is amenorrheic and is fully breastfeeding with no supplemental foods given to the infant (15). For maximum contraceptive reliability, feeding intervals should not exceed 4 hours during the day and 6 hours at night, and supplemental feeding should not exceed 5% to 10% of the total amount of feeding (16). Six-month pregnancy rates of 0.45% to 2.45% are reported for couples relying solely on this method (17). To prevent pregnancy, another method of contraception should be used from 6 months after birth or sooner if menstruation resumes. **Breastfeeding reduces the mother's lifetime risk of breast cancer** (18).

Contraception during Lactation (Lactation amenorrhea)

Use of combination estrogen–progestin hormonal methods (OCs, the patch, and the ring) is generally not advised during lactation because they reduce the amount and quality of breast milk. Combination hormonal methods can be used after 6 weeks, once milk production is established. **Progestin-only OCs, implants, and injectable contraception do not affect milk quality or quantity** (16). Labeling of the U.S. Food and Drug Administration (FDA) and guidelines from the American College of Obstetricians and Gynecologists suggest that progestin-only OCs can be started 2 to 3 days postpartum, whereas depot *medroxyprogesterone acetate (Depo Provera)* injections or implants can begin at 6 weeks (19). These recommendations are not based on any observed adverse effect of early administration, and many maternity programs begin injectable contraception with progestin at the time of hospital discharge. Barrier methods, spermicides, and the *copper T380A* intrauterine device (IUD) (*ParaGard*) are good options for nursing mothers. Because *levonorgestrel* implants have no adverse effect on breastfeeding, none should be expected from the *levonorgestrel T* IUD, which releases *levonorgestrel* but produces lower blood levels than the implants.

Fertility Awareness

Periodic abstinence, described as "natural contraception" or "fertility awareness," requires avoiding intercourse during the fertile period around the time of ovulation. A variety of methods are used: the calendar method, the mucous method (Billings or ovulation method), and the symptothermal method, which is a combination of the first two methods. With the mucous method, the woman attempts to predict the fertile period by feeling the cervical mucus with her fingers. Under estrogen influence, the mucus increases in quantity and becomes progressively more slippery and elastic until a peak day is reached. The mucus then becomes scant and dry under the influence of progesterone until onset of the next menses. Intercourse may be allowed during the "dry days" immediately after menses until mucus is detected. Thereafter, the couple must abstain until the fourth day after the "peak" day.

In the symptothermal method, the first day of abstinence is predicted either from the calendar, by subtracting 21 from the length of the shortest menstrual cycle in the preceding 6 months, or the first day mucus is detected, whichever comes first. The end of the fertile period is predicted by use of basal body temperature. The woman takes her temperature every morning and resumes intercourse 3 days after the thermal shift, the rise in body temperature that signals that the corpus luteum is producing progesterone and that ovulation occurred. The postovulatory method is a variation in which the couple has intercourse only after ovulation is detected.

A system of hormone monitoring designed to better define the fertile period involves placement of disposable test sticks in a small battery-powered device to detect urinary estrone-3 glucuronide and LH. Changes in these hormones reliably predict the fertile period. These devices (*Persona*™ and *Clearblue Easy Fertility Monitor*™) can serve as aids both to becoming pregnant and to avoiding it (20). *Persona*™ is marketed in Europe for contraception. It is reported to have a correct use effectiveness of 94% in avoiding pregnancy. *Clearblue Easy*™ (CEFM) is approved in the United States as an aid to becoming pregnant but is used off label to avoid pregnancy. Exact effectiveness rates are not known. The CEFM is used in the Marquette method, which combines observation of cervical mucus changes with the CEFM results. A correct use pregnancy rate of 2% and a typical use pregnancy rate of 12% were reported (21).

Efficacy

The ovulation method was evaluated by the World Health Organization in a five-country study. Women who successfully completed three monthly cycles of teaching were enrolled in a 13-cycle efficacy study. There was a 3.1% probability of pregnancy in 1 year for the small proportion of couples who used the method perfectly and 86.4% probability of pregnancy for the rest (22). A review of 15 national surveys from developing countries estimated a 12-month gross failure rate of 24 pregnancies per 100 (23).

Risks

Conceptions resulting from intercourse remote from the time of ovulation more often lead to spontaneous abortion than conceptions from midcycle intercourse (24). Malformations are not more common (18).

Condoms

In the 1700s, condoms made of animal intestine were used by the aristocracy of Europe, but condoms were not widely available until the vulcanization of rubber in the 1840s (1). Modern condoms usually are made of latex rubber, although condoms made from animal intestine are still sold and are preferred by some who feel they afford better sensation. New condoms made from nonlatex materials—such as polyurethane or synthetic elastomers that are thin, odorless, transparent, and transmit body heat—are available. Although the nonlatex condoms may break more easily than the latex varieties, substantial numbers of study participants preferred them and would recommend them to others (25).

The risk of condom breakage is about 3% and is related to friction (26). Use of water-based lubricants may reduce the risk of breakage. Petroleum-based products such as mineral oil must be avoided because even brief exposure to them markedly reduces the strength of condoms (27).

Sexually Transmitted Diseases

Gonorrhea, ureaplasma, and pelvic inflammatory disease (PID) and its sequel (tubal infertility) are reduced with consistent use of barrier methods (28–30). Tested *in vitro, Chlamydia trachomatis,* herpes virus type 2, HIV, and hepatitis B did not penetrate latex condoms but did cross through condoms made from animal intestine (31). Follow-up of sexual partners of HIV-infected individuals showed that condom use provides considerable protection (32). Consistent condom use provides more protection than inconsistent use (33). In one study, couples who use condoms 0% to 50% of the time had an HIV seroconversion rate of 20.8 per 100 couple years, whereas those who used condoms 100% of the time had a conversion rate of only 2.3 per 100 couple years (34). *Nonoxynol-9* **should not be used with condoms for HIV protection because it is associated with genital lesions.** *Nonoxynol-9* **does not add to the protection afforded by condoms alone** (35).

Condoms offer protection from cervical neoplasia (36). The relative risk for invasive cervical cancer was 0.4 when those who used condoms or diaphragms were compared with those who never used them (37). The presumed mechanism of protection is reduced transmission of human papillomavirus (HPV).

Risks

Latex allergy could lead to life-threatening anaphylaxis in either partner from latex condoms. Nonlatex condoms of polyurethane and *Tactylon* should be offered to couples who have a history suggestive of latex allergy.

Female Condom

The original female condom introduced in 1992 was a polyurethane vaginal pouch attached to a rim that partly covered the vulva. The recently FDA approved FC2 female condom is an improved version made from softer synthetic latex that does not require hand assembly during manufacture and is therefore less expensive (38). It is recommended for prevention of pregnancy and STDs, including HIV. Breakage may occur less often with the female condom than the male condom; slippage appears to be more common, especially for those new to its use (39). Exposure to seminal fluid is slightly higher than with the male condom (40). Initial US trials showed a pregnancy rate of 15% in 6 months. Subsequent analysis found that with perfect use, the pregnancy rate may be only 2.6%. This rate is comparable to perfect use of the diaphragm and cervical cap, the other female barrier methods (41). As with the male condom, failure rates fall with increasing experience. Colposcopic studies of women using the female condom demonstrate no signs of trauma or change in the bacterial flora (42).

Vaginal Spermicides

Currently available vaginal spermicides combine a spermicidal chemical, either *nonoxynol-9 (N-9)* or *octoxynol,* with a base of cream, jelly, aerosol foam, foaming tablet, film, suppository, or a polyurethane sponge. *Nonoxynol-9* is a nonionic surface-active detergent that immobilizes sperm. *Nonoxynol-9* **spermicides alone appear considerably less effective in preventing pregnancy than condoms or diaphragms.** Women using *nonoxynol-9* spermicides frequently have higher rates of genital lesions than women not using spermicides. These lesions may increase their risk for STDs and HIV (43). In the same studies of serodiscordant couples in which condoms were proven effective in preventing transmission of HIV, *nonoxynol-9* spermicides alone were not effective (34).

Concerns were raised about possible teratogenicity of spermicides. *Nonoxynol-9* is not absorbed from the human vagina (44). Several large studies found no greater risk of miscarriage, birth defects, or low birth weight in spermicide users than in other women (45,46).

Nonoxynol-9 is toxic to the lactobacilli that normally colonize the vagina. Women who use spermicides regularly have increased vaginal colonization with the bacterium *Escherichia coli* and may be predisposed to *E. coli* bacteriuria after intercourse (47).

Vaginal Barriers

At the beginning of the 20th century, four types of vaginal barriers were used in Europe: vaginal diaphragm, cervical cap, vault cap, and Vimule. Vaginal diaphragms, new varieties of cervical caps and the synthetic sponge are used in the United States. When used consistently, vaginal barriers can be reasonably effective. They are safe, and, as with condoms, they have the non-contraceptive benefit of relative protection from STDs, tubal infertility, and cervical neoplasia. A recent search for alternatives to condoms for HIV prevention in high-prevalence areas has rekindled interest in the other vaginal barriers (48).

Diaphragm

The diaphragm consists of a circular spring covered with fine latex rubber (Fig. 10.3). There are several types of diaphragms, as determined by the spring rim: coil, flat, or arcing. Coil-spring and flat-spring diaphragms become a flat oval when compressed for insertion. Arcing diaphragms form an arc or half moon when compressed; they are easiest to insert correctly. **The practitioner must fit the diaphragm for the patient, and instruct her in its insertion and verify by examination that she can insert it correctly to cover the cervix and upper vagina.** Spermicide is always prescribed for use with the diaphragm; whether this practice is necessary is not well studied.

Fitting Diaphragms

Fitting a diaphragm should be performed as follows:

1. **A vaginal examination should be performed.** With the first and second fingers in the posterior fornix, the thumb of the examining hand is placed against the first finger to mark where the first finger touches the pubic bone. The distance from the tip of the middle finger to the tip of the thumb is the diameter of the first diaphragm that should be tried.

2. **A set of test diaphragms of various sizes is used, and the test diaphragm is inserted and checked by palpation.** The diaphragm should open easily in the vagina and fill the fornices without pressure. The largest diaphragm that fits comfortably should be selected. A size 65, 70, or 75 diaphragm will fit most women.

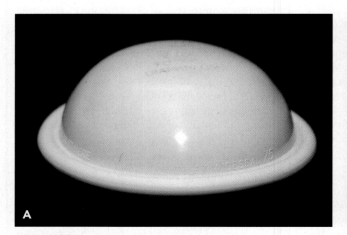 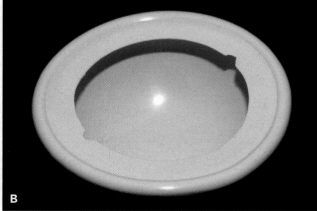

Figure 10.3 **Wide-seal diaphragm.** **A:** Outer caudal side. **B:** Inner cephalad side.

3. **The patient should practice insertion and should be reexamined to confirm proper position of the device.** About 1 teaspoon of water-soluble spermicidal jelly or cream is placed in the cavity of the dome. The diaphragm is inserted with the dome downward so that the cervix will sit in a pool of the spermicide.

4. **The diaphragm can be inserted several hours before intercourse. If intercourse is repeated, additional spermicidal jelly should be inserted into the vagina without removing the diaphragm. The diaphragm should be left in place at least 6 hours after intercourse to allow for immobilization of sperm.** When removed, it is washed with soap and water, allowed to dry, and stored away from heat. It should not be dusted with talc because genital exposure to talc may increase the risk of ovarian cancer.

Risks

Diaphragm use, especially prolonged use during multiple acts of intercourse, appears to increase the risk of bladder infections. The risk of cystitis increases with the numbers of days the diaphragm is used in a week (49). A smaller-sized, wide-seal diaphragm or a cervical cap can be used if recurrent cystitis is a problem, although the problem may relate not only to mechanical obstruction but also to alterations in vaginal flora produced by the spermicide. An epidemiologic study comparing cases of toxic shock with controls found no increased risk from diaphragm use (50).

Other Barriers

The *Prentif* cervical cap made of latex rubber is no longer available in the United States. It was in continuous use for most of the 20th century, but competition from other methods made its continued production impractical.

The *FemCap*

This new version of the cervical cap made of silicone rubber was approved by the FDA in 2003. It looks like a sailor's hat with the dome covering the cervix and the brim fitting into the vaginal fornices (51). It is made in three sizes—22-, 26-, and 30-mm diameter—and is expected to be reusable for 2 years. It is used with spermicide and should be left in place for at least 6 hours after intercourse, but it may be left in place as long as 48 hours at a time. Additional acts of intercourse require insertion of more spermicide. *Femcap* requires a clinician's fitting and prescription for use. The only available efficacy study compared the *FemCap* to the vaginal diaphragm. The 6-month pregnancy rate for the *FemCap* was 13.5%, substantially higher than the 7.9% rate for the diaphragm. Both groups used *N-9* spermicide with the devices (52).

Lea's Shield

Lea's Shield, approved by the FDA in 2002, is another vaginal barrier device made of silicone rubber. It is intended for use with a spermicide. It is shaped like an elliptical bowl with a central air valve approximately the size of a diaphragm, featuring an anterior loop to assist its removal. The posterior end is thicker and therefore less likely to rotate when in place. It comes in one size; proper fitting requires only that it cover the cervix, sit behind the symphysis, and be comfortable. The shield needs to be inserted prior to each act of intercourse and should not be left in the vagina for longer than 48 hours (53). A prescription is required. Approximately 87% of those responding to a question about their use of the shield stated that they would recommend its use to a friend (51). Of 59 women who used the device with *N-9* spermicide, the 6-month pregnancy rate was 15% (54).

The Sponge

The *Today* sponge is a polyurethane dome-shaped device containing *nonoxynol-9*. It is moistened with water and then inserted high in the vagina to cover the cervix. It combines the advantages of a disposable barrier with spermicide and provides protection for 24 hours. The contraceptive efficacy appears to differ with parity. Nulliparous women are reported to have a perfect use pregnancy rate of 9% per year, whereas parous women have a pregnancy rate of 20% (Table 10.2). Rates with typical use are estimated as 16 per year in nullipara and 32% in multipara (55). A trial comparing the sponge with a vaginal spermicide preparation used alone without barrier showed the sponge had a slightly lower pregnancy rate (56).

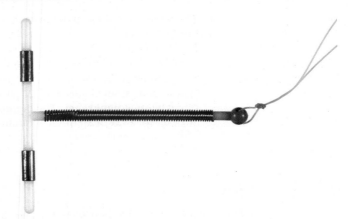

Figure 10.4   *Copper T380A (ParaGard)* intrauterine device.

Intrauterine Contraception

Worldwide over 15% of married women use intrauterine contraception (57). In the United States, usage is increasing, but the estimates are that only 3.4% of women and only 5.0% of married women use intrauterine contraception (4). Candidacy includes nulliparous women, adolescents, and immunocompromised women. Immediate use postpartum or after a first or second trimester abortion broadened usage. **Two IUDs are in use in the United States: the** *copper T380A* **(***ParaGard***) and the** *levonorgestrel***-releasing** *T* **(***Mirena***).** The *copper T380A* has bands of copper on the cross arms of the T in addition to copper wire around the stem, providing a total surface area of 380 mm of copper, almost double the surface area of copper in earlier copper devices (Fig. 10.4). It is approved for up to 10 years of continuous use. The *levonorgestrel T* (Fig. 10.5) is approved in the United States for 5 years of use, although studies through 7 years of use show no loss of efficacy (58). **Both provide safe, long-term contraception with effectiveness equivalent to tubal sterilization.**

Mechanism of Action

Intrauterine devices cause the formation of "biologic foam" within the uterine cavity that contains strands of fibrin, phagocytic cells, and proteolytic enzymes. All IUDs stimulate the formation of prostaglandins within the uterus, consistent with both smooth muscle contraction and inflammation. Copper IUDs continuously release a small amount of the metal, producing an even greater inflammatory response. Scanning electron microscopy studies of the endometrium of women wearing nonmedicated IUDs show alterations in the surface morphology of cells, especially of the microvilli of ciliated cells (59). There are major alterations in the composition of proteins within the uterine cavity and new proteins and proteinase inhibitors are found in washings

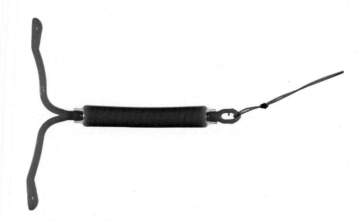

Figure 10.5   *Levonorgestrel T (Mirena*™*)* intrauterine device.

from the uterus (60). The altered intrauterine environment interferes with sperm passage through the uterus, preventing fertilization.

The *levonorgestrel* in the T device is much more potent than natural progesterone and has a strong effect on the endometrium. The hormone is released at an initial rate of 20 μg daily, which declines to half this rate by 5 years. Blood hormone levels are significantly lower than with other progesterone-only contraception and remain stable at approximately 150 to 200 pg/mL (61). About 85% of cycles are ovulatory. The contraceptive effect of the levonorgestrel intrauterine device is a result of thickened and scant cervical mucus, endometrial atrophy, and an intrauterine inflammatory response (62).

The IUD is not an abortifacient. The contraceptive effectiveness does not depend on interference with implantation, although this phenomenon occurs and is the basis for using copper IUDs for emergency contraception. Sperm can be obtained by laparoscopy in washings from the fallopian tubes of control women at midcycle; fewer sperm are present in the tubal washings from women wearing IUDs (63). Ova flushed from the tubes at tubal sterilization showed no evidence of fertilization in women wearing IUDs (64). Studies of serum β-human chorionic gonadotropin (β-HCG) levels in women wearing IUDs do not indicate pregnancy (65).

Effectiveness

The *copper T380A* and the *levonorgestrel T* have remarkably low pregnancy rates, less than 0.2 per 100 woman-years. Total pregnancies over a 7-year period were only 1.1 per 100 for the *levonorgestrel T* and 1.4 for the *copper T380A* (58). Twelve-year data on the *copper T380A* showed a cumulative pregnancy rate of only 1.9 per 100 women and no pregnancies at all after year 8 (66).

Benefits

Modern IUDs provide excellent contraception without continued effort by the user. Both the *copper T380A* and the *levonorgestrel T* protect against ectopic pregnancy. The *levonorgestrel T*, by releasing *levonorgestrel,* reduces menstrual bleeding and cramping. It is used extensively to treat heavy menstrual bleeding and is used in Europe and the United Kingdom as an alternative to hysterectomy for menorrhagia (67). The *levonorgestrel T* also has a beneficial effect on menorrhagia from uterine fibroids; the benefit may be diminished with distorting submucosal fibroids (68,69). The *levonorgestrel T* is an effective way to deliver the necessary progestin therapy in postmenopausal women on estrogen therapy (70). Additional noncontraceptive benefits include a reduced risk of endometrial cancer and improvement in symptoms of endometriosis and adenomyosis (71–74).

Risks

Infection   The Women's Health Study found the *Dalkon Shield* device (now withdrawn from the market) to increase the risk of PID eightfold when women hospitalized for PID were compared with control women hospitalized for other illnesses (75). In contrast, risk from the other IUDs was markedly less. Increased risk was detectable only within 4 months of insertion of the IUD. A prospective World Health Organization study revealed that PID increased only during the first 20 days after insertion. **Thereafter, the rate of diagnosis of PID was about 1.6 cases per 1,000 women per year, the same as in the general population** (76).

Exposure to sexually transmitted pathogens is the more important determinant of PID risk than is wearing an IUD. In the Women's Health Study, women who were married or cohabiting and who said they had only one sexual partner in the past 6 months had no increase in PID (75). In contrast, previously married or single women had marginal increase in risk, even though they had only one partner in the previous 6 months (77). The only pelvic infection that was unequivocally related to IUD use is actinomycosis (78). It appears that PID with actinomycosis was reported only in women wearing an IUD. Rates of colonization with actinomycosis increase with duration of use for plastic devices but appear to be much less for copper-releasing IUDs. Actinomyces may be found in cervical cytology of up to 7% of women with an IUD. Because of the low positive predictive value and a lack of sensitivity and specificity of cervical cytology to diagnose this organism, antibiotic treatment and IUD removal should be reserved for symptomatic women (79).

When PID is suspected in a woman wearing an IUD, appropriate cultures should be obtained, and antibiotic therapy should be administered. Removal of the IUD is not necessary unless symptoms do not improve after 72 hours of treatment (80). Pelvic abscess, if suspected, should be ruled out by ultrasound examination.

Ectopic Pregnancy   All contraceptive methods protect against ectopic pregnancy by preventing pregnancy. But when the method fails and pregnancy occurs, risk of ectopic is affected by the method of contraception. IUDs and tubal sterilization increase the probability of the pregnancy being ectopic when pregnancy occurs, but the rate of any pregnancy is so low that women using either of these methods have much lower rates of ectopic pregnancy than women not using contraception (81). Risk of any pregnancy with a *levonorgestrel* IUD is between 0.1 and 0.2 per 100 woman-years. The rate of an ectopic in wearers of this device is reported as 0.02 per 100 woman-years (82). In a large study of the *copper T380A,* the first-year pregnancy rate was 0.5 per 100 woman-years, and the rate of ectopic was 0.1 per 100 woman-years (83). Ectopic is a very rare event with either IUD, but should a woman wearing one present with pelvic pain and a positive β-HCG, an ectopic must be ruled out. Increased risk of ectopic among past users of older IUDs was reported. The *copper T380A* and the *levonorgestrel T* were not included (81).

Fertility   Tubal factor infertility is not increased among nulligravid women who used copper IUDs, but exposure to sexually transmitted pathogens such as *C. trachomatis* does increase risk (84). The Oxford study found that women gave birth just as promptly after IUD removal as they did after discontinuing use of the diaphragm (85).

Expulsion and Perforation   The rate of expulsion with the *copper T380A* is reported to be 2.5 per 100 woman-years in the first year, and cumulates to 8 per 100 woman-years after 8 years (83). Expulsion rates with the *levonorgestrel T* were reported at 4.2% in years 1 and 2, 1.3% in years 3 through 5, and 0% in years 6 and 7 (86). The risk of uterine perforation associated with insertion is dependent on the inserter. The risk in experienced hands is on the order of 1 per 1,000 insertions or less (87). There are no studies specifically addressing perforation in nulliparous as compared to parous women (88).

Clinical Management

Contraindications to IUD use listed by the World Health Organization include pregnancy, puerperal sepsis, PID, or STDs current or within the past 3 months, endometrial or cervical cancer, undiagnosed genital bleeding, uterine anomalies, and fibroid tumors that distort the endometrial cavity (87). Infection with HIV is not considered a contraindication for IUD use. No increase in pelvic infection, female-to-male transmission, or viral shedding was found among HIV-1 infected women (89,90). Copper allergy and Wilson's disease are contraindications to the use of copper IUDs.

Candidate Selection

IUDs are appropriate for long-term contraception in most women given their ease of use, high efficacy, and favorable side effect profile. Nulliparous women, adolescents, women undergoing a first or second trimester surgical abortion, women with a recent medical abortion, and women immediately postpartum should all be considered candidates for IUDs (91). There is renewed interest in postpartum and postabortal insertion of IUDs. In both circumstances, the woman is clearly no longer pregnant, she may be highly motivated to accept contraception, and the setting is convenient for both the woman and the provider (92,93). Postpartum and postabortal insertions are safe. Complications are not increased by comparison to interval insertion. The only disadvantage is that the expulsion rate is higher. In comparing postpartum to interval insertion, all the women requesting postpartum IUD received the device, but many women scheduled for interval insertion did not return. When surveyed at 6 months postpartum, more women who had postpartum insertion were wearing IUDs than were those who had scheduled for interval insertion (94). Goodman and colleagues found many fewer repeat abortions among women followed after postabortal IUD insertion compared to a cohort of women choosing non-IUD methods of contraception after an induced abortion (94).

Insertion

At the contraceptive visit, the patient's history is obtained and a physical examination, screening for *Neisseria gonorrhoeae* and chlamydia in high-risk women, and detailed counseling regarding risks and alternatives are provided. The IUD usually is inserted during menses to be sure the patient is not pregnant, but it can be inserted at any time in the cycle

if pregnancy can be excluded (95). The *copper-T380A* IUD can be inserted within 5 days of unprotected intercourse for 100% effective emergency contraception.

There are limited data on effective treatment of pain during IUD insertion. One randomized nonblinded study suggested a benefit with 2% lidocaine gel applied to the cervical canal 5 minutes before insertion. Other techniques such as paracervical block were not evaluated. Premedication with oral prostaglandin inhibitors such as *ibuprofen* is strongly advised, although evidence of its benefit with modern IUDs is limited (96).

Antibiotic prophylaxis is not beneficial, probably because the risk of pelvic infection with IUD insertion is so low. A large randomized trial of 1,985 patients receiving either oral *azithromycin* or placebo found no difference in rates of IUD removal during the first 90 days after insertion and no difference in rates of salpingitis (97). These women were screened for STDs only by self-history. Screening for gonorrhea and chlamydia at the time of insertion is recommended for adolescents, but it is not necessary to wait for the results before insertion because patients with positive results have no adverse effects if treated promptly (98). PID, puerperal sepsis, or postabortion sepsis within the past 3 months are considered contraindications and patients with purulent cervicitis should be tested and treated before insertion.

The technique of insertion is as follows:

1. **The cervix is exposed with a speculum.** The vaginal vault and cervix are cleansed with a bacteriocidal solution, such as an iodine-containing solution.
2. **The uterine cavity should be measured with a uterine sound.** The depth of the cavity should measure at least 6 cm from the external os. A smaller uterus is not likely to tolerate currently available IUDs.
3. **Use of a tenaculum for insertion is mandatory to prevent perforation.** The cervix is grasped with a tenaculum and gently pulled downward to straighten the angle between the cervical canal and the uterine cavity. The IUD, previously loaded into its inserter, is then gently introduced through the cervical canal.
4. **With the *copper T380A*, the outer sheath of the inserter is withdrawn a short distance to release the arms of the T and is gently pushed inward again to elevate the now-opened T against the fundus.** The outer sheath and the inner stylet of the inserter are withdrawn, and the strings are cut to project about 2 cm from the external cervical os.
5. **The *levonorgestrel T* IUD is inserted somewhat differently from the *copper T380A*. The inserter tube is introduced into the uterus until the preset sliding flange on the inserter is 1.5 to 2 cm from the external os of the cervix.** The arms of the T device are released upward into the uterine cavity, and the inserter is pushed up under them to elevate the IUD up against the uterine fundus.

In nulliparous women, insertion may be more difficult because of a narrower cervical canal than in parous women. Mechanical dilation may be necessary. Pretreatment with *misoprostol* may be beneficial in difficult IUD insertions (99).

Intrauterine Devices in Pregnancy

If an intrauterine pregnancy is diagnosed and the IUD strings are visible, the IUD should be removed as soon as possible to prevent later septic abortion, premature rupture of the membranes, and premature birth (100). When the strings of the IUD are not visible, an ultrasound examination should be performed to localize the IUD and determine whether expulsion has occurred. **If the IUD is present, there are three options for management:**

1. **Therapeutic abortion**
2. **Ultrasound-guided intrauterine removal of the IUD**
3. **Continuation of the pregnancy with the device left in place**

If the patient wishes to continue the pregnancy, ultrasound evaluation of the location of the IUD should be considered (101). If the IUD is not in a fundal location, ultrasound-guided removal using small alligator forceps may be successful. If the location is fundal, the IUD should be left in place. When pregnancy continues with an IUD in place, the patient must be warned of the symptoms of intrauterine infection and should be cautioned to seek care promptly for fever or flulike symptoms, abdominal cramping, or bleeding. At the earliest sign of infection, high-dose intravenous antibiotic therapy should be given and the pregnancy evacuated promptly.

Duration of Use

Annual rates of pregnancy, expulsions, and medical removals decrease with each year of use (102,103). Therefore, a woman who has no problem by year 5, for example, is very unlikely to experience problems in the subsequent years. The *copper T380A* is FDA approved for 10 years and the *levonorgestrel T* for 5 years, though as previously noted, good data support use of the *copper T380A* through 12 years and of the *levonorgestrel T* through 7 years (66,86).

Choice of Devices

Both of the IUDs available in the United States, the *copper T380A* and the *levonorgestrel T,* provide protection for many years, have remarkably low pregnancy rates, and substantially reduce the risk of ectopic pregnancy. The *levonorgestrel T* reduces the amount of menstrual bleeding and dysmenorrhea. The *copper T380A* initially can be expected to increase menstrual bleeding. It is the most effective means for emergency contraception.

Management of Bleeding and Cramping with Intrauterine Devises

The most important medical reason that women give for requesting removal of an IUD is bleeding and pelvic pain. These symptoms are common in the first few months, but diminish. Nonsteroidal anti-inflammatory drugs are usually helpful. **When pain and bleeding occur later, the patient should be examined for signs of PID, partial expulsion of the device, or an intracavitary fibroid.** Two ultrasonographic studies comparing women with these symptoms after 6 months to women with no bleeding complaints show downward displacement of the IUDs into the cervical canal in many of the symptomatic women and in some cases, intracavitary fibroids (104,105). When the patient wishes to continue with an IUD, removal of the displaced device and insertion of a new one is advisable. In situations where IUDs are inexpensive and ultrasound is expensive or not available, the best course is to offer immediate removal and replacement of the IUD without ultrasound proof of displacement.

Hormonal Contraception

Hormonal contraceptives are female sex steroids, synthetic estrogen and synthetic progesterone (progestin), or progestin-only without estrogen. They can be administered in the form of OCs, patches, implants, and injectables. The most widely used hormonal contraceptive is the combination OC containing both estrogen and progestin. Combination OCs can be monophasic, with the same dose of estrogen and progestin administered each day, or multiphasic, in which varying doses of steroids are given through a 21-day or 24-day cycle. Combination OCs are packaged with 21 active tablets and 7 placebos, or 24 active tablets and 4 placebo tablets. The inclusion of placebos allows the user to take one pill every day without having to count. The medication-free interval while the user takes the placebo tablets allows withdrawal bleeding that mimics a 28-day menstrual cycle. To begin OC use, the user takes the first pill any time from the first day of menses through the Sunday after menstruation begins and thereafter starts a new pack as soon as the first pack is completed. The 7-day medication-free interval was standard for years, but studies showed that a shorter medication-free interval is adequate to trigger cyclic withdrawal bleeding and maintains better suppression of ovulation. Ovarian follicles mature more during the 7-day medication-free interval than during the 4-day interval. Hence the new 24/4 combination theoretically could be more effective in preventing pregnancy than the 21/7 combination, but this has not been demonstrated. Other variations of OC administration are the extended cycle and the continuous cycle methods. Users take active pills containing an estrogen–progestin combination for 3 months at a time (extended cycle) or indefinitely for a year or more (continuous cycle). Users on these regimens have more unscheduled days of spotting or bleeding than those on 28-day cycles in the beginning, but become amenorrheic. As a result they experience fewer cycle triggered symptoms such as headache and menstrual pain. Continuous-combined regimens are preferred for women with chronic pelvic pain or when dysmenorrhea is not relieved by OCs taken in 28-day cycles (106).

Progestin-only OCs are taken every day without interruption. Other forms of hormonal contraception include transdermal administration with the patch, injectable progestins, injectable estrogen–progestin combinations, subdermal implants that release progestin, and vaginal rings that release either estrogen–progestin or progestin alone (107).

Steroid Hormone Action

Sex steroids are characterized by their affinity for specific estrogen, progesterone, or androgen receptors, and by their biologic effects in different systems (108). Steroids are rapidly absorbed in the gut but go directly into the liver through the portal circulation, where they are rapidly metabolized and inactivated. Therefore, large doses of steroids are required when they are administered orally. The addition of the ethinyl group to carbon-17 of the steroid molecule hinders degradation by the liver enzyme 17-hydroxysteroid dehydrogenase and allows potent biological activity after oral doses of only micrograms.

Progestins

Progestins are synthetic compounds that mimic the effect of natural progesterone but differ from it structurally. The progestins differ from one another in their affinities for estrogen, androgen, and progesterone receptors; their ability to inhibit ovulation; and their ability to substitute for progesterone and to antagonize estrogen. Some are directly bound to the receptor (*levonorgestrel, norethindrone*), whereas others require bioactivation as, for example, desogestrel, which is converted in the body to its active metabolite, etonogestrel. The 17-acetoxy progestins (e.g., *medroxyprogesterone acetate*) are bound by the progesterone receptor. *Norgestrel* exists as two stereoisomers, identified as dextronorgestrel and levonorgestrel. Only levonorgestrel is biologically active. Three newer progestins (*norgestimate, desogestrel,* and *gestodene*) are viewed as more "selective" than the other 19-nor progestins, in that they have little or no androgenic effect at doses that inhibit ovulation (109). The FDA approved *norgestimate-* and *desogestrel-*containing OCs, and *gestodene* is available in Europe. *Gestodene* is a derivative of levonorgestrel that is more potent than the other preparations (i.e., very little of it is required for antifertility effects). Similarly, *norelgestromin* is an active metabolite of *norgestimate* and more potent than the parent compound. It is used in the transdermal patch. *Drospirenone,* a progestin introduced in the United States, is a derivative of the diuretic spironolactone. It has high affinity for progesterone receptors, mineralocorticoid receptors, and androgen receptors. It acts as a progesterone agonist but is a mineralocorticoid antagonist and androgen antagonist (110). Comparative studies suggest a small decrease in body weight and in blood pressure, with equivalent cycle control and contraceptive efficacy, in women taking an OC containing 3 mg of *drospirenone*/30 μg *ethinyl estradiol* versus women taking a 150 μg *levonorgestrel*/30 μg *ethinyl estradiol* (*EE*) preparation (111). Pilot studies of women with polycystic ovary syndrome showed good cycle control and reduction in androgen levels with no change in weight, blood pressure, or glucose metabolism (112). The FDA approved the 20 μg *EE*/3 mg *drospirenone* OC for premenstrual dysphoric disorder (PMDD) in women who choose OCs for contraception. When compared to an OC with 30 μg *EE*/150 μg *levonorgestrel,* women taking the *drospirenone* OC had better relief of menstrual symptoms, better improvement in acne, reduction in negative affect during the menstrual phase, and a greater feeling of well-being (113). *Dienogest,* another progestin introduced in the United States, is combined with *estradiol valerate,* not *ethinyl estradiol.* Whether it offers any advantage over already marketed OC combinations is not yet evident. The *dienogest/estradiol valerate* combination is as effective as *levonorgestrel/ethinyl estradiol* as a contraceptive, and in treating abnormal uterine bleeding (114).

Estrogens

In the United States, most OCs contain either of two estrogens: *mestranol* or *ethinyl estradiol* (*EE*). *Mestranol* is *EE* with an extra methyl group. It requires bioactivation in the liver, where the methyl group is cleaved, releasing the active agent, *EE*. Oral contraceptives with 35 μg of *EE* provide the same blood levels of hormone as do OCs containing 50 μg of *mestranol.* (115). *Estradiol cypionate* and *estradiol valerate* are esters of natural 17 β-estradiol also in use for contraception.

Antifertility Effects

Combination Estrogen–Progestin Contraceptives

Ovulation can be inhibited by estrogen or by progestin alone. Pharmacologic synergism is exhibited when the two hormones are combined and ovulation is suppressed at a much lower dose of each agent. Combination OCs, patches, and the *NuvaRing* suppress basal follicle-stimulating hormone (FSH) and LH. They diminish the ability of the pituitary gland to synthesize gonadotropins when it is stimulated by hypothalamic GnRH (116). Ovarian follicles do not mature, little estradiol is produced, and there is no midcycle LH surge. Ovulation does not occur, the corpus luteum does not form, and progesterone is not produced. This blockade of ovulation is dose related. Newer low-dose OCs do not provide as dense a block and allow somewhat higher baseline FSH and LH levels than higher dose formulations (117). This makes ovulation somewhat more likely to occur if pills are missed or if the patient takes another medication that reduces blood levels of the contraceptive steroids.

Progestin-Only Preparations

Highly effective contraception can be provided by progestin alone, thus avoiding the risks of estrogen. The mode of action of progestin-only contraceptives is highly dependent on the dose of the compound (118). With low levels of progestin in the blood, ovulation will occur part of the time. At moderate levels of progestin in the blood, normal basal levels of FSH and LH are present, and some follicle maturation may occur. At higher blood levels as seen with *DepoProvera,* the basal FSH is reduced, and there is less follicular activity, less estradiol production, and no LH surge.

Transdermal Hormonal Contraception

The patch (*OrthoEvra*), which adheres to the user's skin, and the vaginal *NuvaRing* both contain combinations of *EE* and a potent progestin. Both provide sustained release of the steroids and result in relatively constant serum levels that are less than the peak levels seen with OCs but sufficient to prevent ovulation.

Hormonal Implants

With the *levonorgestrel* subdermal implants there is some follicular maturation and estrogen production, but LH peak levels are low and ovulation is often inhibited. In the first year of use, ovulation is believed to occur in about 20% of cycles. The proportion of ovulatory cycles increases with time, probably as a result of the decline in hormone release. By the fourth year of use, 41% of cycles are ovulatory. The more potent progestin released by the *etonogestrel* implant is even more effective at preventing ovulation (119). The mechanisms of action of low-dose progestins include effects on the cervical mucus, endometrium, and tubal motility. The scant, dry cervical mucus that occurs in women using implants inhibits sperm migration into the upper tract. Progestins decrease nuclear estrogen receptor levels, decrease progesterone receptors, and induce activity of the enzyme 17-hydroxysteroid dehydrogenase, which metabolizes natural 17 β-estradiol (118).

The sustained release offered by contraceptive implants allows for highly effective contraception at relatively low steroid blood levels. Figure 10.6 depicts expected steroid blood levels with implants, injectables, and oral contraceptives. An additional mechanism for contraception was discovered with the antiprogesterone *mifepristone (RU486)*. In the normal cycle, there is a small amount of progesterone production from the follicle just before ovulation. This progesterone appears essential to ovulation, because if *mifepristone* is given before ovulation this can be delayed for several days (120,121).

Efficacy of Hormonal Contraception

When used consistently, combination OCs have pregnancy rates as low as 2 to 3 per 100 women per year. Progestin-only OCs are less effective than combination estrogen–progestin preparations, with best results of 3 to 4 pregnancies per 100 woman-years. All methods have the potential for user error; therefore, there may be a 10-fold difference between the best results and results in typical users of OCs. Injectable progestins and implants are much less subject to user error than are OCs. The difference between the best results and results in typical users is small and is comparable to pregnancy rates after tubal sterilization (Table 10.2). Pregnancy rates with the *OrthoEvra* patch and the *NuvaRing* were equivalent to those of OCs; however, because it is easier to use these methods consistently, larger studies may well demonstrate better typical user results than with OCs (122,123). Typical use pregnancy rates with *DMPA* are lower. **The subdermal implants have the lowest rates of any hormonal contraceptive method.**

Hormonal Contraception for Obese Women

The present rate of obesity in Europe and the United States is 30% and is increasing. Most studies of contraceptive efficacy intentionally excluded obese women, so the available information is limited. **Obese women are no less likely than other women to become pregnant, but they do have an increased risk of pregnancy complications** (124). A systematic review of hormonal contraception for overweight and obese women found only seven relevant studies (125). Overweight and obese women appear to be at a similar or slightly higher risk of pregnancy with oral contraceptives. The attributable risk is minimal (124). The efficacy of *DMPA* does not appear to be reduced in heavier women. A possible increase in pregnancies was reported for users of the contraceptive patch who weight more than 90 kg. Heavier women using the vaginal ring

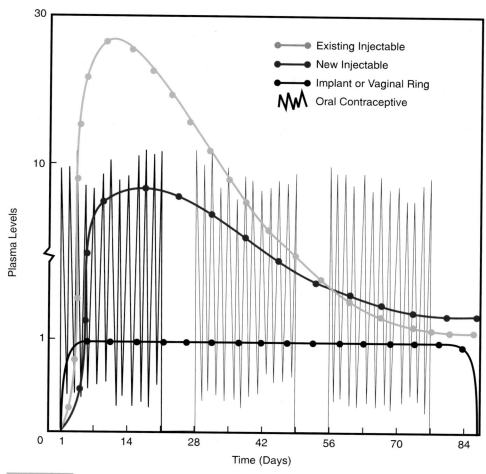

Figure 10.6   **Schematic representation of the expected pharmacokinetic profiles of progestogens administered in different formulations.**   (From **Landgren BM.** Mechanism of action of gestagens. *Int J Gynaecol Obstet* 1990;32:95–110, with permission.)

had no increase in pregnancies. Few heavy women were studied with the etonogestrel implant because the studies excluded women of body weight greater than 130% of ideal body weight. Pregnancy rate does appear to increase with weight in women using the *levonorgestrel* implants at weight 70 kg or more but it is still low. There were no pregnancies in any weight group during the first 3 years of use in a large study (125,126).

Metabolic Effects and Safety

Venous Thrombosis   Women who use estrogen containing hormonal contraceptives are at increased risk for venous thrombosis and thromboembolism. Normally the coagulation system maintains a dynamic balance of procoagulant and anticoagulant systems. Estrogens affect both systems in a dose-related fashion. For most women, fibrinolysis (anticoagulation) is increased as much as coagulation, maintaining the dynamic balance at increased levels of production and destruction of fibrinogen (127,128) (Fig. 10.7). Older studies included women with what are now considered contraindications to use of estrogen-containing hormonal contraceptives: previous thrombosis, preexisting vascular disease, coronary artery disease, cancers, and serious trauma (127,128). Current low-dose OCs have a less measurable effect on the coagulation system, and fibrinolytic factors increase at the same rate as procoagulant factors. Lower estrogen dose (30–35 μg *EE*) OCs reduce the risk of a thromboembolic event when compared with higher dose (50 μg estrogen) OCs (129) (Table 10.5). A very large Danish study showed for the first time that combination OCs with 20 μg of *ethinyl estradiol* have an 18% further reduction in thrombosis risk compared with 30 to 40 μg OCs after adjustment for duration of use (130). The progesterone-only OCs and the *levonorgestrel*-releasing intrauterine device were not associated with venous thrombosis.

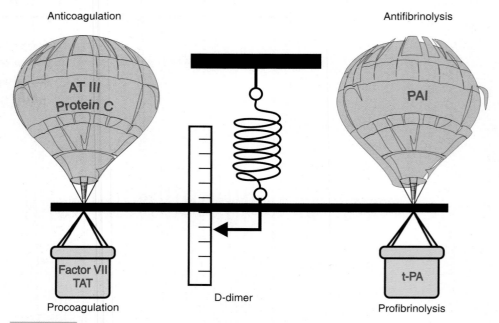

Anticoagulation

Antifibrinolysis

AT III
Protein C

PAI

Factor VII
TAT

t-PA

Procoagulation

D-dimer

Profibrinolysis

Figure 10.7   Dynamic balance of hemostasis. (From **Winkler UH, Buhler K, Schlinder AE.** The dynamic balance of hemostasis: implications for the risk of oral contraceptive use. In: **Runnebaum B, Rabe T, Kissel L, eds.** Female contraception and male fertility regulation. In *Advances in Gynecological and Obstetric Research Series.* Confort, England: Parthenon Publishing Group, 1991:85–92, with permission.)

The absolute risk of deep vein thrombosis was strongly influenced by age, increasing from 1.84 per 10,000 women aged 15 to 19 years to 6.59 per 10,000 for women aged 45 to 49 years with current users, former users, and never users combined. With all types of OCs combined, the overall absolute rate of deep vein thrombosis was 6.29 per 10,000 woman-years for current OC users compared to 3.01 among nonusers, giving an adjusted rate ratio of 2.83 (95% confidence interval [CI], 2.65–3.01) (Table 10.6). This is a higher absolute risk than the 3 per 10,000 woman-years previously estimated and may reflect, among other things, the use of better means for diagnosis of deep vein thrombosis (131). This population-based study includes all Danish women aged 15 to 49, excluding only women with a diagnosis of cancer or of cardiovascular disease diagnosed before the study interval. **Thrombosis risk was highest during the first year of use and decreased thereafter** (Table 10.6).

Thrombophilia   Changes in the coagulation system are detectable in all women, including those taking lower-dose OCs; some women are genetically predisposed to thrombosis when challenged by pregnancy or administration of exogenous estrogen. **Women with inherited deficiencies of antithrombin III, protein C, or protein S are at very high risk for thrombosis with pregnancy or estrogen therapy, but they make up a very small proportion of potential OC users. A much more common variation, factor V Leiden exists in 3% to 5% of the**

Table 10.5 Oral Contraceptive Estrogen Dose and Risk for Deep Vein Thrombosis			
Estrogen (Dose)	*(Rate/10,000 Person Years)*	*Relative Risk (All Cases)*	*Relative Risk (Proven Diagnosis)*
<50 μg	4.2	1.0	1.0[a]
50 μg	7.0	1.5	2.0 (0.0–4.0)
>50 μg	10.0	1.7	3.2 (2.4–4.3)

[a]Baseline risk used to calculate risk for higher doses.
From **Gerstman BB, Piper JM, Tomita DK, et al.** Oral contraceptive dose and the risk of deep venous thrombosis. *Am J Epidemiol* 1991;133:32–37, with permission.

Table 10.6 Crude Incidence Rates and Adjusted Rate Ratios of Venous Thrombosis in Women Using Different Types of Hormonal Contraception

Characteristics	Woman-Years	Number with Venous Thrombosis	Rate per 10,000 Woman-Years	Adjusted Rate Ratio (95% CI)
Age group				
15–19	1,359,821	250	1.84	0.39 (0.33–0.45)[a]
20–24	1,491,764	444	2.98	0.62 (0.54–0.70)[a]
25–29	1,491,959	537	3.60	0.86 (0.76–0.96)[a]
30–34	1,587,896	598	3.77	Reference
35–39	1,628,852	685	4.21	1.18 (1.05–1.32)[a]
40–44	1,518,172	797	5.25	1.57 (1.41–1.74)[a]
45–49	1,368,909	902	6.59	2.09 (1.88–2.32)[a]
Total	10,447,373	4,213	4.03	—
Current Use				
Nonuse (never or former use)	7,194,242	2,168	3.01	Reference Group
Current use	3,253,131	2,045	6.29	2.83 (2.65–3.01)[b]
Duration of Use of Combined OCs				
<one year	684,061	443	6.48	4.17 (3.73–4.66)[b]
1–4 years	1,449,000	787	5.43	2.98 (2.73–3.26)[b]
>4 years	1,031,953	793	7.68	2.76 (2.53–3.02)[b]
Progestogen Only				
Levonorgestrel or *norethindrone*	65,820	12	1.82	0.59 (0.33–1.04)[b]
Desogestrel	9,044	3	3.32	1.10 (0.35–3.41)[b]
Hormone-releasing IUD	101,351	34	3.35	0.89 (0.64–1.26)[b]

OC, oral contraceptive; IUD, intrauterine device.
[a] Adjusted for current use of oral contraceptives, calendar year, and educational level.
[b] Adjusted for age, calendar year, and educational level.
From **Lidegaard O, Lokkegaard E, Svendsen AL, et al.** Hormonal contraception and risk of venous thromboembolism: national follow up study. *BMJ* 2009;339:b2890 [Table I on page 3], with permission.

Caucasian population. It codes for a one amino acid mutation in the factor V protein, inhibiting cleavage of the protein by activated protein C, which is an essential step in maintaining the balance between coagulation and fibrinolysis (109,132). **Risk for a first thromboembolic episode among women using OCs was 2.2 per 10,000 woman-years for women without the factor V mutation and 27.7 per 10,000 woman-years for women with the mutation** (133). Cigarette smoking did not affect this risk. There are pronounced ethnic differences in the presence of this mutation. The Leiden allele is found in 3% to 5% of whites but is rare in Africans, Asians, Amerindians, Eskimos, and Polynesians (134). A similar mutation is found in the prothrombin gene at position 20210 and is described as prothrombin G20210A. This mutation occurs in 3% of the European population and is strongly associated with venous thrombosis in women taking OCs (135). Many more genetic conditions predisposing to thrombosis were described. Pregnancy is an even greater challenge for women with inherited defects of anticoagulation (136). **A woman who sustains a venous event while using OCs should be evaluated thoroughly after she has recovered.** Assessment should include at minimum the measurement of antithrombin III, protein C, and protein S levels, resistance to activated protein C, serum homocysteine, factor V Leiden mutation, the prothrombin G20210A mutation and testing for antiphospholipid syndrome. **It should not be assumed that hormonal contraception was the unique cause of the thrombotic episode.**

Routine screening for all women before prescribing hormonal contraception is not justified because effective contraception would be denied to 5% of Caucasian women, and only a small number of fatal pulmonary emboli would be prevented (137,138). Screening women with a personal or family history of deep vein thrombosis before starting estrogen-containing hormonal contraception or pregnancy is strongly recommended. Women already diagnosed as having factor V Leiden should not receive estrogen-containing contraceptives, i.e., the pill, patch or ring.

Thrombosis and the New Progestins   Several studies found increased risk of venous thrombosis when users of OCs containing the newer progestins *desogestrel* or *gestodene* combined with 20 to 30 μg of *EE* were compared with users of *levonorgestrel* combined with the same doses of estrogen (115). A controversy resulted. It is likely that the biases "attrition of susceptibles," "adverse selection," and "healthy user bias" explain the apparent increase in thrombosis. Most cases of venous thrombosis attributable to OCs occur during the initial months of use (116). Comparing new users to women already taking OCs for some time without incident will demonstrate an apparent increase with the new product that is artificial. Physicians may presume that newer drugs are safer and prescribe them selectively for women with risk factors. Additional **studies have not resolved this controversy.** Heinemann and colleagues found no difference in thrombosis risk in users of OCs containing desogestrel or gestodene compared to users of OCs with other progestins in a large study of cases occurring between 2002 and 2006 in Austria (139). In contrast, both Lidegaard's group in Sweden and van Hylckama Vlieg's group in the Netherlands reported increased risk with the newer progestins (130,140).

Ischemic Heart Disease   Ischemic heart disease and stroke were the major causes of death attributed to OC use in the past. It is known that the principal determinants of risk are advancing age and cigarette smoking (141). With the higher-dose OCs used in the 1980s, smoking had a profound effect on risk. Women smoking 25 or more cigarettes per day had a 30-fold increased risk for myocardial infarction if they used OCs, compared with nonsmokers not using OCs (142). Use of OCs is became safer because most women are taking low-dose pills and because physicians prescribe selectively, excluding women with major cardiovascular risk factors. A very large study in the United States confirmed the safety of OCs as currently prescribed. A total of 187 women aged 15 to 44 years with confirmed myocardial infarction were identified during 3.6 million woman-years of observation in the Kaiser Permanente Medical Care Program in California from 1991 to 1994. This is a rate of 3.2 per 100,000 woman-years (143). Nearly all of the users took OCs with less than 50 μg of *EE*. **After adjusting for age, illness, smoking, ethnicity, and body mass index, risk for myocardial infarction was not increased by OC use (odds ratio [OR], 1.14; 95% CI, 0.27–4.72). Of heart attack victims, 61% smoked; only 7.7% were current users of OCs.** In a later study, the same investigators pooled results from the California study with a similar study from Washington State. The results were the same. **Current users of low-dose OCs had no increased risk for myocardial infarction after adjustment for major risk factors and sociodemographic factors** (144). Past use of OCs does not increase risk for subsequent myocardial infarction (145). These observations are supported by another population-based prospective study. OC use and myocardial infarction were studied prospectively among 48,321 randomly selected women aged 30 to 49 in the Uppsala Health Care Region of Sweden (146). **There was no association between current or past OC use and myocardial infarction.** Most current users were taking low-dose estrogen pills (defined as less than 50 μg of ethinyl estradiol or less than 75 μg of *mestranol*) with second or third generation progestins, more than half were aged 35 or older, and 26% were current cigarette smokers.

Oral Contraceptives and Stroke   In the 1970s, OC use appeared to be linked to risk of both hemorrhagic and thrombotic stroke, but these studies failed to take into consideration preexisting risk factors (147). **A rare form of cerebrovascular insufficiency, moyamoya disease, is linked to OC use, especially among cigarette smokers (148). The present evidence shows no risk of stroke among women who are otherwise healthy and who use low-dose pills.** One study identified all Kaiser Permanente Medical Care Program patients aged 15 to 44 years who sustained fatal or nonfatal stroke in California from 1991 to 1994 (149). **Hypertension, diabetes, obesity, current cigarette smoking, and black ethnicity were strongly associated with stroke risk, but neither current nor past OC use was associated with stroke.** A World Health Organization study of cases from 1989 to 1993 from 17 countries in Europe and the developing world included women taking higher-dose OCs and low-dose OCs. European women using low-dose OCs had no increased risk for either type of stroke, thrombotic or hemorrhagic. Those taking higher-dose OCs did have measurable risk (150,151). Women in developing countries had an apparent modest increase in risk, but this finding was attributed to undetected existing risk factors. Another study from Europe found less stroke risk from low-dose pills than from older, higher-dose pills, and that risk was less if the patient's blood pressure was checked before starting OCs.

Women who smoke and those who have hypertension and diabetes are at increased risk for cardiovascular disease regardless of whether they use oral contraceptives. **The important question is whether risk is further increased if they use low-dose OCs, and if so, by how much.** The World Health Organization study described previously provides some insight: **smokers taking OCs had seven times the risk of ischemic (thrombotic) stroke when compared with smokers who did not use OCs, and hypertensive women had 10-fold increased risk if they took OCs, but a fivefold risk if they did not** (150). Similarly, a study from Denmark found that women with diabetes had a fivefold increase risk for stroke, which increased to 10-fold if they took OCs (152). These data were not limited to low-estrogen OCs. The data suggest that although risk is primarily determined by the predisposing condition—hypertension, diabetes, or cigarette smoking—the risk can be magnified by OC use, even when the OCs are low dose. These observations were confirmed in a recent systematic review (153). Hypertensive women using combination estrogen–progestin oral contraceptives (COCs) had higher risk for ischemic stroke and acute myocardial infarction than hypertensive women not using COCs. **The current US practice of limiting hormonal contraceptives containing estrogen by women older than 35 years of age to nonsmokers without other vascular disease risk factors is prudent** (7).

Blood Pressure   **Oral contraceptives have a dose-related effect on blood pressure.** With the older high-dose pills, as many as 5% of patients could be expected to have blood pressure levels greater than 140/90 mm Hg. The mechanism is believed to be an estrogen-induced increase in renin substrate in susceptible individuals. **Low-dose pills have minimal blood pressure effects, but surveillance of blood pressure is advised to detect the occasional idiosyncratic response.**

Glucose Metabolism   Oral estrogen alone has no adverse effect on glucose metabolism, but progestins exhibit insulin antagonism (154). Older OC formulations with higher doses of progestins produced abnormal glucose tolerance tests with elevated insulin levels in the average patient. The effect on glucose metabolism, similar to the effect on lipids, is related to androgenic potency of the progestin and to its dose.

Lipid Metabolism   Androgens and estrogens have competing effects on hepatic lipase, a liver enzyme critical to lipid metabolism. Estrogens depress low-density lipoproteins (LDL) and elevate high-density lipoproteins (HDL), changes that can be expected to reduce the risk of atherosclerosis (155). Androgens and androgenic progestins can antagonize these beneficial changes, reducing HDL and elevating LDL levels. Estrogens elevate triglyceride levels. Low-dose formulations have minimal adverse effect on lipids, and the newer formulations (with *desogestrel* and *norgestimate* as the progestin) produce potentially beneficial changes by elevating HDL and lowering LDL (156,157). Although average values of a large group show only small lipid changes with the use of current OCs, an occasional patient may have exaggerated effects. Women whose lipid values are higher than the mean before treatment are more likely to experience abnormalities during treatment (156).

Other Metabolic Effects   Oral contraceptives can produce changes in a broad variety of proteins synthesized by the liver. The estrogen in OCs increases circulating thyroid-binding globulin, thereby affecting tests of thyroid function that are based on binding, increasing total thyroxine (T_4) levels, and decreasing triiodothyronine (T_3) resin uptake. The results of actual thyroid function tests, as measured by free T_4 and radioiodine tests, are normal (158).

Oral Contraceptives and Neoplasia

Endometrial Cancer and Ovarian Cancer   **Combination OCs reduce the risk of subsequent endometrial cancer and ovarian cancer** (159,160). Two-year use of OCs reduces the risk of endometrial cancer by 40%, and 4 or more years of use reduces the risk by 60%. The evidence for this benefit continues to accumulate (161). A 50% reduction in ovarian cancer risk for women who took OCs for 3 to 4 years and an 80% reduction with 10 or more years of use was reported (162). There was some benefit from as little as 3 to 11 months of use. A review of all available studies in the world published in English through 2008 concluded that ovarian cancer risk decreased by 20% for each 4 years of use and was seen for carriers of the BRCA1 and 2 mutations as well. The benefit persisted for at least 30 years after last use (163). A similar reduction of risk of ovarian epithelial cancer was found in a prospective study from Norway and Sweden, with borderline tumor risk equally reduced. Combination OCs with less than 50 μg of *EE,* or less than 100 μg of mestranol and reduced doses of progestin, provided as much protection as higher dose pills (164). Today's lower-dose 20 μg *EE* pills were not separately studied. Whether or not they provide the same benefit remains unproven; however, progestin-only contraceptives are reported to provide risk reduction equivalent to that of combined OCs (165).

Cervical Cancer   There may be a weak association between OC use and cancer of the cervix. A systematic review of 28 epidemiologic studies of cervical cancer in OC users compared with those who never used OCs reported summary relative risks of 1.1 (95% CI, 1.1–1.2) at less than 5 years of pill use, 1.6 (1.4–1.7) at 5 to 9 years, and 2.2 (1.9–2.4) at 10 or more years (166). A 2007 update by these same authors reported a pooled relative risk for all studies of 1.9 (95% CI, 1.69–2.13) for invasive cervical cancer or CIN3/carcinoma *in situ* (CIS) with 5 or more years of OC use. Risk declined after use ceased and by 10 years returned to that of never users. Too few had used progestin-only pills to provide a conclusion as to their effect. For injectable progestins, the relative risk was very slightly increased to 1.22 (95% CI, 1.01–1.46), which was just statistically significant (167). Critics of these studies argued that causation is not proven because few adequately control for the key behavioral factors of partners, use of barrier contraception, and adequacy of cervical cancer screening (168). Important risk factors for cervical cancer are early sexual intercourse and exposure to HPV. Women who used OCs typically started sexual relations at younger ages than women who have not used OCs and, in some studies, report having had more partners. These factors increase one's chance of acquiring HPV, the most important risk factor for cervical cancer. Because barrier contraceptives reduce the risk of cervical cancer, use of alternative choices for contraception compounds the difficulty in establishing an association with OC use alone (169). The presence of HPV types 16 or 18 is associated with a 50-fold increase in risk for preneoplastic lesions of the cervix (170). Adenocarcinomas of the cervix are rare, they are not as easily detected as other lesions by screening cervical cytology, and the incidence appears to be increasing. One study found a doubling of risk for adenocarcinoma with OC use that increased with duration of use, reaching a relative risk of 4.4 if total use of OCs exceeded 12 years (171). The results of this study were adjusted for history of genital warts, number of sexual partners, and age at first intercourse. Another summary of case-control studies that includes testing for HPV. HPV types 16 or 18 were present in 82% of the patients, yielding a relative risk of 81.3 (95% CI, 42.0–157.1) for the disease. Cofactors identified with adenocarcinoma included longer-term use of hormonal contraception. **Intrauterine device use was associated with reduced relative risk of 0.41 (95% CI, 0.18–0.93)** (172). Use of hormonal contraception by women from aged 20 to 30 years is estimated to increase the incidence of cervix cancer (any cervix cancer, or CIN3/CIS) diagnosed by age 50 from 7.3 to 8.3 per 1,000 women in lesser-developed countries and from 3.8 to 4.5 in developed countries (172). Use of OCs is, at most, a minor factor in causation of cervical cancer; these findings emphasize the need to immunize against HPV and to provide cervical cancer screening worldwide. To reduce risk, women who are not in mutually monogamous relationships should be advised to use barrier methods in addition to hormonal contraception.

Breast Cancer   There is a large volume of conflicting literature on the relationship between OC use and breast cancer (173). No increase in overall risk is found from OC use, but some studies found that risk may increase in women who used OCs before their first term pregnancy, used OCs for many years, are nulligravid, are young at the time of diagnosis, or continue using OCs in their 40s. A meta-analysis of 54 studies of breast cancer and hormonal contraceptive use reanalyzed data on 53,297 women with breast cancer and 100,239 controls from 25 countries, representing about 90% of the epidemiologic data available worldwide at that time (174). Current use of OCs was associated with a very small, but statistically stable 24% increased relative risk (1.24; 95% CI, 1.15–1.33). The risk fell rapidly after discontinuation, to 16% 1 to 4 years after stopping and to 7% 5 to 9 years after stopping. Risk disappeared 10 years after cessation (relative risk, 1.01; 95% CI, 0.96–1.05). Results did not differ in any important way by ethnic group, reproductive history, or family history. Since the meta-analysis was published, subsequent studies found no increased risk. A case-control study of 4,575 women with breast cancer and 4,682 controls aged 35 to 64 years living in five cities in the United States concluded that **breast cancer risk was not increased for current or past users of OCs and did not increase with prolonged or with higher-estrogen OC use** (175). **Neither family history of breast cancer nor beginning use at a young age was associated with increased risk.** A similar study in Sweden compared 3,016 women aged 50 to 74 years who had invasive breast cancer with 3,263 controls of the same age. No relation was found between past use of OCs and breast cancer (176). Effect of hormone dose was explored in a 2008 US study of 1,469 women with breast cancer who were matched by race, age, and neighborhood to community controls. The investigators then administered questionnaires and performed BRCA1 and 2 testing. Subjects who began OC use during or after 1975 were considered to have used low-dose pills. "Low-dose" was not further defined. Neither OC use overall or "low-dose" OC use was associated with breast cancer risk, among the total group, or within any subset. Women with BRCA1 or 2 did not have higher rates of cancer whether they were OC users or were nonusers (177). The controversy over the association between breast cancer and OC use is likely to continue. The best information available is that there is little or no connection.

Liver Tumors   **Oral contraceptives were implicated as a cause of benign adenomas of the liver.** These hormonally responsive tumors can cause fatal hemorrhage. They usually regress when OC use is discontinued; risk is related to prolonged use (178). The tumors are rare; about 30 cases per 1 million users per year were predicted with older formulations. Presumably, newer low-dose products pose less risk. A link to hepatic carcinoma was proposed. This cancer is closely associated with chronic hepatitis B and C infections and is usually seen in cirrhotic livers. There are case reports of hepatocellular carcinoma in young women with no risk factors other than long-term OC use (179). A large study from six countries in Europe found no association between use of OCs and subsequent liver cancer (180). A systematic review looked for evidence of harm associated with hormonal contraceptive use among women already at risk because of liver disease (181). **The authors concluded from the limited data available that OCs do not affect the course of acute hepatitis or chronic hepatitis, and do not affect the rate of progression or severity of cirrhotic fibrosis, the risk of hepatocellular carcinoma in women with chronic hepatitis, or the risk of liver dysfunction in hepatitis B virus carriers.**

Oral Contraceptives and Sexually Transmitted Infections   Chlamydial colonization of the cervix appears more likely in OC users than in nonusers but, despite this finding, several case-control studies found a reduced risk of acute PID among OC users (182,183). In contrast, a subsequent study found no protection with OC use (184).

Whether hormonal contraceptives influence acquisition of HIV remains uncertain. **The largest study concluded that overall risk was not increased by oral combination OCs or injected DMPA** (185).

Health Benefits of Oral Contraceptives

Oral contraceptives have important health benefits (Table 10.7). **These include contraceptive and noncontraceptive benefits** 182).

Contraceptive Benefits

Oral contraceptives provide highly effective contraception and prevent unwanted pregnancy, an important public health problem. Where safe abortion services are not available, women seek unsafe services and risk death from septic abortion. Combination OCs block ovulation and offer marked protection from ectopic pregnancy. Risk of ectopic pregnancy in a woman taking combination OCs is estimated to be 1/500 of the risk of women not using contraception; progestin-only OCs appear to increase risk of ectopic pregnancy (186).

Noncontraceptive Benefits

As noted earlier, **OC use produces strong and lasting reduced risk for endometrial and ovarian cancer.** In addition, protection was found for women with known hereditary ovarian cancer. **Any past use of OCs conferred a 50% reduction in ovarian cancer risk when women with this history who took OCs were compared with their sisters as controls (OR, 0.5; 95% CI, 0.3–0.8). Protection increased with increasing duration of use** (187). The mechanism of action of OCs in the prevention of ovarian cancer is unknown but may involve selective induction of apoptosis (programmed cell death). Macaques treated with *EE* plus *levonorgestrel* or *levonorgestrel* alone showed an increase in the proportion of ovarian epithelial cells in apoptosis in comparison with animals fed a diet containing no hormones (188).

Other documented benefits of OC use include reduction of benign breast disease (189). Use of OCs helps relieve dysmenorrhea (166). Oral contraceptives offer effective therapy for women with menorrhagia and dysfunctional uterine bleeding (163).

Table 10.7 Established and Emerging Noncontraceptive Benefits of Oral Contraceptives

Established Benefits

Menses-related

Increased menstrual cycle regularity

Reduced blood loss

Reduced iron-deficiency anemia

Reduced dysmenorrhea

Reduced symptoms of premenstrual dysphoric disorder[a]

Inhibition of ovulation

Fewer ovarian cysts

Fewer ectopic pregnancies

Other

Reduced fibroadenomas/fibrocystic breast changes

Reduced acute pelvic inflammatory disease

Reduced endometrial cancer

Reduced ovarian cancer

Emerging Benefits

Increased bone mass

Reduced acne

Reduced colorectal cancer

Reduced uterine leiomyomata

Reduced rheumatoid arthritis

Treatment of bleeding disorders

Treatment of hyperandrogenic anovulation

Treatment of endometriosis

Treatment of perimenopausal changes

[a]Only the low-dose *EE/droperidol* oral contraceptive has U.S. Food and Drug Administration approval for premenstrual dysphoric disorder treatment.
From **Burkman R, Schlesselman JJ, Zieman M.** Safety concerns and health benefits associated with oral contraception. *Am J Obstet Gynecol* 2004;190(Suppl):S12, with permission.

All combination OCs offer some protection from functional ovarian cysts, but this is dose related (190). Although OCs may prevent cyst formation, they are not helpful in treating large functional ovarian cysts and should not be used for this purpose (191). OCs appear to decrease the risk of developing leiomyomata (192).

All combination OCs reduce circulating androgen levels and usually improve acne. Three OCs were specifically FDA approved for acne treatment: the *norgestimate/EE triphasic* (*TriCyclen*), the *norethindrone/EE multiphasic* (*Estrostep*), and the 20 μg *EE* /3 mg droperidol OC.

There is some evidence that OC use is protective against colon cancer. A case-control study in Italy comparing women with colon cancer with controls found a 37% reduction in colon cancer and a 34% reduction in rectal cancer (colon cancer OR, 0.63; 95% CI, 0.45–0.87 and rectal cancer OR, 0.66; 95% CI, 0.43–1.01). Longer use produced more protection against colon cancer (193). Results of the U.S. Nurses Health Study disclosed some degree of protection. Women who used OCs for 96 months or more had a 40% lower risk of colorectal cancer (RR, 0.60; 95% CI, 1.15–2.14) (194). A large case-control study from Wisconsin found most of the benefit limited to women who were less than 14 years since discontinuing OCs (195). The mechanism of protection has not been identified.

Fertility after Oral Contraceptive Use

After discontinuing OCs, return of ovulatory cycles may be delayed for a few months. Women who have amenorrhea more than 6 months after discontinuation of OCs should undergo a full evaluation because of the risk for prolactin-producing pituitary tumors. This risk is not related to OC use but rather to the probability that the slow-growing tumor was already present and produced menstrual irregularity, prompting the patient to take OCs (196).

Sexuality

In a study that recorded all episodes of female-initiated sexual behavior throughout the menstrual cycle, an increase in sexual activity at the time of ovulation was noted. This increase was not present in women who were taking OCs (197). No other study appears to have addressed female initiated sexual activity and OC use. A 2003 study from Spain studied sexual desire in a comparative cohort of women using OCs and a cohort using IUDs. Sexual desire decreased over time, but was not affected by the contraceptive method (198). OCs containing the new progestin *drospirenone* are reported to improve sexual functioning and feelings of well-being (199,200).

Teratogenicity

A meta-analysis of 12 prospective studies, including 6,102 women who used OCs and 85,167 women who did not, revealed no increase in overall risk for malformation, congenital heart defects, or limb reduction defects with the use of OCs (201). Progestins were used to prevent miscarriage. A large study compared women showing signs of threatened abortion who were treated with progestins (primarily oral *medroxyprogesterone acetate*) with women who were not treated. The rate of malformation was the same among the 1,146 exposed infants as among the 1,608 unexposed infants (202). Conversely, estrogens taken in high doses in pregnancy can induce vaginal cancer in female offspring exposed *in utero*. A recent literature search revealed no recent reports linking teratogenicity to hormonal contraception.

Interaction of Oral Contraceptives with Other Drugs

Some drugs (e.g., *rifampin*) reduce the effectiveness of oral contraceptives; conversely, OCs can augment or reduce the effectiveness of other drugs (e.g., *benzodiazepines*) (203,204). Perhaps of greatest clinical significance are six antiepileptic drugs: *phenytoin, phenobarbital, carbamazepine, oxcarbazepine, felbamate,* and *topiramate* (205). These drugs and the antibiotic *rifampin* all induce synthesis of liver cytochrome P450 enzymes and reduce plasma levels of *EE* in women taking OCs, increasing the likelihood of contraceptive failure. Some antiseizure agents have no effect on the levels of contraceptive steroids in the blood. These include *valproic acid, vigabatrin, lamotrigine, gabapentin, tiagabine, levetiracetam, zonisamide, ethosuximide,* and the *benzodiazepines* (205). *St. John's wort* induces cytochrome P450 and is reported to increase clearance of *EE* and *norethindrone* (206). The antifungal agents *griseofulvin, ketoconazole,* and *itraconazole* induce these hepatic enzymes and may reduce OC efficacy (204). *Ampicillin* and *tetracycline* were implicated in numerous case reports of OC failure. They kill gut bacteria (primarily clostridia) that are responsible for hydrolysis of steroid glucuronides in the intestine, which allows reabsorption of the steroid through the enterohepatic circulation. It was not possible to demonstrate reduced plasma levels of *EE* overall or differences in pregnancy rates (207). Some individuals do experience reduced *EE* plasma levels when on *tetracyclines* or *penicillins*; it is best to advise women taking OCs who will be treated with antibiotics to use condoms as well (208). **Certain drugs appear to increase plasma levels of contraceptive steroids. Ascorbic acid (vitamin C) and *acetaminophen* may elevate plasma *EE*, as do the antiretrovirals *efavirenz* and *atazanavir/ritonavir* (7).**

An example of OCs affecting the metabolism of other drugs is seen with *diazepam* and related compounds. Oral contraceptive use reduces the metabolic clearance and increases the half-life of those *benzodiazepines* that are metabolized primarily by oxidation: *chlordiazepoxide, alprazolam, diazepam,* and *nitrazepam*. *Caffeine* and *theophylline* are metabolized in the liver by two of the P450 isozymes, and their clearance is reduced in OC users. *Cyclosporine* is hydroxylated by another of the P450 isozymes, and its plasma concentrations are increased by OCs. Plasma levels of some analgesic drugs are decreased in OC users. *Salicylic acid* and *morphine* clearances are enhanced by OC use; therefore, higher doses could be needed for adequate therapeutic effect. Clearance of *ethanol* may be reduced in OC users.

The interactions of antiretroviral drugs with contraceptive steroids are complex. Some of the drugs increase plasma steroid levels and some reduce them. A complete list of interactions is available in the Centers for Disease Control and Prevention's "U.S. Medical Eligibility for Contraception" (7).

Oral Contraceptives and Clinical Chemistry Alterations

Oral contraceptives have the potential to alter a number of clinical laboratory tests as a result of estrogen-induced changes in hepatic synthesis; however, a large study comparing OC users with pregnant and nonpregnant controls found minimal changes (209). Hormone users took a variety of OCs containing 50 to 100 μg of estrogen, higher doses than are used today. **Compared with nonpregnant women who were not using OCs, the OC users had an increase in T_4 that is explained by increased circulating thyroid-binding protein,** no change in creatinine and globulin levels, slight reduction in mean fasting glucose values and serum glutamic oxaloacetic transaminase, and a decrease in total bilirubin and alkaline phosphatase.

Choice of Oral Contraceptives

Recently introduced OCs include those containing *drosperidol,* more preparations with only 20 μg of *EE,* new multiphasic preparations, cyclic OCs with 24 days of active medication and 4 days of either placebo or 10 μg of *EE,* and extended-cycle and continuous cycle preparations plus branded generic versions of most OCs. A combination OC containing *estradiol valerate* with a new progestin, *dienogest,* was approved in 2010. There is new evidence that 20 μg *EE* pills offer reduced risk for venous thrombosis (130). An approach to OC selection for new patients is to begin with a 20 μg *EE* combination and then adjust depending on the patient's symptoms after the first 2 to 3 months. As reported in a large systematic review of 20 μg *EE* OCs compared to 30 to 35 μg *EE* pills, women taking the lower dose OCs more often report changes in vaginal bleeding, episodes of irregular bleeding and heavy bleeding, and more amenorrhea (210). If a 20 μg pill is offered, the patient should understand that bleeding may be a problem and that she should return if this persists and try a different OC rather than stop the pill. The progestin component may become more important in determining cycle control when 20 μg *EE* is used. A comparison of 20 μg *EE* OCS, one containing 100 μg of *levonorgestrel,* the other with 1 mg of *norethindrone acetate* (*NEA*) found the *NEA* to have about twice as many days of unscheduled vaginal bleeding during the first 3 months, a critical time period for new users, which might be expected to lead to discontinuation (211). In a three-way trial, the 35-μg *EE/norgestimate* triphasic OC (*Tri-Cyclen*) was compared with two 20-μg *EE* pills, one containing 100 μg of *levonorgestrel* (*Alesse*), the other containing 150 μg *desogestrel,* followed by 2 hormone-free days and 5 days of 10 μg *EE* per day (*Mircette*) (212). Contraceptive efficacy was not significantly different. In the first two pill cycles more women taking *Alesse* had breakthrough bleeding and bleeding in the second half of the cycle than those taking the other two OCs in the first two cycles, but thereafter there was little difference. Women taking the higher estrogen *Tri-Cyclen* consistently experienced more frequent estrogenic side effects—bloating, breast tenderness, and nausea—than did women taking either 20-μg *EE* OC. These authors concluded that for the specific OCs evaluated, changing to either one of the 20 μg preparations would be beneficial.

For the average patient, the first choice of preparation for contraceptive purposes is a very low estrogen OC (20 μg *EE*) unless there are other considerations, for example, previous pregnancy while taking the pill. Patients with persistent break-through spotting or bleeding could be offered a pill with the same low estrogen dose, but a more potent progestin, for example *levonorgestrel.* Patients with apparent weight gain from fluid retention while taking OCs, or with hirsutism or acne that did not respond to other OCs, may benefit from a change to the *drospirenone/EE* pill. The lower *estrogen drospirenone* combination is FDA approved for treatment of PMDD and should be considered for women with these symptoms who want hormonal contraception. Women with acne often benefit from the reduction in circulating testosterone that occurs with all combination OCs. Women who experience continuing pelvic pain, dysmenorrhea, or other menstrual triggered symptoms or who simply prefer fewer menstruations may be offered an extended-cycle or continuous cycle-OC regimen.

Alternative Routes for Hormonal Contraception

The *OrthoEvra* patch and the *NuvaRing* both provide combinations of ultrapotent progestins with *EE.* Both patch and ring provide almost constant low levels of the contraceptive steroids that are less than the peak levels seen with OCs. Both offer greater convenience to the user, which improves compliance. The patch has a surface area of 20 cm². It delivers a daily dose of 150 μg *norelgestromin,* the active metabolite of norgestimate, and 20 μg of *EE.* The patch is worn for 1 week then replaced with a new patch for 7 days, continuing for 3 consecutive weeks followed by a week with no patch. The patch was compared with a multiphasic OC containing *levonorgestrel* 50 to 125 μg, and 30 to 40 μg *EE* (*Triphasil*) in a randomized trial of 1,417 women (122). The overall and method failure Pearl indices were 1.24 and 0.99 pregnancies per 100 woman-years in the patch group and 2.18 and 1.23 in the OC group, respectively, numerically less in the patch group but not statistically significant. **Patch users had more breakthrough bleeding**

or spotting in the first two cycles, but thereafter this did not differ from OC users. Patch users reported more breast discomfort, dysmenorrhea, and abdominal pain than the OC users, but other adverse events were uncommon and did not differ. Perfect compliance was reported for 88.2% of patch users' cycles versus 77.7% of the pill users' cycles ($p < .001$). Pregnancy risk with the patch appears to be higher for women weighing more than 90 kg.

The *NuvaRing* is 54 mm in outer diameter and has a cross section of 4 mm. It delivers daily doses of 120 μg of *etonogestrel,* the active metabolite of *desogestrel,* with 15 μg of *EE,* and thus is the lowest estrogen combination hormonal method available in the United States. The soft, flexible ring is worn in the vagina for 3 weeks, and then removed for 1 week, after which time a new ring is inserted. If inserted on the first day of menstruation, no back up method of contraception is needed. It can be inserted on days 2 to 5 and used with a backup method such as condoms for the first week. In a pharmacokinetic study comparing the ring with a combination OC containing 150 μg of *desogestrel* and 30 μg of *EE,* maximum blood levels of *EE* with the ring were about one-third of those seen with the OC, and the *etonogestrel* level was about 40% of that produced by the OC. Despite these findings, ovulation was inhibited in all women studied (213). **Women wearing the ring are reported to have fewer days of irregular bleeding or spotting than women taking an OC** with 150 μg of *levonorgestrel* and 30 μg of *EE* (214). A large study found a total pregnancy rate of 1.18 (95% CI, 0.73–1.80) per 100 woman-years and 0.77 (0.37–1.40) pregnancies per 100 woman-years with perfect use (214). Some women prefer to remove the ring for intercourse, although this is not necessary. It should be reinserted within 3 hours to avoid loss of efficacy.

Patch and Ring and Thrombosis

Since both methods provide constant low blood levels of *EE,* it was hoped that this might reduce risk for thrombosis. The FDA took the unusual step of issuing a "black box warning" for the *EE/norelgestromin* patch after several thrombosis cases were reported, and a small study of pharmacodynamics was interpreted as showing higher mean *EE* blood levels for the patch than with the oral route of administration. A small crossover study found increased activated protein C (APC) resistance when women were changed from a 30 μg *EE*/150 μg *desogestrel* pill to either the patch or the *EE/etonogestrel* ring. This was interpreted as prothrombotic (215). In another study, women on a variety of OCs had baseline measurement of APC resistance, and protein S. The patients were then switched either to the patch or to the ring. Those moving to the patch had changes in laboratory parameters that could be interpreted as prothrombotic, while those moved to the ring showed an improvement in the same studies, theoretically reducing the risk of clotting (216).

Three databased epidemiologic studies looked at thrombosis in patch users compared to oral contraception. The first found no difference, but two subsequent studies did find risk. One study found an overall doubling of the risk of deep vein thrombosis when patch users were compared to users of an OC containing 30 μg *EE*/150 μg *levonorgestrel,* but the risk estimate was of borderline statistical significance and disappeared when the analysis was restricted to women aged 39 or less (217). After publication of this study the FDA issued a new document for consumers suggesting that women concerned about thrombosis and considering the patch discuss the issue with their physicians (218).

No similar FDA warnings were issued about the ring. There are two case reports in the world literature of venous thrombosis with the ring. Both were women in their 30s who sustained cerebral venous thrombosis (219,220). The authors of the fist report note that several other thrombosis cases in women using the ring were reported to Health Canada (220). It is best to assume that the ring has the same risk for thrombosis as the other combination hormonal contraceptives and to counsel women about risk in the same way.

Injectable Hormonal Contraceptives

Depomedroxyprogesterone Acetate

DMPA, a suspension of microcrystals of a synthetic progestin, was approved for contraception in 1992. A single 150-mg intramuscular dose will suppress ovulation in most women for 14 weeks or longer (221). **The regimen of 150 mg every 3 months is highly effective, producing pregnancy rates of about 0.3 per 100 women per year.** Probably because of the high blood levels of the progestin, efficacy appears not to be reduced by administration of other drugs and is not dependent on the patient's weight. Women treated with *DMPA* experience disruption

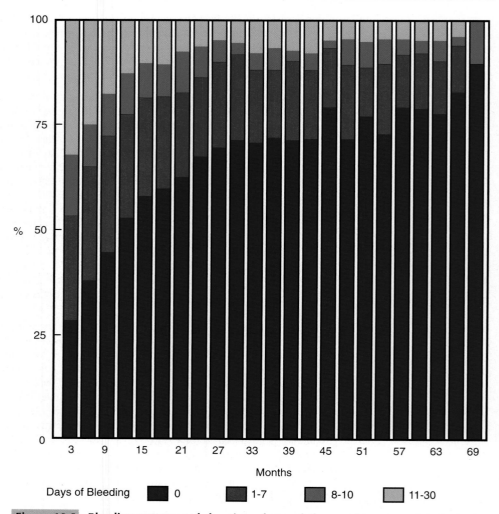

Figure 10.8 Bleeding pattern and duration of use of *depomedroxyprogesterone acetate (DMPA):* percentage of women who have bleeding, spotting, or amenorrhea while taking *DMPA* 150 mg every 3 months. (From **Schwallie PC, Assenzo JR.** Contraceptive use-efficacy study utilizing *medroxyprogesterone acetate* administered as an intramuscular injection once every 90 days. *Fertil Steril* 1973;24:331–339, with permission.)

of the menstrual cycle and have initial spotting and bleeding at irregular intervals. Eventually, total amenorrhea develops in most women who take *DMPA;* with continued administration, amenorrhea develops in 50% of women by 1 year and in 80% by 3 years (Fig. 10.8).

The most important medical reason women discontinue use of *DMPA* and other progestin-only methods is persistent irregular vaginal bleeding. A variety of medications are used to stop this bleeding. Many are effective in terminating individual bleeding episodes, but a systematic review concluded that none improved continuation rates long term (222). New approaches include *mifepristone* and low-dose *doxycycline. Mifepristone* is of interest because irregular bleeding with *DMPA* was related to the down-regulation of endometrial estrogen receptors. Treatment with 50 mg of *mifepristone* every 2 weeks increases endometrial estrogen receptors and reduces breakthrough bleeding in new users of both *DMPA* and the *levonorgestrel* progestin implant (223). Another line of investigation concerns endometrial matrix metalloproteinase, which appears to play a regulatory role in the breakdown of the endometrium to produce normal menstruation. Treatment with *doxycycline* inhibits matrix metalloproteinase production in the endometrium in women after insertion of *levonorgestrel* subdermal implants (224). Five-day courses of either *mifepristone* 25 mg twice a day for one day, followed by *EE* 20 μg per day for 4 days, or *doxycycline* 20 mg twice a day for 5 days, reduced bleeding days by about 50% when compared to placebos during a 6-month randomized trial in women treated for prolonged or frequent bleeding occurring with etonogestrel subdermal implants (225). Capsules of 20 mg *doxycycline* are sold in the United States for treatment of periodontal disease.

DMPA use is commonly associated with weight gain, and that is one of the principal reasons women discontinue use. A large study is representative of the literature. Three cohorts of women who chose their method of contraception were followed for 36 months with measurements of weight and body fat. *DMPA* users gained an average of 5.1 kg. The cohort using OCs over the same interval gained only 1.47 kg, slightly less than the 2.05 kg gained by the cohort not using any hormonal contraception. Total body fat increased 4.14 kg in the *DMPA* cohort, while the increase in the OC users was 1.9 kg, only slightly more than the 1.17 kg in the nonhormonal contraceptive cohort. Many women were followed for 2 years after discontinuing *DMPA*. Those who chose nonhormonal methods after discontinuing *DMPA* lost a mean of 0.42 kg each 6 months. Those who chose to use oral contraceptives gained a mean of 0.43 kg each 6 months during the follow-up interval (226).

Weight gain during the first 6 months and self-reporting of increased appetite are strongly predictive of continued weight gain. Women who gained less than or equal to 5% of body weight in the first 6 months gained a mean of 2.49 kg by 36 months, while those who gained more than 5% by 6 months gained a total mean of 11.08 kg by 36 months (227). Studies are needed of interventions to prevent the weight gain. At minimum, women considering *DMPA* need to know the possibility of significant weight gain and be advised to avoid calorie-dense foods and weigh themselves regularly. Ideally they should be weighed when they return for subsequent injections so they can be counseled about the need for avoiding further gain. Women who gain 5% of body weight by 6 months should consider other contraceptive options.

DMPA persists in the body for several months in women who used it for long-term contraception, and return to fertility may be delayed. It is reassuring that 70% of former users desiring pregnancy conceive within 12 months, and 90% conceive within 24 months after terminating *DMPA* use (228).

Safety

DMPA suppresses ovarian estrogen production. **Prospective studies demonstrated bone loss during *DMPA* therapy, with recovery of bone mass after *DMPA* use is discontinued (229). Similar bone loss and then recovery occurs with lactation.** Adolescents are of special concern because they normally gain bone mass; most of adult bone mass is attained by age 20. Estrogen injections prevent the bone loss and allow adolescent women to gain bone density despite use of *DMPA* (230). A long-term study in adolescents documented bone density loss and confirmed recovery of lumbosacral bone mineral density to baseline by 60 weeks after discontinuation of *DMPA* and significant gain above baseline by 180 weeks. Recovery of density at the hip was slower, 240 weeks to significant gain (231). A systematic review of *DMPA* clinical trials could find no studies where fracture was an outcome, so whether long-term use leads to fractures is still not known (232). The FDA black box warning added to *DMPA* labeling proposes that *DMPA* treatment be limited to 2 years at a time, unless the patient has no other good options for contraception. For many women, especially in third world countries, *DMPA* is often the only option for highly effective contraception because it is inexpensive and easy to administer. The issue should be discussed with women who are considering *DMPA,* but *DMPA* should not be routinely discontinued after 2 years unless the patient wants to conceive or wants to change to another contraceptive method for other reasons.

The effect of *DMPA* on plasma lipids is inconsistent; *DMPA* users appear to have reduced total cholesterol and triglyceride levels, slight reduction in HDL cholesterol, and no change or slight increase in LDL cholesterol, all of which are consistent with a reduction in circulating estrogen levels. In some studies, the decrease in HDL and increase in LDL are statistically significant, although the values remain within normal ranges (233). *DMPA* is not associated with myocardial infarction. Glucose tolerance tests disclose a small elevation of glucose in *DMPA* users.

There is no change in hemostatic parameters, with the exception that antithrombin III levels are sometimes reduced with chronic therapy (233). Venous thrombosis and thromboembolism have occurred in women on *DMPA,* but this is very rare (234). As noted earlier, large epidemiologic studies have not found *DMPA* to be associated with thrombosis (130). Thrombotic episodes occurred in elderly women with advanced cancer who were treated with a variety of agents, including *DMPA* and *tamoxifen* (235). Another episode occurred in a woman with a cerebral metastasis from breast cancer (236). Such patients are at high risk for thrombosis regardless of the use of *DMPA*. Two cases of retinal vein thrombosis were reported. Both women were hypertensive and one of them smoked cigarettes (237).

DMPA is not associated with teratogenesis (238). Nor is it associated with affective disorders or mood changes (239).

DMPA and Lactation

There is widespread support for use of *DMPA* during lactation when the *DMPA* is initiated at or after 6 weeks postpartum. There is good evidence that neither infant growth nor lactation is impaired by *DMPA* or progestin-only oral contraceptives (240). There is continued controversy as to how early *DMPA* should be given after delivery. Because lactation occurs in response to falling maternal estrogen and progesterone levels after birth, administration of *DMPA* in the first few days theoretically might interfere with the initiation of lactation. There is concern about the possible neonatal effects of the progestin, but investigators were unable to demonstrate the presence of *DMPA* or its metabolites in the urine of infants whose mothers received *DMPA* or any other suppression of reproductive hormones (240). In the United States, *DMPA* is commonly started at the time of hospital discharge, 48 to 72 hours after delivery. There is urgent need for controlled trials of immediate *DMPA* compared to other contraceptive options to determine whether this practice has an adverse effect on the initiation of lactation. **The "U.S. Medical Eligibility Criteria for Contraceptive Use 2010" considers *DMPA* use prior to 1 month postpartum as category 2: the benefit is thought to exceed the theoretical risk** (7).

DMPA and Neoplasia

Use of *DMPA* is not associated with cervical cancer (241). **Neither is it associated with ovarian cancer** (242). **Risk of endometrial cancer is substantially reduced by past use of *DMPA*** (243). A large study found no increase in breast cancer risk among *DMPA* users (244).

Benefits

DMPA has many of the noncontraceptive benefits of combination oral contraceptives (245). Decreases in anemia, PID, ectopic pregnancy, and endometrial cancer are reported. *DMPA* is reported to benefit women with sickle cell disease.

Subcutaneous *DMPA*

Depo-subQ Provera 104, a lower-dose *DMPA* preparation for subcutaneous administration, received FDA approval in 2005. The total dose is 30% less than that of the older *DMPA* intramuscular preparation. Because the dose is administered subcutaneously, blood levels are adequate to completely suppress ovulation for more than 13 weeks in all subjects tested, with a mean time of 30 weeks for return to ovulatory function (246). **Contraception efficacy is superb, with no pregnancies in a total of 16,023 woman-cycles in the phase III studies done in the United States** (247). Blood levels were lower in very obese women but still sufficient to completely suppress ovulation. The weight gain reported with the 150 mg *DMPA* remains a problem with the lower dose *DMPA*. Mean weight gain was 1.59 kg in the first year of use. Loss of bone density was observed with this dosage of *DMPA*, as with the larger intramuscular dose.

Once-a-Month Injectable

A once-a-month injectable contraception containing only 25 mg of *DMPA* in combination with 5 mg of the long-acting estrogen *estradiol cypionate* was briefly available in the United States, but was withdrawn by the manufacturer because of a packaging problem (248). Originally developed by the World Health Organization, it is described as *CycloFem* or *CycloProvera* in the literature and was marketed in the United States as *Lunelle* (249). Given once a month, this combination produces excellent contraceptive effects. Monthly withdrawal bleeding is similar to a normal menses, leading to high continuation rates despite the need for a monthly injection. Monthly injectable combinations continue to be widely used outside the United States.

Subdermal Implants

Three progestin-releasing subdermal implants systems are in use worldwide: *Jadelle*™, *Sino-Implant* II™, *and Implanon*™. All three offer long-acting contraception that requires no continuing action by the user and are, hence, forgettable. All are very highly effective and have no serious risk. Each can produce irregular bleeding, which is the principal reason for discontinuation. The mechanism of action is suppression of ovulation in the initial years of use, plus thickening of the cervical mucus that prevents sperm penetration.

The original *levonorgestrel* implant (*Norplant*™) six-rod system was replaced with a two-rod version (*Jadelle*™), which is identical in its release rate and clinical activity to *Norplant*™ and is easier to insert and remove (250). *Jadelle*™ is widely used around the world. It is approved by the FDA but is not marketed in the United States. It is approved for 5 years. The *Sino-Implant II*™ is a less expensive two-rod *levonorgestrel* system manufactured in China and available in several countries. It is effective for 4 years (251). *Implanon*™ is the only subdermal implant sold in the United States. It is a single rod system containing *etonogestrel*, the active metabolite of *desogestrel*. **Because of the greater potency of *etonogestrel*, the single rod releases enough to completely inhibit ovulation for at least 3 years. The single-rod system is most easily inserted and removed. In a United States trial, mean time for insertion was only a half minute and removal required a mean time of 3.5 minutes** (252).

A systematic review of 29,972 women and 28,108 woman-months of follow-up with *Norplant*™, *Jadelle*™, or Implanon™ found no differences in pregnancies or continuation rate over 4 years. No pregnancies occurred in any of the trials. There were no differences in side effects or adverse events. The most common side effect was unpredictable vaginal bleeding (253).

In 923 women followed for 20,648 treatment cycles in 11 studies there were no pregnancies with *Implanon*™ in place. Six pregnancies occurred within 14 days of removal of the devices. When these are included, as required by FDA, the cumulative Pearl index was 0.38 pregnancies per 100 woman-years at 3 years (254). Irregular bleeding was a problem, but occurred most frequently in the first 90 days of use and decreased over time. In a randomized comparison with the six-rod *Norplant*™, *Implanon*™ users had less frequent vaginal bleeding, but more became amenorrheic (255). Other commonly reported side effects are headache, weight gain, acne, breast tenderness, and emotional lability (254). Only 2.3% of subjects discontinued because of weight gain. Most women can use *Implanon*™. The US MEC lists only a small number of conditions as category 3, and these are based on theoretical concerns without actual evidence of harm (7). Insertion in the immediate postpartum period appears to have no adverse effects on mother or infant (256).

Bone density is not affected by *Implanon*™, probably because ovarian follicular activity is not totally suppressed and estradiol synthesis continues (257). Enlarged follicular ovarian cysts are common during the first year of use of *Jadelle*™ or *Implanon*™ and usually resolve spontaneously (258).

A comparative study of coagulation and fibrinolytic factors in users of *etonogestrel* and *levonorgestrel* implants showed no significant changes from baseline, with the exception of a modest increase in antithrombin III (ATIII)and a small decrease in factor VII activity, changes that might reduce coagulability. Lipid levels and liver function studies were not changed, with the exception of small elevations of bilirubin, with somewhat more observed in *levonorgestrel* users than *etonogestrel* users (259). Another study of hemostatic factors found modest decreases in many measurements, within the range of normal, and a modest reduction in the generation of thrombin in users of the *etonogestrel* implant (260). Taken together these studies provide considerable reassurance that the progestin implants do not increase thrombosis risk. With several million women now using the implants, there are no published studies linking either implant to venous thrombosis or myocardial infarction. Strokes were reported in users of *Norplant*™, but case reports do not allow calculation of whether risk is increased from baseline. Attempts to determine stroke risk of users compared to nonusers was inconclusive because so few stroke patients or controls were using the implant (261).

Emergency Contraception

Postcoital use of sex steroids to prevent pregnancy began in the 1960s with high-dose estrogen taken daily for 5 days (262). This was replaced with the combination OC containing *EE* and *levonorgestrel* for greater convenience (263). **More recently *levonorgestrel* alone became the method of choice after the World Health Organization showed its superiority in a large randomized trial with 1,998 women.** The pregnancy rate was 3.2% with the *EE/levonorgestrel* method and only 1.1% with *levonorgestrel* alone (RR for pregnancy, 0.32; 95% CI, 0.18–0.70) for women treated within 72 hours of intercourse. Nausea and vomiting occurred much less frequently with *levonorgestrel* alone (23.1% vs. 50.5%, and 5.6% vs. 18.8%, respectively) (264). The efficacy of both methods declined as the time after intercourse increased. **But even after 72 hours, the pregnancy rate with the *levonorgestrel* treatment was only 2.7%** (Fig. 10.9) (265). A single dose of 1.5 mg *levonorgestrel* is just as effective as two doses of 0.75 mg, has no more side effects, and is more convenient for the patient. Both dosing regimens are FDA approved. Because ***levonorgestrel* is almost as effective at 3 to 5 days after intercourse,**

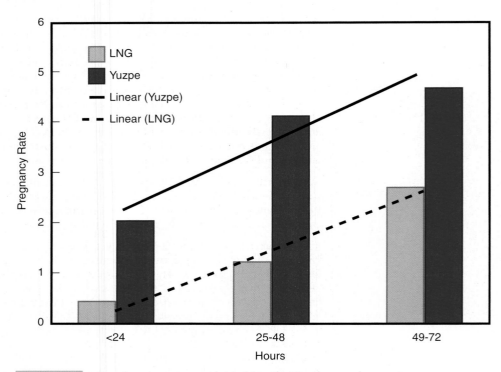

Figure 10.9 **Emergency contraception: pregnancy rates by treatment group and time since unprotected coitus.** LNG, *levonorgestrel,* 0.75 mg × 2. Yuzpe method is ethinyl estradiol, 0.100 mg plus *levonorgestrel* 0.50 mg × 2, 12 hours later. (From Randomized controlled trial of levonorgestrel versus the Yuzpe regimen of combined oral contraceptives for emergency contraception. Task Force on Postovulatory Methods of Fertility Regulation. *Lancet* 1998;352:430 [modified from Table 3], with permission.)

the World Health Organization recommends 1.5 mg of *levonorgestrel* as a single dose, given up to 120 hours after intercourse (266). Research suggests that the main mechanism of action is delay of ovulation. Noe and colleagues established that *levonorgestrel* works only if it is administered prior to the day of ovulation (267). No pregnancies occurred to 87 women who received *levonorgestrel* from 1 to 5 days prior to the day of ovulation. Seven pregnancies occurred to 35 women treated on the day of ovulation or later. **Postcoital *levonorgestrel* is not an abortifacient because it is effective only when taken before ovulation.**

Levonorgestrel alone is safer than the estrogen-containing preparations. There were several case reports of thrombotic events after use of the estrogen/levonorgestrel combination emergency contraception (268). No such complications with *levonorgestrel* alone were published.

Antiprogestins

The antiprogesterone *mifepristone* (*RU486*) is highly effective for postcoital contraception. The usual abortifacient dose is 200 mg, but a dose of only 10 mg is effective for emergency contraception. In one study, 2,065 women were randomized to *mifepristone,* 10 mg, or *levonorgestrel,* two doses of 0.75 mg, including women up to 120 hours after intercourse (269). The crude pregnancy rate was 1.3% for *mifepristone* and 2.0% for *levonorgestrel* ($p = .46$). Side effects were the same, and both methods were judged highly acceptable by the patients. *Mifepristone* is not being developed for this use and is not available at the appropriate dose.

Ulipristal, a new progesterone-receptor modulator developed at the U.S. National Institutes of Health was approved by the FDA and the European Union for emergency contraception to 120 hours after intercourse. **It is at least as effective as *levonorgestrel* 1.5 mg up to 72 hours, and may be superior between 72 and 120 hours** (270). When *Ulipristal* is administered prior to the luteinizing hormone (LH) peak, it delays rupture of the preovulatory follicle for 5 days or more, which may be its primary mechanism of action (271). *Ulipristal* is primarily metabolized by the CYP3A4 enzyme system; hence, patients on drugs such as barbiturates, *rifampin,* and several of the anticonvulsants may have reduced protection from pregnancy with it. It is a prescription drug, while *levonorgestrel* 1.5 mg is available over the counter in the United States for women 18 years of age and over.

The Copper Intrauterine Device for Emergency Contraception

Postcoital insertion of a copper IUD was first reported by Lippes et al. in 1976 (272). In initial trials the device was inserted within 7 days of intercourse and was more effective than steroids for emergency contraception. Studies included women only within 5 days from intercourse. The multicenter trial by Wu and colleagues is an example of the superb efficacy offered by the *copper T380A* (273). Of 1,893 women who returned for a follow-up visit, there were no pregnancies within 1 month of IUD insertion. **Efficacy for emergency contraception is 100% when the device is inserted up to 5 days after intercourse, and almost 100% up to 7 days after intercourse** (273). An added benefit was that 94% of the patients were continuing with the IUD at the 12-month follow-up. There were no uterine perforations. Zhou and colleagues reported similar excellent results in a large study with a different copper device, the *Multiload Cu-375* IUD (274). In much of the world, copper IUDs are very inexpensive. Even in the United States where IUDs are costly, the benefit to the patient of extremely effective emergency contraception, and long-term contraception with one intervention, makes emergency IUDs cost-effective. Whether the *levonorgestrel* IUD would work for emergency contraception is not known.

Hormonal Contraception for Men

The same negative feedback of sex steroids that blocks ovulation in women suppresses spermatogenesis in men, but it will produce loss of libido and potentially extinguish sexual performance. The principle was first demonstrated in 1974 using oral estrogen and methyl testosterone (275). Testosterone given alone can suppress sperm production to very low levels while maintaining normal libido and sexual performance. Over many years investigators have studied long-acting testosterone salts for male contraception (276). Ethnicity is an important predictor of efficacy of sperm suppression with testosterone therapy. Asian men virtually always achieve azoospermia or oligospermia when treated with *testosterone undecanoate* (*TU*) monthly injections, whereas only 86% of Caucasian men achieved azoospermia or oligospermia or with similar testosterone regimens (277). In a Chinese trial, 1,045 men were treated with monthly *TU* 500 mg. Only 4.8% failed to suppress to a sperm count less than 1×10^6 per mL. The cumulative pregnancy rate was only 1.1 per 100 men at 30 months (278). In Caucasian populations testosterone was combined with progestins to further suppress gonadotropin and improve efficacy. In an important trial with Caucasian men, *etonogestrel* subdermal implants and *TU* injections were compared to placebo implants and injections. Only 3% failed to suppress to a sperm count of less than 1×10^6 (279). Side effects that were more common in the medicated group than placebo included acne, night sweats, libido changes (usually increased), and weight gain. Theoretical risks include atherogenesis and prostate cancer but long-term trials will be needed to determine if risk is real. Liver cancer is a concern with long-term androgen therapy (280).

Sterilization

Surgical sterilization is the most common method of fertility control used by couples, with more than 180 million couples having tubal sterilization or vasectomy (4,281) Laparoscopic and hysteroscopic techniques for women and vasectomy for men are safe and readily available throughout the United States. The mean age at sterilization is 30 years. Age younger than 30 years when sterilized, conflict within the marriage, and divorce and remarriage are predictors of sterilization regret, which may lead to a request for reversal of sterilization (281).

Female Sterilization

Hysterectomy is no longer considered for sterilization because morbidity and mortality are too high in comparison with tubal sterilization. Vaginal tubal sterilization, which was associated with occasional pelvic abscess, is rarely performed in the United States. Five procedures are used in the United States.

1. Tubal sterilization at the time of laparotomy for a cesarean delivery or other abdominal operation
2. Postpartum minilaparotomy soon after vaginal delivery
3. Interval minilaparotomy
4. Laparoscopy
5. Hysteroscopy

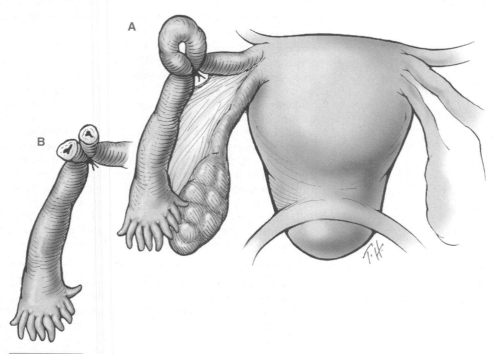

Figure 10.10   Pomeroy technique for tubal sterilization.

Postpartum tubal sterilization at the time of cesarean delivery adds no risk other than a slight prolongation of operating time; cesarean birth poses more risk than vaginal birth, and planned sterilization should not influence the decision to perform a cesarean delivery. Minilaparotomy can be performed in the immediate postpartum state. The uterus is enlarged, and the fallopian tubes lie in the midabdomen, easily accessible through a small, 3- to 4-cm subumbilical incision.

Interval minilaparotomy, first described by Uchida, was rediscovered and popularized in the early 1970s in response to an increased demand for sterilization procedures and a simpler alternative to laparoscopy (282). Still widely practiced in lower resource settings, it is uncommon in the United States because of widespread availability of the endoscopic techniques.

Surgical Technique

The procedure usually elected for tubal sterilization by laparotomy is the Pomeroy or modified Pomeroy technique (Fig. 10.10). In the classic Pomeroy procedure, a loop of tube is excised after ligating the base of the loop with a single absorbable suture. A modification of the procedure is excision of the midportion of the tube after ligation of the segment with two separate absorbable sutures. This modified procedure has several names: *partial salpingectomy, Parkland Hospital technique, separate sutures technique,* and *modified Pomeroy.* In the Madlener technique, now abandoned because of too many failures, a loop of tube is crushed by cross-clamping its base, ligated with permanent suture, and then excised. **Pomeroy and partial salpingectomy procedures have failure rates of 1 to 4 per 1,000 cases** (281). **In contrast, pregnancy is almost unheard of after tubal sterilization by the Irving or Uchida methods.** In the Irving method, the midportion of the tube is excised, and the proximal stump of each tube is turned back and led into a small stab wound in the wall of the uterus and sutured in place, creating a blind loop. With the Uchida method, a *saline-epinephrine* solution (1:1,000) is injected beneath the mucosa of the midportion of the tube, separating the mucosa from the underlying tube. The mucosa is incised along the antimesenteric border of the tube, and a tubal segment is excised under traction so that the ligated proximal stump will retract beneath the mucosa when released. The mucosa is then closed with sutures, burying the proximal stump and separating it from the distal stump. In Uchida's personal series of more than 20,000 cases, there were no pregnancies (282).

Laparoscopy

Laparoscopy is the most common method of interval sterilization in the United States. In the standard laparoscopy technique, the abdomen is inflated with a gas (carbon dioxide) through a special needle inserted at the lower margin of the umbilicus (281). A hollow sheath containing a pointed trocar is then pushed through the abdominal wall at the same location, the trocar is removed, and the laparoscope is inserted into the abdominal cavity through the sheath to visualize the pelvic organs. A second, smaller trocar is inserted in the suprapubic region to allow the insertion of special grasping forceps. Alternatively, an operating laparoscope that has a channel for the instruments can be used; thus, the procedure can be performed through a single small incision. Laparoscopic sterilization is usually performed in the hospital under general anesthesia but can be performed under local anesthesia with conscious sedation. Overnight hospitalization for laparoscopy is rarely needed.

Open Laparoscopy   Standard laparoscopy carries with it a small but definite risk for injury to major blood vessels with insertion of the sharp trocar. With the alternative technique of open laparoscopy, neither needle nor sharp trocar is used; instead, the peritoneal cavity is opened directly through an incision at the lower edge of the umbilicus. A special funnel-shaped sleeve, the Hassan cannula, is inserted, and the laparoscope is introduced through it.

Techniques for Tubal Closure at Laparoscopy   Sterilization is accomplished by any of four techniques: bipolar electrical coagulation, application of a small Silastic rubber band (Falope ring), the plastic and metal Hulka clip, or the Filshie clip. The Filshie clip, first introduced into the United States in 1996 is used extensively in the United Kingdom and Canada (283). It is a hinged device made of titanium with a liner of silicone rubber tubing. Because of its lower pregnancy rate, the Filshie clip has largely supplanted the Hulka clip (284).

In the bipolar electrocoagulation technique, the midisthmic portion of the tube and adjacent mesosalpinx are grasped with special bipolar forceps, and radiofrequency electric current is applied to three adjacent areas, coagulating 3 cm of tube (Fig. 10.11). The tube alone is then recoagulated in the same places. The radiofrequency generator must deliver at least 25 watts into a 100-ohm resistance at the probe tips to ensure coagulation of the complete thickness of the fallopian tube and not just the outer layer; otherwise, the sterilization will fail (285).

To apply the **Falope ring,** the midisthmic portion of the tube is grasped, with tongs advanced through a cylindrical probe that has the ring stretched around it (Fig. 10.12A). A loop of tube is pulled back into the probe, and the outer cylinder is advanced (Fig. 10.12B), releasing the Silastic ring around the base of the loop of tube, producing ischemic necrosis (Fig. 10.12C). If the tube cannot be pulled easily into the applicator, the operator should stop and change to electrical coagulation rather than persist and risk lacerating the tube with the Falope ring applicator. The

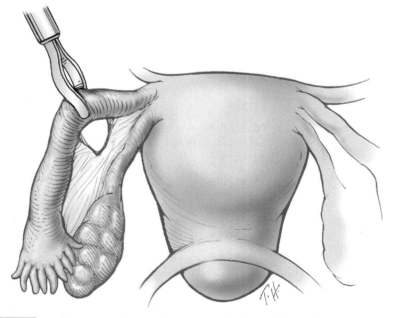

Figure 10.11   **Technique for bipolar electrocoagulation tubal sterilization.**

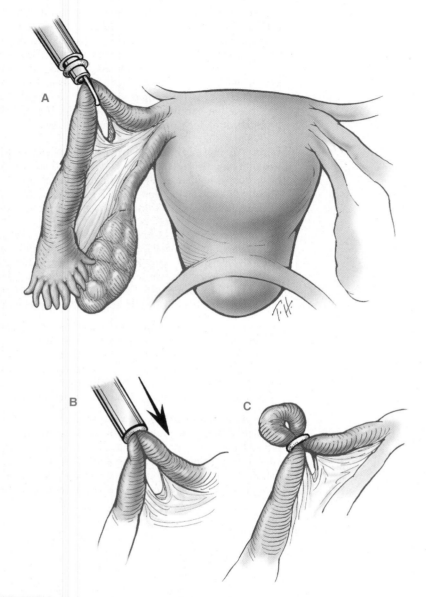

Figure 10.12   Placement of the Falope ring for tubal sterilization.

banded tube must be inspected at close range through the laparoscope to demonstrate that the full thickness of the tube was pulled through the Falope ring.

The **Hulka clip** is placed across the midisthmus, ensuring that the applicator is at right angles to the tube and that the tube is completely contained within the clip before the clip is closed. The **Filshie clip** is placed at right angles across the midisthmus, taking care that the anvil of the posterior jaw can be visualized through the mesosalpinx beyond the tube to ensure that the complete thickness of the tube is completely within the jaws of the clip before it is closed (Fig. 10.13).

The electric plus band or clip techniques each have advantages and disadvantages. Bipolar coagulation can be used with any fallopian tube. The Falope ring and Hulka and Filshie clips cannot be applied if the tube is thickened from previous salpingitis. There is more pain during the first several hours after Falope ring application. This can be prevented by bathing the tubes with a few milliliters of 2% *lidocaine* just before ring placement. Failures of the Falope ring or the clips generally result from misapplication, and pregnancy, if it occurs, is usually

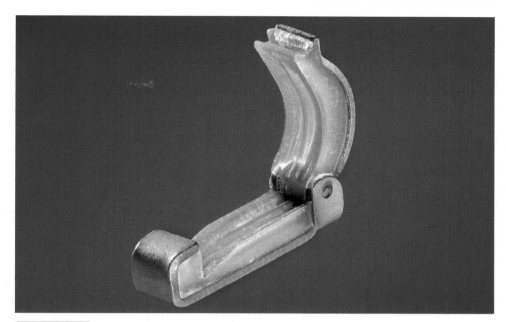

Figure 10.13 **Filshie clip for tubal sterilization.** (Courtesy of CooperSurgical, Inc., Trumbull, CT.)

intrauterine. After bipolar sterilization, pregnancy may result from tuboperitoneal fistula and is ectopic in more than 50% of cases. If inadequate electrical energy is used, a thin band of fallopian tube remains that contains the intact lumen and allows intrauterine pregnancy to occur. Thermocoagulation, the use of heat probes rather than electrical current, is employed extensively in Germany for laparoscopic tubal sterilization but is little used in the United States.

Risks of Tubal Sterilization	**Tubal sterilization is remarkably safe. The Collaborative Review of Sterilization (CREST) study, a 1983 review of 9,475 interval sterilizations from multiple centers in the United States, reported a total complication rate of 1.7 per 100 procedures** (281). Complications were increased by use of general anesthesia, previous pelvic or abdominal surgery, history of PID, obesity, and diabetes mellitus. The most common significant complication was unintended laparotomy for sterilization after intra-abdominal adhesions were found. In another series, 2,827 laparoscopic sterilizations were performed with the Silastic band using local anesthesia and intravenous sedation (286). Only four cases could not be completed (a technical failure rate of 0.14%), and laparotomy was never needed. Rarely, salpingitis can occur as a complication of the surgery. This occurs more often with electric coagulation than nonelectric techniques. Risk of death with female sterilization was 1 to 2 per 100,000 sterilizations in the last national study that was based on data from 1979 to 1980 (281). Almost half of the deaths were from complications of general anesthesia, usually related to the use of mask ventilation. When general anesthesia is used for laparoscopy, endotracheal intubation is mandatory because the pneumoperitoneum increases the risk of aspiration. International data from the Association for Voluntary Surgical Contraception show a similar record of safety from third world programs: 4.7 deaths per 100,000 female sterilizations and 0.5 deaths per 100,000 vasectomies (287).
Sterilization Failure	**Many "failures" occur during the first month after surgery and are the result of a pregnancy already begun when the sterilization was performed. Contraception should be continued until the day of surgery, and a sensitive pregnancy test should be routinely performed on the day of surgery.** Because implantation does not occur until 6 days after conception, a woman could conceive just before the procedure and there would be no way to detect it. Scheduling sterilization early in the menstrual cycle obviates the problem but adds to the logistic difficulty. Another cause of failure is the presence of anatomic abnormalities, usually adhesions surrounding and obscuring one or both tubes. An experienced laparoscopic surgeon with appropriate instruments usually can lyse the adhesions, restore normal anatomic relations, and positively identify the tube. In some circumstances successful sterilization will not be possible by laparoscopy, and the surgeon must know before surgery whether the patient is prepared to undergo laparotomy, if necessary,

Table 10.8 Ten-Year Life-Table Cumulative Probability of Pregnancy per 1,000 Procedures with Different Methods of Tubal Sterilization, United States, 1978–1986

Unipolar coagulation	7.5
Postpartum partial salpingectomy	7.5
Silastic band (Falope or Yoon)	17.7
Interval partial salpingectomy	20.1
Bipolar coagulation	24.8
Hulka-Clemens clip	36.5
Total: all methods	18.5

From **Peterson HB, Xia Z, Hughes JM, et al.** The risk of pregnancy after tubal sterilization: findings from the U.S. Collaborative Review of Sterilization. *Am J Obstet Gynecol* 1996;174:1164 [Table II], with permission.

to accomplish sterilization. The CREST study reported on a cohort of 10,685 women sterilized from 1978 to 1986 at any of 16 participating centers in the United States who were followed from 8 to 14 years (281). The true failure rates for 10 years obtained by the life-table method are given in Table 10.8. Pregnancies resulting from sterilization during the luteal phase of the cycle in which the surgery was performed were excluded. Of all remaining pregnancies, 33% were ectopic. **The most effective methods at 10 years were unipolar coagulation at laparoscopy and postpartum partial salpingectomy, generally a modified Pomeroy procedure. Bipolar tubal coagulation and the Hulka-Clemens clip were least effective.** The Filshie clip was not evaluated because it was not in use in the United States at the time. Younger women had higher risk for failure, as would be expected because of their greater fecundity.

Over the years since the CREST study began, sterilization by unipolar electrosurgery was abandoned because of the risk of bowel burns and was replaced with bipolar electrosurgery or the nonelectric methods (tubal ring, Hulka-Clemens clip, and the Filshie clip). An important later analysis of the CREST data found that bipolar sterilization can have a very low long-term failure rate if an adequate portion of the tube is coagulated. CREST study participants who were sterilized with bipolar electrosurgery from 1985 to 1987 had lower failure rates than those sterilized earlier (1978–1985). **The important difference was in the application technique of the electric energy to the tubes. Women whose bipolar procedure involved coagulation at three sites or more had low 5-year failure rates (3.2 per 1,000 procedures), whereas women who had fewer than three sites of tubal coagulation had a 5-year failure rate of 12.9 per 1,000** ($p = .01$) (288).

Family Health International reported large randomized multicenter trials of the different means of tubal sterilization. The Filshie and Hulka clips were compared in two trials. A total of 2,126 women were studied, of which 878 had either clip placed by minilaparotomy and 1,248 had either clip placed by laparoscopy. The women were evaluated at up to 24 months (289). **Pregnancy rates were 1.1 per 1,000 women with the Filshie clip and 6.9 per 1,000 with the Hulka clip at 12 months, a difference in rates that approached statistical significance** ($p = .06$). This same group compared the Filshie clip with the Silastic tubal ring in a similar study with a total of 2,746 women, of which 915 had the devices placed at minilaparotomy and 1,831 at laparoscopy (290). **Pregnancy rates at 12 months were the same for the Filshie clip and the tubal ring: 1.7 per 1,000 women.** The ring was judged more difficult to apply. The Filshie clip was expelled spontaneously from the vagina by three women during the 12 months of follow-up.

Hysteroscopy

In 2002, the FDA approved *Essure*™, a hysteroscopic method of permanent birth control, and a second hysteroscopy method, *Adiana*™, was approved in 2009. **Both methods can be provided in an office setting, with only local anesthesia or conscious sedation and both offer the prospect of greater safety, lower cost, and greater long-term effectiveness than the best laparoscopy methods.** *Essure*™ is a microinsert consisting of a soft stainless steel inner coil and a dynamic nickel titanium alloy outer coil (Fig. 10.14). Soft fibers of polyethylene terephthalate run along and through the inner coil. To insert the device, a hysteroscope is introduced into the uterine cavity, which is distended with saline. The tubal ostia are visualized. The *Essure*™ device

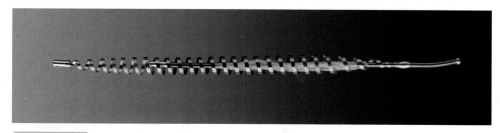

Figure 10.14   *Essure* **device for hysteroscopic sterilization.** (Courtesy of Conceptus, Inc.)

is inserted through the operating channel of the hysteroscope on the end of a slender delivery wire, guided into the tubal opening and advanced into the tube under direct vision (Fig. 10.15). Once in place, an outer sheath is retracted, releasing the outer coils, which expand to anchor the device in the interstitial portion of the tube. The delivery wire is detached and removed and the procedure repeated for the other tube. When properly placed, three to eight of the end coils of the microinsert are visible inside the uterine cavity. The rest are inside the fallopian tube (291,292).

The *Adiana*™ system consists of a catheter electrode that is guided into the interstitial portion of the fallopian tube via the operating channel of a 5-mm hysteroscope (Fig. 10.16). An array of bipolar electrodes on the catheter are used to apply radio frequency electric current for 60 seconds to achieve a temperature of 64°C, creating a superficial injury to the inner surface.

A 3.5-mm flexible cylindrical silicone matrix is deployed from the catheter into the tube at the site of the thermal lesion. The same process is repeated in the other tube. A nonionic medium such as 1.5% *glycine* is used to distend the uterus (293).

Essure™ and *Adiana*™ devices can be installed under local anesthesia in an outpatient setting. No incision is needed. A nonsteroidal anti-inflammatory drug is given 1 to 2 hours before the procedure to decrease tubal spasm. Over time fibrous tissue grows into both devices, occluding the tubes permanently. **Because of this mechanism of action, these methods depend on scar formation, and women who are immunocompromised from HIV infection, medication, or chemotherapy should be advised that their success may be lower** (293,294). **The FDA requires a 3-month follow-up x-ray hysterosalpingography examination to document tubal occlusion for both methods.** The hysterosalpingogram (HSG) for *Essure*™ should document bilateral placement of the devices at the uterotubal junction and a lack of peritoneal spillage of dye. Off-label and outside of the United States, plain x-ray, ultrasound, computerized x-ray tomography, and magnetic resonance imaging were used to confirm the presence and position of the *Essure*™ devices (295,296). The *Adiana*™ matrix is not radio opaque, so successful occlusion is documented only by lack of dye spillage. The patient with transcervical sterilization should continue to use a reliable method of contraception until successful occlusion is documented.

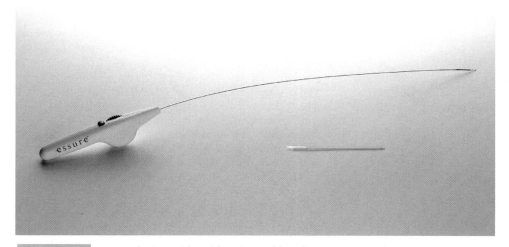

Figure 10.15   *Essure* **device with guide wire and handle.** (Courtesy of Conceptus, Inc.)

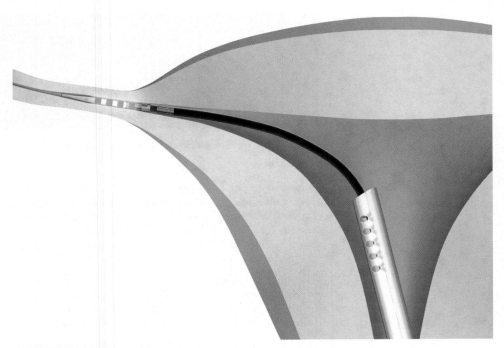

Figure 10.16   *Adiana* **catheter as placed for tubal sterilization.** (Courtesy of Hologic, Inc.)

Risks of Hysteroscopy

Adverse events or side effects were reported on the day of procedure in 3% of the initial *Essure*™ patients. These consisted of vasovagal responses, cramping, nausea, and vaginal spotting (297). Possible but uncommon risks of the hysteroscopic tubal sterilization methods include perforation by the device at insertion and expulsion of the device. In the initial clinical trials tubal perforation was reported in 1% of *Essure*™ placements. None were reported with *Adiana*™. There is theoretical risk of mutagenic or carcinogenic effect to the fetus from nickel alloy in *Essure*™ should pregnancy occur, although no such injury was reported (297). Other potential combinations with transcervical sterilization are related to the hysteroscopy procedure, not the tubal occlusion process. These include hypervolemia, injury to surrounding organs, bleeding, and infection and occur in less than 1% of cases. Excessive fluid absorbance leading to hypervolemia is more of a concern with *Adiana*™ and the nonionic solution that must be used to distend the uterine cavity because of the electrical energy applied. With *Essure*™ the distending medium is normal saline (293,294). An extensive 2009 review of the first 6 years of *Essure*™ use reported in publications, industry sources and the Manufacturer and User Facility Device Experience (MAUDE) database maintained by the FDA, found 20 reports of pelvic pain, which in some cases responded to hysteroscopy or laparoscopic removal of the device. An additional 20 women had second-look hysteroscopy because of persistent abnormal vaginal bleeding. During this time period more than 172,000 *Essure*™ devices were shipped, so such problems are quite rare (298).

Sterilization Failure with Hysteroscopic Methods

The *Essure*™ microinsert was successfully placed in 86% of patients after the first procedure, which increased to 90% after a second procedure using the initial insertion catheter. (298). Reasons for failure of insertion were tubal obstruction, stenosis, or difficulty in accessing the tubal ostia. **Correct placement was confirmed at 3 months in 96%, and complete bilateral occlusion occurred in 92%.** Of those patients with complete occlusion, there were no pregnancies in 5,305 woman-months of use. A subsequent study of an improved catheter design in 2004 reported a 98% successful placement rate (299). The *Adiana*™ trials reported a 94% successful placement rate with the first procedure, which increased to 95% after a second procedure (301).

As of October 2008, 258 *Essure*™-related pregnancies were reported to the manufacturer. Most can be attributed to patient or clinician noncompliance with the manufacturer's instructions, failure to use contraception during the 3-month wait for a HSG, failure to return for the HSG, physician error in interpreting the HSG, and some luteal phase pregnancies. **No known** pregnancies occurred in the clinical trials when the subjects met the criteria to rely on *Essure*™ (297).

In patients with documented occlusion in the *Adiana*™ trials, a 1.1% failure rate was reported in the first year of use and a 1.8% failure rate at 2 years (297). Longer-term data are not yet available for *Adiana*™, but it appears that *Essure*™ will have a lower long-term pregnancy rate than *Adiana*™.

Reversal of Sterilization

Reversal of sterilization is more successful after mechanical occlusion than after electrocoagulation, because the latter method destroys much more of the tube. With modern microsurgical techniques and an isthmus-to-isthmus anastomosis, the first-year pregnancy rate is about 44% (301). A retrospective review comparing microsurgical reanastomosis to *in vitro* fertilization (IVF) found similar total pregnancy rates, but a higher live birthrate with IVF because 10% of the pregnancies after microsurgery were ectopic (301). Hysteroscopic sterilization by the *Essure*™ and *Adiana*™ procedures should be considered irreversible. Reversal was not reported and would have to involve cornual resection and reimplantation of the fallopian tubes, a procedure with a very low success rate. IVF appears to be the only alternative for these women.

Late Sequelae of Tubal Sterilization

Increased menstrual irregularity and pain are attributed to previous tubal sterilization. Study of the problem is complicated by the fact that many women develop these symptoms as they age, even though they did not have tubal surgery and are treated with OCs that reduce pain and create an artificially normal menstrual cycle. Women who discontinue OC use after tubal sterilization will experience more dysmenorrhea and menstrual irregularity, which is unrelated to the sterilization. The best answer available comes from the CREST study (302). A total of 9,514 women who underwent tubal sterilization were compared with 573 women whose partners had undergone vasectomy. Both groups were followed up to 5 years with annual standardized telephone interviews. **Women who underwent tubal sterilization were no more likely to report persistent changes in intermenstrual bleeding or length of the menstrual cycle than women whose partners had vasectomy.** The sterilized women reported decreases in days of bleeding, amount of bleeding, and menstrual pain but were slightly more likely to report cycle irregularity (OR, 1.6; 95% CI, 1.1–2.3). **In summary, the CREST study provided good evidence that there is no posttubal ligation syndrome.**

Noncontraceptive Benefits of Tubal Sterilization

In addition to providing excellent contraception, tubal ligation is associated with reduced risk for ovarian cancer that persists for as long as 20 years after surgery (303).

Vasectomy

About 500,000 vasectomies are performed each year in the United States (281). Vasectomy is a highly effective method. The literature on efficacy is often difficult to interpret because most studies report failure as failure to achieve azoospermia, rather than long-term pregnancy rates among the relevant women. Vasectomy is not effective until all sperm are cleared by the reproductive tract. It is estimated that up to half of pregnancies after vasectomy occur during this time (304). In addition, not all pregnancies after vasectomy can be attributed to the men who had the operation. The best long-term information comes from the CREST study. The cumulative probability of failure was 7.4 per 1,000 procedures at 1 year and 11.3 at year 5, and comparable to the failure rate of tubal sterilization (281).

Vasectomy is usually performed under local anesthesia. The basic technique is to palpate the vas through the scrotum, grasp it with fingers or atraumatic forceps, make a small incision over the vas, and pull a loop of the vas into the incision. A small segment is removed, and then a needle electrode is used to coagulate the lumen of both ends. Improved techniques include the no-scalpel vasectomy, in which the pointed end of the forceps is used to puncture the skin over the vas. This small variation reduces the chance of bleeding and avoids the need to suture the incision. Another variation is the open-ended vasectomy, in which only the abdominal end of the severed vas is coagulated while the testicular end is left open. This is believed to prevent congestive epididymitis (305). Fascial interposition can be used with any of the above techniques and is widely believed to reduce recanalization. This technique involves securing the thin layer of tissue that surrounds the vas over one of the cut ends (306).

| Reversibility | **Vasectomy must be regarded as a permanent means of sterilization; however, with microsurgical techniques, vasovasostomy will result in pregnancy about half of the time. The longer the interval since vasectomy, the poorer is the chance of reversal.** |

Safety   **Operative complications include scrotal hematomas, wound infection, and epididymitis, but serious sequelae are rare.** There were no reports of deaths from vasectomy in the United States in many years, and the death rate in a large third world series was only 0.5 per 100,000. Studies of vasectomized monkeys showed accelerated atherosclerosis, but several large-scale **human studies found no connection between vasectomy and vascular disease** (307). There is no evidence of cardiovascular risk even 20 years after the operation (308). Concerns about long-term safety recurred with the report of a possible association between prostate cancer and vasectomy (309). Recent large studies present the very clear conclusion that vasectomy is not associated with prostate cancer (310–312).

Abortion

It is extremely likely that normal couples will experience at least one unwanted pregnancy at some time during their reproductive years. In third world countries, desired family size is larger, but access to effective contraception is limited. As a result, abortion is common. While there was a decline in the overall number of abortions worldwide from 46 million in 1995 to 42 million in 2003, this decline was greater in developed than in developing countries. About half of induced abortions are illegal and considered "unsafe" by the World Health Organization definition: procedures carried out either by an unskilled person or in unsafe conditions or both (313,314).

As shown in Table 10.9 total abortion rates are quite similar over much of the world. What differs is the rate of safe abortions compared with unsafe abortions. In the developed countries, unsafe abortions are rare. In the developing countries they are very common. The highest rates of unsafe abortion are in Latin America and Africa, where abortion is generally illegal. North America, where abortion is legal and contraceptive use is high, has a lower abortion rate, 21 per 1000 women of reproductive age. Abortion rates are even lower in Western Europe, 12 per 1000 (314). **Where abortion is legal, it is generally safe; where it is illegal, complications are common. Seventy thousand women die every year from complications of unsafe abortion. Societies cannot prevent abortion, but they can determine whether it will be illegal and dangerous or legal and safe.** Death from illegal abortion was once common in the United States. In the 1940s, more than 1,000 women died each year of complications from abortion

Table 10.9 Estimated Numbers and Rates of Safe and Unsafe Abortion Worldwide, by Region and Subregion, 2003

	Number of abortions (millions)			*Abortion rate[a]*		
	Total	*Safe*	*Unsafe*	*Total*	*Safe*	*Unsafe*
World	41.6	21.9	19.7	29	15	14
Developed countries	6.6	6.1	0.5	26	24	2
Developing countries	35.0	15.8	19.2	29	13	16
Africa	5.6	0.1	5.5	29	<0.5	29
Asia	25.9	16.2	9.8	29	18	11
Europe	4.3	3.9	0.5	28	25	3
Latin America & Caribbean	4.1	0.2	3.9	31	1	29
North America	1.5	1.5	<0.05	21	21	<0.5
Oceania	0.1	0.1	0.02	17	15	35

[a]Abortions per 1,000 women aged 15–44.
From **Sedgh G, Henshaw S, Singh S, et al.** Induced abortion: estimated rates and trends worldwide. *Lancet* 2007;370:1338–1345 [Table 2. P1342], with permission.

(315). In 1972, 24 women died of complications of legal abortion and 39 died from known illegal abortions. In 2005, the most recent year for which complete data are available, there were seven deaths from legally induced abortion and no deaths from illegal abortion (abortion induced by a nonprofessional) in the entire United States (316). The American Medical Association's Council on Scientific Affairs reviewed the impact of legal abortion and attributes the decline in deaths during this century to the introduction of antibiotics to treat sepsis; the widespread use of effective contraception beginning in the 1960s, which reduced the number of unwanted pregnancies; and the shift from illegal to legal abortion (317). The United States has a serious problem with teenage pregnancy. Without legal abortion, there would be almost twice as many teenage births each year.

The number of abortions reported each year in the United States—1.2 million in 2006—has been declining since the peak level of 1.61 million in 1990. In 2006, the national abortion ratio was 22.4 abortions for every 1,000 live births, and the national abortion rate was 19.4 per 1,000 women aged 15 to 44 years (318). While abortion rates for all racial and ethnic groups have declined, they are significantly higher for black and Hispanic women. Non-Hispanic white women have 22% of all abortions, black women have 37%, and Hispanic women 22%. Most women who obtain abortions are unmarried, 83.5% in 2006 (316). Use of abortion varies markedly with age. In 2006, 16.9% of women obtaining abortions were between 15 and 19 years of age, and 49.6% were 24 years of age or younger. In 2006, the abortion ratio for women younger than 15 years of age was 759 per 1,000 live births, almost as many abortions as births (Fig. 10.1). The lowest abortion ratio, 141 per 1,000 live births, is for women aged 30 to 34 years.

Regardless of personal feelings about the ethics of interrupting pregnancy, health professionals have a duty to know the medical facts about abortion and to share them with their patients (319). Providers are not required to perform abortions against their ethical principles, but they have a duty to help patients assess pregnancy risks and to make appropriate referrals.

Safety

The overall annual risk of death with legal abortion decreased markedly, from 4.1 per 100,000 in 1972 to 1.8 in 1976, and remained less than 1 per 100,000 since 1987. Risk of death with vacuum curettage was 0.1 per 100,000 at or before 8 weeks in 1993 to 1997 and 0.2 per 100,000 at 9 to 10 weeks (320). Risk increases exponentially with gestational age, reaching 2.7 per 100,000 for dilatation evacuation abortion at 16 to 20 weeks and 7.2 per 100,000 at 21 weeks or more. **The maternal mortality rate in the United States is 12.7 per 100,000 (321); hence, abortion by dilation and evacuation (D&E) through 20 weeks' gestation is safer than continuing pregnancy.** It was estimated that 87% of the legal abortion deaths occurring after 8 weeks would have been prevented had the woman been able get abortion services by 8 weeks (322).

For individual women with high-risk conditions (e.g., cyanotic heart disease), even late abortion is a safer alternative to birth. Because of the availability of low-cost, out-of-hospital, first-trimester abortion, 88% of legal abortions are performed during the first trimester (before 13 weeks of amenorrhea), when abortion is the safest.

Techniques for First-Trimester Abortion

Vacuum Curettage

Most first-trimester abortions are performed by vacuum curettage. Most are performed with local anesthesia with or without conscious sedation, and usually on an outpatient basis in a freestanding specialty clinic or doctor's office (323). Cervical dilatation is accomplished with metal dilators, or by laminaria tents or *misoprostol,* 400 μg, given vaginally or by the buccal route 3 to 4 hours before the procedure (324). A plastic vacuum cannula of 5- to 12-mm diameter is used with a manual vacuum source or an electric vacuum pump. Manual vacuum provided by a modified 50-mL syringe is as effective as the electric pump through 10 menstrual weeks (325). *Doxycycline* is given to prevent infection and has proven effective (326). Complications of a large number of vacuum curettage procedures before 14 weeks of gestation from Planned Parenthood of New York City are presented in Table 10.10. Mild infection not requiring hospitalization and retained tissue or clot requiring resuctioning in the clinic were the most common complications. Somewhat less than 1% experienced any complications, and less than 1 per 1,000

Table 10.10 Complications of 170,000 First-Trimester Abortions		
Number of cases (%)	**Rate**	
Minor complications		
Mild infection	784 (0.46)	1:216
Resuctioned day of surgery	307 (0.18)	1:553
Resuctioned subsequently	285 (0.17)	1:596
Cervical stenosis[a]	28 (0.016)	1:6,071
Cervical tear	18 (0.01)	1:9,444
Underestimation of gestational age	11 (0.006)	1:15,454
Convulsive seizure[b]	5 (0.004)	1:25,086
Total minor complications	1,483 (0.846)	1:118
Complications requiring hospitalization		
Incomplete abortion[c]	47 (0.28)	1:3,617
Sepsis[d]	36 (0.021)	1:4,722
Uterine perforation	16 (0.009)	1:10,625
Vaginal bleeding	12 (0.007)	1:14,166
Inability to complete abortion	6 (0.003)	1:28,333
Combined pregnancy[e]	4 (0.002)	1:42,500
Total requiring hospitalization	121 (0.071)	1:1,405

[a]Causing amenorrhea.
[b]After local anesthesia.
[c]Requiring hospitalization.
[d]Two or more days of fever 40°C or higher.
[e]Intrauterine and tubal pregnancy.
Adapted from **Hakim-Elahi E, Tovel HM, Burnhill HM, et al.** Complications of first trimester abortion: a report of 170,000 cases. *Obstet Gynecol* 1990:76:129–135.

were hospitalized (327). More extensive descriptions of the management of complications are published elsewhere (328,329).

Medical Means for First-Trimester Abortion

Mifepristone (RU486), an analogue of the progestin *norethindrone*, has strong affinity for the progesterone receptor but acts as an antagonist, blocking the effect of natural progesterone. Given alone, the drug was moderately effective in causing abortion of early pregnancy; the combination of *mifepristone* with a low dose of *prostaglandin* proved very effective, producing complete abortion in 96% to 99% of cases (330). The FDA approved a protocol of *mifepristone*, 600 mg orally, followed 2 days later by *misoprostol*, 400 mg, taken orally in women no more than 49 days from start of the last menstrual period. In the years before FDA approval, investigators established the superiority of the evidence-based protocols that are used. These protocols used 200 mg of *mifepristone* rather than 600 mg, because the lower dose is just as effective. Misoprostol, 800 μg is given by vaginal or buccal routes, which provides higher efficacy than the 400 μg oral dose (331–334). The *misoprostol* can be taken at 24, 48, or 72 hours after *mifepristone* with equal efficacy (333). Women may safely self-administer the *misoprostol* at home (334). It can be taken by buccal or vaginal routes with similar blood levels and similar areas under the plasma concentration curve (AUC) (335,336). After case reports of death from *Clostridium sordelli*, a large cohort study was published by Planned Parenthood describing use of prophylactic *doxycycline* 100 mg twice a day for one week, and buccal rather than vaginal administration of *misoprostol* (337).

Contraindications to medical abortion with *mifepristone/misoprostol* include ectopic pregnancy; an IUD in place (remove IUD first); chronic adrenal failure; concurrent long-term corticosteroid therapy; history of allergy to *mifepristone, misoprostol,* or other

prostaglandin; **and the inherited porphyrias (338).** The *mifepristone–misoprostol* combination was studied for gestations at 9 to 13 weeks; although it is almost as effective as earlier in pregnancy, a larger proportion of patients will experience heavy bleeding and require vacuum curettage (339).

Methotrexate/Misoprostol and *Misoprostol* Alone

Alternatives to medical abortion when *mifepristone* is not available include regimens with *methotrexate/misoprostol* and *misoprostol* alone. The antifolate *methotrexate* provides another medical approach to pregnancy termination, but takes longer than the technique using *mifepristone/misoprostol* (340). Medical abortion can be induced with *misoprostol* alone, although it is less effective than the *mifepristone/misoprostol* combination. Vaginal *misoprostol*, 800 μg, repeated in 24 hours if fetal expulsion has not occurred, produces a complete abortion in 91% of pregnancies up to 56 days of amenorrhea (341).

Complications of Medical Abortion

Heavy or prolonged bleeding is the principal complication, with up to 8% of women experiencing some bleeding for as long as 30 days. Need for surgical curettage is predicted by the gestational age when the *mifepristone* is administered. Two percent of women treated at 49 days or less, 3% of those treated at 50 to 56 days, and 5% of those treated at 57 to 63 days needed curettage for bleeding or failed abortion in a large study with 200 mg of *mifepristone* and 800 μg of vaginal *misoprostol* (342). Late bleeding, at 3 to 5 weeks after expulsion of the pregnancy, accounted for more than half of the curettages. The complications reported to the manufacturer of *mifepristone* from the first 80,000 patients treated were published (343). One woman died of ectopic pregnancy after refusing care. Another patient survived severe sepsis, and another, a 21-year-old woman with no risk factors, survived an acute myocardial infarction. Other severe sepsis cases have since occurred. A 27-year-old woman participating in a clinical trial in Canada died of multiple organ system failure from *Clostridium sordelli* sepsis after complete expulsion of a 5.5-week pregnancy despite receiving excellent care (344). Five other similar sepsis deaths were reported in the popular press. **The five deaths in the United States occurred among approximately 500,000 women treated with *mifepristone/misoprostol*, allowing estimation of a case fatality rate of 1 per 100,000, comparable to the rate of death with surgical abortion and much less than the risk of childbirth (345). There were no further cases of clostridial sepsis among the large number of women treated in the Planned Parenthood clinics when the new protocol of buccal *misoprostol* plus routine antibiotic prophylaxis was followed (337).**

Second-Trimester Abortion

Abortions performed after 13 weeks include those done because of fetal defects, medical illness, or psychiatric problems that had not manifested earlier in pregnancy, and changed social circumstances, such as abandonment by the father. Young maternal age is the single greatest factor determining the need for late abortion (317).

Dilation and Evacuation

D&E is the most commonly used method of midtrimester abortion in the United States. Typically, the cervix is prepared by insertion of hygroscopic dilators, stems of the seaweed *Laminaria japonicum* (laminaria), or Dilapan-S hydrophilic polymer rods. Placed in the cervical canal as small sticks, these devices take up water from the cervix and swell, triggering dilation. Laminaria, in addition, induces endogenous prostaglandin synthesis, which aids in cervical softening. When the dilators are removed the following day, sufficient cervical dilation is accomplished to allow insertion of strong forceps and a large-bore vacuum cannula to extract the fetus and placenta (346,348). Ultrasound guidance during the procedure is helpful (348). For more advanced procedures, dilators are inserted sequentially over 2 or more days to achieve a greater degree of cervical dilation (349). At the end of the midtrimester, procedures that combine serial cervical dilation with feticidal injections, induction of labor, and assisted expulsion of the fetus are used (350). Pretreatment for a few hours with buccal or vaginal misoprostol provides sufficient cervical softening and dilatation for early midtrimester D&E, and there is considerable interest in using this as an alternative to overnight laminaria further into the midtrimester (351).

Intact D&E is another modification useful for procedures at the end of the midtrimester. After wide cervical dilatation is achieved with serial placement of cervical dilators, the membranes are ruptured and an assisted breech delivery is performed, with decompression of the after-coming fetal head to allow delivery of the fetus intact (352).

In response to the federal abortion ban of 2003, an increasing number of providers are using feticidal agents prior to late second trimester terminations (353). Intra-amniotic or intrafetal *digoxin* and intracardiac *potassium chloride* are the two most common agents used for this purpose. Both are efficacious with little maternal adverse effects (354,355). The clinical utility of these agents is unproven. The only randomized controlled study looking at clinical outcomes found no change in procedure time or blood loss with the use of *digoxin* (356). Varying doses of *digoxin* were reported. In one study, 1.5 mg intra-amniotic *digoxin* was always successful in inducing fetal demise within 24 hours (357).

Labor-Induction Methods

In Europe and the United Kingdom labor induction is much more common than D&E for midtrimester abortion (358). Induction abortion with hypertonic saline or urea was widely employed for labor induction abortion in the 1970s. These were supplanted by the use of synthetic prostaglandins, and by regimens that combine *mifepristone* and *misoprostol*.

Prostaglandins   Prostaglandins of the E and F series can cause uterine contraction at any stage of gestation. The 15 methyl analogues of prostaglandin $F_2\alpha$ (*carboprost*) and prostaglandin E_2 (*dinoprostone*) are highly effective for midtrimester abortion but frequently produce side effects of vomiting, diarrhea, and with *dinoprostone*, fever. *Misoprostol* a 15 methyl analogue of PGE_1, is much less expensive than other prostaglandins, stable at room temperature, and at doses effective for abortion, produces many fewer side effects (359). Transient fetal survival is not infrequent after prostaglandin inductions. In the United States, it is common to produce fetal demise before induction with regimens similar to those used in late second trimester dilation and evacuation:. intra-amniotic or intrafetal *digoxin*, 1 to 1.5 mg, or fetal intracardiac *potassium chloride* (3 mL of a 2-mmol solution).

Midtrimester Mifepristone/Misoprostol   **Mifepristone pretreatment markedly increases the abortifacient efficacy of *gemeprost* and *misprostol*.** The mean interval from start of the prostaglandin to fetal expulsion is reduced to 6 to 9 hours, much shorter than with *misoprostol* alone (360). *Mifepristone*, 200 mg, is just as effective for this purpose as 600 mg (361). **A common protocol was developed using *mifepristone* and *misoprostol* that is now recommended both by the Royal College of Obstetricians and Gynecologists (RCOG) and the World Health Organization (WHO)** (358,362). Most women are cared for as hospital day-patients without need for overnight admission, a marked improvement over the labor induction methods of the past that often required 2 to 3 days of hospitalization. The protocol involves giving 200 mg of *mifepristone* orally on day 1. The patient returns 36 to 48 hours later for completion of the abortion with *misoprostol*. She is given 800 μg vaginally, and then 3 hours later, 400 μg is given orally and repeated at 3 hour intervals up to four doses. Efficacy is greater when the interval from *mifepristone* to starting *misoprostol* is at least 36 to 38 hours (363). **Mean times from the start of *misoprostol* to fetal expulsion are 5.9 to 6.6 hours** (358,360). The RCOG mandates that legal abortion must not be allowed to terminate in a live birth. Use of a feticide is required at 21 weeks (364). In the series by Ashok et al. of 1,002 women treated with the *mifepristone/misoprostol* protocol, described above, patients who had not expelled the fetus after 24 hours from start of the *misoprostol* were given an additional dose of 200 mg *mifepristone* at midnight, then started on another course of five doses of *misoprostol* the next morning, 800 μg initially, then 400 μg at 3 hour intervals, all given vaginally (360). About 8% needed a curettage procedure for retained placenta. Hemorrhage requiring transfusion occurred in about 1% of patients, usually from retained placenta.

Combination of Induction and Assisted Delivery

Hern developed a procedure that combines a feticidal injection of *digoxin* with serial insertion of multiple laminaria tents over 2 to 3 days, followed by amniotomy, placement of *misoprostol* in the lower uterine segment, and intravenous *oxytocin* to induce labor, and then an assisted delivery (365). The procedure was successful in a large case series at 18 to 34 weeks with very few complications.

High-Dose Oxytocin

***Oxytocin* in very high doses is as effective as *dinoprostone* at 17 to 24 weeks of pregnancy, but is not equal to the *mifepristone/misoprostol* regimen described above** (365). Patients initially receive an infusion of 50 U of *oxytocin* in 500 mL of 5% *dextrose* and normal saline over 3 hours; 1 hour of no *oxytocin*, followed by a 100-U, 500-mL solution over 3 hours; another hour of rest; and then a 150-U, 500-mL solution over 3 hours, alternating 3 hours of *oxytocin*

Table 10.11 Complications of 2,935 Midtrimester Dilation and Evacuation Abortion and Intervention Rates on a Referral Service

	Number (%)	95% Confidence Interval (%)
Complication		
Cervical Laceration	99 (3.3)	2.7–4.0
Atony	78 (2.6)	2.1–3.3
Hemorrhage	30 (1.0)	0.6–1.4
Other	15 (0.5)	0.3–0.8
Disseminated intravascular coagulation	7 (0.2)	0.1–0.4
Retained products	6 (0.2)	0.04–0.4
Perforation	6 (0.2)	0.04–0.4
Treatment of Complications		
Reaspiration	46 (1.5)	1.1–2.0
Hospitalization	42 (1.4)	1.0–1.8
Transfusion	30 (1.0)	0.7–1.4
Uterine artery embolization	21 (0.7)	0.4–1.0
Laparoscopy or laparotomy	13 (0.4)	0.2–0.7

From **Frick AC, Drey EA, Diedrich JT, et al.** Effect of prior cesarean delivery on risk of second-trimester surgical abortion complications. *Obstet Gynecol* 2010;115:762 [Table 2], with permission.

with 1 hour of rest. The *oxytocin* is increased by 50 U in each successive period, until a final concentration of 300 U in 500 mg.

Complications of Second Trimester Abortion

Surgical Abortion Complications

Complications of second trimester surgical abortion are uncommon, but risk increases with gestational age. Complications and their frequency encountered in almost 3,000 midtrimester abortions performed by laminaria followed by D&E on a referral service are listed in Table 10.11. The gestational ages were 14 to 27 weeks and mean gestational age was 20.2 weeks. **The most common complication was a cervical laceration that required suturing.** A major complication, defined as one necessitating transfusion, disseminated intravascular coagulation, reoperations with uterine artery embolization, laparoscopy, or laparotomy, was encountered in 1.3% of patients. History of two or more cesareans, gestational period of 20 weeks or more, and insufficient initial cervical dilation by laminaria were independent risk factors for a major complication in a multivariate analysis (366). The rates of complication in Table 10.11 cannot be directly compared to the rates of complications with labor-induction abortion described below because half of the D&E group were 20 weeks or more gestation, while only a few of the induction patients were more than 20 weeks.

Induction Abortion Complications

The labor-induction methods share common hazards: failure of the primary procedure to produce abortion within a reasonable time, incomplete abortion, retained placenta, hemorrhage, infection, and embolic phenomena. With modern protocols, these are rare. **In a series of 1,002 women treated with *mifepristone* and *misoprostol* at 13 to 21 weeks, 0.7% required a blood transfusion, 0.3% required ergot treatment for hemorrhage, and one required laparotomy for otherwise uncontrollable hemorrhage; 2.6% of patients received antibiotics for presumed pelvic infection after hospital discharge and 7.9% complained of prolonged bleeding** (360). Uterine rupture was reported in women with previous cesarean delivery treated with *misoprostol* in the midtrimester, but in a case series of 101 women with one or more previous cesarean births and three smaller case series totaling 87 patients, no ruptures occurred (367). Larger series are needed to quantify the risk.

Selective Fetal Reduction

Multifetal pregnancies are at risk for extremely preterm birth and major neonatal complications. To prevent this, selective reduction of higher-order multiple gestations often is practiced. The largest series describes 3,513 pregnancies treated with ultrasound-guided fetal intracardiac injection of potassium chloride (0.2–0.4 mL of a 2-mmol solution in the first trimester, 0.5–3.0 mL in the second trimester). The rate of fetal loss fell as operators gained experience. Loss was greater with higher starting number of gestations (starting number greater than six, 15.4% loss, decreasing to 6.2% loss for starting number of two gestations), and greater if more fetuses were left intact (finishing number three, 18.4% loss, decreasing to 7.6% for finishing number of gestations of one) (368). Another indication for selective reduction is the presence of one anomalous fetus in a multifetal gestation. In a series of 402 patients treated for this indication, rates of pregnancy loss after the procedure by gestational age at the time of procedure were 5.4% at 9 to 12 weeks, 8.7% at 13 to 18 weeks, 6.8% at 19 to 24 weeks, and 9.1% at 25 weeks or more (369). No maternal coagulopathy occurred, and no ischemic damages or coagulopathies were seen in the surviving neonates. Maternal serum α-fetoprotein remains elevated into the second trimester after first-trimester procedures (370). Because of the possibility of embolic phenomena and infarction in the surviving twin, a different technique is needed for selective reduction of monoamniotic twins or with monochorionic twin–twin transfusion syndrome. He and colleagues describe ultrasound guided bipolar coagulation of the umbilical cord of the affected twin in such cases (371).

The Future

Spermicides

Research includes efforts to develop spermicides and microbicides that prevent pregnancy and are effective against HIV and STDs. Trials of microbicides such as cellulose sulphate and surfactant were disappointing and showed no efficacy against HIV (371,372). The most promising research includes development of antiretroviral microbicides with alternative delivery systems such as rings and gels. The antiretroviral *tenofovir* has good safety and efficacy in animals and human tissue models and is being evaluated in human effectiveness studies (373).

Intrauterine Devices

The *GyneFix,* a frameless copper IUD available in Europe, consists of a surgical suture with small copper cylinders crimped to it. The knot on the proximal end of the suture is pushed 1 cm into the uterine wall with a special inserter. Comparative trials found it more effective than the *copper T380A* and it requires fewer removals for pain and bleeding (374).

Other ongoing research of IUDs includes a smaller *levonorgestrel* IUD that may be more acceptable to nulliparous women and IUDs that are suitable for irregularly shaped uteri (38).

Vaginal Rings

Silastic vaginal rings releasing either progestin or progestin–estrogen combinations were studied for years. The *NuvaRing* contains both estrogen and progestin, must be changed monthly, and has the same safety concerns as the other estrogen-containing hormonal methods. A new reusable ring, *Nestorone,* contains a nonandrogenic progestin that is inactive orally, and *ethinyl estradiol.* It can be worn for 3 weeks, removed for 1 week, and then reinserted for a total of 13 months of use (375). The advantage of this method is the use of a less androgenic progestin and the elimination of regular trips to the pharmacy. *Progering* contains natural progesterone and no estrogen. It is approved in some countries in Latin America and Asia. It was developed for up to 3 months use by breastfeeding women (376).

Barrier Methods

The *Ovaprene* ring is a nonhormonal "one-size-fits-all" intravaginal organic silicone ring that continuously releases spermiostatic and spermicidal agents over a 4-week period. The phase I trial demonstrated patient acceptability and safety and the product is in phase II trials (377). Under investigation is the SILCS diaphragm, a single-size reusable device with a contoured rim. This device is nonlatex and is available over the counter with no requirement for a pelvic examination (378). Another potential new barrier method under development is a female condom with a dissolvable capsule to ease insertion, a polyurethane vaginal pouch, and a soft outer ring.

Fit and concerns over slippage are improved by urethane foam that allows the condom to cling to the vaginal walls (38).

The Invisible Condom™ is a novel barrier/germicide/spermicide combination in human trials. It is a polymer gel that adheres to the vaginal and cervical mucosa when inserted into the vagina through a special applicator, forming a nondetectable physical barrier. One version has sodium laurel sulfate (SLS) incorporated in to the polymer film. The gel by itself blocks entry of HIV and of herpes virus into target cells *in vitro*. Daily vaginal application of the polymer plus SLS prevents pregnancy in rabbits (379).

Contraceptive Vaccines

Immunologic contraception–sterilization with vaccination against human chorionic gonadotropin was pursued for many years in India but appears to be abandoned (380). Zona pellucida glycoproteins are another target for a potential vaccine, but application in humans appears blocked by the ovarian dysfunction observed in animal studies (381). More promising are efforts that target sperm. Because of the large number of antigens associated with sperm, some of which are found on somatic cells, the challenge lies in choosing the correct antigen (382). The search continues for target proteins unique to reproduction to which a vaccine could be employed without adversely affecting other functions.

Male Contraception

As described earlier, considerable progress was made in hormonal contraception for men based on long-acting androgens in combination with progestins or GnRH antagonists. Nonhormonal male methods are being investigated. These include efforts to target and specifically interfere with spermatogenesis, epididymal sperm maturation, and sperm function (383). The majority of the targets being explored involve inhibiting sperm motility (384). Chinese researchers developed a method of percutaneous occlusion of the vas that was used in more than 100,000 men; it is effective and appears to be reversible. *Polyurethane elastomer* is injected into the vas, where it solidifies and forms a plug, providing an effective block to sperm. The plugs are removed using local anesthesia, and fertility returns in most cases after as long as 4 years with the plugs *in situ* (385).

Another potentially reversible method is the reversible inhibition of sperm under guidance (RISUG). This is a clear polymer gel mixed with dimethyl sulphoxide that solidifies, causing partial obstruction and the rupture of passing sperm membranes, when injected into the vas. Phase II trials demonstrated azoospermia for at least 1 year (38).

Simple Means for Female Sterilization

Another critical area for contraceptive development is nonsurgical means of sterilization of both men and women. Intrauterine quinacrine is the most promising method for nonsurgical female sterilization, but the method is embroiled in controversy because it was developed in the third world and moved quickly to widespread use without adequate proof of safety (386). Approximately 100,000 women were treated with it (387). The technique is very simple: pellets containing 252 mg of *quinacrine* are inserted into the uterus through an IUD inserter during the proliferative phase of the cycle and again 1 month later. Intrauterine *quinacrine* produces sclerosis of the proximal fallopian tube. In a large trial in Vietnam, the cumulative pregnancy rate for 1,335 women who received 2 doses was 3.3 at 1 year, 10.0 at 5 years, and 12.1 at 10 years (388). Another study of almost 25,000 women found the rate of ectopic pregnancy to be 0.26 per 1,000 women treated, which was similar to surgical sterilization and the IUD, OC pills, and condoms (0.42–0.45 per 1,000) and less than nonusers of contraception (1.18 per 1,000) (389). Concern was raised that *quinacrine* would lead to reproductive tract cancers. Two epidemiologic studies found no apparent increased risk for cancer from previous *quinacrine* sterilization in humans (390,391). A study of lifetime risk in rats sterilized with intrauterine *quinacrine* as young adults did find an increase in reproductive tract cancer in those rats treated with eight times the human dose, but not in the rats exposed to lower doses (392).

References

1. **Haymes, NE.** Medical history of contraception. New York: Gamut Press, 1963.
2. **Central Intelligence Agency.** The world factbook. https://www.cia.gov/library/publication/the-world-factbook/geos/xx.html.
3. **Cates W Jr.** Family planning, sexually transmitted diseases and contraceptive choice: a literature update: part I. *Fam Plann Perspect* 1992;24:75–84.
4. **Mosher WD, Jones J.** Use of contraception in the United States 1982–2008. National Survey of Family Growth. *Vital Health Stat* 2010;23:1–44.

5. **Jones RK, Darroch JE, Henshaw SK.** Patterns in the socioeconomic characteristics of women obtaining abortions in 2000–2001. *Perspect Sex Reprod Health* 2002;34:226–235.

6. **Ory, HW.** Mortality associated with fertility and fertility control: 1983. *Fam Plann Perspect* 1983;15:57–63.

7. **Centers for Disease Control and Prevention.** U.S. medical eligibility criteria for contraceptive use, 2010. *MMWR* 2010;59:1–86.

8. **Ashraf, T, Arnold SB, Maxfield, M.** Cost effectiveness of levonorgestrel subdermal implants: comparison with other contraceptive methods available in the United States. *J Reprod Med* 1994;39:791–798.

9. **Brown A.** Long-term contraceptives. *Best Pract Res Clin Obstet Gynaecol* 2010;24:617–631.

10. **Grimes DA.** Forgettable contraception. *Contraception* 2009;80:497–499.

11. **Potts M.** Coitus interruptus. In: Corson SL, Derman RJ, Tyrer L, eds. *Fertility control*. Boston, MA: Little, Brown, 1985:299–306.

12. **DiVincenzi, I (for the European Study Group).** A longitudinal study of human immunodeficiency virus transmission by heterosexual partners. *N Engl J Med* 1994;331:341–346.

13. **Jones RK, Fennell J, Higgins JA, et al.** Better than nothing or savvy risk-reduction practice? The importance of withdrawal. *Contraception* 2009;79:407–410.

14. **McNeilly AS.** Suckling and the control of gonadotropin secretion. In: Kenobi E, Neil JD, Ewing LI, et al., eds. *The physiology of reproduction*. New York: Raven Press, 1988:2323–2349.

15. **Short RV, Lewis PR, Renfree, MB, et al.** Contraceptive effects of extended lactational amenorrhoea: beyond the Bellagio Consensus. *Lancet* 1991;337:715–717.

16. **Queenan JT.** Contraception and breast feeding. *Clin Obstet Gynecol* 2004;47:734–739.

17. **Van der Wijden C, Kleijnen J, Van den Berk T.** Lactational amenorrhea for family planning. *Cochrane Database Syst Rev* 2003;4:CD001329.

18. **Lee SY, Kim MT, Kim SW, et al.** Effect of lifetime lactation on breast cancer risk: a Korean women's cohort study. *Int J Cancer* 2003;105:390–393.

19. **American College of Obstetricians and Gynecologists.** Special Report from ACOG. Breastfeeding: maternal and infant aspects. *ACOG Clinical Review* 2009;12: Supp. 1S-15S.

20. **Genuis SJ, Bouchard TP.** High-tech family planning: reproductive regulation through computerized fertility monitoring. *Eur J Obstet Gynecol Reprod Biol* 2010;153:124–130.

21. **Fehring RJ, Schneider M, Barron ML, et al.** Cohort comparison of two fertility awareness methods of family planning. *J Reprod Med* 2009;54:165–170.

22. **Russell, J, Grummer-Strawn, L.** Contraceptive failure of the ovulation method of periodic abstinence. *Fam Plann Perspect* 1990;22: 65–75.

23. **Che, Y, Cleland JG, Ali MM.** Periodic abstinence in developing countries: an assessment of failure rates and consequences. *Contraception* 2004;69:15–21.

24. **Guerrero R, Rojas OI.** Spontaneous abortion and aging of human ova and spermatozoa. *N Engl J Med* 1975;293.

25. **Gallo MF.** Non-latex versus latex male condoms for contraception. *Cochrane Database Syst Rev* 2003;2:CD003550.

26. **Grady, WR, Tanfer, K.** Condom breakage and slippage among men in the United States. *Fam Plann Perspect* 1994;26:107–112.

27. **Voeller B, Coulson AH, Bernstein GS, et al.** Mineral oil lubricant causes rapid deterioration of latex condoms. *Contraception* 1989;39:95–102.

28. **Stone KM, Grimes DA, Magder LS.** Personal protection against sexually transmitted diseases. *Am J Obstet Gynecol* 1986;155:180–188.

29. **Kelaghan J, Rubin GL, Ory HW, et al.** Barrier-method contraceptives and pelvic inflammatory disease. *JAMA* 1982;248:184–187.

30. **Cramer DW, Goldman MB, Schiff I, et al.** The relationship of tubal infertility to barrier method and oral contraceptive use. *JAMA* 1987;257:2246–2250.

31. **Judson FN, Ehret JM, Bodin GF, et al.** In vitro evaluations of condoms with and without nonoxynol 9 as physical and chemical barrier against *Chlamydia trachomatis,* herpes simplex virus type 2 and human immunodeficiency virus. *Sex Transm Dis* 1989;16: 251–256.

32. **Fischl MA, Dickinson GM, Scott GB, et al.** Evaluation of heterosexual partners, children, and household contacts of adults with AIDS. *JAMA* 1987;257:640–644.

33. **deVincenzi I.** A longitudinal study of human immunodeficiency virus transmission by heterosexual partners. European Study Group on Heterosexual Transmission of HIV. *N Engl J Med* 1994;331:341–346.

34. **Hira SK, Feldblum PJ, Kamanga J, et al.** Condom and nonoxynol-9 use and the incidence of HIV infection in serodiscordant couples in Zambia. *Int J STI AIDS* 1997;8:243–250.

35. **Wilkinson D, Ramjee G, Tholandi M, et al.** Nonoxynol-9 for preventing vaginal acquisition of sexually transmitted infections by women from men. *Cochrane Database Syst Rev* 2002;4:CD003939.

36. **Harris RW, Brinton LA, Cowdell RH, et al.** Characteristics of women with dysplasia or carcinoma in situ of the cervix uteri. *Br J Cancer* 1980;42:359–369.

37. **Parazzini F, Negri E, La Vecchia C, et al.** Barrier methods of contraception and the risk of cervical neoplasia. *Contraception* 1989;40: 519–530.

38. **Rowlands S.** New technologies in contraception. *BJOG* 2009;116: 230–239.

39. **Valappil T, Kelaghan J, Macaluso M, et al.** Female condom and male condom failure among women at high risk for sexually transmitted disease. *Sex Transm Dis* 2005;32:35–43.

40. **Galvao LW, Oliveira LC, Diaz J, et al.** Effectiveness of female condom and male condom in preventing exposure to semen during vaginal intercourse: a randomized trial. *Contraception* 2005;71:130–136.

41. **Trussel J, Sturgen K, Strickler J, et al.** Comparative efficacy of the female condom and other barrier methods. *Fam Plann Perspect* 1994;26:66–72.

42. **Soper DE, Brockwell NJ, Dalton HP.** Evaluation of the effects of a female condom on the female genital tract. *Contraception* 1991;44:21–29.

43. **Wilkinson D, Tholandi M, Ramjee G, et al.** Nonoxynol-9 spermicide for prevention of vaginally acquired HIV and other sexually transmitted infections: systematic review and meta-analysis of randomized controlled trials including more than 5,000 women. *Lancet Infect Dis* 2002;2:613–617.

44. **Malyk B.** *Nonoxynol-9: evaluation of vaginal absorption in humans.* Raritan, NJ: Ortho Pharmaceutical, 1983.

45. **Linn S, Schoenbaum SC, Monson RR, et al.** Lack of association between contraceptive usage and congenital malformation in offspring. *Am J Obstet Gynecol* 1983;147:923–928.

46. **Harlap S, Shiono PH, Ramcharon S, et al.** Chromosomal abnormalities in the Kaiser-Permanente birth defects study, with special reference to contraceptive use around the time of conception. *Teratology* 1985;31:381–387.

47. **Hooton TM, Hillier S, Johnson C, et al.** *Escherichia coli* bacteriuria and contraceptive method. *JAMA* 1991;265:64–69.

48. **van der Straten A, Kang MS, Posner SF, et al.** Predictors of diaphragm use as a potential sexually transmitted disease/HIV prevention method in Zimbabwe. *Sex Transm Dis* 2005;32:64–71.

49. **Hooton TM, Scholes D, Huges JP, et al.** A prospective study of risk factors for symptomatic urinary tract infection in young women. *N Engl J Med* 1996;335:468–474.

50. **Davis JP, Chesney J, Wand PJ, et al.** Toxic shock syndrome: epidemiologic features, recurrence, risk factors and prevention. *N Engl J Med* 1980;303:1429–1435.

51. **Shihata AA, Gollub E.** Acceptability of a new intravaginal barrier contraceptive device (Femcap) *Contraception* 1992;46:511–519.

52. **U.S. Food and Drug Administration.** US FDA FemCap Physician Labeling. Available online at: www.accessdata.fda.gov/cdrh_docs/pdf2/P020041c.pdf

53. **Yranski PA, Gamache ME.** New options for barrier contraception. *JOGNN* 2008; 37:384–89.

54. **U.S. Food and Drug Administration.** US FDA Lea's Shield Physician Labeling. Available online at: www.accessdata.fda.gov/cdrh_docs/pdf/P010043c.pdf

55. **Hatcher RA, Trussell J, Stewart F, et al.** *Contraceptive technology.* New York: Ardent Media, 2004.

56. **Borko E, McIntyre SL, Feldblum PJ.** A comparative clinical trial of the contraceptive sponge and Neo Sampoon tablets. *Obstet Gynecol* 1985;654:511–515.

57. **United Nations.** *World contraceptive use, 2007.* New York: United Nations Publications, 2007.

58. **Sivin I, Stern J.** Health during prolonged use of levonorgestrel 20 micrograms/d and the copper TCu 380A intrauterine contraceptive devices: a multicenter study. *Fertil Steril* 1994;61:70–77.

59. **El Badrawi HH, Hafez ES, Barnhart MI, et al.** Ultrastructural changes in human endometrium with copper and nonmedicated IUDs in utero. *Fertil Steril* 1981;36:41–49.

60. **Umapathysivam K, Jones WR.** Effects of contraceptive agents on the biochemical and protein composition of human endometrium. *Contraception* 1980;22:425–440.

61. Mirena Full Prescribing Information. Bayer Healthcare. Pharmaceuticals, 2009.

62. **Rose S, Chaudhari A, Peterson CM.** Mirena (levonorgestrel intrauterine system): successful novel drug delivery option in contraception. *Adv Drug Del Rev* 2009;61:808–812.

63. **Stanford JB, Mikolajczyk RT.** Mechanism of action of the intrauterine device: update and estimation of post fertilization effect. *Am J Obstet Gynecol* 2002;187:1699–1708.

64. **Alvarez F, Guiloff E, Brache V, et al.** New insights on the mode of action of intrauterine devices in women. *Fertil Steril* 1989;49:768–773.

65. **Segal S, Alvarez-Sanchez F, Adejeuwon CA, et al.** Absence of chorionic gonadotropin in sera of women who use intrauterine devices. *Fertil Steril* 1985;44:214–218.

66. **Anonymous.** Long term reversible contraception. Twelve years experience with the TCU380A and TCU220C. *Contraception* 1997; 56:341–352.

67. **Irvine GA, Campbell-Brown MB, Lumsden MA, et al.** Randomized comparative trial of the levonorgestrel intrauterine system and norethisterone for treatment of idiopathic menorrhagia. *BJOG* 1998;10:592–598.

68. **Magalhaes J, Aldrighi JM, de Lima GR.** Uterine volume and menstrual patters in users of the levonorgestrel-releasing intrauterine system with idiopathic menorrhagia or menorrhagia due to leiomyomas. *Contraception* 2007;75:193–198.

69. **Rizkalla HF, Higgins M, Kelehan P, et al.** Pathological findings associated with the presence of a Mirena intrauterine system at hysterectomy. *Int J Gynecol Pathol* 2008;27:74–78.

70. **Suhonen SP, Holmström T, Allonen HO, et al.** Intrauterine and subdermal progestin administration in postmenopausal hormone replacement therapy. *Fertil Steril* 1995;63:336–342.

71. **Hill DA, Weiss NS, Voigt LF, et al.** Endometrial cancer in relation to intrauterine device use. *Int J Cancer* 1997;70:278–281.

72. **Vercellini P.** A levonorgestrel-releasing intrauterine system for the treatment of dysmenorrheal associated with endometriosis: a pilot study. *Fertil Steril* 1999;72:505–508.

73. **Fedele L.** Use of a levonorgestrel-releasing intrauterine device in the treatment of rectovaginal endometriosis. *Fertil Steril* 2001;75:485–488.

74. **Sheng J, Zhang JP, Lu D.** The LNG-IUS study on adenomyosis: a 3-year follow-up study on the efficacy and side effects of the use of levonorgestrel intrauterine system for the treatment of dysmenorrhea associated with adenomyosis. *Contraception* 2009;79:189–193.

75. **Burkeman RT, for the Women's Health Study.** Association between intrauterine devices and pelvic inflammatory disease. *Obstet Gynecol* 1981;57:269–276.

76. **Farley TMM, Rosenberg MJ, Rowe PJ, et al.** Intrauterine devices and pelvic inflammatory disease: an international perspective. *Lancet* 1992;339:785–788.

77. **Lee NC, Rubin GL, Borucki R.** The intrauterine device and pelvic inflammatory disease revisited: new results from the Women's Health Study. *Obstet Gynecol* 1988;72:721–726.

78. **Kriplani A, Buckshee K, Relan S, et al.** Forgotten intrauterine device leading to actinomycotic pyometra, 13 years after menopause. *Eur J Obstet Gynecol Reprod Biol* 1994;53:215–216.

79. **Westhoff C.** IUDs and colonization or infection with *actinomyces.* *Contraception* 2007;75:S48–S50.

80. **World Health Organization.** *Select practice recommendations for contraceptive use.* Geneva: WHO, 2002.

81. **Mol BW.** Contraception and the risk of ectopic pregnancy. *Contraception* 1995;52:337.

82. **Mikkelsen MS, Højgaard A, Bor P.** [Extrauterine pregnancy with gestagen-releasing intrauterine device in situ] [in Danish]. *Ugeskr Laeger* 2010;172:1304–1305.

83. **Meirik O, Rowe PJ, Peregoudov A, et al.** IUD Research Group at the UNDP/UNFPA/WHO/World Bank Special Programme of Research, Development and Research Training in Human Reproduction. The frameless copper IUD (GyneFix) and the TCu380A IUD: results of an 8-year multicenter randomized comparative trial. *Contraception* 2009;80:133–141.

84. **Hubacher D, Lara-Ricalde R, Taylor D, et al.** Use of copper intrauterine device and the risk of tubal infertility among nulligravid women. *N Engl J Med* 2001;345:561–567.

85. **Vessey M, Doll R, Peto R, et al.** A long term follow up study of women using different methods of contraception—an interim report. *J Biosoc Sci* 1974;8:373–420.

86. **Sivin I, Stern J, Coutinho E, et al.** Prolonged intrauterine contraception: a seven-year randomized study of the levonorgestrel 20 mcg/day (LNg 20) and the Copper T380 Ag IUDS. *Contraception* 1991;44:473–480.

87. **World Health Organization.** *Mechanism of action, safety and efficacy of intrauterine devices.* Technical report series 753. Geneva: World Health Organization, 1987.

88. **Lyus R, Lohr P, Prager S.** Board of the Society of Family Planning. Use of the Mirena LNG-IUS and Paragard CuT380A intrauterine devices in nulliparous women. *Contraception* 2010;81: 367–371.

89. **Sinei SK, Morrison CS, Sekadde-Kigondu C, et al.** Complications of use of intrauterine devices among HIV-1 infected women. *Lancet* 1998;351:1238–1241.

90. **Richardson BA, Morrison CS, Sekadde-Kigondu C, et al.** Effect of intrauterine device on cervical shedding of HIV-1 DNA. *AIDS* 1999;13:2091–2097.

91. **Allen RH, Goldberg AB, Grimes DA.** Expanding access to intrauterine contraception. *Am J Obstet Gynecol* 2009;456:e1–e5.

92. **Grimes DA, Lopez LM, Schulz KF, et al.** Immediate postpartum insertion of intrauterine devices. *Cochrane Database Syst Rev* 2010;5:CD003036.

93. **Grimes DA, Lopez LM, Schulz KF, et al.** Immediate postabortal insertion of intrauterine devices. *Cochrane Database Syst Rev* 2010;6:CD001777.

94. **Goodman S, Hendlish SK, Reeves MF, et al.** Impact of immediate postabortal insertion of intrauterine contraception on repeat abortion. *Contraception* 2008;78:143–148.

95. **White MK, Ory HW, Rooks JB, et al.** Intrauterine device termination rates and the menstrual cycle day of insertion. *Obstet Gynecol* 1980;55:220–224.

96. **Allen RH, Bartz D, Grimes DA, et al.** Interventions for pain with intrauterine device insertion. *Cochrane Database Syst Rev* 2009;3:CD007373.

97. **Walsh T, Grimes D, Frezieres R, et al.** Randomized trial of prophylactic antibiotics before insertion of intrauterine devices. *Lancet* 1998;351:1005–1008.

98. **American College of Obstetricians and Gynecologists.** ACOG Committee Opinion. Intrauterine devices and adolescents. Number 392. December 2007. http://www.acog.org/navbar/current/publications.cfm.

99. **Fiala C, Gemzell-Danielsson K, Tang OS, et al.** Cervical priming with misoprostol prior to transcervical procedures. *Int J Gynaecol Obstet* 2007;99:68–71.

100. **Tatum HJ, Schmidt FH, Jain AK.** Management and outcome of pregnancies associated with copper-T intrauterine contraceptive device. *Am J Obstet Gynecol* 1976;126:869–877.

101. **Stubblefield PG, Fuller AF, Foster SG.** Ultrasound guided intrauterine removal of intrauterine contraceptive device in pregnancy. *Obstet Gynecol* 1988;72:961–964.

102. **Tietze C, Lewit S.** Evaluation of intrauterine devices: ninth progress report of the Cooperative Statistical Program. *Stud Fam Plann* 1970;1:1–40.

103. **Lippes J, Zielezny M.** The loop decade. *Mt Sinai J Med* 1975;4:353–356.

104. **Ronnerdag M, Odlind V.** Late bleeding problems with the levonorgestrel-releasing intrauterine system: evaluation of the endometrial cavity. *Contraception* 2007;75:268–270.

105. **Benaceraf BC, Shipp TD, Bromley B.** Three-dimensional ultrasound detection of abnormally located intrauterine contraceptive

devices which are a source of pelvic pain and abnormal bleeding. *Ultrasound Obstet Gynecol* 2009;34:110–115.

106. **Coffee AL, Kuehl TJ, Willis S, et al.** Oral contraceptives and premenstrual symptoms: comparison of a 21/7 and extended regimen. *Am J Obstet Gynecol* 2006;195:1311–1319.

107. **Johansson EDB, Sitruk-Ware R.** New delivery systems in contraception: vaginal rings. *Am J Obstet Gynecol* 2004;190:S54–S59.

108. **Spelsberg TC, Rories C, Rejman JJ.** Steroid action on gene expression: possible roles of regulatory genes and nuclear acceptor sites. *Biol Reprod* 1989;40:54–69.

109. **Phillips A.** The selectivity of a new progestin. *Acta Obstet Gynecol Scand* 1990;152(Suppl):21–24.

110. **Oelkers W.** Drospirenone, a progestin with antimineralocorticoid properties: a short review. *Mol Cell Endocrinol* 2004;217:255–261.

111. **Suthipongse W, Taneepanichskul S.** An open label randomized comparative study of oral contraceptives between medications containing 3 mg drospirenone/30 microg ethinylestradiol and 150 microg levonorgestrel/30 microg ethinylestradiol in Thai women. *Contraception* 2004;69:23–26.

112. **Guido M, Romualdi D, Guiliani M, et al.** Drospirenone for the treatment of hirsute women with polycystic ovary syndrome: a clinical, endocrinological, metabolic pilot study. *J Clin Endocrinol Metab* 2004;89:2817–2823.

113. **Kelly S, Davies E, Fearns S, et al.** Effects of oral contraceptives containing ethinylestradiol with either drospirenone or levonorgestrel on various parameters associated with well-being in healthy women: a randomized, single-blind, parallel-group, multicentre study. *Clin Drug Investig* 2010;30:325–326.

114. **Jensen JT.** Evaluation of a new estradiol oral contraceptive: estradiol valerate and dienogest. *Expert Opin Pharmacother* 2010;11:1147–1157.

115. **Brody SA, Turkes A, Goldzieher JW.** Pharmacokinetics of three bioequivalent norethindrone/mestranol-50 mcg and three norethindrone/ethinyl estradiol-35 mg formulations: are "low dose" pills really lower? *Contraception* 1989;40:269–284.

116. **Dericks-Tan JSE, Kock P, Taubert HD.** Synthesis and release of gonadotropins: effect of an oral contraceptive. *Obstet Gynecol* 1983;62:687–690.

117. **Gaspard UJ, Dubois M, Gillain D, et al.** Ovarian function is effectively inhibited by a low dose triphasic oral contraceptive containing ethinyl estradiol and levonorgestrel. *Contraception* 1984;29:305–318.

118. **Landgren BM.** Mechanism of action of gestagens. *Int J Gynaecol Obstet* 1990;32:95–110.

119. **Makarainen L, van Beck A, Tuomivaara L, et al.** Ovarian function during the use of a single implant: Implanon compared with Norplant. *Fertil Steril* 1998;69:714–721.

120. **Luukkainen T, Heikinheimo O, Haukkamaa M, et al.** Inhibition of folliculogenesis and ovulation by the antiprogesterone RU 486. *Fertil Steril* 1988;49:961–963.

121. **Van Uem JF, Hsiu JG, Chillik CF, et al.** Contraceptive potential of RU486 by ovulation inhibition. I. Pituitary versus ovarian action with blockade of estrogen-induced endometrial proliferation. *Contraception* 1989;40:171–184

122. **Audet MC, Moreau M, Koltun WD, et al.** Evaluation of contraceptive efficacy and cycle control of a transdermal contraceptive patch vs an oral contraceptive. *JAMA* 2001;285:2347–2354.

123. **Killick S.** Complete and robust ovulation inhibition with the NuvaRing. *Euro J Contraception Reprod Health Care* 2002; 7(Suppl 2):13–18.

124. **Society of Family Planning.** Clinical guidelines: contraceptive considerations in obese women. *Contraception* 2009;80:583–590.

125. **Lopez LM, Grimes DA, Chen-Mok M, et al.** Hormonal contraceptives for contraception in overweight or obese women. *Cochrane Database Syst Rev* 2010;7:CD008452.

126. **Sivin I, Lahteenmaki P, Ranta S, et al.** Levonorgestrel concentrations during use of levonorgestrel rod (LNG ROD) implants. *Contraception* 1997;55:81–85.

127. **Ambrus JL, Mink IB, Courey NG, et al.** Progestational agents and blood coagulation. VII. Thromboembolic and other complications of oral contraceptive therapy in relationship to pretreatment levels of blood coagulation factors: summary report of a ten year study. *Am J Obstet Gynecol* 1976;125:1057–1062.

128. **Winkler UH, Buhler K, Schindler AE.** The dynamic balance of hemostasis: implications for the risk of oral contraceptive use. In: Runnebaum B, Rabe T, Kissel L, eds. *Female contraception and male fertility regulation.* Advances in Gynecological and Obstetric Research Series. Confort, England: Parthenon Publishing Group, 1991:85–92.

129. **Gerstman BB, Piper JM, Tomita DK, et al.** Oral contraceptive dose and the risk of deep venous thromboembolic disease. *Am J Epidemiol* 1991;133:32–37.

130. **Lidegaard O, Lokkegaard E, Svendsen AL, et al.** Hormonal contraception and risk of venous thromboembolism: national follow-up study. *BMJ* 2009;339:b2890.

131. **Farmer RDT, Preston TD.** The risk of venous thromboembolism associated with low oestrogen oral contraceptives. *J Obstet Gynaecol* 1995;15:195–200.

132. **Bertina RM, Koeleman BP, Koster T, et al.** Mutation in blood coagulation factor V associated with resistance to activated protein C. *Nature* 1994;369:64–67.

133. **Vandenbroucke JP, Koster T, Briet E, et al.** Increased risk of venous thrombosis in oral contraceptive users who are carriers of factor V Leiden mutation. *Lancet* 1994;344:1453–1457.

134. **DeStefano V, Chiusolo P, Paciaroni K, et al.** Epidemiology of factor V Leiden: clinical implications. *Semin Thromb Hemost* 1998;24:367–379.

135. **Martinelli I, Sacchi E, Landi G, et al.** High risk of cerebral vein thrombosis in carriers of a prothrombin gene mutation and in users of oral contraceptives. *N Engl J Med* 1988;338:1793–1797.

136. **Trauscht-Van Horn JJ, Capeless EL, Easterling TR, et al.** Pregnancy loss and thrombosis with protein C deficiency. *Am J Obstet Gynecol* 1992;167:968–972.

137. **Vandenbroucke JP, van der Meer FJM, Helmerhorst FM, et al.** Factor V Leiden: should we screen oral contraceptive users and pregnant women? *BMJ* 1996;313:1127–1130.

138. **Comp PC.** Should coagulation tests be used to determine which oral contraceptive users have an increased risk of thrombophlebitis? *Contraception* 2006;73:4–5.

139. **Heinemann LA, Dinger JC, Assmann A, et al.** Use of oral contraceptives containing gestodene and risk of venous thromboembolism: outlook 10 years after the third generation "pill scare." *Contraception* 2010;81:401–405.

140. **van Hylckama Vlieg A, Helmerhorhorst FM, Vandenbroucke JP, et al.** The venous thrombotic risk of oral contraceptives, effects of oestrogen dose and progestogen type: results of the MEGA case-control study. *BMJ* 2009;339:h2921.

141. **Mant D, Villard-Mackintosh L, Vessey MP, et al.** Myocardial infarction and angina pectoris in young women. *J Epidemiol Community Health* 1987;41:215–219.

142. **Rosenberg L, Kaufman DW, Helmrich SP, et al.** Myocardial infarction and cigarette smoking in women younger than 50 years of age. *JAMA* 1985;253:2965–2969.

143. **Sidney S, Petitt DB, Quesenberry CP, et al.** Myocardial infarction in users of low dose oral contraceptives. *Obstet Gynecol* 1996;88:939–944.

144. **Sidney S, Siscovick DS, Petitti DB, et al.** Myocardial infarction and use of low dose oral contraceptives: a pooled analysis of 2 U.S. studies. *Circulation* 1998;98:1058–1063.

145. **Stampfer MJ, Willett WC, Colditz GA, et al.** A prospective study of past use of oral contraceptive agents and risk of cardiovascular diseases. *N Engl J Med* 1988;319:1313–1317.

146. **Margolis KL, Adami H-O, Luo J, et al.** A prospective study of oral contraceptive use and risk of myocardial infarction among Swedish women. *Fertil Steril* 2007;88:310–316.

147. **Vessey MP, Lawless M, Yeates D.** Oral contraceptives and stroke: findings in a large prospective study. *BMJ* 1984;289:530–531.

148. **Levine SR, Fagan SC, Pessin MS, et al.** Accelerated intracranial occlusive disease, oral contraceptives, and cigarette use. *Neurology* 1991;41:1893–1901.

149. **Petitti DB, Sidney S, Bernstein A, et al.** Stroke in users of low dose oral contraceptives. *N Engl J Med* 1996;335:8–15.

150. **World Health Organization Collaborative Study of Cardiovascular Disease and Steroid Hormone Contraception.** Ischaemic stroke and combined oral contraceptives: results of an international, multicenter, case control study. *Lancet* 1996;348:505–510.

151. **World Health Organization Collaborative Study of Cardiovascular Disease and Steroid Hormone Contraception.** Hemorrhagic

stroke, overall stroke risk, and combined oral contraceptives: results of an international, multicenter, case control study. *Lancet* 1996; 348:505–510.

152. **Lidegaard O.** Oral contraceptives, pregnancy and the risk of cerebral thromboembolism: the influence of diabetes, hypertension, migraine and previous thromboembolic disease. *BJOG* 1995;102:153–159.

153. **Curtis KM, Mohllajee AP, Summer LM, et al.** Combined oral contraceptive use among women with hypertension: a systematic review. *Contraception* 2006;73:179–188.

154. **Spellacy WN, Buhi WC, Birk SA.** The effect of estrogens on carbohydrate metabolism: glucose, insulin, and growth hormone studies on 171 women ingesting Premarin, mestranol and ethinyl estradiol for six months. *Am J Obstet Gynecol* 1972;114:378–392.

155. **Knopp RH.** Cardiovascular effects of endogenous and exogenous sex hormones over a woman's lifetime. *Am J Obstet Gynecol* 1988;158:1630–1643.

156. **Burkman RT, Zacur HA, Kimball AW, et al.** Oral contraceptives and lipids and lipoproteins. II. Relationship to plasma steroid levels and outlier status. *Contraception* 1989;40:675–689.

157. **Godsland IF, Crook D, Simpson R, et al.** The effects of different formulations of oral contraceptive agents on lipids and carbohydrate metabolism. *N Engl J Med* 1990;323:1375–1381.

158. **Mishell DR Jr, Colodyn SZ, Swanson LA.** The effect of an oral contraceptive on tests of thyroid function. *Fertil Steril* 1969;20:335–339.

159. **Centers for Disease Control Cancer and Steroid Hormone Study.** Oral contraceptive use and the risk of ovarian cancer. *JAMA* 1983;249:1596–1599.

160. **Centers for Disease Control Cancer and Steroid Hormone Study.** Oral contraceptive use and the risk of endometrial cancer. *JAMA* 1983;249:1600–1604.

161. **Dossus L, Allen N, Kaaks R, et al.** Reproductive risk factors and endometrial cancer: the European Prospective Investigation into Cancer and Nutrition. *Int J Cancer* 2010;127:442–451.

162. **Beral V, Hermon C, Clifford K, et al.** Mortality in relation to oral contraceptive use: 25 year follow-up of women in the Royal College of General Practitioners' Oral Contraception Study. *BMJ* 1999;318:96–100.

163. **Cibula D, Gompel A, Mueck AO, et al.** Hormonal contraception and risk of cancer. *Human Reprod Update* 2010;16:631–650.

164. **Ness RB, Grisso JA, Klapper J, et al.** Risk of ovarian cancer in relation to estrogen and progestin dose and use characteristics of oral contraceptives. *Am J Epidemiol* 2000;152:233–241.

165. **Kumle M, Weiderpass E, Braaten T, et al.** Risk for invasive and borderline epithelial ovarian neoplasias following use of hormonal contraceptives: the Norwegian-Swedish Women's Lifestyles and Health Cohort Study. *Br J Cancer* 2004;90:1386–1391.

166. **Smith JS, Green J, Berrington de Gonzales A, et al.** Cervical cancer and use of hormonal contraceptives: a systematic review. *Lancet* 2003;363:1159–1167.

167. **Appleby P, Beral V, Berrington de Gonzales A, et al.** Cervical cancer and hormonal contraceptives: collaborative reanalysis of individual data for 16,573 women with cervical cancer and 35,509 women without cervical cancer from 24 epidemiological studies. *Lancet* 2007;370:1609–1621.

168. **Miller K, Blumenthal P, Blanchard K.** Oral contraceptives and cervical cancer: critique of a recent review. *Contraception* 2004;69:347–351.

169. **Swann SH, Petitti DB.** A review of problems of bias and confounding in epidemiologic studies of cervical neoplasia and oral contraceptive use. *Am J Epidemiol* 1982;115:10–18.

170. **Schiffman MH, Bauer HM, Hoover RN, et al.** Epidemiologic evidence showing that human papilloma virus infection causes most cervical intraepithelial neoplasia. *J Natl Cancer Inst* 1993;85:958–964.

171. **Ursin G, Peters RK, Henderson BE, et al.** Oral contraceptive use and adenocarcinoma of cervix. *Lancet* 1994;344:1390–1394.

172. **Castellsague X, Diaz M, de Sanjose S, et al.** Worldwide human papilloma virus etiology of cervical adenocarcinoma and its cofactors: implications for screening and prevention. *J Natl Cancer Inst* 2006;98:303–315.

173. **Chilvers C.** Oral contraceptives and cancer. *Lancet* 1994;344:1378–1379.

174. **Collaborative Group on Hormonal Factors in Breast Cancer.** Breast cancer and hormonal contraceptives: collaborative reanalysis of individual data on 53,297 women with breast cancer and 100,239 women without breast cancer from 54 epidemiologic studies. *Lancet* 1996;347:1713–1727.

175. **Marchbanks PA, McDonald JA, Wilson HG, et al.** Oral contraceptives and risk of breast cancer. *N Engl J Med* 2002;346:2025–2032.

176. **Magnusson CM, Persson IR, Baron JA, et al.** The role of reproductive factors and use of oral contraceptives in the aetiology of breast cancer in women aged 50–74 years. *Int J Cancer* 1999;80:231–236.

177. **Lee Huiyan M, McKean-Cowdin R, Van Den Berg D, et al.** Effect of reproductive factors and oral contraceptives on breast cancer risk in BRCA1/2 mutation carriers and noncarriers: results from a population-based study. *Cancer Epidemiol Biomarkers Prev* 2008;17:3170–3178.

178. **Rooks JB, Ory HW, Ishak KG, et al.** Epidemiology of hepatocellular adenoma: the role of oral contraceptive use. *JAMA* 1979;262:644–648.

179. **Fiel MI, Min A, Gerber MA, et al.** Hepatocellular carcinoma in long term oral contraceptive users. *Liver* 1996;16:372–376.

180. **Anonymous.** Oral contraceptives and liver cancer: results from the Multicentre International Liver Tumor Study (MILTS). *Contraception* 1997;56:275–284.

181. **Kapp N, Tilley IB, Curtis KM.** The effects of hormonal contraceptive use among women with viral hepatitis or cirrhosis of the liver: a systematic review. *Contraception* 2009;80:381–386.

182. **Burkman R, Schlesselman JJ, Zieman M.** Safety concerns and health benefits associated with oral contraception. *AM J Obstet Gynecol* 2004;190:S12.

183. **Wolner-Hanssen P, Eschenbach DA, Paavonen J, et al.** Decreased risk of symptomatic chlamydial pelvic inflammatory disease associated with oral contraceptives. *JAMA* 1990;263:54–59.

184. **Ness R, Soper D, Holley R, et al.** Hormonal and barrier contraception and the risk of upper genital tract disease in the PID Evaluation and Clinical Health (PEACH) Study. *Am J Obstet Gynecol* 2001;185:121–127.

185. **Morrison CS, Richardson BA, Mmiro F, et al.** Hormonal contraception and the risk of HIV acquisition. *AIDS* 2007;21:85–95.

186. **Franks AL, Beral V, Cates W Jr, et al.** Contraception and ectopic pregnancy risk. *Am J Obstet Gynecol* 1990;163:1120–1123.

187. **Narod SA, Risch H, Moslehi R, et al.** Oral contraceptives and the risk of hereditary ovarian cancer. Hereditary Ovarian Cancer Clinical Study Group. *N Engl J Med* 1998;339:424–428.

188. **Rodriguez GC, Walmer DK, Cline M, et al.** Effect of progestin on the ovarian epithelium of macaques: cancer prevention through apoptosis. *J Soc Gynecol Investig* 1998;5:271–276.

189. **Vessey M, Yeates D.** Oral contraceptives and benign breast disease: an upate of findings in a large cohort study. *Contraception* 2007;76:418–424.

190. **Lanes SF, Birmann B, Walker AM, et al.** Oral contraceptive type and functional ovarian cysts. *Am J Obstet Gynecol* 1992;166:956–961.

191. **ACOG.** Noncontraceptive use of hormonal contraceptives. Practice Bulletin. No. 110. *Obstet Gynecol* 2010;115:206–218.

192. **Chiaffarino F, Parazzini F, LaVecchia C, et al.** Use of oral contraceptives and uterine fibroids: results from a case-control study. *BJOG* 1999;106:857–860.

193. **Fernandez E, La Vecchia C, Franceschi S, et al.** Oral contraceptives and risk of colorectal cancer. *Epidemiology* 1998;9:295–300.

194. **Martinez ME, Grodstein F, Giovannucci E, et al.** A prospective study of reproductive factors, oral contraceptive use and risk of colorectal cancer. *Cancer Epidemiol Biomarkers Prev* 1997;6:1–5.

195. **Nichols HB, Trentham-Dietz A, Hampton JM, et al.** Oral contraceptive use, reproductive factors, and colorectal cancer risk: findings from Wisconsin. *Cancer Epidemiol Biomarkers Prev* 2005;14:1212–1218.

196. **Shy KK, McTiernan AM, Daling JR, et al.** Oral contraceptive use and the occurrence of pituitary prolactinoma. *JAMA* 1983;249:2204–2207.

197. **Adams DB, Gold AR, Burt AD.** Rise in female initiated sexual activity at ovulation and its suppression by oral contraceptives. *N Engl J Med* 1978;299:1145–1150.

198. **Martin-Loeches M, Ortí RM, Monfort M, et al.** A comparative analysis of the modification of sexual desire of users of oral hormonal

contraceptives and intrauterine contraceptive devices. *Eur J Contracept Reprod Health Care* 2003;8:129–134.

199. **Caruso S, Agnello C, Intelisano G, et al.** Prospective study on sexual behavior of women using 30 microg ethinylestradiol and 3 mg drospirenone oral contraceptives. *Contraception* 2005;72:19–23.

200. **Skrzypulec V, Drosdzol A.** Evaluation of the quality of life and sexual functioning of women using a 30-microg ethinyloestradiol and 3-mg drospirenone combined oral contraceptive. *Eur J Contracept Reprod Health Care* 2008;13:49–57.

201. **Bracken MP.** Oral contraception and congenital malformations in offspring: a review and meta-analysis of the prospective studies. *Obstet Gynecol* 1990;76:552–557.

202. **Katz Z, Lancet M, Skornik J, et al.** Teratogenicity of progestogens given during the first trimester of pregnancy. *Obstet Gynecol* 1985;65:775–780.

203. **Back DJ, Orme ML'E.** Pharmacokinetic drug interactions with oral contraceptives. *Clin Pharmacokinet* 1990;18:472–484.

204. **Shenfield GM.** Oral contraceptives: Are drug interactions of clinical significance? *Drug Saf* 1993;9:21–37.

205. **Crawford P.** Interactions between antiepileptic drugs and hormonal contraception. *CNS Drugs* 2002;16:263–272.

206. **Hall SD, Wang Z, Huang SM, et al.** The interaction between St. John's wort and an oral contraceptive. *Clin Pharmacol Ther* 2003;74:525–535.

207. **Helms SE, Bredle DL, Zajic J, et al.** Oral contraceptive failure rates and oral antibiotics. *J Am Acad Dermatol* 1997;36:705–710.

208. **Dickenson BD, Altman RD, Nielsen NH, et al.** Drug interactions between oral contraceptives and antibiotics. *Obstet Gynecol* 2001;98:53–60.

209. **Knopp RH, Bergelin RO, Wahl PW, et al.** Clinical chemistry alterations in pregnancy and with oral contraceptive use. *Obstet Gynecol* 1985;66:682–690.

210. **Gallo MF, Nanda K, Grimes DA, et al.** 20 mcg versus 20 mcg estrogen combined oral contraceptives for contraception. *Cochrane Database Syst Rev* 2008;4:CD003989.

211. **Del Conte A, Loffer F, Grubb G.** A multicenter, randomized comparative trial of the clinical effects on cycle control of two 21-day regimens of oral contraceptives containing 20 μg EE. *Prim Care Update Obstet Gynecol* 1998;5:173.

212. **Rosenberg MJ, Meyers A, Roy V.** Efficacy, cycle control and side effects of low and lower-dose oral contraceptives: a randomized trial of 20 microgram and 35 microgram estrogen preparations. *Contraception* 1999;60:321–329.

213. **Mulders TM, Dieben TO.** Use of the novel combined contraceptive vaginal ring NuvaRing for ovulation inhibition. *Fertil Steril* 2001;75:865–870.

214. **Dieben TOM, Roumen JME, Apter D.** Efficacy, cycle control and user acceptability of a novel combined contraceptive vaginal ring*bstet Gynecol* 2002;100:585–593.

215. **Fleischer K, van Vliet HA, Rosendaal FR, et al.** Effects of the contraceptive patch, the vaginal ring and an oral contraceptive on APC resistance and SHBG: a cross-over study. *Thromb Res* 2009;123:429–435.

216. **Jensen JT, Burke AE, Barnhart KT, et al.** Effects of switching from oral to transdermal or transvaginal contraception on markers of thrombosis. *Contraception* 2008;78:451–458.

217. **Jick SS, Hagberg KW, Hernandez RK, et al.** Postmarketing study of ORTHO EVRA and levonorgestrel oral contraceptives containing hormonal contraceptives with 30 mcg of ethinyl estradiol in relation to nonfatal venous thromboembolism. *Contraception* 2010;81:16–21.

218. **U.S. Food and Drug Administration.** Ortho Evra questions and answers. January 2008. Available online at: http://www.fda.gov. ezproxy.bu.edu/Drugs/DrugSafety/PostmarketDrugSafety InformationforPatientsandProviders/ucm110403.htm

219. **Dunne C, Malyuk D, Firoz T.** Cerebral venous sinus thrombosis in a woman using the etonogestrel-ethinyl estradiol vaginal contraceptive ring: a case report. *J Obstet Gynaecol Can* 2010;32:270–273.

220. **Fugate JE, Robinson MT, Rabinstein AA, et al.** Cerebral venous sinus thrombosis associated with a combined contraceptive ring. *Neurologist.* 2011;17:105-6.

221. **Kaunitz AM.** Long-acting injectable contraception with depot medroxyprogesterone acetate. *Am J Obstet Gynecol* 1994;170:1543–1549.

222. **Abdel-Aleem H, d'Arcangues C, Vogelsong KM, et al.** Treatment of vaginal bleeding irregularities induced by progestin only contraceptives. *Cochrane Database Syst Rev* 2007;4:CD003449.

223. **Jain JK, Nicosia AF, Nucatola DL, et al.** Mifepristone for the prevention of breakthrough bleeding in new starters of depo-medroxyprogesterone acetate. *Steroids* 2003;68:1115–1119.

224. **Zhao S, Choksuchat C, Zhao Y, et al.** Effects of doxycycline on serum and endometrial levels of MMP-2, MMP-9 and TIMP-1 in women using a levonorgestrel-releasing subcutaneous implant. *Contraception* 2009;79:469–478.

225. **Weisberg E, Hickey M, Palmer D, et al.** A pilot study to assess the effect of three short-term treatments on frequent and/or prolonged bleeding compared to placebo in women using Implanon. *Hum Reprod* 2006;21:295–302.

226. **Berenson AB, Rahman M.** Changes in weight, total fat, percent body fat, and central-to-peripheral fat ratio associated with injectable and oral contraceptive use. *Am J Obstet Gynecol* 2009;200:329.e1–e8.

227. **Le YC, Rahman M, Berenson AB.** Early weight gain predicting later weight gain among depot medroxyprogesterone acetate users. *Obstet Gynecol* 2009;114:279–284.

228. **Pardthaisong T.** Return of fertility after use of the injectable contraceptive Depo-Provera: updated analysis. *J Biosoc Sci* 1984;16:23–34.

229. **Cundy T, Reid OR, Roberts H.** Bone density in women receiving depot medroxyprogesterone acetate for contraception. *BMJ* 1991;303:13–16.

230. **Cromer BA, Lazebnik R, Rome E, et al.** Double-blinded randomized controlled trial of estrogen supplementation in adolescent girls who receive depot medroxyprogesterone acetate for contraception. *Am J Obstet Gynecol* 2005;192:42–47.

231. **Harel Z, Johnson CC, Gold MA, et al.** Recovery of bone mineral density in adolescents following the use of depot medroxyprogesterone acetate contraceptive injections. *Contraception* 2010;81:281–291.

232. **Lopez LM, Grimes DA, Schulz KF, et al.** Steroidal contraceptives: effect on bone fractures in women. *Cochrane Database Syst Rev* 2009;2:CD006033.

233. **Fahmy K, Khairy M, Allam G, et al.** Effect of depomedroxyprogesterone acetate on coagulation factors and serum lipids in Egyptian women. *Contraception* 1991;44:431–434.

234. **Schwallie PG.** Experience with Depo-Provera as an injectable contraceptive. *J Reprod Med* 1974;13:113–117.

235. **Okada Y, Horikawa K.** A case of phlebothrombosis of lower extremity and pulmonary embolism due to progesterone. *Kokyu To Junkan* 1992;40:819–822.

236. **Hitosugi M, Kitamura O, Takatsu A, et al.** A case of dural sinus thrombosis during the medication of medroxyprogesterone acetate. *Nihon Hoigaku Zasshi* 1997;51:452–456.

237. **Deen BF, Shuler BK Jr, Sharon Fekrat S.** Retinal venous occlusion associated with depot medroxyprogesterone acetate. *Br J Ophthalmol* 2007;91:1254.

238. **Kaunitz AM.** Injectable long-acting contraceptives. *Clin Obstet Gynecol* 2001;44:73–91.

239. **Westhoff C.** Depot medroxyprogesterone acetate contraception: metabolic parameters and mood changes. *J Reprod Med* 1996;41:401–406.

240. **Rodriguez MA, Kaunitz AM.** An evidence-based approach to postpartum use of depot medroxyprogesterone acetate in breastfeeding women. *Contraception* 2009;80:4–6.

241. **La Vecchia C.** Depot-medroxyprogesterone acetate, other injectable contraceptives, and cervical cancer. *Contraception* 1994;49:223–229.

242. **World Health Organization.** Depot medroxyprogesterone acetate (DMPA) and the risk of epithelial ovarian cancer. The WHO Collaborative Study of Neoplasia and Steroid Contraceptives. *Int J Cancer* 1991;49:191–195.

243. **Kaunitz AM.** Depot medroxyprogesterone acetate contraception and the risk of breast and gynecologic cancer. *J Reprod Med* 1996;41(5 Suppl):419–427.

244. **Shapiro S, Rosenberg L, Hoffman M, et al.** Risk of breast cancer in relation to the use of injectable progestogen contraceptives and combined estrogen/progestogen contraceptives. *Am J Epidemiol* 2000;151:396–403.

245. **Cullins VE.** Noncontraceptive benefits and therapeutic uses of depot medroxyprogesterone acetate. *J Reprod Med* 1996;41(5 Suppl): 428–433.

246. **Jain J, Dutton C, Nicosia A, et al.** Pharmacokinetics, ovulation suppression and return to ovulation following a lower dose subcutaneous formulation of Depo-Provera. *Contraception* 2004;70:11–18.

247. **Jain J, Jakimiuk AJ, Bode FR, et al.** Contraceptive efficacy and safety of DMPA-SC. *Contraception* 2004;70:269–275.

248. **Guo-wei S.** Pharmacodynamic effects of once a month combined injectable contraceptives. *Contraception* 1994;49:361–385.

249. **Kaunitz AM, Garceau RJ, Cromie MA, et al.** Comparative safety, efficacy and cycle control of Lunelle monthly contraceptive injection (medroxyprogesterone acetate and estradiol cypionate injectable suspension) and Ortho-Novum 7/7/7 oral contraceptive (norethindrone/ethinyl estradiol triphasic). *Contraception* 1999;60(4):179–187.

250. **Gao J, Wang SL, Wu SC, et al.** Comparison of the clinical performance, contraceptive efficacy and acceptability of levonorgestrel releasing IUD, and Norplant 2 implants in China. *Contraception* 1990;41:485–494.

251. **Steiner MJ, Lopez LM, Grimes DA, et al.** Sino-implant (II)—a levonorgestrel-releasing two-rod implant: systematic review of the randomized controlled trials. *Contraception* 2010;81:197–201.

252. **Funk S, Miller MM, Mishell DR Jr, et al.** Safety and efficacy of Implanon™, a single-rod implantable contraceptive containing etonogestrel. *Contraception* 2005;71:319–326.

253. **Power J, French R, Cowan F.** Subdermal implantable contraceptives versus other forms of reversible contraceptives or other implants as effective methods of preventing pregnancy. *Cochrane Database Syst Rev* 2007;3:CD001326.

254. **Darney PD, Patel A, Rosen KM, et al.** Safety and efficacy of a single-rod etonogestrel implant (Implanon): results from 11 international clinical trials. *Contraception* 2009;80:519–526.

255. **Zheng S-S, Zheng H-M, Qian S-Z et al.** A randomized multicenter study comparing the efficacy and bleeding pattern of a single-rod (Implanon) and a six-capsule (Norplant) hormonal contraceptive implant. *Contraception* 1999;60:1–8.

256. **Brito MB, Ferriani RA, Quintana SM, et al.** Safety of the etonogestrel-releasing implant during the immediate postpartum period: a pilot study. *Contraception* 2009;80:519–26.

257. **Beerthuizen R, van Beek A, Massai R, et al.** Bone mineral density during long-tgerm use of the progestogen contraceptive implant Implanon compared to a nonhormonal method of contraception. *Hum Reprod* 2000;15:118–122.

258. **Hidalgo MM, Lisondo C, Juliato CT, et al.** Ovarian cysts in users of Implanon and Jadelle subdermal contraceptive implants. *Contraception* 2006;73:532–536.

259. **Egberg N, van Beek A, Gunnervik C, et al.** Effects on the hemostatic system and liver function in relation to Implanon and Norplant. A prospective randomized clinical trial. *Contraception* 1998;58:93–98

260. **Vieira CS, Ferriani RA, Garcia AA, et al.** Use of the etonogestrel-releasing implant is associated with hypoactivation of the coagulation cascade. *Hum Reprod* 2007;22:2196–2201.

261. **Petitti DB, Siscovick DS, Sidney S, et al.** Norplant implants and cardiovascular disease. *Contraception* 1998;57:361–362.

262. **Haspells AA.** Emergency contraception: a review. *Contraception* 1994;50:101–108.

263. **Yuzpe AA.** Postcoital contraception. *Clin Obstet Gynecol* 1984;11: 787–797.

264. **Anonymous.** Randomized controlled trial of levonorgestrel versus the Yuzpe regimen of combined oral contraceptives for emergency contraception. Task Force on Postovulatory Methods of Fertility Regulation. *Lancet* 1998;352:428–433.

265. **Von Hertzen H, WHO Research Group.** Low dose mifepristone and two regimens of levonorgestrel for emergency contraception: a WHO multicenter randomized trial. *Lancet* 2002;360: 1803–1810.

266. **World Health Organization.** *Fact sheet on the safety of levonorgestrel-alone emergency contraceptive pills (LNG ECPs).* Geneva: WHO, 2010.

267. **Noe G, Croxatto HB, Salvatierra AM, et al.** Contraceptive efficacy of emergency contraception with levonorgestrel given before or after ovulation. *Contraception* 2010;81:414–420.

268. **Horga A, Santamarina E, Quilez A, et al.** Cerebral venous thrombosis associated with repeated use of emergency contraception. *Eur J Neurol* 2007;14:e5.

269. **Hamoda H, Ashok PW, Stalder C, et al.** A randomized trial of mifepristone 10 mg and levonorgestrel for emergency contraception. *Obstet Gynecol* 2004;104:1307–1313.

270. **Glasier AF, Cameron ST, Fine PM, et al.** Uliprostal acetate versus levonorgestrel for emergency contraception, a randomized non inferiority trial. *Lancet* 2010;375:555–562.

271. **Brache V, Cochon L, Jesam C, et al.** Immediate pre-ovulatory administration of 30 mg Ulipristal acetate significantly delays follicular rupture. *Hum Reprod* 2010;25:2256–2263.

272. **Lippes J, Malik T, Tautum HJ.** The postcoital copper-T. *Adv Plann Parent* 1976;11:24–29.

273. **Wu S, Godfrey E, Wojdyla D, et al.** Copper T380A intrauterine device for emergency contraception: a prospective, multicentre, cohort clinical trial. *BJOG* 2010;117:1205–1210.

274. **Zhou L, Xiao B.** Emergency contraception with multiload Cu-375 SL IUD: a multicenter clinical trial. *Contraception* 2001;64:107–112.

275. **Briggs MH, Briggs M.** Oral contraceptives for men. *Nature* 1974;252:585–586.

276. **Wallace EM, Gow SM, Wu FC.** Comparison between testosterone enanthate-induced azoospermia and oligozoospermia in a male contraceptive study. I. Plasma luteinizing hormone, follicle stimulating hormone, testosterone, estradiol, and inhibin concentrations. *J Clin Endocrinol Metab* 1993;77:290–293.

277. **Wang C, Swerdloff RS.** Male hormonal contraception. *Am J Obstet Gynecol* 2004;190:S60–S68.

278. **Gu Y, Gu X, Liang W, et al.** Multicenter contraceptive efficacy trial of injectable testosterone undecanoate in Chinese men. *J Clin Endocrin Metab* 2009;94:1910–1925.

279. **Mommers E, Kersemaekers WM, Elliesen M, et al.** Male hormonal contraception: a double blind, placebo-controlled study. *J Clin Endocrin Metabol* 2008;93:2572–2580.

280. **Murad F, Haynes RC.** Androgens and anabolic steroids. In: Gilman AG, Goodman LS, Gilman A, eds. *Goodman and Gilman's the pharmacological basis of therapeutics.* 6th ed. New York: MacMillan, 1980:1448–1465.

281. **Peterson B.** Sterilization. *Obstet Gynecol* 2008;111:189–203.

282. **Uchida H.** Uchida tubal sterilization. *Am J Obstet Gynecol* 1975;121:153–159.

283. **Filshie GM, Pogmore JR, Dutton AG, et al.** The titanium/silicone rubber clip for female sterilization. *BJOG* 1981;88:655–662.

284. **Penfield AJ.** The Filshie clip for female sterilization: a review of world experience. *Am J Obstet Gynecol* 2000;182:485–489.

285. **Soderstrom RM, Levy BS, Engel T.** Reducing bipolar sterilization failures. *Obstet Gynecol* 1989;74:60–63.

286. **Poindexter AN, Abdul-Malak M, Fast JE.** Laparoscopic tubal sterilization under local anesthesia. *Obstet Gynecol* 1990;75:5–8.

287. **Khairullah Z, Huber DH, Gonzales B.** Declining mortality in international sterilization services. *Int J Gynaecol Obstet* 1992;39:41–50.

288. **Peterson HB, Xia Z, Wilcox LS, et al.** Pregnancy after tubal sterilization with bipolar electrocoagulation. *Obstet Gynecol* 1999;94:163–167.

289. **Dominik R, Gates D, Sokal D, et al.** Two randomized controlled trials comparing the Hulka and Filshie clips for tubal sterilization. *Contraception* 2000;62:169–175.

290. **Sokal D, Gates D, Amatya R, et al.** Two randomized controlled trials comparing the tubal ring and Filshie clip for tubal sterilization. *Fertil Steril* 2000;74:525–533.

291. **Magos A, Chapman L.** Hysteroscopic tubal sterilization. *Obstet Gynecol Clin North Am* 2004;31: 705–719.

292. **Cooper JM, Carignan CS, Cher D, et al.** Micro-insert nonincisional hysteroscopic sterilization. *Obstet Gynecol* 2003;102:59–76.

293. **Adiana Permanent Contraception.** Instructions for use and radiofrequency (RF) generator operator's manual. Hologic, 2009.

294. **Essure Permanent Birth Control System.** Instructions for use. Conceptus, Inc. 2009.

295. **Wittmer MH, Brown DL, Hartman RP, et al.** Sonography, CT, and MRI appearance of the Essure microinsert permanent birth control device. *Am J Roentgenol* 2006;187:959–964.

296. **Teoh M, Meagher S, Kovacs G.** Ultrasound detection of the Essure permanent birth control device: a case series. *Aust N Z J Obstet Gynaecol* 2003;43:378–380.

297. **Smith RD.** Contemporary hysteroscopic methods for female sterilization. *Int J Gynaecol Obstet* 2010;108:79–84.

298. **Connor VF.** Essure: a review six years later. *J Minim Invasive Gynecol* 2009;16:282–290.

299. **Kerin JF, Munday DN, Ritossa MG, et al.** Essure hysteroscopic sterilization: results based on utilizing a new coil catheter delivery system. *J Am Assoc Gynecol Laparosc* 2004;11:388–393.

300. **Palmer SN, Greenberg JA.** Transcervical sterilization: a comparison of Essure ermanent brith control system and Adiana permanent contraception system. *Rev Obstet Gynecol* 2009;2:84–92.

301. **Hirth R, Zbella E, Sanchez M, et al.** Microtubal reanastomosis: success rates as compared to in vitro fertilization. *J Reprod Med* 2010;55:161–165.

302. **Peterson HB, Jeng G, Folger SG, et al.** The risk of menstrual abnormalities after tubal sterilization. *N Engl J Med* 2000;343:1681–1687.

303. **Ness RB, Grisso JA, Cottreau C, et al.** Factors related to inflammation of the ovarian epithelium and risk of ovarian cancer. *Epidemiology* 2000;11:111–117.

304. **Jamieson DJ, Costello C, Trussell J, et al.** The risk of pregnancy after vasectomy. *Obstet Gynecol* 2004;103:848–850.

305. **Hatcher RA, Trussell J, Stewart F, et al.** *Contraceptive technology.* 17th ed. New York: Ardent Media, 1998:567.

306. **Sokal D, Irsula B, Hayes M, et al.** Vasectomy by ligation and excision with or without fascial interposition; a randomized controlled trial. *BMC Med* 2004;2:6.

307. **Goldacre MJ, Holford TR, Vessey MP.** Cardiovascular disease and vasectomy. *N Engl J Med* 1982;308:805–808.

308. **Coady SA, Sharrett AR, Zheng ZJ, et al.** Vasectomy, inflammation, atherosclerosis and long-term followup for cardiovascular diseases: no associations in the atherosclerosis risk in communities study. *J Urol* 2002;167:204–207.

309. **Rosenberg L, Palmer JR, Zauber AG, et al.** Vasectomy and the risk of prostate cancer. *Am J Epidemiol* 1990;132:1051–1055.

310. **John EM, Whittemore AS, Wu AH, et al.** Vasectomy and prostate cancer: results from a multiethnic case-control study. *J Natl Cancer Inst* 1995;87:662–669.

311. **Stanford JL, Wicklund KG, McKnight B, et al.** Vasectomy and risk of prostate cancer. *Cancer Epidemiol Biomarkers Prev* 1999;8:881–886.

312. **Tang LF, Jiang H, Shang XJ, et al.** Vasectomy not associated with prostate cancer: a meta-analysis. *Zhonghua Nan Ke Xue* 2009;15:545–550.

313. **Alan Guttmacher Institute.** *Induced abortion worldwide.* New York: Alan Guttmacher Institute, 2009:1–2.

314. **Sedgh G, Henshaw S, Singh S, et al.** Induced abortion: estimated rates and trends worldwide. *Lancet* 2007;370:1338–1345.

315. **Cates W Jr, Rochat RW.** Illegal abortions in the United States: 1972–1974. *Fam Plann Perspect* 1976;8:86–92.

316. **Pazol K, Gamble SB, Parker WY, et al.** Abortion surveillance—United States 2006. *MMWR Surveil Sum* 2009;58(SS08):1–35.

317. **Council on Scientific Affairs, American Medical Association.** Induced termination of pregnancy before and after Roe v Wade: trends in the mortality and morbidity of women. *JAMA* 1992;268:3231–3239

318. **Jones RK, Zolna MRS, Henshaw SK, et al.** Abortion in the United States: incidence and access to services, 2005. *Perspect Sex Reprod Health* 2008;40:6–16.

319. **Susser M.** Induced abortion and health as a value. *Am J Public Health* 1992;82:1323–1324.

320. **Whitehead SJ, Vartlett LA, Herndon J, et al.** Abortion-related mortality: United States 1993–1997. Paper presented at the National Abortion Federation 26th Annual Meeting; April 15, 2002; San Jose, California.

321. **Xu, J, Kochanek, KD, Murphy, BS, et al.** Deaths: Final Data for 2007. *Nat Vital Stat Rep* 2010;58:19.

322. **Bartlett LA, Berg CJ, Shulman HP, et al.** Risk factors for legal induced abortion-related mortality in the United States. *Obstet Gynecol* 2004;103:729–737.

323. **Stubblefield PG, Carr-Ellis S, Borgatta L.** Methods for induced abortion. *Obstet Gynecol* 2004;104:174–185.

324. **MacIsaac L, Grossman D, Baliestreri E, et al.** A randomized controlled trial of laminaria, oral misoprostol and vaginal misoprostol before abortion. *Obstet Gynecol* 1999;93:766–770.

325. **Goldberg AB, Dean G, Kang MS, et al.** Manual versus electric vacuum aspiration for early first trimester: a controlled study of complication rates. *Obstet Gynecol* 2004;103:101–107.

326. **Sawaya GF, Grady D, Kerlikowske K, et al.** Antibiotics at the time of induced abortion: the case for universal prophylaxis based on a meta-analysis. *Obstet Gynecol* 1996;87:884–890.

327. **Hakim-Elahi E, Tovel HM, Burnhill HM, et al.** Complications of first trimester abortion: a report of 170,000 cases. *Obstet Gynecol* 1990;76:129–135.

328. **Stubblefield PG, Borgatta L.** Complications of induced abortion. In: Pearlman MD, Tintinalli JE, Dyne PL, eds. *Obstetric and gynecological emergencies: diagnosis and management.* New York: McGraw Hill, 2004:65–86.

329. **Paul M, Lichtenberg ES, Borgatta L, et al.** *Management of unintended and abnormal pregnancy. Comprehensive abortion care.* Oxford: Wiley-Blackwell, 2009.

330. **Spitz IM, Bardin CW, Benton L, et al.** Early pregnancy terminations with mifepristone and misoprostol in the United States. *N Engl J Med* 1998;338:1241–1247.

331. **Goldberg AB, Greenberg BS, Darney PD.** Misoprostol and pregnancy. *N Engl J Med* 2001;344:38–47.

332. **Schaff EA, Fielding LS, Eisinger SH, et al.** Low-dose mifepristone followed by vaginal misoprostol at 48 hours for abortion up to 63 days. *Contraception* 2000;61:41–46.

333. **Schaff EA, Fielding SL, Westoff C, et al.** Vaginal misoprostol administered 1, 2, or 3 days after mifepristone for early medical abortion: a randomized trial. *JAMA* 2000;84:1948–1953.

334. **Schaff EA, Stadalius LS, Eisinger SH, et al.** Vaginal misoprostol administered at home after mifepristone (RU486) for abortion. *J Fam Pract* 1997;44:353–360.

335. **Schaff EA, DiDenzo R, Fielding SL.** Comparison of misoprostol plasma concentrations following buccal and sublingual administration. *Contraception* 2005;71:22-5

336. **Zieman M, Fong SK, Benowitz NL, et al.** Absorption kinetics of misoprostol with oral or vaginal administration. *Obstet Gynecol* 1997;90:735–738.

337. **Fjerstad NP, Trussell J, Sivin I et al.** Rates of serious infection after changes in regimens for medical abortion. *N Engl J Med* 2009;361:145–151.

338. **Mifeprex Medication Guide.** New York: Danco Laboratories, LLC.

339. **Ashok PW, Flett GM, Templeton A.** Termination of pregnancy at 9–13 weeks' amenorrhea with mifepristone and misoprostol [Letter]. *Lancet* 1998;352:542–543.

340. **Creinin MD, Vittinghoff E, Keder L, et al.** Methotrexate and misoprostol for early abortion: a multicenter trial. I. Safety and efficacy. *Contraception* 1996;53:321–327.

341. **Borgatta, Mullaly B, Vragovic O, et al.** Misoprostol as the primary agent for medical abortion in a low income urban setting. *Contraception* 2004;70:121–126.

342. **Allen RH, Westhoff C, De Nonno L, et al.** Curettage after mifepristone induced abortion: frequency, timing and indications. *Obstet Gynecol* 2001;98:101–106.

343. **Hausknecht R.** Mifepristone and misoprostol for early medical abortion: 18 months experience in the United States. *Contraception* 2003;67:463-465.

344. **Weibe E, Guilbert E, Jacot F, et al.** A fatal case of *Clostridium sordelli* septic shock syndrome associated with medical abortion. *Obstet Gynecol* 2004;104:1142–1144.

345. **American College of Obstetricians and Gynecologists.** Letter on the safety of RU 486. ACOG news release, December 7, 2004. Washington, DC: American College of Obstetricians and Gynecologists, 2004.

346. **Stubblefield PG.** First and second trimester abortion. In: Nichols DH, Clarke-Pearson DL, eds. *Gynecologic, obstetric and related surgery.* 2nd ed. St. Louis, MO: Mosby, 2000:1033–1045.

347. **Hammond, C, Chason, S.** Dilatation and evacuation. In: Paul M, Lichtenberg ES, Borgatta L, et al., eds. *Management of unintended and abnormal pregnancy. Comprehensive abortion care.* Oxford: Wiley-Blackwell, 2009:157–177.

348. **Darney PD, Sweet RL.** Routine intra-operative ultrasonography for second trimester abortion reduced incidence of uterine perforation. *J Ultrasound Med* 1989;8:71–75.

349. **Hern WM.** *Abortion practice.* Philadelphia, PA: Lippincott, 1984.

350. **Hern WM, Xen C, Ferguson RA, et al.** Outpatient abortion for fetal anomaly and fetal death from 15–34 menstrual weeks gestation: techniques and clinical management. *Obstet Gynecol* 1993;81:301–306.

351. **Patel A, Talmont E, Morfesis J, et al.** Adequacy and safety of buccal misoprostol for cervical preparation of second-trimester pregnancy. *Contraception* 2006;73:420–430.

352. **Chasen ST, Kalish RB, Gupta M, et al.** Dilatation and evacuation at greater than or equal to 20 weeks: comparison of operative techniques. *Am J Obstet Gynecol* 2004;190:1180–1183.

353. **Haddad L, Yanow S, Delli-Bovi L, et al.** Changes in abortion provider practices in response to the Partial-Birth Abortion Ban Act of 2003. *Contraception* 2009;79:379–384.

354. **Drey EA, Thomas LJ, Benowitz NL, et al.** Safety of intra-amniotic digoxin administration before late second-trimester abortion by dilation and evacuation. *Am J Obstet Gynecol* 2000;182:1063–1066.

355. **Pasquini L, Pontello V, Kumar S.** Intracardiac injection of potassium chloride as method for feticide: experience from a single UK tertiary centre. *BJOG* 2008;115:528–531.

356. **Jackson RA, Teplin VL, Drey EA, et al.** Digoxin to facilitate late second-trimester abortion: a randomized, masked, placebo-controlled trial. *Obstet Gynecol* 2001;97:471–476.

357. **Borgatta L, Betstadt SJ, Reed A, et al.** Relationship of intraamniotic digoxin to fetal demise. *Contraception* 2010;81:328–330.

358. **Gemzell-Danielsson K, Lalitkumar S.** Second trimester medical abortion with mifepristone-misoprostol and misoprostol alone: a review of methods and management. *Reprod Health Matters* 2008;16(31 Suppl):162–172.

359. **Jain JK, Mishell DR.** A comparison of intravaginal misoprostol with prostaglandin E for termination of second trimester pregnancy. *N Engl J Med* 1994;331:290–293.

360. **Ashok PW, Templeton A, Wagaarachchi PT, et al.** Midtrimester medical termination of pregnancy: a review of 1002 consecutive cases. *Contraception* 2004;69:51–58.

361. **Webster D, Penny GC, Templeton K.** A comparison of 600 and 200 mg mifepristone prior to second trimester abortion with the prostaglandin misoprostol. *BJOG* 1996;103:706–709.

362. **Royal College of Obstetricians.** *The care of women requesting induced abortion.* Guidelines No. 7. London: Royal College of Obstetricians, 2004.

363. **Chai J, Tang OS, Hong QQ, et al.** A randomized trial to compare two dosing intervals of misoprostol following mifepristone administration in second trimester medical abortion. *Hum Reprod* 2009;24:320–324.

364. **Royal College of Obstetricians and Gynaecologists.** *Termination of pregnancy for fetal abnormality in England, Scotland and Wales.* London: RCOG, 1996.

365. **Hern WM.** Laminaria, induced fetal demise and misoprostol in late abortion. *Int J Gynaecol Obstet* 2001;75:279–286.

366. **Winkler CL, Gray SE, Hauth JC, et al.** Mid-second-trimester labor induction: concentrated oxytocin compared with prostaglandin E₂ suppositories. *Obstet Gynecol* 1991;77:297–300.

367. **Frick AC, Drey EA, Diedrich JT, et al.** Effect of prior cesarean delivery on risk of second-trimester surgical abortion complications. *Obstet Gynecol* 2010;115:760–764.

368. **Dickenson JE.** Misoprostol for second-trimester pregnancy termination in women with a prior cesarean delivery. *Am J Obstet Gynecol* 2005;105:352–356.

369. **Evans MI, Berkowitz RI, Wapner RJ, et al.** Improvements in outcomes of multifetal pregnancy reduction with increased experience. *Am J Obstet Gynecol* 2001;184:97–103.

370. **Evans MI, Goldberg JD, Horenstein J, et al.** Selective termination for structural, chromosomal and mendelian anomalies: international experience. *Am J Obstet Gynecol* 1999;82:61–66.

371. **He ZM, Fang Q, Yang YZ, et al.** Fetal reduction by bipolar cord coagulation in managing complicated monochorionic multiple pregnancies: preliminary experience in China. *Chin Med J (Engl)* 2010;123:549–554.

372. **Morris GC, Lacey CJ.** Microbicides and HIV prevention: lessons from the past, looking to the future. *Curr Opin Infect Dis* 2010;23:57–63.

373. **van Damme L, Govinden R, Mirembe FM, et al.** Lack of effectiveness of cellulose sulfate gel for the prevention of vaginal HIV transmission. *N Engl J Med* 2008;359:463–472.

374. **McGowan I.** Microbicides for HIV prevention: reality or hope? *Curr Opin Infect Dis* 2010;23:26–31.

375. **Wu S, Hu J, Wildemeersch D.** Performance of the frameless GyneFix and theTCU380A IUDs in a three year multicenter randomized comparative trial in parous women. *Contraception* 2000;61:91–98.

376. **Weisberg E, Brache V, Alvarez F, et al.** Clinical performance and menstrual bleeding patterns with three dosage combinations of a Nestorone progestogen/ethinyl estradiol contraceptive vaginal ring used on a bleeding-signaled regimen. *Contraception* 2005;72:46–52.

377. **Upadhyay UD.** New contraceptive choices. *Population Reports,* Series M, No. 19. Baltimore: Johns Hopkins Bloomberg School of Public Health, INFO Project; April 2005. Available at: www.infoforhealth.org/pr/m19

378. **Del Priore G, Malanowska-Stega J, Shalaby SW, et al.** A pilot safety and tolerability study of a nonhormonal vaginal contraceptive ring. *J Reprod Med* 2009;54:685–690.

379. **Coffey PS, Kilbourne-Brook M.** Wear and care of the SILCS diaphragm: experience from three countries. *Sex Health* 2010;7:159–164.

380. **Mbopi-Keou Trottier S, Omar RF, Nkelle NN, et al.** A randomized, double-blind, placebo-controlled safety and acceptability study of two Invisible Condom® formulations in women from Cameroon. *Contraception* 2009;80:484–492.

381. **Talwar GP, Singh O, Pal R, et al.** A birth control vaccine is on the horizon for family planning. *Ann Med* 1993;25:207–212.

382. **McLaughlin EA, Holland MK, Aitken RJ.** Contraceptive vaccines. *Expert Opin Biol Ther* 2003;3:829–841.

383. **Naz RK.** Status of contraceptive vaccines. *Am J Reprod Immunol* 2009;61:11–18.

384. **Lyttle CR, Kopf GS.** Status and future direction of male hormonal contraceptive development. *Curr Opin Pharmacol* 2003;3:667–671.

385. **Blithe D.** Male contraception: what is on the horizon? *Contraception* 2008;78:S23–S27.

386. **Zhao SC.** Vas deferens occlusion by percutaneous injection of polyurethane elastomer plugs: clinical experience and reversibility. *Contraception* 1990;41:453–459.

387. **Potts M, Benagiano G.** Quinacrine sterilization: a middle road. *Contraception* 2001;64:275–276.

388. **Sokal DC, Hieu do T, Loan ND, et al.** Contraceptive effectiveness of two insertions of quinacrine: results from 10-year follow-up in Vietnam. *Contraception* 2008;78:61–65.

389. **Hieu DT, Luong TT.** The rate of ectopic pregnancy for 24,589 quinacrine sterilization (QS) users compared to users of other methods and no method in 4 provinces of Vietnam. 1994–1996.*Int J Gynaecol Obstet* 2003;83(Suppl 2):S35–S43.

390. **Sokal DC, Vach TH, Nanda K, et al.** Quinacrine sterilization and gynecologic cancers: a case-control study in northern Vietnam. *Epidemiology* 2010;21:164–167.

391. **Cancel AM, Dillberger JE, Kelly CM, et al.** A lifetime cancer bioassay of quinacrine administered into the uterine horns of female rats. *Regul Toxicol Pharmacol* 2010;56:156–165.

392. **Sokal DC, Trujillo V, Guzmán SC, et al.** Cancer risk after sterilization with transcervical quinacrine: updated findings from a Chilean cohort. *Contraception* 2010;81:75–78.

11 Sexuality, Sexual Dysfunction, and Sexual Assault

Rosemary Basson
David A. Baram

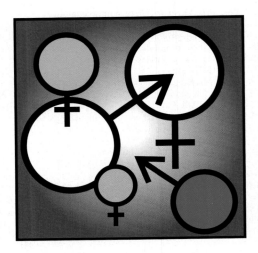

- Most young men and young women have multiple serial sexual partners but use condoms inconsistently, thereby exposing themselves to sexually transmitted diseases (STDs) and unintended pregnancies.

- Sexual response reflects the fundamental interplay between the mind and body: psychological, interpersonal, cultural, environmental, and biological (hormonal, vascular, muscular, neurological) factors interact and modulate sexual experience.

- Factors that can affect sexual response include mood, relationship duration and quality, age and stage in life, past sexual experiences—wanted, coercive, or abusive—personal psychological factors stemming from relationships in childhood with parental figures, previous losses and traumas, and ways of coping with emotions, current and past illness, and use of medication, alcohol, and illicit drugs.

- Physical, emotional, and economic stressors of pregnancy may negatively affect emotional and sexual intimacy.

- Sexual value systems, folklore, religious beliefs, physical changes, and medical restrictions influence sexual attitudes and behavior during pregnancy and postpartum.

- Despite the importance of issues relating to sexuality, many women find it difficult to talk to their physicians about sexual concerns, and many physicians are uncomfortable discussing sexual issues with their patients.

- Asking about sexual concerns gives physicians an opportunity to educate patients about the risk of STDs, encourage safer sex practices, evaluate the need for contraception, dispel sexual misconceptions, and identify sexual dysfunction.

- Many of the sexual problems couples encounter result from a deficit of knowledge or experience, sexual misconceptions, or inability of the couple to communicate about their sexual preferences.

- **Sexual problems are common. Vaginismus is an involuntary reflex precipitated by real or imagined attempts at vaginal entry. Dyspareunia may affect two-thirds of women during their lifetime. Vestibulodynia, the most common type of dyspareunia, has a prevalence of 15%.**

- **Sexual assault of children and adult women has reached epidemic proportions in the United States and is the fastest growing, most frequently committed, and most underreported crime.** The terms *sexual abuse survivor* and *assault survivor* are preferable to *victim.*

- **Childhood sexual abuse has a profound and potentially lifelong effect on the survivor. Although most cases of childhood sexual abuse are not reported by the survivor or her family, it is estimated that as many as one-third of adult women were sexually abused as children.**

- **Women who were sexually abused as children or sexually assaulted as adults often experience sexual dysfunction and difficulty with intimate relationships and parenting.**

- **The National Women's Study revealed that 13%, or one of eight adult women, are survivors of at least one completed rape during their lifetime.**

Most women feel that sexuality is an important part of their lives even when chronic illness is present. Providing patients with information about normal sexual changes that occur with puberty, pregnancy and postpartum, menopause, and older age is part of routine obstetric and gynecologic care.

Sexual dysfunction can arise from gynecologic diseases such as endometriosis, procedures such as those associated with infertility, and treatments such as pelvic radiation, bilateral salpingo-oophorectomy, and use of aromatase inhibitors or gonadotropin-releasing hormone (GnRH) antagonists. Sexual abuse can have long-lasting effects on sexuality and other psychophysiological aspects of a patient's life. Women seen in gynecology clinics may have comorbid illnesses that interrupt their sexual function. Inquiry about sexual concerns and explanation of the implications of a disease and its treatment are integral components of gynecologic care.

Sexuality

The spectrum of normal sexual response varies from one woman to another and throughout a woman's lifetime (1–3). Physicians should be aware of their patients' sexual values, attitudes about specific practices, and concerns about their sexuality. Maintaining open communication with patients about their sexuality allows the physician to counsel them about sexual issues and problems and other aspects of their reproductive health.

Sexual Activity

Sexual activity among adolescents in the United States increased during the past 20 years (3). The average age for first intercourse for both men and women is 16 years. By 19 years of age, as many as three-quarters of women have had intercourse. Most young men and young women have multiple serial sexual partners but use condoms inconsistently, thereby exposing themselves to sexually transmitted diseases (STDs) and unintended pregnancies. A recent study of North American women, using a large and diverse community-based sample, shows that of the 3,205 women aged 30 to 79 years almost one-half were not sexually active in the previous 4 weeks, with 52% of those citing lack of interest and 61% citing lack of partner as the major reasons. Of those who were sexually active recently, 13.7% noted sexual problems and dissatisfaction with their overall sexual lives (4).

Genital Anatomy

For most women, their clitoral tissue is the most sexually sensitive part of their anatomy, and its stimulation produces the most intense sexual feelings and the most intense orgasms. Many women first need to experience both nonphysical and nongenital physical stimulation before clitoral stimulation can be enjoyed. In the absence of arousal, direct clitoral stimulation can be unpleasant and be perceived as too intense and even painful. Immunohistologic studies identified neurotransmitters thought to be associated with sensation concentrated right under the epithelium of the glans clitoris (5). Clitoral tissue extends far beyond the visible portion when the clitoral hood is retracted. It includes the clitoral head, shaft, rami running along the pubic arch, periurethral tissue in front of the anterior vaginal wall, and the bulbar tissue under the superficial perineal muscles surrounding the anterior distal vagina. Other sexually sensitive areas include the nipples, breasts, labia, much of the skin generally, and to some extent, the vagina. **Although the lower third of the vagina is responsive to touch, the upper two-thirds is sensitive primarily to pressure.** The rich supply of nerves in the fascia anterior to the upper vagina (Halban's fascia) and the proximity of the clitoral type of spongy tissue around the urethra anterior to the vagina contribute to the pleasurable sensations of intercourse. Many women experience orgasm more easily from direct clitoral touch, possibly provided at the same time as intercourse.

There is speculation about the existence of a "G-spot," named after Ernest Gräfenberg, who first described it in 1944 (5). This area of the vagina, located anteriorly midway between the symphysis pubis and cervix, is thought to be exquisitely sensitive to deep pressure. Stimulation of this area associated with orgasm and loss of fluid was not scientifically proven to be anything other than dilute urine. Women who are normally continent often leak urine at orgasm; this is not abnormal and does not require medical intervention.

Sexual Response Cycle

Sexual response reflects the fundamental interplay between the mind and body: psychological, interpersonal, cultural, environmental, and biological (hormonal, vascular, muscular, neurological) factors interact and modulate sexual experience. The initial phase of the sexual response cycle may be one of desire, but more often women, particularly those in long-term relationships, are motivated by factors other than sexual desire (3). Women initiate or consent to sex for many reasons, including a wish to increase emotional intimacy with their partners. By directing her attention to sexual stimulation, a woman's subjective sexual arousal/pleasure/excitement triggers sexual desire. Desire and arousal coexist and compound each other (Fig. 11.1). Sexual satisfaction (with one, many, or no orgasms) can be achieved if a woman can stay focused, her pleasure continues, the duration of the stimulation is sufficiently long, and there is no negative outcome (e.g., pain or partner dysfunction). The response is circular, with phases overlapping and in variable order (e.g., desire may follow arousal, and higher arousal may follow the first orgasm). Desire, once triggered, increases the motivation to respond to sexual stimuli and to agree to or ask for more intensely erotic forms of stimulation. Any initial spontaneous desire will augment the response. This circular type of cycle can be experienced a number of times on any one occasion of sexual interaction. This motivation/incentives module reflecting the importance of the mind's appraisal of sexual stimuli is supported by empirical research (6–7).

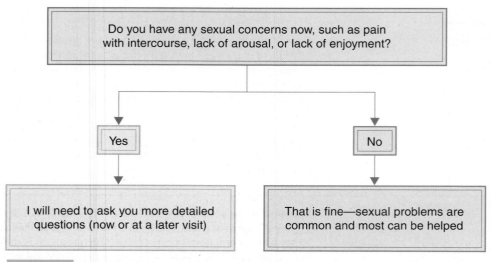

Figure 11.1 The blended sex response cycle showing the many reasons/incentives for initiating/accepting sexual activity.

Physiology

Desire and Arousability

Sexual desire provides one of many motivations to be sexual. Feelings of desire may be triggered by both internal (e.g., fantasies, memories, feelings of arousal) and external (e.g., an interested and interesting partner). Sexual cues are dependent on adequate neuroendocrine function. Multiple neurotransmitters, peptides, and hormones modulate desire and subjective arousal (9). Substances that promote sexual response include norepinephrine, dopamine, oxytocin, melatonin, and serotonin acting on some receptors. Prolactin, serotonin acting on other receptors, endocannabinoids, opioids, and γ-aminobutyric acid inhibit sexual response. These peptides and neurotransmitters are themselves modulated by sex hormones that direct the synthesis of enzymes involved in the production of neurotransmitters and the synthesis of their receptors. Biological factors do not act independently from environmental factors, a finding in human and animal models. Dopamine and progesterone, acting on receptors in the hypothalamus, facilitate sexual behavior in female rats that underwent oophorectomy and received estrogen. The presence of a male animal in an adjacent cage can cause an identical change in sexual behavior (10). Likewise, the ability to be aroused and intensity of response can be increased in some women by giving them a modest dose of testosterone, by administering *bupropion* (dopaminergic), or by a change of partner (11–13). Even in rodents, complex networks exist whereby the female assesses the context of potential sexual activity and relates it to past experience and expectation of reward (14). In women, sexual interest is influenced by their psychological mindset, beliefs and values, expectations, sexual orientation, preferences, and the presence of a safe and erotic environmental setting. Empirical research confirms that an experimentally induced happy or sad mood can impact subjective sexual arousal (but not objective vaginal congestion as measured by a vaginal photoplethysmograph, a tamponlike photoelectric device placed in the vagina) while the woman views an erotic video, with subjects reporting significantly less subjective arousal and marginally significant fewer genital sensations when a negative mood was induced prior to viewing an erotic film clip (15). Moreover, other research concludes that cognitive factors (i.e., lack of erotic thoughts and being distracted or concerned about sexual behavior) were the best predictors of sexual desire: other dimensions including relationship factors, psychopathology, and medical problems appeared to have an indirect impact on sexual desire with the cognitive factors acting as the mediators (16). Sexual desire, interest, and arousability are most strongly influenced by mental health and feelings for the partner, both generally and specifically, at the time of sexual interaction (4,13,17,18). Sexual desire is strongly influenced by fatigue; as a result, sex late at night is not usually attractive to a busy woman. Similarly, chronic illness typically reduces desire and arousability (19).

Sexual Arousal

Recent brain imaging reflects the complexity of sexual arousal, confirming that multiple areas of the brain are involved in sexual response. Brain imaging of healthy people during visual sexual stimulation identifies a model of sexual arousal involving complex brain circuitry, including cortical, limbic, and paralimbic areas known to be involved in cognition, motivation, and emotions linked to changes within the autonomic nervous system (20). Specific inhibitory regions deactivate these sexual responses (21). As demonstrated in this ongoing research, none of this is particularly simple. In a small study, sexually functional surgically menopausal women receiving no hormonal therapy viewed erotic videos during functional magnetic resonance imaging. The women failed to show the brain activation typical of premenopausal women and also typical of themselves when they were treated with both testosterone and estrogen, and yet, they reported sexual arousal from the erotic videos without, and with, hormonal supplementation (22).

Accompanying the subjective excitement and erotic feelings of arousal are a number of physical changes. These changes include genital swelling; increased vaginal lubrication; engorgement of the breasts and nipple erection; increases in skin sensitivity to sexual stimulation; changes in heart rate, blood pressure, muscle tone, breathing, body temperature; mottling of the skin; and a "sex flush" of vasodilatation over the chest, breasts, and face. With sexual stimulation, brain activity in the hypothalamus and other areas influencing the genital response are activated, triggering the autonomic nervous system to allow increased blood flow to the vagina. Vasodilatation of the arterioles in the submucosal vaginal plexus increases transudation of interstitial fluid, which moves from capillaries between the epithelial intercellular spaces and into the vaginal lumen. Simultaneously, the autonomic nervous system allows relaxation of the smooth muscle cells surrounding blood spaces (sinusoids) in the extensive clitoral tissue and labia, causing clitoral swelling and vasodilatation in the labia. Recent immunohistologic studies indicate nerves containing nitric oxide are present in the genital skin covering the clitoris and labia (5).

With arousal, the vagina lengthens, distends, and dilates, and the uterus elevates out of the pelvis. With increased sexual stimulation, vasocongestion reaches a maximum intensity. Genitally, the labia become more swollen and darker red and the lower third of the vagina swells and thickens to form an "orgasmic platform." The clitoris becomes more swollen and elevates to a position near the symphysis pubis, and the uterus elevates fully out of the pelvis. The breasts become more engorged, the skin more mottled, and the nipples more erect.

The neurobiology of arousal is incompletely understood but the genital vasocongestive responses appear to be highly automated, occurring within seconds of an erotic stimulus (23). Parasympathetic nerves release nitric oxide and vasoactive intestinal polypeptide (VIP), mediating vasodilatation (24,25). Acetylcholine (ACh) blocks noradrenergic vasoconstrictive mechanisms and promotes nitric oxide release from endothelium. The parasympathetic and sympathetic nervous systems and the somatic system function less independently than was previously believed. Communication was identified between the cavernous nerves to the clitoris, containing nitric oxide, and the distal portion of the (somatic) dorsal nerve of the clitoris from the pudendal nerve (5). The pelvic sympathetic nerves primarily release (vasoconstrictive) noradrenaline and adenosine triphosphate, but some release ACh, nitric oxide, and VIP. Nitric oxide is thought to be the major neurotransmitter involved in vulvar engorgement (5,25). In the vagina, VIP, nitric oxide, and other unidentified neurotransmitters are involved (25).

Even in women without any sexual dysfunction, there is highly variable correlation between the degree of subjective sexual excitement and the increase in congestion around the vagina (23,26). This poor correlation was shown repeatedly over the past 30 years based on psychophysiologic studies using the vaginal photoplethysmograph. Congestion in response to a sexual video is reduced in women with disruption of the autonomic nerve supplying the vulva and vagina (e.g., from nonnerve-sparing radical hysterectomy). Otherwise healthy women experiencing chronic lack of arousal (including lack of subjective excitement and lack of any awareness of genital congestion) show increases in vaginal congestion from erotic stimuli that are similar those in control women (23,26). With the so-called cervico-motor reflex, cervical touch (in the laboratory with a balloon-tipped catheter to replicate penile pressure) leads to a reduction in pressure in the upper portion of the vagina and an increase in pressure in the middle and lower portions. Simultaneously, an increase in electromyographic activity in the levator ani and puborectalis muscles was recorded. It is thought that during intercourse penile thrusting on the cervix might cause contraction of the pelvic muscles to facilitate "ballooning" of the upper vagina, perhaps to facilitate pooling of semen. The same muscle contraction constricts the lower vagina, which may afford increased stimulation of the partner's penis, thereby maintaining rigidity (27).

A further reflex demonstrated in laboratory studies shows reduced uterine tone in response to mechanical or electrical stimulation of the glans of the clitoris. Background activity of the uterine muscle was abolished by clitoral stimulation if either the glans clitoris or the uterus was anesthetized. Uterine pressure declined on clitoral stimulation. **This reflex may underlie the known increase in size and the elevation of the uterus with sexual arousal** (28).

Orgasm

Orgasms is a brain event, typically triggered by genital stimulation that can occur during sleep or from stimulation of other body parts including the breast and nipple or by fantasy, occasionally by medication, and in spinal cord injured women by vibrostimulation of the cervix. In able-body women, it involves a myotonic response of smooth and striated muscle associated with feelings of sudden release of the sexual tension built up during arousal. It is described as the most intensely pleasurable of the sexual sensations. Reflex rhythmic contractions (3–20 0.8/sec) of the muscles surrounding the vagina and anus occur. Some women may subjectively perceive uterine contractions during orgasm and some may report a difference in their perception of orgasm after hysterectomy, but this is not objectively documented. An objective quantitative measure was established that shows strong correspondence with the subjective experience of orgasm. Analysis of rectal pressure data while volunteers imitated orgasm, tried to achieve orgasm and failed, or experienced orgasm showed a significant and important difference in this analysis between orgasm and both control tasks (29).

Brain imaging studies of women during orgasm showed brain activations and deactivations similar but not identical to those found in men (30). There is profound deactivation in the anterior part of the orbitofrontal cortex (OFC). This area is thought to be involved in urge suppression and behavioral release. This area is activated when experiences are particularly hedonic, with further activation increasing satiation and deactivated with feelings of satiety. The medial OFC is part of the neuronal network underlying self-monitoring and is connected to the amygdala. The latter is deactivated during the genital stimulation and arousal and remains deactivated during orgasm. Deactivation of this network is associated with a more carefree state of mind. The subjective description of orgasm is very much in keeping with this depiction (31).

The majority of women most easily experience orgasm from direct clitoral stimulation. More direct contact with the clitoris is possible from contact of pubis to pubis after the man has ejaculated and penile size is reduced, if the man maintains contact. The bodies are more closely approximated and the woman can move her pelvis on his at a rate that is most conducive to her orgasm. Breast stimulation, kissing, and clitoral stimulation during intercourse are other commons means of experiencing orgasm. **Women are potentially multiorgasmic, capable of experiencing a number of orgasms close together during one sex response cycle and of resuming sexual activity without any refractory period.**

Resolution

Following the sudden release of sexual tension brought about by orgasm, women experience a feeling of relaxation and well-being. The gradual lessening of pelvic engorgement contrasts with the quicker loss of penile firmness in men. Nongenital changes that took place during arousal are reversed, and the body can return to a resting state after some 5 to 10 minutes. With further stimulation, the response can resume before or after this resting state is reached. As depicted in Figure 11.1, the cycle of response can be experienced a number of times during any given sexual encounter. Women who enjoy arousal without orgasm and without any sense that orgasm is very close but frustratingly absent report a similar sense of well-being and relaxation.

Factors Affecting Sexual Response

Numerous factors can affect sexual response (13,19,32–34). These factors include mood; age; relationship duration and quality; personal psychological factors stemming from relationships in childhood with parental figures; previous losses, traumas, and ways of coping with emotions; illness; and use of medication, alcohol, and illicit drugs.

Mental Health

Studies find that mental health has the strongest links to women's sexual function (4,17,35,36). Lack of mental well-being, even if it does not meet the criteria of a clinical diagnosis of mental disorder, is strongly linked to women's symptoms of low desire (37). One study of women, where a diagnosis of clinical depression was excluded, showed a strong association between decreased sexual interest and self-reporting of negative emotional and psychological feelings, including low self-esteem, feelings of insecurity, and lost femininity (18). Impaired sexual desire is noted in most studies of women with depression, even before the administration of antidepressants with sexually negative side effects (35). Paradoxically, depressed women may masturbate more frequently than women who are not depressed, despite an increased prevalence of dyspareunia and difficulties with arousal and orgasm in partnered sex (38). Self-stimulation may cause calmness, relaxation, and improved sleep and in women is often not a consequence of sexual urge or desire.

Aging

The degree to which aging itself, the marked changes in ovarian function associated with menopause, and the marked reduction of adrenal production of prohormones (importantly dehydroepiandrosterone [DHEA]) that can become estrogen and testosterone may affect women's sexual response was addressed in large population studies. **Some studies showned little increase in sexual problems with age, whereas in others almost 40% of the sample reported reductions in responsiveness and an increased desire for nongenital sexual expression (13,39,40).** In one study, the prevalence of reduced desire increased significantly as a function of both menopause status and age, from 22% in the premenopausal group to 32% in the postmenopausal group (41). Low levels of desire were strongly associated with other sexual problems, including difficulties with arousal and orgasm. One large cohort of women studied over 10 years from peri- to postmenopause showed a decline in desire and responsiveness as a function of both age and menopause (42). The independent effect of menopause was indirect. The number of menopausal symptoms experienced influenced well-being, which in turn affected sexual responsiveness and sexual desire and interest.

Many studies of sexuality and aging show that older women report less distress about lack of desire when compared with younger women (17,18,43). In a nonclinical study of 102 women, the determinants of sexual satisfaction in those younger than 45 years of age were compared with those of women older than 45 years of age (18). There was no difference in sexual satisfaction achieved either by intercourse or noncoital sexual activities. Older women reported lower frequency of orgasm and different ratings on certain dimensions of sexual satisfaction. For the older women, the dominant qualities important to their satisfaction were those related to an emotional sense of calm and to factors such as feeling secure with their partner, whereas for younger women the subjective physical experience was more important.

Despite reports of reduced sexual interest and desire by some older women, most retain some interest and maintain the potential for sexual pleasure for their entire lives. In older women, a strong predictor of continued sexual interest is sexual behavior and enjoyment at an earlier age. A discrepancy between sexual interest and actual sexual activity occurs in many cases because an adequate partner is no longer available. In other instances, the cessation of sexual activity with age is more an expression of emotional problems resulting from lack of tenderness, communication, and attraction.

In addition to partner availability, an older woman's sexuality is influenced by her partner's general and sexual health and the relationship itself, which will determine how well the couple can adapt to changes in their sexual function as they age (17,44,45). Although some older women may retain negative societal attitudes toward sex that it is not "natural" (i.e., not focused intercourse), studies show a shift from intercourse to nonpenetrative sex and to a variety of activities that involve affection, romance, affectionate physical intimacy, and companionship (46). For some older women, it is clear that the setting, whether a nursing home or a grown-up child's home, strongly influences the opportunity for sexual expression.

If intercourse is perceived as a necessary component of sexual activity with a partner, some older women will lose motivation and interest as a result of discomfort and dyspareunia associated with lack of estrogen. Although the increase in vaginal congestion in response to visual sexual stimulation is similar in women with and without estrogen, baseline vaginal blood flow is lower in estrogen-deficient women (23). Thus, the increase in lubrication may be insufficient. There may be loss of elasticity and thinning of the vaginal epithelium, which becomes vulnerable to damage from intercourse. Estrogen depletion predisposes women to vulvar vaginitis and urinary tract infections, both of which contribute to dyspareunia and reduce sexual self-image. Women who remain sexually active, alone or with a partner, may have less vulvar and vaginal atrophy than sexually inactive women but may still be symptomatic (47).

Adrenal production of testosterone precursors gradually decreases with age, beginning in the late 30s. Large epidemiological studies have not shown serum levels of testosterone to correlate with women's sexual function (48,49). Available assays were not sufficiently sensitive in the female range of serum testosterone to detect particularly low levels. When mass spectroscopy was used: serum testosterone levels were similar in 121 women carefully assessed and diagnosed with disorders of low desire and arousability to levels in 125 women similarly carefully assessed but to exclude any sexual dysfunction (50). A second difficulty, over and beyond the unreliable assays for serum testosterone, was the fact that intercellular production of testosterone in peripheral tissues (from adrenal and ovarian) precursor hormones—DHEA, DHEA sulfate (DHEAS), and androstenedione (A_4)—previously could not be measured. Total testosterone activity (ovarian and peripherally produced "intracrine production") has been measured using mass spectrometry assays for androgen metabolites, most notably androsterone glucuronide (ADT-G). There appears to be a wide range of ADT-G among women of any given age, and levels decrease with age. **Importantly there were no group differences in ADT-G between 121 women carefully diagnosed with desire and arousal disorders and 124 sexually healthy controls** (50).

Illnesses that accompany aging may have an impact on sexual dysfunction. The association is weaker than that between male erectile dysfunction and hypertension, hyperlipidemia, diabetes, and coronary artery disease. **Depression is the major factor influencing sexual function in women with chronic illness including end-stage renal disease** (51), **multiple sclerosis** (52), **or diabetes** (53). Some sexual activities (e.g., intercourse) or responses (e.g., orgasmic intensity) may be limited by arthritic, cardiac, or respiratory disorders.

Personality Factors

Studies show that, compared with functional women, those who have concerns about low levels of desire and arousability are characterized as having vulnerable self-esteem, high levels of anxiety and guilt, negative body image, introversion, and somatization (18). The clinical impression of women with orgasmic disorder is that many are extremely uncomfortable in conditions in which they are not in control of circumstances or their bodily reactions. **For many women with vaginismus, there is a phobic quality to the fear of vaginal penetration. Many women with provoked vestibulodynia show a marked fear of negative evaluation by others, ultra conscientiousness, and self-criticism, as well as an increase in somatization and anxiety** (54).

Relationships

Most women who report loss of desire and arousability to physicians indicate that their partnerships are stable and satisfactory. An environment free of conflict, abuse, and the threat of separation or divorce is insufficient to nurture a woman's sexual desire. Commonly, the woman reports that her partner is not emotionally intimate with her—not willing to reveal his (or her) feelings, fears, and hopes. Additionally, the woman's need for eroticism and variety of sexual stimulation may not be met. These women frequently classify their relationship as being that of "very good friends." Such a context is insufficiently sexual for nurturing or triggering a woman's sexual desire. Change of partner is shown to be a major factor in increasing women's desire and responsiveness, and there is a lessening of innate desire with the duration of a relationship (13,34). The woman's feelings for her partner is one of the major determinants of lack of distress about sex; similarly, the woman's feelings for her partner, or a change of partner, were major determinants of a woman's desire (13,17,55).

Sexual Dysfunction in the Partner

Multiple aspects of a woman's circumstances can influence her sexual function, and one of the most important aspects is sexual dysfunction in a male partner (56). **Successful treatment of a male partner's erectile dysfunction can result in reversal of the woman's sexual problems, including difficulties with sexual arousal, lubrication, orgasm satisfaction, and pain** (45).

Infertility

Infertility evaluation and assisted reproductive techniques can have negative effects on a woman's body image and feelings of sexual self-worth. Infertility may cause her to feel hopeless and sexually undesirable. The loss of sexual spontaneity resulting from the goal-oriented approach to sex while trying to conceive with scheduled intercourse (coinciding with ovulation naturally or after hormonal stimulation) may lead to sexual dysfunction and is considered a major problem for many women (57). **Erectile dysfunction may be a consequence, compounding the couple's fertility difficulties and the woman's sexual satisfaction** (58). The stress of testing and waiting for results may disrupt emotional intimacy, causing further damage to sexual function. These changes do not always reverse with a successful pregnancy. Often there are unresolved feelings of guilt over personal responsibility for the infertility and feelings of resentment of the multiple procedures required for women compared with one semen analysis for men.

Drugs

Prescription and nonprescription medications, including alcohol and illicit drugs, can alter the normal sexual response (Table 11.1). Adjustments in dosage or formulation of medication may be required. Theoretically, pharmacologic agents might improve or reverse the loss of arousal, desire, and orgasm commonly associated with serotonergic antidepressants (SSRIs). A Cochrane review could make no recommendations for women but did note that *bupropion* may be effective based on the results of one of two randomized controlled trials (43,59). In highly selective women on SSRIs, *sildenafil* may reverse orgasmic dysfunction (60).

Chronic Illness

Chronic illness and living with a cancer diagnosis can affect sexual function in a number of ways (Table 11.2) (20).

Chronic Pelvic Inflammatory Disease and Endometriosis

Chronic dyspareunia, remitting temporarily or not at all with surgical or medical therapy, typically is associated with loss of sexual motivation or interest. Although definitive therapy is the overall goal, encouragement of nonpenetrative sex is very important for preservation of the woman's sexual enjoyment, sexual self-esteem, and relationship. GnRH therapy producing a

Table 11.1 Medications Affecting Sexual Response

Drugs with potential negative sexual effects

- Antihypertensives: β-blockers, thiazides
- Antidepressants: serotonergic antidepressants
- *Lithium*
- Antipsychotics
- Antihistamines
- Narcotics
- Benzodiazepines
- Oral contraceptives and oral estrogen therapy
- Gonadotropin-releasing hormone (GnRH) agonists
- *Spironolactone*
- Cocaine
- Alcohol
- Anticonvulsants

Drugs that appear to be potentially prosexual

- *Danazol*
- *Levadopa*
- Amphetamines
- *Bupropion*

temporary medical menopause can add further difficulties with reduced arousability and vaginal discomfort from the low estrogen state.

Polycystic Ovarian Syndrome

There is no evidence that the higher androgen levels associated with polycystic ovarian syndrome (PCOS) afford protection from low sexual desire or low sexual arousability. Some but not all studies of women with PCOS report reduced sexual satisfaction compared to controls. The limited data suggest that lower satisfaction is related to obesity and cosmetic androgen-related effects of hirsutism and acne. One small case study showed desire to increase in six women with antiandrogen treatment and to decrease in 13 women (61). *Metformin* may improve sexual function in women with PCOS (62).

Recurrent Herpes

Fear of spreading an STD may reduce sexual motivation and arousability. Clear guidance regarding safer sexual practices is needed, along with a discussion of the causes of the woman's

Table 11.2 Sex and Chronic Illness

- Biological disruption of the sexual response, e.g., multiple sclerosis damaging pelvic autonomic nerves
- Negative psychological consequences of the illness affecting sexual response, e.g., feeling sexually unattractive as a result of disfigurement from surgery, medication, stomas
- Increased fatigue
- Chronic pain
- Incontinence or stomas reducing sexual self-confidence
- Accompanying depressive illness
- Treatment of chronic illness, e.g., chemotherapy-inducing ovarian failure
- Limited mobility, e.g., arthritis precluding intercourse, Parkinson's disease precluding masturbation
- Cardiac or respiratory compromise such that orgasm or movements of intercourse cause angina or intense dyspnea

lowered sexual motivation. A recognized difficulty with recurrent herpes is viral shedding despite lack of skin lesions and uncertainty whether long-term antiviral therapy prevents shedding.

Lichen Sclerosis

Tethering of the clitoral hood, which occurs with lichen sclerosis, may cause pain with clitoral stimulation. When this skin disorder involves the introitus, it may cause dyspareunia or prevent entry of penis, dildo, or fingers. Reduced sexual sensitivity of the involved vulvar skin is a common complaint. Topical *corticosteroid* administration is the primary treatment, although topical *testosterone* cream may be beneficial when loss of sexual sensitivity occurs.

Breast Cancer

Sexual dysfunction following breast cancer treatment is likely to persist more than 1 year after diagnosis of breast cancer (63). Chemotherapy appears to be responsible for most of the resulting sexual difficulties, including loss of desire, subjective arousal, vaginal dryness, and dyspareunia (64). A small study of women with past breast cancer and complex endocrine status resulting from ongoing antiestrogen therapy found that, whereas relationship factors predicted desire, history of chemotherapy predicted disorders of arousal lubrication, orgasm, and dyspareunia but there was no connection between sexual function and androgen levels including androgen metabolites (65). A model for predicting sexual interest, function, and satisfaction after breast cancer has evolved from two large independent groups of breast cancer survivors (64). The most important predictors of sexual health were absence of vaginal dryness, presence of emotional well-being, positive body image, better quality of relationship, and lack of partner sexual problems. A temporary "medical menopause" from adjuvant GnRH agonist treatment is associated with reversible sexual dysfunction (66). Use of *tamoxifen* does not consistently alter sexual function, but use of aromatase inhibitors is often associated with severe dyspareunia from the profoundly estrogen-depleted state (67,68).

The optimal management of ongoing dyspareunia from the estrogen deficient state, especially when the woman is on aromatase inhibitors, is unclear. Zero systemic absorption of estrogen from vaginally administered preparations is the goal, and formulations are under investigation for efficacy at lower dosages than are currently available. Some oncologists will permit the use of local estrogen via a Silastic ring that does cause brief, but detectable (although not to premenopausal estrogen levels), systemic absorption. For most of the 3 months that the ring is in place systemic absorption is not detectable. Vaginal moisturizers can allow some benefit but do not restore the full elasticity.

Fertility preservation is considered along with the overall treatment plan for younger women, and a number of options are emerging. One is to delay treatment to undergo a cycle of hormone stimulation and oocyte retrieval, providing the growth of the tumor is not expected to be promoted by exogenous *estrogen*. Other techniques can avoid exposure to exogenous hormones by retrieving ovarian tissue and either aspirating the oocytes or reserving ovarian tissue strips and then using cryopreservation. An even newer technique called *in follicle maturation* involves obtaining immature follicles from the cryopreserved ovarian tissue, maturing them *in vitro*, to be followed by *in vitro* fertilization procedures (20).

Diabetes

The majority of studies clearly identified a strong link between sexual dysfunction and comorbid depression but not with diabetic controls, duration of diabetes, or its complications. Data are limited in quality given that many studies do not clarify estrogen status, different assessments of sexual function are used, and many publications study only the women who do not remain sexually active—those who simply do not have a partner or may have discontinued activity as a result of severe dysfunction (69). Prevalence of low sexual desire is found to be similar in women with and without diabetes, whereas difficulties with lubrication are approximately two times more common in women with diabetes. Some but not all studies show increased prevalence of dyspareunia, orgasmic difficulties, and sexual dissatisfaction (70). A large study involving women enrolled in the long-term Epidemiology of Diabetes Interventions and Complications (EDIC) study neither compared patients with control women nor inquired about dysfunction in those who were not sexually active. Nevertheless, dysfunction was present in 35% of the active women with low desire, and more than half had problems with orgasm arousal and lubrication. In multivariate analysis, only depression and marital status predicted sexual dysfunction (69).

Hysterectomy

Simple Hysterectomy

Despite speculation that there might be different sexual outcomes depending on whether hysterectomy was vaginal, subtotal, or total abdominal, this difference is not supported by study (71,72). In a large prospective observational study of 413 women undergoing three different types of hysterectomy (vaginal, supracervical, and total abdominal hysterectomy), sexual pleasure improved in most women, independent of the type of hysterectomy (72). The prevalence of one or more bothersome sexual problems 6 months after vaginal, supracervical, and total abdominal hysterectomy was 43%, 41%, and 39%, respectively. The results of another prospective trial of 158 women randomized to total abdominal hysterectomy and 161 to supracervical abdominal hysterectomy showed no difference in sexual outcomes (71). A retrospective study of 108 women undergoing classic intrafascial supracervical hysterectomy and 125 undergoing total hysterectomy did not find any sexual benefits of classic intrafascial supracervical hysterectomy over total hysterectomy (73). **There was no difference between groups in time from surgery to first intercourse, change in libido, sexual frequency, or frequency or degree of orgasm.** Overall, two-thirds of the women in the study experienced either no change or an improvement in sexual function, regardless of which procedure was performed. Both this study and a study comparing total laparoscopic hysterectomy with laparoscopically assisted vaginal hysterectomy found similar effects on sexual function (74).

Radical Hysterectomy

Techniques were developed to avoid the portions of the inferior hypogastric plexus in the cardinal and broad ligaments, and preliminary studies suggest minimal reduction of vaginal congestion in response to sexual stimulation in a laboratory setting (75). Only one of two small clinical studies confirmed preservation of sexual function (76,77).

Cancer of the Cervix

Sexual symptoms encountered in women with cancer of the cervix include reduced vaginal lubrication secondary to surgical menopause, radiation damage, and/or interruption of the autonomic nerves. A study conducted in Croatia showed the importance of fear of dyspareunia. Of 210 women treated with combinations of surgery, radiation, and chemotherapy, 50% reported a marked fear of pain. Only six patients identified actual dyspareunia and only three patients found penetration impossible (78).

There is marked synergy between cancer of the cervix and sexual abuse as a cause of sexual dysfunction (79). An absence of sexual satisfaction was reported by 20% of women with neither abuse nor cancer of the cervix, by 31% of women who were sexually abused and did not have cancer of the cervix, by 28% of women with cancer of the cervix and who were not abused, but by 45% of women with a history of both abuse and cancer of the cervix. The lack of sexual satisfaction resulted in a decrease in well-being in 18% of women with neither a history of abuse nor cancer of the cervix, 39% of women who were abused and did not have cancer of the cervix, 23% of women with cancer of the cervix who were not abused, and in 44% of women with a history of both abuse and cancer of the cervix. Dyspareunia was extremely rare in women without cancer of the cervix, but it was reported by 12% of those with cancer of the cervix and by 30% of those with cancer of the cervix and past sexual abuse.

Pregnancy

Physical, emotional, and economic stressors of pregnancy may negatively affect emotional and sexual intimacy. Sexual value systems, folklore, religious beliefs, physical changes, and medical restrictions influence sexual attitudes and behavior during pregnancy and postpartum. In the absence of preterm labor, antepartum bleeding, or an incompetent cervix, there is no evidence that sexual activity, orgasm, or intercourse increases the risk of pregnancy complications. Normal changes that occur with sexual activity during pregnancy include increased breast tenderness, increased sensitivity to uterine contractions with orgasm, general discomfort, less mobility, and fatigue. Sexual satisfaction in pregnancy is closely related to feeling happy about the pregnancy, continuing to feel attractive, and understanding that in a healthy pregnancy sexual activity and orgasm do not harm the fetus.

Toward the end of the third trimester the need for closeness, emotional support, and nurturing may be far greater than any desire for orgasms or intercourse. Nevertheless, a study noted that 39% of 188 women reported being engaged in intercourse during their birth week (80). Difficulties may arise from the partner's reaction to the woman's pregnancy, the physical changes of pregnancy, lack of information regarding sex and pregnancy, and lack of direction from the physician when complications arise. **A general lessening of sexual desire in both pregnancy and the postpartum period is common and considered normal.** A prospective analysis of sexual function of 40 healthy pregnant women showed a reduction in desire and in all aspects of sexual response beginning in the first trimester, changing little in the second, and reducing further in the third trimester (81). **Couples should be encouraged to continue their usual patterns of lovemaking during pregnancy if they are emotionally and physically comfortable and there are no contraindications to either orgasm or intercourse.**

Postpartum

The ongoing vaginal bleeding and discharge, perineal discomfort, hemorrhoids, sore breasts, and decreased vaginal lubrication associated with nursing, compounded by fatigue from disturbed nights, all contribute to decreased motivation for sexual activity. Further complicating factors include fear of waking the baby, a decreased sense of attractiveness, change of body image, or mood change. Many couples resume sexual activity and include intercourse by 6 to 8 weeks postpartum, but some couples wait as long as a year before resuming their prepregnancy level of sexual intimacy. Typically women who nurse report less sexual activity and less sexual satisfaction than those who bottle feed. **The effect of the mode of delivery on sexual function is still unclear. Two studies showed operative vaginal delivery confered the highest risk of dysfunction** (82,83).

Physicians can provide considerable help to patients and their partners by acknowledging and discussing the normal fluctuations in sexual desire and frequency of sexual activity during and after pregnancy.

Assessment of Sexual Problems

Despite the importance of issues relating to sexuality, many women find it difficult to talk to their physicians about sexual concerns and many physicians are uncomfortable discussing sexual issues with their patients. In one survey, 71% of adults said they thought their doctor would dismiss any concerns about sexual problems they might introduce, and 68% said they were afraid that discussing sexuality would embarrass their physician (84). Through the use of a structured questionnaire and review of the records of 1,065 women who consecutively attended 37 family practices in areas of high, medium, and low socioeconomic status, 40% of women had at least one form of sexual dysfunction according to diagnostic criteria of the International Statistical Classification of Disease (ICD-10). Only 4% had a prior entry in their medical record relating to sexual problems (85).

There are numerous reasons physicians are reluctant to discuss issues relating to sexuality with their patients. Anxiety about physicians' perceived inability to treat sexual problems, unwillingness to spend the time required to accurately assess sexual concerns, personal discomfort when discussing sexual matters with patients and distress arising from their patients' history of sexual-related violence are all potential barriers. Not asking about sexual function suggests to patients that sexuality is not important and should not to be discussed. **Moreover, many gynecological interventions and a number of gynecological conditions interrupt sexual function, necessitating the inclusion of sexual health in gynecological assessment. Asking about sexual concerns gives physicians an opportunity to educate patients about the risk of STDs, encourage safer sex practices, evaluate the need for contraception, dispel sexual misconceptions, and identify sexual dysfunction.** Many sexual concerns can be resolved by providing factual information and reassurance. Management of sexual dysfunction requires appropriate biopsychosocial assessment and intervention. Even when patients currently have no sexual problems, when gynecologists routinely inquire about sexual health, they can teach that future sexual issues can be addressed in a professional, confidential, and nonjudgmental setting.

Interviewing Techniques

To be sufficiently comfortable to establish rapport and trust with patients, physicians need to be familiar with the components of a sensitive, detailed, sexual assessment and the general principles of management of dysfunction. Good listening skills and attention to nonverbal cues are helpful. The use of straightforward language that patients can understand and

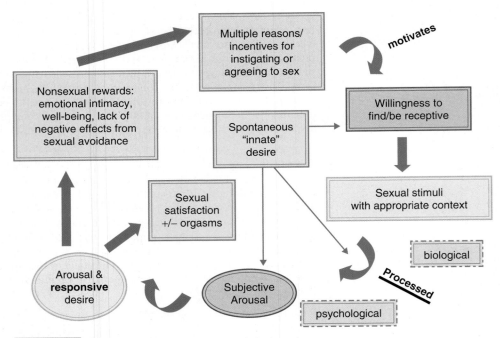

Figure 11.2   **Algorithm for screening sexual dysfunction.**

acknowledge, and the recognition that many people find it difficult to discuss these sensitive, intimate, and extremely common issues are necessary.

A few open-ended questions can initiate the subject of sexual function (Fig. 11.2). Sexual inquiry is part of the medical history taken during a routine gynecologic assessment. There is evidence that an introductory sentence would greatly increase the chance a woman will identify her sexual problem. Listed in Table 11.3 are some examples of screening questions related to particular obstetric–gynecologic circumstances.

Optimally, the detailed assessment is obtained from both partners. Questions can be directed to the couple or the individual partners, depending on the circumstances (Table 11.4). When dyspareunia is present, detailed questioning is necessary (Table 11.5).

Physical Examination

Routine pelvic examination is an essential component of general medical care; this is not the case with women who seek care for sexual concerns. Given the prevalence of negative past sexual experiences, including abuse, **a pelvic examination should be performed only in the presence of a definite indication, and the procedure should be clearly explained to the patient** (Table 11.6). Management of dyspareunia mandates careful vulvar, vaginal, and pelvic examination. A physical examination can confirm normal anatomy and the healthy nonaroused state of the genitalia, it does not confirm healthy sexual function. Nevertheless, such an examination can be both instructive and therapeutic.

Diagnostic Criteria

Just as phases of sexual response overlap, types of women's sexual dysfunctions overlap (18,41). The Second International Consensus on Sexual Dysfunctions in Men and Women provides evidence-based recommendations for the diagnosis of sexual dysfunction and encompasses the proposed revisions to the American Psychiatric Association's *Diagnostic and Statistical Manual,* Fourth Text Revised (DSM-IV-TR) definitions of women's sexual dysfunction (86,87) (Table 11.7).

The official revisions—DSM-V—are due in 2012. Interim publications advocate that desire and arousal disorders are merged (88,89). Increasing evidence indicates that desire ahead of and at the outset of sexual engagement, although probably welcomed by both partners, is not mandatory for women's sexual enjoyment and satisfaction (3). It is the inability to trigger desire and arousal during sexual engagement, and an initial absence of desire, that constitutes disorder. Therefore, merging sexual and desire difficulties into one disorder appears logical.

Table 11.3 Screening for Sexual Problems

Situation in which Screening Question Is Necessary	*Suggested Screening Question*
Before surgery or instituting medication or hormone therapy	*Your surgery or medication is not expected to interfere with your sexual function. I need to check, though, whether you have any difficulties now with sexual desire, arousal, or enjoyment; or is there any pain?*
Routine antenatal visit	*Women's sexual needs can change during pregnancy. Do you have any problems or questions now? There is no evidence that intercourse or orgasm leads to miscarriage. Of course, any bleeding or spotting will require checking and postponing sexual activity until we have evaluated you. Many women find fatigue and/or nausea reduce their sexual life in the first 3 months, but usually things get back to normal for the middle 3 months and sometimes right up to term.*
Complicated antenatal visit	*These complications may well have already caused you to stop being sexual. Specifically, you should not (have intercourse/have orgasms).*
After one or more miscarriages	*Some women temporarily lose desire for sex after a miscarriage—this is quite normal. Many couples concentrate on affectionate touching while they both grieve about what has happened. Do allow yourselves some time. If any sexual problems persist, we can address them.*
Infertility	*All this testing and timed intercourse and disappointment, plus the financial burdens that are coming up, can be very stressful on your sex life. Try to have times when you and your partner are sexual just for pleasure and intimacy's sake—not when you are trying to conceive. Do you have any problems now?*
Postpartum	*It may be some weeks or months before you have the energy to be sexual, especially if your sleep is really interrupted. This is normal. If problems persist, or if you have pain, this can be addressed. Do you have any questions right now?*
Perimenopause or postmenopause	*We know many women have very rewarding sex after menopause—more time, more privacy. If you find the opposite or you begin to have pain or difficulty getting aroused, these things can be addressed. Do you have any concerns now?*
Woman who is depressed	*I know you are depressed right now, but our studies tell us that sex is still important for many women who are depressed. We also know that some of the medications we prescribe interfere with sexual enjoyment. Do you have any problems right now?*
Chronic illness	*Arthritis/multiple sclerosis can interfere with a woman's sex life. Are you having any problems?*
Potential damaging surgery	*Obviously the focus right now is to remove your cancer entirely when we do your surgery. The nerves and blood vessels that allow sexual sensations and lubrication may be temporarily and sometimes permanently damaged. If when you have recovered you notice any sexual problems that persist, they can be addressed. Do you have any sexual concerns now?*
Bilateral oophorectomy	*Your surgery will remove a major source of estrogen and approximately one half of the testosterone your body has been making. Testosterone will still be made by adrenal glands (small glands on top of the kidneys), and some of this gets converted into estrogen. Many women find that these reduced amounts of sex hormones are quite sufficient for sexual enjoyment, but others do not. Any sexual problems that do occur almost certainly can be addressed. Do you have any problems now?*

Each disorder is then further classified by the following descriptors:

1. **Lifelong or acquired**
2. **Generalized or situational**
3. **The degree of distress—mild, moderate, or marked**
4. **Presence of contextual factors**
   A. **Past factors from developmental history affecting psychosexual development**

Table 11.4 Biopsychosocial Assessment of Sexual Dysfunction	
Sexual problem in patient's own words	Clarify further with direct questions; give options rather than leading questions.
Duration, consistency, priority	Duration of problems? Are problems present in all situations? If more than one problem, which is most troubling?
Context of sexual problems	Emotional intimacy with partner, activity/behavior just before sexual activity, privacy, safety, birth control, risk of sexually transmitted disease, usefulness of sexual stimulation, sexual skills of partner, sexual communication, time of day
Rest of each partner's sexual response	Check this currently and before the onset of the sexual problems—sexual motivation, subjective arousal, enjoyment, orgasm, pain, and erection and ejaculation in male partner
Reaction of each partner to sexual problems	How each has reacted emotionally, sexually, and behaviorally
Previous help	Compliance with recommendations and effectiveness
Reason for presenting now	What has precipitated this request for help
Assessment of Each Partner Alone	
Partner's own assessment of the situation	Sometimes it is easier to acknowledge symptoms, e.g., total lack of desire, in the partner's absence
Sex response with self-stimulation	Also ask about sexual thoughts and fantasies
Past sexual experiences[a]	Positive, negative aspects
Developmental history[a]	Relationships to others in the home while growing up, losses, traumas, how they coped. To whom (if anyone) was this person close? Who showed them affection, love, respect? Clarify if some of these themes are playing out now in the current sexual relationship.
Ask about sexual, emotional, and physical abuse[a]	Explain abuse questions are routine and do not necessarily imply causation of the problems.

[a]These items of the single patient interview may sometimes be omitted (e.g., for a recent problem after decades of healthy sexual function).

B. **Present contextual factors—interpersonal, environmental, societal, and cultural**

C. **Medical factors**

Management of Sexual Dysfunction

Many of the sexual problems couples encounter result from a deficit of knowledge or experience, sexual misconceptions, or inability of the couple to communicate about their sexual preferences. Brief counseling and education by the obstetrician–gynecologist regarding the circular sex response cycle can identify the areas where sexual dysfunction can occur.

Table 11.5 Assessment of Dyspareunia: By History
• Ask if vaginal entry is possible at all (i.e., with finger, penis, dildo, speculum, tampon)
• Ask if sexual arousal is experienced when intercourse is attempted and as it progresses
• Ask exactly when the pain is experienced: —With partial entry of the penis/ dildo —With attempted full entry of penile head —With deep thrusting —With penile movement —With the man's ejaculation —With the woman's subsequent urination —For hours or minutes after intercourse attempts
• Ask if on some occasions there is less/no pain, and if so, what is different

Table 11.6 Physical Examination for Sexual Dysfunction	
General examination	Signs of systemic disease leading to low energy, low desire, low arousability, e.g., anemia, bradycardia and slow relaxing reflexes of hypothyroidism. Signs of connective tissue disease, such as scleroderma or Sjögren's, which are associated with vaginal dryness. Disabilities that might preclude movements involved in caressing a partner, self-stimulation, intercourse. Disfigurements/presence of stomas; catheters that may decrease sexual self-confidence, leading to low desire; low arousability.
External genitalia	Sparsity of pubic hair, suggesting low adrenal androgens. Vulval skin disorders, including lichen sclerosis, which may cause soreness with sexual stimulation (e.g., when it involves the clitoral hood). Cracks/fissures in the interlabial folds suggestive of chronic candidiasis. Labial abnormalities that may cause embarrassment/sexual hesitancy (e.g., particularly long labia or asymmetry).
Introitus	Vulval disease involving introitus (e.g., lichen sclerosis). Recurrent splitting of the posterior fourchette manifest as just visible white lines perpendicular to fourchette edge. Abnormalities of the hymen (e.g., hymenal band across the introitus). Adhesions of the labia minora. Swellings in the area of the major vestibular glands. Allodynia (pain sensation from touch stimulus) of the crease between the outer hymenal edge and the inner edge of the labia minora +/− allodynia of the Skene's duct openings (all typical of provoked vestibulodynia). Presence of cystocele, rectocele, or prolapse interfering with the woman's sexual self-image. Inability to tighten and relax perivaginal muscles (often associated with hypertonicity of pelvic muscles and midvaginal dyspareunia). Abnormal vaginal discharge associated with burning dyspareunia.
Internal examination	Pelvic muscle tone. Presence of tenderness or trigger points on palpating deep levator ani as a result of underlying hypertonicity.
Full bimanual examination	Presence of nodules and/or tenderness in the cul-de-sac or vaginal fornix, or along uterosacral ligaments. Retroverted fixed uterus as causes of deep dyspareunia. Tenderness palpating posterior bladder wall from anterior vaginal wall suggestive of bladder pathology.

The PLISSIT Model

Gynecologists may sometimes need to provide detailed management for certain conditions (e.g., for the chronic dyspareunia of provoked vestibulodynia [PVD]), frequently the first two levels of a model, known by its acronym as PLISSIT, are sufficient to address women's sexual problems. The model is as follows:

1. **P**ermission. The concept of permission is the validation of the patient's concerns and confirmation that the gynecologist's office is an appropriate setting to address them.

2. **L**imited **I**nformation. The patient is provided with information about sexual physiology and behavior so misunderstandings, myths, lack of knowledge, and inadequate sexual skills can be addressed.

3. **S**pecific **S**uggestions. This stage may involve altering the problematic sexual context, reeducating patients about specific attitudes and practices, advising different forms of sexual stimulation, screening for mental health issues, identifying interpersonal issues and prescribing hormones and medications.

4. Referral for **I**ntensive **T**herapy. Examples where this step may be necessary include (i) intrapsychological issues stemming from childhood that impair women's ability to be aroused and experience sexual pleasure and satisfaction including past traumas and abuse, (ii) for couples who need more specialized help in sexual communication, and (iii) for male sexual dysfunctions.

As an example of a PLISSIT approach, a woman with chronic dyspareunia from PVD is first given validation of her pain and is provided with the information that PVD is common and many women find that the pain precludes intercourse. The patient and her partner are encouraged to focus on nonpenetrative aspects of lovemaking. The next level is the provision of limited information about chronic pain mechanisms, the role of psychological stress, and genetic and possible immune factors. Specific suggestions could include ongoing encouragement to remove intercourse as one of the ways the couple interact sexually, explanation of basic cognitive behavioral therapy (CBT)

	Table 11.7 Revised DSM-IV Definitions of Women's Sexual Dysfunction	
Diagnosis	*Definition*	*Comments*
Sexual desire/interest disorder	Absent or diminished feelings of sexual interest or desire, absent sexual thoughts or fantasies *and* a lack of responsive desire. Motivations (here defined as reasons/incentives) for attempting to become sexually aroused are scarce or absent. The lack of interest is beyond a normative lessening with life cycle and relationship duration.	Minimal spontaneous sexual thinking or desiring of sex ahead of sexual experiences does not necessarily constitute disorder. Additional lack of responsive desire is integral to the diagnosis.
Combined sexual arousal disorder	Absent or markedly reduced feelings of sexual arousal (sexual excitement and sexual pleasure) from any type of stimulation and absent or impaired genital sexual arousal (vulval swelling and lubrication).	There is minimal sexual excitement (subjective arousal) from any type of stimulation—erotic material, stimulating the partner, genital and nongenital stimulation. There is no awareness of the reflexive genital vasocongestion.
Subjective sexual arousal disorder	Absent or markedly reduced feelings of sexual arousal (sexual excitement and sexual pleasure) from any type of stimulation. Vaginal lubrication and other signs of physical response still occur.	Despite lack of sexual excitement/ subjective arousal, lubrication is noted by the woman or partner. Intercourse is comfortable without use of external lubricant.
Genital arousal disorder	Absent or impaired genital sexual arousal–minimal vulval swelling or vaginal lubrication from any type of sexual stimulation and reduced sexual sensations from caressing genitalia. *Subjective sexual excitement still occurs from nongenital sexual stimuli.*	Subjective arousal (sexual excitement) from nongenital stimuli (erotica, stimulating the partner, receiving breast stimulation, kissing) is key to this diagnosis. Early studies indicate reduced vasocongestion in some but not all cases. Loss of sexual sensitivity of physiologically congested tissues accounts for others.
Orgasmic disorder	Despite the self-report of high sexual arousal/excitement, there is either lack of orgasm, markedly diminished intensity of orgasmic sensations, or marked delay of orgasm from any kind of stimulation.	Women with arousal disorders frequently do not experience orgasm. Their correct diagnosis is one of an arousal disorder.
Vaginismus	Persistent or recurrent difficulties of the women to allow vaginal entry of a penis, finger, or any object despite the woman's expressed wish to do so. There is often (phobic) avoidance and anticipation/fear/experience of pain, along with variable and involuntary pelvic muscle contraction. Structural or other physical abnormalities must be ruled out/addressed.	Confirmation of this diagnosis is not possible until there has been therapy sufficient to allow a careful introital and vaginal examination. It is a presumptive diagnosis initially.
Dyspareunia	Persistent or recurrent pain with attempted or complete vaginal entry and or penile vaginal intercourse	There are many causes, including localized provoked vestibulodynia (vulvar vestibulitis syndrome) and vulvar atrophy from estrogen deficiency.

From **Basson R, Wierman M, van Lankveld J, et al.** Summary on the recommendations on sexual dysfunction in women. *J Sex Med* 2010;7:314–326, with permission.

concepts and/or referral to psychologist or counselor for the same, prescription of medications for chronic pain, prophylaxis for overgrowth of candidiasis when this is relevant, and referral to a pelvic muscle physiotherapist. Referral for intensive therapy may be indicated for further pain management, including learning the skills of mindfulness, further exploration of CBT, for couple counseling if the relationship cannot cope with the stress, or occasionally, to a gynecologist specializing in vulvar surgery if vestibulectomy is considered.

Sexual Dysfunction

The larger surveys find approximately 10% of women report ongoing sexual dysfunction that is particularly upsetting, while a further 20% report sexual problems that are less distressing (4,90). Comorbidity of low desire and subjective arousal along with infrequent or absent orgasm is the most common presentation (18,91). Postmenopausal vaginal dryness and associated dyspareunia affects some 15% to 30% of women with marked cultural differences to the extent that this leads to bothersome sexual difficulties (92). Lack of lubrication and associated dyspareunia is reported by 5% to 25% of younger women with marked cultural differences leading to resulting sexual distress (92). Introital dyspareunia from PVD, the most common cause of dyspareunia in premenopausal women, is thought to affect some 15% of women (93). Isolated lack of orgasm despite high arousal is of unknown prevalence because studies generally include women with low arousal alongside their lack of orgasm.

Management of Sexual Desire and Arousal Disorders

Construction of the woman's sex response cycle showing the various breaks can be highly therapeutic for the woman and her partner. For example, Figure 11.3 shows the various breaks subsequent to infertility testing. The couple learns that it is "normal" for the woman to have low motivation to be sexual when emotional intimacy has suffered. If the issues distancing the couple cannot be addressed in the gynecologist's office (i.e., they extend over and beyond the common reactions to infertility testing and procedures), referral to a relationship counselor may be necessary. The gynecologist can address the sexual context and the type of stimulation that is provided. Often sex has become "mechanical"—intercourse focused to achieve conception. Most women need more nonphysical stimulation, more nongenital physical stimulation, and more nonpenetrative genital sexual stimulation, and this can be stressed. Privacy issues, time of day, and emotional closeness at the time of lovemaking can all be discussed. Factors personal to the woman that may be impairing her ability to be aroused, such as low sexual self-image and distractions, can be identified. Referral for CBT may be necessary when low self-image appears ingrained and stems from developmental factors. Biological factors influencing arousability, including fatigue, medication effect, and depression, may be involved. Fears regarding outcome, such as lack of adequate birth control or partner dysfunction, can be identified. Inquiring about the patient's thoughts at the time of potential lovemaking can be helpful. Some women admit to evoking negative thoughts or allowing spontaneously emerging negative thoughts to intrude

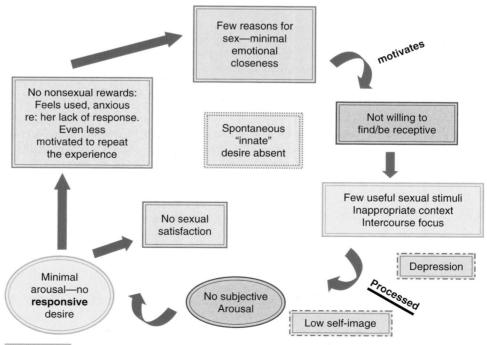

Figure 11.3   **Breaks in the circular sex response cycle subsequent to infertility testing.**

when there is a sexual opportunity. Guilt about sex and about women having sexual pleasure may be present. If the woman is a new mother, she may feel on one level that sex now is "wrong." Experiences of assisted reproduction technique or delivery may lead to the woman feeling loss of control; this in turn may lead to a need to regain control in all aspects of her life, which may suppress her sexual feelings. CBT and mindfulness therapies are recommended (94).

Randomized controlled trials of transdermal *testosterone* for medically and psychiatrically healthy postmenopausal women with low sexual desire were published. Four involved surgically menopausal estrogenized women (95–98). Transdermal *testosterone* (300 μg) daily significantly increased the frequency of sexually satisfying events ($p = .049$) compared to placebo. At baseline, these studies showed that the recruited women reported two to three sexually satisfying experiences per month, and these increased to approximately five per month with active drug (300 μg of *testosterone*), and to four per month with placebo. Using a validated unpublished questionnaire, scores in the desire and arousal scales were significantly increased by active drug in the first three studies (for desire: $p = .05$ in the first study and .006 in the second, .001 in the third). The fourth smaller study of prescribed transdermal *estrogen* recruiting women showed significant increase in desire and response scales, but not in the numbers of sexually satisfying events (98). Results from one study of 549 naturally menopausal women receiving oral *estrogen* and transdermal *testosterone* were similar (99).

Two studies of transdermal *testosterone* to estrogen-deficient women showed benefit (100,101). A previous small study showed minimal or no benefit from transdermal *testosterone* in estrogen-deficient women with past history of cancer (102).

There was minimal benefit from transdermal *testosterone* when given to premenopausal women in another study of 261 premenopausal women recruited on the basis of loss of their former sexual satisfaction (103).

The criteria for recruitment are a major drawback of the *testosterone* patch trials. It is not certain that the recruited women had any sexual disorder: the focus consistently was on the frequency of satisfying events in women able to have such experiences—some 50% (98). The participants did not have consistent difficulties or dysfunctions, pointing against a biological cause or need for a biological remedy and pointing toward psychological, relationship, or contextual factors, which are inherently variable. As noted, there was improvement in the secondary end points of desire and response subscales in the (unpublished) validated questionnaires used in all the trials. Increasing the degree of pleasure and arousal currently experienced may not necessarily imply that absent pleasure and absent arousal would be remedied.

Long-term safety issues include those of the combination of *testosterone* and *estrogen* and concerns about *estrogen* itself. Beginning systemic *estrogen* some 10 years postmenopause is known to increase cardiovascular risk: aromatization of exogenous *testosterone* to estrogen is likely. For postmenopausal women not receiving *estrogen,* long-term sequelae of creating a distinctly nonphysiological profile of the testosterone:estrogen ratio are completely unknown. Endogenously high testosterone along with obesity in older women is associated with insulin resistance and increased cardiovascular morbidity (104).

Genital Arousal Disorder

There are no approved medications for treating desire and arousal disorders in women. Approval was sought from the U.S. Food and Drug Administration (FDA) for transdermal *testosterone* but not granted because of theoretical risks to breast tissue and cardiovascular health with only modest benefit. Approval for phosphodiesterase inhibitors was not sought—the larger studies show no benefit of placebo for women's sexual dysfunction. Off-label use of *sildenafil* when genital congestion is likely to be impaired by an underlying illness such as diabetes, multiple sclerosis, or spinal cord injury showed some modest benefit to lubrication in small studies (33).

Orgasmic Dysfunction

Lifelong orgasmic disorder is more common than acquired loss of orgasm. Some women acquire orgasmic dysfunction in association with relationship problems, depression, substance abuse, medication (especially use of SSRIs), or chronic illness (e.g., multiple sclerosis). Aside from those using SSRIs, most women who experience lack of orgasm are found on careful questioning to have only modest degrees of subjective excitement. Sometimes women respond to reassurance that most couples do not experience orgasm simultaneously, that most women experience orgasm far more easily from direct clitoral stimulation, and that this does not constitute dysfunction.

Common causes of lack of orgasm include obsessive self-observation and monitoring during the arousal phase, sometimes accompanied by anxiety and distracting negative and self-defeating thoughts. The woman may be so intent on monitoring her own and her partner's response and concerned about "failing" that she is unable to allow her natural reflexes to take over and trigger an orgasm. Lack of orgasm may be related to negative feelings toward sexuality, low self-esteem, poor body image, a history of sexual abuse, and fear of losing control, and ineffective sexual technique. **The only evidenced-based therapy is encouragement of self-stimulation, accompanied by erotic fantasy, so-called directed masturbation.** Several excellent self-help books are available to help women become orgasmic through self-stimulation (105). A vibrator may be helpful if the plateau of high arousal is reached but there is still no orgasmic release. When the woman has experienced orgasm with self-stimulation with or without the use of a vibrator, she may or may not be able to teach the technique to her partner. Issues of trust may surface, and more intense psychological help may be needed. To counter the orgasmic delay or absence induced by SSRIs, highly selected women benefited from the prophylactic use of *sildenafil* (61).

Sexual Pain Disorders

Vaginismus

Vaginismus is an involuntary reflexive contraction of pelvic muscle precipitated by real or imagined attempts at vaginal entry. Often other muscles tighten including thighs, abdomen, buttocks, and even jaw, fists, and other muscle groups. It may be generalized—the woman is unable to place anything in her vagina, even her own finger or a tampon—or it may be situational, in which case she can use a tampon and can tolerate a pelvic examination but cannot have intercourse. Couples frequently cope with this difficulty for many years before they seek help and then do so in order to begin a family. Often there are no obvious circumstances predisposing to vaginismus, such as an unpleasant past sexual experience or trauma, sexual abuse, or a painful first pelvic examination. Higher rates of psychopathology were found with regards to agoraphobia without panic disorder and obsessive-compulsive disorder. Some studies showed that women with vaginismus have higher scores on neuroticism, depression, state anxiety, phobic anxiety, social phobia, somatization, and hostility. They were shown to have increased catastrophic thinking compared to those women without dyspareunia and those with other forms of pain (e.g., PVD). Women with vaginismus had higher propensity for disgust (55). Despite the theories, there is no scientific evidence that vaginismus is secondary to religious orthodoxy, negative sexual upbringing, or concerns about sexual orientation. Women with vaginismus typically have an extreme fear of vaginal entry and misconceptions about their anatomy and the size of their vagina. They fear that harm will come from something the size of a penis entering the vagina, and similarly they fear that they would be damaged by vaginal delivery.

Although the term "vaginismus" is often loosely used to refer to reflex tightening secondary to dyspareunia (e.g., from PVD or vaginal atrophy), strictly speaking, the term should only be used when no such pathology is present. Thus, the diagnosis of vaginismus is provisional until a very careful introital and vaginal examination can be done. This is not possible until the woman learns to be able to abduct her thighs, open the labia with her fingers or permit the examiner to do so, and to tolerate introital touch. The therapy for vaginismus must begin before the diagnosis is confirmed:

1. **Encourage the couple to engage in sexual activities that exclude any attempt at intercourse.** They may need to have "dates" and deliberately provide sexual contexts.

2. **Explain to the patient the reflex contraction of pelvic muscles around the vagina to touch, especially when touch was associated only with negative emotions and physical pain.** These women rarely use tampons and avoid the introitus and vagina in sexual play and have not experienced any neutral or positive sensations from this area of their bodies.

3. **Institute self-touch on a daily basis for a few minutes as close to the vaginal opening as possible.** This may be done while the woman is in the bathtub or relaxing by herself on the bed. This is not sexual, and at first it will be highly anxiety provoking. Providing she does this daily, the anxiety will quickly decrease.

4. **Suggest adding visual imagery to the previous exercise** so that she imagines being able to have a limited vaginal examination, sitting up on the examination couch at about

a 70-degree angle to, with the aid of a mirror, view the vaginal opening and separate her labia, and be in control of what happens.

5. **As soon as she is ready, perform the partial vulvovaginal examination as in step 4.** If possible, encourage her to touch the vagina, moving her finger past the hymen, possibly afterward doing the same with the physician's gloved finger.

6. **Once the vagina is adequately examined, prescribe a series of vaginal inserts of gradually increasing diameter.** When symptoms suggestive of PVD are present—especially burning with semen ejaculation, dysuria, or vulvodynia after intercourse attempts—she should use only the smallest insert before a repeat examination takes place.

7. **When it is necessary to exclude PVD, repeat the examination with the woman checking for allodynia with a cotton swab.** Sometimes the physician can do this; it depends entirely on the amount of anxiety and apprehension the woman retains. The number of false-positive findings for allodynia can be limited if the patient touches the rim of the vaginal opening. Provoked vestibulodynia or other gynecologic findings should be treated.

8. Once the patient is able to use larger inserts, the following steps can be undertaken:
   a. **Encourage the woman to allow her partner to assist her in placing the insert in her vagina.**
   b. **Encourage the couple during their sexual times to briefly use the insert**—to prove to her that the insert will still go in when her body is physiologically aroused.
   c. **Once she has used the insert on a number of occasions during sexual play, encourage her to follow it immediately with insertion of her partner's penis.** It is usually preferable for the woman to hold her partner's penis in the same position she used with the insert and to insert the penis herself. He must allow his pelvis to move forward with gentle pressure as she tries to insert it. The use of external lubrication is advised in these first attempts at penile entry.

Phosphodiesterase type 5 inhibitors may be used to treat temporary situational partner erectile dysfunction that occurs at the crucial moment when the woman is finally able to accommodate her partner's penis.

Dyspareunia

Dyspareunia, one of the most common types of sexual dysfunction seen by gynecologists, affects some two-thirds of women during their lifetime. Both psychological and physical factors are involved—the mind being able to powerfully modulate both immune and neurological systems, causing objective changes in the latter. The gynecologist's assessment of dyspareunia needs to be holistic: biological, psychological, and sexual (Fig. 11.4).

There are three aspects to the management of dyspareunia:

1. **Assisting the couple to have rewarding sexual intimacy even if intercourse initially is precluded**

2. **Identifying the psychological issues contributing to and arising from the chronic pain**

3. **Treating, whenever possible, the underlying pathophysiology that triggered the chronic pain circuits**

It is helpful to clarify that the popular depiction of sex as foreplay followed by "real sex" (i.e., intercourse) is not the reality for many sexually satisfied couples. The couple can be encouraged to consider the many varieties of human sexual interaction and ways of giving and receiving genital and nongenital sexual pleasure. It is important for the couple to see removal of intercourse from the menu of sexual activity as an opportunity for more exploration and creativity, and not as a loss. Inclusion of the partner in the assessment and evaluation of chronic dyspareunia allows his feelings to be addressed and his compliance with nonpenetrative sex encouraged. The couple rendered emotionally distant because of chronic dyspareunia may find it difficult to adapt to alternative forms of lovemaking.

Provoked Vestibulodynia

PVD is defined as pain on vestibular touch (from tampon, examining finger, penis, tight seam on clothing, etc.) where physical findings are limited to variable (possibly absent) vestibular erythema and the presence of allodynia (feeling a burning pain from the touch

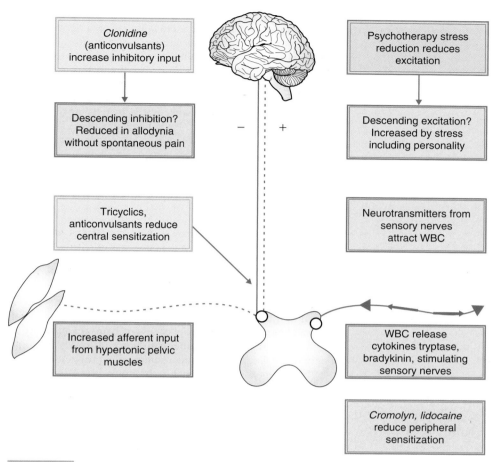

Figure 11.4 Schematic of proposed pathophysiological mechanisms underlying the chronic pain of vulvar vestibulitis syndrome and therapeutic interventions. WBC, white blood cells.

stimulus) on localized areas around the outer edge of the hymen and inner edge of the labia minora where the two meet. The whole introital circumference may be affected: typically the lower part (lower horseshoe or 4 to 8 o'clock location) is involved along with the areas immediately around the openings of Skene's ducts. Typically pelvic muscle tone is heightened. This is the most common cause of dyspareunia seen in clinics, with at least 50% of women reporting lifelong symptoms and others acquiring them after possibly multiple occasions of painless intercourse. **PVD is considered a chronic pain syndrome, with features suggesting both central and peripheral sensitization within the nervous system.** This means that there are physical changes within the nervous system that perpetuate the pain cycles, and these can be targeted both by medications (chronic pain drugs) and mind skills including CBT and mindfulness. **The cause of the sensitization within the nervous system is not established with certainty, but internal stress appears to be a likely cause.** Women with PVD report higher levels of perfectionism, reward dependency, fear of negative evaluation, and harm avoidance, higher levels of trait anxiety, and shyness (55). Higher rates of depression and anxiety disorders are found in women with PVD compared to controls. Women with PVD have more catastrophic thoughts about intercourse pain and the negative consequences on the partner and durability of the relationship than women with other types of dyspareunia (55). There is evidence of hypervigilance for pain. **Many women with PVD have other pain syndromes such as irritable bowel syndrome, temporomandibular joint pain, interstitial cystitis, dysmenorrhea, and, especially for midaged women, fibromyalgia** (55).

The management of PVD includes psychological methods to address the chronic internal stress and possibly adjunctive medications, simultaneously or subsequently. The psychological methods include CBT and mindfulness. Particular attention is paid to the catastrophic thinking. Giving the woman as much information as appropriate on the mechanisms of chronic pain allows her to see the role of the emotions experienced alongside the physical sensation of pain. Realizing that her thoughts can alter her emotions moves her onto understanding how cognitive therapy will change her pain intensity. Mindfulness has been used for 3,500 years for ameliorating chronic pain but only recently in Western medicine. Given its use in other pain conditions, it was added to the holistic treatment of PVD (106). **Chronic pain medications include tricyclic antidepressants and antiseizure drugs. Applications of local anesthetics and or local anti-inflammatories such as *sodium cromoglycate* can be used. Topical steroids need to be avoided because initial benefit moves onto worsening of the presumed neurogenic inflammation.** Evidence-based guidelines suggesting which medical treatment to choose are lacking. A typical outcome of the psychological therapy is that pain intensity and distress lessen sufficiently to allow the woman who regains her sexual confidence with nonpenetrative sex sometimes to begin to include intercourse. Prior to doing so she might use topical local anesthetic on residual areas of allodynia. Her expectation of less pain combines with her expectation of reward to reduce the intensity of the dyspareunia. The local anesthetic may contribute to a positive experience.

Introital pain may be caused by conditions other than PVD. The differential diagnosis includes recurrent tears of the posterior fourchette, which may be treated with the topical application of *estrogen* or *testosterone* and, if necessary, a perineorrhaphy. Other diagnoses are congenital abnormalities, including a hymenal ring that is rigid, scar tissue (e.g., from episiotomy repairs), a vaginal septum, and, much more commonly, vaginitis or vulvitis, sometimes resulting from the use of over-the-counter vaginal sprays and douches. **One important common cause of dyspareunia is friction from inadequate genital sexual arousal. Estrogen deficiency with inadequate lubrication, progressing to loss of elasticity and thinning of the epithelium from vaginal atrophy, is another common cause.** This condition is easily treated with local estrogen therapy. Deep dyspareunia resulting from pelvic disease, including endometriosis, is managed by treatment of the underlying conditions.

Sexual Dysfunction Midlife and Later

Because sexual dysfunction in older women can be related to a variety of factors, broad-spectrum treatment approaches are needed in which individual, interpersonal, and sexual aspects can be addressed simultaneously. The following steps in therapy are recommended:

- **To encourage the woman to take responsibility for discovering what provides sexual pleasure and arousal and to learn to guide her partner toward stimuli and contexts (surroundings and time of day) that are pleasurable to her now, as they may be different and more complicated than when she was a younger woman and possibly her relationship was relatively new.**

- **To assist her to understand that a more rewarding outcome will increase her sexual motivation.** Factors relating to the couple's sexual style and even sexual dysfunction in the partner may need to be addressed.

- **To counsel her that women can begin rewarding sexual experiences in the absence of desire, which can be reassuring and therapeutic.**

- **To acknowledge that resentment, frustration, and disappointment toward her partner will very likely preclude arousal and pleasure: the couple may benefit from referral for relationship counseling.**

- **To advise that deep-seated psychological distress from factors in her development or current refractory mood disorders may require referral to a psychologist or a psychiatrist.**

Practical suggestions for aging patients might include taking a warm bath before lovemaking to loosen stiff joints, making love in the morning when the couple is less fatigued, or having neither intercourse nor orgasm as a necessary goal. Local *estrogen* supplementation can alleviate vaginal dryness, urinary tract symptoms, and dyspareunia, restoring vaginal cell health, decreasing pH, and increasing vulvar and vaginal blood flow. The aging couple can be encouraged to use low-key, more prolonged sexual stimulation because the rate of sexual response is slower.

To relieve sexual symptoms of dyspareunia and lower sexual self-image from estrogen deficiency–associated vaginal dryness and recurrent urinary tract infections, topical vaginal *estrogen* is recommended. There is some evidence topical therapy may be more effective for sexual symptoms than systemic, and when systemic *estrogen* is used for nonsexual reasons, additional topical vaginal *estrogen* may still be required (107).

Ultra low-dose *estrogen* from a Silastic ring or vaginal cream or vaginal pill is an emerging therapy, to avoid the (albeit) small systemic absorption from current formulations of ring (releasing 7.5 μg *estradiol* daily) or *estradiol* tablets (containing 25 μg *estradiol* daily). These ultra low-dose formulations may prove appropriate for women with past history of breast cancer. Every woman with such history currently is treated individually by her oncologist, taking into account her sexual symptoms, the importance to her of penetrative sex, as well as her particular tumor endocrinology.

Investigational local vaginal DHEA may benefit vulvar vaginal atrophy, in the absence of systemic absorption of either DHEA or the intracellularly produced estrogen or testosterone. Early research shows a generalized sexual benefit in terms of coital comfort, ease of orgasm, and sexual motivation (108).

Female Genital Mutilation

Increasing numbers of women who underwent female genital mutilation or female genital cutting (FGC) need gynecologic care in Western counties. This ancient tradition from at least 200 B.C. has cultural rather than religious origins and is not restricted to any particular ethnic group or religious sect. **Type I** FGC involves removing part or all of the clitoris and prepuce, **Type II** is an excision of part or all of the clitoris and the labia minora with or without excision of the labia majora, **Type III** is known as infibulation and is the most extreme form, involving narrowing the vaginal orifice and creating a covering of the adjoined labia minora and or labia majora with or without including the clitoris. There are other "lesser" procedures often noted as **Type IV,** such as pricking of the female genitalia for nonmedical reasons. Although some 85% of FGC are Types I and II and 15% are Type III, recent immigration and refugee resettlement from countries where Type III predominates, including Somalia, resulted in many more women with Type III FGC in North America and Europe.

Sound data are lacking on psychosexual outcome. The taboos against discussing sexual displeasure or pain from FGC limit data collection. Despite this, there is evidence that FGC may not destroy sexual function and prevent enjoyment in all women (109). FGC invariably damages many neural networks associated with the vulvar and perineal areas, potentially altering genital sensation. Neuroplasticity within the brain and spinal cord is thought to account for the fact that some, perhaps even the majority, of women have sexual response, sometimes including that from genital stimulation and other times from stimulation of breasts or other areas of the body.

Results of studies of dyspareunia are somewhat conflicting, some suggesting it is only temporary after first intercourse during the initial period of marriage and after reinfibulation (110). Some studies that noted increased prevalence of dysmenorrhea, vaginal dryness, lack of sexual desire, difficulty reaching orgasm, as compared to noncircumcised women, failed to find increased incidence of dyspareunia.

Surgery is recommended for women with Type III FGC complications such as dysmenorrhea, a desired vaginal birth that would not be possible without surgery, apareunia, dyspareunia, or difficulty voiding. The defibulation should be preformed after counseling regarding risks and benefits, the former including bleeding infections, preterm labor if the woman is already pregnant, and scar formation. The benefits include lower risk of chronic urinary and vaginal infections, voiding difficulties, dysmenorrhea, dyspareunia, and intrapartum complications. Regional or general anesthesia is required, as local anesthesia may allow the sensation of touch to trigger flashbacks to the original traumatic procedure. The surgical technique of defibulation was detailed and summarized (111).

It is apparent to people helping women who underwent FGC that culture plays a very important role in their sexual health. It is imperative that the specific needs of the individual woman with FGC are understood in order to help her. Care should be given in a nonjudgmental manner that encourages trust and open discussion. Her own cultural significance of the FGC should be explored and often an interpreter is necessary to really understand her situation.

Sexual Assault

Sexual assault of children and adult women has reached epidemic proportions in the United States and is the fastest growing, most frequently committed, and most underreported crime (112–114). Sexual assault is a crime of violence, conquest, control, and aggression, not passion, and encompasses a continuum of sexual activity that ranges from sexual coercion to contact abuse (unwanted kissing, touching, or fondling) to forcible rape. **The terms *sexual abuse survivor* and *assault survivor* are preferable to *victim*.**

In a survey of female family practice patients, 47% reported some type of contact sexual victimization during their lifetime; 25% reported attempted rape, and 13% had been forcibly raped, many as children (115). Among battered women, approximately 68% experience marital rape as an element of their repetitive abuse (116). Uninvited sexual attention in the workplace is reported by 50% of women in the United States (117). Spousal rape is reported infrequently because of fear of retribution and economic dependency (118). Obstetrician–gynecologists should routinely inquire about a history of childhood sexual abuse or adult sexual assault. These experiences are common and often have a lasting and profound effect on a woman's mental and sexual function as well as her general health and well-being.

Childhood Sexual Abuse

Childhood sexual abuse has a profound and potentially lifelong effect on the survivor. Although most cases of childhood sexual abuse are not reported by the survivor or her family, it is estimated that as many as one-third of adult women were sexually abused as children. Childhood sexual abuse is often accompanied by another type of household dysfunction, such as physical abuse, violence against other family members, or substance abuse by parental figures (114). **Younger children are more often exposed to genital fondling or noncontact abuse** (exhibitionism, forced observation of masturbation, or posing in child pornography), and **children older than 10 years of age are more likely to be forced to have intercourse or oral sex** (119). **As children age, they are more likely to experience sexual abuse outside the home and more likely to be victimized by strangers. As adolescents, women survivors of childhood sexual abuse are at risk for early unplanned pregnancy, STDs, prostitution, further sexual abuse (revictimization), antisocial behavior, running away from home, lying, stealing, eating disorders and obesity, and multiple somatic symptoms** (120). These women are more likely to engage in health risk behaviors such as smoking, substance abuse, and early sexual activity with multiple partners (121). They may be less likely to use contraception (122). Survivors often avoid pelvic examinations and are less likely to have Papanicolaou (Pap) tests because of the association between vaginal examinations and pain (125). They often receive inadequate prenatal care and are more likely than women who were not abused to experience suicidal ideation and depression during their pregnancies and to deliver smaller and less mature babies (114).

Obstetrician–gynecologists can assist their sexual assault patients by validating their feelings and concerns and giving them control over their examination. It is important to ask the patient for permission to perform the examination, give her the opportunity to have an advocate in the room with her, and let her know that she has the right to stop the examination at any time (114).

Survivors may be unable to trust or establish rapport with adults. Some women blame themselves for the abuse and come to believe that they are not entitled to assistance from others. Thus, they risk continuing to enter abusive relationships. **Women survivors of childhood sexual abuse often develop feelings of powerlessness and helplessness and may become chronically depressed.** They experience a high incidence of self-destructive behavior, including suicide and deliberate self-harm, such as cutting or burning themselves (114,124,125). The most extreme mental health symptoms in assault survivors are associated with the onset of abuse at an early age, frequent abuse over a long period, use of force, or abuse by a parent or other trusted individual. Survivors are at risk for becoming victimized again later in life (126). Of women who report being abused as children, 50% are abused again as adults. Women who are sexually abused as children carry the effects of abuse into adulthood. As adults, they have the same level of physical symptoms and psychological distress as women who do not report childhood sexual abuse but are currently experiencing sexual or physical abuse (127).

Women who were sexually abused as children or sexually assaulted as adults often experience sexual dysfunction and difficulty with intimate relationships and parenting (128).

Chronic sexual concerns may include fear of intimate relationships, lack of sexual enjoyment, difficulty with desire and arousal, and anorgasmia. Compared with women who were not sexually assaulted, they are more likely to experience depression, suicide attempts, chronic anxiety, anger, substance abuse problems, dissociative personality disorder, borderline personality disorder, fatigue, low self-esteem, feelings of guilt and self-blame, and sleep disturbance (127,129–131). They often experience social isolation, phobias, feelings of vulnerability, fear, humiliation, grief, and loss of control (132,133). Survivors of sexual assault represent a disproportionate number of patients with chronic headaches, fibromyalgia, and chronic pelvic pain (they have a lower pain threshold) and are more likely to have somatic symptoms that do not respond to routine medical treatment (130,134). Women with common gynecologic symptoms, such as dysmenorrhea, menorrhagia, and sexual dysfunction, are much more likely to have a history of sexual assault (135). If they were forced to perform oral sex, they may have a dental phobia and avoid preventive dental care.

Survivors may develop posttraumatic stress disorder (PTSD), in which characteristic symptoms are exhibited following a psychologically traumatic event outside of normal human experience. Symptoms of PTSD include blunting of affect, denial of symptoms, intrusive reexperiencing of the incident, avoidance of stimuli associated with the assault, and intense psychological distress and agitation in response to reminders of the event (112,124). Women affected by PTSD are more likely to commit suicide. The cognitive sequelae include flashbacks, nightmares, disturbances in perception, memory loss, and dissociative experiences (136). These women may not be able to tolerate pelvic examinations and may avoid seeking routine gynecologic care because these examinations may remind them of the sexual abuse they experienced as children. They are more likely to use the medical care system for nongynecologic concerns (137). Women with PTSD are at greater risk for being overweight and having gastrointestinal disturbances (121).

Rape

Although the legal definition of sexual assault may vary from state to state, most definitions of rape include the following elements:

1. **The use of physical force, deception, intimidation, or the threat of bodily harm**
2. **Lack of consent or inability to give consent because the survivor is very young or very old, impaired by alcohol or drug use, unconsciousness, or mentally or physically impaired**
3. **Oral, vaginal, or rectal penetration with a penis, finger, or object**

The National Women's Study provides the best statistics available about the incidence of forcible rape in the United States (132). This study revealed that 13%, or **one of eight adult women, are survivors of at least one completed rape during their lifetime.** Of the women they surveyed, 0.7% were raped during the past year, equaling an estimated 683,000 adult women who were raped during a 12-month period. Of the women surveyed, 39% were raped more than once. Most rapes occurred during childhood and adolescence; 29% of all forcible rapes occurred when the survivor was younger than 11 years of age, and 32% occurred between the ages of 11 and 17 years. "Rape in America is a tragedy of youth" (132). Twenty-two percent of rapes occurred between the ages of 18 and 24 years, 7% between the ages of 25 and 29 years, and only 6% occurred when the survivor was older than 30 years of age. Although women of all ages and cultures are vulnerable to sexual assault, prisoners, adolescents, drug users, the elderly, those who experienced sexual assault as children, women in abusive relationships, and women with emotional and physical disabilities are at most risk (138–140).

There are many myths about rape. Perhaps the most common myth is that women are raped by strangers. **Only about 20% to 25% of women are raped by someone they do not know. Most women are raped by a relative or acquaintance (9% by husbands or ex-husbands, 11% by fathers or stepfathers, 10% by boyfriends or ex-boyfriends, 16% by other relatives, and 29% by other nonrelatives)** (132). Acquaintance rape may seem to be less traumatic than stranger rape, but survivors of acquaintance rape often take longer to recover. Another common misconception about rape is that most survivors sustain serious physical or life-threatening injury. Sixty percent of rape survivors report some physical injury. General body injury is more than twice as common as genital and anal injury (141). Serious injury is rare, occurring 4% of the time, although almost half of the rape survivors report being fearful of serious injury or death during the assault (132). The most common genital injuries from a sexual assault are vaginal lacerations resulting in bleeding and pain. Intraperitoneal extension of a vaginal laceration or damage to the anal mucosa is rare (142). Common nongenital injuries in survivors include cuts, bruises, scratches, broken bones and teeth, and knife or gunshot wounds (143). About 0.1% of sexual assaults result in death. Common causes of death during a sexual assault include mechanical asphyxiation, trauma, lacerations, drowning, and gunshot wounds (142).

There are at least four types of rapists (144):

1. *Opportunist rapists* **(30%) exhibit no anger toward the women they assault and usually use little or no force.** These rapes are impulsive and may occur in the context of an existing relationship (date or acquaintance rape). The highest incidence of acquaintance rape is among women in the 12th grade of high school or in the first year of college (145). Approximately one half of female college students report that they were date raped. Many of these women may have been unable to give consent because they were impaired by alcohol or so-called date rape drugs (*Rohypnol* or other benzodiazepines, *ketamine,* or *gamma-hydroxy butyrate* [*GHB*]). Date rape may have even greater psychological consequences than rape by a stranger because it involves a violation of trust (142).

2. *Anger rapists* **(40%) usually batter the survivor and use more physical force than is necessary to overpower her.** This type of sexual assault is episodic, impulsive, and spontaneous. An anger rapist often physically assaults his victim, sexually assaults her, and forces her to perform degrading acts. The rapist is angry or depressed and is often seeking retribution—for perceived wrongs or injustices he imagines were done to him by others, especially women. He may victimize the very young or the very old.

3. *Power rapists* **(25%) do not intend to** *physically* **harm their victim but rather to possess or control her to gain sexual gratification.** A power rapist may use force or the threat of force to overcome his victim. These assaults are premeditated and repetitive, and they may increase in aggression over time. The rapist is usually anxious and may give orders to his victim, ask her personal questions, or inquire about her response during the assault. This assault may occur over an extended period while the victim is held captive. These rapists are insecure about their virility and are trying to compensate for their feelings of inadequacy and low self-esteem.

4. *Sadistic rapists* **(5%) become sexually excited by inflicting pain on their victim.** These rapists may have a thought disorder and often exhibit other forms of psychopathology. This type of assault is calculated and planned. The victim is often a stranger. The rape may involve bondage, torture, or bizarre acts and may occur over an extended period of time. The victim often suffers both genital and nongenital injuries and may be murdered or mutilated. Other rapists may act out of impulse, as when they encounter a victim during the course of another crime such as burglary. Some rapists believe they are entitled to their victim, as in acquaintance rape or father–daughter incest (116). A consistent finding among all types of rapists is a lack of empathy for the survivor.

Even when sexual assaults are reported (only 16% of rapes are reported to the police), few rapists are arrested, and even fewer are brought to trial and convicted. Less than 1% of rapists serve a prison term (144,146). Successful prosecution of rapists is often dependent on the extent of the survivor's injuries and the completion of a detailed forensic examination (147). Many women do not report the assault to the police because they are concerned about their name being disclosed by the news media, they fear retaliation from the perpetrator, are afraid they will not be believed, or do not trust the judicial process (148). Assault is more likely to be repeated if survivors in abusive relationships do not seek medical care, report the incident to police, or seek an order of protection (116).

Only 26% of rape survivors seek medical attention after an assault (116). Women are more likely to immediately seek treatment after sexual assault if weapons were involved, serious physical injury occurred, or physical coercion or confinement was used in the assault (149). Many rape survivors do not inform their physicians about the assault and may never volunteer information about the assault unless they are directly asked. When obtaining a medical history, physicians should routinely ask, "*Has anyone ever forced you to have sexual relations?*"

Effects of Rape

Following sexual assault, women have many concerns, including pregnancy, STDs (including human immunodeficiency virus [HIV] infection), being blamed for the assault, having their name made public, and having their family and friends find out about the assault.

The initial reactions to sexual assault may be shock, numbness, withdrawal, and possibly denial. It is difficult to predict how an assaulted individual will react. Despite their recent trauma, women presenting for medical care may appear calm and detached (147).

The **rape trauma syndrome** is a constellation of physical and psychological symptoms, including fear, helplessness, disbelief, shock, guilt, humiliation, embarrassment, anger, and self-blame. The acute, or disorganization, phase of the syndrome lasts from days to weeks. Survivors may experience intrusive memories of the assault, blunting of affect, and hypersensitivity to environmental stimuli. They are anxious, do not feel safe, have difficulty sleeping and eating, and experience nightmares and a variety of somatic symptoms (116,150,151). They may fear that their assailant will return to retaliate or rape them again.

In the weeks to months following the sexual assault, survivors often return to normal activities and routines. They may appear to have dealt successfully with the assault, but they may be repressing strong feelings of anger, fear, guilt, and embarrassment. In the months following the assault, survivors begin the process of integration and resolution. During this phase, they begin to accept the assault as part of their life experience, and somatic and emotional symptoms may decrease progressively in severity. However, the sequelae of rape are often persistent and long lasting (124). Over the long term, survivors may have difficulty with work and with family relationships. Disruption of existing relationships is not uncommon. Nearly half of the survivors lose their jobs or are forced to quit in the year following the rape, and half change their place of residency (133).

Examination

The responsibilities of physicians providing immediate treatment for sexual assault survivors are listed in Table 11.8. Many health care facilities have trained sexual assault nurse evaluators (SANE). **Because of the legal ramifications, consent must be obtained from the patient before obtaining the history, performing the physical examination, and collecting forensic evidence. Documentation of the handling of specimens is especially important, and the chain of evidence for collected material must be carefully maintained. Everyone who handles the evidence must sign for it and hand it directly to the next person in the chain. The chain of evidence extends from the examiner, to the police detective, to the crime laboratory, and finally to the courtroom.**

Table 11.8 Prophylactic Medications Following Sexual Assault	
Gonorrhea	*Ceftriaxone* 125 mg IM **or** *Ciprofloxacin* 500 mg PO **or** *Spectinomycin* 2 g IM
Chlamydia	*Azithromycin* 1 g PO **or** *Doxycycline* 100 mg PO bid × 7 days **or** *Erythromycin* 500 mg PO qid × 7 days
Trichomoniasis and bacterial vaginosis	*Metronidazole* 2 g PO
Hepatitis B	Vaccine 1.0 mL IM. Repeat in 1 and 6 months.
Tetanus (if indicated)	Td 0.5 mL IM
HIV	*Zidovudine* 300 mg and *Lamivudine* 150 mg (*Combivir*) PO bid for 28 days. Addition of protease inhibitor should be considered for high-risk exposures.
Pregnancy	*Plan B (levonorgestrel* 0.75 mg) 2 tablets immediately **or** *Ovral* 2 tablets immediately, repeat in 12 hours **or** 35 μg combination birth control pill, 4 tablets immediately, repeat in 12 hours **or** *Mifepristone* 10 mg as a single dose **or** Placement of a copper IUD

IM, intramuscularly; PO, by mouth; bid, twice a day; qid, four times a day; Td, tetanus and diphtheria; IUD, intrauterine device.

The patient should be interviewed in a quiet and supportive environment by an examiner who is objective and nonjudgmental. Support personnel and patient advocates, such as family, friends, or, if available, a counselor from a rape crisis service, should be encouraged to accompany the patient. It is important not to leave the survivor alone and to give her as much control as possible over the examination. To provide useful forensic information, the examination should be performed as soon as possible after the incident occurred. Providers in all 50 states are required to report all cases of suspected or known childhood sexual abuse to appropriate authorities.

The history should include the following information:

1. **A general medical history and a gynecologic history must be obtained,** including last menstrual period; prior pregnancies; past gynecologic infections; tetanus immune status; history of liver disease, thrombosis, or hypertension (possible contraindications to emergency contraception with estrogens); contraceptive use; prior sexual assault; and last consensual intercourse before the assault.

2. **It is important to ascertain whether the survivor bathed, douched, used a tampon, urinated, defecated, used an enema, brushed her teeth or used mouthwash, or changed her clothes after the assault. These activities can impair the collection of forensic evidence.**

3. **A detailed description of the sexual assault should be obtained,** including the place, time, and date of the assault; number and appearance of assailants; use of drugs or alcohol in relation to the assault; loss of consciousness; use of weapons, threats, and restraints; and any physical injuries that may have occurred.

4. **A detailed description of the type of sexual contact must be obtained,** including whether vaginal, oral, or anal contact or penetration occurred; insertion of a foreign object with a description of the object; whether the assailant used a condom; and whether there were other possible sites of ejaculation or oral contact, such as the hands, clothes, breasts, or hair of the survivor. Saliva, respiratory spray, or semen recovered from these sites could yield DNA from the assailant.

5. **The emotional state of the survivor should be observed and recorded.**

The physical examination serves to detect, evaluate, and treat all injuries and to collect forensic evidence (152). It is important, when examining survivors, to pay close attention to detail. Examiners should wear powderless gloves at all times in order to prevent contamination of the evidence with their own DNA.

The survivor should undress while standing on clean examination table paper to catch any hair or fibers falling from her clothing. All of her clothing should be placed by the survivor (to avoid DNA contamination from the examiner) in individually labeled paper bags, sealed, and given to the proper authorities. Wet or damp clothing should be air dried before packaging in paper bags because DNA evidence degrades quickly if it is moist (139). During the physical examination, the degree of injury to the survivor should be assessed, and any injuries should be documented for use as evidence. The nature, size, and location of all injuries should be carefully documented, using photographs or body charts (traumagram) if possible. Ultraviolet photography may enable the examiner to record injuries not seen with standard photographic equipment, such as bite marks, stains, blood, or weapon imprints. Nongenital injuries occur in 20% to 50% of all rapes, so it important to carefully examine the entire body (152,153).

The most common injuries are bruises and abrasions of the head, neck, and arms, and genital injuries accompanied by bleeding and pain (150). Hair and skin should be examined for dirt, foreign material, dried blood, and dried semen (152). Ruptured blood vessels in the retina may be the result of trauma from choking. If oral penetration has taken place, injuries of the mouth and pharynx may occur (154). Injury to the oral cavity, including a torn frenulum, broken teeth, trauma to the uvula, and injuries of the hard and soft palate, are related to forced fellatio. Evidence of trauma is more likely when the assault has occurred out of doors or is perpetrated by a stranger (155). **The most common genital findings are erythema and small tears of the vulva, perineum, and introitus.** Genital trauma is more common in postmenopausal women. A Foley catheter, placed in the distal vaginal vault and then inflated, allows for full visualization of hymenal injuries (138). There may be bleeding, mucosal tears, erythema, or a hematoma noted around the rectum if penetration occurred. Identification of small lacerations of the genitalia or rectum may be aided by colposcopy or by staining with *toluidine blue,* which has an affinity for the nuclei of exposed submucosal cells and will make the injuries stand out (153,154,156). *Toluidine blue* should be applied before the speculum examination, as insertion of the speculum itself can cause small lacerations and false-positive results. *Toluidine blue* is spermicidal and should not be applied until all forensic evidence is collected (156). Bite marks are not uncommon and frequently are found on the breasts or genitalia. Impressions and photographs of bite marks can be made and used to help identify the assailant. Foreign bodies may be found in the vagina, rectum, or urethra.

Samples should be obtained from any sites of contact (vagina, rectum, or mouth) and tested for gonorrhea and chlamydia. A vaginal wet prep examination should be performed for evidence of trichomonas. A urine or serum pregnancy test should be performed, and baseline testing for syphilis, hepatitis B (surface antigen and immunoglobulin M antibodies to hepatitis B core antigen), and HIV. Urine and blood samples should be collected to screen for the presence of any date rape drugs.

Evidence must be properly collected for legal purposes according to the following procedures:

1. **Examination of the patient with a Wood light may help identify semen,** which will fluoresce blue-green to orange. Areas of fluorescence should be swabbed with a cotton-tipped applicator moistened with sterile water, then air dried and submitted as evidence. Swabs of the skin, vagina, mouth, breasts, and rectum may be obtained to test for the presence of sperm or semen. In general, use a dry swab to obtain evidence from wet areas, and a wet swab to obtain evidence from dry areas.

2. **A Pap test may be useful to document the presence of sperm.**

3. **A sample of the vaginal secretions should be obtained for examination for motile sperm, semen, or pathogens.** Motile sperm in the vagina indicate ejaculation occurred within 6 hours. Nonmotile sperm can be found in the cervical mucus for as long as 1 week after ejaculation. If ejaculation occurred in the mouth, seminal fluid may be rapidly destroyed by salivary enzymes (142). If the survivor reports an anal assault, specimens can be obtained by washing the rectal vault with 10 mL of normal saline injected with a red rubber catheter. Allow the saline to stand for several minutes, then aspirate the rectal fluid and submit as evidence.

4. **Vaginal secretions should be collected for DNA fingerprinting and to test for the presence of seminal contents,** including acid phosphatase, p30 protein (specific to the prostate), seminal vesicle-specific antigen, and ABO antigens (151).

5. **The survivor's pubic hair should be combed over a sheet of paper in an attempt to obtain pubic hair from the assailant.** Both the comb and the pubic hair should be submitted as evidence. If the pubic hair is matted, it should be clipped, not pulled, and submitted.

6. **Fingernail scrapings from the survivor should be collected** using an orangestick and evaluated for evidence of trace fibers or the assailant's blood, hair, or skin. Use a wet swab to obtain evidence for DNA fingerprinting from between the survivor's fingers.

7. **Saliva should be collected from the survivor** to document whether she is a secretor of major blood group antigens (80% of the population are secretors). If the patient is not a secretor and blood group antigens are found in vaginal washings, the antigens are probably from the semen of the assailant (151).

8. **Respiratory spray from where the assailant placed his face and breathed on the survivor may be collected from her breasts, shoulders, face, or neck. Collect the sample with a moist swab and submit for DNA analysis.**

Treatment

Treatment of sexual assault survivors should be directed to prevention of possible pregnancy and provision of prophylactic treatment for STDs (Table 11.8). About 5% of fertile rape survivors become pregnant as a result of the rape. **All sexual assault survivors of reproductive age should be offered emergency contraception** (157). If the survivor desires emergency contraception, a preexisting pregnancy can usually be ruled out by performing a sensitive human chorionic gonadotropin assay. Pregnancy prophylaxis can be provided by several different regimens (158–160).

1. Administration of one tablet containing 0.75 mg of *levonorgestrel* followed by a second tablet 12 hours later (Plan B). A single 1.5-mg dose of *levonorgestrel* is just as effective as the two-dose regimen and is the preferred method of emergency contraception (159). *Levonorgestrel* is available by prescription for women younger than 17 years, and available over the counter for women 17 years and older. *Levonorgestrel* is more effective than any other emergency contraception method and has the fewest side effects (160)

2. Immediate administration of two tablets of a combination oral contraceptive (each containing 50 μg of *ethinyl estradiol* and 0.5 mg *norgestrel,* such as *Ovral* birth control pills) followed by two more tablets 12 hours later (Yuzpe regimen)

3. Four tablets of a combination birth control pill containing 35 μg of *ethinyl estradiol* and a progesterone followed by four more tablets 12 hours later

4. *Mifepristone* as a single 10 mg dose (161)

5. Placement of a copper-containing intrauterine device

These regimens are highly effective if administered within 120 hours after the sexual assault (159,162). The sooner the medications are taken, the more effective they are. Most regimens have a failure (pregnancy) rate of about 1.5%. Emergency contraception failure poses little teratogenic risk if the pregnancy continues (163). Some patients experience nausea and vomiting when given emergency contraception containing estrogen, which can be controlled with an antiemetic agent such as *promethazine* (12.5 mg every 4–6 hours) or *ondansetron* (4 mg every 6 hours). Emergency contraception should be repeated if vomiting occurs within 2 hours of taking the initial dose. Most women who take emergency contraception usually experience their next menstrual period within 3 days of the expected date. Women using *mifepristone* for emergency contraception may experience delayed onset of the subsequent menstrual period (161). Emergency contraception may delay but not prevent ovulation; for this reason, patients receiving emergency contraception should be encouraged to use contraception if further coital episodes occur during the cycle.

The risk of acquiring an STD from a rape is difficult to assess because the prevalence of preexisting STDs is high (43%) in rape survivors (164–166). The risk is estimated as follows: gonorrhea, 6% to 12%; trichomonas, 12%; chlamydia, 2% to 12%; syphilis, 5%.

1. Because it is difficult to differentiate between a preexisting STD and a newly contracted one attributable to a sexual assault, prophylaxis should be offered to all survivors. This is especially important because most sexual assault patients do not return for follow-up appointments (151). Prophylaxis should cover infections with *Neisseria gonorrhoeae, Chlamydia trachomatis,* trichomonas, bacterial vaginosis, incubating syphilis, and HIV. Recommendations include (165,167):

   a. *Ceftriaxone,* 125 mg intramuscularly for the treatment of gonorrhea (if the patient is allergic to cephalosporins, *spectinomycin,* 2 g intramuscularly, or *ciprofloxacin,* 500 mg orally, may be used), PLUS:

   b. A single dose of 1 g of *azithromycin* orally or 100 mg of *doxycycline* orally twice a day for 7 days for treatment of chlamydia (if the patient is pregnant at the time of the assault, *erythromycin* 500 mg orally four times a day for 7 days may be substituted for *doxycycline*), PLUS:

   c. A single dose of 2 g of *metronidazole* orally for the treatment of trichomoniasis and/or bacterial vaginosis

2. Hepatitis B vaccination should be offered if the sexual assault survivor has experienced vaginal, oral, or anal penetration. Hepatitis B is 20 times more infectious than HIV during intercourse (114). Vaccination is recommended at the time of the initial evaluation. Subsequent doses are provided 1 month and 6 months after the first dose is administered. It is not necessary to treat the patient with hepatitis B immune globulin (167). Vaccination is not necessary if the patient has documented hepatitis B immunity.

3. Tetanus prophylaxis (0.5 mL intramuscularly) should be administered for deep tissue wounds or for bite wounds.

4. Conversion of HIV through sexual assault, although reported, is low and similar to conversion from occupational exposure (0.1% to 0.3% per episode) (168). The probability of transmission depends on the type of assault, presence of trauma and

bleeding, site of ejaculation, HIV viral load in the ejaculate, presence of a concomitant STD or ulcerative lesions in the assailant or survivor, and the community prevalence of HIV/acquired immune deficiency syndrome (153,168). The risk of HIV transmission may be greater in children because of the thinness of the vaginal epithelium. Factors to consider when discussing HIV postexposure prophylaxis with patients include the likelihood of exposure to the virus, the risks and benefits of treatment, the toxicity of routine antiretroviral prophylaxis, the interval between the sexual assault and the initiation of therapy, and the patient's desire to be treated. All survivors of unprotected vaginal or anal sexual assault presenting within 72 hours should be offered HIV prophylaxis unless the assailant is known and tests negative with rapid HIV testing (169). Treatment should be initiated as soon as possible. The usual regimen is *Combivir* or its equivalent (300 mg *zidovudine* [AZT] and 150 mg *lamivudine* [3TC]) administered twice daily for 4 weeks). Administration of a protease inhibitor (*nelfinavir,* five 250 mg tablets twice a day for 28 days) should be considered for high-risk exposures, such as when the assailant is known to be HIV infected. Providers should also consider consulting an HIV specialist or calling the National Clinicians' Post-Exposure Prophylaxis Hotline. Side effects of HIV prophylaxis include nausea, malaise, headache, and anorexia. About 33% of survivors who elect to take antiviral medication discontinue therapy prematurely (168). Patients should be aware that the efficacy of prophylactic treatment for HIV after sexual assault is unknown, and they will have to be carefully monitored if they initiate treatment with antiretroviral medication.

5. **Bite wounds can be treated with *amoxicillin/clavulanate (Augmentin)* 875 mg twice a day for 3 days.**

6. **If prophylactic treatment for gonorrhea, chlamydia, trichomonas, and bacterial vaginosis is not given, the survivor should return in 2 weeks for repeat testing for STDs and pregnancy.** If the initial serologic test results were negative, repeat serologic tests for syphilis, hepatitis B, and HIV should be performed at 6, 12, and 24 weeks after the assault.

7. **Ongoing supportive counseling for the patient should be arranged,** and the patient should be referred to a sexual assault center or a therapist who specializes in the treatment of sexual assault survivors. A number of excellent resources are available for providers caring for women who were sexually assaulted (170). These include a policy statement on treatment of sexual assault survivors from the American Academy of Family Physicians and a national protocol for sexual assault medical forensic evaluations from the U.S. Department of Justice.

References

1. **Hayes RD.** Assessing female sexual dysfunction in epidemiological studies: why is it necessary to measure both low sexual function and sexually related distress? *Sex Health* 2008;5:215–218.
2. **Fugl-Meyer AR, Sjögren Fugl-Meyer K.** Sexual disabilities, problems and satisfaction in 18–74 year old Swedes. *Scand J Sexology* 1999;2:79–105.
3. **Cain VS, Johannes CB, Avis NE.** Sexual functioning and practices in a multi-ethnic study of mid-life women: baseline results from SWAN. *J Sex Res* 2003;40:266–276.
4. **Lutfey KE, Link CL, Rosen RC, et al.** Prevalence and correlates of sexual activity and function in women: results from the Boston Area Community Health (BACH) Survey. *Arch Sex Behav* 2009;38: 514–527.
5. **Yucel S, de Souza A, Baskin LS.** Neuroanatomy of the human female lower urogenital tract. *J Urol* 2004;172:191–195.
6. **Graham CA, Sanders SA, Milhausen RR.** The sexual excitation/sexual inhibition inventory for women: psychometric properties. *Arch Sex Behav* 2006;35:397–409.
7. **Meston CM, Buss DM.** Why humans have sex. *Arch Sex Behav* 2007;36:477–507.
8. **McCall K, Meson C.** Differences between pre- and postmenopausal women in cues for sexual desire. *J Sex Med* 2007;4(2):364–371.
9. **Pfaus JG.** Pathways of sexual desire. *J Sex Med* 2009;6:1506–1533.
10. **Blaustein JD.** Progestin receptors: neuronal integrators of hormonal and environmental stimulation. *Ann N Y Acad Sci* 2003;1007:1–13.
11. **Basson R.** Women's sexual function and dysfunction: current uncertainties, future directions. *Int J Impot Res* 2008;20:466–478.
12. **Segraves RT.** Bupropion sustained release for the treatment of hypoactive sexual desire disorder in premenopausal women. *J Clin Psychopharmacol* 2004;25:339–342.
13. **Dennerstein L, Lehert P.** Modeling mid-aged women's sexual functioning: a prospective, population-based study. *J Sex Marital Ther* 2004;30:173–183.
14. **Pfaus JG, Kippin TE, Centeno S.** Conditioning and sexual behaviour: a review. *Horm Behav* 2001;40:291–321.
15. **ter Kuile MM, Both S, van Uden J.** The effects of experimentally-induced sad and happy mood on sexual arousal in sexually healthy women. *J Sex Med* 2010;7:1177–1184.
16. **Carvalho J, Nobre P.** Sexual desire in women: an integrative approach regarding psychological, medical and relationship dimensions. *J Sex Med* 2010;7:1807–1815.
17. **Bancroft J, Loftus J, Long JS.** Distress about sex: a national survey of women in heterosexual relationships. *Arch Sex Behav* 2003;32:193–211.
18. **Hartmann U, Heiser K, Rüffer-Hesse C, et al.** Female sexual desire disorders: subtypes, classification, personality factors, a new direction for treatment. *World J Urol* 2002;20:79–88.
19. **Basson R.** Sexual function of women with chronic illness and cancer. *Women's Health* 2010;6:407–430.
20. **Basson R, Schultz WW.** Sexual sequelae of general medical disorders. *Lancet* 2007; 369:409–424.

21. **Rees PM, Fowler CJ, Maas CP.** Sexual function men and women with neurological disorders. *Lancet* 2007;369:512–525.

22. **Archer JS, Love-Geffen TE, Herbst-Damm KL, et al.** Effect of estradiol versus estradiol and testosterone on brain activation patterns in postmenopausal women. *Menopause* 2006;13:528–537.

23. **van Lunsen RHW, Laan E.** Genital vascular responsive and sexual feelings in midlife women: psychophysiologic, brain and genital imaging studies. *Menopause* 2004;11:741–748.

24. **Ottesen B, Pedersen B, Neilsen J, et al.** Vasoactive intestinal polypeptide (VIP) provokes vaginal lubrication in normal women. *Peptides* 1987;8:797–800.

25. **Creighton SM, Crouch NS, Foxwell NA, et al.** Functional evidence for nitrergic neurotransmission in human clitoral corpus cavernosum: a case study. *Int J Impot Res* 2004;16:319–324.

26. **Chivers ML, Seto MC, Lalumière ML, et al.** Agreement of self-reported and genital measures of sexual arousal in men and women: a meta-analysis. *Arch Sex Behav* 2010;39:5–56.

27. **Shafik A.** Cervico motor reflex: description of the reflex and role in sexual acts. *J Sex Res* 1996;33:153–157.

28. **Shafik A, El-Sibai O, Mostafa R, et al.** Response of the internal reproductive organs to clitoral stimulation: the clitoro-uterine reflex. *Int J Impot Res* 2005;17:121–126.

29. **van Netten JJ, Georgiadis JR, Nieuwenburg A, et al.** 8-13 Hz fluctuations in rectal pressure are a objective marker of clitorally-induced orgasm in women. *Arch Sex Behav* 2008;37:279–285.

30. **Georgiadis JR, Reinders AATS, Paans AMJ, et al.** Men versus women on sexual brain function: prominent differences during tactile genital stimulation but not during orgasm. *Human Brain Mapping* 2008;30:3089–3101.

31. **Mah K, Binik YM.** Do all orgasms feel alike? Evaluating a two-dimensional model of the orgasmic experience across genders and sexual contexts. *J Sex Res* 2002;39:104–113.

32. **McCabe M, Althof SE, Assalian P, et al.** Psychological and interpersonal dimensions of sexual function and dysfunction. *J Sex Med* 2010;7:327–348.

33. **Basson R.** Clinical practice. Sexual desire and arousal disorders in women. *N Engl J Med* 2006;354:1467–1506.

34. **Klusmann D.** Sexual motivation and the duration of partnership. *Arch Sex Behav* 2002;31:275–287.

35. **Kennedy SH, Dickens SE, Eisfeld BS, et al.** Sexual dysfunction before antidepressant therapy in major depression. *J Affect Disord* 1999;56:201–208.

36. **Avis NE, Zhao X, Johannes CB, et al.** Correlates of sexual function among multi ethnic middle aged women: Results from the study of women's health across the nation (SWAN). *Menopause* 2005;12:385–398.

37. **Davison SL, Bell RJ, LaChina M, et al.** The relationship between self-reported sexual satisfaction and general well-being in women. *J Sex Med* 2009;6:2690–2697.

38. **Frohlich P, Meston C.** Sexual functioning and self-reported depressive symptoms among college women. *J Sex Res* 2002;39:321–325.

39. **Laumann EL, Paik A, Rosen RC.** Sexual dysfunction in United States: prevalence and predictors. *JAMA* 1999;10:537–545.

40. **Mansfield PK, Koch PB.** Qualities midlife women desire in their sexual relationship and their changing sexual response. *Psychol Women Q* 1998;22:282–303.

41. **Leiblum SR, Koochaki PE, Rodenberg CA, et al.** Hypoactive sexual desire disorder in postmenopausal women: US results from the Women's International Study of Health and Sexuality (WISHeS). *Menopause* 2006;13:46–56.

42. **Dennerstein L, Lehert P, Burger H, et al.** Factors affecting sexual functioning of women in the midlife years. *Climacteric* 1999;2:254–262.

43. **Berra M, De Musso F, Matteucci C, et al.** The impairment of sexual function is less distressing for menopausal than for premenopausal women. *J Sex Med* 2010;7:1209–1215.

44. **Sjögren Fugl-Meyer K, Fugl-Meyer AR.** Sexual disabilities are not singularities. *Int J Impot Res* 2002;14:487–493.

45. **Cayan S, Bozlu M, Canpolat B, et al.** The assessment of sexual functions in women with male partners complaining of erectile dysfunction: Does treatment of male sexual dysfunction improve female partner's sexual functions? *J Sex Marital Ther* 2004;30:333–341.

46. **Hajjar RR, Kamel HK.** Sex in the nursing home. *Clin Geriatr Med* 2003;19:575–586.

47. **Santoro N, Komi J.** Prevalence and impact of vaginal symptoms among postmenopausal women. *J Sex Med* 2009;6:2133–2142.

48. **Santoro N, Torrens J, Crawford S, et al.** Correlates of circulating androgens in midlife women: the study of women's health across the nation. *J Clin Endocrinol Metab* 2005;90:4836–4845.

49. **Davis SR, Davison SL, Donath S, et al.** Circulating androgen levels in self-reported sexual function in women. *JAMA* 2005;294:91–96.

50. **Basson R, Brotto LA, Petkau J, et al.** Role of androgens in women's sexual dysfunction. *Menopause* 2010;17:962–971.

51. **Peng YS, Chiang CK, Kao TW, et al.** Sexual dysfunction in female hemodialysis patients: a multicenter study. *Kidney Int* 2005;68:760–765.

52. **Zivadinov R, Zorzon M, Bosco A, et al.** Sexual dysfunction in multiple sclerosis: correlation analysis. *Mult Scler* 1999;5:428–431.

53. **Bhasin S, Enzlin P, Caviello A, et al.** Sexual dysfunction in men and women with endocrine disorders. *Lancet* 2007;369:597–611.

54. **van Lankveld JJDM, Granot M, Weijmar Schultz WCM, et al.** Women's sexual pain disorders. *J Sex Med* 2010;7:615–631.

55. **Avis NE, Stellato R, Crawford S, et al.** Is there an association between menopause status and sexual functioning? *Menopause* 2000;7:297–309.

56. **Öberg K, Sjögern Fugl Myer K.** On Swedish women's distressing sexual dysfunctions: some concomitant conditions and life satisfaction. *J Sex Med* 2005;2:169–180.

57. **Benyamini Y, Gozlan M, Kokia E.** Variability in the difficulties experienced by women undergoing infertility treatments. *Fertil Steril* 2005;83:275–283.

58. **Wischmann TH.** Sexual disorders in infertile couples. *J Sex Med* 2010;7:1868–1876.

59. **Clayton AH, Warnock JK, Kornstein SG, et al.** A placebo-controlled trial of bupropion SR as an antidote for selective serotonin reuptake inhibitor-induced sexual dysfunction. *J Clin Psychiatry* 2004;65:62–67.

60. **Nurnberg HG, Hensley PL, Heiman JR, et al.** Sildenafil treatment of women with antidepressant-associated sexual dysfunction. *JAMA* 2008;300:395–404.

61. **Conaglen HM, Conaglen JV.** Sexual desire in women presenting for antiandrogen therapy. *J Sex Marital Ther* 2003;29:255–267.

62. **Hahn S, Benson S, Elsenbruch S, et al.** Metformin treatment of polycystic ovary syndrome improves health-related quality-of-life, emotional distress and sexuality. *Hum. Reprod* 2006;21:1925–1934.

63. **Ganz PA, Desmond KA, Leedham B, et al.** Quality of life in long-term, disease-free survivors of breast cancer: a follow-up study. *J Natl Cancer Inst* 2002;94:39–49.

64. **Ganz PA, Desmond KA, Belin TR, et al.** Predictors of sexual health in women after a breast cancer diagnosis. *J Clin Oncol* 1999;17:2371–2380.

65. **Adler J, Zanetti R, Wight E, et al.** Sexual dysfunction after premenopausal stage I and II breast cancer: do androgens play a role? *J Sex Med* 2008;5:1898–1906.

66. **Berglund G, Nystedt M, Bolund C, et al.** Effect of endocrine treatment on sexuality in premenopausal breast cancer patient: a prospective randomized study. *J Clin Oncol* 2001;19:2788–2796.

67. **Ganz PA, Rowland JH, Desmond K, et al.** Life after breast cancer: understanding women's health related quality of life and sexual functioning. *J Clin Oncol* 1998;16:501–514.

68. **Fallowfield L, Cella D, Cuzick J, et al.** Quality of life of postmenopausal women in the Arimidex, Tamoxifen, Alone or in Combination (ATAC) Adjuvant Breast Cancer Trial. *J Clin Oncol* 2004;22:4261–4271.

69. **Enzlin P, Rosen R, Wiegl M.** Sexual dysfunction in women with type-I diabetes: long-term findings from the DCCT/EDIC study cohort. *Diabetes Care* 2009;32:780–783.

70. **Wierman ME, Nappi RE, Avis N, et al.** Endocrine aspects of women's sexual function. *J Sex Med* 2010;7:561–585.

71. **Gimbel H, Zobbe V, Andersen BM, et al.** Randomized controlled trial of total compared with subtotal hysterectomy with 1-year follow-up results. *Br J Obstet Gynaecol* 2003;110:1088–1098.

72. **Roovers JPWR, van der Bom JG, Huub van der Vaart C, et al.** Hysterectomy and sexual well being: prospective observational study of vaginal hysterectomy, subtotal abdominal hysterectomy, and total abdominal hysterectomy. *BMJ* 2003;327:774–779.

73. **Kim DH, Lee YS, Lee ES.** Alteration of sexual function after classic

intrafascial supracervical hysterectomy and total hysterectomy. *J Am Assoc Gynecol Laparosc* 2003;10:60–64.

74. **Long CY, Fang JH, Chen WC, et al.** Comparison of total laparoscopic hysterectomy and laparoscopically assisted vaginal hysterectomy. *Gynecol Obstet Invest* 2002;53:214–219.

75. **Pieterse QD, Ter Kuile MM, Deruiter MC, et al.** Vaginal blood flow after radical hysterectomy with and without nerve sparing: a preliminary report. *Int J Gynecol Cancer* 2008;18:576–583.

76. **Jongpipan J, Charoenkwan K.** Sexual function after radical hysterectomy for early-stage cervical cancer. *J Sex Med* 2007;4:1659–1665.

77. **Serati M, Salvatore S, Uccella S, et al.** Sexual function after hysterectomy early-stage cervical cancer: Is there a difference between laparoscopy and laparotomy? *J Sex Med* 2009;6:2516–2522.

78. **Buković D, Strinić T, Habek M, et al.** Sexual life after cervical carcinoma. *Coll Antropol* 2003;27:173–180.

79. **Bergmark K, Avall-Lundqvist E, Dickman PW, et al.** Vaginal changes and sexuality in women with a history of cervical cancer. *N Engl J Med* 1999;340:1383–1389.

80. **Pauleta JR, Pereira NM, Graça LM.** Sexuality during pregnancy. *J Sex Med* 2010;7:136–142.

81. **Asalan G, Asalan D, Kizilyar A, et al.** Prospective analysis of sexual functions during pregnancy. *Int J Impot Res* 2005;17:154–157.

82. **Benedetto C, Marozio L, Prandi G, et al.** Short-term maternal and neonatal outcomes by mood of delivery. A case-controlled study. *Eur J Obstet Gynecol Reprod Biol* 2007;135:35–40.

83. **Safarinejad MR, Kolahi AA, Hosseini L.** The effect of the mode of delivery on the quality of life, sexual function, and sexual satisfaction in primeparous women and their husbands. *J Sex Med* 2009;6:1645–1667.

84. **Marwick C.** Surveys say patients expect little physician help on sex. *JAMA* 1999;281:2173–2174.

85. **Nazareth I, Boynton P, King M.** Problems with sexual function and people attending London general practitioners: Cross-sectional study. *Brit Med J* 327:2003;423-428.

86. **Basson R, Leiblum S, Brotto L, et al.** Revised definitions of women's sexual dysfunction. *J Sex Med* 2004;1:40–48.

87. **Basson R, Leiblum S, Brotto L, et al.** Definitions of women's sexual dysfunctions reconsidered: advocating expansion and revision. *J Psychosom Obstet Gynecol* 2003;24:221–229.

88. **Brotto LA.** The DSM diagnostic criteria for hypoactive sexual desire disorder in women. *Arch Sex Behav* 2010;39:221–239.

89. **Graham CA.** The DSM diagnostic criteria for female sexual arousal disorder. *Arch Sex Behav* 2010;39:240–255.

90. **West SL, D'Aloisio AA, Agans RP, et al.** Prevalence of low sexual desire and hypoactive sexual desire disorder in a nationally representative sample of US women. *Arch Intern Med* 2008;168:1441–1449.

91. **Graziotiin A, Koochaki PE, Rodenberg CA, et al.** The prevalence of hypoactive sexual desire disorder in surgically menopausal women: an epidemiological study of women in four European countries. *J Sex Med* 2009;6:2143–2153.

92. **Leiblum SR, Hayes RD, Wanser RA, et al.** Vaginal dryness: a comparison of prevalence and interventions in 11 countries. *J Sex Med* 2009;6:2425–2433.

93. **Harlow BL, Wise LA, Stewart EG.** Prevalence and predictors of chronic lower genital tract discomfort. *Am J Obset Gynecol* 2001;185:545–550.

94. **Brotto LA, Bitzer J, Laan E, et al.** Women's sexual desire and arousal disorders. *J Sex Med* 2010;7(Pt 2):586–614.

95. **Braunstein G, Sundwall DA, Katz M, et al.** Safety and efficacy of a testosterone patch for the treatment of hypoactive sexual disorder in surgically menopausal women: a randomized, placebo-controlled trial. *Arch Intern Med* 2005;165:1582–1589.

96. **Buster JE, Kingsberg SA, Aguirre O, et al.** Testosterone patch for low sexual desire in surgically menopausal women: a randomized trial. *Obstet Gynecol* 2005;105:944–952.

97. **Simon J, Braunstein G, Nachtigall L, et al.** Testosterone patch increases sexual activity and desire in surgically menopausal women with hypoactive sexual desire disorder. *J Clin Endocrinol Metab* 2005;90:5226–5233.

98. **Davis SR, van der Mooren MJ, van Lunsen RHW, et al.** Efficacy and safety of a testosterone patch for the treatment of hypoactive sexual desire disorder in surgically menopausal women: a randomized, placebo controlled trial. *Menopause* 2006;13:387–396.

99. **Shifren JL, Davis SR, Moreau M, et al.** Testosterone patch for the treatment of hypoactive sexual desire disorder in naturally menopausal women: results from the INTIMATE NM1 STUDY. *Menopause* 2006;13:770–779.

100. **Davis S, Moreau M, Kroll R, et al.** Testosterone for low libido in postmenopausal women not taking estrogen. *N Engl J Med* 2008;359:2005–2017.

101. **Panay N, Al-Azzawi F, Bouchard C, et al.** Testosterone treatment of HSDD in naturally menopausal women: the ADORE study. *Climacteric* 2010;13:121–131.

102. **Barton DL, Wender DB, Sloan JA, et al.** Randomized controlled trial to evaluate transdermal testosterone in female cancer survivors with decreased libido: North Central Cancer Treatment Group Protocol N02C3. *J Nat Cancer Inst* 2007;99:672–679.

103. **Davis S, Papalia MA, Norman RJ, et al.** Safety and efficacy of a testosterone metered-dose transdermal spray for treatment of decreased sexual satisfaction in premenopausal women: a placebo-controlled randomized, dose ranging study. *Ann Intern Med* 2008;148:569–577.

104. **Wild RA.** Endogenous androgens and cardiovascular risk. *Menopause* 2007;14:609–610.

105. **Barbach L.** *For yourself: the fulfillment of female sexuality.* New York: Signet, 2000.

106. **Fortney L, Taylor M.** Meditation in medical practices: a review of the evidence and practice. *Prim Care Clin Office Pract* 2010;37:81–90.

107. **Long CY, Liu CM, Hsu SC, et al.** A randomized comparative study of the effects of oral and topical estrogen therapy on the vaginal vascularization and sexual function in hysterectomized postmenopausal women. *Menopause* 2006;13;737–743.

108. **Labrie F, Archer D, Bouchard C, et al.** Effect on intravaginal dehydroepiandrosterone (Prasterone) on libido and sexual dysfunction in postmenopausal women. *Menopause* 2010;16:923–931.

109. **Obermeyer CM.** The consequences of female circumcision for health and sexuality: an update on the evidence. *Cult Health Sex* 2005;7:443–461.

110. **Elnashar A, Abelhady R.** The impact of female genital cutting on health of newly married women. *Int J Gynaecol Obstet* 2007;97:238–244.

111. **Johnson C, Nour NM.** Surgical techniques: defibulation of type III female genital cutting. *J Sex Med* 2007;4:1544–1547.

112. **Dunn SFM, Gilchrist VJ.** Sexual assault. *Prim Care* 1993;20:359–373.

113. **Sorenson SB, Stein JA, Siegel JM, et al.** The prevalence of adult sexual assault. *Am J Epidemiol* 1987;126:1154–1164.

114. **American College of Obstetricians and Gynecologists.** *Sexual assault.* Technical bulletin no. 242. Washington, DC: ACOG, 1997.

115. **McGrath ME, Hogan JW, Peipert JF.** A prevalence survey of abuse and screening for abuse in urgent care patients. *Obstet Gynecol* 1998;91:511–514.

116. **McFarlane J, Malecha A, Watson K, et al.** Intimate partner assault against women: frequency, health consequences, and treatment outcomes. *Obstet Gyncol* 2005;105:99–108.

117. **Walch AG, Broadhead WE.** Prevalence of lifetime sexual victimization among female patients. *J Fam Pract* 1992;35:511–516.

118. **DeLahunta EA, Baram DA.** Sexual assault. *Clin Obstet Gynecol* 1997;40:648–660.

119. **Bachman GA, Moeller TP, Bennet J.** Childhood sexual abuse and the consequences in adult women. *Obstet Gynecol* 1988;71:631–642.

120. **Campbell R.** The psychological impact of rape victims. *Am Psychol* 2008;63:702–717.

121. **Springs FE, Friedrich WN.** Health risk behaviors and medical sequelae of childhood sexual abuse. *Mayo Clin Proc* 1992;67:527–532.

122. **Lang AJ, Rodgers CS, Laffaye C, et al.** Sexual trauma, posttraumatic stress disorder, and health behavior. *Behav Med* 2003;28:150–158.

123. **Weitlauf JC, Finney JW, Ruzek JI, et al.** Distress and pain during pelvic examinations: effect of sexual violence. *Obstet Gynecol* 2008;112:1343–1350.

124. **Council on Scientific Affairs, American Medical Association.** Violence against women: relevance for medical practitioners. *JAMA* 1992;267:3184–3189.

125. **Wyatt GE, Guthrie D, Notgrass CM.** Differential effects of

women's child sexual abuse and subsequent sexual revictimization. *J Consult Clin Psychol* 1992;60:167–173.

126. **Polit DF, White CM, Morton TD.** Child sexual abuse and premarital intercourse among high-risk adolescents. *J Adolesc Health* 1990;11:231–234.

127. **McCauley J, Kern DE, Kolodner K, et al.** Clinical characteristics of women with a history of childhood abuse: unhealed wounds. *JAMA* 1997;277:1362–1368.

128. **Mackey TF, Hacker SS, Weissfeld LA, et al.** Comparative effects of sexual assault on sexual functioning of child sexual abuse survivors and others. *Issues Ment Health Nurs* 1991;12:89–112.

129. **Laws A.** Does a history of sexual abuse in childhood play a role in women's medical problems? A review. *J Womens Health* 1993;2:165–172.

130. **American College of Obstetricians and Gynecologists.** *Adult manifestations of childhood sexual abuse.* Technical Bulletin No. 259. Washington, DC: ACOG, 2000.

131. **Danielson CK, Holmes MM.** Adolescent sexual assault: an update of the literature. *Curr Opin Obstet Gynecol* 2004;16:383–388.

132. **Kilpatrick DG, Edmunds CN, Seymour AK.** *Rape in America.* New York: National Victim Center, 1992.

133. **Ellis E, Atkeson B, Calhoun K.** An assessment of long term reaction to rape. *J Abnorm Psychol* 1981;90:263–266.

134. **Walling MK, Reiter RC, O'Hara MW, et al.** Abuse history and chronic pain in women. 1. Prevalences of sexual abuse and physical abuse. *Obstet Gynecol* 1994;84:193–199.

135. **Golding JM, Wilsnack SC, Learman LA.** Prevalence of sexual assault history among women with common gynecologic symptoms. *Am J Obstet Gynecol* 1998;179:1013–1019.

136. **Hendricks-Matthews MK.** Survivors of abuse. *Prim Care* 1993;20:391–406.

137. **Felitti VJ.** Long-term medical consequences of incest, rape, and molestation. *South Med J* 1991;84:328–331.

138. **Jones JS, Rossman L, Wynn BN, et al.** Comparative analysis of adult versus adolescent sexual assault: epidemiology and patterns of anogenital injury. *Acad Emerg Med* 2003;10:872–877.

139. **Mein JK, Palmer CM, Shand MC, et al.** Management of acute adult sexual assault. *Med J Aust* 2003;178:226–230.

140. **Eckert LO, Sugar NF.** Older victims of sexual assault: an unrecognized population. *Am J Obstet Gynecol* 2008;198:688.e1–688.e7.

141. **Sugar NF, Fine DN, Eckert LO.** Physical injury after sexual assault: findings of a large case series. *Am J Obstet Gynecol* 2004;190:71–76.

142. **Hampton HL.** Care of the women who has been raped. *N Engl J Med* 1995;332:234–237.

143. **Linden JA.** Sexual assault. *Emerg Med Clin North Am* 1999;17:685–697.

144. **Groth AN.** *Men who rape: the psychology of the offender.* New York: Plenum, 1979.

145. **Bechtel K, Podrazik M.** Evaluation of the adolescent rape victim. *Pediatr Clin North Am* 1999;46:809–822.

146. **Wiley J, Sugar N, Fine D, Eckert LO.** Legal outcomes of sexual assault. *Am J Obstet Gynecol* 2003;188:1638–1641.

147. **McGregor MJ, Du Mont J, Myhr TL.** Sexual assault forensic medical examination: is evidence related to successful prosecution? *Ann Emerg Med* 2002;39:639–647.

148. **Williams A.** *Managing adult sexual assault. Aust Fam Physician* 2004;33:825–828.

149. **Millar G, Stermac L, Addison M.** Immediate and delayed treatment seeking among adult sexual assault victims. *Women Health* 2002;35:53–64.

150. **Burgess A, Holmstrom L.** Rape trauma syndrome. *Am J Psychol* 1974;131:981–986.

151. **Holmes MM, Resnick HS, Frampton D.** Follow-up of sexual assault victims. *Am J Obstet Gynecol* 1998;179:336–342.

152. **Patel M, Minshall L.** Management of sexual assault. *Emerg Med Clin North Am* 2001;19:817–831.

153. **Geist F.** Sexually related trauma. *Emerg Med Clin North Am* 1988;6:439–466.

154. **Dupre AR, Hampton HL, Morrison H, et al.** Sexual assault. *Obstet Gynecol Surv* 1993;48:640–647.

155. **Maguire W, Goodall E, Moore T.** Injury in adult female sexual assault complainants and related factors. *Eur J Obstet Gynecol Reprod Biol* 2009;142:149–153.

156. **Jones JS, Dunnuck C, Rossman L, et al.** Significance of toluidine blue positive findings after speculum examination for sexual assault. *Am J Emerg Med* 2004;22:201–203.

157. **Beckmann CR, Groetzinger LL.** Treating sexual assault victims: a protocol for health professionals. *Female Patient* 1989;14:78–83.

158. **Glasier A.** Emergency postcoital contraception. *N Engl J Med* 1997;337:1058–1064.

159. **Von Hertzen H, Piaggio G, King J, et al.** Low dose mifepristone and two regimens of levonorgestrel for emergency contraception: a WHO multicentre randomised trial. *Lancet* 2002;360:1803–1810.

160. **American College of Obstetricians and Gynecologists.** *Emergency contraception.* Practice Bulletin No 112. Washington, DC: ACOG, 2010.

161. **Hamoda H, Ashok PW, Stalder C, et al.** A randomized trial of mifepristone (10 mg) and levonorgestrel for emergency contraception. *Obstet Gynecol* 2004;104:1307–1313.

162. **Ellertson C, Evans M, Ferden S, et al.** Extending the time limit for starting the Yuzpe regimen of emergency contraception to 120 hours. *Am J Obstet Gynecol* 2003;101:1168–1171.

163. **Beebe DK.** Emergency management of the adult female rape victim. *Am Fam Physician* 1991;43:2041–2046.

164. **Jenny C, Hooton TM, Bowers A, et al.** Sexually transmitted diseases in victims of rape. *N Engl J Med* 1990;322:713–716.

165. **Reynolds MW, Peipert JF, Collins B.** Epidemiologic issues of sexually transmitted diseases in sexual assault victims. *Obstet Gynecol Surv* 2000;55:51–57.

166. **Kawsar M, Anfield A, Walters E, et al.** Prevalence of sexually transmitted infections and mental health needs of female child and adolescent survivors of rape and sexual assault attending a specialist clinic. *Sex Transm Infect* 2004;80:138–141.

167. **Centers for Disease Control and Prevention.** 2006 guidelines for sexually transmitted diseases. *MMWR* 2006;55(RR11):1–94

168. **Weinberg GA.** Postexposure prophylaxis against human immunodeficiency virus infections after sexual assault. *Pediatr Infect Dis J* 2002;21:959–960.

169. **Merchant RC, Keshavarz R, Low C.** HIV post-exposure prophylaxis provided at an urban paediatric emergency department to female adolescents after sexual assault. *Emerg Med J* 2004;21:449–451.

170. **Luce H, Schrager S.** Sexual assault of women. *Am Fam Phys* 2010;81:489–495.

12 Common Psychiatric Problems

Nada Logan Stotland

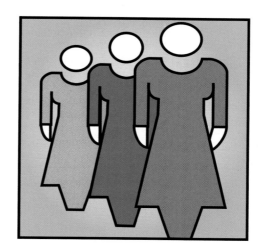

- **Major depression, anxiety disorders, and other specific disorders are common and therefore are seen in general gynecologic practice.**

- **Appropriate referral to mental health specialists must be made in a sensitive manner.**

- **Suicidal and homicidal behaviors are absolute indications for referral.**

- **Alcohol and other substance abuse needs prompt recognition and intervention.**

- **Some women are vulnerable to mood symptoms at times of hormonal change. However, menopausal hormone levels are not correlated with depression, and premenstrual syndrome should not be diagnosed without 2 months of prospective daily ratings.**

- **Personality disorders and somatizing disorders rarely can be cured, but informed management can greatly decrease the suffering of the patient**

- **Withdrawal of successful psychotropic treatment is very likely to lead to relapse.**

- **Psychotic disorders should nearly always be managed by psychiatrists.**

Psychiatric problems are a central or complicating factor for many patients who seek care on an outpatient basis (1,2). Psychiatric diagnoses are extremely common and account for considerable morbidity and mortality in the general population (3). Despite their prevalence, psychiatric disorders are often undiagnosed or misdiagnosed (4–7). **Clinical depression affects up to one-fourth of women during their lives, but probably more than half of those women are neither diagnosed nor treated** (8–11). More than half of the patients who commit suicide have seen a nonpsychiatric physician during the previous 3 months (12).

Psychiatry in the Gynecology Office

Many gynecologists feel uncomfortable diagnosing and treating psychiatric illnesses. The practice of gynecology is demanding, and patients with psychological problems can evoke a variety of negative reactions in physicians (Table 12.1). Some physicians, and some members of the public, have the misconception that psychiatric diagnoses are vague and ill-defined. Current diagnostic criteria and categories of psychiatric disorders are supported by empirical evidence

Table 12.1 Practitioners' Negative Reactions Toward Patients with Psychiatric Problems

1. Social stigma attached to psychiatric diagnoses, patients, and practitioners.

2. Belief that individuals with psychiatric disorders are weak, unmotivated, manipulative, or defective.

3. Belief that the criteria for psychiatric diagnoses are intuitive rather than empirical.

4. Belief that psychiatric treatments are ineffective and unsupported by medical evidence.

5. Fear that patients with psychiatric problems will demand and consume inordinate and limitless time from a medical practice.

6. Precipitation in others, including doctors, of feelings that are complementary to the strong and unpleasant emotions experienced by patients with psychiatric disorders.

7. Gynecologists' own uncertainty about their skills at psychiatric diagnosis, referral, and treatment.

8. Failure to acknowledge psychiatric problems as legitimate grounds for medical attention.

that is as reliable and valid as those used in most medical treatment. Physicians are naturally reluctant to uncover problems for which there seems to be no solutions. There are effective treatments for psychiatric disorders, and they are straightforward to use in clinical practice. Although the newly enacted parity laws forbid discrimination by insurers against mental health care, gynecologists and their patients may have difficulty accessing mental health services. It is sometimes necessary for the physician and family to advocate strongly for necessary care. By incorporating the management strategies in this chapter into their practice, gynecologists can reduce clinical frustration and play a major role in improving the health and well-being of their patients.

Psychiatric Assessment

In the past, the diagnosis of psychiatric disorders was based partially on hypotheses about a patient's unconscious psychological conflicts, which cannot be verified (13). **Current psychiatric diagnosis, as codified in the *Diagnostic and Statistical Manual of Mental Disorders*, fourth edition, text revision (DSM-IV-TR), produced and published by the American Psychiatric Association, is based on empirical, valid, and reliable evidence** (9). The DSM-IV yields reliability comparable to that of diagnostic systems used in other areas of medicine, and its diagnoses strongly correlate with response to treatment. The criteria in DSM-IV are the basis for the diagnostic entities described in this chapter. The new edition, DSM-IV-TR, differs only in the explanations of some of the diagnoses and not in the diagnostic criteria themselves. **The DSM-IV-PC is a special edition designed for the primary care provider. This volume is organized by initial signs and symptoms rather than psychiatric categories and uses algorithms and decision trees to facilitate the diagnostic process** (9). The fifth edition of the DSM is scheduled for publication in 2013, and it might not contain changes of major importance for gynecology practice. Accurate diagnosis is absolutely critical to successful management, whether care is provided by a gynecologist or through referral to a mental health expert.

Approach to the Patient

Although diagnostic criteria list signs and symptoms, the interaction with a patient should not be reduced to a series of rapid-fire questions and answers. **A wealth of valuable information can be obtained from the patient's spontaneous description of her concerns and from her responses to the physician's open-ended questions** (14). A patient who is encouraged to speak for several minutes before being asked to respond to specific questions will reveal information that is useful, even vital, to her care: a thought disorder, a predominant mood, abnormally high anxiety, a personality style or disorder, and attitudes toward her diagnosis and treatment. Such information may emerge only much later, or not at all, in a question-and-answer format (15,16). **It is critical that the gynecologist neither jumps to diagnostic conclusions nor proceeds directly to therapeutic interventions.** One study revealed that many primary care physicians, feeling that they have too little time or training to assess psychological symptoms, tend to minimize verbal interactions with patients and to rely on the prescription of psychotropic medications (17). Allowing a few moments for open-ended discussion does not mean that the physician and the other patients awaiting care are to be held hostage by an overly talkative patient. The clinician can tell the patient with multiple, detailed symptoms how much time is available for the current appointment, invite her to focus on her most pressing problem, and offer a future appointment to continue the account.

Psychiatric Referral

Many gynecologists consider referral to a mental health professional, particularly a psychiatrist, to be a delicate matter. The first question is when to refer, followed by how to refer and to whom. Most mild psychiatric disorders are treated by nonpsychiatric physicians, who often prescribe antidepressants and anxiolytic medications (18). Psychiatric disorders often are overlooked, misdiagnosed, or mistreated in primary care practice. The factors that determine the decision to refer are the:

- Nature and severity of the patient's disorder

- Expertise of the gynecologist

- Time available in the gynecologic practice

- Patient's preference

- Gynecologist's degree of comfort with the patient and the disorder

- Availability of mental health professionals

Patients who are suicidal, homicidal, or acutely psychotic should be referred immediately to a psychiatrist, and often are accompanied to the appointment (19). The primary provider should refer patients for psychiatric evaluation when the diagnosis is not clear or when the patient fails to respond to initial treatment. The gynecologist can resume responsibility for ongoing care of many patients after their initial or periodic assessment by a psychiatrist.

How to Refer

Some clinicians fear that patients will be insulted or alarmed by a psychiatric referral. Following are techniques that decrease the discomfort of both the gynecologist and the patient and enhance the likelihood of success (19). **The referral should be explained on the basis of the patient's own signs, symptoms, and level of distress.** For a patient suffering from clinical depression, for example, this might be difficulty sleeping, loss of appetite, and lack of energy. For a patient with an anxiety disorder, it might be palpitations, shortness of breath, and nervousness. For a patient with mild Alzheimer's disease, it might be forgetfulness or frightening episodes in which she finds herself in a neighborhood she does not recognize. With the advent of treatments that may slow dementia, these referrals are easier and more meaningful because there is now some hope for effective intervention.

When a somatizing (psychosomatic) disorder is suspected, the gynecologist should emphasize the difficulty of living with symptoms in the absence of a definitive diagnosis and treatment rather than the hypothesis that the symptoms have a psychological basis (19):

1. *"It is very stressful to be suffering while we can't pinpoint the problem. I would like you to see one of our staff who specializes in helping people cope with these difficult situations."*

2. *"It must be difficult to function when you have been so sickly all your life, have seen so many doctors, have had so many diagnostic tests and medical treatments, and still don't have an answer or feel well."*

It is counterproductive to convey the idea that because the diagnostic process has not revealed a specific disorder, the problem must be "in the patient's head." It alienates the patient. It is never possible to rule out an organic cause with absolute certainty; and diseases "in the head" are real diseases (19).

Although suicidal and homicidal behaviors are absolute indications for referral, many physicians fear that questioning patients about these behaviors will provoke them. That is not the case (12). An open discussion of impulses to hurt oneself or someone else helps the patient to regain control, recognize the need for mental health care, or agree to emergency interventions such as psychiatric hospitalization, whereas avoiding the subject intensifies the patient's feelings of isolation. The management of suicidal behavior is addressed later in this chapter in the section on mood disorders.

Likewise, the possibility of psychosis need not be avoided. **Most patients with psychotic disorders have had previous experience with psychiatric referral. Their psychotic symptoms are often distressing, so treatment is an appealing option** (19). They can discuss hallucinations and delusions quite matter-of-factly. The rare patient who comes to a gynecologist in the midst of a first episode of psychosis is likely to be frightened by her symptoms and willing to accept expert consultation.

Despite increasing public sophistication about mental illnesses and psychiatric care, some patients believe that any mention of mental health intervention implies that they are either "crazy" or that the referring physician is convinced that their physical symptoms are imaginary or feigned. It is helpful to state explicitly that this is not the case. Making the real reason for the referral clear and founded in signs and symptoms obvious to the patient will nearly always allay anxiety over a psychiatric referral (19).

It is not acceptable to refer a patient to a psychiatrist without informing her in advance and obtaining her consent, unless she is acutely psychotic, functionally incompetent, or in the throes of a suicidal or homicidal emergency. Even under those circumstances, it is highly preferable to be straightforward. A referral that begins with an unexpected clinical encounter with a psychiatrist is unfair to both the psychiatrist and the patient and is unlikely to result in a satisfactory outcome (17–19).

To allay any concern a patient may have that a mental health referral is an indication of the gynecologist's disdain or disinterest, and to promote good patient care in general, the referring gynecologist should make it clear to the patient that he or she will remain involved in the patient's care. The mental health professional should be introduced as a member of the health care team, and the gynecologist should ask the patient to call after the mental health appointment to report on how it went. The patient should be given a follow-up appointment with the gynecologist at the time of the referral (19).

Making a Mental Health Professional Referral

Mental disorders are treated by social workers, psychologists, members of the clergy (often the first to be consulted), and various kinds of counselors as well as by psychiatrists (17–19). The lay public or even some medical professionals may not understand the distinctions between types of mental health professionals. The criteria for membership in each profession can vary by region and institution. Social workers and psychologists can receive degrees at the bachelor, master, or doctoral level. In some states, licensure is required. Social workers require a master's degree and psychologists receive a doctoral degree, in addition to supervised clinical experience to qualify for licensure. The category of counselor includes a wide variety of practitioners, such as marriage counselors, pastoral counselors, school counselors, and family counselors. The training of social workers may focus on social policy, institutional care, psychosocial aspects of medical illness, or individual treatment (17–19).

Practitioners of all these disciplines may or may not be trained in psychotherapy. For a patient whose symptoms do not meet criteria for a major psychiatric disorder and who is able to eat, sleep, and carry out her regular duties, supportive psychotherapy provided by a trained mental health professional may suffice. Supportive psychotherapy calls on a patient's existing coping mechanisms to combat a stressful situation. Doctoral-level psychologists and neuropsychologists can perform testing that can be helpful in establishing a diagnosis. Such testing is especially useful in identifying and localizing brain pathology and in defining intelligence levels. Undiagnosed cognitive deficits may contribute to noncompliance with gynecologic care as well as other problems (17–19).

Trained social workers are often knowledgeable about community resources for patients and their families and about the impact of gynecologic diseases and treatments on the patients. Self-help or professionally led therapy groups can be helpful for patients reacting to gynecologic problems such as infertility or malignancy. Participation in a supportive group was said to lengthen the survival time and improve the quality of life for some patients with cancer, although this assertion is controversial (20–26).

Psychiatrists are the only medically trained mental health professionals. They play a particularly important role in resolving diagnostic dilemmas, especially when questions arise about the psychological or behavioral manifestations of medical illness and pharmacologic treatment;

when a medical understanding of the gynecologic condition and treatment is essential to the care of the patient; and when such issues as drug–drug interactions must be considered (19). **Psychiatrists are the only mental health professionals trained to prescribe psychoactive medications and other biologic interventions and provide psychotherapy.** The legislatures of New Mexico and Louisiana have conferred prescribing rights on doctoral-level psychologists with additional training but have not defined the limits of the prescribing authority. It is highly likely that psychiatrists will continue to treat the most seriously ill patients and take ultimate responsibility for psychiatric emergencies (19).

Because psychiatric problems frequently present in gynecologic practice, it is worthwhile for the gynecologist to develop an ongoing relationship with one or more local mental health professionals. The state psychiatric society may have a list of subspecialists in "consultation liaison" psychiatry; this is an official subspecialty of the American Board of Psychiatry and Neurology. Many psychiatrists without specific fellowship training offer consultative services. The availability of familiar and trusted resources enhances the likelihood that problems will be identified and addressed. An ongoing relationship with a mental health professional allows the gynecologist to familiarize that professional with relevant developments in gynecology. **It is important to keep up-to-date information on local suicide prevention hotlines and other kinds of resources for battered women and for mothers who may pose a danger to their children.** Local laws may require that physicians report to the authorities their knowledge of mothers in this situation (19).

Whenever a patient's thinking, emotions, or behaviors cause concern, the gynecologist should first consider a nonpsychiatric medical disorder or a reaction to prescribed or illicit drugs. Psychiatric disorders frequently coexist with these conditions (19). HIV/AIDS infection, some malignancies, hypothyroidism, and other diseases can present with psychiatric symptoms.

Psychiatric conditions are extremely common in gynecologic practice. Some are primary and some are related to reproductive events. **All patients should be screened for depression, anxiety, domestic violence, and substance abuse, each of which can be diagnosed and treated, either by the gynecologist or by referral to a social resource or a mental health specialist (16–19).**

Mood Disorders

Mood is the emotional coloration of a person's experience. **Mood may be pathologically elevated (mania) or lowered (depression) or may alternate between the two (bipolar or manic-depressive disorder)** (26). Mood disorders are different from, but frequently confused with, the inevitable ups and downs of everyday life, such as the reactions to difficult situations, including gynecologic conditions. In the English language, *depression* is used to describe both a transient mood and a psychiatric disorder. Because of this confusion, both patients and their loved ones become frustrated when well-meaning attempts to reason with them, distract them, or do thoughtful things for them in a manner that would affect a self-limited reaction to a difficult situation, fail to influence their protractedly disturbed moods.

Mania is characterized by the following behavior (26):

1. **Elevated mood, with euphoria or without irritability**
2. **Grandiosity**
3. **Pressured, accelerated speech and physical activity**
4. **Increased energy**
5. **Decreased sleep**
6. **Reckless and potentially damaging behaviors, such as wild expenditures and promiscuity**

Mania can be acute or subacute (hypomania). Hypomania can produce self-confidence, ebullience, energy, and productivity that are the envy of others, making the patient reluctant to relinquish this mood by undergoing treatment. It can be particularly difficult to arrest the condition before it progresses to full-blown mania. Acute mania is a life-threatening condition; without treatment, patients fail to maintain essential sleep and nutrition levels and literally exhaust themselves with frantic activity. Patients with bipolar illness must be taught and encouraged, and often learn from bitter experience, to recognize the early signs of disturbed mood so that treatment or treatment changes can be initiated (16).

Depression

The overall lifetime prevalence of affective disorders is 8.3%; the 6-month prevalence is 5.8%. **During the reproductive years, depression is two to three times more common in women than in men** (26–32). The highest incidence of depression is in the age group of 25 to 44 years, but depression occurs in every age group, from toddlers to the aged. Women have a lifetime risk of 10% to 25% and a point prevalence of 5% to 9% (33–36). **Although public understanding and acceptance of mental illnesses has significantly increased, patients may have difficulty accepting, and telling others, that they are suffering from depression.**

Depression is the single most common reason for psychiatric hospitalization in the United States. **As many as 15% of individuals with severe depressive disorders eventually commit suicide** (37). Depression is a significant risk factor for cardiovascular disease and for noncompliance with essential treatments for other diseases, including diabetes. Depression is a recurrent disorder; of those who experience a major depressive episode, 50% have a second one. Of these, 70% have a third, and the incidence continues to increase with each subsequent episode. In the past diagnostic criteria were not standardized, so it is difficult to know whether the incidence of depression has increased over recent years, as has been asserted in the popular press.

Because women's roles in society changed a great deal over the past few decades, there is a temptation to postulate a higher rate of depression attributable to women's work outside the home. **There is no evidence that employment outside the home increases women's vulnerability to depression.** Multiple life roles actually contribute to life satisfaction, although the need to carry out multiple roles in the absence of adequate social support, as is all too common in women's lives, is stressful (38–40).

Depression is characterized by the following (9,19):

1. **Sad mood or irritability**
2. **Hopelessness**
3. **Helplessness**
4. **Decreased ability to concentrate**
5. **Decreased energy**
6. **Interference with sleep, generally with early awakening, inability to return to sleep, and failure to feel rested; atypically, with increased sleep**
7. **Decreased appetite and weight; atypically, increased food intake**
8. **Withdrawal from social relationships**
9. **Inability to enjoy previously gratifying activities**
10. **Loss of libido**
11. **Guilt**
12. **Psychomotor retardation or agitation**
13. **Thoughts of death or suicide**

The patient who has five or more of the signs and symptoms of depression for most of each day for 2 weeks or more fulfills the criteria for the diagnosis of clinical depression (36–38). **Depression may be acute or chronic (dysthymic disorder).** Like many diseases, it is caused by genetic, neurophysiologic, and environmental factors. Trauma in early life plays a role. Serotonin is a major mediator of mood. Treatment, whether pharmacologic or psychotherapeutic, is effective for depression. **The average duration of a major depressive episode is approximately 9 months** (36). **Patients must be cautioned to continue treatment at least that long, even if symptoms remit; relapse is common.**

Depression may be precipitated by an adverse life event such as an interpersonal loss, economic reversal, or serious illness (41,42). When there is an identifiable precipitant, there is a danger that the depression will be written off as the inevitable reaction to the event rather than considered properly as a complication that requires active treatment, similar to infection or pneumonia complicating a surgical procedure. When a patient's symptoms meet criteria for the diagnosis, treating the depression will relieve symptoms and will enable her to cope more successfully with the precipitating situation (43).

Paradoxically, patients in happy life situations, and their loved ones, may have resistance to the idea that they are depressed. They need to understand that depression is not a sign of ingratitude or lack of appreciation for their life advantages, but a disease, like any other, that can strike even otherwise fortunate people.

Concomitant gynecologic or other medical illness can cause signs and symptoms similar to those of depression—loss of energy, sleep, and appetite—but does not cause guilt, hopelessness, or helplessness (44). These observations are helpful in differentiating depression from the malaise associated with other disease states.

Gynecologic Issues

The incidence of depression peaks, and the gender difference prevails, during the reproductive years (45). Connections between female reproductive functions and mood changes have been posited for centuries. When it first became possible to determine circulating hormone levels, researchers expected to find specific relationships between psychological and physiological changes. These expectations were uniformly discounted. **There is no serum hormone level associated with premenstrual dysphoria, postpartum depression, or depression at menopause** (46). There is a subgroup of women who are vulnerable, not to absolute circulating hormone levels, but to hormonal changes (47–50). There is a correlation between the degree of hormonal change, pre- and postpartum, and the incidence of postpartum mood disorder. **Women who are vulnerable to hormonal changes may experience severe premenstrual mood symptoms, postpartum depression, and, possibly, depression in association with hormonal influences such as hormonal contraceptive methods, menopause, and hormone treatments** (51).

Premenstrual Syndrome

Depending on the methodology used to gather the data, most women report mood and behavioral changes associated with the menstrual cycle. Although there are both ups and downs associated with the cycle, it is the more problematic parts of the cycle that are characterized, as premenstrual syndrome, or PMS. **An estimated 3% to 5% of ovulating women appear to suffer from symptoms so marked that they qualify for a diagnosis of premenstrual dysphoric disorder (PMDD)** (52–54).

PMDD is included in DSM-IV-TR as an example of a depressive disorder, not otherwise specified, and as a category requiring additional research (9). Provisional diagnostic criteria are provided to standardize this research.

In most cycles over the past year, the patient had at least five of the following symptoms for most of the time during the premenstrual week, with symptoms remitting completely in the postmenstrual week (54):

- **Depressed mood, hopelessness, self-deprecation**

- **Anxiety, tension**

- **Affective lability**

- **Anger, irritability, interpersonal conflict**

- **Decreased interest in usual activities**

- **Difficulty concentrating**

- **Decreased energy**

- **Appetite changes or cravings**

- **Changes in sleep**

- **Feeling overwhelmed or out of control**

- **Physical symptoms such as breast tenderness, headache, bloating**

The symptoms markedly interfere with work, family, or academic responsibilities; are not exacerbations of another existing disorder; and are corroborated by at least 2 months of prospective daily ratings (54).

Premenstrual syndrome, as differentiated from premenstrual dysphoric disorder, has been characterized by more than 100 different physical and psychological signs and symptoms, making it difficult to define scientifically. Methodological problems further complicate the situation; in the United States, the prevalence of attitudes linking the menstrual cycle to adverse mood and behavioral changes is so high that it skews women's perceptions, the way they report symptoms to researchers, and the factors to which they attribute negative feelings. No specific circulating hormone levels or markers are associated with premenstrual symptoms (55). When prospective daily ratings are obtained systematically, the symptoms of most women who seek care for PMS are not related to the menstrual cycle (56,57). Therefore, careful assessment is essential. Before the diagnosis of PMS or PMDD can be established, a woman must record symptom ratings daily for at least two full cycles. Records of emotions and behaviors should be kept separate from menstrual records to avoid confounding patients' perceptions. At the same time, the patient must be screened for other psychiatric disorders, including depression and personality disorders, and for domestic abuse and other life circumstances that may contribute to her psychological state (58).

No treatment for PMS has been validated by empirical studies (59). Studies of St. John's wort, possibly the most popular alternative treatment, are contradictory (60). A number of lifestyle changes and other benign interventions alleviate symptoms for some patients with PMS (61):

- Elimination of caffeine from the diet

- Smoking cessation

- Regular exercise

- Regular meals and a nutritious diet

- Adequate sleep

- Stress reduction

Stress reduction can be accomplished by reducing or delegating responsibilities, insofar as that is possible, and devoting part of every day to relaxation techniques such as meditation and yoga. Many women experience stress factors over which they have no control (59).

For premenstrual dysphoric disorder, several selective serotonin reuptake inhibitors (SSRIs) proved effective in clinical trials (62–65). Although SSRIs and all other antidepressants require about 2 weeks of daily administration to achieve therapeutic effect for other depressive disorders, it appears that *fluoxetine* is effective for PMDD when taken in the usual daily doses for the 1 to 2 weeks preceding menstruation. The medication is packaged for this specific indication and dosage. It is thought that the mode of action of SSRIs when used in this fashion differs from that which alleviates major depression (65). Other medications for the treatment of PMS and PMDD are shown in Table 12.2. There is some interest in the role of oral contraceptives in management of PMDD, and for patients interested in contraception, trials of oral contraceptives are a reasonable approach (66). Symptoms must be carefully monitored to determine whether the hormonal intervention improves or exacerbates the problem mood changes.

Other Reproductive Events

Infertility is described by most women who undergo treatment for it as the most stressful event of their lives. Each unsuccessful treatment episode is experienced as the loss of a hoped-for pregnancy (67). The loss of a fetus or newborn induces grief, with some of the same symptoms as depression. Depression is associated with guilt, whereas bereavement is not. However, women who lose pregnancies or infants often do feel guilty, regardless of whether these feelings are logically justified. Patients should not be pressed to "put the loss behind them" or expected to be "over it" within several months. Some feelings of sadness may persist for years. However, their sleep, appetite, and other vital functions and behaviors should begin to improve after a few weeks (68). Grief that persists and interferes with normal function is characterized as pathologic. Depression can complicate grief and should be treated (69).

Table 12.2 Scientific Basis of Selected Medications Used to Treat Premenstrual Syndrome

Treatment	Scientific Basis	Advantages	Disadvantages	Notes
Alprazolam	Several double-blind, placebo-controlled, randomized crossover studies. Results were mixed. Placebo was as effective as *alprazolam* in some studies.	Oral medication appears to be more effective in alleviating depression and anxiety symptoms than physical symptoms.	Potential for dependence; requires tapering; drowsiness reported by many subjects; long-term effects unknown; safety during pregnancy unknown.	The studies involved highly selective groups of women. There was a high dropout rate in one of the positive studies. In one study that found *alprazolam* effective, 87% of the women had a history of major depression or an anxiety disorder. Different doses were used in the studies (0.75–2.25 mg); the standard effective dosage is unknown.
Fluoxetine (Prozac)	Several double-blind, randomized, placebo-controlled, crossover trials. All found *fluoxetine* effective.	Well tolerated; single daily oral dose. Significant decrease in psychic and behavioral symptoms.	Long-term effects unknown. Safety during pregnancy unknown. Appears less effective in controlling physical symptoms.	Trials involved very small, highly select groups of women. Duration of treatment did not exceed 3 months. All trials used 20 mg orally daily.
Gonadotropin-releasing hormone agonist	Several small, double-blind, randomized, placebo-controlled, crossover trials. Most patients experienced improvement.	Rapidly reversible; many patients report being virtually symptom-free during therapy.	Produces pseudomenopause; expensive; risk for osteoporosis, hypoestrogenic symptoms. Usually given for only short periods of time.	An add-back regimen of estrogen-progestin in addition to gonadotropin-releasing hormone agonist has been reported. If replicated, it may have potential for an effective, long-term treatment for premenstrual syndrome.
Spironolactone	Several double-blind, randomized, placebo-controlled trials. Mixed results.	May alleviate bloating and improve symptoms related to mood. Oral medication taken once or twice a day. Nonaddictive.	Effectiveness not proven consistently across studies.	*Spironolactone* is the only diuretic that has shown effectiveness in treating premenstrual syndrome in controlled, randomized trials. Method of action may be antiandrogen properties.
Vitamin B_6	Ten randomized double-blind trials. About one-third of the trials reported positive results, one-third reported negative results, and one-third reported ambiguous results.		No conclusive evidence that vitamin B_6 is more effective than placebo.	Doses ranged from 50 to 500 mg. Only one study involved more than 40 participants. The large multicenter trial (N = 204) reported similar results for placebo and vitamin B_6.

From **The American College of Obstetricians and Gynecologists.** *Committee opinion.* Washington, DC: ACOG, 1995, with permission.

There is no convincing evidence that induced abortion causes clinical depression or any other negative psychiatric sequelae. Studies purporting to demonstrate negative sequelae fail to take into account the circumstances under which women conceive unintended pregnancies and elect to terminate them—abuse, abandonment, poverty, rape, and incest—or the circumstances in which they occur—familial pressure or disapproval, the presence of clinic demonstrators (70).

Peripartum Psychiatric Disorders

The incidence of depression in women during their reproductive years is approximately 10%. The incidence of depression does not decrease during pregnancy; most postpartum depression is a continuation of antepartum depression (71–73). Although there are some cross-cultural variations under study, postpartum depression is found around the globe (74). Risk factors include social isolation, lack of social supports, history of depression, and past or present victimization (75). **It is important to remember that women without risk factors may become depressed.** Postpartum depression must be distinguished from the transitory, self-limited, and very common "baby blues," which are associated with changes in hormone levels and are better characterized as mood intensity and lability rather than depression. Mild depression can be managed with psychotherapy (76). Moderate to severe cases often require antidepressant medications (77). Electroconvulsive treatment acts rapidly and effectively, appears to be safe during and after pregnancy, and can be a life-saving option for the most severe cases (78). Treatment with artificial light may alleviate milder symptoms (79). Although no agent can be declared perfectly safe for use during pregnancy and lactation, older SSRI agents are well studied, yielding little or no evidence of adverse effects on the fetus or nursing infant (80–82). These agents are used in the treatment of obsessive-compulsive disorder (83).

Medication should not be stopped arbitrarily, nor should breastfeeding be prohibited. **The withdrawal of antidepressant medication during pregnancy is very likely to result in postpartum depression; both antenatal and postnatal depression have demonstrable, long-term ill effects for mother and child** (84–91). There is concern about withdrawal syndromes in neonates whose mothers took SSRIs (92). These concerns arise from anecdotal reports and do not include data about the number of births from which the reports emerged, nor about confounding variables. Some observers recommended that pregnant women be withdrawn from SSRIs some days or weeks before delivery. However, delivery dates are often uncertain; maternal withdrawal might subject the fetus, rather than the newborn, to withdrawal symptoms; and the likelihood of postpartum depression, with its effects on both mother and infant, would be greatly increased. Researchers are exploring ways to prevent postpartum depression, but thus far nothing has proved effective (93,94).

Sertraline appears to be the safest medication for pregnant and lactating women, and *paroxetine* is the cause of most concern. If treatment is begun during pregnancy or lactation *sertraline* is the reasonable choice. Switching a patient successfully treated with another antidepressant to *sertraline* is not indicated. The fetus would be exposed to a second medication, and the patient may not respond as well to *sertraline* as to the currently effective antidepressant (80–82).

Hysterectomy

Studies of the relationship between hysterectomy and mental illnesses are contradictory (95,96). Probably the determining factors in psychiatric outcomes are the reason for the procedure and the context, whether the patient loses valued fertility as a result, including the reactions of significant others and cultural beliefs about the importance of an intact uterus (97).

Menopause

Although menopause was assumed for many years to be associated with an increased incidence of depression, empirical studies led to conflicting results and controversy. Menopause appears to have mood effects in some women that can be differentiated from the secondary effects, such as hot flashes interfering with sleep. Psychosocial studies indicate that some patients are upset by their loss of fertility or the departure of grown children from the home (*empty nest syndrome*), but many women find menopause liberating (98,99). For some women the return of adult children to the maternal home, or responsibilities for the care of grandchildren, seems to be a precipitating factor for depression. Patients who suffered PMS or postpartum depression may be vulnerable to a recurrence of depression at this new time of hormonal change. Patients with depression at the time of menopause should be assessed for psychosocial precipitants and domestic abuse. There are conflicting reports on the effectiveness of hormones for treatment of mood symptoms during menopause (100–105). Treatment with SSRIs may ameliorate hot flashes (106).

Depression in elderly patients can cause a *pseudodementia*, characterized by decreased activity and interest and what appears to be forgetfulness. Unlike patients with genuine dementia, these patients report memory loss rather than trying to compensate and cover up for it. The early stages of dementia can precipitate depression as patients react to the loss of cognitive abilities (107).

Approach to the Patient

The severity of depression is determined by the patient's emotional pain and the degree of interference with her normal functioning. Depression is an agonizingly painful and disabling, but readily diagnosable and treatable, disease (108). Nevertheless, it shares the stigma of all psychiatric disorders. Patients and their families often attribute the signs and symptoms of depression to life circumstances or to a medical condition, either diagnosed or undiagnosed. The persistence of symptoms in the face of a pleasant life situation or the failure of the patient to respond to attempts at cheering, such as changes of scene, often exacerbate suffering by provoking guilt in the patient and frustration in her significant others. Some patients report low energy and general malaise rather than depressed mood. Physical symptoms are especially common in Asian and some other cultures and in the elderly (107). Some patients with severe depression continue to function and can appear normal and cheerful. **The only way to rule out depression is by asking about symptoms and using the diagnostic criteria** (108).

Management

Both antidepressant medication and psychotherapy are effective treatments for depression. There is evidence that a combination of the two produces the best outcomes (109–111). Reports about the efficacy of alternative treatments, the most common of which is St. John's wort, are conflicting, but mostly negative (112). Patients should be specifically questioned about their use of herbal and other preparations and encouraged to use those whose components are standardized. Transcranial magnetic stimulation is a promising research intervention (113,114).

There are many forms of psychotherapy. Those that were specifically studied for efficacy in the treatment of depression are cognitive-behavioral therapy and interpersonal therapy. These forms of therapy are focused on present thoughts, feelings, relationships, and behaviors. Therapy continues for a set number of sessions, usually no more than 16 weekly sessions, in a prescribed, predetermined progression (115). **There is increasing evidence that supportive and psychodynamic psychotherapy is effective.**

It is especially important for the patient to have the opportunity to work out her feelings about having a psychiatric disorder, understand how it has affected her life, and feel comfortable taking medication or undergoing psychotherapy (115). Patients often attribute depression to weakness, laziness, or immorality, and they often confuse antidepressants with stimulants, tranquilizers, and other psychoactive drugs. Although written materials cannot substitute entirely for verbal instruction, it is useful to provide the patient with written material about depression so that she can review it at her leisure and with her family and friends if they have difficulty understanding her condition. There is widespread difficulty understanding written information, especially about medicine. **Many or most antidepressant prescriptions are either not filled or not taken as prescribed** (116).

Depression in one individual has a powerful effect on other members of the family, particularly children. This can be a motivating factor for patients who are reluctant to accept treatment.

The types and characteristics of antidepressants are presented in Table 12.3. **All antidepressants have comparable therapeutic efficacy, and all require up to 2 to 4 weeks to take full effect.** It is not yet possible to identify those patients who will respond best to certain medications, but there is early evidence that depression may be related to specific neurotransmitters and respond differentially to medications affecting a given neurotransmitter. The response to treatment may differ with gender, but the data are not sufficient to drive clinical decisions (117).

It is sensible to use a more activating agent (*fluoxetine*) in a lethargic patient and a more sedating agent (*paroxetine*) in an agitated patient (118). Nonetheless, responses vary on an individual basis, even within the same class of medications. The choice of antidepressant is based on side effects, dosage, cost, and the physician's clinical experience (Table 12.4). Patients tend to respond to medications that worked for them in the past and to those that worked for depressed family members. **Many patients require successive trials of two or more antidepressants before the one that is effective for them is identified. It is essential to continue active management through the usual duration of a depressive episode—9 to 12 months for major depression,**

Table 12.3 Pharmacology of Antidepressant Medications

Drug	Therapeutic Dosage Range (mg/day)	Average (range) of Elimination Half-Lives (hours)[a]	Potentially Fatal Drug Interactions
Tricyclics			
Amitriptyline (Elavil, Endep)	75–300	24 (16–46)	Antiarrhythmics, MAO inhibitors
Clomipramine (Anafranil)	75–300	24 (20–40)	Antiarrhythmics, MAO inhibitors
Desipramine (Norpramin, Pertofrane)	75–300	18 (12–50)	Antiarrhythmics, MAO inhibitors
Doxepin (Adapin, Sinequan)	75–300	17 (10–47)	Antiarrhythmics, MAO inhibitors
Imipramine (Janimine, Tofranil)	75–300	22 (12–34)	Antiarrhythmics, MAO inhibitors
Nortriptyline (Aventyl, Pamelor)	40–200	26 (18–88)	Antiarrhythmics, MAO inhibitors
Protriptyline (Vivactil)	20–60	76 (54–124)	Antiarrhythmics, MAO inhibitors
Trimipramine (Surmontil)	75–300	12 (8–30)	Antiarrhythmics, MAO inhibitors
Heterocyclics			
Amoxapine (Asendin)	100–600	10 (8–14)	MAO inhibitors
Maprotiline (Ludiomil)	100–225	43 (27–58)	MAO inhibitors
Selective serotonin reuptake inhibitors			
Citalopram (Celexa)	20–40	4–6	MAO inhibitors
Escitalopram (Lexapro)	20–40	5	MAO inhibitors
Fluvoxamine	100–200	2–8	MAO inhibitors
Fluoxetine (Prozac) (now available in a once-a-week preparation)	10–40	168 (72–360)[b]	MAO inhibitors
Paroxetine (Paxil)	20–50	24 (3–65)	MAO inhibitors[c]
Sertraline (Zoloft)	50–150	24 (10–30)	MAO inhibitors
Monoamine oxidase inhibitors (MAO inhibitors) [d]			
Isocarboxazid (Marplan)	30–50	Unknown	For all three MAO inhibitors: vasoconstrictors,[e] decongestants,[e] meperidine, and possibly other narcotics
Phenelzine (Nardil)	45–90	2 (1.5–4.0)	
Tranylcypromine (Parnate)	20–60	2 (1.5–3.0)	
5-HT2 Antagonists			
Trazodone (Desyrel)	150–600	8 (4–14)	
Nefazodone (Serzone)	300–500	3	
Others			
Bupropion (Wellbutrin, Wellbutrin SR, Wellbutrin XL)	225–450	14 (8–24)	MAO inhibitors (possibly)
Mirtazapine (Remeron)	15–45	20–40	
Venlafaxine (Effexor, Effexor-XR)	75–375	5	
Duloxetine (Cymbalta)	20–60 bid	8–17	

MAO, monoamine oxidase; bid, two times a day.
[a]Half-lives are affected by age, gender, race, concurrent medications, and length of drug exposure.
[b]Includes both *fluoxetine* and *norfluoxetine*.
[c]By extrapolation from *fluoxetine* data.
[d]MAO inhibition lasts longer (7 days) than drug half-life.
[e]Including *pseudoephedrine, phenylephrine, phenylpropanolamine, epinephrine, norepinephrine,* and others.
Modified From **Depression Guideline Panel.** *Depression in primary care: detection, diagnosis, and treatment.* Quick reference guide for clinicians, no. 5. Rockville, MD: U.S. Department of Health and Human Services, Public Health Service, Agency for Health Care Policy and Research; 1993:15; AHCPR pub. no. 93-0552, with permission.

Table 12.4 Side-Effect Profiles of Antidepressant Medications

		Central Nervous System		Cardiovascular			
	Anticholinergic[b]	Drowsiness	Insomnia Agitation	Orthostatic Hypotension	Cardiac Arrhythmia	Gastrointestinal Distress	Weight Gain (more than 6 kg)
Amitriptyline	4+	4+	0	4+	3+	0	4+
Citalopram	0.5	0.5	0.5	0	0	1.5	0
Desipramine	1+	1+	1+	2+	2+	0	1+
Doxepin	3+	4+	0	2+	2+	0	3+
Imipramine	3+	3+	1+	4+	3+	1+	3+
Mirtazapine	0.5–1	4	0.5	0.5	0	0	4
Nortriptyline	1+	1+	0	2+	2+	0	1+
Protriptyline	2+	1+	1+	2+	2+	0	0
Trimipramine	1+	4+	0	2+	2+	0	3+
Venlafaxine	0.5	0.5	2	0	0.5	3	0
Amoxapine	2+	2+	2+	2+	3+	0	1+
Maprotiline	2+	4+	0	0	1+	0	2+
Nefazodone	0.5	0.5	0	2	0.5	2	0.5
Trazodone	0	4+	0	1+	1+	1+	1+
Bupropion	0	0	2+	0	1+	1+	0
Fluoxetine	0	0	2+	0	0	3+	0
Paroxetine	0	0	2+	0	0	3+	0
Sertraline	0	0	2+	0	0	3+	0
Monoamine oxidase inhibitors	1	1+	2+	2+	0	1+	2+

[a]Numerals indicate the likelihood of side effect occurring ranging from 0 (for absent or rare) to 4+ (for relatively common).
[b]Dry mouth, blurred vision, urinary hesitancy, constipation.
From **Depression Guideline Panel.** Depression in primary care: detection, diagnosis, and treatment. Quick reference guide for clinicians, no. 5. Rockville, MD: U.S. Department of Health and Human Services, Public Health Service, Agency for Health Care Policy and Research; 1993:14;AHCPR pub. no. 93-0553, with permission.

until the patient has responded sufficiently that she has returned to her previous level of mood and function. If the patient does not recover completely, she should be referred to a psychiatrist (118).

Tricyclic Antidepressants

Tricyclic antidepressants are the oldest antidepressants still in use and are available in generic preparations (118–122). They all have significant anticholinergic side effects that may be problematic in medically ill and elderly patients. They are associated with some slowing of intracardiac conduction; this side effect can be tolerated and managed in all but a few patients, and it can be therapeutic for those with hyperconductibility. **Tricyclic antidepressants should be taken in divided doses through the day, although bedtime dosing may help patients who have difficulty sleeping.** Some tricyclic agents, such as *nortriptyline,* have "therapeutic windows"—blood levels above or below which they are not effective—that must be monitored. **The average dose for tricyclic agents is 225 mg per day in divided doses (122). The most important drawback of tricyclic medications is their lethality in overdose, which is especially important because they are used with depressed patients who are already at risk for suicide. In the rare event** that they must be used by a potentially suicidal patient, the patient must be given only a few pills at a time (121). Some medication plans, private or public, require that treatment begin with the least expensive generic medication, and that the patient first fail with that medication before a newer compound will be provided. The clinician may have to serve as advocate for the patient when this is not a clinically acceptable approach.

Monoamine Oxidase Inhibitors

Monoamine oxidase (MAO) inhibitors are especially effective for atypical depression, which is associated with abnormally increased, rather than decreased, sleep and appetite. They require dietary restrictions and can be used only in patients who are able to understand and comply with those restrictions to avoid hypertensive crises (117).

Selective Serotonin Reuptake Inhibitors

SSRIs pose few risks of medical complications. Side effects include anxiety, tremor, headache, and gastrointestinal upset (either diarrhea or constipation), and usually abate within a few days of the onset of treatment. **A more serious side effect is loss of libido and interference with orgasm** (119). Patients may be reluctant to report sexual side effects, but they may discontinue treatment because of them. Some women are willing to accept the sexual side effects of SSRIs as an acceptable price to pay for recovery, especially considering that depression already interferes with their sexual functioning. Female patients are frequently concerned about weight gain. In one study, it appeared that a weight gain of 5 to 7 pounds might be attributed to an SSRI; the return of normal appetite may lead to weight gain. Concerned patients should be advised to watch their diets carefully while taking the medication. There is some evidence that *bupropion* causes less weight gain than SSRIs. **SSRIs appear to interfere with the efficacy of *tamoxifen*, resulting in excess mortality from breast cancer** (120).

SSRIs are administered in a once-a-day regimen, with little need for dosage adjustments in most cases. SSRIs have long half-lives, so occasional late or missed doses do not constitute a problem. Withdrawal, especially sudden withdrawal, from SSRIs causes flulike symptoms and sleep problems in a small proportion of patients (121). Patients should be cautioned not to discontinue their medications without consulting the physician, and only then by gradually decreasing the dose. As with most medications, antidepressants were not initially tested in older women, but several are under consideration by the U.S. Food and Drug Administration (FDA) for use in this age group (122). The FDA mandated so-called black box warnings on SSRIs when used in adolescents and young adults. This decision is highly controversial. The studies upon which the decision was based included no subject who had committed suicide. Suicidal thoughts, which are extremely common, were conflated with serious attempts, all lumped together as *suicidality*. SSRI prescriptions decreased after the warning was imposed, and there is some evidence that suicides have gone up as a result (123–125).

Atypical Agents

Medications considered atypical include *venlafaxine, lithium* salts, and anticonvulsants, which are effective mood stabilizers used for bipolar disorders (126–130). *Bupropion* is available in a once-a-day preparation. It lowers the seizure threshold slightly more than other antidepressants and should be avoided or used with caution in patients who have a history of head trauma. It is used, under a separate trade name, for smoking cessation, and is particularly useful for smokers who are depressed. *Bupropion* seems to cause fewer sexual side effects than the SSRIs and may decrease these side effects when added to an SSRI regimen.

Suicide

The most acute issue in the assessment and referral of depressed patients is the possibility of suicide (131). Following are the risk factors for suicide:

- **Depression**

- **Recent losses**

- **Previous suicide attempts, even if seemingly not serious**

- **Impulsivity**

- **Concurrent alcohol or substance abuse**

- **Current or past physical or sexual abuse**

- **Family history of suicide**

- **A plan to commit suicide**

- **Access to the means to carry out the plan**

Women attempt suicide more frequently than men, but men complete the act more frequently than women (131,132). This is probably because men use more drastic or irreversible means, such as firearms, whereas women tend to overdose, which can be treated if discovered. It might seem that someone who repeatedly makes suicidal gestures is more interested in the responses of others than in ending her life. However, **past attempts or gestures increase the risk of completed suicide. Patients who made a suicide attempt should be queried about the following risk factors: the intent to die (rather than escape, sleep, or make people understand her distress); increasing numbers or doses of drugs taken in a progression of attempts; and drug or alcohol misuse, especially if it, too, is increasing. Inquiry about suicidal ideation and behavior is an inherent part of every mental status examination and is mandatory for every patient with past or current depression or evidence of self-destructive behavior.** The inquiry can follow from discussion of difficulties in the patient's life or mood or be introduced with a comment that almost everyone has thoughts of death at one time or another. Nonsuicidal patients will immediately volunteer that they have had such thoughts and that they have no intention of acting on them. They will often add reasons: they have too much to look forward to, it is against their religion, or it would hurt their family.

It is important to distinguish among thoughts of death, the wish to be dead, and the intention to kill oneself (132). A patient in a painful life situation—a chronic, painful, or terminal medical condition, the birth of a severely damaged child, or a grievous loss—may express a wish to die, and even refuse recommended medical care but emphatically and honestly disavow any intention of actively harming herself. The patient must be directly asked (132).

If the patient previously engaged in impulsive self-destructive behavior, without a plan or warning, it is wise to consult a psychiatrist. If a patient is actively contemplating suicide, she must see a psychiatrist immediately (132,133). Other mental health professionals may be helpful but are less likely to have dealt extensively with and assumed responsibility for suicidal patients, to be able to determine whether the patient should be hospitalized, and to have admitting privileges. Until she is in the physical presence of a psychiatrist, or in a safe environment such as a hospital emergency room, a suicidal patient should be observed and protected at all times—every second—whether she is in the consulting room or the bathroom. The staff member assigned to remain with her may not leave to make a telephone call, go to the bathroom, or get a cup of coffee. Family members may offer to monitor the patient and can sometimes be effective, but the health care professional is responsible for ensuring that they understand and implement this level of supervision. **It is better to risk inconvenience and possible embarrassment to both the gynecologist and the patient than to risk a fatal outcome. When suicide is an immediate consideration, only a psychiatrist can make the decision that a patient is safe** (133). Psychiatric referral can be useful in less dramatic cases: when the gynecologist lacks experience or is overloaded with patients, when a first trial of treatment is unsuccessful or there is uncertainty about the diagnosis, when domestic violence or substance abuse may be present, and when the depression is recurrent.

Many people are not aware that approximately half of suicides are not associated with depression. Suicide can occur in the context of an anxiety disorder, personality disorder, psychotic illnesses, or as an impulsive response to an adverse life event (133). Suicide is not an inevitable consequence of any of these conditions, including depression. Most people rescued from potentially lethal suicide attempts do not ultimately commit suicide. That is why barriers on bridges and other devices to prevent impulsive suicides are necessary.

Alcohol and Substance Abuse

Alcohol and substance abuse are major causes of morbidity and mortality (134). **The essential feature of substance dependence, or addiction, is the continued use of the substance despite serious resulting problems. Alcohol and substance abuse are among the most common—and most frequently overlooked—conditions in medical practice.**

In the DSM-IV-TR, the term "substance" can mean a medication, a toxin, or a drug of abuse. **Nicotine is included among "substances," and women appear to be more susceptible to** nicotine addiction than men, but smoking cessation is more a topic for general medicine than for psychiatry (9,135).

Substance abuse leads to major complications, including intoxication and withdrawal. Withdrawal is major problem because, as mentioned in this chapter in the section on benzodiazepines, patients often fail to inform clinicians of their alcohol and substance use before being hospitalized or undergoing procedures, when they may experience unanticipated undiagnosed withdrawal (136–138).

Significant problems caused by continued use of the substance may include symptoms of withdrawal, interference with family and work obligations, and the depletion of, or criminal activity to obtain, resources to obtain the substance. **Other features include tolerance, or the need to consume more of the substance to obtain the same effect, and compulsive use** (139).

Patients frequently use alcohol along with other substances of abuse. The abuse of prescription medication, especially in younger populations, has increased (140). Patients should be advised to take care that their medications are not accessible to others.

Alcohol is the most frequent substance of abuse. Legal and accepted by society, it nevertheless causes a high proportion of morbidity, mortality, and life complications. **Women's alcohol abuse is more likely to take place in private than is men's; society frowns more on women who are drunk or create disturbances in public than on men who do the same. Women are more likely than men to use a substance because an intimate partner uses or abuses that substance, and to trade sexual favors for access to the substance (141). There is strong evidence for a genetic link for alcoholism, but not for the other substances of abuse.**

The most successful treatment for substance abuse disorders is a so-called 12-step program such as Alcoholics Anonymous. **Most of the programs for the treatment of substance abuse were developed for men. Women are less responsive to the usual confrontational approach** (142,143). Many women with substance abuse issues have children. Such women, and women who are pregnant, are often reluctant to enter treatment for fear of prosecution or losing custody. **Treatment programs for women with primary responsibility for children must include arrangements for child care.** Recidivism after treatment is very common, but that does not mean that treatment is useless. **On average, patients require three episodes of treatment before achieving sobriety** (139). **The essential obligation of the primary physician is to ask each patient about substance consumption and any problems arising from it** (141). *Buprenorphine* is a useful adjunct medication; physicians are required to undergo specific training in order to prescribe *buprenorphine* (144).

Anxiety Disorders

Anxiety is a sense of dread without objective cause for fear, accompanied by the usual physical concomitants of fear. Although every human being has anxious feelings from time to time, anxiety disorders are diagnosed when anxiety becomes disabling or so painful as to interfere with an individual's quality of life. **Anxiety disorders place patients at risk for suicide (145).**

Diagnosis

The anxiety disorders include generalized anxiety disorder, panic disorder, agoraphobia, specific phobias, obsessive-compulsive disorder, and posttraumatic stress disorder (146–148).

Generalized Anxiety Disorder

Generalized anxiety disorder is a condition in which anxiety pervades every aspect of a patient's life. She suffers from restlessness, easy fatigability, difficulty concentrating, irritability, muscle tension, and sleep disturbances. **Whereas depressed patients fall asleep more or less normally and then awaken earlier than intended, anxious patients tend to have difficulty falling asleep** (146,147).

Panic Disorder

Panic disorder is characterized by panic attacks: acute periods, generally lasting about 15 minutes, with intense fear and at least four of the following symptoms (146–152):

- **Diaphoresis**
- **Trembling**

- Shortness of breath

- A choking sensation

- Chest discomfort

- Gastrointestinal distress

- Lightheadedness

- A sense of unreality

- Fear of going crazy or dying

- Paresthesias

- Chills or hot flashes

The attacks can recur with or without specific precipitating events (148). The patient is preoccupied with them and makes behavioral changes she hopes will avert future attacks: avoiding specific situations, assuring herself there is an escape route from certain situations, or refusing to be alone.

The symptoms of panic attacks are often confused with the symptoms of cardiac or pulmonary disease. They lead to many fruitless trips to the emergency department and to costly, even invasive, medical investigations. A careful history can establish the correct diagnosis in most cases (153–155).

Agoraphobia	**Agoraphobia is the avoidance of situations in which the patient fears she may be trapped, such as the center of a row in the theater or driving over a bridge.** She fears that such a situation will trigger anxiety or a panic attack and therefore tends more and more to stay at home or limit her sphere of activity to an increasingly short list of venues. Agoraphobia and panic disorder can occur separately or together (150–154).
Specific Phobias	**Specific phobias are irrational fears of certain objects or situations, although the patient recognizes that the object or situation poses no real danger.** Of particular concern in gynecology are fear of needles and fear of vomiting (150).
	Social phobia causes the patient to fear and avoid situations in which the patient anticipates, without rational cause, that she will be perceived in a humiliating light. Such situations include giving a business-related presentation, making an announcement at a meeting, and having a casual dinner with friends. Patients may alter their lives to avoid these anxieties, interfering with their interpersonal relationships and their ability to carry out their responsibilities, or they may manage to carry on despite considerable psychological pain (150).
Obsessive-Compulsive Disorder	**Obsessive-compulsive disorder (OCD) is characterized by obsessions: recurrent impulses, images, or thoughts that the patient recognizes as her own, but dislikes and cannot control; or compulsions: intrusive, repetitive behaviors that the patient feels she must perform to prevent some dire consequence** (155–157). The disorder can be mild or totally crippling; in half of the cases, it becomes chronic. This disorder is classified as an anxiety disorder because the obsessions are anxiety provoking, and the compulsions are performed to avoid overwhelming anxiety. The term OCD has made its way into popular parlance to describe people who focus on petty details and have trouble making up their minds. This is an incorrect use of the term.
Posttraumatic Stress Disorder	**Posttraumatic stress disorder (PTSD) is the result of exposure to an event that threatens the life or bodily integrity of the patient or others.** At the time of the trauma, the patient experiences horror, terror, or a sense of helplessness. Afterward, the patient may lose conscious memory of all or part of the event, avoid situations reminiscent of it, and become acutely distressed when she cannot avoid them. She feels numb and detached, without a sense of the future. She is hyperarousable and irritable and has difficulty sleeping and concentrating. She re-experiences the event in nightmares, flashbacks, and intrusive thoughts (149).
Epidemiology	**Panic disorder without agoraphobia is twice as common in women as it is in men; panic disorder with agoraphobia is three times more common in women** (149). Onset is

generally in young adulthood, often following a stressful event. The lifetime prevalence is 1.5% to 3.5%; the 1-year prevalence is 1% to 2%. A substantial percentage of patients experience depressive episodes as well. Phobias are somewhat more common in women, depending on the object of the phobia. The 1-year prevalence is 9%, and the lifetime prevalence is 10% to 11%. Obsessive-compulsive disorder is equally common in women and men, with evidence of familial transmission. Prevalence is 2.5% for lifetime and 1.5% to 2.1% for 1 year. Posttraumatic stress disorder has a lifetime prevalence of 1% to 14%; victims of violence (including child abuse and wife battering) and war are at increased risk. Men and women differ in the types of violence to which they tend to be exposed. Rape, for example, poses a similarly high risk of PTSD in both men and women, but women are more often the victims of rape (149).

Assessment

Given the relationship between anxiety disorders and traumatic experiences, the presence of signs and symptoms of anxiety disorders should trigger inquiries about abuse (146,147). Before making attempts to treat these disorders, it is important to know how long the patient has suffered from the disorder, what previous attempts were made to diagnose and treat it, and the effect it had on her psychological development, life choices, lifestyle, and relationships. In some cases, the entire family will have organized their schedules and activities around the patient's symptoms and limitations; they may not volunteer this information.

Management

Treatment should not be limited to antianxiety medications. Managing, even tolerating, patient anxiety is an anxiety-provoking process; anxiety is contagious and raises the specter of unlimited demands on the gynecologist's time and energy. Prescribing medication is a familiar and comfortable, if not optimal, way to end a medical interview. Overprescribing benzodiazepines is a cause for medical and media concern. It is useful to defer the administration of anxiolytic medications until the impact of the physician's support and interest can be assessed (150). Treatment should address the effects on the patient's life and family and the signs and symptoms of the specific disease (151).

Benzodiazepines are most useful in acute situations (150). Use can quickly become chronic, with escalating dosages, diminishing therapeutic effects, and increasing demands on the physician. Women taking benzodiazepines may forget to include them in their medical history. When admitted to the hospital, they may suffer unrecognized withdrawal symptoms, complicating their treatment, or may continue to take medications from a personal supply without informing the medical staff (150).

There are many patients who could benefit from anxiolytics but who are inordinately worried about becoming dependent or addicted. A patient with no history of addictive behaviors is unlikely to get into trouble with a standard dose of medication (156,157). **It is important to ascertain the source of anxiety or obsessive behavior.** Many patients and their families are anxious because of misinformation or misunderstanding about a medical problem or treatment. Few patients can absorb all the information about significant gynecologic conditions at a single visit, but many feel that asking questions will burden the physician or make the patient appear stupid. Patients suffer anxiety when there is disagreement among family members or medical staff about the diagnosis or recommended treatment. Many patients dread certain aspects of care, sometimes on the basis of past experience or outdated information (157). A simple explanation or alteration in procedure can alleviate the anxiety. For example, a reassuring family member or friend can be allowed to stay with the patient during a diagnostic test, sedation can be administered orally or by inhalation before an intravenous line is inserted, or the patient can be allowed control over her own analgesia.

Behavioral interventions are extremely useful in managing anxiety disorders without problematic side effects. They include hypnosis, desensitization, and relaxation techniques (152–163). These techniques provide a patient with tools to cope with her own anxiety. Specialists in behavioral medicine, usually psychologists, are expert in these techniques. A local medical school department of psychiatry or behavioral medicine is a good source for referrals. Interested gynecologists can master some of the techniques.

It is easy to be trapped into a cat-and-mouse game with an anxious and needy patient who has an anxiety or personality disorder (153). **Faced with an obsessive or anxious, talkative, and needy patient in the midst of bedside rounds, clinic, or office hours, the clinician can develop a pattern of avoidance, sometimes alternating with overindulgence**

stemming from feelings of guilt. **This kind of behavior results in sporadic, unpredictable reinforcement of the patient's symptoms and demands for attention and is very likely to increase them.** Attempting to escape by appearing distracted or harassed or yielding with despair to the destruction of the day's schedule and the care of other patients simply heightens the patient's anxiety (154–160).

It is preferable to develop a prospective approach (153,162,163). **Gynecologists tend to underrate the power of their personal interactions with patients and their own ability to structure and limit those interactions appropriately. A patient with a long list of symptoms can be informed at the beginning of the visit how much time is available and asked to focus on her most important problem, with other problems to be discussed at future, scheduled appointments** (162). Instead of scheduling appointments and returning telephone calls grudgingly in response to patient demands, the gynecologist should inform the patient that her condition requires brief regular scheduled visits. If she is contacting the office more often than visits can reasonably be scheduled, she should be asked to call between visits, at prearranged times, to advise the staff of her progress. There are useful self-help groups for patients with various psychiatric conditions and their families. Although groups focused only on victimization can validate patients' experiences and pain and help them build new lives, they may interfere with their motivation to find other ways to identify themselves and obtain gratification (159). The gynecologist can monitor the patient's responses to the self-help group interaction.

Medication does have a place in the management of anxiety disorders (164–166). Table 12.5 describes many of these agents. SSRIs are effective for a variety of anxiety disorders, sometimes

Table 12.5 Compounds Used for Anxiety

Medication	Trade Name	Rate of Absorption[a]	Half-Life[b]	Active Long-Acting Metabolite	Comments
Benzodiazepines					Metabolism of benzodiazepines is inhibited by *cimetidine, disulfiram, isoniazid,* and oral contraceptives. Metabolism of benzodiazepines is enhanced by *rifampin.*
Alprazolam	*Xanax*	Intermediate	Intermediate	No	Preferred in elderly patients or patients with poor hepatic functions.
Chlordiazepoxide	*Librium, others*	Intermediate	Intermediate	Yes	
Clonazepam	*Klonopin*	Long	Long	No	
Clorazepate	*Tranxene, others*	Short	Short	Yes	
Diazepam	*Valium, others*	Short	Long	Yes	Half-life increased three or four times in elderly patients.
Lorazepam	*Ativan, others*	Intermediate	Intermediate	No	Preferred in elderly patients or patients with poor hepatic function.
Oxazepam	*Serax*	Long	Intermediate	No	Preferred in elderly patients or patients with poor hepatic function.
Prazepam	*Centrax*	Long	Short	Yes	
Atypical agent					
Buspirone	*BuSpar*				Not effective in panic disorder, little sedation, little risk of dependence or tolerance.

[a]Long ≥2 hours; Intermediate = 1–2 hours; Short ≤1 hour.
[b]Long >20 hours; Intermediate = 6–20 hours; Short <6 hours.
From **Gilman AG, Rall TW, Nies AS, et al.** *The pharmacological basis of therapeutics.* 8th ed. New York: McGraw-Hill, 1990; **Stotland NL.** Psychiatric and psychosocial issues in primary care for women. In: **Seltzer VL, Pearse WH, eds.** *Women's primary health care: office practice and procedures.* New York: McGraw-Hill, 1995.

in different dosage regimens than those used for depression. Benzodiazepines are effective when taken for acute anxiety or during relatively brief, time-limited (several days) stressful situations. The specific agent should be chosen on the basis of onset of action and half-life. The patient must be admonished to avoid concomitant use of alcohol and to exercise extreme care about driving or engaging in other activities requiring attention, concentration, and coordination.

Patients who fail to respond to a trial of office counseling or medication, who are unable to fulfill their responsibilities, who exhaust the patience and resources of significant others, who pose a diagnostic dilemma, who consume inordinate quantities of medical resources, or whose symptoms are becoming increasingly worse should be evaluated by a psychiatrist (166).

Somatizing Disorders

Diagnosis

Somatizing disorders are those in which psychological conflicts are expressed in the form of physical symptoms. There is a spectrum of somatizing disorders based on the degree to which the patient is aware of or responsible for the onset of the symptoms. The spectrum ranges from the deliberate malingerer to the so-called hysteric, who is completely unaware of the link between her psyche and her physical symptom (167).

Malingering

Malingering is the deliberate mimicking of signs and symptoms of physical or mental illness to achieve a tangible personal gain, such as exemption from dangerous military duties or exoneration from criminal responsibility. Factitious disorder, or *Munchausen syndrome*, is a poorly understood condition in which the patient actively causes physical damage to herself or feigns somatic symptoms that result in repeated hospital admissions and painful, dangerous, invasive diagnostic and therapeutic procedures (167). These patients may introduce feces or purulent material into wounds or intravenous lines, inject themselves with insulin, or produce hemorrhages. Given enough diagnostic and therapeutic interventions, significant iatrogenic conditions, such as adhesions from surgery or Cushing syndrome from the administration of steroids, may develop in these patients (167).

These patients are initially engaging but eventually frustrate the medical staff. Declaring that the patient "only wants attention" is not helpful (167). Most people want attention, but very few are willing to go to these lengths to get it. Confirming the diagnosis is a delicate process. When staff members become suspicious, they will be tempted to validate their suspicions by spying on the patient or sending her out of her hospital room on a pretext and then searching her belongings. The latter is illegal, and either action, followed by a confrontation, will end the therapeutic relationship and provoke the patient to flee rather than addressing the problem. Calls for a psychiatric consultation may provoke resentment in the patient and family. Patients soon reappear in another medical facility. As a result, there are few data about the etiology, incidence, and management of this condition. Often these patients are medically sophisticated because they or their family members had some kind of medical training or they gained knowledge during previous hospitalizations. Mothers may enact this disorder through their children by deliberately making them ill, a condition called **Munchausen's by proxy** (167). Munchhausen's by proxy gained some popular notoriety, and it resulted in accusations and loss of custody for some mothers whose children had serious, chronic diseases requiring multiple medical interventions. Shared electronic records might affect the occurrence of these conditions.

Somatization Disorder

Somatization disorder consists of multiple physical symptoms for which adequate medical bases cannot be established, with these symptoms leading either to numerous medical visits or to impairment in the patient's function (168). Symptoms begin before age 30 and continue for many years thereafter. The diagnosis requires symptoms of pain related to at least four different anatomic sites or physiologic functions: two gastrointestinal symptoms, one sexual or reproductive symptom, and one pseudoneurologic symptom or deficit other than pain (seizures, paresis). The patient's perception is that she is "sickly" (168). She responds accurately to questions about her past symptoms and treatments but may not volunteer information about them unless she is asked.

Conversion Disorder

Conversion disorder is the condition formerly called hysteria. The patient's loss of a voluntary motor or sensory function cannot be explained by medical illness, is not deliberately produced by the patient, and appears to be related to psychological stress or conflict. The prognosis is directly related to the length of time from onset to diagnosis and treatment (169–172).

Other Somatizing Disorders

Pain disorder **is a conversion condition with pain as the only symptom.** *Body dysmorphic disorder* **is preoccupation with a trivial or imagined defect in bodily appearance, a preoccupation that is not alleviated by the many medical and surgical treatments that the patient pursues (167,173).** The gynecologist should hesitate to refer such a patient to a plastic or cosmetic surgeon, although specialists tend to be familiar with the condition and should hesitate to perform procedures on these patients.

Hypochondriasis **is not a matter of a particular number or type of symptoms. It is a patient's (nonpsychotic) conviction or fear that she suffers from a serious disease despite evidence and reassurance to the contrary (167).** When one disease is ruled out, the patient is either convinced that the diagnosis was overlooked or switches her concerns to some other disease.

Epidemiology

Somatization is believed to be among the most common and most difficult psychological conditions in office practice. It is estimated that 60% to 80% of the general population experiences one or more somatic symptoms in a given week, providing an ample substrate for the patient preoccupied with her health (167). **Somatization disorder occurs almost exclusively in women;** menstrual symptoms may be an early sign. Lifetime prevalence in women is 0.2% to 2.0%. **Conversion disorder occurs 2 to 10 times more frequently in women than in men** (there is no difference for gender in children), and it is more common in rural and disadvantaged populations with little medical sophistication (167). Cases have become relatively rare. Conversion disorder may develop into somatization disorder. Reported rates of somatization disorder range from 11 to 300 per 100,000. Pain disorder is extremely common in both genders. Hypochondriasis is equally distributed between men and women; prevalence in general medical practice is estimated to be 4% to 9%. There are few statistics about body dysmorphic disorder, but it seems to be equally distributed between men and women, with an average age of onset of about 30 years (167).

Assessment

Most somatizing disorders are chronic. The goal of treatment in primary care is not to eliminate all the somatic symptoms but to help the patient cope with them and minimize their effect on her relationships and responsibilities (167). Because patients often seek care simultaneously or sequentially from several physicians, it is crucial to ask about all past and current diagnostic procedures, diagnoses, treatments, and responses. Patients' level of function over the years is important; prognosis is inversely related to chronicity. Chronicity should not be an excuse for a failure to treat the patient. The impact on the lives of patients and their families can be mitigated even if the condition is not entirely eliminated. For these and most other patients, the gynecologist needs to know what the patient believes is wrong with her and what she believes she needs in the way of diagnostic and therapeutic interventions. When the patient does not receive what she expects or desires, she is unlikely to comply with the recommended course of action, although she may accept it and pretend to be following it so as to avoid criticism from the physician. This behavior is actually very common among patients in general (167).

Management

The management of somatizing disorders is focused on the avoidance of unnecessary medical interventions, iatrogenic medical or psychological complications, and disability. It is never possible to rule out all potential medical causes of a symptom. The literature is full of case presentations of patients with multiple sclerosis, brain tumors, and intermittently flaring infections that for years were mislabeled as psychosomatic until a correct diagnosis of the condition was made (167,173). Organic pathology can befall patients with somatizing disorders. Patients who have benign gastrointestinal symptoms for extended periods can get appendicitis. Often a difficult differentiation must be made in each specific case and presentation.

Patients who have a somatizing disorder often approach each new clinician as the one who, "*unlike the incompetent and insensitive physicians consulted in the past,*" will finally get to the bottom of her troubles and cure her symptoms. The gynecologist must not get caught up in these expectations, but rather remind the patient that symptoms that have resisted diagnosis and treatment for many years are likely to be challenging ones. As with anxious patients, it is important to structure the doctor–patient relationship to avoid giving the patient attention inconsistently and only in response to escalating symptoms and demands (173). It is best to schedule frequent, brief office visits during which the clinician allots a small amount of time to listen to and sympathize with the patient's somatic symptoms and spends the bulk of the time reinforcing the patient's efforts to function despite her symptoms. Family members should be encouraged to facilitate functionality rather than invalidism.

Unmasking patently psychologically based symptoms by tricking the patient (shouting "Fire!" in the vicinity of a "paralyzed" patient), or documenting the patient's behavior when she does not realize she is being observed, is momentarily gratifying for medical staff but humiliating for the patient. It may force her to relinquish a symptom, at least temporarily, but she will seek care elsewhere, exacerbating her dysfunction, distrust, and demands on the health care system (173).

Patients with conversion, somatization, and hypochondriacal disorders often benefit from prescriptive behavioral regimens aimed at saving face and improving function (174). It was once believed that a patient relieved of one symptom would soon substitute another, but this assumption is not confirmed by empirical evidence. The behavioral regimen should consist of health-promoting activities relevant to the target symptoms, planned in a stepwise progression, and recommended with reasonable medical conviction and authority. For example, the patient with psychogenic difficulty swallowing could be advised to drink only clear liquids, at specified intervals, for a specified number of days, and then go on similarly to full liquids, purees, soft foods, and finally a regular diet. The patient with difficulties in the extremities can undertake an exercise regimen. The patient's preoccupation with her symptoms can be channeled into documentation of her progress in a log that she brings to her medical appointments. The physician is not bound to peruse the entire document at each visit. If it is too long, the patient can be asked to prepare a summary. This process may enlighten both her and the physician to the relationships between her symptoms and her diet, relationships, or activities. She should be advised not to dwell on her symptoms apart from this important notation (174).

It is critical to remember that patients whose somatic symptoms result from depression, posttraumatic stress disorder and other anxiety disorders, and domestic violence frequently seek care from gynecologists. In the case of domestic violence, the gynecologist is often the only human contact the abuser allows the patient outside the domestic situation (175–177). These possibilities must be ruled out before care is directed to symptom management. **Several medical associations have drawn attention to the need to screen women for domestic violence and the infrequency with which this is actually done. It appears that screening alone does not significantly change outcomes. Acknowledging domestic violence and finding and accessing resources are part of an often prolonged and incremental process—of which screening can be an important first step** (178).

There is considerable cross-cultural variation in the extent to which feelings and psychological conflicts are somatized. In many Asian cultures, for example, presenting problems with feelings, behaviors, and interpersonal relationships are almost unheard of; these problems are expressed, diagnosed, and treated somatically. Conversely, some very sophisticated and psychologically informed patients in Western society may dismiss serious somatic signs and symptoms as indications of psychological conflict (177).

Referral

Patients with somatizing disorders may resist mental health referral more adamantly than any other single class of patients (167). Focused as they are on physical symptoms, these patients can regard referral as a message that their symptoms are not being taken seriously and as a sign of contempt and rejection by the gynecologist. It is particularly useful with these patients to emphasize that distinctions between mind and body are artificial. The brain is part of the body. Our language expresses this synthesis; anxiety causes "butterflies in the stomach," aggravation "gives us a headache," and unwelcome news "gives us a heart attack."

The referral should be framed as support for the patient's suffering rather than as a statement that her problems are "all in her head" (168). The mental health professional should be introduced as a member of the medical team. Some medical institutions have dedicated psychiatric consultation, medical psychiatry, or behavioral medicine services offering expertise in the psychological complications of disease and in somatization disorders. Because so-called somatic and psychological symptoms often coexist and interact, the gynecologist should work in collaboration with the mental health professional. Patients should be given a return appointment with the primary physician, or a request for a telephone contact, at the time of the original mental health referral to reassure them that they are not being dismissed and to inform the primary physician of the results of the consultation (168).

Personality Disorders

Personality disorders are pervasive, lifelong, maladaptive patterns of perception and behavior (177–179). Patients with personality disorders believe that whatever unpleasant feelings they have are caused by the behavior of others. They view their own behaviors, which can wreak havoc in the health care setting as well as in patients' lives, as normal, expectable, inevitable reactions to these perceived circumstances. To make matters worse, their behaviors tend to provoke in others the very responses that confirm their expectations; for example, a patient who is convinced that people always abandon her will cling desperately to others, eventually driving them away.

Diagnosis

Personality disorders are organized into clusters in DSM-IV (9). Patients often manifest characteristics of several disorders within a cluster and between clusters.

Cluster A

> **Paranoid personality disorder**
> **Schizoid personality disorder**
> **Schizotypal personality disorder**

Cluster B

> **Narcissistic personality disorder**
> **Histrionic personality disorder**
> **Borderline personality disorder**
> **Antisocial personality disorder**

Cluster C

> **Avoidant personality disorder**
> **Dependent personality disorder**
> **Obsessive-compulsive personality disorder**

Individuals with Cluster A disorders are isolated, suspicious, detached, and odd. Narcissistic patients are grandiose, arrogant, envious, and entitled. Histrionic individuals are flamboyant and provocative. Antisocial patients disregard laws and rules of common decency toward others. Borderline personality disorder causes patients to have difficulty controlling their impulses and maintaining stable moods and relationships (177). They engage in self-destructive behaviors. They fluctuate between overvaluation and castigation of the same person or direct these feelings alternately between one person and another. When this happens on a gynecology service or in the office, it can precipitate significant tensions among the staff. There is one caveat: **research reveals that many women who were abused are diagnosed as borderline when posttraumatic stress disorder more accurately fits their symptoms (175–178). Posttraumatic stress disorder** is a less stigmatizing and more treatable condition than borderline personality disorder.

Epidemiology

Lifetime prevalence of personality disorders as a group is 2.5% (177–179). Cluster A disorders are more common in men. Within Cluster B disorders, 75% of cases are women; the prevalence in the general population is 2%. Personality disorders such as narcissistic personality are more common in the clinical population than in the general population. Among Cluster C disorders, dependent personality is one of the most frequently diagnosed. Obsessive-compulsive personality is twice as common in men as in women. It is important to distinguish the personality disorder from the symptomatic obsessive-compulsive disorder. There is a strong association between personality disorders and a history of childhood abuse. The possibility of an ongoing abusive situation should be considered. There is so much overlap among the clusters that the diagnostic structure may well change in the forthcoming DSM revision (179).

Assessment

The impact of personality disorders ranges widely (177–179). At one end of the spectrum, the disorder is an exaggerated personality style. At the other end of the spectrum, the individual suffers terrible emotional pain and is unable to function in work roles or relationships, spending significant periods of time in psychiatric hospitals. She characterizes her symptoms of despair as inevitable responses to abandonment or other mistreatment. As the definition implies, the patient will not seek treatment for the signs and symptoms listed in the diagnostic criteria but instead will have complaints about her treatment by others, their responses to her, and the unfairness and difficulties of life in general. Taking the history, the clinician should frame questions in those same terms: *How long have these troubles gone on, and how much do they interfere with her ability to work and relate to others?* Personality disorders do not bring patients to gynecologists' offices directly, but they greatly complicate things when patients arrive.

Management

Intense and lengthy psychotherapy is required to effect significant improvement in patients who have personality disorders (177). There is increasing evidence that expert, targeted therapeutic interventions can be successful and that the long-term prognosis is more hopeful than previously believed. The challenge in the gynecology setting is to minimize contention and drain on medical staff while maximizing the likelihood of effective diagnosis and treatment of the patient's medical problems. **The most helpful single step is the identification of the personality disorder.** Diagnosis enables the gynecologist to recognize the reasons for a patient's problem behaviors, to avoid becoming entangled in fruitless interactions with the patient, and to set appropriate limits.

There is increasing evidence that psychotropic medications are useful adjuncts in the treatment of personality disorders (179). Treatment should be provided in consultation with a psychiatrist. The patient's ability to use the medication can be compromised by impulsivity, self-destructive tendencies, and unstable relationships. Low doses of major tranquilizers are sometimes helpful, especially when the patient has brief psychotic episodes. Minor tranquilizers or anxiolytics pose significant risk of overdose and physical and psychological habituation (179). They can be prescribed for temporary stresses, but only in a quantity sufficient for several days and with no refill allowed. Some patients' anxiety, demands, and power struggles are eased when they are given control over their own use of medication. Such an approach requires enough familiarity with the patient to ensure her safety and should be managed by an expert. Because the patient with a personality disorder attributes her problems to others, her symptoms cannot be adduced as reasons for psychiatric referral, but her suffering can be. If a diagnosis of a personality disorder absolutely must be noted in the patient's chart or on insurance forms, it is essential that she be so informed. It is useful to review the DSM-IV-TR criteria with her so that she understands the basis for the diagnosis (9). **All psychiatric diagnoses, but particularly personality disorders, carry a significant stigma.**

Adjustment Disorders

Diagnosis

Adjustment disorders are temporary, self-limited responses to life stressors that are part of the normative range of human experience (unlike those that precipitate posttraumatic stress disorder) (180). The patient has mood or anxiety symptoms that are sufficient to lead her to seek medical care but that do not meet criteria of sufficient quantity or quality to qualify for psychiatric diagnosis. The diagnosis requires an identifiable stressor, onset within 3 months after the stress begins, and spontaneous resolution within 6 months after the stressor ends. Obviously the latter cannot be determined until the symptoms resolve—but they do rule out the disorder if the symptoms persist beyond that time (180,181).

Adjustment disorders can be distinguished from normal grieving (180,181). Grieving produces symptoms similar to those of depression, although depression is more likely to cause guilt. Interference with function should not persist beyond several months, but some degree of sadness and preoccupation with the lost loved one often goes on for years. Patients with persistently disabling grief should be referred to a mental health professional.

Epidemiology

Adjustment disorders affect men and women equally. An estimated 5% to 20% of patients undergoing outpatient mental health treatment suffer from adjustment disorders. There is little literature on the subject; one study reported a prevalence of 2.3% among a sample of patients receiving care in a walk-in general health clinic (180).

Management

Patients with adjustment disorders can be treated effectively with brief counseling in the primary care setting (180). The counseling can be provided by the gynecologist or by a nurse clinician, social worker, or psychologist, preferably a member of the office or hospital staff who is familiar with the gynecologist and the practice. The medical setting is sometimes the only place where the patient can vent her feelings and think through her situation. Counseling is aimed at facilitating the patient's own coping skills and helping her to make thoughtful decisions about her situation. The gynecologist should follow the patient's progress and facilitate referral to a psychiatrist if symptoms do not resolve.

Eating Disorders

The etiology of eating disorders is neurobiological as well as psychosocial (182). **Preoccupation with thinness, sometimes to the point of pathology, is a major problem for women in North America** (183). Only a small number of women profess to be satisfied with their weights and body shapes. Nearly all admit to current or recent attempts to limit food intake. Physicians often share social prejudices against overweight patients and can easily exacerbate patients' concerns by making chance comments. In some cases, such comments by the physician or others can precipitate, if not cause, an eating disorder.

Diagnosis

Anorexia nervosa **is characterized by severe restrictions on food intake, often accompanied by excessive physical exercise and the use of diuretics or laxatives.** Clinical features include menstrual irregularities or amenorrhea, intense and irrational fear of becoming fat, preoccupation with body weight as an indicator of self-worth, and inability to acknowledge the realities and dangers of the condition. Some patients approach gynecologists for treatment of infertility (184).

Bulimia **is characterized by eating binges followed by self-induced vomiting or purging.** Patients' weights may be normal or somewhat higher than normal. Patients have drastically low self-esteem, and the condition frequently coexists with depression (185).

Obesity **is an increasingly frequent health problem, and there is little evidence that any nonsurgical approach is effective over time.** Sensible eating should be encouraged, and fad or crash diets, which are rampant, are medically and psychologically counterproductive (186). Given the stigma against being overweight in our society, patients may avoid the doctor's office just because they will be weighed there. **The best approach with overweight patients is to acknowledge that being overweight is detrimental to health but that changing one's diet and lifestyle, and losing weight, is very difficult. Primary care physicians should indicate that they are not going to judge the patient, but are available to provide support and information at the patient's request.**

Epidemiology

More than 90% of cases of anorexia and bulimia occur in female patients. The prevalence is 0.5% to 1.0% in late adolescence and 1% to 3% in early adulthood. There is some evidence of familial transmission (182–185).

Assessment

The clinician treating the anorexic patient needs to know how much insight she has into her problem and to assess her mood, relationships, and general level of function. Anorexia poses significant risks of severe metabolic complications and death, often from cardiac consequences of electrolyte abnormalities. Thorough physical and laboratory examination is critical; immediate hospitalization may be necessary (182–185).

Management

Patients with anorexia or bulimia should be treated by mental health professionals, preferably those with subspecialization in this area. The conditions are highly refractory to treatment; patients can resort to elaborate subterfuges to conceal their failure to eat and gain weight (185–187). There are Web sites dedicated to anorexia, with information about the minimum calories necessary to sustain life, and photographs of individuals who seem pleased with their skeletal appearance. Up to 50% of cases will become chronic, and approximately 10% of those will ultimately die of the disease. Antidepressant medication is sometimes helpful. Amenorrheic patients should not be treated with ovulation induction. Evaluation for osteopenia and osteoporosis is necessary (187).

Psychotic Disorders

Schizophrenia affects approximately 1% of persons worldwide (188). Since the deinstitutionalization of persons with severe and persistent mental illnesses several decades ago, most affected individuals live in the community. Often health care and other services are inadequate, leaving these women vulnerable to sexual abuse and involuntary impregnation. Overall, the fertility of women with schizophrenia approximates that of matched populations. Schizophrenia is not an absolute contraindication to successful parenting, but there is considerable stigma against psychotic disorders, and patients may avoid prenatal care because they fear loss of custody (189,190).

Diagnosis

Psychotic disorders are characterized by major distortions of thinking and behavior. They include schizophrenia, schizophreniform disorders, schizoaffective disorders, delusional disorders, and brief psychotic disorders. General medical and toxic conditions must be ruled out in determining the diagnosis. Distinctions between the disorders are based on symptoms, time course, severity, and associated affective symptoms. **The hallmark of psychosis is the presence of delusions or hallucinations. Hallucinations are sensory perceptions in the absence of external sensory stimuli. Delusions are bizarre beliefs about the nature of motivation of external events** (188). Because there is no reliable definition of "bizarre," a physician working with a patient from an unfamiliar culture must determine whether a given belief is normal in that culture. Delusions and hallucinations are the positive symptoms of schizophrenia. The negative symptoms include apathy and loss of connection to others and to interests. The negative symptoms may be more disabling than the positive. There is increasing evidence that schizophrenia is associated with cognitive deficits (191).

Epidemiology

Onset of schizophrenia is in the late teens to mid-30s. Women succumb later in life and have more prominent mood symptoms and a better prognosis than men (191,192). The risk is 10 times greater for first-degree biologic relatives and for individuals of low socioeconomic status (192). It is unclear whether indigent status is a precipitating stress or a result of psychotic illness, but, especially as extremely few individuals have private or public coverage for adequate treatment, most people with schizophrenia are indigent.

Assessment

There is wide variability in the functional impact of psychotic disorders. Patients must not be assumed to be incompetent to make medical decisions or lead independent lives, especially if they comply with treatment. Patients must be asked specifically about their living situations and coping skills. When psychotic women have responsibility for the care of children, their ability to do so should be assessed in consultation with a mental health expert. Motherhood and child custody are exceedingly sensitive matters for these vulnerable patients (191).

A relentlessly downhill course is not inevitable; remissions and recovery can occur (192). Therefore, the patient's mental status must be examined carefully. Under the pressures of a busy medical setting, psychotic illnesses can be overlooked, only to erupt in the labor room, operating room, or recovery room. Patients who believe that conspiracies or aliens are responsible for their symptoms can answer yes-or-no medical questions without revealing their delusions. Open-ended questions (*"Tell me about your symptoms"*) are more useful (191).

Sensationalized media accounts of violent crimes committed by psychotic patients exacerbate public misconceptions about these diseases. Statistically, individuals with psychoses are more likely to be victims than perpetrators of crime. Untreated patients, especially when under the influence of alcohol or other substances, are at somewhat increased risk of violent behavior; treated patients are no more violent than the general public (192).

Management

Psychotic illnesses are usually managed by psychiatrists. A primary care practitioner can assume responsibility, in consultation with a psychiatrist, for a stable patient who complies with treatment. When a patient expresses delusions, the clinician may indicate that he or she does not share these delusions, but should not debate with the patient (193–195). It is important to concentrate on the patient's strengths. She can be humiliated easily by thoughtless epithets or behaviors that betray the expectation of violence or incompetence. Patients with severe cases must be treated with an integrated system of social services, family support, rehabilitation, general medical care, psychotherapy, and psychopharmacology. In the process of referral to a mental health professional, the primary clinician should be clear, matter-of-fact, open, and confident of the possibility of successful treatment (192).

References

1. **Schurman RA, Kramer PD, Mitchell JB.** The hidden mental health network: treatment of mental illness by nonpsychiatrist physicians. *Arch Gen Psychiatry* 1985;42:89–94.

2. **Dubovsky SL.** *Psychotherapeutics in primary care.* New York: Grune & Stratton, 1981.

3. **Berndt ER, Koran LM, Finkelstein SN, et al.** Lost human capital from early-onset chronic depression. *Am J Psychiatry* 2000;157:940–947.

4. **Smith I, Adkins S, Walton J.** *Pharmaceuticals: therapeutic review.* New York: Shearson, Lehman, Hutton International Research, 1988.

5. **Pierce C.** Failure to spot mental illness in primary care is a global problem. *Clin Psychiatry News* 1993;21:5.

6. **Margolis RL.** Nonpsychiatric house staff frequently misdiagnose psychiatric disorders in general hospital inpatients. *Psychosomatics* 1994;35:485–491.

7. **Perez-Stable EJ, Miranda J, Munoz RF, et al.** Depression in medical outpatients: underrecognition and misdiagnosis. *Arch Intern Med* 1990;150:1083–1088.

8. **American Psychiatric Association.** *Diagnostic and statistical manual of mental disorders,* 4th ed. Washington, DC: American Psychiatric Press, 1994.

9. **American Psychiatric Association.** *Diagnostic and statistical manual of mental disorders,* 4th ed. Text revision. Washington, DC: American Psychiatric Association, 2000.

10. **Depression Guideline Panel.** *Depression in primary care:* Vol. 1, *detection and diagnosis.* Clinical practice guideline no 5. AHCPR, Publication No 93-0550. Rockville, MD: U.S. Department of Health and Human Services, Public Health Service, Agency for Health Care Policy and Research, 1993.

11. **Cassem NH.** Depression. In: **Cassem NH, ed.** *Massachusetts General Hospital handbook of general hospital psychiatry.* St. Louis, MO: Mosby Year Book, 1991:237–268.

12. **Murphy GE.** The physician's responsibility for suicide. II: Errors of omission. *Ann Intern Med* 1975;82:305–309.

13. **Veith I.** *Hysteria: the history of a disease.* Chicago: University of Chicago Press, 1965.

14. **Roter DL, Hall JA, Kern DE, et al.** Improving physicians' interviewing skills and reducing patients' emotional distress: a randomized clinical trial. *Arch Intern Med* 1995;155:1877–1884.

15. **Beckman HB, Frankel RM.** The effect of physician behavior on the collection of data. *Ann Intern Med* 1984;101:692–696.

16. **Scheiber SC.** The psychiatric interview, psychiatric history, and mental status examination. In: **Hales RE, Yudofsky SC, Talbott JA, eds.** *Textbook of psychiatry,* 2nd ed. Washington, DC: American Psychiatric Press, 1994:187–219.

17. **Orleans CT, George LK, Houpt JL, et al.** How primary care physicians treat psychiatric disorders: a national survey of family practitioners. *Am J Psychiatry* 1985;142:52–57.

18. **Dubovsky SL, Weissberg MP.** *Clinical psychiatry in primary care,* 3rd ed. Baltimore, MD: Williams & Wilkins, 1986.

19. **Stotland NL, Garrick TR.** *Manual of psychiatric consultation.* Washington, DC: American Psychiatric Press, 1990.

20. **Spiegel D, Bloom JR, Kraemer HL, et al.** Effect of psychosocial treatment on survival of patients with metastatic breast cancer. *Lancet* 1989;2:888–891.

21. **Fawzy FI, Cousins NI, Fawzy NW, et al.** A structured psychiatric intervention for cancer patients. I: Changes over time in methods of coping and affective disturbance. *Arch Gen Psychiatry* 1990;47:720–725.

22. **Cunningham AJ, Edmonds CV, Jenkins GP, et al.** A randomized controlled trial of the effects of group psychological therapy on survival in women with metastatic breast cancer. *Psychooncology* 1998;7:508–517.

23. **Maunsell E, Brisson J.** Social support and survival among women with breast cancer. *Cancer* 1995;76:631–637.

24. **Gellert GA, Maxwell RM, Siegel BS.** Survival of breast cancer patients receiving adjunctive psychosocial support therapy: a 10-year follow-up study. *J Clin Oncol* 1993;11:66–69.

25. **Blake-Mortimer J, Gore-Felton C, Kimerling R, et al.** Improving the quality and quantity of life among patients with cancer: a review of the effectiveness of group psychotherapy. *Eur J Cancer* 1999;35:1581–1586.

26. **Goldman N, Ravid R.** Community surveys: sex differences in mental illness. In: **Guttentag M, Salasin S, Belle D, eds.** *The mental health of women.* New York: Academic Press, 1980.

27. **Nolen-Hoeksema S.** *Sex differences in depression.* Stanford, CA: Stanford University Press, 1990.

28. **Weissman MM, Leaf PJ, Holzer CE, et al.** The epidemiology of depression: an update on sex differences in rates. *J Affect Disord* 1984;7:179–188.

29. **Leibenluft E, ed.** *Gender differences in mood and anxiety disorders: from bench to bedside.* Washington, DC: American Psychiatric Press, 1999.

30. **Kornstein SG, Schatzberg AF, Thase ME, et al.** Gender differences in chronic major and double depression. *J Affect Disord* 2000;60:1–11.

31. **Sloan DM, Kornstein SG.** Gender differences in depression and response to anti-depressant treatment. *Psychiatr Clin North Am* 2003;26:581–594.

32. **Kornstein SG.** Gender differences in depression: implications for treatment. *J Clin Psychiatry* 1997;58:12–18.

33. **Regier DA, Boyd JK, Burke JD Jr, et al.** One-month prevalence of mental disorders in the United States—based on five epidemiologic catchment area sites. *Arch Gen Psychiatry* 1988;45:977–985.

34. **Robins LN, Helzer JE, Weissman MN, et al.** Lifetime prevalence of specific psychiatric disorders in three sites. *Arch Gen Psychiatry* 1984;41:949–958.

35. **Boyd JH, Weissman MM.** Epidemiology of affective disorders: a reexamination and future directions. *Arch Gen Psychiatry* 1981;38:1039–1046.

36. **Andrade L, Caraveo-Anduaga JJ, Berglund P, et al.** The epidemiology of major depressive episodes: results from the International Consortium of Psychiatric Epidemiology (ICPE) surveys. *Int J Methods Psychiatr Res* 2003;12:3–21.

37. **Bolton JM, Pagura J, Enns MW, et al.** A population-based longitudinal study of risk factors for suicide attempts in major depressive disorder. *J Psychiatry Res* 2010;44:817–826.

38. **Sainsbury P.** Depression, suicide, and suicide prevention. In: **Baltimore RA, ed.** *Suicide.* Baltimore, MD: Williams & Wilkins, 1990:17–38.

39. **Radloff LS.** Sex differences in depression: the effects of occupation and marital status. *Sex Roles* 1975;1:249–265.

40. **Roberts RE, O'Keefe SJ.** Sex differences in depression reexamined. *J Health Soc Behav* 1981;22:394–399.

41. **Swanson KM.** Predicting depressive symptoms after miscarriage: a path analysis based on the Lazarus paradigm. *J Womens Health Gend Based Med* 2000;9:191–206.

42. **Dugan E, Cohen SJ, Bland DR, et al.** The association of depressive symptoms and urinary incontinence among older adults. *J Am Geriatr Soc* 2000;48:413–416.

43. **Schwenk TL, Evans DL, Laden SK, et al.** Treatment outcome and physician-patient communication in primary care patients with chronic, recurrent depression. *Am J Psychiatry* 2004;161:1892–1901.

44. **McGrath E, Keita GP, Strickland BR, et al.** *Women and depression: risk factors and treatment issues.* Final report of the American Psychological Association's National Task Force on Women and Depression. Washington, DC: American Psychological Association, 1990.

45. **Born L, Steiner M.** The relationship between menarche and depression in adolescence. *CNS Spectrums* 2001;6:126–138.

46. **Pearlstein TB.** Hormones and depression: what are the facts about premenstrual syndrome, menopause, and hormone replacement therapy? *Am J Obstet Gynecol* 1995;173:646–653.

47. **Freeman EW, Sammel MD, Liu L, et al.** Hormones and menopausal status as predictors of depression in women in transition to menopause. *Arch Gen Psychiatry* 2004;61:62–70.

48. **Harlow BL, Wise LA, Otto MW, et al.** Depression and its influence on reproductive endocrine and menstrual cycle markers associated with perimenopause: the Harvard Study of Moods and Cycles. *Arch Gen Psychiatry* 2003;60:29–36.

49. **Soares CN, Cohen LS, Otto MW, et al.** Characteristics of women with premenstrual dysphoric disorder (PMDD) who did or did not report history of depression: a preliminary report from the Harvard Study of Moods and Cycles. *J Womens Health Gend Based Med* 2001;10:873–878.

50. **Schmidt PJ, Haq N, Rubinow DR.** A longitudinal evaluation of the relationship between reproductive status and mood in perimenopausal women. *Am J Psychiatry* 2004;161:2238–2244.

51. **Oinonen KA, Mazmanian D.** To what extent do oral contraceptives influence mood and affect? *J Affect Disord* 2002;70:229–240.

52. **Endicott J, Amsterdam J, Eriksson E, et al.** Is premenstrual dysphoric disorder a distinct clinical entity? *J Womens Health Gend Based Med* 1999;8:663–679.

53. **Halbreich U, Borenstein J, Pearlstein T, et al.** The prevalence, impairment, impact, and burden of premenstrual dysphoric disorder (PMS/PMDD). *Psychoneuroendocrinology* 2003;28:1023–1030.

54. **Freeman EW.** Premenstrual syndrome and premenstrual dysphoric disorder: definitions and diagnosis. *Psychoneuroendocrinology* 2003;28:25–37.

55. **Hamilton JA, Parry BL, Blumenthal SL.** The menstrual cycle in context: I. Affective syndromes associated with reproductive hormonal changes. *J Clin Psych* 1988;49:474–480.

56. **Jensvold MF.** Psychiatric aspects of the menstrual cycle. In: **Stewart DE, Stotland NL, eds.** *Psychological aspects of women's health care.* Washington, DC: American Psychiatric Press, 1993:165–192.

57. **Bailey JW, Cohen LS.** Prevalence of mood and anxiety disorders in women who seek treatment for premenstrual syndrome. *J Womens Health Gend Based Med* 1999;8:1181–1184.

58. **Brand B.** Trauma and women. *Psychiatr Clin North Am* 2003;26:759–779.

59. **Rapkin A.** A review of treatment of premenstrual syndrome and premenstrual dysphoric disorder. *Psychoneuroendocrinology* 2003;28:39–53.

60. **Canning S, Waterman M, Orsi N, et al.** The efficacy of *Hypericum perforatum* (St. John's wort) for the treatment of premenstrual syndrome: a randomized, double-blind, placebo-controlled trial. *CNS Drugs* 2010;24:207–225

61. **Wyatt KM, Dimmock PW, Jones PW, et al.** Efficacy of vitamin B6 in the treatment of premenstrual syndrome: a systematic review. *BMJ* 1999;318:1375–1381.

62. **Pearlstein TB, Halbreich U, Batzar ED, et al.** Psychosocial functioning in women with premenstrual dysphoric disorder before and after treatment with sertraline or placebo. *J Clin Psychiatry* 2000;61:101–109.

63. **Freeman EW, Rickels K, Sondheimer SJ, et al.** Differential response to antidepressants in women with premenstrual syndrome/premenstrual dysphoric disorder: a randomized controlled trial. *Arch Gen Psychiatry* 1999;56:932–939.

64. **Romano S, Judge R, Dillon J, et al.** The role of fluoxetine in the treatment of premenstrual dysphoric disorder. *Clin Ther* 1999;21:615–633.

65. **Young SA, Hurt PH, Benedek DM, et al.** Treatment of premenstrual dysphoric disorder with sertraline during the luteal phase: a randomized, double-blind, placebo-controlled crossover trial. *J Clin Psych* 1998;59:76–80.

66. **Freeman EW, Kroll R, Rapkin A, et al.** Evaluation of a unique oral contraceptive in the treatment of premenstrual dysphoric disorder. *J Womens Health Gend Based Med* 2001;10:561–569.

67. **Anderson KM, Sharpe M, Rattray A, et al.** Distress and concerns in couples referred to a specialist infertility clinic. *J Psychosom Res* 2003;54:353–355.

68. **Perlin LI.** Sex roles and depression. In: **Datan N, Ginsberg L, eds.** *Life-span developmental psychology: normative life crises.* New York: Academic Press, 1975:191–207.

69. **Najib A, Lorberbaum JP, Kose S, et al.** Regional brain activity in women grieving a romantic relationship breakup. *Am J Psychiatry* 2004;161:2245–2256.

70. **Major B, Cozzarelli C, Cooper ML, et al.** Psychological responses of women after first-trimester abortion. *Arch Gen Psychiatry* 2000;57:777–784.

71. **Wisner KL, Parry BL, Piontek CM.** Postpartum depression. *N Engl J Med* 2002;347:194–199.

72. **Evans J, Heron J, Francomb H, et al.** Cohort study of depressed mood during pregnancy and after childbirth. *BMJ* 2001;323:257–260.

73. **Bennett HA, Einarson A, Taddio A, et al.** Prevalence of depression during pregnancy: systematic review. *Obstet Gynecol* 2004;103:698–709.

74. **Oates MR, Cox JL, Neema S, et al.** Postnatal depression across countries and cultures: a qualitative study. *Br J Psychiatry* 2004;184[Suppl 46]:S10–S16.

75. **Robertson E, Grace S, Wallington T, et al.** Antenatal risk factors for postpartum depression: a synthesis of recent literature. *Gen Hosp Psychiatry* 2004;26:289–295.

76. **Segre LS, Stuart S, O'Hara MW.** Interpersonal psychotherapy for antenatal and postpartum depression. *Primary Psychiatry* 2004;11:52–56.

77. **Spinelli MG, Endicott J.** Controlled clinical trial of interpersonal psychotherapy versus parenting education program for depressed pregnant women. *Am J Psychiatry* 2003;160:555–562.

78. **Miller LJ.** Use of electroconvulsive therapy during pregnancy. *Hosp Commun Psychiatry* 1994;45:444–450.

79. **Oren DA, Wisner KL, Spinelli M, et al.** An open trial of morning light therapy for treatment of antepartum depression. *Am J Psychiatry* 2002;159:666–669.

80. **Miller LJ.** Postpartum depression. *JAMA* 2002;287:762–765.

81. **Iqbal MM.** Effects of antidepressants during pregnancy and lactation. *Ann Clin Psychiatry* 1999;11:237–256.

82. **Wisner KL, Gelenberg AJ, Leonard H, et al.** Pharmacologic treatment of depression during pregnancy. *JAMA* 1999;282:1264–1269.

83. **Abramowitz JS, Schwartz SA, Moore KM, et al.** Obsessive-compulsive symptoms in pregnancy and the puerperium: a review of the literature. *J Anxiety Disord* 2003;17:461–478.

84. **Suri R, Altshuler L, Hendrick V, et al.** The impact of depression and fluoxetine treatment on obstetrical outcome. *Arch Women Ment Health* 2004;7:193–200.

85. **Hendrick V, Smith LM, Suri R, et al.** Birth outcomes after prenatal exposure to antidepressant medication. *Am J Obstet Gynecol* 2003;188:812–815.

86. **Gold LH.** Use of psychotropic medication during pregnancy: risk management guidelines. *Psychiatr Ann* 2000;30:421–432.

87. **Casper RC, Fleisher BE, Lee-Ancajas JC, et al.** Follow-up of children of depressed mothers exposed or not exposed to antidepressant drugs during pregnancy. *J Pediatr* 2003;142:402–408.

88. **Chung TK, Lau TK, Yip AS, et al.** Antepartum depressive symptomatology is associated with adverse obstetric and neonatal outcomes. *Psychosom Med* 2001;63:830–834.

89. **Nulman I, Rovet J, Stewart DE, et al.** Child development following exposure to tricyclic antidepressants or fluoxetine throughout fetal life: a prospective, controlled study. *Am J Psychiatry* 2002;159:1889–1895.

90. **Andersson L, Sundstrom-Poromaa I, Wulff M, et al.** Neonatal outcome following maternal antenatal depression and anxiety: a population-based study. *Am J Epidemiol* 2004;159:872–881.

91. **Smith MV, Shao L, Howell H, et al.** Perinatal depression and birth outcomes in a Healthy Start Project. *Matern Child Health* 2011;15:401–409.

92. **Koren G.** Discontinuation syndrome following late pregnancy exposure to antidepressants. *Arch Pediatr Adolesc Med* 2004;158:307–308.

93. **Kumar C, McIvor RJ, Davies T, et al.** Estrogen administration does not reduce the rate of recurrence of affective psychosis after childbirth. *J Clin Psychiatry* 2003;64:112–118.

94. **Wisner KL, Perel JM, Peindl KS, et al.** Prevention of recurrent postpartum depression. *J Clin Psychiatry* 2001;62:82–86.

95. **Cooper R, Mishra G, Hardy R, et al.** Hysterectomy and subsequent psychological health: findings from a British birth cohort study. *J Affect Disord* 2009;115:122–130.

96. **Bhattacharya SM, Jha A.** A comparison of health-related quality of life (HRQOL) after natural and surgical menopause. *Maturitas* 2010;66:431–434.

97. **Cabness J.** The psychosocial dimensions of hysterectomy: private places and the inner spaces of women at midlife. *Soc Work Health Care* 2010;49:211–226.

98. **McKinlay JB, McKinlay SM, Brambilla DJ.** Health status and utilization behavior associated with menopause. *Am J Epidemiol* 1987;125:110–121.

99. **Hamilton JA.** Psychobiology in context: reproductive-related events in men's and women's lives (review of motherhood and mental illness). *Contemp Psych* 1984;3:12–16.

100. **Rossouw JE, Anderson GL, Prentice RL, et al.** Risks and benefits of estrogen plus progestin in healthy postmenopausal women: principal results from the Women's Health Initiative randomized controlled trial. *JAMA* 2002;288:321–333.

101. **Anderson GL, Limacher M, Assaf AR, et al.** Effects of conjugated estrogen in postmenopausal women with hysterectomy: the Women's Health Initiative randomized controlled trial. *JAMA* 2004;291:1701–1712.

102. **Hays J, Ockene JK, Brunner RL, et al.** Effects of estrogen plus progestin on health-related quality of life. *N Engl J Med* 2003;348:1839–1854.

103. **Cohen LS, Soares CN, Poitras JR, et al.** Short-term use of *estradiol* for depression in perimenopausal and postmenopausal women: a preliminary report. *Am J Psychiatry* 2003;160:1519–1522.

104. **Kugaya A, Epperson CN, Zoghbi S, et al.** Increase in prefrontal cortex serotonin 2A receptors following estrogen treatment in postmenopausal women. *Am J Psychiatry* 2003;160:1522–1524.

105. **Soares CN, Almeida OP, Joffe H, et al.** Efficacy of *estradiol* for the treatment of depressive disorders in perimenopausal women: a double-blind, randomized, placebo-controlled trial. *Arch Gen Psychiatry* 2001;58:529–534.

106. **Stearns V, Beebe KL, Iyengar M, et al.** *Paroxetine* controlled release in the treatment of menopausal hot flashes: a randomized controlled trial. *JAMA* 2003;289:2827–2834.

107. **Drayer RA, Mulsant BH, Lenze EJ, et al.** Somatic symptoms of depression in elderly patients with medical comorbidities. *Int J Geriatr Psychiatry* 2005;20:973–982.

108. **Jefferson JW, Greist JH.** Mood disorders. In: **Hales RE, Yudofsky SC, Talbott JA, eds.** *Textbook of psychiatry*, 2nd ed. Washington, DC: American Psychiatric Press, 1994:465–494.

109. **Altshuler LL, Cohen LS, Moline ML, et al.** The Expert Consensus Guideline Series. Treatment of depression in women. *Postgrad Med* 2001 [Spec No]:1–107.

110. **Nemeroff CB, Heim CM, Thase ME, et al.** Differential responses to psychotherapy versus pharmacotherapy in patients with chronic forms of major depression and childhood trauma. *Natl Acad Sci U S A* 2003;100:14293–14296.

111. **Charney DS, Berman RM, Miller HL.** Treatment of depression. In: **Schatzberg AF, Nemeroff CB, eds.** *Essentials of clinical psychopharmacology.* Washington, DC: American Psychiatric Publishing, 2005:353–386.

112. **Linde K, Berner M, Egger M, et al.** St. John's wort for depression: meta-analysis of randomised controlled trials. *Br J Psychiatry* 2005;186:99–107.

113. **Janicak PG, Dowd SM, Strong MJ, et al.** The potential role of repetitive transcranial magnetic stimulation in treating severe depression. *Psychiatr Ann* 2005;35:138–145.

114. **Kozel FA, Nahas Z, Bohning DE, et al.** Functional magnetic resonance imaging and transcranial magnetic stimulation for major depression. *Psychiatr Ann* 2005;35:130–136.

115. **Wright JK, Beck AT.** Cognitive therapy. In: **Hales RE, Yudofsky SC, Talbott JA, eds.** *Textbook of psychiatry*, 2nd ed. Washington, DC: American Psychiatric Press, 1994:1083–1114.

116. **Akincigil A, Bowblis JR, Levin C, et al.** Adherence to antidepressant treatment among privately insure patients diagnosed with depression. *Med Care* 2007;45:363–369.

117. **Quitkin FM, Stewart JW, McGrath PJ, et al.** Are there differences between women's and men's antidepressant responses? *Am J Psychiatry* 2002;159:1848–1854.

118. **Druss BG, Hoff RA, Rosenheck RA.** Underuse of antidepressants in major depression: prevalence and correlates in a national sample of young adults. *J Clin Psychiatry* 2000;61:234–237.

119. **Kennedy SH, Eisfeld BS, Dickens SE, et al.** Antidepressant-induced sexual dysfunction during treatment with *moclobemide, paroxetine, sertraline,* and *venlafaxine. J Clin Psychiatry* 2000;61:276–281.

120. **Kelly CM, Juurlink DN, Gomes T, et al.** Selective serotonin reuptake inhibitors and breast cancer mortality in women receiving *tamoxifen:* a population-based cohort study. *BMJ* 2010;340:693.

121. **Tollefson GD, Rosenbaum JF.** Selective serotonin reuptake inhibitors. In: **Schatzberg AF, Nemeroff CB, eds.** *Essentials of clinical psychopharmacology.* Washington, DC: American Psychiatric Publishing, 2005:27–42.

122. **Masand PS, Gupta S.** Selective serotonin-reuptake inhibitors: an update. *Harvard Rev Psychiatry* 1999;7:69–84.

123. **Schneeweiss S, Patrick AR, Slolmon DH, et al.** Variation in the risk of suicide attempts and completed suicides by antidepressant agent in adults: a propensity score-adjusted analysis of 9 years' data. *Arch Gen Psychiatry* 2010;67:497–506.

124. **Singh T, Prakash A, Rais T, et al.** Decreased use of antidepressants in youth after US Food and Drug Administration black box warning. *Psychiatry (Edgmont)* 2009;6:30–34.

125. **Libby AM, Orton HD, Valuck RJ.** Persisting decline in depression treatment after FDA warnings. *Arch Gen Psychiatry* 2009;66:633–639.

126. **Kent JM.** SNaRIs, NaSSAs, and NaRIs: new agents for the treatment of depression. *Lancet* 2000;355:911–918.

127. **Horst WD, Preskorn SH.** Mechanisms of action and clinical characteristics of three atypical antidepressants: *venlafaxine, nefazodone, bupropion. J Affect Disord* 1998;51:237–254.

128. **Montgomery SA.** New developments in the treatment of depression. *J Clin Psychiatry* 1999;60[Suppl 14]:10–15.

129. **Goodwin FK, Jamison KR.** Medical treatment of manic episodes. In: **Goodwin FK, Jamison KR, eds.** *Manic-depressive illness.* New York: Oxford University Press, 1990:603–629.

130. **Goodwin FK, Jamison KR.** Medical treatment of acute bipolar depression. In: **Goodwin FK, Jamison KR, eds.** *Manic-depressive illness.* New York: Oxford University Press, 1990:630–664.

131. **Klerman GL.** Clinical epidemiology of suicide. *J Clin Psychiatry* 1987;48[Suppl]:33–38.

132. **Buda M, Tsuang MT.** The epidemiology of suicide: implications for clinical practice. In: **Blumenthal SJ, Kupfer DJ, eds.** *Suicide over the life cycle: risk factors, assessment, and treatment of suicidal patients.* Washington, DC: American Psychiatric Press, 1990:17–38.

133. **Pilowsky DJ, Olfson M, Gameroff MJ, et al.** Panic disorder and suicidal ideation in primary care. *Depress Anxiety* 2006;23:11–16.

134. **Han B, Gfroerer JC, Colliver JD.** Associations between duration of illicit drug use and health conditions: results from the 2005–2007 national surveys on drug use and health. *Ann Epidemiol* 2010;20:289–297.

135. **Croghan IT, Ebbert JO, Hurt RD, et al.** Gender difference among smokers receiving interventions for tobacco dependence in a medical setting. *Addict Behav* 2009;34:61–67.

136. **Rockett IR, Putnam SL, Jia H, et al.** Declared and undeclared substance abuse among emergency department patients: a population-based study. *Addiction* 2006;101:706–712.

137. **Haber PS, Demirkol A, Lange K, et al.** Management of injecting drug users admitted to hospital. *Lancet* 2009;374:1284–1293.

138. **Smith PC, Schmidt SM, Allensworth-Davies D, et al.** A single-question screening test for drug use in primary care. *Arch Inter Med* 2010;170:1155–1160.

139. **Clay SW, Allen J, Parran T.** A review of addiction. *Postgrad Med* 2008;120:1–7.

140. **Boyd CJ, Teter CJ, West BT, et al.** Non-medical use of prescription analgesics: a three-year national longitudinal study. *J Addict Dis* 2009;28:232–242.

141. **Ahern J, Galea S, Hubbard A, et al.** "Culture of drinking" and individual problems with alcohol use. *Am J Epidemiol* 2008;167:1041–1049.

142. **Tuchman E.** Women and addiction: the importance of gender issues in substance abuse research. *J Addict Dis* 2010;29:127–138.

143. **Lefebvre L, Midmer D, Boyd JA, et al.** Participant perception of an integrated program for substance abuse in pregnancy. *J Obstet Gynecol Neonatal Nurs* 2010;39:46–52.

144. **Wakhlu S.** Buprenorphine: a review. *J Opioid Manag* 2009;5:59–64.

145. **Nepon J, Belik SL, Bolton J, et al.** The relationship between anxiety disorders and suicide attempts: findings from the National Epidemiologic Survey on Alcohol and Related Conditions. *Depress Anxiety* 2010;27:791–798.

146. **Rosenbaum JF, Pollack MH.** Anxiety. In: **Cassem NH, ed.** *Massachusetts General Hospital handbook of general hospital psychiatry.* St. Louis, MO: Mosby Year Book, 1991:159–190.

147. **Hollander E, Simeon D, Gorman JM.** Anxiety disorders. In: **Hales RE, Yudofsky SC, Talbott JA, eds.** *Textbook of psychiatry*, 2nd ed. Washington, DC: American Psychiatric Press, 1994:495–564.

148. **Sheikh JI, Leskin GA, Klein DF.** Gender differences in panic disorder: findings from the National Comorbidity Survey. *Am J Psychiatry* 2002;159:55–58.

149. **Yehuda R.** Post-traumatic stress disorder. *N Engl J Med* 2002;346:108–114.

150. **Baldessrini RJ.** Drugs and the treatment of psychiatric disorders. In: **Gilman AG, Rall TW, Nies AS, et al, eds.** *Goodman and Gilman's the pharmacological basis of therapeutics*, 8th ed. New York: Pergamon, 1990:383–435.

151. **Bakish D.** The patient with comorbid depression and anxiety: the unmet need. *J Clin Psychiatry* 1999;60[Suppl 6]:20–24.

152. **Barlow DH, Craske MG, Cerny JA, et al.** Behavioral treatment of panic disorder. *Behav Ther* 1989;20:261–282.

153. **Taylor S, Wald J.** Expectations and attributions in social anxiety disorder: diagnostic distinctions and relationship to general anxiety and depression. *Cogn Behav Ther* 2003;32:166–178.

154. **Pollack MH, Simon NM, Zalta AK, et al.** *Olanzapine* augmentation of *fluoxetine* for refractory generalized anxiety disorder: a placebo controlled study. *Biol Psychiatry* 2006;59:211–215.

155. **van Oppen P, van Balkom AJ, de Haan E, et al.** Cognitive therapy and exposure in vivo alone and in combination with *fluvoxamine* in obsessive-compulsive disorder: a 5-year follow-up. *J Clin Psychiatry* 2005;66:1415–1422.

156. **Moritz S, Rufer M, Fricke S, et al.** Quality of life in obsessive-compulsive disorder before and after treatment. *Compr Psychiatry* 2005;46:453–459.

157. **Cottraux J, Bouvard MA, Milliery M.** Combining pharmacotherapy with cognitive-behavioral interventions for obsessive-compulsive disorder. *Cogn Behav Ther* 2005;34:185–192.

158. **Furukawa TA, Watanabe N, Churchill R.** Combined psychotherapy and antidepressants for panic disorder with or without agoraphobia. *Cochrane Database Syst Rev* 2007;1:CD004364.

159. **Schnurr PP, Friedman MJ, Engel CC, et al.** Cognitive behavioral therapy for posttraumatic stress disorder in women: a randomized controlled trial. *JAMA* 2007;297:820–830.

160. **Foa EB, Steketee G, Grayson JB, et al.** Deliberate exposure and blocking of obsessive-compulsive rituals: immediate and long-term effects. *Behav Ther* 1984;15:450–472.

161. **Cooper NA, Clum GA.** Imaginal flooding as a supplementary treatment for PTSD in combat veterans: a controlled study. *Behav Ther* 1989;20:381–391.

162. **Butler G.** Issues in the application of cognitive and behavioral strategies to the treatment of social phobia. *Clin Psychol Rev* 1989;9:91–106.

163. **Craske MG, Brown TA, Barlow DH.** Behavioral treatment of panic disorder: a two-year followup. *Behav Ther* 1991;22:289–304.

164. **Roy-Byrne PP, Cowley DS.** *Benzodiazepines in clinical practice: risks and benefits.* Washington, DC: American Psychiatric Press, 1991.

165. **Jenike MA, Baer L, Summergrad P, et al.** Obsessive-compulsive disorder: a double-blind, placebo-controlled trial of *clomipramine* in 27 patients. *Am J Psychol* 1989;146:1328–1330.

166. **Jenike MA, Baer L.** An open trial of *buspirone* in obsessive-compulsive disorder. *Am J Psychol* 1988;145:1285–1286.

167. **Cassem NH, Barsky AJ.** Functional symptoms and somatoform disorders. In: **Cassem NH, ed.** *Massachusetts General Hospital handbook of general hospital psychiatry.* St. Louis, MO: Mosby Year Book, 1991:131–157.

168. **Frostholm L, Fink P, Christensen KS, et al.** The patients' illness perceptions and the use of primary health care. *Psychosom Med* 2005;67:997–1005.

169. **Ford CV, Folks DG.** Conversion disorders: an overview. *Psychosomatics* 1985;26:371–377,380–383.

170. **Ljundberg L.** Hysteria: clinical, prognostic, and genetic study. *Acta Psychol Scand* 1957;32:1–162.

171. **Stefansson JH, Messina JA, Meyerowitz S.** Hysterical neurosis, conversion type: clinical and epidemiological considerations. *Acta Psychiatr Scand* 1976;59:119–138.

172. **Toone BK.** Disorders of hysterical conversion. In: **Bass C, ed.** *Physical symptoms and psychological illness.* London, Engl.: Blackwell Science, 1990:207–234.

173. **Strassnig M, Stowell KR, First MB, et al.** General medical and psychiatric perspectives on somatoform disorders: separated by an uncommon language. *Curr Opin Psychiatry* 2006;19:194–200.

174. **Ruddy R, House A.** Psychosocial interventions for conversion disorder. *Cochrane Database Syst Rev* 2005;19:CD005331.

175. **Koss MP.** The women's mental health research agenda: violence against women. *Am Psychol* 1990;45:257–263.

176. **Bryer JB, Nelson BA, Miller JB, et al.** Childhood sexual and physical abuse as factors in adult psychiatric illness. *Am J Psychol* 1987;114:1426–1430.

177. **Warshaw C.** Women and violence. In: **Stotland NL, Stewart DE, eds.** *Psychological aspects of women's health care*, 2nd ed. Washington, DC: American Psychiatric Press, 2001:477–548.

178. **MacMillan HL, Wathen CN, Jamieson E, et al.** Screening for intimate partner violence in health care settings: a randomized trial. *JAMA* 2009;302:493–501.

179. **Clark LA.** Assessment and diagnosis of personality disorder: perennial issues and an emerging reconceptualization. *Ann Rev Psychol* 2007;58:227–257.

180. **Andreasen NC, Wasek P.** Adjustment disorders in adolescents and adults. *Arch Gen Psychiatry* 1980;37:1166–1170.

181. **Fabrega H Jr, Mezzich JE, Mezzich AC.** Adjustment disorder as a marginal or transitional illness category in DSM-III. *Arch Gen Psychol* 1987;44:567–572.

182. **Kaye W, Strober M, Jimerson D.** The neurobiology of eating disorders. In: **Charney DS, Nestler EJ, eds.** *The neurobiology of mental illness.* New York: Oxford University Press, 2004:1112–1128.

183. **Mickley D.** Are you overlooking eating disorders among your patients? *Womens Health in Primary Care* 2000;3:40–52.

184. **Strober M, Morell W, Burroughs J, et al.** A controlled family study of anorexia nervosa. *J Psych Res* 1985;19:329–346.

185. **Stewart DE, Robinson GE.** Eating disorders and reproduction. In: **Stotland NL, Stewart DE, eds.** *Psychological aspects of women's health care*, 2nd ed. Washington, DC: American Psychiatric Press, 2001:411–456.

186. **VanItallie TB.** Health implications of overweight and obesity in the United States. *Ann Intern Med* 1985;103:983–1038.

187. **Bulik CM, Berkman ND, Brownley KA, et al.** Anorexia nervosa treatment: a systematic review of randomized controlled trials. *Int J Eat Discord* 2007;40:310–320.

188. **Von Korff M, Nestadt G, Romanoski A, et al.** Prevalence of treated and untreated DSM-III schizophrenia: results of a two-stage community survey. *J Nerv Ment Dis* 1985;173:577–581.

189. **Nilsson E, Lichtenstein P, Cnattinguis S, et al.** Women with schizophrenia: pregnancy outcome and infant death among their offspring. *Schizophr Res* 2002;58:221–229.

190. **Jablensky AV, Morgan V, Zubrick SR, et al.** Pregnancy, delivery and neonatal complications in a population cohort of women with schizophrenia and major affective disorders. *Am J Psychiatry* 2005;162:79–91.

191. **Goff DC, Manschreck TC, Groves JE.** Psychotic patients. In: **Cassem NH, ed.** *Massachusetts General Hospital handbook of general hospital psychiatry.* St. Louis, MO: Mosby Year Book, 1991:217–236.

192. **Black DW, Andreasen NC.** Schizophrenia, schizophreniform disorder, and delusional (paranoid) disorder. In: **Hales RE, Yudofsky SC, Talbott JA, eds.** *Textbook of psychiatry*, 2nd ed. Washington, DC: American Psychiatric Press, 1994:411–463.

193. **Beiser M, Iacono WG.** Update on the epidemiology of schizophrenia. *Can J Psychiatry* 1990;35:657–668.

194. **Michels R, Marzuk PM.** Progress in psychiatry. *N Engl J Med* 1993;329:552–560.

195. **Stotland NL.** Psychiatric and psychosocial issues in primary care for women. In: **Seltzer VL, Pearse WH, eds.** *Women's primary health care: office practice and procedures.* New York: McGraw-Hill, 1995.

13

Complementary Therapy

Tracy W. Gaudet

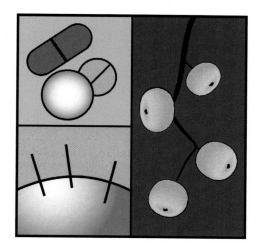

- The spectrum of complementary and alternative approaches is broad and includes methods worthy of integration into our current practice, and ineffective or fraudulent practices that should be avoided.

- A complete history should include the patient's use of complementary and alternative medicine (CAM), particularly botanicals and supplements, as these can have actions ranging from estrogenic to anticoagulant.

- The U.S. Food and Drug Administration does not currently regulate botanicals and supplements, so extra steps must be taken to ensure the quality of such products.

- The management of many women's health issues can be enhanced by the integration of selected CAM approaches.

- Perceived congruency of values around life and health with CAM providers was predictive of use of these approaches; dissatisfaction with conventional medicine is not a predictor of use of CAM.

- Acupuncture is of benefit in a variety of conditions, including pain, nausea and vomiting of pregnancy, and secondary to chemotherapy.

- Mind–body approaches such as stress reduction, visualization, and hypnosis are gaining evidence as valuable adjuncts in a spectrum of women's health concerns, from surgery to fertility.

The use of complementary and alternative medicine (CAM) for health maintenance and disease management is on a steady rise in the United States, and for nearly 15 years, the number of visits to alternative care providers exceeded the number of visits to primary care providers. Although evidence exists to support many of these approaches, some approaches are used in the absence of any documented benefit and can be potentially dangerous and fraudulent (1). The primary users are women, who are frequently making decisions regarding treatment options without the advice of their physicians. Obstetrician–gynecologists are in an excellent position to help guide patients in their treatment choices, counseling them about potentially dangerous alternative treatments and supporting their use of potentially beneficial ones. The most significant challenge is the lack of training that most obstetrician–gynecologists have in this area; thus, this chapter reviews the domains of CAM as they apply to the practice of gynecology.

Table 13.1 The Five Domains of Complementary and Alternative Medicine

Domains	Examples
Alternative Medical Systems	Homeopathic medicine, naturopathic medicine, traditional Chinese medicine, Ayurveda
Mind–Body Interventions	Meditation, prayer, mental healing, creative outlets (art, music, dance)
Biologically Based Therapies	Dietary supplements, herbal products
Manipulative and Body-Based Methods	Chiropractic or osteopathic manipulation, massage
Energy Therapies	Biofield therapies, such as qi gong, Reiki, therapeutic touch Bioelectromagnetic therapies, such as pulsed fields, magnetic fields, AC or DC fields

Adapted from **National Institutes of Health.** National Center for Complementary and Alternative Medicine. What is complementary and alternative medicine? Available online at: http://nccam.nih.gov/health/whatiscam/

Definitions

The concept of complementary and alternative medicine is by definition a relative one. In a landmark publication, CAM was defined as "medical interventions not taught widely at U.S. medical schools or generally available at U.S. hospitals" (2). As practices or therapies move in or out of the mainstream in this country, the definition of CAM will change. The spectrum of therapies, practitioners, and products that fall into this category are extremely broad and include everything from botanical medicine to "crystal gazing." The five domains of CAM are listed in Table 13.1.

The amount of evidence on the use of these approaches varies widely. A significant number of randomized controlled trials, including those with sufficient quantity and quality to allow meta-analyses in some areas, were done to assess the efficacy of acupuncture, botanical medicine, nutritional approaches, manual therapies, and mind–body medicine. Research in the other domains is much more limited. Many culturally based practices such as shamanism and curanderismo have virtually no research basis. A growing number of randomized controlled trials are being done in spiritual healing and homeopathy, but these techniques remain controversial based on the lack of understood biophysical mechanisms to justify their efficacy.

Integrative medicine **is a distinct entity separate from the practice of CAM.** Integrative medicine neither blindly advocates CAM nor rejects conventional medicine. Integrative medicine is healing oriented and patient centered and adopts a whole-person approach to the treatment of disease and the maintenance of health. It draws on the best practices of medicine, regardless of system of origin. Typically, **integrative medicine would include, in addition to conventional medicine, CAM techniques that may be of benefit, including nutrition, movement and exercise, mind–body approaches, and spirituality.** As the paradigm of conventional medicine broadens to include other therapeutic modalities that previously were considered "alternative," and the focus of our system becomes more accepting of health optimization and disease management, we will see greater integration of these philosophies, approaches, and providers. The distinction of "complementary and alternative therapies" may ultimately no longer be useful, nor will integrative medicine. This approach, which is inclusive of effective philosophies and approaches that can improve the health and healing of women, will simply become the standard for U.S. health care.

Demographic Data

The first national survey assessing the use of CAM in the United States was done in 1990. This study revealed that 34% of the 1,539 individuals who responded to the survey had used

CAM in the previous 12 months and that most of these users were women. When extrapolated, these results suggested 425 million visits to alternative care providers occurred that year, which exceeded the number of visits to primary care providers in the same year (388 million visits). An estimated $13.7 million was spent, $10.3 million of which was spent out of pocket. This expenditure is comparable to the $12.8 billion spent out of pocket for all hospitalizations in the United States that same year. Only 28.5% of individuals disclosed this usage to their physician. Of note to conventional health care providers, 71.5% of individuals using these approaches did *not* inform their physicians of their use (2).

This national survey was repeated 7 years later and established the use of CAM in the United States as a significant and growing trend (N = 2,055). When compared with use in 1990, the use of CAM increased from 33.8% to 42.1%. Extrapolations suggest a 47.3% increase in total visits to alternative medicine providers, from 427 million in 1990 to 629 million visits in 1997, again exceeding visits to primary care providers. Most of these users again were women, with 48.9% of women having used CAM that year, compared with 37.8% of men (1). There was no significant improvement in disclosure, with only 39.8% of users disclosing this information to their physicians. Most users were again found to be paying entirely out of pocket, with no significant change between 1990 (64%) and 1997 (58.3%). Estimated expenditures for alternative medicine services increased 45.2%, and total 1997 out-of-pocket expenditures related to alternative therapies were conservatively estimated at $27 billion, which is comparable to the out-of-pocket expenditures for all physician services that year. More recently, the CDC reported that in 2002, 75% of adult Americans reported having used CAM approaches, and 62% had used them in the past year (3). A study of gynecologic oncology patients revealed that 56% were using CAM, and surveys of menopausal women showed that 80% were using "nonprescriptive therapies" (4). **The Study of Women's Health Across the Nation (SWAN) found that approximately one-half of women were actively using herbal, spiritual, or manipulative therapies** (4). A study examining the use of CAM by women suffering from nausea and vomiting during pregnancy found that 61% reported using CAM therapies, with the most popular being ginger, vitamin B_6, and acupressure (5). A study evaluating the use of CAM therapies by women with advanced-stage breast cancer revealed that 73% of patients used CAM, with relaxation or meditation techniques and botanicals being used most often (6). The reason most often given for the use of CAM was immune support, followed by the second treatment of cancer. A survey in Washington state exploring use of alternative therapies for menopause revealed that 76% of women were using alternative approaches, with 43% of these women using stress-reduction techniques, 37% using over-the-counter alternative approaches, 32% using chiropractic medicine, 30% massage therapy, 23% dietary soy, 10% acupuncture, 9% naturopathy or homeopathy, and 5% herbalists (7). Of these women, 89% to 100% found these approaches to be somewhat or very helpful. Current users of hormone therapy were 50% more likely to use CAM than those who never used hormone therapy. **Following the results of the Women's Health Initiative indicating the risks associated with hormone therapy, interest in the use of CAM for management of menopausal symptoms increased.**

The Attraction

A national survey published in 1998 was the first to explore the very intriguing question of *why* so many patients were turning to CAM (8). Three hypotheses were proposed:

1. Dissatisfaction with conventional medicine.
2. Personal control in their health care.
3. Philosophical congruence of values around life, health, and wellness.

Surprisingly, **dissatisfaction with conventional medicine was *not* predictive of use of CAM. Patients turn to CAM because they are seeking greater congruency of values regarding life, health, and wellness** (8). The message is, that people are happy to use conventional medicine when they have a diseased or injured body part, but when their goal is to improve their health or manage a chronic condition or lifestyle issue, they turn to alternative care providers. Establishing a partnership with patients can help them explore all of the options for maximizing their health. The Centers for Disease Control and Prevention (CDC) reported that the majority (55%) of people stated that their reason for using CAM therapies was that they thought combining these approaches with conventional ones would help them. It is interesting to note that 26% reported they tried these approaches because medical professionals had recommended them (3).

The reluctance of patients to inform their physicians of their use of CAM creates barriers to the best practice of medicine. Included in the realm of CAM are potentially harmful practices and products and potential interactions between effective CAM and conventional approaches. In a 5-year prospective cohort study following women in San Francisco with newly diagnosed breast cancer, 72% were using at least one form of CAM in the management or treatment of their breast cancer. Of these women, 54% disclosed their use to their physician (much higher than the national average), whereas 94% discussed their conventional treatment with their CAM provider (9). Three reasons were given for the patients' lack of disclosure:

1. Women anticipated physician disinterest, negative response, or unwillingness or inability to contribute useful information
2. Women believed their use of CAM to be irrelevant to their biomedical treatment
3. Women did not view disclosure as appropriate coordination of disparate healing strategies

This study highlighted the fact that the use of conventional approaches is well integrated into CAM patient visits, whereas the history of use of CAM is poorly integrated into the conventional medical encounter. Overall, patients' disclosure to their physicians is very cautious, even when the physicians involved would welcome the discussion.

The Challenge

The demographics and trends associated with CAM use create challenges for physicians and dangers for patients. A huge market demand exists, and with it comes an opportunity for products and therapies that may be ineffective, dangerous, or fraudulently marketed. The development of the patient demand preceded the incorporation of education regarding CAM for medical students, residents, and practicing physicians. As a result, patients make decisions regarding their care without the benefit of medical advice or the coordination of their care by one provider. The best practice of medicine necessitates the integration of all therapies that can benefit the patient and the exclusion of those that can cause harm. Integration of these techniques will require the collaborative, concerted effort of physicians, CAM providers, and patients.

Complementary and Alternative Medicine Techniques

The many types of CAM techniques can be organized by categories as outlined by the National Institutes of Health (NIH). Each type is associated with some risk or complication. Licensing and certification requirements vary widely from state to state, but most techniques have a formal structure for training and accreditation (Table 13.2).

Biologically Based Therapies: Botanical Medicine

Botanical or herbal therapies use botanicals singly or in combination for therapeutic value. A botanical is a plant or plant part that contains chemical substances that act on the body. Botanical or herbal medicines were studied extensively in Europe, and large multicenter trials are beginning to provide more robust evidence in this country.

Botanical medicine is the area of CAM most conceptually accessible to patients. Botanicals are the source of the active agents in approximately 25% of prescription drugs and 60% of over-the-counter drugs. In the United States these products are often not perceived as active and are regulated as "dietary supplements," that are not under the direction of the U.S. Food and Drug Administration (FDA). The most popular botanicals used in the United States are listed in Table 13.3.

Complications and Risks

Botanical medicines are being used by an increasing number of patients, and they often do not advise their clinicians of this use. Certain patients are at risk for drug–botanical interactions or adverse reactions, and patients should be questioned about them (Tables 13.4 and 13.5). Mega doses of vitamins and supplements have associated risks and complications, and their use is increasing.

Because botanicals are regulated as dietary supplements, quality control is challenging. In 1994, the Dietary Supplement Health and Education Act (DSHEA) was enacted (10). This act makes it legal to refer to the supplement's effect on the body's structure or function or to

Therapy	Training	Licensure
Botanical/herbal medicine	None standardized	Written examination developed by the National Certification Commission for Acupuncture and Oriental Medicine tests for entry-level capabilities in oriental herbal medicine. Passage allows practitioners to call themselves Diplomates of Chinese Herbology (Dipl CH).
Chiropractic	Must complete a 4-year chiropractic college program of study accredited by the Council on Chiropractic Education (CCE)	National
Massage therapy and bodywork	The American Massage Therapy Association (AMTA) accredits 25% of massage training schools. The National Certification Board for Therapeutic Massage and Bodywork (NCBTMB) administers a certification examination used by 35 states. Certification from NCBTMB requires passing this examination and the completion of a minimum of 500 in-class hours of formal education and training.	Offered at the state level in 40 states.
Hypnotherapy		The International Medical and Dental Hypnotherapy Association will certify hypnotherapists if they meet the minimum eligibility requirements and provide referrals.
Clinical hypnosis	Basic certification requires a minimum of 40 hours of ASCH approved workshop training, 20 hours of individualized training, and a minimum of 2 years of independent practice using clinical hypnosis. The advanced level, called approved consultant, requires a minimum of 60 additional hours of ASCH-approved workshop training and 5 years of independent practice using clinical hypnosis.	American Society of Clinical Hypnosis (ASCH) Certification in clinical hypnosis ensures that the certified individual is a bona fide health care professional who is licensed in that state to provide medical, dental, or psychotherapeutic services.
Meditation and stress reduction	None	None
Acupuncture	Schools provide 3- or 4-year training programs in oriental medicine that consist of about 2,500 to 3,200 hours.	In most states, the practitioner must provide proof that he/she has attended and graduated from an accredited school or from a school that is in the process of being accredited by the Accreditation Commission for Acupuncture and Oriental Medicine (ACAOM).
		Forty states either license or register acupuncturists as Doctors of Oriental Medicine or Acupuncture Physicians, and about two-thirds of these states grant licenses.
	The National Certification Commission for Acupuncture and Oriental Medicine (NCCAOM) tests entry-level capabilities with a comprehensive written examination, point location examination, and clean needle technique. Medical doctors can be certified by the American Board of Medical Acupuncture by taking a minimum 300 hours in training.	An acupuncturist must pass this examination and meet continuing education requirements every 4 years to retain certification and licensure.
Naturopathic medicine		Currently only 15 states have licensing laws, and they differ considerably. There are seven accredited, 4-year naturopathic medical schools.

Table 13.3 Top-Selling Herbal Dietary Supplements in the Food, Drug, and Mass Market Retail Channels in 2009 (for 52 Weeks Ending December 27, 2009)

Rank/Herb	Dollar Sales	% Change vs. 1 Year Ago
1. Cranberry	$31,314,220	23.28
2. Soy	$19,647,980	−12.35
3. Saw palmetto	$18,813,300	7.09
4. Garlic	$17,908,530	−7.66
5. Echinacea	$16,230,560	6.94
6. Ginkgo	$16,011,830	−8.10
7. Milk thistle	$11,162,670	19.72
8. St. John's wort	$8,758,233	5.90
9. Ginseng	$8,292,474	1.65
10. Black cohosh	$8,123,878	−0.29
11. Green tea	$6,715,113	21.71
12. Evening primrose	$4,259,037	9.17
13. Valerian	$4,142,234	24.76
14. Horny goat weed	$2,819,403	16.94
15. Bilberry	$1,983,723	7.41
16. Elderberry	$1,837,587	−0.42
17. Grape seed	$1,783,874	−3.78
18. Ginger	$1,183,641	24.81
19. Aloe vera	$646,164	−4.81
20. Horse chestnut seed	$558,946	−28.79
Total All Herb Supplements (including herbs not shown)	$335,585,700	14.38

From **Cavaliere C, Rea P, Lynch ME, et al.** Herbal supplement sales rise in all channels in 2009. American Botanical Council. *Herbalgram* 2010;86:62. Available online at: http://cms.herbalgram.org/herbalgram/issue86/article3530.html?Issue=86.

a person's well-being. Products within the jurisdiction of DSHEA are easily recognized by the following statement on their labels: "This product is not intended to diagnose, treat, cure, or prevent any disease." Because the FDA does not regulate these products, the potential for lack of standardization of products, as well as adulteration or mislabeling, exists. Pharmacokinetic evaluation is lacking.

Botanicals can cause toxicity in one of three ways: (i) the products can be adulterated; (ii) the labels can recommend dosages that exceed appropriate use and cause toxicity even when the product is safe in appropriate dosages; and (iii) even when they are of good quality and taken in the correct dosage, these products can interact with other supplements and pharmaceutical agents. The Institute of Medicine recommended the following measures: seed-to-shelf quality control, accuracy and comprehensiveness in labeling and other disclosure, enforcement against inaccurate and misleading claims, research into consumer use, incentives for privately funded research, and consumer protection against all potential hazards.

Training and Licensure in Biologically Based Therapies

There is no national licensure for botanical or herbal medicine, and there is no national or professional organization that regulates or accredits Western and Ayurvedic herbal medicine education. In 1996, the National Certification Commission for Acupuncture and Oriental Medicine developed a national certification written examination, which tests for entry-level capabilities in oriental herbal medicine. Passage of this examination allows practitioners to call themselves

Table 13.4 Botanicals: Potential for Interactions with Drugs

Drug Class	Herb	Potential Interactions
Anticoagulants	Bilberry	Increased risk of bleeding (high dose)
	Chamomile	Increased risk of bleeding
	Coenzyme Q-10	Decreased effectiveness
	Danshen	Increased risk of bleeding
	Dong quai	Increased risk of bleeding
	Feverfew	Increased risk of bleeding
	Garlic	Increased risk of bleeding
	Ginger	Increased risk of bleeding
	Ginkgo	Increased risk of bleeding
	Ginseng	Increased risk of bleeding
	Kava	Increased risk of bleeding
	St. John's wort	Decreased effectiveness
Anticonvulsants	Borage	Decreased seizure threshold
	Comfrey	Increased risk of phenobarbital toxicity
	Evening primrose oil	Decreased seizure threshold
	Valerian	Increased effects of barbiturates
Antidepressants	Ephedra	Increased effect of monoamine oxidase inhibitors
	Ginseng	Increased risk of monoamine oxidase inhibitors
	Kava	Hypertension
	St. John's wort	Monoamine oxidase inhibitors; increased blood pressure level
	Yohimbine	Tricyclics—hypertension; selective serotonin reuptake inhibitors; increased serotonin levels
Diuretics	Aloe	Increased risk of hypokalemia
	Cascara sagrada	Increased risk of hypokalemia
	Licorice	Increased risk of hypokalemia
	Senna	Increased risk of hypokalemia
Hypoglycemic agents	Ginseng	Risk of hypoglycemia
	Stinging nettle	Potential elevation of blood glucose level
Sedatives	Chamomile	Increased drowsiness
	Kava	Increased risk of sedation
	Valerian	Increased risk of sedation

Data from **O'Mathuna DP.** Herb-drug interactions. *Altern Med Alert* 2003;6:37–43.

Table 13.5 Selected Risk Factors for Adverse Reactions or Drug Interactions with Botanicals

- Bleeding disorders or anticoagulation
- Seizure disorders
- Radiation with or without chemotherapy
- Immunosuppression
- Diabetes
- Pregnancy
- Renal insufficiency
- Liver disease
- Heart failure
- Electrolyte imbalances
- Taking sedatives/anxiolytics/central nervous system depressants, oral contraceptives, diuretics, monoamine oxidase inhibitors, antiretroviral drugs
- Undiagnosed medical conditions

Diplomats of Chinese Herbology (Dipl CH). The Commission's website contains a searchable directory of certified practitioners (11).

Manipulative and Body-Based Methods

Chiropractic Medicine

Chiropractic medicine focuses on the relationship between structure (primarily the spine) and function, and how that relationship affects the preservation and restoration of health. It uses manipulative therapy as an integral tool. Chiropractors can legally do more than manipulate and align the spine, including taking a medical history, performing a physical examination, and ordering lab tests and x-rays to determine a diagnosis. The spectrum of chiropractors varies in terms of the conditions treated with manipulation. Although some practitioners limit their practice primarily to musculoskeletal problems, others claim to offer effective treatment for virtually any medical condition. They are referred to as doctors, which can be misleading to patients.

Complications and Risks

The most significant risk associated with chiropractic medicine is stroke. Vertebrobasilar accidents occur mainly after a cervical manipulation with a rotatory component. The average age of patients with a vertebrobasilar accident is 38 years. The frequency of serious adverse events varied from 1 stroke per 20,000 manipulations to 1.46 serious adverse events per 10 million manipulations and 2.68 deaths per 10 million manipulations (12). The true incidence of these risks is not known and more data are needed.

Training and Licensure

There is a national process for licensure for chiropractic medicine to which all 50 states adhere. Chiropractors must complete a 4-year chiropractic college program of study accredited by the Council on Chiropractic Education (CCE).

Massage Therapy and Bodywork

Massage therapy involves manipulation of the soft tissues of the body to normalize those tissues. A wide variety of approaches are available that include deep-tissue massage, Swedish massage, reflexology, Rolfing, and many others. A number of randomized controlled trials documented the value of massage therapy, particularly in pediatric conditions such as childhood asthma. Some studies show an increase in dopamine and serotonin, and an increase in natural killer cells and lymphocytes with regular massage therapy.

Massage therapy and bodywork are used by a wide array of people seeking the benefits of massage, which include physical relaxation, reduced anxiety, increased circulation, and pain relief. Specific indications for massage include treatment of acute low-back pain and lymphatic massage for patients with lymphedema from conditions such as postmastectomy extremity edema. Massage is used by various practitioners, including physicians, physical therapists, osteopathic physicians, chiropractors, acupuncturists, nurses, and massage therapists.

Complications and Risks

Massage should not be used in the presence of bleeding disorders, phlebitis and thrombophlebitis, edema that is caused by heart or kidney failure, fever or infections that can be spread by blood or lymph circulation, and leukemia or lymphoma. Massage should not be performed on or near malignant tumors and bone metastases; over bruises, unhealed scars, or open wounds; on or near recent fracture sites; or over joints or other tissues that are acutely inflamed.

Training and Licensure

There is no national licensure in massage therapy, but licensure is offered in 40 states. One-fourth of the massage training schools are accredited by the American Massage Therapy Association (AMTA). The National Certification Board for Therapeutic Massage and Bodywork (NCBTMB) administers a certification examination, and 35 states use it for licensure. The NCBTMB is an independent, private, nonprofit organization, founded in 1992, that fosters high standards for therapeutic massage and bodywork professionals. There are more than 90,000 nationally certified massage therapists and bodyworkers in the United States. Certification by NCBTMB requires successful completion of the examination and the completion of a minimum of 500 in-class hours of formal education and training (13).

Mind–Body Interventions

Clinical Hypnosis and Imagery

Hypnosis involves the induction of trance states and the use of therapeutic suggestions. Hypnosis has documented value for a variety of psychological conditions and pain control and recovery from surgery.

Complications and Risks

Hypnotized persons occasionally report unanticipated negative effects during and after hypnosis. The spectrum of reported effects encompassed minor transient symptoms such as headaches, dizziness, or nausea in experimental situations to less frequent symptoms of anxiety or panic, unexpected reactions to an inadvertently given suggestion, and difficulties in awakening from hypnosis. More serious reactions following hypnosis are attributed to the misapplication of hypnotic techniques, failure to prepare the participant, and preexisting psychopathology or personality factors. There are no known deaths attributed to the use of hypnosis.

False memories of suggested events that did not occur in reality, particularly when legal and interpersonal battles are involved, can be viewed as an untoward reaction to psychotherapeutic procedures. In hypnotic and nonhypnotic situations, leading and suggestive overtures can produce false memories. Because hypnosis involves direct and indirect suggestions, some of which may be leading in nature, and because hypnosis can increase confidence of recalled events with little or no change in the level of accuracy, therapists must be attentive to the problem of creating false memories.

Training and Licensure

There is no national or state licensure for hypnotherapists. The International Medical and Dental Hypnotherapy Association will certify hypnotherapists if they meet the minimum eligibility requirements and will provide referrals.

American Society of Clinical Hypnosis (ASCH) certification in clinical hypnosis is distinct from other certification programs in that it ensures that the certified individual is a health care professional who is licensed in his or her state to provide medical, dental, or psychotherapeutic services. Certification by ASCH distinguishes the professional practitioner from the lay hypnotist. There are two levels of certification, each is simply called *certification,* which requires, among other things, a minimum of 40 hours of ASCH-approved workshop training, 20 hours of individualized training, and a minimum of 2 years of independent practice using clinical hypnosis. An advanced level, called *approved consultant,* recognizes individuals who obtained advanced training in clinical hypnosis and who have extensive experience in using hypnosis within their professional practices. Certification at this level requires a minimum of 60 additional hours of ASCH-approved workshop training and 5 years of independent practice using clinical hypnosis (14).

Meditation and Stress Reduction

Meditation is a self-directed practice that can relax the body and calm the mind. Most meditative techniques came to the West from religious practices in the East, particularly India, China, and Japan, but it can be found in all cultures of the world. A National Institutes of Health Consensus Panel in 1996 concluded that **mind–body and behavioral techniques were effective in the treatment of stress-related conditions and insomnia, and since then evidence for their effectiveness has continued to grow.** *Mindfulness-based stress reduction* (MBSR), based on *Vipassana meditation* from India, is promoted in this country. This technique is based on the cultivation of mindfulness, an intentional, focused awareness of nonjudgmental attentiveness to experiences in the present moment. Vipassana meditation, one of India's most ancient techniques of meditation, was taught more than 2,500 years ago as a remedy for universal ills.

Transcendental meditation (TM) is a simple, natural, effortless procedure practiced for 15 to 20 minutes in the morning and evening while sitting comfortably with the eyes closed. During this technique, the individual experiences a unique state of restful alertness. Transcendental meditation is useful in the treatment of hypertension.

The relaxation response, which can be elicited by any number of techniques, is a physical state of deep rest that changes the physical and emotional responses to stress (e.g., decrease in heart rate, blood pressure, and muscle tension). If practiced regularly, it can have lasting effects when encountering stress throughout the day.

Complications and Risks

Meditation rarely may lead to a "spiritual emergency," defined as a crisis during which the process of growth and change becomes chaotic and overwhelming as individuals enter new realms of spiritual experience. It is included in the *Diagnostic and Statistical Manual of Mental Disorders,* fourth edition (DSM-IV) diagnostic category "religious or spiritual problem." Types of spiritual emergency include but are not limited to loss or change of faith, existential or spiritual crisis, experience of unitive consciousness or altered states, psychic openings, possession, near-death experience, kundalini, shamanic journey, or difficulties with a meditation practice.

Training and Licensure in Meditation and Stress Reduction

There is no nationally recognized licensing or certification procedure for teachers of meditation. Many mental health care professionals are trained in a variety of stress reduction techniques.

Energy Therapies

Energy therapies involve the use of energy fields. They are of two categories:

1. *Biofield therapies* are intended to affect energy fields that purportedly surround and penetrate the human body. Some forms of energy therapy attempt to manipulate biofields by applying pressure or manipulating the body by placing the hands in, or through, these fields. Examples include qi gong, Reiki, and therapeutic touch.
2. *Bioelectromagnetic-based therapies* involve the unconventional use of electromagnetic fields, such as pulsed fields, magnetic fields, or alternating current or direct current fields.

Complications and Risks

Energy-based therapies are the least well researched and the most diverse of all CAM modalities. It is not possible to address potential complications and risks.

Training and Licensure in Energy-Based Therapies

Given the wide array of therapies that fall under this category, the levels of training vary tremendously from modality to modality.

Alternative Medical Systems

Oriental Medicine and Acupuncture

Acupuncture is a therapeutic intervention that is used in many Asian systems of medicine. It is based on the theory that there are energy channels called meridians that run throughout the body, and that disease results from blockages of this energy. Acupuncture is used as one approach to release these blockages. It involves stimulating specific anatomic points in the body along these meridians by puncturing the skin with a very fine needle (32 gauge or smaller). There are many distinct styles of acupuncture, which include traditional oriental medicine, Japanese manaka style, Korean hand acupuncture, and the Worsley five-element method.

Given the Western, biomedical model, acupuncture is difficult to comprehend. There is, however, an intriguing and growing body of research on this technique. In one study involving stimulation of an acupuncture point located on the lateral aspect of the foot that corresponds to the visual cortex, magnetic resonance imaging detected activity of the visual cortex of the brain equivalent to the activity seen when a light is shone in the eye. No activity was seen when an acupuncture needle was placed 1 cm away from the designated acupuncture point (15). Many of the CAM approaches that claim to have an effect and yet seem to be inconsistent with the biomedical model deserve further investigation.

A 1997 National Institutes of Health Consensus Panel established that there was convincing evidence for the use of acupuncture in the treatment of postoperative dental pain as well as nausea and vomiting (16). Other indications that were considered promising and worthy of more research included headache, low-back pain, stroke, addiction, asthma, premenstrual syndrome, osteoarthritis, carpal tunnel syndrome, and tennis elbow. There is an extensive body of animal research supporting the neurophysiologic effects of acupuncture on the endorphin system.

Complications and Risks

Bruising and minor bleeding are the most common complications of acupuncture and occur in about 2% of all needles placed (17). They rarely require treatment other than local pressure to the needle site. The most significant risk of acupuncture is infection, and cases of hepatitis have been documented when needles were reused. The risk of transmissible infection is eliminated by onetime use of disposable needles, which is now standard practice in the United States. Pneumothorax is the second most significant risk of acupuncture. The needles used are 32 gauge or smaller; therefore, a chest tube usually is not required for treatment.

Training and Licensure

Currently there is no national licensure for acupuncture. Educational requirements for state licensure for acupuncture vary. Forty states either license or register acupuncturists as *doctors of oriental medicine* or *acupuncture physicians*. About two-thirds of these states grant licenses. To get licensed in most states, the practitioner must provide proof that he or she has attended and graduated from an accredited school or from a school that is in the process of being accredited by the Accreditation Commission for Acupuncture and Oriental Medicine (ACAOM) (18). These schools provide 3- or 4-year training programs in oriental medicine. The National Certification Commission for Acupuncture and Oriental Medicine (NCCAOM) administers a standardized examination to test entry-level capabilities in acupuncture that consists of a comprehensive written examination, point location examination, and demonstration of clean needle technique (11). An acupuncturist must pass this examination and meet continuing education requirements every 4 years to retain certification and licensure. In the US, many states adopted this examination as the basis for licensure. Medical doctors can practice acupuncture. Physician acupuncture practitioners may not be as fully trained in the art as nonphysician licensed acupuncturists. To be certified by the American Board of Medical Acupuncture, physicians must take a minimum of 300 hours in training (19).

Homeopathy

Homeopathic medicine is a CAM alternative medical system based on the work of the German physician and chemist Samuel Hahnemann approximately 200 years ago. **In homeopathic medicine, there is a belief in "the law of infinitesimals" and that "like cures like."** Small, highly diluted quantities of medicinal substances are given to cure symptoms when the same substances given at higher or more concentrated doses would actually cause those symptoms.

Naturopathic Medicine

Unlike oriental medicine or homeopathy, naturopathy does not have a long history of traditional use, nor is it based in a comprehensive system. **Naturopathy views disease as a manifestation of alterations in the processes by which the body naturally heals itself and emphasizes health restoration rather than disease treatment.** Naturopathic physicians employ an array of healing practices, including diet and clinical nutrition; homeopathy; acupuncture; herbal medicine; hydrotherapy (the use of water in a range of temperatures and methods of applications); spinal and soft-tissue manipulation; physical therapies involving electric currents, ultrasonography, and light therapy; therapeutic counseling; and pharmacology.

Training and Licensure

There is no national licensure for naturopathy, and licensure at the state level is inconsistent. Only 15 states have licensing laws, and those laws differ considerably. Seven 4-year naturopathic medical schools are accredited by the Council on Naturopathic Medical Education (20). This training focuses on outpatient medicine and does not require a residency. Although the 4-year programs are rigorous, it is possible to get a naturopathic degree online.

Patient Care Issues

The Placebo Effect

The role of the placebo effect in various CAM approaches needs to be further elucidated with rigorous scientific research. Just as with conventional medicine, the effects of certain approaches are more likely than others to be associated with a placebo response. After exposure to a stimulus believed by both the patient and the practitioner to be an active intervention, the body responds physiologically in an equivalent manner. **Approximately one-third of patients in placebo-controlled trials of conventional methods experience a placebo response.** It would be of great value to medicine if the placebo response were better understood and could be activated more reliably in patients. There is no evidence that the placebo response is more active in CAM than in conventional approaches.

Quality Control

Quality control issues in CAM are very challenging for several reasons. First, the market demand is huge and is far ahead of the health care system's ability to address issues of regulation, education, or research. Because CAM, by definition, is inclusive of everything that conventional medicine is not, issues of quality control are extremely difficult. The Federation of State Medical Boards developed the "Model Guidelines for the Use of Complementary and Alternative Therapies in Medical Practice," approved by the House Delegates of the Federation of State Medical Boards of the United States, Inc., as policy in April 2002 (21). The intention of this initiative was to provide guidelines that are clinically responsible, ethically appropriate, and consistent with what state medical boards consider to be within the boundaries of professional practice and accepted standard of care.

Potential Misuse

In addition to physical risks, patients and physicians alike should be aware of other areas of potential misuse. Two areas are of particular concern. First, given that the dollars being spent out of pocket are so significant, there are some products and some providers whose primary motivation is monetary. Patients can spend significant dollars based on false promises or claims. Second, patients can postpone effective therapy or treatment by turning to CAM modalities exclusive of conventional approaches. This time can be significant in the treatment of many patients' diseases. Factors that should increase suspicion for potential misuse are listed in Table 13.6.

The Potential Benefits: Therapeutic Opportunities

Given all of the risks and uncertainties, it is appropriate to ask the question: Why should physicians educate themselves regarding CAM? The most basic answer is commitment to the best practice of medicine. If patients are using therapies that are potentially dangerous in their action or in their interaction, physicians should be aware of this possibility and counsel them accordingly. Physicians have a commitment to offer their patients the best treatment options, regardless of their system of origin. If there are CAM therapies that can benefit patients, the physician should be knowledgeable about them and be willing to discuss them with patients.

In addition to this most fundamental of reasons, there are additional therapeutic opportunities offered by CAM, as shown by the following examples:

Table 13.6 Factors that Should Increase Suspicion for Potential Misuse
1. Providers or products that make claims that are grandiose and dubious, for example; chiropractors who claim to cure insulin-dependent diabetes or offer alternative approaches to cure cancer.
2. Providers or products who foster dependence, for example, therapists who recommend multiple visits per week or frequent visits for an unlimited period.
3. Providers who recommend products that they sell and from which they profit.
4. Providers or products that support the use of alternative approaches exclusive of conventional medicine or conventional providers.

- Decreased harm of interventions: Chiropractic medicine to treat acute low-back pain and potentially avoid surgery; mind–body approaches to decrease anxiety and need for medical management

- Treatment of conditions when conventional approaches fail: Treatment of nausea and vomiting of pregnancy with acupuncture, vitamin B_6, and ginger

- Prevention: Increased intake of isoflavones to potentially decrease the risk of breast cancer

- Improved outcomes: Successful management of menopausal symptoms in patients at risk for breast cancer

Doctor–Patient Interaction

One of the greatest barriers regarding issues of CAM is a lack of communication. As multiple studies show, most patients do not tell their physicians of their use of CAM. Often, this is the case even when the physicians are receptive to the topic. Given the prevalence of use and the potential for interactions with conventional approaches, it is imperative that questions regarding CAM be integrated into the patient history. Many patients simply do not think of sharing this information with their physicians, so direct and specific inquiry is necessary. Many practices incorporate this information in a separate sheet for patients to fill out and for physicians to review and add to the chart. It is useful to know all CAM therapies that patients used in the past or are using presently, particularly anything ingestible. If a patient is seeing a CAM practitioner, it is best to specifically ask if they recommended any supplements or botanicals. Oriental medicine practitioners or acupuncturists, for example, often treat with botanical products or herbal teas. Naturopaths and chiropractors often recommend vitamins and supplements. When patients are asked this history directly in an atmosphere of respect, they usually are very forthcoming, and the most significant barrier is broken.

Three factors contribute to an interesting dynamic that often arises when discussing issues of CAM with patients. This is an area in which (i) very few physicians received formal training, (ii) there is little (albeit increasing) research in the mainstream medical journals, and (iii) there is a tremendous amount of information, of variable quality, in the lay press. All of these factors contribute to a circumstance that often is uncomfortable for physicians. This discomfort is important to recognize because it can contribute to avoidance of the topic altogether. The development of CAM therapies and their integration into the treatment plans is a new and evolving area. It is appropriate to begin the conversation with a patient by explaining that this is new territory in conventional medicine and that you are not an expert. Most patients have assumed this to be the case, appreciate the honesty, and value the opportunity to discuss these dilemmas. This is a significant step in building a trusting and therapeutic relationship with patients interested in CAM.

It is useful to share the following decision tree with patients when making decisions regarding the use of CAM (Fig. 13.1).

Step One: Assess Potential Harm

Although research regarding CAM approaches is often less than optimal, the potential for any therapy to do harm should be thoroughly evaluated (to the best of available knowledge). It is necessary to evaluate the potential to cause both direct harm and indirect harm.

Potential for Direct Harm   This should include any evidence regarding potential harm directly from the therapy or potential interactions. When lacking good evidence, assessment of the invasiveness of the therapy is a strong predictor of risk.

Potential for Indirect Harm   This should include an assessment of potential harm caused by postponing effective treatments, and by financial exploitation. Many CAM approaches are costly, and the patient usually assumes all of the cost. Marketing can prey on vulnerable patients and result in significant and unnecessary expenditures.

Step Two: Assess Potential Benefits

The potential for any approach to be of benefit should be assessed on several levels.

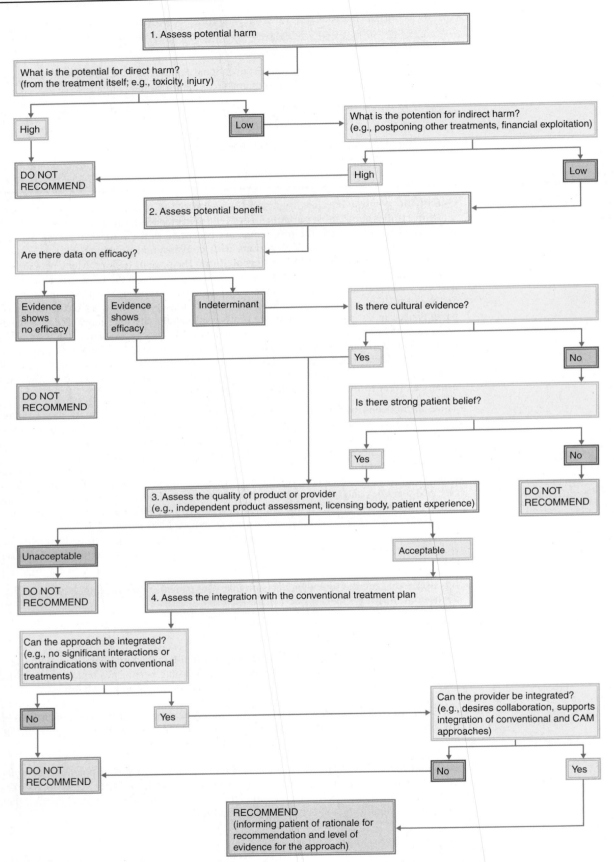

Figure 13.1   **Decision Tree for Integrating Complementary and Alternative Medicine Approaches.**

Scientific Evidence   A review of the peer-reviewed literature should certainly be conducted for evidence of the effectiveness of the approach under consideration.

Cultural Evidence   Another form of useful information is the historic or cultural use of the approach. For example, it is valuable to consider whether a therapy has a long history of use within a given culture. If, on the other hand, the approach has no historic use, this is important to recognize. Examples include the use of black cohosh for menopausal symptoms, which was used for centuries with reported safety and effectiveness, compared with red clover, which has no historic use or track record. Another example would be acupuncture, with thousands of years of use, compared with chelation, which was in use for a relatively short time and is associated with considerable debate regarding its benefit.

Personal Belief   Another part of the assessment of benefit is to recognize the patient's belief system as it pertains to the approach. If the patient has a strong belief in the approach, and there is no evidence of potential harm, it is often reasonable to support its use. Activating a healing response or a placebo effect can often be very therapeutic.

Step Three: Assess the "Delivery System"

When assessing the delivery system, both products and providers must be considered.

Product   Assessing the history of the manufacturing company and understanding its process of quality assurance can be useful. Referral to independent sources for determining the quality of product and accuracy of labeling may be useful.

Provider   It can be difficult to assess the skill level of CAM providers. Inquiring about the education of a given provider and his or her licensing status (if there is a licensing body for the field) is an important place to start. It is useful to talk to other patients who used these services. Finally, one's own sense of a provider is extremely important.

Step Four: Assess the Integration

Although the individual CAM therapy may have no evidence of harm and can be of potential benefit, the way in which it is integrated into the patient's overall treatment plan is important. The same is true for CAM providers.

Approaches   The therapy or approach should be integrated into the overall treatment plan. For example, large doses of antioxidant vitamins should not be used in patients undergoing radiation therapy, as they may counteract the action of the radiation. Likewise, patients with Down syndrome should not undergo chiropractic manipulation.

Providers   Perhaps most importantly, the potential for integration of the providers is essential to assess. If the intention is to offer the patient the best possible care, all providers, conventional and CAM alike, should be assessed for their willingness to integrate their care for the benefit of their patients. If any providers are unsupportive of conventional medicine, it is critical to recognize this and look for a provider who supports integration of care.

It is useful for each physician to recognize his or her own biases about CAM and willingness to learn about the techniques. At a minimum, physicians should know the basics about which CAM approaches may be of benefit to patients and which may be of harm. Familiarity with resources in the community that are more focused on these areas can serve physician and patient alike.

Specific Gynecologic Issues

Menstrual Disorders

Biologically Based Therapies: Supplements and Botanicals

Premenstrual Symptoms

In a recent review of randomized controlled trials of biologically based approaches for premenstrual symptoms (PMS), the authors concluded that data supported the use of calcium for PMS and suggests that vitamin B_6 and chasteberry may be effective (22). Preliminary data revealed some benefit with magnesium, St. John's wort, and vitamin E. There was no benefit in their review of evening primrose oil. A meta-analysis reviewing the data on supplements for dysmenorrheal concluded there was effectiveness for magnesium, vitamin B_1, and vitamin B_6, and data for magnesium was promising (23).

Calcium   Calcium, 900 to 1,200 mg per day in divided doses, has at least some effect on the symptoms of PMS, premenstrual dysphoric disorder, and dysmenorrheal, specifically negative affect (mood swings, depression, tension, anxiety, crying spells), water retention (edema of extremities, breast tenderness, abdominal bloating, headache, fatigue), food cravings (changes in appetite, cravings for sweet or salt), and pain (lower abdominal cramping, generalized aches and pains, low backache) (22). One of the largest studies to date examined the effect of calcium, 1,200 mg per day, and reported a 50% decrease in PMS symptoms (24). In addition, the Women's Health Study showed that higher intakes of calcium and vitamin D may be associated with a lower risk of developing breast cancer in premenopausal women, particularly with more aggressive breast tumors (25).

Vitamin B_6   Vitamin B_6 binds to estrogen and progesterone receptors and was the subject of most of the randomized controlled trials regarding CAM and PMS. Evidence suggests some benefit over placebo for the symptoms of mastalgia, swollen breasts, pain, and depression. Another review of randomized controlled trials indicated that although most of these trials demonstrated some benefit, definite clinical recommendations could not be made (26). While most controlled studies on vitamin B_6 in the treatment of PMS had limited numbers of patients, which makes the evidence of positive effects fairly weak, this is a benign therapy in doses of 100 mg or less and is reasonable to support. Vitamin B_6 for the treatment of dysmenorrheal was more effective at reducing pain than both placebo and a combination of magnesium plus vitamin B_6 (23). It is important to note that peripheral neuropathies can be seen in doses of 200 mg per day or higher, as well as interaction with other medications, specifically anti-Parkinson's disease drugs.

Magnesium   Magnesium has less evidence for efficacy in treating the symptoms of PMS than calcium, although low magnesium levels were reported in women who have PMS. Whereas the evidence is less strong, several studies show a significant decrease in PMS symptoms (27,28). In the three randomized controlled trials, only the study using magnesium pyrrolidone carboxylic acid showed significant effect. One with no effect was limited by only 1 month of supplementation. In research on its effectiveness for dysmenorrheal, magnesium was more effective than placebo for pain relief, and the need for additional medication was less. There was no significant difference in the number of adverse effects experienced (23).

Although more studies are needed to clearly determine effectiveness and which formulation is most efficacious, use of magnesium is reasonable to support clinically and counteracts the constipating effects of calcium. Magnesium can be taken in 200 to 400 mg per day divided doses, either cyclically during the luteal phase or continuously.

Vitamin E   Studies performed in the 1940s suggested that vitamin E might be effective in the treatment of menstrual disorders such as PMS. Recent studies for PMS were mixed. Two randomized controlled trials investigating vitamin E (in d-alpha tocopherol form) showed promising results in the treatment of PMS over placebo (29). A randomized controlled trials studying the effect of vitamin E on dysmenorrhea showed decreases in both severity and duration of pain, as well as blood loss (30). The dosing regimen used was 200 IU twice a day beginning 2 days before the expected menses and continued for the first 3 days of menstruation. It is believed that the mechanism of action of vitamin E is an inhibition of arachidonic acid release with a consequential decrease in prostaglandin formation. Vitamin E with mixed tocopherols at 400 IU per day with meals is considered safe and may be of benefit.

Most controlled studies on vitamin B_6 in the treatment of PMS have limited numbers of patients; therefore, the evidence of positive effects is fairly weak (31). This is a benign therapy in doses of 100 mg or less. A systematic review of nine trials indicated significant benefit over placebo for the symptoms of mastalgia, swollen breasts, pain, and depression (32).

Omega-3 Fatty Acids   There are two major types of omega-3 fatty acids: eicosapentaenoic acid (EPA) and docosahexaenoic acid (DHA). Omega-3 fatty acids act as anti-inflammatory agents in that they shift arachidonic acid metabolism away from prostaglandin $F_{2\alpha}$ ($PgF_{2\alpha}$) and increase levels of the less inflammatory PgE_1. Omega-3 fatty acids are essential foods, and levels are extremely low in the average diet of individuals in the United States. They can be increased through dietary means as well as supplements (Table 13.7). One study looked at essential fatty

Table 13.7 Omega-3 Content of Foods[a]				
All Fish	*ALA (g)*	*EPA (g)*	*DHA (g)*	*Total (g)*
Trout, rainbow	–	0.1	0.4	0.5
Sea bass, Japanese	–	0.1	0.3	0.4
Halibut, Pacific	–	0.1	0.3	0.4
Bass, fresh water	–	0.1	0.2	0.3
Carp	–	0.2	0.1	0.3
Catfish, channel	–	0.1	0.2	0.3
Cod, Atlantic	–	0.1	0.2	0.3
Ocean perch	–	0.2	0.1	0.3
Pike, walleye	–	0.1	0.2	0.3
Flounder	–	0.1	0.1	0.2
Haddock	–	0.1	0.1	0.2
Snapper, red	–	Trace	0.2	0.2
Sole	–	Trace	0.1	0.1
DHA enriched eggs	–	Varied	Varied	–

[a]For general health, individuals should try to consume 7–10 g of omega-3 fatty acids weekly.
Data from United States Department of Agriculture. USDA national nutrient database.
Beltsville, MD: USDA; 2004. Available online at http://www.nal.usda.gov/fnic/foodcomp/search

acids (EFA) and PMS and showed no effect. There are some positive studies looking at the effectiveness of omega-3 fatty acids in treating mild depression with fish oils. This may be a reasonable approach to try if one of the patient's primary symptoms is mood depression (3 g, divided with meals) (33). Side effects are rare, but occasionally patients will experience nausea, diarrhea, belching, or an unpleasant taste in the mouth. Omega-3 fatty acids have an anticoagulant effect and are relatively high in calories.

Chasteberry   Chasteberry (*Vitex agnus-castus*) is a botanical with a long history of use for "menstrual disorders." Many small studies have shown promising results, and one larger study examined the effectiveness of chasteberry on PMDD (34,35). In this randomized controlled trial, the active arm received 20 mg of chasteberry daily. Compared with placebo, the patients receiving chasteberry had a significant improvement in the combined symptom score (35). A multicenter noninterventional trial examined the experience and tolerance of chasteberry in 1,634 patients. After use in three cycles, 93% of women reported a decrease in or cessation of symptoms, and 94% of patients reported good or very good tolerance to this botanical. Adverse drug reactions were suspected by physicians in 1.2% of patients, but there were no serious adverse reactions (36). A randomized, single-blind trial comparing *Vitex* and *fluoxetine* showed equal symptom reduction at 2 months (58% and 68%, respectively) (37). **In both arms, there were significantly improved symptoms. Two of the three randomized controlled trials evaluating chasteberry for PMS showed some benefit on symptoms such as irritability, mood swings, anger, breast tenderness, and headaches. In the study with no benefit, the placebo arm was a soy-based product, which may reduce symptoms of PMS.** Because chasteberry contains iridoids and flavonoids, the mechanism of action is believed to be stimulation of dopamine D_2 receptors, which decrease prolactin levels. *In vitro*, it inhibits opioid, mu, and kappa receptors. It has no effect on luteinizing hormone or follicle-stimulating hormone levels (38). *Vitex* restores progesterone levels and in Germany is used to treat menstrual irregularities and undiagnosed infertility. No significant toxicities were reported with *Vitex* extracts when used in appropriate dosages.

St. John's Wort   St. John's wort (*Hypericum perforatum*) is recognized as an effective antidepressant for the treatment of mild to moderate depression. One open trial of 19 women found that this compound, when used at a dose of 300 mg per day of a 0.3% hypericin standardized extract, showed a 51% improvement in mood disturbances in PMS/PMDD (39). This dose is one-third of that typically used for depression. The most recent randomized controlled trial showed a "nonsignificant trend for SJW to be superior to placebo." This trial did not use a product that contains both active ingredients, namely hypericin and hyperforin (22). Although adverse reactions occur less frequently than with prescription antidepressants, care must be exercised with the use of this product. Most common side effects include gastrointestinal upset, headache, and agitation. Rare but severe phototoxicity was reported. Because St. John's wort induces the cytochrome P450 complex, significant drug interactions can occur. Specifically, reduced levels of birth control pills, *theophylline, cyclosporine,* and antiretroviral drugs were reported. Interactions were described with *buspirone,* statins, calcium channel blockers, *digoxin,* and *carbamazepine.* There are no apparent significant interactions with *Coumadin.* The mechanism of action for its efficacy in the treatment of PMS is not elucidated. There were two isolated reports of pregnancy occurring in women who were taking oral contraceptives in conjunction with St. John's wort. If patients choose to take St. John's wort, they may want to use a backup method of birth control or change to a different method.

Ginkgo Ginkgo (*Ginkgo biloba*) traditionally was used to relieve breast tenderness and discomfort, improve concentration, and enhance sexual function. Its vascular effects, particularly with regard to dementia and peripheral vascular disease, were studied. One large study examined the effectiveness of ginkgo in the treatment of women with PMS and found that after two cycles with treatment, breast symptoms were significantly improved in the ginkgo group. The effectiveness in terms of concentration or libido was not examined (40). In doses ranging from 60 to 240 mg of standardized extract per day, ginkgo showed some clinical efficacy in the treatment of breast pain, tenderness, and fluid retention. In at least one study, ginkgo was effective in the relief of symptoms related to emotional distress (41). Ginkgo is promoted as an agent that can increase libido, but the methodology of these studies was criticized, and further studies are required to better define the botanical's role in these areas. Side effects include gastrointestinal upset and headache. High doses can cause nausea, vomiting, diarrhea, restlessness, or insomnia. Ginkgo has anticoagulant activity, and care must be taken when used with anti-inflammatory drugs and with *warfarin.* The underlying mechanism of action is believed to be dilation of vessels and increased blood flow.

Other products that are used to treat symptoms of PMS and PMDD but are not recommended are listed in Table 13.8.

Dysmenorrhea

Although dysmenorrhea is managed more effectively than PMS and PMDD with conventional approaches, treatment still has a failure rate of approximately 20% to 25%, and many patients seek

Table 13.8 Other Products Often Used to Treat Symptoms of PMS And PMDD (Not Recommended)

- **Tryptophan,** an amino acid that is a precursor of serotonin, has been shown in several trials to improve the symptoms of PMS and PMDD. Impurities in one product made in Japan have been associated with the development of eosinophilia–myalgia syndrome (EMS), which can be fatal. It is unclear if all the cases were related to impurities or if some were related simply to the active ingredients. Until this is clearly understood, tryptophan should be avoided.

- **Dehydroepiandrosterone (DHEA),** a hormone secreted by the adrenal glands and often used for depression, has not been shown to be of benefit in PMS/PMDD.

- **Melatonin,** a hormone that regulates sleep–wake cycles and often is used to prevent jet lag, has been used for the treatment of PMS. There is no evidence of efficacy, and it can worsen depression in some patients.

- **Black cohosh** (*Cimicifuga racemosa*) has been well studied in the treatment of menopausal symptoms, but it has not been studied in the treatment of PMS/PMDD. Although it may prove to be beneficial, data are needed.

- **Evening primrose oil** is frequently used for PMS, but with the exception of cyclic mastalgia, research has failed to show benefit beyond placebo.

- **Dong quai** is an oriental herb often used in combination with other herbs for the treatment of menstrual disorders and menopausal symptoms. Its effectiveness has not been researched.

- **Kava** has been used to treat anxiety and irritability, and several studies have documented its effectiveness. It has, however, been associated with hepatotoxicity, even necessitating liver transplant. It is unclear whether this effect was related to drug or alcohol interactions, contaminants, or the kava itself.

PMS, premenstrual syndrome; PMDD, premenstrual dysphoric disorder.

Table 13.9 Findings on Alternative Treatments

- **Magnesium** Three small trials were included that compared magnesium with placebo. Overall, magnesium was more effective than placebo for pain relief, and the need for additional medication was lessened. There was no significant difference in the number of adverse effects experienced.

- **Vitamin B$_6$** One small trial showed vitamin B$_6$ to be more effective at reducing pain than both placebo and a combination of magnesium and vitamin B$_6$.

- **Vitamin B$_1$** One large trial showed that vitamin B$_1$ was more effective than placebo in reducing pain.

- **Vitamin E** One small trial comparing daily vitamin E with *ibuprofen* taken during menses showed no difference in pain relief.

- **Omega-3 fatty acids** One small trial showed fish oil to be more effective than placebo in pain relief. A number of studies have found that the intake of marine origin omega-3 fatty acids (such as salmon and sardines) decrease symptoms of dysmenorrhea. Given the established benefits of omega-3 fatty acids in other conditions such as heart disease, high intake of these compounds can be recommended throughout the cycle.

Adapted from **Proctor ML, Murphy PA.** Herbal and dietary therapies for primary and secondary dysmenorrhea. *Cochrane Database Syst Rev* 2001;3:CD002124.

alternatives. Table 13.9 lists findings by a Cochrane review study on alternative treatments. **The review concluded that vitamin B$_1$ is effective in the treatment of dysmenorrhea when taken at 100 mg daily, although this finding is based on only one large randomized controlled trial** (23). The results further suggested that magnesium is a promising treatment, but it is unclear what dose or treatment regimen should be used (23). The addition of fish oils showed promising results. The concentration of omega-6 fatty acid derived eicosanoids such as PgE$_2$ are elevated during menstruation in women who experience dysmenorrhea. Dysmenorrhea was associated with low dietary intake of omega-3 fatty acids. Several studies showed supplementation to be effective in the management of dysmenorrheal (42). Krill omega-3 phospholipids, which contain phosphatidylcholine with DHA/EDA, outperformed conventional fish oil DHA/EDP in double blind studies on PMS and dysmenorrhea (43). Given the established benefits of omega-3 fatty acids in other conditions, such as heart disease, high intake of these compounds can be recommended throughout the menstrual cycle.

Manipulative and Body-Based Methods

Premenstrual Symptoms

Massage relieves anxiety, sadness, and pain immediately after the therapy, but it does not reduce symptoms of PMS/PMDD overall.

There is no evidence to support the effectiveness of chiropractic manipulation in these conditions. One small (N = 25) placebo-controlled crossover study showed the group receiving chiropractic treatment had a significant improvement in symptoms, but the group that received placebo first improved over baseline with the placebo and experienced no further improvement when they received the active treatment (44).

Dysmenorrhea

A Cochrane review of the use of spinal manipulation for primary and secondary dysmenorrhea concluded that overall there is no evidence to suggest that spinal manipulation is effective in the treatment of primary or secondary dysmenorrhea. In four trials, high-velocity, low-amplitude manipulation was no more effective than sham manipulation, although it was possibly better than no treatment (45). Three of the smaller trials indicated a difference in favor of the manipulation; the one trial with sufficient sample size found no difference. There was no difference in adverse effects between the two groups (45).

Mind–Body Interventions

Relaxation techniques showed some very promising results for women with PMS/PMDD. One study examined the effect of the relaxation response for 15 minutes, twice a day, for 3 months, compared with women who read for the same amount of time, and women who charted their symptoms. Of women in the relaxation response group, 58% experienced improvement in their symptoms, compared with 27% for the reading group, and 17% for the charting group (46). Given that there are many other health benefits to the relaxation response, with no cost and no risk, it is a good technique to recommend to patients. Cognitive-behavioral therapy (CBT) and group therapy were of benefit in several small studies. In one study, CBT was effective in reducing psychological and somatic symptoms and impairment of functioning when compared to controls. In two additional studies, the authors found that CBT reduced PMS symptoms compared to the control group (47).

Alternative Medical Systems

Oriental Medicine and Acupuncture

Oriental medicine and acupuncture were used traditionally for thousands of years for myriad menstrual symptoms, PMS and PMDD among them. The effectiveness in this domain is not well studied. In one small study (n = 35), there was a 78% reduction in PMS symptoms in the acupuncture arm compared to 6% in the placebo arm (48). There were studies showing the effectiveness of acupuncture in the treatment of mild depression and generalized anxiety, although not all results were positive. There was a Cochrane review on the use of Chinese herbal medicine on PMS, and one on dysmenorrheal. In the review on PMS, the efficacy of Chinese herbal preparations, a randomized controlled trial of Jingqianping showed significant reductions in eliminations of symptoms (49).

There was one small but methodologically sound trial of acupuncture in the treatment of primary dysmenorrhea. This trial followed 43 women for 1 year and showed significant effectiveness of acupuncture when compared with placebo (91% of women showed improvement, compared with 10% to 36%, 18%, and 10% in the other groups) (23). In a study that randomized 201 patients, acupuncture improved dysmenorrheal and quality of life compared to usual care (50). In addition, there is some preliminary evidence that acupressure can be an effective, cost-free, and safe therapy for menstrual pain and anxiety. The study taught patients to self-administer 20 minutes of acupressure on Sanyinjian (SP6), which is an acupressure point located above the ankle. In a review on Chinese herbal presentations and their effectiveness on dysmenorrhea, 39 randomized controlled trials were included, involving 3,475 women. Chinese herbal medicine resulted in pain relief, and a decrease in overall symptoms and use of additional medications when compared to the use of pharmaceutical drugs. Individualized Chinese formulations resulted in significant improvement when compared to Chinese health products. Chinese herbal medicine produced better pain relief than acupuncture (51). More research is needed, but this is a promising and safe modality, and if a woman is fully informed and interested in pursing these approaches and has access to a qualified provider, it is appropriate to support.

Homeopathy

The use of homeopathy in the treatment of PMS and PMDD is not well studied, and neither is its effectiveness in the treatment of related disorders such as depression or anxiety. One study did claim positive results but was fairly weak in design and in showing improvement (46). In one small but well-done study on individualized homeopathic remedies, 90% of patients had at least 30% improvement in their symptoms, compared to 37.5% having that degree of improvement in the placebo arm (47).

Infertility

Mind–Body Interventions

Mind–body approaches are of particular interest in the infertility patient. The treatments for infertility stress inducing, and increased stress is associated with decreased fertility (and increased risk of such things as gestational diabetes, preterm labor and delivery, and prolonged labor).

In a study of infertility patients, two group psychological interventions were compared with routine care. The two groups who received group support and cognitive behavioral therapy had fertility rates of 54% and 55%, respectively, compared with the control group, which had a pregnancy rate of 20%. There were large and disparate dropout rates, which complicate the interpretation of these results (52). In Austria, physicians are required to prescribe psychotherapeutic therapy for every patient undergoing assisted reproductive techniques. These approaches include psychotherapy, hypnotherapy, relaxation, and physical perception exercises. A review of its success associated with pregnancy rates found that of the 1,156 women, the cumulative pregnancy rate of those who utilized the mind–body techniques was 56% and in those who intended to use these approaches were 41.9%, higher than those who refused (53). In a case control study examining the impact of hypnosis on pregnancy rate in *in vitro* fertilization (IVF), the pregnancy rate in those cycles where hypnosis was used was 53% versus 28% in the controls, and the implantation rate 30% versus 14% (54).

Mind–body therapies, such as relaxation techniques and hypnosis, are reasonable to recommend to relieve a wide variety of issues that can arise with infertility patients.

Alternative Medical Systems

The use of acupuncture was studied in the treatment of infertility and overall shows promise. Auricular acupuncture was studied as an alternative therapy for female infertility secondary to oligomenorrhea or luteal insufficiency, and the authors concluded it was a valuable therapy (55). Another study used electroacupuncture in anovulatory women with polycystic ovarian syndrome and found that regular ovulation was induced in more than one-third of the women. After early positive results, there were several recent studies on acupuncture and IVF. In a study of 228 women examining acupuncture and IVF, while the difference did not reach statistical significance, the pregnancy rate in the acupuncture arm was 31% versus 23% in the control arm, and ongoing pregnancy rates at 18 weeks gestation was 28% versus 18% (56). In a randomized controlled trial of 225, women undergoing IVF or intracytoplasmic sperm injection (ICSI) with acupuncture had clinical pregnancy rates of 33.6% versus 15.6% in the control group, and ongoing pregnancy rates of 28.4% versus 13.8% (57). In a trial of 182 women comparing usual care versus acupuncture 25 minutes before and after embryo transfer versus acupuncture before and after transfer and 2 days after the transfer, there was again a significant increase in pregnancy rates with acupuncture, but no additional benefit was found in the patients who also received acupuncture 2 days after transfer. The clinical pregnancy rates in the acupuncture group were 39% versus 26% in the controls, and the ongoing pregnancy rate was 36% versus 22% (58).

In a randomized controlled trial comparing usual care to usual care plus 25 minutes of a standard acupuncture treatment pre- and postembryo transfer, the pregnancy rates were 43% in the intervention arm as opposed to 26% in the control arm (59). In a meta-analysis including seven trials and 1,366 women, the authors concluded that the evidence suggests that embryo transfer done with acupuncture improved pregnancy rates and live births among women undergoing IVF (60). At the same time, a meta-analysis including 13 trials and 2,500 women concluded there was not sufficient evidence to conclude that acupuncture improves IVF clinical pregnancy rates (61). The acupuncture protocols are typically designed to promote sedation, uterine relaxation, and increased uterine blood flow. The basis for the effect of acupuncture is hypothesized to be potentially related to modulating neuroendocrinological factors, increases in uterine and ovarian blood flow, modulating cytokines, and reducing stress, anxiety or depression. Blood flow impedance in uterine arteries, measured as the pulsatility index, was considered useful in assessing endometrial receptivity to embryo transfer. A study was performed assessing the effect of electroacupuncture on the pulsatility index of infertile women. After treatment twice a week for 4 weeks, the mean pulsatility index was significantly reduced both shortly after the last treatment and also 10 to 14 days after the treatments. The skin temperature of the forehead was increased significantly, suggesting a central inhibition of sympathetic activity (62). In a study of women undergoing IVF, the women who received acupuncture had increased cortisol levels and increased prolactin levels when compared to the controls, trending toward more normal cycle dynamics (63). More studies are needed both in the efficacy of acupuncture and infertility and in the mechanisms of action. Clinically speaking, there is provocative evidence that acupuncture appears safe in early pregnancy and is reasonable to support if patients are interested.

Menopause

Before the release of the results of the Women's Health Initiative, 80% of women in the United States were using "nonprescriptive therapies" to help manage their menopausal symptoms, and many of these therapies were CAM approaches. In a study examining the use of CAM during menopause, a group of 3,302 women were followed across 6 years, and 80% of them used some form of CAM (64). In a study examining women's treatment choices after discontinuing hormone therapy (HT), 76% of women reported using nonhormonal alternative therapies, and of these 68% found them helpful (65). In a study exploring women's beliefs about "natural hormones," women using compounding pharmacies believed that compared with standard hormones, natural hormones are safer, cause fewer side effects, and are equally or more effective for symptom relief. Many women believed natural hormone therapy was equally or more effective for long-term protection of bones and lipid levels (66). It is reasonable to assume that women are exploring and choosing such therapies in ever increasing numbers, often without being accurately or fully informed. This expanded market generates more products and promotion of alternatives. It is imperative that physicians be informed about these options so they can help patients make medically sound choices.

Biologically Based Therapies

The list of botanicals promoted and used for the treatment of menopausal symptoms is extensive. Following is a review of the products most commonly used and recommended based on research evidence.

Vitamin E

Since the 1940s, vitamin E has been studied for the treatment of hot flashes. Although some early studies showed promising results, other studies evaluating 200- to 600-IU doses failed to show an effect. There was one small trial with 51 women that showed an effect on hot flashes of 400 IU daily, but it was suggested that up to 1,200 IU may be necessary to have an effect, doses which are too high to recommend. Vitamin E is an anticoagulant, and spontaneous subarachnoid hemorrhages were reported. One study examining vitamin E in menopausal patients with breast cancer found that after 4 weeks of 800 IU daily, the patients in the treatment arm had on average one less hot flash per day. Although this finding was statistically significant, it was not significant clinically (67).

Black Cohosh

Premenstrual Symptoms and Menopause   Black cohosh (*Cimicifuga racemosa*) has traditionally been used for relief of both PMS and menopause symptoms. It has been used in the Native American population for centuries and in Germany since 1950. Its most studied form is a brand called *Remifemin,* which is standardized to 1 mg of *deoxyactein* and is administered in a dose of 40 mg two times daily. Most early studies were uncontrolled, but later studies were more methodologically sound. Initially, it was felt that black cohosh decreased luteinizing hormone levels, but it is believed that it may behave like a selective estrogen receptor modulator (SERM), and act at serotonin receptors. It does not contain phytoestrogens and does not have an estrogenic effect on vaginal cytology. Additionally, there are no changes in hormone levels in women taking black cohosh. In laboratory studies, black cohosh actually suppresses rather than stimulates breast cells (68). Women taking black cohosh show significant improvement in menopausal symptoms, anxiety, and vaginal epithelium. It is well tolerated with no side effects noted. When compared with hormone therapy, black cohosh has comparable results, and women show improvements in hot flashes, fatigue, irritability, and vaginal dryness. In a meta-analysis of randomized controlled trials of black cohosh, the authors concluded that there was a trend in reducing vasomotor symptoms. One study of 304 women demonstrated a decrease in the number and intensity of hot flashes, improvement in mood, sleep, sweating, and sexual disorders. In a double-blind, placebo-controlled trial, black cohosh, 40 mg, was compared with conjugated estrogen, 0.6 mg, and placebo (69). The researchers monitored 62 women for 3 months and black cohosh was found to have effects equal to conjugated estrogen and to be superior to placebo in decreasing climacteric symptoms. Black cohosh had no effect on endometrial thickening as measured by vaginal ultrasonography, unlike conjugated estrogen, which had a significant increase in endometrial thickening. Additionally, both black cohosh and conjugated estrogen increased the vaginal superficial cells. In a trial comparing black cohosh to placebo and to estrogen over 12 months, black cohosh was found to be effective (70). In a large-scale, controlled, observational study of black cohosh alone and black cohosh in combination with St. John's wort involving 6,141 women, both therapies were effective and well tolerated. For psychological symptoms, the combination was superior to black cohosh alone (71). Although many published studies have design weaknesses and more research is needed, black cohosh appears to be safe and may be efficacious for the treatment of menopausal symptoms. It should be started at 20 to 40 mg twice daily, standardized to 2.5 triterpenes The Commission E recommends 40 to 200 mg (72).

Patients should be informed that it might take 4 to 8 weeks to feel an effect. Side effects are rare and include gastrointestinal upset, headache, and dizziness. While the longest study in the literature lasted 12 months, there is no indication that longer use is unsafe.

Breast Cancer Multiple studies showed that black cohosh has an inhibitory effect on estrogen receptor breast cancer cells. One study showed augmentation of the antiproliferative effects of *tamoxifen*. In a study that looked at the effectiveness of black cohosh in reducing menopausal symptoms for breast cancer patients, both the placebo group and the group receiving black cohosh had a 27% reduction in the number and intensity of hot flashes. Only sweating was significantly more improved in the black cohosh arm (73). In another study, 136 breast cancer survivors were randomized either to *tamoxifen* alone or *tamoxifen* plus black cohosh. At 6 months, there were no significant differences, but at 1 year, 47% of women in the intervention arm versus none in the control group were free of hot flashes. Severe hot flashes were reduced in the intervention arm (24%) compared with the *tamoxifen*-alone arm (74%) (74). Although it is useful to know that black cohosh is not estrogenic, its efficacy in this group of patients is not established.

Ginseng

Many different botanicals use the name *ginseng*. The two most common are Siberian ginseng (*Eleuthero*) and oriental or Korean ginseng (*Panax*). Both of these agents are extracted from the root of their respective plants, and both are used to combat fatigue or to restore "vital force" for performance enhancement.

Panax ginseng is a small perennial that grows in northeast Asia. One study of 12 patients examined its effect on menopausal women, both with and without the symptoms of fatigue, insomnia, and depression. At baseline, the patients with symptoms had significantly higher anxiety states. The dehydroepiandrosterone-sulfate was one-half that of those in the control group, and the cortisol/dehydroepiandrosterone-sulfate ratio was significantly higher in the symptomatic patients. After treatment, the Cornell Medical Index and anxiety state decreased to that of the controls, and the cortisol/dehydroepiandrosterone-sulfate ratio decreased significantly, although not to the level of the control group (75).

In terms of the physiologic symptoms, a randomized, multicenter, double-blind parallel group study compared a standard ginseng extract with placebo. Quality of life and physiologic parameters were assessed at baseline and after 16 weeks of treatment. There was no significant difference in symptom relief and no significant difference in the physiologic parameters of follicle-stimulating hormone, estradiol, endometrial thickening, maturity index, or vaginal pH. Patients did experience significant improvement in depression, sense of well-being, and health (76). A second study demonstrated improvement in fatigue, insomnia, mood, and depression (70).

There is no evidence to support the use of ginseng for relief of physiologic symptoms. If patients are suffering from psychological symptoms of menopause, they may benefit from *Panax* ginseng. Although its mechanism of action is not clear, *Panax* ginseng does not appear to be estrogenic. Use of *Panax* ginseng should be avoided with stimulants, and it may cause headaches, breast pain, diarrhea, or bleeding. The recommended dose is 100 mg of a standardized extract two times daily for 3 of 4 weeks.

The estrogenic effect of black cohosh, dong quai, ginseng, and licorice root was evaluated by (i) an examination of the effect on cell proliferation of MCF-7 cells (a human breast cancer cell line), (ii) transient gene expression assay, and (iii) a bioassay in mice. The authors concluded that dong quai and ginseng stimulate growth of MCF-7 cells independent of estrogenic activity, and that black cohosh and licorice root do not have estrogenic activity or stimulate the breast cell line (68).

Red Clover

Red clover (*Trifolium pratense*) is a member of the legume family, with brand names including *Promensil* and *Rimostil*. It contains at least four estrogenic isoflavones and is promoted as a source of phytoestrogens. Red clover is a medicinal herb with no traditional long-term use in menopause. Its estrogenic effects were first discovered by observing its effects on sheep. The term *Clover syndrome* is used to describe the symptoms frequently seen in sheep that consume large amounts of red clover. **This syndrome is characterized by reproductive complications, including infertility.** Despite its presumed estrogenic activity, several studies, including two double-blind, placebo-controlled trials, failed to show an effect over placebo in the treatment of menopausal symptoms (77). A number of meta-analyses concluded that overall red clover was not clinically better than placebo for relief of vasomotor symptoms (70). In a trial involving 252 women, two red clover supplements were compared with placebo across 12 weeks (*Promensil*, containing 82 mg isoflavones, and *Rimostil*, containing 57 mg isoflavones) (78). Although *Promensil* did reduce hot flashes more quickly than *Rimostil* or placebo, all three groups had the same reduction of hot flashes at the end of 12 weeks. Another large trial of 205 women had similar results. While this does supply some evidence for a biological effect of *Promensil*, neither of the red clover supplements had a clinically significant effect when compared with placebo. Its effect on the endometrium must be further delineated.

Red clover has no clear demonstrable effect, it is believed to be estrogenic, and its effect on the breast and endometrium is not adequately studied. Coumarins are present in some clover species.

Dong Quai

Dong quai (*Angelica sinensis*) has a long history of traditional use in menopause and in the treatment of menstrual problems. Traditionally, in the oriental system of medicine, it is used in combination with other botanicals. Several studies of the effectiveness of dong quai in treating the symptoms of menopause failed to show its effectiveness (79). No evidence exists to support the use of dong quai as a single agent in the treatment of menopausal symptoms. The use of dong quai in combination with other herbs, as is done traditionally, is not well studied. It is important to note that dong quai contains coumarin derivatives.

Kava

Kava (*Piper methysticum*) is native to the South Pacific, and one of its traditional uses is to reduce anxiety. It is often recommended for menopausal symptoms, particularly irritability, insomnia, and anxiety. Studies showed that 100 to 200 mg, three times daily, standardized to 30% kavalactones, decreases irritability and insomnia associated with menopause. It often is used in combination with other components, such as black cohosh and valerian, for the management of menopausal symptoms. One study that examined the use of kava in addition to hormone therapy for the treatment of anxiety showed that the combined use resulted in a significant decrease in anxiety when compared with hormone therapy alone (80).

Kava has the potential for significant, albeit rare, side effects. Cases of hepatotoxicity severe enough to require transplant were reported (81). Other side effects include dermatitis, and a movement disorder similar to Parkinson's disease but reversible. It was removed from many European markets. The use of kava is not recommended, but if patients are using this botanical (which is available over the counter), they should be informed of the risks, and advised to avoid taking kava in conjunction with other anxiety-reducing agents, with alcohol, or *acetaminophen*, and have liver function tests performed periodically.

St. John's Wort

The leaves and the tips of the flowers of the plant St. John's wort (*Hypericum perforatum*) have been used medicinally, primarily as an antidepressant. It is used for anxiety, and in Germany, it is used to treat menopausal mood swings.

Although its mechanism of action is unclear, St. John's wort does appear to be beneficial in relieving mild to moderate depression, with 60% improvement in mood, energy, and sleep with a dose of 300 mg three times daily. Standardization is controversial, but it is believed to have at least two active ingredients, namely hypericin and hyperforin. Most research was done on products standardized to 0.3% hypericin. The first trial to examine its use for menopausal symptoms was done in 1999. Patients not taking hormone therapy were given 300 mg of St. John's wort three times daily, and symptoms were evaluated at baseline and at 5, 8, and 12 weeks by both the patients and physicians. At baseline, 80% to 90% of all symptoms were moderate to marked in severity. By 12 weeks, 20% to 30% remained at this level, whereas most patients had only slight symptoms or were symptom free. There was no change in vasomotor symptoms; 80% of patients reported that their sexuality was substantially enhanced. Of 106 patients, 4 reported adverse effects. These effects included skin rash with sun exposure, gastrointestinal upset, headache, and fatigue (82). In a randomized trial of 301 women using a combination of black cohosh and St. John's wort, the treatment was superior to placebo for both climacteric and psychological symptoms

(83). St. John's wort induces the cytochrome P450 complex. Specifically, lower levels of oral contraceptives, *theophylline, cyclosporine,* and antiretroviral drugs were reported. Interactions were described with *buspirone,* statins, calcium channel blockers, *digoxin,* and *carbamazepine.* There are no apparent significant interactions with *Coumadin.*

Chasteberry

Chasteberry (*Vitex agnes*) has a long history of uses by civilizations ranging from Greeks to the monks of medieval times. Among the uses is treatment of menopausal symptoms. Although its use was recommended for this indication, the efficacy of chasteberry in menopause is not demonstrated.

Ginkgo Biloba

Ginkgo biloba is often promoted for the improvement of libido in menopausal women. Muira puama plus ginkgo had a significant effect in 65% of the patients in one study (84). Side effects include gastrointestinal upset and headaches, and drug interactions can occur with estrogens, statins, and calcium channel blockers. Ginkgo has an anticoagulant effect.

Phytoestrogens

Phytoestrogens are plant-based compounds that have weak estrogenic activity. They appear to have SERM activity with modest agonist effect at the beta estrogen receptor. Phytoestrogens are categorized as isoflavones, coumestans, lignans, or flavonoids. The most promoted of these groups is isoflavones, which are genistein, daidzein, or glycitein. Soybeans and soy products are a rich source of isoflavones. Several reviews and meta-analyses found mixed results on menopausal symptoms (70,85). Women who want to consume phytoestrogens should do so through food products rather than supplements, and should aim for 100 mg of isoflavones a day, or 25 g of soy protein. One randomized controlled trial of 366 women demonstrated endometrial hyperplasia in 3.8% of women who consumed 150 mg per day of isoflavones for 5 years versus 0% in the placebo arm (85).

Mind–Body Interventions

Mind–body therapies for the treatment of menopausal symptoms were studied in several domains, but the trials are often small and not always high quality. In a small prospective trial of 30 women, applied relaxation was compared to *estradiol*. The women in the relaxation group had a 76% reduction in hot flashes at 6-month follow-up versus 90% in the *estradiol* arm, which was reached at 12 weeks (86). In another study by Nedstrand et al., 38 women with breast cancer showed improvement in vasomotor symptoms with both applied relaxation and electro-acupuncture (86). In one randomized controlled trial, symptomatic menopausal patients who had at least five hot flashes per 24 hours were randomized to either the relaxation response, to reading, or to a control group. The relaxation response group had significant reductions in hot flash intensity, tension–anxiety levels, and depression compared with the control group, which had no significant changes (87). In another randomized controlled trial of symptomatic menopausal patients, women with frequent hot flashes were randomized to paced respiration, muscle relaxation, and alpha-wave feedback. In the paced respiration group, there was significant reduction in the hot flash frequency, whereas muscle relaxation and biofeedback showed no differences. The proposed mechanism of action is decreased central sympathetic activity (88). In a trial with 76 breast cancer patients, an intervention of counseling and emotional support was associated with an improvement in both menopausal symptoms and sexual function compared to the control arm (89). In a trial of 102 women the effect of acupuncture, applied relaxation, estrogens, and placebo were examined. Both acupuncture and applied relaxation reduced the number of hot flashes significantly better than placebo (90).

Insomnia, which is another frequent symptom of menopause, is a complex, multifactorial problem. Optimal treatment is described as incorporating the following components: stress management, coping strategies, enhancement of relationships, and lifestyle changes that facilitate sleep (91).

Overall, mind–body techniques are a low- or no-cost, low-risk intervention that can decrease central nervous system adrenergic tone. They are reported to decrease hot flashes and other menopausal symptoms, and provide general health benefits.

Alternative Medical Systems

Oriental medicine was used for more than 2,500 years and includes treatment with acupuncture, herbs, and movement. Although diagnosis and treatment are highly individualized, from the perspective of oriental medicine, menopause is often associated with deficiencies in qi, blood, and jing. Acupuncture is one of the best-studied CAM modalities, but more studies of higher quality are needed regarding its application to the menopausal patient. The existing studies on acupuncture and menopausal symptoms are mixed. In a systematic review, which included 11 trials and 763 women, concluded that while some studies showed greater benefit with acupuncture than hormone therapy for reducing vasomotor symptoms, many showed no benefit (92). Another systematic review drew the same conclusions (93). In a randomized controlled trial of 267 women comparing individualized acupuncture plus self-care to self-care alone, both the frequency and the intensity of hot flashes significantly decreased in the acupuncture arm. Overall, this group had significant improvement in vasomotor, sleep, and somatic symptoms (94). One uncontrolled study, which explored the experience of more than 300 women, found that 97% of women reported that acupuncture improved their symptoms, and 51% reported being symptom free (95). In a pilot study looking at the use of acupuncture in patients being treated with *tamoxifen,* 15 patients were followed for 6 months (96). Patients were evaluated before and after 1, 3, and 6 months of treatment. There was significant improvement in anxiety, depression, and somatic and vasomotor symptoms. Libido was not affected. A study with 45 women with breast cancer found significantly decreased hot flashes with electroacupuncture (97). This is a promising area for those patients whose options for treatment of these symptoms are limited.

In the hands of a competent practitioner, acupuncture is a safe CAM modality. If menopausal patients are interested in exploring this technique as part of their plan for managing symptoms and understand the lack of comprehensive studies, it is reasonable to support a trial of acupuncture with a qualified practitioner. Because many of the herbal treatments in oriental medicine can be estrogenic, it is best to avoid them if the patient is taking any form of hormonal therapy.

"Natural" Hormones

There is increasing confusion around the myriad hormonal options for patients. Because many hormonally active compounds are available over the counter, physician awareness about these issues is essential, especially in light of the findings of the Women's Health Initiative and the large number of women seeking "alternatives."

Natural versus Bioidentical Hormones

There is a dominant belief in the culture that natural is "good" and synthetic is "bad." A natural product is any product with principal ingredients that are of animal, mineral, or vegetable origins. Natural products may have no resemblance to the ingredients in their natural state. For example, conjugated equine estrogens are natural products. They do not resemble anything natural or native to the human body. It is useful to make this distinction with patients. Very often patients requesting "natural hormones" are uncertain about what they are actually requesting. Most patients, when using this term, are looking for bioidentical hormones, or hormones that are molecularly identical to the hormones their ovaries produce.

The ovaries produce three types of estrogen: 17 beta-estradiol, estrone, and estriol. Premenopausally, the predominant estrogen produced by the ovary is 17-beta estradiol, or E_2. It is converted back and forth to estrone, E_1, which is made in the fat and is the predominant estrogen postmenopausally. All of the patches, and several oral formulations such as *Estrace,* are E_2. When E_2 is taken orally, much of it is converted to E_1 in the gut. E_1 and E_2 essentially are equivalent in their level of estrogenic activity. Estriol, E_3, is the weakest of the three estrogens and is predominantly made in the placenta during pregnancy. It is not conventionally prescribed and is available only through compounding pharmacies. *Estriol* is the predominant form of estrogen in *Tri-Est* and *Bi-Est. Estriol, Tri-est,* and *Bi-est* are frequently used and recommended by the alternative medicine community.

Conjugated equine estrogens are composed of more than 10 different molecules extracted from the urine of pregnant mares. This is a natural product but is not bioidentical or native. In addition to animal conjugated equine estrogen, a synthetic version, such as *Cenestin,* is available.

It is difficult to draw conclusions regarding options for the use of these hormones. The reasons for this are listed in Table 13.10.

Table 13.10 Reasons for Difficulty in Drawing Conclusions Regarding Use of Hormones

Drawing conclusions regarding options for the use of these hormones is challenging for a variety of reasons:

1. **It is essential to reinforce to patients that all hormones are not created equal.** Different hormones have different effects. For example, *estriol* is often promoted as a hormone that does everything that conjugated equine estrogen does but with none of the risks. Given that it is a significantly weaker estrogen than conjugated equine estrogen, this is dubious and is not based in scientific evidence.

2. **Native or bioidentical hormones are rarely included in research protocols.** The Women's Health Initiative studied only conjugated equine estrogen (*Premarin*) and MPA (*Provera*). The Postmenopausal Estrogen-Progestin Intervention (PEPI) used only conjugated equine estrogen, but did compare it with micronized *progesterone* (and showed micronized *progesterone* to be as effective as *medroxyprogesterone acetate* at protecting the endometrium and better than *medroxyprogesterone acetate* at protecting the lipid benefits of estrogen).

3. **All forms of hormone therapy frequently are clumped together as one entity.** The distinctions between the types of hormones studied are rarely made in the media and often not clear even in the medical literature. The coverage of the Women's Health Initiative is a perfect example, as the media generalized its findings to hormone therapy, and even most information released by and for doctors did not clarify that the findings were regarding one specific form of estrogen combined with one specific form of progestin.

Bioidentical Hormones

Progestins   Bioidentical *progesterone* is available either through compounding pharmacies or through retail pharmacies as micronized *progesterone*, natural *progesterone*, or *progesterone* USP (brand name *Prometrium*). *Medroxyprogesterone acetate* (MPA) is a nonbioidentical progestin (i.e., its molecular structure is foreign to the body).

Bioidentical Estrogens E_2, or 17 beta-estradiol, often is used interchangeably with *conjugated equine estrogen*. It is effective in relieving vasomotor symptoms, helps maintain bone, and improves the lipid profile. It is most bioidentical when delivered in the form of the patch because its oral form is converted to estrone in the gut. (The patch bypasses the liver and is not as beneficial in its effects on high-density lipoprotein and low-density lipoprotein, but it increases triglycerides to a lesser extent.) No comprehensive long-term data regarding its use are available.

Estriol, or E_3, the weakest of the estrogens that occurs naturally only in high circulating levels during pregnancy, is very popular in the alternative community. It is often promoted as the ideal estrogen, a natural alternative providing all of the benefits of hormone therapy with none of the risks. This assumption is not supported by the literature, as the research on *estriol* is limited. In one study examining the use of *estriol* over 12 months, 53 women were given 2 mg daily. They reported good symptom relief and satisfaction, and histologic evaluation of the endometrium revealed no hyperplasia or atypia. Bone mineral density showed no change (98). In another study examining the effect of *estriol*, 64 women were followed for 24 months. There were four treatment arms: 2.0 mg E_3 plus 2.5 mg *medroxyprogesterone acetate*, 0.625 mg of *conjugated estrogen* plus 2.5 mg *medroxyprogesterone acetate*, 1 μg of 1-alpha hydroxy vitamin D_3, and 1.8 g calcium lactate containing 250 mg of elemental calcium. Outcome measures were taken at baseline, 6, 12, 18, and 24 months, and included the following assessments: bone mineral density at third lumbar vertebrae, serum levels of osteocalcin, total alkaline phosphatase, and urinary ratios of calcium/creatinine and hydroxyproline/creatinine. The findings revealed decreased bone mineral density in the vitamin D and calcium groups and no decrease in the *conjugated estrogen* and E_3 groups. Osteocalcin and alkaline phosphate was decreased or without change in the conjugated estrogen and E_3 groups, and was increased in the vitamin D_3 and calcium groups. Urinary calcium/creatinine ratios were decreased with E_3 and conjugated estrogen, and there was no decrease with the use of vitamin D_3 and calcium. Urinary hydroxyproline/creatinine ratios were decreased in the conjugated estrogen group, unchanged in the E_3 and vitamin D_3 groups, and increased in the calcium group. Uterine bleeding was significantly less in the E_3 group compared with the conjugated estrogen group, with 2.4 days compared with 13 days per person. In conclusion, the study supported the finding that a bone-preserving effect occurred with E_3 when compared with *conjugated estrogen* (99).

It was proposed that *estriol* might have anticarcinogenic activity. Unlike *estradiol, estriol* is not carcinogenic in rodent models, reduces uterine growth, and enhances phagocytic activity. After one or more pregnancy, *estriol* excretion significantly increases in comparison with nulliparous women. This may or may not be linked to the increased risk of breast and ovarian cancer in nulliparous women. In a study following over 84,000 Finnish women, oral and transdermal estradiol was associated with a slightly increased risk of breast cancer (2 to 3 additional cases per 1,000 women across 10 years), while oral estriol and vaginal estrogens were not associated with an increased risk (100).

Oral *estriol* appears to provide symptom relief and to stimulate breast and endometrial tissue less than estradiol (101). It may prove to have mildly beneficial effects on bone. It appears to exert estrogenic effects on the endometrium and to have no effect or mild effects on lipids. No clinical interventional trials exist on the effect of oral *estriol* use on the breast.

Tri-est and Bi-est   *Tri-est* and *Bi-est* are formulations in which the predominant *estrogen* is *estriol*. The typical formulations contain 80% *estriol*. Typically *Tri-est* contains 2 mg of *estriol*, 0.25 mg of *estradiol*, and 0.25 mg of *estrone*, and *Bi-est* contains 2 mg of *estriol* and 0.5 mg of *estradiol*. It should be noted that these names refer only to the types of *estrogen* used, and the specific amounts of each can vary. These particular formulations are often marketed as the most "natural" form of estrogen therapy because they contain either two or all three forms of naturally occurring estrogens. The following factors should be noted:

- *Tri-est* and *Bi-est* are not formulated in naturally occurring ratios or quantities.

- Although *Tri-est* and *Bi-est* are only 20% E_2 or E_2 plus E_3, the dose of these more potent estrogens are significant (i.e., 0.5 mg).

- Although a certain combination of $E_1/E_2/E_3$ may prove to have benefits over other forms of hormone therapy and should be explored, this research does not exist.

Estriol Vaginal Cream   *Estriol* vaginal cream was studied in women who had recurrent urinary tract infections. This randomized controlled trial compared vaginal *estriol* cream with placebo for 8 months of treatment and showed a significant reduction in urinary tract infections (0.5 vs. 5.9 per patient year). In the treatment arm, there was a reduction in vaginal pH from 5.5 to 3.8 compared with no decline in the placebo group (101). In a randomized controlled trial of 27 women on hormone therapy with urogenital atrophy, the addition of vaginal estriol shortened the latency period for urinary symptoms (102).

The effect of vaginal *estriol* cream on the endometrium was evaluated in a study examining long-term use for urogenital atrophy. Patients were given 0.5 mg of *estriol* cream vaginally for 21 days, then twice weekly for 12 months. Hysteroscopic and histologic examinations were performed at baseline, 6 months, and 12 months. Complete endometrial atrophy occurred in all patients (N = 23) (103). This pilot study needs to be performed in a larger patient population, but its findings are promising.

Bioidentical Progestins   The Postmenopausal Estrogen-Progestin Intervention (PEPI) trials provided a multicentered, randomized controlled trial that, among other things, compared *conjugated equine estrogen* plus *medroxyprogesterone acetate* with *conjugated equine estrogen* plus natural or micronized *progesterone* (104). The trial compared 12 days of 10 mg of *medroxyprogesterone acetate* with 200 mg of micronized *progesterone*. The micronized *progesterone* provided equal protection of the endometrium and was better at protecting the beneficial effects of the *conjugated equine estrogen* on the lipid profile. Patients reported that micronized *progesterone* had significantly fewer side effects than *medroxyprogesterone acetate*. This was the case in several other trials (105,106). Given these data, there is no reason not to prescribe micronized *progesterone*. The arm of the Women's Health Initiative that was prematurely discontinued was the conjugated equine *estrogen/medroxyprogesterone acetate* arm. The *conjugated equine estrogen*–alone arm was continued. The role and the effect of *medroxyprogesterone acetate* should be closely examined. In ovariectomized rhesus monkeys, E_2 plus *medroxyprogesterone acetate* interfered with ovarian estrogen protection against coronary vasospasm. E_2 plus *micronized progesterone* protected against coronary vasospasm. Given the increased cardiovascular risks in women taking *conjugated equine estrogen* and *medroxyprogesterone acetate*, combined with the positive data from PEPI, micronized *progesterone* is an excellent choice for patients who are taking systemic estrogen who still have a uterus.

Table 13.11 Progesterone and Wild Yam Creams	
400–700 mg progesterone per ounce	Pro-Gest Bio Balance Progonol Ostaderm Pro-Alo
2–15 mg progesterone per ounce	PhytoGest Pro-Dermex Endocreme Life Changes Yamcon Wild Yam Extract PMS Formula Menopause Formula Femarone-Nutri-Gest
Less than 2 mg progesterone per ounce	Progerone Wild Yam Cream Progestone-HP

Natural *progesterone* was used as a single agent in the treatment of menopausal symptoms. The typical dose is 100 mg per day. More research is needed to demonstrate efficacy.

Yam Creams, Progesterone Creams   Yam creams and *progesterone* creams, which are both sold over the counter, are distinctly different products. Yam creams should, by definition, not contain *progesterone,* but rather should contain phytoprogesterones, plant products that are *progesterone*-like (Table 13.11). *Progesterone* creams, by contrast, should contain progesterone. Part of the challenge is that there is a large media presence asserting that *progesterone* creams can solve all that ails menopausal women. These creams are not regulated by the FDA. Their content is highly variable, ranging from 700 mg *progesterone* per ounce to less than 2 mg per ounce in products whose names imply that they are progesterone creams, not yam creams. The absorption of these products is highly variable.

Wild yam creams (which refer to the genus name *Dioscorea villosa,* rather than the fact that they are grown in the wild) are applied topically. They contain steroidal saponins, including diosgenin, and claim to affect estrogen steroidogenesis. Although these are interesting products, studies of their safety and efficacy are needed. In one double-blind, placebo-controlled crossover study, after a 4-week baseline period, patients received 3 months of active treatment and 3 months of placebo. Symptom diaries were maintained at baseline and then for 1 week of each month. Blood and salivary hormone levels as well as serum lipids were assessed at baseline, 3 months, and 6 months. At 3 months there were no significant side effects and no change in levels of blood pressure, weight, lipid levels, follicle-stimulating hormone, glucose, estradiol, or progesterone. In terms of symptom relief, the placebo and yam cream had a minor effect on the number and severity of flashes. Wild yam creams appear to be free of side effects, and they appear to have little effect on menopausal symptoms (107).

In terms of *progesterone* creams, a randomized controlled trial of 223 women with severe menopausal symptoms using progesterone cream found the progesterone arm to be no more effective than placebo (108). In another randomized controlled trial, transdermal *progesterone* was compared to placebo. One-quarter teaspoon of 20 mg of *progesterone* was used daily for 12 months. In addition, all patients took a multivitamin plus 1,200 mg of calcium. Outcomes evaluated included dual-energy x-ray absorptiometry (DEXA) results, serum thyroid-stimulating hormone, follicle-stimulating hormone, lipids, chemistry, and symptom diary. The group that received the progesterone cream reported 83% improvement in hot flashes compared with 19% improvement in the placebo group. There was no difference in bone density (109).

Given the data currently available, *progesterone* or yam creams should not be considered adequate to protect the uterus in a woman taking systemic estrogen. *Progesterone* cream may be useful for symptom relief in women not taking systemic hormone therapy, and it may prove to have other benefits and risks.

Table 13.12 Unknown Aspects of Hormone Therapy
• Risks and benefits of bioidentical hormone therapy (i.e., how the results of the Women's Health Initiative translate to bioidentical hormones)
• Role of *medroxyprogesterone acetate* in increasing certain risks
• Long-term risks and benefits of *estriol*
• Effects of different doses of hormones
• Correlation of circulating hormone levels to different doses, and the correlation of different hormone levels to risks and benefits
• Effect of lifelong hormonal exposure
• Risks and benefits of hormone therapy when initiated at the age of menopause

Counseling Patients

It's important to communicate to patients what is known regarding hormone therapy and what is not known. Some of the unknown aspects of hormone therapy are listed in Table 13.12.

Given the present state of the medical knowledge, the need to individualize treatment plans in menopausal women cannot be overemphasized. It is essential to clarify patient goals, and individual health risks, history of hormonal exposure (both length and time), family history, and personal preferences.

Surgery and Complementary and Alternative Medicine

Studies showed that most surgical patients use some form of CAM. There are special considerations regarding CAM and the surgical patient. These issues primarily fall into two domains:

1. Supplements that, when used perioperatively, may affect the patient's course
2. CAM approaches that may be of benefit to the surgical patient

When examining what patients are using that may affect their surgical course, the greatest concern and awareness needs to be in the domain of biologically based therapies. A survey of 2,560 surgical patients in five California hospitals revealed that 68% of patients were using botanicals, 44% of them did not consult their physician, 56% did not inform their anesthesiologists, and 47% did not stop them before their surgery. Variables that were associated with use included female gender, age 35 to 49 years, higher income, Caucasian race, higher education, and problems with sleep, joints, back, allergies, and addiction (110). A survey based in a tertiary care center examined the use of botanicals and vitamins in patients preoperatively (N = 3,106). Of the patients studied, 22% were using botanicals and 51% were using vitamins. The typical users were women in the age range of 40 to 60 years. The most commonly used compounds were echinacea, ginkgo biloba, St. John's wort, garlic, and ginseng (111). In another study based in a university medical center that surveyed patients undergoing outpatient surgery, 64% of patients were using supplements: 90% of them were using vitamins, 43% were using garlic extracts, 32% ginkgo biloba, 30% St. John's wort, 18% ma huang, 12% echinacea, and others were using aloe, cascara, and licorice (112).

Effects on Surgery

Many of the most commonly used substances have effects of which surgeons and anesthesiologists should be aware. Botanicals used with anesthesia can lead to the following complications:

- Prolongation of anesthetic agents
- Coagulations disorders
- Cardiovascular effects
- Electrolyte disturbances

- Hepatotoxicity

- Endocrine effects

The American Society of Anesthesiologists does not have an official guideline, but it recommends that all natural products be discontinued 2 to 3 weeks before elective surgery.

Prolongation of Anesthetic Agents

Valerian, kava, ginseng, and St. John's wort are among the more commonly used botanicals that may prolong the effects of anesthetic agents. Valerian has sedative effects that are believed to be mediated by *benzodiazepine* and γ-aminobutyric acid (GABA) receptors. For patients who use valerian on a daily basis, it is suggested that it be tapered off over the weeks preceding the surgery. Kava is mediated by GABA receptors and potentiates the sedative effects of anesthetics. The general recommendation is to discontinue its use 24 hours before surgery. St. John's wort induces cytochrome P450 enzymes (*cyclosporin, indinavir,* and *warfarin*). It modulates the GABA receptor and inhibits the reuptake of serotonin, dopamine, and noradrenaline. The recommendation is to discontinue it 5 days preoperatively.

Coagulation Effects

Some of the more commonly used supplements and botanicals that are reported to have anticoagulative properties include fish oil, ginseng (Asian and American), ginkgo, garlic, vitamin E, ginger, feverfew, dong quai, saw palmetto, and chondroitin. Coenzyme Q-10, fish oil, and flax seed can have this effect.

Cardiovascular Effects

Licorice root contains glycyrrhizic acid, which has an aldosteronelike effect and can result in hypertension, hyperkalemia, and edema. Glycyrrhizic acid is used in manufactured foods as a sweetener. Ma huang (ephedra) is associated with arrhythmias and hypertension, and ginseng is associated with hypertension. Fish oil, coenzyme Q-10, and garlic are associated with hypotension. There were case reports of reversible episodes of hypertension and palpitations with glucosamine. Occasional occurrences of hypertension, tachycardia, and other cardiac complaints of unknown causality were reported with saw palmetto.

Electrolyte Disturbances

Licorice root was associated with hypernatremia and hypokalemia. Goldenseal can reduce the effect of antihypertensives. Saw palmetto, ginseng, and green tea can cause electrolyte disturbances.

Hepatotoxicity and Endocrine Effects

The following botanicals are associated with hepatotoxicity: kava, red yeast rice (which contains the ingredient in *lovastatin*), chaparral, valerian, and echinacea. In terms of endocrinologic effects, both chromium and ginseng can cause hypoglycemia. Table 13.13 highlights some of the more commonly used botanicals and vitamins and their possible effects in the surgical patient.

Complementary and Alternative Medicine Approaches that May Benefit the Surgical Patient

The two domains in which there is the most research and the most promise with regard to surgical patients are mind–body-based therapies and approaches based in complete systems, specifically oriental medicine and acupuncture.

Oriental Medicine and Acupuncture

A review of the use of acupuncture as the sole source of anesthesia for patients undergoing cesarean delivery in China reviewed 12 years of experience with success rates of 92% to 99%. Blood pressure, heart rate, and respiratory rate remained stable throughout the surgery, which is a significant advantage over pharmaceutical anesthesia (113). Although it is unlikely that acupuncture will readily be used as the only source of anesthesia in this country, it demonstrates the effectiveness of this approach and encourages its consideration as an adjunct. In one randomized controlled trial in patients undergoing upper- and lower-abdominal (gastrointestinal) surgery, acupuncture was given 2.5 cm lateral to the spine before induction. Postoperatively, patients who received the acupuncture had decreased postoperative pain, nausea and vomiting, analgesic requirement, and sympathoadrenal responses. Supplemental morphine use dropped by 50%, and postoperative nausea was reduced by 30%. Cortisol and epinephrine levels were reduced 30% to 50% during the recovery phase and the first postoperative day (114). Several studies specifically looking at nausea and vomiting in women undergoing gynecologic surgeries showed benefit in both acupuncture and acupressure (115–117).

Table 13.13 Commonly Used Botanicals and Vitamins and Their Possible Effects in the Surgical Patient

Substance	Potential Negative Effects
Chaparral	Hepatotoxicity
Chondroitin	Anticoagulative properties
Chromium	Hypoglycemia
Coenzyme Q-10	Hypotension; cardiac effects; anticoagulative properties
Dong quai	Anticoagulative properties
Echinacea	Hepatotoxicity
Feverfew	Anticoagulative properties
Fish Oil	Anticoagulative properties; hypotension
Garlic	Anticoagulative properties
Ginger	Anticoagulative properties
Ginkgo	Anticoagulative properties
Ginseng	Anticoagulative properties Hypertension Hypoglycemia
Glucosamine	Hypoglycemia
Goldenseal	Can reduce effect of antihypertensives
Green tea	Anticoagulative properties; cardiac effects
Flax seed	Anticoagulative properties
Kava	Potentiates the sedative effects of anesthetics Hepatotoxicity
Licorice root	Hypertension Hyperkalemia Hypokalemia Hypernatremia Edema
Ma huang (ephedra)	Arrhythmias Hypertension
Red yeast rice	Hepatotoxicity
Saw palmetto	Anticoagulative properties; cardiac effects; electrolyte disturbances
St. John's wort	Prolongation of anesthetic effects Inhibits reuptake of serotonin, dopamine, and noradrenaline
Valerian	Prolongation of anesthetic effects Hepatotoxicity
Vitamin E	Anticoagulative properties

In a sham-controlled trial, the intensity of transcutaneous acupoint electrical stimulation (TAES) was studied in women undergoing lower-abdominal surgery. In patients receiving high-intensity TAES (9–12 mA), there was a 65% decrease in analgesia requirement, decreased duration in patient-controlled anesthesia therapy, and decrease in nausea, vomiting, and pruritus (118).

In Germany, auricular electrically stimulated anesthesia is frequently used. Review of one randomized controlled trial in patients anesthetized with *desflurane* with and without auricular acupuncture revealed significantly reduced anesthetic requirement (the amount of anesthesia required to prevent purposeful movements) (119).

Acupuncture warrants further investigation as an adjunct to anesthesia in gynecologic patients. Even simple adjuncts, such as the use of acupressure bands or electroacupressure bands, are reasonable to support as they are safe and showed some efficacy in decreasing nausea and vomiting postoperatively.

Mind–Body Interventions

Mental preparation for surgery results in psychological, physiologic, and economic benefit. Higher levels of anxiety are associated with a greater risk of complications, depression, and increased need for anesthesia, decreased immune function, and a longer time to heal. Many different physiologic aspects are affected, including decreased chemotaxis and phagocytosis and decreased inflammatory factors such as cytokines. One study examining wound healing took healthy dental students and made a standardized scalpel incision in the palate at two times: one right before examinations and one during summer vacation. The incisions in these healthy students took 3 days (40%) longer to heal during times of stress versus times of decreased stress (120). The power of the spoken word was explored as long ago as 1964, when a study randomized patients to a preoperative visit characterized by sympathetic, caring, and informative communication versus an interchange characterized by cursory remarks. The patients receiving the sympathetic preoperative visit required half the pain medicines and had a two-and-a-half-day decreased hospital stay (121).

A meta-analysis of mind–body interventions and surgery included 191 studies and more than 8,600 patients. **The use of mind–body approaches, including such interventions as hypnosis, imagery, and relaxation, was associated with reduced blood loss, decreased pain, decreased medication use, increased return of bowel function, decreased psychological stress, and decreased hospital stay by 1.5 days.** In a study of 241 patients undergoing invasive medical procedures randomized to standard care versus structured attention versus self-hypnosis, the hypnosis has the most pronounced effects on pain and anxiety and improved hemodynamic stability (122). In a study designed to examine the impact of preoperative instructions, patients undergoing spinal procedures involving fusions or instrumentation (surgeries associated with significant blood loss) were enrolled. All subjects received a 15-minute interaction with a psychologist. The subjects were randomized into one of three groups receiving either direct simple information alone, information plus instruction in muscle relaxation, or information plus instruction in previsualization of the blood moving away from the surgical site during surgery. Controlling for the length of surgery and incision length, the estimated blood loss in the first two groups averaged 900 mL and in the third group was 500 mL (123).

In a study of ambulatory surgery patients receiving spinal anesthesia, patients who were randomized to listening to soothing music had decreased sedative requirements both during the surgery and in the perioperative period (124). Patients undergoing cataract surgery were randomized to receive a 5-minute hand massage preoperatively or to the control group. When compared with the control group, the intervention group had significantly decreased levels of anxiety, systolic blood pressure, diastolic blood pressure, heart rate, and epinephrine and norepinephrine (125).

In a study of women undergoing hysterectomy, patients received standardized anesthesia and were randomized to music during surgery, music plus positive suggestions, or the sounds of the operating room. On the day of surgery, both the music group and the music-plus-suggestion groups received significantly less rescue anesthesia. On postoperative day 1, the patients who had heard music during surgery had more effective analgesia and early mobilization. At the time of discharge, both intervention groups had less fatigue. There was no change in nausea and vomiting, bowel function, or length of stay (126).

In another study with patients undergoing abdominal hysterectomy, patients were randomized to listen intraoperatively to one of four tapes: positive suggestions regarding pain, or nausea and vomiting, or both, or white noise. The positive suggestions had no beneficial effects in reducing nausea and vomiting or the consumption of analgesics or antiemetics (127). In another randomized controlled trial in patients undergoing thyroidectomy under general anesthesia, patients were randomized to listen to taped positive suggestions during surgery versus a blank tape. The group receiving the suggestions had less nausea and vomiting (47% vs. 85%), and less antiemetic treatment (30% vs. 68%) (128). In a study exploring the timing of listening to taped suggestions, patients who received the suggestions preoperatively had a 30% decrease in estimated blood loss. Patients receiving the suggestions both pre- and perioperatively had a 26% decrease in blood loss, and in the group listening to the suggestions only intraoperatively, there was a 9%

decrease in blood loss. The authors suggest that the preoperative suggestions may be the critical factor (129).

In a retrospective study examining the use of hypnosis plus conscious sedation for plastic surgery, the patients who received hypnosis had better pain and anxiety relief, decreased nausea and vomiting, and a significant reduction in *midazolam* and *alfentanil* requirements and patient satisfaction was significantly increased (130).

Although the studies and interventions in mind–body approaches in the surgical patient are varied, these interventions are low cost and low risk and may offer very real benefits for the patient, as well as a greater sense of empowerment.

Conclusion

As physicians driven by our desire and commitment to provide the best possible care, we have a responsibility to inform our patients of all therapies that can be of benefit, regardless of their system of origin. In practice this is challenging, because there are many unanswered questions in the use of complementary and alternative modalities, and because there is no established standard of care. Each physician, together with his or her patient, needs to form his or her own opinions regarding the appropriate integration of CAM therapies. Many patients will want conclusive evidence of any therapy before using it. Others, assured of the relative safety of a therapy, may require less conclusive evidence. Illustrating this dilemma, in a systematic review of randomized trials regarding CAM approaches to PMS, the authors concluded that "despite some positive findings, the evidence was not compelling for any of these therapies, with most trials suffering from various methodological limitations. On the basis of current evidence, no complementary or alternative therapy can be recommended as a treatment for premenstrual syndrome" (131). Although this concept certainly is appealing in its simplicity, it may not be in the best interest of patients. We need to be consistent in our requirement of evidence, using the same levels of evidence for incorporating interventions from CAM as from conventional approaches. As with many clinical decisions we are forced to make with incomplete data, many factors must be considered. The potential risks and benefits must be weighed carefully, and *primum non nocere* must certainly be our guide.

In many regards, we are in the most challenging time as it relates to integrating appropriate CAM approaches into the practice of gynecology. As more research is done and as medical schools and residency programs incorporate education about these approaches, the gap between our patients' desires and our standard practices will decrease as appropriate therapies are seamlessly incorporated and ineffective and fraudulent ones are discarded.

References

1. **Eisenberg DM, Davis RB, Ettner SL, et al.** Trends in alternative medicine use in the United States, 1990–1997: results of a follow-up national survey. *JAMA* 1998;280:1569–1575.
2. **Eisenberg DM, Kessler RC, Foster C, et al.** Unconventional medicine in the United States. Prevalence, costs, and patterns of use. *N Engl J Med* 1993;328:246–252.
3. **Barnes PM, Powell-Griner E, McFann K, et al.** Complementary and alternative medicine use among adults: United States, 2002. *Adv Data* 2004;343:1–19.
4. **Bair YA, Gold EB, Greendale GA, et al.** Ethnic differences in use of complementary and alternative medicine at midlife: longitudinal results from SWAN participants. *Am J Public Health* 2002;92:1832–1840.
5. **Hollyer T, Boon H, Georgouis A, et al.** The use of CAM by women suffering from nausea and vomiting during pregnancy. *BMC Complement Altern Med* 2002;2:5.
6. **Shen J, Andersen R, Albert PS, et al.** Use of complementary/alternative therapies by women with advanced-stage breast cancer. *BMC Complement Altern Med* 2002;2:8.
7. **Newton KM, Buist DS, Keenan NL, et al.** Use of alternative therapies for menopause symptoms: results of a population-based survey. *Obstet Gynecol* 2002;100:18–25.
8. **Astin JA.** Why patients use alternative medicine: results of a national study. *JAMA* 1998;279:1548–1553.
9. **Adler SR, Fosket JR.** Disclosing complementary and alternative medicine use in the medical encounter: a qualitative study in women with breast cancer. *J Fam Pract* 1999;48:453–458.
10. **U.S. Food and Drug Administration (USFDA).** Dietary supplements. www.fda.gov/food/dietarysupplements.
11. **National Certification Commission for Acupuncture and Oriental Medicine (NCCAOM).** http://www.nccaom.org/.
12. **Gouveia LO, Castanho P, Ferreira JJ.** Safety of chiropractic interventions: a systematic review. *Spine (Phila Pa 1976)* 2009;34:E405–E413.
13. **National Certification Board for Theraputic Massage and Bodywork (NCBTMB).** www.ncbtmb.org/.
14. **American Society of Clinical Hypnosis (ASCH).** www.asch.net.
15. **Cho ZH, Chung SC, Jones JP, et al.** New findings of the correlation between acupoints and corresponding brain cortices using functional MRI. *Proc Natl Acad Sci U S A* 1998;95:2670–2673.
16. **National Institutes of Health Consensus Panel.** Acupuncture. http://consensus.nih.gov/1997/1997acupuncture107html.htm.
17. **National Center for Complementary and Alternative Medicine.** Acupuncture for pain. Available online at: http://nccam.nih.gov/health/acupuncture/acupuncture-for-pain.htm. Accessed Sept. 18, 2009.
18. **Accreditation Commission for Acupuncture and Oriental Medicine (ACAOM).** http://www.acaom.org/.

19. **American Board of Medical Acupuncture.** http://www.dabma. org/.

20. **Council on Naturopathic Medical Education.** http://www.cnme. org/.

21. **Federation of State Medical Boards.** Model Guidelines for the Use of Complementary and Alternative Therapies in Medical Practice. Available online at: http://www.fsmb.org/pdf/2002_grpol_ Complementary_Alternative_Therapies.pdf.

22. **Whelan AM, Jurgens TM, Naylor H.** Herbs, vitamins and minerals in the treatment of premenstrual syndrome: a systematic review. *Can J Clin Pharmacol* 2009;16:e407–e429.

23. **Proctor M, Murphy PA.** Herbal and dietary therapies for primary and secondary dysmenorrhoea. *Cochrane Database Syst Rev* 2001;3:CD002124.

24. **Thys-Jacobs S, Starkey P, Bernstein D, et al.** Calcium carbonate and the premenstrual syndrome: effects on premenstrual and menstrual symptoms. Premenstrual Syndrome Study Group. *Am J Obstet Gynecol* 1998;179:444–452.

25. **Bertone-Johnson ER, Hankinson SE, Bendich A, et al.** Calcium and vitamin D intake and risk of incident premenstrual syndrome. *Arch Intern Med* 2005;165:1246–1252.

26. **Fugh-Berman A, Kronenberg F.** Complementary and alternative medicine (CAM) in reproductive-age women: a review of randomized controlled trials. *Reprod Toxicol* 2003;17:137–152.

27. **Walker AF, DeSouza MC, Vickers MF, et al.** Magnesium supplementation alleviates premenstrual symptoms of fluid retention. *J Womens Health* 1998;7:1157–1165.

28. **Facchinetti F, Borella P, Sances G, et al.** Oral magnesium successfully relieves premenstrual mood changes. *Obstet Gynecol* 1991;78:177–181.

29. **London RS, Murphy L, Kitlowski KE, et al.** Efficacy of alpha-tocopherol in the treatment of the premenstrual syndrome. *J Reprod Med* 1987;32:400–404.

30. **Ziaei S, Zakeri M, Kazemnejad A.** A randomised controlled trial of vitamin E in the treatment of primary dysmenorrhoea. *BJOG* 2005;112:466–469.

31. **Kleijnen J, Ter Riet G, Knipschild P.** Vitamin B6 in the treatment of the premenstrual syndrome—a review. *Br J Obstet Gynaecol* 1990;97:847–852.

32. **Wyatt KM, Dimmock PW, Jones PW, et al.** Efficacy of vitamin B-6 in the treatment of premenstrual syndrome: systematic review. *BMJ* 1999;318:1375–1781.

33. **Dell DL, Svec C.** *The PMDD phenomenon: breakthrough treatments for premenstrual dysphoric disorder (PMDD) and extreme premenstrual syndrome (PMS).* New York: McGraw-Hill, 2002.

34. **Berger D, Schaffner W, Schrader E, et al.** Efficacy of *Vitex agnus castus* L. extract Ze 440 in patients with pre-menstrual syndrome (PMS). *Arch Gynecol Obstet* 2000;264:150–153.

35. **Schellenberg R.** Treatment for the premenstrual syndrome with agnus castus fruit extract: prospective, randomised, placebo controlled study. *BMJ* 2001;322:134–137.

36. **Loch EG, Selle H, Boblitz N.** Treatment of premenstrual syndrome with a phytopharmaceutical formulation containing *Vitex agnus castus*. *J Womens Health Gend Based Med* 2000;9:315–320.

37. **Atmaca M, Kumru S, Tezcan E.** *Fluoxetine* versus *Vitex agnus castus* extract in the treatment of premenstrual dysphoric disorder. *Hum Psychopharmacol* 2003;18:191–195.

38. **Meier B, Berger D, Hoberg E, et al.** Pharmacological activities of *Vitex agnus-castus* extracts in vitro. *Phytomedicine* 2000;7:373–381.

39. **Stevinson C, Ernst E.** A pilot study of *Hypericum perforatum* for the treatment of premenstrual syndrome. *BJOG* 2000;107:870–876.

40. **Tamborini A, Taurelle R.** Value of standardized ginkgo biloba extract (EGb 761) in the management of congestive symptoms of premenstrual syndrome). *Rev Fr Gynecold Obstet* 1993;88:447–457.

41. **Ashton AK.** Antidepressant-induced sexual dysfunction and ginkgo biloba. *Am J Psychiatry* 2000;157:836–837.

42. **Saldeen P, Saldeen T.** Women and omega-3 fatty acids. *Obstet Gynecol Surv* 2004;59:722–730; quiz 745–746.

43. **Kidd PM.** Omega-3 DHA and EPA for cognition, behavior, and mood: clinical findings and structural-functional synergies with cell membrane phospholipids. *Altern Med Rev* 2007;12:207–227.

44. **Walsh MJ, Polus BI.** A randomized, placebo-controlled clinical trial on the efficacy of chiropractic therapy on premenstrual syndrome. *J Manipulative Physiol Ther* 1999;22:582–585.

45. **Proctor ML, Hing W, Johnson TC, et al.** Spinal manipulation for primary and secondary dysmenorrhoea. *Cochrane Database Syst Rev* 2006;3:CD002119.

46. **Goodale IL, Domar AD, Benson H.** Alleviation of premenstrual syndrome symptoms with the relaxation response. *Obstet Gynecol* 1990;75:649–655.

47. **Girman A, Lee R, Kligler B.** An integrative medicine approach to premenstrual syndrome. *Am J Obstet Gynecol* 2003; 188[Suppl]:S56–S65.

48. **Habek D, Habek JC, Barbir A.** Using acupuncture to treat premenstrual syndrome. *Arch Gynecol Obstet* 2002;267:23–26.

49. **Jing Z, Yang X, Ismail KM, et al.** Chinese herbal medicine for premenstrual syndrome. *Cochrane Database Syst Rev* 2009;1: CD006414.

50. **Witt CM, Reinhold T, Brinkhaus B, et al.** Acupuncture in patients with dysmenorrhea: a randomized study on clinical effectiveness and cost-effectiveness in usual care. *Am J Obstet Gynecol* 2008;198: e1–e8.

51. **Zhu X, Proctor M, Bensoussan A, et al.** Chinese herbal medicine for primary dysmenorrhoea. *Cochrane Database Syst Rev* 2008; 2:CD005288.

52. **Domar AD, Seibel MM, Benson H.** The mind/body program for infertility: a new behavioral treatment approach for women with infertility. *Fertil Steril* 1990;53:246–249.

53. **Poehl M, Bichler K, Wicke V, et al.** Psychotherapeutic counseling and pregnancy rates in in vitro fertilization. *J Assist Reprod Genet* 1999;16:302–305.

54. **Levitas E, Parmet A, Lunenfeld E, et al.** Impact of hypnosis during embryo transfer on the outcome of in vitro fertilization-embryo transfer: a case-control study. *Fertil Steril* 2006;85:1404–1408.

55. **Gerhard I, Postneek F.** Auricular acupuncture in the treatment of female infertility. *Gynecol Endocrinol* 1992;6:171–181.

56. **Smith C, Coyle M, Norman RJ.** Influence of acupuncture stimulation on pregnancy rates for women undergoing embryo transfer. *Fertil Steril* 2006;85:1352–1358.

57. **Dieterle S, Ying G, Hatzmann W, et al.** Effect of acupuncture on the outcome of in vitro fertilization and intracytoplasmic sperm injection: a randomized, prospective, controlled clinical study. *Fertil Steril* 2006;85:1347–1351.

58. **Westergaard LG, Mao Q, Krogslund M, et al.** Acupuncture on the day of embryo transfer significantly improves the reproductive outcome in infertile women: a prospective, randomized trial. *Fertil Steril* 2006;85:1341–1346.

59. **Paulus WE, Zhang M, Strehler E, et al.** Influence of acupuncture on the pregnancy rate in patients who undergo assisted reproduction therapy. *Fertil Steril* 2002;77:721–724.

60. **Manheimer E, Zhang G, Udoff L, et al.** Effects of acupuncture on rates of pregnancy and live birth among women undergoing in vitro fertilisation: systematic review and meta-analysis. *BMJ* 2008;336:545–549.

61. **El-Toukhy T, Sunkara SK, Khairy M, et al.** A systematic review and meta-analysis of acupuncture in in vitro fertilisation. *BJOG* 2008;115:1203–1213.

62. **Stener-Victorin E, Waldenström U, Andersson SA, et al.** Reduction of blood flow impedance in the uterine arteries of infertile women with electro-acupuncture. *Hum Reprod* 1996;11:1314–1317.

63. **Magarelli PC, Cridennda DK, Cohen M.** Changes in serum cortisol and prolactin associated with acupuncture during controlled ovarian hyperstimulation in women undergoing in vitro fertilization-embryo transfer treatment. *Fertil Steril* 2009;92:1870–1879.

64. **Bair YA, Gold EB, Zhang G, et al.** Use of complementary and alternative medicine during the menopause transition: longitudinal results from the Study of Women's Health Across the Nation. *Menopause* 2008;15:32–43.

65. **Shrader SP, Ragucci KR.** Life after the women's health initiative: evaluation of postmenopausal symptoms and use of alternative therapies after discontinuation of hormone therapy. *Pharmacotherapy* 2006;26:1403–1409.

66. **Adams C, Cannell S.** Women's beliefs about "natural" hormones and natural hormone replacement therapy. *Menopause* 2001;8:433–440.

67. **Barton DL, Loprinzi CL, Quella SK, et al.** Prospective evaluation of vitamin E for hot flashes in breast cancer survivors. *J Clin Oncol* 1998;16:495–500.

68. **Amato P, Christophe S, Mellon PL.** Estrogenic activity of herbs commonly used as remedies for menopausal symptoms. *Menopause* 2002;9:145–150.

69. **Wuttke W, Seidlova-Wuttke D, Gorkow C.** The Cimicifuga preparation BNO 1055 vs. conjugated estrogens in a double-blind placebo-controlled study: effects on menopause symptoms and bone markers. *Maturitas* 2003;44[Suppl 1]:S67–S77.

70. **Wong VC, Lim CE, Luo X, et al.** Current alternative and complementary therapies used in menopause. *Gynecol Endocrinol* 2009;25:166–174.

71. **Briese V, Stammwitz U, Friede M, et al.** Black cohosh with or without St. John's wort for symptom-specific climacteric treatment—results of a large-scale, controlled, observational study. *Maturitas* 2007;57:405–414.

72. **Blumenthal M, ed.** *The Complete German Commission E Monographs: Therapeutic Guide to Herbal Medicines.* Austin, TX, American Botanical Council; 1998.

73. **Jacobson JS, Troxel AB, Evans J, et al.** Randomized trial of black cohosh for the treatment of hot flashes among women with a history of breast cancer. *J Clin Oncol* 2001;19:2739–2745.

74. **Hernandez Munoz G, Pluchino S.** *Cimicifuga racemosa* for the treatment of hot flushes in women surviving breast cancer. *Maturitas* 2003;44[Suppl 1]:S59–S65.

75. **Tode T, Kikuchi Y, Hirata J, et al.** Effect of Korean red ginseng on psychological functions in patients with severe climacteric syndromes. *Int J Gynaecol Obstet* 1999;67:169–174.

76. **Wiklund IK, Mattsson LA, Kindgren R, et al.** Effects of a standardized ginseng extract on quality of life and physiological parameters in symptomatic postmenopausal women: a double-blind, placebo-controlled trial. Swedish Alternative Medicine Group. *Int J Clin Pharmacol Res* 1999;19:89–99.

77. **Knight DC, Howes JB, Eden JA.** The effect of *promensil*, an isoflavone extract, on menopausal symptoms. *Climacteric* 1999;2:79–84.

78. **Tice JA, Ettinger B, Ensrud K, et al.** Phytoestrogen supplements for the treatment of hot flashes: the Isoflavone Clover Extract (ICE) study: a randomized controlled trial. *JAMA* 2003;290:207–214.

79. **Hirata JD, Swiersz LM, Zell B, et al.** Does dong quai have estrogenic effects in postmenopausal women? A double-blind, placebo-controlled trial. *Fertil Steril* 1997;68:981–986.

80. **De Leo V, La Marca A, Lanzetta D, et al.** Assessment of the association of Kava-Kava extract and hormone replacement therapy in the treatment of postmenopause anxiety. *Minerva Ginecol* 2000;52(6):263–267.

81. **Teschke R, Schulze J.** Risk of kava hepatotoxicity and the FDA consumer advisory. *JAMA* 2010;304(19):2174–2145.

82. **Grube B, Walper A, Wheatley D.** St. John's wort extract: efficacy for menopausal symptoms of psychological origin. *Adv Ther* 1999;16:177–186.

83. **Uebelhack R, Blohmer JU, Graubaum HJ, et al.** Black cohosh and St. John's wort for climacteric complaints: a randomized trial. *Obstet Gynecol* 2006;107[Pt 1]:247–255.

84. **Waynberg J, Brewer S.** Effects of Herbal vX on libido and sexual activity in premenopausal and postmenopausal women. *Adv Ther* 2000;17:255–262.

85. **Dennehy CE.** The use of herbs and dietary supplements in gynecology: an evidence-based review. *J Midwifery Womens Health* 2006;51:402–409.

86. **Nedstrand E, Wijma K, Wyon Y, et al.** Applied relaxation and oral estradiol treatment of vasomotor symptoms in postmenopausal women. *Maturitas* 2005;51:154–162.

87. **Irvin JH, Domar AD, Clark C, et al.** The effects of relaxation response training on menopausal symptoms. *J Psychosom Obstet Gynaecol* 1996;17:202–207.

88. **Freedman RR, Woodward S.** Behavioral treatment of menopausal hot flushes: evaluation by ambulatory monitoring. *Am J Obstet Gynecol* 1992;167:436–439.

89. **Ganz PA, Greendale GA, Petersen L, et al.** Managing menopausal symptoms in breast cancer survivors: results of a randomized controlled trial. *J Natl Cancer Inst* 2000;92:1054–1064.

90. **Zaborowska E, Brynhildsen J, Damberg S, et al.** Effects of acupuncture, applied relaxation, estrogens and placebo on hot flushes in postmenopausal women: an analysis of two prospective, parallel, randomized studies. *Climacteric* 2007;10:38–45.

91. **Jones CR, Czajkowski L.** Evaluation and management of insomnia in menopause. *Clin Obstet Gynecol* 2000;43:184–197.

92. **Cho SH, Whang WW.** Acupuncture for vasomotor menopausal symptoms: a systematic review. *Menopause* 2009;16:1065–1073.

93. **Lee MS, Shin BC, Ernst E.** Acupuncture for treating menopausal hot flushes: a systematic review. *Climacteric* 2009;12:16–25.

94. **Borud EK, Alraek T, White A, et al.** The Acupuncture on Hot Flushes Among Menopausal Women (ACUFLASH) study, a randomized controlled trial. *Menopause* 2009;16:484–493.

95. **Borud E, Grimsgaard S, White A.** Menopausal problems and acupuncture. *Auton Neurosci* 2010;157(1-2):57–62.

96. **Porzio G, Trapasso T, Martelli S, et al.** Acupuncture in the treatment of menopause-related symptoms in women taking *tamoxifen.* *Tumori* 2002;88:128–130.

97. **Frisk J, Carlhäll S, Källström AC, et al.** Long-term follow-up of acupuncture and hormone therapy on hot flushes in women with breast cancer: a prospective, randomized, controlled multicenter trial. *Climacteric* 2008;11:166–174.

98. **Takahashi K, Okada M, Ozaki T, et al.** Safety and efficacy of oestriol for symptoms of natural or surgically induced menopause. *Hum Reprod* 2000;15:1028–1036.

99. **Itoi H, Minakami H, Sato I.** Comparison of the long-term effects of oral estriol with the effects of conjugated estrogen, 1-alpha-hydroxyvitamin D3 and calcium lactate on vertebral bone loss in early menopausal women. *Maturitas* 1997;28:11–17.

100. **Lyytinen H, Pukkala E, Ylikorkala O.** Breast cancer risk in postmenopausal women using estrogen-only therapy. *Obstet Gynecol* 2006;108:1354–1360.

101. **Raz R, Stamm WE.** A controlled trial of intravaginal estriol in postmenopausal women with recurrent urinary tract infections. *N Engl J Med* 1993;329:753–756.

102. **Palacios S, Castelo-Branco C, Cancelo MJ, et al.** Low-dose, vaginally administered estrogens may enhance local benefits of systemic therapy in the treatment of urogenital atrophy in postmenopausal women on hormone therapy. *Maturitas* 2005;50:98–104.

103. **Gerbaldo D, Ferraiolo A, Croce S, et al.** Endometrial morphology after 12 months of vaginal oestriol therapy in post-menopausal women. *Maturitas* 1991;13:269–274.

104. **The Writing Group for the PEPI Trial.** Effects of estrogen or estrogen/progestin regimens on heart disease risk factors in postmenopausal women. The Postmenopausal Estrogen/Progestin Interventions (PEPI) trial. *JAMA* 1995;273:199–208.

105. **Ryan N, Rosner A.** Quality of life and costs associated with micronized progesterone and medroxyprogesterone acetate in hormone replacement therapy for nonhysterectomized, postmenopausal women. *Clin Ther* 2001;23:1099–1115.

106. **Fitzpatrick LA, Pace C, Wiita B.** Comparison of regimens containing oral micronized progesterone or medroxyprogesterone acetate on quality of life in postmenopausal women: a cross-sectional survey. *J Womens Health Gend Based Med* 2000;9:381–387.

107. **Komesaroff PA, Black CVS, Cable V, et al.** Effects of wild yam extract on menopausal symptoms, lipids and sex hormones in healthy menopausal women. *Climacteric* 2001;4:144–150.

108. **Benster B, Carey A, Wadsworth F, et al.** Double-blind placebo-controlled study to evaluate the effect of pro-juven progesterone cream on atherosclerosis and bone density. *Menopause Int* 2009;15:100–106.

109. **Leonetti HB, Longo S, Anasti JN.** Transdermal progesterone cream for vasomotor symptoms and postmenopausal bone loss. *Obstet Gynecol* 1999;94:225–228.

110. **Leung JM, Dzankic S, Manku K, et al.** The prevalence and predictors of the use of alternative medicine in presurgical patients in five California hospitals. *Anesth Analg* 2001;93:1062–1068.

111. **Tsen LC, Segal S, Pothier M, et al.** Alternative medicine use in presurgical patients. *Anesthesiology* 2000;93:148–151.

112. **Kaye AD, Clarke RC, Saber R, et al.** Herbal medicines: current trends in anesthesiology practice—a hospital survey. *J Clin Anesth* 2000;12:468–471.

113. **Wang DW, Jin YH.** Present status of cesarean section under acupuncture anesthesia in China. *Fukushima J Med Sci* 1989;35:45–52.

114. **Kotani N, Hashimoto H, Sato Y, et al.** Preoperative intradermal acupuncture reduces postoperative pain, nausea and vomiting,

analgesic requirement, and sympathoadrenal responses. *Anesthesiology* 2001;95:349–356.

115. **Frey UH, Scharmann P, Löhlein C, et al.** P6 acustimulation effectively decreases postoperative nausea and vomiting in high-risk patients. *Br J Anaesth* 2009;102:620–625.

116. **Streitberger K, Diefenbacher M, Bauer A, et al.** Acupuncture compared to placebo-acupuncture for postoperative nausea and vomiting prophylaxis: a randomised placebo-controlled patient and observer blind trial. *Anaesthesia* 2004;59:142–149.

117. **Turgut S, Ozalp G, Dikmen S, et al.** Acupressure for postoperative nausea and vomiting in gynaecological patients receiving patient-controlled analgesia. *Eur J Anaesthesiol* 2007;24:87–91.

118. **Wang B, Tang J, White PF, et al.** Effect of the intensity of transcutaneous acupoint electrical stimulation on the postoperative analgesic requirement. *Anesth Analg* 1997;85:406–413.

119. **Greif R, Laciny S, Mokhtarani M, et al.** Transcutaneous electrical stimulation of an auricular acupuncture point decreases anesthetic requirement. *Anesthesiology* 2002;96:306–312.

120. **Marucha PT, Kiecolt-Glaser JK, Favagehi M.** Mucosal wound healing is impaired by examination stress. *Psychosom Med* 1998;60:362–365.

121. **Egbert LD.** Reduction of postoperative pain by encouragement and instruction of patients. A study of doctor-patient rapport. *N Engl J Med* 1964;270:825–827.

122. **Lang EV, Benotsch EG, Fick LJ, et al.** Adjunctive non-pharmacological analgesia for invasive medical procedures: a randomised trial. *Lancet* 2000;355:1486–1490.

123. **Bennett HL, Benson DR, Kuiken DA.** Preoperative instructions for decreased bleed during spine surgery. *Anesthesiology* 1986;65:A245.

124. **Lepage C, Drolet P, Girard M, et al.** Music decreases sedative requirements during spinal anesthesia. *Anesth Analg* 2001;93:912–916.

125. **Kim MS, Cho KS, Woo H, et al.** Effects of hand massage on anxiety in cataract surgery using local anesthesia. *J Cataract Refractive Surg* 2001;27:884–890.

126. **Nilsson U, Rawal N, Unestáhl LE, et al.** Improved recovery after music and therapeutic suggestions during general anaesthesia: a double-blind randomised controlled trial. *Acta Anaesthesiol Scand* 2001;45:812–817.

127. **Dawson P, Van Hamel C, Wilkinson D, et al.** Patient-controlled analgesia and intra-operative suggestion. *Anaesthesia* 2001;56:65–69.

128. **Eberhart LH, Doring HJ, Holzrichter P, et al.** Therapeutic suggestions given during neurolept-anaesthesia decrease post-operative nausea and vomiting. *Eur J Anaesthesiol* 1998;15:446–452.

129. **Enqvist B, von Konow L, Bystedt H.** Pre- and perioperative suggestion in maxillofacial surgery: effects on blood loss and recovery. *Int J Clin Exp Hypn* 1995;43:284–294.

130. **Faymonville ME, Fissette J, Mambourg PH, et al.** Hypnosis as adjunct therapy in conscious sedation for plastic surgery. *Reg Anesth* 1995;20:145–151.

131. **Stevinson C, Ernst E.** Complementary/alternative therapies for premenstrual syndrome: a systematic review of randomized controlled trials. *Am J Obstet Gynecol* 2001;185:227–235.

GENERAL GYNECOLOGY

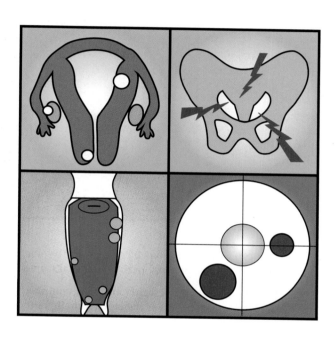

14 Benign Diseases of the Female Reproductive Tract

Paula J. Adams Hillard

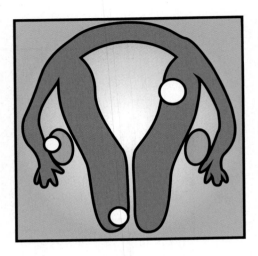

- The causes of abnormal bleeding vary by age, with anovulatory bleeding most likely in adolescents and perimenopausal women.

- Pelvic masses in adolescents are most commonly functional or benign neoplastic ovarian masses, whereas the risks of malignant ovarian tumors increase with age.

- Although pelvic ultrasonography is an excellent technique for imaging pelvic masses and ultrasonographic characteristics may suggest reassuring characteristics of an ovarian mass, the possibility of malignancy must be kept in mind.

- Vulvovaginal symptoms of any sort in a young child should prompt the consideration of possible sexual abuse.

- Most uterine leiomyomas are asymptomatic, although bleeding, pressure symptoms, or pain may necessitate medical or surgical management.

Benign gynecologic conditions can present with a variety of signs and symptoms that vary by age. In this chapter, the most likely causes of specific signs and symptoms, as well as diagnosis and management, are described for each age group: prepubertal, adolescent, reproductive age, and postmenopausal women. **The common gynecologic problems include those that cause pain, bleeding, pelvic masses (which may be symptomatic or asymptomatic), as well as vulvar and vaginal symptoms.** Benign conditions of the female genital tract include anatomic lesions of the uterine corpus and cervix, ovaries, fallopian tubes, vagina, and vulva. A classification of benign lesions of the vulva, vagina, and cervix appears in Table 14.1. Leiomyoma, polyps, and hyperplasia are the most common benign conditions of the uterus in adult women. Benign uterine leiomyoma (uterine fibroids) are presented in Chapter 15. Benign tumors of the ovaries are listed in Table 14.2. Malignant diseases are presented in Chapters 35–40.

Prepubertal Age Group

Prepubertal Bleeding

Prior to menarche, which normally does not occur before nine years of age, *any* bleeding requires evaluation. To appropriately evaluate a young girl with vaginal bleeding, a practitioner should understand the events of puberty (1–4). The hormonal changes that control the

Table 14.1 Classification of Benign Conditions of the Vulva, Vagina, and Cervix

Vulva

Skin conditions

Pigmented lesions

Tumors and cysts

Ulcers

Nonneoplastic epithelial disorders

Vagina

Embryonic origin

    Mesonephric, paramesonephric, and urogenital sinus cysts

    Adenosis (related to in utero diethylstilbestrol exposure)

    Vaginal septa or duplications

Pelvic organ prolapse/Disorders of pelvic support

    Anterior vaginal prolapse

        Cystourethrocele

        Cystocele

    Apical vaginal prolapse

        Uterovaginal

        Vaginal vault

    Posterior vaginal prolapse

        Enterocele

        Rectocele

Other

    Condyloma

    Urethral diverticula

    Fibroepithelial polyp

    Vaginal endometriosis

Cervix

Infectious

    Condyloma

    Herpes simplex virus ulceration

    Chlamydial cervicitis

    Other cervicitis

Other

    Endocervical polyps

    Nabothian cysts

    Columnar epithelium eversion

Table 14.2 Benign Ovarian Tumors

Functional

Follicular

Corpus luteum

Theca lutein

Inflammatory

Tubo-ovarian abscess or complex

Neoplastic

Germ cell

Benign cystic teratoma

Other and mixed

Epithelial

Serous cystadenoma

Mucinous cystadenoma

Fibroma

Cystadenofibroma

Brenner tumor

Mixed tumor

Other

Endometrioma

cyclic functioning of the hypothalamic–pituitary–ovarian axis are described in Chapter 7. An understanding of the normal sequence and timing of these events is critical to an appropriate assessment of a girl at the onset of bleeding (see Chapter 29). Menarche typically occurs when an adolescent has reached Tanner stage 3 or 4 of breast development (Fig. 14.1). Bleeding in the absence of breast development must be evaluated.

Differential Diagnosis of Prepubertal Vaginal Bleeding

Slight vaginal bleeding can occur within the first few days of life because of withdrawal from exposure to high levels of maternal estrogen. New mothers of female infants should be informed of this possibility to preclude unnecessary anxiety. After the neonatal period, a number of causes of bleeding should be considered in the prepubertal age group (Table 14.3). Menses rarely occur before breast budding (5,6). Vaginal bleeding in the absence of secondary sexual characteristics should be evaluated carefully.

The causes of bleeding in this age group range from the medically mundane to malignancies that may be life threatening. The source of the bleeding is sometimes difficult to identify, and parents who observe blood in a child's diapers or panties may be unsure of the source— whether from the urinary tract, the vagina, or the rectum. Pediatricians usually look for urinary causes of bleeding, and gastrointestinal factors such as constipation and or anal fissure or inflammatory bowel disease should be considered. The possibility of abuse should always be considered in girls with any vulvovaginal symptoms, particularly if bleeding is present. Failure to diagnose sexual abuse may leave a child in significant danger.

Vulvar Lesions   Vulvar irritation can lead to pruritus with excoriation, maceration of the vulvar skin, or fissures that can bleed. Other visible external causes of bleeding in this age group include urethral prolapse, condylomas, lichen sclerosus, or molluscum contagiosum. **Urethral prolapse can present acutely with a tender mass that may be friable or bleed slightly; it is most common in African American girls and may be confused with a vaginal mass** (Fig. 14.2). The classic presentation is a mass symmetrically surrounding the urethra. This condition can be managed medically with the topical application of estrogens (7). The presence of condyloma should prompt questioning about abuse, although it was suggested that **condyloma that appears**

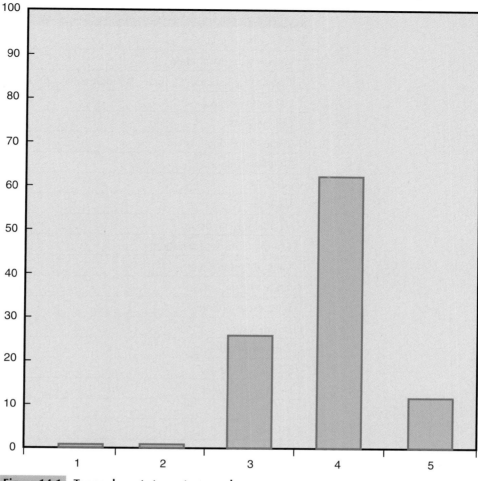

Figure 14.1   Tanner breast stage at menarche.

during the first 2 to 3 years of life may be acquired perinatally from maternal infection with human papillomavirus (Fig. 14.3) (8,9). Excoriation and subepithelial hemorrhage ("blood blisters") into the skin can cause external bleeding in the presence of prepubertal lichen sclerosus; this finding may mistakenly be identified as abuse, and the conditions are not mutually exclusive (Fig. 14.4) (10). **Although most gynecologists recognize the appearance of lichen sclerosus in postmenopausal women, the condition can occur in prepubertal girls and may not be recognized by clinicians who are unfamiliar with this condition.** As with adults, the cause of lichen sclerosus remains uncertain; a familial incidence was identified (11).

Foreign Body   **A foreign body in the vagina is a common cause of vaginal discharge, which may appear purulent or bloody.** Young children explore all orifices and may place all varieties of small objects inside their vaginas (Fig. 14.5). An object, such as a small plastic toy, can sometimes be palpated on rectal examination, and occasionally "milked" toward the vaginal introitus to allow removal. The most common foreign bodies found in the vagina are small pieces of toilet paper (12). Although it was suggested that the presence of vaginal foreign bodies might be a marker for sexual abuse, this is not always the case; but the possibility of abuse should always be considered.

Precocious Puberty   **Vaginal bleeding in the absence of other secondary sexual characteristics may result from precocious puberty** (see Chapter 29), although as with normal puberty, the onset of breast budding or pubic hair growth are more likely to occur before vaginal bleeding. A large observational study suggested that the onset of pubertal changes—breast budding and pubic hair—might occur earlier than previously thought (2). Evaluation for precocious puberty was recommended for girls with pubertal development younger than age 8 years. Guidelines proposed evaluation of white girls younger than age 7 years and African American girls younger

Table 14.3 Causes of Vaginal Bleeding in Prepubertal Girls
Vulvar and external
Vulvitis with excoriation
Trauma (e.g., accidental injury [straddle injury] or sexual abuse)
Lichen sclerosus
Condylomas
Molluscum contagiosum
Urethral prolapse
Vaginal
Vaginitis
Vaginal foreign body
Trauma (abuse, penetration)
Vaginal tumor
Uterine
Precocious puberty
Ovarian tumor
Granulosa cell tumor
Germ cell tumor
Exogenous estrogens
Topical
Enteral
Other
McCune-Albright syndrome

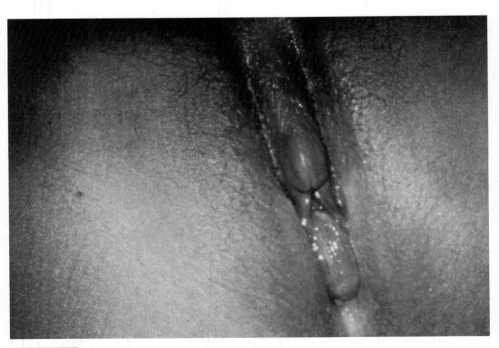

Figure 14.2   Urethral prolapse in prepubertal girl.

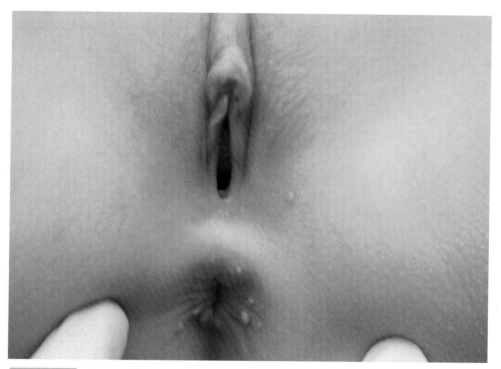

Figure 14.3   Perianal condyloma in prepubertal girl.

than age 6 years who have either breast development or pubic hair, rather than the traditional age of 8 (13). An expert panel concluded that there is reasonable evidence that pubertal milestones are occurring at a younger age in girls (3).

Trauma   Trauma can be a cause of genital bleeding. **A careful history should be obtained from one or both parents or caretakers and the child herself, because trauma caused by sexual abuse often is not recognized. Trauma can be characterized as accidental or nonaccidental, which is described as child abuse.** Physical findings that are inconsistent with the description of the alleged accident should prompt consideration of abuse and appropriate consultation or referral to an experienced social worker or sexual abuse team. **All states impose a mandatory legal obligation to report suspected child physical abuse;** most states specifically require reporting child sexual abuse, but even in those that do not, the laws are broad enough to encompass sexual abuse implicitly (14,15). Notification is required even with the suspicion of sexual abuse. In general, a straddle injury occurring with accidental trauma affects the anterior and lateral vulvar area, whereas penetrating injuries with lesions of the fourchette or lesions that extend through the hymenal ring are less likely to occur as a result of accidental trauma (Fig. 14.6) (16).

Abuse   **The medical evaluation of suspected child sexual abuse is best managed by individuals who have experience in assessing the physical findings, laboratory results, and the children's statements and behaviors.** Genital findings are categorized as follows (17):

1. Normal, normal variants, and other conditions
2. Nonspecific findings that may be the result of abuse, depending on the timing of the examination, but that may be due to other causes
3. Concerning for abuse or trauma, including findings that were noted with documented abuse and that may be concerning for abuse, but for which insufficient data exist to determine that abuse is the only cause
4. Clear evidence of blunt force or penetrating trauma.

The overall classification of the likelihood for abuse can be categorized as follows (17):

1. No evidence of abuse
2. Possible abuse

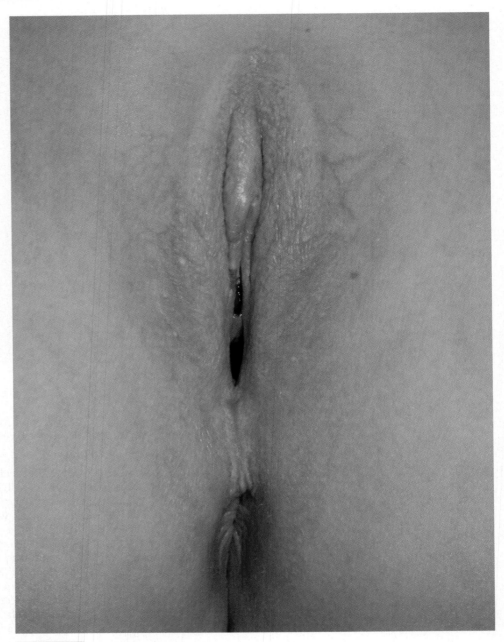

Figure 14.4 Prepubertal lichen sclerosus.

3. Probable abuse

4. Definitive evidence of abuse or sexual contact.

Most cases of child sexual abuse do not come to light with an acute injury and instead are associated with normal or nonspecific genital findings (17,18). Forms of abuse such as fondling or digital penetration may not result in visible genital lesions.

Other Causes   **Other serious but rare causes of vaginal bleeding include vaginal tumors. The most common tumor in the prepubertal age group is a rhabdomyosarcoma (sarcoma botryoides), which is associated with bleeding and a grapelike clustered mass** (see Chapter 36). Other forms of vaginal tumor are rare but should be ruled out with a thorough examination under anesthesia with vaginoscopy if no other obvious external source of bleeding is found.

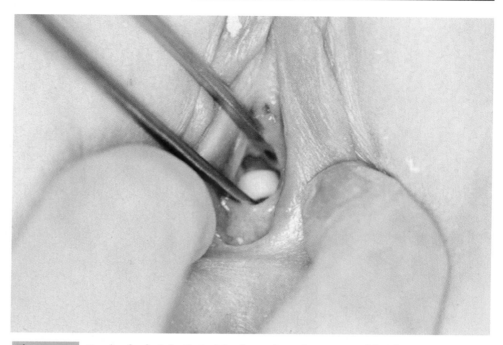

Figure 14.5   Foreign body (plastic toy) in the vagina of an 8-year-old girl.

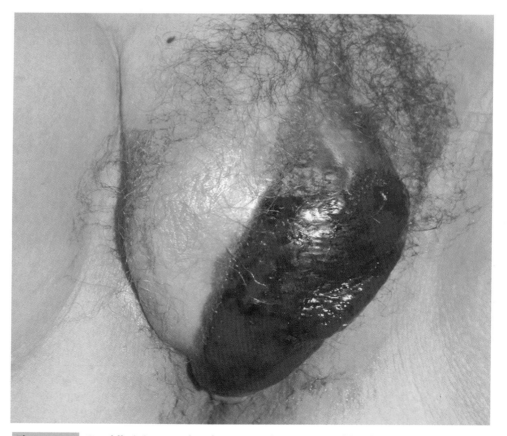

Figure 14.6   Straddle injury—vulvar hematoma in a 13-year-old girl.

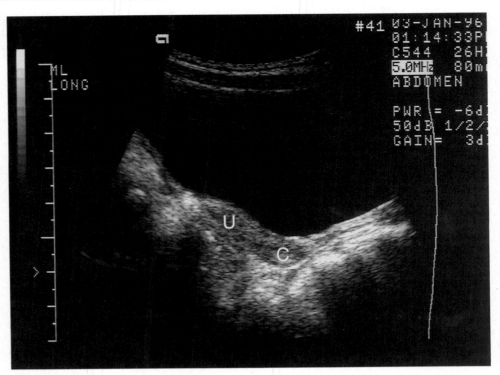

Figure 14.7   Pelvic ultrasound (transabdominal) of a premenarchal 10-year-old girl.

Hormonally active ovarian tumors can cause endometrial proliferation and bleeding. Likewise, exogenously administered estrogens can result in bleeding. Rarely, bleeding can result from the prolonged use of topical estrogens prescribed as therapy for vulvovaginitis or labial adhesions or from accidental ingestion of prescription estrogens.

Diagnosis of Prepubertal Bleeding

Examination   A careful examination is indicated when a child has genital symptoms. The technique of examining the prepubertal child is described in Chapter 1. **If no obvious cause of bleeding is visible externally or within the distal vagina, an examination can be performed using anesthesia with vaginoscopy to completely visualize the vagina and cervix. This examination should be performed by a clinician who has experience in pediatric and adolescent gynecology.**

Imaging   If an ovarian or vaginal mass is suspected, a transabdominal pelvic ultrasonographic examination can provide useful information. The appearance of the ovaries (normal prepubertal size and volume, follicular development, cystic, or solid) can be noted, as well as the size and configuration of the uterus. **The prepubertal uterus has a distinctive appearance, with equal proportions of cervix and fundus and a size of approximately 2 to 3.5 cm in length and 0.5 to 1 cm in width** (Fig. 14.7). The uterine fundus enlarges with estrogen stimulation, resulting in the postmenarchal appearance in which the uterine fundus is larger than the cervix (19). An ultrasonographic examination should be the first imaging study performed; more sophisticated imaging techniques, such as magnetic resonance imaging (MRI) or computed tomography (CT) scanning, are rarely indicated as initial diagnostic modalities, and they add unnecessary expense and radiation exposure with CT.

Management of Prepubertal Vaginal Bleeding

The management of bleeding in prepubertal-age girls is directed toward the cause of bleeding. If bloody discharge believed to result from nonspecific vulvovaginitis persists despite therapy, further evaluation may be necessary to rule out the presence of a foreign body. Skin lesions (chronic irritation) and lichen sclerosus may be difficult to manage but can be treated with a course of topical steroids; lichen sclerosus often requires the use of ultrahigh-potency topical steroids and ongoing maintenance therapy. **Vaginal and ovarian tumors should be managed in consultation with a gynecologic oncologist.**

Table 14.4 Causes of Pelvic Mass by Approximate Frequency and Age					
Infancy	*Prepubertal*	*Adolescent*	*Reproductive*	*Perimenopausal*	*Postmenopausal*
Functional cyst	Functional cyst	Functional cyst	Functional cyst	Fibroids	Ovarian tumor (malignant of benign)
Germ cell tumor	Germ cell tumor	Pregnancy	Pregnancy	Epithelial ovarian tumor	Functional cyst
		Benign cystic teratoma /other germ cell tumors	Uterine fibroids	Functional cyst	Bowel, malignant tumor or inflammatory
		Obstructing vaginal or uterine anomalies	Epithelial ovarian tumor		Metastases
		Epithelial ovarian tumor			

Prepubertal Pelvic Masses

Presentation of Prepubertal Pelvic Masses

The probable causes of a pelvic mass found on physical examination or through radiologic studies are vastly different in prepubertal children than they are in adolescents or post-menopausal women (Table 14.4). **A pelvic mass may be gynecologic in origin, or it may arise from the urinary tract or bowel. The gynecologic causes of a pelvic mass may be uterine, adnexal, or more specifically ovarian.** Because of the small pelvic capacity of a prepubertal child, a pelvic mass very quickly becomes abdominal in location as it enlarges and may be palpable on abdominal examination. Ovarian masses in this age group may be asymptomatic, associated with chronic pressure-related bowel or bladder symptoms, or may present with acute pain caused by rupture or torsion. Abdominal or pelvic pain is one of the most frequent initial symptoms. The diagnosis of ovarian masses in prepubertal girls is difficult because the condition is rare in this age group and, consequently, there is a low index of suspicion. Many symptoms are nonspecific, and acute symptoms are more likely to be attributed to more common entities such as appendicitis. **Abdominal palpation and bimanual rectoabdominal examination are important in any child who has nonspecific abdominal or pelvic symptoms.** An ovarian mass that is abdominal in location can be confused with other abdominal masses occurring in children, such as Wilms' tumor or neuroblastoma. Acute pain is often associated with torsion. The ovarian ligament becomes elongated as a result of the abdominal location of ovarian tumors, thus creating a predisposition to torsion. Adnexal torsion is more likely to occur with an ovarian mass than with a normal size ovary. While torsion of a normal ovary is rare in adolescents and adults, it is more likely to occur in prepubertal girls.

Diagnosis of Prepubertal Pelvic Masses

Ultrasonography is the most valuable tool for diagnosing ovarian masses. The characteristics of a pelvic mass can be determined. Whereas both unilocular and multilocular cysts frequently resolve with observation, the finding of a solid component mandates surgical assessment because of the high risk of a germ cell tumor (20). Additional imaging studies, such as CT scanning, MRI, or Doppler flow studies, may be helpful in establishing the diagnosis (21).

Differential Diagnosis

Fewer than 2% of ovarian malignancies occur in children and adolescents (22). Ovarian tumors account for approximately 1% of all malignant tumors in these age groups. Germ cell tumors make up one-half to two-thirds of ovarian neoplasms in individuals younger than 20 years of age. A review of studies conducted from 1940 until 1975 concluded that 35% of all ovarian neoplasms occurring during childhood and adolescence were malignant (23). **In girls younger than 9 years of age, approximately 80% of the ovarian neoplasms were malignant.** Germ cell tumors account for approximately 60% of ovarian neoplasms in children and adolescents compared with 20% of these tumors in adults (23). Epithelial neoplasms are rare in the prepubertal age group; thus, data usually are reported from referral centers. Some reports include only neoplastic masses, whereas others include nonneoplastic masses; some series combine data from prepubertal and adolescent girls. One community survey of ovarian masses revealed that the frequency of malignancy was much lower than previously reported; **of all ovarian masses confirmed surgically in childhood and adolescence, only 6% of patients with ovarian enlargement had malignant neoplasms, and only 10% of neoplasms were malignant** (24). Surgical decision making influences the statistics on incidence; the surgical excision of functional masses that would resolve in time inflates the percentage of benign masses. In one series, nonneoplastic masses in young women and girls younger than 20 years of age constituted two-thirds of the total (25). Even in girls younger than 10 years of age, 60% of the masses were nonneoplastic, and two-thirds of the neoplastic masses were benign. Authors of older case series were less aware of the benign and functional masses that are now found incidentally with routine sonographic images. Functional, follicular cysts can occur in fetuses, newborns, and prepubertal children (26). Rarely, they may be associated with sexual precocity.

Management of Prepubertal Pelvic Masses

A plan for the management of pelvic masses in prepubertal age girls is shown in Figure 14.8. **Unilocular cysts are virtually always benign, even in this age group, and will regress in**

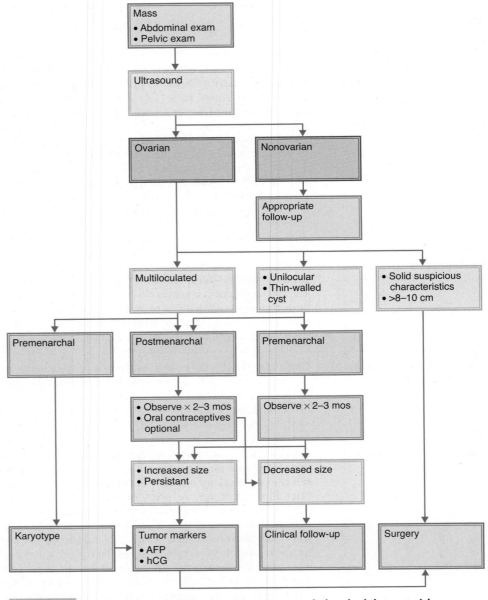

Figure 14.8   Management of pelvic masses in premenarchal and adolescent girls.

3 to 6 months; thus, they do not require surgical management with oophorectomy or oophorocystectomy. Close observation is recommended, and there is a risk of ovarian torsion that must be discussed with the child's parents (27). Recurrence rates after cyst aspiration (either ultrasonographically guided or with laparoscopy) may be as high as 50%. Attention should be directed to long-term effects on endocrine function and future fertility; preservation of ovarian tissue is a priority for patients with benign tumors. Oophorectomy should be avoided if at all possible for benign masses (28). **Premature surgical therapy for a functional ovarian mass can result in ovarian and tubal adhesions that can adversely affect future fertility.** Solid masses, those larger than approximately 8 cm, and enlarging masses require surgical intervention, as the likelihood of neoplasm is high.

Prepubertal Vulvar Conditions

Neonatal Vulvar Conditions

Various developmental and congenital vulvovaginal abnormalities occur in the neonatal age group. Whereas an extensive discussion of these abnormalities is beyond the scope of this text, obstetrician-gynecologists will recognize that they must be prepared to deal with the parents and family when an infant is born with ambiguous genitalia. The etiology of these problems, and intersex disorders (now termed disorder of sex development [DSD]) that may be discovered in an older child can be complex (29). Chromosomal abnormalities, enzyme deficiencies (including 17- or 21-hydroxylase deficiency as causes of congenital adrenal hyperplasia), or prenatal masculinization of a female fetus resulting from maternal androgen-secreting ovarian tumors or, rarely, drug exposure can all result in genital abnormalities that are noted at birth. These abnormalities are described in Chapter 31

Ambiguous genitalia represent a social and potential medical urgency that is best handled by a team of specialists, which may include urologists, neonatologists, endocrinologists, and pediatric gynecologists (30). The first question parents ask after a baby is born "is it a boy or a girl?" In the case of ambiguous genitalia, the parents should be informed that the baby's genitals are not fully developed and, therefore, a simple examination of the external genitalia cannot determine the actual sex. The parents should be told that data will be collected but that it may take several days or longer to determine the baby's intended sex. In some situations, it may be best to state simply that the baby has some serious medical complications. The issues of sex assignment and appropriateness or timing of surgical therapy are controversial and should be managed by clinicians with extensive experience in this area (29,30).

Other genital abnormalities may be noted at birth, although few obstetricians or pediatricians carefully examine the external genitalia of female neonates. It is argued that **careful inspection of the external genitalia of all female infants should be performed, with gentle probing of the introitus and anus to determine the patency of the hymen or a possible imperforate anus.** If patency is in doubt, a rectal thermometer may be used to gently test the patency. It is suggested that this examination should be performed on all female infants in the delivery room (31,32). Various types of hymenal configurations in the newborn are described, ranging from imperforate to microperforate, to cribriform, to hymenal bands, and to hymens with central anterior, posterior, or eccentric orifices (33). An examination during the neonatal period would prevent the discovery of an imperforate hymen or vaginal septum after a young woman experiences periodic pelvic and abdominal pain with the development of a large hematometra or hematocolpos (34).

Congenital vulvar tumors may include strawberry hemangiomas, which are relatively superficial vascular lesions, and large cavernous hemangiomas. Treatment is controversial; many lesions will spontaneously regress. Some clinicians have used interferon-α therapy (35,36).

Childhood Vulvar Conditions

Vulvar and vaginal symptoms, such as burning, dysuria, itching, or a rash, are common initial symptoms among children that are reported to gynecologists. It may be difficult for a young child to describe vulvar sensations. Parents may notice the child crying during urination, scratching herself repeatedly, or complaining of vague symptoms. Often, the child's pediatrician will have evaluated the child for urinary tract infection. Evaluation for pinworms is warranted, because pinworms can cause severe itching in the vulvar as well as perianal area. **Vulvovaginitis is the most common gynecologic problem of childhood.** Prepubertally, the vulva, vestibule, and vagina are anatomically and histologically vulnerable to bacterial infection, with the bacteria

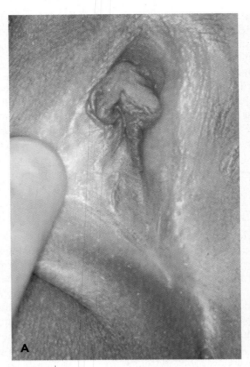
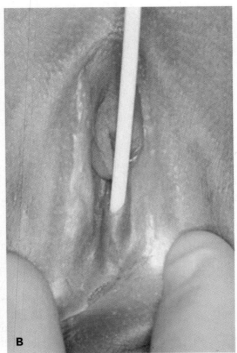

Figure 14.9   A: Labial adhesions B: Cotton-tipped applicator placed inside the labial adhesions shown in (A).

typically present in the perianal area. The physical proximity of the vagina and vestibule to the anus can result in overgrowth of bacteria that can cause primary vulvitis and secondary vaginitis. Yeast infections are rare in prepubertal children who are toilet trained and out of diapers (37).

The clinician should be familiar with normal prepubertal genital anatomy and hymenal configuration (38,39). **The unestrogenized vulvar vestibule is mildly erythematous and can be confused with infection. In addition, smegma around and beneath the prepuce may resemble patches of candida vulvitis. In prepubertal girls, the vulvar area is quite susceptible to chemical irritants.**

Chronic skin conditions such as lichen sclerosus, psoriasis, seborrheic dermatitis, and atopic vulvitis may occur in children (40). Lichen sclerosus, the cause of which is not well established, has a characteristic "cigarette paper" appearance in a keyhole distribution (around the vulva and anus) (Fig. 14.4). Lichen sclerosus should be treated in pediatric patients as it is in adults; there is some evidence that the condition may regress as the child progresses through adrenarche and menarche, although this appears to be infrequent. The use of ultrapotent steroids topically has been successful in children and adults (41).

Labial agglutination or adhesions may occur as a result of chronic vulvar inflammation from any cause (Fig. 14.9A). The treatment of labial adhesions consists of a brief course (2 to 6 weeks) of externally applied estrogen cream. The area of agglutination (adhesion) will become thin as a result, and separation can usually be performed in the office with the use of a topical anesthetic (e.g., lidocaine jelly) (Fig. 14.9B). Manual separation in the office without pretreatment with topical estrogen and without anesthesia is discouraged, as this practice may be so traumatic to the child that she will not allow subsequent examination. In the absence of a previously traumatic examination or previous surgical separation with recurrence, surgical separation frequently is not required (42). Treatment with a topical emollient (such as petrolatum) is indicated after lysis to prevent recurrent adhesions. Urethral prolapse may cause acute pain or bleeding, or the presence of a mass may be noted (Fig. 14.2).

Vulvovaginal symptoms of any sort in a young child should prompt the consideration of possible sexual abuse. Sexually transmitted infections may occur in prepubertal children (43).

Although vulvar condyloma presenting before age 2 to 3 years can be transmitted during vaginal delivery from the mother or from warts on caretakers' hands, the possibility of abuse should be considered in all children with genital warts (44,45). Condyloma in older girls may be spread in a nonsexual manner, but was classified as "indeterminant" in classification findings that may be associated with sexual abuse (44). Sensitive, but direct, questioning of the parent or caretaker and the child should be a part of the evaluation; if sexual abuse is suspected, the incident must be reported to the appropriate social services agency.

Nonsexually transmitted vulvar ulcers can occur in peripubertal and adolescent girls, often in association with systemic symptoms suggestive of a viral illness (46). Herpes simplex virus, syphilis, and Behçet's disease can cause vulvar ulcers, and they may occur as a form of genital aphthosis (Fig. 14.10).

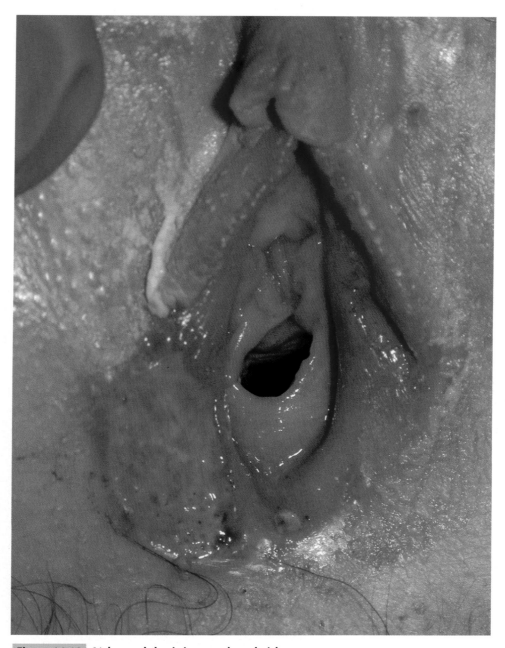

Figure 14.10 **Vulvar aphthosis in prepubertal girl.**

Prepubertal Vaginal Conditions

Vaginal Discharge in Prepubertal Girls

The symptom of vaginal discharge in the prepubertal age group is almost always caused by inflammation and irritation. In prepubertal girls, the primary site typically is the vulva, with vaginitis following secondarily, whereas in adolescents and adults, vaginitis typically is the primary finding with vulvitis occurring secondarily. **Sexual abuse should always be considered in prepubertal children with vaginal discharge or a foreign body** (47). Although the routine use of cultures to detect sexually transmitted diseases (STDs) in girls with a history of sexual abuse was questioned, vaginal culture for gonorrhea and chlamydia should be performed in girls who have symptoms that include vaginal discharge (48). In prepubertal girls, vulvovaginitis is usually caused by multiple organisms that are present in the perineal area, although a single organism such as *Streptococcus,* or even rarely *Shigella,* may be causative (49). When the cause is related to poor perineal hygiene, cultures often reveal a mixture of bacterial organisms. In this situation, the typical history is intermittent symptoms of irritation, itching, discharge, and odor over many months to years. Treatment should be initiated with a focus on hygiene and cleansing measures (40). A short-term (less than 4 weeks) course of treatment with topical estrogens and broad-spectrum antibiotics may be necessary. The problem is frequently recurrent. In girls who have a relatively acute onset of vaginal discharge and vulvovaginal symptoms, a single bacterial organism is more likely to be the cause of their symptoms.

Pokorny and Stormer described a technique for obtaining vaginal cultures and for performing vaginal irrigation (50). A catheter within a catheter can be fashioned using the tubing from an intravenous butterfly setup within a sterile urethral catheter. Nonbacteriostatic saline (1–3 mL) can be injected, aspirated, and sent for culture (Fig. 14.11). Cultures taken in this manner are almost always better tolerated than cultures obtained using a cotton-tipped applicator. A larger quantity of saline can be used to irrigate the vagina while the catheter is still within the vagina. Small foreign bodies can often be flushed from the vagina in this manner. The most common foreign body is a small piece of toilet paper, although children will place other objects (toys, beans, coins) within their vaginas (Fig. 14.5). **A persistent vaginal discharge after treatment or a discharge that is bloody or brown in color without other obvious external lesions should prompt vaginal irrigation or vaginoscopy to rule out a foreign body** (12).

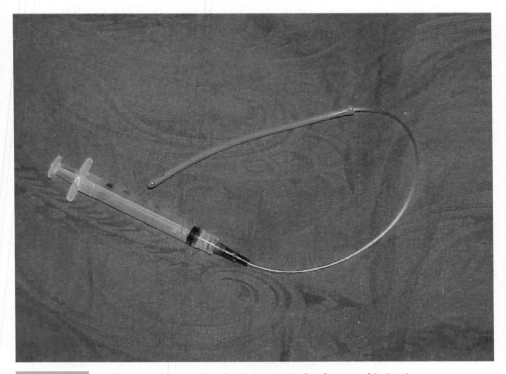

Figure 14.11   Catheter technique for obtaining vaginal culture and irrigation.

Adolescent Age Group

The adolescent's experience and expression of illness and pain should be viewed within the context of her life experiences. Most adolescents have limited life experiences with problems such as pain, discomfort, or bleeding. An adolescent may state that she is experiencing the "worst pain of her life" and yet may appear to be reasonably comfortable. She may well be stating the truth about this experience, which the clinician must still interpret differently from the symptoms of an adult woman who, for instance, may be in active labor. It should be remembered that an individual's response to illness and pain is to some extent a learned behavior.

Adolescent Abnormal Bleeding

Normal Menses in Adolescents

To assess vaginal bleeding during adolescence, it is necessary to understand the range of normal menstrual cycles (see Chapter 7). **During the first 2 to 5 years after menarche, most cycles are anovulatory. Despite this, they are somewhat regular, within a range of approximately 21 to 45 days, in contrast to adult women, whose cycles typically range between 21 and 38 days** (51–55). In more than one-fourth of girls, a pattern of plus or minus 10 days and a cycle length of 21 to approximately 45 days are established within the first three cycles; in one-half of girls, the pattern is established by the seventh cycle; and in two-thirds of girls, such a pattern is established within 2 years of menarche (53) (Table 14.5).

The mean duration of menses is 4.7 days; 89% of cycles last 7 days. The average blood loss per cycle is 35 mL, and the major component of menstrual discharge is endometrial tissue (56). **An 80 mL/cycle is used as a definition of heavy menstrual bleeding and recurrent bleeding in excess of 80 mL/cycle results in anemia, although the clinical utility of the 80 mL/cycle is questioned** (57,58).

The common clinical practice of asking how many pads or tampons are soaked on a heavy day or per cycle can give a rough approximation of blood loss (three to five pads per day is typical). Individual variations in fastidiousness, lack of familiarity with the volume of blood loss other than one's own, and errors in estimation or recollection result in inaccuracies in estimations of menstrual volume. One study found that one-third of individuals who estimated their cycles to be moderate or light had bleeding in excess of 80 mL/cycle, whereas nearly one-half of those who described the bleeding as heavy had flow less than 80 mL/cycle (59). In addition, the amount of menstrual blood contained in each tampon or pad may vary both within brands as well as from one brand to another (57). However, changing a pad hourly, clots larger than "50 pence size," and requiring a change overnight are associated with a measured volume of greater than 80 mL (58).

The transition from anovulatory to ovulatory cycles during adolescence takes place during the first several years after menarche. It results from the so-called *maturation of the hypothalamic–pituitary–ovarian axis,* characterized by positive feedback mechanisms in which a rising estrogen level triggers a surge of luteinizing hormone and ovulation. **Most adolescents have ovulatory cycles by the end of their second year of menstruation, although most cycles (even anovulatory ones) remain within a rather narrow range of approximately 21 to 42 days.**

Table 14.5 Parameters for Normal Menstrual Cycles in Adolescents	
	Normal
Menstrual Cycle Frequency	21–45 days
Cycle Variation from cycle to cycle	Less than in adults
Duration of flow	4–8 days
Volume of flow	4–80 mL

From **Hillard PJ.** Menstruation in young girls: a clinical perspective. *Obstet Gynecol* 2002;99:655–662.

Table 14.6 Conditions Associated with Anovulation and Abnormal Bleeding
Eating disorders
Anorexia nervosa
Bulimia nervosa
Excessive physical exercise
Chronic illness
Primary ovarian insufficiency—POI (previously termed premature ovarian failure [POF])
Alcohol and other drug abuse
Stress
Thyroid disease
Hypothyroidism
Hyperthyroidism
Diabetes mellitus
Androgen excess syndromes (e.g., polycystic ovary syndrome [PCOS])

Differential Diagnosis of Adolescent Abnormal Bleeding

Cycles that are longer than 42 days, bleeding that occurs more frequently than 21 days, and bleeding that lasts more than 7 days should be considered abnormal, particularly after the first 2 years from the onset of menarche. Bleeding occurring less frequently than an internal of 90 days is abnormal, even in the first gynecologic year after menarche (51). The variability in cycle length is greater during adolescence than adulthood; thus, greater irregularity is acceptable if neither significant anemia nor hemorrhage is present. However, consideration should be given to an evaluation of possible causes of abnormal menses (particularly underlying causes of anovulation such as androgen excess syndromes or causes of oligomenorrhea such as eating disorders) for girls whose cycles are consistently outside normal ranges or whose cycles were previously regular and become irregular (60,61). Conditions that are associated with abnormal bleeding are listed in Table 14.6 and more fully discussed in Chapters 29–31.

Anovulation **Anovulatory bleeding can be too frequent, prolonged, or heavy, particularly after a long interval of amenorrhea.** The physiology of this phenomenon relates to a failure of the feedback mechanism in which rising estrogen levels result in a decline in follicle-stimulating hormone (FSH) with subsequent decline of estrogen levels. In anovulatory cycles, estrogen secretion continues, resulting in endometrial proliferation with subsequent unstable growth and incomplete shedding. The clinical result is irregular, prolonged, and heavy bleeding.

Studies of adolescent menses show differences in rates of ovulation based on the number of months or years postmenarche. **The younger the age at menarche, the sooner regular ovulation is established.** In one study, the time from menarche until 50% of the cycles were ovulatory was 1 year for girls whose menarche occurred when they were younger than 12 years of age, 3 years for girls whose menarche occurred between 12 and 12.9 years of age, and 4.5 years for girls whose menarche occurred at 13 years of age or older (62).

Pregnancy-Related Bleeding **The possibility of pregnancy must be considered when an adolescent seeks treatment for abnormal bleeding** (Table 14.7). Bleeding in pregnancy can be associated with a spontaneous abortion, ectopic pregnancy, or other pregnancy-related complications, such as a molar pregnancy. In the United States, 30% of 15- to 17-year-old adolescent girls have had sexual intercourse, as have 70.6% of those 18 to 19 years old (63). Issues of confidentiality for adolescent health care are critical to an adolescent's willingness to seek appropriate reproductive health care (see Chapter 1).

Exogenous Hormones The cause of abnormal bleeding that is experienced while an individual is taking exogenous hormones usually is very different from bleeding that occurs without hormonal manipulation (64). **Oral contraceptive use is associated with breakthrough bleeding, which occurs in as many as 30% to 40% of individuals during the first cycle of combination pill use. In addition, irregular bleeding can result from missed pills** (65,66). Strict

Table 14.7 Causes of Bleeding by Approximate Frequency and Age Group

Infancy	Prepubertal	Adolescent	Reproductive	Perimenopausal	Postmenopausal
Maternal estrogen withdrawal	Vulvovaginitis	Anovulation	Exogenous	Anovulation	Atrophy
	Vaginal foreign body	Exogenous hormone use	Pregnancy	Fibroids	Endometrial polyps
	Precocious puberty	Pregnancy	Anovulation	Cervical and endometrial polyps	Endometrial cancer
	Tumor	Coagulopathy	Fibroids	Thyroid dysfunction	Hormonal therapy
			Cervical and endometrial polyps		Other tumor—vulvar, vaginal, cervical
			Thyroid dysfunction		

compliance with correct and consistent pill taking is difficult for many individuals who take oral contraceptives; one study reported that only 40% of women took a pill every day (67). Other studies suggest that adolescents have an even more difficult time taking oral contraceptives than do adults, missing an average of three pills per month (68). A study of urban teens reported approximately two episodes of three or more consecutive missed pills occurring during each 3-month interval (69). With this many missed pills, it is not surprising that some individuals experience irregular bleeding. The solution is to emphasize consistent pill taking; if the individual is unable to comply with daily pill use, an alternative contraceptive method may be preferable.

All forms of hormonal contraception, from combination and progestin-only minipills, to contraceptive patches, rings, intrauterine devices, and injectable and implantable contraception, can be associated with abnormal bleeding, although studies assessing bleeding have not used uniform methodologies and thus comparisons are difficult (70–72). Irregular bleeding occurs frequently in users of *depomedroxyprogesterone acetate* (*DMPA*), although at the end of 1 year, more than 50% of users will be amenorrheic (73,74). The mechanism of bleeding associated with these hormonal methods is not well established; an atrophic endometrium or factors related to angiogenesis may be involved, suggesting options for therapy (64,75). It should not be assumed that any bleeding occurring while an individual is using a hormonal method of contraception is caused by that method. Other local causes of bleeding, such as cervicitis or endometritis, can occur during use of hormone therapy and may be particularly important to consider in adolescents who are at risk for STDs (76,77).

Hematologic Abnormalities   In the adolescent age group, the possibility of a hematologic cause of abnormal bleeding must be considered. One classic study reviewed all visits by adolescent patients to an emergency room with the symptom of excessive or abnormal bleeding (75,78). The most common coagulation abnormality diagnosed was idiopathic thrombocytopenic purpura, followed by von Willebrand disease. Subsequent studies confirmed this association, particularly with excessive bleeding at the time of menarche. Von Willebrand's disease occurs in approximately 1% of women in the United States and, in its mildest form, menorrhagia may be the only symptom (79–81). **Adolescents who have severe menorrhagia, especially at menarche, should be screened for coagulation abnormalities, including von Willebrand disease.**

Infections   Irregular or postcoital bleeding can be associated with chlamydial cervicitis. **Adolescents have the highest rates of chlamydial infections of any age group, and sexually active teens should be screened routinely for chlamydia (82). Menorrhagia can be the initial sign in patients infected with sexually transmissible organisms.** Adolescents have the highest rates of pelvic inflammatory disease (PID) of any age group of sexually experienced individuals (see Chapter 18) (83).

Other Endocrine or Systemic Problems   Abnormal bleeding can be associated with thyroid dysfunction. Signs and symptoms of thyroid disease can be somewhat subtle in teens (see

Chapter 31). Hepatic dysfunction should be considered because it can lead to abnormalities in clotting factor production. Hyperprolactinemia can cause amenorrhea or irregular bleeding.

Polycystic ovary syndrome (PCOS) can occur during adolescence, and manifestations of excess androgen (hirsutism, acne) should prompt evaluation, although the diagnostic criteria for PCOS during adolescence are not well established (84). **Androgen disorders occur in about 5% to 10% of adult women, making them the most common endocrine disorders in women** (see Chapter 31). **Classic PCOS, functional ovarian hyperandrogenism, or partial late-onset congenital adrenal hyperplasia can occur in adolescence. These disorders often are overlooked, unrecognized, or untreated.** Women with even mild disorders are candidates for intervention, including lifestyle interventions to normalize weight, and pharmacologic interventions to manage abnormal bleeding or hirsutism. These disorders may be a harbinger of type 2 diabetes, endometrial cancer, and cerebrovascular disease. **Acne, hirsutism, and menstrual irregularities are often dismissed as normal during adolescence but may be manifestations of hyperandrogenism** (52,85). Androgen abnormality can persist beyond adolescence. Obesity, hirsutism, and acne should be evaluated to minimize the significant psychosocial costs. Androgenic changes are partially reversible if detected early and managed appropriately. Behavioral changes in lifestyle (diet and exercise) should be strongly encouraged but are often difficult to achieve. Signs of insulin resistance (acanthosis nigricans) should be evaluated and managed appropriately (86).

Anatomic Causes   **Obstructive or partially obstructive genital anomalies typically present during adolescence.** Complex müllerian abnormalities, such as obstructing longitudinal vaginal septa or uterus didelphys, can cause hematocolpos or hematometra (Fig. 14.12). If these obstructing anomalies have or develop a small outlet, persistent dark-brownish discharge (old blood) may appear instead of or in addition to a pelvic mass. Many varieties of uterine and vaginal anomalies exist, and clinicians who have expertise with these anomalies should be involved in their management. Figure 14.13 illustrates situations in which abnormal bleeding can result from partially obstructing septa.

Diagnosis of Adolescent Abnormal Bleeding

Examination   A careful general physical examination can reveal signs of androgen excess such as acanthosis nigricans or facial, chest or periareolar, or abdominal terminal hair growth. Because body hair is felt by many to be culturally unacceptable in women and girls, sensitive questioning about specific hair removal techniques (bleaching, waxing, use of depilatories, shaving, plucking, threading) is warranted during an examination. A complete pelvic examination is appropriate in patients who are sexually active, are having severe pain, or may have an anatomic anomaly. Testing for gonorrhea and *Chlamydia trachomatis* infection is appropriate during a speculum examination if the patient is sexually active. Some young teens who have a history that is classic

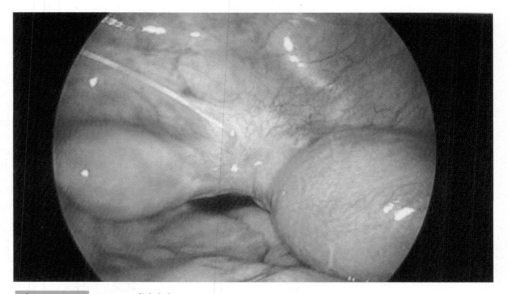

Figure 14.12   Uterus didelphys.

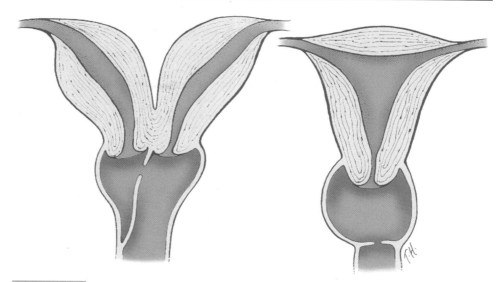

Figure 14.13   The types of obstructive or partially obstructive genital anomalies that can occur during adolescence.

for anovulation, who deny sexual activity, and who agree to return for follow-up evaluation may be managed with a limited gynecologic examination supplemented with pelvic ultrasonography.

Laboratory Testing   **Any adolescent with abnormal bleeding should undergo sensitive pregnancy testing, regardless of whether she states that she has had intercourse.** The medical consequences of failing to diagnose a pregnancy are too severe to risk missing the diagnosis. Complications of pregnancy should be managed accordingly. In addition to a pregnancy test, laboratory testing should include a complete blood count with platelet count and screening tests for coagulopathies and platelet dysfunction. An international expert panel made recommendations about when a gynecologist should suspect a bleeding disorder and pursue a diagnosis (Table 14.8). The consensus report recommends measurement of complete blood cell count (CBC), platelet count and function, prothrombin time (PT), activated partial thromboplastin time (PTT),

Table 14.8 When Should a Gynecologist Suspect a Bleeding Disorder
Heavy menstrual bleeding since menarche
Family history of bleeding disorder
Personal history of any of the following:
Epistaxis in the last year
Bruising without injury >2 cm diameter
Minor wound bleeding
Oral or gastrointestinal bleeding without anatomic lesion
Prolonged or heavy bleeding after dental extraction
Unexpected postoperative bleeding
Hemorrhage from ovarian cyst
Hemorrhage requiring blood transfusion
Postpartum hemorrhage, especially delayed >24 h
Failure to respond to conventional management of menorrhagia

From **James AH, Kouides PA, Abdul-Kadir R, et al.** Von Willebrand disease and other bleeding disorders in women: consensus on diagnosis and management from an international expert panel. *Am J Obstet Gynecol* 2009;201:12e1–e8.

von Willebrand factor (VWF) (measured with ristocetin cofactor activity and antigen, factor VIII), and fibrinogen to be assessed in collaboration with a hematologist (81).

Thyroid studies may be relevant. Testing for STDs may be performed as warranted on either a cervical or a urine specimen using DNA amplification techniques. Cervical cytology testing is generally not appropriate for adolescents, particularly at an emergency or urgent visit for excessive bleeding (87).

Imaging Studies   If the pregnancy test results are positive, pelvic imaging using ultrasonography may be necessary to confirm a viable intrauterine pregnancy and rule out a spontaneous abortion or ectopic pregnancy. If a pelvic mass is suspected on examination, or if the examination is inadequate (more likely to be the case in an adolescent than an older woman) and additional information is required, pelvic ultrasonography may be helpful. **Although transvaginal ultrasonographic examination can be more helpful than transabdominal ultrasonography in ascertaining details of pelvic anatomy, the use of the vaginal probe may not be possible in a young girl or one who has not used tampons or had intercourse.** Direct communication between the clinician and the radiologist can be helpful in identifying patients who are appropriate candidates for transvaginal ultrasonographic examination, such as those who are sexually active, rather than a blanket prohibition against transvaginal ultrasound examination in adolescents.

Other imaging studies are not indicated as initial testing but may be helpful in selected instances. **If a pelvic ultrasonographic examination does not lead to clarification of the anatomy when vaginal septa, uterine septa, uterine duplication, or vaginal agenesis is suspected, MRI can be helpful in delineating anatomic abnormalities** (88). This imaging technique is useful in the evaluation of uterine and vaginal developmental anomalies, although laparoscopy can still play a role in the clarification of abnormal anatomy (89). CT scanning may be helpful in detecting nongenital intra-abdominal abnormalities.

Management of Abnormal Bleeding

Management of bleeding abnormalities related to pregnancy, thyroid dysfunction, hepatic abnormalities, hematologic abnormalities, or androgen excess syndromes should be directed to treating the underlying condition. Oral contraceptives can be extremely helpful in managing androgen excess syndromes, inherited bleeding disorders, and anovulation, although an appropriate evaluation should be performed prior to initiation of hormonal contraception (90–92).

Treatment with *mefenamic acid* and other nonsteroidal anti-inflammatory agents (NSAIDs) results in decreased menstrual bleeding when compared with placebo (93). *Tranexamic acid,* an antifibrinolytic agent, is more effective in decreasing heavy menstrual bleeding, and was approved by the U.S. Food and Drug Administration (FDA) for this indication in late 2009 (93a). After specific diagnoses are ruled out by appropriate laboratory testing, this condition can be managed either expectantly or with hormone therapy, depending on the clinical presentation and other factors, such as the need for contraception.

Anovulation: Mild Bleeding

Adolescents who have mildly abnormal bleeding, as defined by adequate hemoglobin levels and minimal disruption of daily activities, are best managed with prospective menstrual charting, frequent reassurance, close follow-up, and supplemental iron. If the patient is bleeding heavily or for a prolonged interval, an apparent decrease in the bleeding does not necessarily mean that therapy is not required. Intermittent bleeding characterizes anovulatory bleeding and is likely to continue in the absence of therapy.

A patient who is mildly anemic will benefit from hormone therapy. If the patient is not bleeding at the time of evaluation and has no contraindications to the use of estrogen, **a combination low-dose oral contraceptive can be prescribed for use in the manner in which it is used for contraception.** If the patient is not sexually active, she should be reevaluated after three to six cycles to determine whether she desires to continue this regimen. Parents may sometimes object to the use of oral contraceptives if their daughter is not sexually active (or if they believe her not to be or even if they would like her not to be). These objections are frequently based on misconceptions about the potential risks of the pill and can be overcome by careful explanation of the pill's role as medical therapy. Objections may be based on concerns that hormonal therapy for medical indications is likely to hasten the onset of coitarche or sexual debut, although no data support this fear. If the medication is discontinued when the young woman is not sexually active and she subsequently becomes sexually active and requires contraception, it may be difficult to explain the reinstitution of oral contraceptives to the parents. If there is no significant medical or family history that would preclude their use, combination oral contraceptives are especially appropriate for the management of abnormal bleeding in adolescents for a number of reasons:

1. **Approximately 50% of high schools juniors in the United States are sexually experienced** (63).

2. **Adolescents typically wait many months after initiating sexual activity to seek medical contraception.**

3. **At least 80% of adolescent pregnancies are unintended** (94).

4. **Approximately one-quarter of adolescent pregnancies end in abortion** (95).

5. **Approximately one in three young women will experience a pregnancy before age 20** (96).

Thus, consideration should certainly be given to continuing the oral contraception use, and parents should be reassured that the medical risks are small in otherwise healthy adolescents and that there are no significant risks associated with prolonged use. Individuals may choose to continue oral contraceptives for contraception or their noncontraceptive benefits (improvement of acne, decreased dysmenorrhea, and lighter, more regular menstrual flow, protective effect for endometrial and ovarian cancer).

Sometimes, providing parents with accurate information about the safety of oral contraceptives, emphasizing that currently available oral contraceptive preparations contain lower doses of estrogens and progestins than those used in the 1960s and 1970s, and emphasizing the hormonal rather than contraceptive function may not be persuasive. In such cases, cyclic progestins are an alternative. A systematic review of the use of combination hormonal therapy versus progestins alone for the treatment of anovulatory bleeding found a paucity of evidence supporting the efficacy of one management regimen over another (97). ***Medroxyprogesterone acetate*, 5 to 10 mg/day for 10 to 13 days every 1 to 2 months, prevents excessive endometrial buildup and irregular shedding caused by unopposed estrogen stimulation.** This therapy should be reevaluated regularly and accompanied by oral administration of iron. Eventual maturation of the hypothalamic–pituitary–ovarian axis usually will result in the establishment of regular menses unless there are underlying conditions such as hyperandrogenism.

Acute Bleeding

Moderate   **Patients who are bleeding acutely but in a stable condition and do not require hospital admission will require doses of hormones that are higher than those in oral contraceptives to effectively stop anovulatory bleeding. An effective regimen is the use of combination monophasic oral contraceptives (every 6 hours for 4 to 7 days).** After that time, the dose should be tapered or stopped to allow shedding of the dyssynchronous endometrium and withdrawal bleeding. With this therapy, the patient and her parents should be given specific written and oral instructions warning them about the potential side effects of high-dose hormone therapy—nausea, breast tenderness, and breakthrough bleeding. The patient should be instructed to call with any concerns rather than discontinue the pills, and she must understand that stopping the prescribed regimen may result in a recurrence of heavy bleeding. Both the patient and her mother should be warned to expect heavy withdrawal flow for the first period. It will be controlled by the institution of combination low-dose oral contraceptive therapy, given once daily and continued for three to six cycles, to allow regular withdrawal flow. If the patient is not sexually active, the pill may be discontinued after the recommended course of therapy and the menstrual cycles may be reassessed.

Emergency Management   **The decision to hospitalize a patient depends on the rate of current bleeding and the severity of any existing anemia. The actual acute blood loss may not be reflected adequately in the initial blood count but will be revealed with serial hemoglobin assessments. The cause of acute menorrhagia may be a primary coagulation disorder; thus, measurements of coagulation and hemostasis, including screening for coagulopathy, should be performed for any adolescent patients with acute menorrhagia, as noted above in the recommendations of an international panel** (81). Von Willebrand disease, platelet disorders, or hematologic malignancies can cause menorrhagia. Depending on the patient's level of hemodynamic stability or compromise, a blood sample can be analyzed for type and screen. The decision to transfuse must be considered carefully, and the benefits and risks should be discussed with the adolescent and her parents. Generally, there is no need for transfusion unless the patient is hemodynamically unstable.

In patients who, by exclusion, are diagnosed as having anovulatory bleeding, hormone therapy usually makes it possible to avoid surgical intervention (dilation and curettage [D&C], operative hysteroscopy, or laparoscopy). A patient who is hospitalized for severe bleeding requires aggressive management as follows:

1. **After stabilization, when appropriate laboratory assessment and an examination established a working diagnosis of anovulation, hormonal management will usually control bleeding.**

2. Estrogen-progestin therapy in the form of combined oral contraceptives given as one or two pills twice a day for 5 to 7 days is typically effective within 12 to 24 hours. Alternatively, *conjugated estrogens,* **either 25 to 40 mg given intravenously every 6 hours or 2.5 mg given orally every 6 hours, will usually be effective** (98).

3. **If this hormonal therapy is not effective, the patient should be reevaluated and the diagnosis should be reassessed.** The failure of hormonal management suggests that a local cause of bleeding is more likely. In this event, consideration should be given to a pelvic ultrasonographic examination to determine any anatomic causes of bleeding (such as uterine leiomyomas, endometrial polyps, or endometrial hyperplasia) and to assess the presence of intrauterine clots that may impair uterine contractility and prolong the bleeding episode. Although anatomic causes of heavy menstrual bleeding are rare in adolescents, they become increasingly common in women of reproductive age.

4. **If intrauterine clots are detected, evacuation of the clots (suction curettage or D&C) is indicated.** Although a D&C will provide effective immediate control of the bleeding, it is unusual to reach this step in adolescents.

More drastic forms of treatment other than a D&C (such as ablation of the endometrium by laser or cryotherapy) are considered inappropriate for adolescents because of concerns about future fertility.

If intravenous or oral administration of hormonal therapy controls the bleeding, oral progestin therapy should be instituted and continued for several days to stabilize the endometrium. This therapy can be accomplished by using a combination oral contraceptive, usually one with 30 to 35 mg of estrogen, or by using the tapering regimen previously described. The medication can be tapered and ultimately must be stopped to allow withdrawal bleeding, which may be heavy, given an excessively built-up endometrium. Low-dose combination oral contraception once daily should be continued for three to six cycles, or longer if desired, to provide normal menstrual cycles. Manipulation of the regimen by increasing or decreasing the dose of oral contraceptives to twice a day or three times a day after the initial high dose therapy should be discouraged.

In general, the prognosis for regular ovulatory cycles and subsequent normal fertility in young women who experience an episode of abnormal bleeding is good, particularly for patients who develop abnormal bleeding as a result of anovulation within the first years after menarche and in whom there are no signs of other specific conditions. Some girls, including those in whom there is an underlying medical cause, such as PCOS, will continue to have abnormal bleeding into middle and late adolescence and adulthood and will benefit from the ongoing use of oral contraceptives to manage hirsutism, acne, and irregular periods. Ovulation induction may ultimately be necessary to achieve fertility in these individuals, although teens should be advised that they should not assume that they are infertile. Individuals with coagulopathies may benefit from ongoing oral contraceptive use, use of *tranexamic acid,* or intranasal *desmopressin* (99).

A progestin-releasing intrauterine device (IUD) can be effective in managing heavy bleeding, and may be appropriate for adolescent use (100,101). The *levonorgestrel* IUD is approved by the FDA for treatment of heavy menstrual bleeding in women requiring contraception and is recommended as first-line medical therapy for this group of women (102).

Long-Term Menstrual Suppression

For patients with underlying medical conditions, such as coagulopathies, a malignancy requiring chemotherapy, or developmental disabilities, long-term therapeutic amenorrhea with menstrual suppression using the following regimens may be necessary or helpful (103):

1. Progestins such as oral *norethindrone, norethindrone acetate,* or *medroxyprogesterone acetate* on a continuous daily basis (104).

2. Continuous (noncyclic) combination regimens of oral estrogen and progestins (birth control pills) or other forms of combination estrogen/progestins (transdermal patch, vaginal ring) that do not include a withdrawal bleeding–placebo week (105,106).

3. Depot formulations of progestins (*DMPA*), with or without concurrent estrogens (104).

4. Gonadotropin-releasing hormone (GnRH) analogues with or without estrogen add-back therapy (105).

5. *Levonorgestrel* intrauterine system (IUS) (107).

The choice of regimen depends on the presence of any contraindications (such as active liver disease precluding the use of estrogens) and the clinician's experience. **Although the goal of these long-term suppressive therapies is amenorrhea, all of these regimens may be accompanied by breakthrough bleeding.** At 1 year, rates of amenorrhea approach 90% with extended cycle combination oral contraceptives, 50% with *DMPA,* and 50% with the *levonorgestrel* IUS (73,108,109). Because both *DMPA* and GnRH analogues are associated with disadvantageous effects on bone mineral density, the potential risks must be weighed against their medical benefits. Regular follow-up visits and continued patient encouragement are required with all of these options. Episodes of spotting and breakthrough bleeding that do not result in a lowered hemoglobin level may be managed expectantly. When breakthrough bleeding affects the hemoglobin level, it should be evaluated with respect to the underlying disease. For example, in a patient with underlying platelet dysfunction, breakthrough bleeding may reflect a lowered platelet count. Bleeding in a patient with hepatic disease may reflect worsening hepatic function. NSAIDs and supplemental low-dose hormonal therapy can be helpful in the management of excessive breakthrough bleeding that has no specific cause other than the hormone therapy (110).

Adolescent Pelvic Masses

Presentation

Adolescents with pelvic masses may be asymptomatic or may have chronic or acute symptoms. An ovarian mass may be discovered incidentally when an ultrasonographic examination is performed to evaluate the urinary system or when imaging is performed to evaluate pelvic pain. The mere presence of a mass on imaging studies does not always indicate that the mass is the cause of pelvic pain. **A "ruptured ovarian cyst" is a classic diagnosis when an adolescent presents with pelvic pain, even if ultrasonography findings suggest only a simple cystic follicle and a physiologic amount of pelvic fluid that are unlikely to cause pain.** Alternatively, ovarian masses can cause severe acute or intermittent symptoms caused by torsion, intraperitoneal rupture, or bleeding into the ovarian tissue (Fig. 14.14). These conditions can represent a true surgical emergency or urgency, and their diagnoses can be challenging. The pressure of an enlarging ovarian mass can cause bowel-related symptoms such as constipation, vague discomfort, and early satiety; urinary frequency; or even ureteral or bladder neck obstruction.

Diagnosis

The history and pelvic examination are critical in the diagnosis of a pelvic mass. Considerations in adolescents include the anxiety associated with a first pelvic examination, as well as issues of confidentiality related to questions about sexual activity. Techniques for history taking and the performance of the first examination are discussed in Chapter 1.

Laboratory studies should always include a pregnancy test (regardless of stated sexual activity), and a complete blood count may be helpful in diagnosing inflammatory masses. Tumor markers, including α-fetoprotein and human chorionic gonadotropin (hCG), may be elaborated by germ cell tumors and can be useful in preoperative diagnosis and follow-up (see Chapter 37).

As in all other age groups, the primary diagnostic technique for evaluating pelvic masses in adolescents is ultrasonography. Although transvaginal ultrasonographic examinations may provide more detail than transabdominal ultrasonography, particularly with inflammatory masses, a transvaginal examination may not be well tolerated by adolescents (111). Ultrasonography usually is the most helpful imaging technique for assessing ovarian masses. **For cases in which the suspected diagnosis is appendicitis or another nongynecologic condition, or if the results of the ultrasonographic examination are inconclusive, CT or MRI may be helpful.** An accurate preoperative assessment of anatomy is critical, particularly in cases of uterovaginal

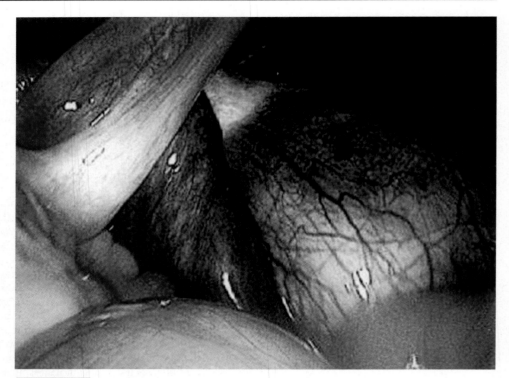

Figure 14.14   Adnexal mass with torsion.

malformations. MRI can be useful for evaluating this group of rare anomalies (88). Adolescents who present with abdominal pain should be evaluated with some type of imaging procedure because an unexpected finding of a complex uterine or vaginal anomaly requires careful surgical planning and management.

Differential Diagnosis of Adolescent Pelvic Masses

Ovarian Masses in Adolescents **Many studies of ovarian tumors in the pediatric and adolescent age group do not distinguish between prepubertal or premenarchal girls and menarchal adolescents. The findings of some reports are based on age group, although this is less helpful than a distinction by pubertal development. In evaluating a pelvic or abdominal mass, the clinician must take into consideration the patient's pubertal status because the likelihood of functional masses increases after menarche** (Table 14.4). The risk of malignant neoplasms is lower among adolescents than among younger children. Germ cell tumors are the most common tumors of the first decade of life but occur less frequently during adolescence (see Chapter 37). Mature cystic teratoma is the most frequent neoplastic tumor of children and adolescents, accounting for more than one-half of ovarian neoplasms in women younger than 20 years of age (112). Epithelial neoplasms occur with increasing frequency beyond adolescence.

It is well established that neoplasia can arise in dysgenetic gonads. The risk of malignant tumors in dysgenetic gonads of patients with a Y chromosome depends on the nature of the disorder of sex development, the presence of the gonadoblastoma region of the Y chromosome, and other factors—both established and as yet unknown (113). A number of genes involved in gonadal differentiation were described. In the past, it was stated that the risk of malignant tumors is approximately 25%, and thus gonadectomy was recommended (114). Other perspectives suggest that a gonadal biopsy may allow the estimation of individual risk and permit a more conservative approach to gonadectomy. A multidisciplinary approach to diagnosis of disorders of sex development with attention to biological, genetic, and psychological factors is advocated (115). **Functional ovarian cysts occur frequently in adolescence.** They may be an incidental finding on examination or may be associated with pain caused by torsion, leakage, or rupture. Paratubal cysts represent embryologic remnants that may be confused with an ovarian mass; they are typically asymptomatic, but can be associated with adnexal torsion (Fig. 14.14). Adnexal or ovarian torsion is a challenging diagnosis to make in prepubertal girls or adolescents; torsion of a mass is more likely to occur than is torsion of normal adnexa, although this can occur. Doppler ultrasound examination may not predict the presence of torsion, although discrepancy in ovarian volume and large volume of the torsed adnexa may be helpful in making the diagnosis (116,117). Management should consist of detorsion rather than oophorectomy, even if the mass appears to have no blood flow, as recovery of ovarian function is likely (118).

Endometriosis is less common during adolescence than in adulthood, although it can occur during adolescence. In one study of adolescents referred with chronic pain, 50% to 65% had endometriosis (119). Although endometriosis can occur in young women with obstructive genital anomalies (presumably as a result of retrograde menstruation), most adolescents with endometriosis do not have associated obstructive anomalies. In young women, endometriosis may have an atypical appearance characterized by nonpigmented or vesicular lesions, peritoneal windows, and puckering (120).

Uterine Masses in Adolescents

Other causes of pelvic masses, such as uterine abnormalities, are rare in adolescence. Uterine leiomyomas are not often seen in this age group. Obstructive uterovaginal anomalies occur during adolescence, at the time of menarche, or shortly thereafter. Frequently, the correct diagnosis either is not suspected or is delayed (121). A wide range of anomalies can occur, from imperforate hymen to transverse vaginal septa; from vaginal agenesis with a normal uterus and functional endometrium to vaginal duplications with obstructing longitudinal septa, and obstructed uterine horns (Fig. 14.13). Patients may seek treatment for cyclic pain, amenorrhea, vaginal discharge, or an abdominal, pelvic, or vaginal mass. A hematocolpos, hematometra, or both frequently will be present, and the resulting mass can be quite large (34).

Inflammatory Masses in Adolescents

Of all age groups of sexually active women, adolescents have the highest rates of PID (83). Thus, an adolescent who has pelvic pain may have an inflammatory mass. Such masses may consist of a tubo-ovarian complex (a mass of matted bowel, tube, and ovary), tubo-ovarian abscess (a mass consisting primarily of an abscess cavity within an anatomically defined structure such as the ovary), pyosalpinx, or, chronically, hydrosalpinx.

The diagnosis of PID is primarily a clinical one based on the presence of lower abdominal, pelvic, and adnexal tenderness; cervical motion tenderness; a mucopurulent discharge; and elevated temperature, white blood cell count, or sedimentation rate (see Chapter 18). The risk of PID is clearly associated with that of acquiring STDs, and methods of contraception may either decrease the risk (male latex condoms) or increase it (the intrauterine device in the interval immediately after insertion) (122,123).

Pregnancy

In adolescents, pregnancy should always be considered as a cause of a pelvic mass. In the United States, nearly half of adolescent women have experienced sexual intercourse (124). Most pregnancies in adolescents are unintended; 100% of pregnancies in adolescents younger than age 15, 87% in women aged 15 to 17, and 79% in women aged 18 to 19 are unintended (94). Adolescents may be more likely than adults to deny the possibility of pregnancy because of wishful thinking, anxiety about discovery by parents or peers, or unfamiliarity with menstrual cycles and information about fertility. Ectopic pregnancies may cause pelvic pain and an adnexal mass. The increasing incidence of ectopic pregnancies in the United States is strongly associated with rising rates of PID. With the availability of quantitative measurements of β-hCG, more ectopic pregnancies are being discovered before rupture, allowing conservative management with laparoscopic surgery or medical therapy (see Chapter 20). The risk of ectopic pregnancy varies by method of contraception; users of no contraception have the highest risk, whereas oral contraceptive users have the lowest risk (125). As with older patients, paraovarian cysts and nongynecologic masses can appear as a pelvic or abdominal mass in adolescents (Fig. 14.15).

Management of Pelvic Masses in Adolescents

The management of masses in adolescents depends on the suspected diagnosis and the initial symptom. Figure 14.8 outlines a plan of management for pelvic masses in adolescents. **Asymptomatic unilocular cystic masses are best managed conservatively because the likelihood of malignancy is low. If surgical management is required based on symptoms or uncertainty of diagnosis, attention should be directed to minimizing the risks of subsequent**

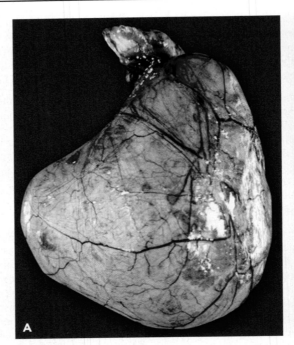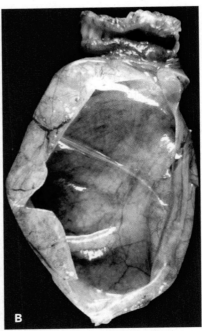

Figure 14.15 A: Paratubal cyst. B: Paratubal cyst, incised.

infertility resulting from pelvic adhesions. In addition, every effort should be made to conserve ovarian tissue. In the presence of a malignant unilateral ovarian mass, management may include unilateral oophorectomy rather than more radical surgery, even if the ovarian tumor metastasized (see Chapter 37). Analysis of frozen sections may not be reliable. In general, conservative surgery is appropriate; further surgery can be performed, if necessary, after an adequate histologic evaluation of the ovarian tumor.

When symptoms persist in a patient with the clinical diagnosis of PID or tubo-ovarian abscess, laparoscopy should be considered to confirm the diagnosis. A clinical diagnosis may be incorrect in as many as one-third of patients (118). The surgical management of inflammatory masses is rarely necessary in adolescents, except to treat rupture of tubo-ovarian abscess or failure of medical management with broad-spectrum antibiotics (see Chapter 18). Some surgeons advocated laparoscopy to perform irrigation, lysis of adhesions, drainage of unilateral or bilateral pyosalpinx or tubo-ovarian abscess, or extirpation of significant disease (126). If surgical management is required because of failed medical therapy, conservative, unilateral adnexectomy usually can be performed in these situations, rather than a pelvic clean-out, thereby maintaining reproductive potential. Percutaneous drainage, transvaginal ultrasonographic drainage, and laparoscopic management of tubo-ovarian abscesses are being done more often, although evidence supporting this approach is sparse. As with the laparoscopic management of ovarian masses, the surgeon's skill and experience with this procedure are critical, and prospective studies on its effectiveness are lacking (127). Laparoscopic management is associated with a risk of major complications, including bowel obstruction and bowel or vessel injury (128).

Adolescent Vulvar Conditions

Disorders of sex development may cause genital ambiguity, typically noted at birth, although virilization may occur at puberty (29). Adolescents with gonadal dysgenesis or androgen insensitivity may have abnormal pubertal development and primary amenorrhea (see Chapters 29 and 30). Various developmental anomalies—vaginal agenesis, imperforate hymen, transverse and longitudinal vaginal septa, vaginal and uterine duplications, hymenal bands, and septa—most frequently are diagnosed in early adolescents with amenorrhea (for the obstructing abnormalities) or with concerns such as inability to use tampons (for hymenal and

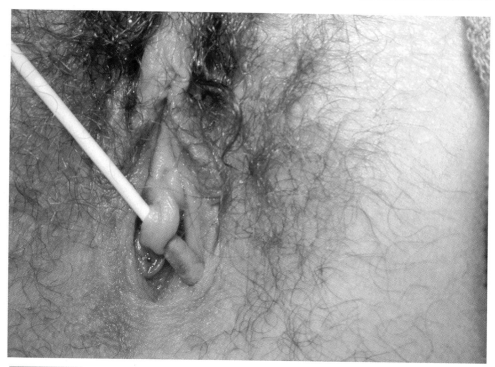

Figure 14.16   Hymenal band.

vaginal bands and septa). These developmental abnormalities must be evaluated carefully to determine both external and internal anatomy.

A tight hymenal ring may be discovered when the patient seeks care because of concerns about the inability to use tampons or have intercourse. Both manual dilation and small relaxing incisions at 6 o'clock and 8 o'clock in the hymenal ring can be effective. This procedure can sometimes be done in the office using local anesthesia but may require conduction or general anesthesia in the operating room. Hymenal bands are not rare and lead to difficulty in using tampons; they usually can be incised in the office using local anesthetic (Fig. 14.16). Hypertrophy of the labia minora may be considered a variant of normal, and reassurance rather than a cosmetic surgical reduction is appropriate as the primary therapy. Surgical management is described, although the procedure could be considered to be esthetic rather than medically mandated. Genital ulcerations may occur in girls with leukemia or other cancers requiring chemotherapy (129,130). Vulvar ulcerations in the absence of sexual activity or infectious etiology are described as vulvar aphthosis (46) (Fig. 14.10). The possibility of sexual abuse, incest, or involuntary intercourse should be considered for young adolescents with vulvovaginal symptoms, STDs, or pregnancy.

The presence of vulvar symptoms such as itching or burning may prompt a patient to seek care; however, this anatomic site is not one that is easily inspected by the patient. Thus, vulvar lesions may be found on examination that were not noticed by the patient. **Vulvar self-examination should be encouraged and could potentially result in the earlier diagnosis of vulvar lesions such as melanoma.** Adolescents presenting with vulvar itching may have lichen sclerosus; this condition can be relatively asymptomatic, even when an examination reveals loss of anatomic structures and scarring (11) (Fig. 14.4).

Adolescents and adults often incorrectly self-diagnose vulvovaginal candidiasis; in one study, only one-third of women with self-diagnosed yeast vaginitis were found to have this infection (131) (see Chapter 18). A clinical examination and appropriate testing can be performed even on young adolescents using a clinician or self-obtained cotton swab to obtain vaginal secretions for pH testing and microscopic examination (Fig. 14.17).

Vulvar condyloma is an extremely common cause of vulvar lesions in adolescents (see Chapter 18). Genital warts can affect the vulva, perineum, and perianal skin, and the vagina,

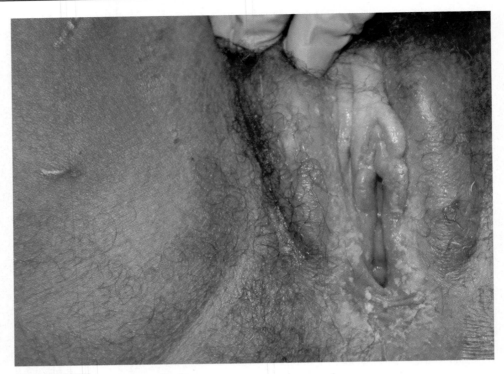

Figure 14.17   Candidal vulvitis.

urethra, and anus (Fig. 14.18). Condyloma in adolescents typically is sexually transmitted. It may be asymptomatic or cause symptoms of itching, irritation, or bleeding. Symptomatic, enlarging, or extensive vulvar condyloma can be managed with topical medication applied by the patient or clinician. The choice of treatment should be guided by patient preference, available resources, and the clinician's experience; no one treatment is superior to the others (132). The

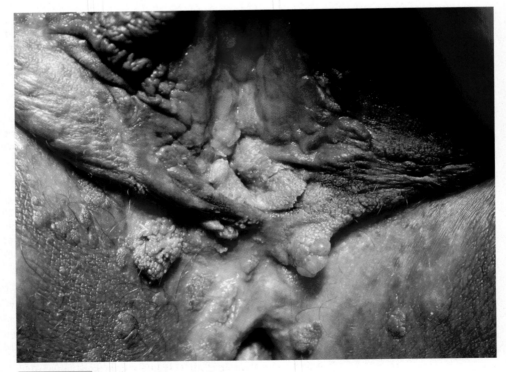

Figure 14.18   Extensive vulvar condyloma.

availability of a quadrivalent human papillomavirus (HPV) vaccine that includes HPV types 6 and 11 potentially will have a beneficial impact on the incidence of vulvar condyloma and HPV-related vulvar intraepithelial neoplasia (VIN) (133).

Adolescent Vaginal Conditions

Vulvovaginal symptoms in adolescents may be caused by a variety of conditions, ranging from vulvar lichen sclerosus to urinary tract infection to *C. trachomatis* to non-STD-related vaginitis. Urinary or vaginal symptoms do not differentiate well between urinary tract infections (UTIs) and vaginitis. Adolescent girls who are screened for both *C. trachomatis* and UTI have high rates of concurrent disease (134). Because clinical diagnosis based on symptoms is imprecise, female adolescents with vaginal or urinary symptoms should be tested for both *C. trachomatis* and UTI. Testing with DNA-based procedures may be performed on samples obtained from the cervix, from swabs of vaginal secretions (either clinician or patient obtained), and from urine specimens. Testing that does not involve a speculum examination may be particularly helpful for adolescents; a rigorous review concluded that noninvasive chlamydia testing was comparable to cervical or urethral screening, although this was not the case with testing for gonorrhea (126,135).

Discharge is one of the most common vaginal symptoms. Conditions ranging from vaginal candidiasis to chlamydia cervicitis to bacterial vaginosis may cause vaginal discharge in adolescents. Infectious vaginal conditions are described in more detail in Chapter 18. The risks of self-diagnosis of vaginal discharge in adolescents may be greater than in adult women, as infection with STDs—including *Neisseria gonorrhoea, Trichomonas vaginalis, C. trachomatis,* herpes simplex, and *Condyloma acuminata*—are common in adolescents and may be less likely recognized.

Use of tampons is associated with both microscopic and macroscopic ulcerations. Healing of the macroscopic ulcerations occurs within several weeks without specific therapy if tampon use is suspended. A follow-up examination to demonstrate healing is appropriate, with biopsy of any persistent ulcerations to rule out other lesions.

Toxic shock syndrome (TSS) is associated with tampon use and vaginal exotoxins produced by *Staphylococcus aureus*. This syndrome consists of fever, hypotension, a diffuse erythroderma with desquamation of the palms and soles, plus involvement of at least three major organ systems (136). Vaginal involvement includes mucous membrane inflammation. The frequency of TSS appears to be declining, and an increasing percentage of cases are not associated with menses. Approximately one-half of all cases of TSS are menstrual related (137). Epidemiologic studies suggest that adolescents are at greater risk of menstrual TSS than older women; however, this finding does not appear to be explained by differences in the detection of antibodies to the TSST-1 toxin-producing strain of *S. aureus* or in *S. aureus* vaginal colonization rates (138).

Abscesses of Bartholin and Skene's glands are related to both aerobic and anaerobic organisms, with mixed infections accounting for approximately 60% of these and other vulvar and labial abscesses, although the possibility of methicillin-resistant *S. aureus* (MRSA) infections must be kept in mind (139,140). Therapy consists of surgical drainage, with use of antibiotics as a secondary measure. In younger adolescents, incision and drainage with insertion of a Word indwelling catheter may require general anesthesia (140).

Reproductive-Age Group

Reproductive-Age Abnormal Bleeding

Normal Menses

After adolescence, menstrual cycles generally conform to a cycle length of 21 to 38 days, with menstrual flow duration of fewer than 7 days (Table 14.9). **As a woman approaches menopause, cycle length becomes more irregular as fewer cycles are ovulatory** (51,141). The most frequent cause of irregular bleeding in the reproductive age group is hormonal, although other causes such as pregnancy-related bleeding (spontaneous abortion, ectopic pregnancy) should always be considered (Table 14.4). A variety of terms are used to describe abnormal menses; it is strongly recommended by an international panel of experts that the confusing terms noted in Table 14.10 be abandoned in favor of a much simpler system with description of cycle

Table 14.9 Parameters for Normal Menstrual Cycles in Women of Reproductive Age	
	Normal
Menstrual cycle frequency	24–38
Cycle variation from cycle to cycle	2–20 days
Duration of flow	4–8 days
Volume of flow	4–80 mL

Data from **Fraser IS, Critchley HO, Munro MG.** Abnormal uterine bleeding: getting our terminology straight. *Curr Opin Obstet Gynecol* 2007;19:591–595.

regularity (irregular, regular, or absent), frequency (frequent, normal, or infrequent), duration (prolonged, normal, or shortened), and heaviness of bleeding episodes (heavy, normal, or light) (Table 14.11) (141). Prospective charting of bleeding can be helpful in characterizing abnormal bleeding. **The mean duration of menses is 4.7 days; 89% of cycles last 7 days or longer. The average blood loss per cycle is 35 mL (56). Menses is a suspension of blood- and tissue-derived solids within a mixture of serum and cervicovaginal fluid; the blood content of menses varies over the days of bleeding, but on average is close to 50%** (142). **Recurrent bleeding in excess of 80 mL/cycle results in anemia.**

Differential Diagnosis of Abnormal Bleeding in Reproductive-Age Women

Dysfunctional Uterine Bleeding   **The term *dysfunctional uterine bleeding* (DUB) is used to describe abnormal bleeding for which no specific cause was found. It is used as a diagnosis rather than a symptom; although there is no agreement about a simpler term to replace the phrase, *idiopathic heavy, regular bleeding, idiopathic heavy, irregular bleeding,* and *idiopathic prolonged, irregular bleeding* were suggested** (141). **DUB is often used as a diagnosis of exclusion, which is probably more confusing than enlightening. Other terms that are commonly used to describe bleeding abnormalities include *anovulatory uterine bleeding* and *abnormal uterine bleeding*** (143).

Most anovulatory bleeding results from what is termed *estrogen breakthrough*. In the absence of ovulation and the production of progesterone, the endometrium responds to estrogen stimulation with proliferation. This endometrial growth without periodic shedding results in eventual breakdown of the fragile endometrial tissue. Healing within the endometrium is irregular and dyssynchronous. Relatively low levels of estrogen stimulation will result in irregular and prolonged bleeding, whereas higher sustained levels result in episodes of amenorrhea followed by acute, heavy bleeding.

Pregnancy-Related Bleeding   Spontaneous abortion can be associated with excessive or prolonged bleeding. A woman may be unaware that she conceived and may seek care because of abnormal bleeding. In the United States, more than 50% of pregnancies are unintended, and about 7% of women are at risk for unintended pregnancy but use no method of contraception (94,144). These women may be at particular risk for bleeding related to an unsuspected pregnancy. About one-half of unintended pregnancies result from nonuse of contraception; the other

Table 14.10 Abnormal Menses—Terminology			
Term	*Interval*	*Duration*	*Amount*
Menorrhagia	Regular	Prolonged	Excessive
Metrorrhagia	Irregular	±Prolonged	Normal
Menometrorrhagia	Irregular	Prolonged	Excessive
Hypermenorrhea	Regular	Normal	Excessive
Hypomenorrhea	Regular	Normal or less	Less
Oligomenorrhea	Infrequent or irregular	Variable	Scanty
Amenorrhea	Absent	No menses for 90 days	Absent

Cycle		Normal	
Regularity	Absent	Regular	Irregular
Frequency of menstruation	Infrequent	Normal	Frequent
Duration of menstrual flow	Shortened	Normal	Prolonged
Volume of menstrual flow	Light	Normal	Heavy

Table 14.11 Menstrual Terminology

one-half result from contraceptive failures (145). **Unintended pregnancies are most likely to occur among adolescents and women older than 40 years of age** (see Chapter 10). If an ectopic pregnancy is ruled out, the management of spontaneous abortion may include either observation, if the bleeding is not excessive; medical or pharmacologic uterine evacuation (with *misoprostol*); or surgical management with suction curettage or D&C, depending on the clinician's judgment and the patient's preference (146–148). Surgical management appears to be the most likely technique to result in complete evacuation; lower rates of success are seen with both medical and expectant management, although the type of miscarriage and gestational age affect these rates (149) (see Chapter 20).

Exogenous Hormones   **Irregular bleeding that occurs while a woman is using contraceptive hormones should be considered in a different context than bleeding that occurs in the absence of exogenous hormone use. Breakthrough bleeding during the first 1 to 3 months of oral contraceptive use occurs in as many as 30% to 40% of users; it should almost always be managed expectantly with reassurance because the frequency of breakthrough bleeding decreases with each subsequent month of use** (66). Irregular bleeding can result from inconsistent use (150–152). Other estrogen-progestin delivery systems, including the contraceptive patch, vaginal ring, and intramuscular regimens, are associated with irregular breakthrough bleeding. These nondaily contraceptive regimens may promote successful use, making irregular bleeding a less important factor for some women in assessing the balance of risks versus benefits (see Chapter 10).

Use of progestin-only methods—including *DMPA,* progestin-only pills, the contraceptive implant, and the *levonorgestrel* IUS—is associated with relatively high rates of initial irregular and unpredictable bleeding; rates of amenorrhea vary over time and by method (142,153). Because irregular bleeding is so often present with these methods of contraception, counseling before their use is imperative. Women who do not believe that they can cope with irregular, unpredictable bleeding may not be good candidates for these methods. Hormonal implants and IUDs releasing progestins do offer significant benefits of high efficacy and ease of use (154). **The management of irregular bleeding with hormonal contraceptive use can range from reassurance and initial expectant management to recommendations for a change in the hormonal delivery system or regimen.** The use of additional oral estrogen improves bleeding with both *DMPA* and the subdermal *levonorgestrel*. The use of NSAIDs results in decreased breakthrough bleeding. The development of a better understanding of the mechanisms causing irregular bleeding will likely result in more effective and acceptable management strategies (153).

Not all bleeding that occurs while an individual is using hormonal contraception is a consequence of hormonal factors. In one study, women who experienced irregular bleeding while taking oral contraceptives had a higher frequency of *C. trachomatis* infection (76). Thus, screening should be considered in women presenting with irregular bleeding while using hormonal contraception.

Endocrine Causes   **Both hypothyroidism and hyperthyroidism can be associated with abnormal bleeding. With hypothyroidism, menstrual abnormalities, including menorrhagia, are common** (see Chapter 31). The most common cause of thyroid hyperfunctioning in premenopausal women is Graves disease, which occurs four to five times more often in women than men. Hyperthyroidism can result in oligomenorrhea or amenorrhea, and it can lead to elevated levels of plasma estrogen (155). Other causes of anovulation include hypothalamic dysfunction, hyperprolactinemia, premature ovarian failure, and primary pituitary disease (Table 14.6) (143). These conditions often are considered causes of amenorrhea, and they may cause irregular bleeding (see Chapter 30). The rare and unusual causes of abnormal bleeding should not be overlooked. Women with primary ovarian insufficiency (POI; previously termed premature ovarian failure [POF]) frequently see several clinicians with symptoms of oligomenorrhea or amenorrhea prior to receiving a diagnosis; the diagnosis of POI is often delayed during waning ovarian function and insufficiency (156,157). POI is thought to occur in approximately 1 of 100 women by age 40, 1 of 1,000 women by age 30, and 1 of 10,000 women by age 20. Women should be encouraged to track their menstrual cyclicity and to consider that the menstrual cycle can be a "vital sign" that reflects overall health (61).

Diabetes mellitus can be associated with anovulation, obesity, insulin resistance, and androgen excess. Androgen disorders are very common among women of reproductive age and should be evaluated and managed accordingly. PCOS is present in 5% to 8% of adult women and undiagnosed in many of them (158). Because androgen disorders are associated with significant cardiovascular disease, the condition should be diagnosed promptly and treated. This condition becomes of more immediate concern in older women of reproductive age. Management of bleeding disorders associated with androgen excess consists of an appropriate diagnostic evaluation followed by the use of oral contraceptives (in the absence of significant contraindications or the desire for conception) or the use of insulin-sensitizing agents, coupled with dietary and exercise modification (159–161).

Anatomic Causes   **Anatomic causes of abnormal bleeding occur more frequently in women of reproductive age than in women in other age groups. Uterine leiomyomas and endometrial polyps are common conditions that most often are asymptomatic; however, they remain important causes of abnormal bleeding** (162). Uterine leiomyomas occur in as many as one-half of all women older than age 35 years and are the most common tumors of the genital tract (151,152,162). The incidence varies from 30% to 70%, depending on criteria for study, whether clinical symptoms, ultrasound, or histologic assessment (163). One study of a randomly selected population estimated a cumulative prevalence of greater than 80% in black women and nearly 70% in white women (164). Abnormal bleeding is the most common symptom for women with leiomyomas. Although the number and size of uterine leiomyomas do not appear to influence the occurrence of abnormal bleeding, submucosal myomas are the most likely to cause bleeding. The mechanism of abnormal bleeding related to leiomyomas is not well established (see Chapter 15 for further discussion of uterine fibroids).

Endometrial polyps are a cause of intermenstrual bleeding, heavy menstrual bleeding, irregular bleeding, and postmenopausal bleeding and are associated with the use of *tamoxifen* and with dysmenorrhea and infertility. As with leiomyomas, most endometrial polyps are asymptomatic. The incidence of endometrial polyps increases with age throughout the reproductive years (162). The diagnosis may be suspected on the basis of endometrial thickening on transvaginal pelvic ultrasound, and patterns of feeder blood vessels may aid in distinguishing endometrial polyps from intracavity fibroids and from endometrial malignancy (162,165,166). Visualization with hysteroscopy or sonohysterography or the microscopic assessment of tissue obtained by a biopsy done in the office or a curettage specimen is required for confirmation. Whether and when to recommend removal is not well established, particularly if a polyp is asymptomatic and is found incidentally. One study of randomly selected Danish women using transvaginal ultrasound and sonohysterography found polyps in 5.8% of asymptomatic premenopausal women and 11.8% of asymptomatic postmenopausal women, In this study abnormal bleeding was present in 38% of those without polyps versus 13% with polyps (167). Endometrial polyps can regress spontaneously, although it is not clear how frequently this occurs. In one study of asymptomatic women, the 1-year regression rate was 27% (168). Smaller polyps are more likely to resolve, and larger polyps may be more likely to result in abnormal bleeding (169). Whereas polyps may resolve spontaneously over time, a clinically important question is whether they are likely to undergo malignant transformation. Because even asymptomatic polyps usually are removed at the time of identification, this question is difficult to answer. The chance of malignancy or premalignant changes in endometrial polyps appears to be quite low in premenopausal women and higher among postmenopausal women, with bleeding reports range from premalignant change in 0.2% to 24% and malignancy in 0% to 13% (170).

Abnormal bleeding, either intermenstrual or postcoital, can be caused by cervical lesions. Bleeding can result from endocervical polyps and infectious cervical lesions, such as condylomata, herpes simplex virus ulcerations, chlamydial cervicitis, or cervicitis caused by other organisms. Other benign cervical lesions, such as wide eversion of endocervical columnar epithelium or nabothian cysts, may be detected on examination but rarely cause bleeding.

Coagulopathies and Other Hematologic Causes of Abnormal in Reproductive-Age Women   As with adolescents, hematologic causes of abnormal bleeding should be considered in women with heavy menstrual bleeding, particularly in those who had abnormal bleeding since menarche. **Of all women with menorrhagia, 5% to 20% have a previously undiagnosed bleeding disorder, primarily von Willebrand's disease** (171). Table 14.8 presents guidelines for a gynecologist's suspicion of a bleeding disorder and pursuit of a diagnosis (81). Abnormal liver function, which can be seen with alcoholism or other chronic liver diseases, results in inadequate production of clotting factors and can lead to excessive menstrual bleeding.

Infections Causes   **As in adolescents, menorrhagia can be the first sign of endometritis in women infected with sexually transmissible organisms. Women with cervicitis, particularly chlamydial cervicitis, can experience irregular bleeding and postcoital spotting** (see Chapter 18). Therefore, cervical testing for *C. trachomatis* should be considered, especially for adolescents, women in their 20s, and women who are not in a monogamous relationship. Endometritis can cause excessive menstrual flow. Thus, a woman who seeks treatment for menorrhagia and increased menstrual pain and has a history of light-to-moderate previous menstrual flow may have an upper genital tract infection or PID (endometritis, salpingitis, oophoritis). Occasionally, chronic endometritis will be diagnosed when an endometrial biopsy is obtained for evaluation of abnormal bleeding in a patient without specific risk factors for PID.

Neoplasia   **Abnormal bleeding is the most frequent symptom of women with invasive cervical cancer.** A visible cervical lesion should be evaluated by biopsy rather than awaiting the results of cervical cytology testing, because the results of cervical cytology testing may be falsely negative with invasive lesions as a result of tumor necrosis. Unopposed estrogen is associated with a variety of abnormalities of the endometrium, from cystic hyperplasia to adenomatous hyperplasia, hyperplasia with cytologic atypia, and invasive carcinoma. Although vaginal neoplasia is uncommon, the vagina should be evaluated carefully when abnormal bleeding is present. Attention should be directed to all surfaces of the vagina, including anterior and posterior areas that may be obscured by the vaginal speculum on examination.

Diagnosis of Abnormal Bleeding in Reproductive-Age Women

For all women, the evaluation of excessive and abnormal menses includes a thorough medical and gynecologic history, the exclusion of pregnancy, the consideration of possible malignancy, and a careful gynecologic examination. For women of normal weight between the ages of approximately 20 and 35 years who do not have clear risk factors for STDs, who have no signs of androgen excess, who are not using exogenous hormones, and who have no other findings on examination, management may be based on a clinical diagnosis. Additional laboratory or imaging studies may be indicated if the diagnosis is not apparent on the basis of examination and history.

Laboratory Studies   **In any patient with heavy menstrual bleeding, an objective measurement of hematologic status should be performed with a complete blood count to detect anemia or thrombocytopenia. A pregnancy test should be performed to rule out pregnancy-related problems. In addition, because of the possibility of a primary coagulation problem, screening coagulation studies should be considered** (Table 14.8). The consensus report of an international expert panel recommends measurement of CBC, platelet count and function, PT, activated PTT, VWF (measured with ristocetin cofactor activity and antigen, factor VIII) and fibrinogen to be assessed in collaboration with a hematologist (81).

Imaging Studies   **Women with abnormal bleeding who have a history consistent with chronic anovulation, who are obese, or who are older than 35 to 40 years of age require further evaluation.** A pelvic ultrasonographic examination may be helpful in delineating anatomic abnormalities if the examination results are suboptimal or if an ovarian mass is suspected. A pelvic ultrasonographic examination is the best initial technique for evaluating the uterine contour, endometrial thickness, and ovarian structure (172,173). The use of a vaginal probe transducer allows assessment of endometrial and ovarian disorders, particularly in women who are obese. **Because of variation in endometrial thickness with the menstrual cycle, measurements of endometrial stripe thickness are significantly less useful in premenopausal than postmenopausal women** (174). Sonohysterography is especially helpful in visualizing intrauterine problems such as polyps or submucous leiomyoma. Although these sonographic techniques are helpful in visualizing intrauterine pathology, histologic evaluation is required to rule out malignancy. Other techniques, such as CT scanning and MRI, are not as helpful in the initial evaluation of causes of abnormal bleeding and should be reserved for specific indications,

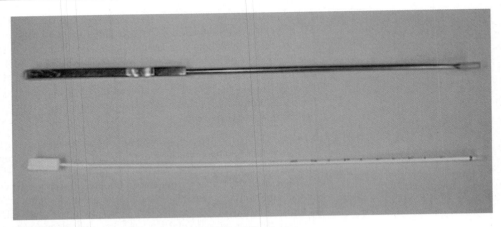

Figure 14.19 **Devices used for sampling endometrium.**
Top: Kevorkian Curette. **Bottom:** Pipelle.

such as exploring the possibility of other intra-abdominal pathology or adenopathy. MRI can be a secondary step in evaluating location of uterine fibroids with relationship to the endometrial cavity, staging and preoperative evaluation of endometrial cancer, detecting adenomyosis, and delineating adnexal and ovarian pathology (175).

Endometrial Sampling   **Endometrial sampling should be performed to evaluate abnormal bleeding in women who are at risk for endometrial pathology, including polyps, hyperplasia, or carcinoma. Such sampling is mandatory in the evaluation of anovulatory bleeding in women older than 35 to 40 years of age, in younger women who are obese, and in those who do not respond to medical therapy or those with a history of prolonged anovulation (143). The technique of D&C, which was used extensively for the evaluation of abnormal bleeding, was largely replaced by endometrial biopsy in the office.** The classic study in which a D&C was performed before hysterectomy with the conclusion that less than one-half of the endometrium was sampled in more than one-half of the patients led to questioning the use of D&C for endometrial diagnosis (176,177). Hysteroscopy, either diagnostic or operative, with endometrial sampling, can be performed either in the office or operating room (178).

A number of devices are designed for endometrial sampling, including a commonly used, inexpensive, disposable flexible plastic sheath with an internal plunger that allows tissue aspiration; disposable plastic cannulae of varying diameters that attach to a manually locking syringe that allows the establishment of a vacuum; and cannulae (both rigid metal and plastic) with tissue traps that attach to an electric vacuum pump (Fig. 14.19). Several studies comparing the adequacy of sampling using these devices with D&C showed a comparable ability to detect abnormalities. It should be noted that these devices are designed to obtain a tissue sample rather than a cytologic washing. The diagnostic accuracy of endometrial biopsy for endometrial malignancy and hyperplasia is good, although persistent bleeding should prompt further testing (179,180).

Management

Attention should be directed to establishing a cause of abnormal bleeding. In most cases, medical therapy is effective in managing abnormal bleeding and should be attempted before surgical management. Medical management with either oral contraceptives or progestogens is the preferred therapy of anovulatory bleeding in women of reproductive age (143). Progestin-releasing IUDs are effective in treating heavy menstrual bleeding and demonstrate comparable benefits for quality of life (181). **It is argued that the IUD should be offered prior to consideration of hysterectomy, as there are comparable benefits on heavy menstrual bleeding and clear cost benefits** (182). When medical therapy fails in women with anovulatory uterine bleeding and without the desire for future childbearing, the surgical options of endometrial ablation or hysterectomy can be considered. Endometrial ablation is an efficient and cost-effective alternative to hysterectomy, although this therapy may not be definitive, with increasing rates of repeat ablation and hysterectomy over time (143). In women with leiomyomas, hysterectomy provides a definitive cure. A variety of surgical alternatives to hysterectomy are available to women with symptomatic uterine leiomyomas.

Nonsurgical Management   **Most bleeding problems, including anovulatory bleeding, can be managed nonsurgically.** Treatment with NSAIDs, such as *ibuprofen* and *mefenamic acid,* decreases menstrual flow by 30% to 50%, but is less effective than *tranexamic acid, danazol, or levonorgestrel* IUD (93). Antifibrinolytics such as *tranexamic acid* were effective in reducing menstrual blood loss, and this indication was approved by the FDA in late 2008 (183).

Hormonal management of abnormal bleeding frequently can control excessive or irregular bleeding. The treatment of choice for anovulatory bleeding is medical therapy with oral contraceptives (143). Oral contraceptives are used clinically to decrease menstrual flow, although supporting data from prospective clinical trials are sparse (184). Low-dose oral contraceptives may be used by reproductive-age women without medical contraindications and during the perimenopausal years in healthy nonsmoking women who have no major cardiovascular risk factors. The benefits of menstrual regulation in such women often override the potential risks. The medical treatment of acute abnormal bleeding in reproductive-age women is the same as that described for adolescents.

For patients in whom estrogen use is contraindicated, progestins, both oral and parenteral, can be used to control excessive bleeding. Cyclic oral *medroxyprogesterone acetate,* administered from day 15 or 19 to day 26 of the cycle, reduces menstrual flow and offers no advantages over other medical therapies such as NSAIDs, *tranexamic acid, danazol,* or the *levonorgestrel* IUD; progestogen therapy for 21 days of the cycle reduces menstrual flow, although women found the treatment less acceptable than the *levonorgestrel* IUD (97). The benefits of progestins to the patient with oligomenorrhea and anovulation include a regular flow and the prevention of long intervals of amenorrhea, which may end in unpredictable, profuse bleeding. This therapy reduces the risk of hyperplasia resulting from persistent, unopposed estrogen stimulation of the endometrium. Depot formulations of *medroxyprogesterone acetate* are used to establish amenorrhea in women at risk of excessive bleeding. Oral, parenteral, or intrauterine delivery of progestins are used in selected women with endometrial hyperplasia or early endometrial cancer who wish to maintain their fertility (185). Continued monitoring is indicated. *Danazol* is effective in decreasing bleeding and inducing amenorrhea; it is used rarely for ongoing management of abnormal bleeding because of its androgenic side effects, including weight gain, hirsutism, alopecia, and irreversible voice changes. GnRH analogues are used for short-term treatment of abnormal bleeding, either alone or with add-back therapy consisting of combined estrogen/progestogen or progestogen alone (186).

Surgical Therapy **The surgical management of abnormal bleeding should be reserved for situations in which medical therapy is unsuccessful or is contraindicated. Although sometimes appropriate as a diagnostic technique, D&C is questionable as a therapeutic modality.** One study reported a measured reduction in menstrual blood loss for the first menstrual period only (187). Other studies suggest a longer-lasting benefit (188).

The surgical options range from a variety of techniques for endometrial ablation or resection to hysterectomy to a variety of conservative surgical techniques for management of uterine leiomyoma, including hysteroscopy with resection of submucous leiomyomas, laparoscopic techniques of myomectomy, uterine artery embolization, and magnetic resonance–guided focused ultrasonography ablation (see Chapters 23 and 24) (143,189). The choice of procedure depends on the cause of the bleeding, the patient's preferences, the physician's experience and skills, the availability of newer technologies, and a careful assessment of risks versus benefits based on the patient's medical condition, concomitant gynecologic symptoms or conditions, and desire for future fertility. The assessment of the relative advantages, risks, benefits, complications, and indications of these procedures is a subject of ongoing clinical research. Various techniques of endometrial ablation were compared with the gold standard of endometrial resection, and the evidence suggests comparable success rates and complication profiles (190). The advantages of techniques other than hysterectomy include a shorter recovery time and less early morbidity. However, symptoms can recur or persist; repeat procedures or subsequent hysterectomy may be required if conservative options are chosen. Additional studies that include quality-of-life outcomes will be helpful. Collaborative decision making, taking into account individual patient preferences, should follow a thorough discussion of options, risks, and benefits (191). Much is written about the psychologic sequelae of hysterectomy, and some of the aforementioned surgical techniques were developed in an effort to provide less drastic management options. **Most well-controlled studies suggest that, in the absence of preexisting psychopathology, indicated but elective surgical procedures for hysterectomy have few, if any, significant psychologic sequelae (including depression)** (see Chapter 12 and 24) (192,193).

Table 14.12 Conditions Diagnosed as a Pelvic Mass in Women of Reproductive Age
Full urinary bladder
Urachal cyst
Sharply anteflexed or retroflexed uterus
Pregnancy (with or without concomitant leiomyomas)
Intrauterine
Tubal
Abdominal
Ovarian or adnexal masses
Functional cysts
Inflammatory masses
Tubo-ovarian complex
Diverticular abscess
Appendiceal abscess
Matted bowel and omentum
Peritoneal cyst
Stool in sigmoid
Neoplastic tumors
Benign
Malignant
Paraovarian or paratubal cysts
Intraligamentous myomas
Less common conditions that must be excluded:
Pelvic kidney
Carcinoma of the colon, rectum, appendix
Carcinoma of the fallopian tube
Retroperitoneal tumors (anterior sacral meningocele)
Uterine sarcoma or other malignant tumors

Reproductive-Age Pelvic Masses

Conditions diagnosed as a pelvic mass in women of reproductive age are presented in Table 14.12.

Differential Diagnosis

It is difficult to determine the frequency of diagnoses of pelvic mass in women of reproductive age because many pelvic masses are not treated with surgery. **Nonovarian or nongynecologic conditions may be confused with an ovarian or uterine mass** (Table 14.12). The frequency of masses found at laparotomy was studied, although the percentages are affected by varying indications for surgery, indications for referral, type of practice (gynecologic oncology vs. general gynecology), and patient populations (a higher percentage of African Americans with uterine leiomyomas, for example). Benign masses, such as functional ovarian cysts or asymptomatic uterine leiomyoma, typically do not require or warrant surgery (Table 14.4).

Age is an important determinant of the likelihood of malignancy. In one study of women who underwent laparotomy for pelvic mass, malignancy was seen in only 10% of those younger than 30 years of age, and most of these tumors had low malignancy potential (194). The most common tumors found during laparotomy for pelvic mass are mature

cystic teratomas or dermoids (seen in one-third of women younger than 30 years of age) and endometriomas (approximately one-fourth of women 31 to 49 years of age) (194,195).

Uterine Masses

Uterine leiomyomas, commonly termed uterine fibroids, are by far the most common benign uterine tumors and are usually asymptomatic (195). Other benign uterine growths, such as uterine vascular tumors, are rare. See Chapter 15 for discussion of diagnosis, types and locations of fibroids, incidence, symptoms, causes, natural history, pathology, and management.

Ovarian Masses

During the reproductive years, the most common ovarian masses are benign. Ovarian masses can be functional or neoplastic, and neoplastic tumors can be benign or malignant. Functional ovarian masses include follicular and corpus luteal cysts. About two-thirds of ovarian tumors are encountered during the reproductive years. Most ovarian tumors (80% to 85%) are benign, and two-thirds of these occur in women between 20 and 44 years of age. **The chance that a primary ovarian tumor is malignant in a patient younger than 45 years of age is less than 1 in 15.** Most tumors produce few or only mild, nonspecific symptoms. The most common symptoms include abdominal distension, abdominal pain or discomfort, lower abdominal pressure sensation, and urinary or gastrointestinal symptoms. If the tumor is hormonally active, symptoms of hormonal imbalance, such as vaginal bleeding related to estrogen production, may be present. Acute pain may occur with adnexal torsion, cyst rupture, or bleeding into a cyst. Pelvic findings in patients with benign and malignant tumors may differ. Masses that are unilateral, cystic, mobile, and smooth are most likely to be benign, whereas those that are bilateral, solid, fixed, irregular, and associated with ascites, *cul-de-sac* nodules, and a rapid rate of growth are more likely to be malignant (196).

In assessing ovarian masses, the distribution of primary ovarian neoplasms by decade of life can be helpful (197). Ovarian masses in women of reproductive age are most likely benign, but the possibility of malignancy must be considered (Fig. 14.20) (196).

Nonneoplastic Ovarian Masses **Functional ovarian cysts include follicular cysts, corpus luteum cysts, and theca lutein cysts. All are benign and usually do not cause symptoms or require surgical management.** Cigarette and marijuana smoking are associated with an increased risk of functional cysts, although the increased risk may be attenuated in overweight or obese women (198). **Oral contraceptive use is associated with a decreased risk of developing ovarian cysts, although low-dose pills may have a smaller benefit, and oral contraceptives do not hasten the resolution of ovarian cysts** (199,200). The annual rate of hospitalization for functional ovarian cysts is estimated to be as high as 500 per 100,000 woman-years in the United States, although little is known about the epidemiology of the condition. **The most common functional cyst is the follicular cyst, which rarely is larger than 8 cm.** A cystic follicle can be defined as a follicular cyst when its diameter is greater than 3 cm. These cysts usually are found incidental to pelvic examination, although they may rupture or torse, causing pain and peritoneal signs. They can resolve in 4 to 8 weeks with expectant management (201).

Corpus luteum cysts are less common than follicular cysts. Corpus luteum cysts may rupture, leading to a hemoperitoneum and requiring surgical management. Patients taking anticoagulant therapy or with bleeding diatheses are at particular risk for hemorrhage and rupture. Rupture of these cysts occurs more often on the right side and may occur during intercourse. **Most ruptures occur on cycle days 20 to 26** (202). Unruptured corpus luteum cysts can cause pain, presumably because of bleeding into the enclosed ovarian cyst cavity. They can produce symptoms that can be difficult to discern from adnexal torsion.

Theca lutein cysts are the least common of functional ovarian cysts. They are usually bilateral and occur with pregnancy, including molar pregnancies. They may be associated with multiple gestations, molar pregnancies, choriocarcinoma, diabetes, Rh sensitization, clomiphene citrate use, human menopausal gonadotropin–human chorionic gonadotropin ovulation induction, and the use of GnRH analogues. Theca lutein cysts may be quite large (up to 30 cm), are multicystic, and regress spontaneously (203).

Combination monophasic oral contraceptive therapy is reported to reduce the risk of functional ovarian cysts (204). It appears that, in comparison with previously available higher-dose pills, the effect of cyst suppression with low-dose oral contraceptives is attenuated (205,206).

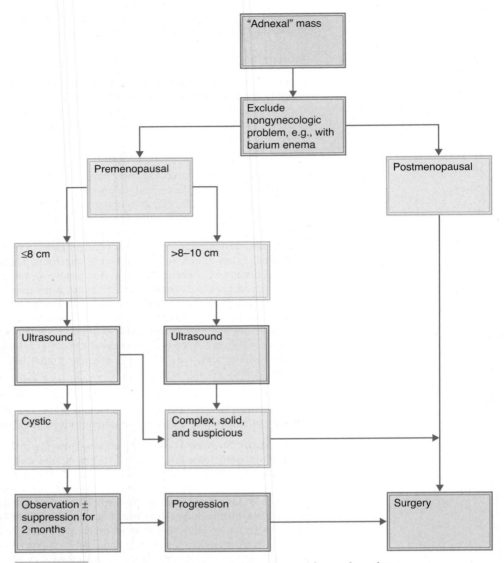

Figure 14.20 **Preoperative evaluation of the patient with an adnexal mass.**

The use of triphasic oral contraceptives is not associated with an appreciable increased risk of functional ovarian cysts (207).

Other Benign Masses Women with endometriosis may develop ovarian endometriomas ("chocolate" cysts), which can enlarge to 6 to 8 cm in size. A mass that does not resolve with observation may be an endometrioma (see Chapter 17). Excision is preferable to ablative techniques with regard to resolution of pain, achievement of spontaneous pregnancy, and risk of recurrence (208).

Although enlarged, polycystic ovaries were originally considered the *sine qua non* of PCOS, and are included among the Rotterdam diagnostic criteria, they are not always present with other features of the syndrome (209). An enlarged ovarian volume is suggested as an alternative diagnostic criterion, although whether the threshold should be 10 cm^3 or 7 cm^3 is debated (210). The prevalence of PCOS among the general population depends on the diagnostic criteria used. In one study, 257 volunteers were examined with ultrasonography; 22% were found to have polycystic ovaries (211). The finding of generously sized ovaries on examination or polycystic ovaries on ultrasonographic examination should prompt evaluation for the full-blown syndrome, which includes hyperandrogenism, chronic anovulation, and polycystic ovaries (159). Therapy

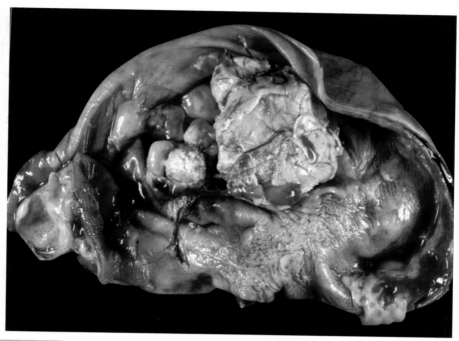

Figure 14.21   **Mature cystic teratoma (dermoid cyst) of the ovary.**

for PCOS is medical and generally not surgical, with lifestyle modification and weight loss playing a potentially important role (212).

Neoplastic Masses   **Most benign cystic teratomas (dermoid cysts) occur during the reproductive years, although dermoid cysts have a wider age distribution than other ovarian germ cell tumors; in some case series, up to 25% of dermoids occur in postmenopausal women, and they can occur in newborns** (213). Histologically, benign cystic teratomas have an admixture of elements (Fig. 14.21). In one study of ovarian masses that were surgically excised, dermoid cysts represented 62% of all ovarian neoplasms in women younger than 40 years of age (197). Malignant transformation occurs in less than 2% of dermoid cysts in women of all ages; most cases occur in women older than 40 years of age. The risk of torsion with dermoid cysts is approximately 15%, and it occurs more frequently than with ovarian tumors, perhaps because of the high fat content of most dermoid cysts, allowing them to float within the abdominal and pelvic cavity. As a result of this fat content, on pelvic examination a dermoid cyst frequently is described as anterior in location. They are bilateral in approximately 10% of cases, although many have advanced the argument against bivalving a normal-appearing contralateral ovary because of the risk of adhesions, which may result in infertility. **An ovarian cystectomy is almost always possible, even if it appears that only a small amount of ovarian tissue remains.** Preserving a small amount of ovarian cortex in a young patient with a benign lesion is preferable to the loss of the entire ovary (214). Laparoscopic cystectomy often is possible, and intraoperative spill of tumor contents is rarely a cause of complications, although granulomatous peritonitis was reported (215–217). Laparoscopic removal may be associated with a higher risk of recurrence (216).

The risk of epithelial tumors increases with age. Although serous cystadenomas are often considered the more common benign neoplasm, in one study, benign cystic teratomas represented 66% of benign tumors in women younger than 50 years of age; serous tumors accounted for only 20% (197). **Serous tumors are generally benign; 5% to 10% have borderline malignant potential, and 20% to 25% are malignant.** Serous cystadenomas are often multilocular, sometimes with papillary components (Fig. 14.22). The surface epithelial cells secrete serous fluid, resulting in a watery cyst content. Psammoma bodies, which are areas of fine calcific granulation, may be scattered within the tumor and are visible on radiograph. A frozen section is necessary to distinguish between benign, borderline, and malignant serous tumors because this distinction cannot be made on gross examination alone. Mucinous ovarian tumors may grow to large dimensions. Benign mucinous tumors typically have a lobulated, smooth surface, are multilocular, and may be bilateral in up to 10% of cases. Mucoid material is present within the

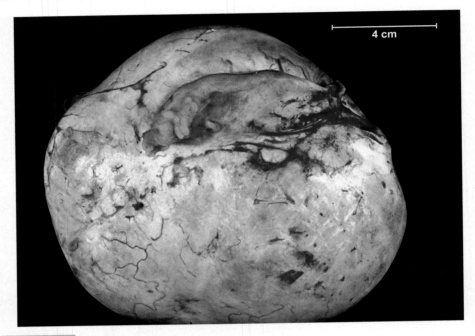

Figure 14.22   **Serous cystadenoma.**

cystic loculations. **Five to 10% of mucinous ovarian tumors are malignant.** They may be difficult to distinguish histologically from metastatic gastrointestinal malignancies. Other benign ovarian tumors include fibromas (a focus of stromal cells), Brenner tumors (which appear grossly similar to fibromas and are frequently found incidentally), and mixed forms of tumors, such as the cystadenofibroma.

Uterine, gastric, breast, and colorectal malignancies can metastasize to the ovaries and should be considered, although as with many malignancies, these tumors are more common in postmenopausal-aged women.

Other Adnexal Masses

Masses that include the fallopian tube are related primarily to inflammatory causes in the reproductive age group. A tubo-ovarian abscess can be present in association with PID (see Chapter 18). In addition, a complex inflammatory mass consisting of bowel, tube, and ovary may be present without a large abscess cavity. Ectopic pregnancies can occur in the reproductive age group and must be excluded when a patient presents with pain, a positive pregnancy test, and an adnexal mass (see Chapter 20). Paraovarian cysts may be noted either on examination or on imaging studies. In many instances, a normal ipsilateral ovary can be visualized using ultrasonography. The frequency of malignancy in paraovarian tumors is quite low and may be more common in paraovarian masses larger than 5 cm (218).

Diagnosis

A complete pelvic examination, including rectovaginal examination and Papanicolaou (Pap) test, should be performed. **Estimations of the size of a mass should be presented in centimeters** rather than in comparison to common objects or fruit (e.g., orange, grapefruit, tennis ball, golf ball). After pregnancy is excluded, one simple office technique that can help determine whether a mass is uterine or adnexal includes sounding and measuring the depth of the uterine cavity. Pelvic imaging can confirm the characteristics of the adnexal mass—whether solid or cystic or mixed echogenicity. Diagnosis of uterine leiomyomas usually is based on the characteristic finding of an irregularly enlarged uterus. The size and location of the usually multiple leiomyomas can be confirmed and documented with pelvic ultrasonography (Fig. 14.23). If the examination is adequate to confirm uterine leiomyoma and symptoms are absent, ultrasonography is not always necessary unless an ovarian mass cannot be excluded.

Other Studies   **Endometrial sampling with an endometrial biopsy or hysteroscopy is mandatory when both pelvic mass and abnormal bleeding are present.** An endometrial lesion—carcinoma or hyperplasia—may coexist with a benign mass such as a leiomyoma. In

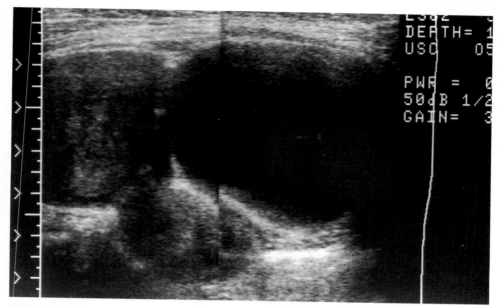

Figure 14.23   Transvaginal pelvic ultrasound demonstrating multiple uterine leiomyomas.

a woman with leiomyomas, abnormal bleeding cannot be assumed to be caused solely by the fibroids. Clinicians differ in recommendations about the need for endometrial biopsy when the diagnosis is leiomyomas with regular menses.

If urinary symptoms are prominent, studies of the urinary tract may be necessary, including urodynamic testing, if incontinence or symptoms of pelvic pressure are present. Cystoscopy may be necessary or appropriate to rule out intrinsic bladder lesions.

Laboratory Studies   Laboratory studies that are indicated for women of reproductive age with a pelvic mass include pregnancy test, cervical cytology, and complete blood count. The value of tumor markers, such as CA125 in distinguishing malignant from benign adnexal masses in *premenopausal* women with a pelvic mass, is questioned. **A number of benign conditions, including uterine leiomyomas, PID, pregnancy, and endometriosis can cause elevated CA125 levels in premenopausal women; thus, measurement of CA125 levels is not useful in premenopausal women with adnexal masses, because it may lead to unnecessary surgical intervention. Ultrasonographic characteristics are more helpful than CA125 in suggesting risks of malignancy in premenopausal women** (219).

Imaging Studies   Other studies may be necessary or appropriate. The most commonly indicated study is pelvic ultrasonography, which will help document the origin of the mass to determine whether it is uterine, adnexal, bowel, or gastrointestinal. The ultrasonographic examination provides information about the size of the mass and its consistency—unilocular cyst, mixed echogenicity, multiloculated cyst, or solid mass—which can help determine management (Figs. 14.24 and 14.25). Solid components, mural nodules, papillary excrescences, and ascites increase the suspicion of malignancy (220). A number of different ultrasound scoring systems were developed in an effort to quantify risks of malignancy.

Transvaginal and transabdominal ultrasonography are complementary in the diagnosis of pelvic masses, particularly those that have an abdominal component. Transvaginal ultrasonography has the advantage of providing additional information about the internal architecture or anatomy of the mass. Heterogeneous pelvic masses, described as tubo-ovarian abscesses on transabdominal ultrasonography, can be differentiated as pyosalpinx, hydrosalpinx, tubo-ovarian complex, and tubo-ovarian abscess with transvaginal ultrasonography (Fig. 14.26).

The diagnostic accuracy of transvaginal ultrasonography in diagnosing endometrioma can be quite high (Fig. 14.27). Endometriomas can have a variety of ultrasonographic appearances, from purely cystic to varying degrees of complexity with septation or debris to a solid appearance. A variety of scoring systems were developed with the intent of predicting benign versus malignant

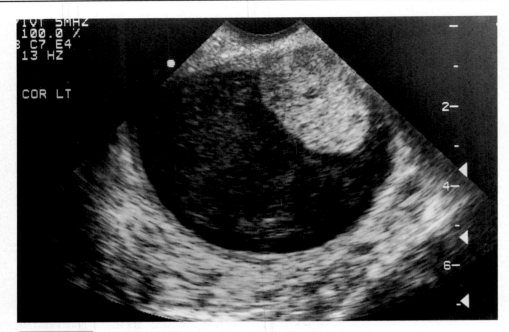

Figure 14.24   **Transvaginal ultrasound of a unilocular ovarian cyst.**

adnexal masses using ultrasound; the ultrasonographic morphologic characteristics used in many types of scoring systems are listed in Table 14.13 (220). Color flow Doppler was added to other sonographic characteristics to predict risk of malignancy; ultrasound techniques are comparable to CT and MRI in differentiating benign from malignant masses (221,222). Although an analysis of such features may be helpful, histologic confirmation of surgically removed persistent masses remains the standard of care.

CT seldom is indicated as a primary diagnostic procedure, although it may be helpful in planning treatment when a malignancy is strongly suspected or when a nongynecologic disorder may be

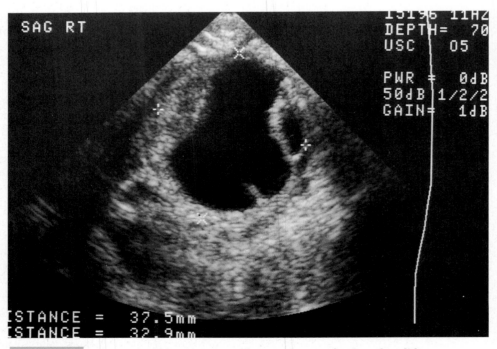

Figure 14.25   **Transvaginal ultrasonogram of a complex, predominantly solid mass.**

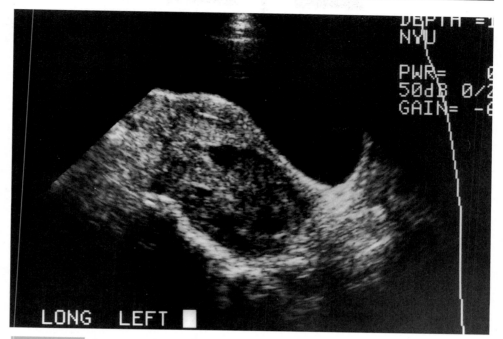

Figure 14.26   Transvaginal ultrasonogram of bilateral tubo-ovarian abscesses.

present. Abdominal flat-plate radiography is not a primary diagnostic procedure, although if used for other indications, it may reveal calcifications that can assist in the discovery or diagnosis of a mass. Pelvic calcifications (teeth) consistent with a benign cystic teratoma, a calcified uterine fibroid, or scattered calcifications consistent with psammoma bodies of a papillary serous cystadenoma can be seen with abdominal radiography (Fig. 14.28).

Ultrasonography or CT imaging may be appropriate to demonstrate ureteral deviation, compression, or dilation in the presence of moderately large and laterally located fibroids or other

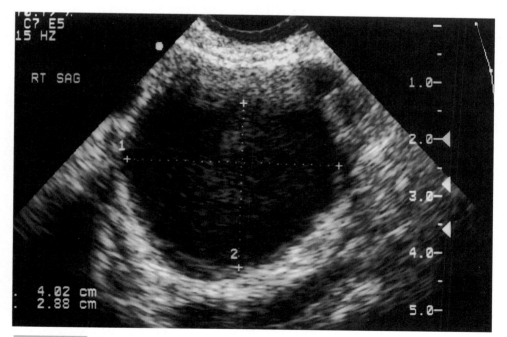

Figure 14.27   Transvaginal ultrasonogram of an endometrioma of the ovary.

Table 14.13 Ultrasonographic Characteristics of Adnexal Masses That May Be Useful in Predicting Malignancy

Unilocular cyst vs. multilocular vs. solid components
Regular contour vs. irregular border
Smooth walls vs. nodular vs. irregular
Presence or absence of ascites
Unilateral vs. bilateral
Wall thickness
Internal echogenicity and septations (including thickness)
Presence of other intra-abdominal pathology (liver, etc.)
Vascular characteristics and color flow Doppler pattern

pelvic mass. Such findings rarely provide an indication for surgical intervention for otherwise asymptomatic leiomyomas.

Hysteroscopy provides direct evidence of intrauterine pathology or submucous leiomyomas that distort the uterine cavity (see Chapter 23). Hysterosalpingography will demonstrate indirectly the contour of the endometrial cavity and any distortion or obstruction of the uterotubal junction secondary to leiomyomas, an extrinsic mass, or peritubal adhesions. The techniques combining hysterosalpingography, in which fluid is instilled into the uterine cavity, with transvaginal ultrasonography are helpful in the diagnosis of intrauterine pathology. Hysterosalpingography or sonohysterography may be indicated in women with infertility and uterine leiomyoma (193).

MRI may be most useful in the diagnosis of uterine anomalies, although its value rarely justifies the increased cost of the procedure over ultrasonography for the diagnosis of other pelvic masses (88).

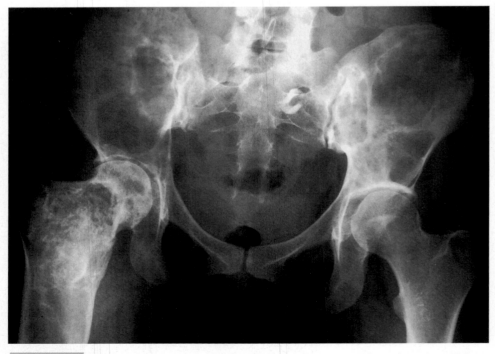

Figure 14.28   Benign cystic teratoma (dermoid cyst) of the ovary with teeth seen on abdominal radiograph.

Management of Pelvic Mass in Reproductive-Age Women

The management of a pelvic mass is based on an accurate diagnosis. An explanation of this diagnosis should be conveyed to the patient, along with a discussion of the likely course of the disease (e.g., growth of uterine leiomyomas, regression of fibroids at menopause, regression of a follicular cyst, the uncertain malignant potential of an ovarian mass). All options for management should be presented and discussed, although it is appropriate for the physician to state a recommended approach with an explanation of the reasons for the recommendation. Management should be based on the primary symptoms and may include observation with close follow-up, temporizing surgical therapies, medical management, or definitive surgical procedures.

Leiomyomas

The management of uterine leiomyomas is dependent on the patient's age and proximity to anticipated menopause, symptoms, patient preference, and the experience and skills of the clinician. Variability in reporting data regarding severity of symptoms, uterine anatomy, and response to therapy makes it difficult to compare different types of therapies, which include observation, medical, surgical, and radiologic-based techniques (see Chapter 15 for discussion of uterine fibroids).

Ovarian Masses

The now-routine application of ultrasound technology to gynecologic examinations led to the more frequent detection of ovarian cysts, sometimes as an incidental finding. Ultrasonography is a relatively easy diagnostic study to perform, but this ease led to the labeling of physiologic ovarian morphology and cystic follicles, as pathologic and the subsequent referral of patients for therapies, including surgery, without indications. **Treatment of ovarian masses that are suspected to be functional tumors is expectant** (Fig. 14.24). **A number of randomized prospective studies showed no acceleration of the resolution of functional ovarian cysts** (some of which were associated with the use of *clomiphene citrate* or human menopausal gonadotropins) **with oral contraceptives compared with observation alone** (200). **Oral contraceptives are effective in reducing the risk of subsequent ovarian cysts and may be appropriate for women who desire both contraception and their noncontraceptive benefits.**

Symptomatic cysts should be evaluated promptly, although mildly symptomatic masses suspected to be functional should be managed with analgesics rather than surgery to avoid the risk of surgical complications, including the development of adhesions that may impair subsequent fertility. Surgical intervention is warranted in the presence of severe pain or the suspicion of malignancy or torsion. **On ultrasonography, large cysts and those that have multiloculations, solid components, septa, papillae, and increased blood flow should be suspected of neoplasia** (219) (Fig. 24.25). **If a malignant mass is suspected at any age, surgical evaluation should be performed promptly.**

Ovarian or adnexal torsion is suspected on the basis of peritoneal signs and the acuity of onset. Doppler flow studies suggesting abnormal flow are predictive of torsion, although torsion can be seen with normal flow (223). The absence of internal ovarian flow is not specific to torsion and may be seen with cystic lesions, although in these situations peripheral flow usually can be visualized.

The management of suspected ovarian torsion, which can occur at any age from prepubertal to postmenopausal, is surgical. When torsion is confirmed by laparoscopy, untwisting of the mass and ovarian preservation rather than extirpation are generally indicated (224,225). The value of oophoropexy in preventing recurrent torsion is not well established.

Ultrasonographic or CT-directed aspiration procedures of ovarian masses should not be used in women in whom there is a suspicion of malignancy. In the past, laparoscopic surgery for ovarian masses was reserved for diagnostic or therapeutic purposes in patients at very low risk for malignancy. Although it is feasible to perform laparoscopic surgical staging and treatment of ovarian low-malignant-potential tumors and early-stage ovarian cancer safely, the role of laparoscopy versus laparotomy in a woman with ovarian cancer is debated (226). Concerns related to laparoscopy in managing gynecologic malignancy include the accuracy of intraoperative diagnosis, inadequate resection, significance of tumor spillage, inaccurate or delayed surgical staging, delay in therapy, and the possibility of port-site metastasis. In laparoscopic oophorectomy for presumed benign disease, there is a possibility of a missed diagnosis of malignancy, even with frozen section, which would necessitate reexploration. Whether laparoscopic management results in long-term compromise of outcome or significant benefits remains unclear and, consequently, so does the role of laparoscopic management of complex masses that may be malignant (227,228).

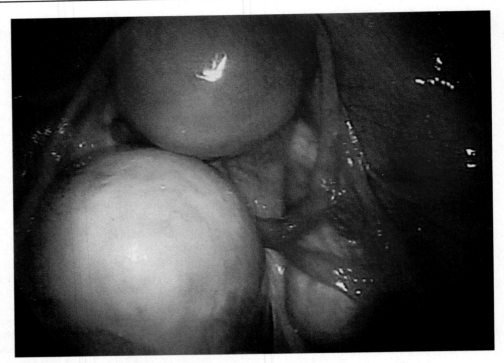

Figure 14.29   Laparoscopic appearance of benign ovarian mass (dermoid cyst).

The management of presumed benign ovarian masses with operative laparoscopy is now routine, although complication rates may be higher with complicated operative laparoscopic procedures such as those required for extensive endometriosis (Fig. 14.29) (229). **The choice of surgical approach (laparotomy or laparoscopy) should be based on the surgical indications, the patient's condition, the surgeon's expertise and training, informed patient preference, and the most recent data supporting the chosen approach.** The advantage of this technique is the shorter hospital stay, shorter recovery time, and lessened postoperative pain. A Cochrane review concluded that these findings should be interpreted with caution, given the small numbers of high-quality studies that provide comparisons (230).

The role of laparoscopy is even more controversial in the removal of dermoid cysts than with other benign masses. Concern focuses on preventing the spill of the cyst contents. Randomized clinical trials reported variable findings regarding spill; some studies suggest that cyst contents are more likely to spill with laparoscopy, whereas others do not find a difference or note no increase in morbidity when spillage occurred. Culdotomy and the use of an endoscopic specimen bag are associated with lower rates of tumor spillage (217).

Reproductive-Age Vulvar Conditions

In postmenarchal individuals, vulvar symptoms are most often related to a primary vaginitis and a secondary vulvitis. The mere presence of vaginal discharge can lead to vulvar irritative symptoms, or candidal vulvitis may be present (Fig. 14.17). The causes of vaginitis and cervicitis are covered in Chapter 18. Adult women describe vulvar symptoms using a variety of terms (itching, pain, discharge, discomfort, burning, external dysuria, soreness, pain with intercourse or sexual activity). **Burning with urination from noninfectious causes may be difficult to distinguish from a urinary tract infection, although some women can distinguish pain when the urine hits the vulvar area (an external dysuria) from burning pain (often suprapubic in location) during urination.** Itching is a very common vulvar symptom. A variety of vulvar conditions and lesions can present with pruritus. As in adolescents, vulvovaginal symptoms may be caused by STDs, nonsexually transmitted vaginitis, or UTIs. The distinction between symptoms related to a UTI and those of vaginitis is difficult, and consideration should be given to testing for both *C. trachomatis* and obtaining a urine culture, particularly in young reproductive-age women (134).

Table 14.14 Subacute and Chronic Skin Recurrent Conditions of the Vulva

Noninfectious	*Infectious*
Acanthosis nigricans	Cellulitis
Atopic dermatitis	Folliculitis
Behçet's disease	Furuncle/carbuncle
Contact dermatitis	Insect bites (e.g., chiggers, fleas)
Crohn's disease	Necrotizing fasciitis
Diabetic vulvitis[a]	Pubic lice
Hidradenitis suppurativa[a]	Scabies
	Tinea
Lichen sclerosus	Condyloma
Paget's disease	Vulvar candidiasis
"Razor bumps"—folliculitis or pseudofolliculitis	HSV
Psoriasis	
Seborrheic dermatitis	
Vulvar aphthous ulcer	
Vulvar intraepithelial neoplasia	

[a]Etiology unknown, often secondarily infected.

A number of skin conditions that occur on other areas of the body may occur on the vulvar area. Table 14.14 contains a list of these conditions classified by either infectious or noninfectious causes. Whereas the diagnosis of some of these conditions is apparent from inspection alone (e.g., a skin tag), any lesions that appear atypical or in which the diagnosis is not clear should be analyzed by biopsy, because the risks of malignant lesions increases with age (Fig. 14.30).

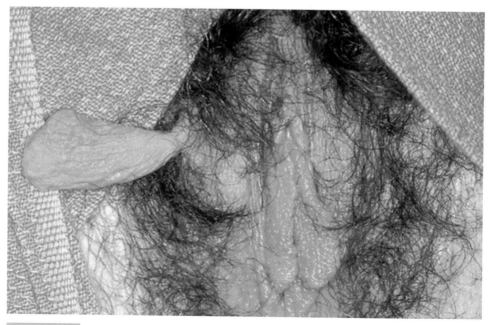

Figure 14.30   **Large benign skin tag from left labium majus.**

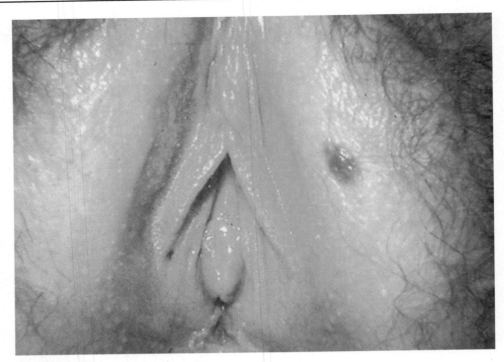

Figure 14.31   **Pigmented vulvar lesion.**

Pigmented vulvar lesions include benign nevi, lentigines, melanosis, seborrheic keratosis, condyloma, and some VINs, especially multifocal VIN-3 (Fig. 14.31). **Suspicious pigmented vulvar lesions in particular should warrant biopsy to rule out VIN or malignant melanoma** (231). Approximately 10% of white women have a pigmented vulvar lesion; some of these lesions may be malignant (see Chapter 38) or have the potential for progression (VIN) (see Chapter 19). There is an increase in rates of VIN in women younger than age 50, along with increasing rates of vulvar squamous cell carcinoma *in situ,* possibly related to increasing rates of HPV infection. Heightened awareness among clinicians may play a role in the increasing frequency of diagnosis; suspicious lesions warrant vulvar biopsy. Pigmented lesions include common nevi, lentigines, melanomas, dysplastic nevi, blue nevi, and a lesion termed atypical melanocytic nevi of the genital type (AMNGT) (232). AMNGTs have some histologic features that may overlap with those of melanoma, but with a benign prognosis.

Vulvar Biopsy

A vulvar biopsy is essential in distinguishing benign from premalignant or malignant vulvar lesions, especially because many types of lesions may have a somewhat similar appearance. Vulvar biopsies should be performed liberally in women of reproductive age to ensure that these lesions are diagnosed and treated appropriately. A prospective study of vulvar lesions evaluated by biopsy in a gynecologic clinic found lesions occurring in the following order of frequency: epidermal inclusion cyst, lentigo, Bartholin duct obstruction, carcinoma *in situ,* melanocytic nevi, acrochordon, mucous cyst, hemangiomas, postinflammatory hyperpigmentation, seborrheic keratoses, varicosities, hidradenomas, verruca, basal cell carcinoma, and unusual tumors such as neurofibromas, ectopic tissue, syringomas, and abscesses (233). Clearly, the frequency with which a lesion would be reported after a tissue biopsy is related to the frequency with which all lesions of a given pathology are evaluated in this manner. Thus, this listing probably underrepresents such common lesions as condylomata (Fig. 14.18).

Biopsy is easily performed in the office using a local anesthetic. Typically, 1% *lidocaine* **is infiltrated beneath the lesion using a small (25- to 27-gauge) needle.** Disposable punch biopsy instruments come in a variety of sizes from 2 to 6 mm in diameter. These skin biopsy instruments, along with fine forceps, scissors, and a scalpel, should be available in all outpatient gynecologic settings. For smaller biopsies, it is usually not necessary to place a suture. Topical *silver nitrate* can be used for hemostasis. Multiple tissue samples may be appropriate to obtain representative areas of a lesion if the lesion has a variable appearance or is multifocal. Although the vulvar biopsy procedure involves minimal discomfort, the biopsy sites will be painful for several days after the procedure. The prescription of a topical anesthetic such as 2% *lidocaine* jelly, to be applied periodically and before urinating, is appreciated by patients who require this procedure. Infection of the site can occur, and patients should be cautioned to report excessive erythema or purulent drainage.

Other Vulvar Conditions

Classification and description of intraepithelial lesions of the vulva are presented in Chapter 19.

Pseudofolliculitis or Mechanical Folliculitis   This is similar to what is described as pseudofolliculitis barbae (razor bumps) and may occur in women who follow the popular practice of shaving pubic hair (234). **Pseudofolliculitis consists of an inflammatory reaction surrounding an ingrown hair and occurs most commonly among individuals with curly hair, particularly African Americans.**

Infectious Folliculitis   Shaving may be associated with an infectious folliculitis, commonly caused by *Staphylococcus aureus* and *Streptococcus pyogenes*. Shaving and other methods of pubic hair removal are associated with razor burn, contact dermatitis, and the transmission of other infectious agents such as *Molluscum contagiosum,* HPV, and herpes simplex along with other bacteria including *Pseudomonas aeruginosa* (234).

Fox-Fordyce Disease   This condition is characterized by a chronic, pruritic eruption of small papules or cysts formed by keratin-plugged apocrine glands. It is commonly present over the lower abdomen, mons pubis, labia majora, and inner portions of the thighs. **Hidradenitis suppurativa is a chronic condition involving the apocrine glands with the formation of multiple deep nodules, scars, pits, and sinuses that occur in the axilla, vulva, and perineum.** Hyperpigmentation and secondary infection are often seen. Hidradenitis suppurativa can be extremely painful and debilitating. In the past, it was treated with antibiotics, isotretinoin, or steroids; surgical therapy with wide local excision may be necessary. Tumor necrosis factor-α inhibitors show promise in treatment (235).

Acanthosis Nigricans   This disease involves widespread velvety pigmentation in skin folds, particularly the axillae, neck, thighs, submammary area, and vulva and surrounding skin (Fig. 14.32). It is of particular interest to gynecologists because of its association with hyperandrogenism and PCOS; as such, it is associated with obesity, chronic anovulation, acne, glucose

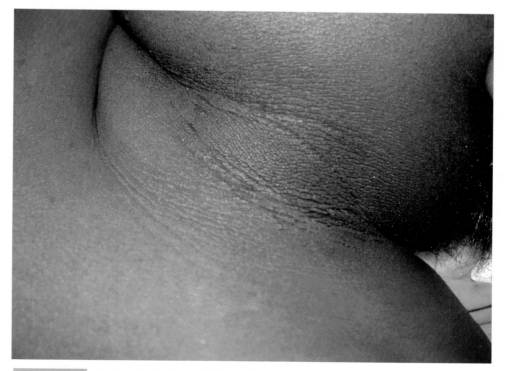

Figure 14.32   **Acathosis nigricans of the neck.**

intolerance, insulin resistance, and cardiovascular disease (159,236). Topical and oral retinoids are used to treat the acanthosis nigricans, along with management of the underlying conditions including obesity and insulin resistance or diabetes (237).

Extramammary Paget's Disease   This is an intraepithelial neoplasia containing vacuolated Paget's cells (see Chapter 19). Clinically, the appearance of Paget's disease is variable, and it may have an appearance varying from moist, oozing ulcerations to an eczematoid lesion with scaling and crusting to a grayish lesion (238). It may be confused with candidiasis, psoriasis, seborrheic dermatitis, contact dermatitis, and VIN. A biopsy to confirm the diagnosis is mandatory.

Vulvar Intraepithelial Neoplasia   **VIN is associated with HPV infection and is increasing in frequency, particularly among young women** (see Chapter 19). Diagnosis requires biopsy of any suspicious vulvar lesions, particularly those that are pigmented or discolored. The increasing frequency of this entity dictates a careful vulvar inspection during annual gynecologic examinations.

Vulvar Tumors, Cysts, and Masses

Condylomata Acuminata   **These are very common vulvar lesions and are usually easily recognized and treated with topical therapies such as *trichloroacetic* and *bichloracetic acid*. Other sexually transmitted organisms, such as the virus responsible for molluscum contagiosum and the lesions of syphilis and condylomata lata, may occasionally be mistaken for vulvar condylomata acuminata caused by HPV** (see Chapter 18). A summary of benign vulvar tumors is listed in Table 14.15. There is argument regarding whether sebaceous cysts exist on the vulva or whether these lesions are histopathologically epidermal or epidermal inclusion cysts (238). So-called sebaceous cysts are clinically indistinguishable from epidermal inclusion cysts that may result from the burial of fragments of skin after the trauma of childbirth or episiotomy or that arise from occluded pilosebaceous ducts. These cysts are seldom symptomatic, although if infection develops, incision and drainage may be required acutely, and ultimately complete excision is indicated.

Bartholin Duct Cysts   These are common vulvar lesions in reproductive-age women. They result from occlusion of the duct with accumulation of mucus and may be asymptomatic. Infection of the gland can result in the accumulation of purulent material, with the formation of a

Table 14.15 Types of Vulvar Tumors	
1. Cystic lesions	*3. Anatomic*
Bartholin duct cyst	Hernia
Cyst in the canal of Nuck (hydrocele)	Urethral diverticulum
Epithelial inclusion cyst	Varicosities
Skene duct cyst	*4. Infections*
2. Solid tumors	Abscess—Bartholin, Skene, periclitoral, other
Acrochordon (skin tag)	Condyloma lata
Angiokeratoma	Molluscum contagiosum
Bartholin gland adenoma	Pyogenic granuloma
Cherry angioma	*5. Ectopic*
Fibroma	Endometriosis
Hemangioma	Ectopic breast tissue
Hidradenoma	
Lipoma	
Granular cell myoblastoma	
Neurofibroma	
Papillomatosis	

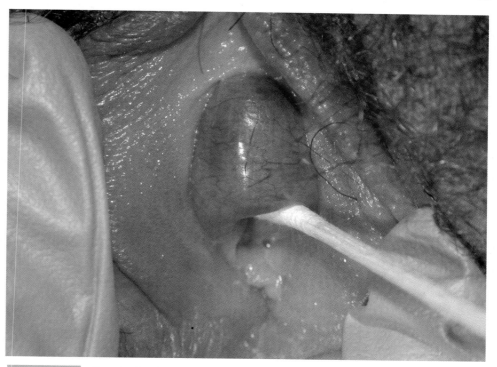

Figure 14.33 **Skene's gland cyst.**

rapidly enlarging, painful, inflammatory mass (a Bartholin abscess). An inflatable bulb-tipped catheter was described by Word and is quite easy to use (239). The small catheter is inserted through a small stab wound into the abscess after infiltration of the skin with local anesthesia; the balloon of the catheter is inflated with 2 to 3 mL of saline and the catheter remains in place for 4 to 6 weeks, allowing epithelialization of a tract and the creation of a permanent gland opening.

Skene's Duct Cysts   These are cystic dilations of the Skene glands, typically located adjacent to the urethral meatus within the vulvar vestibule. Although most are small and often asymptomatic, they may enlarge and cause urinary obstruction, requiring excision (Fig 14.33).

Painful Intercourse

Painful intercourse (dyspareunia) may be caused by many different vulvovaginal conditions, including common vaginal infections and vaginismus (see Chapters 11 and 18). A careful sexual history is essential, as is a careful examination of the vulvar area and vagina. *Vulvodynia* is the term used to describe unexplained vulvar pain, sexual dysfunction, and the resultant psychological disability (240,241). **The term *vulvar vestibulitis* was previously used to describe a situation in which there is pain during intercourse or when attempting to insert an object into the vagina; pain on pressure to the vestibule on examination and vestibular erythema (known as Friedrich's triad); this entity is now described as localized provoked vulvodynia in the International Society for the Study of Vulvovaginal Disease (ISSVD)** (240–243) (see Chapter 16). A number of recent studies failed to demonstrate a consistent relationship with any genital infectious organism, including *C. trachomatis,* gonorrhea, *Trichomonas,* mycoplasma, *Ureaplasma, Gardnerella,* candida, or HPV, and the condition has been characterized as multifactorial, with both inflammatory, neuropathic, and functional components. Although the symptoms of dyspareunia with insertion can be disabling, no curative therapies were found. Both medical and behavioral therapies are of some benefit, and some authors encourage surgery, but the role of this treatment and newer therapies such as the injection of botulinum toxin A is not well established (241).

Vulvar Ulcers

A number of STDs can cause vulvar ulcers, including herpes simplex virus, syphilis, lymphogranuloma venereum, and granuloma inguinale (see Chapter 18). *Crohn's disease* can include vulvar involvement with abscesses, fistulae, sinus tracts, fenestrations, and other scarring. Although medical treatment, with systemic steroids and other systemic agents, is the standard therapy, surgical therapy for both intestinal and vulvar disease may be required.

Behçet's Disease   This systemic condition is characterized by genital and oral ulcerations with ocular inflammation and many other manifestations (244). The cause and the most effective therapy are not well established, although anti-inflammatory and immunosuppressive therapies may be effective (245).

Lichen Planus   This condition causes oral and genital ulcerations. Typically, there is desquamative vaginitis with erosion of the vestibule. Treatment is based on the use of both topical and systemic steroids. Plasma cell mucositis appears as erosions in the vulvar area, particularly the vestibule. Biopsy is essential in establishing the diagnosis.

Reproductive-Age Vaginal Conditions

Vaginal discharge is one of the most common vaginal symptoms. Conditions ranging from vaginal candidiasis to chlamydia cervicitis to bacterial vaginosis to cervical carcinoma may cause vaginal discharge. Infectious vaginal conditions are addressed more completely in Chapter 18. Vaginal lesions may occasionally be palpable to a woman. More commonly, vaginal lesions are discovered on examination by a clinician. They may contribute to symptoms (such as bleeding or discharge) or they may be entirely asymptomatic. Vaginitis, cervicitis, and vaginal or cervical lesions (including malignancies) can be causes of vaginal discharge. Other noninfectious causes of discharge are as follows:

1. **Retained foreign body—tampon, pessary**
2. **Ulcerations—tampon-induced, lichen planus, herpes simplex infection**
3. **Malignancy—cervical, vaginal**

Some vaginal lesions are asymptomatic and are noted incidentally on examination. Fibroepithelial polyps consist of polypoid folds of connective tissue, capillaries, and stroma covered by vaginal epithelium. Although they can be excised easily in the office, their vascularity can be troublesome, and excision is not necessary unless the diagnosis is in question. **Cysts of embryonic origin can arise from mesonephric, paramesonephric, and urogenital sinus epithelium. Gartner's duct cysts are of mesonephric origin and are usually present on the lateral vaginal wall.** They rarely cause symptoms and, therefore, do not require treatment. Other embryonic cysts can arise anterior to the vagina and beneath the bladder. Cysts that arise from the urogenital sinus epithelium are located in the area of the vulvar vestibule. Vaginal adenosis, the presence of epithelial-lined glands within the vagina, is associated with *in utero* exposure to *diethylstilbestrol*. No therapy is necessary other than close observation and periodic palpation to detect nodules that may need to be evaluated by biopsy to rule out vaginal clear cell adenocarcinoma (see Chapter 36).

Women will sometimes describe a bulging lesion of the vagina and vulvar area, variably associated with symptoms of pressure or discomfort. The most common cause of such a lesion is one of the disorders of vaginal support. Management of these conditions is discussed in Chapter 27. Other genital lesions, such as urethral diverticula or embryonic cysts, may cause similar symptoms.

Postmenopausal Age Group

Postmenopausal Abnormal Bleeding

Differential Diagnosis

The causes of postmenopausal bleeding and the percentage of patients who seek treatment for different conditions are presented in Table 14.16.

Benign Disorders

Hormone therapy may be used to manage troublesome menopausal symptoms; it is recommended to treat with the lowest effective dose with the risks versus benefits regularly reviewed by a woman and her doctor (246). Women who are taking hormone therapy during menopause may be using a variety of hormonal regimens that can result in bleeding (see Chapter 34). Because unopposed estrogen therapy can result in endometrial hyperplasia, various regimens of progestins are typically added to the estrogen regimen; they are given in a continuous fashion, although they may be given in a sequential fashion for women within 1 year of menopause (246).

Table 14.16 Etiology of Postmenopausal Bleeding	
Factor	*Approximate Percentage*
Exogenous estrogens	30
Atrophic endometritis/vaginitis	30
Endometrial cancer	15
Endometrial or cervical polyps	10
Endometrial hyperplasia	5
Miscellaneous (e.g., cervical cancer, uterine sarcoma, urethral caruncle, trauma)	10

From **Hacker NF, Moore JG.** *Essentials of obstetrics and gynecology,* 3rd ed. Philadelphia: WB Saunders, 1998:635, with permission.

Endometrial sampling is indicated for any unexpected bleeding that occurs with hormonal therapy. **A significant change in withdrawal bleeding or breakthrough bleeding (e.g., absence of withdrawal bleeding for several months followed by resumption of bleeding or a marked increase in the amount of bleeding) should prompt endometrial sampling.**

Patient adherence to hormonal regimens is a significant issue with hormone therapy, with the challenges of oral therapy mitigated by nonoral routes of administration (247). Missed doses of oral medication and failure to take the medication in the prescribed fashion can lead to irregular bleeding or spotting that is benign in origin but that can result in patient dissatisfaction (248).

The problems that women most often report with hormone therapy include vaginal bleeding and weight gain. The use of a continuous low-dose combined regimen has the advantage that for many women, bleeding will ultimately cease after several months, during which irregular and unpredictable bleeding may occur (248,249). Some women are unable to tolerate these initial months of irregular bleeding. The risk of endometrial hyperplasia or neoplasia with this regimen is low.

Other benign causes of bleeding include atrophic vaginitis and endometrial and cervical polyps, which may become apparent as postcoital bleeding or spotting. Women who experience bleeding after menopause may attempt to minimize the extent of the problem; they may describe it as "spotting" or "pink or brownish discharge." However, any indication of bleeding or spotting should be evaluated. **In the absence of hormone therapy, any bleeding after menopause (classically defined as absence of menses for 1 year) should prompt evaluation with endometrial sampling.** Studies of transvaginal ultrasonography revealing an endometrial thickness 4 mm or less correlate with a low risk of endometrial malignancy, and thus endometrial sampling is not required (250). Endometrial polyps and other abnormalities can be seen in women who are taking *tamoxifen.* These polyps are more likely to involve cystic dilation of glands, stromal condensation around the glands, and squamous metaplasia of the overlying epithelium (251). These polyps can be benign, although they must be distinguished from endometrial malignancies, which may occur when taking *tamoxifen.* The incidence of endometrial polyps not associated with *tamoxifen* increases with age during the reproductive years; it is not clear whether the incidence subsequently peaks or decreases during the postmenopausal years (162). Endometrial polyps are more likely to be malignant in postmenopausal women, and hypertension is associated with an increased risk of malignancy (252).

Neoplasia

Endometrial, cervical, and ovarian malignancies must be ruled out in the presence of postmenopausal bleeding. One series found a malignancy (endometrial or cervical) in approximately 10% of women with postmenopausal bleeding (253). **A Pap test is essential when postmenopausal bleeding is noted, although the Pap test is an insensitive diagnostic test for detecting endometrial cancer.** The Pap test results are negative in some cases of invasive cervical carcinoma because of tumor necrosis.

Cervical malignancy is diagnosed by cervical biopsy of grossly visible lesions and colposcopically directed biopsy for women with abnormal Pap test results (see Chapter 19). Functional ovarian tumors may produce estrogen and lead to endometrial hyperplasia or carcinoma, which may cause bleeding.

Diagnosis of Postmenopausal Abnormal Bleeding

Pelvic examination to detect local lesions and a Pap test to assess cytology are essential first steps in finding the cause of postmenopausal bleeding. Pelvic ultrasonographic examination and, in particular, transvaginal ultrasonography or sonohysterography can suggest the cause of bleeding (250,254). **Endometrial sampling, through office biopsy, hysteroscopy, or D&C, is usually considered essential.** An endometrial thickness of less than 5 mm measured by transvaginal ultrasonography is unlikely to indicate endometrial cancer, although some authors suggest that the diagnostic accuracy is overestimated and recommend a cutoff of 3 mm (250,255).

Management of Postmenopausal Abnormal Bleeding

Benign Disorders   The management of bleeding caused by atrophic vaginitis includes topical (vaginal) or systemic use of estrogens after other causes of abnormal bleeding are excluded. Such therapy can provide significant benefits in terms of quality of life, but must be weighed with each individual, considering contraindications and patient preferences (256,257). Serum levels appear to be lower with vaginal administration using creams, tablets, or rings (258). Cervical polyps can easily be removed in the office.

Endometrial Hyperplasia   The terminology used to describe endometrial hyperplasia is confusing, and the clinician must consult with the pathologist to ensure an understanding of the diagnosis. **The World Health Organization (WHO) system classifies endometrial hyperplasia as simple hyperplasia, complex hyperplasia, simple atypical hyperplasia, and complex atypical hyperplasia** (259). Approximately 40% to 50% of women with atypical hyperplasia have concurrent carcinoma. **The management of endometrial hyperplasia is based on an understanding of the natural history of the lesion involved.** The risk of progression of hyperplasia without atypia is low but is approximately 30% among those with atypical hyperplasia (259). Hysterectomy is recommended for treatment of atypical endometrial hyperplasia in postmenopausal women. Management of endometrial cancer with surgical staging and multidisciplinary review of pathology and treatment planning is addressed in Chapter 35.

Progestin therapy (oral, parenteral, or intrauterine device delivery) may be used in women with atypical endometrial hyperplasia who are poor operative candidates. These women should have an endometrial biopsy every 3 months to check for recurrence, with recurrence risks approaching 50% (185). A suggested scheme of management is outlined in Figure 14.34. This treatment is discussed in more detail in Chapter 35.

Postmenopausal Pelvic Mass

Differential Diagnosis

Ovarian Masses   **During the postmenopausal years, the ovaries become smaller.** Ovarian volume is related to age, menopausal status, weight, height, and use of exogenous hormones (260). A large body habitus and uterine size make it more difficult to palpate and assess ovarian size, particularly among postmenopausal women, and transvaginal ultrasonography is significantly more accurate than clinical examination. Transvaginal ultrasonography is suggested in addition to annual pelvic examination among overweight postmenopausal women (261). Although ovarian cancer is notoriously difficult to diagnose at any early stage, the concept that it is frequently asymptomatic is challenged. Symptoms may include back pain, fatigue, bloating, constipation, abdominal pain, and urinary symptoms; these symptoms are of greater severity and more recent onset in women with ovarian malignancy (262). Thus it is argued that among primary clinicians, the possibility of an ovarian mass (either benign or malignant) in women with these symptoms warrants further diagnostic investigation. However, the positive predictive value of these symptoms is not high for the prediction of early-stage disease, and the use of symptoms to trigger an evaluation for ovarian cancer is noted to result in diagnosis of the disease in only 1 in 100 women in the general population with such symptoms (263). Ovarian cancer is predominantly a disease of postmenopausal women; the incidence increases with age, and the average patient age is about 56 to 60 years (see Chapter 37).

With increased use of pelvic ultrasonographic evaluation, a new problem arose in postmenopausal women: the discovery of a small ovarian cyst. This is particularly troublesome in

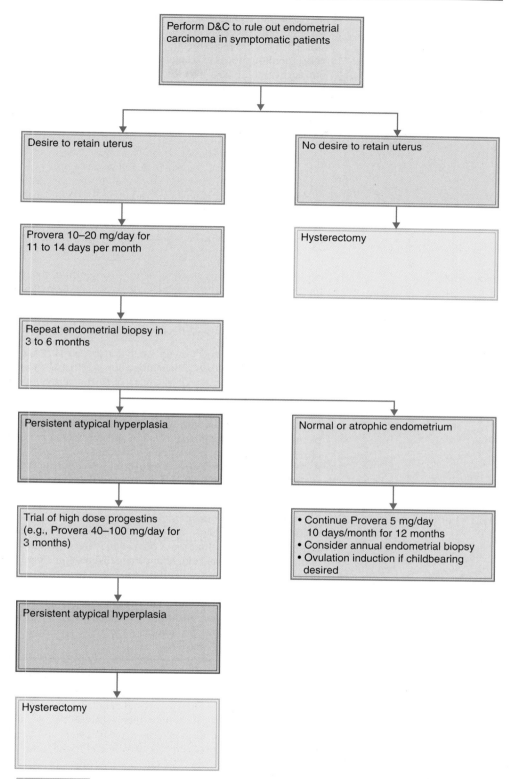

Figure 14.34   Management of endometrial hyperplasia. (Reproduced with permission from Berek & Hacker's Gynecologic Oncology, 5th edition, Lippincott Williams & Wilkins, 2010, p 410.)

a woman who is entirely asymptomatic and whose ultrasonographic examination was performed for indications unrelated to pelvic pathology. It is suggested that **when the cyst is asymptomatic, small (<5–10 cm in diameter), unilocular, and thin walled, with a normal CA125 level, the risk of malignancy is extremely low and these masses can be followed conservatively, without surgery** (220,264,265). Surgery may be indicated in some women with a strong family history of ovarian, breast, endometrial, or colon cancer, or with a mass that appears to be enlarging (see Chapter 37). The addition of color flow Doppler examination and other ultrasonographic characteristics may be helpful in distinguishing benign from malignant masses, although the role of Doppler ultrasonography remains somewhat controversial (Tables 14.4 and 14.13) (220).

Uterine and Other Masses   Many postmenopausal women have not had regular gynecologic care, and the discovery of a pelvic mass may reflect the persistence of a uterine leiomyoma that previously was not discovered. The possibility of transient ovarian cysts is noted above, and it may be difficult to distinguish an ovarian from a uterine mass. Some women may not remember having been told they had a pelvic mass. Thus, **a review of medical records may be helpful in determining the preexistence of a benign pelvic mass.** Uterine leiomyomas are hormonally responsive and typically decrease in size or resolve after menopause (see Chapter 15).

Diagnosis

A personal and family medical history is helpful in detecting individuals at increased risk for the development of ovarian cancer. Several hereditary family cancer syndromes involve ovarian neoplasms (see Chapter 37). However, **patients with hereditary forms of epithelial ovarian cancer account for only a small percentage of all cases; 90% to 95% of cases of ovarian cancer are sporadic and without identifiable heritable risk.**

In postmenopausal women with a pelvic mass, a CA125 measurement may be helpful in predicting a higher likelihood of a malignancy, which may guide decisions regarding management, consultation, or referral. A high index of suspicion by both women and their clinicians represents the best way to detect early ovarian cancer. Persistent symptoms such as an increase in abdominal size, bloating, fatigue, abdominal pain, indigestion, inability to eat normally, urinary frequency, pelvic pain, constipation, back pain, new onset of urinary incontinence, or unexplained weight loss require evaluation and consideration of the possibility of ovarian cancer. A physical examination, transvaginal ultrasonography, and CA125 measurement are appropriate. **A normal CA125 level does not rule out ovarian cancer; up to 50% of early-stage ovarian malignancies and 20% to 25% of advanced cancers have normal values of CA125** (266).

Management

The use of improved imaging techniques may allow the nonoperative management of ovarian masses that are probably benign (Table 14.13). **A suspicious or persistent complex mass requires surgical evaluation. A physician trained to appropriately stage and debulk ovarian cancer, such as a gynecologic oncologist, should perform the surgery in a hospital with the necessary support and consultative services to optimize the patient's outcome** (266). **When a malignant ovarian mass is discovered and the appropriate surgical staging and debulking procedure cannot be performed by the generalist obstetrician-gynecologist, a gynecologic oncologist should be consulted. Comprehensive surgical staging facilitates appropriate therapy and optimizes prognosis.**

Postmenopausal Vulvar Conditions

Anatomic changes that occur in postmenopausal women include atrophy of the labia majora and increasing prominence of the labia minora. The epithelium of the hymen and vestibule become thin; there is a shift in vaginal cellular maturation in response to estrogen deprivation, with resultant thinning. Although these changes lead to minimal symptoms in most women, external dysuria, pruritus, tenderness, dyspareunia, and bleeding can result from fissuring and excoriations. **Because of the risk of VIN and malignancy, suspicious lesions require vulvar biopsy.**

Vulvar Dermatoses

Several vulvar conditions occur most commonly in postmenopausal women. Symptoms are primarily itching and vulvar soreness, in addition to dyspareunia.

In the past, numerous terms were used to describe disorders of vulvar epithelial growth that produce a number of nonspecific gross changes. These terms included *leukoplakia, lichen sclerosus* and *atrophicus, atrophic* and *hyperplastic vulvitis,* and *kraurosis vulvae.* The ISSVD in 2006 recommended a classification of vulvar dermatoses based on histologic patterns, listed with the likely clinical diagnoses, rather than on the basis of clinical morphology as in the previous categorization (see Chapter 19) (267). This classification system excludes neoplastic and infectious conditions. Vulvar conditions that are described in this classification system include atopic, allergic, and irritant contact dermatitis, psoriasis, lichen simplex chronicus, lichen sclerosus, lichen planus, pemphigoid, aphthous ulcers, Behçet's disease, and Crohn's disease.

Lichen Sclerosus

Lichen sclerosus is the most common white lesion of the vulva. Lichen sclerosus can occur at any age, although it is most common among postmenopausal women and prepubertal girls (Fig. 14.4). The symptoms are pruritus, dyspareunia, and burning. Lichen sclerosus characteristically is associated with decreased subcutaneous fat to the extent that the vulva is atrophic, with small or absent labia minora, obliteration of the anatomic landmarks, thin labia majora, and sometimes phimosis of the prepuce. The surface is pale with a shiny, crinkled pattern (described as having characteristics like "cigarette paper"), often with fissures and excoriation. The lesion tends to be symmetric and often extends to the perineal and perianal areas. The diagnosis is confirmed by biopsy. Invasive cancer is associated with lichen sclerosus, although the significance of this association is unclear in terms of causation (289).

Treatment is with an ultrapotent topical steroid such as 0.05% *clobetasol.* **Approximately 93% of patients respond satisfactorily** (269). Maintenance therapy is frequently required, and a graduated reduction from ultrapotent to medium- and low-potency topical steroids can help to maintain remission of symptoms (269–271). The topical calcineurin inhibitors *pimecrolimus* and *tacrolimus* were effective in individuals not responding to topical steroids, although the FDA approved a warning suggesting possible risk of cancer from this class of drugs and caution is thus advised with long-term use avoided (272).

Premalignant Vulvar Lesions

Squamous vulvar intraepithelial neoplasia is seen most often in postmenopausal women but may occur during the reproductive years. Pruritus is the most common symptom, although "lumps" may be described and are sometimes confused with condyloma (268). Current terminology describes two types of VINs: VIN, usual type, that is typically HPV-related and encompassing former VIN-2 and -3 with warty, basaloid, and mixed types; and VIN, differentiated type (273). The lesion appears thickened and hyperkeratotic, and there may be excoriation. Lesions may be discrete but may be symmetric and multiple. About one-third of women will have a history of HPV related cervical disease or condyloma (268). Most women with VIN are smokers. Biopsy is necessary to confirm the diagnosis and to exclude malignancy. See Chapter 19 for management of VIN.

Urethral Lesions

The urethra and vagina have a common embryonic origin and are steroid-dependent tissues. Urethral caruncles and prolapse of the urethral mucosa are examples of vulvar lesions that may be seen in other age groups but that occur more commonly among older women. Both conditions can be treated with topical or systemic estrogen preparations. Various vulvar skin lesions, including seborrheic keratoses and cherry hemangiomas (senile hemangiomas), occur more commonly on aging skin.

Postmenopausal Vaginal Conditions

Up to 50% of postmenopausal women have symptoms of atrophic vaginitis (257). Symptoms include an external dysuria, pruritus, tenderness, dyspareunia, and bleeding from fissuring or ulcerations. In addition to the clinical findings of a shiny, flat, thin-appearing vaginal mucosa without rugae, microscopic examination of vaginal secretions reveals an increased number of white blood cells. **Treatment with local or systemic estrogens effectively manages the symptoms and restores normal pH levels with ongoing therapy** (274,275). Systemic absorption does occur with topical estrogen therapy, and rates of absorption differ depending on the degree of atrophy. Topical emollients may be helpful if estrogens are not desired or are contraindicated. Vaginal lubricants are universally useful in minimizing symptoms of dyspareunia for postmenopausal women (275).

References

1. **Biro FM, Lucky AW, Simbartl LA, et al.** Pubertal maturation in girls and the relationship to anthropometric changes: pathways through puberty. *J Pediatr* 2003;142:643–646.

2. **Herman-Giddens ME, Slora EJ, Wasserman RC, et al.** Secondary sexual characteristics and menses in young girls seen in office practice: a study from the Pediatric Research in Office Settings network. *Pediatrics* 1997;99:505–512.

3. **Euling SY, Herman-Giddens ME, Lee PA, et al.** Examination of US puberty-timing data from 1940 to 1994 for secular trends: panel findings. *Pediatrics.* 2008;121(Suppl 3):S172–S191.

4. **Apter D, Hermanson E.** Update on female pubertal development. *Curr Opin Obstet Gynecol* 2002;14:475–481.

5. **Marshall WA, Tanner JM.** Variations in pattern of pubertal changes in girls. *Arch Dis Child* 1969;44:291–303.

6. **Harlan WR, Harlan EA, Grillo GP.** Secondary sex characteristics of girls 12 to 17 years of age: the U.S. Health Examination Survey. *J Pediatr* 1980;96:1074–1078.

7. **Anveden-Hertzberg L, Gauderer MW, Elder JS.** Urethral prolapse: an often misdiagnosed cause of urogenital bleeding in girls. *Pediatr Emerg Care* 1995;11:212–214.

8. **Allen AL, Siegfried EC.** The natural history of condyloma in children. *J Am Acad Dermatol* 1998;39:951–955.

9. **Siegfried E, Rasnick-Conley J, Cook S, et al.** Human papillomavirus screening in pediatric victims of sexual abuse. *Pediatrics* 1998;101(Pt 1):43–47.

10. **Powell J, Wojnarowska F.** Childhood vulval lichen sclerosus and sexual abuse are not mutually exclusive diagnoses. *BMJ* 2000;320:311.

11. **Powell J, Wojnarowska F.** Childhood vulvar lichen sclerosus: an increasingly common problem. *J Am Acad Dermatol* 2001;44:803–806.

12. **Smith YR, Berman DR, Quint EH.** Premenarchal vaginal discharge: findings of procedures to rule out foreign bodies. *J Pediatr Adolesc Gynecol* 2002;15:227–230.

13. **Kaplowitz PB, Oberfield SE.** Reexamination of the age limit for defining when puberty is precocious in girls in the United States: implications for evaluation and treatment. Drug and Therapeutics and Executive Committees of the Lawson Wilkins Pediatric Endocrine Society. *Pediatrics* 1999;104(Pt 1):936–941.

14. **Flinn S.** Child sexual abuse I: an overview. Advocates for Youth 1995 available at http://www.advocatesforyouth.org/index.php?option=com_content&task=view&id=410&Itemid=336.

15. **Anonymous.** American Medical Association Diagnostic and Treatment Guidelines on Child Sexual Abuse. *Arch Fam Med* 1993;2:19–27.

16. **Iqbal CW, Jrebi NY, Zielinski MD et al.** Patterns of accidental genital trauma in young girls and indications for operative management. *J Pediatr Surg* 2010;45:930–933.

17. **Adams JA.** Evolution of a classification scale: medical evaluation of suspected child sexual abuse. *Child Maltreat* 2001;6:31–36.

18. **Sapp MV, Vandeven AM.** Update on childhood sexual abuse. *Curr Opin Pediatr* 2005;17:258–264.

19. **Holm K, Laursen EM, Brocks V, et al.** Pubertal maturation of the internal genitalia: an ultrasound evaluation of 166 healthy girls. *Ultrasound Obstet Gynecol* 1995;6:175–181.

20. **Oltmann SC, Garcia N, Barber R, et al.** Can we preoperatively risk stratify ovarian masses for malignancy? *J Pediatr Surg* 2010;45:130–134.

21. **Servaes S, Victoria T, Lovrenski J, et al.** Contemporary pediatric gynecologic imaging. *Semin Ultrasound CT MR* 2010;31:116–140.

22. **Stepanian M, Cohn DE.** Gynecologic malignancies in adolescents. *Adolesc Med Clin* 2004;15:549–568.

23. **Breen JL, Maxson WS.** Ovarian tumors in children and adolescents. *Clin Obstet Gynecol* 1977;20:607–623.

24. **Diamond MP, Baxter JW, Peerman CG Jr, et al.** Occurrence of ovarian malignancy in childhood and adolescence: a community-wide evaluation. *Obstet Gynecol* 1988;71(Pt 1):858–860.

25. **van Winter JT, Simmons PS, Podratz KC.** Surgically treated adnexal masses in infancy, childhood, and adolescence. *Am J Obstet Gynecol* 1994;170:1780–1789.

26. **Helmrath MA, Shin CE, Warner BW.** Ovarian cysts in the pediatric population. *Semin Pediatr Surg* 1998;7:19–28.

27. **Warner BW, Kuhn JC, Barr LL.** Conservative management of large ovarian cysts in children: the value of serial pelvic ultrasonography. *Surgery* 1992;112:749–755.

28. **Hernon M, McKenna J, Busby G, et al.** The histology and management of ovarian cysts found in children and adolescents presenting to a children's hospital from 1991 to 2007: a call for more paediatric gynaecologists. *BJOG* 2010;117:181–184.

29. **Lee PA, Houk CP, Ahmed SF, et al.** Consensus statement on management of intersex disorders. International Consensus Conference on Intersex. *Pediatrics* 2006;118:e488–e500.

30. **Consortium on the Management of Disorders of Sex Development.** Clinical guidelines for the management of disorders of sex development in childhood. Intersex Society of North America. Available at http://dsdguidelines.org/files/clinical.pdf.

31. **Muram D, Buxton BH.** The importance of the gynecologic examination in the newborn. *J Tenn Med Assoc* 1983;76:239.

32. **Posner JC, Spandorfer PR.** Early detection of imperforate hymen prevents morbidity from delays in diagnosis. *Pediatrics* 2005;115:1008–1012.

33. **Berenson AB.** A longitudinal study of hymenal morphology in the first 3 years of life. *Pediatrics* 1995;95:490–496.

34. **Hillard PJ.** Imperforate hymen. *eMedicine* 2010. Available online at: http://emedicine.medscape.com/article/269050-overview

35. **Garmendia G, Miranda N, Borroso S, et al.** Regression of infancy hemangiomas with recombinant IFN-alpha 2b. *J Interferon Cytokine Res* 2001;21:31–38.

36. **Bouchard S, Yazbeck S, Lallier M.** Perineal hemangioma, anorectal malformation, and genital anomaly: a new association? *J Pediatr Surg* 1999;34:1133–1135.

37. **Stricker T, Navratil F, Sennhauser FH.** Vulvovaginitis in prepubertal girls. *Arch Dis Child* 2003;88:324–326.

38. **Pokorny SF.** The genital examination of the infant through adolescence. *Curr Opin Obstet Gynecol* 1993;5:753–757.

39. **Emans SJ.** Office Evaluation of the Child and Adolescent in **Emans, SJ, Laufer MR, Goldstein DP, eds.** *Pediatric and adolescent gynecology.* 5th ed. Philadelphia: Lippincott Williams & Wilkins, 2005: 1–50

40. **Van Eyk N, Allen L, Giesbrecht E, et al.** Pediatric vulvovaginal disorders: a diagnostic approach and review of the literature. *J Obstet Gynaecol Can* 2009;31:850–862.

41. **Garzon MC, Paller AS.** Ultrapotent topical corticosteroid treatment of childhood genital lichen sclerosus. *Arch Dermatol* 1999;135:525–528.

42. **Muram D.** Treatment of prepubertal girls with labial adhesions. *J Pediatr Adolesc Gynecol* 1999;12:67–70.

43. **Shapiro RA, Makoroff KL.** Sexually transmitted diseases in sexually abused girls and adolescents. *Curr Opin Obstet Gynecol* 2006;18:492–497.

44. **Adams JA.** Medical evaluation of suspected child sexual abuse. *J Pediatr Adolesc Gynecol* 2004;17:191–197.

45. **Sinal SH, Woods CR.** Human papillomavirus infections of the genital and respiratory tracts in young children. *Semin Pediatr Infect Dis* 2005;16:306–316.

46. **Huppert JS, Gerber MA, Deitch HR, et al.** Vulvar ulcers in young females: a manifestation of aphthosis. *J Pediatr Adolesc Gynecol* 2006;19:195–204.

47. **Herman-Giddens ME.** Vaginal foreign bodies and child sexual abuse. *Arch Pediatr Adolesc Med* 1994;148:195–200.

48. **Siegel RM, Schubert CJ, Myers PA, et al.** The prevalence of sexually transmitted diseases in children and adolescents evaluated for sexual abuse in Cincinnati: rationale for limited STD testing in prepubertal girls. *Pediatrics* 1995;96:1090–1094.

49. **Herbst R.** Perineal streptococcal dermatitis/disease: recognition and management. *Am J Clin Dermatol* 2003;4:555–560.

50. **Pokorny SF, Stormer J.** Atraumatic removal of secretions from the prepubertal vagina. *Am J Obstet Gynecol* 1987;156:581–582.

51. **Treloar AE, Boynton RE, Behn BG, et al.** Variation of the human menstrual cycle through reproductive life. *Int J Fertil* 1967;12(Pt 2):77–126.

52. **Hillard PJ.** Menstruation in young girls: a clinical perspective. *Obstet Gynecol* 2002;99:655–662.

53. **Flug D, Largo RH, Prader A.** Menstrual patterns in adolescent Swiss girls: a longitudinal study. *Ann Hum Biol* 1984;11:495–508.

54. **World Health Organization Task Force on Adolescent Reproductive Health.** Longitudinal study of menstrual patterns in the early postmenarcheal period. Duration of bleeding episodes and menstrual cycles. *J Adolesc Health Care* 1986;7:236–244.

55. **Fraser IS, Critchley HO, Munro MG, et al.** A process designed to lead to international agreement on terminologies and definitions used to describe abnormalities of menstrual bleeding. *Fertil Steril* 2007;87:466–476.

56. **Fraser IS, McCarron G, Markham R, et al.** Blood and total fluid content of menstrual discharge. *Obstet Gynecol* 1985;65:194–198.

57. **Warner PE, Critchley, HO, Lumsden, MA, et al.** Menorrhagia II: is the 80-mL blood loss criterion useful in management of complaint of menorrhagia? *Am J Obstet Gynecol* 2004;190:1224–1229.

58. **Warner PE, Critchley HO, Lumsden MA, et al.** Menorrhagia I: measured blood loss, clinical features, and outcome in women with heavy periods: a survey with follow-up data. *Am J Obstet Gynecol* 2004;190:1216–1223.

59. **Fraser IS, McCarron G, Markham R.** A preliminary study of factors influencing perception of menstrual blood loss volume. *Am J Obstet Gynecol* 1984;149:788–793.

60. **Venturoli S, Porcu E, Fabbri R, et al.** Menstrual irregularities in adolescents: hormonal pattern and ovarian morphology. *Horm Res* 1986;24:269–279.

61. **ACOG Committee Opinion No. 349.** Menstruation in girls and adolescents: using the menstrual cycle as a vital sign. *Obstet Gynecol* 2006;108:1323–1328.

62. **Apter D, Vihko R.** Early menarche, a risk factor for breast cancer, indicates early onset of ovulatory cycles. *J Clin Endocrinol Metab* 1983;57:82–86.

63. **Gavin L, MacKay AP, Brown K, et al.** Sexual and reproductive health of persons aged 10–24 years—United States, 2002–2007. *MMWR Surveill Summ* 2009;58:1–58.

64. **Fraser IS, Hickey M, Song JY.** A comparison of mechanisms underlying disturbances of bleeding caused by spontaneous dysfunctional uterine bleeding or hormonal contraception. *Hum Reprod* 1996;11(Suppl 2):165–178.

65. **Rosenberg MJ, Burnhill MS, Waugh MS, et al.** Compliance and oral contraceptives: a review. *Contraception* 1995;52:137–141.

66. **Rosenberg MJ, Long SC.** Oral contraceptives and cycle control: a critical review of the literature. *Adv Contracept* 1992;8(Suppl 1):35–45.

67. **Oakley D, Sereika S, Bogue EL.** Oral contraceptive pill use after an initial visit to a family planning clinic. *Fam Plann Perspect* 1991;23:150–154.

68. **Balassone ML.** Risk of contraceptive discontinuation among adolescents. *J Adolesc Health Care* 1989;10:527–533.

69. **Woods JL, Shew ML, Tu W, et al.** Patterns of oral contraceptive pill-taking and condom use among adolescent contraceptive pill users. *J Adolesc Health* 2006;39:381–387.

70. **Mishell DR Jr, Guillebaud J, Westhoff C, et al.** Combined hormonal contraceptive trials: variable data collection and bleeding assessment methodologies influence study outcomes and physician perception. *Contraception* 2007;75:4–10.

71. **Fraser IS.** Bleeding arising from the use of exogenous steroids. *Baillieres Best Pract Res Clin Obstet Gynaecol* 1999;13:203–222.

72. **Abdel-Aleem H, d'Arcangues C, Vogelsong KM, et al.** Treatment of vaginal bleeding irregularities induced by progestin only contraceptives. *Cochrane Database Syst Rev* 2007;4:CD003449.

73. **Kaunitz AM.** Long-acting injectable contraception with depot medroxyprogesterone acetate. *Am J Obstet Gynecol* 1994;170(Pt 2):1543–1549.

74. **Kaunitz AM.** Current concepts regarding use of DMPA. *J Reprod Med* 2002;47(Suppl):785–789.

75. **Lockwood CJ, Schatz F, Krikun G.** Angiogenic factors and the endometrium following long term progestin only contraception. *Histol Histopathol* 2004;19:167–172.

76. **Krettek JE, Arkin SI, Chaisilwattana P, et al.** Chlamydia trachomatis in patients who used oral contraceptives and had intermenstrual spotting. *Obstet Gynecol* 1993;81(Pt 1):728–731.

77. **Ferenczy A.** Pathophysiology of endometrial bleeding. *Maturitas* 2003;45:1–14.

78. **Claessens EA, Cowell CA.** Acute adolescent menorrhagia. *Am J Obstet Gynecol* 1981;139:277–280.

79. **Philipp CS, Faiz A, Dowling N, et al.** Age and the prevalence of bleeding disorders in women with menorrhagia. *Obstet Gynecol* 2005;105:61–66.

80. **James AH.** Bleeding disorders in adolescents. *Obstet Gynecol Clin North Am* 2009;36:153–162.

81. **James AH, Kouides PA, Abdul-Kadir R, et al.** Von Willebrand disease and other bleeding disorders in women: consensus on diagnosis and management from an international expert panel. *Am J Obstet Gynecol* 2009;201:12e1–e8.

82. **Workowski KA, Berman SM.** Sexually transmitted diseases treatment guidelines, 2006. *MMWR Recomm Rep* 2006;55(RR11):1–94.

83. **Gray-Swain MR, Peipert JF.** Pelvic inflammatory disease in adolescents. *Curr Opin Obstet Gynecol* 2006;18:503–510.

84. **Carmina E, Oberfield SE, Lobo RA.** The diagnosis of polycystic ovary syndrome in adolescents. *Am J Obstet Gynecol* 2010;203:201e1–e5.

85. **Rosenfield RL, Lucky AW.** Acne, hirsutism, and alopecia in adolescent girls. Clinical expressions of androgen excess. *Endocrinol Metab Clin North Am* 1993;22:507–532.

86. **Legro RS.** Detection of insulin resistance and its treatment in adolescents with polycystic ovary syndrome. *J Pediatr Endocrinol Metab* 2002;15(Suppl 5):1367–1378.

87. **ACOG Practice Bulletin No. 109.** Cervical cytology screening. *Obstet Gynecol* 2009;114:1409–1420.

88. **Church DG, Vancil JM, Vasanawala SS.** Magnetic resonance imaging for uterine and vaginal anomalies. *Curr Opin Obstet Gynecol* 2009;21:379–389.

89. **Economy KE, Barnewolt C, Laufer MR.** A comparison of MRI and laparoscopy in detecting pelvic structures in cases of vaginal agenesis. *J Pediatr Adolesc Gynecol* 2002;15:101–104.

90. **Warren-Ulanch J, Arslanian S.** Treatment of PCOS in adolescence. *Best Pract Res Clin Endocrinol Metab* 2006;20:311–330.

91. **Demers C, Derzko C, David M, et al.** Gynaecological and obstetric management of women with inherited bleeding disorders. *Int J Gynaecol Obstet* 2006;95:75–87.

92. **Parker MA, Sneddon AE, Arbon P.** The menstrual disorder of teenagers (MDOT) study: determining typical menstrual patterns and menstrual disturbance in a large population-based study of Australian teenagers. *BJOG* 2010;117:185–192.

93. **Lethaby A, Augood C, Duckitt K, et al.** Nonsteroidal anti-inflammatory drugs for heavy menstrual bleeding. *Cochrane Database Syst Rev* 2007;4:CD000400.

93a. **U.S. Food and Drug Adminstration.** FDA approves lysteda to treat heavy menstrual bleeding. http://www.fda.gov/AboutFDA/StayInformed/RSSFeeds/ucm144575.htm

94. **Finer LB, Henshaw SK.** Disparities in rates of unintended pregnancy in the United States, 1994 and 2001. *Perspect Sex Reprod Health* 2006;38:90–96.

95. **Anonymous.** *Facts on American teens' sexual and reproductive health.* New York: Guttmacher Institute, 2010.

96. **Anonymous.** How is the 3 in 10 statistic calculated? Fact Sheet, The National Campaign to Prevent Teen Pregnancy. Pregnancy. Washington, DC: 2008. Available at http://www.thenationalcampaign.org/resources/pdf/FastFacts_3in10.pdf

97. **Lethaby A, Irvine G, Cameron I.** Cyclical progestogens for heavy menstrual bleeding. *Cochrane Database Syst Rev* 2008;1:CD001016.

98. **Speroff L, Fritz MA.** Dysfunctional uterine bleeding. In *Clinical gynecologic endocrinology and infertility.* New York: Lippincott Williams & Wilkins, 2005:558–559.

99. **Fraser IS, Porte RJ, Kouides PA, et al.** A benefit-risk review of systemic haemostatic agents: part 2: in excessive or heavy menstrual bleeding. *Drug Saf* 2008;31:275–282.

100. **Lethaby AE, Cooke I, Rees M.** Progesterone or progestogen-releasing intrauterine systems for heavy menstrual bleeding. *Cochrane Database Syst Rev* 2005;4:CD002126.

101. **Yen S, Saah T, Hillard PJ.** IUDs and adolescents—an under-utilized opportunity for pregnancy prevention. *J Pediatr Adolesc Gynecol* 2010;23:123–128.

102. **Nelson AL.** Levonorgestrel intrauterine system: a first-line medical treatment for heavy menstrual bleeding. *Womens Health (Lond)* 2010;6:347–356.

103. **ACOG Committee Opinion No. 448.** Menstrual manipulation for adolescents with disabilities. *Obstet Gynecol* 2009;114:1428–1431.

104. **Kucuk T, Ertan K.** Continuous oral or intramuscular medroxyprogesterone acetate versus the levonorgestrel releasing intrauterine system in the treatment of perimenopausal menorrhagia: a randomized, prospective, controlled clinical trial in female smokers. *Clin Exp Obstet Gynecol* 2008;35:57–60.

105. **Martin-Johnston MK, Okoji OY, Armstrong A.** Therapeutic amenorrhea in patients at risk for thrombocytopenia. *Obstet Gynecol Surv* 2008;63:395–402; quiz 405.

106. **Legro RS, Pauli LG, Kunselman AR, et al.** Effects of continuous versus cyclical oral contraception: a randomized controlled trial. *J Clin Endocrinol Metab* 2008;93:420–429.

107. **Pillai M, O'Brien K, Hill E.** The levonorgestrel intrauterine system (Mirena) for the treatment of menstrual problems in adolescents with medical disorders, or physical or learning disabilities. *BJOG* 2010;117:216–221.

108. **Miller L, Hughes JP.** Continuous combination oral contraceptive pills to eliminate withdrawal bleeding: a randomized trial. *Obstet Gynecol* 2003;101:653–661.

109. **Baldaszti E, Wimmer-Puchinger B, Loschke K.** Acceptability of the long-term contraceptive levonorgestrel-releasing intrauterine system (Mirena): a 3-year follow-up study. *Contraception* 2003;67:87–91.

110. **Diaz S, Croxatto HB, Pavez M, et al.** Clinical assessment of treatments for prolonged bleeding in users of Norplant implants. *Contraception* 1990;42:97–109.

111. **Bulas DI, Ahlstrom PA, Sivit CJ, et al.** Pelvic inflammatory disease in the adolescent: comparison of transabdominal and transvaginal sonographic evaluation. *Radiology* 1992;183:435–439.

112. **Kozlowski KJ.** Ovarian masses. *Adolesc Med* 1999;10:337–350, vii.

113. **Looijenga LH, Hersmus R, de Leeuw BH, et al.** Gonadal tumours and DSD. *Best Pract Res Clin Endocrinol Metab* 2010;24:291–310.

114. **Schellhas HF.** Malignant potential of the dysgenetic gonad. Part 1. *Obstet Gynecol* 1974;44:298–309.

115. **Cools M, Looijenga LH, Wolfenbuttel KP, et al.** Disorders of sex development: update on the genetic background, terminology and risk for the development of germ cell tumors. *World J Pediatr* 2009;5:93–102.

116. **Linam LE, Darolia R, Nafaa LN, et al.** US findings of adnexal torsion in children and adolescents: size really does matter. *Pediatr Radiol* 2007;37:1013–1019.

117. **Servaes S, Zurakowski D, Laufer MR, et al.** Sonographic findings of ovarian torsion in children. *Pediatr Radiol* 2007;37:446–451.

118. **Breech LL, Hillard PJ.** Adnexal torsion in pediatric and adolescent girls. *Curr Opin Obstet Gynecol* 2005;17:483–489.

119. **Laufer MR, Goltein L, Bush M, et al.** Prevalence of endometriosis in adolescent girls with chronic pelvic pain not responding to conventional therapy. *J Pediatr Adolesc Gynecol* 1997;10:199–202.

120. **Laufer MR, Sanfilippo J, Rose G.** Adolescent endometriosis: diagnosis and treatment approaches. *J Pediatr Adolesc Gynecol* 2003;16(Suppl):S3–S11.

121. **Capito C, Echaleb A, Lortat-Jacob S, et al.** Pitfalls in the diagnosis and management of obstructive uterovaginal duplication: a series of 32 cases. *Pediatrics* 2008;122:e891–e897.

122. **Martinez F, Lopez-Arregui E.** Infection risk and intrauterine devices. *Acta Obstet Gynecol Scand* 2009;88:246–250.

123. **Baeten JM, Nyange PM, Richardson BA, et al.** Hormonal contraception and risk of sexually transmitted disease acquisition: results from a prospective study. *Am J Obstet Gynecol* 2001;185:380–385.

124. **Eaton DK, Kann L, Kinchen S, et al.** Youth risk behavior surveillance—United States, 2009. *MMWR Surveill Summ* 2010;59:1–142.

125. **Mol BW, Ankum WM, Bossuyt PM, et al.** Contraception and the risk of ectopic pregnancy: a meta-analysis. *Contraception* 1995;52:337–341.

126. **Molander P, Cacciatore B, Sjoberg J, et al.** Laparoscopic management of suspected acute pelvic inflammatory disease. *J Am Assoc Gynecol Laparosc* 2000;7:107–110.

127. **Aboulghar MA, Mansour RT, Serour GI.** Ultrasonographically guided transvaginal aspiration of tuboovarian abscesses and pyosalpinges: an optional treatment for acute pelvic inflammatory disease. *Am J Obstet Gynecol* 1995;172:1501–1503.

128. **Buchweitz O, Malik E, Kressin P, et al.** Laparoscopic management of tubo-ovarian abscesses: retrospective analysis of 60 cases. *Surg Endosc* 2000;14:948–950.

129. **Muram D, Gold SS.** Vulvar ulcerations in girls with myelocytic leukemia. *South Med J* 1993;86:293–294.

130. **Reddy J, Laufer MR.** Hypertrophic labia minora. *J Pediatr Adolesc Gynecol* 2010;23:3–6.

131. **Ferris DG, Nyirjesy P, Sobel JD, et al.** Over-the-counter antifungal drug misuse associated with patient-diagnosed vulvovaginal candidiasis. *Obstet Gynecol* 2002;99:419–425.

132. **Workowski KA, Berman S.** Sexually transmitted diseases Treatment guidelines 2010. *MMWR Recomm Rep* 2010;59(RR12):1–110.

133. **Majewski S, et al.** The impact of a quadrivalent human papillomavirus (types 6, 11, 16, 18) virus-like particle vaccine in European women aged 16 to 24. *J Eur Acad Dermatol Venereol* 2009;23:1147–1155.

134. **Huppert JS, Biro FM, Mehrabi J, et al.** Urinary tract infection and chlamydia infection in adolescent females. *J Pediatr Adolesc Gynecol* 2003;16:133–137.

135. **Cook RL, Hutchison SL, Ostergaard L, et al.** Systematic review: noninvasive testing for *Chlamydia trachomatis* and *Neisseria gonorrhoeae*. *Ann Intern Med* 2005;142:914–925.

136. **Schuchat A, Broome CV.** Toxic shock syndrome and tampons. *Epidemiol Rev* 1991;13:99–112.

137. **Hajjeh RA, Reingold A, Weil A, et al.** Toxic shock syndrome in the United States: surveillance update, 1979–1996. *Emerg Infect Dis* 1999;5:807–810.

138. **Hochwalt A, Parsonnet J, Modern P.** Vaginal *S. aureus* and TSST-1 antibody prevalence among teens. Poster presentation at North American Society for Pediatric and Adolescent Gynecology, 2005. New Orleans, LA.

139. **Reichman O, Sobel JD.** MRSA infection of buttocks, vulva, and genital tract in women. *Curr Infect Dis Rep* 2009;11:465–470.

140. **Brook I.** Microbiology and management of polymicrobial female genital tract infections in adolescents. *J Pediatr Adolesc Gynecol* 2002;15:217–226.

141. **Fraser IS, Critchley HO, Munro MG.** Abnormal uterine bleeding: getting our terminology straight. *Curr Opin Obstet Gynecol* 2007;19:591–595.

142. **Fraser IS, Warner P, Marantos PA.** Estimating menstrual blood loss in women with normal and excessive menstrual fluid volume. *Obstet Gynecol* 2001;98(Pt 1):806–814.

143. **ACOG Practice Bulletin.** Management of anovulatory bleeding. *Int J Gynaecol Obstet* 2001;72:263–271.

144. **Mosher WD, Jones J.** Use of contraception in the United States: 1982–2008. *Vital Health Stat* 2010;23:1–44.

145. **Henshaw SK.** Unintended pregnancy in the United States. *Fam Plann Perspect* 1998;30:24–29, 46.

146. **Moodliar S, Bagratee JS, Moodley J.** Medical vs. surgical evacuation of first-trimester spontaneous abortion. *Int J Gynaecol Obstet* 2005;91:21–26.

147. **Ballagh SA, Harris HA, Demasio K.** Is curettage needed for uncomplicated incomplete spontaneous abortion? *Am J Obstet Gynecol* 1998;179:1279–1282.

148. **Fontanarosa M, Galiberti S, Fontanarosa N.** Fertility after non-surgical management of the symptomatic first-trimester spontaneous abortion. *Minerva Ginecol* 2007;59:591–594.

149. **Sotiriadis A, Makrydimas G, Papatheodorou S, et al.** Expectant, medical, or surgical management of first-trimester miscarriage: a meta-analysis. *Obstet Gynecol* 2005;105(Pt 1):1104–1113.

150. **Stubblefield PG.** Menstrual impact of contraception. *Am J Obstet Gynecol* 1994;170(Pt 2):1513–1522.

151. **Rosenberg MJ, Waugh MS, Burnhill MS.** Compliance, counseling and satisfaction with oral contraceptives: a prospective evaluation. *Fam Plann Perspect* 1998;30:89–92, 104.

152. **Rosenberg MJ, Waugh MS, Meehan TE.** Use and misuse of oral contraceptives: risk indicators for poor pill taking and discontinuation. *Contraception* 1995;51:283–288.

153. **Bachmann G, Korner P.** Bleeding patterns associated with non-oral hormonal contraceptives: a review of the literature. *Contraception* 2009;79:247–258.

154. **ACOG Committee Opinion No. 450.** Increasing use of contraceptive implants and intrauterine devices to reduce unintended pregnancy. *Obstet Gynecol* 2009;114:1434–1438.

155. **Krassas GE.** Thyroid disease and female reproduction. *Fertil Steril* 2000;74:1063–1070.

156. **Rebar RW.** Premature ovarian failure. *Obstet Gynecol* 2009;113: 1355–1363.

157. **Nelson LM.** Clinical practice. Primary ovarian insufficiency. *N Engl J Med* 2009;360:606–614.

158. **Azziz R, Woods KS, Reyna R, et al.** The prevalence and features of the polycystic ovary syndrome in an unselected population. *J Clin Endocrinol Metab* 2004;89:2745–1749.

159. **Guzick DS.** Polycystic ovary syndrome. *Obstet Gynecol* 2004;103: 181–193.

160. **Palomba S, Falbo A, Russo T, et al.** Systemic and local effects of metformin administration in patients with polycystic ovary syndrome (PCOS): relationship to the ovulatory response. *Hum Reprod* 2010;25:1005–1013.

161. **Cibula D, Fanta M, Vrbikova J, et al.** The effect of combination therapy with metformin and combined oral contraceptives (COC) versus COC alone on insulin sensitivity, hyperandrogenaemia, SHBG and lipids in PCOS patients. *Hum Reprod* 2005;20:180–184.

162. **Ryan GL, Syrop CH, Van Voorhis BJ.** Role, epidemiology, and natural history of benign uterine mass lesions. *Clin Obstet Gynecol* 2005;48:312–324.

163. **Okolo S.** Incidence, aetiology and epidemiology of uterine fibroids. *Best Pract Res Clin Obstet Gynaecol* 2008;22:571–588.

164. **Day Baird D, Dunson DB, Hill MC, et al.** High cumulative incidence of uterine leiomyoma in black and white women: ultrasound evidence. *Am J Obstet Gynecol* 2003;188:100–107.

165. **Tamura-Sadamori R, Emoto M, Naganuma Y, et al.** The sonohysterographic difference in submucosal uterine fibroids and endometrial polyps treated by hysteroscopic surgery. *J Ultrasound Med* 2007;26:941–948.

166. **Lieng M, Qvigstad E, Dahl GF, et al.** Flow differences between endometrial polyps and cancer: a prospective study using intravenous contrast-enhanced transvaginal color flow Doppler and three-dimensional power Doppler ultrasound. *Ultrasound Obstet Gynecol* 2008;32:935–940.

167. **Dreisler E, Stampe Sorenson S, Ibsen PH, et al.** Prevalence of endometrial polyps and abnormal uterine bleeding in a Danish population aged 20–74 years. *Ultrasound Obstet Gynecol* 2009;33:102–108.

168. **Lieng M, Istre O, Sandvik L, et al.** Prevalence, 1-year regression rate, and clinical significance of asymptomatic endometrial polyps: cross-sectional study. *J Minim Invasive Gynecol* 2009;16:465–471.

169. **DeWaay DJ, Syrop CH, Nygaard IE, et al.** Natural history of uterine polyps and leiomyomata. *Obstet Gynecol* 2002;100:3–7.

170. **Lieng M, Istre O, Qvigstad E.** Treatment of endometrial polyps: a systematic review. *Acta Obstet Gynecol Scand* 2010;89:992–1002.

171. **James AH, Manco-Johnson MJ, Yawn BP, et al.** Von Willebrand disease: key points from the 2008 National Heart, Lung, and Blood Institute guidelines. *Obstet Gynecol* 2009;114:674–678.

172. **Dubinsky TJ.** Value of sonography in the diagnosis of abnormal vaginal bleeding. *J Clin Ultrasound* 2004;32:348–353.

173. **Bignardi T, Van den Bosch T, Condous G.** Abnormal uterine and post-menopausal bleeding in the acute gynaecology unit. *Best Pract Res Clin Obstet Gynaecol* 2009;23:595–607.

174. **Breitkopf DM, Frederickson RA, Snyder RR.** Detection of benign endometrial masses by endometrial stripe measurement in premenopausal women. *Obstet Gynecol* 2004;104:120–125.

175. **Lane BF, Wong-You-Cheong JJ.** Imaging of endometrial pathology. *Clin Obstet Gynecol* 2009;52:57–72.

176. **Stock RJ, Kanbour A.** Prehysterectomy curettage. *Obstet Gynecol* 1975;45:537–541.

177. **Grimes DA.** Diagnostic dilation and curettage: a reappraisal. *Am J Obstet Gynecol* 1982;142:1–6.

178. **van Dongen H, de Kroon CD, Jacobi CE, et al.** Diagnostic hysteroscopy in abnormal uterine bleeding: a systematic review and meta-analysis. *BJOG* 2007;114:664–675.

179. **Clark TJ, Mann CH, Shah N, et al.** Accuracy of outpatient endometrial biopsy in the diagnosis of endometrial cancer: a systematic quantitative review. *BJOG* 2002;109:313–321.

180. **Clark TJ, Mann CH, Shah N, et al.** Accuracy of outpatient endometrial biopsy in the diagnosis of endometrial hyperplasia. *Acta Obstet Gynecol Scand* 2001;80:784–793.

181. **Heliovaara-Peippo S, Halmesmaki K, Hurskainen R, et al.** The effect of hysterectomy or levonorgestrel-releasing intrauterine system on lower abdominal pain and back pain among women treated for menorrhagia: a five-year randomized controlled trial. *Acta Obstet Gynecol Scand* 2009;88:1389–1396.

182. **Dueholm M.** Levonorgestrel-IUD should be offered before hysterectomy for abnormal uterine bleeding without uterine structural abnormalities: there are no more excuses! *Acta Obstet Gynecol Scand* 2009;88:1302–1304.

183. **ACOG Practice Bulletin.** Alternatives to hysterectomy in the management of leiomyomas. *Obstet Gynecol* 2008;112(Pt 1):387–400.

184. **Farquhar C, Brown J.** Oral contraceptive pill for heavy menstrual bleeding. *Cochrane Database Syst Rev* 2009;4:CD000154.

185. **ACOG Practice Bulletin.** Clinical management guidelines for obstetrician-gynecologists, management of endometrial cancer. *Obstet Gynecol* 2005106: 413–425.

186. **Cetin NN, Karabacak O, Korucuoglu U, et al.** Gonadotropin-releasing hormone analog combined with a low-dose oral contraceptive to treat heavy menstrual bleeding. *Int J Gynaecol Obstet* 2009;104:236–239.

187. **Haynes PJ, Hodgson H, Anderson AB, et al.** Measurement of menstrual blood loss in patients complaining of menorrhagia. *BJOG* 1977;84:763–788.

188. **Nickelsen C.** Diagnostic and curative value of uterine curettage. *Acta Obstet Gynecol Scand* 1986;65:693–697.

189. **Banu NS, Manyonda IT.** Alternative medical and surgical options to hysterectomy. *Best Pract Res Clin Obstet Gynaecol* 2005;19:431–449.

190. **Lethaby A, Shepperd S, Cooke I, et al.** Endometrial resection/ablation techniques for heavy menstrual bleeding. *Cochrane Database Syst Rev* 2009;4:CD001501.

191. **Kuppermann M, Learman LA, Schembri M, et al.** Predictors of hysterectomy use and satisfaction. *Obstet Gynecol* 2010;115:543–551.

192. **Persson P, Brynhildsen J, Kjolhede P.** Short-term recovery after subtotal and total abdominal hysterectomy—a randomised clinical trial. *BJOG* 2010;117:469–478.

193. **Yen JY, Chen YH, Long CY, et al.** Risk factors for major depressive disorder and the psychological impact of hysterectomy: a prospective investigation. *Psychosomatics* 2008;49:137–142.

194. **Hernandez E, Miyazawa K.** The pelvic mass. Patients' ages and pathologic findings. *J Reprod Med* 1988;33:361–364.

195. **Wallach EE, Vlahos NF.** Uterine myomas: an overview of development, clinical features, and management. *Obstet Gynecol* 2004; 104:393–406.

196. **Cannistra SA.** Cancer of the ovary. *N Engl J Med* 2004;351:2519–2529.

197. **Koonings PP, Campbell K, Mishell DR Jr, et al.** Relative frequency of primary ovarian neoplasms: a 10-year review. *Obstet Gynecol* 1989;74:921–926.

198. **Holt VL, Cushing-Haugen KL, Daling JR.** Risk of functional ovarian cyst: effects of smoking and marijuana use according to body mass index. *Am J Epidemiol* 2005;161:520–525.

199. **Christensen JT, Boldsen JL, Westergaard JG.** Functional ovarian cysts in premenopausal and gynecologically healthy women. *Contraception* 2002;66:153–157.

200. **Cochrane Update.** Oral contraceptives for functional ovarian cysts. *Obstet Gynecol* 2009;114:679–680.

201. **Grimes DA, Hughes JM.** Use of multiphasic oral contraceptives and hospitalizations of women with functional ovarian cysts in the United States. *Obstet Gynecol* 1989;73: 1037–1039.

202. **Hallatt JG, Steele CH Jr, Snyder M.** Ruptured corpus luteum with hemoperitoneum: a study of 173 surgical cases. *Am J Obstet Gynecol* 1984;149:5–9.

203. **Joshi R, Dunaif A.** Ovarian disorders of pregnancy. *Endocrinol Metab Clin North Am* 1995;24:153–169.

204. **Vessey M, Metcalfe A, Wells C, et al.** Ovarian neoplasms, functional ovarian cysts, and oral contraceptives. *Br Med J (Clin Res Ed)* 1987;294:1518–1520.

205. **Holt VL, Daling JR, McKnight B, et al.** Functional ovarian cysts in relation to the use of monophasic and triphasic oral contraceptives. *Obstet Gynecol* 1992;79:529–533.

206. **Lanes SF, Birmann B, Walker AM, et al.** Oral contraceptive type and functional ovarian cysts. *Am J Obstet Gynecol* 1992;166:956–961.

207. **Grimes DA, Godwin AJ, Rubin A, et al.** Ovulation and follicular development associated with three low-dose oral contraceptives: a randomized controlled trial. *Obstet Gynecol* 1994;83:29–34.

208. **Hart RJ, Hickey M, Maouris P, et al.** Excisional surgery versus ablative surgery for ovarian endometriomata. *Cochrane Database Syst Rev* 2008;2:CD004992.

209. **Anonymous.** Revised 2003 consensus on diagnostic criteria and long-term health risks related to polycystic ovary syndrome. *Fertil Steril* 2004;81:19–25.

210. **Jonard S, Robert Y, Dewailly D.** Revisiting the ovarian volume as a diagnostic criterion for polycystic ovaries. *Hum Reprod* 2005;20:2893–2898.

211. **Polson DW, Adams J, Wadsworth J, et al.** Polycystic ovaries—a common finding in normal women. *Lancet* 1988;1:870–872.

212. **Karimzadeh MA, Javedani M.** An assessment of lifestyle modification versus medical treatment with clomiphene citrate, metformin, and clomiphene citrate-metformin in patients with polycystic ovary syndrome. *Fertil Steril* 2010;94:216–220.

213. **Kurman R, ed.** *Blaustein's pathology of the female genital track.* Vol. 5. New York: Springer, 2005.

214. **Templeman CL, Fallat ME, Lam AM, et al.** Managing mature cystic teratomas of the ovary. *Obstet Gynecol Surv* 2000;55:738–745.

215. **Milingos S, Protopapas A, Drakakis P, et al.** Laparoscopic treatment of ovarian dermoid cysts: eleven years' experience. *J Am Assoc Gynecol Laparosc* 2004;11:478–485.

216. **Laberge PY, Levesque S.** Short-term morbidity and long-term recurrence rate of ovarian dermoid cysts treated by laparoscopy versus laparotomy. *J Obstet Gynaecol Can* 2006;28:789–793.

217. **Kondo W, Bourdel N, Cotte B, et al.** Does prevention of intraperitoneal spillage when removing a dermoid cyst prevent granulomatous peritonitis? *BJOG* 2010;117:1027–1030.

218. **Stein AL, Koonings PP, Schlaerth JB, et al.** Relative frequency of malignant parovarian tumors: should parovarian tumors be aspirated? *Obstet Gynecol* 1990;75:1029–1031.

219. **Van Calster B, Timmerman D, Bourne T, et al.** Discrimination between benign and malignant adnexal masses by specialist ultrasound examination versus serum CA-125. *J Natl Cancer Inst* 2007;99:1706–1714.

220. **ACOG Practice Bulletin.** Management of adnexal masses. *Obstet Gynecol* 2007;110:201–214.

221. **Liu J, Xu Y, Wang J.** Ultrasonography, computed tomography and magnetic resonance imaging for diagnosis of ovarian carcinoma. *Eur J Radiol* 2007;62:328–334.

222. **Medeiros LR, Rosa DD, da Rosa MI, et al.** Accuracy of ultrasonography with color Doppler in ovarian tumor: a systematic quantitative review. *Int J Gynecol Cancer* 2009;19:1214–1220.

223. **Huchon C, Staraci S, Fauconnier A.** Adnexal torsion: a predictive score for pre-operative diagnosis. *Hum Reprod* 2010;25:2276–2280.

224. **Huchon C, Fauconnier A.** Adnexal torsion: a literature review. *Eur J Obstet Gynecol Reprod Biol* 2010;150:8–12.

225. **Bottomley C, Bourne T.** Diagnosis and management of ovarian cyst accidents. *Best Pract Res Clin Obstet Gynaecol* 2009;23:711–724.

226. **Vaisbuch E, Dgani R, Ben-Arie A, et al.** The role of laparoscopy in ovarian tumors of low malignant potential and early-stage ovarian cancer. *Obstet Gynecol Surv* 2005;60:326–330.

227. **Cho JE, Liu C, Gossner G, et al.** Laparoscopy and gynecologic oncology. *Clin Obstet Gynecol* 2009;52:313–326.

228. **Mettler L, Meinhold-Heerlein I.** The value of laparoscopic surgery to stage gynecological cancers: present and future. *Minerva Ginecol* 2009;61:319–337.

229. **Minelli L, Ceccaroni M, Ruffo G, et al.** Laparoscopic conservative surgery for stage IV symptomatic endometriosis: short-term surgical complications. *Fertil Steril* 2010;94:1218–1222.

230. **Medeiros LR, Rosa DD, Bozzetti MC, et al.** Laparoscopy versus laparotomy for benign ovarian tumour. *Cochrane Database Syst Rev* 2009;2:CD004751.

231. **Ragnarsson-Olding BK, Kanter-Lewensohn LR, Lagerlof B, et al.** Malignant melanoma of the vulva in a nationwide, 25-year study of 219 Swedish females: clinical observations and histopathologic features. *Cancer* 1999;86:1273–1284.

232. **Ribe A.** Melanocytic lesions of the genital area with attention given to atypical genital nevi. *J Cutan Pathol* 2008;35(Suppl 2):24–27.

233. **Hood AF, Lumadue J.** Benign vulvar tumors. *Dermatol Clin* 1992;10:371–385.

234. **Trager JD.** Pubic hair removal—pearls and pitfalls. *J Pediatr Adolesc Gynecol* 2006;19:117–123.

235. **Alikhan A, Lynch PJ, Eisen DB.** Hidradenitis suppurativa: a comprehensive review. *J Am Acad Dermatol* 2009;60:539–563.

236. **Hermanns-Le T, Scheen A, Pierard GE.** Acanthosis nigricans associated with insulin resistance: pathophysiology and management. *Am J Clin Dermatol* 2004;5:199–203.

237. **Higgins SP, Freemark M, Prose NS.** Acanthosis nigricans: a practical approach to evaluation and management. *Dermatol Online J* 2008;14:2.

238. **Kaufman R, Faro S, Brown D, eds.** Cystic tumors in Benign diseases of the vulva and vagina. 5 ed. Philadelphia: Elsevier Mosby, 2005:449.

239. **Word B.** Office treatment of cysts and abscess of Bartholin's gland duct. *South Med J* 1968;61(5): 514-8.

240. **Farage MA, Galask RP.** Vulvar vestibulitis syndrome: a review. *Eur J Obstet Gynecol Reprod Biol* 2005;123:9–16.

241. **Petersen CD, Lundvall L, Kristensen E, et al.** Vulvodynia. Definition, diagnosis and treatment. *Acta Obstet Gynecol Scand* 2008; 87:893–901.

242. **Moyal-Barracco M, Lynch PJ.** 2003 ISSVD terminology and classification of vulvodynia: a historical perspective. *J Reprod Med* 2004;49:772–777.

243. **Friedrich EG Jr.** Vulvar vestibulitis syndrome. *J Reprod Med* 1987;32:110–114.

244. **Sakane T, Takeno M, Suzuki N, et al.** Behçet's disease. *N Engl J Med* 1999;341:1284–1291.

245. **Gul A.** Standard and novel therapeutic approaches to Behçet's disease. *Drugs* 2007;67:2013–2022.

246. **Furness S, Roberts H, Marjoribanks J, et al.** Hormone therapy in postmenopausal women and risk of endometrial hyperplasia. *Cochrane Database Syst Rev* 2009;2:CD000402.

247. **Sitruk-Ware R.** New hormonal therapies and regimens in the postmenopause: routes of administration and timing of initiation. *Climacteric* 2007;10:358–370.

248. **Kenemans P, van Unnik GA, Mijatovic V, et al.** Perspectives in hormone replacement therapy. *Maturitas* 2001;38(Suppl 1):S41–S48.

249. **Shoupe D.** HRT dosing regimens: continuous versus cyclic-pros and cons. *Int J Fertil Womens Med* 2001;46:7–15.

250. **ACOG Committee Opinion No. 426.** The role of transvaginal ultrasonography in the evaluation of postmenopausal bleeding. *Obstet Gynecol* 2009;113(Pt 1):462–464.

251. **Hann LE, Kim CM, Gonen M, et al.** Sonohysterography compared with endometrial biopsy for evaluation of the endometrium in tamoxifen-treated women. *J Ultrasound Med* 2003;22:1173–1179.

252. **Savelli L, De Iaco P, Santini D, et al.** Histopathologic features and risk factors for benignity, hyperplasia, and cancer in endometrial polyps. *Am J Obstet Gynecol* 2003;188:927–931.

253. **Karlsson B, Granberg S, Wikland M, et al.** Transvaginal ultrasonography of the endometrium in women with postmenopausal bleeding—a Nordic multicenter study. *Am J Obstet Gynecol* 1995;172:1488–1494.

254. **Epstein E, Valentin L.** Managing women with post-menopausal bleeding. *Best Pract Res Clin Obstet Gynaecol* 2004;18:125–143.

255. **Timmermans A, Opmeer BC, Khan KS, et al.** Endometrial thickness measurement for detecting endometrial cancer in women with postmenopausal bleeding: a systematic review and meta-analysis. *Obstet Gynecol* 2010;116:160–167.

256. **Castelo-Branco C, Cancelo MJ, Villero J, et al.** Management of post-menopausal vaginal atrophy and atrophic vaginitis. *Maturitas* 2005;52(Suppl 1):S46–S52.

257. **Santoro N, Komi J.** Prevalence and impact of vaginal symptoms among postmenopausal women. *J Sex Med* 2009;6:2133–2142.

258. **Dorr MB, Nelson AL, Mayer PR, et al.** Plasma estrogen concentrations after oral and vaginal estrogen administration in women with atrophic vaginitis. *Fertil Steril* 2010;94:2365–2368.

259. **Lacey JV Jr, Chia VM.** Endometrial hyperplasia and the risk of progression to carcinoma. *Maturitas* 2009;63:39–44.

260. **Pavlik EJ, DePriest PD, Gallion HH, et al.** Ovarian volume related to age. *Gynecol Oncol* 2000;77:410–412.

261. **Ueland FR, DePriest PD, Desimone CP, et al.** The accuracy of examination under anesthesia and transvaginal sonography in evaluating ovarian size. *Gynecol Oncol* 2005;99:400–403.

262. **Goff BA, Mandel LS, Melancon CH, et al.** Frequency of symptoms of ovarian cancer in women presenting to primary care clinics. *JAMA* 2004;291:2705–2712.

263. **Rossing MA, Wicklund KG, Cushing-Haugen KL, et al.** Predictive value of symptoms for early detection of ovarian cancer. *J Natl Cancer Inst* 2010;102:222–229.

264. **Greenlee RT, Kessel B, Williams CR, et al.** Prevalence, incidence, and natural history of simple ovarian cysts among women >55 years old in a large cancer screening trial. *Am J Obstet Gynecol* 2010;202:373e1–e9.

265. **Modesitt SC, Pavlik EJ, Ueland FR, et al.** Risk of malignancy in unilocular ovarian cystic tumors less than 10 centimeters in diameter. *Obstet Gynecol* 2003;102:594–599.

266. **ACOG Committee Opinion No. 280.** The role of the generalist obstetrician-gynecologist in the early detection of ovarian cancer. *Obstet Gynecol* 2002;100:1413–1416.

267. **Lynch PJ, Moyal-Barracco M, Bogliatto F, et al.** 2006 ISSVD classification of vulvar dermatoses: pathologic subsets and their clinical correlates. *J Reprod Med* 2007;52:3–9.

268. **Maclean AB, Jones RW, Scurry J, et al.** Vulvar cancer and the need for awareness of precursor lesions. *J Low Genit Tract Dis* 2009;13:115–117.

269. **Ayhan A, Guven ES, Guven S, et al.** Testosterone versus clobetasol for maintenance of vulvar lichen sclerosus associated with variable degrees of squamous cell hyperplasia. *Acta Obstet Gynecol Scand* 2007;86:715–719.

270. **Sinha P, Sorinola O, Luesley DM.** Lichen sclerosus of the vulva. Long-term steroid maintenance therapy. *J Reprod Med* 1999;44:621–624.

271. **Bradford J, Fischer G.** Long-term management of vulval lichen sclerosus in adult women. *Aust N Z J Obstet Gynaecol* 2010;50:148–152.

272. **Yesudian PD.** The role of calcineurin inhibitors in the management of lichen sclerosus. *Am J Clin Dermatol* 2009;10:313–318.

273. **Sideri M, Jones RW, Wilkinson EJ, et al.** Squamous vulvar intraepithelial neoplasia: 2004 modified terminology, ISSVD Vulvar Oncology Subcommittee. *J Reprod Med* 2005;50:807–810.

274. **Ballagh SA.** Vaginal hormone therapy for urogenital and menopausal symptoms. *Semin Reprod Med* 2005;23:126–140.

275. **Palacios S.** Managing urogenital atrophy. *Maturitas* 2009;63:315–318.

15 Uterine Fibroids

William H. Parker

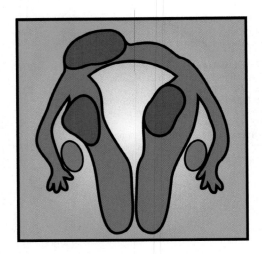

- Fibroids are very common and most are asymptomatic and can be managed expectantly.

- There is no definite relationship between oral contraceptives and the presence of fibroids.

- First-degree relatives of women with fibroids have a 2.5 times increased risk of developing fibroids.

- The risk of having fibroids is 2.9 times greater in African American women than in white women.

- Women with fibroids are only slightly more likely to experience pelvic pain than women without fibroids.

- Rapid uterine growth is not well defined, and almost never indicates sarcoma in premenopausal women; sarcomas are rare and more likely occur in postmenopausal women with symptoms of pain and bleeding.

- Sonography is the most readily available and least costly imaging technique to differentiate fibroids from other pelvic pathology; however, MRI permits more precise evaluation of the number, size and position of fibroids and can better evaluate the proximity to the endometrial cavity.

- The presence of submucosal fibroids decreases fertility and removing them can increase fertility; subserosal fibroids do not affect fertility and removing them does not increase fertility; and intramural fibroids may slightly decrease fertility, but removal does not increase fertility.

- Most fibroids do not increase in size during pregnancy.

- For women who are mildly or moderately symptomatic with fibroids, watchful waiting may allow treatment to be deferred, perhaps indefinitely.

- As women approach menopause watchful waiting may be considered because there is limited time to develop new symptoms, and after menopause bleeding stops and fibroids decrease in size.

- Surgical treatment options include abdominal myomectomy, laparoscopic myomectomy, hysteroscopic myomectomy, endometrial ablation, and abdominal, vaginal, or laparoscopic hysterectomy.

- An inability to evaluate the ovaries on pelvic examination is not an indication for surgery.

- Myomectomy should be considered as a safe alternative to hysterectomy, even for those women who have large uterine fibroids and wish to retain their uterus.

- Submuccous fibroids, sometimes associated with increased menstrual bleeding or infertility, often can be removed hysteroscopically.

- Routine ultrasound follow-up is sensitive, but may detect many clinically insignificant fibroids.

- Uterine artery embolization (UAE) is an effective treatment for selected women with uterine fibroids. The effects of UAE on early ovarian failure, fertility, and pregnancy are unclear.

Fibroids (leiomyomas, myomas) are an important health care concern because they are the most frequent indication for the performance of hysterectomy, accounting for nearly 240,000 such procedures in the United States (1). In comparison, approximately 30,000 myomectomies were performed that year. Inpatient surgery for fibroids costs $2.1 billion per year in the United States, and the cost of outpatient surgeries, medical and nonmedical costs, and time away from work or family add significantly to these expenditures (2).

Origins of Uterine Fibroids

Fibroids are benign, monoclonal tumors of the smooth muscle cells of the myometrium and contain large aggregations of extracellular matrix composed of collagen, elastin, fibronectin, and proteoglycan (3).

Incidence

Fibroids are remarkably common. Fine serial sectioning of uteri from 100 consecutive women subjected to hysterectomy discovered fibroids in 77%, some as small as 2 mm (4). A random sampling of women ages 35 to 49, screened by self-report, medical record review, and sonography, found that among African American women by age 35 the incidence of fibroids was 60%, and it was over 80% by age 50 (Fig. 15.1). White women have an incidence of 40% at age 35 and almost 70% by age 50 (5).

Etiology

Although the precise causes of fibroids are unknown, advances have been made in understanding the molecular biology of these benign tumors and their hormonal, genetic, and growth factors (6).

Genetics

Fibroids are monoclonal and about 40% have chromosomal abnormalities that include translocations between chromosomes 12 and 14, deletions of chromosome 7, and trisomy of chromosome 12 (7,8). Cellular, atypical, and large fibroids are most likely to show chromosomal abnormalities. The remaining 60% may have as yet undetected mutations. More than 100 genes were found to be up- or down-regulated in fibroid cells (9). Many of these genes appear to regulate cell growth, differentiation, proliferation, and mitogenesis (9). Collagen types I and III are abundant, but collagen fibrils are in disarray, much like the collagen found in keloid formation (10).

Genetic differences between fibroids and leiomyosarcomas indicate that leiomyosarcomas do not result from the malignant degeneration of fibroids. Cluster analysis of 146 genes found that the majority is down-regulated in leiomyosarcomas but not in fibroids or myometrium. Comparative genomic hybridization did not find specific anomalies shared by fibroids and leiomyosarcomas (11).

Hormones

Both estrogen and progesterone appear to promote the development of fibroids. Fibroids are rarely observed before puberty, are most prevalent during the reproductive years, and regress after menopause. Factors that increase overall lifetime exposure to estrogen, such as obesity and early menarche, increase the incidence. Decreased exposure to estrogen found with smoking, exercise, and increased parity is protective (12).

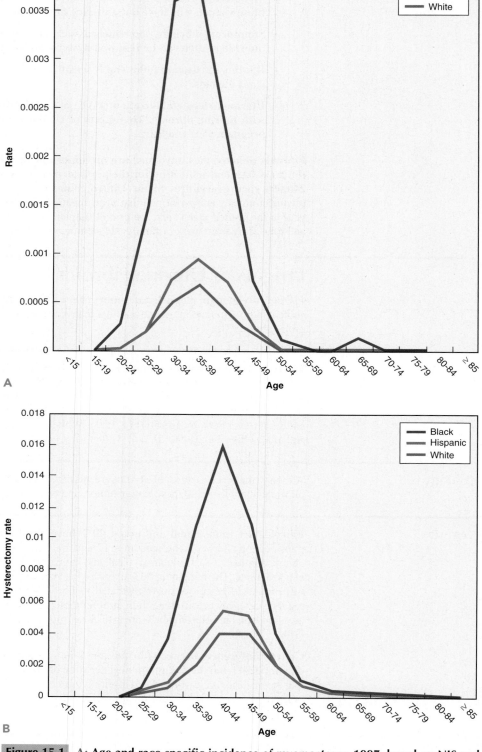

Figure 15.1 A: Age-and race-specific incidence of myomectomy, 1997, based on NIS and U.S. Census Bureau estimates. B: Age- and race-specific incidence of hysterectomy for fibroids, 1997, based on NIS and U.S. Census Bureau estimates. (From **Health Services/ Technology Assessment Tests (HSTAT).** Available at http://www.ncbi.nlm.nih.gov/books/ bv.fcgi?rid=hstat1.section.48317.)

Serum levels of estrogen and progesterone are similar in women with and without clinically detectable fibroids. However, as a result of increased levels of aromatase within fibroids, *de novo* production of estradiol is higher than in normal myometrium (12). Progesterone is important in the pathogenesis of fibroids, which have increased concentrations of progesterone receptors A and B compared with normal myometrium (13,14). The highest mitotic counts are found in fibroids at the peak of progesterone production (15). Gonadotropin-releasing hormone (GnRH) agonists decrease the size of fibroids, but progestin given concurrently with GnRH prevents a decrease in size (14).

Human fibroid tissue, grafted to immunodeficient mice, increased in size in response to estradiol plus progesterone, but the growth was blocked by the antiprogestin *RU486* (16). The volume of grafted fibroid tissue decreased after progesterone withdrawal. Treatment with estradiol alone did not increase the graft size, but did induce expression of progesterone receptors and supported the action of progesterone on the grafts (16).

Growth Factors

Growth factors, proteins, or polypeptides, produced locally by smooth muscle cells and fibroblasts, appear to stimulate fibroid growth primarily by increasing extracellular matrix (6). Many of these growth factors are overexpressed in fibroids and either increase smooth muscle proliferation (transforming growth factor-β [TGF-β, basic fibroblast growth factor [bFGF]), increase DNA synthesis (epidermal growth factor [EGF], platelet-derived growth factor [PDGF]), stimulate synthesis of extracellular matrix (TGF-β), promote mitogenesis (TGF-β, EGF, insulin-like growth factor [IGF], prolactin [PRL]), or promote angiogenesis (bFGF, vascular endothelial growth factor [VEGF]).

Risk Factors

Prospective, longitudinal studies characterize the factors that influence the development of uterine fibroids (4,17,18). Although selection bias may limit epidemiologic studies, the risk factors discussed below are considered.

Age

The incidence of fibroids increases with age, 4.3 per 1,000 woman-years for 25 to 29 year olds and 22.5 for 40 to 44 year olds. African American women develop fibroids at an earlier age than white women (17).

Endogenous Hormonal Factors

Greater exposure to endogenous hormones, as found with early menarche (younger than 10 years of age) increases and late menarche decreases the likelihood of having uterine fibroids (18). Fibroids are smaller, less numerous, and have smaller cells in hysterectomy specimens from postmenopausal women, when endogenous estrogen levels are low (4,19).

Family History

First-degree relatives of women with fibroids have a 2.5 times increased risk of developing fibroids (20). Monozygous twins are reportedly hospitalized for treatment of fibroids more often than heterozygous twins, but these findings may be the result of reporting bias (21).

Ethnicity

African American women have a 2.9 times greater risk of having fibroids than white women, unrelated to other known risk factors (22). African American women have fibroids develop at a younger age and have more numerous, larger, and more symptomatic fibroids (23). It is unclear whether these differences are genetic or result from known differences in circulating estrogen levels, estrogen metabolism, diet, or environmental factors.

Weight

A prospective study found that the risk of fibroids increased 21% with each 10 kg increase in body weight, and with increasing body mass index (BMI) (24). Similar findings were reported in women with greater than 30% body fat (25). Obesity increases conversion of adrenal androgens to estrone and decreases sex hormone binding globulin. The result is an increase in biologically available estrogen, which may explain an increase in fibroid prevalence and/or growth.

Diet

Few studies examined the association between diet and the presence or growth of fibroids (26). A diet rich in beef, other red meat, and ham increased the incidence of fibroids, while a diet rich in green vegetables decreased this risk. These findings are difficult to interpret because calorie and fat intake were not measured.

Exercise

Women in the highest category of physical activity (approximately 7 hours per week) were significantly less likely to have fibroids than women in the lowest category (less than 2 hours per week) (27).

Oral Contraceptives

There is no definite relationship between oral contraceptives and the presence of fibroids. An increased risk of fibroids with oral contraceptive use was reported, but a subsequent study found no increased risk with use or duration of use (28,29). Studies in women with known fibroids who were prescribed oral contraceptives showed no increase in fibroid growth (24,30). The formation of new fibroids does not appear to be influenced by oral contraceptive use (31).

Menopausal Hormone Therapy

For the majority of postmenopausal women with fibroids, hormone therapy will not stimulate fibroid growth. If fibroids do grow, progesterone is likely to be the cause (32). One study evaluated postmenopausal women with fibroids who were given 2 mg of oral *estradiol* daily and randomized to 2.5 or 5 mg of *medroxyprogesterone acetate* (*MPA*) per day (32). One year after starting treatment, 77% of women taking 2.5 mg *MPA* had either no change or a decrease in fibroids diameters and 23% had a slight increase. However, 50% of women taking 5 mg *MPA* had an increase in fibroid size (mean diameter increase of 3.2 cm).

Postmenopausal women with fibroids treated with 0.625 of *conjugated equine estrogen* (*CEE*) and 5 mg *MPA* were compared over 3 years to a similar group of women not taking hormone therapy (33). By the end of the third year, only 3 of 34 (8%) treated and 1 of 34 (3%) untreated women had any increase in fibroid volume over baseline (32). Postmenopausal women with known fibroids, followed with sonography, were noted to have an average 0.5 cm increase in the diameter of fibroid after using transdermal *estrogen* patches plus oral *progesterone* for 12 months (33). Women taking oral *estrogen* and *progesterone* had no increase in fibroid size (34).

Pregnancy

Increasing parity decreases the incidence and number of clinically apparent fibroids (35–37). The remodeling process of the postpartum myometrium, a result of apoptosis and dedifferentiation, may be responsible for the involution of fibroids (38). Another theory postulates that the vessels supplying fibroids regress during involution of the uterus, depriving fibroids of their source of nutrition (39).

Smoking

Smoking reduces the incidence of fibroids. Reduced conversion of androgens to estrone, caused by inhibition of aromatase by nicotine, increased 2-hydroxylation of estradiol, and stimulation of higher levels of sex hormone–binding globulin (SHBG) decrease bioavailability of estrogen (40–42).

Tissue Injury

Cellular injury or inflammation resulting from an environmental agent, infection, or hypoxia was proposed as a mechanism for initiation of fibroid formation (43). Repetitive tissue injury to the endometrium and endothelium might promote the development of monoclonal smooth muscle proliferations in the muscular wall. Frequent mucosal injury with stromal repair (menstruation) may release growth factors that promote the high frequency of uterine fibroids (43).

No increased incidence was found in women with prior sexually transmitted infections, prior intrauterine device (IUD) use or prior talc exposure (35). Herpes simplex virus (HSV) I or II, cytomegalovirus (CMV), Epstein-Barr virus (EBV), and chlamydia were not found in fibroids.

Symptoms

Fibroids are almost never associated with mortality, but they may cause morbidity and significantly affect quality of life (44). **Women who have hysterectomies because of fibroid-related symptoms have significantly worse scores on SF-36 quality-of-life questionnaires than women diagnosed with hypertension, heart disease, chronic lung disease, or arthritis** (44).

Of 116 women with fibroids larger than 5 cm on sonographic examination and uterine size greater than 12 cm on pelvic examination, 42% were satisfied with their initial level of symptoms, including stress, bleeding, and pain (45). Most of the 48 women who chose to have treatment within 1 year were more likely to have higher scores on bleeding and pain scales and be more concerned about their symptoms. Most women chose myomectomy (n = 20), hysterectomy (n = 15), or hysteroscopic myomectomy (n = 4), and symptoms scores improved markedly during the 7.5 months (mean) of follow-up.

Abnormal Bleeding

The association of fibroids with menorrhagia is not clearly established. Therefore, other possible etiologies, including coagulopathies such as von Willebrand's disease, should be considered in a woman with heavy menstrual bleeding (46).

A random sample of women aged 35 to 49 was evaluated by self-reported bleeding patterns and by abdominal and transvaginal sonography to determine the presence, size, and location of fibroids (47). Of the 878 women screened, 564 (64%) had fibroids and 314 (36%) did not. Forty-six percent of women with fibroids reported, "gushing blood" during menstrual periods, compared with 28% without fibroids. Gushing blood and length of periods were related to the size of fibroids but not to the presence of submucous fibroids or multiple fibroids.

Another study found that women with fibroids used 7.5 pads or tampons on the heaviest day of bleeding compared with 6.1 pads or tampons used by women without fibroids (48). Women with fibroids larger than 5 cm had slightly more gushing and used about three more pads or tampons on the heaviest day of bleeding than women with smaller fibroids.

Pain

Women with fibroids are only slightly more likely to experience pelvic pain than women without fibroids. Transvaginal sonography was performed on a population-based cohort of 635 non-care-seeking women with an intact uterus to determine the presence of uterine fibroids (49). Dyspareunia, dysmenorrhea, or noncyclic pelvic pain was measured by visual analog scales. The 96 women found to have fibroids were only slightly more likely to report moderate or severe dyspareunia or noncyclic pelvic pain and had no higher incidence of moderate or severe dysmenorrhea than women without fibroids. Neither the number nor the total volume of fibroids was related to pain. However, women who present for clinical evaluation for fibroid-associated pain may be different from those in the general population (49).

Fibroid degeneration may cause pelvic pain. As fibroids enlarge, they may outgrow their blood supply, with resulting cell death (50). Types of degeneration determined both grossly and microscopically include hyaline degeneration, calcification, cystic degeneration, and hemorrhagic degeneration. The type of degeneration appears to be unrelated to the clinical symptoms (50). Pain from fibroid degeneration is often successfully treated with analgesics and observation. Torsion of a pedunculated subserosal fibroid may produce acute pelvic pain that requires surgical intervention (51).

Urinary Symptoms

Fibroids may cause urinary symptoms, although few studies examined this association. Following uterine artery embolization with a 35% reduction in mean uterine volume, frequency and urgency were greatly or moderately improved in 68% of women, slightly improved in 18%, and unchanged or worse in only 14% (52). This finding suggests that **increased uterine volume associated with fibroids is related to urinary symptoms.**

Fourteen women with large fibroids and urinary symptoms were given six monthly injections of GnRH agonist (GnRH-a) with a resulting 55% decrease in uterine volume (53). Following therapy, urinary frequency, nocturia, and urgency decreased. There were no changes in urge or stress incontinence as measured by symptoms or urodynamic studies. It is not clear whether these findings are related to a decrease in uterine volume or to other effects of GnRH treatment.

Natural History of Fibroids

Most fibroids grow slowly. A prospective, longitudinal study of 72 premenopausal women (38 black, 34 white) using computer analysis of serial MRI found that the median growth rate was 9% over 12 months (17). However, multiple fibroids in the same individual were found to have highly variable growth rates, suggesting that growth results from factors other than hormone levels. After age 35, growth rates declined with age for white women but not for black women, which likely explains the increased fibroid-related symptoms noted in black women. Seven percent of fibroids regressed over the study period. Continued follow-up of these women is planned and should provide a better understanding of this important issue.

Rapid Fibroid Growth

In premenopausal women, "rapid uterine growth" almost never indicates presence of uterine sarcoma. One study found only 1 sarcoma among 371 (0.26%) women operated on for rapid growth of presumed fibroids (54). No sarcomas were found in the 198 women who had a 6-week increase in uterine size over 1 year, which is the definition of rapid growth that was used in the past.

Uterine Sarcoma

Women found to have uterine sarcoma are often clinically suspected of having a pelvic malignancy (54,55). Women with pain and bleeding and who are closer to menopause or postmenopausal may have a rare sarcoma. Of nine women found to have uterine sarcomas, all were postmenopausal and eight were admitted with abdominal pain and vaginal bleeding (55). All eight had presumed gynecologic malignancies: uterine sarcoma in four, endometrial carcinoma in three, and ovarian cancer in one. One additional woman had surgery for prolapse and a sarcoma was found incidentally (55). Between 1989 and 1999, the Surveillance, Epidemiology, and End Results (SEER) database reported 2,098 women with uterine sarcomas with an average age of 63 years, whereas a literature review found a mean age of 36 years in women subjected to myomectomy (54,56).

Diagnosis

Pelvic Examination

Clinically significant subserosal and intramural fibroids can usually be diagnosed by pelvic examination based on findings of an enlarged, irregularly shaped, firm and nontender uterus (57). Uterine size assessed by bimanual examination, even for most women with BMI greater than 30, correlates well with uterine size and weight at pathological examination (58). Routine sonographic examination is not necessary when the diagnosis is almost certain. However, a definite diagnosis of submucous fibroids often requires saline-infusion sonography, hysteroscopy, or magnetic resonance imaging (MRI) (59).

Fibroid Location

The FIGO fibroid classification system categorizes submucous, intramural, subserosal, and transmural fibroids.

Type 0 - **intracavitary (e.g., a pedunculated submucosal fibroid entirely within the cavity)**
Type 1 - **less than 50% of the fibroid diameter within the myometrium**
Type 2 - **50% or more of the fibroid diameter within the myometrium**
Type 3 - **abut the endometrium without any intracavitary component**
Type 4 - **intramural and entirely within the myometrium, without extension to either the endometrial surface or to the serosa**
Type 5 - **subserosal at least 50% intramural**
Type 6 - **subserosal less than 50% intramural**
Type 7 - **subserosal attached to the serosa by a stalk**
Type 8 - **no involvement of the myometrium; includes cervical lesions, those in the round or broad ligaments without direct attachment to the uterus, and "parasitic" fibroids**

Transmural fibroids are categorized by their relationship to both the endometrial and the serosal surfaces, with the endometrial relationship noted first, e.g., type 2–3 (Table 15.1; Fig 15.2) (60).

Imaging

For symptomatic women, consideration of medical therapy, noninvasive procedures, or surgery often depends on an accurate assessment of the size, number, and position of fibroids. Transvaginal sonography (TVS), saline-infusion sonography (SIS), hysteroscopy, and MRI were all performed on 106 women scheduled for hysterectomy and the findings were compared to pathologic examination (59). Submucous fibroids were best identified with MRI (100% sensitivity, 91% specificity). Identification was about equal with transvaginal sonography (sensitivity 83%, specificity 90%), saline-infusion sonography (sensitivity 90%, specificity

Table 15.1 FIGO Leiomyoma Classification System		
SM – Submucosal	0	Pedunculated intracavitary
	1	<50% intramural
	2	≥50% intramural
O – Other	3	Contacts endometrium; 100% intramural
	4	Intramural
	5	Subserosal ≥50% intramural
	6	Subserosal <50% intramural
	7	Subserosal pedunculated
	8	Other (specify e.g. cervical, parasitic)
Hybrid leiomyomas (impact both endometrium and serosa)		Two numbers are listed separated by a hyphen. By convention, the first refers to the relationship with the endometrium while the second refers to the relationship to the serosa. One example is below
	2–5	Submucosal and subserosal, each with less than half the diameter in the endometrial and peritoneal cavities, respectively.

89%), and hysteroscopy (sensitivity 82%, specificity 87%). MRI is not technique dependent and has low interobserver variability for diagnosis of submucous fibroids, intramural fibroids, and adenomyosis when compared with TVS, SIS, and hysteroscopy (61,62).

The presence of adenomyosis is associated with junctional zone thickness of more than 15 mm (or 12 mm in a nonuniform junctional zone). Focal, not well-demarcated, and high or low intensity areas in the myometrium correlate with adenomyosis (63).

MRI allows evaluation of the number, size, and position of submucous, intramural, and subserosal fibroids and can evaluate their proximity to the bladder, rectum, and endometrial cavity. MRI helps define what can be expected at surgery and might help the surgeon avoid missing fibroids during surgery (64). For women who wish to preserve fertility, MRI to document location and position relative to the endomyometrium may be helpful prior to hysteroscopic, laparoscopic, or abdominal myomectomy.

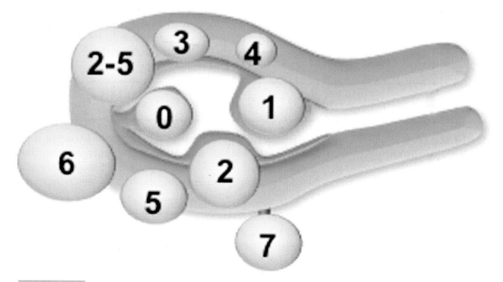

Figure 15.2   FIGO Leiomyoma Classification System.

Sonography is the most readily available and least costly imaging technique to differentiate fibroids from other pelvic pathology and is reasonably reliable for evaluation of uterine volume less than 375 cc and containing four or fewer fibroids (61). Sonographic appearance of fibroids can be variable, but often they appear as symmetrical, well-defined, hypoechoic and heterogenous masses. Areas of calcification or hemorrhage may appear hyperechoic, while cystic degeneration may appear anechoic. SIS utilizes saline inserted into the uterine cavity to provide contrast and better defines submucous fibroids (61).

Imaging of Uterine Sarcomas

The preoperative diagnosis of leiomyosarcoma may be possible. Diagnosis with total serum lactate dehydrogenase (LDH) and LDH isoenzyme 3 measurements along with gadolinium-enhanced diethylenetriamine penta-acetic acid (Gd-DTPA) dynamic MRI was reported to be highly accurate (65). MRI images are taken during the arterial phase, between 40 and 60 seconds after infusion of gadolinium. Sarcomas have increased vascularity and show increased enhancement with gadolinium, while degenerating fibroids have decreased perfusion and exhibit decreased enhancement. Using LDH measurements and Gd-DTPA, a study of 87 women with uterine fibroids, 10 women with leiomyosarcomas, and 130 women with degenerating fibroids reported 100% specificity, 100% positive predictive value, 100% negative predictive value, and 100% diagnostic accuracy for leiomyosarcoma (Fig. 15.3).

Fertility

The presence of submucous fibroids decreases fertility rates and removing them increases fertility rates. Subserosal fibroids do not affect fertility rates but removing them does increase fertility. Intramural fibroids may slightly decrease fertility, but removal does not increase fertility (66). A meta-analysis of the effect of fibroids on fertility and the effect of myomectomy on fertility found that submucous fibroids that distort the uterine cavity appear to decrease fertility, with ongoing pregnancy/live birth rates decreased by about 70% (relative risk [RR] 0.32; 95% confidence interval [CI], 0.12–0.85) (66). Resection of submucous fibroids slightly increased fertility relative to infertile controls without fibroids (ongoing pregnancy/live birth rate, RR 1.13; 95% CI, 0.96–1.33).

Analysis of studies that routinely used hysteroscopy to confirm clear nondistortion of the cavity by intramural fibroids found ongoing pregnancy/live birth rates were not significantly different compared to controls (RR 0.73; 95% CI, 0.38–1.40) (66). Importantly, removal of intramural or subserosal fibroids did not improve ongoing pregnancy/live birth rates (RR 1.67; 95% CI, 0.75–3.72).

Myomectomy may involve operative and anesthetic risks, risks of infection or postoperative adhesions, a slight risk of uterine rupture during pregnancy, an increased likelihood that a cesarean section will be recommended for delivery, and the expense of surgery and time for recovery. Therefore, until intramural fibroids are shown to decrease and myomectomy to increase fertility rates, surgery should be undertaken with reluctance (66). Randomized studies are needed to clarify the relative risks and benefits of surgical intervention.

Fibroids and Pregnancy

Incidence of Fibroids during Pregnancy

The prevalence of fibroids among pregnant women is 18% in African American women, 8% in white women, and 10% in Hispanic women, based on first trimester sonography (67). Mean size of the fibroids was 2.5 cm. Clinical examination detects 42% of fibroids greater than 5 cm during pregnancy, but only 12.5% when they are less than 5 cm (68).

Effect of Pregnancy on Fibroids

Most fibroids do not increase in size during pregnancy. Pregnancy has a variable, and unpredictable, effect on fibroid growth, likely dependent on individual differences in fibroid gene expression, circulating growth factors, and fibroid-localized receptors (68,69). A prospective study of 36 pregnant women with a single fibroid discovered during routine first trimester sonographic screening and examined by sonography at 2- to 4-week intervals found that 69% of the

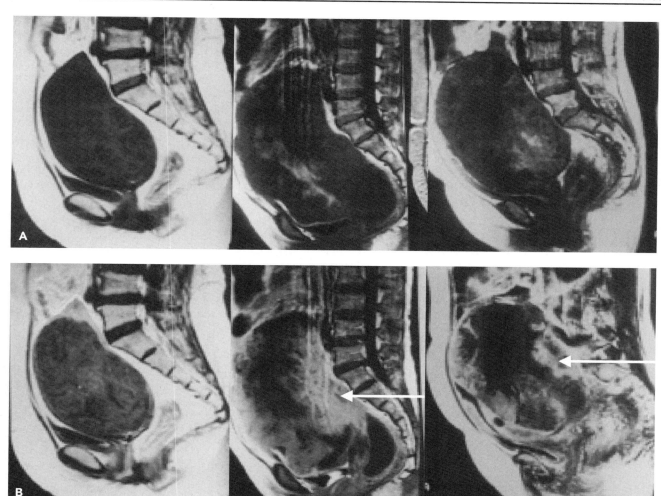

Figure 15.3   **MR images.** **A: Degenerating fibroid.** Left to right. Preenhanced T1 image, T2 image, and no enhancement on T1 Gd-DPTA at 60 seconds. **B: Leiomyosarcoma.** Left to right, preenhanced T1 image, T2 image (arrow to dorsal part of tumor), and enhancement of dorsal part of tumor (*arrow*) on T1 Gd-DPTA at 60 seconds. (From **Goto A, Takeuchi S, Sugimura K, et al.** Usefulness of Gd-DTPA contrast-enhanced dynamic MRI and serum determination of LDH and its isozymes in the differential diagnosis of leiomyosarcoma from degenerated leiomyoma of the uterus. *Int J Gynecol Cancer* 2002;12:354–361.)

women had no increase in fibroid volume throughout pregnancy (69). In the 31% of women noted to have an increase in volume, the greatest increase occurred before the 10th week of gestation. There was no relationship between initial fibroid volume and fibroid growth during gestational periods. A reduction in fibroid size toward baseline measurements was observed 4 weeks after delivery.

Fibroid Degeneration during Pregnancy

In women noted to have fibroids during pregnancy, clinical symptoms and sonographic evidence of fibroid degeneration occurs in about 5% (70). Among 113 women followed during pregnancy with serial sonography, 10 (9%) developed anechoic spaces or coarse heterogenous patterns consistent with fibroid degeneration. Seven of 10 women had severe abdominal pain requiring hospitalization, consistent with clinical symptoms of degeneration. No sonographic changes were noted in the other 103 women, and only 11.7% had similar abdominal pain. A small study of women with fibroid-associated pain during pregnancy found use of *ibuprofen* shortened the hospital stay and decreased the rate of readmission (71).

Influence of Fibroids on Pregnancy

Very rarely does the presence of a fibroid during pregnancy lead to an unfavorable outcome. Research was conducted on large populations of pregnant women examined with routine second trimester sonography with follow-up care and delivery at the same institution (72,73). In a study of 12,600 pregnant women, the outcomes of 167 women with fibroids were no different with regard to the incidence of preterm delivery, premature rupture of membranes, fetal growth restriction, placenta previa, placental abruption, postpartum hemorrhage, or retained placenta (72). Cesarean section was more common among women with fibroids (23% vs. 12%).

The other study of 15,104 pregnancies, including 401 women with fibroids, found no increased risk of premature rupture of membranes, operative vaginal delivery, chorioamnionitis, or endometritis (73). However, there were increased risks of preterm delivery (19.2% vs. 12.7%), placenta previa (3.5% vs. 1.8%), and postpartum hemorrhage (8.3% vs. 2.9%). Cesarean section was again more common (49.1% vs. 21.4%).

Fetal injury attributed to mechanical compression by fibroids is uncommon. A search of the PubMed database from 1980 to 2010 revealed one case of fetal head anomalies with fetal growth restriction, one case of a postural deformity, one case of a limb reduction, and one case of fetal head deformation with torticollis (74–75).

Any decision to perform a myomectomy in order to prevent problems during pregnancy should take into account the risks of surgery, anesthesia, postoperative adhesions, and an increased likelihood of subsequent cesarean delivery, along with concerns about discomfort, expense, and time away from work or family.

Rupture of Myomectomy Scar during Pregnancy

Following abdominal myomectomy, uterine rupture during pregnancy appears to be a rare event. Two studies comprising 236,454 deliveries reported 209 instances of uterine rupture, with only 4 cases attributable to prior myomectomy (78,79). Because the number of women who had a previous myomectomy was not known, the incidence of rupture in these studies could not be determined. However, a retrospective study of 412 women who had abdominal myomectomies reported only one woman with uterine rupture (0.2%) (80).

Operative techniques, instruments, and energy sources used during laparoscopic myomectomy may differ from those employed during laparotomy. A study of 19 published and unpublished cases of uterine rupture during pregnancy following laparoscopic myomectomy found that almost all cases involved deviations from standard surgical technique as described for abdominal myomectomy (81). In seven cases, the uterine defect was not repaired; in three cases it was repaired with a single suture; in four cases it was repaired with only one layer of suture; and in one case only the serosa was closed. In only three cases was a multilayered closure employed. In 16 of the cases, monopolar or bipolar energy was used for hemostasis.

Although definite conclusions and recommendations regarding appropriate technique for laparoscopic myomectomy must await proper study of myometrial wound healing, it appears prudent for surgeons to adhere to time-tested techniques developed for abdominal myomectomy, including multilayered closure of myometrium (for other than superficial uterine defects) and limited use of electro-surgery for hemostasis. Yet, even with ideal surgical technique, individual wound healing characteristics may predispose to uterine rupture.

Treatment

The development of new treatments for fibroids is slow, perhaps because many women with fibroids are asymptomatic, fibroids are benign, and mortality is very low (82). **If offered hysterectomy as a first, and sometimes only, treatment option, some women choose to accommodate to symptoms and stop seeking treatment.** This may lead physicians to underestimate the true impact of the condition, despite the fact that women who have hysterectomies as a result of fibroid-related symptoms have significantly worse scores on SF-36 quality-of-life questionnaires than women diagnosed with hypertension, heart disease, chronic lung disease, or arthritis (44).

After an exhaustive review of the medical literature published between 1975 and 2000, with evaluation of 637 relevant articles and careful study of 200 articles, the authors found no satisfactory answers to fundamental question about fibroid treatments (83). Women and their physicians need information on which to base decisions regarding possible treatments.

This section summarizes the literature regarding the management of fibroids. Treatment options include observation, medical therapy, hysteroscopic myomectomy, laparoscopic myomectomy, hysterectomy, uterine artery embolization, and focused ultrasound.

Watchful Waiting

Not having treatment for fibroids rarely results in harm, except for women with severe anemia from fibroid-related menorrhagia or hydronephrosis from ureteric obstruction from an massively enlarged fibroid uterus. Predicting future fibroid growth or onset of new symptoms is not possible (84). During observation, the average fibroid volume increases 9% per year with a range of −25% to +138% (84). A nonrandomized study of women with uterine size 8 weeks or greater who chose watchful waiting found that 77% of women had no significant changes in the self-reported amount of bleeding, pain, or degree of bothersome symptoms at the end of 1 year (85). Furthermore, mental health, general health, and activity indexes were also unchanged. Of the 106 women who initially chose watchful waiting, 23% opted for hysterectomy during the course of the year.

Therefore, for women who are mildly or moderately symptomatic with fibroids, watchful waiting may allow treatment to be deferred, perhaps indefinitely. As women approach menopause, watchful waiting may be considered, because there is limited time to develop new symptoms and after menopause, bleeding stops and fibroids decrease in size (19). Although not specifically studied, the incidence of hysterectomy for fibroids declines considerably after menopause, suggesting that there is a significant decline in symptoms.

Medical Therapy

Nonsteroidal Anti-inflammatory Medication

Nonsteroidal anti-inflammatory drugs (NSAIDs) were not shown to be effective for the treatment of menorrhagia in women with fibroids. A placebo-controlled, double-blind study of 25 women with menorrhagia, 11 of whom also had fibroids, found a 36% decrease in blood loss among women with idiopathic menorrhagia, but no decrease in women with fibroids. No other studies examined this treatment (86).

Gonadotropin-Releasing Hormone Agonists

Treatment with GnRH-a decreases uterine volume, fibroid volume, and bleeding. However, the benefits of GnRH-a are limited by side effects and risks associated with long-term use (87,88). Monthly GnRH-a given for 6 months reduced fibroid volume by 30% and total uterine volume by 35% (87). Reduction in uterine size occurs mostly within the first 3 months of treatment (88). Menorrhagia responds well to GnRH-a; 37 of 38 women had resolution by 6 months. Following discontinuation of GnRH-a, menses returns in 4 to 8 weeks and uterine size returns to pretreatment levels within 4 to 6 months (89). In this study 64% of women remained asymptomatic 8 to 12 months after treatment.

Side effects occur in 95% of women treated with GnRH-a (89). Seventy-eight percent experience hot flushes, 32% vaginal dryness, and 55% have transient frontal headaches. However, during 6 months of treatment only 8% of women discontinued GnRH-a because of the side effects. Arthralgia, myalgia, insomnia, edema, emotional lability, depression, and decreased libido are reported. **The hypoestrogenic state induced by GnRH-a causes significant bone loss after 6 months of therapy** (90).

In an effort to reduce side effects, inhibit bone loss, and allow longer-term use of GnRH-a, low doses of *estrogen* and *progestins* may be added while continuing GnRH-a. However, a study of long-term use of GnRH-a over 6 years found a wide range of reduction in bone density among women and no difference in bone loss between groups given *estrogen* and *progestin* versus those treated with GnRH-a alone (91).

Gonadotropin-Releasing Hormone Agonist as Temporary Treatment for Perimenopausal Women

Women in late perimenopause who are symptomatic from uterine fibroids may consider short-term use of GnRH-a. Thirty-four perimenopausal women with symptomatic fibroids were treated with GnRH-a for 6 months, 12 of whom required repeat treatment 6 months after discontinuation of the medication (92). Thirty-one women avoided surgery; 15 of the women went into natural menopause. Although not specifically studied, add-back therapy might be considered in this setting.

Gonadotropin-Releasing Hormone Antagonist

The immediate suppression of endogenous GnRH by daily subcutaneous injection of the GnRH antagonist *ganirelix* results in a 29% reduction in fibroid volume within 3 weeks (93). Treatment is accompanied by hypoestrogenic symptoms. When long-acting compounds are available, a GnRH antagonist might be considered for medical treatment prior to surgery.

Progesterone-Mediated Medical Treatment

The reduction in uterine size following treatment with the progesterone-blocking drug *mifepristone* is similar to that found with GnRH-a (94). A prospective, randomized, controlled trial of *mifepristone* treatment found a 48% decrease in mean uterine volume after 6 months (95). *Mifepristone* blocks progesterone, and the unopposed exposure of the endometrium to estrogen may lead to endometrial hyperplasia. A systematic review found endometrial hyperplasia in 10 of 36 (28%) women screened with endometrial biopsies (96).

Progesterone-Releasing Intrauterine Device

The *levonorgestrel*-releasing intrauterine system (LNG-IUS) may be reasonable treatment for selected women with fibroid-associated menorrhagia. In women with fibroids, uterine size no larger than 12 weeks, and a normal uterine cavity, LNG-IUS substantially reduces menstrual bleeding (97). Twenty-two of 26 (85%) women with documented fibroid-related menorrhagia returned to normal bleeding within 3 months. By 12 months, 27 of 67 (40%) women had amenorrhea and 66 women had hemoglobin levels above 12 g/dL.

One study examined 32 women with at least one fibroid less than 5 cm in diameter and less than 50% of the tumor volume projecting into the endometrial cavity (type II) who had insertion of an LNG-IUS (98). After 12 months, mean estimated blood loss, measured by pictorial blood loss assessment, decreased from 392 to 37 mL with an associated increase in hemoglobin levels. There was no change in uterine volume over the course of the study. Some studies show that LNG-IUS expulsion rates are higher in women with fibroids than in women without fibroids (99).

Alternative Medicine Treatment

A nonrandomized, nonblinded study compared fibroid growth in 37 women treated with Chinese medicine, body therapy, and guided imagery to 37 controls treated with nonsteroidal anti-inflammatory medications, progestins, or oral contraceptive pills (100). After 6 months, sonographic evaluation demonstrated that fibroids stopped growing or shrank in 22 of 37 (59%) women treated with Chinese medicine compared to 3 of 37 (8%) controls. Although symptoms responded equally well in both groups, satisfaction was higher in the Chinese medicine group. Participants actively sought alternative therapy, however, and assessment of satisfaction may reflect selection bias.

An uncontrolled study reported treatment of 110 women with fibroids smaller than 10 cm with the Chinese herbal medicine kuei-chih-fu-ling-wan for at least 12 weeks (101). Clinical and sonographic evaluation found complete resolution of fibroids in 19% of women, a decrease in size in 43%, no change in 34%, and an increase in 4%. Menorrhagia improved in 60 of 63 (95%) of women and dysmenorrhea improved in 48 of 51 (94%). Fifteen of the 110 (14%) women chose to have a hysterectomy during the 4 years of the study.

Surgical Treatment Options

Surgical treatment options currently include abdominal myomectomy, laparoscopic myomectomy, hysteroscopic myomectomy, endometrial ablation, and abdominal, vaginal, or laparoscopic hysterectomy.

Serious medical conditions, such as severe anemia or ureteral obstruction, often need to be addressed surgically. Pain from fibroid degeneration is usually successfully treated with analgesics until symptoms resolve, but if severe the patient may opt for surgery. Torsion of a pedunculated subserosal fibroid may produce acute pain that requires surgical intervention. Surgical intervention may be indicated in women with fibroids associated with menorrhagia, pelvic pain or pressure, urinary frequency, or incontinence that compromises quality of life (102).

Abdominal myomectomy was long employed as a conservative treatment for uterine fibroids, and much of the literature predates the use of prospective, randomized controlled trials. Although myomectomy is stated to relieve symptoms in 80% of women, there is scant literature documenting its efficacy and many large series have not reported data for relief of symptoms following surgery (102–104). A prospective, nonrandomized study comparing myomectomy with uterine artery embolization did report that 75% of women in the myomectomy group had a significant decrease in symptom scores after 6 months (105).

Back pain may, on occasion, be related to the presence of fibroids, but other possible causes should be considered. **Inability to evaluate the ovaries on pelvic examination is not an indication for surgery** (106). There is no evidence that pelvic examination increases early detection or decreases the mortality related to ovarian cancer, and sonography can be used to evaluate the adnexa should symptoms develop.

Treating Preoperative Anemia

Recombinant Erythropoietin

Severe anemia can be rapidly corrected using recombinant forms of *erythropoietin* and iron supplementation. *Erythropoietin alfa* and *epoetin* are commonly used to increase preoperative hemoglobin concentrations in cardiac, orthopaedic, and neurologic surgery. A randomized study showed that use of *epoetin* 250 IU/kg (approximately 15,000 U) per week for 3 weeks prior to elective orthopaedic or cardiac surgery increased the hemoglobin concentrations by 1.6 g/dL and significantly reduced transfusion rates when compared to controls (107). No side effects were experienced. A prospective, nonrandomized study of *epoetin* given preoperatively found a significant increase in hemoglobin concentrations prior to, and following, gynecologic surgery (108). For best results, iron stores should be increased with supplemental iron. Vitamin C, 1,000 IU per day, increases iron absorption in the intestines.

Gonadotropin-Releasing Hormone Agonist

GnRH-a may be used preoperatively to mitigate abnormal bleeding, with a resultant increase of hemoglobin concentration. Women with fibroids and initial mean hemoglobin concentrations of 10.2 g were randomized preoperatively to GnRH-a plus oral *iron* or placebo plus oral *iron* (109). After 12 weeks, 74% of the women treated with GnRH-a and *iron* had hemoglobins greater than 12 g compared with 46% of the women treated with *iron* alone.

A Cochrane review found that women with fibroids treated preoperatively with 3 to 4 months of GnRH-a had improved preoperative hemoglobins (110). Although operative blood loss was less for abdominal myomectomy patients treated with GnRH, there was no significant difference in transfusion rates compared with untreated women.

Abdominal Myomectomy

Myomectomy should be considered a safe alternative to hysterectomy. Victor Bonney, an early advocate of abdominal myomectomy, stated in 1931 that "The restoration and maintenance of physiologic function is, or should be, the ultimate goal of surgical treatment." Case-controlled studies suggest that there may be less risk of intraoperative injury with myomectomy when compared with hysterectomy (111). A retrospective review of 197 women who had myomectomies and 197 women who underwent hysterectomies with similar uterine size (14 versus 15 weeks) found operating times were longer in the myomectomy group (200 versus 175 minutes), but estimated blood loss was greater in the hysterectomy group (227 versus 484 mL) (111). The risks of hemorrhage, febrile morbidity, unintended surgical procedure, life-threatening events, and rehospitalization were no different between groups. However, 26 (13%) women in the hysterectomy group suffered complications, including 1 bladder injury, 1 ureteral injury, 3 bowel injuries, 8 women with ileus, and 6 women with pelvic abscesses. In contrast, complications occurred in 11 (5%) of the myomectomy patients, including 1 bladder injury, 2 women with reoperation for small bowel obstruction, and 6 women with ileus.

Myomectomy may be considered even for those women who have large uterine fibroids and wish to retain their uterus. A study of 91 women with uterine size larger than 16 cm (range 16–36 cm) reported one bowel injury, one bladder injury, and one reoperation for bowel obstruction, but no women had conversion to hysterectomy (112). The cell saver, which is a devise used to collect blood intraoperatively and reinfuse, was used in 70 women, and only 7 required homologous blood transfusion. A retrospective cohort study compared 89 women having abdominal hysterectomy for fibroids (mean uterine size 15 cm) to abdominal myomectomy in 103 women (mean uterine size 12 cm) (113). Although selection bias was likely, the hysterectomy group suffered two ureteral, one bladder, one bowel, and one nerve injury and two reoperations for bowel obstruction, while there were no visceral injuries in the myomectomy group.

Cesarean Section and Concurrent Myomectomy

In carefully selected women, myomectomy may be safely accomplished at the time of cesarean section by experienced surgeons. One series reported 25 women with removal of 84 fibroids (2 to 10 cm) at the time of cesarean section without the need for cesarean hysterectomy (114). Estimated blood loss was 876 mL (range 400 to 1,700 mL) and five women required blood transfusion. Another study compared 111 women who had myomectomy at the time of cesarean section with 257 women with fibroids who were not subjected to myomectomy during cesarean section (115). Only one of the women in the myomectomy group required transfusion and none required hysterectomy or embolization. There were no differences in mean operative times, incidence of fever, or length of hospital stay between the two groups. Although the cases were likely selected carefully, the authors concluded that, in experienced hands, myomectomy might be safely performed in selected women during cesarean section.

Surgical Technique for Abdominal Myomectomy

Managing Blood Loss

Available surgical techniques allow safe removal of even large fibroids. Use of tourniquets or vasoconstrictive agents may be used to limit blood loss. *Vasopressin,* an antidiuretic hormone, causes constriction of smooth muscle in the walls of capillaries, small arterioles and venules. Synthetic *vasopressin* (*Pitressin,* Parke-Davis, NJ) decreases blood loss during myomectomy and in a prospective, randomized study was as effective as mechanical occlusion of the uterine and ovarian vessels (116,117). Rare cases of bradycardia and cardiovascular collapse were reported; intravascular injection should be carefully avoided and patients should be carefully monitored (118). The use of *vasopressin* to decrease blood loss during myomectomy is an off-label use of this drug.

Cell savers may be considered for use during myomectomy. Use of the cell saver avoids the risks of infection and transfusion reaction, the oxygen transport capacity of salvaged red blood cells is equal to or better than stored allogeneic red cells, and the survival of red blood cells appears to be at least as good as transfused allogeneic red cells (119). The device suctions blood from the operative field, mixes it with heparinized saline, and stores the blood in a canister. If the patient requires blood reinfusion, the stored blood is washed with saline, filtered, centrifuged to a hematocrit of approximately 50%, and given back to the patient intravenously. Consequently, the need for preoperative autologous blood donation or heterologous blood transfusion often can be avoided (120). In a study of 92 women who had myomectomy for uterine size greater than 16 cm the cell saver was used for 70 women with a mean volume of reinfused packed red blood cells of 355 mL (121).

The cost of using a cell saver compared with donation of autologous blood was not studied for abdominal myomectomy. However, economic models suggest it is cost effective (121). Most hospitals charge a minimal fee for having the cell saver available "on-call" and charge an additional fee if it is used. Assuming that most women who donate autologous blood prior to myomectomy do not require blood transfusion, availability of the cell saver should spare many women the time and expense of donating, storing, and processing autologous blood. For a cohort of women, the cost of using the cell saver should, therefore, be significantly lower than the cost of autologous blood.

When heavy bleeding is anticipated or if copious bleeding is encountered, ligation of both uterine arteries can be performed (122). Uterine artery embolization was used successfully to control bleeding at the time of, or following, myomectomy (123). Because the uterine arteries recanulate, future fertility should not be compromised. These techniques often obviate the need for hysterectomy.

Uterine incisions can be made either vertically or transversely, because fibroids distort normal vascular architecture, making attempts to avoid the arcuate vessels impossible (124). However,

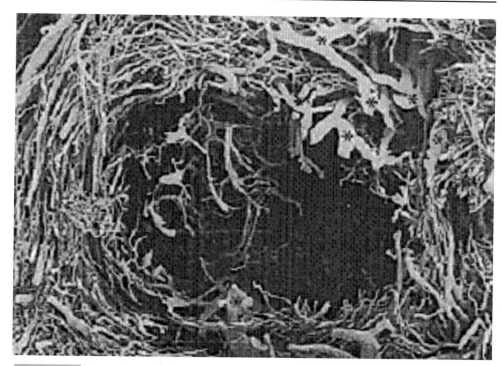

Figure 15.4   Corrosion casting of fibroid vessels.

careful planning and placement of uterine incisions can avoid inadvertent extension of the incision to the uterine cornua or ascending uterine vessels.

Based on vascular corrosion casting and examination by electron microscopy, fibroids are completely surrounded by a dense blood supply and no distinct vascular pedicle exists at the base of the fibroid (125) (Fig. 15.4). Extending the uterine incisions through the myometrium and entire pseudocapsule until the fibroid is clearly distinguished identifies a less vascular surgical plane, which is deeper than commonly recognized.

Limiting the number of uterine incisions has been suggested in order to reduce the risk of adhesions to the uterine serosa (126). However, in this manner tunnels must be created within the myometrium in order to extract distant fibroids, making hemostasis more difficult within these defects. Hemostasis is important in order to avoid adhesion formation, and fibrin, leucocytes, and platelets in the presence of erythrocytes leads to adhesion formation. If tunneling incisions are avoided and hemostasis secured immediately, the risk of adhesion formation should be lessened. Therefore, if incisions are made directly over the fibroids and only those fibroids that are easily accessed are removed, the defects can be promptly closed and hemostasis can be secured immediately (112). Multiple uterine incisions may be needed, but adhesion barriers may help limit adhesion formation (127).

Laparoscopic Myomectomy

Currently available instruments make laparoscopic myomectomy feasible, although the size and number of fibroids reasonably removed limits the wide application of this approach because of the technical difficulty of both the procedure and laparoscopic suturing (128). Although microprocessor-assisted myomectomy (robotic) may obviate some of these technical problems, the added cost and longer operating times associated with this approach must be considered (see Chapter 25).

A systematic review of randomized controlled trials of laparoscopic versus open myomectomy included six studies with a total of 576 patients (129). Laparoscopic myomectomy was associated with longer operating times but reduced operative blood loss, less postoperative decline in hemoglobin levels, reduced postoperative pain, more patients fully recuperated at day 15, and fewer overall complications. Major complications, pregnancy rates, and new appearance of fibroids were comparable in the two groups.

Case series without controls show the feasibility of laparoscopic surgery in women with large fibroids. In a series of 144 women with mean fibroid diameter of 7.8 cm (range, 5 to 18 cm), only 2 women required conversion to laparotomy (130). In another series of 332 consecutive women undergoing laparoscopic myomectomy for symptomatic fibroids as large as 15 cm, only 3 women required conversion to laparotomy (131).

Surgical Technique for Laparoscopic Myomectomy

Port placement should be based on the position and size of the fibroids to be removed (Fig. 15.5). Laparoscopic suturing may be more ergonomic if there are two ports on either the patient's right side for right-handed surgeons or left side for left-handed surgeons; a 12-mm port about 2 cm medial to the iliac crest for suture access, and another 5-mm lateral port near the level of the umbilicus (132). A left upper quadrant approach may be used for initial access when uterine size is near or above the umbilicus (133).

Pitressin is injected into the fibroid. An incision is made directly over the fibroid and carried deeply until definite fibroid tissue and the avascular surgical plane is noted. Transverse incisions permit more ergonomic suturing. The fibroid is grasped with a tenaculum for traction and the plane between the myometrium and fibroid is dissected until the fibroid is free. Bleeding vessels in the myometrial defect are desiccated sparingly with bipolar electrosurgical paddles, taking care not to devascularize the myometrium and interfere with wound healing. Delayed absorbable sutures are placed in one, two, or three layers, as needed, adhering to accepted surgical technique at laparotomy. Morcellation of the fibroid with an electromechanical device is accomplished under direct vision. The pelvis and abdomen are irrigated, the fluid suctioned, and an adhesion barrier may be placed.

Myolysis and Cryomyolysis

A number of energy sources including bipolar electrosurgery, Nd:YAG laser and cryogenic probes were used under laparoscopic direction to reduce fibroid size by means of fibroid destruction and interference with local vascular supply (134). Although uterine and fibroid volumes decreased by approximately 50%, there were dense adhesions to the uterine serosa in 6 of 15 (53%) women undergoing subsequent laparoscopic evaluations for other reasons (135). Myolysis is not recommended for women who wish future fertility.

Adhesions Following Myomectomy

Adhesion formation after myomectomy is well documented (136). A Cochrane review found that *Interceed* reduced the incidence of adhesion formation, both *de novo* and reformation, at laparoscopy and laparotomy (137). Data were insufficient, however, to support its use to improve pregnancy rates. There was limited evidence of effectiveness of *Seprafilm* (Genzyme, Cambridge, MA) in preventing adhesion formation in a prospective study that randomized 127 women undergoing abdominal myomectomy to treatment or no treatment with *Seprafilm* (127). During second-look laparoscopy, women treated with *Seprafilm* had significantly fewer adhesions and lower adhesion severity scores than untreated women. This study and others find an increased incidence of adhesions with posterior uterine incisions compared to anterior incisions (138).

Hysteroscopic Myomectomy

Submucous fibroids, sometimes associated with increased menstrual bleeding or infertility, often can be removed hysteroscopically. Classification of submucous fibroids is based on the degree of the fibroid within the cavity; class 0 fibroids are intracavitary; class I have 50% or more of the fibroid within the cavity; and class II have less than 50% of the fibroid within the cavity (60) (Fig. 15.6). A meta-analysis of the effect of fibroids on fertility found that submucous fibroids with distortion of the uterine cavity decreased ongoing pregnancy/live birth rates by 70% (RR 0.32; 95% CI, 0.12–0.850) and resection increased ongoing pregnancy/live birth rates (RR 1.13; 95% CI, 0.96–1.33) (66).

No meta-analysis of the association of submucous fibroids and abnormal uterine bleeding was performed. However, most studies show a reduction in bleeding following resection. Using pictorial assessment to estimate menstrual blood loss prior to and for 41 months following hysteroscopic resection of submucous fibroids, a significant decrease in bleeding was reported in 42 of 51 (82%) women with submucous pedunculated (type 0), 24 of 28 (86%) with sessile (type I), and 15 of 22 (68%) with intramural fibroids (type II) (140). A study of 285 consecutive women with menorrhagia or metrorrhagia who had hysteroscopic resection of submucous fibroid(s) found that additional surgery was required for 9.5% at 2 years, 10.8% at 5 years, and 26.7% at 8 years (141).

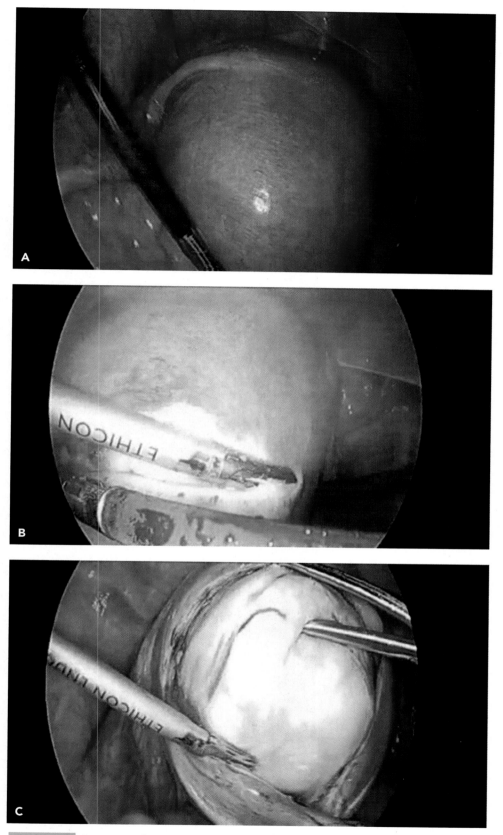

Figure 15.5 **Laparoscopic myomectomy. A.** 7 cm. posterior intramural fibroid. **B.** Transverse incision through myometrium until fibroid reached. **C.** Traction on fibroid and counter-traction on myometrium to tease fibroid away from myometrium.

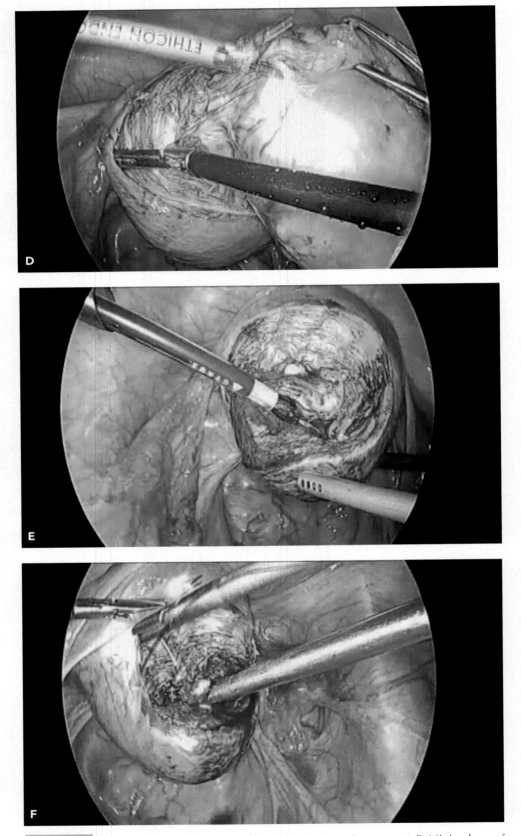

Figure 15.5 *(Continued)* **D.** Adherent attachments to myometrium are cut. **E.** Minimal use of bipolar electrosurgery to control larger vessels. **F.** Three layer suture close of myometrium.

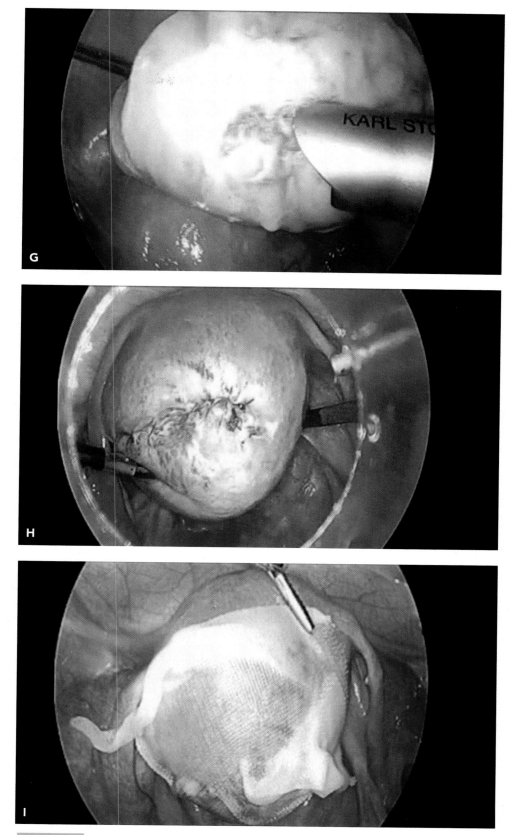

Figure 15.5 *(Continued)* **G.** Morcellator used to remove fibroid from abdominal cavity. **H.** Pelvis irrigated and suctioned. **I.** Adhesion barrier placed over uterine incision.

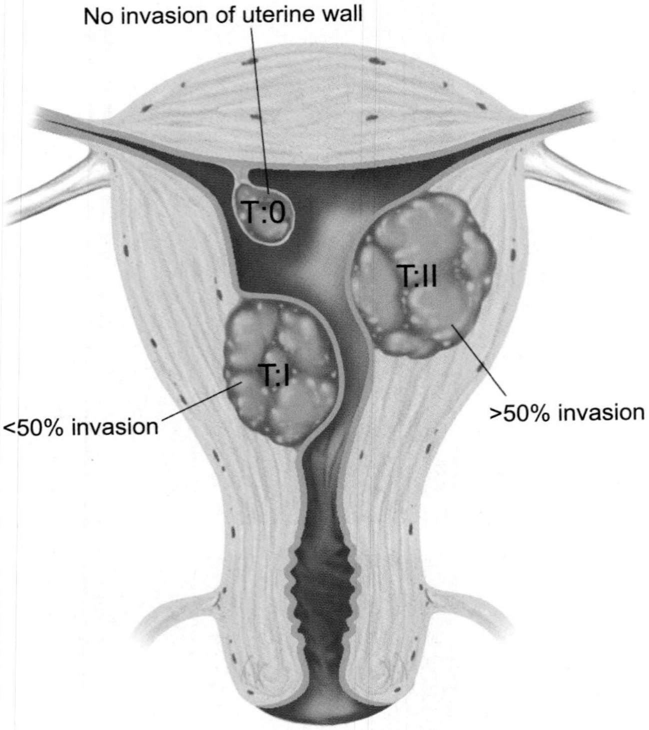

Figure 15.6 **Fibroid classification.** (From **Munro MG, Critchley HO, Broder MS, et al.** FIGO Working Group on Menstrual Disorders. FIGO classification system (PALM-COEIN) for causes of abnormal uterine bleeding in nongravid women of reproductive age. *Int J Gynaecol Obstet* 2011;113:3–13)

Surgical Technique for Hysteroscopic Myomectomy

Hysteroscopic resection of a submucous fibroid can be accomplished under visual control using a telescope and continuous flow of distension fluid through the uterine cavity. The electrosurgical working element uses monopolar or bipolar electrodes. Monopolar electrodes require nonconducting distending solution (sorbitol 5%, sorbitol 3% with mannitol 0.5%, or glycine 1.5%), while bipolar electrodes can be used with saline.

Cervical dilation is usually required prior to insertion of the hysteroscope. *Cytotec* may facilitate easier dilation (142). The cutting loop is passed beyond the fibroid and cutting activated only when the loop is moving toward the surgeon and in direct view. Fibroids should be resected down to the level of the surrounding myometrium and, if fertility is desired, care should be taken to avoid excessive thermal damage to normal myometrium. Often, the remaining portion of the fibroid will be expressed into the uterine cavity by uterine contractions, allowing further resection. Fragments of fibroid are removed from the cavity with a grasping forceps or by capturing the fragments with the loop and extracting the telescope. G0 and G1 fibroids up to about 5 cm may be resected hysteroscopically.

G2 fibroids require careful preoperative evaluation with saline-infusion sonography or MRI to gauge the thickness of normal myometrium between the fibroid and the serosa in order to assess the potential risk of uterine perforation with the loop electrode. The risk of perforation increases with deeper myometrial involvement of the fibroid (143). In some cases, repeat resection may be required after a few weeks, as the remaining portion of the fibroid is expressed into the uterine cavity by uterine contractions.

Procedure-Specific Risks

Cervical dilatation or insertion of the hysteroscope can cause uterine perforation, as can deep myometrial resection. Often the first sign of perforation is a rapid increase in the fluid deficit. Careful inspection of the uterine cavity should be undertaken to look for brisk bleeding or bowel injury. If no injury is apparent, the procedure should be terminated and the patient should be observed and may be discharged if stable (144). If a perforation occurs during activation of the electrode, then laparoscopy should be performed to carefully inspect for bowel or bladder injury.

Fluid Absorption and Electrolyte Imbalance

Intravascular absorption of distending media is a potentially dangerous complication that can result in pulmonary edema, hyponatremia, heart failure, cerebral edema, and even death (145). Careful monitoring of the fluid deficit is important and a fluid deficit of 750 mL during surgery should serve as a warning sign, with planned termination of the procedure. **Many authors suggest termination of the procedure when the fluid deficit exceeds 1,000 mL, although other guidelines suggest termination after introduction of 1,500 mL of a nonelectrolyte solution or 2,000 mL of an electrolyte solution** (145). Electrolytes should be assessed and corrected if necessary and diuretics considered. Risk factors for fluid overload include resection of fibroids with deep intramural extension or prolonged operating time. The use of normal saline combined with bipolar energy reduces the risk of hyponatremia, but a fluid deficit over 1,500 mL can lead to cardiac overload (146).

Endometrial Ablation for Abnormal Bleeding Associated with Fibroids

In selected women not desiring future childbearing, endometrial ablation with or without hysteroscopic myomectomy may be efficacious. Pad counts following ablation with or without fibroid resection found that 48 of 51 (94%) women had resolution of abnormal bleeding after a mean follow-up of 2 years (range, 1 to 5 years) (147). A study of 62 women followed for an average of 29 months (range, 12 to 60 months) found that 74% of the women had hypomenorrhea or amenorrhea, and only 12% required a hysterectomy (148).

Hydrothermal ablation was used to treat 22 women with known submucous fibroids up to 4 cm, with 91% reporting amenorrhea, hypomenorrhea, or eumenorrhea after a minimum of 12 months' follow-up (149). In a study of 65 women with menometrorrhagia and type I or II submucous myomas up to 3 cm, after treatment with *NovaSure* endometrial ablation device (Hologic, Bedford, MA), normal bleeding or amenorrhea was observed in most women at 1 year (150).

New Appearance of Fibroids

Although new fibroids may sometimes develop following myomectomy, most women will not require additional treatment. If the first surgery is performed in the presence of a single fibroid, only 11% of women will need subsequent surgery (151). If multiple fibroids are removed during the initial surgery, only 26% will need subsequent surgery (mean follow-up 7.6 years). Individual fibroids, once removed, do not grow back. Fibroids detected after myomectomy, often referred to as "recurrence," result either from failure to remove fibroids at the time of surgery or they are newly developed fibroids. Perhaps this circumstance is best designated "new appearance" of fibroids (152).

Sonography found that 29% of women had persistent fibroids 6 months after myomectomy (153). Additionally, the background formation of new fibroids in the general population should be considered. As previously noted, a hysterectomy study found fibroids in 77% of specimens from women who did not have a preoperative diagnosis of fibroids (4).

Incomplete follow-up, insufficient length of follow-up, the use of either transabdominal or transvaginal sonography (with different sensitivity), detection of very small clinically insignificant fibroids, or use of calculations other than life-table analysis confound many studies of new fibroid appearance (154).

Clinical Follow-Up

Self-reported diagnosis based on symptom questionnaires has reasonably good correlation with sonographic or pathologic confirmation of significant fibroids and may be the most appropriate method of gauging clinical evidence of new appearance (22). One study of 622 patients ages 22 to 44 at the time of surgery and followed over 14 years found the cumulative new appearance rate based on clinical examination and confirmed by ultrasound was 27% (155) (Fig. 15.7). An excellent review of life-table analysis studies found a cumulative risk of clinically significant new appearance of 10% 5 years after abdominal myomectomy (156).

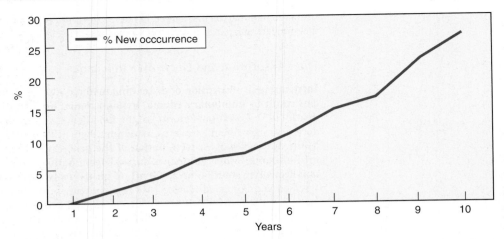

Figure 15.7 **Overall 10-year new appearance after initial myomectomy.** (From **Candiani G, Fedele L, Parazzini F, et al.** Risk of recurrence after myomectomy. *Br J Obsete Gynecol* 1991;98:385–389.)

Sonographic Follow-Up	**Routine ultrasound follow-up is sensitive but detects many clinically insignificant fibroids.** One hundred forty-five women, mean age 38 (range, 21 to 52), were followed after abdominal myomectomy with clinical evaluation every 12 months and transvaginal sonography at 24 and 60 months (sooner, with clinical suspicion of new fibroids) (153). However, no lower size limit was used for the sonographic diagnosis of fibroids and, thus, the cumulative probability of new appearance was 51% at 5 years. A study of 40 women who had a normal sonogram 2 weeks following abdominal myomectomy found that the cumulative risk of sonographically detected new fibroids larger than 2 cm was 15% over 3 years (157).
Need for Subsequent Surgery	Meaningful information for a woman considering treatment for her fibroids is the approximate risk of developing symptoms that would require yet additional treatment. A study of 125 women followed by symptoms and clinical examination after a first abdominal myomectomy found that a second surgery was required during the follow-up period (average 7.6 years) for 11% of women who had one fibroid removed initially and for 26% of women who had multiple fibroids removed (151). Crude rates of hysterectomy after myomectomy vary from 4% to 16% over 5 years (158,159).

Prognostic Factors Related to New Appearance of Fibroids

Age	Given that the incidence of fibroids increases with increasing age, 4 per 1,000 woman-years for 25- to 29-year-olds and 22 per 1,000 for 40- to 44-year-olds, new fibroids would be expected to form as age increases, even following myomectomy (17).
Subsequent Childbearing	The 10-year clinical new appearance rate for women who subsequently gave birth was 16%, but for those women who did not the rate was 28% (155).
Number of Fibroids Initially Removed	After at least 5 years of follow-up, 27% of women who initially had a single fibroid removed had clinically detected new fibroids and 59% of women with multiple fibroids initially removed had new fibroids (151).
Gonadotropin-Releasing Hormone Agonists	Preoperative treatment with GnRH-a decreases fibroid volume and may make smaller fibroids harder to identify during surgery. A randomized study found that 3 months following abdominal myomectomy, 5 (63%) of 8 women in the GnRH group had fibroids less than 1.5 cm detected sonographically, while only 2 of 16 (13%) untreated women had small fibroids detected (153).

Laparoscopic Myomectomy	**New appearance of fibroids is not more common following laparoscopic myomectomy when compared with abdominal myomectomy.** Eighty-one women randomized to either laparoscopic or abdominal myomectomy were followed with transvaginal sonography every 6 months for at least 40 months (160). Fibroids larger than 1 cm were detected in 27% of women following laparoscopic myomectomy compared to 23% in the abdominal myomectomy group, and no woman in either group required any further intervention.

Uterine Artery Embolization

Uterine artery embolization (UAE) is an effective treatment for selected women with uterine fibroids. The effects of UAE on early ovarian failure, fertility and pregnancy are unclear. Therefore, many interventional radiologists advise against the procedure for women considering future fertility. Appropriate candidates for UAE include women who have bothersome enough symptoms to warrant hysterectomy or myomectomy. Although extremely rare, complications of UAE may necessitate life-saving hysterectomy, and women who would not accept hysterectomy even for a life-threatening complication should not undergo UAE. Contraindications to treatment of fibroids with UAE include women with active genital infection, genital tract malignancy, diminished immune status, and severe vascular disease limiting access to the uterine arteries, contrast allergy, or impaired renal function (161).

UAE outcomes are well studied and documented. A validated fibroid-specific quality-of-life questionnaire was used to measure outcome data on UAE patients (162). **The American College of Obstetricians and Gynecologists recommends that women considering UAE have a thorough evaluation with a gynecologist to help facilitate collaboration with the interventional radiologist and that responsibility of caring for the patient be clear** (163).

Uterine Artery Embolization Technique	Percutaneous cannulation of the femoral artery is performed by a properly trained and experienced interventional radiologist (164) (Fig. 15.8). Embolization of the uterine artery and its branches is accomplished by injecting gelatin sponges, polyvinyl alcohol particles (PVA), or tris-acryl gelatin microspheres via the catheter until occlusion, or slow flow, is documented. Total radiation exposure (approximately 15 cGy) is comparable to one or two computed tomography scans or barium enemas (165).
	Tissue hypoxia secondary to UAE causes postprocedural pain that usually requires pain management in the hospital for 1 day. NSAID medications are usually taken for 1 to 2 weeks, and many women return to normal activity within 1 to 3 weeks. Approximately 5% to 10% of women have pain for longer than 2 weeks (165). Ten percent of women require readmission to the hospital for postembolization syndrome, characterized by diffuse abdominal pain, nausea, vomiting, low-grade fever, malaise, anorexia, and leucocytosis. Treatment with intravenous fluids, NSAID medications, and pain management usually leads to resolution of symptoms within 2 to 3 days (165). **Persistent fever should be managed with antibiotics. Failure to respond to antibiotics may indicate sepsis, which needs to be aggressively managed with hysterectomy.**

Uterine Artery Embolization Outcomes	The largest prospective study reported to date includes 555 women ages 18 to 59 (mean, 43), 80% of whom had heavy bleeding, 75% had pelvic pain, 73% had urinary frequency or urgency, and 40% of women had required time off work due to fibroid-related symptoms (166). Telephone interviews 3 months after UAE found that menorrhagia improved in 83% of women, dysmenorrhea improved in 77%, and urinary frequency in 86%. Mean fibroid volume reduction of the dominant fibroid was 33% at 3 months, but improvement in menorrhagia was not related to preprocedural uterine volume (even >1,000 cm^3) or to the degree of volume reduction obtained. Of note, two women (0.4%) had continued uterine growth and worsening pain and were found to have sarcomas. The hysterectomy rate due to complications was 1.5%. Within the follow-up period, 3% of women under 40, but 41% of women over 50, had amenorrhea.
	A prospective, randomized trial comparing hysterectomy and UAE in 177 women with symptomatic fibroids found that major complications were rare (167). Hospital stay was significantly shorter for UAE (2 versus 5 days), but UAE was associated with more readmissions (9 versus 0) for pain and/or fever in the 6-week postoperative period. Significant complications included

461

one woman who required resection of a submucous fibroid and one who had sepsis in the UAE group and one woman who had a vesico-vaginal fistula following hysterectomy.

Estimates suggest that more than 100,000 UAE procedures have been performed worldwide with 12 deaths Therefore, the estimated mortality rate of 1/10,000 compares well with the mortality rate of approximately 3/10,000 for a similar group of women under age 50 and without malignancy or compromised immunity undergoing hysterectomy (168).

Early Ovarian Failure

The risk of premature ovarian failure following UAE needs further study. Transient amenorrhea was reported in as many as 15% of women. Ovarian arterial perfusion as measured by Doppler sonography immediately following UAE shows that 35% of women had decreased ovarian perfusion and 54% had complete loss of perfusion (169). However, basal follicle-stimulating hormone (FSH) and antimüllerian hormone levels indicated decreased ovarian reserve in all women in one study (170).

Although normal FSH, estradiol, ovarian volume and antral follicle counts were documented in most women following UAE, these tests cannot predict earlier onset of menopause (171).

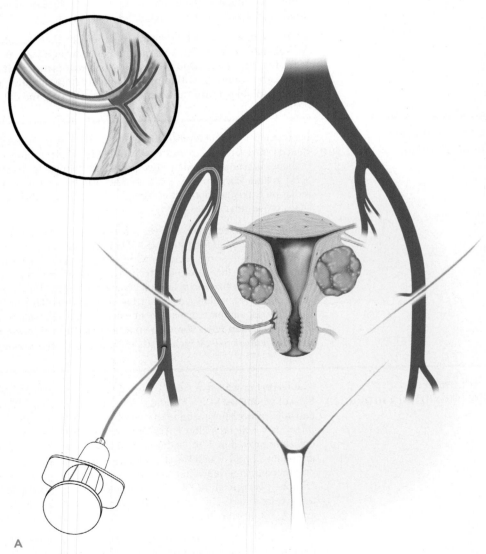

A

Figure 15.8 A–C: UAE techniques. A. A catheter is threaded to the uterine arteries and embolic material injected to block off blood flow to the uterus.

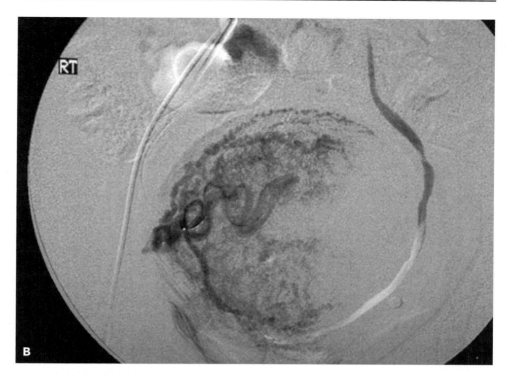

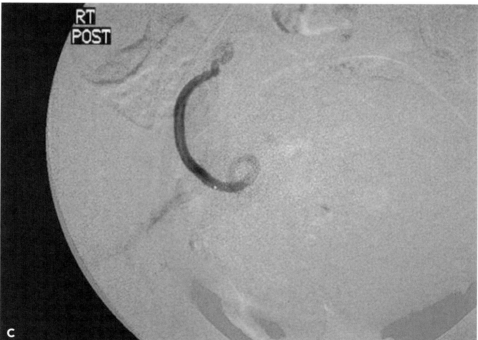

Figure 15.8   *(Continued)* B. Contrast dye shows the vessels supplying the fibroid prior to UAE. C. Following UAE, embolic material blocks blood flow to the fibroid.

Younger women, whose ovaries contain a large number of follicles, are likely to maintain a normal FSH despite destruction of a significant number of follicles, but it is not clear if future fertility will be impaired. Loss of follicles might cause menopause at an age earlier than would otherwise be expected. Long-term follow-up of women having UAE will be necessary to answer this important question.

Fertility and Pregnancy Following Uterine Artery Embolization

Because of the possibility of decreased ovarian function, and the potential for increased pregnancy complications, women who wish to conceive should not be treated with UAE (172). Although the risk appears to be low for women younger than 40 years old, premature ovarian failure would be devastating in this setting. Potential fertility following UAE is uncertain. A prospective trial of women with intramural fibroids larger than 4 cm, randomly selected for either UAE or myomectomy, reported there were more pregnancies and fewer abortions after surgery than after UAE (173). Obstetrical and perinatal results were similar.

Of 34 pregnancies subsequent to UAE, 32% of women had a spontaneous abortion (174). In a report of 164 women desiring future fertility prior to UAE, 21 women achieved pregnancy, 4 (24%) had a spontaneous abortion, 2 had elective terminations, and 18 had live births during 24 months of follow-up (175). For women achieving pregnancy, one study reported that 6% had postpartum hemorrhage, 16% had premature delivery, and 11% had malpresentation (174). Another study reported eight term and six preterm deliveries, but two women had placenta previa and one woman had a membranous placenta. It is not clear whether this high incidence of abnormalities is related to an effect of UAE on the endometrium or a placental problem inherently found in women with uterine fibroids. As a result, some authors recommend early pregnancy sonography to look for placenta accreta (175). Uterine wall defects, necrosis, and fistula have been reported following UAE, and the integrity of the uterine wall during pregnancy and childbirth remains unknown (176).

Uterine Artery Occlusion

Alternative methods of uterine artery occlusion were developed, both more and less invasive than UAE, including laparoscopic uterine artery occlusion and nonincisional transvaginal uterine artery occlusion. Fifty-eight patients were randomized to UAE or laparoscopic uterine artery occlusion (177). After a median follow-up time of 48 months clinical failures and symptom recurrence occurred in 14 women after laparoscopy (48%) and in five women after UAE (17%). Laparoscopic occlusion requires general anesthesia, is invasive, and requires a skilled laparoscopic surgeon. Transvaginal occlusion is performed by placing a specially designed clamp in the vaginal fornices and, guided by Doppler ultrasound auditory signals, is positioned to occlude the uterine arteries (178). The clamp is left in place for 6 hours and then removed. Results of this approach are not yet known.

Magnetic Resonance–Guided Focused Ultrasound

Ultrasound energy can be focused to create sufficient heat at a focal point so that protein is denatured and cell death occurs. Concurrent MRI allows precise targeting of tissue and monitoring of therapy by assessing the temperature of treated tissue (179). The advantages of this procedure are a very low morbidity and a very rapid recovery, with return to normal activity in one day. The procedure is not recommended for women wishing future fertility (179). Initial studies had treatment limited by the U.S. Food and Drug Administration to approximately 10% of fibroid volume, and while a 15% reduction in fibroid size was reported 6 months following treatment, only a 4% reduction was noted at 24 months (180). More recent studies with larger treatment areas reported better results; 6 months after treatment, the average volume reduction was 31% (+/−28%) (181).

An evaluation of clinical outcomes 6 months after treatment found that 71% of women had significant symptom reduction, but at 12 months about 50% still had significant symptom reduction (180). Twenty-three of 82 (28%) evaluable patients had undergone subsequent hysterectomy, myomectomy, or UAE. Women actively sought out magnetic resonance–guided focused ultrasound (MRgFUS), and no control group (sham MRgFUS) was included, so a placebo effect cannot be ruled out. One woman had a sciatic nerve injury caused by ultrasound energy and 5% had superficial skin burns. It remains to be seen whether increased treatment volumes will be associated with increased risks. As the technology continues to develop, further studies will be needed to evaluate the risks and efficacy of MRgFUS in the treatment of uterine fibroids.

Management Summary

A woman's individual circumstance, including fibroid-related symptoms and their effect on quality of life, desire (or not) to preserve fertility, and her wishes regarding treatment

options should be considered when discussing possible treatments. Multiple treatment options usually exist and the following points might be considered.

For an asymptomatic woman diagnosed with fibroids who desires fertility in the near future, evaluation of the uterine cavity with saline infusion sonography, hysteroscopy, or MRI provides useful information regarding the presence of submucous fibroids and their potential impact on fertility. If the cavity is not deformed, fibroids need not be treated and conception may be attempted. If the cavity is deformed, myomectomy (hysteroscopic or abdominal) can be considered. An experienced laparoscopic surgeon may offer laparoscopic myomectomy, with a multilayered myometrial closure.

For an asymptomatic woman who does not desire future fertility, observation (watchful waiting) should be considered. A periodic review of the patient's symptoms and a pelvic examination to evaluate uterine size should be accomplished. In the presence of very large fibroids, renal ultrasound or computed tomography urogram can be considered to rule out significant hydronephrosis.

For a symptomatic woman who desires future fertility and her primary symptom is abnormal bleeding, baseline hemoglobin measurement should be considered because accommodation to anemia can occur. If indicated, further evaluation of the endometrium with endometrial biopsy can be performed. Evaluation of the uterine cavity with saline-infusion sonography, hysteroscopy, or MRI can help determine the appropriate treatment options.

If the cavity is deformed, myomectomy (hysteroscopic or abdominal) should be considered. An experienced laparoscopic surgeon may offer laparoscopic myomectomy. If the symptoms of pain or pressure (bulk symptoms) are present, and if the uterine cavity is not deformed, myomectomy (abdominal or laparoscopic) can be considered.

For a symptomatic woman who does not desire future fertility, observation (watchful waiting) can be considered if no treatment is desired at that time. A symptomatic perimenopausal woman may desire observation until she enters menopause, when symptoms often diminish. Baseline hemoglobin measurements should be obtained and if a significant anemia exists, then treatment should be considered. If metrorrhagia is present, evaluation of the endometrium with sonography or endometrial biopsy should be considered. If the endometrium is normal, a *levonorgestrel*-IUS or endometrial ablation may be appropriate treatment. Myomectomy (hysteroscopic, abdominal, or laparoscopic), hysterectomy (vaginal, laparoscopic, or abdominal), or uterine artery embolization can be considered.

For a woman with primarily fibroid-related pain or pressure symptoms (bulk symptoms), myomectomy, hysterectomy, and uterine artery embolization or focused ultrasound (presently limited by size and number of fibroids) may be considered.

References

1. **Whiteman MK, Hillis SD, Jamieson DJ, et al.** Inpatient hysterectomy surveillance in the United States, 2000–2004. *Am J Obstet Gynecol* 2008;198:34.e1–34.e7.
2. **Myers E, Barber M, Couchman G, et al.** Management of uterine fibroids. AHRQ Evidence Reports Volume 1, Number 34. 2001. http://www.ncbi.nlm.nih.gov/books/NBK33649/#A48853
3. **Leppert PC, Catherino WH, Segars JH.** A new hypothesis about the origin of uterine fibroids based on gene expression profiling with microarrays. *Am J Obstet Gynecol* 2006;195:415–420.
4. **Cramer SF, Patel A.** The frequency of uterine leiomyomas. *Am J Clin Pathol* 1990;94:435–438.
5. **Day Baird D, Dunson DB, Hill MC, et al.** High cumulative incidence of uterine leiomyoma in black and white women: ultrasound evidence. *Am J Obstet Gynecol* 2003;188:100–107.
6. **Flake GP, Andersen J, Dixon D.** Etiology and pathogenesis of uterine leiomyomas: a review. *Environ Health Perspect* 2003;111:1037–1054.
7. **Hashimoto K, Azuma C, Kamiura S, et al.** Clonal determination of uterine leiomyomas by analyzing differential inactivation of the X-chromosome-linked phosphoglycerokinase gene. *Gynecol Obstet Invest* 1995;40:204–208.
8. **Ligon AH, Morton CC.** Genetics of uterine leiomyomata. *Genes Chromosomes Cancer* 2000;28:235–245.
9. **Lee EJ, Kong G, Lee SH, et al.** Profiling of differentially expressed genes in human uterine leiomyomas. *Int J Gynecol Cancer* 2005;15:146–154.
10. **Ferenczy A, Richart RM, Okagaki T.** A comparative ultrastructural study of leiomyosarcoma, cellular leiomyoma, and leiomyoma of the uterus. *Cancer* 1971;28:1004–1018.
11. **Quade BJ, Wang TY, Sornberger K, et al.** Molecular pathogenesis of uterine smooth muscle tumors from transcriptional profiling. *Genes Chromosomes Cancer* 2004;40:97–108.
12. **Cook JD, Walker CL.** Treatment strategies for uterine leiomyoma: the role of hormonal modulation. *Semin Reprod Med* 2004;22:105–111.
13. **Englund K, Blanck A, Gustavsson I, et al.** Sex steroid receptors in human myometrium and fibroids: changes during the menstrual cycle and gonadotropin-releasing hormone treatment. *J Clin Endocrinol Metab* 1998;83:4092–4096.
14. **Nisolle M, Gillerot S, Casanas-Roux F, et al.** Immunohistochemical study of the proliferation index, oestrogen receptors and progesterone receptors A and B in leiomyomata and normal myometrium during the menstrual cycle and under gonadotrophin-releasing hormone agonist therapy. *Hum Reprod* 1999;14:2844–50.

15. **Kawaguchi K, Fujii S, Konishi I, et al.** Mitotic activity in uterine leiomyomas during the menstrual cycle. *Am J Obstet Gynecol* 1989;160:637–641.

16. **Ishikawa H, Ishi K, Serna VA, et al.** Progesterone is essential for maintenance and growth of uterine leiomyoma. *Endocrinology.* 2010;151:2433–2442.

17. **Peddada SD, Laughlin SK, Miner K, et al.** Growth of uterine leiomyomata among premenopausal black and white women. *Proc Natl Acad Sci U S A* 2008;105:19887–19892.

18. **Marshall LM, Spiegelman D, Goldman MB, et al.** A prospective study of reproductive factors and oral contraceptive use in relation to the risk of uterine leiomyomata. *Fertil Steril* 1998;70:432–439.

19. **Cramer SF, Marchetti C, Freedman J, et al.** Relationship of myoma cell size and menopausal status in small uterine leiomyomas. *Arch Pathol Lab Med* 2000;124:1448–1453.

20. **Vikhlyaeva EM, Khodzhaeva ZS, Fantschenko ND.** Familial predisposition to uterine leiomyomas. *Int J Gynaecol Obstet* 1995;51:127–131.

21. **Treloar SA, Martin NG, Dennerstein L, et al.** Pathways to hysterectomy: insights from longitudinal twin research. *Am J Obstet Gynecol* 1992;167:82–88.

22. **Marshall LM, Spiegelman D, Barbieri RL, et al.** Variation in the incidence of uterine leiomyoma among premenopausal women by age and race. *Obstet Gynecol* 1997;90:967–973.

23. **Kjerulff KH, Langenberg P, Seidman JD, et al.** Uterine leiomyomas. Racial differences in severity, symptoms and age at diagnosis. *J Reprod Med* 1996;41:483–490.

24. **Ross RK, Pike MC, Vessey MP, et al.** Risk factors for uterine fibroids: reduced risk associated with oral contraceptives. *BMJ (Clin Res Ed)* 1986;293:359–362.

25. **Shikora SA, Niloff JM, Bistrian BR, et al.** Relationship between obesity and uterine leiomyomata. *Nutrition* 1991;7:251–255.

26. **Chiaffarino F, Parazzini F, La Vecchia C, et al.** Diet and uterine myomas. *Obstet Gynecol* 1999;94:395–398.

27. **Baird D, Dunson D, Hill M, et al.** Association of physical activity with development of uterine leiomyoma. *Am J Epidemiol* 2007;165:157–163.

28. **Parazzini F, Negri E, La Vecchia C, et al.** Oral contraceptive use and risk of uterine fibroids. *Obstet Gynecol* 1992;79:430–433.

29. **Samadi AR, Lee NC, Flanders WD, et al.** Risk factors for self-reported uterine fibroids: a case-control study. *Am J Public Health* 1996;86:858–862.

30. **Ratner H.** Risk factors for uterine fibroids: reduced risk associated with oral contraceptives. *BMJ* 1986;293:1027.

31. **Orsini G, Laricchia L, Fanelli M.** Low-dose combination oral contraceptives use in women with uterine leiomyomas. *Minerva Ginecol* 2002;54:253–261.

32. **Palomba S, Sena T, Morelli M, et al.** Effect of different doses of progestin on uterine leiomyomas in postmenopausal women. *Eur J Obstet Gynecol Reprod Biol* 2002;102:199–201.

33. **Yang CH, Lee JN, Hsu SC, et al.** Effect of hormone replacement therapy on uterine fibroids in postmenopausal women—a 3-year study. *Maturitas* 2002;43:35–39.

34. **Reed SD, Cushing-Haugen KL, Daling JR, et al.** Postmenopausal estrogen and progestogen therapy and the risk of uterine leiomyomas. *Menopause* 2004;11:214–222.

35. **Parazzini F, Negri E, La Vecchia C, et al.** Reproductive factors and risk of uterine fibroids. *Epidemiology* 1996;7:440–442.

36. **Lumbiganon P, Rugpao S, Phandhu-fung S, et al.** Protective effect of depot-medroxyprogesterone acetate on surgically treated uterine leiomyomas: a multicentre case-control study. *Br J Obstet Gynaecol* 1996;103:909–914.

37. **Baird DD, Dunson DB.** Why is parity protective for uterine fibroids? *Epidemiology* 2003;14:247–250.

38. **Cesen-Cummings K, Houston KD, Copland JA, et al.** Uterine leiomyomas express myometrial contractile-associated proteins involved in pregnancy-related hormone signaling. *J Soc Gynecol Investig* 2003;10:11–20.

39. **Burbank F.** Childbirth and myoma treatment by uterine artery occlusion: do they share a common biology? *J Am Assoc Gynecol Laparosc* 2004;11:138–152.

40. **Barbieri RL, McShane PM, Ryan KJ.** Constituents of cigarette smoke inhibit human granulosa cell aromatase. *Fertil Steril* 1986;46:232–236.

41. **Michnovicz JJ, Hershcopf RJ, Naganuma H, et al.** Increased 2-hydroxylation of estradiol as a possible mechanism for the anti-estrogenic effect of cigarette smoking. *N Engl J Med* 1986;315:1305–1309.

42. **Daniel M, Martin AD, Drinkwater DT.** Cigarette smoking, steroid hormones, and bone mineral density in young women. *Calcif Tissue Int* 1992;50:300–305.

43. **Cramer SF, Mann L, Calianese E, et al.** Association of seedling myomas with myometrial hyperplasia. *Hum Pathol* 2009;40:218–225.

44. **Rowe MK, Kanouse DE, Mittman BS, et al.** Quality of life among women undergoing hysterectomies. *Obstet Gynecol* 1999;93:915–921.

45. **Davis BJ, Haneke KE, Miner K, et al.** The fibroid growth study: determinants of therapeutic intervention. *J Womens Health (Larchmt)* 2009;18:725–732.

46. **Munro MG, Lukes AS.** Abnormal uterine bleeding and underlying hemostatic disorders: report of a consensus process. *Fertil Steril* 2005;84:1335–1337.

47. **Marino JL, Eskenazi B, Warner M, et al.** Uterine leiomyoma and menstrual cycle characteristics in a population-based cohort study. *Hum Reprod* 2004;19:2350–2355.

48. **Wegienka G, Baird DD, Hertz-Picciotto I, et al.** Self-reported heavy bleeding associated with uterine leiomyomata. *Obstet Gynecol* 2003;101:431–437.

49. **Lippman SA, Warner M, Samuels S, et al.** Uterine fibroids and gynecologic pain symptoms in a population-based study. *Fertil Steril* 2003;80:1488–1494.

50. **Murase E, Siegelman ES, Outwater EK, et al.** Uterine leiomyomas: histopathologic features, MR imaging findings, differential diagnosis, and treatment. *Radiographics* 1999;19:1179–1197.

51. **Gaym A, Tilahun S.** Torsion of pedunculated subserous myoma—a rare cause of acute abdomen. *Ethiop Med J* 2007;45:203–207.

52. **Pron G, Bennett J, Common A, et al.** The Ontario Uterine Fibroid Embolization Trial. Part 2. Uterine fibroid reduction and symptom relief after uterine artery embolization for fibroids. *Fertil Steril* 2003;79:120–127.

53. **Langer R, Golan A, Neuman M, et al.** The effect of large uterine fibroids on urinary bladder function and symptoms. *Am J Obstet Gynecol* 1990;163:1139–1141.

54. **Parker W, Fu Y, Berek J.** Uterine sarcoma in patients operated on for presumed leiomyoma and rapidly growing leiomyoma. *Obstet Gynecol* 1994;83:414–418.

55. **Boutselis J, Ullery J.** Sarcoma of the uterus. *Obstet Gynecol* 1962;20:23–35.

56. **Brooks SE, Zhan M, Cote T, et al.** Surveillance, epidemiology, and end results analysis of 2677 cases of uterine sarcoma 1989–1999. *Gynecol Oncol* 2004;93:204–208.

57. **American College of Obstetricians and Gynecology.** Surgical Alternatives to Hysterectomy in the Management of Leiomyomas. ACOG Practice Bulletin 16. *Int J Gynaecol Obstet* 2001;73:285–294.

58. **Cantuaria GH, Angioli R, Frost L, et al.** Comparison of bimanual examination with ultrasound examination before hysterectomy for uterine leiomyoma. *Obstet Gynecol* 1998;92:109–112.

59. **Dueholm M, Lundorf E, Hansen ES, et al.** Evaluation of the uterine cavity with magnetic resonance imaging, transvaginal sonography, hysterosonographic examination, and diagnostic hysteroscopy. *Fertil Steril* 2001;76:350–357.

60. **Munro MG, Critchley HO, Broder MS, et al.** FIGO classification system (PALM-COEIN) for causes of abnormal uterine bleeding in nongravid women of reproductive age. *Int J Gynaecol Obstet* 2011;113:3–13.

61. **Dueholm M, Lundorf E, Hansen ES, et al.** Accuracy of magnetic resonance imaging and transvaginal ultrasonography in the diagnosis, mapping, and measurement of uterine myomas. *Am J Obstet Gynecol* 2002;186:409–415.

62. **Dueholm M, Lundorf E, Sorensen JS, et al.** Reproducibility of evaluation of the uterus by transvaginal sonography, hysterosonographic examination, hysteroscopy and magnetic resonance imaging. *Hum Reprod* 2002;17:195–200.

63. **Dueholm M, Lundorf E, Hansen ES, et al.** Magnetic resonance imaging and transvaginal ultrasonography for the diagnosis of adenomyosis. *Fertil Steril* 2001;76:588–594.

64. **Dueholm M, Lundorf E, Olesen F.** Imaging techniques for evaluation of the uterine cavity and endometrium in premenopausal patients

before minimally invasive surgery. *Obstet Gynecol Surv* 2002;57:388–403.

65. **Goto A, Takeuchi S, Sugimura K, et al.** Usefulness of Gd-DTPA contrast-enhanced dynamic MRI and serum determination of LDH and its isozymes in the differential diagnosis of leiomyosarcoma from degenerated leiomyoma of the uterus. *Int J Gynecol Cancer* 2002;12:354–361.

66. **Pritts E, Parker W, Olive D.** Fibroids and infertility: an updated systematic review of the evidence. *Fertil Steril* 2009;91:1215–1223.

67. **Laughlin S, Baird D, Savitz D, et al.** Prevalence of uterine leiomyomas in the first trimester of pregnancy: an ultrasound-screening study. *Obstet Gynecol* 2009;113:630–635.

68. **Muram D, Gillieson M, Walters JH.** Myomas of the uterus in pregnancy: ultrasonographic follow-up. *Am J Obstet Gynecol* 1980;138:16–19.

69. **Rosati P, Exacoustos C, Mancuso S.** Longitudinal evaluation of uterine myoma growth during pregnancy. A sonographic study. *J Ultrasound Med* 1992;11:511–515.

70. **Lev-Toaff AS, Coleman BG, Arger PH, et al.** Leiomyomas in pregnancy: sonographic study. *Radiology* 1987;164:375–380.

71. **Katz VL, Dotters DJ, Droegemueller W.** Complications of uterine leiomyomas in pregnancy. *Obstet Gynecol* 1989;73:593–596.

72. **Vergani P, Ghidini A, Strobelt N, et al.** Do uterine leiomyomas influence pregnancy outcome? *Am J Perinatol* 1994;11:356–358.

73. **Qidwai GI, Caughey AB, Jacoby AF.** Obstetric outcomes in women with sonographically identified uterine leiomyomata. *Obstet Gynecol* 2006;107:376–382.

74. **Chuang J, Tsai HW, Hwang JL.** Fetal compression syndrome caused by myoma in pregnancy: a case report. *Acta Obstet Gynecol Scand* 2001;80:472–473.

75. **Joo JG, Inovay J, Silhavy M, et al.** Successful enucleation of a necrotizing fibroid causing oligohydramnios and fetal postural deformity in the 25th week of gestation. A case report. *J Reprod Med* 2001;46:923–925.

76. **Graham JM** Jr. The association between limb anomalies and spatially-restricting uterine environments. *Prog Clin Biol Res* 1985;163C:99–103.

77. **Romero R, Chervenak FA, DeVore G, et al.** Fetal head deformation and congenital torticollis associated with a uterine tumor. *Am J Obstet Gynecol* 1981;141:839–840.

78. **Palerme GR, Friedman EA.** Rupture of the gravid uterus in the third trimester. *Am J Obstet Gynecol* 1966;94:571–576.

79. **Garnet J.** Uterine rupture during pregnancy. An analysis of 133 patients. *Obstet Gynecol* 1964;23:898–905.

80. **Obed J, Omigbodun A.** Rupture of the uterus in patients with previous myomectomy and primary caesarean section scars: a comparison. *J Obstet Gynaecol* 1996;1:1621.

81. **Parker W, Einarsson J, Istre O, et al.** Risk factors for uterine rupture following laparoscopic myomectomy. *J Minim Invasive Gynecol* 2010;17:551–554.

82. **Walker CL, Stewart EA.** Uterine fibroids: the elephant in the room. *Science* 2005;308:1589–1592.

83. **Myers ER, Barber MD, Gustilo-Ashby T, et al.** Management of uterine leiomyomata: what do we really know? *Obstet Gynecol* 2002;100:8–17.

84. **Parker WH.** Etiology, symptomatology, and diagnosis of uterine myomas. *Fertil Steril* 2007;87:725–736.

85. **Carlson KJ, Miller BA, Fowler FJ Jr.** The Maine Women's Health Study: II. Outcomes of nonsurgical management of leiomyomas, abnormal bleeding, and chronic pelvic pain. *Obstet Gynecol* 1994;83:566–572.

86. **Ylikorkala O, Pekonen F.** Naproxen reduces idiopathic but not fibromyoma-induced menorrhagia. *Obstet Gynecol* 1986;68:10–12.

87. **Schlaff WD, Zerhouni EA, Huth JA, et al.** A placebo-controlled trial of a depot gonadotropin-releasing hormone analogue leuprolide in the treatment of uterine leiomyomata. *Obstet Gynecol* 1989;74:856–862.

88. **Friedman AJ, Hoffman DI, Comite F, et al.** Treatment of leiomyomata uteri with leuprolide acetate depot: a double-blind, placebo-controlled, multicenter study. The Leuprolide Study Group. *Obstet Gynecol* 1991;77:720–725.

89. **Letterie GS, Coddington CC, Winkel CA, et al.** Efficacy of a gonadotropin-releasing hormone agonist in the treatment of uterine leiomyomata: long-term follow-up. *Fertil Steril* 1989;51:951–956.

90. **Leather AT, Studd JW, Watson NR, et al.** The prevention of bone loss in young women treated with GnRH analogues with "add-back" estrogen therapy. *Obstet Gynecol* 1993;81:104–107.

91. **Pierce SJ, Gazvani MR, Farquharson RG.** Long-term use of gonadotropin-releasing hormone analogs and hormone replacement therapy in the management of endometriosis: a randomized trial with a 6-year follow-up. *Fertil Steril* 2000;74:964–968.

92. **de Aloysio D, Altieri P, Pretolani G, et al.** The combined effect of a GnRH analog in premenopause plus postmenopausal estrogen deficiency for the treatment of uterine leiomyomas in perimenopausal women. *Gynecol Obstet Invest* 1995;39:115–119.

93. **Flierman PA, Oberye JJ, van der Hulst VP, et al.** Rapid reduction of leiomyoma volume during treatment with the GnRH antagonist ganirelix. *BJOG* 2005;112:638–642.

94. **Murphy AA, Morales AJ, Kettel LM, et al.** Regression of uterine leiomyomata to the antiprogesterone RU486: dose-response effect. *Fertil Steril* 1995;64:187–190.

95. **Fiscella K, Eisinger SH, Meldrum S, et al..** Effect of mifepristone for symptomatic leiomyomata on quality of life and uterine size: a randomized controlled trial. *Obstet Gynecol* 2006;108:1381–1387.

96. **Steinauer J, Pritts EA, Jackson R, et al.** Systematic review of mifepristone for the treatment of uterine leiomyomata. *Obstet Gynecol* 2004;103:1331–1336.

97. **Grigorieva V, Chen-Mok M, Tarasova M, et al.** Use of a levonorgestrel-releasing intrauterine system to treat bleeding related to uterine leiomyomas. *Fertil Steril* 2003;79:1194–1198.

98. **Soysal S, Soysal M.** The efficacy of levonorgestrel-releasing intrauterine device in selected cases of myoma-related menorrhagia: a prospective controlled trial. *Gynecol Obstet Invest* 2005;59:29–35.

99. **Mercorio F, De Simone R, Di Spiezio Sardo A, et al.** The effect of a levonorgestrel-releasing intrauterine device in the treatment of myoma-related menorrhagia. *Contraception* 2003;67:277–280.

100. **Mehl-Madrona L.** Complementary medicine treatment of uterine fibroids: a pilot study. *Altern Ther Health Med* 2002;8:34–36.

101. **Sakamoto S, Yoshino H, Shirahata Y, et al.** Pharmacotherapeutic effects of kuei-chih-fu-ling-wan (keishi-bukuryo-gan) on human uterine myomas. *Am J Chin Med* 1992;20:313–317.

102. **Buttram VC Jr, Reiter RC.** Uterine leiomyomata: etiology, symptomatology, and management. *Fertil Steril* 1981;36:433–445.

103. **Sirjusingh A, Bassaw B, Roopnarinesingh S.** The results of abdominal myomectomy. *West Indian Med J* 1994;43:138–139.

104. **Vercellini P, Maddalena S, De Giorgi O, et al.** Determinants of reproductive outcome after abdominal myomectomy for infertility. *Fertil Steril* 1999;72:109–114.

105. **Goodwin SC, Bradley LD, Lipman JC, et al.** Uterine artery embolization versus myomectomy: a multicenter comparative study. *Fertil Steril* 2006;85:14–21.

106. **Reiter RC, Wagner PL, Gambone JC.** Routine hysterectomy for large asymptomatic uterine leiomyomata: a reappraisal. *Obstet Gynecol* 1992;79:481–484

107. **Wurnig C, Schatz K, Noske H, et al.** Subcutaneous low-dose epoetin beta for the avoidance of transfusion in patients scheduled for elective surgery not eligible for autologous blood donation. *Eur Surg Res* 2001;33:303–310.

108. **Sesti F, Ticconi C, Bonifacio S, et al.** Preoperative administration of recombinant human erythropoietin in patients undergoing gynecologic surgery. *Gynecol Obstet Invest* 2002;54:1–5.

109. **Stovall TG, Muneyyirci-Delale O, Summitt RL Jr, et al.** GnRH agonist and iron versus placebo and iron in the anemic patient before surgery for leiomyomas: a randomized controlled trial. Leuprolide Acetate Study Group. *Obstet Gynecol* 1995;86:65–71.

110. **Lethaby A, Vollenhoven B, Sowter M.** Efficacy of pre-operative gonadotrophin hormone releasing analogues for women with uterine fibroids undergoing hysterectomy or myomectomy: a systematic review. *BJOG* 2002;109:1097–1108.

111. **Sawin SW, Pilevsky ND, Berlin JA, et al.** Comparability of perioperative morbidity between abdominal myomectomy and hysterectomy for women with uterine leiomyomas. *Am J Obstet Gynecol* 2000;183:1448–1455.

112. **West S, Ruiz R, Parker WH.** Abdominal myomectomy in women with very large uterine size. *Fertil Steril* 2006;85:36–39.

113. **Iverson RE Jr, Chelmow D, Strohbehn K, et al.** Relative morbidity of abdominal hysterectomy and myomectomy for management of uterine leiomyomas. *Obstet Gynecol* 1996;88:415–419.

114. **Ehigiegba AE, Ande AB, Ojobo SI.** Myomectomy during cesarean section. *Int J Gynaecol Obstet* 2001;75:21–25.

115. **Roman AS, Tabsh KM.** Myomectomy at time of cesarean delivery: a retrospective cohort study. *BMC Pregnancy Childbirth* 2004;4:14.

116. **Frederick J, Fletcher H, Simeon D, et al.** Intramyometrial vasopressin as a haemostatic agent during myomectomy. *Br J Obstet Gynaecol* 1994;101:435–437.

117. **Ginsburg ES, Benson CB, Garfield JM, et al.** The effect of operative technique and uterine size on blood loss during myomectomy: a prospective randomized study. *Fertil Steril* 1993;60:956–962.

118. **Hobo R, Netsu S, Koyasu Y, et al.** Bradycardia and cardiac arrest caused by intramyometrial injection of vasopressin during a laparoscopically assisted myomectomy. *Obstet Gynecol* 2009;113(Pt 2):484–486.

119. **Goodnough L, Monk T, Brecher M.** Autologous blood procurement in the surgical setting: lessons learned in the last 10 years. *Vox Sang* 1996;71:133–141.

120. **Yamada T, Ikeda A, Okamoto Y, et al.** Intraoperative blood salvage in abdominal simple total hysterectomy for uterine myoma. *Int J Gynaecol Obstet* 1997;59:233–236.

121. **Davies L, Brown TJ, Haynes S, et al.** Cost-effectiveness of cell salvage and alternative methods of minimising perioperative allogeneic blood transfusion: a systematic review and economic model. *Health Technol Assess* 2006;10:1–210.

122. **Helal AS, Abdel-Hady el-S, Refaie E, et al.** Preliminary uterine artery ligation versus pericervical mechanical tourniquet in reducing hemorrhage during abdominal myomectomy. *Int J Gynaecol Obstet* 2010;108:233–235.

123. **Dumousset E, Chabrot P, Rabischong B, et al.** Preoperative uterine artery embolization (PUAE) before uterine fibroid myomectomy. *Cardiovasc Intervent Radiol* 2008;31:514–520.

124. **Discepola F, Valenti DA, Reinhold C, et al.** Analysis of arterial blood vessels surrounding the myoma: relevance to myomectomy. *Obstet Gynecol* 2007;110:1301–1303.

125. **Walocha JA, Litwin JA, Miodonski AJ.** Vascular system of intramural leiomyomata revealed by corrosion casting and scanning electron microscopy. *Hum Reprod* 2003;18:1088–1093.

126. **Guarnaccia MM, Rein MS.** Traditional surgical approaches to uterine fibroids: abdominal myomectomy and hysterectomy. *Clin Obstet Gynecol* 2001;44:385–400.

127. **Diamond MP.** Reduction of adhesions after uterine myomectomy by Seprafilm membrane (HAL-F): a blinded, prospective, randomized, multicenter clinical study. Seprafilm Adhesion Study Group. *Fertil Steril* 1996;66:904–910.

128. **Parker WH, Rodi IA.** Patient selection for laparoscopic myomectomy. *J Am Assoc Gynecol Laparosc* 1994;2:23–26.

129. **Jin C, Hu Y, Chen X, et al.** Laparoscopic versus open myomectomy-a meta-analysis of randomized controlled trials. *Eur J Obstet Gynecol Reprod Biol* 2009;145:14–21.

130. **Malzoni M, Rotond M, Perone C, et al.** Fertility after laparoscopic myomectomy of large uterine myomas: operative technique and preliminary results. *Eur J Gynaecol Oncol* 2003;24:79–82.

131. **Andrei B, Crovini G, Rosi A.** Uterine myomas: pelviscopic treatment. *Clin Exp Obstet Gynecol* 1999;26:44–46.

132. **Koh C, Janik G.** Laparoscopic myomectomy: the current status. *Curr Opin Obstet Gynecol* 2003;15:295–301.

133. **Agarwala N, Liu CY.** Safe entry techniques during laparoscopy: left upper quadrant entry using the ninth intercostal space–a review of 918 procedures. *J Minim Invasive Gynecol* 2005;12:55–61.

134. **Zupi E, Marconi D, Sbracia M, et al.** Directed laparoscopic cryomyolysis for symptomatic leiomyomata: one-year follow up. *J Minim Invasive Gynecol* 2005;12:343–346.

135. **Donnez J, Squifflet J, Polet R, et al.** Laparoscopic myolysis. *Hum Reprod Update* 2000;6:609–613.

136. **Dubuisson JB, Fauconnier A, Chapron C, et al.** Second look after laparoscopic myomectomy. *Hum Reprod* 1998;13:2102–2106.

137. **Farquhar C, Vandekerckhove P, Watson A, et al.** Barrier agents for preventing adhesions after surgery for subfertility. *Cochrane Database Syst Rev* 2000;2:CD000475.

138. **Tulandi T, Murray C, Guralnick M.** Adhesion formation and reproductive outcome after myomectomy and second-look laparoscopy. *Obstet Gynecol* 1993;82:213–215.

139. **Wamsteker K, Emanuel MH, de Kruif JH.** Transcervical hysteroscopic resection of submucous fibroids for abnormal uterine bleeding:

results regarding the degree of intramural extension. *Obstet Gynecol* 1993;82:736–740.

140. **Vercellini P, Zaina B, Yaylayan L, et al.** Hysteroscopic myomectomy: long-term effects on menstrual pattern and fertility. *Obstet Gynecol* 1999;94:341–347.

141. **Emanuel MH, Wamsteker K, Hart AA, et al.** Long-term results of hysteroscopic myomectomy for abnormal uterine bleeding. *Obstet Gynecol* 1999;93:743–748.

142. **Darwish AM, Ahmad AM, Mohammad AM.** Cervical priming prior to operative hysteroscopy: a randomized comparison of laminaria versus misoprostol. *Hum Reprod* 2004;19:2391–2394.

143. **Murakami T, Hayasaka S, Terada Y, et al.** Predicting outcome of one-step total hysteroscopic resection of sessile submucous myoma. *J Minim Invasive Gynecol* 2008;15:74–77.

144. **Indman PD.** Hysteroscopic treatment of submucous myomas. *Clin Obstet Gynecol* 2006;49:811–820.

145. **Loffer FD, Bradley LD, Brill AI, et al.** Hysteroscopic fluid monitoring guidelines. The ad hoc committee on hysteroscopic training guidelines of the American Association of Gynecologic Laparoscopists. *J Am Assoc Gynecol Laparosc* 2000;7:167–168.

146. **Murakami T, Tamura M, Ozawa Y, et al.** Safe techniques in surgery for hysteroscopic myomectomy. *J Obstet Gynaecol Res* 2005;31:216–223.

147. **Indman PD.** Hysteroscopic treatment of menorrhagia associated with uterine leiomyomas. *Obstet Gynecol* 1993;81:716–720.

148. **Mints M, Radestad A, Rylander E.** Follow up of hysteroscopic surgery for menorrhagia. *Acta Obstet Gynecol Scand* 1998;77:435–438.

149. **Glasser MH, Zimmerman JD.** The HydroThermAblator system for management of menorrhagia in women with submucous myomas: 12- to 20-month follow-up. *J Am Assoc Gynecol Laparosc* 2003;10:521–527.

150. **Sabbah R, Desaulniers G.** Use of the NovaSure impedance controlled endometrial ablation system in patients with intracavitary disease: 12-month follow-up results of a prospective, single-arm clinical study. *J Minim Invasive Gynecol* 2006;13:467–471.

151. **Malone L.** Myomectomy: recurrence after removal of solitary and multiple myomas. *Obstet Gynecol* 1969;34:200–203.

152. **Parker WH.** Uterine myomas: management. *Fertil Steril* 2007;88:255–271.

153. **Fedele L, Parazzini F, Luchini L, et al.** Recurrence of fibroids after myomectomy: a transvaginal ultrasonographic study. *Hum Reprod* 1995;10:1795–1796.

154. **Olive DL.** Review of the evidence for treatment of leiomyomata. *Environ Health Perspect* 2000;108(Suppl 5):841–843.

155. **Candiani GB, Fedele L, Parazzini F, et al.** Risk of recurrence after myomectomy. *Br J Obstet Gynaecol* 1991;98:385–389.

156. **Fauconnier A, Chapron C, Babaki-Fard K, et al.** Recurrence of leiomyomata after myomectomy. *Hum Reprod Update* 2000;6:595–602.

157. **Vavala V, Lanzone A, Monaco A, et al.** Postoperative GnRH analog treatment for the prevention of recurrences of uterine myomas after myomectomy. A pilot study. *Gynecol Obstet Invest* 1997;43:251–254.

158. **Dadak C, Feiks A.** [Organ-sparing surgery of leiomyomas of the uterus in young females]. *Zentralbl Gynakol* 1988;110:102–106.

159. **Rosenfeld DL.** Abdominal myomectomy for otherwise unexplained infertility. *Fertil Steril* 1986;46:328–330.

160. **Rossetti A, Sizzi O, Soranna L, et al.** Long-term results of laparoscopic myomectomy: recurrence rate in comparison with abdominal myomectomy. *Hum Reprod* 2001;16:770–774.

161. **Society of Obstetricians and Gynaecologists of Canada.** Clinical practice guidelines. *Int J Gynecol Obstet* 2005;89:305–318.

162. **Harding G, Coyne KS, Thompson CL, et al.** The responsiveness of the uterine fibroid symptom and health-related quality of life questionnaire (UFS-QOL). *Health Qual Life Outcomes* 2008;6:99.

163. **American College of Obstetricians and Gynecologists.** ACOG committee opinion. Uterine artery embolization. *Obstet Gynecol* 2004;103:403–404.

164. **Spies JB, Sacks D.** Credentials for uterine artery embolization. *J Vasc Interv Radiol* 2004;15:111–113.

165. **Zupi E, Pocek M, Dauri M, et al.** Selective uterine artery embolization in the management of uterine myomas. *Fertil Steril* 2003;79:107–111.

166. **Pron G, Cohen M, Soucie J, et al.** The Ontario Uterine Fibroid Embolization Trial. Part 1. Baseline patient characteristics, fibroid burden, and impact on life. *Fertil Steril* 2003;79:112–119.

167. **Hehenkamp WJ, Volkers NA, Donderwinkel PF, et al.** Uterine artery embolization versus hysterectomy in the treatment of symptomatic uterine fibroids (EMMY trial): peri- and postprocedural results from a randomized controlled trial. *Am J Obstet Gynecol* 2005;193:1618–1629.

168. **Agency for Healthcare Research and Quality.** National inpatient sample of the HCUP database of the Agency for HealthCare Research and Quality. http://hcupnet.ahrq.gov/HCUPnet.jsp

169. **Ryu RK, Chrisman HB, Omary RA, et al.** The vascular impact of uterine artery embolization: prospective sonographic assessment of ovarian arterial circulation. *J Vasc Interv Radiol* 2001;12:1071–1074.

170. **Hehenkamp WJ, Volkers NA, Broekmans FJ, et al.** Loss of ovarian reserve after uterine artery embolization: a randomized comparison with hysterectomy. *Hum Reprod* 2007;22:1996–2005.

171. **Tropeano G, Di Stasi C, Litwicka K, et al.** Uterine artery embolization for fibroids does not have adverse effects on ovarian reserve in regularly cycling women younger than 40 years. *Fertil Steril* 2004;81:1055–1061.

172. **Tulandi T, Salamah K.** Fertility and uterine artery embolization. *Obstet Gynecol* 2010;115:857–860.

173. **Mara M, Maskova J, Fucikova Z, et al.** Midterm clinical and first reproductive results of a randomized controlled trial comparing uterine fibroid embolization and myomectomy. *Cardiovasc Intervent Radiol* 2008;31:73–85.

174. **Goldberg J, Pereira L, Berghella V, et al.** Pregnancy outcomes after treatment for fibromyomata: uterine artery embolization versus laparoscopic myomectomy. *Am J Obstet Gynecol* 2004;191:18–21.

175. **Pron G, Mocarski E, Bennett J, et al.** Pregnancy after uterine artery embolization for leiomyomata: the Ontario multicenter trial. *Obstet Gynecol* 2005;105:67–76.

176. **Godfrey CD, Zbella EA.** Uterine necrosis after uterine artery embolization for leiomyoma. *Obstet Gynecol* 2001;98:950–952.

177. **Hald K, Noreng HJ, Istre O, et al.** Uterine artery embolization versus laparoscopic occlusion of uterine arteries for leiomyomas: long-term results of a randomized comparative trial. *J Vasc Interv Radiol* 2009;20:1303–1310.

178. **Vilos GA, Vilos EC, Romano W, et al.** Temporary uterine artery occlusion for treatment of menorrhagia and uterine fibroids using an incisionless Doppler-guided transvaginal clamp: case report. *Hum Reprod* 2006;21:269–271.

179. **Stewart EA, Gedroyc WM, Tempany CM, et al.** Focused ultrasound treatment of uterine fibroid tumors: safety and feasibility of a noninvasive thermoablative technique. *Am J Obstet Gynecol* 2003;189:48–54.

180. **Stewart EA, Rabinovici J, Tempany CM, et al.** Clinical outcomes of focused ultrasound surgery for the treatment of uterine fibroids. *Fertil Steril* 2006;85:22–29.

181. **LeBlang SD, Hoctor K, Steinberg FL.** Leiomyoma shrinkage after MRI-guided focused ultrasound treatment: report of 80 patients. *AJR Am J Roentgenol* 2010;194:274–280.

Pelvic Pain and Dysmenorrhea

Andrea J. Rapkin

Leena Nathan

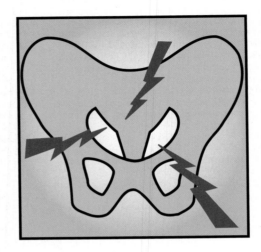

- Acute pelvic pain is rapid in onset, often associated with unstable vital signs and obvious abnormalities on physical examination and laboratory assessment. Improper diagnosis can result in significant morbidity and even mortality.

- Timely and thorough assessment, guided by organ system (reproductive, gastrointestinal, urinary) and category of pathology will ensure effective diagnosis and management of infection, obstruction, ischemia (torsion), leakage of irritating substance (viscus or cyst rupture), neoplasia, or pregnancy-related pain.

- Chronic pelvic pain is a multifaceted disorder characterized by changes in the processing of afferent signaling in the pelvic organs, the surrounding somatic tissues, and the spinal cord and brain. The shared thoracolumbar and sacral innervations of the pelvic structures and the up-regulation processing of neural input in the central nervous system account for the multiplicity of somatic and psychological symptoms experienced by women with chronic pelvic pain.

- A thorough history and physical examination are important for successful management of both chronic and acute pain. The ancillary laboratory and diagnostic procedures performed to assess acute, life-threatening processes differ from those focused on chronic pain conditions. Chronic pelvic pain requires a multidisciplinary approach for both diagnosis and management.

Definitions

Acute pain is intense and characterized by sudden onset, sharp rise, and short course. *Cyclic pain* refers to pain that occurs with a definite association to the menstrual period. *Dysmenorrhea*, or painful menstruation, is the most common cyclic pain phenomenon and is classified as *primary* or *secondary* on the basis of associated anatomic pathology (1). *Chronic pelvic pain* is defined as pain of greater than 6 months in duration, localized to the anatomic pelvis, and severe enough to cause functional disability or necessitating medical care (2).

Whereas acute pain is generally associated with autonomic reflex responses, such as nausea, emesis, diaphoresis, and apprehension, such autonomic reflex responses are not present in women with chronic pelvic pain. Acute pain is affiliated with signs of inflammation or infection, such as fever and leukocytosis, which are absent in chronic pain states. The pathophysiology of acute pelvic pain involves mediators of inflammation present in high concentration as a result of infection, ischemia, or chemical irritation.

By contrast, the etiology of chronic pelvic pain often involves changes in modulation or "up-regulation" of normally nonpainful stimuli. Pain is out of proportion to the degree of tissue damage (3). Chronic pain is thus characterized by physiologic, affective, and behavioral responses that differ from those associated with acute pain (4). An inflammatory lesion, such as endometriosis, for example, can set up an environment of chronic neurogenic inflammation or stimulation, which can result in "plastic" changes in the peripheral and central nervous system and the persistence of chronic pain (5–7). Moreover, genetic predisposition, adverse environmental pressures, and hormonal milieu are thought to increase the vulnerability and predisposition for chronic pain disorders (8).

Acute Pain

The differential diagnosis of acute pelvic pain is outlined in Table 16.1. Assessing the character of the pain helps create a differential diagnosis. **Rapid onset of pain is most consistent with perforation or rupture of a hollow viscus or ischemia following the torsion of a vascular pedicle. Colic or severe cramping pain is commonly associated with muscular contraction or obstruction of a hollow viscus, such as intestine, ureter, or uterus. Pain perceived over the entire abdomen suggests a generalized reaction to an irritating fluid within the peritoneal cavity such as blood, purulent fluid, or contents of an ovarian cyst.**

The first perception of visceral pain is a vague, deep, poorly localizable sensation associated with autonomic reflex responses. When the pain becomes localized to a region of the abdominal wall, the pain is called referred pain. Referred pain is well localized and more superficial and is appreciated within the nerve distribution or dermatome of the spinal cord segment innervating the involved viscus. The location of the referred pain provides insight into the location of the primary disease process (9). The innervations of the pelvic organs are outlined in Table 16.2. The upper vagina, cervix, uterus, and adnexa share the same visceral innervations with the large intestine, rectum, bladder, lower ureter, and lower small intestine. Pain from the reproductive organs, genitourinary (GU), and gastrointestinal (GI) tracts are therefore referred to the same dermatomes (10,11).

Evaluation of Acute Pelvic Pain

In the evaluation of acute pelvic pain, early diagnosis is critical because significant delay increases morbidity and mortality. Central to correct diagnosis is an accurate history. The date and character of the last and previous menstrual periods and the presence of abnormal bleeding or discharge should be ascertained. The menstrual, sexual, and contraceptive history and any history of sexually transmitted conditions and previous gynecologic disorders are relevant. Pain history should include how and when the pain started, pregnancy-related symptoms (amenorrhea, irregular bleeding, nausea, breast tenderness), GI symptoms (anorexia, nausea, vomiting, constipation, obstipation, absence of flatus, hematochezia), urinary symptoms (dysuria, urgency frequency, hesitancy, hematuria), signs of infection (fever, chills, purulent vaginal discharge), and symptoms attributable to a hemoperitoneum (orthostasis, abdominal distention, and right upper quadrant or shoulder pain). Document any past medical and surgical history, and current medications.

Baseline laboratory studies will include, at the least, a complete blood count with differential (CBC), clean catch mid-stream routine urine analysis (RUA), sensitive urine or serum pregnancy test, gonorrhea and chlamydia screening, and a transvaginal pelvic ultrasound. Other tests such as computerized tomography (CT) with and without contrast, chemistry panel, or blood type and screen (if transfusion is likely) may be indicated depending on the patient's symptoms and the specific differential diagnosis.

Table 16.1 Differential Diagnosis of Acute Pelvic Pain

Gynecologic

Acute Pain

1. **Complication of pregnancy**
   a. Ectopic pregnancy
   b. Abortion, threatened or incomplete

2. **Acute infections**
   a. Endometritis
   b. Pelvic inflammatory disease (acute PID) or salpingo-oophoritis
   c. Tubo-ovarian abscess

3. **Adnexal disorders**
   a. Hemorrhagic functional ovarian cyst
   b. Torsion of adnexa
   c. Rupture of functional, neoplastic, or inflammatory ovarian cyst

Recurrent Pelvic Pain

1. Mittelschmerz (midcycle pain)
2. Primary dysmenorrhea
3. Secondary dysmenorrhea

Gastrointestinal

1. Gastroenteritis
2. Appendicitis
3. Bowel obstruction
4. Diverticulitis
5. Inflammatory bowel disease
6. Irritable bowel syndrome

Genitourinary

1. Cystitis
2. Pyelonephritis
3. Ureteral lithiasis

Musculoskeletal

1. Abdominal wall hematoma
2. Hernia

Other

1. Acute porphyria
2. Pelvic thrombophlebitis
3. Aortic aneurysm
4. Abdominal angina

Table 16.2 Nerves Carrying Painful Impulses from the Pelvic Organs		
Organ	*Spinal Segments*	*Nerves*
Abdominal wall	T12–L1	Iliohypogastric, ilioinguinal, genitofemoral
Lower abdominal wall, anterior vulva, urethra, clitoris	L1–L2	Ilioinguinal, genitofemoral
Lower back	L1–L2	
Pelvic floor, anus, perineum, and lower vagina	S2–S4	Pudendal, inguinal, genitofemoral, posterofemoral cutaneous
Upper vagina, cervix, uterine corpus, inner third of fallopian tubes, broad ligament, upper bladder, terminal ileum, and terminal large bowel	T11–L2 S2–S4	Thoracolumbar autonomics (sympathetics) via hypogastric plexus; sacral autonomics (parasympathetics) via pelvic nerve
Ovaries, outer two-thirds of fallopian tubes, and upper ureter	T9–T10	Thoracic autonomics (sympathetics) via renal and aortic plexus and celiac and mesenteric ganglia, aortic and superior mesenteric plexuses

Reproductive Tract Causes of Acute Pelvic Pain

Ectopic Pregnancy

All reproductive-aged women presenting with acute pain should be screened for pregnancy.

An ectopic pregnancy is defined as implantation of the fetus in a site other than the uterine cavity (see Chapter 20).

Symptoms of Ectopic Pregnancy

Implantation of the fetus in the fallopian tube produces pain with acute dilation of the tube. If tubal rupture occurs, localized abdominal pain tends to be temporarily relieved and is replaced by generalized pelvic and abdominal pain and dizziness with the development of a hemoperitoneum. A period of amenorrhea followed by irregular bleeding and acute onset of pain compose the classic triad of symptoms. A mass in the cul-de-sac may produce an urge to defecate. Referred pain to the right shoulder often develops if the intra-abdominal blood collection transverses the right colic gutter and irritates the diaphragm (C3 to C5 innervation).

Signs

Vital signs often reveal orthostatic changes in the case of a ruptured ectopic. Orthostasis is diagnosed by obtaining a patient's pulse and blood pressure while they are supine, then after sitting for 3 minutes, and finally after standing for 3 minutes. If the systolic blood pressure decreases by 20 mm Hg or the diastolic blood pressure decreases by 10 mm Hg when standing from a supine position, orthostasis is confirmed. Although pulse rate is not specifically included in the definition of orthostasis, it is easy to obtain and an increase in pulse rate can be suggestive of orthostasis. Elevated temperature is generally absent with an ectopic.

Abdominal examination is notable for tenderness and guarding in one or both lower quadrants. With the development of hemoperitoneum, generalized abdominal distention and rebound tenderness are prominent and bowel sounds are decreased. Pelvic examination generally reveals mild tenderness on motion of the cervix. Adnexal tenderness is present, usually more pronounced on the side of the ectopic pregnancy, and a mass may be palpated. The diagnostic approach and the medical and surgical management of ectopic pregnancy are discussed in Chapter 20 (12,13).

Leaking or Rupture of an Ovarian Cyst

Functional cysts (e.g., follicle or corpus luteum) are the most common ovarian cysts and are more likely to rupture than benign or malignant neoplasms. The pain associated with rupture of the ovarian follicle at the time of ovulation is called *mittelschmerz*. The small amount of blood leaking into the peritoneal cavity and high concentration of follicular fluid prostaglandins contribute to this midcycle pelvic pain. The pain is usually mild to moderate and self-limited, and with an intact coagulation system, hemoperitoneum is unlikely.

A hemorrhagic corpus luteum cyst develops during the luteal phase of the menstrual cycle. The rapidly expanding ovarian capsule or, with rupture, the blood in the peritoneal cavity is responsible for the acute pain. Rupture of this cyst can produce either a small amount of intraperitoneal bleeding or frank hemorrhage, resulting in significant blood loss and hemoperitoneum.

Cystic ovarian neoplasms or inflammatory ovarian masses, such as endometriomas or abscesses, can leak or rupture. A history of a dermoid cyst or endometrioma that has not yet undergone surgical extirpation is not uncommon. **Surgical exploration is indicated if the rupture leads to significant hemoperitoneum (corpus luteum) or chemical peritonitis (endometrioma or dermoid), which could impair future fertility, or an acute abdomen (abscess), which is life threatening.**

Symptoms

An ovarian cyst that is not undergoing torsion, rapidly enlarging, infected, or leaking does not usually cause acute pain. **A corpus luteum cyst is the most common cyst to rupture and leads to hemoperitoneum. Symptoms of a ruptured corpus luteum cyst are similar to those of a ruptured ectopic pregnancy.** The patient is in the luteal phase or can have delayed menses due to the persistently functioning corpus luteum. The onset of pain is usually sudden and is associated with increasing pelvic then generalized abdominal pain and dizziness or syncope with development of significant hemoperitoneum.

A ruptured endometrioma or benign cystic teratoma (dermoid cyst) produces similar symptoms; however, dizziness and signs of hypovolemia are not present because blood loss is minimal.

Signs

Orthostasis resulting from hypovolemia is present only when there is intravascular volume depletion, such as with a hemoperitoneum. Fever is rare. **The most important sign is the presence of significant abdominal tenderness, often associated with localized or generalized lower quadrant rebound tenderness because of peritoneal irritation.** The abdomen can be moderately distended with decreased bowel sounds. On pelvic examination, a mass is often palpable if the cyst is leaking and has not completely ruptured.

Diagnosis

The diagnosis and the type of ruptured cyst are ascertained by blood tests and transvaginal ultrasound. Pregnancy test, complete blood count, and, if orthostasis is present, type and screening should be ordered. Leukocytosis is uncommon. The hematocrit is decreased if active bleeding is present. If ultrasound is not available, a culdocentesis will reveal the nature of the intraperitoneal fluid. If orthostasis is absent and the peripheral hematocrit is relatively normal, clinically significant hemoperitoneum is unlikely. This conclusion is supported by culdocentesis findings of clear or blood-tinged fluid with a fluid hematocrit under 16% or transvaginal ultrasound revealing only a small amount of free intraperitoneal fluid.

Culdocentesis is very helpful in determining the cause of peritonitis: fresh blood suggests a corpus luteum; chocolate "old" blood, an endometrioma; oily sebaceous fluid, a benign teratoma; purulent fluid, pelvic inflammatory disease (PID) or tubo-ovarian abscess. A skillful reading of transvaginal ultrasound images can help to characterize a cystic structure in the pelvis as a dermoid, endometrioma, corpus luteum, or pelvic abscess and quantify the amount of intraperitoneal fluid.

Management

Orthostasis, significant anemia, hematocrit of the culdocentesis fluid of greater than 16%, or a large amount of free peritoneal fluid on ultrasound suggests significant hemoperitoneum and usually requires surgical management by laparoscopy or laparotomy. Patients who are not orthostatic or febrile, who are not pregnant or anemic, and who have only a small amount of fluid in the cul-de-sac can often be observed in the hospital, without surgical intervention, or even discharged home from the emergency room after observation.

Adnexal Torsion

Torsion (twisting) of the vascular pedicle of an ovary, ovary with cyst, fallopian tube, paratubal cyst, or rarely a pedunculated uterine myoma results in ischemia of the structures distal to the twisted pedicle and acute onset of pain. A benign cystic teratoma is the most common neoplasm to undergo torsion. Because of adhesions, ovarian carcinoma and inflammatory masses such as endometriomas or abscesses rarely undergo torsion. It is unusual for a normal tube and ovary to torque, although a polycystic ovary can undergo torsion. Diagnosis of adnexal torsion is challenging. The clinician must base the diagnosis on history, clinical examination, and additional investigations such as pelvic ultrasound (14). There is no specific size criteria for ovarian torsion, but one study found that 83% of torsion occurred in ovaries that were 5 cm or larger (15).

Symptoms

The pain of torsion is usually severe and constant or, if the torsion is partial and intermit, the pain can wax and wane. The onset of the torsion and subsequent abdominal pain frequently coincides with activity such as lifting, exercise, or intercourse. Autonomic reflex responses (e.g., nausea, emesis, tachycardia, and apprehension) are usually present.

Signs

Mild temperature elevation, tachycardia, and leukocytosis may accompany the necrosis of tissue. Pregnancy test is negative unless there is a co-existent pregnancy. The diagnosis must be suspected in any woman with acute pain and unilateral adnexal mass.

On examination, the localized direct and rebound tenderness can be noted in the lower quadrant(s). Another important sign is the presence of a large pelvic mass on bimanual examination.

Diagnosis

The process of torsion occludes the lymphatic and venous drainage of the involved adnexa; therefore, the torqued viscus rapidly increases in size and can be easily palpated on examination or visualized by ultrasound. However, the presence of Doppler blood flow to the ovary on ultrasound does not definitely rule out torsion.

Management

Adnexal torsion must be treated surgically. The adnexa may be untwisted and a cystectomy performed if appropriate. Even if it appears that necrosis occurred, there is evidence that it remains functional and sparing the adnexa can preserve its hormonal and reproductive function (16). Treatment can be accomplished by laparoscopy or laparotomy, depending on the size of the mass.

Acute Salpingo-oophoritis and Pelvic Inflammatory Disease

The diagnosis and management of acute salpingo-oophoritis and PID are discussed in Chapter 18 (17,18)

Symptoms

All cases of PID are polymicrobial, involving gram-negative and -positive aerobic and anaerobic bacteria; however, PID initiated by *Neisseria gonococcus* or chlamydia is manifested by the acute onset of pelvic pain that increases with movement, fever, purulent vaginal discharge, and sometimes nausea and emesis. Subclinical PID can be seen with chlamydial salpingo-oophoritis, with more insidious symptoms that can be confused with the symptoms of irritable bowel syndrome. Bacterial vaginosis has been commonly associated with PID (19).

Signs

Elevated temperature and tachycardia are typical. Abdominal examination may show distention and decreased bowel sounds caused by secondary ileus. Direct and rebound abdominal tenderness with palpation are marked. **The most important signs of acute salpingo-oophoritis are cervical motion tenderness and bilateral adnexal tenderness.** Evaluation of the pelvis may be difficult because of pain and guarding, but lack of a discrete mass or masses differentiates acute salpingo-oophoritis from tubo-ovarian abscess or torsion. Right upper quadrant can be a distinct sign of PID-related perihepatitis involving the liver capsule and peritoneal surfaces, called Fitz-Hugh–Curtis syndrome.

Diagnosis

Leukocytosis and elevated erythrocyte sedimentation rate (ESR), a nonspecific, although more sensitive, sign of inflammation, are found in patients with acute PID. Pregnancy test is usually negative because PID as co-existent intrauterine pregnancy (IUP) is rare. If the pregnancy test is positive, an infected or very inflamed ectopic pregnancy, or instrumented IUP or infected, incomplete abortion should be suspected. Appendicitis and diverticulitis can be mistaken for PID. Laparoscopy can be useful if the diagnosis is uncertain. The Centers for Disease Control and Prevention guidelines for diagnosing PID state that PID should be suspected and treatment started if the patient is at risk for PID and she has uterine, cervical, or adnexal motion tenderness without any apparent cause (19a). Findings that support the diagnosis include cervical or vaginal mucopurulent discharge, elevated ESR or C-reactive protein (CRP), laboratory confirmation of gonorrhea or chlamydia, oral temperature of 38.3°C or higher, or white blood cells on wet mount of vaginal secretions or culdocentesis fluid. Most specific criteria for the diagnosis include endometritis on endometrial biopsy, laparoscopic evidence of PID (tubal edema, erythema, and purulent discharge), or thickened, fluid-fluid fallopian tubes on pelvic ultrasound or magnetic resonance imaging (MRI).

Tubo-Ovarian Abscess

Tubo-ovarian abscesses, a complication of acute salpingo-oophoritis, are usually unilateral and multilocular (20). The symptoms and signs are similar to those of acute salpingitis. A ruptured tubo-ovarian abscess is a life-threatening surgical emergency because gram-negative endotoxic shock can develop rapidly.

Signs

Vital signs reveal fever, tachycardia, and low blood pressure if the patient is septic. Tubo-ovarian abscesses can often be palpated on bimanual examination as firm, exquisitely tender, bilateral fixed masses. The abscesses can be palpated or "point" in the pelvic cul-de-sac and are appreciated on rectovaginal examination. Approximately 90% of patients will have abdominal or pelvic pain and 60% to 80% will present with fever and/or leukocytosis (21).

Diagnosis

The diagnostic imaging of choice for tubo-ovarian abscesses is ultrasound. CT with and without contrast can be used to establish the diagnosis. The differential diagnosis of a unilateral mass includes tubo-ovarian abscess and adnexal torsion, ectopic pregnancy, endometrioma, leaking ovarian cyst, and periappendiceal or diverticular abscess. If physical and ultrasound examination results are not definitive, laparoscopy or laparotomy must be performed.

Management

Tubo-ovarian abscesses should always be treated as an inpatient, and conservative medical therapy with broad spectrum antibiotics can be attempted (see Chapter 18). **In one study, this yielded a treatment success rate of 75%** (22). **If the patient is persistently febrile or not improving clinically, CT or ultrasound-guided drainage of the abscesses should be undertaken. CT-guided percutaneous drainage can be achieved transabdominally or transvaginally. Drainage along with intravenous antibiotics is considered first-line therapy** (23). If fertility is not desired, bilateral salpingo-oophorectomy and hysterectomy will provide definitive therapy.

A ruptured tubo-ovarian abscess rapidly leads to diffuse peritonitis, evidenced by tachycardia and rebound tenderness in all four quadrants of the abdomen. With endotoxic shock, hypotension and oliguria ensue, and the result can be fatal. Exploratory laparotomy with resection of infected tissue is mandatory (24) (see Chapter 18).

Uterine Leiomyomas

Leiomyomas (fibroids) are uterine smooth muscle tumors, as discussed in detail in Chapter 15. Discomfort may be present when myomas are in the broad ligament or encroaching on adjacent bladder, rectum, or supporting ligaments of the uterus. The discomfort is usually reported as noncyclic pressure or pain symptoms and less often, urinary frequency, dysmenorrhea, dyspareunia, or constipation. There is no association between degree of pain and fibroid volume or number (25).

Acute pelvic pain caused by uterine leiomyomas is rare but can develop if the myoma undergoes degeneration or torsion (26). Degeneration of myomas occurs secondary to loss of blood supply, usually attributable to rapid growth associated with pregnancy. **In a nonpregnant woman, degenerating uterine leiomyoma is often a misdiagnosis, because it can be confused with subacute salpingo-oophoritis.** A pedunculated subserosal leiomyoma can undergo torsion with ischemic necrosis and can be associated with pain similar to that of adnexal torsion. When a submucous leiomyoma becomes pedunculated within the endometrial cavity, the uterus contracts forcefully as if to expel a foreign body and the resulting pain is similar to that of labor. The cramping pain is usually associated with vaginal hemorrhage.

Signs

Vital signs are usually normal, although a low-grade temperature and mild tachycardia can be present with degeneration. Abdominal or bimanual examination and ultrasound reveal an irregular solid mass or masses arising from the uterus. If degeneration occurs, the inflammation can cause abdominal tenderness in response to palpation and mild localized rebound tenderness.

Diagnosis and Management

With degeneration there is usually leukocytosis. **Ultrasound can distinguish adnexal from uterine etiology of an eccentric mass.** If diagnosis is still uncertain, a pelvic MRI is more accurate (27). The fibroid can be excised laparoscopically; however, surgery is not mandatory. A submucous leiomyoma with pain and hemorrhage should be excised transcervically with hysteroscopic guidance.

Endometriosis-Related Acute Pain

In women with endometriosis, endometrial glands and stroma implant outside the uterine cavity, most commonly at the cul-de-sac, ovaries, or pelvic visceral and parietal peritoneum. Each menstrual cycle potentially results in further proliferation, causing inflammation, scarring, fibrosis, and adhesion formation. Women with endometriosis often experience dysmenorrhea, dyspareunia, and dyschezia, irregular bleeding, or subfertility. Acute pain attributable to endometriosis is usually premenstrual and menstrual; if nonmenstrual acute generalized pain occurs, a ruptured endometrioma (chocolate endometriotic cyst within the ovary) should be considered. **The management of endometriosis is discussed under dysmenorrhea and chronic pelvic pain** (see also Chapter 17).

Diagnosis

The abdomen is often tender in one or both the lower quadrants. Significant distention or rebound tenderness may be present if there is there is a ruptured endometrioma. Bimanual and rectovaginal examinations can reveal a fixed, retroverted uterus with tender nodules in the uterosacral region or thickening of the cul-de-sac. An adnexal mass, if present, usually is fixed to the broad ligament and cul-de-sac. The clinical diagnosis of endometriosis is accurate approximately 50% of the time. Definitive diagnosis is made by laparoscopy or laparotomy. In the setting of chronic pain symptoms, as noted above, with an acute exacerbation a leaking endometrioma should be suspected. If there is a characteristic mass on ultrasound, laparoscopy is indicated.

Gastrointestinal Tract Causes of Acute Pelvic Pain

Appendicitis

The most common intestinal source of acute pelvic pain in women is appendicitis. Lifetime incidence in the United States is 7%, and it is the most common cause of emergent abdominal surgery (28). The symptoms and signs of appendicitis can be similar to those of PID, but the nausea and emesis are often more prominent with appendicitis.

Symptoms

The first symptom of appendicitis is typically diffuse abdominal pain, periumbilical pain, followed by anorexia, nausea, and vomiting. Within a matter of hours, the pain generally shifts to the right lower quadrant. Fever, chills, emesis, and obstipation (no flatus or stool per rectum) may ensue. However, this classic symptom pattern is often absent. Atypical abdominal pain can occur when the appendix is retrocecal or entirely within the true pelvis (which occurs in 15% of the population). In this setting, tenesmus and diffuse suprapubic pain may occur.

Signs

A low-grade fever is generally present, but the temperature may be normal. High temperatures are typically seen with appendiceal perforation. **Local tenderness is usually elicited on palpation of the right lower quadrant (McBurney point). The appearance of severe generalized muscle guarding, abdominal rigidity, rebound tenderness, right-sided mass, tenderness on rectal examination, positive psoas sign (pain with forced hip flexion or passive extension of hip), and obturator signs (pain with passive internal rotation of flexed thigh) indicate appendicitis.** The pelvic examination usually does not show cervical motion or bilateral adnexal tenderness, but right-sided unilateral adnexal area tenderness can be present.

Diagnosis

Many patients with acute appendicitis have normal total leukocyte counts but a left shift is usually present. Ultrasound examination of the pelvic organs is normal, whereas the appendix may appear abnormal on ultrasound or CT with contrast. CT with oral contrast with normal filling of the appendix rules out appendicitis. Diagnostic laparoscopy can be useful to rule out other sources of pelvic pathology, but it may be difficult to visualize the appendix sufficiently to rule out early appendiceal inflammation, so appendectomy can be indicated if the diagnosis is uncertain.

Management

Initial management is intravenous administration of fluids, strict restriction of any oral intake, and preoperative antibiotics followed by laparoscopy or laparotomy. **Surgery with a false-positive rate of 15% is considered acceptable and is preferable to prolonged observation with the risk of rupture and peritonitis. Not only is a ruptured appendix life threatening, but it can have profound consequences for the fertility of women of reproductive age. With the advent of imaging, negative appendectomy rates are less than 10% (29).**

Acute Diverticulitis

Acute diverticulitis is a condition in which there is inflammation of a diverticulum or outpouching of the wall of the colon, usually involving the sigmoid colon. Diverticulitis typically affects postmenopausal women but can occur in women during their 30s and 40s.

Symptoms

The severe, left lower quadrant pain of diverticulitis can occur following a long history of symptoms of irritable bowel (bloating, constipation, and diarrhea), although diverticulosis usually is asymptomatic. Diverticulitis is less likely to lead to perforation and peritonitis than is appendicitis. Fever, chills, and constipation typically are present, but anorexia and vomiting are uncommon.

Signs

Bowel sounds are hypoactive and are substantially decreased with peritonitis related to a ruptured diverticular abscess. Abdominal examination reveals distention with left lower quadrant tenderness on direct palpation and localized rebound tenderness. Abdominal and bimanual rectovaginal examinations may reveal a poorly mobile, doughy inflammatory mass in the left lower quadrant. Leukocytosis and fever are common. Stool guaiac may be positive as a result of inflammation of the colon or microperforation.

Diagnosis and Management

CT with and without contrast is an important adjunct to history and physical examination (30). It will reveal a swollen, edematous bowel and can rule out an abscess. A barium enema is contraindicated. Diverticulitis is initially managed medically with intravenous administration of fluids, strict restriction of oral intake, and broad-spectrum intravenous antibiotics. A diverticular abscess, obstruction, fistula, or perforation requires general surgical intervention.

Intestinal Obstruction

The most common causes of intestinal obstruction in women are postsurgical adhesions, hernia formation, inflammatory bowel disease, or carcinoma of the bowel or ovary.

Symptoms

Intestinal obstruction is heralded by the onset of colicky abdominal pain followed by abdominal distention, vomiting, constipation, and obstipation. Higher and more acute obstruction results in early vomiting. Colonic obstruction presents with a greater degree of abdominal distention and obstipation. Vomiting first consists of gastric contents, followed by bile, then material with feculent odor, depending on the level of obstruction.

Signs

Fever is often present in the late stages. At the onset of mechanical obstruction, bowel sounds are high pitched and maximal during an episode of colicky pain. As the obstruction progresses, bowel sounds decrease and, when absent, suggest ischemic bowel. Marked abdominal distention often ensues.

Diagnosis and Management

An upright abdominal x-ray series shows a characteristic gas pattern, distended loops of bowel, and air fluid levels; and it helps to determine whether obstruction is partial or complete (no colonic gas seen). CT can be useful. White blood cell count will be elevated in patients with ischemic bowel. Complete obstruction requires surgical management, whereas partial obstruction often can be managed with intravenous fluids, bowel rest, and selective use of nasogastric suction. The cause of the obstruction should be determined and treated if possible. Underlying GI or reproductive tract malignancy may be present.

Urinary Tract Causes of Acute Pelvic Pain

Ureteral colic due to ureteral lithiasis is caused by a sudden increase in intraluminal pressure and associated inflammation. Urinary tract infections producing acute pain include cystitis and pyelonephritis. The most common microbes causing urinary tract infections are *Escherichia coli* followed by *Proteus*, *Klebsiella*, and *Pseudomonas* (31).

Symptoms and Signs

The pain of lithiasis is typically severe and crampy; it can radiate from the costovertebral angle to the groin. Hematuria is often present. Urinary tract infection (UTI) comprises bladder or kidney infection. Cystitis is associated with dull suprapubic pain, urinary frequency, urgency, dysuria, and occasionally hematuria. Pyelonephritis is associated with flank and costovertebral angle (CVA) pain, although lateralizing lower abdominal pain occasionally is present. Urethritis due to chlamydia or gonorrhea infection can have similar symptoms to those of a UTI. These infections must be ruled out if relevant.

Diagnosis

Diagnosis of stone can be made by urinalysis revealing red blood cells and demonstration of the stone via abdominal ultrasound, CT urography, or intravenous pyelography (uric acid stones may not be detected by CT). There is pain with firm pressure over the costovertebral angle in the case of lithiasis or pyelonephritis. Peritoneal signs are absent. Suprapubic tenderness may accompany cystitis.

The diagnosis of UTI is based on RUA revealing bacteria and leukocytes with or without leukocyte esterase and nitrites, in the absence of squamous epithelial cells. Findings can subsequently be confirmed by culture. The diagnostic thresholds for white blood cell count (WBC) and vaginal squamous cells vary with each laboratory. An elevated number of squamous cells in the urinary specimen suggests contamination of the urine specimen with vaginal secretions and can result in false-positive urine analysis and culture.

Management

Expectant medical treatment consists of oral hydration or intravenous fluids (if the patient is unable to tolerate oral intake), antibiotics for UTI, and pain control. Surgical management, such as lithotripsy or open surgery, is an option for renal and urethral lithiasis. Nonpregnant women (and pregnant women who are afebrile with a normal WBC count) with pyelonephritis and all women with cystitis can be treated on an outpatient basis. Nonpregnant women with pyelonephritis can be treated with a 14-day course of a *fluoroquinolone* or *trimethoprim/ sulfamethoxazole* (some recommend one intravenous dose of a third-generation cephalosporin before discharging patients with oral antibiotics) (see Chapter 18) (32). Caution should be used with *trimethoprim/sulfamethoxazole* given rising resistance patterns. It is important to follow up urine culture sensitivities and treat accordingly. If there is no improvement, raising concerns for patient compliance, inability to tolerate oral medications and fluids, or whether the patient may be immunocompromised as related to AIDS, intravenous drug use/abuse, diabetes, pregnancy, or chronic steroid use, then the patient should be hospitalized and given intravenous antibiotics.

Tuberculosis should be excluded as a cause of pyelonephritis if the characteristic sterile pyuria is present and the patient's condition does not improve with antibiotics.

Acute Pelvic Pain: Summary

All women of reproductive age with acute pelvic pain should have a complete blood count with differential, ESR, urinalysis, and a sensitive qualitative urine or serum pregnancy test. If not diagnosed expeditiously, an acute process can often result in significant morbidity or mortality. For patients who have chronic pelvic pain and develop acute exacerbation, it is important to rule out a superimposed acute process. Symptoms of fever, chills, diaphoresis, abnormal vaginal bleeding, dizziness, syncope, emesis, significant diarrhea, obstipation, dysuria, hematuria, and hematochezia, and/or signs of elevated temperature, tachycardia, orthostasis, abdominal distention, abnormal bowel sounds, ascites, peritonitis, or abnormal pregnancy are all indicative of an acute process.

Laboratory tests for the evaluation of acute pelvic pain include a CBC with differential, erythrocyte sedimentation rate, clean catch midstream RUA, gonorrhea and chlamydia nucleic acid amplification testing (NAAT) from cervix or urine, and urine or serum pregnancy test. The sedimentation rate is nonspecific, but often is the only abnormal laboratory finding in women with subacute PID. If the pregnancy test is positive, a quantitative β-human chorionic gonadotropin (βhCG) should be ordered. Other studies that are recommended include transvaginal pelvic ultrasound, or if imaging is not available, culdocentesis. The fluid from culdocentesis can be sent for hematocrit if bloody fluid is obtained or Gram stain with culture if the fluid is purulent. The presence of a mass in the cul-de-sac precludes culdocentesis. CT with and without contrast, abdominal x-rays, or upper or lower Gastrografin studies help rule out gastrointestinal pathology when gastrointestinal symptoms predominate. CT is useful for evaluation of retroperitoneal masses or abscesses related to the gastrointestinal tract. Pelvic MRI can be diagnostic if the pelvic ultrasound cannot determine whether a mass is uterine or adnexal.

Diagnostic laparoscopy is reserved for establishing the diagnosis in patients who have acute abdomen of uncertain cause, for elucidating the nature of an ambiguous adnexal mass, or for delineating whether a pregnancy is intrauterine or extrauterine (if ultrasound results and βhCG are equivocal). Visualization is hampered if diagnostic laparoscopy is performed for a large pelvic mass (>12 cm) and is relatively contraindicated in patients with peritonitis, severe ileus, or bowel obstruction. In these settings, laparotomy is preferable. The majority of patients with pelvic pain and a normal pelvic ultrasound have improvement or resolution of symptoms with conservative therapy and do not require surgical intervention (33).

Cyclic Pain: Primary and Secondary Dysmenorrhea

Dysmenorrhea is a common gynecologic disorder affecting as many as 60% of menstruating women (34). Primary dysmenorrhea refers to menstrual pain without pelvic pathology, whereas secondary dysmenorrhea is defined as painful menses associated with underlying pathology. Primary dysmenorrhea usually appears within 1 to 2 years of menarche, when ovulatory cycles are established. The disorder affects younger women but may persist into their 40s. Secondary dysmenorrhea usually develops years after menarche and can occur with anovulatory cycles. The differential diagnosis of secondary dysmenorrhea is outlined in Table 16.3 (2).

Primary Dysmenorrhea

The etiology of primary dysmenorrhea includes excessive or imbalanced amount of prostanoids secreted from the endometrium during menstruation. The prostanoids result in increased uterine contractions with a dysrhythmic pattern, increased basal tone and increased active pressure. Uterine hypercontractility, decreased uterine blood flow, and increased peripheral nerve hypersensitivity contribute to pain (35,36). Prostaglandin compounds are found in higher concentrations in secretory endometrium than in proliferative endometrium. The decline of progesterone levels in the late luteal phase triggers lytic enzymatic action, resulting in a release of phospholipids with the generation of arachidonic acid and activation of the cyclo-oxygenase (COX) pathway. The biosynthesis and metabolism of prostaglandins and thromboxane derived from arachidonic acid are depicted in Figure 16.1. Increased synthesis of prostanoids in women with primary dysmenorrhea results in higher uterine tone with high-amplitude contractions causing dysmenorrhea (36). It is theorized that women suffering from dysmenorrhea have up-regulated COX enzyme activity and prostanoid synthase activity. This led to the use of nonsteroidal anti-inflammatory drugs (NSAIDs), which act as COX enzyme inhibitors, for therapy (37).

Symptoms

The pain of primary dysmenorrhea usually begins a few hours before or just after the onset of a menstrual period and may last 48 to 72 hours. The pain is similar to labor, with suprapubic cramping, and may be accompanied by lumbosacral backache, pain radiating down the anterior thigh, nausea, vomiting, diarrhea, and rarely syncopal episodes. The pain of dysmenorrhea is colicky in nature and, unlike abdominal pain that is caused by chemical or infectious peritonitis, is relieved by abdominal massage, counter-pressure, or movement of the body.

Signs

On examination, the vital signs are normal. The suprapubic region may be tender to palpation. Bowel sounds are normal, and there is no upper abdominal tenderness and no abdominal rebound tenderness. **Bimanual examination at the time of the dysmenorrheic episode often reveals uterine tenderness; severe pain does not occur with movement of the cervix or palpation of the adnexal structures.** The pelvic organs are normal in primary dysmenorrhea.

Diagnosis

To diagnose primary dysmenorrhea, it is necessary to clinically rule out underlying pelvic pathology and confirm the cyclic nature of the pain. During the pelvic examination, the size, shape, and mobility of the uterus; the size and tenderness of adnexal structures; and the nodularity or fibrosis of uterosacral ligaments or rectovaginal septum should be assessed. NAAT for gonorrhea and chlamydia and if relevant, CBC and ESR, help rule out endometritis and subacute PID. Pelvic ultrasound should be performed if symptoms do not resolve with NSAIDs. If no abnormalities are found, a tentative diagnosis of primary dysmenorrhea can be established. Laparoscopy is not necessary at this point.

Table 16.3 Differential Diagnosis of Chronic Pelvic Pain

Gynecologic	Genitourinary
Noncyclic	Recurrent or relapsing cystourethritis
Adhesions	Urethral syndrome
Endometriosis	Interstitial cystitis/bladder pain syndrome
Salpingo-oophoritis	Ureteral diverticuli or polyps
Ovarian remnant or retained ovary syndrome	Carcinoma of the bladder
Pelvic congestion	Ureteral obstruction
Ovarian neoplasm benign or malignant	*Neurologic*
Pelvic relaxation	Nerve entrapment syndrome, neuroma, or other neuropathies
Cyclic	Trigger points
Primary dysmenorrhea	*Musculoskeletal*
Mittelschmerz	Myofascial pain and trigger points
Secondary dysmenorrhea	*Low-back pain syndrome*
Endometriosis/adenomyosis	Congenital anomalies
Uterine or vaginal anomalies with obstruction of menstrual outflow	Scoliosis and kyphosis
Intrauterine synechiae (Asherman syndrome)	Spondylolysis
Endometrial polyps or nonhormonal intrauterine device (IUD)	Spondylolisthesis
Uterine leiomyomata	Spinal injuries
Pelvic congestion syndrome	Inflammation
Gastrointestinal	Tumors
Irritable bowel syndrome	Osteoporosis
Ulcerative colitis	Degenerative changes
Crohn's disease	Coccydynia
Carcinoma	Myofascial syndrome
Infection	*Systemic*
Recurrent partial bowel obstruction	Fibromyalgia
Diverticulitis	Acute intermittent porphyria
Hernia	Abdominal migraine
Abdominal angina	Connective tissue disease including systemic lupus erythematosus
	Lymphoma
	Neurofibromatosis

Management

Prostaglandin synthase inhibitors, also called nonsteroidal anti-inflammatory agents, are effective for the treatment of primary dysmenorrhea (38). The inhibitors should be taken up to 1 to 3 days before or, if menses are irregular, at the first onset of even minimal pain or bleeding and then continuously every 6 to 8 hours to prevent reformation of prostaglandin by-products. The medication should be taken for the first few days of menstrual flow.

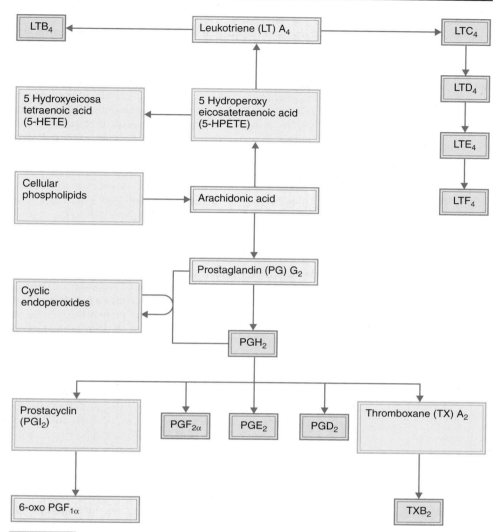

Figure 16.1   **The biosynthesis and metabolism of prostaglandins and thromboxane derived from arachidonic acid.**   (From **Chaudhuri G.** Physiologic aspects of prostaglandins and leukotrienes. *Semin Reprod Endocrinol* 1985;3:219, with permission.)

A 4- to 6-month course of therapy is warranted to determine whether the patient will respond to treatment. Changes in dosages and types of NSAIDs should be attempted if initial treatment is not successful. The medication may be contraindicated in patients with gastrointestinal ulcers or bronchospastic hypersensitivity to aspirin. Side effects are usually mild and include nausea, dyspepsia, diarrhea, and occasionally fatigue.

Hormonal contraceptives are indicated for primary dysmenorrhea unresponsive to NSAIDs or for patients with primary dysmenorrhea who have no contraindications to hormonal contraceptive and who desire contraception. Hormonal contraceptive agents (such as combined estrogen and progestin) or progesterone only oral contraceptives (either cyclic or continuous regimens), transdermal patch, vaginal ring, injectable progestin preparations, or levonorgestrel-releasing intrauterine devices are more effective than placebo alone and result in less absence from work or school (39). Continuous or extended cycle combined oral contraceptive pills are just as efficacious for this pain syndrome (40). Hormonal contraceptives inhibit ovulation, decrease endometrial proliferation, and create an endocrine milieu similar to the early proliferative phase of the menstrual cycle, when prostaglandin levels are lowest. Decreased prostaglandin levels result in less uterine cramping.

If the patient does not respond to this regimen, hydrocodone or codeine may be added for 2 to 3 days per month; before addition of the narcotic medication, psychological factors should be evaluated, and diagnostic laparoscopy to rule out pathology should be considered.

Nonpharmacologic pain management, in particular heat, acupuncture, or transcutaneous electrical nerve stimulation (TENS), may be useful (41–43). Acupuncture is thought to excite receptors or nerve fibers, blocking pain impulses through interactions with mediators like serotonin and endorphins. The perception of pain signals is altered with TENS. It does not directly affect uterine contractions. Abdominal electrical or chemical heating pads are effective in treating primary dysmenorrhea. A Cochrane review evaluated seven randomized controlled trials that used herbal and dietary therapies such as vitamins, minerals proteins, herbs, and fatty acids for relief of dysmenorrhea. There are insufficient data to support any herbal or vitamin regimen (42).

Methods used only rarely to treat primary dysmenorrhea include surgical laparoscopic uterine nerve ablation and presacral neurectomy and hysterectomy (44).

Secondary Dysmenorrhea

Secondary dysmenorrhea is cyclic menstrual pain that occurs in association with underlying pelvic pathology. The pain of secondary dysmenorrhea often begins 1 to 2 weeks before menstrual flow and persists until a few days after the cessation of bleeding. Underlying causes include endometriosis, adenomyosis, subacute endometritis and pelvic inflammatory disease, copper intrauterine devices (IUDs), ovarian cysts, congenital pelvic malformations, and cervical stenosis. Whereas the diagnosis of primary dysmenorrhea is based on history and presence of a normal pelvic examination and ultrasound, the diagnosis of secondary dysmenorrhea may require review of a pain diary to confirm cyclicity and, in addition to a transvaginal ultrasound examination, laparoscopy and/or hysteroscopy may be indicated.

The most common cause of secondary dysmenorrhea is endometriosis, followed by adenomyosis and nonhormonal intrauterine devices. NSAIDs and hormonal contraceptives are less likely to provide pain relief in women with secondary dysmenorrhea than in those with primary dysmenorrhea. The differential diagnosis of secondary dysmenorrhea is outlined in Table 16.3. The management of secondary dysmenorrhea is treatment of the underlying disorder.

Adenomyosis

Adenomyosis is defined as presence of endometrial stroma and glands within the myometrium, at least one low-power field from the basis of the endometrium, whereas endometriosis is characterized by ectopic endometrium appearing within the peritoneal cavity. Adenomyosis, endometriosis, and uterine leiomyomas frequently coexist. Although occasionally noted in women in their younger reproductive years, the average age of symptomatic women is usually older than 40 years. Increasing parity, early menarche, and shorter menstrual cycles may all be risk factors according to one study (45–47).

Symptoms

Symptoms typically associated with adenomyosis include excessively heavy or prolonged menstrual bleeding, dyspareunia, and dysmenorrhea. Symptoms often begin up to 2 weeks before the onset of a menstrual flow and may not resolve until after the cessation of menses.

Signs

The uterus is typically diffusely enlarged, although usually less than 14 cm in size, and is often soft and tender, particularly at the time of menses. Mobility of the uterus is not restricted, and there is no associated adnexal pathology (48).

Diagnosis

Adenomyosis is a clinical diagnosis. Imaging studies including pelvic ultrasound or MRI, although helpful, are not definitive. Because of the cost of MRI and negligible improvement in diagnostic accuracy, this study is not recommended routinely. In women with diffuse uterine enlargement and negative pregnancy test results, secondary dysmenorrhea may be attributed to adenomyosis; however, the pathologic confirmation of suspected adenomyosis can be made only at the time of hysterectomy.

Management

The management of adenomyosis depends on the patient's age and desire for future fertility. Relief of secondary dysmenorrhea caused by adenomyosis can be ensured after hysterectomy, but less invasive approaches can be tried initially. NSAIDs, hormonal contraceptives, and menstrual suppression using oral, intrauterine, or injected progestins or gonadotropin-releasing hormone agonists are all useful. Treatment follows the same protocol as treatment for endometriosis. Uterine artery embolization can be effective (49).

Endometriosis

In women with endometriosis, endometrial glands and stroma are found outside the uterine cavity, especially at the cul-de-sac, ovaries, and pelvic visceral and parietal peritoneum. Given that confirmation requires visual diagnosis, the prevalence of endometriosis is unknown. It is thought to occur in approximately 10% of the general female population, 15% to 20% of infertile women, and more than 30% of women with chronic pelvic pain. In some cases, regression can occur spontaneously (50). (See the section below on endometriosis under the heading of chronic pelvic pain and also Chapter 17.)

Symptoms

Patients typically complain of severe dysmenorrhea and cyclic pelvic pain that starts up to 2 weeks prior to menses. The pain can be sharp or pressurelike, localized to the midline or involving the lower abdomen, back, and rectum. Other symptoms include deep thrust dyspareunia, subfertility, irregular bleeding despite ovulatory cycles, and nongynecologic symptoms such as cyclic dyschezia, urinary urgency, frequency, bloating, and rarely hematochezia or hematuria.

Signs

Bimanual and rectovaginal examinations may reveal uterosacral nodularity and focal tenderness. Fibrosis resulting from endometriosis can cause a fixed retroverted uterus or laterally deviated cervix or uterus. Bimanual examination can demonstrate a fullness consistent with ovarian cystic endometrioma. Patients can have focal uterosacral or broad ligament area tenderness.

Diagnosis

The clinical diagnosis of endometriosis is accurate in approximately 50% of cases. Though a definitive diagnosis of endometriosis cannot be made on image studies, endometriomas are generally distinguishable from hemorrhagic corpus lutea by the appearance on ultrasound. Homogenous hemorrhagic appearing cysts that fail to resolve after one to two menstrual cycles are suspicious for endometriomas. CA125 can be elevated but is a nonspecific and nonsensitive marker for endometriosis. Definitive diagnosis is made by direct operative visualization either laparoscopically or via laparotomy. Active red flame, or colorless vesicles or petechial lesions usually indicate early disease, while powder-burn, fibrotic lesions suggest more longstanding lesions. Suspicious findings should be biopsied for confirmation. Deep infiltrating lesions and peritoneal windows are most often found within the posterior cul-de-sac, especially at the uterosacral ligaments, and may cause pain by penetrating the many nerve endings in this area (51). Patients with endometriosis have nerve fibers in their endometrial tissue, and studies show endometrial biopsy is a potential but as yet unproven diagnostic tool. A double-blind study of 99 women undergoing laparoscopy and endometrial biopsy for evaluation of endometrial nerve fibers found that the biopsy was just as effective as laparoscopy for diagnosing endometriosis (52).

Management of Secondary Dysmenorrhea Due to Endometriosis: Pharmacologic

Medications can be used to reduce the cyclic hormonal stimulation of these lesions and eventually decidualize or atrophy the lesions. No studies directly compared medical versus surgical management of endometriosis. However, given the excellent response rate, relatively low cost, and fair tolerability with hormonal therapy, an expert consensus panel recommended that women with suspected endometriosis who are not actively trying to conceive and who do not have an adnexal mass start with first-line medical management before laparoscopy. First-line treatment consists of a trial of NSAIDs with or without combined estrogen-progestin formulations (53). Both cyclic and continuous combined oral contraceptives (OCs) can be used with equal efficacy (54). Most studies used OCs containing low-dose estrogen and more androgenic progestins; however, newer generation progestins are also effective. For women who continue to have dysmenorrhea after using hormonal contraceptives in a cyclical fashion, continuous OCs regimen can be tried, without a hormonal break or with menstruation every 3 months.

Second-line medical therapy involves high-dose progestins or gonadotropin-releasing hormone (GnRH) analogues. This can be initiated for refractory symptoms or for patients with contraindication to estrogen. Progestins alone are associated with few metabolic concerns and are safe and inexpensive alternatives to surgical intervention. Progestins or progestins plus estrogen effectively manage pain symptoms in approximately three-quarters of the women with endometriosis (55). High-dose *medroxyprogesterone acetate* and *norethindrone acetate* are equally effective to the GnRH analogues (56). Progestins should be given at a dose to achieve amenorrhea, then the dose can be tapered to control symptoms.

A randomized controlled trial comparing *levonorgestrel* intrauterine system (LNG-IUS) with depot GnRH for the treatment of endometriosis-related chronic pain found that both were effective treatments (57).

Androgenic hormones such as danazol are thought to inhibit the luteinizing hormone surge and steroidogenesis and may have anti-inflammatory effects. These medications increase free testosterone, resulting in possible side effects such as deepening of voice, weight gain, acne, and hirsutism. Vaginal *danazol* in lower doses may be effective.

GnRH agonist and add-back treatment can be used as pharmacologic treatments for endometriosis (58). A randomized-controlled trial of GnRH agonist therapy for 6 months in cases of confirmed endometriosis showed decreased size of endometriotic lesions and pain symptoms. Side effects are related to the hypoestrogenic state and include vasomotor symptoms, mood swings, vaginal dryness, decreased libido, myalgias, and, eventually, bone loss. These side effects can be reduced with supplemental calcium and hormonal add-back therapy with *norethindrone acetate* 2 to 5 mg daily with or without low-dose estrogen (0.625 mg of conjugated estrogen or 1 mg of 17 β-estradiol) (58). Given the side effects, GnRH agonists usually are not used for more than 8 to 12 months, but with add-back hormones and/or bisphosphonate, GnRH therapy can be considered for use for more than 1 year. Recurrence of symptoms after discontinuation of GnRH agonist ranges from 36% to 70% 5 years after completion of treatment.

Aromatase p-450 and prostaglandin E2 (PgE_2) pathways are thought to be involved in the genesis of endometriotic implants. Aromatase plays an important role in estrogen biosynthesis by catalyzing the conversion of androstenedione and testosterone to estrone and estradiol. Although aromatase activity is not detectable in normal endometrium, it is found in eutopic endometrium and endometriotic lesions. Thus, aromatase inhibitors (AIs) are now being used as adjunctive therapy with medical therapies in refractory cases (59). A 2008 review of eight studies evaluated AIs for management of endometriosis and found that AIs combined with progestins or OCs or GnRH analogues decreased mean pain scores and lesion size and improved quality of life. In the only randomized controlled trial (97 women) evaluated in this meta-analysis, aromatase inhibitor (*anastrozole*) in combination with GnRH agonist significantly improved pain ($P <0.0001$) compared with GnRH agonist alone at 6-month follow-up, and there was no significant reduction in spine or hip bone density (60).

Management of Endometriosis: Surgical

Laparoscopy and laparotomy are appropriate and for some patients, they are the preferred treatment for the management of secondary dysmenorrheal pain related to endometriosis that is unresponsive to hormonal agents (see also Chapter 17). Excellent operative skill is required to manage endometriosis surgically. Endometriotic lesions should be ablated or resected. Endometriomas must be removed with their capsule. Resection of endometriomas by ovarian cystectomy improves pain and fertility in women with chronic pelvic pain and endometriosis when compared to fenestration, drainage, and coagulation. In a randomized controlled trial of laser ablation for minimal to moderate endometriosis, over 90% of women felt improved at 1-year follow-up, and 87% of women with stage III to IV endometriosis were satisfied with the results at 1-year follow-up. Recurrent pain after 24 months is close to 50% (61).

In women who no longer desire fertility with severe secondary dysmenorrhea, hysterectomy with bilateral salpingo-oophorectomy (BSO) and removal of endometriosis lesions is the preferred treatment. Hysterectomy without BSO results in a higher rate of disease recurrence and a 30% reoperation rate. The risk of recurrent endometriosis with hormone replacement is small if combined estrogen-progestin preparations are used and unopposed estrogen is avoided.

There are limited data regarding outcomes for repeated conservative surgical procedures, including pelvic denervating procedures (61). The authors conclude that although re-operation is often considered the best option, the long-term outcome appears suboptimal with a cumulative probability of recurrent pain between 20% and 40% and of a further surgical procedure of at least 20%. Hysterectomy with BSO decreased the need for re-operation to treat pelvic pain by sixfold. Postoperative medical treatment with OCs can be effective (62). Re-operation in a symptomatic patient after previous conservative surgery should take into account the psychological state of the patient, desire for future fertility, and whether the pain responded to prior surgical therapy with at least 1, but preferably 3 to 5 years of pain relief.

Rectovaginal endometriosis is often deeply infiltrating, highly innervated, and associated with severe cyclic pelvic pain and dyspareunia (see also Chapter 17). These lesions can be surgically challenging for laparoscopic resection. Hormonal therapy can be effective. Vercellini et al. (63) reviewed hormonal therapy in 217 patients: 68 in five observational studies, 59 in a cohort study, and 90 in a randomized controlled trial (63). The study compared aromatase inhibitor, vaginal *danazol*, GnRH agonist, intrauterine progestin, and two estrogen-progestin combinations, transvaginally or transdermally and an oral progestin. With the exception of an aromatase inhibitor used alone, the pain relief with medical therapies was satisfactory over the 6- to 12-month course of the treatment, with 60% to 90% of women reporting substantial decrease or complete relief from pain symptoms.

Chronic Pelvic Pain

Chronic pelvic pain (CPP) is defined as pelvic pain that persists in the same location for greater than 6 months' duration, causing functional disability or requiring treatment (64). **CPP is an inclusive, general term that encompasses many more specific causes, ranging from reproductive, gastrointestinal, and urinary tract etiologies to myofascial pain and nerve entrapment syndromes.** Chronic pelvic pain affects 12% to 20% of women in the United States. The differential diagnosis of CPP is outlined in Table 16.3. Nongynecologic causes of pain, such as irritable bowel syndrome, interstitial cystitis/bladder pain syndrome, abdominal wall or pelvic floor myofascial syndrome, or neuropathy, are frequently overlooked but common causes of chronic pelvic pain. This can in part explain why 60% to 80% of patients undergoing laparoscopy for chronic pelvic pain have no intraperitoneal pathology (2).

Patients with CPP are often anxious and depressed. Their marital, sexual, social, and occupational lives are disrupted. These patients frequently have poor treatment outcomes from traditionally effective gynecologic and medical therapy and may undergo multiple unsuccessful surgical procedures for pain. About 12% to 19% of hysterectomies are performed for pelvic pain, and 30% of patients who present to pain clinics have had a hysterectomy (65).

CPP states are characterized by up-regulation of central nervous system (CNS) responsiveness to peripheral stimuli. **The relationship between the pain and pathology, such as endometriosis, adhesions, or venous congestion, is inconsistent and treatment is associated with pain recurrence. Recent investigations suggest that "plasticity" of the nervous system or alterations in signal processing may be involved in the maintenance of chronic pain states** (2,6). Maladaptive changes within the peripheral and central nervous system predispose to allodynia (pain with usually nonpainful stimuli), hyperalgesia (excessive pain with a potentially painful stimulus), widening of the receptive field (pain experienced over a larger territory), and abnormal reflex responses in surrounding musculature (5–7).

The spinal cord is not a simple conduit between the periphery and the brain. It is an important site of "gating" mechanisms, such as excitation, inhibition, convergence, and summation of neural stimuli (66). With visceral tissue injury, a subset of nociceptive C-fibers that are usually dormant, called "silent" afferents, can become activated. The dorsal horn of the spinal cord is then flooded with noxious chemical stimuli that, over time, can lead to up-regulation of the signaling in the dorsal horn and brain, and pain sensation can be persistent and amplified, even after the peripheral pathology has resolved. The dorsal horn neurons demonstrate a number of electrophysiologic changes in this setting, such as the development of spontaneous activity, enlarged receptive fields, and lowered threshold for firing.

In chronic pain states, the pain is no longer adaptive. The initial painful input produces a persistent abnormal state of increased responsiveness called central sensitization (67). It is not known why in some individuals or in certain settings, prolonged stimuli or injury will result in sensitization. Different regions of the CNS are important in modulating the sensory and affective components of the pain response. Pain persistence is fostered by adverse or traumatic early experience, conditioning, fear, arousal, depression, and anxiety.

Evaluation of Chronic Pelvic Pain

On the first visit, a thorough pain history should be performed, taking into consideration the nature of each pain symptom: location, radiation, severity, aggravating and alleviating factors; effect of menstrual cycle, stress, work, exercise, intercourse, and orgasm; the context in which pain arose; and the social and occupational toll of the pain (Table 16.4). A visual or verbal analog pain scale to record pain severity 0 through 10 and stating "no pain" and "worst possible pain" is important in assessing the severity of pain and comparing the changes in severity over subsequent visits. The evaluation should include a comprehensive questionnaire that addresses depression, anxiety, emotional, physical and sexual trauma, quality of life, and criteria to assist with the diagnosis of irritable bowel syndrome and interstitial cystitis or bladder pain syndrome. The International Pelvic Pain Society published a comprehensive pain assessment tool in order to facilitate the history and physical examination, which can be found on the International Pelvic Pain Society's Web site and reprinted and reproduced (68).

Diagrams of a woman's abdomen, back, and genital area should be used to help the patient define the location of pain (2). The patient should be questioned about symptoms specific to the types of pathology listed in Table 16.3.

1. **Genital** (abnormal vaginal bleeding, abnormal vaginal discharge, dysmenorrhea, dyspareunia, sub-fertility, sexual functioning)
2. **Enterocoelic** (constipation, diarrhea, flatulence, hematochezia, and relationship of pain to times of altered bowel function or form and pain relief with bowel movements)
3. **Musculoskeletal/neuropathic** (physical trauma—surgical or injury, exacerbation with exercise or postural changes, weakness, numbness, lancinating pain)

Table 16.4 Pain History Mneumonic	
OLD CAARTS	Pain History
Onset	When and how did pain start? Did it change over time?
Location	Localize specifically. Can you put a finger on it?
Duration	How long does it last?
Characteristic	Cramping, aching, stabbing, burning. "like lightening," tingling, itching
Alleviating/Aggravating factors	What makes it better (medication, stress reduction, heat/ice, position change) or worse (specific activity, stress, menstrual cycle)?)
Associated symptoms	Gynecologic (dyspareunia, dysmenorrhea, abnormal bleeding, discharge, infertility), GI (constipation, diarrhea, bloating, gas, rectal bleeding), GU (frequency, dysuria, urgency, incontinence), Neurologic (specific nerve distribution)
Radiation	Does it move to other areas (dermatomal)?
Temporal	What time of day (elation to menstrual cycle and activities of daily living)?
Severity	Scale of 0–10

GI, gastrointestinal; GU, genitourinary. From **Rapkin AJ, Howe CN.** Chronic pelvic pain: a review. In: *Family practice recertification.* Monroe Township, New Jersey: Medical World Communications, 2006; 28:59–67.

4. **Urologic** (urgency, frequency, nocturia, hesitancy, dysuria, hematuria, incontinence)

5. **Psychological** (previous diagnoses, hospitalizations, and medications, current depression, anxiety, panic, including suicidal ideation, past and current emotional, physical, or sexual trauma)

Record a thorough gynecological, medical, and surgical history; medication, ethanol, or recreational drug intake; prior evaluations for pain with outcome; and review prior operative and pathology reports. Prior physical, emotional, and sexual trauma or abuse should be ascertained (69–71). The attitude of the patient and her family toward the pain, resultant behavior of the patient and her family, and current upheavals in the patient's life should be discussed. The part of the history relating to sensitive issues may have to be revisited after establishing rapport with the patient.

Whatever the original cause of the pain, when pain has persisted for any length of time, it is likely that other psychosocial factors are now contributing to the maintenance of the pain. Pain is commonly accompanied by anxiety and depression, and these conditions need to be carefully assessed and treated (2,72,73). In a typical gynecologic setting, referral to a psychologist or psychiatrist for parallel evaluation can evoke resistance. The inference is drawn that the referring physician is ascribing the pain to psychological causes. The patient needs to understand the reason for this referral and to be reassured that it is a routine and necessary part of the evaluation. **A psychologist is one of the key personnel in a multidisciplinary pain clinic.**

A complete physical examination should be performed, with particular attention directed to the abdominal and lumbosacral areas, vulva, pelvic floor, and internal organs via vaginal, bimanual, and rectovaginal examination. The examination should include the *Carnett test,* which is an evaluation of the painful sites on the abdominal wall before and after tensing of the abdominal muscles (head raised off the table or with bilateral straight leg raise) to differentiate abdominal wall and visceral sources of pain. Abdominal wall pain is augmented and visceral pain is diminished with palpating the tender points after these maneuvers (74). While standing, the patient should be examined for hernias, both abdominal (inguinal and femoral) and pelvic (cystocele and enterocele). An attempt should be made to locate by palpation the tissues that reproduce the patient's pain. If abdominal wall sources of pain are noted, it is useful to block these areas with injection of local anesthetics and then perform the pelvic examination (74). Neuropathic symptoms (sharp or lancinating or electrical pain, burning, or tingling sensations) should be localized to the peripheral nerve subserving the involved area.

Reproductive Tract

The most common findings noted at the time of laparoscopy for CPP are endometriosis and adhesions. Patients with other gynecologic pathology, such as benign or malignant ovarian cysts, uterine leiomyomas of size sufficient to encroach on supporting ligaments or other somatic structures, or significant pelvic relaxation should be evaluated and treated in a manner that is appropriate for the underlying condition. Pain associated with these latter conditions is generally not severe, and appropriate surgical management is therapeutic.

Endometriosis

See the section on secondary dysmenorrhea above and for a more thorough discussion of the diagnosis and management of endometriosis refer to Chapter 17.

Endometriosis can be demonstrated in 15% to 40% of patients undergoing laparoscopy for chronic pelvic pain. Endometriosis is a surgical diagnosis based on identification and histology of characteristic lesions (75). Endometriosis produces a low-grade inflammatory reaction; over time this results in adhesions between confluent pelvic organs (76). However, the cause of the pain is not well established. **There is no correlation between the location of disease and pain symptoms** (77,78). **There appears to be no relationship between the incidence and severity of pain or the stage of the endometriotic lesions, and as many as 30% to 50% of patients have no pain regardless of stage. Similarly, 40% to 60% of patients have no tenderness on examination regardless of stage** (78). Deeply infiltrating endometriosis lesions that involve the rectovaginal septum and the bowel, ureters, and bladder are strongly associated with pain (76,79,80). Pelvic adhesions related to endometriosis are a predictor of pelvic pain (81). Vaginal and uterosacral deep lesions are associated with dyspareunia and dyschezia.

Prostaglandin E and $F_{2\alpha}$ production from explants of petechial lesions present in mild, low-stage disease was found to be significantly greater than from the explants of powder-burn or black lesions, which are more common in patients with higher-stage endometriosis. Prostaglandin and cytokine production may account for severe pain in some patients with mild disease. More importantly, endometriotic implants acquire a vascular and nerve supply that may contribute to peripheral and central nervous system sensitization and persistence of pain even after surgical therapy (82–84).

Endometriosis-related pain syndrome is a new and evolving concept that is defined as pain that does not respond adequately to appropriate medical and surgical therapy, especially in the setting of minimal or mild disease. In this situation, neural plasticity results from central sensitization, hypothetically initiated by the peripheral inflammatory insult (83). The disease is no longer just the endometriosis, but is fostered by the alterations in the peripheral and CNS. Endometriosis-related pain syndrome is often co-existent or "co-morbid" with other chronic conditions such as bladder pain syndrome/interstitial cystitis (BPS/IC), irritable bowel syndrome (IBS), myofascial pain, fibromyalgia and vulvodynia, and anxiety disorders. These disorders need to be managed concurrently.

Adhesions

Adhesions noted at the time of laparoscopy may be in the same general region of the abdomen as the source of the pelvic pain; however, neither the specific location (i.e., adnexa structures, parietal, visceral peritoneum, or bowel) nor density of the adhesions correlates consistently with the presence of pain symptoms (85,86). In one nonrandomized, noncontrolled study of adhesion lysis, a subgroup of women with anxiety, depression, multiple somatic symptoms, and social and occupational disruption responded poorly to adhesiolysis. The group without these characteristics had significant improvement in pain (87). Prospective randomized controlled trials do not support adhesiolysis for women with CPP. A randomized controlled trial of laparoscopic adhesiolysis showed an improvement in both the groups (i.e., laparoscopy with and laparoscopy without lysis of adhesions), suggesting a large placebo effect (88–90). One randomized controlled trial that did not consistently demonstrate a significant long-term reduction in pain did find some improvement if the adhesions were dense and involved the small bowel (91).

Most women with adhesions had a prior surgical procedure with possible injury to abdominal wall nerves, such as the iliohypogastric or ilioinguinal nerves, and those are more likely to be the cause of the pain. The abdominal wall must be carefully evaluated for myofascial or nerve injury, or entrapment, as the source of pain before assuming that adhesions contribute to the genesis of pain.

Diagnosis

Diagnostic laparoscopy is recommended if GI, GU, and myofascial and neuropathic causes are ruled out or treated and the results of the psychological evaluation are negative. Mini-laparoscopy using local anesthesia and conscious sedation is used to perform "conscious pain mapping," whereby specific adhesions are tweaked and pelvic pain response is recorded (92). In an observational study of 50 women using local anesthesia, manipulation of appendiceal and pelvic adhesions contributed to pelvic pain. However, lysis of these adhesions did not improve outcomes over traditional laparoscopic therapy (2,11).

Management

The causal role of adhesions in the genesis of pelvic pain is uncertain, and surgery will lead to further adhesion formation and perhaps organ injury. Therefore, lysis is not recommended unless there is intermittent partial bowel obstruction or infertility. Although some observational studies showed that laparoscopic lysis of adhesions can alleviate chronic pelvic pain, randomized controlled trials have not revealed any long-term benefit. If surgery is performed, barrier materials such as oxidized regenerated cellulose or hyaluronic acid with carboxymethylcellulose can be used for prevention of adhesion re-formation. Repeated surgical procedures for lysis of adhesions are not indicated.

Pelvic Congestion

Pelvic congestion syndrome involves congestion or dilation of uterine and/or ovarian venous plexuses (93–97). First proposed in the 1950s, this condition was a suggested result of emotional stress that could lead to smooth muscle spasm and congestion of ovarian and uterine pelvic venous plexuses. A subsequent blind study was undertaken to compare results of transuterine venography in patients with unexplained CPP and negative laparoscopy with controls (97). This study demonstrated that women with CPP had a larger mean ovarian vein diameter, delayed disappearance of contrast medium, and greater ovarian plexus congestion compared to controls. The existence of this condition is controversial.

Signs and Symptoms

Pelvic congestion affects women of reproductive age. Typical symptoms include bilateral lower abdominal and back pain that is increased with standing for long periods, secondary dysmenorrhea, dyspareunia, abnormal uterine bleeding, chronic fatigue, and irritable bowel symptoms (97). Pain usually begins with ovulation and lasts until the end of menses. The uterus is often bulky, and the ovaries are enlarged with multiple functional cysts. The uterus, parametria, and uterosacral ligaments are tender.

Diagnosis

Transuterine venography is the primary method for diagnosis, although other modalities, such as pelvic ultrasound, magnetic resonance imaging, and laparoscopy, may disclose varicosities (93). Because of the cost and possible side effects of treatment, further management should be based on related symptoms and not simply on the presence of varicosities.

Management

Treatment of suspected pelvic congestion ranges from the less invasive hormonal suppression and cognitive behavioral pain management to the more invasive ovarian vein embolization or hysterectomy and salpingo-oophorectomy (93–97). Low-estrogen, progestin-dominant continuous oral contraceptives, high-dose progestins, and GnRH analogues often provide pain relief (94). Hormonal suppression should be the initial mode of treatment for women with suspected pelvic congestion. *Medroxyprogesterone acetate,* 30 mg daily, is useful (95). A multidisciplinary approach incorporating psychotherapy, behavioral pain management, or both is highly recommended. Percutaneous transcatheter embolization can be considered for women who do not respond to medical or hormonal therapy (96,97). Technically more invasive, transcatheter embolotherapy selectively catheterizes the ovarian and internal iliac veins, followed by contrast venography and embolization. This treatment showed some promise in small uncontrolled studies, but larger randomized controlled trials are necessary to validate its benefits. For women who have completed their childbearing, hysterectomy with oophorectomy is a reasonable option if multidisciplinary management has failed (97).

Subacute Salpingo-oophoritis

Patients with salpingo-oophoritis usually present with symptoms and signs of acute infection. Atypical or partially treated infection may not be associated with fever or peritoneal signs. Subacute or atypical salpingo-oophoritis is often a sequel of chlamydia or mycoplasma infection. Abdominal tenderness, cervical motion, and bilateral adnexal tenderness are typical of pelvic infection (see Chapter 18).

Ovarian Remnant and Residual Ovary Syndromes

In a reproductive-aged patient who has had a bilateral salpingo-oophorectomy, with or without a hysterectomy, for severe endometriosis or PID, chronic pelvic pain may be caused by ovarian remnant syndrome. **This syndrome results from residual ovarian cortical tissue that is left in situ after a difficult dissection in an attempt to perform an oophorectomy. This tissue can become encased in adhesions and result in painful cysts.** Often, the patient had multiple pelvic operations with the uterus and adnexa removed sequentially. Laparoscopic oophorectomy, combined with a difficult dissection, is a strong risk factor.

Residual ovary syndrome is uncommon considering the number of women undergoing hysterectomy with ovarian preservation. **Theoretically, after a hysterectomy with one or both ovaries intentionally left in situ, adhesions develop and encase the ovaries, then cyclical expansion of the ovaries can result in pain and, in some cases, a tender persistent mass.**

Symptoms

The patient usually reports lateralizing pelvic pain, often cycling with ovulation or the luteal phase that is described as sharp and stabbing or constant, dull, and nonradiating, occasionally with associated genitourinary or gastrointestinal symptoms. Symptoms tend to arise 2 to 5 years after initial oophorectomy. A tender mass in the lateral region of the pelvis is pathognomonic. The patient may report deep dyspareunia, constipation, or flank pain.

Diagnosis

Ultrasonography usually confirms a mass with the characteristics of ovarian tissue. The accuracy of ultrasound can be improved by treating the patient with a 5- to 10-day course of *clomiphene citrate*, 100 mg daily, to stimulate follicular development. In a patient who has had bilateral salpingo-oophorectomy and is not taking hormone therapy, estradiol and follicle-stimulating hormone (FSH) assays reveal a characteristic premenopausal picture (FSH <40 mIU/mL and estradiol >20 pg/mL), although on occasion the remaining ovarian tissue may not be active enough to suppress FSH levels (98). The patient may have a persistent estrogenized state based on the vulvar and vaginal examination and lack postmenopausal symptoms such as hot flashes, night sweats, and mood changes. Medical therapy that suppresses ovarian function can be diagnostic and therapeutic.

Management

Initial medical treatment with high-dose progestins or oral contraceptives usually provides good results. Patients also experience pain relief with a GnRH agonist, although these medications are impractical for long-term therapy. Those who achieve relief with GnRH agonists also experience relief with subsequent surgery (99). Laparoscopic examination usually is not productive because the ovarian mass may be missed or adhesions may prevent accurate diagnosis. A few articles documented successful laparoscopic treatment of this condition (100,101). Removal of the remnant ovarian tissue is necessary for treatment, and the corrective surgery tends to be arduous, with risks of cystotomy, enterotomy, and postoperative small bowel obstruction (98). Surgical pathology usually reveals the presence of ovarian tissue, sometimes with endometriosis, corpus lutea or follicle cysts, and fibrous adhesions. *Clomiphene citrate* can be used 7 to 10 days before surgery to induce folliculogenesis, allowing ovarian tissue to be more easily detected.

Gastroenterologic Etiology

The uterus, cervix, and adnexa share visceral innervation with the lower ileum, sigmoid colon, and rectum. These pain signals travel through sympathetic nerves to spinal cord segments T10 to L1. It is often difficult, therefore, to determine whether lower abdominal pain is of gynecologic or enterocoelic origin. Skillful medical history and examination are necessary to distinguish gynecologic from gastrointestinal causes of pain. Inflammatory bowel disease, such as Crohn's disease or ulcerative colitis, infectious enterocolitis, intestinal neoplasms, appendicitis, and hernia must be ruled out with appropriate history and physical examination, complete blood cell count, and stool cultures and visualization of colonic mucosa when appropriate.

IBS is one of the more common causes of lower abdominal pain and may account for up to 60% of referrals to the gynecologist for chronic pelvic pain. An estimated 35% of patients with chronic pelvic pain have a concurrent diagnosis of IBS (102,103). Women who had a hysterectomy for chronic pelvic pain are twice as likely to have IBS. The pathophysiology of IBS appears to be influenced by central nervous system sensitization and decreased descending inhibition, which ultimately leads to the visceral hypersensitivity. Visceral hypersensitivity and abnormal reflex responses, demonstrated in both animal and human studies, results in an increased intensity of pain, lowered threshold for sensation, and an enlarged viscera-somatic region of pain referral, all of which lead to the IBS symptoms (104,105).

Symptoms

The predominant symptom of IBS is abdominal pain. Other symptoms include abdominal distention, excessive flatulence, alternating diarrhea and constipation, increased pain before a bowel movement, decreased pain after a bowel movement, and pain exacerbated by events that increase gastrointestinal motility, such as eating, stress, anxiety, depression, and menses. The pain is usually intermittent, occasionally constant, cramp-like, and more likely to occur in the left lower quadrant. The patient with IBS can be placed into one of three categories: constipation-predominant, diarrhea-predominant, and pain-predominant (alternating bowel habits) depending on their main symptoms. The new Rome III criteria for diagnosis

Table 16.5 Rome III Criteria for Irritable Bowel Syndrome

At least 3 days per month of recurrent abdominal pain or discomfort for the previous 3 months, has associated with two of three features:

1. Relieved with defecation; and/or
2. Onset associated with a change in frequency of stool; and/or
3. Onset associated with a change in form (appearance) of stool.

(Table 16.5) includes at least 3 days of recurrent abdominal pain or discomfort per month over the past 3 months with at least two of the following features: relief with defecation, onset associated with change in stool frequency, or onset associated with change in form and appearance of stool (106).

Signs

On physical examination, the findings of a palpable tender sigmoid colon or discomfort during insertion of the finger into the rectum and hard feces in the rectum are suggestive of IBS.

Diagnosis

The diagnosis of IBS is usually based on history and physical examination, and although suggestive, especially in young women, the findings are not specific. A CBC, thyroid function study, stool sample to test for white cells and occult blood, and sigmoidoscopy or colonoscopy or barium enema are usually required, particularly in older individuals and in young individuals who have not responded to initial treatment. The results of these studies are all normal in patients with IBS.

Management

Treatment consists of reassurance, education, stress reduction, bulk-forming agents and other symptomatic treatments, and low-dose tricyclic antidepressants. A multidisciplinary management approach consisting of medical and psychological approaches is recommended. Patients should eliminate triggers in their diet, such as food containing lactose, sorbitol, alcohol, fat, and fructose. Products that contain caffeine can cause abdominal bloating, cramping, and more frequent bowel movements. After the patient has tried these lifestyle changes, if she remains symptomatic, a short-term trial of antispasmodics such as *dicyclomine* or *hyoscyamine* can be given (105). Multidisciplinary therapy addresses the cognitive, affective, and behavioral components of the pain. Therapy may decrease the intensity of nociceptor stimulation as well as change the patient's interpretation of the meaning of pain (105).

Antispasmodic agents relax the smooth muscle and reduce contractility of the gastrointestinal tract. While antispasmodics and laxatives may produce symptomatic relief of bowel symptoms, the pain symptoms of IBS may respond to antidepressants. Low-dose tricyclic antidepressants (TCAs) can alleviate the pain of IBS as shown in a number of randomized controlled trials. TCAs can also reduce excessive gastrointestinal contractility and are approved for use as antispasmodics. TCAs may be used for women with moderate to severe pain, who were refractory to other therapies. Although the dose to achieve the analgesic response is much lower than that used for antidepressive effects, TCAs may be increased to higher dosages in patients with co-existing depression. Selective serotonin reuptake inhibitors (SSRIs) and serotonin/norepinephrine reuptake inhibitors (SNRIs) were used successfully in the treatment of IBS and can be used in those patients failing TCA treatment or those who are depressed or are unable to tolerate the side effects of TCAs.

Urologic Etiology

Chronic pelvic pain of urologic origin may be related to recurrent cystourethritis, urethral syndrome, sensory urgency of uncertain cause, and interstitial cystitis/bladder pain. With an appropriate diagnostic workup, infiltrating bladder tumors, ureteral obstruction, renal lithiasis, and endometriosis can easily be ruled out as possible causes.

Urethral Syndrome

Urethral syndrome is defined as a symptom complex including dysuria, frequency and urgency of urination, suprapubic discomfort, and often dyspareunia in the absence of any abnormality of the urethra or bladder (107). The cause of urethral syndrome is uncertain and is attributed to a subclinical infection, urethral obstruction, and psychogenic and allergic factors. The symptoms of urethral syndrome may actually evolve into the initial stages of interstitial cystitis.

Symptoms

Urinary urgency, frequency, suprapubic pressure, and other less frequent symptoms such as bladder or vaginal pain, urinary incontinence, postvoid fullness, dyspareunia, and suprapubic pain are commonly observed.

Signs

Physical and neurologic examinations should be performed. Anatomic abnormalities, including pelvic relaxation, urethral caruncle, and hypoestrogenism, should be evaluated. The patient should be evaluated for vaginitis. The urethra should be carefully palpated to detect purulent discharge.

Diagnosis

A clean catch or catheterized urine specimen for routine urinalysis and culture should be obtained to rule out urinary tract infection. As indicated, urethral and cervical studies for chlamydia should be obtained, and a wet prep for vaginitis should be performed. Urethral syndrome should be considered if infection is ruled out, the evaluation does not disclose vulvovaginitis, and no allergic phenomenon causing contact dermatitis of the urethra can be detected. The possibility of ureoplasma, chlamydia, candida, trichomonas, gonorrhea, and herpes should be eliminated. Cystoscopic evaluation should be performed to rule out urethral diverticulum, stones, and cancer. Pelvic floor muscles should be evaluated, as spasm of these muscles can lead to urethral pain and tenderness. The urethral pain can also be a manifestation of bladder pain syndrome.

Management

Various forms of therapy are suggested for urethral syndrome. Those patients in whom no infectious agent is present but who have sterile pyuria may respond to a 2- to 3-week course of *doxycycline* or *erythromycin*. Long-term, low-dose antimicrobial prophylaxis often is used in women with urgency and frequency symptoms who had careful documentation of recurrent urinary tract infections. Some of these women may continue to have symptoms when their urine is not infected, and bacterial infection redevelops over time. Posttreatment test of cure cultures are useful. It is recommended that all postmenopausal women with this condition be given a trial of local estrogen therapy for at least 2 months. If there is no improvement after antibiotic or estrogen therapy, physical therapy, and cognitive-behavioral therapy, then urethral dilation can be considered but recent studies are lacking. Positive results were noted with biofeedback techniques. Other treatments including acupuncture and laser therapy proved successful (108). Psychological support is very important in this group of women. Management requires a multidisciplinary approach, as is true of chronic pelvic pain in general.

Interstitial Cystitis/ Bladder Pain Syndrome or Painful Bladder Syndrome

Interstitial cystitis (IC)/bladder pain syndrome occurs more often in women than men. Most patients are between 40 and 60 years of age. In 2002, painful bladder disorders were defined by the International Continence Society (ICS) in a set of new recommendations (109). The most widely used definition, **painful bladder syndrome (PBS) is described as a clinical syndrome (i.e., a complex of symptoms) consisting of "suprapubic pain related to bladder filling, accompanied by other symptoms, such as increased daytime and nighttime frequency in the absence of proven infection or other obvious pathology." By comparison, the term "interstitial cystitis" refers to patients who have PBS symptoms, but who also have "typical cystoscopic and histological features" during bladder hydrodistension** (109).

The etiology of IC/PBS is unknown, but several hypotheses exist. A defective glycosaminoglycan (GAG) epithelial layer, which allows irritating substances in the urine to penetrate the urothelium to the subepithelial nerve endings, may be responsible for the syndrome (110). This theoretical mechanism is based on the fact that many IC sufferers have a positive potassium diffusion test and are sensitive to certain foods and beverages. Immunological mechanisms were proposed because abnormal mast cell activity, increased substance P expressing nerve fibers and increased nerve growth factor, were all found in bladder biopsies of IC affected individuals (110). Autoimmune mechanisms may be responsible in some individuals given that there is a higher incidence of systemic lupus erythematosus, allergies, inflammatory bowel and irritable bowel disease, and fibromyalgia in patients with bladder symptoms. Another possible mechanism is central sensitization with altered sympathetic and hypothalamic adrenal axis, substantiated by the existence of "phantom" bladder pain even after surgical removal of the bladder (110).

Symptoms

Symptoms include severe and disabling urinary frequency and urgency, nocturia, and occasional dysuria and hematuria. Suprapubic, pelvic, urethral, vaginal, vulvar, or perineal pain is common and can be relieved to some extent by emptying of the bladder (111).

Signs

Pelvic examination usually reveals anterior vaginal wall and suprapubic tenderness. Pelvic floor muscles are invariably involved, and tender to palpation. Urinalysis may reveal microhematuria without pyuria, although results are usually normal.

Diagnosis

The diagnosis is one of exclusion and is no longer based on cystoscopy. Patients who should be excluded include those younger than 18 years, those with symptoms for less than 9 months, absence of nocturia, frequency less than eight times per day, genitourinary infection (including bacterial cystitis, vaginitis, herpes), radiation- or chemotherapy-induced cystitis, bladder calculi, genitourinary cancers, lack of urgency with bladder filling greater than 350 cm^3, involuntary bladder contractions, or relief with antibiotics, antispasmodic, or anticholinergics.

National Institutes of Health (NIH) Consensus Criteria for diagnosis of IC states that patients must have at least two of the following: (i) pain on bladder filling relieved by emptying, (ii) pain in suprapubic, pelvic, urethral, vaginal, or perineal region, (iii) glomerulations on endoscopy or decreased compliance on cystometrogram (111a).

Patients can be evaluated with cystoscopy with hydrodistension and biopsy. Petechial bladder mucosal hemorrhages (glomerulations) are characteristic of IC. The use of a pelvic pain and urgency or frequency symptom scale and a bladder potassium intravesical test can promote early diagnosis; it is still debatable whether a positive potassium test is definitive for interstitial cystitis or if a positive test is a manifestation of bladder hyperalgesia (112).

Management

Although there is no definitive cure for IC/BPS, patients can achieve remission with multidisciplinary therapy. First-line treatments are primarily behavioral modification such as bladder training and stress management, cognitive-behavioral therapy, dietary modifications or restriction of acidic, spicy, and fermented foods, and pelvic floor muscle physical therapy. Urinary alkalinization can be useful (113). TCAs have been efficacious. *Amitriptyline* 10 mg can be taken at bedtime and titrated as tolerated up to 150 mg or to relief of symptoms. *Amitriptyline* has antihistaminic, anticholinergic, and sodium channel blocking properties that are potentially therapeutic for opposing the histamine from mast cell degranulation, the urinary frequency, and the neuropathic pain, respectively. Oral *pentosan polysulfate sodium* (PPS) is the only U.S. Food and Drug Administration (FDA) approved oral therapy for IC and is modestly beneficial (114). *Pentosan polysulfate* is a heparinlike moiety that resembles the GAG layer, but should not be used with NSAIDs because of the bleeding risk.

Intravesical therapy can be first or second-line. With an intravesical mixture of *lidocaine,* bicarbonate, and *heparin* instilled three times a week for 3 weeks, 57% of women reported resolution of pain (115). *Dimethylsulfoxide (DMSO)* is the only FDA approved intravesical treatment of IC. Intravesical 50% *DMSO* showed significant symptomatic improvement compared to placebo in two randomized controlled trials. Intravesical solutions containing dissolved PPS showed some promise but are not FDA approved and are under investigation (116).

Sacral neuromodulation is an invasive, yet promising, technique under investigation for treatment of refractory IC (117). Sacral neuromodulation is not FDA approved for IC, and larger studies are required to confirm efficacy.

Neurologic and Musculoskeletal Causes

Nerve Entrapment

Abdominal cutaneous nerve injury or entrapment may occur spontaneously or within weeks to years after transverse suprapubic skin or laparoscopy incisions. The ilioinguinal (T12 and L1, L2) or iliohypogastric (T12 and L1, L2) nerves may become trapped between the transverse and internal oblique muscles, especially when the muscles contract. Alternatively, the nerve may be ligated or traumatized during the surgery (118).

Femoral nerve injury, one of the most commonly injured nerves in gynecologic laparotomy, can result when deep lateral retractor blades compress the nerve between the blade and the lateral pelvic side wall (119). Symptoms of nerve entrapment include sharp, burning, aching pain and paresthesias in the dermatomal distribution of the involved nerve. Femoral nerve damage results in an inability to flex at the hip joint or to extend at the knee (119). With nerve entrapment, hip flexion and exercise or activity exacerbates pain and rest or infiltration with a local anesthetic relieves pain (120). The pain is usually judged as coming from the abdomen, not the skin.

Pudendal neuropathy is another form of nerve pain that can result from vaginal surgery, especially with lateral mesh attachments, childbirth, and even chronic constipation or pelvic floor muscle abnormalities. Vulvar surgical procedures including episiotomies, laser hair removal, and Bartholin's gland removal may injure branches of the pudendal nerve, namely the vestibular, rectal, or clitoral branches (121).

Nantes criteria for pudendal neuropathy are: (i) pain in the area innervated by the pudendal nerve (i.e., ipsilateral clitoris/penis, distal urethra, labia/scrotum, perineum, and anus); (ii) pain is increased while sitting; (iii) patient is not awakened by pain; (iv) no sensory loss on clinical examination (sensory deficits are suggestive of a sacral nerve root lesion); (v) resolution of pain with administration of pudendal nerve block (122).

Signs

On examination, the point of maximal tenderness or pain should be localized with the fingertip. The maximal point of tenderness in an iliohypogastric or ilioinguinal injury is usually at the rectus margin, medial and inferior to the anterior iliac spine. For the pudendal nerve the maximal tenderness is usually near the ischial spine. A tentative diagnosis can be confirmed by a diagnostic nerve block with 3 to 5 mL of 0.25% *bupivacaine*. Patients usually report immediate relief of symptoms after injection, and at least 50% of patients experience relief lasting longer than a few hours over a week or two.

Management

Many patients may require no further intervention after a series of weekly nerve blocks, although some patients require physical therapy or the addition of medications that down-regulate nerve firing. If injection successfully produces only limited pain relief and there are no contributory visceral or psychological factors, radiofrequency nerve ablation or surgical decompression of the involved nerve may be recommended. Medication for neuropathic pain, such as topical local anesthetics, anticonvulsants or antidepressants, often is effective.

Myofascial Pain

Myofascial syndrome is documented in about 15% of patients with chronic pelvic pain (120). **These patients are noted to have numerous trigger points, hyperirritable areas within a tight band of skeletal muscle or within its fascia** (123,124). Trigger points are possibly initiated by pathogenic autonomic reflex of visceral or muscular origin and are painful on compression (124–126). The referred pain of the trigger point occurs in a dermatomal distribution and may be caused by nerves from the muscle or deeper structures sharing a common second-order neuron in the spinal cord. The patient can experience weakness and restriction in range of motion of the affected muscle. Physical therapy is a mainstay (127). Painful trigger points characteristically can be abolished with the injection of local anesthetic into the painful area, and topical *lidocaine* patches or creams can be useful (123). Trigger points can be present in women with chronic pelvic pain irrespective of presence or type of underlying pathology. In one study, 89% of women with chronic pelvic pain had abdominal, vaginal, or lumbosacral trigger points (123). In the absence of the initial or ongoing organic pathology, various factors are theorized to predispose to the chronicity of the myofascial syndrome, including psychological, hormonal, and biomechanical factors (124). A multidisciplinary approach to myofascial pain must include cognitive behavioral and relaxation approaches.

Symptoms

Abdominal wall and pelvic floor myofascial pain is often exacerbated during the premenstrual period or by stimuli to the dermatome of trigger points (e.g., full bladder, bowel, or any stimulation to organs that share the dermatome of the involved nerve) (125).

Signs

On examination, fingertip pressure on the trigger points evokes local and referred pain. Tensing of the muscles by either straight leg lifting or raising the head off the table or palpation increases the pain. A specific jump sign can be elicited by palpation with fingertip or a cotton swab. An electric (tingling) sensation confirms correct needle placement (123).

Management

Massage therapy can help relieve the pain in some cases. "Myofascial release" is a special vigorous message that can be effective (124). Depending on the location of the myofascial trigger points, pelvic floor physical therapy is indicated (128). Sustained pressure with adequate force to a trigger point for a specified period can inactivate the irritable nerve (129). NSAIDs, *gabapentin, pregabalin,* low-dose TCAs, and benzodiazepines may be useful in patients requiring pharmacologic interventions. Injection of the trigger point with 3 mL of 0.25% *bupivacaine* provides relief that usually outlasts the duration of the anesthetic action. After four to five biweekly injections, the procedure should be abandoned if long-lasting relief is not obtained. A 60-patient randomized controlled trial compared *lidocaine* patch and placebo patch versus anesthetic injection for the treatment of myofascial pain syndrome. The study revealed similar efficacy of anesthetic patch to the gold standard treatment with trigger point injection and was associated with less discomfort than injection therapy (126). Acupuncture can be effective (130). Concomitant with injection at trigger points; relaxation, stress reduction, and cognitive-behavioral pain management should be undertaken, especially if anxiety, depression, history of emotional trauma, physical or sexual abuse, sexual dysfunction, or social or occupational disruption are present.

Fibromyalgia	**Fibromyalgia is a *myofascial pain syndrome,* made up of the triad of diffuse pain, fatigue, and nonrestorative sleep. Women with abdominal wall or pelvic floor myofascial pain, bladder pain syndrome or interstitial cystitis and IBS often have *fibromyalgia.* Women are affected more commonly than men. To diagnose the syndrome, the patient must have tender points in all four quadrants. The cause is thought to be a central nervous system sensitization that results in abnormal perception of chronic pain. Fibromyalgia is closely associated with *chronic fatigue syndrome,* a combination of regional myofascial problems including infections and autoimmune disorders or dysautonomias.** The management includes education, environmental changes (well-balanced diet, adequate time for sleep, and an environment conducive to restful sleep), exercise and stretching, and counseling or cognitive behavioral therapy for relaxation and maximizing coping mechanisms. Medications used include NSAIDs, low-dose TCAs, selective serotonin/norepinephrine reuptake inhibitors, anticonvulsants, and benzodiazepines to improve sleep (129).
Low-Back Pain Syndrome	**In women who experience lower-back pain without pelvic pain, gynecologic pathology rarely is the cause of their pain. However, low-back pain may accompany gynecologic pathology. Back pain may be caused by gynecologic, vascular, neurologic, psychogenic, or spondologenic (related to the axial skeleton and its structure) pathology** (131).

Symptoms

Women with low-back pain syndrome often have pain occurring after trauma or physical exertion, in the morning on arising, or with fatigue. Nongynecologic low-back pain can intensify with the menstrual cycle.

Signs

Examination consists of inspection, evaluation with movement, and palpation. Various anatomic structures in the spine should be considered as sources of pain. Muscles, vertebral joints, and discs (including lumbosacral junction, paravertebral sacrospinal muscles, and sacroiliac joints) are common sources of spondylogenic pain that must be examined carefully (2).

Diagnosis

Diagnostic imaging studies performed while the patient is standing, lying, and sitting with maximal flexion can be helpful. An elevated ESR suggests pain of inflammatory or neoplastic origin. Though most patients with acute back pain do not require imaging, plain films can be obtained to evaluate for infection, fracture, malignancy, spondylolisthesis, degenerative changes, disc space narrowing, and prior surgery. For patients who require advanced imaging, MRI without contrast is considered to be the best imaging modality.

Management

Consultation with the patient's primary care provider should be sought before initiating management for back pain unless the source could be referred gynecologic pain. For more complex cases, an orthopaedic or neurosurgery consult may be required.

Psychological Factors

From a psychological perspective, various factors may promote the chronicity of pain, including the meaning attached to the pain, anxiety, the ability to redirect attention, personality, mood state, past experience, and reinforcement contingencies that may amplify or attenuate pain (132). The Minnesota Multiphasic Personality Inventory (MMPI) studies of women with chronic pelvic pain reveal a high prevalence of a convergence "V" profile (elevated scores on the hypochondriasis, hysteria, and depression scales). Treatment that results in subjective improvement in pain severity and increased activity level produces a significant improvement in personality profile (133).

There is also a close relationship between depression and pain (73). Both give rise to similar behavior, such as behavioral and social withdrawal and decreased activity, and may be mediated by the same neurotransmitters, including norepinephrine, serotonin, and endorphins. The Beck Depression Inventory can be used as a tool for evaluation; a score over 12 suggests dysphoria and over 18, depression (133a). Antidepressants, particularly serotonin norepinephrine reuptake inhibitors (SNRIs) often relieve both depression and pain.

Childhood physical abuse has been noted to be more prevalent in women with chronic pelvic pain than in those with other types of pain (39% vs. 18.4%) (71). In a comparison of women with chronic pelvic pain, women with nonpelvic chronic pain (headache), and pain-free women, a higher lifetime prevalence of major sexual abuse and physical abuse was found in the chronic pelvic pain group. Childhood traumas may lead to an increased vulnerability to psychosocial stress and impaired coping strategies and promote chronicity of pain after an injury.

If patients are taught self-efficacy and adaptive pain coping skills through psychological treatment interventions, pain can be reduced and functioning improved. Cognitive behavioral therapy can be useful in treating chronic pelvic pain (134). Dramatizing the pain is a coping mechanism that is used by pain sufferers to generate support from others around them (135). This practice, combined with pain-related anxiety and fear, propagates pain (133).

Management of Chronic Pelvic Pain

Multidisciplinary Approach

The approach to women with chronic pain must be therapeutic, optimistic, supportive, and sympathetic. The patient should be instructed to complete a daily pain ratings form after her first office visit. This form provides the clinician and patient with important information for pain management. Pain level (0–10), vaginal bleeding, and events that trigger pain such as stress, foods, and certain physical activities are recorded. The pain ratings can encourage the patient's sense of control and decrease feelings of helplessness. Daily recording improves self-efficacy and compliance, allows for diagnosis of atypical cyclic pain (luteal as opposed to menstrual), and helps the patient to recognize the connection between pain and stressors. The ratings should be reviewed at follow-up visits.

Offering regular follow-up appointments is preferable to asking the patient to return only if pain persists because the latter reinforces pain behavior. Specific pain management skills should be taught using cognitive-behavioral approaches by a psychologist or using such techniques as mindfulness-based meditation or yoga. Patients should be taught ways to enhance opportunities for control of pain. Psychotherapy is indicated for women who have pronounced depression, sexual difficulties, or indications of past trauma. Various strategies, including relaxation techniques, stress management, sexual and marital counseling, hypnosis, and other psychotherapeutic approaches probably increase CNS descending inhibition of peripheral pain signals. Psychological group treatment is a very cost-effective approach for helping patients learn stress reduction techniques and develop coping behavioral mechanisms (136). Acupuncture can be helpful (138). Physical therapy evaluation and treatment are important.

Various studies of multidisciplinary pain management were performed. This approach incorporates the skills of the gynecologist, psychologist, and physical therapist, and may include an anesthesiologist for specialized nerve blocks. Retrospective, uncontrolled studies revealed relief of pain in 85% of the participants (137). One prospective randomized study revealed a similar response rate, which was significantly better than that of traditional therapy for pain and associated symptom reduction, improvement of daily functioning, and quality of life (138).

The following groups of patients should be considered for multidisciplinary therapy early in the management process: (i) no obvious pathology, (ii) pathology that has an equivocal role in pain production, (iii) poor response to traditionally effective medical or surgical management, (iv) more than one visceral or somatic structure involved in the production of pain (i.e., more than one "pain generator"), (v) significant stress, anxiety, posttraumatic stress disorder, or depression, (vi) history of past or current physical, emotional, or sexual trauma.

Pharmacologic Interventions

Any patients with dysmenorrhea or pain that worsens in the luteal or menstrual phase should be given hormonal agents to suppress ovulation and/or menses, as discussed above.

Patients with neuropathic pain or those with evidence of central sensitization or myofascial pain benefit from agents that alter neural processing. A low dose of a tricyclic antidepressant, various anticonvulsants, or selective serotonin/norepinephrine reuptake inhibitors are often effective, especially if combined with cognitive behavioral therapy. These pharmacologic agents lower the threshold for nerve firing and can help reduce reliance on narcotic pain medication, increasing activity and relieving the impact the pain has on the women's overall lifestyle (11). Only one small, randomized controlled trial looked at the effect of selective serotonin reuptake inhibitors on pelvic pain, and failed to show a significant difference in pain or functional ability in a short follow-up period (138).

Anticonvulsants such as *gabapentin* or *pregabalin* are useful for treatment of chronic pelvic pain. *Gabapentin* plus *amitriptyline* was more efficacious than *amitriptyline* alone (139).

Local anesthetics are sodium channel blockers and they downgrade nerve firing. Ilioinguinal iliohypogastric, pudendal, nerve blocks and trigger point injections can be easily learned by the gynecologist and used liberally where appropriate to down-regulate neural signaling (11).

Women with depression should be treated with an appropriate therapeutic dose of antidepressant medication. Psychiatry can be consulted in this setting.

The role of opioid therapy in chronic pain is controversial and randomized controlled trials are lacking. Long-term management of chronic pelvic pain with narcotic medications is considered a last resort after failure of all other treatment modalities. Opioids should be given on a scheduled basis, and patients should have consistent follow-up with evaluation of the extent of pain relief, level of function, and quality of life. Physicians should carefully document failure of other treatment options and patient counseling. Narcotics should be prescribed only with a narcotic contract. The patient should sign a written contract agreeing to obtain pain medications from only one provider and describing other expectations with respect to treatment. Some other points that the patient should agree to include no early refills or increasing dosage of medication without discussion with the doctor, no alcohol or illegal drugs, random blood or urine drug screens if needed, and psychiatric or psychological evaluation if needed (140).

Physical Therapy

Physical therapy (PT) procedures restore tissue and joint flexibility, improve posture and body mechanics, restore strength and coordination, reduce nervous system irritability, and restore function. PT is an important component of the management of patients with myofascial pain in the abdominal wall, pelvic floor, or lower back (141).

Laparoscopy

Women with disabling pain that is premenstrual and or menstrual and that does not respond to NSAIDs or hormonal contraceptives should be considered for laparoscopic evaluation. Diagnostic laparoscopy is a standard procedure in the evaluation of patients with chronic noncyclic pelvic pain; however, laparoscopy is generally withheld until other nongynecologic somatic or visceral causes of pain are excluded. Nonrandomized retrospective and prospective studies suggest that diagnostic laparoscopy provides a positive psychological effect on the treatment of chronic pelvic pain, but this should not be the main goal of laparoscopy (142). During diagnostic laparoscopy, endometriotic lesions should be excised for biopsy, and if infection is suspected, cultures should be performed. The laparoscopy is essentially a debulking procedure, and all visible endometriosis may not be able to be removed safely; but if possible the implants should be excised or electrocoagulated.

Presacral neurectomy and laparoscopic uterosacral nerve ablation (LUNA) are techniques to interrupt the nerve supply to the uterus. A large study showed that LUNA was no more effective for chronic pelvic pain than laparoscopy alone (143). A Cochrane database review revealed that there is insufficient evidence to recommend pelvic nerve disruption for the treatment of dysmenorrhea (45).

The role of pelvic adhesions in pain is unclear, and the efficacy of lysis of adhesions is even more in doubt. Adhesiolysis, even via laparoscopy, is frequently complicated by adhesion reformation and may not be effective for relief of pain in controlled trials (90,144). Other causes must be treated first, and psychological consultation and management should precede or accompany the lysis of adhesions.

Hysterectomy

Although 19% of hysterectomies are performed to cure pelvic pain, 30% of patients presenting to pain clinics have already undergone hysterectomy without experiencing pain relief. A multidisciplinary approach including a gynecologist, physical therapist, and a psychologist decreased the frequency of hysterectomy in one study from 16.3% of patients with chronic pelvic pain to 5.8% (145).

Hysterectomy is particularly useful for women who have completed childbearing and have secondary dysmenorrhea or chronic pain related to endometriosis, to uterine pathology, such as adenomyosis, or to pelvic congestion. Before recommending hysterectomy for pain or unilateral adnexectomy for unilateral pain, it is useful to apply the **PREPARE** mnemonic in discussions with the patient (146): the **P**rocedure that is being done, **R**eason or indication, **E**xpectation or desired outcome of the procedure, **P**robability that the outcome will be achieved, **A**lternatives and nonsurgical options, and **R**isks as well as **E**xpense (see Chapter 3). Hysterectomy for central pelvic pain in women with dysmenorrhea, dyspareunia, and uterine tenderness provided relief of pain in 77% of women in one retrospective study and in 74% of women in one prospective cohort study (147,148). Nevertheless, 25% of women in the retrospective study noted that pain persisted or worsened at 1-year follow-up (147). Persistent pain in the prospective study was associated with multiparity, prior history of PID, absence of pathology, and Medicaid payer status (148). The Maine Women's Health Study, a prospective cohort study, studied outcomes of 199 women with frequent pain at baseline who underwent hysterectomy. In this cohort, only 11% reported persistent symptoms after their surgery (149).

The American College of Obstetricians and Gynecologists outlined criteria that should be met before performing a hysterectomy for pelvic pain (150). They require at least 6 months of pelvic pain without any otherwise correctable pathology. When deciding on the surgical approach, consideration should be given to a vaginal or laparoscopic hysterectomy over an abdominal approach if there are no extensive adhesions expected or large uterine/fibroid size does not preclude it. There are many studies that confirm less morbidity and shorter hospital stays with vaginal compared with abdominal hysterectomies (151). A prospective study of abdominal versus vaginal versus laparoscopically assisted surgery did not find any statistical difference or worsening of outcomes of urinary or sexual function between the different approaches at 6 months (151).

References

1. **Dawood MY.** Dysmenorrhea. *Clin Obstet Gynecol* 1990;3:168–178.
2. **Howard FM.** Chronic pelvic pain. *Obstet Gynecol* 2003;101:594–611.
3. **Wesselmann U.** Neurogenic inflammation and chronic pelvic pain. *World J Urol* 2001;19:180–185.
4. **Nijenhuis ER, van Dyck R, ter Kuile MM, et al.** Evidence for associations among somatoform dissociation, psychological dissociation and reported trauma in patients with chronic pelvic pain. *J Psychosom Obstet Gynecol* 2003;24:87–98.
5. **Giamberardino MA, De Laurentis S, Affaitati G, et al.** Modulation of pain and hyperalgesia from the urinary tract by algogenic conditions of the reproductive organs in women. *Neurosci Lett* 2001;304:61–64.
6. **Doggweiler-Wiygul R.** Chronic pelvic pain. *World J Urol* 2001;19:155–156.
7. **Bajaj P, Bajaj P, Madsen H, et al.** Endometriosis is associated with central sensitization: a psychophysical controlled study. *J Pain* 2003;4:372–380.
8. **Diatchenko L, Nackley AG, Slade GD, et al.** Idiopathic pain disorders pathways of vulnerability. *Pain* 2006;123:226–230.
9. **Woolf CJ.** Central sensitization: implications for the diagnosis and treatment of pain. *Pain* 2011;152[Suppl]:S2–S15
10. **Winnard KP, Dmitrieva N, Berkley KJ.** Cross-organ interactions between reproductive, gastrointestinal, and urinary tracts: modulation by estrous stage and involvement of the hypogastric nerve. *Am J Physiol Regul Integr Comp Physiol* 2006;291:R1592–R1601.
11. **Howard FM.** The role of laparoscopy in the chronic pelvic pain patient. *Clin Obstet Gynecol* 2003;4:749–766.
12. **Bouyer J, Job-Spira N, Pouly J, et al.** Fertility following radical, conservative-surgical or medical treatment for tubal pregnancy: a population-based study. *Br J Obstet Gynaecol* 2000;107:714–721.
13. **Murray H, Baakdah H, Bardell T, et al.** Diagnosis and treatment of ectopic pregnancy. *CMAJ* 2005;173:905–912.
14. **Huchon C, Fauconnier A.** Adnexal torsion: a literature review. *Eur J Obstet Gynecol Reprod Biol* 2010;150:8–12.
15. **Oltmann SC, Fischer A, Barber R, et al.** Cannot exclude torsion—a 15-year review. *J Pediatr Surg* 2009;44:1212.
16. **Oelsner G, Cohen S, Soriano D, et al.** Minimal surgery for the twisted ischaemic adnexa can preserve ovarian function. *Human Reprod* 2003;18:2599–2602.
17. **Cates W Jr, Wasserheit JN.** Genital chlamydial infections: epidemiology and reproductive sequelae. *Am J Obstet Gynecol* 1991;164:1771–1781.
18. **Ness RB, Hillier SL, Kipp K, et al.** Bacterial vaginosis and risk of pelvic inflammatory disease. *Obstet Gynecol* 2004;104:761–769.
19. **Ness RB, Kip KE, Hillier SL, et al.** A cluster analysis of bacterial vaginosis-associated microflora and pelvic inflammatory disease. *Am J Epidemiol* 2005;162:585–590.
19a. **Centers for Disease Control and Prevention.** Update to CDC's Sexually Trnasmitted Diseases Treatment Guideline, 2006. *MMWR* 2006;55:RR-11.
20. **Hiller N, Sella T, Lev-Sagi A, et al.** Computed tomographic features of tuboovarian abscess. *J Reprod Med* 2005;50:203.
21. **Landers DV, Sweet RL.** Tubo-ovarian abscess: contemporary approach to management. *Rev Infect Dis* 1983;5:876–884.
22. **Reed SD, Landers DV, Sweet RL.** Antibiotic treatment of tuboovarian abscess: comparison of broad-spectrum beta-lactam agents versus clindamycin-containing regimens. *Am J Obstet Gynecol* 1991;164:1556.
23. **Gjelland K, Ekerhovd E, Granberg S.** Transvaginal ultrasound-guided aspiration for treatment of tubo-ovarian abscess: a study of 302 cases. *Am J Obstet Gynecol* 2005;193:1323.
24. **Krivak TC, Cooksey C, Propst A.** Tubo-ovarian abscess: diagnosis, medical and surgical management. *Compr Ther* 2004;30:93–100.
25. **Ferrero S, Abbamonte LH, Giordano M, et al.** Uterine myomas, dyspareunia, and sexual function. *Fertil Steril* 2006;86:1504.
26. **Lippman SA, Warner M, Samuels S, et al.** Uterine fibroids and gynecologic pain symptoms in a population-based study. *Fertil Steril* 2003;80:1488–1494.
27. **Dueholm M, Lundorf E, Hansen ES, et al.** Accuracy of magnetic resonance imaging and transvaginal ultrasonography in the diagnosis, mapping, and measurement of uterine myomas. *Am J Obstet Gynecol* 2002;186:409–415.
28. **Addiss DG, Shaffer N, Fowler BS, et al.** The epidemiology of appendicitis and appendectomy in the United States. *Am J Epidemiol* 1990;132:910–925.
29. **SCOAP Collaborative, Cuschieri J, Florence M, et al.** Negative appendectomy and imaging accuracy in the Washington State Surgical Care and Outcomes Assessment Program. *Ann Surg* 2008;248:557–563.
30. **Rao PM, Rhea JT.** Colonic diverticulitis: evaluation of the arrowhead sign and the inflamed diverticulum for CT diagnosis. *Radiology* 1998;209:775–779.
31. **Echols RM, Tosiello RL, Haverstock DC, et al.** Demographic, clinical, and treatment parameters influencing the outcome of acute cystitis. *Clin Infect Dis* 1999;29:113–119.
32. **Takahashi S, Hirose T, Satoh T, et al.** Efficacy of a 14-day course of oral ciprofloxacin therapy for acute uncomplicated pyelonephritis. *J Infect Chemother* 2001;7:255–257.
33. **Harris RD, Holtzman SR, Poppe AM.** Clinical outcome in female patients with pelvic pain and normal pelvic US findings. *Radiology* 2000;216:440–443.
34. **Burnett MA, Antao V, Black A, et al.** Prevalence of primary dysmenorrhea in Canada. *J Obstet Gynaecol Can* 2005;27:765–770.
35. **Dawood MY.** Primary dysmenorrhea: advances in pathogenesis and management. *Obstet Gynecol* 2006;108:428.
36. **Jabbour HN, Sales KJ.** Prostaglandin receptor signaling and function in human endometrial pathology. *Trends Endocrinol Metab* 2004;15:398–404.
37. **Milsom I, Minic M, Dawood MY, et al.** Comparison of the efficacy and safety of nonprescription doses of naproxen and naproxen sodium with ibuprofen, acetaminophen, and placebo in the treatment of primary dysmenorrhea: a pooled analysis of five studies. *Clin Ther* 2002;24:1384.
38. **Marjoribanks J, Proctor ML, Farquhar C.** Nonsteroidal anti-inflammatory drugs for primary dysmenorrhoea. *Cochrane Database Syst Rev* 2003;4:CD001751.
39. **Proctor ML, Roberts H, Farquhar C.** Combined oral contraceptive pill (OCP) as treatment for primary dysmenorrhoea. *Cochrane Database Syst Rev* 2001;4:CD002120.

40. **Edelman AB, Gallo MF, Jensen JT, et al.** Continuous or extended cycle vs. cyclic use of combined oral contraceptives for contraception. *Cochrane Database Syst Rev* 2005;3:CD004695.

41. **White AR.** A review of controlled trials of acupuncture for women's reproductive health care. *J Fam Plan Reprod Health Care* 2003;29:233–236.

42. **Proctor ML, Smith CA, Farquhar C, et al.** Transcutaneous electrical nerve stimulation and acupuncture for primary dysmenorrhoea. *Cochrane Database Syst Rev* 2002;1:CD002123.

43. **Akin MD, Weingand KW, Hengehold DA, et al.** Continuous low-level topical heat in the treatment of dysmenorrhea. *Obstet Gynecol* 2001;97:343–349.

44. **Proctor ML, Latthe PM, Farquhar CM, et al.** Surgical interruption of pelvic nerve pathways for primary and secondary dysmenorrhoea. *Cochrane Database Syst Rev* 2005;4:CD001896.

45. **Vercellini P, Parazzini F, Oldani S, et al.** Adenomyosis at hysterectomy: a study on frequency distribution and patient characteristics. *Hum Reprod* 1995;10:1160–1162.

46. **Lee NC, Dikcer RC, Rubin GL, et al.** Confirmation of the preoperative diagnoses for hysterectomy. *Am J Obstet Gynecol* 1984;150:283–287.

47. **Templeman C, Marshall SF, Ursin G, et al.** Adenomyosis and endometriosis in the California Teachers Study. *Fertil Steril* 2008;90:415.

48. **Levgur M.** Diagnosis of adenomyosis: a review. *J Reprod Med* 2007;52:177.

49. **Kim MD, Kim S, Kim NK, et al.** Long-term results of uterine artery embolization for symptomatic adenomyosis. *AJR Am J Roentgenol* 2007;188:176.

50. **Giudice LC, Kao LC.** Endometriosis. *Lancet* 2004;364:1789–1799.

51. **Cornillie FJ, Oosterlynck D, Lauweryns JM, et al.** Deeply infiltrating pelvic endometriosis: histology and clinical significance. *Fertil Steril* 1990;53:978–983.

52. **Al-Jefout M, Dezarnaulds G, Cooper M, et al.** Diagnosis of endometriosis by detection of nerve fibres in an endometrial biopsy: a double blind study. *Hum Reprod* 2009;24:3019–3024.

53. **Allen C, Hopewell S, Prentice A.** Non-steroidal anti-inflammatory drugs for pain in women with endometriosis. *Cochrane Database Syst Rev* 2005;4:CD004753.

54. **Hughes E, Brown J, Collins JJ, et al.** Ovulation suppression for endometriosis. *Cochrane Database Syst Rev* 2007;3:CD000155.

55. **Vercellini P, Frontino G, De Giorgi O, et al.** Comparison of a levonorgestrel-releasing intrauterine device versus expectant management after conservative surgery for symptomatic endometriosis: a pilot study. *Fertil Steril* 2003;80:305.

56. **Somigliana E, Vigano P, Barbara G, et al.** Treatment of endometriosis-related pain: options and outcomes. *Front Biosci (Elite Ed)* 2009;1:455–465.

57. **Petta CA, Ferriani RA, Abrao MS, et al.** Randomized clinical trial of a levonorgestrel-releasing intrauterine system and a depot GnRH analogue for the treatment of chronic pelvic pain in women with endometriosis. *Hum Reprod* 2005;20:1993.

58. **Hornstein MD, Surrey ES, Weisberg GW, et al.** Leuprolide acetate depot and hormonal add-back in endometriosis: a 12-month study. *Obstet Gynecol* 1998;91:16–24.

59. **Ferrero S, Camerini G, Seracchioli R, et al.** Letrozole combined with norethisterone acetate compared with norethisterone acetate alone in the treatment of pain symptoms caused by endometriosis. *Hum Reprod* 2009;24:3033–3041.

60. **Eastell R, Adams JE, Coleman RE, et al.** Effect of anastrozole on bone mineral density: 5-year results from the anastrozole, tamoxifen, alone or in combination trial 18233230. *J Clin Oncol* 2008;26:1051–1057.

61. **Vercellini P, Barbara G, Abbiati A, et al.** Repetitive surgery for recurrent symptomatic endometriosis: what to do? *Eur J Obstet Gynecol Reprod Biol* 2009;146:15–21.

62. **Seracchioli R, Mabrouk M, Manuzzi L, et al.** Post-operative use of oral contraceptive pills for prevention of anatomical relapse or symptom-recurrence after conservative surgery for endometriosis. *Hum Reprod* 2009;24:2729–2735.

63. **Vercellini P, Crosignani PG, Somigliana E, et al.** Medical treatment for rectovaginal endometriosis: what is the evidence? *Hum Reprod* 2009;24:2504–2514.

64. **ACOG Committee on Practice Bulletins.** ACOG Practice Bulletin No. 51. Chronic pelvic pain. *Obstet Gynecol* 2004;103:589–605.

65. **Farquhar CM, Steiner CA.** Hysterectomy rates in the United States 1990–1997. *Obstet Gynecol* 2002;99:229–234.

66. **Cervero F, Laird JM.** Understanding the signaling and transmission of visceral nociceptive events. *J Neurobiol* 2004;61:45–54.

67. **Latremoliere A, Woolf CJ.** Central sensitization: a generator of pain hypersensitivity by central neural plasticity. *J Pain* 2009;10:895–926.

68. **International Pelvic Pain Society.** Pelvic pain assessment form. Available at http://www.pelvicpain.org/pdf/History_and_Physical_Form/IPPS-H&PformR-MSW.pdf. Accessed April 27, 2011.

69. **Meltzer-Brody S, Leserman J, Zolnoun D, et al.** Trauma and post-traumatic stress disorder in women with chronic pelvic pain. *Obstet Gynecol* 2007;109:902–908.

70. **Walling MK, O'Hara MW, Reiter RC, et al.** Abuse history and chronic pain in women: II. A multivariate analysis of abuse and psychological morbidity. *Obstet Gynecol* 1994;84:200–206.

71. **Rapkin AJ, Kames LD, Darke LL, et al.** History of physical and sexual abuse in women with chronic pelvic pain. *Obstet Gynecol* 1990;76:92–96.

72. **Lorençatto C, Petta CA, Navarro MJ, et al.** Depression in women with endometriosis with and without chronic pelvic pain. *Acta Obstet Gynecol Scand* 2006;85:88–92.

73. **Randolph ME, Reddy DM.** Sexual functioning in women with chronic pelvic pain: the impact of depression, support, and abuse. *J Sex Res* 2006;43:38–45.

74. **Srinivasan R, Greenbaum DS.** Chronic abdominal wall pain: a frequently overlooked problem. Practical approach to diagnosis and management. *Am J Gastroenterol* 2002;97:3207.

75. **Wykes CB, Clark TJ, Khan KS.** Accuracy of laparoscopy in the diagnosis of endometriosis: a systematic quantitative review. *BJOG* 2004;111:1204–1212.

76. **Vercellini P, Frontino G, Pietropaolo G, et al.** Deep endometriosis: definition, pathogenesis, and clinical management. *J Am Assoc Gynecol Laparosc* 2004;11:153–161.

77. **Fedele L, Parazzini F, Bianchi S, et al.** Stage and localization of pelvic endometriosis and pain. *Fertil Steril* 1990;53:155–158.

78. **Fukaya T, Hoshiai H, Yajima A.** Is pelvic endometriosis always associated with chronic pain? A retrospective study of 618 cases diagnosed by laparoscopy. *Am J Obstet Gynecol* 1993;169:719–722.

79. **Donnez J, Squifflet J.** Laparoscopic excision of deep endometriosis. *Obstet Gynecol Clin North Am* 2004;31:567–580, ix.

80. **Konincky RP, Meuleman C, Demeyere S, et al.** Suggestive evidence that pelvic endometriosis is a progressive disease, whereas deeply infiltrating endometriosis is associated with pelvic pain. *Fertil Steril* 1991;55:759–765.

81. **Porpora MG, Koninckx PR, Piazze J, et al.** Correlation between endometriosis and pelvic pain. *J Am Assoc Gynecol Laparosc* 1999;6:429–434.

82. **Berkley KJ, Rapkin AJ, Papka RE.** The pains of endometriosis. *Science* 2005;308:1587–1589.

83. **Stratton P, Berkley K.** Chronic pelvic pain and endometriosis: translational evidence of the relationship and implications. *Hum Reprod Update* 2011;17:327–346.

84. **Tokushige N, Markham R, Russell P, et al.** Different types of small nerve fibers in eutopic endometrium and myometrium in women with endometriosis. *Fertil Steril* 2007;88:795–803.

85. **Stout AL, Steege JF, Dodson WC, et al.** Relationship of laparoscopic findings to self-report of pelvic pain. *Am J Obstet Gynecol* 1991;164[Pt 1]:73–79.

86. **Rapkin AJ.** Adhesions and pelvic pain: a retrospective study. *Obstet Gynecol* 1986;68:13–15.

87. **Steege JF, Scott AL.** Resolution of chronic pelvic pain after laparoscopic lysis of adhesions. *Am J Obstet Gynecol* 1991;165:278–283.

88. **Swank DJ, Swank-Bordewijk SC, Hop W, et al.** Laparoscopic adhesiolysis in patients with chronic abdominal pain: a blinded randomized controlled multi-centre trial. *Lancet* 2003;361:1247–1251.

89. **Swank DJ, Van Erp WF, Repelaer Van Driel O, et al.** A prospective analysis of predictive factors on the results of laparoscopic adhesiolysis in patients with chronic abdominal pain. *Surg Laparosc Endosc Percutan Tech* 2003;13:88–94.

90. **Hammoud A, Gago LA, Diamond M.** Adhesions in patients with chronic pelvic pain: a role for adhesiolysis? *Fertil Steril* 2004;82:1483–1491.

91. **Peters AAW, Trimbos-Kemper GCM, Admiral C, et al.** A randomized clinical trial on the benefit of adhesiolysis in patients with intraperitoneal adhesions and chronic pelvic pain. *Br J Obstet Gynaecol* 1992;99:59–62.

92. **Howard FM, El-Minawi AM, Sanchez R.** Conscious pain mapping by laparoscopy in women with chronic pelvic pain. *Obstet Gynecol* 2000;96:934–939.

93. **Gupta A, McCarthy S.** Pelvic varices as a cause for pelvic pain: MRI appearance. *Magn Reson Imaging* 1994;12:679–681.

94. **Soysal ME.** A randomized controlled trial of goserelin and medroxyprogesterone acetate in the treatment of pelvic congestion. *Hum Reprod* 2001;16:931–939.

95. **Farquhar CM, Rogers V, Franks S, et al.** A randomized controlled trial of medroxyprogesterone acetate and psychotherapy for the treatment of pelvic congestion. *Br J Obstet Gynaecol* 1989;96:1153–1162.

96. **Kim HS, Malhotra AD, Rowe PC, et al.** Embolotherapy for pelvic congestion syndrome: long-term results. *J Vasc Interv Radiol* 2006;17:289.

97. **Tu FF, Hahn D, Steege JF.** Pelvic congestion syndrome-associated pelvic pain: a systematic review of diagnosis and management. *Obstet Gynecol Surv* 2010;65:332–340.

98. **Magtibay PM, Nyholm JL, Hernandez JL, et al.** Ovarian remnant syndrome. *Am J Obstet Gynecol* 2005;193:2062–2066.

99. **Carey MP, Slack MC.** GnRH analogue in assessing chronic pelvic pain in women with residual ovaries. *BJOG* 1996;103:150–153.

100. **Kho RM, Magrina JF, Magtibay PM.** Pathologic findings and outcomes of a minimally invasive approach to ovarian remnant syndrome. *Fertil Steril* 2007;87:1005.

101. **Nezhat C, Kearney S, Malik S, et al.** Laparoscopic management of ovarian remnant. *Fertil Steril* 2005;83:973.

102. **Williams RE, Hartmann KE, Sandler R, et al.** Prevalence and characteristics of irritable bowel syndrome among women with chronic pelvic pain. *Obstet Gynecol* 2004;104:452–458.

103. **Williams RE, Hartmann KE, Sandler RS, et al.** Recognition and treatment of irritable bowel syndrome among women with chronic pelvic pain. *Am J Obstet Gynecol* 2005;192:761

104. **Mertz HR.** Irritable bowel syndrome. *N Engl J Med* 2003;349:2136–2146.

105. **Mayer EA.** Irritable bowel syndrome. *N Engl J Med* 2008;358:1692–1699.

106. **Drossman DA.** Rome III: the new criteria. *Chin J Dig Dis* 2006;7:181–185.

107. **Kaur H, Arunkalaivanan AS.** Urethral pain syndrome and its management. *Obstet Gynecol Surv* 2007;62:348–351.

108. **Costantini E, Zucchi A, Del Zingaro M, et al.** Treatment of urethral syndrome: a prospective randomized study with Nd:YAG laser. *Urol Int* 2006;76:134–138.

109. **Abrams P, Cardozo L, Fall M, et al.** The standardisation of terminology of lower urinary tract function: report from the Standardisation Sub-committee of the International Continence Society. *Neurourol Urodyn* 2002;21:167.

110. **Parsons CL.** The role of the urinary epithelium in the pathogenesis of interstitial cystitis/prostatitis/urethritis. *Urology* 2007;69:S9.

111. **Wesselmann U.** Interstitial cystitis: a chronic visceral pain syndrome. *Urology* 2001;57:32.

111a. **Chancellor MB.** A Multidisciplinary Consensus Meeting on IC/PBS Outcome of the Consensus Meeting on Interstitial Cystitis/Painful Bladder Syndrome, February 10, 2007, Washington, DC. *Rev Urol* 2007 9: 81–83.

112. **Parsons CL.** The potassium sensitivity test: a new gold standard for diagnosing and understanding the pathophysiology of interstitial cystitis. *J Urol* 2009;182:432–434.

113. **Chancellor MB, Yoshimura N.** Neurophysiology of stress urinary incontinence. Rev Urol 2004;6[Suppl 3]:S19–S28.

114. **Dimitrakov J, Kroenke K, Steers WD, et al.** Pharmacologic management of painful bladder syndrome/interstitial cystitis: a systematic review. Arch Intern Med 2007;167:1922.

115. **Welk BK, Teichman JM.** Dyspareunia response in patients with interstitial cystitis treated with intravesical lidocaine, bicarbonate, and heparin. *Urology* 2008;71:67–70.

116. **Moldwin RM, Evans RJ, Stanford EJ, et al.** Rational approaches to the treatment of patients with interstitial cystitis. *Urology* 2007;69[Suppl]:73–81.

117. **Maher CF, Carey MP, Dwyer PL, et al.** Percutaneous sacral nerve root neuromodulation for intractable interstitial cystitis. *J Urol* 2001;165:884–886.

118. **Rahn DD, Phelan JN, Roshanravan SM, et al.** Anterior abdominal wall nerve and vessel anatomy: clinical implications for gynecologic surgery. *Am J Obstet Gynecol* 2010;202:234.e1–5.

119. **Fardin F, Benettello P, Negrin P.** Iatrogenic femoral neuropathy: considerations on its prognosis. *Electromyogr Clin Neurophysiol* 1980;20:153–155.

120. **Reiter RC.** Occult somatic pathology in women with chronic pelvic pain. *Clin Obstet Gynecol* 1990;33:154–160.

121. **Bohrer JC, Chen CC, Walters MD.** Pudendal neuropathy involving the perforating cutaneous nerve after cystocele repair with graft. *Obstet Gynecol* 2008;112:496.

122. **Labat JJ, Riant T, Robert R, et al.** Diagnostic criteria for pudendal neuralgia by pudendal nerve entrapment (Nantes criteria). *Neurourol Urodyn* 2008;27:306.

123. **Slocumb JC.** Neurological factors in chronic pelvic pain: trigger points and the abdominal pelvic pain syndrome. *Am J Obstet Gynecol* 1984;149:536–543.

124. **Travell J.** Myofascial trigger points: clinical view. *Adv Pain Res Ther* 1976;1:919–926.

125. **Doggweiler-Wiygul R.** Urologic myofascial pain syndromes. *Curr Pain Headache Rep* 2004;8:445–451.

126. **Affaitati G, Fabrizio A, Savini A, et al.** A randomized, controlled study comparing a lidocaine patch, a placebo patch, and anesthetic injection for treatment of trigger points in patients with myofascial pain syndrome: evaluation of pain and somatic pain thresholds. *Clin Ther* 2009;31:705–720.

127. **Butrick CW.** Pelvic floor hypertonic disorders: identification and management. *Obstet Gynecol Clin North Am* 2009;36:707–722.

128. **FitzGerald MP, Anderson RU, Potts J, et al.** Randomized multicenter feasibility trial of myofascial physical therapy for the treatment of urological chronic pelvic pain syndromes. *J Urol* 2009;182:570.

129. **Goldenberg DL, Burckhardt C, Crofford L.** Management of fibromyalgia syndrome. *JAMA* 2004;292:2388.

130. **Tough EA, White AR, Cummings TM, et al.** Acupuncture and dry needling in the management of myofascial trigger point pain: a systematic review and meta-analysis of randomised controlled trials. *Eur J Pain* 2009;13:3–10.

131. **Chou R, Qaseem A, Snow V, et al.** Diagnosis and treatment of low back pain: a joint clinical practice guideline from the American College of Physicians and the American Pain Society. *Ann Intern Med* 2007;147:478.

132. **Keefe FJ, Rumble ME, Scipio CD, et al.** Psychological aspects of persistent pain: current state of the science. *J Pain* 2004;5:195–211.

133. **Duleba AJ, Jubanyik KJ, Greenfield DA, et al.** Changes in personality profile associated with laparoscopic surgery for chronic pelvic pain. *J Am Assoc Gynecol Laparosc* 1998;5:389–395.

133a. **Beck AT.** Depression: Causes and Treatment. Philadelphia: University of Pennsylvania Press. 2006;ISBN0-8122-1032-8.

134. **Masheb RM, Kerns RD, Lozano C, et al.** A randomized clinical trial for women with vulvodynia: cognitive-behavioral therapy vs. supportive psychotherapy. *Pain* 2009;141:31–40.

135. **Sullivan M, Thorn B, Haythornthwaite J, et al.** Theoretical perspectives on the relation between catastrophizing and pain. *Clin J Pain* 2001;17:5–64.

136. **Albert H.** Psychosomatic group treatment helps women with chronic pelvic pain. *J Psychosom Obstet Gynecol* 1999;20:216–225.

137. **Rapkin AJ, Kames LD.** The pain management approach to chronic pelvic pain. *J Reprod Med* 1987;32:323–327.

138. **Peters AAW, van Dorst E, Jellis B, et al.** A randomized clinical trial to compare two different approaches in women with chronic pelvic pain. *Obstet Gynecol* 1991;77:740.

139. **Sator-Katzenschlager SM, Scharbert G, Kress HG, et al.** Chronic pelvic pain treated with gabapentin and amitriptyline: a randomized controlled pilot study. *Wien Klin Wochenschr* 2005;117:761–768.

140. **Rapkin AJ, Hartshorn TG, Partownavid P.** Pain management. *Clin Update Womens Health Care* 2011; in press.

141. **Tu FF, Holt J, Gonzales J, et al.** Physical therapy evaluation of patients with chronic pelvic pain: a controlled study. *Am J Obstet Gynecol* 2008;198:272.e1–7.

142. **Elcombe S, Gath D, Day A.** The psychological effects of laparoscopy on women with chronic pelvic pain. *Psychol Med* 1997; 27:1041–1050.

143. **Daniels J, Gray R, Hills RK, et al.** LUNA Trial Collaboration. Laparoscopic uterosacral nerve ablation for alleviating chronic pelvic pain: a randomized controlled trial. *JAMA* 2009;302:955–961.

144. **Swank DJ, Jeekel H.** Laparoscopic adhesiolysis in patients with chronic abdominal pain. *Curr Opin Obstet Gynecol* 2004;16:313–318.

145. **Reiter RC, Gambone JC, et al.** Availability of a multidisciplinary pelvic pain clinic and frequency of hysterectomy for pelvic pain. *J Psychosom Obstet Gynecol* 1991;12[Suppl]:109.

146. **Reiter RC, Lench JB, Gambone JC.** Clinical commentary: consumer advocacy, elective surgery, and the "golden era of machine." *Obstet Gynecol* 1989;74:815–817.

147. **Stovall TG, Ling FW, Crawford DA.** Hysterectomy for chronic pelvic pain of presumed uterine etiology. *Obstet Gynecol* 1990;75:676–679.

148. **Hillis SD, Marchbanks PA, Peterson HB.** The effectiveness of hysterectomy for chronic pelvic pain. *Obset Gynecol* 1995;86:941–945.

149. **Carlson KJ, Miller BA, Fowler FJ Jr.** The Maine Women's Health Study: I. Outcomes of hysterectomy. *Obstet Gynecol* 1994;83:556–565.

150. **ACOG Criteria Set.** Hysterectomy, abdominal or vaginal for chronic pelvic pain. Number 29, November 1997. Committee on Quality Assessment. American College of Obstetricians and Gynecologists. *Int J Gynaecol Obstet* 1998;60:316–317.

151. **El-Toukhy TA, Hefni M, Davies A, et al.** The effect of different types of hysterectomy on urinary and sexual functions: a prospective study. **J Obstet Gynaecol** 2004;24:420–425.

17 Endometriosis

Thomas M. D'Hooghe

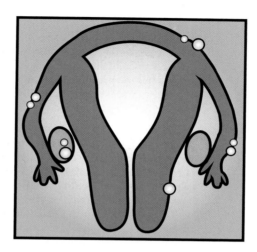

- Endometriosis is diagnosed by visual inspection of the pelvis during laparoscopy, ideally with histological confirmation; positive histology confirms the diagnosis, but negative histology does not exclude it.

- Endometriosis can be associated with subfertility, pelvic pain, i.e., dysmenorrhea, dyspareunia and nonmenstrual pain, and reduced quality of life.

- Severe or deeply infiltrating endometriosis should be managed in a facility with the necessary expertise to provide treatment in a multidisciplinary context, including advanced laparoscopic surgery and laparotomy.

- Classification systems for endometriosis are subjective and correlate poorly with pain symptoms, but have some value in determining the prognosis and management of infertility.

- Suppression of ovarian function for 6 months reduces pain associated with endometriosis. Hormonal drugs are equally effective in reducing pain but have differing side effects and cost.

- Ablation of endometriotic lesions with laparoscopic uterine nerve ablation (LUNA) in minimal to moderate disease reduces pain associated with endometriosis; however, because LUNA used alone has no effect on dysmenorrhea associated with endometriosis, there is no evidence that LUNA is a necessary component of treatment.

- Ablation of endometriotic lesions plus adhesiolysis in minimal to mild endometriosis is more effective than diagnostic laparoscopy alone in improving fertility.

- Suppression of ovarian function is not effective in improving subsequent fertility in patients with endometriosis.

Endometriosis is defined as the presence of endometrial tissue (glands and stroma) outside the uterus. The most frequent sites of implantation are the pelvic viscera and the peritoneum. Endometriosis varies in appearance from a few minimal lesions on otherwise intact pelvic organs, to massive ovarian endometriotic cysts that distort tubo-ovarian anatomy and extensive adhesions involving bowel, bladder, and ureter. It is estimated to occur in 10% of reproductive-age women and is associated with pelvic pain and infertility. Considerable progress in understanding the pathogenesis, spontaneous evolution, diagnosis, and treatment of endometriosis has occurred. **The European Society for Human Reproduction and Embryology (ESHRE) guidelines for the clinical management of endometriosis are published and regularly updated to present emerging clinical evidence** (1).

Epidemiology

Prevalence

Endometriosis is found predominantly in women of reproductive age but is reported in adolescents and in postmenopausal women receiving hormonal replacement (2). It is found in women of all ethnic and social groups. **Estimates of the frequency of endometriosis vary widely, but the prevalence of the condition is assumed to be around 10%** (3,4). Although no consistent information is available on the incidence of the disease, temporal trends suggest an increase among women of reproductive age (4).

In women with pelvic pain or infertility, a high prevalence of endometriosis (from a low of 20% to a high of 90%) is reported (5,6). **In women with unexplained subfertility with or without pain (regular cycle, partner with normal sperm), the prevalence of endometriosis is reported to be as high as 50%** (7). **In asymptomatic women undergoing tubal ligation (women of proven fertility), the prevalence of endometriosis ranges from 3% to 43%** (8–13). This variation in the reported prevalence may be explained by several factors. First, it may vary with the diagnostic method used: laparoscopy, the operation of choice for diagnosis, is a better method than laparotomy for diagnosing minimal to mild endometriosis. Second, minimal or mild endometriosis may be more thoroughly evaluated in a symptomatic patient given general anesthesia than in an asymptomatic patient during tubal sterilization. Third, the interest and experience of the surgeon is important because there is a wide variation in the appearance of subtle endometriosis implants, cysts, and adhesions. Most studies that evaluate the prevalence of endometriosis in women of reproductive age lack histologic confirmation (8–10,14–19).

Risk and Protective Factors

The following are identified risk factors for endometriosis: infertility, red hair, early age at menarche, shorter menstrual cycle length, hypermenorrhea, nulliparity, müllerian anomalies, birth weight (less than 7 pounds), one of multiple fetal gestation, diethylstilbestrol (DES) exposure, endometriosis in first-degree relative, tall height, dioxin or polychlorinated biphenyls (PCB) exposure, a diet high in fat and red meat, and prior surgeries or medical therapy for endometriosis (20). Prior use of contraception or intrauterine device (IUD), or smoking is not associated with increased risk of endometriosis (21,22). **Protective factors against the development of endometriosis include multiparity, lactation, tobacco exposure *in utero*, increased body mass index, increased waist-to-hip ratios and exercise, and diet high in vegetables and fruits** (20). Some evidence suggests that women with a "pinpoint cervix" have an increased risk for endometriosis, but more studies are needed to confirm this observation (23).

Endometriosis and Cancer

Several publications link endometriosis with an increased risk for certain gynecologic and nongynecologic cancers (24,25). These associations are controversial and no data exist to inform clinicians regarding the best management of patients who might be at risk of developing such cancers (1). Endometriosis should not be considered a medical condition associated with a clinically relevant risk of any specific cancer (26). **Data from large cohort and case-control studies indicate an increased risk of ovarian cancers in women with endometriosis. The observed effect sizes are modest, varying between 1.3 and 1.9** (27). **Evidence from clinical series consistently demonstrates that the association is confined to the endometrioid and clear-cell histologic types of ovarian cancer** (28). A causal relationship between endometriosis and these specific histotypes of ovarian cancer should be recognized, but the low magnitude of the risk observed is consistent with the view that ectopic endometrium undergoes malignant transformation with a frequency similar to its eutopic counterpart (29). Evidence for an association with melanoma and non-Hodgkin's lymphoma is increasing but needs to be verified, whereas an increased risk for other gynecologic cancer types is not supported (28).

Etiology

Although signs and symptoms of endometriosis were described since the 1800s, its widespread occurrence was acknowledged only during the 20th century. Endometriosis is an estrogen-dependent disease. **Three theories were proposed to explain the histogenesis of endometriosis:**

1. **Ectopic transplantation of endometrial tissue**
2. **Coelomic metaplasia**
3. **The induction theory**

No single theory can account for the location of endometriosis in all cases.

Transplantation Theory **The transplantation theory, originally proposed by Sampson in the mid-1920s, is based on the assumption that endometriosis is caused by the seeding or implantation of endometrial cells by transtubal regurgitation during menstruation** (30). **Substantial clinical and experimental data support this hypothesis** (5,31). Retrograde menstruation occurs in 70% to 90% of women, and it may be more common in women with endometriosis than in those without the disease (8,32). The presence of endometrial cells in the peritoneal fluid, indicating retrograde menstruation, is reported in 59% to 79% of women during menses or in the early follicular phase, and these cells can be cultured *in vitro* (33,34). The presence of endometrial cells in the dialysate of women undergoing peritoneal dialysis during menses supports the theory of retrograde menstruation (35). Endometriosis is most often found in dependent portions of the pelvis—the ovaries, the anterior and posterior cul-de-sac, the uterosacral ligaments, the posterior uterus, and the posterior broad ligaments (36). The menstrual reflux theory combined with the clockwise peritoneal fluid current explains why endometriosis is predominantly located on the left side of the pelvis (refluxed endometrial cells implant more easily in the rectosigmoidal area) and why diaphragmatic endometriosis is found more frequently on the right side (refluxed endometrial cells implant there by the falciform ligament) (37,38).

Endometrium obtained during menses can grow when injected beneath abdominal skin or into the pelvic cavity of animals (39,40). Endometriosis was found in 50% of *Rhesus* monkeys after surgical transposition of the cervix to allow intra-abdominal menstruation (41). Increased retrograde menstruation by obstruction of the outflow of menstrual fluid from the uterus is associated with a higher incidence of endometriosis in women and in baboons (42–44). Women with shorter intervals between menstruation and longer duration of menses are more likely to have retrograde menstruation and are at higher risk for endometriosis (45). Menstruation is associated with intraperitoneal inflammation in both women and baboons, but a limited quantity of endometrial cells can be identified in peritoneal fluid during menstruation in women, possibly because endometrial–peritoneal attachment is reported to occur within 24 hours (46–48). Ovarian endometriosis may be caused by either retrograde menstruation or by lymphatic flow from the uterus to the ovary; metaplasia and bleeding from a corpus luteum may be a critical event in the development of some endometriomas (49–51).

Deeply infiltrative endometriosis, with a depth of at least 5 mm beneath the peritoneum, can present as nodules in the cul-de-sac, rectosigmoid, and bladder area and occurs with other forms of peritoneal or ovarian endometriosis (52). According to anatomic, surgical, and pathologic findings, deep endometriotic lesions originate intraperitoneally rather than extraperitoneally. The lateral asymmetry in the occurrence of ureteral endometriosis is compatible with the menstrual reflux theory and with the anatomic differences of the left and right hemipelvis (37). Adolescents and young women can have peritoneal disease (53). This observation, together with evidence from the development and spontaneous evolution of endometriosis in baboons, supports the notion that endometriosis starts as peritoneal disease and that the three different phenotypes and locations of endometriosis (peritoneal, ovarian, and deep) represent a homogenous disease continuum with a single origin (i.e., regurgitated endometrium), rather than three different disease entities, as advocated by some investigators (37,54,55).

Extrapelvic endometriosis, although rare (1% to 2%), may result from vascular or lymphatic dissemination of endometrial cells to many gynecologic (vulva, vagina, cervix) and nongynecologic sites. The latter include bowel (appendix, rectum, sigmoid colon, small intestine, hernia sacs), lungs and pleural cavity, skin (episiotomy or other surgical scars, inguinal region, extremities, umbilicus), lymph glands, nerves, and brain (56).

Coelomic Metaplasia   **The transformation (metaplasia) of coelomic epithelium into endometrial tissue is a proposed mechanism for the origin of endometriosis.** One study evaluating structural and cell surface antigen expression in the rete ovarii and epoophoron reported little commonality between endometriosis and ovarian surface epithelium, suggesting that serosal metaplasia is unlikely in the ovary (57). The results of another study involving the genetic induction of endometriosis in mice suggest that ovarian endometriotic lesions may arise directly from the ovarian surface epithelium through a metaplastic differentiation process induced by activation of an oncogenic *K-ras* allele (50).

Induction Theory   **The induction theory is an extension of the coelomic metaplasia theory. It proposes that an endogenous (undefined) biochemical factor can induce undifferentiated peritoneal cells to develop into endometrial tissue.** This theory is supported by experiments in rabbits but is not substantiated in women or nonhuman primates (58,59).

Genetic Factors

Increasing evidence suggests that endometriosis is partially a genetic disease. Recent findings that support this association include evidence of familial clustering in humans and in *Rhesus* monkeys, a founder effect detected in the Icelandic population, concordance in monozygotic twins, a similar age at onset of symptoms in affected nontwin sisters, a six- to nine-times increased prevalence of endometriosis among first-degree relatives of women compared with the general population, and a 15% prevalence of magnetic resonance imaging (MRI) findings suggestive of endometriosis in the first-degree relatives of women with stage III or IV disease based on the classification of the American Society of Reproductive Medicine (60). **The induction of humanlike endometriosis by genetic activation of an oncogenic *K-ras* allele lends further support to the genetic basis of this disorder** (50).

Population Studies

The risk of endometriosis is seven times greater if a first-degree relative is affected by endometriosis (61). **Because no specific Mendelian inheritance pattern is identified, multifactorial inheritance is postulated.** A relative risk for endometriosis of 7.2 was found in mothers and sisters, and a 75% (six in eight) incidence was noted in homozygotic twins of patients with endometriosis (62). In another study of twins, 51% of the variance of the latent liability to endometriosis may be attributable to additive genetic influences (63). Other investigators reported that 14 monozygotic twin pairs were concordant for endometriosis, and two pairs were discordant (64). Of these twin pairs, nine had moderate to severe endometriosis. A relationship was shown between endometriosis and systematic lupus erythematosus, dysplastic nevi, and a history of melanoma in women of reproductive age (65,66). Endometriosis is linked to the presence of individual human leukocyte antigens (67–69). Genome-wide association studies show that the risk of endometriosis is associated with a mutation on the short arm of chromosome 7 (7p15.2) in women of European ancestry and that this association is the strongest for moderate to severe disease (70).

Genetic Polymorphisms and Endometriosis

A number of studies investigated genetic polymorphisms as a possible factor contributing to the development of endometriosis. About 50% of the studies in one review demonstrated positive correlations between different polymorphisms and endometriosis (71). This relation was seen most clearly in groups 1 (cytokines and inflammation), 2 (steroid-synthesizing enzymes and detoxifying enzymes and receptors), 4 (estradiol metabolism), 5 (other enzymes and metabolic systems), and 7 (adhesion molecules and matrix enzymes). Group 8 (apoptosis, cell-cycle regulation, and oncogenes) seemed to be negatively correlated with the disease, whereas groups 3 (hormone receptors), 6 (growth factor systems), and especially 9 (human leukocyte antigen system components) showed a relatively strong correlation. As many results were contradictory, the review concluded that genetic polymorphisms might have a limited value in assessing possible development of endometriosis (71). Future studies should include large numbers of women with laparoscopically and histologically confirmed endometriosis and women with a laparoscopically confirmed normal pelvis as controls, taking into account ethnic variability.

Aneuploidy

Epithelial cells of endometriotic cysts are monoclonal on the basis of phosphoglycerate kinase gene methylation, and normal endometrial glands are monoclonal (72,73). In a comparison of endometriotic tissue with eutopic endometrium, flow cytometric DNA analysis failed to show aneuploidy (74). Studies using comparative genomic hybridization, or multicolor *in situ* hybridization, showed aneuploidy for chromosomes 11, 16, and 17, increased heterogeneity of chromosome 17 aneuploidy, and losses of 1p and 22q (50%), 5p (33%), 6q (27%), 70 (22%), 9q (22%), and 16 (22%) of 18 selected endometriotic tissues (75–77). In another study, trisomies 1 and 7, and monosomies 9 and 17 were found in endometriosis, ovarian endometrioid adenocarcinoma, and normal endometrium (78). The proportions of aneusomic cells were significantly higher in ovarian endometriosis compared with extragonadal endometriosis and normal endometrium (*p* <0.001), suggesting a role of the ovarian stromal milieu in the induction of genetic changes, which may lead to invasive cancer in isolated cases (78).

Microsatellite DNA assays reveal an allelic imbalance (loss of heterozygosity) in *p16 (Ink4)*, *GALT, p53,* and *APOA2* loci in patients with endometriosis and in stage II of endometriosis (79). Another report found a loss of heterozygosity in 28% of endometriotic lesions at one or more sites: chromosomes 9p (18%), 11q (18%), and 22q (15%) (73).

Immunologic Factors and Inflammation

Although retrograde menstruation appears to be a common event in women, not all women who have retrograde menstruation develop endometriosis. The immune system may be altered in women with endometriosis, and it is hypothesized that the disease may develop as a result of reduced immunologic clearance of viable endometrial cells from the pelvic cavity (80,81). Endometriosis can be caused by decreased clearance of peritoneal fluid endometrial cells resulting from reduced natural killer (NK) cell activity or decreased macrophage activity (82). Decreased cell-mediated cytotoxity toward autologous endometrial cells is associated with endometriosis (82–86). These studies used techniques that have considerable variability in target cells and methods (87,88). Whether NK cell activity is lower in patients with endometriosis than in those without endometriosis is controversial. Some reports demonstrate reduced NK activity and others found no increase in NK activity in women with moderate to severe disease (84–86,89–94). There is great variability in NK cell activity among normal individuals that may be related to variables such as smoking, drug use, and exercise (87).

In contrast, endometriosis can be considered a condition of immunologic tolerance, as opposed to ectopic endometrium, which essentially is self-tissue (80). It can be questioned why viable endometrial cells in the peritoneal fluid would be a target for NK cells or macrophages. Auto-transplantation of blood vessels, muscles, skin grafts, and other tissues is extremely successful (83–85). There is no *in vitro* evidence that peritoneal fluid macrophages actually attack and perform phagocytosis of viable peritoneal fluid endometrial cells. High-dose immunosuppression can increase slightly the progression of spontaneous endometriosis in baboons (95). There is no clinical evidence that the prevalence of endometriosis is increased in immunosuppressed patients. The fact that women with kidney transplants, who undergo chronic immunosuppression, are not known to have increased infertility problems can be considered indirect evidence that these patients do not develop extensive endometriosis.

Substantial evidence suggests that endometriosis is associated with a state of subclinical peritoneal inflammation, marked by an increased peritoneal fluid volume, increased peritoneal fluid white blood cell concentration (especially macrophages with increased activation status), and increased inflammatory cytokines, growth factors, and angiogenesis-promoting substances. It is reported in baboons that subclinical peritoneal inflammation occurs during menstruation and after intrapelvic injection of endometrium (93). A higher basal activation status of peritoneal macrophages in women with endometriosis may impair fertility by reducing sperm motility, increasing sperm phagocytosis, or interfering with fertilization, possibly by increased secretion of cytokines such as tumor necrosis factor-α (TNF-α) (96–100). Tumor necrosis factor may facilitate the pelvic implantation of ectopic endometrium (99,100). The adherence of human endometrial stromal cells to mesothelial cells *in vitro* is increased by the pretreatment of mesothelial cells with physiologic doses of TNF-α (101). Macrophages or other cells may promote the growth of endometrial cells by secretion of growth and angiogenetic factors such as epidermal growth factor (EGF), macrophage-derived growth factor (MDGF), fibronectin, and adhesion molecules such as integrins (101–107). After attachment of endometrial cells to the peritoneum, subsequent invasion and growth appear to be regulated by matrix metalloproteinases (MMP) and their tissue inhibitors (108,109).

There is increasing evidence that local inflammation and secretion of prostaglandins (PG) is related to differences in endometrial aromatase activity between women with and without endometriosis. Expression of aromatase cytochrome P450 protein and mRNA is present in human endometriotic implants but not in normal endometrium, suggesting that ectopic endometrium produces estrogens, which may be involved in the tissue growth interacting with the estrogen receptor (110). Inactivation of 17β-estradiol is impaired in endometriotic tissues because of deficient expression of 17β-hydroxysteroid dehydrogenase type 2, which is normally expressed in eutopic endometrium in response to progesterone (111). The inappropriate aromatase expression in endometriosis lesions can be stimulated by prostaglandin E_2 (PGE_2). This reaction leads to local production of E_2, which stimulates PGE_2 production, resulting in a positive-feedback system between local inflammation and estrogen-driven local growth of ectopic endometrium (112).

The subclinical pelvic inflammatory status associated with endometriosis is reflected in the systemic circulation. Increased concentrations of C-reactive protein, serum amyloid A (SAA), TNF-α, membrane cofactor protein-1, interleukin-6 (IL-6), IL-8, and chemokine (C-C motif) receptor 1 (CCR1) are observed in peripheral blood samples of patients with endometriosis when compared with controls (113). This observation offers a basis for the development of noninvasive diagnostic tests.

Both hypothesis-driven research and system biology approaches using mRNA microarray and proteomic techniques studies show that eutopic endometrium is biologically different in women with endometriosis when compared to controls with respect to proliferation, apoptosis, angiogenesis, and inflammatory pathways (114–117). Several studies show a higher prevalence of nerve fibers and neurotrophic factors in the eutopic endometrium from women with endometriosis when compared to controls (46,118).

Environmental Factors and Dioxin

There is an increasing awareness of potential links between reproductive health, infertility, and environmental pollution. Attention was directed toward the potential role of dioxins in the pathogenesis of endometriosis, but the issue remains controversial. A meta-analysis concluded that there is insufficient evidence in women or in nonhuman primates that endometriosis is caused by dioxin exposure (119).

Human Data

A 1976 explosion of a factory in Seveso, Italy, resulted in the highest recorded levels of dioxin exposure in humans, but data are not published (120). The Seveso Women's Health Study will correlate prospective individual data on exposure to dioxin with reproductive endpoints such as the incidence of endometriosis, infertility, and decreased sperm quality. One case-control study failed to show an association in the general population between endometriosis and exposure to PCB and chlorinated pesticides during adulthood. No differences in mean plasma concentrations of 14-PCB and 11-chlorinated pesticides were found between women with and those without endometriosis (121). In another study, increased exposure to dioxin-like compounds is associated with (moderate to severe) endometriosis in a case-control study in women (122). Genetic mechanisms may play a role in dioxin exposure and the development of endometriosis. Transcripts of the *CYP1A1* gene, a dioxin-induced gene, are significantly higher (nine times higher) in endometriotic tissues than in eutopic endometrium (112). Other investigators report a similar expression of arylhydrocarbon receptor and dioxin-related genes (using semiquantitative reverse transcriptase polymerase chain reaction) in the endometrium from women with or without endometriosis (123). In Japanese women, no association was found between endometriosis prevalence or severity and polymorphisms for arylhydrocarbon receptor repressor, arylhydrocarbon (x2) receptor, and arylhydrocarbon nuclear translocator or *CYP1A1* genes (124). Based on these data, there is insufficient evidence supporting the association between endometriosis and dioxin exposure in humans.

Primates

An initial retrospective case-control study reported that the prevalence of endometriosis was not statistically different ($p = 0.08$) between monkeys chronically exposed to dioxin during 4 years (11 of 14, 79%) and unexposed animals (2 of 6, 33%) after a period of 10 years. A positive correlation was found between the severity of endometriosis and dioxin dose, serum levels of dioxin, and dioxin-like chemicals (125,126). Two prospective studies evaluated the association between dioxin exposure and development of endometriosis in *Rhesus* monkeys. In one study, monkeys exposed over 12 months to low-dose dioxin (0.71 ng/kg/day) had endometriosis implants with smaller maximal and minimal diameters and similar survival rate when compared with endometriotic lesions in unexposed controls, suggesting no effect of dioxin on endometriosis (127). After 12 months of exposure to high-dose dioxin (17.86 ng/kg/day), larger diameters and a higher survival rate of endometriosis implants were observed in exposed *Rhesus* monkeys compared with unexposed controls. The second randomized study performed in 80 *Rhesus* monkeys compared those with no treatment with those treated with 0, 5, 20, 40, and 80 μg of *Aroclor* (1,254 kg per day) for 6 years. Endometriosis occurred in 37% of controls and in 25% of treated monkeys as determined by laparoscopy and necropsy data (128). No association was observed between endometriosis severity and PCB exposure. These data question the importance of dioxin exposure, except at high doses, in the development of endometriosis in primates.

Rodents

Continuous exposure to 2,3,7,8-tetrachlorodibenzo-P-dioxin inhibited the growth of surgically induced endometriosis in ovariectomized mice treated with high-dose estradiol. No correlation was observed between the dose of dioxin and survival of endometrial implants, adhesions, and serum E_2 levels (129). In ovariectomized mice induced with endometriosis, similar stimulating effects of estrone and 4-chlorodiphenyl ether (4-CDE) were observed on survival rates of endometriotic mice, suggesting an estrogen-like effect of 4-CDE (130). Potential mechanisms mediating dioxin action to promote endometriosis in rodents are complex and probably different in rats and mice, and furthermore in women. The mouse appears to be a better model to elucidate these mechanisms, but both models have important limitations (131,132).

Stem Cells

Endometrial stem cells are identified, are bone marrow derived, can differentiate into neurogenic or pancreatic-β cells, may contribute to the development of endometriosis in a murine model, and their potential role in the pathogenesis of endometriosis needs to be investigated (133–136).

Future Research

The study of endometriosis is compounded by the need to determine the presence or absence of pathology. The pathogenesis of endometriosis, the pathophysiology of related infertility, and the spontaneous evolution of endometriosis are being studied. At the time of diagnosis, most patients with endometriosis had the disease for an unknown period, making it difficult to initiate clinical experiments that would determine the etiology or progression of the disease (31). Because endometriosis occurs naturally only in women and nonhuman primates, and invasive experiments cannot be performed easily, it is difficult to undertake properly controlled studies. There is a need for the development of a good animal model with spontaneous endometriosis. The main advantage of the rat and rabbit models used to study endometriosis is their low cost relative to primates, but the disadvantages are numerous (137–140). In both models, the type of lesion appears to be quite different from the variety of pigmented and nonpigmented lesions observed in women (137–139). Primates are phylogenetically close to humans, have a comparable menstrual cycle, are afflicted with spontaneous endometriosis, and when induced with endometriosis, develop macroscopic lesions that are similar to those found in human disease (41,141–145). Spontaneous endometriosis in the baboon is minimal and disseminated, similar to the different stages of endometriosis in women (141,146–148).

Immunomodulatory drugs inhibiting pelvic inflammation associated with endometriosis may offer new approaches to medical treatment and can be studied in these models (149–153). In a consensus workshop following the 10th World Congress on Endometriosis in 2008, it was agreed that multidisciplinary expertise is required to advance our understanding of this disease, and 25 recommendations for research were developed (154).

Diagnosis

Clinical Presentation

Endometriosis should be suspected in women with subfertility, dysmenorrhea, dyspareunia, or chronic pelvic pain, although these symptoms can be associated with other diseases.

Endometriosis may be asymptomatic, even in women with more advanced disease, (i.e., ovarian endometriosis or deeply invasive rectovaginal endometriosis).

Risk factors for endometriosis include short cycle length, heavier menstruation, and longer flow duration, probably related to a higher incidence of retrograde menstruation (45,155,156). Patient height and weight are positively and negatively, respectively, associated with the risk of endometriosis (157).

Endometriosis can be associated with significant gastrointestinal symptoms (pain, nausea, vomiting, early satiety, bloating and distention, altered bowel habits). A characteristic motility change (ampulla of Vater–duodenal spasm, a seizure equivalent of the enteric nervous system, along with bacterial overgrowth), is documented in most women with the disease (158). Women of reproductive age with endometriosis are not osteopenic (159).

The average delay between onset of pain symptoms and surgically confirmed endometriosis is quite long: 8 years or longer in the United Kingdom and 9 to 12 years in the United States (160). Similar durations were observed in Scandinavia and in Brazil (161,162). A delay in diagnosis of endometriosis of 6 and 3 years in women with pain and women with infertility, respectively, was reported. Over the past two decades, there was a steady decrease in the delay in diagnosis and a decline in the prevalence of advanced endometriosis at first diagnosis (163). Patient awareness of endometriosis was increased. Many patients' quality of life is affected by pain, emotional impact of subfertility, anger about disease recurrence, and uncertainty about the future regarding repeated surgeries or long-term medical therapy and its side effects (164). Endometriosis should be perceived as a chronic disease, at least in a subset of highly symptomatic women, and quality-of-life issues should be evaluated using reliable and valid questionnaires (165).

Pain

In adult women, dysmenorrhea may be especially suggestive of endometriosis if it begins after years of pain-free menses. Dysmenorrhea often starts before the onset of menstrual bleeding and continues throughout the menstrual period. In adolescents, the pain may be present after menarche without an interval of pain-free menses. Evidence suggests that absenteeism from school and both the incidence and duration of oral contraceptive use for severe primary dysmenorrhea during adolescence is higher in women who later develop deeply infiltrative endometriosis than in women without deeply infiltrative endometriosis (166).

The distribution of pain is variable but most often is bilateral. Local symptoms can arise from rectal, ureteral, and bladder involvement, and lower back pain can occur. Some women with extensive disease have no pain, whereas others with only minimal to mild disease may experience severe pelvic pain. All endometriosis lesion types are associated with pelvic pain, including minimal to mild endometriosis (167). Endometriomas are not associated with dysmenorrheal severity, and dysmenorrhea is less frequent in women with only ovarian endometriomas compared with other locations (168,169). Endometriomas can be considered a marker for greater severity of deeply infiltrative lesions (170). Deeply infiltrative lesions are consistently associated with pelvic pain, gastrointestinal symptoms, and painful defecation (171). The role of adhesions in pain and endometriosis is poorly understood (172).

Many studies failed to detect a correlation between the degree of pelvic pain and the severity of endometriosis (11,169,173). Some studies reported a positive correlation between endometriosis stage and endometriosis-related dysmenorrhea or chronic pelvic pain (174,175). In one study, a significant but weak correlation was observed between endometriosis stage and severity of dysmenorrhea and nonmenstrual pain, whereas a strong association was found between posterior cul-de-sac lesions and dyspareunia (176).

Possible mechanisms causing pain in patients with endometriosis include local peritoneal inflammation, deep infiltration with tissue damage, adhesion formation, fibrotic thickening, and collection of shed menstrual blood in endometriotic implants, resulting in painful traction with the physiologic movement of tissues (177,178). The character of pelvic pain is related to the anatomic location of deeply infiltrating endometriotic lesions (171). Severe pelvic pain and dyspareunia may be associated with deep infiltrating subperitoneal endometriosis (6,177,179). In rectovaginal endometriotic nodules, a close histologic relationship was observed between nerves and endometriotic foci and between nerves and the fibrotic component of the nodule (180). Increasing evidence suggests a close relationship between the density of innervation of endometriotic lesions and pain symptoms (176).

Subfertility

Many arguments support the hypothesis that there is a causal relationship between the presence of endometriosis and subfertility (181). The following factors have been reported:

1. Increased prevalence of endometriosis in subfertile women (33%) when compared to women of proven fertility (4%), a reduced monthly fecundity rate (MFR) in baboons with mild to severe (spontaneous or induced) endometriosis when compared to those with minimal endometriosis or a normal pelvis.

2. Trend toward a reduced monthly fecundity rate in infertile women with minimal to mild endometriosis when compared to women with unexplained infertility.

3. Endometriotic ovarian cysts that negatively affect the rate of spontaneous ovulation (182).

4. Dose–effect relationship: a negative correlation between the r-AFS stage of endometriosis and the monthly fecundity rate and cumulative pregnancy rate (181,183).

5. Reduced monthly fecundity rate and cumulative pregnancy rate after donor sperm insemination in women with minimal to mild endometriosis when compared to those with a normal pelvis.

6. Reduced monthly fecundity rate after husband sperm insemination in women with minimal to mild endometriosis when compared to those with a normal pelvis.

7. Reduced implantation rate per embryo after *in vitro* fertilization (IVF) in women with endometriosis when compared to women with tubal factor infertility (181,184).

8. Increased monthly fecundity rate and cumulative pregnancy rate after surgical removal of minimal to mild endometriosis.

When endometriosis is moderate or severe, involving the ovaries and causing adhesions that block tubo-ovarian motility and ovum pickup, it is associated with subfertility (182,185). This effect was shown in primates, including cynomolgus monkeys and baboons (144,186). Numerous mechanisms (ovulatory dysfunction, luteal insufficiency, luteinized unruptured follicle syndrome, recurrent abortion, altered immunity, and intraperitoneal inflammation) are proposed as explanations, but an association between fertility and minimal or mild endometriosis remains controversial (187).

Spontaneous Abortion   A possible association between endometriosis and spontaneous abortion was suggested in uncontrolled or retrospective studies. Some controlled studies evaluating the association between endometriosis and spontaneous abortion have important methodologic shortcomings: heterogeneity between cases and controls, analysis of the abortion rate before the diagnosis of endometriosis, and selection bias of study and control groups (80,188,189). **Based on controlled prospective studies, there is no evidence that endometriosis is associated with (recurrent) pregnancy loss or that medical or surgical treatment of endometriosis reduces the spontaneous abortion rate** (190–192). Some data suggest that miscarriage rates may be increased after treatment with assisted reproductive technology (193).

Endocrinologic Abnormalities

Endometriosis is associated with anovulation, abnormal follicular development with impaired follicle growth, reduced circulating E_2 levels during the preovulatory phase, disturbed luteinizing hormone (LH) surge patterns, premenstrual spotting, luteinized unruptured follicle syndrome, and galactorrhea and hyperprolactinemia (194). Increased incidence and recurrence of the luteinized unruptured follicle syndrome is reported in baboons with mild endometriosis, but not in primates with minimal endometriosis or a normal pelvis (195). Luteal insufficiency with reduced circulating E_2 and progesterone levels, out-of-phase endometrial biopsies, and aberrant integrin expression was reported in the endometrium of women with endometriosis by some researchers, but these findings were not confirmed by other investigators (194,196,197). No convincing data exist to conclude that the incidence of these endocrine abnormalities is increased in women who have endometriosis.

Extrapelvic Endometriosis

Extrapelvic endometriosis, although often asymptomatic, should be suspected when symptoms of pain or a palpable mass occur outside the pelvis in a cyclic pattern. Endometriosis involving the intestinal tract (especially colon and rectum) is the most common site of extrapelvic disease and may cause abdominal and back pain, abdominal distention, cyclic rectal bleeding, constipation, and obstruction. Ureteral involvement can lead to obstruction and result in cyclic pain, dysuria, and hematuria. Pulmonary endometriosis can manifest as pneumothorax, hemothorax, or hemoptysis during menses. Umbilical endometriosis should be suspected when a patient has a palpable mass and cyclic pain in the umbilical area (56).

Treatment of extragenital endometriosis will depend on the site. If complete excision is possible, this is the treatment of choice; when this is not possible, long-term medical treatment is necessary using the same principles of medical treatment for pelvic endometriosis (1). Appendicular endometriosis is usually treated by appendectomy. Surgical treatment of bladder endometriosis is usually in the form of excision of the lesion and primary closure of the bladder wall. Ureteral lesions may be excised after stenting the ureter; in the presence of intrinsic lesions or significant obstruction, segmental excision with end-to-end anastomosis or reimplantation may be necessary. Abdominal wall and perineal endometriosis is usually treated by complete excision of the nodule (1).

Clinical Examination

In many women with endometriosis, no abnormality is detected during the clinical examination. However, the vulva, vagina, and cervix should be inspected for any signs of endometriosis, although the occurrence of endometriosis in these areas is rare (e.g., episiotomy scar). The presence of a narrow pinpoint cervical ostium can be a risk factor for endometriosis (23). **Other signs of possible endometriosis include uterosacral or cul-de-sac nodularity, lateral or cervical displacement caused by uterosacral scarring, painful swelling of the rectovaginal septum, and unilateral ovarian cystic enlargement** (198). In more advanced disease, the uterus is often in fixed retroversion, and the mobility of the ovaries and fallopian tubes is reduced. Evidence of deeply infiltrative endometriosis (deeper than 5 mm under the peritoneum) in the rectovaginal septum with cul-de-sac obliteration or cystic ovarian endometriosis should be suspected when there is clinical documentation of uterosacral nodularities during menses, especially if CA125 serum levels are higher than 35 IU/mL (199–201). In these cases, black-blue colored lesions can sometimes be observed in the vagina during speculum examination.

The clinical examination may have false-negative results. The diagnosis of endometriosis should be confirmed by visual inspection during laparoscopy and by histological confirmation of endometriosis in biopsied lesions.

Imaging

Ultrasound

Peritoneal endometriosis cannot be reliably visualized by imaging techniques. Compared to laparoscopy, transvaginal ultrasound has no value in diagnosing peritoneal endometriosis, but it is useful in making or excluding the diagnosis of an ovarian endometrioma (1,202). Either transvaginal or transrectal ultrasonography can be used with high sensitivity and specificity for the diagnosis of ovarian endometrioma (202–204). The typical ultrasound features of an endometriotic ovarian cyst in premenopausal women were described as "ground glass echogenicity of the cyst fluid, one to four locules and no solid parts" (205). Transvaginal ultrasound may have a role in the diagnosis of endometriosis nodules with a diameter of 1 cm involving the bladder or rectum, but this is dependent on the interest and experience of the ultrasonographer and the quality and resolution of the ultrasound equipment.

Local guidelines for the management of suspected ovarian malignancy should be followed in cases of ovarian endometrioma (1). Ultrasound scanning with or without serum CA125 testing is usually used to try to identify rare instances of ovarian cancer; however, CA125 levels are frequently elevated in the presence of endometriomas, so this approach is often not useful (1).

Other Imaging

Other imaging techniques, including **computed tomography (CT) and MRI,** can be used to provide additional and confirmatory information, but they cannot be used for primary diagnosis (1,206). These techniques **are more costly than ultrasonography, and their added value is unclear.**

Hysterosalpingography is not recommended as a diagnostic test for endometriosis, although the presence of filling defects (presence of hypertrophic or polypoid endometrium) has a significant positive correlation with endometriosis (positive and negative predictive values of 84% and 75%, respectively) (207).

Imaging to Assess Intestinal and Urologic Involvement

If there is clinical evidence of deeply infiltrating endometriosis, ureteral, bladder, and bowel involvement should be assessed. Ureteral involvement may be asymptomatic in up to 50% of patients with deeply infiltrative endometriosis (208). Consideration should be given to performing ultrasound (transrectal, transvaginal or renal), a CT urogram, or an MRI. A barium enema study might be useful, depending on the individual circumstances, to map the extent of disease present, which may be multifocal (1). There is no proof that one technique is superior to another; it is recommended that the technique that is most familiar to the radiologist involved be used.

Blood and Other Tests

There is no specific blood test for the diagnosis of endometriosis. A general endometriosis screening test may be neither appropriate (risk for overdiagnosis) nor feasible. A blood test with a high sensitivity would be useful if that would identify women with symptomatic endometriosis (pelvic pain, infertility) that is not detectable by ultrasound imaging (209). This would include all cases of minimal to mild endometriosis and those cases of moderate to severe endometriosis without detectable ovarian endometriotic cysts or nodules (210). These are patients who could benefit from laparoscopic surgery to reduce endometriosis-associated pain and infertility or to diagnose and treat other pelvic causes of pelvic pain or infertility, like pelvic adhesions. From that perspective, a lower specificity would be acceptable because the main goal of such a test would be to rule in all women with potential endometriosis or other pelvic disease who might benefit from surgery (211).

CA125

Levels of CA125, a glycoprotein from coelomic epithelium and common to most nonmucinous epithelial ovarian carcinomas, are significantly higher in women with moderate or severe endometriosis and normal in women with minimal or mild disease (212,213). It is presumed that endometriosis lesions produce peritoneal irritation and inflammation and this leads to an increased shedding of CA125 (213). During menstruation, an increase in CA125 levels was shown in women with and without endometriosis (214–218). Other studies did not find an increase during menses, or found an increase only with moderate to severe endometriosis (219–222). The levels of CA125 vary widely: in patients without endometriosis (8–22 U/mL in the nonmenstrual phase), in those with minimal to mild endometriosis (14–31 U/mL in the nonmenstrual phase), and in those with moderate to severe disease (13–95 U/mL in the nonmenstrual phase). **Compared with laparoscopy, measurement of serum CA125 levels has no value as a diagnostic tool** (223).

The specificity of CA125 is reported to be higher than 80% in most studies. This high level of specificity is achieved in selected women with infertility or pain, who are known to be at risk for endometriosis. **The low level of sensitivity of CA125 (20% to 50% in most studies) poses limitations for the clinical use of this test for diagnosis of endometriosis.** Theoretically, the sensitivity might increase during the menstrual period, when the increase in CA125 level is more pronounced in women who have endometriosis. Studies using cutoff levels of 35 U/mL or 85 U/mL did not find a significant improvement in sensitivity (221,222,224). A sensitivity of 66% was found when the CA125 level was determined during both the follicular phase and the menstrual phase in each patient and when the ratio of menstrual versus follicular values (>1.5) was used instead of one CA125 level (222). Other studies reported that the value of CA125 in diagnosis of endometriosis is limited but higher for moderate to severe disease, especially if serum CA125 concentrations are measured during the midfollicular phase (223,225).

Serial CA125 determinations may be useful to predict the recurrence of endometriosis after therapy (226,227). CA125 levels decrease after combined medical and surgical therapy or during medical treatment of endometriosis with *danazol,* gonadotropin-releasing hormone (GnRH) analogues, or *gestrinone,* but not with *medroxyprogesterone acetate* (*MPA*) or placebo (228–230). Levels of CA125 are reported to increase to pretreatment levels as early as 3, 4, or 6 months after the cessation of therapy with *danazol,* GnRH analogues, or *gestrinone* (218,229–233). Posttreatment increases in CA125 levels are reported to correlate with endometriosis recurrence (217,227,234). Other studies did not substantiate a correlation between posttreatment CA125 levels and disease recurrence (228,231,235).

Other Tests

It is not possible to diagnose endometriosis in a noninvasive way based on the increased concentration of cytokines and growth factors in peripheral blood or on endometrial biopsy analysis (46,236).

Laparoscopy

General Considerations

Unless disease is visible in the vagina or elsewhere, laparoscopy is the standard technique for visual inspection of the pelvis and establishment of a definitive diagnosis (1). There is insufficient evidence to justify timing the laparoscopy at a specific time in the menstrual cycle, but it should not be performed during or within 3 months of hormonal treatment so as to avoid underdiagnosis (1). Laparoscopic recognition of endometriosis will vary with the experience of the surgeon, especially for subtle bowel, bladder, ureteral, and diaphragmatic lesions (1). A meta-analysis of its value against a histological diagnosis showed (assuming a 10% pretest probability of endometriosis) that a positive laparoscopy increases the likelihood of disease to 32% (95% confidence interval [CI], 21%–46%) and a negative laparoscopy decreases the likelihood to 0.7% (95% CI, 0.1%–5.0%) (1,237). Diagnostic laparoscopy is associated with an approximately 3% risk of minor complications (e.g., nausea, shoulder tip pain) and a risk of major complications (e.g., bowel perforation, vascular damage) of 0.6 to 1.8 per 1,000 cases (1,238,239). Endometriosis can be treated during laparoscopy, thus combining diagnosis and therapy.

Laparoscopic Technique

During diagnostic laparoscopy, the pelvic and abdominal cavity should be systematically investigated for the presence of endometriosis. This examination should include a complete inspection in a clockwise or counterclockwise fashion with a blunt probe, with palpation of lesions to check for nodularity as a sign of deeply infiltrative endometriosis of the bowel, bladder, uterus, tubes, ovaries, cul-de-sac, or broad ligament (Fig. 17.1). The type, location, and extent of all lesions and adhesions should be documented in the operative notes; ideally, the findings should be recorded with photographs or on video such as a DVD (1).

Laparoscopic Findings

The laparoscopic findings of endometriosis include peritoneal lesions, ovarian endometriotic cysts, and deeply infiltrative endometriosis invading the peritoneal surface with a depth of at least 5 mm. **Most patients with ovarian endometriotic cysts or deeply infiltrative endometriosis also have peritoneal disease.**

Peritoneal Endometriosis

Characteristic findings include typical ("powder-burn" or "gunshot") lesions on the serosal surfaces of the peritoneum. These lesions are black, dark brown, or bluish nodules or small cysts containing old hemorrhage surrounded by a variable degree of fibrosis (Fig. 17.2). Endometriosis can appear as subtle lesions, including red implants (petechial, vesicular, polypoid, hemorrhagic, red flamelike), serous or clear vesicles, white plaques or scarring, yellow-brown discoloration of the peritoneum, and subovarian adhesions (Fig. 17.3) (138,139,141,240,241). Histologic confirmation of the laparoscopic impression is essential for the diagnosis of endometriosis, for subtle lesions, and for the typical lesions reported to be histologically negative in 24% of cases (242,243).

Deeply Infiltrative Endometriosis

Mild forms of deep endometriosis may be detected only by palpation under an endometriotic lesion or by discovery of a palpable mass beneath visually normal peritoneum, most notably in the posterior cul-de-sac (Fig. 17.4) (200). **At laparoscopy, deeply infiltrating endometriosis may have the appearance of minimal disease, resulting in an underestimation of disease severity** (200). Reduced size of the cul-de-sac in women with deep endometriosis suggests that such lesions develop not in the rectovaginal septum but intraperitoneally and that burial of anterior rectal wall adhesions creates a false bottom, giving an erroneous impression of extraperitoneal origin (244).

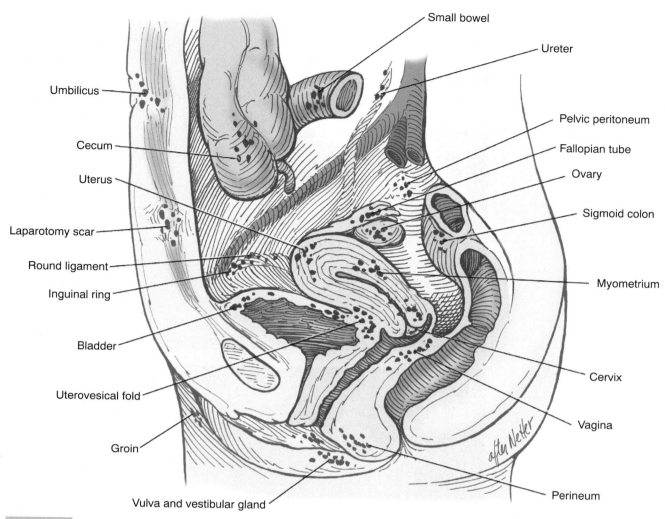

Figure 17.1 Pelvic endometriosis.

Ovarian Endometriosis

The diagnosis of ovarian endometriosis is facilitated by careful inspection of all sides of both ovaries, which may be difficult when adhesions are present in more advanced stages of disease (Fig. 17.5). With superficial ovarian endometriosis, lesions can be both typical and subtle. Larger ovarian endometriotic cysts (i.e., endometriomas) usually are located on the anterior surface of the ovary and are associated with retraction, pigmentation, and adhesions to the posterior peritoneum. **These ovarian endometriotic cysts often contain a thick, viscous dark brown fluid (i.e., "chocolate fluid"), composed of hemosiderin derived from previous intraovarian hemorrhage.** Because this fluid may be found in other conditions, such as in hemorrhagic corpus luteum cysts or neoplastic cysts, **biopsy and preferably removal of the ovarian cyst for histologic confirmation are necessary for the diagnosis** in the revised endometriosis classification of the American Society for Reproductive Medicine (ASRM). If that is not possible, the presence of an ovarian endometriotic cyst should be confirmed by the following features: cyst diameter of less than 12 cm, adhesion to pelvic sidewall or broad ligament, endometriosis on surface of ovary, and tarry, thick, chocolate-colored fluid content (245). Ovarian endometriosis appears to be a marker for more extensive pelvic and intestinal disease. Exclusive ovarian disease is found in only 1% of endometriosis patients, with the remaining patients having extensive pelvic or intestinal endometriosis (246).

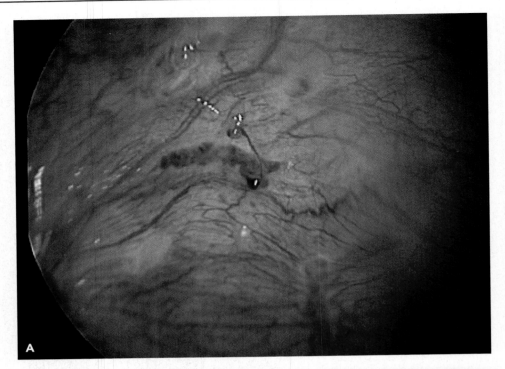

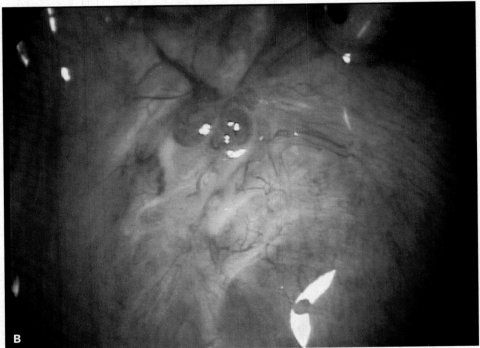

Figure 17.2   Typical and subtle endometriotic lesions on peritoneum. A: Typical black-puckered lesions with hypervascularization and orange polypoid vesicles. **B:** Red polypoid lesions with hypervascularization. (Photographs from Dr. Christel Meuleman, Leuven University Fertility Center, Leuven University Hospitals, Leuven, Belgium.)

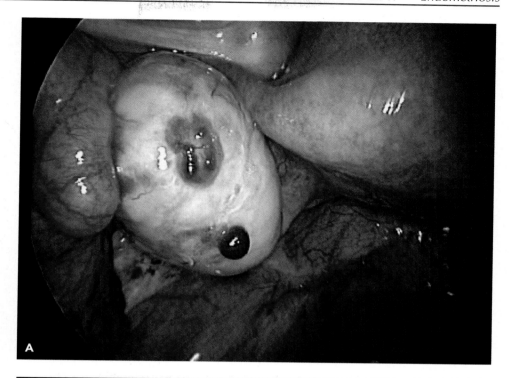

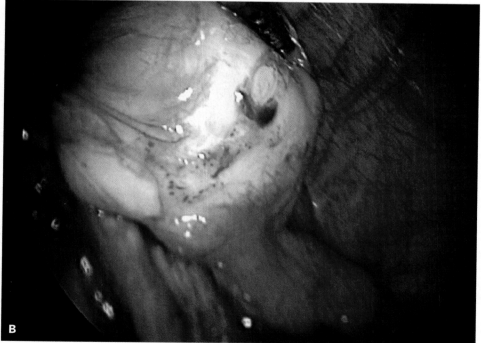

Figure 17.3 **Ovarian endometriosis.** (Photographs from Dr. Christel Meuleman, Leuven University Fertility Center, Leuven University Hospitals, Leuven, Belgium.) **A:** Superficial ovarian endometriosis. **B:** Superficial ovarian endometriosis and endometrioma—laparoscopic image prior to adhesiolysis.

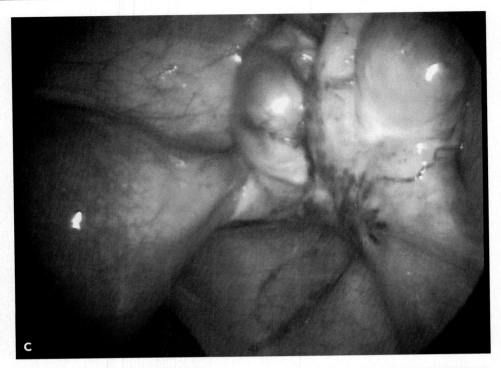

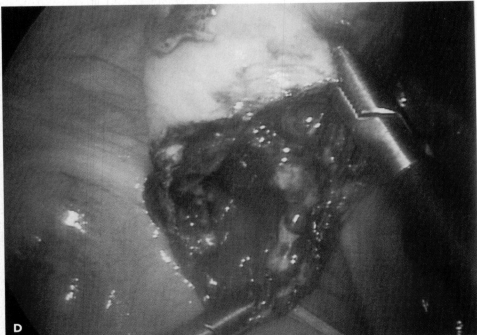

Figure 17.3   (*continued*) **C:** Laparoscopic image of uterus and right ovary with dark endometrioma. **D:** Ovarian endometriotic cystectomy

Histologic Confirmation   Positive histology confirms the diagnosis of endometriosis; negative histology does not exclude it (1). Whether histology should be obtained when peritoneal disease alone is present is controversial; visual inspection is usually adequate but histological confirmation of at least one lesion is ideal (1). In cases of ovarian endometrioma (>4 cm in diameter) and in deeply infiltrating disease, histology is recommended to exclude rare instances of malignancy (1).

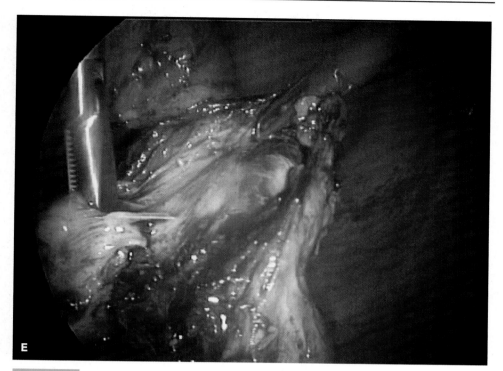

Figure 17.3   *(continued)* E: Ovarian endometriotic cystectomy.

In a study of 44 patients with chronic pelvic pain, endometriosis was laparoscopically diagnosed in 36%, but histologic confirmation was obtained in only 18%. This approach resulted in a low diagnostic accuracy of laparoscopic inspection with a positive predictive value of only 45%, explained by a specificity of only 77% (247).

Microscopically, endometriotic implants consist of endometrial glands and stroma, with or without hemosiderin-laden macrophages (Fig. 17.6). It is suggested that using these stringent and unvalidated histologic criteria may result in significant underdiagnosis of endometriosis (5). Problems in obtaining biopsies (especially small vesicles) and variability in tissue processing (step or partial instead of serial sectioning) may contribute to false-negative results. Endometrioid stroma may be more characteristic of endometriosis than endometrioid glands (248). The presence of stromal endometriosis, which contains endometrial stroma with hemosiderin-laden macrophages or hemorrhage, was reported in women and in baboons and may represent a very early event in the pathogenesis of endometriosis (147,242,243). Isolated endometrial stromal cell nodules and immunohistochemically positive for vimentin and estrogen receptor can be found in the absence of endometrial glands along blood or lymphatic vessels (249).

Different types of lesions may have different degrees of proliferative or secretory glandular activity (248). Vascularization, mitotic activity, and the three-dimensional structure of endometriosis lesions are key factors (177,250,251). **Deep endometriosis is described as a specific type of pelvic endometriosis characterized by proliferative strands of glands and stroma in dense fibrous and smooth muscle tissue** (19). Smooth muscles are frequent components of endometriotic lesions on the peritoneum, ovary, rectovaginal septum, and uterosacral ligaments (252).

Microscopic endometriosis is defined as the presence of endometrial glands and stroma in macroscopically normal pelvic peritoneum. It is important in the histogenesis of endometriosis and its recurrence after treatment (253,254). The clinical relevance of microscopic endometriosis is controversial because it is not observed uniformly. Using undefined criteria for what constitutes normal peritoneum, peritoneal biopsy specimens of 1 to 3 cm were obtained during laparotomy from 20 patients with moderate to severe endometriosis (254). Examination of the biopsy results with low-power scanning electron microscopy revealed unsuspected microscopic endometriosis in 25% of cases not confirmed by light microscopy. Peritoneal endometriotic foci were demonstrated by light microscopy in areas that showed no obvious evidence of disease (255).

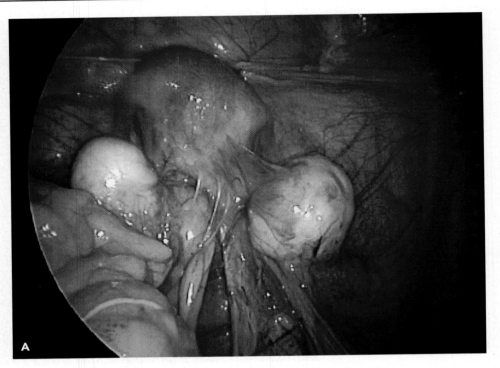

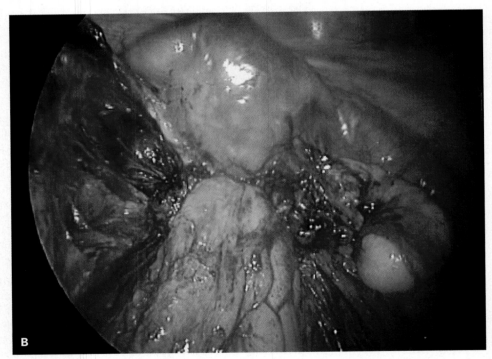

Figure 17.4   Laparoscopic excision of deep endometriosis from the cul-de-sac. (Photographs from Dr. Christel Meuleman, Leuven University Fertility Center, Leuven University Hospitals, Leuven, Belgium.) **A:** Extensive endometriosis with deep nodule at the right uterosacral ligament, masked by adhesions. **B:** Deep nodule still present in dense adhesion between rectum and uterosacral ligaments.

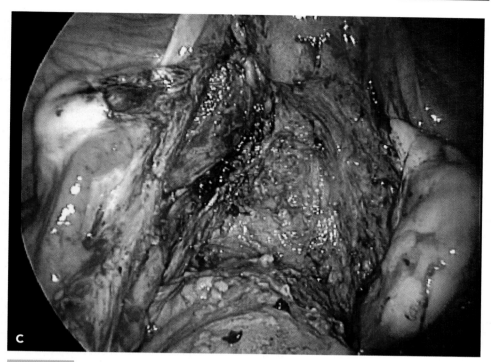

Figure 17.4   (*continued*) **C:** Cul-de-sac after resection of deep nodule with CO_2 laser.

In serial sections of laparoscopic biopsies of normal peritoneum, 10% to 15% of women had microscopic endometriosis, and endometriosis was found in 6% of those without macroscopic disease (241,256,257). Other studies were unable to detect microscopic endometriosis in 2-mm biopsy specimens of visually normal peritoneum (258–261). Examination of larger samples (5–15 mm) of visually normal peritoneum revealed microscopic endometriosis in only 1 of 55 patients studied (262). A histologic study of serial sections through the entire pelvic peritoneum of visually normal peritoneum from baboons with and without disease indicated that microscopic endometriosis is a rare occurrence (95). **Macroscopically appearing normal peritoneum rarely contains microscopic endometriosis** (262).

Laparoscopic Classification

Many classification systems were proposed, but only one was accepted. This system is the revised American Fertility Society (AFS) system, which is based on the appearance, size, and depth of peritoneal and ovarian implants; the presence, extent, and type of adnexal adhesions; and the degree of cul-de-sac obliteration (185,210). **In this ASRM classification system, the morphology of peritoneal and ovarian implants should be categorized as red (red, red-pink, and clear lesions), white (white, yellow-brown, and peritoneal defects), and black (black and blue lesions), according to color photographs provided by ASRM.**

This system reflects the extent of endometriotic disease but has considerable intraobserver and interobserver variability (263,264). Like all classification systems, the ASRM classification for endometriosis is subjective and correlates poorly with pain symptoms, but may be of value in infertility prognosis and management (181). Because this ASRM revised classification of endometriosis is the only internationally accepted system, it is the best available tool to describe objectively the extent of endometriosis and relate it to spontaneous evolution. More outcome-based research is needed to discover whether it is possible to improve the standardization and positive correlation of the ASRM classification of endometriosis with symptoms (pain, infertility) and with therapeutic outcome (pain relief, enhancement of fertility) after medical or surgical treatment. More variables than only the stage of endometriosis may have to be entered in such prediction models. Evidence suggests that endometriosis with an ASRM score of 16 or more, together with other variables like age, duration of infertility, and least functional score for ovaries and fallopian tubes after endometriosis surgery, is predictive of pregnancy (183).

American Society for Reproductive Medicine
Revised Classification of Endometriosis

Patient's Name _____ Date _____

Stage I (Minimal) - 1-5
Stage II (Mild) - 6-15   Laparoscopy_____ Laparotomy_____ Photography_____
Stage III (Moderate) - 16-40   Recommended Treatment_____
Stage IV (Severe) - >40   _____
Total_____   Prognosis_____

PERITONEUM	ENDOMETRIOSIS		<1cm	1-3cm	>3cm
		Superficial	1	2	4
		Deep	2	4	6
OVARY	R	Superficial	1	2	4
		Deep	4	16	20
	L	Superficial	1	2	4
		Deep	4	16	20

	POSTERIOR CUL-DE-SAC OBLITERATION	Partial	Complete
		4	40

	ADHESIONS		<1/3 Enclosure	1/3-2/3 Enclosure	>2/3 Enclosure
OVARY	R	Filmy	1	2	4
		Dense	4	8	16
	L	Filmy	1	2	4
		Dense	4	8	16
TUBE	R	Filmy	1	2	4
		Dense	4*	8*	16
	L	Filmy	1	2	4
		Dense	4*	8*	16

*If the fimbriated end of the fallopian tube is completely enclosed, change the point assignment to 16.

Additional Endometriosis: _____   Associated Pathology: _____
_____   _____
_____   _____

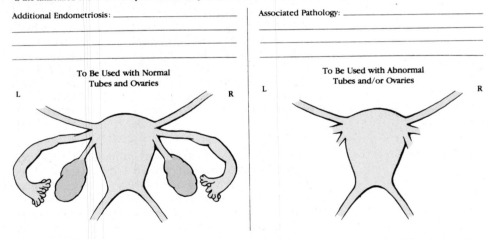

To Be Used with Normal   To Be Used with Abnormal
Tubes and Ovaries   Tubes and/or Ovaries
L   R   L   R

Figure 17.5 Revised American Society for Reproductive Medicine Classification. (From the American Society for Reproductive Medicine. Revised American Society for Reproductive Medicine classification of endometriosis. *Am Soc Reprod Med* 1997;5:817–821.)

Spontaneous Evolution

Endometriosis appears to be a progressive disease in a significant proportion (30% to 60%) of patients. During serial observations, deterioration (47%), improvement (30%), or elimination (23%) was documented over a 6-month period (265,266). In another study, endometriosis progressed in 64%, improved in 27%, and remained unchanged in 9% of patients over 12 months (267). A third study of 24 women reported 29% with disease progression, 29% with disease regression, and 42% with no change over 12 months. Follow-up studies in both baboons and women with spontaneous endometriosis over 24 months demonstrated disease progression in

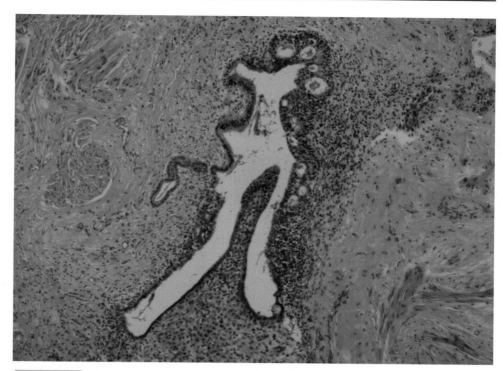

Figure 17.6 **Histologic appearance of endometriosis: endometrial glandular epithelium, surrounded by stroma in typical lesion and clear vesicle.**

all baboons and in 6 of 7 women (268–270). Several studies reported that subtle lesions and typical implants may represent younger and older types of endometriosis, respectively. In a cross-sectional study, the incidence of subtle lesions decreased with age (271). This finding was confirmed by a 3-year prospective study that reported that the incidence, overall pelvic area involved, and volume of subtle lesions decreased with age, but in typical lesions, these parameters and the depth of infiltration increased with age (6). Remodeling of endometriotic lesions (transition between typical and subtle subtypes) is reported to occur in women and in baboons, indicating that endometriosis is a dynamic condition (272,273). Several studies in women, cynomolgus monkeys, and rodents showed that endometriosis is ameliorated after pregnancy (273–276).

The characteristics of endometriosis are variable during pregnancy, and lesions tend to enlarge during the first trimester but regress thereafter (277). Studies in baboons revealed no change in the number or surface area of endometriosis lesions during the first two trimesters of pregnancy (278). These results do not exclude a beneficial effect that may occur during the third trimester or in the immediate postpartum period. Establishment of a "pseudopregnant state" with exogenously administered estrogen and progestins is based on the belief that symptomatic improvement may result from decidualization of endometrial implants during pregnancy (279). This hypothesis is not substantiated, and it is possible that amenorrhea can explain the beneficial effect of pregnancy and lactation on endometriosis-associated pain symptoms.

Management

Prevention

No strategies to prevent endometriosis are uniformly successful. A reduced incidence of endometriosis was reported in women who engaged in aerobic activity from an early age, but the possible protective effect of exercise was not investigated thoroughly (45). There is insufficient evidence that oral contraceptive use offers protection against the development of endometriosis. One report showed an increased risk for endometriosis in a select population of women taking oral contraceptives, possibly explained by the observation that dysmenorrhea as a reason to initiate estroprogestins is significantly more common in women with endometriosis than in women without the disease (280,281). Oral contraceptives (OCs) inhibit ovulation, substantially reduce the volume of menstrual flow, and may interfere with implantation of refluxed endometrial cells, but the hypothesis of recommending OCs for primary prevention of endometriosis is not sufficiently substantiated (282). Although the risk of endometriosis appears reduced during OC use, it is possible that this effect results from postponement of surgical evaluation caused by temporary suppression of pain symptoms (283). Confounding by selection and indication biases may explain the trend toward an increase in risk of endometriosis observed after discontinuation, but further clarification is needed (283).

Principles of Treatment

Treatment of endometriosis must be individualized, taking into consideration the clinical problem in its entirety, including the impact of the disease and the effect of its treatment on quality of life. Evidence-based recommendations that are continuously updated can be found in the ESHRE guidelines for the clinical management of endometriosis (1).

In most women with endometriosis, preservation of reproductive function is desirable (1). Many women with endometriosis have pain and subfertility at the same time or may desire children after sufficient pain relief, which complicates the choice of treatment. Endometriosis surgery should be considered as reproductive surgery, recently defined by the World Health Organization (WHO) as "all surgical procedures carried out to diagnose, conserve, correct and/or improve reproductive function" (284). The least invasive and least expensive approach that is effective with the least long-term risks should be chosen (1). **Symptomatic endometriosis patients can be treated with analgesics, hormones, surgery, assisted reproduction, or a combination of these modalities (1). Regardless of the clinical profile (subfertility, pain, asymptomatic findings), treatment of endometriosis may be justified because endometriosis appears to progress in 30% to 60% of patients within a year of diagnosis and it is not possible to predict in which patients it will progress** (267). Elimination of the endometriotic implants by surgical or medical treatment often provides only temporary relief. In addition to eliminating the endometriotic lesions, the goal should be to treat the sequelae (pain and subfertility) often associated with this disease and to prevent recurrence of endometriosis (1). **Endometriosis is a chronic disease and the recurrence rate is high after both hormonal and surgical treatment (1).**

It is important to involve the patient in all decisions, to be flexible in considering diagnostic and therapeutic approaches, and to maintain a good relationship. It may be appropriate to seek advice from more experienced colleagues or to refer the patient to a center with the necessary expertise to offer treatments in a multidisciplinary context, including advanced laparoscopic surgery and laparotomy (1,285). Because the management of severe or deeply infiltrating endometriosis is complex, referral is strongly recommended when disease of such severity is suspected or diagnosed (1).

Treatment of Endometriosis-Associated Pain

Pain may persist despite seemingly adequate medical or surgical treatment of the disease. A multidisciplinary approach involving a pain clinic and counseling should be considered early in the treatment plan. The least invasive and least expensive approach that is effective should be used (1).

Surgical Treatment

Depending on the severity of disease, diagnosis and removal of endometriosis should be performed simultaneously at the time of surgery, provided preoperative consent was obtained (1,286–289). **The goal of surgery is to excise all visible endometriotic lesions and associated adhesions—peritoneal lesions, ovarian cysts, deep rectovaginal endometriosis—and to restore normal anatomy** (1). In most women, laparoscopy can be used, and this technique decreases cost, morbidity, and the possibility of recurrence of adhesions postoperatively (1). **Laparotomy should be reserved for patients with advanced-stage disease who cannot undergo a laparoscopic procedure and for those in whom fertility conservation is not necessary** (1).

Peritoneal Endometriosis **Endometriosis lesions can be removed during laparoscopy** by surgical excision with scissors, bipolar coagulation, or laser methods (CO_2 laser, potassium-titanyl-phosphate laser, or argon laser). Some surgeons claim that the CO_2 laser is superior because it causes only minimal thermal damage, but **no evidence is available to show the superiority of one technique over another.** Comparable cumulative pregnancy rates were reported after treatment of mild endometriosis with laparoscopic excision and electrocoagulation (290). Ablation of endometriotic peritoneal lesions plus laparoscopic uterine nerve ablation (LUNA) in minimal to moderate disease reduces endometriosis-associated pain at 6 months compared to diagnostic laparoscopy; the smallest effect is seen in patients with minimal disease (1,291). **There is no evidence that LUNA is a necessary component, and LUNA by itself has no effect on dysmenorrhoea associated with endometriosis** (1,292,293). The effectiveness of surgical ablation of peritoneal endometriosis is convincingly shown in two randomized trials where the control group underwent a laparoscopy without surgical ablations of lesions. The treated group had a significant reduction of symptoms that persisted for 12 months and 18 months, respectively (268,294,295). The effectiveness of surgical treatment by laparotomy was not investigated by a randomized trial, although many published observational studies claim a high percentage of success (1).

Adhesiolysis   The removal of endometriosis-related adhesions (adhesiolysis) should be performed carefully. Adhesions lysed at surgery can form again (296). **Routine use of pharmacologic or liquid agents to prevent postoperative adhesions after fertility surgery cannot be recommended based on a systematic review, including 16 randomized controlled trials,** with the following indications for surgery included myomectomy (five trials), ovarian surgery (five trials), pelvic adhesions (four trials), endometriosis (one trial), and mixed (one trial) (297). No studies reported pregnancy or reduction in pain as outcomes (297). The absorbable adhesion barrier Interceed reduced the incidence of adhesion formation following laparoscopy and laparotomy, but there are insufficient data to support its use to improve pregnancy rates (297). The substance expanded polytetrafluoroethylene (Gore-Tex Surgical Membrane, Preclude; WL Gore, Flagstaff, AZ) may be superior to Oxidised regenerated cellulose (Interceed; Gynecare, Somerville, NJ) in preventing adhesion formation, but its usefulness is limited by the need for suturing and later removal (297). There was no evidence of effectiveness of chemically derived sodium hyaluronate and carboxymethylcellulose (Seprafilm, Genzyme Corporation, Cambridge, USA) or sheet-type fibrin sealant (Fibrin sheet, Tacho Comb, Tokyo, Japan) in preventing adhesion formation (297). In a randomized trial in patients with surgically treated stages I to III endometriosis without endometrioma, postoperative adnexal application of Oxiplex/AP (FzioMed, San Luis Obispo, California) gel treatment was superior to surgery alone (control group) with respect to postoperative adhesion formation (defined as secondary outcome) 6 to 8 weeks later in a subgroup of patients with red lesions (298). This observation needs to be confirmed in other randomized trials with postoperative adhesion formation as primary outcome. In the same study, control patients with at least 50% red lesions had a greater increase in ipsilateral adnexal adhesion scores than patients with mostly black or white and/or clear lesions (298).

Ovarian Endometriosis

Surgical Technique

Superficial ovarian lesions can be vaporized. The surgical management of ovarian endometriotic cysts is controversial. The primary indication for extirpation of an endometrioma is to ensure it is not malignant (1). The laparoscopic approach to the management of endometriomata is favored over a laparotomy approach because it offers the advantage of a shorter hospital stay, faster patient recovery, and decreased hospital costs (299). **The most common procedures for the treatment of ovarian endometriomas are either excision of the cyst capsule or drainage and electrocoagulation of the cyst wall.** During excision, the ovarian endometrioma is aspirated, followed by incision and removal of the cyst wall from the ovarian cortex with maximal preservation of normal ovarian tissue. During drainage and electrocoagulation, the ovarian endometrioma is aspirated and irrigated, its wall can be inspected with ovarian cystoscopy for intracystic lesions, and it is vaporized to destroy the mucosal lining of the cyst. Small ovarian endometriomata (less than 3-cm diameter) can be treated by drainage and electrocoagulation (1). Ovarian endometriomata larger than 3 cm should be removed completely (1,300). In cases where excision is technically difficult without removing a large part of the ovary, a three-step procedure (marsupialization and rinsing followed by hormonal treatment with GnRH analogues and cyst wall electrocoagulation or laser vaporization 3 months later) should be considered (1,301).

Outcome after Cystectomy

Although as little as one-tenth of an ovary may be enough to preserve function and fertility, at least for a while, there is increasing concern that ovarian cystectomy with concomitant removal or destruction of normal ovarian tissue may reduce ovarian follicle reserve and reduce fertility (302). One study reported reduced follicular response in natural and clomiphene citrate–stimulated cycles, but not in gonadotropin-stimulated cycles, in women younger than 35 years of age who underwent cystectomy compared with controls of similar age with normal ovaries (302). **According to a systematic review, there is good evidence that excisional surgery for endometriomas with a diameter of 3 cm provides a more favorable outcome than drainage and ablation with regard to the recurrence of the endometrioma, recurrence of pain symptoms, and in women who were previously subfertile or had subsequent spontaneous pregnancy** (299). **This approach should be the favored surgical approach, based on two randomized studies of the laparoscopic management of ovarian endometriomata of greater than 3 cm in size for the primary symptom of pain** (303,304). Laparoscopic excision of the cyst wall of the endometrioma was associated with a reduced recurrence rate of the symptoms of dysmenorrhea (odds ratio [OR] 0.15; 95% CI, 0.06–0.38), dyspareunia (OR 0.08; 95% CI, 0.01–0.51), and nonmenstrual pelvic pain (OR 0.10; 95% CI, 0.02–0.56), a reduced rate of recurrence of the endometrioma (OR 0.41; 95% CI, 0.18–0.93), and with a reduced requirement for further surgery (OR 0.21; 95% CI, 0.05–0.79) than surgery to ablate the endometrioma. For those women subsequently attempting to conceive, it was associated with an increased spontaneous pregnancy rate in women who had documented prior subfertility (OR 5.21; 95% CI, 2.04–13.29).

A randomized study demonstrated an increased ovarian follicular response to gonadotrophin stimulation for women who underwent excisional surgery when compared to ablative surgery (weighted mean difference (WMD) 0.6; 95% CI, 0.04–1.16) (305). There is insufficient evidence to favor excisional surgery over ablative surgery with respect to the chance of pregnancy after controlled ovarian stimulation and intrauterine insemination (OR 1.40; 95% CI, 0.47–4.15) or treatment with assisted reproductive technology (299). It is controversial whether there is a potential negative effect of ovarian cystectomy on reproductive function. In a small prospective randomized clinical trial, 10 patients assigned to undergo laparoscopic cystectomy had a lower antral follicle count and a more pronounced reduction in serum anti-müllerian hormone (AMH) levels (from 3.9 to 2.9 ng/mL) 6 months after surgery when compared to the 10 patients treated with a "three-stage procedure" as described above (reduction in AMH levels from 4.5 to 3.99 ng/mL) (306,307). More randomized trials are needed to assess the effect of ovarian cystectomy on ovarian reserve and on reproductive function, especially with respect to conception after treatment with medically assisted reproduction.

It is possible that the surgical techniques used to treat ovarian endometriotic cysts may influence postoperative adhesion formation and/or ovarian function. In a randomized study comparing surgical methods to achieve ovarian hemostasis after laparoscopic endometriotic ovarian cystectomy, closure of the ovary with an intraovarian suture resulted in a lower rate and extension of postsurgical ovarian adhesions at 60 to 90 days follow-up when compared to only bipolar coagulation on the internal ovarian surface (308).

Deeply Infiltrating Rectovaginal and Rectosigmoid Endometriosis

Deeply infiltrating endometriosis is usually multifocal and complete surgical excision must be performed in a one-step surgical procedure in order to avoid more than one surgery, provided the patient is fully informed (1,179,287). Because management of deeply infiltrating endometriosis is complex, referral to a center with sufficient expertise to offer all available treatments in a multidisciplinary approach is strongly recommended (1). Surgical management is only for symptomatic deeply infiltrating endometriosis. Asymptomatic patients must not undergo surgery. Progression of the disease and appearance of specific symptoms rarely occurred in patients with asymptomatic rectovaginal endometriosis (288). When surgical treatment is decided, the treatment must be radical with excision of all infiltrating lesions (1). It is difficult to perform randomized studies to detect the best surgical technique to treat deeply infiltrative endometriosis because these severe cases are all managed individually and not all surgeons are familiar with all treatment options (1). Complete excision while preserving the uterus and ovarian tissue might include the resection of the uterosacral ligaments, the resection of the upper part of the posterior vaginal wall, and urological and bowel operations.

Preoperative Preparation

The patients' surgical agreement must be obtained preoperatively to perform this difficult and high-risk procedure, especially in cases of expected or possible bowel or urological surgery.

Preoperative imaging is necessary to assess bowel and urological impact of deeply infiltrative endometriosis, as described above. CT urogram to exclude ureteral endometriosis and flexible sigmoidoscopy or double-contrast colon radiography to exclude transmural rectosigmoidal endometriosis, supplemented with MRI in selected cases, are preferred (285). As endometriosis sometimes involves nongynecologic organs (i.e., the bowel, the urinary tract, or pelvic bones), other surgical specialists should be consulted as appropriate. These severe cases should be handled in centers with special expertise. Preoperative intestinal preparation may be recommended. Placement of ureteric catheters may facilitate the excision of periureteral endometriosis to facilitate ureterolysis and end-to-end ureteral reanastomosis that may be needed in cases of infiltrative periureteral endometriosis causing ureteral obstruction. The pattern of pain in endometriosis is complicated and pain does not always respond to treatment, so consultation with pain specialists may be useful.

Removal of full-thickness bladder detrusor endometriosis entails excision of the bladder dome or posterior wall, generally well above the trigone. Transurethral resection is contraindicated. A radical approach to obstructive uropathy is suggested, with resection of the stenotic ureteral tract and reimplantation with antireflux vesicoureteral plasty (309).

Surgical excision of deep rectovaginal and rectosigmoidal endometriosis is difficult and can be associated with major complications such as bowel perforations with resulting peritonitis (310). It is debated whether this type of endometriosis is best treated by shaving, conservative excision or resection reanastomosis, by laparoscopy and laparotomy, or laparoscopically assisted vaginal technique (311).

In a randomized study comparing colorectal resection for endometriosis by laparoscopy or laparotomy, clinical outcome was similar with respect to dyschezia, bowel pain and cramping, and dysmenorrhea and dyspareunia, but laparoscopy was associated with less blood loss, fewer complications, and a higher pregnancy rate than laparotomy (312).

There are very few methodologically valid studies evaluating clinical outcome after deeply infiltrative with colorectal extension, as demonstrated in a systematic review (313). In a review on the clinical outcome of surgical treatment of deeply infiltrating endometriosis with colorectal involvement, most of the 49 reviewed studies included complications (94%) and pain (67%); few studies reported recurrence (41%), fertility (37%), and quality of life (10%); only 29% reported (loss of) follow-up. Of 3,894 patients, 71% underwent bowel resection and anastomosis, 10% had full-thickness excision, and 17% were treated with superficial surgery. Comparison of clinical outcome between different surgical techniques was not possible. Postoperative complications were present in 0% to 3% of the patients. Although pain improvement was reported in most studies, pain evaluation was patient based in less than 50% (visual analog scale [VAS] in only 18%). Although quality of life was improved in most studies, prospective data were available for only 149 patients. Pregnancy rates were 23% to 57% with a cumulative pregnancy rate of 58% to 70% within 4 years. The overall endometriosis recurrence rate in studies (longer than 2 years follow-up) was 5% to 25%, with most of the studies reporting 10%. Owing to highly variable study design and data collection, a Consolidated Standards of Reporting Trials (CONSORT)-inspired checklist was developed for future studies (313). Prospective studies reporting standardized and well-defined clinical outcome after surgical treatment of deeply invasive endometriosis with colorectal involvement with long-term follow-up are needed (313).

Surgical Treatment of Pain

The outcome of surgical therapy in patients with endometriosis and pain is influenced by many psychological factors relating to personality, depression, and marital and sexual problems. It is difficult to evaluate scientifically the objective effect of different surgical approaches because the extirpation and destruction of the pathological tissue can impact the results as can surgery *per se*, the doctor–patient relationship, complications, and other factors. There is a significant placebo response to surgical therapy: diagnostic laparoscopy without complete removal of endometriosis may alleviate pain in 50% of patients (295,314,315). Similar results were reported using oral placebos (316). Although some reports claimed pain relief with laser laparoscopy in 60% to 80% of patients with very low morbidity, none was prospective or controlled or allowed a definitive conclusion regarding treatment efficacy (200,317–320). The longstanding effect of surgery on pain is difficult to evaluate because the follow-up time is too short, usually just a few months. The major shortcoming of surgical treatment in endometriosis related pain is the lack of prospective randomized studies with sufficient follow-up time to draw clear clinical conclusions.

Laparoscopic Uterine Nerve Ablation

In a prospective, controlled, randomized, study, surgical therapy with ablation of endometriotic lesions and LUNA was shown to be superior to expectant management 6 months after treatment of mild and moderate endometriosis (295). In women with mild and moderate disease treated with laser, 74% achieved pain relief. Treatment was least effective in women with minimal disease. There were no reported operative or laser complications (295). One year later, symptom relief was still present in 90% of those who responded initially (268,295). Patients with severe disease were not included because surgery resulted in pain relief in 80% of patients who did not respond to medical therapy (295,319). There is randomized evidence that LUNA is not a necessary part of this treatment because addition of uterosacral ligament resection to conservative laparoscopic surgery for endometriosis stages I to IV did not reduce the medium- or long-term frequency and severity of recurrence of dysmenorrhea (292,293). These data were confirmed in a second randomized trial in women with chronic pelvic pain lasting longer than 6 months without or with minimal endometriosis, adhesions, or pelvic inflammatory disease, where LUNA did not result in improvements in pain, dysmenorrhea, dyspareunia, or quality of life compared with laparoscopy without pelvic denervation (321).

In a randomized crossover study, laparoscopic excision of endometriosis was found to be more effective than placebo in reducing pain and improving quality of life (294). These results suggest that laparoscopic surgery may be effective for the treatment of pain associated with mild to severe endometriosis. In women with minimal endometriosis, laser treatment may limit progression of disease.

Meta-analysis and Systematic Review

In a systematic review assessing the efficacy of laparoscopic surgery in the treatment of pelvic pain associated with endometriosis and including five randomized controlled studies, meta-analysis demonstrated an advantage of laparoscopic surgery when compared to diagnostic laparoscopy only at 6 months (OR 5.72; 95%CI, 3.09–10.60; 171 participants, three trials) and 12 months (OR 7.72; 95%CI, 2.97–20.06; 33 participants, one trial) after surgery (291). Few women diagnosed with severe endometriosis were included in the meta-analysis and any conclusions from this meta-analysis regarding treatment of severe endometriosis should be made with caution. It was not possible to draw conclusions from the meta-analysis which specific laparoscopic surgical intervention is most effective (291).

The extent and duration of the therapeutic benefit of surgery for endometriosis-related pain are poorly defined, and the expected benefit is operator dependent (322). In a systematic review based on three randomized controlled studies, the absolute benefit increase of destruction of lesions compared with diagnostic only operation in terms of proportion of women reporting pain relief was between 30% and 40% after short follow-up periods (322). The pain relief ended to decrease with time, and the reoperation rate, based on long-term follow-up studies, was as high as 50% (322). In most case series on excisional surgery for rectovaginal endometriosis, substantial short-term pain relief was experienced by approximately 70% to 80% of the patients who continued the study. At 1-year follow-up, approximately 50% of the women needed analgesics or hormonal treatments (322). Medium-term recurrence of lesions was observed in approximately 20% of the cases, and approximately 25% of the women underwent repetitive surgery (322). It appears that pain recurrence and reoperation rates after conservative surgery for symptomatic endometriosis are high and probably underestimated (322).

Preoperative Hormonal Treatment

In patients with severe endometriosis, it is recommended that surgical treatment be preceded by a 3-month course of medical treatment to reduce vascularization and nodular size (200). A randomized controlled study comparing presurgical medical therapy (3 months of GnRH agonists) with surgery alone in women with moderate to severe endometriosis showed a significant improvement in AFS scores in the medical therapy group (WMD −9.60; 95% CI, −11.42 to −7.78), without significant difference in ease of surgery between the two groups and without documentation of improved outcomes for the patients (323). **Hormonal therapy prior to surgery improves r-AFS scores, but there is insufficient evidence of any effect on outcome measures such as pain relief** (1,324).

Oophorectomy and Hysterectomy

Radical procedures such as oophorectomy or total hysterectomy are indicated only in severe situations and can be performed laparoscopically or by laparotomy. Women aged 30 years or younger at the time of hysterectomy for endometriosis-associated pain are more likely than older women to have residual symptoms, to report a sense of loss, and to report more disruption from pain in different aspects of their lives (325). If a hysterectomy is performed, all visible endometriotic tissue should be removed. Although associated with improved pain relief and a reduced chance of future surgery, a bilateral salpingo-oophorectomy in young women should be considered in only the most severe or recurrent cases (326,327). Resection is an effective treatment for rectovaginal endometriosis, in combination with hysterectomy (328).

Hormone Therapy after Bilateral Oophorectomy

When postoperative hormone therapy with *estrogen* is used after bilateral oophorectomy, there is a negligible risk for renewed growth of residual endometriosis (329). **To reduce this risk, hormone therapy should be withheld until 3 months after surgery. The addition of *progestins* to this regimen protects the endometrium.** The decision to start hormone therapy with a combination of *estrogen* and *progestin* should be balanced against the increased risk of breast cancer and heart disease associated with hormone therapy. Some cases of adenocarcinoma were reported, presumably arising from endometriosis lesions remaining in women treated with unopposed estrogen (330).

Recurrence after Postoperative Treatment

Systemic Medical Therapy

In a systematic review published in 2004 to determine the effectiveness of systemic medical therapies used for hormonal suppression before or after surgery for endometriosis, or before and after surgery for the eradication of endometriosis, improvement of symptoms, pregnancy rates, and overall tolerability, by comparing them with no treatment or placebo, 11 trials were included (324). **Five trials compared postsurgical medical therapy with surgery alone (without medical therapy) and assessed the outcomes of pain recurrence, disease recurrence, and pregnancy rates** (331–334). There was no statistically significant reduction in pain recurrence at 12 months (relative risk [RR] 0.76; 95% CI, 0.52–1.10), but the difference at 24 months approached statistical significance (RR 0.70; 95% CI, 0.47–1.03). **There was no statistically significant difference between the use of these medical therapies after surgery compared to surgery alone with regard to disease recurrence** (RR 1.02; 95% CI, 0.27–3.84) or pregnancy rates (RR 0.78; 95% CI, 0.50–1.22). Postsurgical medical therapy was compared to surgery plus placebo in three studies (332,335,336). There was no difference between medical therapy and placebo with regard to the measures for pain; multidimensional pain score (WMD −0.40; 95% CI, −2.15–1.35); linear scale score (0.10; 95% CI, −2.24–2.44); or change in pain (−0.40; 95% CI, −1.48–0.68). There was no difference between medical therapy and placebo for pregnancy rates (RR 1.05; 95% CI, 0.44–2.51) or total AFS scores (WMD −2.10; 95% CI, −4.56–0.36). There was no significant difference between presurgery hormonal suppression and postsurgery hormonal suppression for the outcome of pain in one trial (323).

These results were confirmed in another randomized controlled trial with 5 years of follow-up, showing that GnRH analogue treatment with *triptorelin* depot 3.75 intramuscular after operative laparoscopy for stages III and IV endometriosis was comparable to placebo injections with respect to time to relapse of endometrioma, pain recurrence, and time to pregnancy (337).

There is circumstantial evidence that regular postoperative use of OCs effectively prevents endometrioma recurrence (338). In a prospective controlled cohort study with a median follow-up of 28 months after laparoscopic excision of ovarian endometriomata, the 36-month cumulative proportion of subjects free from endometrioma recurrence was 94% in women who always used cyclic oral contraception compared with 51% in those who never used it ($p <.001$; adjusted incidence rate ratio [IRR[0.10; 95% CI, 0.04–0.24) (338).

Some randomized controlled studies suggest that postoperative hormonal treatment can be useful in delaying the recurrence of endometriosis and/or pelvic pain. One study supported the long-term postoperative use of OCs to reduce the frequency and the severity of recurrent endometriosis-related dysmenorrhea (339). The prevention of endometriosis-related pain recurrence by postoperative long-term (24 months) cyclic and continuous administration of OCs was compared to no treatment in women after surgery for ovarian endometrioma. A significant reduction in recurrence rate and VAS scores for dysmenorrhea was evident in the continuous users versus the other groups at 6 months, and in cyclic users versus nonusers at 18 months postoperatively. No significant differences in recurrence rate and VAS scores for dyspareunia and chronic pelvic pain were demonstrated among the groups. The increase of VAS scores for dysmenorrhea, dyspareunia, and chronic pelvic pain during the postoperative follow-up of 6 to 24 months was significantly higher in nonusers than in the users (339).

In a second study, **long-term cyclic and continuous postoperative use of OCs was shown to effectively reduce and delay endometrioma recurrence** (340). The crude recurrence rate within 24 months was significantly lower in cyclic (14.7%) and continuous users (8.2%) compared with nonusers (29%). The recurrence-free survival was significantly lower in nonusers compared with cyclic and continuous users. The mean recurrent endometrioma diameter at first observation and the mean diameter increase every 6 months of follow-up were significantly lower in cyclic and continuous users compared with nonusers, whereas **no significant differences between cyclic users and continuous users in terms of endometrioma recurrence were demonstrated** (340).

In a third study, women who underwent conservative pelvic surgery for symptomatic endometriosis stages III and IV (r-AFS) were treated postoperatively during 6 months with either placebo, GnRH agonist (*triptorelin* or *leuprorelin*, 3.75 mg every 28 days), continuous estroprogestin (*ethinylestradiol*, 0.03 mg plus *gestodene*, 0.75 mg) or dietary therapy (vitamins, minerals salts, lactic ferments, fish oil) (341). At 12 months after surgery, patients treated with postoperative hormonal suppression therapy showed a lower VAS score for dysmenorrhea than patients in the other groups. Hormonal suppression therapy and dietary supplementation were equally effective in reducing nonmenstrual pelvic pain. **Postoperative medical and dietary therapy allowed a better quality of life when compared to placebo treatment** (341).

Local Treatment

In a systematic review to determine whether postoperative use of an *levonorgestrel* intrauterine system in women with endometriosis improves pain symptoms associated with menstruation and reduces recurrence compared with surgery only, placebo, or systemic hormones, one small randomized controlled trial was identified showing a statistically significant reduction in the recurrence of painful periods in the *levonorgestrel* intrauterine system treated group compared with the control group receiving a GnRH agonist (OR 0.14; 95% CI, 0.02–0.75) (342,343). The proportion of women who were satisfied with their treatment was higher in the *levonorgestrel* intrauterine system treated group than in the control group, but this difference did not reach statistical difference (OR 3.00; 95% CI, 0.79–11.44) (342,343). In another small randomized trial, postsurgical treatment with either *levonorgestrel* intrauterine system or depot *MPA* for 3 years indicated symptom control and recurrence were comparable, but compliance and change in bone mineral density were better in the *levonorgestrel* intrauterine system treated group than in the depot *MPA* group (344).

Medical Treatment	**If the patient desires treatment of pain symptoms that are suggestive of endometriosis in the absence of a definitive diagnosis, empirical treatment is appropriate and includes counseling, analgesia, nutritional therapy, progestins, or combined oral contraceptives. It is unclear whether oral contraceptives should be taken in a conventional, continuous, or tricycle regimen. A GnRH agonist may be taken, but is not recommended,** because this class of drug is more expensive and associated with more side effects and concerns about bone density than oral contraceptives (1).
Primary Dysmenorrhea	**Analgesics** Women suffering from dysmenorrhea are treated with analgesics; many women treat themselves with over-the-counter oral analgesics. Primary dysmenorrhea is defined as menstrual pain without organic pathology, based on physical examination alone, and it can be argued that some women

with so-called primary dysmenorrhea probably have endometriosis (345). In a systematic review it was concluded that **nonsteroidal anti-inflammatories (NSAIDs), except *niflumic acid*, were more effective than placebo for relief of primary dysmenorrhea, but there was insufficient evidence to suggest whether any individual NSAID was more effective than another** (345). In another review, selective cyclo-oxygenase-2 inhibitors *rofecoxib* and *valdecoxib* were as effective as *naproxen* and more effective than placebo for the treatment of primary dysmenorrhea (346). Concerns were raised about the safety of these medications, and its manufacturers withdrew *rofecoxib* from the market.

According to another systematic review based on two relatively small, randomized controlled trials comparing *paracetamol* and *coproxamol* with placebo, *coproxamol* (*paracetamol* 650 mg and *dextropropoxyphene* 65 mg) but not *paracetamol* (500 mg 4 times daily) was more effective than placebo in reducing primary dysmenorrhea (346). This observation may be explained by the suboptimal dosage of *paracetamol* used. A small randomized trial demonstrated that *paracetamol* (*acetaminophen*) 1,000 mg four times daily was superior to placebo for the treatment of primary dysmenorrhea (347).

Oral Contraceptives

There is a paucity of information for the use of modern OCs for primary dysmenorrhea. A Cochrane review suggested that first- and second-generation OCs with 50 μg or more estrogen may be more effective than placebo treatment for dysmenorrhea. It concluded that the studies included for analysis were of poor quality and heterogenous so that no recommendation could be made regarding the efficacy of modern, lower dose OCs (evidence level 1a) (348). A randomized controlled trial comparing a low-dose oral contraceptive containing 20 μg *ethinyl estradiol* and 100 μg *levonorgestrel* with placebo showed better pain relief in adolescent girls with dysmenorrhea using the OC than placebo (349).

There is some evidence in general populations that OCs can effectively treat dysmenorrhea (350). OCs have the advantage of long-term safety; hence they can be used indefinitely in low-risk women. In clinical practice, when they are used for menstrual pain, they may be taken tricyclicly or continuously to reduce the number of periods or avoid them altogether (evidence level 4). There is no direct comparison of these options with the conventional approach.

Other Treatments

Several Cochrane reviews and one clinical-evidence review suggest that other treatment modalities that might be helpful in primary dysmenorrhea include supplemental thiamine or vitamin E, high frequency transcutaneous nerve stimulation, topical heat and herbal remedy *toki-shakuyaku-san*. They suggest that treatment modalities with unknown benefit are vitamin B12, fish oil, magnesium, acupuncture, other herbal remedies and behavioral interventions, and that spinal manipulation is unlikely to be beneficial (348,350–352).

Treatment of Endometriosis-Associated Pain

Nonsteroidal Anti-inflammatory Drugs

Considering that endometriosis is a chronic inflammatory disease, anti-inflammatory drugs would appear to be effective for treatment of endometriosis-related dysmenorrhea. Although NSAIDs are used extensively and are often the first-line therapy for reduction of endometriosis-related pain, the analgesic effect of NSAIDs was not studied extensively. Only one small, double-blind, placebo-controlled, four-period, crossover clinical study was published (353). This study claimed complete or substantial pain relief of endometriosis-related dysmenorrhea in 83% of cases treated with *naproxen* compared with 41% in cases treated with placebo. A different analysis of the data from the same study by **the Cochrane Collaborative Network did not confirm a positive effect of *naproxen* on pain relief** (OR 3.27; 95% CI. 0.61–17.69) **in women with endometriosis** (354). There was inconclusive evidence to indicate whether women taking NSAIDs (*naproxen*) were less likely to require additional analgesia (OR 0.12; 95% CI, 0.01–1.29) or to experience side effects (OR 0.46; 95% CI, 0.09–2.47) when compared to placebo (354).

Endometriosis-related pain is nociceptive, but persistent nociceptive input from endometriotic lesions leads to central sensitization manifested by somatic hyperalgesia and increased referred pain (355). The potential effectiveness of NSAIDs in the reduction of endometriosis-related pain may be explained by a local antinociceptive effect and a reduced central sensitization in addition to the anti-inflammatory effect. NSAIDs have significant side effects, including gastric ulceration and possible inhibition of ovulation. Prostaglandins are involved in the follicle rupture mechanism at ovulation, which is why women who wish to become pregnant should not take NSAIDs at the time of ovulation (356).

Hormonal Treatment

Effect of Hormonal Treatment on Pain   Because estrogen is known to stimulate the growth of endometriosis, hormonal therapy is designed to suppress estrogen synthesis, thereby inducing atrophy of ectopic endometrial implants or interrupting the cycle of stimulation and bleeding (1). Implants of endometriosis react to gonadal steroid hormones in a manner similar, but not identical, to normally stimulated ectopic endometrium. Ectopic endometrial tissue displays histologic and biochemical differences from normal ectopic endometrium in characteristics such as glandular activity (proliferation, secretion), enzyme activity (17β-hydroxysteroid dehydrogenase), and steroid (estrogen, progestin, and androgen) hormone receptor levels. Withdrawal of estrogen stimulation causes cellular inactivation and degeneration of endometriotic implants but not their disappearance.

There is strong evidence that suppression of ovarian function for 6 months reduces pain associated with endometriosis. Combined oral contraceptives *danazol, gestrinone, medroxyprogesterone acetate,* and GnRH agonists are all equally effective but their side effects and cost profiles differ (1). **Pain relief may be of short duration, presumably because endometriosis and endometriosis-associated pain recur after the cessation of medical treatment.** The use of *diethylstilbestrol, methyltestosterone,* or other androgens is no longer advocated because they lack efficacy, have significant side effects, and pose risks to the fetus if pregnancy occurs during therapy. A new generation of aromatase inhibitors, estrogen receptor modulators, and progesterone antagonists may offer new hormonal treatment options.

Hormonal Treatment for Pain from Rectovaginal Endometriosis   Surgical treatment may reduce the pain associated with rectovaginal endometriosis, but it is associated with a high risk of morbidity and major complications. The effect of medical treatment in terms of pain relief in women with rectovaginal endometriosis appears to be substantial (357). In a systematic review including 217 cases of medically treated rectovaginal endometriosis, the antalgic effect of the considered medical therapies (vaginal danazol, GnRH agonist, progestin, and estrogen-progestin combinations used transvaginally, transdermally, or orally) for the entire treatment period (from 6 to 12 months) was 60% to 90%, with patients reporting considerable reduction or complete relief from pain symptoms, with the exception of when an aromatase inhibitor was used alone (357).

Oral Contraceptives

Although oral contraceptives are effective in inducing a decidualized endometrium, the estrogenic component in oral contraceptives may stimulate endometrial growth and increase pelvic pain in the first few weeks of treatment. The long-term significance of this effect is undetermined. Oral contraceptives are less costly than other treatments and may be helpful in the short-term management of endometriosis with potential long-term benefits in some women.

The use of cyclic oral contraceptives may provide prophylaxis against the development or recurrence of endometriosis. Estrogens in oral contraceptives may stimulate the proliferation of endometriosis. The reduced menstrual bleeding that often occurs in women taking oral contraceptives may be beneficial to women with prolonged, frequent menstrual bleeding, which is a known risk factor for endometriosis (45).

Further research is warranted to assess the effect of low-dose oral contraceptives in preventing endometriosis and treating associated pain, because the evidence for its efficacy is limited. In a systematic review to assess the effects of OC's in comparison to other treatments for painful symptoms of endometriosis in women of reproductive age, only one study met the inclusion criteria (all truly randomized controlled trials of the use of OCs in the treatment of women of reproductive age with symptoms ascribed to the diagnosis of endometriosis and made visually at surgical procedure were included) (358,359). In this study, a total of 57 women were allocated to two groups to compare an OC to a GnRH analogue (359). Methods of randomization and allocation concealment were unclear and the analogue group became amenorrheic during the treatment period of 6 months, while women in the OC group reported a decrease in dysmenorrhea (358,359). No evidence of a significant difference between the two groups was observed in terms of dysmenorrhea at 6 months follow-up after stopping treatment (OR 0.48; 95% CI, 0.08–2.90). Some evidence for a decrease in dyspareunia was found at the end of treatment in women in the GnRH analogue group; although no evidence of a significant difference in dyspareunia was observed at the end of the 6 months follow-up (OR 4.87; 95% CI, 0.96–24.65). According to these data, there is no evidence of a difference in outcomes between the OC studied and GnRH analogue in the treatment of endometriosis-associated painful symptoms (358). The lack of studies with larger sample sizes or studies focusing on other comparable treatments is concerning, and further research is needed to evaluate the role of OCs in managing symptoms associated with management of endometriosis (358).

In a recent double-blind, randomized, placebo-controlled trial, patients with suspected or surgically proven endometriosis were randomly assigned to receive either monophasic OC (*ethinylestradiol* plus *norethisterone*) or placebo during four cycles (360). Total dysmenorrhea scores assessed by verbal rating scale were significantly decreased at the end of treatment in both groups. From the first cycle through the end of treatment, dysmenorrhea in the OC group was significantly milder than in the placebo group. The volume of ovarian endometrioma was significantly decreased in the OC group but not in the placebo group (360).

Continuous Contraceptives

The treatment of endometriosis with continuous low-dose monophasic oral contraceptives (one pill per day for 6 to 12 months) was originally used to induce pseudopregnancy caused by the resultant amenorrhea and decidualization of endometrial tissue (279). The concept was to induce an adynamic endometrium through elimination of the normal cyclic hormonal changes characteristic of the menstrual cycle (361). This induction of a pseudopregnancy state with combination oral contraceptive pills is effective in reducing dysmenorrhea and pelvic pain. The subsequent amenorrhea induced by oral contraceptives could decrease the risk for disease progression by preventing or reducing (retrograde) menstruation. Pathologically, oral contraceptive use is associated with decidualization of endometrial tissue, necrobiosis, and possibly absorption of the endometrial tissue (362). **There is no convincing evidence that medical therapy with oral contraceptives offers definitive therapy. Instead, the endometrial implants survive the induced atrophy and, in most patients, reactivate after termination of treatment.**

Any low-dose OC containing 30 to 35 μg of *ethinyl estradiol* used continuously can be used for the management of endometriosis. The objective of the treatment is the induction of amenorrhea, which should be continued for 6 to 12 months. Continuous or extended cyclic use of oral contraceptives is well tolerated when compared to the cyclic use of OCs for contraceptive purposes (363). In a randomized controlled trial of women with recurrent moderate or severe pelvic pain after unsuccessful conservative surgery for symptomatic rectovaginal endometriosis, continuous treatment with oral *ethinyl E2*, 0.01 mg plus *cyproterone acetate*, 3 mg per day, or *norethindrone acetate*, 2.5 mg per day during 12 months resulted in substantially reduced dysmenorrhea, deep dyspareunia, nonmenstrual pelvic pain, and dyschezia scores without major between-group differences in patient satisfaction rates (62% and 73%, respectively) (364).

In a patient preference cohort study to evaluate the efficacy and tolerability of a contraceptive vaginal ring (supplying 15 μg of *ethinyl E* and 120 μg per day of *etonogestrel*) and transdermal patch (delivering 20 μg of *ethinyl E* and 150 μg per day *norelgestromin*) in the treatment of women with recurrent moderate or severe pelvic pain after conservative surgery for symptomatic endometriosis and endometriosis-associated pain, patients who preferred the ring were significantly more likely to be satisfied and to comply with treatment than those who chose the patch (282). Both systems were associated with poor bleeding control when used continuously.

Progestins

Progestins may exert an antiendometriotic effect by causing initial decidualization of endometrial tissue followed by atrophy. They can be considered as the first choice for the treatment of endometriosis because they are as effective as *danazol* or GnRH analogues and have a lower cost and possibly a lower incidence of side effects than these agents (365).

Table 17.1 Medical Treatment of Endometriosis-Associated Pain: Effective Regimens (Usual Duration: 6 Months)

	Administration	Dose	Frequency
Progestogens			
Medroxyprogesterone acetate	PO	30 mg	Daily
Dienogest	PO	2 mg	Daily
Megestrol acetate	PO	40 mg	Daily
Lynestrenol	PO	10 mg	Daily
Dydrogesterone	PO	20–30 mg	Daily
Antiprogestins			
Gestrinone	PO	1.25 or 2.5 mg	Twice weekly
Danazol	PO	400 mg	Daily
Gonadotropin-Releasing Hormone			
Leuprolide	SC	500 mg	Daily
	IM	3.75 mg	Monthly
Goserelin	SC	3.6 mg	Monthly
Buserelin	IN	300 μg	Daily
	SC	200 μg	Daily
Nafarelin	IN	200 μg	Daily
Triptorelin	IM	3.75 mg	Monthly

PO, oral; SC, subcutaneous; IM, intramuscular; IN, intranasal.

There is no evidence that any single agent or any particular dose is preferable to another. The effective doses of several progestins are summarized in Table 17.1. In most studies, the effect of treatment was evaluated after 3 to 6 months of therapy. Progestins appear to be an effective therapy for the painful symptoms associated with endometriosis (366).

Medroxyprogesterone Acetate   *MPA* is the most studied agent. It is effective in relieving pain starting at a dose of 30 mg per day, increasing the dose based on the clinical response and bleeding patterns according to data from nonrandomized trials (367,368). A randomized placebo-controlled study reported a significant reduction in stages and scores of endometriosis in both the placebo group and the group treated with *MPA* 50 mg per day and placebo at laparoscopy within 3 months after cessation of therapy (369). These findings raise questions about the need for medical therapy with *MPA* in this dose.

Evidence suggests a possible role for depot *MPA* in the treatment of endometriosis. In a randomized controlled study, depot *MPA* (150 mg every 3 months) was more effective in the relief of dysmenorrhea than treatment with a cyclic 21-day oral contraceptive (*ethinyl estradiol* 20 μg plus *desogestrel* 0.15 mg) combined with very low-dose *danazol* (50 mg per day) (370). In another multicenter, randomized, evaluator-blinded, comparator-controlled trial, depot *MPA* (150 mg) or *leuprolide acetate* (11.25 mg), given every 3 months for 6 months were equivalent in reducing endometriosis-associated pain during the study and the 12-month posttreatment follow-up period, with less impact on bone mineral density and fewer hypoestrogenic side effects but more bleeding being observed in the depot *MPA* treated group (371). Add-back therapy would prevent the negative effects on bone density and hypoestrogenic side effects associated with GnRH-agonist therapy. In a pilot study, pain relief, side effects, and treatment satisfaction were comparable during a 12-month treatment with *etonogestrel* implantate subcutaneous (68 mg) or depot *medroxyprogesterone acetate* 150 mg intramuscular depot *MPA* in 41 patients with dysmenorrhea, nonmenstrual pelvic pain, and dyspareunia associated with histologically proven endometriosis (372). **Although depot *MPA* treatment is effective for the treatment of pain associated with endometriosis, it is not indicated in infertile women because it induces**

profound amenorrhea and anovulation, and a varying length of time is required for ovulation to resume after discontinuation of therapy.

Dienogest   In two randomized noninferiority trials, treatment during 6 months with *dienogest* 2 mg per day orally demonstrated equivalent efficacy to depot *leuprolide acetate* (3.75 mg, depot intramuscular injection, every 4 weeks) or intranasal *buserelin acetate* (900 μg per day, intranasally) in relieving the pain associated with endometriosis, offering a different safety and tolerability profile (less bone loss, fewer hot flushes, more irregular genital bleeding) (373,374). *Dienogest* treatment was not compared to the recommended treatment of GnRH agonist combined with add-back (see discussion above) in these two trials.

Other Progestins

Megestrol Acetate   *Megestrol acetate* was administered in a dose of 40 mg per day with good results (370). Pain was reduced significantly during luteal phase treatment with 60 mg *dydrogesterone,* and this improvement was still evident at 12-month follow-up (316). Other treatment strategies included *dydrogesterone* (20 to 30 mg per day, either continuously or on days 5 to 21) and *lynestrenol* (10 mg per day).

Side effects of progestins include nausea, weight gain, fluid retention, and breakthrough bleeding caused by hypoestrogenemia. Breakthrough bleeding, although common, is usually corrected by short-term (7-day) administration of *estrogen.* Depression and other mood disorders are a significant problem in about 1% of women taking these medications.

Intrauterine Progesterone

The *levonorgestrel* intrauterine system releasing 20 μg per day of *levonorgestrel* reduces endometriosis-associated pain caused by peritoneal and rectovaginal endometriosis and reduces the risk of recurrence of dysmenorrhea after conservative surgery (375). *Levonorgestrel* induces endometrial glandular atrophy and decidual transformation of the stroma, reduces endometrial cell proliferation, and increases apoptotic activity (375). A systematic review identified two randomized trials and three prospective observational studies, all involving small numbers and a heterogeneous group of patients (376). The evidence suggests that the *levonorgestrel* intrauterine system reduces endometriosis associated pain with symptom control maintained over 3 years (377–380). Twelve months of treatment results in a significant reduction in dysmenorrhea, pelvic pain, and dyspareunia; a high degree of patient satisfaction; and a significant reduction in the volume of rectovaginal endometriotic nodules (377,378). After the first year of use, a 70% to 90% reduction in menstrual blood loss is observed.

Progesterone Antagonists

Progesterone antagonists and progesterone receptor modulators may suppress endometriosis based on their antiproliferative effects on the endometrium, without the risk for hypoestrogenism or bone loss that occurs with GnRH treatment. These products are not available in the United States, and their clinical effectiveness is unproven.

Mifepristone   *Mifepristone* (RU-486) is a potent antiprogestagen with a direct inhibitory effect on human endometrial cells and, in high doses, an antiglucocorticoid action (381). The recommended dose for endometriosis is 25 to 100 mg per day. In uncontrolled studies, *mifepristone,* 50 to 100 mg per day, reduced pelvic pain and induced 55% regression of the lesions without significant side effects (382,383). In an uncontrolled pilot study, low-dose *mifepristone,* 5 mg per day, resulted in pain improvement, without change in endometriosis lesions, suggesting that this dosage was probably too low (384).

Onapristone   The progesterone antagonists *onapristone* (ZK98299) and *ZK136799,* used in the treatment of rats with surgically induced endometriosis, resulted in a remission in 40% to 60% of treated animals. In animals with persistent endometriosis, growth inhibition was obtained in 48% and 85% of endometriotic lesions after therapy with *onapristone* and *ZK136799,* respectively (385).

Other Progesterone Antagonists   The chemical synthesis and pharmacologic characterization of a highly potent progesterone antagonist, *ZK230211,* were reported, with little or no other endocrinologic effects. *ZK230211* is active on progesterone receptors A and B (386). In primates, this drug blocks ovulation and menstruation at all effective doses, whereas another progesterone antagonist, *ZK137316,* allowed ovulation but blocked menstruation in a dose-dependent fashion (387). All progesterone antagonist–treated animals maintained normal follicular phase concentration of estradiol and returned to menstrual cyclicity within 15 to 41 days after treatment (387). Both progesterone antagonists block unopposed estrogen action on the endometriosis through their antiproliferative effect.

Gestrinone

Gestrinone is a 19-nortestosterone derivative with androgenic, antiprogestagenic, antiestrogenic, and antigonadotropic properties. It acts centrally and peripherally to increase free testosterone and reduce sex hormone–binding globulin levels (androgenic effect), reduce serum estradiol values to early follicular phase levels (antiestrogenic effect), reduce mean LH levels, and obliterate the LH and follicle-stimulating hormone (FSH) surge (antigonadotropic effect). *Gestrinone* causes cellular inactivation and degeneration of endometriotic implants but not their disappearance (388). Amenorrhea occurs in 50% to 100% of women and is dose dependent.

Resumption of menses generally occurs 33 days after discontinuing the medication (389,390). An advantage of *gestrinone* is its long half-life (28 hours) when given orally. The standard dose is 2.5 mg twice a week. Although 1.25 mg twice weekly is effective, a randomized study demonstrated in women with mild to moderate endometriosis that 2.5 mg *gestrinone* twice weekly for 24 weeks is more effective and has a better effect on bone mass (+7% vs. −7%) when compared with 1.25 mg *gestrinone* twice weekly for 24 weeks (391). The clinical side effects of *gestrinone* are dose dependent and similar to but less intense than those caused by *danazol* (391). They include nausea, muscle cramps, and androgenic effects such as weight gain, acne, seborrhea, and oily hair and skin.

In a multicenter, randomized, double-blind study, *gestrinone* was as effective as GnRH for the treatment of pelvic pain associated with endometriosis, with fewer side effects and the added advantage of twice-weekly administration (392). Pregnancy is contraindicated while taking *gestrinone* because of the risk for masculinization of the fetus.

Danazol

Recognized pharmacologic properties of *danazol* include suppression of GnRH or gonadotropin secretion, direct inhibition of steroidogenesis, increased metabolic clearance of estradiol and progesterone, direct antagonistic and agonistic interaction with endometrial androgen and progesterone receptors, and immunologic attenuation of potentially adverse reproductive effects (98,393). The multiple effects of *danazol* produce a high-androgen, low-estrogen environment (estrogen levels in the early follicular to postmenopausal range) that does not support the growth of endometriosis, and the amenorrhea that is produced prevents new seeding of implants from the uterus into the peritoneal cavity.

The immunologic effects of *danazol* were studied in women with endometriosis and adenomyosis and include a decrease in serum immunoglobulins, a decrease in serum C3, a rise in serum C4 levels, decreased serum levels of autoantibodies against various phospholipid antigens, and decreased serum levels of CA125 during treatment (218,230–234,394,395). *Danazol* inhibits peripheral blood lymphocyte proliferation in cultures activated by T-cell mitogens but does not affect macrophage-dependent T-lymphocyte activation of B lymphocytes (396). *Danazol* inhibits IL-1 and TNF production by monocytes in a dose-dependent manner and suppresses macrophage- and monocyte-mediated cytotoxicity of susceptible target cells in women with mild endometriosis (397,398). These immunologic findings may be important in the remission of endometriosis with *danazol* treatment and may offer an explanation of the effect of *danazol* in the treatment of a number of autoimmune diseases, including hereditary angioedema, autoimmune hemolytic anemia, systemic lupus erythematosus, and idiopathic thrombocytopenic purpura (399–403). Doses of 800 mg per day are used frequently in North America, whereas 600 mg per day is prescribed in Europe and Australia. It appears that the absence of menstruation is a better indicator of response than drug dose. A practical strategy for the use of *danazol* is to start treatment with 400 mg daily (200 mg twice a day) and increase the dose, if necessary, to achieve amenorrhea and relieve symptoms (393).

In a systematic review to determine the effectiveness of *danazol* compared to placebo or no treatment in the treatment of the symptoms and signs, other than infertility, of endometriosis in women of reproductive age, five randomized trials were included in which *danazol* (alone or as adjunctive therapy to surgery) was compared to placebo or no therapy (404). Treatment with *danazol* (including adjunctive to surgical therapy) was effective in relieving painful symptoms related to endometriosis when compared to placebo (404). Laparoscopic scores improved with *danazol* treatment (including as adjunctive therapy) when compared with either placebo or no treatment (404). Side effects were more commonly reported in those patients receiving *danazol* than for placebo (404).

The significant adverse side effects of *danazol* are related to its androgenic and hypoestrogenic properties. The most common side effects include weight gain, fluid retention, acne, oily skin, hirsutism, hot flashes, atrophic vaginitis, reduced breast size, reduced libido, fatigue, nausea, muscle cramps, and emotional instability. Deepening of the voice is another potential side effect that is nonreversible. *Danazol* can cause increased cholesterol and low-density lipoprotein levels and decreased high-density lipoproteins levels, but it is unlikely that these short-term effects are clinically important. *Danazol* is contraindicated in patients with liver disease because it is largely metabolized in the liver and may cause hepatocellular damage. *Danazol* is contraindicated in patients with hypertension, congestive heart failure, or impaired renal function because it can cause fluid retention. The use of *danazol* is contraindicated in pregnancy because of its androgenic effects on the fetus.

Because of the many side effects of oral *danazol,* alternative routes of administration were studied. In an uncontrolled pilot study, local *danazol* treatment using a vaginal *danazol* ring (1,500 mg) was effective for pain relief in deeply infiltrative endometriosis. This treatment did not cause the classic *danazol* side effects or detectable serum *danazol* levels, and it allowed ovulation and conception to occur (405).

Gonadotropin-Releasing Hormone Agonists

Gonadotropin-releasing hormone agonists bind to pituitary GnRH receptors and stimulate LH and FSH synthesis and release. The agonists have a much longer biologic half-life (3 to 8 hours) than endogenous GnRH (3.5 minutes), resulting in the continuous exposure of GnRH receptors to GnRH-agonist activity. This exposure causes a loss of pituitary receptors and downregulation of GnRH activity, resulting in low FSH and LH levels. Ovarian steroid production is suppressed, providing a medically induced and reversible state of pseudomenopause. A direct effect of GnRH agonists on ectopic endometrium is possible, because expression of the GnRH receptor gene is documented in ectopic endometrium and because direct inhibition of endometriosis cells was shown *in vitro* (406). In rat models used to study surgical adhesion formation and endometriosis, GnRH-agonist therapy decreased activity of plasminogen activators and matrix MMPs and increased the activity of their inhibitors, suggesting potential GnRH-agonist–regulated mechanisms for reducing adhesion formation (407).

Various GnRH agonists were developed and used in treating endometriosis. These agents include *leuprolide, buserelin, nafarelin, histrelin, goserelin, deslorelin,* and *triptorelin*. These drugs are inactive orally and must be administered intramuscularly, subcutaneously, or by intranasal absorption. The best therapeutic effect is often associated with an *estradiol* dose of 20 to 40 pg/mL (75–150 pmol/L). These so-called depot formulations are attractive because of the reduced frequency of administration and because nasal administration can be complicated by variations in absorption rates and problems with patient compliance (390). The results with GnRH agonists are similar to those with oral contraceptive *progestin* or *gestrinone* therapy. **Treatment for 3 months with a GnRH agonist is effective in improving pain for 6 months** (332).

Although GnRH agonists do not have an adverse effect on serum lipids and lipoproteins levels, their side effects are caused by hypoestrogenism and include hot flashes, vaginal dryness, reduced libido, and osteoporosis (6% to 8% loss in trabecular bone density after 6 months of therapy). Reversibility of bone loss is equivocal and therefore of concern, because treatment periods of longer than 6 months may be required (408,409). The goal is to suppress endometriosis and maintain serum estrogen levels of 30 to 45 pg/mL. More extreme estradiol suppression will induce bone loss (408). **The dose of daily GnRH agonist can be regulated by monitoring estradiol levels, by the addition of low-dose *progestin* or *estrogen–progestin* in an add-back regimen, or by draw-back therapy.**

The goal of add-back therapy is to treat endometriosis and endometriosis-associated pain effectively while preventing vasomotor symptoms and bone loss related to the hypoestrogenic state induced by GnRH analogues. Add-back therapy can be achieved by administering progestins only, including *norethisterone,* 1.2 mg, and *norethindrone acetate,* 5 mg, but bone loss is not prevented by *medrogestone,* 10 mg per day (409–411). Add-back therapy can be achieved by *tibolone,* 2.5 mg per day, or by an estrogen–progestin combination (i.e., *conjugated estrogens,* 0.625 mg, combined with *medroxyprogesterone acetate,* 2.5 mg, or with *norethindrone acetate,* 5 mg; *estradiol,* 2 mg, combined with *norethisterone acetate,* 1 mg) (405,408,410–414). Treatment for up to 2 years with combined estrogen and progestagen add-back appears to be effective and safe in terms of pain relief and bone density protection; progestagen only add-back is not protective (415).

GnRH agonists should not be prescribed to girls who have not yet attained their maximal bone density, as some concern remains about the long-term effects of GnRH analogues on bone loss. In one report, bone mineral density reduction occurred during long-term GnRH-agonist use and was not fully recovered up to 6 years after treatment (416). Use of add-back therapy (2 mg *estradiol* and 1 mg *norethisterone acetate*) did not affect this process (416). Draw-back therapy was suggested as an alternative in a study showing that 6 months of intake of 400 μg per day of *nafarelin* was as effective as a draw-back regimen consisting of 1 month of intake of 400 μg per day of *nafarelin* followed by 5 months of 200 μg per day of *nafarelin,* with similar estradiol levels (30 pg/mL) but less loss of bone mineral density (417).

Aromatase Inhibitors

Treatment of rats with induced endometriosis using the nonsteroidal aromatase inhibitor *fadrozole hydrochloride* or *YM511* resulted in a dose-dependent volume reduction of endometriosis transplants (418,419). In one case report, treatment of severe postmenopausal endometriosis with an aromatase inhibitor, *anastrozole,* 1 mg per day, and elemental *calcium,* 1.5 g per day for 9 months resulted in hypoestrogenism, pain relief after 2 months, and after 9 months a 10-fold reduction in the 30-mm diameter size of red, polypoid vaginal lesions, along with remodeling to gray tissue (420).

There is concern with the use of aromatase inhibitors such as *anastrozole* or *letrozole* in the treatment of menopausal women because these drugs are known to stimulate ovulation and continuous administration can result in the development of functional ovarian cysts. This side effect can be prevented by combining aromatase inhibitors with ovarian suppressing drugs such as OCs or *progestins* in premenopausal women. A systematic review assessing the effects of aromatase inhibitors in women symptomatic of pain with endometriosis included eight studies including 137 women (421). In case series (seven studies, 40 women), aromatase inhibitors combined with progestins or OCs or GnRH analogues reduced mean pain scores and lesion size and improved quality of life (421). A randomized controlled trial including 97 women demonstrated that aromatase inhibitors in combination with GnRH analogues significantly improved pain (p <0.0001), compared with GnRH analogues alone, with significant improvement in multidimensional patient scores (p <0.0001), without significant reduction in spine or hipbone densities (422). Aromatase inhibitors appear to have a promising effect on pain associated with endometriosis, but the strength of this inference is limited because of a dearth of evidence and because aromatase inhibitors need to be combined with other hormonal medication (421).

Selective Estrogen Receptor Modulators

The role of selective estrogen receptor modulators (SERMs) in the treatment of endometriosis is unclear. In animal models, *raloxifene* therapy resulted in regression of endometriosis. The effect was seen in a surgically prepared, rat uterine explant model and in *Rhesus* macaques diagnosed with spontaneous endometriosis before exposure (423). In a placebo-controlled randomized trial in women with chronic pelvic pain and surgically treated biopsy-proven endometriosis, postoperative treatment with *raloxifene* during 6 months resulted in a shortened time to return of pain (defined as 2 months of pain equal to or more severe than that at study entry) and to repeat laparoscopy, suggesting that *raloxifene* is not effective in the treatment of endometriosis-associated pain (424). Biopsy-proven endometriosis was not associated with return of pain, suggesting that other factors were implicated in recurrent pelvic pain after surgery in this study (424).

Nonhormonal Medical Therapy

Recent progress in understanding the pathogenesis of endometriosis led to the expectation that new pharmaceutic agents affecting inflammation and angiogenesis activity may prevent or inhibit the development of endometriosis. Most of these compounds were tested only in rodent models, and more research is needed in the baboon model for endometriosis and in women to ensure their safety and efficacy, as they may interfere with normal physiological processes like ovulation, menstruation, and implantation (54).

Selective Inhibition of Tumor Necrosis Factor-α   In rats with experimental endometriosis, recombinant human TNF-α–binding protein can reduce 64% of the size of endometriosis-like peritoneal lesions (425). Several prospective randomized placebo- and drug-controlled studies in baboons showed that TNF-α antagonists effectively prevent and treat induced endometriosis and endometriosis-related adhesions and are effective in the treatment of spontaneous endometriosis in baboons (54). These results were not confirmed in a small placebo-controlled randomized trial in women with deeply infiltrative endometriosis awaiting surgery, possibly because the endometriosis phenotype in these women (deeply infiltrative and fibrotic disease) was different from the endometriosis phenotype in the baboon studies (inflammatory peritoneal disease with adhesions) (426). TNF-α antagonists are less effective in fibrotic inflammatory bowel disease than in earlier nonfibrotic inflammatory bowel disease.

Pentoxifylline   In a systematic review determining the effectiveness and safety of *pentoxifylline,* which has anti-inflammatory effects in the management of endometriosis in subfertile, premenopausal women, four trials involving 334 participants were included (427). *Pentoxifylline* had no significant effect on reduction in pain (one randomized trial, MD −1.60; 95% CI, −3.32–0.12), improvement of fertility (three randomized trials, OR 1.54; 95% CI, 0.89–2.66) or recurrence of endometriosis (one randomized trial, OR 0.88; 95% CI, 0.27–2.84) (427). No trials reported the effects of *pentoxifylline* on the odds of live birth rate per woman, improvement of endometriosis-related symptoms, or adverse events (427).

Peroxisome Proliferator Activated Receptor-γ Agonists   Peroxisome proliferator activated receptor-γ (PPAR-γ) agonists prevent and treat endometriosis in both rodent and baboon models for endometriosis and show promise for treatment of human endometriosis (152,153,428,429).

Many substances potentially capable of modulating immunologic or inflammatory mechanisms involved in the onset or progression of the disease could be the targets for future research in endometriosis (430,431). Preliminary trials with cyclooxygenase-2 (COX-2) inhibitors, leukotriene receptor antagonists, TNF-α inhibitors, antiangiogenic agents and kinase inhibitors show promising results *in vitro* in rodent and in nonhuman primate models, but their safety is an important issue regarding human use (432).

Chinese Herbal Medicine

In China, treatment of endometriosis using herbal medicines is routine, and considerable research into the role of herbal medicines in alleviating pain, promoting fertility, and preventing relapse has occurred (433). A systematic review of the effectiveness and safety of herbal medicines in alleviating endometriosis-related pain and infertility, including two Chinese randomized trials involving 158 women, concluded that postsurgical administration of herbal medicines may have comparable benefits to hormonal treatment with *gestrinone* but with fewer side effects (433). Oral herbal medicines might have a better overall treatment effect than *danazol;* it could be more effective in relieving dysmenorrhea and shrinking adnexal masses when used in conjunction with an herbal enema (433). More rigorous research is required to accurately assess the potential role of herbal medicines in treating endometriosis (433).

Treatment of Endometriosis-Associated Subfertility

Surgical Treatment

The treatment of endometriosis-related infertility is dependent on the age of the woman, the duration of infertility, the stage of endometriosis, the involvement of ovaries, tubes, or both in the endometriosis process, previous therapy, associated pain symptoms, and the priorities of the patient, taking into account her attitude toward the disease, the cost of treatment, her

financial means, and the expected results. If surgery is performed and spontaneous pregnancy does not occur within 2 years of surgery, there is little chance of subsequent natural conception (434).

Surgery for Minimal to Mild Endometriosis

Surgical management of infertile women with minimal to mild endometriosis is controversial. Based on the results of a meta-analysis of two randomized trials, ablation of endometriotic lesions plus adhesiolysis to improve fertility in minimal to mild endometriosis is effective compared to diagnostic laparoscopy alone (191,192,435). One Canadian study reported that laparoscopic surgery enhanced fecundity in infertile women with minimal or mild endometriosis (191). They studied 341 infertile women, 20 to 39 years of age, with minimal or mild endometriosis. During diagnostic laparoscopy, the women were randomly assigned to undergo resection or ablation of visible endometriosis or diagnostic laparoscopy only. **They found that resection or ablation of minimal and mild endometriosis increased the likelihood of pregnancy in infertile women.** They were followed for 36 weeks after the laparoscopy or, for those who became pregnant during that interval, for up to 20 weeks of pregnancy. The study participants were recruited among infertile women scheduled for diagnostic laparoscopy with strict eligibility criteria. The women in the study had no previous surgical treatment for endometriosis, no medical treatment for endometriosis in the previous 9 months, and no other medical or surgical treatment for infertility in the previous 3 months. They had no history of pelvic inflammatory disease and no severe pelvic pain precluding expectant management. The diagnosis of endometriosis required the presence of one or more typical bluish or black lesions. The stage of endometriosis was determined according to the revised American Society of Reproductive Medicine classification. Both the monthly fecundity rate and the cumulative pregnancy rate after 36 weeks were significantly higher and twice as high after surgical excision of minimal to mild endometriosis (4.7% and 30.7%, respectively) than after diagnostic laparoscopy (2.4% and 17.7%, respectively). In the treated group, 31% of the patients became pregnant, compared with 18% in the nontreated group ($p = 0.006$). Limitations of this study include the lack of blinding of the patients, and the fecundity rate after surgery was below that observed in control groups from other studies (1,436).

In a multicenter study in Italy, a similar study design was used to compare the effect of diagnostic laparoscopy with surgical resection and ablation of visible endometriosis (on fertility parameters) in infertile women with minimal to mild endometriosis (192). Eligible patients were less than 36 years old, were trying to conceive, and had a laparoscopically confirmed diagnosis of minimal or mild endometriosis. None of the women had therapy for endometriosis or infertility. Treatment was randomly allocated during laparoscopy. There was a follow-up period of 1 year after the laparoscopy. **The results of this study did not show a beneficial effect of surgery regarding fertility.** During the follow-up period after laparoscopy, no statistically significant differences in conception and live birth rates were observed in the treated group (24% and 20%, respectively) or in the control group (29% and 22%, respectively). The methodological quality of the Italian study was inferior to the Canadian study, as reviewed before (181,191,192). First, the study was underpowered, including only 91 patients, compared to 341 patients in the Canadian study. Second, it is remarkable and unexplained that the Italian study included after randomization more patients undergoing surgical excision of endometriosis (n = 54) than patients undergoing diagnostic laparoscopy (n = 47). Third, the duration of infertility was longer in the Italian study (4 years) than in the Canadian study (32 months). Duration of infertility is an important factor influencing both monthly fecundity rate and cumulative pregnancy rates independently from other causes of infertility. The bias introduced by the long duration of infertility in couples participating in the Italian trial may have reduced the possibility to find any significant effect of surgical treatment, especially in view of the lack of proper power calculation in the Italian study. Fourth, the Italian study did not present any data on monthly fecundity rate or cumulative pregnancy rates using life table analysis, but only published the crude live birth rate per patient, not controlled for number of cycles per patient. Fertility outcome should be measured by more controlled variables such as monthly fecundity rate and the cumulative pregnancy rates or time to pregnancy. Fifth, 41 of 91 patients in the Italian study had received GnRH analogue treatment after surgery (18 from the surgical excision group, 23 from the diagnostic laparoscopy group) (192). There was no specification for how long this medical treatment was given and how ovarian function was affected. The lack of this information introduces another bias influencing fertility outcome. Taking into account the relative methodological weaknesses of the Italian study when compared to the Canadian study, extreme caution is needed before combining these two studies in a meta-analysis, especially because the fertility outcome data are reported so differently. It seems preferable to use the data of the better study demonstrating that **surgical treatment of minimal to mild endometriosis appears to offer a small, but significant, benefit with regard to fertility outcome** (1,181,191,437). The surgical removal of peritoneal endometriosis may be important to prevent progression of endometriosis. Care is needed to prevent adhesion formation that could result as a consequence of overenthusiastic excision of minimal to mild endometriosis.

Surgery for Moderate to Severe Endometriosis

When endometriosis causes mechanical distortion of the pelvis, surgery should be performed to achieve reconstruction of normal pelvic anatomy. No randomized trials or meta-analyses are available to answer the question of whether surgical excision of moderate to severe endometriosis enhances pregnancy rate (1). Most studies present only crude pregnancy rates without detailed information regarding time of follow-up and are therefore not relevant (1).

Based on three studies, there seems to be a negative correlation between the stage of endometriosis and the spontaneous cumulative pregnancy rate after surgical removal of endometriosis, but statistical significance was reached in only one study (438–440).

Other studies reported a significant negative correlation between endometriosis stage and pregnancy rate and decreased pregnancy rates when the revised scores exceeded 15 or 70 (183,438,441). Data from different studies cannot be compared easily because of retrospective design, lack of a control group, significant variability and lack of standardization with respect to inclusion criteria, surgical procedures, extent of surgery, skill of the surgeon, variable duration of follow-up without life table analysis, postoperative hormonal suppression or medically assisted reproduction, and lack of control for other infertility-related factors such as male infertility or ovarian dysfunction. These limitations explain why management differed and was not standardized, and why the cumulative pregnancy rates 9 to 12 months after surgery for moderate to severe endometriosis vary between 24% and 30% (1,442–444).

Surgery for Ovarian Endometriomas in Subfertile Patients

Laparoscopic cystectomy for ovarian endometriomas greater than 4 cm diameter improves fertility compared with drainage and coagulation (300,303).

Perioperative Medical Treatment	Preoperative medical treatment with *danazol,* GnRH agonists, or progestins may be useful to reduce the extent of endometriosis in patients with advanced disease. **Postoperative medical treatment is rarely indicated because it is ineffective based on randomized trials, prevents pregnancy, and because the highest spontaneous pregnancy rates occur during the first 6 to 12 months after conservative surgery** (333,335).
Hormonal Treatment	**Conception is either impossible or contraindicated during medical treatment of endometriosis. There is no evidence that medical treatment of minimal to mild endometriosis leads to better chances of pregnancy than expectant management** (436). The published evidence does not comment on more severe disease (1).
Medically Assisted Reproduction	Medically assisted reproduction—including controlled ovarian hyperstimulation with intrauterine insemination, IVF, and gamete intrafallopian transfer—may be an option for infertility treatment in addition to surgical reconstruction and expectant management (284). Assisted reproductive technology (ART) is the method of choice when distortion of the tubo-ovarian anatomy contraindicates the use of superovulation with intrauterine insemination or gamete intrafallopian transfer (284). The role of ART in the treatment of endometriosis-associated infertility may be limited in large tertiary care and referral centers for surgical treatment of endometriosis (445). After conservative surgery for endometriosis, 44% conceived *in vivo* (44%), and 51% of those who failed to conceive *in vivo* did not undergo ART treatment with the cumulative rate of IVF use at 36 months of infertility at 33%. The live birth/ongoing pregnancy rate per started cycle and per patient was 10% and 20%, respectively (445). For a full discussion on the application of ART infertility, see Chapter 32.

Management of Adolescents

The most common presenting symptom in adolescents with endometriosis is cyclic pain (1). Less commonly acyclic pain, dyspareunia, gastrointestinal symptoms, irregular menses, urinary symptoms, and vaginal discharge are described (1,446–449). Similar presenting symptoms occur in adolescent patients evaluated for pelvic pain with and without endometriosis (449,450). **It is hard to predict the presence of endometriosis in adolescents with pelvic pain merely from the presenting symptoms, because similar symptoms occur in patients evaluated laparoscopically for pelvic pain with and without endometriosis** (1,449,450). Laparoscopy should be considered for adolescents with chronic pelvic pain who do not respond to medical treatment (NSAIDs, OCs) because endometriosis is very common (up to 70%) under these circumstances (446,449–456). **Minimal and mild endometriosis, according to the revised ASRM classification, are the most common stages of the disease in adolescents.** Gynecologic surgeons should pay special attention to red, clear, or white lesions, which are more prevalent in adolescents than in adults with endometriosis (1,446–458). Mild disease can be treated by laparoscopic surgical removal of implants at the time of diagnosis, followed by continuous administration of low-dose combination OCs to prevent recurrence. More advanced disease can be treated medically for 6 months, followed by continuous OCs to prevent progression of disease. Surgery is indicated if this hormonal treatment is not effective. **GnRH agonists with add-back therapy can only be considered for adolescents older than 17 years of age who have completed pubertal and bone maturation, and then only if symptoms persist during other forms of hormonal suppression** (1,459–461).

Menstrual outflow obstructions such as müllerian anomalies may cause early development of endometriosis in adolescents. Regression of the disease was observed when surgical correction of the anomaly was accomplished (462–464).

Evidence suggests that **absenteeism from school and the incidence and duration of OC use for severe primary dysmenorrhea during adolescence is higher in women who later develop deeply infiltrative endometriosis than in women without deeply infiltrative endometriosis** (166).

Physicians treating adolescents with endometriosis should adopt a multidimensional approach, where surgery, hormonal manipulation, pain medication, mental health support, complementary and alternative therapies, and education in self-management strategies are useful components (1).

Management of Postmenopausal Women

Despite available studies supporting standard hormone therapy for women with endometriosis and postsurgical menopause, there is still concern that *estrogens* may induce a recurrence of the disease and its symptoms. The evidence in the literature is insufficient to suggest depriving symptomatic patients of this treatment. In a systematic review evaluating pain and disease recurrence in women with endometriosis who used hormone therapy for postsurgical menopause, two randomized trials were included (465). In one trial, recurrence of pain in women with a conserved uterus was not significantly different in 1 of 11 women treated with continuous *tibolone* (2.5 mg per day), or in 4 of 10 women receiving nonstop transdermal application of *17-β estradiol* (0.05 mg per day) combined with cyclic *medroxyprogesterone acetate* (10 mg per day) for 12 days per month (466). In the second trial, recurrence of pain was not significantly different in any of 57 patients in the no-treatment arm, or in 4 of 115 women receiving sequential administration of *estrogens* and *progesterone* with two 22-cm patches applied weekly to produce a controlled release of 0.05 mg per day, combined with oral administration of micronized *progesterone* administered orally (200 mg per day) for 14 days with a 16-day interval free of treatment (5,329). In this study, the endometriosis recurrence and reoperation rate were comparable in both groups (2 of 115 of the treatment group; 0 of 57 of the no-treatment group) (329).

Recurrent Endometriosis After Treatment

Recurrence After Medical Treatment

Because hormonal suppressive treatment does not cure endometriosis (it only suppresses the activity of endometriotic lesions during the treatment), "recurrence," or rather persistence, of endometriosis can be expected in nearly all patients within 6 months to 2 years after the cessation of medical treatment, and this is positively correlated with the severity of endometriosis.

Recurrence After Conservative Surgery

Endometriosis tends to recur unless definitive surgery is performed. Pain recurs within 5 years in about one in five patients with pelvic pain treated by complete laparoscopic excision of visible endometriotic lesions (467). The endometriosis recurrence rate is about 5% to 20% per year, reaching a cumulative rate of 40% after 5 years. Medical treatment appears to have limited and inconsistent effects when used for only a few months after conservative procedures (468). Data on the benefit of prolonged drug regimens with OCs or *progestogen* are lacking. The current ASRM classification system has low value to predict pain recurrence and endometriosis relapse after conservative surgical treatment (469).

Recurrence After Hysterectomy

The medium-term outcome of hysterectomy for endometriosis-associated pain is satisfactory; the probability of pain persistence after hysterectomy is 15% and risk of pain worsening is 3% to 5%, with a six times higher risk of further surgery in patients with ovarian preservation as compared to concomitant bilateral ovarian removal (470). At least one ovary should be preserved in young women, especially in those who cannot or will not receive *estrogen-progestin* therapy (471). The risk of recurrence of endometriosis during hormonal therapy seems marginal if combined preparations or *tibolone* are used and *estrogen*-only treatments are avoided (471).

Risk Factors for Recurrence

The rate of recurrence increases with the stage of disease, the duration of follow-up, and the occurrence of previous surgery (14,472–475). The likelihood of recurrence appears to be lower when endometriosis is located only on the right side of the pelvis than when the left side is involved (475). The risk of endometriosis recurrence is significantly correlated to the age of the patient. The younger the patient is at the moment of the diagnosis the higher the risk of recurrence. Higher recurrence rates in younger patients seem to justify a more radical treatment in this group (288). Persistence of dysmenorrheal and nonmenstrual pelvic pain after excision of endometriosis can be related to adenomyosis as defined by a thickened (>11 mm) uterine junctional zone on MRI (476). More data are needed to define the best therapeutic option in women with recurrent endometriosis, in terms of pain relief, pregnancy rate, and patient compliance (470).

Prevention of Recurrence

After first-line surgery for endometriosis, women should be invited to seek conception as soon as possible. Alternatively, OC use until pregnancy is desired should be considered because several lines of evidence suggest that ovulation inhibition reduces the risk of endometriosis recurrence (477). A recurrent endometrioma developed in 26 of 250 regular users (10%; 95% CI, 7%–15%) compared with 46 of 115 never users (40%; 95% CI, 31%–50%), with a common odds ratio of 0.16 (95% CI, 0.04–0.65) (477).

Medical Treatment of Recurrence

In a randomized prospective clinical study, continuous treatment for 6 months with *desogestrel* (75 μg per day) (n = 20) versus a combined oral contraceptive (*ethinyl estradiol* 20 μg plus *desogestrel* 150 μg) resulted in a significant and comparable improvement of both pelvic pain and dysmenorrhea with breakthrough bleeding in 20% of the *desogestrel*-treated patients, and a significant body weight increase in 15% of the OC-treated women (478).

Surgical Treatment of Recurrence

The optimal surgical solution in women with recurrent symptoms after previous conservative procedures for endometriosis should be based on the desire for conception and on psychological characteristics (479). Studies on surgical management of recurrent rectovaginal endometriosis are warranted because of the peculiar technical difficulties and the high risk of complications associated with this challenging disease (479).

Conservative Surgery

According to review papers, the long-term probability of pain recurrence after repeat conservative surgery for recurrent endometriosis varies from 20% to 40%, and a further surgical procedure will occur in 15% to 20% of the cases (470,479). These figures are probably an underestimate related to drawbacks in study design, exclusions of dropouts, and publication bias and should be considered with caution (479). No studies evaluated the association of presacral neurectomy to the surgical treatment of recurrent endometriosis among patients with recurrent disease (470). The spontaneous conception rate among women undergoing repetitive surgery for recurrent endometriosis associated with infertility is 20% (12- and 24-month cumulative pregnancy rates of 14% and 26%), whereas the overall crude pregnancy rate after a primary surgical procedure is 40% (12- and 24-month cumulative pregnancy rates of 32% and 38%) (470,479). Among infertile patients treated with repetitive surgery for recurrent endometriosis the spontaneous pregnancy rate was 19% (12- and 24-month cumulative pregnancy rates), whereas it was 34% for those untreated (12- and 24-month cumulative pregnancy rates of 25% and 30%). The probability of conception after IVF is not significantly lower after repetitive surgery (20%) when compared to primary surgery (30%) (hazard ratio [HR] 1.51; 95% CI, 0.58–3.91%) (479).

Hysterectomy

The outcome of hysterectomy for endometriosis-associated pain at medium-term follow-up seems satisfactory. About 15% of patients had persistent symptoms and 3% to 5% experienced worsening of pain (479).

Coping with Disease

Coping with endometriosis as a chronic disease is an important component of management. According to guidelines for the management of endometriosis, evidence from two systematic reviews suggests that high frequency transcutaneous electrical nerve stimulation (TENS), acupuncture, vitamin B_1, and magnesium may help to relieve dysmenorrhea (1,348,351). Whether such treatments are effective in endometriosis-associated dysmenorrhea is unknown. Many women with endometriosis report that nutritional and complementary therapies such as reflexology, traditional Chinese medicine, herbal treatments, and homeopathy improve pain symptoms. Although there is no evidence from randomized controlled trials to support the effectiveness of these treatments in endometriosis, they should not be ruled out if the woman feels they work in conjunction with more traditional therapies or that they could be beneficial to her overall pain management and quality of life. Patient self-help groups can provide invaluable counseling, support, and advice. ESHRE provides a comprehensive international list of self-help groups on their web site (1).

References

1. **Kennedy S, Bergqvist A, Chapron C, et al.** On behalf of the ESHRE Special Interest Group for Endometriosis and Endometrium Guideline Development Group. ESHRE guideline for the diagnosis and treatment of endometriosis. *Hum Reprod* 2005;20:2698–2704. www.endometriosis.org/support.html.

2. **Sanfilippo JS, Williams RS, Yussman MA, et al.** Substance P in peritoneal fluid. *Am J Obstet Gynecol* 1992;166:155–159.

3. **Eskenazi B, Warner ML.** Epidemiology of endometriosis. *Obstet Gynecol Clin North Am* 1997;24:235–258.

4. **Viganò P, Parazzini F, Somigliana E, et al.** Endometriosis: epidemiology and aetiological factors. *Best Pract Res Clin Obstet Gynaecol* 2004;18:177–200.

5. **Haney AF.** Endometriosis: pathogenesis and pathophysiology. In: **Wilson EA, ed.** *Endometriosis*. New York: AR Liss, 1987:23–51.

6. **Koninckx PR, Meuleman C, Demeyere S, et al.** Suggestive evidence that pelvic endometriosis is a progressive disease, whereas deeply infiltrating endometriosis is associated with pelvic pain. *Fertil Steril* 1991;55:759–765.

7. **Meuleman C, Vandenabeele B, Fieuws S, et al.** High prevalence of endometriosis in infertile women with normal ovulation and normospermic partners. *Fertil Steril* 2009;92:68–74.

8. **Liu DTY, Hitchcock A.** Endometriosis: its association with retrograde menstruation, dysmenorrhoea and tubal pathology. *Br J Obstet Gynecol* 1986;93:859–862.

9. **Moen MH.** Endometriosis in women at interval sterilization. *Acta Obstet Gynecol Scand* 1987;66:451–454.

10. **Kirshon B, Poindexter AN, Fast J.** Endometriosis in multiparous women. *J Reprod Med* 1989;34:215–217.

11. **Mahmood TA, Templeton A.** Prevalence and genesis of endometriosis. *Hum Reprod* 1991;6:544–549.

12. **Moen MH, Muus KM.** Endometriosis in pregnant and non-pregnant women at tubal sterilization. *Hum Reprod* 1991;6:699–702.

13. **Waller KG, Lindsay P, Curtis P, et al.** The prevalence of endometriosis in women with infertile partners. *Eur J Obstet Gynecol Reprod Biol* 1993;48:135–139.

14. **Waller KG, Shaw MD.** Gonadotropin-releasing hormone analogues for the treatment of endometriosis: long term follow-up. *Fertil Steril* 1993;59:511–515.

15. **Strathy JH, Molgaard CA, Coulam CB, et al.** Endometriosis and infertility: a laparoscopic study of endometriosis among fertile and infertile women. *Fertil Steril* 1982;38:667–672.

16. **Fakih HN, Tamura R, Kesselman A, et al.** Endometriosis after tubal ligation. *J Reprod Med* 1985;30:939–941.

17. **Dodge ST, Pumphrey RS, Miyizawa K.** Peritoneal endometriosis in women requesting reversal of sterilization. *Fertil Steril* 1986;45:774–777.

18. **Trimbos JB, Trimbos-Kemper GCM, Peters AAW, et al.** Findings in 200 consecutive asymptomatic women having a laparoscopic sterilization. *Arch Gynecol Obstet* 1990;247:121–124.

19. **Cornillie FJ, Oosterlynck D, Lauweryns JM, et al.** Deeply infiltrating pelvic endometriosis: histology and clinical significance. *Fertil Steril* 1990;53:978–983.

20. **McLeod BS, Retzloff MG.** Epidemiology of endometriosis: an assessment of risk factors. *Clin Obstet Gynecol* 2010;53:389–396.

21. **Hemmings R, Rivard M, Olive DL, et al.** Evaluation of risk factors associated with endometriosis. *Fertil Steril* 2004;81:1513–1521.

22. **Chapron C, Souza C, de Ziegler D, et al.** Smoking habits of 411 women with histological proven endometriosis and 567 affected women. *Fertil Steril* 2010;94:2353–2355.

23. **Barbieri RL.** Stenosis of the external cervical os: an association with endometriosis in women with chronic pelvic pain. *Fertil Steril* 1998;70:571–573.

24. **Baldi A, Campioni M, Signorile PG.** Endometriosis: pathogenesis, diagnosis, therapy and association with cancer [review]. *Oncol Rep* 2008;19:843–846.

25. **Nezhat F, Datta MS, Hanson V, et al.** The relationship of endometriosis and ovarian malignancy [review]. *Fertil Steril* 2008;90:1559–1570.

26. **Somigliana E, Vercellini P, Viganó P, et al.** Should endometriomas be treated before IVF-ICSI cycles? *Hum Reprod Update* 2006;12:57–64.

27. **Somigliana E, Infantino M, Benedetti F, et al.** The presence of ovarian endometriomas is associated with a reduced responsiveness to gonadotropins. *Fertil Steril* 2006;86:192–196.

28. **Somigliana E, Viganò P, Parazzini F, et al.** Association between endometriosis and cancer: a comprehensive review and a critical analysis of clinical and epidemiological evidence. *Gynecol Oncol* 2006;101:331–341.

29. **Viganò P, Somigliana E, Parazzini F, et al.** Bias versus causality: interpreting recent evidence of association between endometriosis and ovarian cancer. *Fertil Steril* 2007;88:588–593.

30. **Sampson JA.** Peritoneal endometriosis due to menstrual dissemination of endometrial tissue into the pelvic cavity. *Am J Obstet Gynecol* 1927;14:422–469.

31. **Ramey JW, Archer DF.** Peritoneal fluid: its relevance to the development of endometriosis. *Fertil Steril* 1993;60:1–14.

32. **Halme J, Becker S, Hammond MG, et al.** Retrograde menstruation in healthy women and in patients with endometriosis. *Obstet Gynecol* 1984;64:151–154.

33. **Koninckx PR, De Moor P, Brosens IA.** Diagnosis of the luteinized unruptured follicle syndrome by steroid hormone assays in peritoneal fluid. *Br J Obstet Gynecol* 1980;87:929–934.

34. **Kruitwagen RFPM, Poels LG, Willemsen WNP, et al.** Endometrial epithelial cells in peritoneal fluid during the early follicular phase. *Fertil Steril* 1991;55:297–303.

35. **Blumenkrantz MJ, Gallagher N, Bashore RA, et al.** Retrograde menstruation in women undergoing chronic peritoneal dialysis. *Obstet Gynecol* 1981;57:667–670.

36. **Jenkins S, Olive DL, Haney AG.** Endometriosis: pathogenetic implications of the anatomic distribution. *Obstet Gynecol* 1986;67:355–358.

37. **Vercellini P, Frontino G, Pietropaolo G, et al.** Deep endometriosis: definition, pathogenesis, and clinical management. *J Am Assoc Gynecol Laparosc* 2004;11:153–161.

38. **Vercellini P, Abbiati A, Viganò P, et al.** Asymmetry in distribution of diaphragmatic endometriotic lesions: evidence in favour of the menstrual reflux theory. *Hum Reprod* 2007;22:2359–2367.

39. **Scott RB, TeLinde RW, Wharton LR Jr.** Further studies on experimental endometriosis. *Am J Obstet Gynecol* 1953;66:1082–1099.

40. **D'Hooghe TM, Bambra CS, Isahakia M, et al.** Intrapelvic injection of menstrual endometrium causes endometriosis in baboons (*Papio cynocephalus, Papio anubis*). *Am J Obstet Gynecol* 1995;173:125–134.

41. **TeLinde RW, Scott RB.** Experimental endometriosis. *Am J Obstet Gynecol* 1950;60:1147–1173.

42. **Olive DL, Martin DC.** Treatment of endometriosis-associated infertility with CO_2 laser laparoscopy: the use of one- and two-parameter exponential models. *Fertil Steril* 1987;48:18–23.

43. **Pinsonneault O, Goldstein DP.** Obstructing malformations of the uterus and vagina. *Fertil Steril* 1985;44:241–247.

44. **D'Hooghe TM, Bambra CS, Suleman MA, et al.** Development of a model of retrograde menstruation in baboons (*Papio anubis*). *Fertil Steril* 1994;62:635–638.

45. **Cramer DW, Wilson E, Stillman RJ, et al.** The relation of endometriosis to menstrual characteristics, smoking and exercise. *JAMA* 1986;355:1904–1908.

46. **Bokor A, Kyama CM, Vercruysse L, et al.** Density of small diameter sensory nerve fibres in endometrium: a semi-invasive diagnostic test for minimal to mild endometriosis. *Hum Reprod* 2009;24: 3025–3032.

47. **D'Hooghe TM, Bambra CS, Xiao L, et al.** The effect of menstruation and intrapelvic injection of endometrium on peritoneal fluid parameters in the baboon. *Am J Obstet Gynecol* 2001;184:917–925.

48. **Witz CA, Cho S, Centonze VE, et al.** Time series analysis of transmesothelial invasion by endometrial stromal and epithelial cells using three-dimensional confocal microscopy. *Fertil Steril* 2003;79:770–778.

49. **Ueki M.** Histologic study of endometriosis and examination of lymphatic drainage in and from the uterus. *Am J Obstet Gynecol* 1991;165:201–209.

50. **Dinulescu DM, Ince TA, Quade BJ, et al.** Role of K-*ras* and P*ten* in the development of mouse models of endometriosis and endometrioid ovarian cancer. *Nat Med* 2005;11:63–70.

51. **Vercellini P, Somigliana E, Vigano P, et al.** "Blood on the tracks" from corpora lutea to endometriomas. *BJOG* 2009;116:366–371.

52. **Somigliana E, Vercellini P, Gattei U, et al.** Bladder endometriosis: getting closer and closer to the unifying metastatic hypothesis. *Fertil Steril* 2007;87:1287–1290.

53. **Laufer MR, Sanfilippo J, Rose G.** Adolescent endometriosis: diagnosis and treatment approaches. *J Pediatr Adolesc Gynecol* 2003;16:S3–S11.

54. **D'Hooghe TM, Kyama CK, Mihalyi AM, et al.** The baboon model for translational research in endometriosis. *Reprod Sci* 2009;16:152–161.

55. **Nisolle M, Donnez J.** Peritoneal endometriosis, ovarian endometriosis, and adenomyotic nodules of the rectovaginal septum are three different entities [review]. *Fertil Steril* 1997;68:585–596.

56. **Rock JA, Markham SM.** Extra pelvic endometriosis. In: **Wilson EA, ed.** *Endometriosis.* New York: AR Liss, 1987:185–206.

57. **Russo L, Woolmough E, Heatley MK.** Structural and cell surface antigen expression in the rete ovarii and epoophoron differs from that in the fallopian tube and in endometriosis. *Histopathology* 2000;37:64–69.

58. **Levander G, Normann P.** The pathogenesis of endometriosis: an experimental study. *Acta Obstet Gynecol Scand* 1955;34:366–398.

59. **Merrill JA.** Endometrial induction of endometriosis across millipore filters. *Am J Obstet Gynecol* 1966;94:780–789.

60. **Kennedy SH.** Genetics of endometriosis. In: **Tulandi T, Redwine D, eds.** *Endometriosis: advances and controversies.* New York: Dekker, 2004:55–68.

61. **Simpson JL, Elias S, Malinak LR, et al.** Heritable aspects of endometriosis. I. Genetics studies. *Am J Obstet Gynecol* 1980;137: 327–331.

62. **Moen MH, Magnus P.** The familial risk of endometriosis. *Acta Obstet Gynecol Scand* 1993;72:560–564.

63. **Treloar SA, O'Connor DT, O'Connor VM, et al.** Genetic influences on endometriosis in an Australian twin sample. *Fertil Steril* 1999;71:701–710.

64. **Hadfield RM, Mardon HJ, Barlow DH, et al.** Endometriosis in monozygotic twins. *Fertil Steril* 1997;68:941–942.

65. **Grimes DA, LeBolt SA, Grimes KR, et al.** Systemic lupus erythematosus and reproductive function: a case-control study. *Am J Obstet Gynecol* 1985;153:179–186.

66. **Hornstein MD, Thomas PP, Sober AJ, et al.** Association between endometriosis, dysplastic naevi and history of melanoma in women of reproductive age. *Hum Reprod* 1997;12:143–145.

67. **Simpson JL, Malinak LR, Elias S, et al.** HLA associations in endometriosis. *Am J Obstet Gynecol* 1984;148:395–397.

68. **Moen M, Bratlie A, Moen T.** Distribution of HLA-antigens among patients with endometriosis. *Acta Obstet Gynecol Scand Suppl* 1984;123:25–27.

69. **Maxwell C, Kilpatrick DC, Haining R, et al.** No HLA-DR specificity is associated with endometriosis. *Tissue Antigens* 1989;34:145–147.

70. **Painter JN, Anderson CA, Nyholt DR, et al.** Genome-wide association study identifies a locus at 7p15.2 associated with endometriosis. *Nat Genet* 2011;43:51–54.

71. **Falconer H, D'Hooghe T, Fried G.** Endometriosis and genetic polymorphisms [review]. *Obstet Gynecol Surv* 2007;62:616–628.

72. **Tamura M, Fukaya T, Murakami T, et al.** Analysis of clonality in human endometriotic cysts based on evaluation of X chromosome inactivation in archival formalin-fixed, paraffin-embedded tissue. *Lab Invest* 1998;78:213–218.

73. **Jiang X, Hitchcock A, Bryan E, et al.** Microsatellite analysis of endometriosis reveals loss of heterozygosity at candidate ovarian tumor suppressor gene loci. *Cancer Res* 1996;56:3534–3539.

74. **Bergqvist A, Baldetorp B, Ferno M.** Flow cytometric DNA analysis in endometriotic tissue compared to normal tissue EM. *Hum Reprod* 1996;11:1731–1735.

75. **Gogusev J, Bouquet de Joliniere J, Telvi L, et al.** Detection of DNA copy number changes in human endometriosis by comparative genomic hybridisation. *Hum Genet* 1999;105:444–451.

76. **Shin JC, Ross HL, Elias S, et al.** Detection of chromosomal aneuploidy in endometriosis by multicolor in situ hybridization. *Hum Genet* 1997;100:401–406.

77. **Kosugi Y, Elias S, Malinak LR, et al.** Increased heterogenecity of chromosome 17 aneuploidy in endometriosis. *Am J Obstet Gynecol* 1999;180:792–797.

78. **Körner M, Burckhardt E, Mazzucchelli L.** Higher frequency of chromosomal aberrations in ovarian endometriosis compared to extragonadal endometriosis: a possible link to endometrioid adenocarcinoma. *Mod Pathol* 2006;19:1615–1623.

79. **Goumenou AG, Arvanitis DA, Matalliotakis IM, et al.** Microsatellite DNA assays reveal an allelic imbalance in p16Ink4, GALT, p53, and APOA2 loci in patients with endometriosis. *Fertil Steril* 2001;75:160–165.

80. **D'Hooghe TM, Hill JA.** Immunobiology of endometriosis. In: **Bronson RA, Alexander NJ, Anderson DJ, et al., eds.** *Immunology of reproduction.* Cambridge, MA: Blackwell, 1996;322–358.

81. **Dmowski WP, Steele RN, Baker GF.** Deficient cellular immunity in endometriosis. *Am J Obstet Gynecol* 1981;141:377–383.

82. **Oosterlynck D, Cornillie FJ, Waer M, et al.** Women with endometriosis show a defect in natural killer cell activity resulting in a decreased cytotoxicity to autologous endometrium. *Fertil Steril* 1991;56:45–51.

83. **Steele RW, Dmowski WP, Marmer DJ.** Immunologic aspects of endometriosis. *Am J Reprod Immunol* 1984;6:33–36.

84. **Viganò P, Vercillini P, Di Blasio AM, et al.** Deficient antiendometrium lymphocyte-mediated cytotoxicity in patients with endometriosis. *Fertil Steril* 1991;56:894–899.

85. **Melioli G, Semino C, Semino A, et al.** Recombinant interleukin-2 corrects *in vitro* the immunological defect of endometriosis. *Am J Reprod Immunol* 1993;30:218–277.

86. **D'Hooghe TM, Scheerlinck JP, Koninckx PR, et al.** Antiendometrial lymphocytotoxicity and natural killer activity in baboons with endometriosis. *Hum Reprod* 1995;10:558–562.

87. **Hill JA.** Immunology and endometriosis. *Fertil Steril* 1992;58:262–264.

88. **Hill JA.** "Killer cells" and endometriosis. *Fertil Steril* 1993;60:928–929.

89. **Oosterlynck DJ, Meuleman C, Waer M, et al.** The natural killer activity of peritoneal fluid lymphocytes is decreased in women with endometriosis. *Fertil Steril* 1992;58:290–295.

90. **Iwasaki K, Makino T, Maruyama T, et al.** Leukocyte subpopulations and natural killer activity in endometriosis. *Int J Fertil Menopausal Stud* 1993;38:229–234.

91. **Garzetti GG, Ciavattini A, Provinciali M, et al.** Natural killer activity in endometriosis: correlation between serum estradiol levels and cytotoxicity. *Obstet Gynecol* 1993;81:665–668.

92. **Tanaka E, Sendo F, Kawagoe S, et al.** Decreased natural killer activity in women with endometriosis. *Gynecol Obstet Invest* 1992;34:27–30.

93. **D'Hooghe TM, Nugent N, Cuneo S, et al.** Recombinant human TNF binding protein (r-hTBP-1) inhibits the development of endometriosis in baboons: a prospective, randomized, placebo- and drug-controlled study. Accepted for oral presentation at the annual meeting of the American Society for Reproductive Medicine, Orlando, Florida, October 22–24, 2001.

94. **Hirata J, Kikuchi Y, Imaizumi E, et al.** Endometriotic tissues produce immunosuppressive factors. *Gynecol Obstet Invest* 1993;37:43–47.

95. **D'Hooghe TM, Bambra CS, De Jonge I, et al.** A serial section study of visually normal posterior pelvic peritoneum from baboons with

and without spontaneous endometriosis. *Fertil Steril* 1995;63:1322–1325.

96. **Zeller JM, Henig I, Radwanska E, et al.** Enhancement of human monocyte and peritoneal macrophage chemiluminescence activities in women with endometriosis. *Am J Reprod Immunol Microbiol* 1987;13:78–82.

97. **Halme J, Becker S, Haskill S.** Altered maturation and function of peritoneal macrophages: possible role in pathogenesis of endometriosis. *Am J Obstet Gynecol* 1987;156:783–789.

98. **Hill JA, Barbieri RL, Anderson DJ.** Immunosuppressive effects of *danazol in vitro.* *Fertil Steril* 1987;48:414–418.

99. **Halme J.** Release of tumor necrosis factor-a by human peritoneal macrophages *in vivo* and *in vitro.* *Am J Obstet Gynecol* 1989;161:1718–1725.

100. **Hill JA, Cohen J, Anderson DJ.** The effects of lymphokines and monokines on human sperm fertilizing ability in the zona-free hamster egg penetration test. *Am J Obstet Gynecol* 1989;160:1154–1159.

101. **Zhang R, Wild RA, Ojago JM.** Effect of tumor necrosis factor-alpha on adhesion of human endometrial stromal cells to peritoneal mesothelial cells: an *in vitro* system. *Fertil Steril* 1993;59:1196–1201.

102. **Sillem M, Prifti S, Monga B, et al.** Integrin-mediated adhesion of uterine endometrial cells from endometriosis patients to extracellular matrix proteins is enhanced by TNF-alpha and IL-1. *Eur J Obstet Gynecol* 1999;87:123–127.

103. **Olive DL, Montoya I, Riehl RM, et al.** Macrophage-conditioned media enhance endometrial stromal cell proliferation *in vitro.* *Am J Obstet Gynecol* 1991;164:953–958.

104. **Sharpe KL, Zimmer RL, Khan RS, et al.** Proliferative and morphogenic changes induced by the coculture of rat uterine and peritoneal cells: a cell culture model for endometriosis. *Fertil Steril* 1992;58:1220–1229.

105. **Halme J, White C, Kauma S, et al.** Peritoneal macrophages from patients with endometriosis release growth factor activity *in vitro.* *J Clin Endocrinol Metab* 1988;66:1044–1049.

106. **Kauma S, Clark MR, White C, et al.** Production of fibronectin by peritoneal macrophages and concentration of fibronectin in peritoneal fluid from patients with or without endometriosis. *Obstet Gynecol* 1988;72:13–18.

107. **van der Linden PJQ, de Goeij APFM, Dunselman GA, et al.** Expression of integrins and E-cadherin in cells from menstrual effluent, endometrium, peritoneal fluid, peritoneum, and endometriosis. *Fertil Steril* 1994;61:85–90.

108. **Sharpe-Timms KL, Keisler LW, McIntush EW, et al.** Tissue inhibitor of metalloproteinase-1 concentrations are attenuated in peritoneal fluid and sera of women with endometriosis and restored in sera by gonadotropin-releasing hormone agonist therapy. *Fertil Steril* 1998;69:1128–1134.

109. **Kokorine I, Nisolle M, Donnez J, et al.** Expression of interstitial collagenase (MMP-1) is related to the activity of human endometriotic lesions. *Fertil Steril* 1997;68:246–251.

110. **Kitawaki J, Noguchi T, Amatsu T, et al.** Expression of aromatase cytochrome P450 protein and messenger ribonucleic acid in human endometriotic and adenomyotic tissues but not in normal endometrium. *Biol Reprod* 1997;57:514–519.

111. **Zeitoun K, Takayama K, Sasano H, et al.** Deficient 17beta-hydroxysteroid dehydrogenase type 2 expression in endometriosis: failure to metabolize 17beta-estradiol. *J Clin Endocrinol Metab* 1998;83:4474–4480.

112. **Bulun SE, Zeitoun K, Takayama K, et al.** Molecular basis for treating endometriosis with aromatase inhibitors. *Hum Reprod Update* 2000;6:413–418.

113. **Agic A, Xu H, Finas D, et al.** Is endometriosis associated with systemic subclinical inflammation? *Gynecol Obstet Invest* 2006;62:139–147.

114. **Kao LC, Germeyer A, Tulac S, et al.** Expression profiling of endometrium from women with endometriosis reveals candidate genes for disease-based implantation failure and infertility. *Endocrinology* 2003;144:2870–2881.

115. **Kyama CM, Mihalyi A, Simsa P, et al.** Role of cytokines in the endometrial-peritoneal cross-talk and development of endometriosis [review]. *Front Biosci* (Elite Ed) 2009;1:444–454.

116. **Nasu K, Yuge A, Tsuno A, et al.** Involvement of resistance to apoptosis in the pathogenesis of endometriosis [review]. *Histol Histopathol* 2009;24:1181–1192.

117. **Kyama CM, Mihalyi A, Gevaert O, et al.** Evaluation of endometrial biomarkers for semi-invasive diagnosis of endometriosis. *Fertil Steril* 2010;95:1338–1348e1–e3.

118. **Al-Jefout M, Dezarnaulds G, Cooper M, et al.** Diagnosis of endometriosis by detection of nerve fibres in an endometrial biopsy: a double blind study. *Hum Reprod* 2009;24:3019–3024.

119. **Guo SW.** The link between exposure to dioxin and endometriosis: a critical reappraisal of primate data. *Gynecol Obstet Invest* 2004;57:157–173.

120. **Eskenazi B, Mocarelli P, Warner M, et al.** Seveso Women's Health Study: a study of the effects of 2,3,7,7-tetrachlorodibenzo-p-dioxin on reproductive health. *Chemosphere* 2000;40:1247–1253.

121. **Lebel G, Dodin S, Ayotte P, et al.** Organochlorine exposure and the risk of endometriosis. *Fertil Steril* 1998;69:221–228.

122. **Simsa P, Kyama C, Mihalyi A, et al.** Increased exposure to dioxin-like compounds is associated with endometriosis in a case-control study in women. *Reprod Biomed Online* 2010;20:681–688.

123. **Igarashi T, Osuga Y, Tsutsumi O, et al.** Expression of Ah receptor and dioxin-related genes in human uterine endometrium in women with or without endometriosis. *Endocr J* 1999;46:765–772.

124. **Watanabe T, Imoto I, Losugi Y, et al.** Human arylhydrocarbon receptor repressor (AHRR) gene: genomic structure and analysis of polymorphism in endometriosis. *J Hum Genet* 2001;46:342–346.

125. **Rier SE, Martin DC, Bowman RE, et al.** Endometriosis in rhesus monkeys (*Macaca mulatta*) following chronic exposure to 2,3,7,8-tetrachlorodibenzo-p-dioxin. *Fund Appl Toxicol* 1993;21:433–441.

126. **Rier SE, Turner WE, Martin DC, et al.** Serum levels of TCDD and dioxin-like chemicals in rhesus monkeys chronically exposed to dioxin: correlation of increased serum PCB levels with endometriosis. *Toxicol Sci* 2001;59:147–159.

127. **Yang Y, Degranpre P, Kharfi A, et al.** Identification of macrophage migration inhibitory factor as a potent endothelial cell growth promoting agent released by ectopic human endometrial cells. *J Clin Endocrinol Metab* 2000;85:4721–4727.

128. **Arnold DL, Nera EA, Stapley R, et al.** Prevalence of endometriosis in rhesus (*Macaca mulatta*) monkeys ingesting PCB (Aroclor 1254): review and evaluation. *Fund Appl Toxicol* 1996;31:42–55.

129. **Yang JZ, Foster WG.** Continuous exposure of 2,3,7,8 tetrachlorodibenzo-p-dioxin inhibits the growth of surgically induced endometriosis in the ovariectomized mouse treated with high dose estradiol. *Toxicol Ind Health* 1997;13:15–25

130. **Yang JZ, Yagminas AL, Foster WG.** Stimulating effects of 4-chlorodiphenyl ether on surgically induced endometriosis in the mouse. *Reprod Toxicol* 1997;11:69–75.

131. **Cummings AM, Metcalf JL, Birnbaum L.** Promotion of endometriosis by 2,3,7,8-tetrachlorodibenzo-p-dioxin in rats and mice: time-dose dependence and species comparison. *Toxicol Appl Pharmacol* 1996;138:131–139.

132. **Smith EM, Hammonds EM, Clark MK, et al.** Occupational exposures and risk of female infertility. *J Occup Environ Med* 1997;39:138–147.

133. **Gargett CE, Masuda H.** Adult stem cells in the endometrium. *Mol Hum Reprod* 2010;16:818–834.

134. **Simon C, Guttierez A, Vidal A, et al.** Outcome of patients with endometriosis in assisted reproduction: results from *in vitro* fertilization and oocyte donation. *Hum Reprod* 1994;9:725–729.

135. **Du H, Taylor HS.** Stem cells and reproduction. *Curr Opin Obstet Gynecol* 2010;22:235–241.

136. **Du H, Taylor HS.** Contribution of bone marrow-derived stem cells to endometrium and endometriosis. *Stem Cells* 2007;25:2082–2086.

137. **Jansen RPS, Russell P.** Nonpigmented endometriosis: clinical, laparoscopic and pathologic definition. *Am J Obstet Gynecol* 1986;155:1160–1163.

138. **Stripling MC, Martin DC, Chatman DL, et al.** Subtle appearance of pelvic endometriosis. *Fertil Steril* 1988;49:427–431.

139. **Martin DC, Hubert GD, Vander Zwaag R, et al.** Laparoscopic appearances of peritoneal endometriosis. *Fertil Steril* 1989;51:63–67.

140. **Grümmer R.** Animal models in endometriosis research [review]. *Hum Reprod Update* 2006;12:641–649.

141. **D'Hooghe TM, Bambra CS, Cornillie FJ, et al.** Prevalence and laparoscopic appearances of endometriosis in the baboon (*Papio cynocephalyus, Papio anubis*). *Biol Reprod* 1991;45:411–416.

142. **Schenken RS, Williams RF, Hodgen GD.** Experimental endometriosis in primates. *Ann N Y Acad Sci* 1991;622:242–255.

143. **DiZerega GS, Barber DL, Hodgen GD.** Endometriosis: role of ovarian steroids in initiation, maintenance and suppression. *Fertil Steril* 1980;649–653.

144. **Schenken RS, Asch RH, Williams RF, et al.** Etiology of infertility in monkeys with endometriosis: luteinized unruptured follicles, luteal phase defects, pelvic adhesions, and spontaneous abortions. *Fertil Steril* 1984;41:122–130.

145. **Mann DR, Collins DC, Smith MM, et al.** Treatment of endometriosis in Rhesus monkeys: effectiveness of a gonadotropin-releasing hormone agonist compared to treatment with a progestational steroid. *J Clin Endocrinol Metab* 1986;63:1277–1283.

146. **Da Rif CA, Parker RF, Schoeb TR.** Endometriosis with bacterial peritonitis in a baboon. *Lab Anim Sci* 1984;34:491–493.

147. **Cornillie FJ, D'Hooghe TM, Lauweryns JM, et al.** Morphological characteristics of spontaneous pelvic endometriosis in the baboon (*Papio anubis* and *Papio cynocephalus*). *Gynecol Obstet Invest* 1992;34:225–228

148. **D'Hooghe TM.** Clinical relevance of the baboon as a model for the study of endometriosis. *Fertil Steril* 1997;68:613–625.

149. **D'Hooghe TM, Debrock S.** Future directions in endometriosis research. *Obstet Gynecol Clin North Am* 2003;30:221–244.

150. **D'Hooghe TM, Nugent N, Cuneo S, et al.** Recombinant human TNF binding protein (r-hTBP-1) inhibits the development of endometriosis in baboons: a prospective, randomized, placebo- and drug-controlled study. *Biol Reprod* 2006;74:131–136.

151. **Falconer H, Mwenda JM, Chai DC, et al.** Treatment with anti-TNF monoclonal antibody (c5N) reduces the extent of induced endometriosis in the baboon. *Hum Reprod* 2006;21:1856–1862.

152. **Lebovic DI, Mwenda JM, Chai DC, et al.** PPAR-gamma receptor ligand induces regression of endometrial explants in baboons: a prospective, randomized, placebo- and drug-controlled study. *Fertil Steril* 2007;88:1108–1119.

153. **Lebovic DI, Mwenda JM, Chai DC, et al.** PPAR-gamma receptor ligand partially prevents the development of endometrial explants in baboons: a prospective, randomized, placebo-controlled study. *Endocrinology* 2010;151:1846–1852.

154. **Rogers PAW, D'Hooghe TM, Fazleabas AG, et al.** Priorities for endometriosis research: recommendations from an international consensus workshop. *Reprod Sci* 2009;16:335–346.

155. **Arumugam K, Lim JMH.** Menstrual characteristics associated with endometriosis. *Br J Obstet Gynecol* 1997;104:948–950.

156. **Vercellini P, De Giorgi O, Aimi G, et al.** Menstrual characteristics in women with and without endometriosis. *Obstet Gynecol* 1997;90:264–268.

157. **Signorello LB, Harlow BL, Cramer DW, et al.** Epidemiologic determinants of endometriosis: a hospital-based control study. *Ann Epidemiol* 1997;7:267–274.

158. **Mathias JR, Franklin R, Quast DC, et al.** Relation of endometriosis and neuromuscular disease of the gastrointestinal tract: new insights. *Fertil Steril* 1998;70:81–88.

159. **Ulrich U, Murano R, Skinner MA, et al.** Women of reproductive age with endometriosis are not osteopenic. *Fertil Steril* 1998;69:821–825.

160. **Hadfield RM, Mardon H, Barlow D, et al.** Delay in the diagnosis of endometriosis: a survey of women from the USA and the UK. *Hum Reprod* 1996;11:878–880.

161. **Husby GK, Haugen RS, Moen MH.** Diagnostic delay in women with pain and endometriosis. *Acta Obstet Gynecol Scand* 2003;82:649–653.

162. **Arruda MS, Petta CA, Abras MS, et al.** Time elapsed from onset of symptoms to diagnosis of endometriosis in a cohort study of Brazilian women. *Hum Reprod* 2003;18:756–759.

163. **Dmowski WP, Lesniewicz R, Rana N, et al.** Changing trends in the diagnosis of endometriosis: a comparative study of women with endometriosis presenting with chronic pain or infertility. *Fertil Steril* 1997;67:238–243.

164. **Gao X, Outley J, Botteman M, et al.** Economic burden of endometriosis [review]. *Fertil Steril* 2006;86:1561–1572.

165. **Colwell HH, Mathias SD, Pasta DJ, et al.** A health-related quality-of-life instrument for symptomatic patients with endometriosis: a validation study. *Am J Obstet Gynecol* 1998;179:47–55.

166. **Chapron C, Lafay-Pillet MC, Monceau E, et al.** Questioning patients about their adolescent history can identify markers associated with deep infiltrating endometriosis. *Fertil Steril* 2010;95:877–881.

167. **Fauconnier A, Chapron C.** Endometriosis and pelvic pain: epidemiological evidence of the relationship and implications [review]. *Hum Reprod Update* 2005;11:595–606.

168. **Chopin N, Ballester M, Borghese B, et al.** Relation between severity of dysmenorrhea and endometrioma. *Acta Obstet Gynecol Scand* 2006;85:1375–1380.

169. **Vercellini P, Cortesi I, Trespidi L, et al.** Endometriosis and pelvic pain: relation to disease stage and localization. *Fertil Steril* 1996;65:299–304.

170. **Chapron C, Pietin-Vialle C, Borghese B, et al.** Associated ovarian endometrioma is a marker for greater severity of deeply infiltrating endometriosis. *Fertil Steril* 2009;92:453–457.

171. **Fauconnier A, Chapron C, Dubuisson JB, et al.** Relation between pain symptoms and the anatomic location of deep infiltrating endometriosis. *Fertil Steril* 2002;78:719–726.

172. **Stratton P, Berkley KJ.** Chronic pelvic pain and endometriosis: translational evidence of the relationship and implications. *Hum Reprod Update* 2010;17:327–346.

173. **Fedele L, Bianchi S, Bocciolone L, et al.** Pain symptoms associated with endometriosis. *Obstet Gynecol* 1992;79:767–769.

174. **Muzii L, Marano R, Pedulla S, et al.** Correlation between endometriosis-associated dysmenorrhea and the presence of typical and atypical lesions. *Fertil Steril* 1997;68:19–22.

175. **Stovall DW, Bowser LM, Archer DF, et al.** Endometriosis-associated pain: evidence for an association between the stage of disease and a history of chronic pelvic pain. *Fertil Steril* 1997;68:13–18.

176. **Vercellini P, Fedele L, Aimi G, et al.** Association between endometriosis stage, lesion type, patient characteristics and severity of pelvic pain symptoms: a multivariate analysis of over 1000 patients. *Hum Reprod* 2007;22:266–271.

177. **Cornillie FJ, Vasquez G, Brosens IA.** The response of human endometriotic implants to the anti-progesterone steroid *R2323*: a histologic and ultrastructural study. *Pathol Res Pract* 1990;180:647–655.

178. **Barlow DH, Glynn CJ.** Endometriosis and pelvic pain. *Baillieres Clin Obstet Gynaecol* 1993;7:775–790.

179. **Chapron C, Fauconnier A, Dubuisson JB, et al.** Deep infiltrating endometriosis: relation between severity of dysmenorrhoea and extent of disease. *Hum Reprod* 2003;18:760–766.

180. **Anaf V, Simon P, El Nakadi I, et al.** Relationship between endometriotic foci and nerves in rectovaginal endometriotic nodules. *Hum Reprod* 2000;15:1744–1750.

181. **D'Hooghe TM, Debrock S, Hill JA, et al.** Endometriosis and subfertility: is the relationship resolved? *Sem Reprod Med* 2003;21:243–254.

182. **Benaglia L, Somigliana E, Vercellini P, et al.** Endometriotic ovarian cysts negatively affect the rate of spontaneous ovulation. *Hum Reprod* 2009;24:2183–2186.

183. **Adamson GD, Pasta DJ.** Endometriosis fertility index: the new, validated endometriosis staging system. *Fertil Steril* 2010;94:1609–1615.

184. **Barnhart K, Dunsmoor-Su R, Coutifaris C.** Effect of endometriosis on *in vitro* fertilization. *Fertil Steril* 2002;77:1148–1155.

185. **American Fertility Society.** Classification of endometriosis. *Fertil Steril* 1979;32:633–634.

186. **D'Hooghe TM, Bambra CS, Raeymaekers BM, et al.** A prospective controlled study over 2 years shows a normal monthly fertility rate (MFR) in baboons with stage I endometriosis and a decreased MFR in primates with stage II–IV disease. *Fertil Steril* 1994;5(Suppl):1–113.

187. **Haney AF.** Endometriosis-associated infertility. *Baillieres Clin Obstet Gynaecol* 1993;7:791–812.

188. **Metzger DA, Olive DL, Stohs GF, et al.** Association of endometriosis and spontaneous abortion: effect of control group selection. *Fertil Steril* 1986;45:18–22.

189. **Vercammen E, D'Hooghe TM, Hill JA.** Endometriosis and recurrent miscarriage. *Semin Reprod Med* 2000;18:363–368.

190. **Matorras R, Rodriguez F, Gutierrez de Teran G, et al.** Endometriosis and spontaneous abortion rate: a cohort study in infertile women. *Eur J Obstet Gynecol Reprod Biol* 1998;77:101–105.

191. **Marcoux S, Maheux R, Bérubé S, et al.** Laparoscopic surgery in infertile women with minimal or mild endometriosis. *N Engl J Med* 1997;337:217–222.

192. **Gruppo Italiano per lo Studio dell' Endometriosi.** Ablation of lesions or no treatment in minimal-mild endometriosis in infertile women: a randomized trial. *Hum Reprod* 1999;14:1332–1334.

193. **Bokor A, D'Hooghe TM.** Endometriosis and miscarriage: is there any association? In: *Endometriosis: current management and future trends.* New Delhi: Jaypee Medical Publishers, 2011:136–142.

194. **Cahill DJ, Hull MGR.** Pituitary-ovarian dysfunction and endometriosis. *Hum Reprod Update* 2000;6:56–66.

195. **D'Hooghe TM, Bambra CS, Raeymaekers BM, et al.** Increased incidence and recurrence of recent corpus luteum without ovulation stigma (luteinized unruptured follicle-syndrome?) in baboons (*Papio anubis, Papio cynocephalus*) with endometriosis. *J Soc Gynecol Invest* 1996;3:140–144.

196. **Lessey BA, Castelbaum AJ, Sawin SW, et al.** Aberrant integrin expression in the endometrium of women with endometriosis. *J Clin Endocrinol Metab* 1994;79:643–649.

197. **Matorras R, Rodriguez F, Perez C, et al.** Infertile women with and without endometriosis: a case-control study of luteal phase and other infertility conditions. *Acta Obstet Gynecol Scand* 1996;75:826–831.

198. **Propst AM, Storti K, Barbieri RL.** Lateral cervical displacement is associated with endometriosis. *Fertil Steril* 1998;70:568–570.

199. **Koninckx PR, Martin DC.** Deep endometriosis: a consequence of infiltration or retraction or possibly adenomyosis externa? *Fertil Steril* 1992;58:924–928.

200. **Koninckx PR, Oosterlynck D, D'Hooghe T, et al.** Deeply infiltrating endometriosis is a disease whereas mild endometriosis could be considered a non-disease. *Ann N Y Acad Sci* 1994;734:333–341.

201. **Koninckx PR, Meuleman C, Oosterlynck D, et al.** Diagnosis of deep endometriosis by clinical examination during menstruation and plasma CA 125 concentration. *Fertil Steril* 1996;65:280–287.

202. **Moore J, Copley S, Morris J, et al.** A systematic review of the accuracy of ultrasound in the diagnosis of endometriosis. *Ultrasound Obstet Gynecol* 2002;20:630–634.

203. **Guerriero S, Paoletti AM, Mais V, et al.** Transvaginal ultrasonography combined with CA125 plasma levels in the diagnosis of endometrioma. *Fertil Steril* 1996;65:293–298.

204. **Fedele L, Bianchi S, Portuese A, et al.** Transrectal ultrasonography in the assessment of rectovaginal endometriosis. *Obstet Gynecol* 1998;91:444–448.

205. **Van Holsbeke C, Van Calster B, Guerriero S, et al.** Endometriomas: their ultrasound characteristics. *Ultrasound Obstet Gynecol* 2010;35:730–740.

206. **Kinkel K, Chapron C, Balleyguier C, et al.** Magnetic resonance imaging characteristics of deep endometriosis. *Hum Reprod* 1999;14:1080–1086.

207. **McBean JH, Gibson M, Brumsted JR.** The association of intrauterine filling defects on HSG with endometriosis. *Fertil Steril* 1996;66:522–526.

208. **Carmignani L, Vercellini P, Spinelli M, et al.** Pelvic endometriosis and hydroureteronephrosis. *Fertil Steril* 2010;93:1741–1744.

209. **Somigliana E, Vercellini P, Vigano' P, et al.** Non-invasive diagnosis of endometriosis: the goal or own goal? *Hum Reprod* 2010;25:1863–1868.

210. **American Society for Reproductive Medicine.** Revised American Society for Reproductive Medicine classification of endometriosis. *Am Soc Reprod Med* 1997;5:817–821.

211. **D'Hooghe TM, Mihalyi AM, Simsa P, et al.** Why we need a non-invasive diagnostic test for minimal to mild endometriosis with a high sensitivity [editorial and opinion paper]. *Gynecol Obstet Invest* 2006;62:136–138.

212. **Bast RC, Klug TL, St. John E, et al.** A radio-immunoassay using a monoclonal antibody to monitor the course of epithelial ovarian cancer. *N Engl J Med* 1983;309:883–887.

213. **Barbieri RL, Niloff JM, Bast RC Jr, et al.** Elevated serum concentrations of CA125 in patients with advanced endometriosis. *Fertil Steril* 1986;45:630–634.

214. **Pittaway DE, Fayez JA.** The use of CA125 in the diagnosis and management of endometriosis. *Fertil Steril* 1986;46:790–795.

215. **Pittaway DE, Fayez JA.** Serum CA125 levels increase during menses. *Am J Obstet Gynecol* 1987;156:75–76.

216. **Masahashi T, Matsuzawa K, Ohsawa M, et al.** Serum CA125 levels in patients with endometriosis: changes in CA125 levels during menstruation. *Obstet Gynecol* 1988;72:328–331.

217. **Takahashi K, Abu Musa A, Nagata H, et al.** Serum CA125 and 17-b-estradiol in patients with external endometriosis on *danazol*. *Gynecol Obstet Invest* 1990;29:301–304.

218. **Franssen AMHW, van der Heijden PFM, Thomas CMG, et al.** On the origin and significance of serum CA125 concentrations in 97 patients with endometriosis before, during, and after *buserelin acetate, nafarelin*, or *danazol*. *Fertil Steril* 1992;57:974–979.

219. **Moloney MD, Thornton JG, Cooper EH.** Serum CA125 antigen levels and disease severity in patients with endometriosis. *Obstet Gynecol* 1989;73:767–769.

220. **Nagamani M, Kelver ME, Smith ER.** CA125 levels in monitoring therapy for endometriosis and in prediction of recurrence. *Int J Fertil* 1992;37:227–231.

221. **Hornstein M, Thomas PP, Gleason RE, et al.** Menstrual cyclicity of CA125 in patients with endometriosis. *Fertil Steril* 1992;58:279–283.

222. **O'Shaughnessy A, Check JH, Nowroozi K, et al.** CA125 levels measured in different phases of the menstrual cycle in screening for endometriosis. *Obstet Gynecol* 1993;81:99–103.

223. **Mol BW, Bayram N, Lijmer JG, et al.** The performance of CA-125 measurement in the detection of endometriosis: a meta-analysis. *Fertil Steril* 1998;70:1101–1108.

224. **Pittaway DE.** CA125 in women with endometriosis. *Obstet Gynecol Clin North Am* 1989;16:237–252.

225. **Hompes PGA, Koninckx PR, Kennedy S, et al.** Serum CA-125 concentrations during midfollicular phase, a clinically useful and reproducible marker in diagnosis of advanced endometriosis. *Clin Chem* 1996;42:1871–1874.

226. **Pittaway DE, Douglas JW.** Serum CA125 in women with endometriosis and chronic pain. *Fertil Steril* 1989;51:68–70.

227. **Pittaway DE.** The use of serial CA125 concentrations to monitor endometriosis in infertile women. *Am J Obstet Gynecol* 1990;163:1032–1037.

228. **Kauppila A, Telimaa S, Ronnberg L, et al.** Placebo-controlled study on serum concentrations of CA125 before and after treatment with *danazol* or high-dose medroxyprogesterone acetate alone or after surgery. *Fertil Steril* 1988;49:37–41.

229. **Dawood MY, Khan-Dawood FS, Wilson L Jr.** Peritoneal fluid prostaglandins and prostanoids in women with endometriosis, chronic pelvic inflammatory disease, and pelvic pain. *Am J Obstet Gynecol* 1984;148:391–395.

230. **Bischof P, Galfetti MA, Seydoux J, et al.** Peripheral CA125 levels in patients with uterine fibroids. *Hum Reprod* 1992;7:35–38.

231. **Ward BG, McGuckin MA, Ramm L, et al.** Expression of tumour markers CA125, CASA and OSA in minimal/mild endometriosis. *Aust N Z J Obstet Gynaecol* 1991;31:273–275.

232. **Fraser IS, McCarron G, Markham R.** Serum CA125 levels in women with endometriosis. *Aust N Z J Obstet Gynaecol* 1989;29:416–420.

233. **Acien P, Shaw RW, Irvine L, et al.** CA125 levels in endometriosis patients before, during and after treatment with *danazol* or LHRH agonists. *Eur J Obstet Gynecol* 1989;32:241–246.

234. **Takahashi K, Yoshino K, Kusakari M, et al.** Prognostic potential of serum CA125 levels in *danazol*-treated patients with external endometriosis: a preliminary study. *Int J Fertil* 1990;35:226–229.

235. **Fedele L, Arcaini L, Vercellini P, et al.** Serum CA125 measurements in the diagnosis of endometriosis recurrence. *Obstet Gynecol* 1988;72:19–22.

236. **May KE, Conduit-Hulbert SA, Villar J, et al.** Peripheral biomarkers of endometriosis: a systematic review. *Hum Reprod Update* 2010;16:651–674.

237. **Wykes CB, Clark TJ, Khan KS.** Accuracy of laparoscopy in the diagnosis of endometriosis: a systematic quantitative review. *BJOG* 2004;111:1204–1212.

238. **Chapron C, Querleu D, Bruhat MA, et al.** Surgical complications of diagnostic and operative gynaecological laparoscopy: a series of 29,966 cases. *Hum Reprod* 1998;13:867–872.

239. **Harkki-Siren P, Sjoberg J and Kurki T.** Major complications of laparoscopy: a follow-up Finnish study. *Obstet Gynecol* 1999;94:94–98.

240. **Vasquez G, Cornillie F, Brosens IA.** Peritoneal endometriosis: scanning electron microscopy and histology of minimal pelvic endometriotic lesions. *Fertil Steril* 1984;42:696–703.

241. **Nisolle M, Paindaveine B, Bourdin A, et al.** Histological study of peritoneal endometriosis in infertile women. *Fertil Steril* 1990;53:984–988.

242. **Clement PB.** Pathology of endometriosis. *Pathol Annu* 1990;25 (Pt 1):245–295.

243. **Moen MH, Halvorsen TB.** Histologic confirmation of endometriosis in different peritoneal lesions. *Acta Obstet Gynecol Scand* 1992;71:337–342.

244. **Vercellini P, Aimi G, Panazza S, et al.** Deep endometriosis conundrum: evidence in favor of a peritoneal origin. *Fertil Steril* 2000;73:1043–1046.

245. **Vercellini P, Vendola N, Bocciolone L, et al.** Reliability of the visual diagnosis of endometriosis. *Fertil Steril* 1991;56:1198–2000.

246. **Redwine DB.** Ovarian endometriosis: a marker for more extensive pelvic and intestinal disease. *Fertil Steril* 1999;72:310–315.

247. **Walter AJ, Hentz JG, Magtibay PM, et al.** Endometriosis: correlation between histologic and visual findings at laparoscopy. *Am J Obstet Gynecol* 2001;184:1407–1413.

248. **Czernobilsky B.** Endometriosis. In: **Fox H, ed.** *Obstetrical and gynecological pathology.* New York: Churchill Livingstone, 1987:763–777.

249. **Mai KT, Yazdi HM, Perkins DG, et al.** Pathogenetic role of the stromal cells in endometriosis and adenomyosis. *Histopathology* 1997;30:430–442.

250. **Donnez J, Nisolle M, Casanas-Roux F.** Three-dimensional architectures of peritoneal endometriosis. *Fertil Steril* 1992;57:980–983.

251. **Nisolle M, Casanas-Roux F, Anaf V, et al.** Morphometric study of the stromal vascularization in peritoneal endometriosis. *Fertil Steril* 1993;59:681–684.

252. **Anaf V, Simon Ph, El Nakadi I, et al.** Relationship between endometriotic foci and nerves in rectovaginal endometriotic nodules. *Hum Reprod* 2000;15:1744–1750.

253. **Wardle PG, Hull MGR.** Is endometriosis a disease? *Baillieres Clin Obstet Gynecol* 1993;7:673–685.

254. **Murphy AA, Green WR, Bobbie D, et al.** Unsuspected endometriosis documented by scanning electron microscopy in visually normal peritoneum. *Fertil Steril* 1986;46:522–524.

255. **Steingold KA, Cedars M, Lu JKH, et al.** Treatment of endometriosis with a long-acting gonadotropin-releasing hormone agonist. *Obstet Gynecol* 1987;69:403–411.

256. **Nezhat F, Allan CJ, Nezhat F, et al.** Nonvisualized endometriosis at laparoscopy. *Int J Fertil* 1991;36:340–343.

257. **Balasch J, Creus M, Fabregeus F, et al.** Visible and non-visible endometriosis at laparoscopy in fertile and infertile women and in patients with chronic pelvic pain: a prospective study. *Hum Reprod* 1996;11:387–391.

258. **Jansen RPS.** Minimal endometriosis and reduced fecundability: prospective evidence from an artificial insemination by donor program. *Fertil Steril* 1986;46:141–143.

259. **Hayata T, Matsu T, Kawano Y, et al.** Scanning electron microscopy of endometriotic lesions in the pelvic peritoneum and the histogenesis of endometriosis. *Int J Gynecol Obstet* 1992;39:311–319.

260. **Murphy AA, Guzick DS, Rock JA.** Microscopic peritoneal endometriosis. *Fertil Steril* 1989;51:1072–1074.

261. **Redwine DB.** Is "microscopic" peritoneal endometriosis invisible? *Fertil Steril* 1988;50:665–666.

262. **Redwine DB, Yocom LB.** A serial section study of visually normal pelvic peritoneum in patients with endometriosis. *Fertil Steril* 1990;54:648–651.

263. **Hornstein MD, Gleason RE, Orav J, et al.** The reproducibility of the revised American Fertility Society classification of endometriosis. *Fertil Steril* 1993;59:1015–1021.

264. **Lin SY, Lee RKK, Hwu YM, et al.** Reproducibility of the revised American Fertility Society classification of endometriosis during laparoscopy or laparotomy. *Int J Gynecol Obstet* 1998;60:265–269.

265. **Thomas EJ, Cooke ID.** Impact of *gestrinone* on the course of asymptomatic endometriosis. *BMJ* 1987;294:272–274.

266. **Thomas EJ, Cooke ID.** Successful treatment of asymptomatic endometriosis: does it benefit infertile women? *BMJ* 1987;294:1117–1119.

267. **Mahmood TA, Templeton A.** The impact of treatment on the natural history of endometriosis. *Hum Reprod* 1990;5:965–970.

268. **Sutton CJ, Pooley AS, Ewen SP, et al.** Follow-up report on a randomized controlled trial of laser laparoscopy in the treatment of pelvic pain associated with minimal to moderate endometriosis. *Fertil Steril* 1997;68:1070–1074.

269. **D'Hooghe TM, Bambra CS, Raeymaekers BM, et al.** Serial laparoscopies over 30 months show that endometriosis is a progressive disease in captive baboons (*Papio anubis*, *Papio cynocephalus*). *Fertil Steril* 1996;65:645–649.

270. **Hoshiai H, Ishikawa M, Yoshiharu S, et al.** Laparoscopic evaluation of the onset and progression of endometriosis. *Am J Obstet Gynecol* 1993;169:714–719.

271. **Redwine DB.** Age-related evolution in color appearance of endometriosis. *Fertil Steril* 1987;48:1062–1063.

272. **D'Hooghe TM, Bambra CS, Isahakia M, et al.** Evolution of spontaneous endometriosis in the baboon (*Papio anubis*, *Papio cynocephalus*) over a 12-month period. *Fertil Steril* 1992;58:409–412.

273. **Wiegerinck MAHM, Van Dop PA, Brosens IA.** The staging of peritoneal endometriosis by the type of active lesion in addition to the revised American Fertility Society classification. *Fertil Steril* 1993;60:461–464.

274. **Hanton EM, Malkasian GD Jr, Dockerty MB, et al.** Endometriosis associated with complete or partial obstruction of menstrual egress. *Obstet Gynecol* 1966;28:626–629.

275. **Schenken RS, Williams RF, Hodgen G.** Effect of pregnancy on surgically induced endometriosis in cynomolgus monkeys. *Am J Obstet Gynecol* 1987;157:1392–1396.

276. **Vernon MW, Wilson EA.** Studies on the surgical induction of endometriosis in the rat. *Fertil Steril* 1985;44:684–694.

277. **McArthur JW, Ulfelder H.** The effect of pregnancy upon endometriosis. *Obstet Gynecol Surv* 1965;20:709–733.

278. **D'Hooghe TM, Bambra CS, De Jonge I, et al.** Pregnancy does not affect endometriosis in baboons (*Papio anubis*, *Papio cynocephalus*). *Arch Gynecol Obstet* 1997;261:15–19.

279. **Kistner RW.** The treatment of endometriosis by inducing pseudopregnancy with ovarian hormones: a report of fifty-eight cases. *Fertil Steril* 1959;10:539–556.

280. **Italian Endometriosis Study Group.** Oral contraceptive use and risk of endometriosis. *Br J Obstet Gynecol* 1999;106:695–699.

281. **Somigliana E, Vercellini P, Vigano P, et al.** Endometriosis and estroprogestins: the chicken or the egg causality dilemma. *Fertil Steril* 2010;95:431–433.

282. **Vercellini P, Barbara G, Somigliana E, et al.** Comparison of contraceptive ring and patch for the treatment of symptomatic endometriosis. *Fertil Steril* 2010;93:2150–2161.

283. **Vercellini P, Eskenazi B, Consonni D, et al.** Oral contraceptives and risk of endometriosis: a systematic review and meta-analysis. *Hum Reprod Update* 2010;17:159–170.

284. **Zegers-Hochschild F, Adamson GD, de Mouzon J, et al.** International Committee for Monitoring Assisted Reproductive Technology (ICMART) and the World Health Organization (WHO) revised glossary of ART terminology, 2009. *Fertil Steril* 2009;92:1520–1524.

285. **Meuleman C, D'Hoore A, Van Cleynenbreugel B, et al.** Outcome after multidisciplinary CO_2 laser laparoscopic excision of deep infiltrating colorectal endometriosis. *Reprod Biomed Online* 2009;18:282–289.

286. **Abbott JA, Hawe J, Clayton RD, et al.** The effects and effectiveness of laparoscopic excision of endometriosis: a prospective study with 2–5 year follow-up. *Hum Reprod* 2003;18:1922–1927.

287. **Chapron C, Fauconnier A, Vieira M, et al.** Anatomical distribution of deeply infiltrating endometriosis: surgical implications and proposition for a classification. *Hum Reprod* 2003;18:157–161.

288. **Fedele L, Bianchi S, Zanconato G, et al.** Long-term follow-up after conservative surgery for rectovaginal endometriosis. *Am J Obstet Gynecol* 2004;190:1020–1024.

289. **Redwine DB, Wright JT.** Laparoscopic treatment of complete obliteration of the cul-de-sac associated with endometriosis: long-term follow-up of en bloc resection. *Fertil Steril* 2001;76:358–365.

290. **Tulandi T, Al Took S.** Reproductive outcome after treatment of mild endometriosis with laparoscopic excision and electrocoagulation. *Fertil Steril* 1998;69:229–231.

291. **Jacobson TZ, Duffy JM, Barlow D, et al.** Laparoscopic surgery for pelvic pain associated with endometriosis. *Cochrane Database Syst Rev* 2009;4:CD001300.

292. **Sutton C, Pooley AS, Jones KD, et al.** A prospective, randomized, double-blind controlled trial of laparoscopic uterine nerve ablation in the treatment of pelvic pain associated with endometriosis. *Gynaecol Endoscopy* 2001;10:217–222.

293. **Vercellini P, Aimi G, Busacca M, et al.** Laparoscopic uterosacral ligament resection for dysmenorrhea associated with endometriosis: results of a randomized, controlled trial. *Fertil Steril* 2003;80:310–19.

294. **Abbott J, Hawe J, Hunter D, et al.** Laparoscopic excision of endometriosis: a randomized, placebo-controlled trial. *Fertil Steril* 2004;82:878–884.

295. **Sutton CJ, Ewen SP, Whitelaw N, et al.** Prospective, randomized, double-blind, controlled trial of laser laparoscopy in the treatment of pelvic pain associated with minimal, mild, and moderate endometriosis. *Fertil Steril* 1994;62:696–700.

296. **Parker JD, Sinaii N, Segars JH, et al.** Adhesion formation after laparoscopic excision of endometriosis and lysis of adhesions. *Fertil Steril* 2005;84:1457–1461.

297. **Farquhar C, Vandekerckhove P, Watson A, et al.** Barrier agents for preventing adhesions after surgery for subfertility. *Cochrane Database Syst Rev* 2000;2:CD000475. Update in: *Cochrane Database Syst Rev* 2008;2:CD000475.

298. **DiZerega GS, Coad J, Donnez J.** Clinical evaluation of endometriosis and differential response to surgical therapy with and without application of Oxiplex/AP* adhesion barrier gel. *Fertil Steril* 2007;87:485–489.

299. **Hart RJ, Hickey M, Maouris P, Buckett W.** Excisional surgery versus ablative surgery for ovarian endometriomata. *Cochrane Database Syst Rev* 2008;2:CD004992.

300. **Chapron C, Vercellini P, Barakat H, et al.** Management of ovarian endometriomas. *Hum Reprod Update* 2002;8:6–7.

301. **Donnez J, Nisolle M, Gillet N, et al.** Large ovarian endometriomas. *Hum Reprod* 1996;11:641–646.

302. **Loh FH, Tan AT, Kumar J, et al.** Ovarian response after laparoscopic ovarian cystectomy for endometriotic cysts in 132 monitored cycles. *Fertil Steril* 1999;72:316–321.

303. **Beretta P, Franchi M, Ghezzi F, et al.** Randomized clinical trial of two laparoscopic treatments of endometriosis: cystectomy versus drainage and coagulation. *Fertil Steril* 1998;70:1176–1180.

304. **Alborzi S, Momtahan M, Parsanezhad ME, et al.** A prospective, randomized study comparing laparoscopic ovarian cystectomy versus fenestration and coagulation in patients with endometriomas. *Fertil Steril* 2004;82:1633–1617.

305. **Alborzi S, Ravanbakhsh R, Parsanezhad ME, et al.** Comparison of follicular response of ovaries to ovulation induction after laparoscopic ovarian cystectomy or fenestration and coagulation versus normal ovaries in patients with endometrioma. *Fertil Steril* 2007;88:507–509.

306. **Pados G, Tsolakidis D, Assimakopoulos E, et al.** Sonographic changes after laparoscopic cystectomy compared with three-stage management in patients with ovarian endometriomas: a prospective randomized study. *Hum Reprod* 2010;25:672–677.

307. **Tsolakidis D, Pados G, Vavilis D, et al.** The impact on ovarian reserve after laparoscopic ovarian cystectomy versus three-stage management in patients with endometriomas: a prospective randomized study. *Fertil Steril* 2010;94:71–77.

308. **Pellicano M, Bramante S, Guida M, et al.** Ovarian endometrioma: postoperative adhesions following bipolar coagulation and suture. *Fertil Steril* 2008;89:796–799.

309. **Vercellini P, Carmignani L, Rubino T, et al.** Surgery for deep endometriosis: a pathogenesis-oriented approach. *Gynecol Obstet Invest* 2009;68:88–103.

310. **Koninckx PR, Timmermans B, Meuleman C, et al.** Complications of CO-2 laser endoscopic excision of deep endometriosis. *Hum Reprod* 1996;11:2263–2268.

311. **Redwine DB, Koning M, Sharpe DR.** Laparoscopically assisted transvaginal segmental resection of the rectosigmoid colon for endometriosis. *Fertil Steril* 1996;65:193–197.

312. **Daraï E, Dubernard G, Coutant C, et al.** Randomized trial of laparoscopically assisted versus open colorectal resection for endometriosis: morbidity, symptoms, quality of life, and fertility. *Ann Surg* 2010;251:1018–1023.

313. **Meuleman C, Tomassetti C, D'Hoore A, et al.** Surgical treatment of deeply infiltrating endometriosis with colorectal involvement. *Hum Reprod Update* 2011;17:311–326.

314. **Candiani GB, Fedele L, Vercellini P, et al.** Presacral neurectomy for the treatment of pelvic pain associated with endometriosis: a controlled study. *Am J Obstet Gynecol* 1992;167:100–103.

315. **Fedele L, Bianchi S, Bocciolone L, et al.** *Buserelin acetate* in the treatment of pelvic pain associated with minimal and mild endometriosis: a controlled study. *Fertil Steril* 1993;59:516–521.

316. **Overton CE, Lindsay PC, Johal B, et al.** A randomized, double-blind, placebo-controlled study of luteal phase *dydrogesterone* (*Duphaston*) in women with minimal to mild endometriosis. *Fertil Steril* 1994;62:701–707.

317. **Feste JR.** Laser laparoscopy: a new modality. *J Reprod Med* 1985;30:413–417.

318. **Nezhat C, Winer W, Crowgey S, et al.** Video laparoscopy for the treatment of endometriosis associated with infertility. *Fertil Steril* 1989;51:237–240.

319. **Sutton CJG, Hill D.** Laser laparoscopy in the treatment of endometriosis: a 5 year study. *Br J Obstet Gynecol* 1990;97:181–185.

320. **Daniell JF.** Fiberoptic laser laparoscopy. *Baillieres Clin Obstet Gynaecol* 1989;3:545–562.

321. **Daniels J, Gray R, Hills RK, et al.** LUNA trial collaboration. Laparoscopic uterosacral nerve ablation for alleviating chronic pelvic pain: a randomized controlled trial. *JAMA* 2009;302:955–961.

322. **Vercellini P, Crosignani PG, Abbiati A, et al.** The effect of surgery for symptomatic endometriosis: the other side of the story. *Hum Reprod Update* 2009;15:177–188.

323. **Audebert A, Descampes P, Marret H, et al.** Pre or post operative medical treatment with nafarelin in stage III–IV endometriosis: a French multicentered study. *Eur J Obstet Gynecol Reprod Biol* 1998;79:145–148.

324. **Yap C, Furness S, Farquhar C.** Pre and post operative medical therapy for endometriosis surgery. *Cochrane Database Syst Rev* 2004;3:CD003678.

325. **MacDonald SR, Klock SC, Milad MP.** Long-term outcome of non-conservative surgery (hysterectomy) for endometriosis-associated pain in women <30 years old. *Am J Obstet Gynecol* 1999;180:1360–1363.

326. **Lefebvre G, Allaire C, Jeffrey J, et al.** SOGC clinical guidelines: hysterectomy. *J Obstet Gynaecol Can* 2002;24:37–61.

327. **Namnoum AB, Hickman TN, Goodman SB, et al.** Incidence of symptom recurrence after hysterectomy for endometriosis. *Fertil Steril* 1995;64:898–902.

328. **Ford J, English J, Miles WA, et al.** Pain, quality of life and complications following the radical resection of rectovaginal endometriosis. *BJOG* 2004;111:353–356.

329. **Matorras R, Elorriaga MA, Pijoan JI, et al.** Recurrence of endometriosis in women with bilateral adnexectomy (with or without total hysterectomy) who received hormone replacement therapy. *Fertil Steril* 2002;77:303–308.

330. **Heaps JM, Berek JS, Nieberg RK.** Malignant neoplasms arising in endometriosis. *Obstet Gynecol* 1990;75:1023–1028.

331. **Bianchi S, Busacca M, Agnoli B, et al.** Effects of 3 month therapy with *danazol* after laparoscopic surgery for stage III/IV endometriosis: a randomized study. *Hum Reprod* 1999;14:1335–1337.

332. **Hornstein MD, Hemmings R, Yuzpe AA, et al.** Use of *nafarelin* versus placebo after reductive laparoscopic surgery for endometriosis. *Fertil Steril* 1997;68:860–864.

333. **Vercellini P, Crosignani PG, Fadini R, et al.** A gonadotropin-releasing hormone agonist compared with expectant management after conservative surgery for symptomatic endometriosis. *Br J Obstet Gynecol* 1999;106:672–677.

334. **Busacca M, Somigliana E, Bianchi S, et al.** Post-operative GnRH analogue treatment after conservative surgery for symptomatic endometriosis stage III–IV: a randomized controlled trial. *Hum Reprod* 2001;16:2399–2402.

335. **Parazzini F, Fedele L, Busacca M, et al.** Postsurgical treatment of advanced endometriosis: results of a randomized clinical trial. *Am J Obstet Gynecol* 1994;171:1205–1207.

336. **Telimaa S, Ronnberg L, Kauppila A.** Placebo-controlled comparison of *danazol* and high-dose *medroxyprogesterone acetate* in the treatment of endometriosis after conservative surgery. *Gynecol Endocrinol* 1987;1:363–371.

337. **Loverro G, Carriero C, Rossi AC, et al.** A randomized study comparing *triptorelin* or expectant management following conservative laparoscopic surgery for symptomatic stage III–IV endometriosis. *Eur J Obstet Gynecol Reprod Biol* 2008;136:194–198.

338. **Vercellini P, Somigliana E, Daguati R, et al.** Postoperative oral contraceptive exposure and risk of endometrioma recurrence. *Am J Obstet Gynecol* 2008;198:504.e1–e5.

339. **Seracchioli R, Mabrouk M, Frascà C, et al.** Long-term oral contraceptive pills and postoperative pain management after laparoscopic excision of ovarian endometrioma: a randomized controlled trial. *Fertil Steril* 2010;94:464–471.

340. **Seracchioli R, Mabrouk M, Frascà C, et al.** Long-term cyclic and continuous oral contraceptive therapy and endometrioma recurrence: a randomized controlled trial. *Fertil Steril* 2010;93:52–56.

341. **Sesti F, Pietropolli A, Capozzolo T, et al.** Hormonal suppression treatment or dietary therapy versus placebo in the control of painful symptoms after conservative surgery for endometriosis stage III–IV. A randomized comparative trial. *Fertil Steril* 2007;88:1541–1547.

342. **Abou-Setta AM, Al-Inany HG, Farquhar CM.** *Levonorgestrel*-releasing intrauterine device (LNG-IUD) for symptomatic endometriosis following surgery. *Cochrane Database Syst Rev* 2006;4:CD005072.

343. **Vercellini P, Frontino G, De Giorgi O, et al.** Comparison of a *levonorgestrel*-releasing intrauterine device versus expectant management after conservative surgery for symptomatic endometriosis: a pilot study. *Fertil Steril* 2003;80:305–309.

344. **Wong AY, Tang LC, Chin RK.** *Levonorgestrel*-releasing intrauterine system (*Mirena*) and depot *medroxyprogesterone acetate* (*Depo-Provera*) as long-term maintenance therapy for patients with moderate and severe endometriosis: a randomised controlled trial. *Aust N Z J Obstet Gynaecol* 2010;50:273–279.

345. **Marjoribanks J, Proctor ML, Farquhar C.** Nonsteroidal anti-inflammatory drugs for primary dysmenorrhoea. *Cochrane Database Syst Rev* 2003;4:CD001751.

346. **Zhang WY, Li Wan Po A.** Efficacy of minor analgesics in primary dysmenorrhoea: a systematic review. *Br J Obstet Gynecol* 1998;105:780–789.

347. **Dawood MY, Khan-Dawood FS.** Clinical efficacy and differential inhibition of menstrual fluid prostaglandin F2alpha in a randomized, double-blind, crossover treatment with placebo, *acetaminophen*, and *ibuprofen* in primary dysmenorrhea. *Am J Obstet Gynecol* 2007;196:35.e1–e5.

348. **Proctor ML, Smith CA, Farquhar CM, et al.** Transcutaneous electrical nerve stimulation and acupuncture for primary dysmenorrhoea (Cochrane Review). In: *The Cochrane Library, Issue 3*. Chichester, UK: Wiley, 2004.

349. **Davis AR, Westhoff C, O'Connell K, et al.** Oral contraceptives for dysmenorrhea in adolescent girls: a randomized trial. *Obstet Gynecol* 2005;106:97–104.

350. **Proctor M, Farquhar C.** Dysmenorrhoea. *Clin Evid* 2006;12:2429–2448.

351. **Proctor ML, Murphy PA.** Herbal and dietary therapies for primary and secondary dysmenorrhoea (Cochrane Review). In: *The Cochrane Library, Issue 3*. Chichester, UK: Wiley, 2004.

352. **Proctor ML, Hing W, Johnson TC, et al.** Spinal manipulation for primary and secondary dysmenorrhoea. *Cochrane Database Syst Rev* 2006;3:CD002119.

353. **Kauppila A, Ronnberg L.** *Naproxen sodium* in dysmenorrhea secondary to endometriosis. *Obstet Gynecol* 1985;65:379–383.

354. **Allen C, Hopewell S, Prentice A, et al.** Nonsteroidal anti-inflammatory drugs for pain in women with endometriosis. *Cochrane Database Syst Rev* 2009;2:CD004753.

355. **Bajaj P, Bajaj P, Madsen J, et al.** Endometriosis is associated with central sensitization: a psychophysical controlled study. *J Pain* 2003;4:372–380.

356. **Kauppila A, Puolakka J, Ylikorkala O.** Prostaglandin biosynthesis inhibitors and endometriosis. *Prostaglandins* 1979;18:655–661.

357. **Vercellini P, Crosignani PG, Somigliana E, et al.** Medical treatment for rectovaginal endometriosis: what is the evidence? *Hum Reprod* 2009;24:2504–2514.

358. **Moore J, Kennedy SH, Prentice A.** Modern combined oral contraceptives for pain associated with endometriosis (Cochrane Review). In: *The Cochrane Library, Issue 3*. Chichester, UK: Wiley, 2004.

359. **Prentice A, Deary AJ, Goldbeck WS, et al.** Gonadotrophin-releasing hormone analogues for pain associated with endometriosis. In: *The Cochrane Library, Issue 3*. Chichester, UK: Wiley, 2004.

360. **Harada T, Momoeda M, Taketani Y, et al.** Low-dose oral contraceptive pill for dysmenorrhea associated with endometriosis: a placebo-controlled, double-blind, randomized trial. *Fertil Steril* 2008;90:1583–1588.

361. **Nothnick WB, D'Hooghe TM.** New developments in the medical treatment of endometriosis. *Gynecol Obstet Invest* 2003;55:189–198.

362. **Kyama CM, Mihalyi A, Mwenda JM, et al.** The role of immunologic factors in the development of endometriosis: indications for treatment strategies. *Therapy* 2005;4:623–639.

363. **Edelman AB, Gallo MF, Jensen JT, et al.** Continuous or extended cycle vs. cyclic use of combined oral contraceptives for contraception. *Cochrane Database Syst Rev* 2005;3:CD004695.

364. **Vercellini P, Pietropaolo G, De Giorgi O, et al.** Treatment of symptomatic rectovaginal endometriosis with an estrogen-progestogen combination versus low-dose *norethindrone acetate*. *Fertil Steril* 2005;84:1375–1387.

365. **Kistner RW.** The use of progestins in the treatment of endometriosis. *Am J Obstet Gynecol* 1958;75:264–278.

366. **Prentice A, Deary AJ, Bland E.** Progestagens and anti-progestagens for pain associated with endometriosis. *Cochrane Database Syst Rev* 2000;2:CD002122.

367. **Moghissi KS.** Pseudopregnancy induced by estrogen-progestogen or progestogens alone in the treatment of endometriosis. *Prog Clin Biol Res* 1990;323:221–232.

368. **Telimaa S, Puolakka J, Ronnberg L, et al.** Placebo-controlled comparison of *danazol* and high-dose *medroxyprogesterone acetate* in the treatment of endometriosis. *Gynecol Endocrinol* 1987;1:13–23.

369. **Harrison RF, Barry-Kinsella C.** Efficacy of *medroxy-progesterone* treatment in infertile women with endometriosis: a prospective, randomized, placebo-controlled study. *Fertil Steril* 2000;74:24–30.

370. **Vercellini P, De Giorgi O, Oldani S, et al.** Depot *medroxyprogesterone acetate* versus an oral contraceptive combined with very-low-dose *danazol* for long-term treatment of pelvic pain associated with endometriosis. *Am J Obstet Gynecol* 1996;175:396–341.

371. **Schlaff WD, Carson SA, Luciano A, et al.** Subcutaneous injection of depot *medroxyprogesterone acetate* compared with *leuprolide acetate* in the treatment of endometriosis-associated pain. *Fertil Steril* 2006;85:314–325.

372. **Walch K, Unfried G, Huber J, et al.** *Implanon* versus *medroxyprogesterone acetate*: effects on pain scores in patients with symptomatic endometriosis—a pilot study. *Contraception* 2009;79:29–34.

373. **Strowitzki T, Marr J, Gerlinger C, et al.** *Dienogest* is as effective as *leuprolide acetate* in treating the painful symptoms of endometriosis: a 24-week, randomized, multicentre, open-label trial. *Hum Reprod* 2010;25:633–641.

374. **Harada T, Momoeda M, Taketani Y, et al.** Dienogest is as effective as intranasal buserelin acetate for the relief of pain symptoms associated with endometriosis—a randomized, double-blind, multicenter, controlled trial. *Fertil Steril* 2009;91:675–681.

375. **Viganò P, Somigliana E, Vercellini P.** *Levonorgestrel*-releasing intrauterine system for the treatment of endometriosis: biological and clinical evidence. *Womens Health* 2007;3:207–214.

376. **Varma R, Sinha D, Gupta JK.** Non-contraceptive uses of *levonorgestrel*-releasing hormone system (LNG-IUS)—a systematic enquiry and overview. *Eur J Obstet Gynecol Reprod Biol* 2006;125:9–28.

377. **Vercellini P, Aimi G, Panazza S, et al.** A *levonorgestrel*-releasing intrauterine system for the treatment of dysmenorrhea associated with endometriosis: a pilot study. *Fertil Steril* 1999;72:505–508.

378. **Fedele L, Bianchi S, Zanconato G, et al.** Use of a *levonorgestrel*-releasing intrauterine device in the treatment of rectovaginal endometriosis. *Fertil Steril* 2001;75:485–488.

379. **Petta CA, Ferriani RA, Abrao MS, et al.** Randomized clinical trial of a *levonorgestrel*-releasing intrauterine system and a depot GnRH analogue for the treatment of chronic pelvic pain in women with endometriosis. *Hum Reprod* 2005;20:1993–1998.

380. **Lockhat FB, Emembolu JO, Konje JC.** The efficacy, side-effects and continuation rates in women with symptomatic endometriosis undergoing treatment with an intra-uterine administered progestogen (*levonorgestrel*): a 3-year follow-up. *Hum Reprod* 2005;20:789–793.

381. **Murphy AA, Zhou MH, Malkapuram S, et al.** *RU486*-induced growth inhibition of human endometrial cells. *Fertil Steril* 2000;74:1014–1019.

382. **Koide SS.** *Mifepristone*: auxiliary therapeutic use in cancer and related disorders. *J Reprod Med* 1998;43:551–560.

383. **Kettel LM, Murphy AA, Morales AJ, et al.** Treatment of endometriosis with the antiprogesterone *mifepristone* (*RU486*). *Fertil Steril* 1996;65:23–28.

384. **Kettel LM, Murphy AA, Morales AJ, et al.** Preliminary report on the treatment of endometriosis with low-dose *mifepristone* (*RU486*). *Am J Obstet Gynecol* 1998;178:1151–1156.

385. **Stoeckemann K, Hegele-Hartung C, Chwalisz K.** Effects of the progesterone antagonists *onapristone* (*ZK 98 299*) and *ZK 136 799* on surgically induced endometriosis in intact rats. *Hum Reprod* 1995;10:3264–3271.

386. **Fuhrmann U, Hess Stummp H, Cleve A, et al.** Synthesis and biological activity of a novel, highly potent progesterone receptor antagonist. *J Med Chem* 2000;43:5010–5016.

387. **Slayden OD, Chwalisz K, Brenner RM.** Reversible suppression of menstruation with progesterone antagonists in rhesus macaques. *Hum Reprod* 2001;8:1562–1574.

388. **Brosens IA, Verleyen A, Cornillie FJ.** The morphologic effect of short-term medical therapy of endometriosis. *Am J Obstet Gynecol* 1987;157:1215–1221.

389. **Fedele L, Bianchi S, Viezzoli T, et al.** *Gestrinone* versus *danazol* in the treatment of endometriosis. *Fertil Steril* 1989;51:781–785.

390. **Wingfield M, Healy DL.** Endometriosis: medical therapy. *Bailliers Clin Obstet Gynecol* 1993;7:813–838.

391. **Hornstein MD, Gleason RE, Barbieri RL.** A randomized double-blind prospective trial of two doses of *gestrinone* in the treatment of endometriosis. *Fertil Steril* 1990;53:237–241.

392. **Gestrinone Italian Study Group.** Gestrinone versus a GnRHa for the treatment of pelvic pain associated with endometriosis: a multicenter, randomized, double-blind study. *Fertil Steril* 1996;66:911–919.

393. **Barbieri RL, Ryan KJ.** *Danazol*: endocrine pharmacology and therapeutic applications. *Am J Obstet Gynecol* 1981;141:453–463.

394. **El-Roeiy A, Dmowski WP, Gleicher N, et al.** *Danazol* but not gonadotropin-releasing hormone agonists suppresses autoantibodies in endometriosis. *Fertil Steril* 1988;50;864–871.

395. **Ota H, Maki M, Shidara Y, et al.** Effects of *danazol* at the immunologic level in patients with adenomyosis, with special reference to autoantibodies: a multi-center cooperative study. *Am J Obstet Gynecol* 1992;167:481–486.

396. **Hill JA, Haimovici F, Politch JA, et al.** Effects of soluble products of activated macrophages (lymphokines and monokines) on human sperm motion parameters. *Fertil Steril* 1987;47:460–465.

397. **Mori H, Nakagawa M, Itoh N, et al.** Danazol suppresses the production of interleukin-1b and tumor necrosis factor by human monocytes. *Am J Reprod Immunol* 1990;24:45–50.

398. **Braun DP, Gebel H, Rotman C, et al.** The development of cytotoxicity in peritoneal macrophages from women with endometriosis. *Fertil Steril* 1992;1203:1203–1210.

399. **Gelfand JA, Sherins RJ, Alling DW, et al.** Treatment of hereditary angioedema with *danazol*. *N Engl J Med* 1976;295:1444–1448.

400. **Ahn YS, Harrington WJ, Mylvaganam R, et al.** *Danazol* therapy for autoimmune hemolytic anemia. *Ann Intern Med* 1985;102:298–301.

401. **Agnello V, Pariser K, Gell J, et al.** Preliminary observations on *danazol* therapy of systemic lupus erythematosus: effect on DNA antibodies, thrombocytopenia and complement. *J Rheumatol* 1983;10:682–687.

402. **Schreiber AD, Chien P, Tomaski A, et al.** Effect of *danazol* in immune thrombocytopenic purpura. *N Engl J Med* 1987;316:503–508.

403. **Mylvaganam R, Ahn YS, Harrington WJ, et al.** Immune modulation by *danazol* in autoimmune thrombocytopenia. *Clin Immunol Immunopathol* 1987;42:281–287.

404. **Selak V, Farquhar C, Prentice A, et al.** Danazol for pelvic pain associated with endometriosis. *Cochrane Database Syst Rev* 2007;4:CD000068.

405. Igarashi M, Iizuka M, Abe Y, et al. Novel vaginal *danazol* ring therapy for pelvic endometriosis, in particular deeply infiltrating endometriosis. *Hum Reprod* 1998;13:1952–1956.

406. Borroni R, Di Blasio AM, Gaffuri B, et al. Expression of GnRH receptor gene in human ectopic endometrial cells and inhibition of their proliferation by leuprolide acetate. *Mol Cell Endocrinol* 2000;159:37–43

407. Sharpe-Timms KL, Zimmer RL, Jolliff WJ, et al. GnRHa therapy alters activity of plasminogen activators, matrix metalloproteinases, and their inhibitors in rat models for adhesion formation and endometriosis: potential GnRHa regulated mechanisms reducing adhesion formation. *Fertil Steril* 1998;68:916–923.

408. Barbieri RL. Hormone treatment of endometriosis: the estrogen threshold hypothesis. *Am J Obstet Gynecol* 1992;166:740–745.

409. Riis BJ, Christiansen C, Johansen JS, et al. Is it possible to prevent bone loss in young women treated with luteinizing hormone-releasing agonists? *J Clin Endocrinol Metab* 1990;70:920–924.

410. Hornstein MD, Surrey ES, Weisberg GW, et al. *Leuprolide acetate* depot and hormonal add-back in endometriosis: a 12-month study. *Obstet Gynecol* 1998;91:16–24.

411. Sillem M, Parviz M, Woitge HW, et al. Add-back *medrogestone* does not prevent bone loss in premenopausal women treated with goserelin. *Exp Clin Endocrinol Diabetes* 1999;107:379–385.

412. Taskin O, Uryan I, Yalcinoglu I, et al. Effectiveness of *tibolone* on hypoestrogenic symptoms induced by *goserelin* treatment in patients with endometriosis. *Fertil Steril* 1997;67:40–45.

413. Lindsay PC, Shaw RW, Bennink HJC, et al. The effect of add-back treatment with *tibolone* (*Livial*) on patients treated with the GnRHa *triptorelin* (*Decapeptyl*). *Fertil Steril* 1996;65:342–348.

414. Franke HR, van de Weijere PHM, Pennings TMM, et al. Gonadotropin-releasing hormone agonist plus "add-back" hormone replacement therapy for treatment of endometriosis: a prospective randomized placebo-controlled double-blind trial. *Fertil Steril* 2000;74:534–539.

415. Sagsveen M, Farmer JE, Prentice A, et al. Gonadotrophin-releasing hormone analogues for endometriosis: bone mineral density. *Cochrane Database Syst Rev* 2003;4:CD001297.

416. Pierce SJ, Gazvani MR, Farquharson RG. Long-term use of gonadotropin-releasing hormone analogs and hormone replacement therapy in the management of endometriosis: a randomized trial with a 6-year follow-up. *Fertil Steril* 2000;74:964–968.

417. Tahara M, Matsuoka T, Yokoi T, et al. Treatment of endometriosis with a decreasing dosage of gonadotropin-releasing hormone agonist (*nafarelin*): a pilot study with low-dose agonist therapy ("draw-back" therapy). *Fertil Steril* 2000;73:799–804

418. Yano S, Ikegami Y, Nakao K. Studies on the effect of the new non-steroidal aromatase inhibitor *fadrozole hydrochloride* in an endometriosis model in rats. *Arzneimittelforschung* 1996;46:192–195.

419. Kudoh M, Susaki Y, Ideyama Y, et al. Inhibitory effects of a novel aromatase inhibitor, YM511, in rats with experimental endometriosis. *J Steroid Biochem Mol Biol* 1997;63:1–3.

420. Takayama K, Zeitoun K, Gunby RT, et al. Treatment of severe postmenopausal endometriosis with an aromatase inhibitor. *Fertil Steril* 1998;69:709–713.

421. Nawathe A, Patwardhan S, Yates D, et al. Systematic review of the effects of aromatase inhibitors on pain associated with endometriosis. *BJOG* 2008;115:818–822.

422. Soysal S, Soysal M, Ozer S, et al. The effects of post-surgical administration of *goserelin* plus *anastrazole* compared to *goserelin* alone in patients with severe endometriosis: a prospective randomised trial. *Hum Reprod* 2004;19:160–167.

423. Buelke SJ, Bryant HU, Francis PC. The selective estrogen receptor modulator, *raloxifene*: an overview of nonclinical pharmacology and reproductive and developmental testing. *Reprod Toxicol* 1998;12:217–221.

424. Stratton P, Sinaii N, Segars J, et al. Return of chronic pelvic pain from endometriosis after raloxifene treatment: a randomized controlled trial. *Obstet Gynecol* 2008;111:88–96.

425. D'Antonio M, Martelli F, Peano S, et al. Ability of recombinant human TNF binding protein-1 (r-hTBP-1) to inhibit the development of experimentally induced endometriosis in rats. *J Reprod Immunol* 2000;48:81–98.

426. Koninckx PR, Craessaerts M, Timmerman D, et al. Anti-TNF-alpha treatment for deep endometriosis-associated pain: a randomized placebo-controlled trial. *Hum Reprod* 2008;23:2017–2023.

427. Lv D, Song H, Li Y, et al. *Pentoxifylline* versus medical therapies for subfertile women with endometriosis. *Cochrane Database Syst Rev* 2009;3:CD007677.

428. Lebovic DI, Kir M, Casey CL, et al. Peroxisome proliferator-activated receptor-gamma induces regression of endometrial explants in a rat model of endometriosis. *Fertil Steril* 2004;82:1008–1013.

429. Moravek MB, Ward EA, Lebovic DI. Thiazolidinediones as therapy for endometriosis: a case series. *Gynecol Obstet Invest* 2009;68:167–170.

430. Ingelmo JM, Quereda F, Acien P. Intraperitoneal and subcutaneous treatment of experimental endometriosis with recombinant human interferon-alpha-2b in a murine model. *Fertil Steril* 1999;71:907–911.

431. Keenan JA, Williams-Boyce PK, Massey PJ, et al. Regression of endometrial explants in a rat model of endometriosis treated with immune modulators *loxoribine* and *levamisole*. *Fertil Steril* 2000;72:135–141.

432. Kyama CM, Mihalyi A, Simsa P, et al. Non-steroidal targets in the diagnosis and treatment of endometriosis [review]. *Curr Med Chem* 2008;15:1006–1017.

433. Flower A, Liu JP, Chen S, et al. Chinese herbal medicine for endometriosis. *Cochrane Database Syst Rev* 2009;3:CD006568.

434. Olive DL, Lee KL. Analysis of sequential treatment protocols for endometriosis-associated infertility. *Am J Obstet Gynecol* 1986;154:613–619.

435. Jacobson TZ, Barlow DH, Koninckx PR, et al. Laparoscopic surgery for subfertility associated with endometriosis (Cochrane Review). In: *The Cochrane Library, Issue 3*. Chichester, UK: Wiley, 2004.

436. Hughes E, Brown J, Collins JJ, et al. Ovulation suppression for endometriosis. *Cochrane Database Syst Rev* 2007;3:CD000155.

437. Arumugam K, Urquhart R. Efficacy of laparoscopic electrocoagulation in infertile patients with minimal or mild endometriosis. *Acta Obstet Gynecol Scand* 1991;70:125–127.

438. Adamson GD, Hurd SJ, Pasta DJ, et al. Laparoscopic endometriosis treatment: is it better? *Fertil Steril* 1993;59:35–44.

439. Guzick DS, Canis M, Silliman NP, et al. Prediction of pregnancy in infertile women based on the ASRM's revised classification for endometriosis. *Fertil Steril* 1997;67:822–836.

440. Osuga Y, Koga K, Tsutsumi O, et al. Role of laparoscopy in the treatment of endometriosis-associated infertility. *Gynecol Obstet Invest* 2002;53(Suppl 1):33–39.

441. Canis M, Pouly JL, Wattiez A, et al. Incidence of bilateral adnexal disease in severe endometriosis (revised American Fertility Society [AFS] stage IV): should a stage V be included in the AFS classification? *Fertil Steril* 1992;57:691–692.

442. Chapron C, Fritel X, Dubuisson JB. Fertility after laparoscopic management of deep endometriosis infiltrating the uterosacral ligaments. *Hum Reprod* 1999;14:329–332.

443. Pagidas K, Falcone T, Hemmings R, et al. Comparison of reoperation for moderate (stage III) and severe (stage IV) endometriosis-related infertility. *Fertil Steril* 1996;65:791–795.

444. Rock JA, Guzick DS, Dengos C, et al. The conservative surgical treatment of endometriosis: evaluation of pregnancy success with respect to the extent of disease as categorized using contemporary classification systems. *Fertil Steril* 1981;35:131–137.

445. Somigliana E, Daguati R, Vercellini P, et al. The use and effectiveness of in vitro fertilization in women with endometriosis: the surgeon's perspective. *Fertil Steril* 2009;91:1775–1779.

446. Goldstein DP, De Cholnoky C, Emans SJ. Adolescent endometriosis. *J Adolesc Health Care* 1980;1:37–41.

447. Bai SW, Cho HJ, Kim JY, et al. Endometriosis in an adolescent population: the severance hospital in Korean experience. *Yonsei Med J* 2002;43:48–52.

448. Ballweg ML. Big picture of endometriosis helps provide guidance on approach to teens: comparative historical data show endo starting younger, is more severe. *J Pediatr Adolesc Gynecol* 2003;16:S21–A26.

449. Reese KA, Reddy S, Rock JA. Endometriosis in an adolescent population: the Emory experience. *J Pediatr Adolesc Gynecol* 1996;9:125–128.

450. **Laufer MR, Goitein L, Bush M, et al.** Prevalence of endometriosis in adolescent girls with chronic pelvic pain not responding to conventional therapy. *J Pediatr Adolesc Gynecol* 1997;10:199–202.

451. **Vercellini P, Fedele L, Arcaini L, et al.** Laparoscopy in the diagnosis of chronic pelvic pain in adolescent women. *J Reprod Med* 1989;34:827–830.

452. **Emmert C, Romann D, Riedel HH.** Endometriosis diagnosed by laparoscopy in adolescent girls. *Arch Gynecol Obstet* 1998;261:89–93.

453. **Hassan E, Kontoravdis A, Hassiakos D, et al.** Evaluation of combined endoscopic and pharmaceutical management of endometriosis during adolescence. *Clin Exp Obstet Gynecol* 1999;26:85–87.

454. **Kontoravdis A, Hassan E, Hassiakos D, et al.** Laparoscopic evaluation and management of chronic pelvic pain during adolescence. *Clin Exp Obstet Gynecol* 1999;26:76–77.

455. **Shin SY, Lee YY, Yang SY, et al.** Characteristics of menstruation-related problems for adolescents and premarital women in Korea. *Eur J Obstet Gynecol Reprod Biol* 2005;121:236–242.

456. **Stavroulis AI, Saridogan E, Creighton SM, et al.** Laparoscopic treatment of endometriosis in teenagers. *Eur J Obstet Gynecol Reprod Biol* 2006;125:248–250.

457. **Davis GD, Thillet E, Lindemann J.** Clinical characteristics of adolescent endometriosis. *J Adolesc Health* 1993;14:362–368.

458. **Marsh EE, Laufer MR.** Endometriosis in premenarcheal girls who do not have an associated obstructive anomaly. *Fertil Steril* 2005;83:758–760.

459. **Evers JLH.** The pregnancy rate of the no-treatment group in randomized clinical trials of endometriosis therapy. *Fertil Steril* 1989;52:906–909.

460. **Propst AM, Laufer M.** Endometriosis in adolescents: incidence, diagnosis and treatment. *J Reprod Med* 1999;44:751–758.

461. **American College of Obstetricians and Gynecologists.** ACOG Committee Opinion. No. 310. Endometriosis in adolescents. *Obstet Gynecol* 2005;105:921–927.

462. **Sanfilippo JS, Wakim NG, Schikler KN, et al.** Endometriosis in association with uterine anomaly. *Am J Obstet Gynecol* 1986;154:39–43.

463. **Uğur M, Turan C, Mungan T, et al.** Endometriosis in association with mullerian anomalies. *Gynecol Obstet Invest* 1995;40:261–264.

464. **Hur JY, Shin JH, Lee JK, et al.** Septate uterus with double cervices, unilaterally obstructed vaginal septum, and ipsilateral renal agenesis: a rare combination of müllerian and wolffian anomalies complicated by severe endometriosis in an adolescent. *J Minim Invasive Gynecol* 2007;14:128–131.

465. **Al Kadri H, Hassan S, Al-Fozan HM, et al.** Hormone therapy for endometriosis and surgical menopause. *Cochrane Database Syst Rev* 2009;1:CD005997.

466. **Fedele L, Bianchi S, Rafaelli R, et al.** Comparison of transdermal *estradiol* and *tibolone* for the treatment of oophorectomized women with deep residual endometriosis. *Maturitas* 1999;32:189–193.

467. **Redwine DB.** Conservative laparoscopic excision of endometriosis by sharp dissection: life table analysis of reoperation and persistent of recurrent disease. *Fertil Steril* 1991;56:628–634.

468. **Vercellini P, Barbara G, Abbiati A, et al.** Repetitive surgery for recurrent symptomatic endometriosis: what to do? *Eur J Obstet Gynecol Reprod Biol* 2009;146:15–21.

469. **Vercellini P, Fedele L, Aimi G, et al.** Reproductive performance, pain recurrence and disease relapse after conservative surgical treatment for endometriosis: the predictive value of the current classification system. *Hum Reprod* 2006;21:2679–2685.

470. **Berlanda N, Vercellini P, Fedele L.** The outcomes of repeat surgery for recurrent symptomatic endometriosis. *Curr Opin Obstet Gynecol* 2010;22:320–325.

471. **Vercellini P, Somigliana E, Viganò P, et al.** The effect of second-line surgery on reproductive performance of women with recurrent endometriosis: a systematic review. *Acta Obstet Gynecol Scand* 2009;88:1074–1082.

472. **Busacca M, Marana R, Caruana P, et al.** Recurrence of ovarian endometrioma after laparoscopic excision. *Am J Obstet Gynecol* 1999;180:519–523.

473. **Schindler AE, Foertig P, Kienle E, et al.** Early treatment of endometriosis with GnRH-agonists: impact on time to recurrence. *Eur J Obstet Gynecol* 2000;93:123–125.

474. **Dmowski WP, Cohen MR.** Antigonadotropin (*danazol*) in the treatment of endometriosis: evaluation of posttreatment fertility and three-year follow-up data. *Am J Obstet Gynecol* 1978;130:41–48.

475. **Ghezzi F, Beretta P, Franchi M, et al.** Recurrence of endometriosis and anatomical location of the primary lesion. *Fertil Steril* 2001;75:136–140.

476. **Parker JD, Leondires M, Sinaii N, et al.** Persistence of dysmenorrhea and nonmenstrual pain after optimal endometriosis surgery may indicate adenomyosis. *Fertil Steril* 2006;86:711–715.

477. **Vercellini P, Somigliana E, Viganò P, et al.** Post-operative endometriosis recurrence: a plea for prevention based on pathogenetic, epidemiological and clinical evidence. *Reprod Biomed Online* 2010;21:259–265.

478. **Razzi S, Luisi S, Ferretti C, et al.** Use of a progestogen only preparation containing *desogestrel* in the treatment of recurrent pelvic pain after conservative surgery for endometriosis. *Eur J Obstet Gynecol Reprod Biol* 2007;135:188–190.

479. **Vercellini P, Somigliana E, Daguati R, et al.** The second time around: reproductive performance after repetitive versus primary surgery for endometriosis. *Fertil Steril* 2009;92:1253–1255.

18 Genitourinary Infections and Sexually Transmitted Diseases

David E. Soper

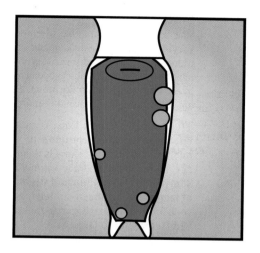

- Vaginitis is diagnosed by office-based testing.

- More prolonged antifungal therapy is indicated for women with complicated vulvovaginal candidiasis (VVC) than for those with uncomplicated disease.

- Women with normal physical examination findings and no evidence of fungal infection disclosed by microscopy are unlikely to have VVC and should not be treated empirically unless results of a vaginal yeast culture are positive.

- Cervicitis is commonly associated with bacterial vaginosis (BV), which, if not treated concurrently, leads to significant persistence of the symptoms and signs of cervicitis.

- Women with mild-to-moderate pelvic inflammatory disease (PID) can be treated as outpatients.

- Trocar drainage, with or without placement of a drain, is successful in as many as 90% of patients with PID complicated by tubo-ovarian abscess that fails to respond to antimicrobial therapy within 72 hours.

- Because false-negative results are common with herpes simplex virus (HSV) cultures, especially in patients with recurrent infections, type-specific glycoprotein G-based antibody assay tests are useful in confirming a clinical diagnosis of genital herpes.

- Suppressive treatment partially decreases symptomatic and asymptomatic viral shedding and the potential for transmission.

Genitourinary tract infections are among the most frequent disorders for which patients seek care from gynecologists. By understanding the pathophysiology of these diseases and having an effective approach to their diagnosis, physicians can institute appropriate antimicrobial therapy to treat these conditions and reduce long-term sequelae.

The Normal Vagina

Normal vaginal secretions are composed of vulvar secretions from sebaceous, sweat, Bartholin, and Skene glands; transudate from the vaginal wall; exfoliated vaginal and cervical cells; cervical mucus; endometrial and oviductal fluids; and micro-organisms and their metabolic products. The type and amount of exfoliated cells, cervical mucus, and upper genital tract fluids are determined by biochemical processes that are influenced by hormone levels (1). Vaginal secretions may increase in the middle of the menstrual cycle because of an increase in the amount of cervical mucus. These cyclic variations do not occur when oral contraceptives are used and ovulation does not occur.

The vaginal desquamative tissue is made up of vaginal epithelial cells that are responsive to varying amounts of estrogen and progesterone. Superficial cells, the main cell type in women of reproductive age, predominate when estrogen stimulation is present. Intermediate cells predominate during the luteal phase because of stimulation by progesterone. Parabasal cells predominate in the absence of either hormone, a condition that may be found in postmenopausal women who are not receiving hormonal therapy.

The normal vaginal flora is mostly aerobic, with an average of six different species of bacteria, the most common of which is hydrogen peroxide–producing lactobacilli. The microbiology of the vagina is determined by factors that affect the ability of bacteria to survive (2). These factors include vaginal pH and the availability of glucose for bacterial metabolism. **The pH level of the normal vagina is lower than 4.5, which is maintained by the production of lactic acid.** Estrogen-stimulated vaginal epithelial cells are rich in glycogen. Vaginal epithelial cells break down glycogen to monosaccharides, which can be converted by the cells themselves, and lactobacilli to lactic acid.

Normal vaginal secretions are floccular in consistency, white in color, and usually located in the dependent portion of the vagina (posterior fornix). Vaginal secretions can be analyzed by a wet-mount preparation. A sample of vaginal secretions is suspended in 0.5 mL of normal saline in a tube, transferred to a slide, covered with a slip, and assessed by microscopy. Some clinicians prefer to prepare slides by suspending secretions in saline placed directly on the slide. Secretions should not be placed on the slide without saline because this method causes drying of the vaginal secretions and does not result in a well-suspended preparation. Microscopy of normal vaginal secretions reveals many superficial epithelial cells, few white blood cells (less than 1 per epithelial cell), and few, if any, clue cells. **Clue cells are superficial vaginal epithelial cells with adherent bacteria, usually *Gardnerella vaginalis*, which obliterates the crisp cell border when visualized microscopically.** Potassium hydroxide 10% (KOH) may be added to the slide, or a separate preparation can be made, to examine the secretions for evidence of fungal elements. The results are negative in women with normal vaginal microbiology. Gram stain reveals normal superficial epithelial cells and a predominance of gram-positive rods (lactobacilli).

Vaginal Infections

Bacterial Vaginosis

Bacterial vaginosis (BV) is an alteration of normal vaginal bacterial flora that results in the loss of hydrogen peroxide–producing lactobacilli and an overgrowth of predominantly anaerobic bacteria (3,4). **The most common form of vaginitis in the United States is BV** (5). Anaerobic bacteria can be found in less than 1% of the flora of normal women. In women with BV, however, the concentration of anaerobes, and *G. vaginalis* and *Mycoplasma hominis*, is 100 to 1,000 times higher than in normal women. Lactobacilli are usually absent.

It is not known what triggers the disturbance of normal vaginal flora. It is postulated that repeated alkalinization of the vagina, which occurs with frequent sexual intercourse or use of douches, plays a role. After normal hydrogen peroxide–producing lactobacilli disappear, it is difficult to reestablish normal vaginal flora, and recurrence of BV is common.

Numerous studies show an association of BV with significant adverse sequelae. Women with BV are at increased risk for pelvic inflammatory disease (PID), postabortal PID, postoperative cuff infections after hysterectomy, and abnormal cervical cytology (6–9). Pregnant women with BV are at risk for premature rupture of the membranes, preterm

labor and delivery, chorioamnionitis, and postcesarean endometritis (10,11). In women with BV who are undergoing surgical abortion or hysterectomy, perioperative treatment with *metronidazole* eliminates this increased risk (12,13).

Diagnosis

Office-based testing is required to diagnose BV. It is diagnosed on the basis of the following findings (14):

1. **A fishy vaginal odor, which is particularly noticeable following coitus, and vaginal discharge are present.**

2. **Vaginal secretions are gray and thinly coat the vaginal walls.**

3. **The pH of these secretions is higher than 4.5 (usually 4.7 to 5.7).**

4. **Microscopy of the vaginal secretions reveals an increased number of clue cells, and leukocytes are conspicuously absent. In advanced cases of BV, more than 20% of the epithelial cells are clue cells.**

5. **The addition of KOH to the vaginal secretions (the "whiff" test) releases a fishy, aminelike odor.**

Clinicians who are unable to perform microscopy should use alternative diagnostic tests such as a pH and amines test card, detection of *G. vaginalis* ribosomal RNA, or Gram stain (15). Culture of *G. vaginalis* is not recommended as a diagnostic tool because of its lack of specificity.

Treatment

Ideally, treatment of BV should inhibit anaerobes but not vaginal lactobacilli. **The following treatments are effective:**

1. *Metronidazole*, **an antibiotic with excellent activity against anaerobes but poor activity against lactobacilli, is the drug of choice for the treatment of BV.** A dose of 500 mg administered orally twice a day for 7 days should be used. Patients should be advised to avoid using alcohol during treatment with oral *metronidazole* and for 24 hours thereafter.

2. *Metronidazole* **gel, 0.75%, one applicator (5 g) intravaginally once daily for 5 days, may also be prescribed.**

The overall cure rates range from 75% to 84% with the aforementioned regimens (16). ***Clindamycin* in the following regimens is effective in treating BV:**

1. *Clindamycin* **ovules, 100 mg, intravaginally once at bedtime for 3 days**

2. *Clindamycin* **bioadhesive cream, 2%, 100 mg intravaginally in a single dose**

3. *Clindamycin* **cream, 2%, one applicator full (5 g) intravaginally at bedtime for 7 days**

4. *Clindamycin,* **300 mg, orally twice daily for 7 days**

Many clinicians prefer intravaginal treatment to avoid systemic side effects such as mild to moderate gastrointestinal upset and unpleasant taste. Treatment of the male sexual partner does not improve therapeutic response and therefore is not recommended (16).

Trichomonas Vaginitis

Trichomonas vaginitis is caused by the sexually transmitted, flagellated parasite, *Trichomonas vaginalis*. The transmission rate is high; 70% of men contract the disease after a single exposure to an infected woman, which suggests that the rate of male-to-female transmission is even higher. The parasite, which exists only in trophozoite form, is an anaerobe that has the ability to generate hydrogen to combine with oxygen to create an anaerobic environment. It often accompanies BV, which can be diagnosed in as many as 60% of patients with trichomonas vaginitis (17).

Diagnosis

Local immune factors and inoculum size influence the appearance of symptoms. Symptoms and signs may be much milder in patients with small inocula of trichomonads, and trichomonas vaginitis often is asymptomatic (17,18).

1. **Trichomonas vaginitis is associated with a profuse, purulent, malodorous vaginal discharge that may be accompanied by vulvar pruritus.**

2. **A purulent vaginal discharge may exude from the vagina.**

3. **In patients with high concentrations of organisms, a patchy vaginal erythema and colpitis macularis ("strawberry" cervix) may be observed.**

4. **The pH of the vaginal secretions is usually higher than 5.0.**

5. **Microscopy of the secretions reveals motile trichomonads and increased numbers of leukocytes.**

6. **Clue cells may be present because of the common association with BV.**

7. **The whiff test may be positive.**

Morbidity associated with trichomonal vaginitis may be related to BV. Patients with trichomonas vaginitis are at increased risk for postoperative cuff cellulitis following hysterectomy (8). **Pregnant women with trichomonas vaginitis are at increased risk for premature rupture of the membranes and preterm delivery.** Because of the sexually transmitted nature of trichomonas vaginitis, women with this infection should be tested for other sexually transmitted diseases (STDs), particularly *Neisseria gonorrhoeae* and *Chlamydia trachomatis*. Serologic testing for syphilis and HIV infection should be considered.

Treatment

The treatment of trichomonal vaginitis can be summarized as follows:

1. *Metronidazole* **is the drug of choice for treatment of vaginal trichomoniasis.** Both a single-dose (2 g orally) and a multidose (500 mg twice daily for 7 days) regimen are highly effective and have cure rates of about 95%.

2. **The sexual partner should be treated.**

3. *Metronidazole* **gel, although effective for the treatment of BV, should not be used for the treatment of vaginal trichomoniasis.**

4. **Women who do not respond to initial therapy should be treated again with** *metronidazole*, **500 mg, twice daily for 7 days.** If repeated treatment is not effective, the patient should be treated with a single 2-g dose of *metronidazole* once daily for 5 days or *tinidazole*, 2 g, in a single dose for 5 days.

5. **Patients who do not respond to repeated treatment with** *metronidazole* **or** *tinidazole* **and for whom the possibility of reinfection is excluded should be referred for expert consultation.** In these uncommon refractory cases, an important part of management is to obtain cultures of the parasite to determine its susceptibility to *metronidazole* and *tinidazole*.

Vulvovaginal Candidiasis

An estimated 75% of women experience at least one episode of vulvovaginal candidiasis (VVC) during their lifetimes (19). Nearly 45% of women will experience two or more episodes (20). Few are plagued with a chronic, recurrent infection. *Candida albicans* is responsible for 85% to 90% of vaginal yeast infections. Other species of *Candida*, such as *C. glabrata* and *C. tropicalis*, can cause vulvovaginal symptoms and tend to be resistant to therapy. Candida are dimorphic fungi existing as blastospores, which are responsible for transmission and asymptomatic colonization, and as mycelia, which result from blastospore germination and enhance colonization and facilitate tissue invasion. The extensive areas of pruritus and inflammation often associated with minimal invasion of the lower genital tract epithelial cells suggest that an extracellular toxin or enzyme may play a role in the pathogenesis of this disease. A hypersensitivity phenomenon may be responsible for the irritative symptoms associated with VVC, especially for patients with chronic, recurrent disease. Patients with symptomatic disease usually have an increased concentration of these micro-organisms ($>10^4$ per mL) compared with asymptomatic patients ($<10^3$ per mL) (21).

Factors that predispose women to the development of symptomatic VVC include antibiotic use, pregnancy, and diabetes (22–25). Pregnancy and diabetes are associated with a qualitative decrease in cell-mediated immunity, leading to a higher incidence of candidiasis.

Table 18.1 Classification of Vulvovaginal Candidiasis	
Uncomplicated	*Complicated*
Sporadic or infrequent in occurrence	Recurrent symptoms
Mild to moderate symptoms	Severe symptoms
Likely to be *Candida albicans*	Non-albicans Candida
Immunocompetent women	Immunocompromised, e.g., diabetic women

From **Sobel JD, Faro S, Force RW,** et al. Vulvovaginal candidiasis: epidemiologic, diagnostic, and therapeutic considerations. *Am J Obstet Gynecol* 1998;178:203–211.

It is helpful to categorize women with VVC as having either uncomplicated or complicated disease (Table 18.1)

Diagnosis

The symptoms of VVC consist of vulvar pruritus associated with a vaginal discharge that typically resembles cottage cheese.

1. **The discharge can vary from watery to homogeneously thick.** Vaginal soreness, dyspareunia, vulvar burning, and irritation may be present. External dysuria ("splash" dysuria) may occur when micturition leads to exposure of the inflamed vulvar and vestibular epithelium to urine. Examination reveals erythema and edema of the labia and vulvar skin. Discrete pustulopapular peripheral lesions may be present. The vagina may be erythematous with an adherent, whitish discharge. The cervix appears normal.

2. **The pH of the vagina in patients with VVC is usually normal (<4.5).**

3. **Fungal elements, either budding yeast forms or mycelia, appear in as many as 80% of cases.** The results of saline preparation of the vaginal secretions usually are normal, although there may be a slight increase in the number of inflammatory cells in severe cases.

4. **The whiff test is negative.**

5. **A presumptive diagnosis can be made in the absence of fungal elements confirmed by microscopy if the pH and the results of the saline preparation evaluations are normal *and* the patient has increased erythema based on examination of the vagina or vulva. A fungal culture is recommended to confirm the diagnosis. Conversely, women with a normal physical examination findings and no evidence of fungal elements disclosed by microscopy are unlikely to have VVC and should not be empirically treated unless a vaginal yeast culture is positive.**

Treatment

The treatment of VVC is summarized as follows:

1. **Topically applied azole drugs are the most commonly available treatment for VVC and are more effective than *nystatin* (16) (Table 18.2).** Treatment with azoles results in relief of symptoms and negative cultures in 80% to 90% of patients who have completed therapy. Symptoms usually resolve in 2 to 3 days. Short-course regimens up to 3 days are recommended. Although the shorter period of therapy implies a shortened duration of treatment, the short-course formulations have higher concentrations of the antifungal agent, causing an inhibitory concentration in the vagina that persists for several days.

2. **The oral antifungal agent, *fluconazole*, used in a single 150-mg dose, is recommended for the treatment of VVC.** It appears to have equal efficacy when compared with topical azoles in the treatment of mild to moderate VVC (26). Patients should be advised that their symptoms will persist for 2 to 3 days so they will not expect additional treatment.

3. **Women with complicated VVC (Table 18.1) benefit from an additional 150-mg dose of *fluconazole* given 72 hours after the first dose. Patients with complications can be treated with a more prolonged topical regimen lasting 10 to 14 days. Adjunctive**

Table 18.2 Vulvovaginal Candidiasis—Topical Treatment Regimens
Butoconazole
2% cream, 5 g intravaginally for 3 days[a,b]
Clotrimazole
1% cream, 5 g intravaginally for 7–14 days[a,b]   2% cream 5 g intravaginally for 3 days
Miconazole
2% cream, 5 g intravaginally for 7 days[a,b]   200-mg vaginal suppository for 3 days[a]   100-mg vaginal suppository for 7 days[a,b]   4% cream 5 g intravaginally for 3 days   1,200 mg vaginal suppository, one suppository for one day
Nystatin
100,000-U vaginal tablet, one tablet for 14 days
Tioconazole
6.5% ointment, 5 g intravaginally, single dose[a]
Terconazole
0.4% cream, 5 g intravaginally for 7 days[a]   0.8% cream, 5 g intravaginally for 3 days[a]   80-mg suppository for 3 days[a]

[a]Oil-based, may weaken latex condoms.
[b]Available as over-the-counter preparation.
Adapted from **Centers for Disease Control and Prevention.** The sexually transmitted diseases treatment guidelines. *MMWR* 2006;55:[RR-11]:1–94.

treatment with a weak topical steroid, such as **1%** *hydrocortisone* cream, may be helpful in relieving some of the external irritative symptoms.

Recurrent Vulvovaginal Candidiasis

A small number of women develop recurrent VVC (RVVC), defined as four or more episodes in a year. These women experience persistent irritative symptoms of the vestibule and vulva. Burning replaces itching as the prominent symptom in patients with RVVC. The diagnosis should be confirmed by direct microscopy of the vaginal secretions and by fungal culture. **Many women with RVVC presume incorrectly they have a chronic yeast infection. Many of these patients have chronic atopic dermatitis or atrophic vulvovaginitis.**

The treatment of patients with RVVC consists of inducing a remission of chronic symptoms with *fluconazole* (**150 mg every 3 days for three doses). Patients should be maintained on a suppressive dose of this agent (***fluconazole*, **150 mg weekly) for 6 months.** On this regimen, 90% of women with RVVC will remain in remission. After suppressive therapy, approximately half will remain asymptomatic. Recurrence will occur in the other half and should prompt reinstitution of suppressive therapy (27).

Inflammatory Vaginitis

Desquamative inflammatory vaginitis **is a clinical syndrome characterized by diffuse exudative vaginitis, epithelial cell exfoliation, and a profuse purulent vaginal discharge** (28). The cause of inflammatory vaginitis is unknown, but Gram stain findings reveal a relative absence of normal long gram-positive bacilli (lactobacilli) and their replacement with gram-positive cocci, usually streptococci. Women with this disorder have a purulent vaginal discharge, vulvovaginal burning or irritation, and dyspareunia. A less frequent symptom is vulvar pruritus. Vaginal erythema is present, and there may be an associated vulvar erythema, vulvovaginal ecchymotic spots, and colpitis macularis. The pH of the vaginal secretions is uniformly higher than 4.5 in these patients.

Initial therapy is the use of 2% *clindamycin* cream, one applicator full (5 g) intravaginally once daily for 7 days. Relapse occurs in about 30% of patients, who should be retreated with intravaginal 2% *clindamycin* cream for 2 weeks. When relapse occurs in postmenopausal patients, supplementary hormonal therapy should be considered (28).

Atrophic Vaginitis

Estrogen plays an important role in the maintenance of normal vaginal ecology. **Women undergoing menopause, either naturally or secondary to surgical removal of the ovaries, may develop inflammatory vaginitis, which may be accompanied by an increased, purulent vaginal discharge. In addition, they may have dyspareunia and postcoital bleeding resulting from atrophy of the vaginal and vulvar epithelium.** Examination reveals atrophy of the external genitalia, along with a loss of the vaginal rugae. The vaginal mucosa may be somewhat friable in areas. Microscopy of the vaginal secretions shows a predominance of parabasal epithelial cells and an increased number of leukocytes.

Atrophic vaginitis is treated with topical *estrogen* vaginal cream. Use of 1 g of *conjugated estrogen* cream intravaginally each day for 1 to 2 weeks generally provides relief. Maintenance *estrogen* therapy, either topical or systemic, should be considered to prevent recurrence of this disorder.

Cervicitis

The cervix is made up of two different types of epithelial cells: squamous epithelium and glandular epithelium. The cause of cervical inflammation depends on the epithelium affected. The ectocervical epithelium can become inflamed by the same micro-organisms that are responsible for vaginitis. In fact, the ectocervical squamous epithelium is an extension of and is continuous with the vaginal epithelium. Trichomonas, candida, and herpes simplex virus (HSV) can cause inflammation of the ectocervix. Conversely, *N. gonorrhoeae* and *C. trachomatis* infect only the glandular epithelium (29).

Diagnosis

The diagnosis of cervicitis is based on the finding of a purulent endocervical discharge, generally yellow or green in color and referred to as "mucopus" (30).

1. **After removal of ectocervical secretions with a large swab, a small cotton swab is placed into the endocervical canal and the cervical mucus is extracted. The cotton swab is inspected against a white or black background to detect the green or yellow color of the mucopus.** In addition, the zone of ectopy (glandular epithelium) is friable or easily induced to bleed. This characteristic can be assessed by touching the ectropion with a cotton swab or spatula.

2. **Placement of the mucopus on a slide that can be Gram stained will reveal the presence of an increased number of neutrophils (>30 per high-power field).** The presence of intracellular gram-negative diplococci, leading to the presumptive diagnosis of gonococcal endocervicitis, may be detected. If the Gram stain results are negative for gonococci, the presumptive diagnosis is chlamydial cervicitis.

3. **Tests for gonorrhea and chlamydia, preferably using nucleic acid amplification tests, should be performed.** The microbial etiology of endocervicitis is unknown in about 50% of cases in which neither gonococci nor chlamydia is detected.

Treatment

Treatment of cervicitis consists of an antibiotic regimen recommended for the treatment of uncomplicated lower genital tract infection with both chlamydia and gonorrhea (16) (Table 18.3). Fluoroquinolone resistance is common in *Neisseria gonorrhoeae* isolates, and, therefore, these agents are no longer recommended for the treatment of women with gonococcal cervicitis. It is imperative that all sexual partners be treated with a similar antibiotic regimen. Cervicitis is commonly associated with BV, which, if not treated concurrently, leads to significant persistence of the symptoms and signs of cervicitis.

Table 18.3 Treatment Regimens for Gonococcal and Chlamydial Infections

Neisseria gonorrhoeae endocervicitis

Ceftriaxone, 250 mg IM in a single dose, *or, if not an option*
Cefexime, 400 mg in a single dose

Chlamydia trachomatis endocervicitis

Azithromycin, 1 g orally (single dose), *or*
Doxycycline, 100 mg orally twice daily for 7 days

Adapted from **Centers for Disease Control and Prevention.** Sexually transmitted diseases treatment guidelines, 2010. Workowski KA, Berman S; Centers for Disease Control and Prevention (CDC). *MMWR Recomm Rep.* 2010 Dec 17;59(RR-12):1–110. Erratum in: *MMWR Recomm Rep.* 2011 Jan 14;60(1):18. Dosage error in article text.

Pelvic Inflammatory Disease

PID is caused by micro-organisms colonizing the endocervix and ascending to the endometrium and fallopian tubes. It is a clinical diagnosis implying that the patient has upper genital tract infection and inflammation. The inflammation may be present at any point along a continuum that includes endometritis, salpingitis, and peritonitis (Fig. 18.1).

PID is commonly caused by the sexually transmitted micro-organisms *N. gonorrhoeae* and *C. trachomatis* (31–33). Recent evidence suggests that *Mycoplasma genitalium* can cause PID and presents with mild clinical symptoms similar to chlamydial PID (34). Endogenous micro-organisms found in the vagina, particularly the BV micro-organisms, are often isolated from the upper genital tract of women with PID. The BV micro-organisms include anaerobic bacteria such as *Prevotella* and peptostreptococci as well as *G. vaginalis*. BV often occurs in women with

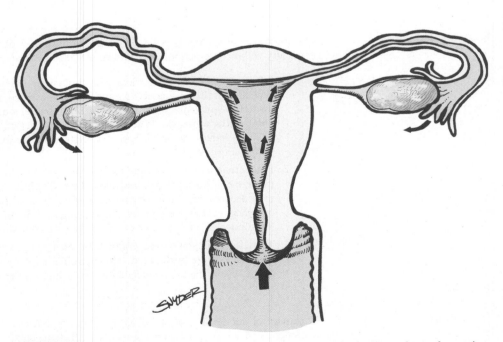

Figure 18.1   **Micro-organisms originating in the endocervix ascend into the endometrium, fallopian tubes, and peritoneum, causing pelvic inflammatory disease (endometritis, salpingitis, peritonitis).**   (From **Soper DE.** Upper genital tract infections. In: Copeland LJ, ed. *Textbook of gynecology*. Philadelphia, PA: Saunders, 1993:521, with permission.)

PID, and the resultant complex alteration of vaginal flora may facilitate the ascending spread of pathogenic bacteria by enzymatically altering the cervical mucus barrier (35). Less frequently, respiratory pathogens such as *Haemophilus influenzae*, group A streptococci, and pneumococci can colonize the lower genital tract and cause PID.

Diagnosis

Traditionally, the diagnosis of PID is based on a triad of symptoms and signs, including pelvic pain, cervical motion and adnexal tenderness, and the presence of fever. It is recognized that there is wide variation in many symptoms and signs among women with this condition, which makes the diagnosis of acute PID difficult. Many women with PID exhibit subtle or mild symptoms that are not readily recognized as PID. Consequently, delay in diagnosis and therapy probably contributes to the inflammatory sequelae in the upper reproductive tract (36).

In the diagnosis of PID, the goal is to establish guidelines that are sufficiently sensitive to avoid missing mild cases but sufficiently specific to avoid giving antibiotic therapy to women who are not infected. Genitourinary tract symptoms may indicate PID; therefore, the diagnosis of PID should be considered in women with any genitourinary symptoms, including, but not limited to, lower abdominal pain, excessive vaginal discharge, menorrhagia, metrorrhagia, fever, chills, and urinary symptoms (37). **Some women may develop PID without having any symptoms.**

Pelvic organ tenderness, either uterine tenderness alone or uterine tenderness with adnexal tenderness, is present in patients with PID. Cervical motion tenderness suggests the presence of peritoneal inflammation, which causes pain when the peritoneum is stretched by moving the cervix and causing traction of the adnexa on the pelvic peritoneum. Direct or rebound abdominal tenderness may be present.

Evaluation of both vaginal and endocervical secretions is a crucial part of the workup of a patient with PID (38). In women with PID, an increased number of polymorphonuclear leukocytes may be detected in a wet mount of the vaginal secretions or in the mucopurulent discharge.

More elaborate tests may be used in women with severe symptoms because an incorrect diagnosis may cause unnecessary morbidity (39) (Table 18.4). These tests include endometrial biopsy to confirm the presence of endometritis, ultrasound or radiologic tests to characterize a tubo-ovarian abscess, and laparoscopy to confirm salpingitis visually.

Treatment

Therapy regimens for PID must provide empirical, broad-spectrum coverage of likely pathogens, including *N. gonorrhoeae*, *C. trachomatis*, *M. genitalium*, gram-negative

Table 18.4 Clinical Criteria for the Diagnosis of Pelvic Inflammatory Disease

Symptoms

None necessary

Signs

Pelvic organ tenderness
Leukorrhea and/or mucopurulent endocervicitis

Additional criteria to increase the specificity of the diagnosis

Endometrial biopsy showing endometritis
Elevated C-reactive protein or erythrocyte sedimentation rate
Temperature higher than 38°C (100.4°F)
Leukocytosis
Positive test for gonorrhea or chlamydia

Elaborate criteria

Ultrasound documenting tubo-ovarian abscess
Laparoscopy visually confirming salpingitis

Table 18.5 Guidelines for Treatment of Pelvic Inflammatory Disease

Outpatient Treatment

Cefoxitin, 2 g intramuscularly, plus *probenecid*, 1 g orally concurrently, *or*

Ceftriaxone, 250 mg intramuscularly, *or*

Equivalent cephalosporin

Plus:

Doxycycline, 100 mg orally 2 times daily for 14 days, *or*

Azithromycin, 500 mg initially and then 250 mg daily for a total of 7 days

Inpatient Treatment

Regimen A

Cefoxitin, 2 g intravenously every 6 hours, *or*

Cefotetan, 2 g intravenously every 12 hours

Plus:

Doxycycline, 100 mg orally or intravenously every 12 hours

Regimen B

Clindamycin, 900 mg intravenously every 8 hours

Plus:

Ceftriaxone, *1–2 g* intravenously every 12 hours, *or*
Gentamicin, loading dose intravenously or intramuscularly (2 mg/kg of body weight)
followed by a maintenance dose (1.5 mg/kg) every 8 hours

[a]Outpatient treatment only, i.e., women treated for PID as an outpatient should also receive *metronidazole* gel for BV if they have BV.
Adapted from **Soper DE.** Pelvic inflammatory disease. *Obstet Gynecol* 2010;116:419–428.

facultative bacteria, anaerobes, and streptococci (16,40). Recommended regimens for the treatment of PID are listed in Table 18.5. **An outpatient regimen of *cefoxitin* and *doxycycline* is as effective as an inpatient parenteral regimen of the same antimicrobials** (41). **Therefore, hospitalization is recommended only when the diagnosis is uncertain, pelvic abscess is suspected, clinical disease is severe, or compliance with an outpatient regimen is in question. Hospitalized patients can be considered for discharge when their fever has lysed ($<99.5°$F for more than 24 hours), the white blood cell count has become normal, rebound tenderness is absent, and repeat examination shows marked amelioration of pelvic organ tenderness** (42).

Sexual partners of women with PID should be evaluated and treated for urethral infection with chlamydia or gonorrhea (Table 18.3). One of these STDs usually is found in the male sexual partners of women with PID not associated with chlamydia or gonorrhea (43,44).

Tubo-ovarian Abscess

An end-stage process of acute PID, tubo-ovarian abscess is diagnosed when a patient with PID has a pelvic mass that is palpable during bimanual examination. The condition usually reflects an agglutination of pelvic organs (tube, ovary, bowel) forming a palpable complex. Occasionally, an ovarian abscess can result from the entrance of micro-organisms through an ovulatory site. **Tubo-ovarian abscess is treated with an antibiotic regimen administered in a hospital** (Table 18.5). **About 75% of women with tubo-ovarian abscess respond to antimicrobial therapy alone. Failure of medical therapy suggests the need for drainage of the abscess** (45). Although drainage may require surgical exploration, percutaneous drainage guided by imaging studies (ultrasound or computed tomography) should be used as an initial option if possible. Trocar drainage, with or without placement of a drain, is successful in up to 90% of cases in which the patient failed to respond to antimicrobial therapy after 72 hours (46).

Other Major Infections

Genital Ulcer Disease

In the United States, most patients with genital ulcers have genital HSV or syphilis (47–50). **Chancroid is the next most common cause of sexually transmitted genital ulcers, followed by the rare occurrence of lymphogranuloma venereum (LGV) and granuloma inguinale (donovanosis). These diseases are associated with an increased risk for HIV infection.** Other infrequent and noninfectious causes of genital ulcers include abrasions, fixed drug eruptions, carcinoma, and Behçet's disease.

Diagnosis

A diagnosis based on history and physical examination alone is often inaccurate. Therefore, **all women with genital ulcers should undergo a serologic test for syphilis** (50). Because of the consequences of inappropriate therapy, such as tertiary disease and congenital syphilis in pregnant women, diagnostic efforts are directed at excluding syphilis. Optimally, the evaluation of a patient with a genital ulcer should include dark-field examination or direct immunofluorescence testing for *Treponema pallidum*, culture or antigen testing for HSV, and culture for *Haemophilus ducreyi*. Dark-field or fluorescent microscopes and selective media to culture for *H. ducreyi* often are not available in most offices and clinics. Even after complete testing, the diagnosis remains unconfirmed in one-fourth of patients with genital ulcers. For this reason, most clinicians base their initial diagnosis and treatment recommendations on their clinical impression of the appearance of the genital ulcer (Fig. 18.2) and knowledge of the most likely cause in their patient population (48).

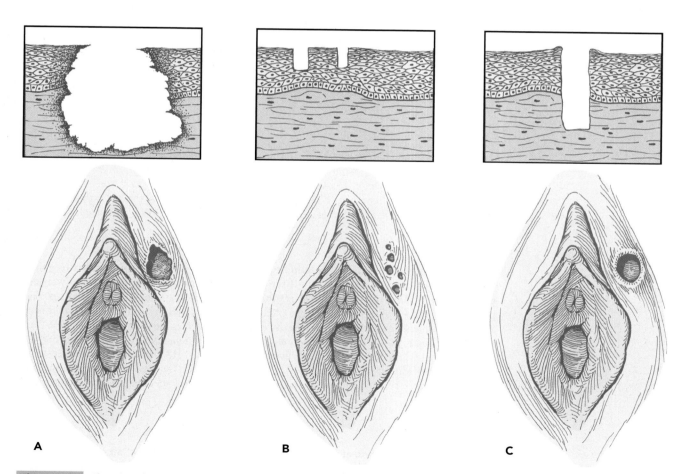

A   B   C

Figure 18.2   **Showing the appearance of the ulcers of chancroid (A), herpes (B), and syphilis (C).** The ulcer of chancroid has irregular margins and is deep with undermined edges. The syphilis ulcer has a smooth, indurated border and a smooth base. The genital herpes ulcer is superficial and inflamed. (Modified from **Schmid GP, Shcalla WO, DeWitt WE.** Chancroid. In: Morse SA, Moreland AA, Thompson SE, eds. *Atlas of sexually transmitted diseases.* Philadelphia, PA: Lippincott, 1990.)

Several clinical presentations are highly suggestive of specific diagnoses:

1. **A painless and minimally tender ulcer, not accompanied by inguinal lymphadenopathy, is likely to be syphilis, especially if the ulcer is indurated.** A nontreponemal rapid plasma reagin (RPR) test, or venereal disease research laboratory (VDRL) test, and a confirmatory treponemal test—fluorescent treponemal antibody absorption (FTA ABS) or microhemagglutinin–*T. pallidum* (MHA TP)—should be used to diagnose syphilis presumptively. Some laboratories screen samples with treponemal enzyme immunoassay (EIA) tests, the results of which should be confirmed with nontreponemal tests. The results of nontreponemal tests usually correlate with disease activity and should be reported quantitatively.

2. **Grouped vesicles mixed with small ulcers, particularly with a history of such lesions, are almost always pathognomonic of genital herpes.** Nevertheless, laboratory confirmation of the findings is recommended because the diagnosis of genital herpes is traumatic for many women, alters their self-image, and affects their perceived ability to enter new sexual relationships and bear children. A culture test is the most sensitive and specific test; sensitivity approaches 100% in the vesicle stage and 89% in the pustular stage and drops to as low as 33% in patients with ulcers. Nonculture tests are about 80% as sensitive as culture tests. Because false-negative results are common with HSV cultures, especially in patients with recurrent infections, type-specific glycoprotein G-based antibody assays are useful in confirming a clinical diagnosis of genital herpes.

3. **One to three extremely painful ulcers, accompanied by tender inguinal lymphadenopathy, are unlikely to be anything except chancroid.** This is especially true if the adenopathy is fluctuant.

4. **An inguinal bubo accompanied by one or several ulcers is most likely chancroid. If no ulcer is present, the most likely diagnosis is LGV.**

Treatment

Chancroid

Recommended regimens for the treatment of chancroid include *azithromycin,* 1 g orally in a single dose; *ceftriaxone,* 250 mg intramuscularly in a single dose; *ciprofloxacin,* 500 mg orally twice a day for 3 days; or *erythromycin* base, 500 mg orally four times daily for 7 days. Patients should be reexamined 3 to 7 days after initiation of therapy to ensure the gradual resolution of the genital ulcer, which can be expected to heal within 2 weeks unless it is unusually large.

Herpes

A first episode of genital herpes should be treated with *acyclovir*, 400 mg orally three times a day; or *famciclovir*, 250 mg orally three times a day; or *valacyclovir*, 1.0 orally twice a day for 7 to 10 days or until clinical resolution is attained. Although these agents provide partial control of the symptoms and signs of clinical herpes, it neither eradicates latent virus nor affects subsequent risk, frequency, or severity of recurrences after the drug is discontinued. Daily suppressive therapy (*acyclovir*, 400 mg orally twice daily; or *famciclovir*, 250 mg twice daily; or *valacyclovir*, 1.0 g orally once a day) reduces the frequency of HSV recurrences by at least 75% among patients with six or more recurrences of HSV per year. Suppressive treatment partially, but not totally, decreases symptomatic and asymptomatic viral shedding and the potential for transmission (49).

Syphilis

Parenteral administration of *penicillin G* is the preferred treatment of all stages of syphilis. *Benzathine penicillin G*, 2.4 million units intramuscularly in a single dose, is the recommended treatment for adults with primary, secondary, or early latent syphilis. The Jarisch-Herxheimer reaction—an acute febrile response accompanied by headache, myalgia, and other symptoms—may occur within the first 24 hours after any therapy for syphilis; patients should be advised of this possible adverse reaction.

Table 18.6 Treatment Options for External Genital and Perianal Warts		
Modality	*Efficacy (%)*	*Recurrence Risk*
Cryotherapy	63–88	21–39
Imiquimod 5% cream[a]	33–72	13–19
Podophyllin 10%–25%	32–79	27–65
Podofilox 0.5%[a]	45–88	33–60
Trichloroacetic acid 80%–90%	81	36
Electrodesiccation or cautery	94	22
Laser[b]	43–93	29–95
Interferon	44–61	0–67
Sinecatechin 15% ointment	60	ND

ND, no data.
[a]May be self-applied by patients at home.
[b]Expensive; reserve for patients who have not responded to other regimens.

Latent syphilis is defined as those periods after infection with *T. pallidum* when patients are seroreactive but show no other evidence of disease. Patients with latent syphilis of longer than 1 year's duration or of unknown duration should be treated with *benzathine penicillin G*, 7.2 million units total, administered as three doses of 2.4 million units intramuscularly each, at 1-week intervals. All patients with latent syphilis should be evaluated clinically for evidence of tertiary disease (e.g., aortitis, neurosyphilis, gumma, and iritis). Quantitative nontreponemal serologic tests should be repeated at 6 months and again at 12 months. An initially high titer (1:32) should decline at least fourfold (two dilutions) within 12 to 24 months.

Genital Warts

External genital warts are a manifestation of human papillomavirus (HPV) infection (51). The nononcogenic HPV types 6 and 11 are usually responsible for external genital warts. The warts tend to occur in areas most directly affected by coitus, namely the posterior fourchette and lateral areas on the vulva. Less frequently, warts can be found throughout the vulva, in the vagina, and on the cervix. Minor trauma associated with coitus can cause breaks in the vulvar skin, allowing direct contact between the viral particles from an infected man and the basal layer of the epidermis of his susceptible sexual partner. Infection may be latent or may cause viral particles to replicate and produce a wart. External genital warts are highly contagious; more than 75% of sexual partners develop this manifestation of HPV infection when exposed.

The goal of treatment is removal of the warts; it is not possible to eradicate the viral infection. Treatment is most successful in patients with small warts that were present for less than 1 year. It is not determined whether treatment of genital warts reduces transmission of HPV. Selection of a specific treatment regimen depends on the anatomic site, size, and number of warts, and expense, efficacy, convenience, and potential adverse effects (Table 18.6). **Recurrences more often result from reactivation of subclinical infection than reinfection by a sex partner; therefore, examination of sex partners is not absolutely necessary.** However, many of these sex partners may have external genital warts and may benefit from therapy and counseling concerning transmission of warts. HPV infection with types 6, 11, 16, and 18 can be prevented by vaccination.

Human Immunodeficiency Virus

It is estimated that almost 40% to 50% of individuals with HIV are women. Intravenous drug use and heterosexual transmission are responsible for most of the cases of AIDS in women in the United States (52). Infection with HIV produces a spectrum of disease that progresses from an asymptomatic state to full-blown AIDS. The pace of disease progression in untreated adults is variable. The median time between infection with HIV and the development of AIDS is 10 years, with a range from a few months to more than 12 years. In a study of adults infected with HIV, symptoms developed in 70% to 85% of infected adults, and AIDS developed in 55% to 60% within 12 years after infection. The natural history of the disease can be significantly altered by antiretroviral therapy. Women with HIV-induced altered immune function are at increased risk for infections such as tuberculosis (TB), bacterial pneumonia, and *Pneumocystis jiroveci* pneumonia (PCP). Because of its impact on the immune system, HIV affects the diagnosis, evaluation, treatment, and follow-up of many other diseases and may decrease the efficacy of antimicrobial therapy for some STDs.

Diagnosis

Infection is most often diagnosed by HIV antibody tests. Antibody testing begins with a sensitive screening test such as enzyme-linked immunosorbent assay (ELISA) or a rapid assay. If confirmed by Western blot, a positive antibody test result confirms that a person is infected with HIV and is capable of transmitting the virus to others. HIV antibody is detectable in more than 95% of patients within 6 months of infection. Women diagnosed with any STI, particularly genital ulcer disease, should be offered HIV testing (48). **Routine HIV screening is recommended for women aged 19 to 64 years and targeted screening for women with risk factors outside of that age range, for example, sexually active adolescents** (53).

The initial evaluation of an HIV-positive woman includes screening for diseases associated with HIV such as TB and STIs, administration of recommended vaccinations (hepatitis B, pneumococcal, meningococcal and influenza), and behavioral and psychosocial counseling. Intraepithelial neoplasia is strongly associated with HPV infection and occurs in high frequency in women with both HPV and HIV.

Treatment

Decisions regarding the initiation of antiretroviral therapy should be guided by monitoring the laboratory parameters of HIV RNA (viral load) and CD4$^+$ T-cell count, and the clinical condition of the patient. The primary goals of antiretroviral therapy are maximal and durable suppression of viral load, restoration or preservation of immunologic function, improvement of quality of life, reduction of HIV-related morbidity and mortality, and prevention of HIV transmission. **Antiretroviral therapy should be initiated in all women with a history of an AIDS-defining illness or with a CD4 count less than 350 cells per mm^3.** Antiretroviral treatment should be started regardless of CD4 count in women with the following conditions: pregnancy, HIV-associated nephropathy, and hepatitis B coinfection when treatment of hepatitis B is indicated. Patients must be willing to accept therapy to avoid the emergence of resistance caused by poor compliance. Dual nucleoside regimens used in addition to a protease inhibitor or nonnucleoside reverse transcriptase inhibitor provide a better durable clinical benefit than monotherapy.

Patients with less than 200 CD4$^+$ T cells per μL should receive prophylaxis against opportunistic infections, such as *trimethoprim/sulfamethoxazole* or aerosol *pentamidine* for the prevention of PCP pneumonia. Those with less than 50 CD4$^+$ T cells per uL should receive *azithromycin* prophylaxis for mycobacterial infections (54).

Urinary Tract Infection

Acute Cystitis

Women with acute cystitis generally have an abrupt onset of multiple, severe urinary tract symptoms including dysuria, frequency, and urgency associated with suprapubic or low-back pain. Suprapubic tenderness may be noted on physical examination. Urinalysis reveals pyuria and sometimes hematuria. Several factors increase the risk for cystitis, including sexual intercourse, the use of a diaphragm and a spermicide, delayed postcoital micturition, and a history of a recent urinary tract infection (55–57).

Diagnosis

***Escherichia coli* is the most common pathogen isolated from the urine of young women with acute cystitis, and it is present in 80% of cases** (58). *Staphylococcus saprophyticus* is present in an additional 5% to 15% of patients with cystitis. The pathophysiology of cystitis in women involves the colonization of the vagina and urethra with coliform bacteria from the rectum. For this reason, the effects of an antimicrobial agent on the vaginal flora play a role in the eradication of bacteriuria.

Treatment

High concentrations of *trimethoprim* and *fluoroquinolone* in vaginal secretions can eradicate *E. coli* while minimally altering normal anaerobic and microaerophilic vaginal flora. An increasing linear trend in the prevalence of resistance of *E. coli* (>10%) to the fluoroquinolones (e.g., *ciprofloxacin*) was noted. Despite a similar increase in *E. coli* resistance (9%–18%) to *trimethoprim/sulfamethoxazole*, therapeutic efficacy remains stable. In contrast, no such increase in resistance was noted with *nitrofurantoin*. *Nitrofurantoin* (macrocrystals, 100 mg orally twice daily for 5 days) or *trimethoprim/sulfamethoxazole* 160/800 mg orally twice daily for 3 days) are the optimal choices for empirical therapy for uncomplicated cystitis (59).

In patients with typical symptoms, an abbreviated laboratory workup followed by empirical therapy is suggested. The diagnosis can be presumed if pyuria is detected by microscopy or leukocyte esterase testing. Urine culture is not necessary, and a short course of antimicrobial therapy should be given. No follow-up visit or culture is necessary unless symptoms persist or recur.

Recurrent Cystitis

About 20% of premenopausal women with an initial episode of cystitis have recurrent infections. More than 90% of these recurrences are caused by exogenous reinfection. Recurrent cystitis should be documented by culture to rule out resistant micro-organisms. Patients may be treated by one of three strategies: (i) continuous prophylaxis, (ii) postcoital prophylaxis, or (iii) therapy initiated by the patient when symptoms are first noted.

Postmenopausal women may have frequent reinfections. **Hormonal therapy or topically applied estrogen cream, along with antimicrobial prophylaxis, is helpful in treating these patients.**

Urethritis

Women with dysuria caused by urethritis have a more gradual onset of mild symptoms, which may be associated with abnormal vaginal discharge or bleeding related to concurrent cervicitis. Patients may have a new sex partner or experience lower abdominal pain. Physical examination may reveal the presence of mucopurulent cervicitis or vulvovaginal herpetic lesions. *C. trachomatis*, *N. gonorrhoeae*, or genital herpes may cause acute urethritis. Pyuria is present on urinalysis, but hematuria is rarely seen. Treatment regimens for chlamydia and gonococcal infections are presented in Table 18.3.

Occasionally, vaginitis caused by *C. albicans* or trichomonas is associated with dysuria. On careful questioning, patients generally describe external dysuria, sometimes associated with vaginal discharge, and pruritus and dyspareunia. They usually do not experience urgency or frequency. Pyuria and hematuria are absent.

Acute Pyelonephritis

The clinical spectrum of acute, uncomplicated pyelonephritis in young women ranges from gram-negative septicemia to a cystitislike illness with mild flank pain. *E. coli* accounts for more than 80% of these cases (58). Microscopy of unspun urine reveals pyuria and gram-negative bacteria. A urine culture should be obtained in all women with suspected pyelonephritis; blood cultures should be performed in those who are hospitalized because results are positive in 15% to 20% of cases. In the absence of nausea and vomiting and severe illness, outpatient oral therapy can be given safely. Patients who have nausea and vomiting, are moderately to severely ill, or are pregnant should be hospitalized. Outpatient treatment regimens include *trimethoprim/sulfamethoxazole* (160/800 mg every 12 hours for 14 days) or a quinolone (e.g., *levofloxacin*, 750 mg daily for 7 days). Inpatient treatment regimens include the use of parenteral *levofloxacin* (750 mg daily), *ceftriaxone* (1–2 g daily), *ampicillin* (1 g every 6 hours), and *gentamicin* (especially if *Enterococcus* species are suspected) or *aztreonam* (1 g every 8–12 hours). Symptoms should resolve after 48 to 72 hours. If fever and flank pain persist after 72 hours of therapy, ultrasound or computed tomography should be considered to rule out a perinephric or intrarenal abscess or ureteral obstruction. A follow-up culture should be obtained 2 weeks after the completion of therapy (60).

References

1. **Huggins GR, Preti G.** Vaginal odors and secretions. *Clin Obstet Gynecol* 1981;24:355–377.

2. **Larsen B.** Microbiology of the female genital tract. In: Pastorek J, ed. Obstetric and gynecologic infectious disease. New York: Raven Press, 1994:11–26.

3. **Eschenbach DA, Davick PR, Williams BL, et al.** Prevalence of hydrogen peroxide-producing Lactobacillus species in normal women and women with vaginal vaginosis. *J Clin Microbiol* 1989;27:251–256.

4. **Spiegel CA, Amsel R, Eschenbach DA, et al.** Anaerobic bacteria in nonspecific vaginitis. *N Engl J Med* 1980;303:601–607.

5. **Kent HL.** Epidemiology of vaginitis. *Am J Obstet Gynecol* 1991;165:1168–1176.

6. **Eschenbach DA, Hillier S, Critchlow C, et al.** Diagnosis and clinical manifestations of bacterial vaginosis. *Am J Obstet Gynecol* 1988;158:819–828.

7. **Larsson P, Platz-Christensen JJ, Thejls H, et al.** Incidence of pelvic inflammatory disease after first trimester legal abortion in women with bacterial vaginosis after treatment with metronidazole: a double-blind randomized study. *Am J Obstet Gynecol* 1992;166:100–103.

8. **Soper DE, Bump RC, Hurt WG.** Bacterial vaginosis and trichomoniasis vaginitis are risk factors for cuff cellulitis after abdominal hysterectomy. *Am J Obstet Gynecol* 1990;163:1016–1023.

9. **Platz-Christensen JJ, Sundstrom E, Larsson PG.** Bacterial vaginosis and cervical intraepithelial neoplasia. *Acta Obstet Gynecol Scand* 1994;73:586–588.

10. **Martius J, Eschenbach DA.** The role of bacterial vaginosis as a cause of amniotic fluid infection, chorioamnionitis and prematurity: a review. *Arch Gynecol Obstet* 1900;247:1–13.

11. **Watts DH, Krohn MA, Hillier SL, et al.** Bacterial vaginosis as a risk factor for postcesarean endometritis. *Obstet Gynecol* 1990;75:52–58.

12. **Larsson PG, Carlsson B.** Does pre- and postoperative metronidazole treatment lower vaginal cuff infection rate after abdominal hysterectomy among women with bacterial vaginosis? *Infect Dis Obstet Gynecol* 2002;10:133–140.

13. **Larsson PG, Platz-Christensen JJ, Thejls H, et al.** Incidence of pelvic inflammatory disease after first-trimester legal abortion in women with bacterial vaginosis after treatment with metronidazole: a double-blind, randomized study. *Am J Obstet Gynecol* 1992;166:100–103.

14. **Amsel R, Totten PA, Spiegel CA, et al.** Nonspecific vaginitis: diagnostic criteria and microbial and epidemiologic associations. *Am J Med* 1983;74:14–22.

15. **Soper DE.** Taking the guesswork out of vaginitis. *Contemp Obstet Gynecol* 2005;50:32–39.

16. **Centers for Disease Control and Prevention.** The sexually transmitted diseases treatment guidelines. *MMWR* 2006;55:[RR-11]:1–94.

17. **Wolner-Hanssen P, Krieger JN, Stevens CE, et al.** Clinical manifestations of vaginal trichomoniasis. *JAMA* 1989;261:571–576.

18. **Krieger JN, Tam MR, Stevens CE, et al.** Diagnosis of trichomoniasis: comparison of conventional wet-mount examination with cytologic studies, cultures, and monoclonal antibody staining of direct specimens. *JAMA* 1988;259:1223–1227.

19. **Hurley R, De Louvois J.** Candida vaginitis. *Postgrad Med J* 1979;55:645–647.

20. **Hurley R.** Recurrent Candida infection. *Clin Obstet Gynecol* 1981;8:208–213.

21. **Sobel JD, Faro S, Force RW, et al.** Vulvovaginal candidiasis: epidemiologic, diagnostic, and therapeutic considerations. *Am J Obstet Gynecol* 1998;178:203–211.

22. **Caruso LJ.** Vaginal moniliasis after tetracycline therapy. *Am J Obstet Gynecol* 1964;90:374.

23. **Oriel JD, Waterworth PM.** Effect of minocycline and tetracycline on the vaginal yeast flora. *J Clin Pathol* 1975;28:403.

24. **Morton RS, Rashid S.** Candidal vaginitis: natural history, predisposing factors and prevention. *Proc R Soc Med* 1977;70[Suppl 4]:3–12.

25. **McClelland RS, Richardson BA, Hassan WM, et al.** Prospective study of vaginal bacterial flora and other risk factors for vulvovaginal candidiasis. *J Infect Dis* 2009;199:1883–1890.

26. **Brammer KW.** Treatment of vaginal candidiasis with a single oral dose of fluconazole. *Eur J Clin Microbiol Infect Dis* 1988;7:364–367.

27. **Sobel JD, Wiesenfeld HC, Martens M, et al.** Maintenance fluconazole therapy for recurrent vulvovaginal candidiasis. *N Engl J Med* 2004;351:876–883.

28. **Sobel JD.** Desquamative inflammatory vaginitis: a new subgroup of purulent vaginitis responsive to topical 2% clindamycin therapy. *Am J Obstet Gynecol* 1994;171:1215–1220.

29. **Kiviat NB, Paavonen JA, Wolner-Hanssen P, et al.** Histopathology of endocervical infection caused by *Chlamydia trachomatis*, herpes simplex virus, *Trichomonas vaginalis*, and *Neisseria gonorrhoeae*. *Hum Pathol* 1990;21:831–837.

30. **Brunham RC, Paavonen J, Stevens CE, et al.** Mucopurulent cervicitis: the ignored counterpart in women of urethritis in men. *N Engl J Med* 1984;311:1–6.

31. **Soper DE, Brockwell NJ, Dalton HP.** Microbial etiology of urban emergency department acute salpingitis: treatment with ofloxacin. *Am J Obstet Gynecol* 1992;167:653–660.

32. **Sweet RL, Draper DL, Schachter J, et al.** Microbiology and pathogenesis of acute salpingitis as determined by laparoscopy: what is the appropriate site to sample? *Am J Obstet Gynecol* 1980;138:985–989.

33. **Wasserheit JN, Bell TA, Kiviat NB, et al.** Microbial causes of proven pelvic inflammatory disease and efficacy of clindamycin and tobramycin. *Ann Intern Med* 1986;104:187–193.

34. **Short VL, Totten PA, Ness RB, et al.** Clinical presentation of *Mycoplasma genitalium* infection versus *Neisseria gonorrhoeae* infection among women with pelvic inflammatory disease. *Clin Infect Dis* 2009;48:41–47.

35. **Soper DE, Brockwell NJ, Dalton HP, et al.** Observations concerning the microbial etiology of acute salpingitis. *Am J Obstet Gynecol* 1994;170:1008–1017.

36. **Hillis SD, Joesoef R, Marchbanks PA, et al.** Delayed care of pelvic inflammatory disease as a risk factor for impaired fertility. *Am J Obstet Gynecol* 1993;168:1503–1509.

37. **Wolner-Hanssen P, Kiviat NB, Holmes KK.** Atypical pelvic inflammatory disease: subacute, chronic, or subclinical upper genital tract infection in women. In: **Holmes KK, March P-A, Sparking PF, eds.** *Sexually transmitted diseases*, 2nd ed. New York: McGraw-Hill, 1990:614–620.

38. **Westrom L.** Diagnosis and treatment of salpingitis. *J Reprod Med* 1983;28:703–708.

39. **Soper DE.** Diagnosis and laparoscopic grading of acute salpingitis. *Am J Obstet Gynecol* 1991;164:1370–1376.

40. **Peterson HB, Walker CK, Kahn JG, et al.** Pelvic inflammatory disease: key treatment issues and options. *JAMA* 1991;266:2605–2611.

41. **Ness RB, Soper DE, Holley RL, et al.** Effectiveness of inpatient and outpatient treatment strategies for women with pelvic inflammatory disease: results from the Pelvic Inflammatory Disease Evaluation and Clinical Health (PEACH) randomized trial. *Am J Obstet Gynecol* 2002;186:929–937.

42. **Soper DE.** Pelvic inflammatory disease. *Obstet Gynecol* 2010;116:419–428.

43. **Gilstrap LC 3rd, Herbert WN, Cunningham FG, et al.** Gonorrhea screening in the male consorts of women with pelvic infection. *JAMA* 1977;238:965–966.

44. **Potterat JJ, Phillips L, Rothenberg RB, et al.** Gonococcal pelvic inflammatory disease: case-finding observations. *Am J Obstet Gynecol* 1980;138:1101–1104.

45. **Reed SD, Landers DV, Sweet RL.** Antibiotic treatment of tuboovarian abscesses: comparison of broad-spectrum B-lactam agents versus clindamycin-containing regimens. *Am J Obstet Gynecol* 1991;164:1556–1562.

46. **Varghese JC, O'Neill MJ, Gervais DA, et al.** Transvaginal catheter drainage of tuboovarian abscess using the trocar method: technique and literature review. *AJR Am J Roentgenol* 2001;177:139–144.

47. **Corey L, Adams HG, Brown ZA, et al.** Genital herpes simplex virus infection: clinical manifestations, course, and complications. *Ann Intern Med* 1983;98:958–972.

48. **Schmid GP.** Approach to the patient with genital ulcer disease. *Med Clin North Am* 1990;74:1559–1572.

49. **Corey L, Wald A, Patel R, et al. HSV Transmission Study Group.** Once-daily valacyclovir to reduce the risk of transmission of genital herpes. *N Engl J Med* 2004;350:11–20.

50. **Hutchinson CM, Hook EW.** Syphilis in adults. *Med Clin North Am* 1990;74:1389–1416.

51. **Beutner KR, Richwald GA, Wiley DJ, et al.** External genital warts: report of the American Medical Association Consensus Conference. AMA Expert Panel on External Genital Warts. *Clin Infect Dis* 1998;27:796–806.

52. **Anderson JR, ed.** *A guide to the clinical care with women with HIV/AIDS.* Washington, DC: DHHS, HRSA, HAB.

53. **American College of Obstetrics and Gynecology.** Routine human immunodeficiency virus screening (Committee Opinion). No. 411. August 2008. http://www.acog.org/publications/committee_opinions/co411.cfm.

54. **Department of Health and Human Services.** Panel on antiretroviral guidelines for adults and adolescents. Guidelines for the use of antiretroviral agents in HIV-1 infected adults and adolescents.. December 1, 2009. Available online at: http://www.aidsinfo.nih.gov/ContentFiles/AdultandAdolescentGL.pdf

55. **Remis RS, Gurwith MJ, Gurwith D, et al.** Risk factors for urinary tract infection. *Am J Epidemiol* 1987;126:685–694.

56. **Fihn SD, Latham RH, Roberts P, et al.** Association between diaphragm use and urinary tract infection. *JAMA* 1985;254:240–245.

57. **Strom BL, Collins M, West SL, et al.** Sexual activity, contraceptive use, and other risk factors for symptomatic and asymptomatic bacteriuria: a case-control study. *Ann Intern Med* 1987;107:816–823.

58. **Stamm WE, Counts GW, Running KR, et al.** Diagnosis of coliform infection in acutely dysuric women. *N Engl J Med* 1982;307:463–468.

59. **Gupta K, Scholes D, Stamm WE.** Increasing prevalence of antimicrobial resistance among uropathogens causing acute uncomplicated cystitis in women. *JAMA* 1999;281:736–738.

60. **Gupta K, Hooten TM, Naber KG,** et al. International clinical practice guidelines for the treatment of acute uncomplicated cystitis and pyelonephritis in women: a 2010 update by the Infectious Disease Society of America and the European Society for Microbiology and Infectious Diseases. *Clin Infect Dis* 2011;52:e103–e120.

19 Intraepithelial Disease of the Cervix, Vagina, and Vulva

Francisco Garcia
Kenneth D. Hatch
Jonathan S. Berek

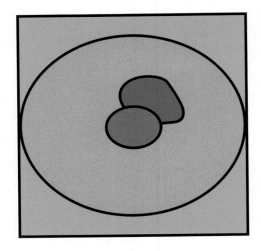

- Cervical intraepithelial neoplasia (CIN) most often arises in an area of metaplasia in the transformation zone at the advancing squamocolumnar junction (SCJ). Metaplasia advances from the original SCJ inward, toward the external os and over the columnar villi, to establish the *transformation zone*. CIN is most likely to begin either during menarche or after pregnancy, when metaplasia is most active; after menopause, metaplasia is less active and a woman has a lower risk of developing CIN.

- Untreated, most CIN 1 and some CIN 2 lesions spontaneously regress; nevertheless, CIN refers to a lesion that may progress to invasive carcinoma. This term is equivalent to the term *dysplasia*, which means abnormal maturation; consequently, proliferating metaplasia without atypical mitotic activity should not be called dysplasia. Squamous metaplasia should not be diagnosed as dysplasia (or CIN) because it does not progress to invasive cancer.

- More than 90% of CIN is attributed to human papillomavirus (HPV) infection. Only certain types of HPV cause high-grade intraepithelial lesions and cancer (HPV-16, -18, -31, -33, -35, -39, -45, -51, -52, -56, -58, -59, -68). Type 16 is the most common form of HPV found in invasive cancer and in CIN 2 and CIN 3; it is found in 47% of women with cancer.

- Potentially premalignant squamous lesions fall into three categories: (i) *atypical squamous cells* (ASC), (ii) *low-grade squamous intraepithelial lesions* (LSIL), and (iii) *high-grade squamous intraepithelial lesions* (HSIL). The ASC category is subdivided into two categories: those of unknown significance (ASC-US) and those in which high-grade lesions must be excluded (ASC-H).

- The LSIL category includes CIN 1 (mild dysplasia) and the changes of HPV, termed *koilocytotic atypia*. The HSIL category includes CIN 2 and CIN 3 (moderate dysplasia, severe dysplasia, and carcinoma *in situ*).

- The spontaneous regression rate of biopsy-proven CIN 1 is 60% to 85% in prospective studies. The regressions typically occur within a 2-year follow-up with cytology and colposcopy. For LSIL that persists longer than 2 years, the choice of treatment is optional. Expectant management is still appropriate in some patients, and ablative therapies, including cryotherapy and laser ablation, are acceptable treatment modalities.

- When a cytologic specimen suggests the presence of HSIL, colposcopy and directed biopsy should be performed. Although high-grade CIN can be treated with a variety of techniques, the preferred treatment for CIN 2 or 3 in nonadolescent patients is loop electrosurgical excision procedure (LEEP).

- Atypical endocervical cells pose a risk for adenocarcinoma *in situ* (AIS), which must be considered a precursor of adenocarcinoma.

- After sampling to rule out invasive disease, vaginal intraepithelial neoplasia (VAIN 3 lesions can be treated with laser or outpatient excisional therapy. Patients with vaginal intraepithelial neoplasia (VAIN 1 and most VAIN 2 and HPV infection do not require treatment. These lesions are multifocal and often regress, but may recur after ablative therapy.

- Vulvar intraepithelial neoplasia, grade 3 (VIN 3), is treated by simple excision, laser ablation, or superficial (partial) vulvectomy, with or without split-thickness skin grafting. Excision of small foci of disease produces excellent results, and although multifocal or extensive lesions may be difficult to treat by this approach, it offers the most cosmetic result. VIN 1 or 2 is generally associated with dystrophic changes or HPV and can be managed expectantly.

- Intraepithelial disease frequently occurs in the cervix, vagina, and vulva, and it may coexist in these areas. The cause and epidemiologic basis are common to all three locations, and treatment typically is ablative, excisional, and conservative. Early diagnosis and management are essential to prevent disease from progressing to invasive cancer.

Cervical Intraepithelial Neoplasia

The concept of *preinvasive disease* of the cervix was introduced in 1947, when it was recognized that epithelial changes could be identified that had the appearance of invasive cancer but were confined to the epithelium (1). Subsequent studies showed that these lesions, if left untreated, could progress to cervical cancer (2). Improvements in cytologic assessment led to the identification of early precursor lesions called *dysplasia,* a name that acknowledges the malignant potential of these lesions. Historically carcinoma *in situ* (CIS) was treated very aggressively (most often with hysterectomy), whereas dysplasias were believed to be less significant and were not treated or were treated by colposcopic biopsy and cryosurgery. The concept of *cervical intraepithelial neoplasia* (CIN) was introduced in 1968, when Richart suggested that dysplasias have the potential for progression (3). **Most untreated CIN 1 and some CIN 2 lesions regress spontaneously; nevertheless, high-grade CIN refers to a lesion that may progress to invasive carcinoma when left untreated (4). Proliferating metaplasia without mitotic activity should not be called dysplasia or CIN because it does not progress to invasive cancer.**

The criteria for the diagnosis of intraepithelial neoplasia may vary according to the pathologist, but the significant features are cellular immaturity, cellular disorganization, nuclear abnormality, and increased mitotic activity. The extent of the mitotic activity, immature cellular proliferation, and nuclear atypia identifies the degree of neoplasia. If the presence of mitoses and immature cells is limited to the lower third of the epithelium, the lesion usually is designated as CIN 1. Involvement of the middle and upper thirds is diagnosed as CIN 2 and CIN 3, respectively (Fig. 19.1).

Cervical Anatomy

The cervix is composed of *columnar epithelium,* which lines the endocervical canal, and *squamous epithelium,* which covers the exocervix (5). The point at which they meet is called the *squamocolumnar junction* (SCJ) (Figs. 19.2 and 19.3).

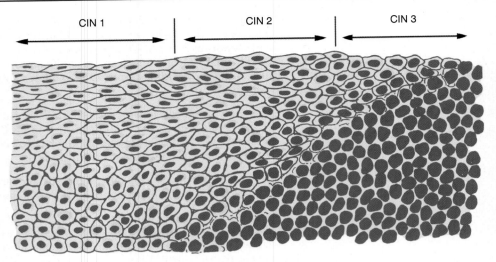

Figure 19.1   Diagram of cervical intraepithelial neoplasia compared with normal epithelium.

The Squamocolumnar Junction

The SCJ rarely remains restricted to the external os. Instead, it is a dynamic point that changes in response to puberty, pregnancy, menopause, and hormonal stimulation (Fig. 19.4). In neonates, the SCJ is located on the exocervix. At menarche, the production of estrogen causes the vaginal epithelium to fill with glycogen. Lactobacilli act on the glycogen to lower the pH, stimulating the subcolumnar reserve cells to undergo *metaplasia* (5).

Metaplasia advances from the original SCJ inward, toward the external os and over the columnar villi. This process establishes an area called the *transformation zone*. The transformation zone extends from the original SCJ to the physiologically active SCJ, as

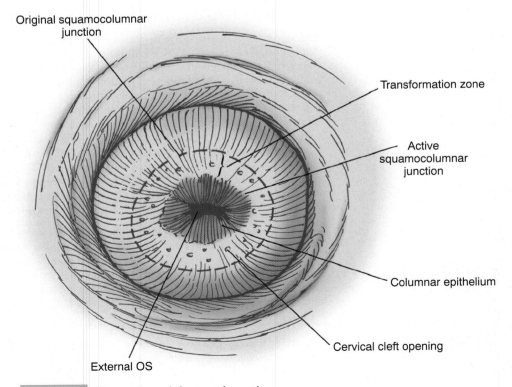

Figure 19.2   The cervix and the transformation zone.

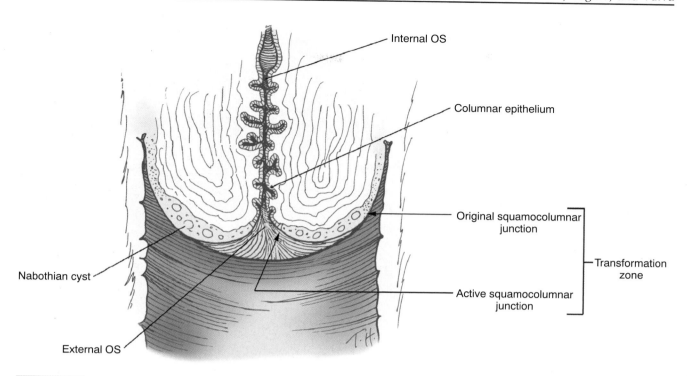

Figure 19.3   Diagram of the cervix and the endocervix.

demarcated by the squamocolumnar junction. As the metaplastic epithelium in the transformation zone matures, it begins to produce glycogen and eventually resembles the original squamous epithelium, both colposcopically and histologically (Fig. 19.5A and B).

In most cases, CIN is believed to originate as a single focus in the transformation zone at the advancing SCJ. The anterior lip of the cervix is twice as likely to develop CIN as the posterior lip, and CIN rarely originates in the lateral angles. Once CIN occurs, it can progress horizontally to involve the entire transformation zone, but it usually does not replace the original squamous epithelium. This progression usually results in CIN with a sharp external border. Proximally, CIN involves the cervical clefts, and this area tends to have the most severe CIN lesions. The extent of involvement of these cervical glands has significant therapeutic implications because the entire gland must be destroyed to ensure elimination of the CIN (5). The only way to determine where the original SCJ was located is to look for nabothian cysts or cervical cleft openings, which indicate the presence of columnar epithelium. After the metaplastic epithelium matures and forms glycogen, it is called the *healed* transformation zone and is relatively resistant to oncogenic stimuli. The entire SCJ with early metaplastic cells is susceptible to oncogenic factors, which may cause these cells to transform into CIN. Therefore, **CIN is most likely to begin either during menarche or after pregnancy, when metaplasia is most active. Conversely, after menopause a woman undergoes little metaplasia and is at a lower risk of developing CIN from *de novo* human papillomavirus (HPV) infection.** Oncogenic factors are introduced through sexual contact in general and intercourse in particular. Although several agents, including sperm, seminal fluid histones, trichomonas, chlamydia, and herpes simplex virus, were studied, it is established that persistent high-risk oncogenic HPV infection is the overwhelming risk factor for the development of CIN.

Normal Transformation Zone

The original squamous epithelium of the vagina and exocervix has four layers (5):

1. The *basal layer* is a single row of immature cells with large nuclei and a small amount of cytoplasm.

2. The *parabasal layer* includes two to four rows of immature cells that have normal mitotic figures and provide the replacement cells for the overlying epithelium.

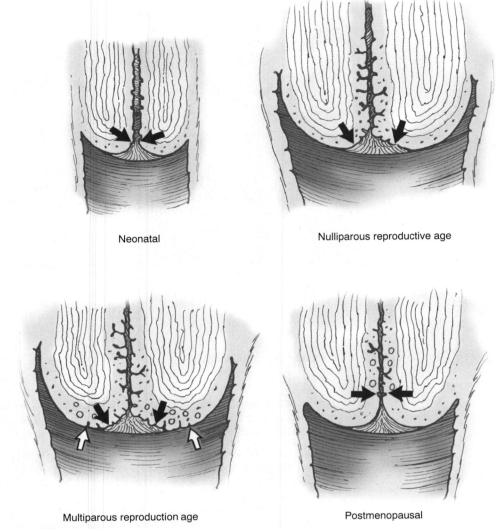

Neonatal

Nulliparous reproductive age

Multiparous reproduction age

Postmenopausal

Figure 19.4   Different locations of the transformation zone and the squamocolumnar junction during a woman's lifetime. The *arrows* mark the active transformation zone.

3. The *intermediate layer* includes four to six rows of cells with larger amounts of cytoplasm in a polyhedral shape separated by an intercellular space. Intercellular bridges, where differentiation of glycogen production occurs, can be identified with light microscopy.

4. The *superficial layer* includes five to eight rows of flattened cells with small uniform nuclei and a cytoplasm filled with glycogen. The nucleus becomes pyknotic, and the cells detach from the surface (exfoliation). These cells form the basis for Papanicolaou (Pap) testing.

Columnar Epithelium   Columnar epithelium has a single layer of columnar cells with mucus at the top and a round nucleus at the base. The glandular epithelium is composed of numerous ridges, clefts, and infoldings and, when covered by squamous metaplasia, leads to the appearance of gland openings. Technically, the endocervix is not a gland, but often the term *gland openings* is used.

Metaplastic Epithelium   Metaplastic epithelium, found at the SCJ, begins in the subcolumnar reserve cells (Fig. 19.4). Under stimulation of lower vaginal acidity, the reserve cells proliferate, lifting the columnar epithelium. The immature metaplastic cells have large nuclei and a small amount of cytoplasm without glycogen. As the cells mature normally, they produce glycogen,

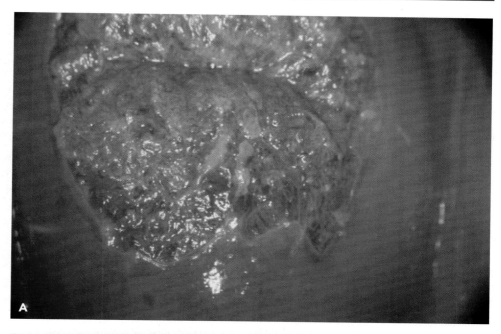

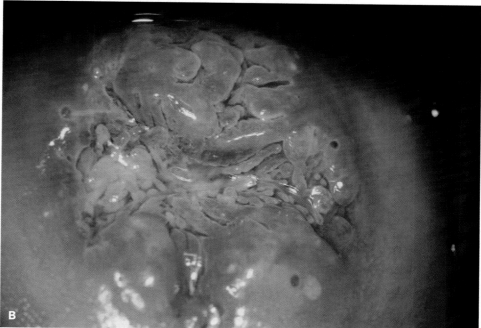

Figure 19.5   A: Active metaplasia in the transformation zone. B: Maturing metaplasia in the transformation zone.

eventually forming the four layers of epithelium. The metaplastic process begins at the tips of the columnar villi, which are exposed first to the acid vaginal environment. As the metaplasia replaces the columnar epithelium, the central capillary of the villus regresses, and the epithelium flattens out, leaving the epithelium with its typical vascular network. As metaplasia proceeds into the cervical clefts, it replaces columnar epithelium and similarly flattens the epithelium. The deeper clefts may not be completely replaced by the metaplastic epithelium, leaving mucus-secreting columnar epithelium trapped under the squamous epithelium. Some of these glands open onto the surface; others are completely encased, with mucus collecting in nabothian cysts. **Gland openings and nabothian cysts mark the original SCJ and the outer edge of the original transformation zone** (5) (Fig. 19.5A and B).

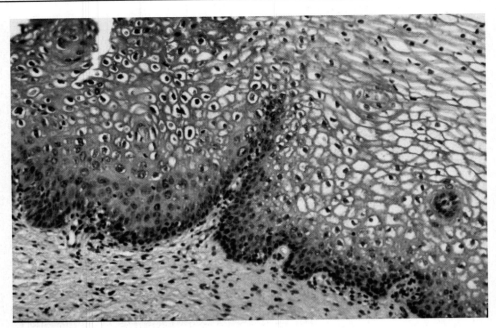

Figure 19.6   Cervical intraepithelial neoplasia grade 1 (CIN 1) with koilocytosis. The normal maturation process and differentiation from the basal and parabasal layers to the intermediate and superficial layers are maintained. In the upper layers, koilocytes are characterized by perinuclear halos, well-defined cell borders, and nuclear hyperchromasia, irregularity, and enlargement.

Human Papillomavirus

The cytologic changes of HPV were first recognized by Koss and Durfee in 1956 and given the term *koilocytosis* (6). Their significance was not recognized until 20 years later, when Meisels and colleagues reported these changes in mild dysplasia (7) (Fig. 19.6). Molecular biologic studies showed high levels of HPV DNA and capsid antigen, indicating productive viral infection in these koilocytic cells (8). The HPV genome is found in all grades of cervical neoplasia (9). Infection with HPV is the primary cause of cervical cancer (10). As the CIN lesions become more severe (Fig. 19.7), the koilocytes disappear, the HPV copy numbers decrease, and the capsid antigen disappears, indicating that the virus is not capable of reproducing in less differentiated cells (11). Instead, portions of the HPV DNA become integrated into the host cell. Integration of the transcriptionally active DNA into the host cell appears to be essential for malignant transformation (12). **Malignant transformation requires the expression of E6 and E7 HPV oncoproteins** (13). Because HPV will not grow in cell culture, there is no direct evidence of the carcinogenesis of HPV. However, a cell culture system for growing keratinocytes was described that allows for stratification and differentiation of specific keratinase types (14). When normal cells are transfected with the plasmid-containing HPV-16, the transfected cells produce cytologic abnormalities identical to those seen in intraepithelial neoplasia. The E6 and E7 oncoproteins are identifiable in the transfected cell lines, providing strong laboratory evidence of a cause-and-effect relationship (15). Cervical cancer cell lines that contain active copies of HPV-16 or -18 (SiHa, HeLa, C 4-11, Ca Ski) express HPV-16 E6 and E7 oncoproteins (16).

HPV DNA can be detected in most women with cervical neoplasia (17,18). There are more than 120 types of HPV identified, with 30 of these HPV types primarily infecting the squamous epithelium of the lower anogenital tract of men and women (19,20). Detection of HPV is associated with a 250-fold increase risk of high-grade CIN (21). **The percentage of intraepithelial neoplasia attributed to HPV infection approaches 90%** (18).

Only certain types of HPV account for about 90% of high-grade intraepithelial lesions and cancer (HPV-16, -18, -31, -33, -35, -39, -45, -51, -52, -56, -58, -59 and -68) (18). **Type 16 is the most common HPV found in invasive cancer and in CIN 2 and CIN 3, and it is found in 47% of women with cancer in all stages** (22). It is the most common HPV type found in women with normal cytology.

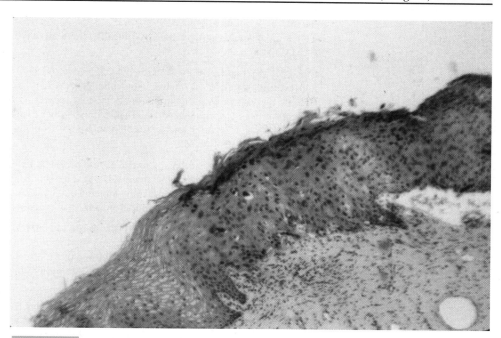

Figure 19.7   Cervical biopsy showing normal cells, cervical intraepithelial neoplasia 2 and 3 (CIN 2, CIN 3). In CIN 3, the normal maturation is lost.

HPV-16 infection is not very specific; it can be found in 16% of women with low-grade lesions and in up to 14% of women with normal cytology. **Human papillomavirus type-18 is found in 23% of women with invasive cancers, 5% of women with CIN 2 and CIN 3, 5% of women with HPV and CIN 1, and fewer than 2% of patients with negative findings** (18). **Therefore, HPV-18 is more specific than HPV-16 for invasive tumors.**

Usually, HPV infections do not persist. Those that do persist may remain latent for many years. Most women who are exposed have no clinical evidence of disease, and the infection is eventually suppressed or eliminated (17). Other women exhibit low-grade cervical lesions that mostly regress spontaneously. **In the vast majority of cases, the infection will clear in 9 to 15 months** (23). A small minority of women exposed to HPV develops persistent infection that may progress to CIN (17,24). Persistent high-risk HPV infection increases the risk of high-grade disease 300-fold and is required for the development and maintenance of CIN 3 (25,26). Factors that may have a role in persistence and progression include smoking, contraceptive use, infection with other sexually transmitted diseases, or nutrition (17,22). Any factor that influences the integration of HPV DNA into the human genome may cause progression to invasive disease (27).

Human Papillomavirus Vaccine

Because HPV infection is a necessary factor in the development of cervical neoplasia, an important step in primary prevention was the development of a prophylactic vaccine to protect against HPV infection. The development of prophylactic vaccination became possible through the development of protein mimics that simulate the outermost protein capsid of the virus and are termed viruslike particles (VLPs) (28). *Gardasil* (Merck, NJ, USA), a quadrivalent vaccine containing the VLPs for HPV-6, -11, -16, and -18, was approved by the U.S. Food and Drug Administration (FDA) in 2006; and *Cervarix* (GlaxoSmithKline, Middlesex, U.K.), a bivalent vaccine, was approved in 2009, and contains the VLPs to types 16 and 18. **Clinical trials demonstrated that both the bivalent and quadrivalent vaccines are highly efficient in preventing CIN 2, CIN 3, or adenocarcinoma *in situ* caused by HPV-16 and -18 in women from 15 to 26 years of age** (29,30). **For the population who are seronegative and HPV DNA negative for HPV-16 and -18 at vaccination and received all three vaccinations, the efficacy is 100%** (31,32). **This protection is documented to last as long as 6.4 years after vaccination** (31).

In a small subset of women who were seropositive for HPV-16 or -18, but DNA negative, the vaccine efficacy remained at 100% (29,30). This suggests that past exposure and clearance of the virus does not reduce the efficacy of the vaccine. On the other hand, the vaccines do not show efficacy in women who are HPV-16 and -18 DNA positive at the time of entry onto the study. This indicates that the **vaccines are not able clear an active infection and cannot be used to treat CIN.**

Since HPV-16 and -18 are contained in 52% of CIN and 70% of invasive cancers, the data concerning cross-protection from the other high-risk types are important (33). The bivalent vaccine demonstrates protection from persistent infection with HPV types 31, 33, and 45 and protection from CIN-related HPV-31 (29). Quadrivalent vaccine data showing cross-protection against CIN 2 or greater and against HPV 31 exist, but this indication is not included in the FDA-approved labeling (34).

The 3-year follow-up studies of both vaccine products exhibit a reduction in referrals to colposcopy by 26% and 20%, respectively (29,35). This is accompanied by a reduction in excisional procedures of 69% and 42% for the bivalent and quadrivalent products, respectively (29,35). The additional reduction may come from cross-protection against nonvaccine specific HPV types.

The quadrivalent vaccine prevents HPV-6 and -11 infections that cause genital warts. The clinical trials for women show a 99% efficacy in protection from HPV-6, -11, -16, and -18 caused external warts in women who received all three of the vaccine shots and 80% of those who did not (36). In the vaccine trials in men and boys the protection was 89% at 29 months, leading to approval of this quadrivalent vaccine in males (37).

The quadrivalent vaccine trials evaluated the protection from vulva intraepithelial neoplasia (VIN) and vaginal intraepithelial neoplasia (VAIN). The women who were HPV negative at vaccination and followed the protocol had a 100% reduction in HPV-16, -18 caused VIN 2 or 3, and VAIN 2 or 3 lesions compared to placebo (38). When the entire vaccinated population was evaluated, the reduction in VIN 2 or 3 and VAIN 2 or 3 was 50% (38). These data demonstrate that high-risk HPV types other than 16 and 18 are responsible for a significant proportion of VIN and VAIN. It reveals that women who were already positive for HPV-16 and -18 were not protected from VIN and VAIN. The bivalent trials were not designed to assess vulvar or vaginal end points.

Duration of vaccine efficacy is important because we know that HPV infection peaks in the early 20s and cervical cancer occurs in the 40s. The vaccines are approved for women up to 26 years of age and to be protective they should be effective beyond 10 years. In order to induce a significant antibody response to the antigen, it is combined with an adjuvant. The quadrivalent adjuvant is aluminum hydroxyphosphate sulfate, which proved to be superior to a simple aluminum adjuvant in binding to HPV-16 in mice. By contrast, the bivalent adjuvant is an aluminum hydroxide combined with a monophosphoryl lipid A. This is theorized to function as a link between the HPV and the activation of the innate immune system. This adjuvant produced higher antibody titers than aluminum-induced titers at the 4-year follow-up visit (39). It remains unclear whether a booster shot will be needed as the adolescent cohort reaches its mid-20s where the exposure to HPV peaks. Because the first vaccinations were given less than 10 years ago, the studies to determine the advisability of a booster are ongoing.

The American Committee on Immunization Practices developed recommendations for the utilization of both the quadrivalent and bivalent vaccines in young girls and women. In 2007 the American Cancer Society issued a set of clinical guidelines that remain relevant to the use of these agents (40). Under these guidelines, **routine HPV vaccination is recommended for girls at 11 to 12 years of age, but may be provided as early as 9 years and as late as 18 years. For young women between the ages of 19 to 26, there are insufficient data to determine the value of universal vaccination.** A decision to vaccinate a woman in that age group should be based on an informed discussion with her health care provider regarding her risk of previous HPV exposure and potential benefit and harm from the vaccination (41–44). **Screening practices for cervical intraepithelial neoplasia and cancer should remain unchanged in both vaccinated and unvaccinated women.**

Screening

Pap Test Classification: The Bethesda System

In 1988, the first National Cancer Institute (NCI) workshop held in Bethesda, Maryland, resulted in the development of the Bethesda System for cytologic reporting (45). A standardized method of reporting cytology findings facilitated peer review and quality assurance. **The terminology**

Table 19.1 Comparison of Cytology Classification Systems

Bethesda System	Dysplasia/CIN System	Papanicolaou System
Within normal limits	Normal	I
Infection (organism should be specified)	Inflammatory atypia (organism)	II
Reactive and reparative changes		
Squamous cell abnormalities Atypical squamous cells (1) of undetermined significance (ASC-US) (2) exclude high-grade lesions (ASC-H)	Squamous atypia HPV atypia, exclude **LSIL** Exclude HSIL HPV atypia	IIR
Low-grade squamous intraepithelial lesion (LSIL)	Mild dysplasia **CIN 1**	
High-grade squamous intraepithelial lesion (HSIL)	Moderate dysplasia **CIN 2** Severe dysplasia **CIN 3** Carcinoma *in situ*	III IV
Squamous cell carcinoma	Squamous cell carcinoma	V

CIN, cervical intraepithelial neoplasia, HPV, human papillomavirus.

was refined in the Bethesda III System (2001). According to this system, potentially premalignant squamous lesions fall into three categories: (i) *atypical squamous cells* (ASC), (ii) *low-grade squamous intraepithelial lesions* (LSIL), and (iii) *high-grade squamous intraepithelial lesions* (HSIL) (46). The ASC category is subdivided into two categories: those of unknown significance (ASC-US), and those in which high-grade lesions must be excluded (ASC-H). Low-grade squamous intraepithelial lesions include CIN 1 (mild dysplasia) and the changes of HPV, termed *koilocytotic atypia*. The HSIL category includes CIN 2 and CIN 3 (moderate dysplasia, severe dysplasia, and carcinoma *in situ*). A comparison of the various terms is shown in Table 19.1.

Cellular changes associated with HPV (i.e., koilocytosis and CIN 1) are incorporated within the category of LSIL because the natural history, distribution of various HPV types, and cytologic features of both of these lesions are the same (27). **Long-term follow-up studies showed that lesions properly classified as koilocytosis progress to high-grade intraepithelial neoplasia in 14% of cases and that lesions classified as mild dysplasia progress to severe dysplasia or CIS in 16% of cases** (4,46). It was initially thought that lesions classified as koilocytosis would contain only low-risk HPV types, such as HPV-6 and -11, whereas high-risk HPV types, such as HPV-16 and -18, would be limited to true neoplasms, including CIN 1, thus justifying the distinction. Histopathologic and molecular virologic correlation showed a similar heterogeneous distribution of low- and high-risk HPV types in both koilocytosis and CIN 1 (47). Studies evaluating the dysplasia, CIS, and CIN terminology consistently demonstrated problems with interobserver and intraobserver reproducibility (48). The greatest lack of reproducibility is between koilocytosis and CIN 1 (49). **On the basis of clinical behavior, molecular biologic findings, and morphologic features, HPV changes and CIN 1 appear to be the same disease.** The rationale for combining CIN 2 and CIN 3 into the category of HSIL is similar. The biologic studies reveal a comparable mix of high-risk HPV types in the two lesions, and the separation of the lesions is not reproducible (48,49). The management of CIN 2 and CIN 3 is similar.

Pap Test Accuracy

Screening for cervical cancer precursors using exfoliative cervico-vaginal cytology, the Pap test was successful in reducing the incidence of cervical cancer by 79% and the mortality by 70% since 1950 (50). **However, 20% of women in the United States do not undergo regular screening and have not had a Pap test in the previous 3 years.** The annual incidence rate dropped from 8 to 5 cases per 100,000 women, so approximately 8,200 women per year are diagnosed with cervical cancer (50–52). Some cases of cervical cancer continue to occur in patients who have regular Pap tests. A literature review of cervical cytology testing techniques was conducted by the Agency for Healthcare Research and Quality (53). The conclusion was that the sensitivity of conventional cytologic testing in detecting cervical cancer precursor lesions was

51%, with an estimated false-negative rate of 49%. **In three reviews of the accuracy of cervical cytology assessment, the sensitivity of the Pap test in detecting CIN 2 or 3 ranged from 47% to 62% and the specificity ranged from 60% to 95% (54–56). Nearly 30% of new cancer cases each year occur among women who underwent Pap testing. Errors of sampling, fixation, interpretation, or follow-up may be responsible for the missed cases** (57). Prior overestimates of Pap test sensitivity of approximately 80% led to erroneous recommendations of screening frequency (58).

The conventional Pap test technique needs to be improved in order to reduce false-negative errors. Sampling errors occur because a lesion is too small to exfoliate cells or the device did not pick up the cells and transfer them to the fixation media. Historically, preparation errors occurred because of poor fixation on the glass slide, leading to air drying and its consequences for interpretation. The slide preparations could be too thick and obscured by vaginal discharge, blood, or mucus. These problems were obviated with the widespread utilization of liquid-based media. Interpretive errors may still occur when the slide contains diagnostic cells that the screening technician or automated detection device fails to identify.

The ubiquitous use of liquid-based medium to collect the cytologic sample and preserve the collected cervical cells significantly decreased specimen sampling and preparation errors. With this technique, liquid samples are processed to provide a uniform, thin layer of cervical cells without debris on a glass slide. The Agency for Healthcare Research and Quality assessment of liquid-based cytology improved the sensitivity of the Pap test to the stated goal of 80%. The cell sample is collected with an endocervical brush used in combination with a plastic spatula or with a plastic broom. The sample is rinsed in a vial containing liquid alcohol-based preservative. With this technique, 80% to 90% of the cells are transferred to the liquid media, as compared with the 10% to 20% transferred to the glass slide with conventional cytologic testing. Using liquid-based media eliminates air drying. The cells are retrieved from the vial by passing the liquid through a filter, which traps the larger epithelial cells, separating them from the small blood and inflammatory cells. This process yields a thin layer of diagnostic cells properly preserved and more easily interpreted by the cytologist. This technique reduces by 70% to 90% the rate of unsatisfactory samples encountered with conventional cytologic testing (59). Liquid-based cytology is commonly performed by most of the laboratories in the United States.

Another technology approved by the FDA for primary screening and rescreening samples of cervical cytology initially interpreted as normal is the automated image-guided slide screening system. This technique uses an automated microscope coupled to a special digital camera. The system scans the slide and uses computer imaging techniques to analyze each field of view on the slide. Computer algorithms rank each slide on the probability that the sample may contain an abnormality. The selected slides are reviewed by a cytotechnologist or a cytopathologist. This technique reduced the false-negative rate by 32% (60).

Bethesda System Modifications

The Bethesda System for reporting the results of cervical cytology developed as a uniform system of cytology reporting that would provide clear guidance for clinical management (45). It creates a standardized framework for laboratory reports that includes a descriptive diagnosis and an evaluation of specimen adequacy. The Bethesda System was modified to reflect the development of new technologies and research findings.

In the Bethesda System, specimen adequacy is categorized as *satisfactory* or *unsatisfactory* for evaluation. If a specimen is found to be unsatisfactory, cervical cytology is repeated promptly. Otherwise the specimen is classified as *satisfactory*. If sampling of the transformation zone is inadequate or obscuring factors are present, cervical cytology can be repeated in 6 to 12 months. The general categorizations are (i) negative for intraepithelial lesion or malignancy, (ii) epithelial cell abnormality, and (iii) other. In the category of *negative for intraepithelial lesions or malignancy,* evidence for the presence of *trichomonas vaginalis,* candida, bacterial vaginosis, actinomyces, and herpes simplex virus may be noted. Included in this category are reactive cellular changes, glandular cells status after hysterectomy, and atrophy. The category *epithelial cell abnormality* includes squamous cell and glandular cell abnormalities. The rest of the categories of ASC, LSIL and HSIL remain unchanged from the classification noted above (Table 19.2).

The group of glandular cell abnormalities includes atypical glandular cells (AGC), which are further described by the terms endocervical, endometrial, or glandular cells not

Table 19.2 Bethesda System 2001

Specimen Type: *Indicate conventional smear (Pap smear) vs. liquid based vs. other*

Specimen Adequacy

- Satisfactory for evaluation (describe presence or absence of endocervical/transformation zone component and any other quality indicators, e.g., partially obscuring blood, inflammation, etc.)
- Unsatisfactory for evaluation... (*specify reason*)
  - Specimen rejected/not processed (*specify reason*)
  - Specimen processed and examined, but unsatisfactory for evaluation of epithelial abnormality because of (*specify reason*)

General Categorization (*optional*)

- Negative for intraepithelial lesion or malignancy
- Epithelial cell abnormality: See Interpretation/Result (*specify "squamous" or "glandular" as appropriate*)
- Other: See Interpretation/Result (*e.g., endometrial cells in a woman 40 years of age*)

Automated Review

If case examined by automated device, specify device and result.

Ancillary Testing

Provide a brief description of the test methods and report the result so that it is easily understood by the clinician.

Interpretation/Result

Negative for Intraepithelial Lesion or Malignancy (*when there is no cellular evidence of neoplasia, state this in the General Categorization above and/or in the Interpretation/Result section of the report, whether or not there are organisms or other nonneoplastic findings*)

Organisms

- Trichomonas vaginalis
- Fungal organisms morphologically consistent with *Candida* spp.
- Shift in flora suggestive of bacterial vaginosis
- Bacteria morphologically consistent with *Actinomyces* spp.
- Cellular changes consistent with herpes simplex virus

Other Nonneoplastic Findings (*optional to report; list not inclusive*):

- Reactive cellular changes associated with:
  - inflammation (includes typical repair)
  - radiation
  - intrauterine contraceptive device (IUD)
- Glandular cells status posthysterectomy
  - Atrophy

Other

- Endometrial cells (*in a woman 40 years of age*)
  (*specify if "negative for squamous intraepithelial lesion"*)

Epithelial Cell Abnormalities

Squamous Cell

- Atypical squamous cells
  - of undetermined significance (ASC-US)
  - cannot exclude HSIL (ASC-H)
- Low-grade squamous intraepithelial lesion (LSIL) encompassing: HPV/mild dysplasia/CIN 1
- High-grade squamous intraepithelial lesion (HSIL) encompassing: moderate and severe dysplasia, CIS/CIN 2 and CIN 3
  - with features suspicious for invasion (*if invasion is suspected*)
- Squamous cell carcinoma

(Continued)

Table 19.2 (*Continued*)

Glandular Cell

- Atypical
  - endocervical cells (not otherwise specified [NOS] *or specify in comments*)
  - endometrial cells (NOS *or specify in comments*)
  - glandular cells (NOS *or specify in comments*)
- Atypical
  - endocervical cells, favor neoplastic
  - glandular cells, favor neoplastic
- Endocervical adenocarcinoma *in situ*
- Adenocarcinoma
  - endocervical
  - endometrial
  - extrauterine
- NOS

Other Malignant Neoplasms (*specify*)

Educational Notes and Suggestions (*optional*)

Suggestions should be concise and consistent with clinical follow-up guidelines published by professional organizations (references to relevant publications may be included).

From **Solomon D, Davey D, Kurman R, et al.** The 2001 Bethesda System: terminology for reporting results of cervical cytology. *JAMA* 2002; 287:2114–2119. Available online at: www.bethesda2001.cancer.gov www.cancer.gov/newscenter/pressreleases/2002/bethesda2001

otherwise specified, depending on the presumptive origin, or modified to atypical *glandular cells favor neoplasia* in the presence of evidence of their origin (Table 19.2).

Cervical Cancer Precursors

Guidelines based on the literature were developed to guide cervical cancer screening, follow-up, and treatment. The evolving state of the science and our improved understanding of HPV and cervical carcinogenesis, and clinical practice and liability considerations, occasionally lead to subtle differences in the interpretation of these guidelines. Ultimately guidelines cannot substitute for an informed discussion of risks and benefits between a patient and health care provider in order to make decisions about treatment.

The 2002 American Cancer Society (ACS) recommended that screening with conventional Pap testing should occur every year. If liquid-based cytology is being used, screening can be extended to every 2 years. Beginning at the age of 30, women may be screened every 3 years using a combination of cytology and a high-risk HPV DNA test. **Screening should begin at the age of 21 or within 3 years of the onset of sexual activity, and screening can stop at age 70 if there were no abnormal Pap test result in the previous 10 years. Under these recommendations, screening after hysterectomy for benign (non-HPV related) disease is not necessary** (61).

The American College of Obstetricians and Gynecologists (ACOG) updated its guidelines (62). The ACOG recommends that women not initiate cervical cancer screening until they are 21, regardless of the onset of sexual activity. This acknowledges the very low prevalence of invasive cancer in very young women, the long multiyear process of cervical carcinogenesis, and the very low but real risks for preterm birth associated with outpatient excisional procedures. Likewise screening frequency was revised to every 2 years from age 21 to 29 (with either conventional slide or liquid-based cytology), and every 3 years for women after age 30 years if three consecutive negative, i.e., negative for intraepithelial lesion or malignancy (NILM) Pap tests can be documented. More frequent screening continues to be recommended for HIV-positive women (twice first year and annually after), those who are immune-suppressed, *diethylstilbestrol* (DES) daughters, and for those with a history of CIN 2 or greater (screen annually for 20 years). Discontinuation of screening is reasonable between 65 to 70 years, with reassessment of risk factors annually to determine if reinitiating screening is appropriate. Likewise in the setting of posthysterectomy for benign indications it is reasonable to discontinue screening in the absence of a history of high-grade CIN or cancer (Table 19.3).

Table 19.3 Comparison of Screening Guidelines from the American Cancer Society and the American College of Obstetricians and Gynecologists		
Comparison of Cervical Cytology Screening		
Guideline	*American Cancer Society*	*American College of Obstetricians and Gynecologists*
Initial screening	• Age 21 or 3 y after vaginal sex	• Age 21 or 3 y after vaginal sex
Interval	• Every year for conventional Pap • Every 2 years for liquid-based Pap • Every 2–3 y after age 30 with 3 consecutive normals	• Every year for either liquid-based Pap or conventional • Every 2–3 y after age 30 with 3 consecutive normals
Discontinue	• Age 70 if 3 consecutive normals in 10 y	• No upper limit of age

In 2003, the FDA approved **HPV DNA testing combined with cervical cytology as a screening technique for women older than age 30. When the results of both tests are negative, the woman does not have to be retested for 3 years. The negative predictive value of a double negative test exceeds 99%** (19). Because most HPV infections are transient, clear spontaneously, and do not lead to real cancer precursors (especially in young women), it should not be used for screening in women younger than 30 (63). Women who have negative test results for both cytology and HPV have a 1 in 1,000 chance of having CIN 2 or worse detected in the following 6 months (64). Prospective studies report less than 2 per 1,000 women will develop CIN 2 or greater in the following 3 years (64–66).

Atypical Squamous Cells

The ASC category is restricted to those test results disclosing abnormal cells that are truly of unknown significance. The ASC category does not include benign, reactive, and reparative changes, which are classified as normal in the Bethesda system. Because of the subjective diagnostic criteria and the fear of medical–legal action, the diagnosis is relatively common, ranging from 3% to 25% in some centers (67). When standardized diagnostic criteria are used, the rate of ASC results should be 3% to 5% (68). **The ASC category is subdivided into ASC-US and ASC-H.**

The cytologic diagnosis of ASC-US is associated with a 10% to 20% incidence of CIN 1 and a 3% to 5% risk for CIN 2 or 3 (69–72). It is apparent that CIN 1 is most often a benign HPV infection and will regress spontaneously in more than 60% of cases; therefore, the goal of triage of an ASC-US Pap test result is to identify more advanced CIN 2 and 3 lesions (73).

The option of repeat Pap testing is suboptimal because of a false-negative rate of 20% to 50% for identifying CIN lesions and practical issues with patient compliance. About 50% of patients will undergo colposcopy because of subsequent abnormal Pap test results, making this option nearly as costly as immediate colposcopy (69). **Immediate colposcopy is assumed to be the most sensitive method of detecting CIN 2 or 3** (69,72). Because 80% of patients will not have significant lesions, it is important to avoid overinterpretation of the colposcopic findings and to be conservative in performing biopsies. There is the risk that pathologists will overinterpret the biopsy results and the patient will be diagnosed with CIN when metaplasia is the only finding.

Several studies documented the usefulness of HPV testing in the assessment of ASC-US Pap test results (74–76). These studies demonstrate that HPV testing can identify 90% of the patients with CIN 2 or 3 lesions. To compare the aforementioned triage method in a prospective, randomized fashion, the NCI funded an ASC-US/LSIL Triage Study (ALTS) (77). Patients with ASC-US or LSIL were randomized to three triage arms: (i) immediate colposcopy, (ii) HPV test, and (iii) conservative management by repeat Pap test. There were 1,163 women in the immediate colposcopy group, and 14 refused the examination. The results of colposcopy are assumed to reflect the prevalent disease rates, which were as follows: CIN 1, 14.3%; CIN 2, 16.1%; and CIN 3, 5%. Thus, 75% of the women with ASC-US had negative colposcopy results and either did not have a biopsy (25%) or had a biopsy with negative results. The HPV test results were positive in 56.1% of the patients, and 6.1% of the patients did not return for colposcopy. Of the 494 who underwent colposcopy, the results were as follows: CIN 1, 22.5%; CIN 2, 11.9%;

587

and CIN 3, 15.6%. The sensitivity of HPV test was 95.9% for the detection of CIN 2 and 96.3% for the detection of CIN 3.

In the conservatively managed group, only one follow-up Pap test was reported. To be effective, Pap testing must be done every 6 months. Despite this, the results of the single follow-up Pap test were included. Using a cutoff that includes any positive finding of ASC-US or greater, the sensitivity is 85% for CIN 2 and 85.3% for CIN 3, with 58.6% of patients being referred for colposcopy. If LSIL is used as a cutoff, 26.2% of the patients are referred, with sensitivity of 64.0% for both CIN 2 and 3. Using HSIL as the cutoff, 6.9% are referred, and the sensitivity falls to 44%. **The conclusion of the ALTS trial is that HPV triage is highly sensitive in identifying CIN 2 and 3 lesions and that it cuts the rate of referral for colposcopy by approximately one-half** (78). When mathematical models are used to simulate the natural history of HPV and cervical cancer in a cohort of U.S. women, a 2- to 3-year screening strategy that uses cytologic assessment in combination with either HPV DNA testing or reflex HPV testing appears more effective and less costly in reducing the rate of cancer than annual conventional cytology (79).

Low-Grade Squamous Intraepithelial Lesions

The cytologic diagnosis of LSIL is reproducible and accounts for 1.6% of cytologic diagnoses (68). About 75% of the patients have CIN, with 20% being CIN 2 or 3 (69–71). These patients require additional evaluation. The ALTS trial closed the HPV test arm early because the HPV positivity rate was 82% and was not a valid discriminator in determining the presence of disease. The ALTS trial found that a cytology interpretation of LSIL is associated with a 25% risk of histologic CIN 2 or 3 within 2 years. No effective triage strategy was identified to spare many women from colposcopic referral without increasing their risk of CIN 3 and invasive carcinoma (80). **Guidelines confirm the validity of the current practice of performing colposcopy to evaluate a single LSIL result** (75).

High-Grade Squamous Intraepithelial Lesions

Any woman with a cytologic specimen suggesting the presence of HSIL should undergo colposcopy and directed biopsy (75). This is because two-thirds of patients with this cytologic finding will have CIN 2 or greater. After colposcopically directed biopsy and determination of the distribution of the lesion, excisional or ablative therapy that addresses the entire transformation zone should be performed.

Diagnosis

Colposcopy Findings

Acetowhite Epithelium   **Epithelium that turns white after application of acetic acid (3%–5%) is called *acetowhite epithelium* (53). The application of acetic acid coagulates the proteins of the nucleus and cytoplasm and makes the proteins opaque and white (5).**

The acetic acid does not affect mature, glycogen-producing epithelium because the acid does not penetrate below the outer one-third of the epithelium. The cells in this region have very small nuclei and a large amount of glycogen (not protein). These areas appear pink during colposcopy. Dysplastic cells are those most affected. They contain large nuclei with abnormally large amounts of chromatin (protein). The columnar villi become "plumper" after acetic acid is applied, making these cells easier to see. They appear slightly white, particularly in the presence of the beginning signs of metaplasia. The immature metaplastic cells have larger nuclei and show some effects of the acetic acid. Because the metaplastic epithelium is very thin, it is not as white or opaque as CIN but instead appears gray and filmy (5).

Leukoplakia   Translated literally, *leukoplakia* is white plaque (5). In colposcopic terminology, this plaque is white epithelium, visible before application of acetic acid. Leukoplakia is caused by a layer of keratin on the surface of the epithelium. Immature squamous epithelial cells have the potential to develop into keratin-producing cells or glycogen-producing cells. In the vagina and on the cervix, the normal differentiation is toward glycogen. Keratin production is abnormal in the cervicovaginal mucosa. Leukoplakia can be caused by HPV; keratinizing CIN; keratinizing carcinoma; chronic trauma from diaphragm, pessary, or tampon use; and radiotherapy.

Leukoplakia should not be confused with the white plaque of a monilial infection, which can be completely wiped off with a cotton-tipped applicator. The most common reason for leukoplakia is HPV infection (Fig. 19.8). Because it is not possible to see through the thick keratin layer

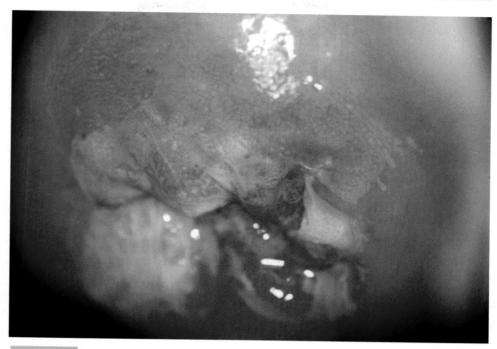

Figure 19.8 Colposcopy of cervical intraepithelial neoplasia 2 (CIN 2) associated with human papillomavirus (HPV) infection of the cervix.

to the underlying vasculature during colposcopy, such areas should undergo biopsy to rule out keratinizing carcinoma.

Punctation   Dilated capillaries terminating on the surface appear from the ends as a collection of dots and are referred to as punctation (Fig. 19.9). When these vessels occur in a well-demarcated area of acetowhite epithelium, they indicate an abnormal epithelium—

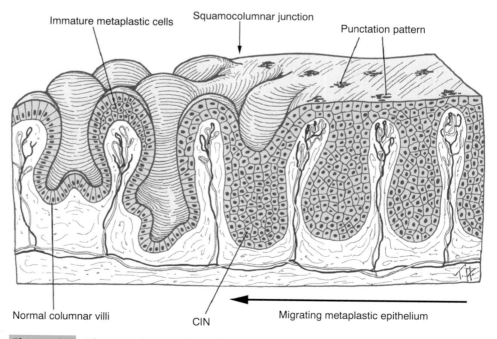

Figure 19.9 **Diagram of punctation.** The central capillaries of the columnar villi are preserved and produce the punctate vessels on the surface.

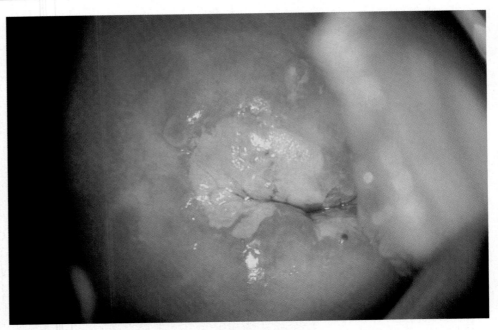

Figure 19.10 Human papillomavirus (HPV)/cervical intraepithelial neoplasia 2 (CIN 2) presents as a white lesion with surface spicules.

most often CIN (5) (Fig. 19.10). The punctate vessels are formed as the metaplastic epithelium migrates over the columnar villi. Normally, the capillary regresses; however, when CIN occurs, the capillary persists and appears more prominent.

Mosaic **Terminal capillaries surrounding roughly circular or polygonal-shaped blocks of acetowhite epithelium crowded together are called mosaic because their appearance is similar to mosaic tile** (Fig. 19.11). These vessels form a "basket" around the blocks of abnormal epithelium. They may arise from a coalescence of many terminal punctate vessels or from the vessels that surround the cervical gland openings (5). Mosaicism tends to be associated with higher-grade lesions and CIN 2 (Fig. 19.12) and CIN 3 (Fig. 19.13).

Atypical Vascular Pattern **Atypical vascular patterns are characteristic of invasive cervical cancer** and include looped vessels, branching vessels, and reticular vessels.

Endocervical Curettage **ASCCP guidelines do not require endocervical curettage. In cases when an endocervical sample is needed, a cytobrush is sufficient for sampling the endocervical canal.**

Cervical Biopsy **The cervical biopsy is performed at the area most likely to have dysplasia. If the lesion is large or multifocal, multiple biopsies may be necessary to ensure a complete sample of the affected tissue.**

Correlation of Findings **Ideally, both the pathologist and colposcopist should review the colposcopic findings and the results of cytologic assessment, cervical biopsy, and endocervical sample before deciding therapy.** This is particularly valuable when operators are learning the technique of colposcopy. Cytology results should not be sent to one laboratory and the histology results to another. When the cytology and biopsy results correlate, the colposcopist can be reasonably certain that the worst lesion was identified. If the cytology indicates a more significant lesion than the histology, the patient may require further evaluation, including repeat colposcopy, additional biopsies, and excisional diagnostic procedures under certain circumstances. An algorithm for the evaluation, treatment, and follow-up of abnormal Pap test results is presented in Figure 19.14.

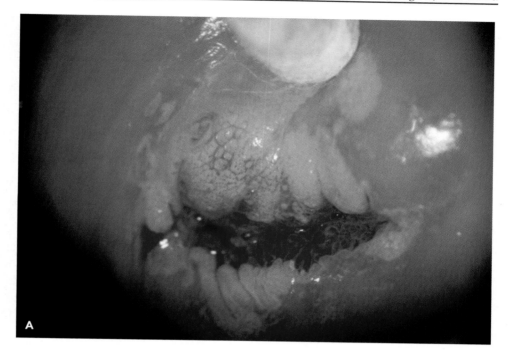

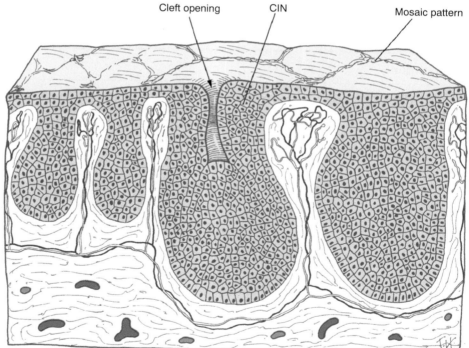

Figure 19.11   A: Mosaic pattern and punctation. This pattern develops as islands of dysplastic epithelium proliferate and push the ends of the superficial blood vessels away, creating a pattern that looks like mosaic tiles. **B:** Diagram of mosaic pattern.

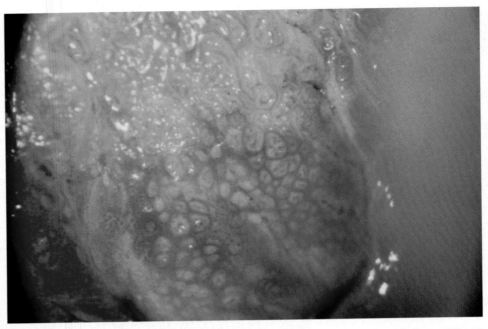

Figure 19.12   Human papillomavirus (HPV)/cervical intraepithelial neoplasia 3 (CIN 3). Cribriform pattern of HPV at periphery with mosaicism and punctation near the squamo-columnar junction.

Management

ASCCP 2006 Consensus Guidelines

The American Society for Colposcopy and Cervical Pathology (ASCCP) Consensus Guidelines were developed in 2001 for women with cytologic abnormalities and cervical cancer precursors and to incorporate the 2001 Bethesda System (46,81,82). Improved understanding of the pathogenesis and natural history of cervical HPV infection and cervical cancer precursors, combined with an appreciation of the impact of treatment of CIN on future pregnancy among young

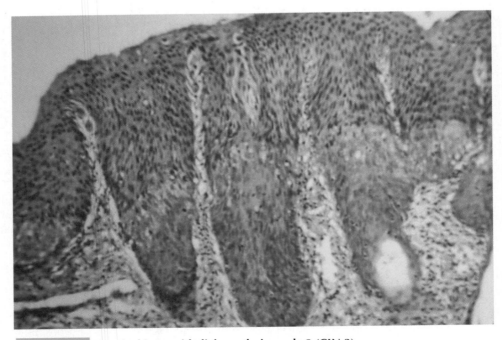

Figure 19.13   Cervical intraepithelial neoplasia grade 3 (CIN 3).

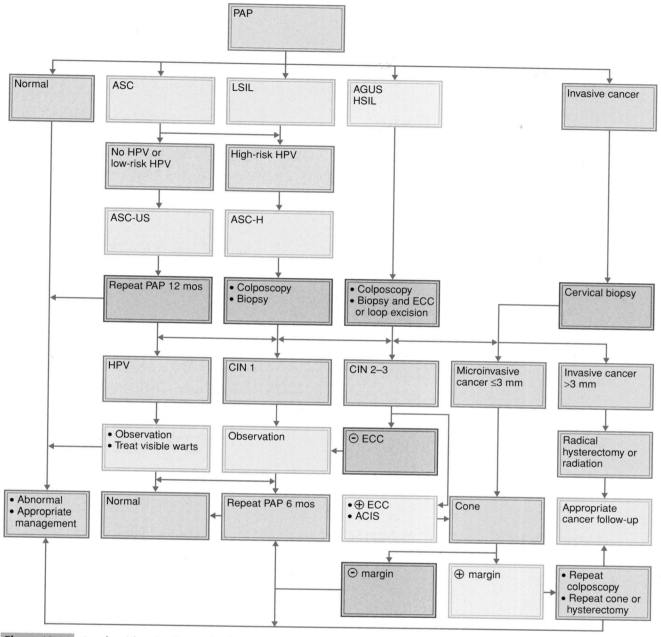

Figure 19.14 An algorithm for the evaluation, treatment, and follow-up of an abnormal Pap test.

women, and the management of adenocarcinoma *in situ* led to a critical review of the Guidelines (75,83).

In 2006, the **American Society for Colposcopy and Cervical Pathology (ASCCP) and the NCI sponsored a consensus conference** to update evidence-based guidelines for abnormal cervical cancer screening. **Comprehensive and specific guidelines for the management of cervical cytologic and histologic entities are available on the Web** (84). The ASCCP 2006 Consensus Guidelines for management based on cytologic findings are presented in Figure 19.15 and those based on histologic findings are in Figure 19.16.

Atypical Squamous Cells

Based on these recommendations, **women with ASC-US should be managed initially with either (i) two repeat Pap tests with referral for colposcopy for any significant abnormality, (ii) immediate colposcopy, or (iii) testing for high-risk type HPV** (Fig. 19.15A).

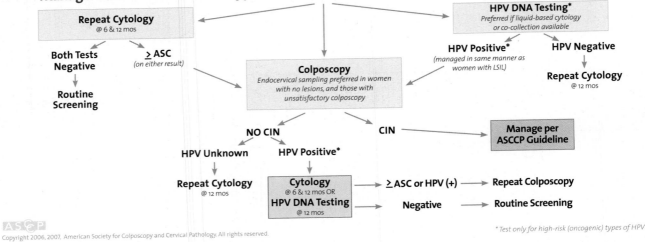

A **Management of Women with Atypical Squamous Cells of Undetermined Significance (ASC-US)**

HPV DNA Testing*
Preferred if liquid-based cytology or co-collection available

Repeat Cytology
@ 6 & 12 mos

HPV Positive*
(managed in same manner as women with LSIL)

HPV Negative

Both Tests Negative

≥ ASC
(on either result)

Colposcopy
Endocervical sampling preferred in women with no lesions, and those with unsatisfactory colposcopy

Repeat Cytology
@ 12 mos

Routine Screening

NO CIN

CIN

Manage per ASCCP Guideline

HPV Unknown

HPV Positive*

Repeat Cytology
@ 12 mos

Cytology
@ 6 & 12 mos OR
HPV DNA Testing
@ 12 mos

≥ ASC or HPV (+)

Repeat Colposcopy

Negative

Routine Screening

* Test only for high-risk (oncogenic) types of HPV

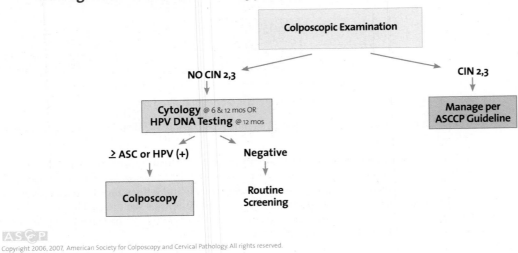

B **Management of Adolescent Women with Either Atypical Squamous Cells of Undetermined Significance (ASC-US) or Low-grade Squamous Intraepithelial Lesion (LSIL)**

Adolescent Women with ASC-US OR LSIL
(females 20 years and younger)

Repeat Cytology
@ 12 months

< HSIL

≥ HSIL

Repeat Cytology
@ 12 mos later

Colposcopy

Negative

≥ ASC

Routine Screening

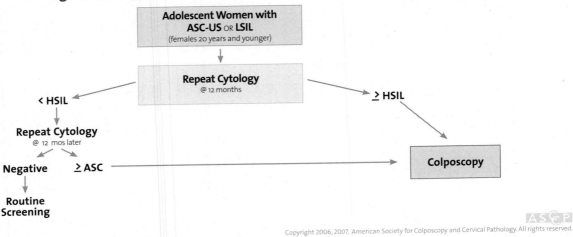

C **Management of Women with Atypical Squamous Cells: Cannot Exclude High-grade SIL (ASC - H)**

Colposcopic Examination

NO CIN 2,3

CIN 2,3

Cytology @ 6 & 12 mos OR
HPV DNA Testing @ 12 mos

Manage per ASCCP Guideline

≥ ASC or HPV (+)

Negative

Colposcopy

Routine Screening

Figure 19.15 **A–J: Algorithms from the 2006 Consensus Guidelines for the Management of Women with Cervical Cytologic Abnormalities.** Reprinted from the *Journal of Lower Tract Disease,* vol. 11, issue 4, with the permission of the ASCCP (© American Society for Colposcopy and Cervical Pathology 2007. No copies of the algorithms may be made without the prior consent of the ASCCP.)

D

Management of Women with Low-grade Squamous Intraepithelial Lesion (LSIL) *

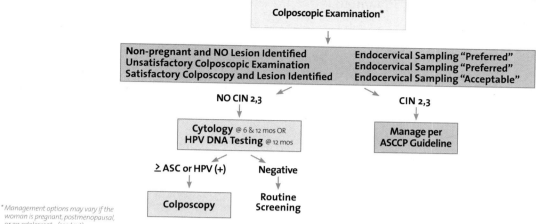

Management options may vary if the woman is pregnant, postmenopausal, or an adolescent - (see text)

E

Management of Pregnant Women with Low-grade Squamous Intraepithelial Lesion (LSIL)

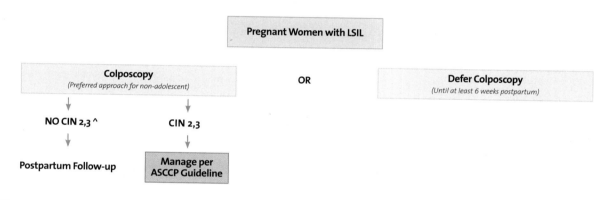

^ In women with no cytological, histological, or suspected CIN 2,3 or cancer

F

Management of Women with High-grade Squamous Intraepithelial Lesion (HSIL) *

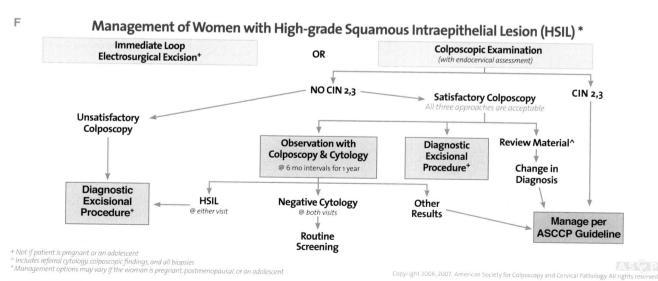

+ *Not if patient is pregnant or an adolescent*
^ *Includes referral cytology, colposcopic findings, and all biopsies*
* *Management options may vary if the woman is pregnant, postmenopausal, or an adolescent*

Figure 19.15 *(continued)*

G

Management of Adolescent Women (20 Years and Younger) with High-grade Squamous Intraepithelial Lesion (HSIL)

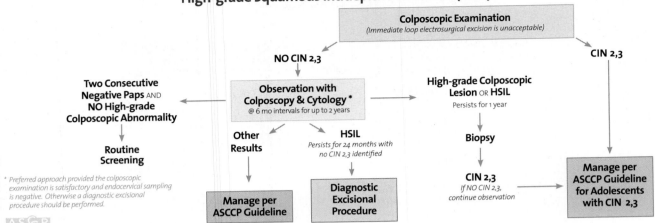

Colposcopic Examination
(Immediate loop electrosurgical excision is unacceptable)

NO CIN 2,3

CIN 2,3

Two Consecutive Negative Paps AND **NO High-grade Colposcopic Abnormality**

Observation with Colposcopy & Cytology *
@ 6 mo intervals for up to 2 years

High-grade Colposcopic Lesion OR **HSIL**
Persists for 1 year

Routine Screening

Other Results

HSIL
Persists for 24 months with no CIN 2,3 identified

Biopsy

Manage per ASCCP Guideline for Adolescents with CIN 2,3

* *Preferred approach provided the colposcopic examination is satisfactory and endocervical sampling is negative. Otherwise a diagnostic excisional procedure should be performed.*

Manage per ASCCP Guideline

Diagnostic Excisional Procedure

CIN 2,3
If NO CIN 2,3, continue observation

H

Initial Workup of Women with Atypical Glandular Cells (AGC)

All Subcategories
(except atypical endometrial cells)

Atypical Endometrial Cells

Colposcopy *(with endocervical sampling)*
AND **HPV DNA Testing** ^
AND **Endometrial Sampling**
(if > 35 yrs or at risk for endometrial neoplasia)*

Endometrial AND **Endocervical Sampling**

NO Endometrial Pathology

Colposcopy

^ *If not already obtained. Test only for high-risk (oncogenic) types.*
* *Includes unexplained vaginal bleeding or conditions suggesting chronic anovulation.*

I

Subsequent Management of Women with Atypical Glandular Cells (AGC)

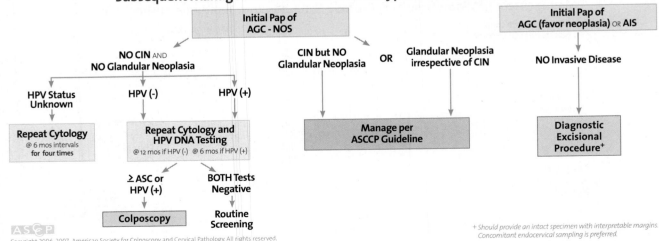

Initial Pap of AGC - NOS

Initial Pap of AGC (favor neoplasia) OR **AIS**

NO CIN AND **NO Glandular Neoplasia**

CIN but NO Glandular Neoplasia   OR   **Glandular Neoplasia irrespective of CIN**

NO Invasive Disease

HPV Status Unknown

HPV (-)

HPV (+)

Repeat Cytology
@ 6 mos intervals for four times

Repeat Cytology and HPV DNA Testing
@ 12 mos if HPV (-) @ 6 mos if HPV (+)

Manage per ASCCP Guideline

Diagnostic Excisional Procedure⁺

≥ ASC or HPV (+)

BOTH Tests Negative

Colposcopy

Routine Screening

+ *Should provide an intact specimen with interpretable margins. Concomitant endocervical sampling is preferred.*

Figure 19.15   *(continued)*

J

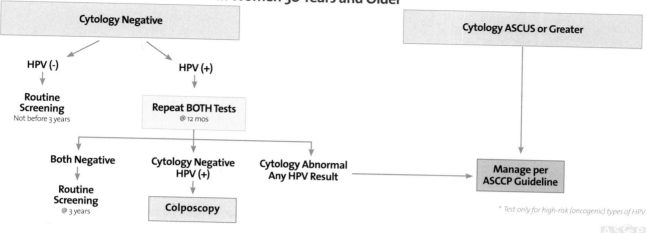

Figure 19.15   (*continued*)

Testing for HPV DNA is the preferred method when liquid-based cytology is used or when co-collection is feasible. Women who have positive test results should be referred for colposcopy, and those with negative results should receive yearly cytology assessment (75). Adolescent women with ASC-US or LSIL should have a repeat cytology in 12 months (Fig. 19.15B). **Women with ASC-H should be referred to colposcopy, they do not benefit from triage with high-risk HPV testing** (Fig 19.15C). The management of cytologic abnormalities with findings of LSIL and HSIL are presented in Figure 19.15 D–F, and AGC in Figures 19.15H and 19.15I, and for adolescent women with HSIL in Figure 19.15H.

CIN 1

The spontaneous regression rate of biopsy-proven CIN 1 is 60% to 85% in prospective studies. The regressions typically occur within a 2-year follow-up with cytology and colposcopy (4,75,85–88). **Patients who have biopsy proven CIN 1 (after a cytologic finding of ASC, ASC-H, LSIL) with satisfactory colposcopy and who agree to the evaluation every 6 months may be followed with Pap testing performed at 6 and 12 months or HPV DNA testing at 12 months. After two negative test results or a single negative HPV DNA test, routine screening may be resumed** (75). **Colposcopy and repeat cytology at 12 months or a diagnostic excisional procedure may be necessary if the CIN 1 biopsy was preceded by an HSIL or AGC cytology** (75). Regression of CIN 1 decreases after 24 months, with the regression rate becoming the same as for CIN 2 by 5 years (89).

For patients with persistent CIN 1 after 24 months, the choice of treatment is optional. Expectant management is acceptable, as long as the patient is cooperative with follow-up. Patients with chronic systemic disease associated with immunosuppression, such as those requiring steroids, chemotherapy, or antirejection drugs, may have chronically persistent low-grade abnormalities. Ablative therapies, including cryotherapy or laser ablation, seem preferable to excisional procedures including loop electrosurgical excision procedure (LEEP) (75). A randomized prospective trial comparing cryosurgery with laser and LEEP showed no difference in persistent disease rate (4%) or recurrent disease rate (17%). Cryosurgery has the advantage of low cost and ease of use. The disadvantages are lack of tissue specimen, inability to adapt to lesion size, and posttreatment vaginal discharge. If colposcopy findings are unsatisfactory, ablative therapy should be avoided.

CIN 2 and 3

All CIN 2 and 3 lesions require treatment in women 21 years of age and older (75). **This recommendation is based on a meta-analysis showing that CIN 2 progresses to CIS in 20% of cases and to invasion in 5%. Progression of CIS to invasion is 5%** (90).

Management of Women with a Histological Diagnosis of Cervical Intraepithelial Neoplasia Grade 1 (CIN 1) Preceded by ASC-US, ASC-H, or LSIL Cytology

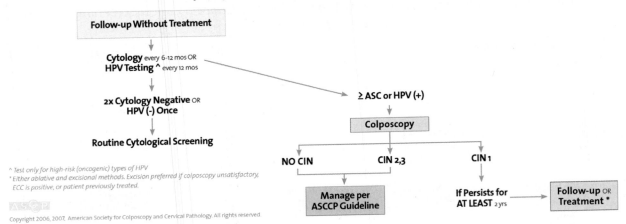

Follow-up Without Treatment

↓

Cytology every 6-12 mos OR
HPV Testing ^ every 12 mos

↓

2x Cytology Negative OR
HPV (-) Once

↓

Routine Cytological Screening

→ **≥ ASC or HPV (+)**

↓

Colposcopy

NO CIN   **CIN 2,3**   **CIN 1**

Manage per ASCCP Guideline

If Persists for AT LEAST 2 yrs → **Follow-up** OR **Treatment ***

^ Test only for high-risk (oncogenic) types of HPV
* Either ablative and excisional methods. Excision preferred if colposcopy unsatisfactory, ECC is positive, or patient previously treated.

Management of Women with a Histological Diagnosis of Cervical Intraepithelial Neoplasia - Grade 1 (CIN 1) Preceded by HSIL or AGC-NOS Cytology

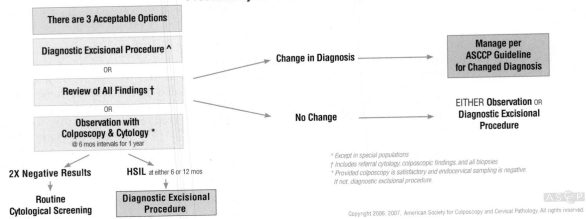

There are 3 Acceptable Options

Diagnostic Excisional Procedure ^

OR

Review of All Findings †

OR

Observation with Colposcopy & Cytology *
@ 6 mos intervals for 1 year

→ **Change in Diagnosis** → **Manage per ASCCP Guideline for Changed Diagnosis**

→ **No Change** → EITHER **Observation** OR **Diagnostic Excisional Procedure**

2X Negative Results   **HSIL** at either 6 or 12 mos

↓   ↓

Routine Cytological Screening   **Diagnostic Excisional Procedure**

^ Except in special populations
† Includes referral cytology, colposcopic findings, and all biopsies
* Provided colposcopy is satisfactory and endocervical sampling is negative. If not, diagnostic excisional procedure.

Management of Adolescent Women (20 Years and Younger) with a Histological Diagnosis of Cervical Intraepithelial Neoplasia - Grade 1 (CIN 1)

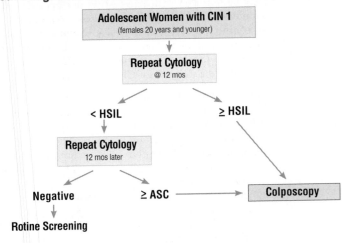

Adolescent Women with CIN 1
(females 20 years and younger)

↓

Repeat Cytology
@ 12 mos

< HSIL   **≥ HSIL**

↓

Repeat Cytology
12 mos later

Negative   **≥ ASC** → **Colposcopy**

↓

Rotine Screening

Figure 19.16   A–F: Algorithms from the 2006 Consensus Guidelines for the Management of Women with Cervical Histologic Abnormalities.   Reprinted from the *Journal of Lower Tract Disease,* vol. 11, issue 4, with the permission of the ASCCP (© American Society for Colposcopy and Cervical Pathology 2007. No copies of the algorithms may be made without the prior consent of the ASCCP.)

D

Management of Women with a Histological Diagnosis of Cervical Intraepithelial Neoplasia - (CIN 2,3) *

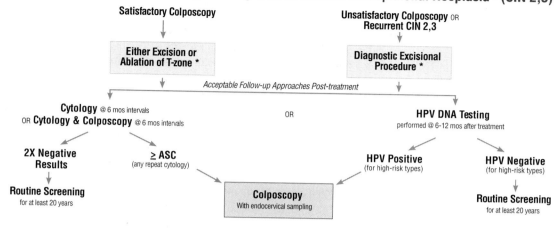

Satisfactory Colposcopy

Unsatisfactory Colposcopy OR Recurrent CIN 2,3

Either Excision or Ablation of T-zone *

Diagnostic Excisional Procedure *

Acceptable Follow-up Approaches Post-treatment

Cytology @ 6 mos intervals OR **Cytology & Colposcopy** @ 6 mos intervals

OR

HPV DNA Testing performed @ 6-12 mos after treatment

2X Negative Results

≥ ASC (any repeat cytology)

HPV Positive (for high-risk types)

HPV Negative (for high-risk types)

Routine Screening for at least 20 years

Colposcopy With endocervical sampling

Routine Screening for at least 20 years

* Management options will vary in special circumstances

E

Management of Adolescent and Young Women with a Histological Diagnosis of Cervical Intraepithelial Neoplasia - Grade 2,3 (CIN 2,3)

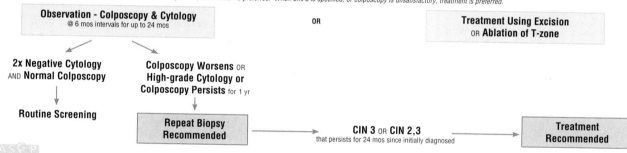

Adolescents and Young Women with CIN 2,3

Either treatment or observation is acceptable, provided colposcopy is satisfactory.
When CIN 2 is specified, observation is preferred. When CIN 3 is specified, or colposcopy is unsatisfactory, treatment is preferred.

Observation - Colposcopy & Cytology @ 6 mos intervals for up to 24 mos

OR

Treatment Using Excision OR **Ablation of T-zone**

2x Negative Cytology AND **Normal Colposcopy**

Colposcopy Worsens OR **High-grade Cytology or Colposcopy Persists** for 1 yr

Routine Screening

Repeat Biopsy Recommended

CIN 3 OR **CIN 2,3** that persists for 24 mos since initially diagnosed

Treatment Recommended

F

Management of Women with Adenocarcinoma *in-situ* (AIS) Diagnosed from a Diagnostic Excisional Procedure

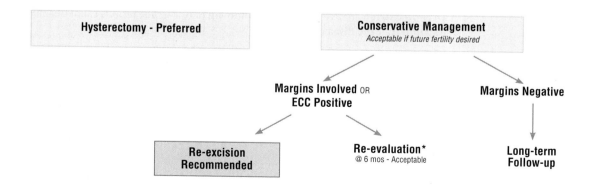

Hysterectomy - Preferred

Conservative Management
Acceptable if future fertility desired

Margins Involved OR **ECC Positive**

Margins Negative

Re-excision Recommended

Re-evaluation* @ 6 mos - Acceptable

Long-term Follow-up

* Using a combination of cytology, HPV testing, and colposcopy with endocervical sampling

Figure 19.16 *(continued)*

In recognition of the small but real risk for preterm birth, young women less than 20 years may be offered a program of surveillance with cytology and colposcopy at 6-month intervals with treatment only for persistence at 24 months (75). The heterogeneity of CIN 2 lesions is significant and regression rates are higher than for CIN 3. The histological distinction between CIN 2 and CIN 3 remains subjective and these diagnoses are combined in the 2006 Consensus Guidelines.

Although CIN can be treated with a variety of techniques, the preferred treatment for CIN 2 and 3 is LEEP. This allows a specimen to be sent for evaluation and enables the pathologist to identify occult microinvasive cancer or adenomatous lesions to ensure these lesions were treated adequately. The persistent and recurrent disease rate posttreatment is estimated at 4% to 10% (91,92).

Most of the excisional and ablative techniques used to treat CIN can be performed in an outpatient setting, which is one of the main objectives in the management of this disease.

Because all therapeutic modalities carry an inherent recurrence rate of up to 10%, surveillance at 6-month intervals with cytology and colposcopy or alternatively with high-risk HPV testing at 6 to 12 months is required (75). Surveillance is continued until two consecutive negative results occur. Referral to colposcopy for any abnormal results is mandatory.

Ablative therapy is appropriate when the following conditions exist:

1. There is no evidence of microinvasive or invasive cancer on cytology, colposcopy, endocervical curettage, or biopsy.
2. The lesion is located on the ectocervix and can be seen entirely.
3. There is no involvement of the endocervix with high-grade dysplasia as determined by colposcopy and endocervical curettage.

Management Summary

This summary of the management of these histologic lesions is based on ASCCP 2006 Consensus Guidelines (adapted from MJ Campion [93]) (Fig 19.16):

CIN 1 Preceded by ASC-US, ASC-H or LSIL Cytology

1. **Women with a histologic diagnosis of CIN 1 preceded by ASC-US, ASC-H or LSIL cytology should be followed by yearly HPV-DNA testing or Pap tests every 6–12 months** (Fig. 19.16A). If HPV DNA testing remains positive or if repeat cytology is reported as ASC-US or greater, repeat colposcopy is recommended.
2. **If the HPV DNA test is negative or two consecutive Pap smears are reported as negative, return to routine screening is recommended.**
3. **If CIN 1 persists for 2 years or more, continued follow-up or treatment is appropriate. Treatment can be ablative or excisional.**
4. **If colposcopy is unsatisfactory or the endocervical sample is positive for a high-grade CIN, a diagnostic excisional procedure is recommended.**
5. **Two consecutive negative Pap tests in follow-up of low-grade lesions is not absolute indication that the disease regressed.**

CIN 1 Preceded by HSIL or AGC-NOS Cytology

1. **Women with a histologic diagnosis of CIN 1 diagnosed during the assessment of pap tests showing HSIL (CIN 2 or 3) or atypical glandular cells-not otherwise specified (AGC-NOS) can be managed by either an excisional diagnostic procedure or 6-monthly colposcopy and cytology for 1 year** (Fig 19.16B). Those with a cytological finding of AGC-NOS must have a satisfactory colposcopic examination and negative endocervical sampling.
2. **If the patient is followed expectantly, a diagnostic excisional procedure is recommended if the repeat cytology at either 6 or 12 months is HSIL or AGC-NOS.** If the histology of a colposcopically directed biopsy confirms high-grade CIN, the management is according to guidelines regardless of the cytology result.
3. **After two consecutive *negative for intraepithelial neoplasia or malignancy* results in follow-up, routine cytologic screening can be resumed.**

4. **If CIN 1 is preceded by HSIL or AGC-NOS cytology and colposcopy is unsatisfactory, a diagnostic excisional procedure is recommended, except in special circumstances** (e.g., pregnancy).

CIN 1 in Adolescents and Pregnancy

1. **For adolescents with CIN 1, follow-up with annual cytology is recommended** (Fig 19.16C). Only those with HSIL or greater at 12 months should be referred for colposcopy.

2. **At 24-months, those with ASC-US or greater should be referred.**

3. **Prospective follow-up by HPV DNA testing in this age group is not useful because of the high rate of positive results.**

CIN 2 or 3

1. **Both excisional and ablative procedures are acceptable treatment modalities for women with histologically proven CIN 2 or 3 with satisfactory colposcopy** (Fig. 19.16D). An excisional procedure is recommended for residual/recurrent CIN 2 or 3.

2. **Ablation is unacceptable for women with a histologic diagnosis of CIN 2 or 3 and unsatisfactory colposcopy.**

3. **Cytologic and colposcopic follow-up of CIN 2 or 3 is necessary only in specific circumstances.** Acceptable posttreatment follow-up options include cytology alone, every 6 months, combined cytology and colposcopy every 6 months, and HPV DNA testing at 6 to 12 months.

4. **If HPV DNA testing is positive or if the repeat cytology is ASC-US or greater, referral for colposcopy and endocervical sampling is recommended.**

5. **If HPV DNA testing is negative or if two consecutive posttreatment cytology results are *negative for intraepithelial lesion or malignancy*, routine screening for at least 20 years is recommended, and should be annual for at least 5 years.** A negative HPV DNA test is an excellent predictor of a normal posttreatment for CIN 2 or 3.

6. **If CIN 2 or 3 is histologically found at the margins of an excised specimen or in an endocervical sample obtained immediately after the procedure, cytologic follow-up with endocervical sampling every 4 to 6 months is preferred.** The role of colposcopy in this follow-up option is not clearly defined in the Guidelines, although in practice, cytology and colposcopy will be performed in most clinical settings.

7. **A repeat diagnostic excisional procedure is acceptable.** The Guidelines allow for hysterectomy if a repeat diagnostic excisional procedure is not feasible. An undisclosed invasive cancer within the endocervical canal must be excluded prior to hysterectomy.

8. **For women with histologically proven residual/recurrent CIN 2 or 3, the Guidelines permit a repeat excisional procedure or hysterectomy.**

CIN 2 or 3 in Adolescence and Pregnancy

1. **For adolescents with a histological diagnosis of CIN 2 or 3 not otherwise specified, the Guidelines state that either treatment or observation by cytology and colposcopy every 6 months for up to 24 months is acceptable provided colposcopy is satisfactory** (Fig 19.16E). **Allowing for the subjectivity in this histological distinction, observation is preferred for a diagnosis of CIN 2 alone, but treatment is acceptable.**

2. **Treatment is recommended for a histologic diagnosis of CIN 3 or if colposcopy is unsatisfactory.** Although invasive cervical cancer is very rare in this age group, prospective follow-up of a histological diagnosis of CIN 2 or 3, not otherwise specified, in young women should be limited to those women likely to be compliant with the recommendations.

3. **After 2 consecutive *negative for intraepithelial lesion or malignancy results*, implying negative cytology and colposcopy with satisfactory colposcopic examinations, adolescents and young women can return to routine cytologic screening.** An annual screening interval should be recommended.

4. **Treatment is recommended if CIN 3 is diagnosed histologically or if CIN 2 or 3 persists for 24 months.**

Cervical Adenocarcinoma *in situ* (AIS)

1. **Hysterectomy remains the preferred management recommendation for women with a histological diagnosis of AIS on a specimen from a diagnostic excisional procedure** (Fig 19.16F).

2. **A histologic diagnosis of AIS from a punch biopsy or a cytological diagnosis of AIS is not sufficient to justify hysterectomy without a diagnostic excisional procedure.** The difficulty in defining colposcopic limits of AIS lesions, the frequent extension of disease within the endocervical canal and the presence of multifocal, "skip-lesions" (i.e., lesions that are not contiguous) compromise conservative excisional procedures.

3. **Negative margins in an excisional specimen do not mean the lesion is completely excised.**

4. **If future fertility is desired, conservative excisional management is acceptable.** The overall failure rate of excision is less than 10%. Margin status is a useful clinical predictor of residual disease as is endocervical sampling at the time of excision.

5. **If a conservative excisional procedure is performed and margins are involved or the endocervical sample at the time of excision shows AIS or CIN, reexcision is recommended.**

6. **A reassessment at 6 months using a combination of cytology, colposcopy, HPV DNA testing, and endocervical sampling is acceptable. Long-term follow-up is recommended for women who do not undergo hysterectomy for AIS.**

Treatment Modalities

Cryotherapy

Cryotherapy destroys the surface epithelium of the cervix by crystallizing the intracellular water, resulting in the eventual destruction of the cell. The temperature needed for effective destruction must be in the range of ($-20°$ to $-30°C$). Nitrous oxide ($-89°C$) and carbon dioxide ($-65°C$) produce temperatures below this range and, therefore, are the most commonly used gases for this procedure.

The technique believed to be most effective is a freeze-thaw-freeze method in which an ice ball is achieved 5 mm beyond the edge of the probe. The time required for this process is related to the pressure of the gas; the higher the pressure, the faster the ice ball is achieved. Cryotherapy is an effective treatment for CIN with very acceptable failure rates under certain conditions (94–97). It is a relatively safe procedure with few complications. Cervical stenosis is rare but can occur. Posttreatment bleeding is uncommon and is usually related to infection.

Cure rates are related to the grade of the lesion; CIN 3 has a greater chance of treatment failure (Table 19.4). Townsend showed that cures are related to the size of the lesion; those covering most of the ectocervix have failure rates as high as 42%, compared with a 7% failure rate for lesions less than 1 cm in diameter (99). Positive findings on endocervical curettage can reduce the cure rate significantly. Endocervical gland involvement is important because the failure rate

Table 19.4 Results of Cryotherapy for Cervical Intraepithelial Neoplasia (CIN) Compared with Grade of CIN

Author (ref. no.)	CIN 1		CIN 2		CIN 3	
	No.	Failure (%)	No.	Failure (%)	No.	Failure (%)
Ostergard (95)	13/205	6.3	7/93	7.5	9/46	19.6
Creasman et al. (96)	15/276	5.4	17/235	7.2	46/259	17.8
Benedet et al. (97)	7/143	4.9	19/448	4.2	65/1,003	6.5
Anderson and Hartley (98)			9/123	7.3	17/74	23.0
Total	35/624	5.6	50/899	5.6	137/1,382	9.9

Table 19.5 Success Rate for Laser Vaporization

Author (ref. no.)	CIN 1		CIN 2		CIN 3	
	No.	NED (%)	No.	NED (%)	No.	NED (%)
Burke (100)	49	41 (83.6)	42	36 (85.7)	40	31 (77.5)
Wright et al. (101)	110	108 (98.2)	140	133 (95)	190	179 (94.2)
Rylander et al. (102)	22	21 (95.5)	49	48 (97.9)	133	116 (87.2)
Jordan et al. (103)	142	140 (98.6)	153	145 (94.7)	416	390 (93.8)
Benedet et al. (104)	312	301 (96.5)	472	428 (90.7)	773	702 (90.8)
Baggish et al. (105)	741	675 (91.1)	1,048	978 (93.3)	1,281	1,228 (96)
TOTAL	1,376	1,286 (93.5)	1,904	1,768 (92.9)	2,833	2,646 (93.4)

NED, no evidence of disease.

in women with gland involvement was 27%, compared with 9% in those who did not have such involvement (98).

Cryotherapy should be considered acceptable therapy when the following criteria are met:

1. CIN 1 that has persisted for 24 months, or CIN 2
2. Small lesion
3. Ectocervical location only
4. Negative endocervical sample
5. No endocervical gland involvement on biopsy

Laser Ablation

Although rarely used in practice, laser ablation was used effectively for the treatment of CIN (Table 19.5). The expense of the equipment combined with the necessity for special training limited the use of laser ablation. Most early CIN is now managed expectantly, so the need for ablation is decreasing.

Loop Electrosurgical Excision

Loop electrosurgical excision is a valuable tool for the diagnosis and treatment of CIN (106–116). It offers the advantage of performing an operation that is simultaneously diagnostic and therapeutic during one outpatient visit (100–105,117–122).

The tissue effect of electricity depends on the concentration of electrons (size of the wire), the power (watts), and the water content of the tissue. If low power or a large-diameter wire is used, the effect will be electrocautery, and the thermal damage to tissue will be extensive. If the power is high (35–55 watts) and the wire loop is small (0.5 mm), the effect will be electrosurgical, and the tissue will have little thermal damage. The actual cutting is a result of a steam envelope developing at the interface between the wire loop and the water-laden tissue. This envelope is pushed through the tissue, and the combination of electron flow and acoustical events separates the tissue. After the excision, a 5-mm diameter ball electrode is used, and the power is set at 50 watts. The ball is placed near the surface so that a spark occurs between the ball and the tissue. This process is called *electrofulguration,* and it results in some thermal damage that leads to hemostasis. If too much fulguration occurs, the patient will develop an eschar with more discharge, and the risk for infection and late bleeding will be higher.

Research shows that LEEP is associated with an increased risk of overall preterm delivery, preterm delivery after premature rupture of membranes, and low-birth-weight infants in subsequent pregnancies at greater than 20 weeks gestation (123). **Loop excision should not be used before an intraepithelial lesion is identified with histopathology. Although "see and treat" may be appropriate in certain settings and among populations for whom follow-up is not possible, the potential excision of the entire transformation zone along with varying amounts of the cervical canal, may compromise birth outcomes (114,116). This is particularly true for young women, who may have large, immature transformation zones with**

Table 19.6 Therapeutic Efficiency of Cervical Conization: Comparison between Laser and Knife Techniques

Percentage of patients who are "cured" by conization

Author (ref. no.)	Laser (%)	Author (ref. no.)	Knife (%)
Wright et al. (101)	96.2	**Larsson et al.** (118)	94.0
Baggish et al. (105)	97.5	**Bostofte et al.** (119)	90.2
Larsson et al. (118)	95.6	**Bjerre et al.**[a] (120)	94.8
Bostofte et al. (119)	93.2	**Kolstad and Klem**[a] (121)	97.6

[a]Patients had negative cone margins.

extensive acetowhite areas. Complications following loop electrosurgical excision are minimal and compare favorably with those following laser ablation and conization. Intraoperative hemorrhage, postoperative hemorrhage, and cervical stenosis can occur but at low rates, as noted in Table 19.6. The SCJ is visible in more than 90% of patients after this procedure. Effectiveness of LEEP and comparison of LEEP to other excision procedures are shown in Tables 19.7 through 19.9.

Conization

Conization of the cervix plays an important role in the management of CIN. Before the availability of colposcopy, conization was the standard method of evaluating an abnormal Pap test result. **Conization is both a diagnostic and therapeutic procedure and has the advantage over ablative therapies of providing tissue for further evaluation to rule out invasive cancer** (117,118,120,124).

Conization is indicated for diagnosis in women with HSIL or AGC-adenocarcinoma *in situ* and may be considered under the following conditions:

1. **Limits of the lesion cannot be visualized with colposcopy.**
2. **The SCJ is not seen at colposcopy.**
3. **Endocervical curettage (ECC) histologic findings are positive for CIN 2 or CIN 3.**
4. **Substantial lack of correlation between cytology, biopsy, and colposcopy results.**
5. **Microinvasion is suspected based on biopsy, colposcopy, or cytology results.**
6. **The colposcopist is unable to rule out invasive cancer.**

Lesions with positive margins are more likely to recur after conization (117,118,120) (Table 19.10). Endocervical gland involvement is predictive of recurrence (23.6% with gland involvement compared with 11.3% without gland involvement) (125). When compared with conization, LEEP is the simpler technique, and short-term results are similar to those obtained with conization or laser excision (91,126). **In a prospective study examining the long-term effects of LEEP, conization, and laser excision, no difference in recurrence of dysplasia or in pregnancy outcomes was found** (127) (Tables 19.11 and 19.12).

Table 19.7 Perioperative and Postoperative Bleeding from Cervical Conization: Comparison between Laser and Knife Techniques

Percentage of patients undergoing conization who develop significant vaginal bleeding

Author (ref. no.)	Laser (%)	Author (ref. no.)	Knife (%)
Wright et al. (101)	12.2	**Larsson et al.** (118)	14.8
Baggish (117)	2.5	**Bostofte et al.** (119)	17.0
Larsson et al. (118)	2.3	**Jones** (122)	10.0
Bostofte et al. (119)	5.0	**Luesley et al.** (124)	13.0

Table 19.8 Complications of Electrosurgical Excision

Author (ref. No.)	No. of Patients	Operative Hemorrhage	Postoperative Hemorrhage	Cervical Stenosis
Prendiville et al. (106)	111	2	2	—
Whiteley et al. (107)	80	0	3	—
Mor-Yosef et al. (108)	50	1	3	—
Bigrigg et al. (109)	1,000	0	6	—
Gunasekera et al. (110)	98	0	0	—
Howe and Vincenti (111)	100	0	1	—
Minucci et al. (112)	130	0	1	2
Wright et al. (113)	432	0	8	2
Luesley et al. (114)	616	0	24	7
TOTAL	2,617	3 (0.001%)	48 (1.8%)	11/6178 (1.0%)

Hysterectomy

Hysterectomy is considered a treatment of last resort for recurrent high-grade CIN. In a study of 38 cases of invasive cancer occurring after hysterectomy among 8,998 women (0.4%), the incidence of significant bleeding, infection, and other complications, including death, is higher with hysterectomy than with other means of treating CIN (128). There are some situations in which hysterectomy remains a valid and appropriate (although not mandatory) method of treatment for CIN:

1. Microinvasion
2. CIN 3 at the endocervical limits of conization specimen in selected patients
3. Poor compliance with follow-up
4. Other gynecologic problems requiring hysterectomy, such as fibroids, prolapse, endometriosis, and pelvic inflammatory disease
5. Histologically confirmed recurrent high-grade CIN

Glandular Cell Abnormalities

Atypical Glandular Cells

The Bethesda System created the term *atypical glandular cells* to describe the spectrum of glandular cell abnormalities. This classification is subdivided with the qualifier into the categories

Table 19.9 Unsuspected Invasion in Electrosurgical Excision Specimens

Author (ref. no.)	Patients	Microinvasive	Invasive
Prendiville et al. (106)	102	1	—
Bigrigg et al. (109)	1,000	5	—
Gunasekera et al. (110)	98	—	1
Howe and Vincenti (111)	100	1	—
Wright et al. (113)	141	3	—
Luesley et al. (114)	616	1	—
Chappatte et al. (116)	100	4	6 (adenocarcinoma *in situ*)
TOTAL	2,157	15 (0.7%)	1 (0.04%)

Table 19.10 Grade of Discomfort of Large-Loop Excision versus Laser Conization

Side Effect	Loop Excision (n = 98)	Laser (n = 101)
Not unpleasant	80 (92%)	32 (32%)
Moderately unpleasant	16 (16%)	50 (50%)
Very unpleasant	2 (2%)	19 (18%)
Operative time	20–50 sec (mean, 16 sec)	4–15 min (mean, 6.5 min)

From **Gunasekera PC, Phipps JH, Lewis BV.** Large loop excision of the transformation zone (LLETZ) compared to carbon dioxide laser in the treatment of CIN: a superior mode of treatment. *Br J Obstet Gynaecol* 1990;97:995–998, with permission.

favor neoplasia and *not otherwise specified* (NOS). The latter qualified with the cell of origin when identifiable as either endocervical or endometrial origin. Included in the glandular cell category is endocervical carcinoma *in situ* and adenocarcinoma (129).

Atypical glandular cells are important because of their risk for significant disease. In a series of 63 patients from whom subsequent cervical biopsy or hysterectomy specimens were evaluated, 17 women had CIN 2 or 3, five women had adenocarcinoma *in situ*, and two women had invasive adenocarcinoma (125). An additional eight patients had CIN 1, and two women had endometrial hyperplasia. Overall, 32 patients (50.8%) had significant cervical lesions. This is a much higher positive rate than that for ASC-US Pap test results.

Adenocarcinoma

In adenocarcinoma *in situ* (AIS), the endocervical glandular cells are replaced by tall columnar cells with nuclear stratification, hyperchromasia, irregularity, and increased mitotic activity (130). Cellular proliferation results in crowded, cribriform glands. The normal branching pattern of the endocervical glands is maintained. Most neoplastic cells resemble those of the endocervical mucinous epithelium. Endometrioid and intestinal cell types occur less often. About 50% of women with cervical AIS have squamous CIN. Some of the AIS lesions represent incidental findings in specimens removed for treatment of squamous neoplasia. **Because AIS is located near or above the transformation zone, conventional cervical specimens may not be effective for detecting glandular disease. Obtaining good endocervical specimens by cytobrush may improve detection of AIS.** If the focus of AIS is small, cervical biopsy and endocervical curettage may have negative findings. In such cases, a more comprehensive survey of the cervix by diagnostic conization may be necessary. This type of specimen allows exclusion of coexisting invasive adenocarcinoma. **The term *microinvasion* should not be used to describe adenocarcinomas.** After the gland is invaded, it is methodologically problematic to estimate a true "depth of invasion" because the invasion may have originated from the mucosal surface or the periphery of the underlying glands. The "breakthrough" of the basement membrane cannot be described; therefore, the tumor is either AIS or invasive adenocarcinoma.

Table 19.11 Results of Loop Electrosurgical Excision

Author (ref. no.)	Patients Treated	Patients Recurred
Prendiville et al. (106)	102	2
Whiteley et al. (107)	80	4
Bigrigg et al. (109)	1,000	41
Gunasekera et al. (110)	98	7
Luesley et al. (114)	616	27
Murdoch et al. (115)	600	16
Total	2,496	97 (3.9%)

Table 19.12 Recurrence of Cervical Intraepithelial Neoplasia After Cone Biopsy			
Author (ref. no.)	*No. of Patients*	*Negative Margins*	*Positive Margins*
Larsson et al. (118)	683	56	246
Bjerre et al. (120)	1,226	64	429
Kolstad and Klem (121)	1,121	27	291
TOTAL	3,030	147 (4.9%)	966 (31.9%)

With the recent apparent increase in invasive adenocarcinoma of the endocervix, more attention is directed toward AIS. There is evidence that AIS may progress to invasive cancer (108). In a series of 52 cases of adenocarcinoma of the uterine cervix, the results of 18 endocervical biopsies were interpreted as negative 3 to 7 years before the presentation with cancer (130). In five of these cases, AIS was found. In a study of the anatomic distribution of AIS in 23 women, all patients had AIS involving both the surface and the glandular endocervical epithelium, often with the deepest glandular cleft involved (131). The entire endocervical canal was at risk; nearly one-half of the patients had lesions 1.5 to 3 cm from the external os. Overall, 15 patients had unifocal disease, 3 had multifocal disease, and 5 had AIS of undermined type; 11 of the 23 patients had squamous intraepithelial lesions and AIS. In a study of 40 patients with AIS who had cervical conization, 23 of 40 patients (58%) had coexisting squamous intraepithelial lesions and 2 had invasive squamous cell carcinoma (128). Of the 22 patients who underwent hysterectomy, the margins on the cone specimen were positive in 10 patients, and 70% had residual AIS, including 2 patients with foci of invasive adenocarcinoma. One of the 12 patients with negative margins had focal residual adenocarcinoma in the hysterectomy specimen, and 18 women had conization only with negative margins and no relapse of disease after a medium interval of 3 years. Thus, positive margins on the conization specimen are significant findings in these patients (132).

In a more alarming study of 28 patients with AIS, of the 8 patients with positive margins who underwent repeat conization or hysterectomy, 3 had residual AIS and 1 patient had invasive adenocarcinoma (133). Of 10 patients with negative margins who underwent hysterectomy or repeat conization, 4 had residual AIS. One patient in whom the cone margin could not be evaluated had invasive adenocarcinoma. Of the 15 patients treated conservatively with repeat conization of the cervix and close follow-up, 7 (47%) had a recurrent glandular lesion detected after the conization, including invasive adenocarcinoma in 2 women. A glandular lesion was not suspected in 48% of the patients, based on Pap test and endocervical curettage results obtained before conization of the cervix.

AIS must be considered a serious cancer precursor of adenocarcinoma. The entire endocervical canal is at risk, and detection of the lesion with cytologic assessment or endocervical curettage may not be reliable. Any patient with a positive cone margin should undergo repeat conization. If fertility is not desired, a hysterectomy should be performed because of the risk of recurrence, even in the presence of negative margins.

Vaginal Intraepithelial Neoplasia

VAIN often accompanies CIN and is believed to share a common etiology (134). Such lesions may be extensions onto the vagina from the CIN, or they may be satellite lesions occurring mainly in the upper vagina. **Because the vagina does not have a transformation zone with immature epithelial cells to be infected by HPV, the mechanism of entry for HPV is by way of microabrasions resulting primarily from insertional sexual activity.** As these abrasions heal with metaplastic squamous cells, the HPV may begin its growth in a manner similar to that in the cervical transformation zone. VAIN lesions are asymptomatic. Because they often accompany active HPV infection, the patient may report vulvar warts or an odoriferous vaginal discharge from vaginal warts.

Screening

Women with an intact cervix should undergo routine cytologic screening. **Because VAIN is nearly always accompanied by CIN, the Pap test result is likely to be positive when VAIN is**

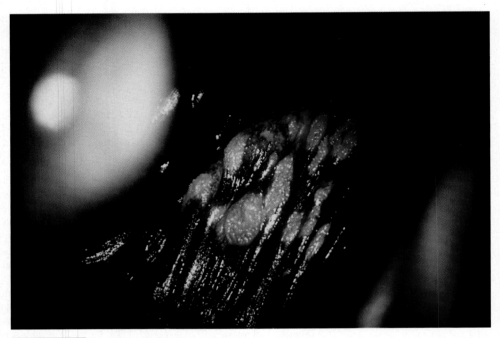

Figure 19.17 Human papillomavirus (HPV)/vaginal intraepithelial neoplasia grade 1 (VAIN 1). Note the surface spicules with partial uptake of Lugol's stain.

present. The vagina should be carefully inspected by colposcopic examination at the time of colposcopy for any CIN lesion. Particular attention should be paid to the upper vagina. **Women who have persistent abnormal Pap tests without evident cervical pathology and those with abnormal cytology after treatment of CIN should be examined carefully for VAIN.** For women in whom the cervix was removed for high-grade cervical neoplasia, Pap testing should be performed at regular intervals (e.g., yearly), depending on the diagnosis and severity of lesion.

Diagnosis

Colposcopic examination and directed biopsy are the mainstays of diagnosis of VAIN. Typically, the lesions are located along the vaginal ridges, are ovoid in shape and slightly raised, and often have surface spicules. VAIN 1 lesions usually are accompanied by a significant amount of koilocytosis, indicating their HPV origin (Fig. 19.17). VAIN 2 exhibits a thicker acetowhite epithelium, a more raised external border, and less iodine uptake (Fig. 19.18A). When VAIN 3 occurs, the surface may become papillary, and the vascular patterns of punctation and mosaic may occur (Fig. 19.18B). Early invasion is typified by vascular patterns similar to those of the cervix.

Treatment

Patients with VAIN 1 and HPV infection do not require treatment. These lesions often regress, are multifocal, and recur quickly when treated with ablative therapy. VAIN 2 lesions can be managed expectantly or treated by ablation. VAIN 3 lesions are more likely to harbor an early invasive lesion. In a study of 32 patients who underwent upper vaginectomy for VAIN 3, occult invasive carcinoma was found in 9 patients (28%) (135). It is recommended in older patients that VAIN 3 lesions located in the dimples of the vaginal cuff be excised to rule out occult invasive cancer. **VAIN 3 lesions that are adequately sampled to rule out invasive disease can be treated with laser therapy. The major advantage of laser vaporization therapy is the ability to control the depth and width of destruction by direct vision through the colposcope.** The other advantage of laser therapy is the rapid posttreatment healing phase. This process takes about 3 to 4 weeks, after which time a new epithelium has formed completely and, in most cases, has a mature glycogen-containing epithelium.

Tissue Interaction   When the laser beam contacts tissue, its energy is absorbed by the water in the cells, causing it to boil instantly. The cells explode into a puff of vapor (thus the term *laser*

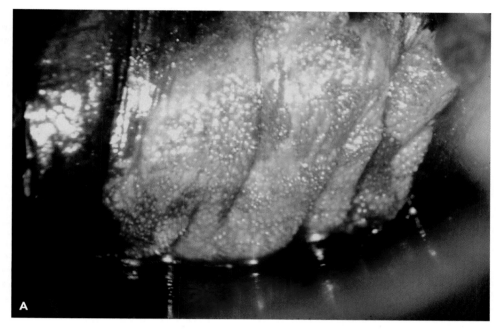

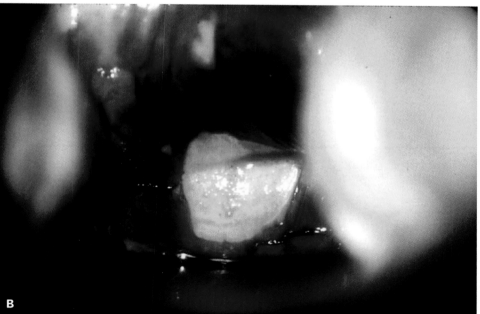

Figure 19.18   A: Vaginal intraepithelial neoplasia grade 2 (VAIN 2). B: Vaginal intraepithelial neoplasia grade 3 (VAIN 3).

vaporization). The protein and mineral content is incinerated by the heat and leaves a charred appearance at the base of the exposed area. The depth of laser destruction is a function of the power of the beam (in watts), the area of the beam (in millimeters squared), and the length of time the laser remains in the tissue. The beam must be moved uniformly across the tissue surface to prevent deep destruction. The laser beam vaporizes a central area and leaves a narrow zone of heat necrosis surrounding the laser crater. The goal of laser vaporization is to minimize the area of tissue necrosis. This goal is accomplished by using high wattage (20 watts) with medium beam size (1.5 mm) and moving the beam uniformly but quickly over the surface. The zone of thermal necrosis will be 0.1 mm when the laser is used in this manner. Some lasers have a function called *super pulse,* in which the laser beam is electronically switched off and on thousands of times per second, thereby allowing the tissue to cool between pulses to create less thermal necrosis.

Cryosurgery should not be used in the vagina because the depth of injury cannot be controlled and inadvertent injury to the bladder or rectum may occur. Superficial fulguration with electrosurgical ball cautery may be used under colposcopic control to observe the depth of destruction by wiping away the epithelial tissue as it is ablated. Excision is an excellent method for treatment of upper vaginal lesions in a small area. Occasionally, total vaginectomy will be required for a VAIN 3 lesion occupying the entire vagina. It should be accompanied by a split-thickness skin graft. This aggressive treatment for widespread vaginal lesions should not be used for VAIN 2.

The malignant potential of VAIN appears to be less than that of CIN. In a review of 136 cases of CIS of the vagina over a 30-year period, 4 cases (3%) progressed to invasive vaginal cancer despite the use of various treatment methods (134).

Vulvar Intraepithelial Disease

Vulvar Dystrophies

In the past, terms such as *leukoplakia, lichen sclerosis et atrophicus, primary atrophy, sclerotic dermatosis, atrophic and hyperplastic vulvitis,* and *kraurosis vulvae* were used to denote disorders of epithelial growth and differentiation (136). In 1966, Jeffcoate suggested that these terms did not refer to separate disease entities because their macroscopic and microscopic appearances were variable and interchangeable (137). He assigned the generic term *chronic vulvar dystrophy* to the entire group of lesions.

The International Society for the Study of Vulvar Disease (ISSVD) recommended that the old *dystrophy* terminology be replaced by a new classification under the pathologic heading *nonneoplastic epithelial disorders of skin and mucosa.* This classification is shown in Table 19.13. In all cases, diagnosis requires biopsy of suspicious-looking lesions, which are best detected by careful inspection of the vulva in a bright light aided, if necessary, by a magnifying glass (138).

The malignant potential of these nonneoplastic epithelial disorders is low, particularly now that the lesions with atypia are classified as VIN. Patients with lichen sclerosis and concomitant hyperplasia may be at particular risk (139).

Vulvar Intraepithelial Neoplasia

As with the vulvar dystrophies, there is confusion regarding the nomenclature for VIN. Four major terms are used: *erythroplasia of Queyrat, Bowen's disease, carcinoma in situ simplex,* and *Paget's disease.* In 1976, the ISSVD decreed that the first three lesions were merely gross variants

Table 19.13 Classification of Epithelial Vulvar Diseases
Nonneoplastic epithelial disorders of skin and mucosa
Lichen sclerosis (lichen sclerosis et atrophicus)   Squamous hyperplasia (formerly hyperplastic dystrophy)   Other dermatoses
Mixed nonneoplastic and neoplastic epithelial disorders
Intraepithelial neoplasia

Squamous intraepithelial neoplasia
  VIN 1
  VIN 2
  VIN 3 (severe dysplasia or carcinoma *in situ*)
 Nonsquamous intraepithelial neoplasia
  Paget's disease
  Tumors of melanocytes, noninvasive

Invasive tumors

VIN, vulvar intraepithelial neoplasia.
From **Committee on Terminology, International Society for the Study of Vulvar Disease.** New nomenclature for vulvar disease. *Int J Gynecol Pathol* 1989;8:83, with permission.

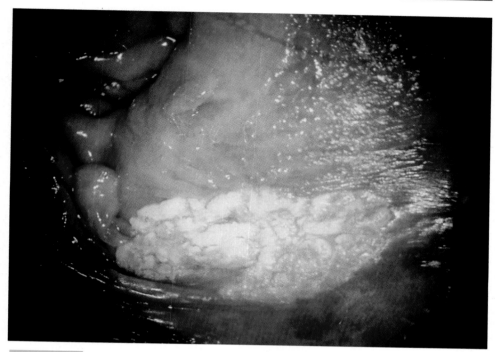

Figure 19.19 Carcinoma *in situ* of the vulva (vulvar intraepithelial neoplasia grade 3, VIN 3).

of the same disease process and that all of these entities should be included under the umbrella term *squamous cell carcinoma in situ* (stage 0) (114). In 1986, the ISSVD recommended the term *vulvar intraepithelial neoplasia* (Table 19.13).

VIN is graded as 1 (mild dysplasia), 2 (moderate dysplasia), or 3 (severe dysplasia or CIS) on the basis of cellular immaturity, nuclear abnormalities, maturation disturbance, and mitotic activity. In VIN 1, immature cells, cellular disorganization, and mitotic activity occur predominantly in the lower one-third of the epithelium, whereas in VIN 3, immature cells with scanty cytoplasm and severe chromatinic alterations occupy most of the epithelium (Fig. 19.19). Dyskeratotic cells and mitotic figures occur in the superficial layer. The appearance of VIN 2 is intermediate between VIN 1 and VIN 3. Additional cytopathic changes of HPV infection, such as perinuclear halos with displacement of the nuclei by the intracytoplasmic viral protein, thickened cell borders, binucleation, and multinucleation, are common in the superficial layers of VIN, especially in VIN 1 and VIN 2. These viral changes are not definitive evidence of neoplasia but are indicative of viral exposure (140). Most vulvar condylomas are associated with HPV-6 and -11, whereas HPV-16 is detected in more than 80% of VIN cases by molecular techniques.

VIN 3 can be unifocal or multifocal. Typically, multifocal VIN 3 presents with small hyperpigmented lesions on the labia majora (Fig. 19.20). Some cases of VIN 3 are more confluent, extending to the posterior fourchette and involving the perineal tissues. The term *bowenoid papulosis (bowenoid dysplasia)* was used to describe multifocal VIN lesions ranging from grade 1 to 3. Clinically, patients with bowenoid papulosis present with multiple small pigmented papules (40% of cases) that are usually less than 5 mm in diameter. Most women with these lesions are in their 20s, and some are pregnant. After childbirth, the lesions may regress spontaneously. The term *bowenoid papulosis* is no longer recommended by the ISSVD.

Paget's Disease of the Vulva

Extramammary Paget's disease of the vulva (AIS) was described 27 years after the description by Sir James Paget of the mammary lesion that now bears his name (141). Some patients with vulvar Paget's disease have an underlying adenocarcinoma, although the precise frequency is difficult to ascertain.

Histology

Most cases of vulvar Paget's disease are intraepithelial. Because these lesions demonstrate apocrine differentiation, the malignant cells are believed to arise from undifferentiated basal

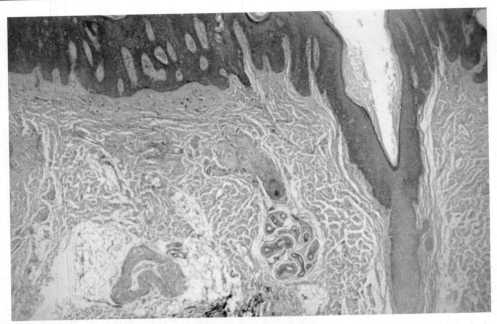

Figure 19.20 Vulvar carcinoma *in situ:* carcinoma *in situ* (VIN 3) extending into the hair follicle.

cells, which convert into an appendage type of cell during carcinogenesis (Fig. 19.21). The "transformed cells" spread intraepithelially throughout the squamous epithelium and may extend into the appendages. In most patients with an underlying invasive carcinoma of the apocrine sweat gland, Bartholin gland, or anorectum, the malignant cells are believed to migrate through the dermal ductal structures and reach the epidermis. In such cases, metastasis to the regional lymph nodes and other sites can occur.

Paget's disease must be distinguished from superficial spreading melanoma. All sections should be studied thoroughly using differential staining, particularly periodic acid–Schiff (PAS) and mucicarmine stains. Mucicarmine has routinely positive results in the cells of Paget's disease and negative results in melanotic lesion.

Clinical Features

Paget's disease of the vulva predominantly affects postmenopausal white women, and the presenting symptoms are usually pruritus and vulvar soreness. The lesion has an eczematoid appearance macroscopically and usually begins on the hair-bearing portions of the vulva (Fig. 19.22). It may extend to involve the mons pubis, thighs, and buttocks. Extension to the mucosa of the rectum, vagina, or urinary tract is described (142). The more extensive lesions are usually raised and velvety in appearance.

A second synchronous or metachronous primary neoplasm is associated with extramammary Paget's disease in about 4% of patients, which is much less common than previously believed (143). Associated carcinomas were reported in the cervix, colon, bladder, gallbladder, and breast. When the anal mucosa is involved, there usually is an underlying rectal adenocarcinoma (139).

Treatment

VIN   The treatment of VIN 3 varies from wide excision to the performance of a superficial or "skinning" vulvectomy (144–147). Although the treatment originally recommended for CIS of the vulva was wide excision, fears that the disease is preinvasive led to the widespread use of superficial vulvectomy (146). **Because progression is relatively uncommon, typically occurring in 5% to 10% of cases, extensive surgery is not warranted** (144). This is particularly important because many VIN 3 lesions are found in premenopausal women.

The therapeutic alternatives for VIN 3 are simple excision, laser ablation, and superficial vulvectomy with or without split-thickness skin grafting.

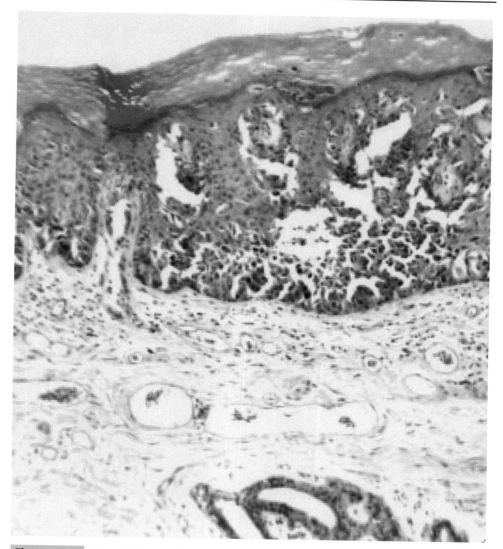

Figure 19.21 **Paget's disease of vulva.** The epidermis is permeated by abnormal cells with vacuolated cytoplasm and atypical nuclei. This heavy concentration of abnormal cells in the parabasal layers is typical of Paget's disease.

Excision of small foci of disease produces excellent results and has the advantage of providing a histopathologic specimen. Although multifocal or extensive lesions may be difficult to treat by this approach, it offers the potential for the most cosmetic result. Repeat excision is often necessary but can usually be accomplished without vulvectomy (145,147).

The carbon dioxide laser can be used for multifocal lesions but is unnecessary for unifocal disease. The disadvantages are that it can be painful and costly and does not provide a histopathologic specimen (148).

Superficial vulvectomy is appropriate to treat extensive and recurrent VIN 3 (147). The goal of the surgery is to extirpate all of the disease while preserving as much of the normal vulvar anatomy as possible. The anterior vulva and the clitoris should be preserved if possible. In some patients, the disease extends up the anus, which must be resected. An effort should be made to close the vulvar defect primarily, reserving the use of skin grafts for instances in which the vulvar defect cannot be closed because the resection is so extensive. Split-thickness skin grafts can be harvested from the thighs or buttocks, but the latter is more easily concealed (149).

Paget's Disease **Unlike squamous cell VIN 3, in which the histologic extent of disease correlates closely with the macroscopic lesion, Paget's disease usually extends well beyond**

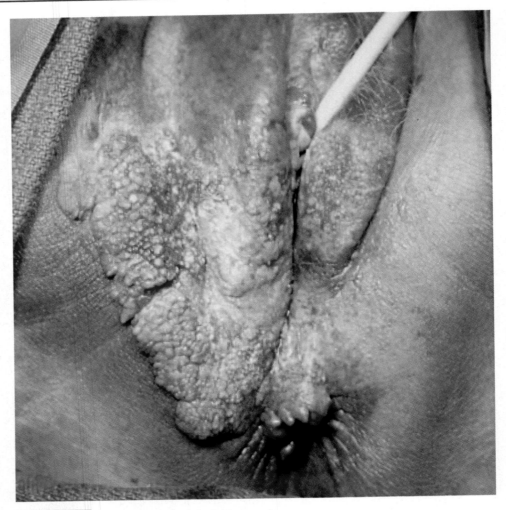

Figure 19.22   **Paget's disease of the labium majus.**

the gross lesion (150). This extension results in positive surgical margins and frequent local recurrence unless a wide local excision is performed (151). **Underlying adenocarcinomas are apparent clinically, but this finding does not occur invariably; therefore, the underlying dermis should be removed for adequate histologic evaluation.** For this reason, laser therapy is unsatisfactory in treating primary Paget's disease. If underlying invasive carcinoma is present, it should be treated in the same manner as a squamous vulvar cancer. This treatment usually requires radical vulvectomy and at least an ipsilateral inguinal-femoral lymphadenectomy.

Recurrent lesions are almost always *in situ,* although there was at least one report of an underlying adenocarcinoma in recurrent Paget's disease (143). It is reasonable to treat recurrent lesions with surgical excision.

References

1. **Pund ER, Nieburgs H, Nettles JB, et al.** Preinvasive carcinoma of the cervix uteri: seven cases in which it was detected by examination of routine endocervical smears. *Arch Pathol Lab Med* 1947;44:571–577.
2. **Koss LG, Stewart FW, Foote FW, et al.** Some histological aspects of behavior of epidermoid carcinoma in situ and related lesions of the uterine cervix: a long-term prospective study. *Cancer* 1963;16:1160–1211.
3. **Richart RM.** Natural history of cervical intraepithelial neoplasia. *Clin Obstet Gynecol* 1968;10:748.
4. **Nasiell K, Roger V, Nasiell M.** Behavior of mild cervical dysplasia during long-term follow-up. *Obstet Gynecol* 1986;67:665–669.
5. **Hatch KD.** *Handbook of colposcopy: diagnosis and treatment of lower genital tract neoplasia and HPV infections.* Boston, MA: Little Brown, 1989.
6. **Koss LG, Durfee GR.** Unusual patterns of squamous epithelium of the uterine cervix: cytologic and pathologic study of koilocytotic atypia. *Ann N Y Acad Sci* 1956;63:1245–1261.
7. **Meisels A, Fortin R, Roy M.** Condylomatous lesions of the cervix.

II. Cytologic, colposcopic and histopathologic study. *Acta Cytol* 1977;21:379–390.

8. **Beckmann AM, Myerson D, Daling JR, et al.** Detection and localization of human papillomavirus DNA in human genital condylomas by in situ hybridization with biotinylated probes. *J Med Virol* 1985;16:265–273.

9. **Schneider A, Oltersdorf T, Schneider V, et al.** Distribution pattern of human papilloma virus 16 genome in cervical neoplasia by molecular in situ hybridization of tissue sections. *Int J Cancer* 1987;39:717–721.

10. **Walboomers JM, Jacobs MV, Manos MM, et al.** Human papillomavirus is a necessary cause of invasive cervical cancer worldwide. *J Pathol* 1999;189:12–19.

11. **Crum CP, Mitao M, Levine RU, et al.** Cervical papillomaviruses segregate within morphologically distinct precancerous lesions. *J Virol* 1985;54:675–681.

12. **Durst M, Kleinheinz A, Hotz M, et al.** The physical state of human papillomavirus type 16 DNA in benign and malignant genital tumours. *J Gen Virol* 1985;66:1515–1522.

13. **Munger K, Phelps WC, Bubb V, et al.** The E6 and E7 genes of the human papillomavirus type 16 together are necessary and sufficient for transformation of primary human keratinocytes. *J Virol* 1989;63:4417–4421.

14. **McCance DJ, Kopan R, Fuchs E, et al.** Human papillomavirus type 16 alters human epithelial cell differentiation in vitro. *Proc Natl Acad Sci U S A* 1988;85:7169–7173.

15. **Dyson N, Howley PM, Munger K, et al.** The human papilloma virus-16 E7 oncoprotein is able to bind to the retinoblastoma gene product. *Science* 1989;243:934–937.

16. **Yee CL, Krishnan-Hewiett I, Baker CC, et al.** Presence and expression of human papillomavirus sequences in human cervical carcinoma cell lines. *Am J Pathol* 1985;119:361–366.

17. **Koutsky LA, Holmes KK, Critchlow CW, et al.** A cohort study of the risk of cervical intraepithelial neoplasia grade 2 or 3 in relation to papillomavirus infection. *N Engl J Med* 1992;327:1272–1278.

18. **Lorincz AT, Reid R, Jenson AB, et al.** Human papillomavirus infection of the cervix: relative risk associations of 15 common anogenital types. *Obstet Gynecol* 1992;79:328–337.

19. **Lorincz AT, Richart RM.** Human papillomavirus DNA testing as an adjunct to cytology in cervical screening programs. *Arch Pathol Lab Med* 2003;127:959–968.

20. **Association of Reproductive Health Professionals.** Managing HPV a new era in patient care http://www.arhp.org/Professional-Education/Programs/HPV.

21. **Liaw KL, Glass AG, Manos MM, et al.** Detection of human papillomavirus DNA in cytologically normal women and subsequent cervical squamous intraepithelial lesions. *J Natl Cancer Inst* 1999;91:954–960.

22. **Bauer HM, Ting Y, Greer CE, et al.** Genital human papillomavirus infection in female university students as determined by a PCR-based method. *JAMA* 1991;265:472–477.

23. **Ho GY, Bierman R, Beardsley L, et al.** Natural history of cervicovaginal papillomavirus infection in young women. *N Engl J Med* 1998;338:423–428.

24. **Ley C, Bauer HM, Reingold A, et al.** Determinants of genital human papillomavirus infection in young women. *J Natl Cancer Inst* 1991;83:997–1003.

25. **Bory JP, Cucherousset J, Lorenzato M, et al.** Recurrent human papillomavirus infection detected with the hybrid capture II assay selects women with normal cervical smears at risk for developing high grade cervical lesions: a longitudinal study of 3,091 women. *Int J Cancer* 2002;102:519–525.

26. **Nobbenhuis MA, Walboomers M, Helmerhorst TJ, et al.** Relation of human papillomavirus status to cervical lesions and consequences for cervical-cancer screening: a prospective study. *Lancet* 1999;354:20–25.

27. **Shiffman MH.** Recent progress in defining the epidemiology of human papilloma virus infection and cervical cancer. *J Natl Cancer Inst* 1992;84:398–399.

28. **Chen XS, Garcea RL, Goldberg I, et al.** Structure of small virus-like particles assembled from the L1 protein of human papillomavirus 16. *Mol Cell* 2000;5:557–567.

29. **Paavonen J, Naud P, Salmerón J.** Efficacy of human papillomavirus (HPV)-16118 AS04-adjuvanted vaccine against cervical infection and precancer caused by oncogenic HPV types (PATRICIA): final analysis of a double-blind, randomized study in young women. *Lancet* 2009;374:301–314.

30. **Koutsky LA, for the FUTURE II Study Group.** Quadrivalent vaccine against human papillomavirus to prevent high-grade cervical lesions. *N Engl J Med* 2007;356:1915–1927.

31. **The GlaxoSmithKline Vaccine HPV-007 Study Group.** Sustained efficacy and immunogenicity of the HPV-16/18 AS04-adjuvanted vaccine: analysis of a randomised placebo-controlled trial up to 6.4 years. *Lancet* 2009;374:1975–1985.

32. **Villa LL, Costa RLR, Petta CA, et al.** High sustained efficacy of a prophylactic quadrivalent human papillomavirus types 6111/16/18 L1 virus-like particle vaccine through 5 years of follow-up. *Br J Cancer* 2006;95:1459–1466.

33. **Moscicki AB, Schiffman M, Kjaer S, et al.** Chapter 5: Updating the natural history of HPV and anogenital cancer. *Vaccine* 2006;24[Suppl 3]:S42–51.

34. **Brown DR, Kjaer SK, Sigurdson K, et al.** The impact of quadrivalent human papillomavirus (HPV; types 6, 11, 16, and 18) L1 virus-like particle vaccine on infection and disease due to oncogenic nonvaccine HPV types in generally HPV-naive women aged 16–26 years. *J Infect Dis* 2009;199:926–935.

35. **Olsson S-E, Paavonen J.** Impact of HPV 6/11/16/18 vaccine on abnormal Pap tests and procedures. Presented at: 25th International Papillomavirus Conference. Malmo, Sweden, 8-12 May 2009 (Abstract 0-01.08).

36. **FUTURE I/II Study Group.** Four year efficacy of prophylactic human papillomavirus quadrivalent vaccine against low grade cervical, vulvar, and vaginal intraepithelial neoplasia and anogenital warts: randomised controlled trial. *BMJ* 2010;341:c3493.

37. **U.S. Food and Drug Administration.** Clinical review of biologics license application for human papillomavirus 6, 11, 16, 18 L1 virus like particle vaccine (*S. cerevisiae*) (STN 125126 GARDASIL), manufactured by Merck, Inc. Available online at: www.fda.gov/downloads/biologicsbloodvaccines/vaccines/approvedproducts/ucm 111287.pdf

38. **Muñoz N, Kjaer SK, Sigurdsson K, et al.** Impact of human papillomavirus (HPV)-6/11/16/18 vaccine on all HPV-associated genital diseases in young women. *J Natl Cancer Inst* 2010;102:325–339.

39. **Giannini SL, Hanon E, Moris P, et al.** Enhanced humoral and memory B cellular immunity using HPV16/18 L1 VLP vaccine formulated with the MPL/aluminum salt combination (AS04) compared to aluminum salt only. *Vaccine* 2006;24:5937–5949.

40. **Saslow D, Castle PE, Cox JT, et al.** American Cancer Society guideline for human papillomavirus (HPV) vaccine use to prevent cervical cancer and its precursors. *CA Cancer J Clin* 2007;57:7–28.

41. **Lowy DR, Frazer IH.** Prophylactic human papillomavirus vaccines. *J Natl Cancer Inst Monogr* 2003;31:111–116.

42. **Koutsky LA, Ault KA, Wheeler CM, et al.** A controlled trial of a human papillomavirus type 16 vaccine. *N Engl J Med* 2002;347:1645–1651.

43. **Harper DM, Franco EL, Wheeler CM, et al.** Efficacy of a bivalent L1 virus-like particle vaccine in prevention of infection with human papillomavirus types 16 and 18 in young women: a randomised controlled trial. *Lancet* 2004;364:1757–1765.

44. **Villa LL, Costa RL, Petta CA, et al.** Prophylactic quadrivalent human papillomavirus (types 6, 11, 16, and 18) L1 virus-like particle vaccine in young women: a randomised double-blind placebo-controlled multicentre phase II efficacy trial. *Lancet Oncol* 2005;6:271–278.

45. **National Cancer Institute Workshop.** The 1988 Bethesda System for reporting cervical/vaginal cytological diagnoses. *JAMA* 1989;262:931–934.

46. **Solomon D, Davey D, Kurman R, et al.** The 2001 Bethesda System: terminology for reporting results of cervical cytology. *JAMA* 2002;287:2114–2119.

47. **Willett GD, Kurman RJ, Reid R, et al.** Correlation of the histologic appearance of intraepithelial neoplasia of the cervix with human papillomavirus types: emphasis on low grade lesions including so-called flat condyloma. *Int J Gynecol Pathol* 1989;8:18–25.

48. **Ismail SM, Colclough AB, Dinnen JS, et al.** Reporting cervical intra-epithelial neoplasia (CIN): intra- and interpathologist variation and factors associated with disagreement. *Histopathology* 1990;16:371–376.

49. **Sherman ME, Schiffman MH, Erozan YS, et al.** The Bethesda System: a proposal for reporting abnormal cervical smears based on the reproducibility of cytopathologic diagnoses. *Arch Pathol Lab Med* 1992;116:1155–1158.

50. **Ries L, Eisner MP, Kosary CL, et al.** *SEER Cancer Statistics Review, 1975–2002.* Bethesda, MD: National Cancer Institute, 2004.

51. **Jemal A, Siegel R, Ward E, et al.** Cancer statistics, 2006. *CA Cancer J Clin* 2006;56:106–130.

52. **U.S. Department of Health and Human Services.** *Healthy people 2010.* Washington, DC: U.S. Government Printing Office, 2000.

53. **McCrory DC, Matchar DB, Bastian L, et al.** Evaluation of cervical cytology. Evidence Report/Technology Assessment No. 5. (Prepared by Duke University under Contract No. 290-97-0014.) AHCPR Publication No. 99-E010. Rockville, MD: Agency for Health Care Policy and Research. February 1999.

54. **Fahey MT, Irwig L, Macaskill P.** Meta-analysis of Pap test accuracy. *Am J Epidemiol* 1995;141:680–689.

55. **Mitchell MF, Schottenfeld D, Tortolero-Luna G, et al.** Colposcopy for the diagnosis of squamous intraepithelial lesions: a meta-analysis. *Obstet Gynecol* 1998;91:626–631.

56. **Nanda K, McCrory DC, Myers ER, et al.** Accuracy of the Papanicolaou test in screening for and follow-up of cervical cytologic abnormalities: a systematic review. *Ann Intern Med* 2000;132:810–819.

57. **Sawaya GF, Grimes DA.** New technologies in cervical cytology screening: a word of caution. *Obstet Gynecol* 1999;94:307–310.

58. **Wright TC Jr, Cox JT, Massad LS, et al.** ASCCP-Sponsored Consensus Conference. 2001 Consensus Guidelines for the management of women with cervical cytological abnormalities. *JAMA* 2002;287:2120–2129.

59. **Bolick DR, Hellman DJ.** Laboratory implementation and efficacy assessment of the ThinPrep cervical cancer screening system. *Acta Cytol* 1998;42:209–213.

60. **McQuarrie HG, Ogden J, Costa M.** Understanding the financial impact of covering new screening technologies: the case of automated Pap smears. *J Reprod Med* 2000;45:898–906.

61. **Saslow D, Runowicz CD, Solomon D, et al.** American Cancer Society guideline for the early detection of cervical neoplasia and cancer. *CA Cancer J Clin* 2002;52:342–362.

62. **American College of Obstetricians and Gynecologists.** Cervical cytology screening. ACOG Practice Bulletin. Number 109, December 2009. *Obstet Gynecol* 2009;149:1409–1420.

63. **Wright TC Jr, Schiffman M, Solomon D, et al.** Interim guidance for the use of human papillomavirus DNA testing as an adjunct to cervical cytology for screening. *Obstet Gynecol* 2004;103:304–309.

64. **Sherman ME, Lorincz AT, Scott DR, et al.** Baseline cytology, human papillomavirus testing, and risk for cervical neoplasia: a 10-year cohort analysis. *J Natl Cancer Inst* 2003;95:46–52.

65. **Clavel C, Masure M, Bory JP, et al.** Human papillomavirus testing in primary screening for the detection of high-grade cervical lesions: a study of 7932 women. *Br J Cancer* 2001;84:1616–1623.

66. **Castle PE, Wacholder S, Lorincz AT, et al.** A prospective study of high-grade cervical neoplasia risk among human papillomavirus-infected women. *J Natl Cancer Inst* 2002;94:1406–1414.

67. **Davey DD, Naryshkin S, Nielsen ML, et al.** Atypical squamous cells of undetermined significance: interlaboratory comparison and quality assurance monitors. *Diagn Cytopathol* 1994;11:390–396.

68. **Kurman RJ, Henson DE, Herbst AL, et al.** Interim guidelines for management of abnormal cervical cytology. The 1992 National Cancer Institute Workshop. *JAMA* 1994;271:1866–1869.

69. **Wright TC, Sun XW, Koulos J.** Comparison of management algorithms for the evaluation of women with low-grade cytologic abnormalities. *Obstet Gynecol* 1995;85:202–210.

70. **Lonky NM, Navarre GL, Sanders S, et al.** Low-grade Papanicolaou smears and the Bethesda system: a prospective cytohistopathologic analysis. *Obstet Gynecol* 1995;85:716–720.

71. **Kinney WK, Manos MM, Hurley LB, et al.** Where's the high-grade cervical neoplasia? The importance of minimally abnormal Papanicolaou diagnoses. *Obstet Gynecol* 1998;91:973–976.

72. **Cox JT, Lorincz AT, Schiffman MH, et al.** Human papillomavirus testing by hybrid capture appears to be useful in triaging women with a cytologic diagnosis of atypical squamous cells of undetermined significance. *Am J Obstet Gynecol* 1995;172:946–954.

73. **Melnikow J, Nuovo J, Willan AR, et al.** Natural history of cervical squamous intraepithelial lesions: a meta-analysis. *Obstet Gynecol* 1998;92:727–735.

74. **Wright TC Jr, Lorincz A, Ferris DG, et al.** Reflex human papillomavirus deoxyribonucleic acid testing in women with abnormal Papanicolaou smears. *Am J Obstet Gynecol* 1998;178:962–966.

75. **Wright TC Jr, Massad LS, Dunton CJ, et al.** 2006 consensus guidelines for the management of women with abnormal cervical cancer screening tests. *Am J Obstet Gynecol* 2007;197:346–355.

76. **Manos MM, Kinney WK, Hurley LB, et al.** Identifying women with cervical neoplasia: using human papillomavirus DNA testing for equivocal Papanicolaou results. *JAMA* 1999;281:1605–1610.

77. **Solomon D, Schiffman M, Tarone R.** Comparison of three management strategies for patients with atypical squamous cells of undetermined significance: baseline results from a randomized trial. *J Natl Cancer Inst* 2001;93:293–299.

78. **ASCUS-LSIL Traige Study (ALTS) Group.** Results of a randomized trial on the management of cytology interpretations of atypical squamous cells of undetermined significance. *Am J Obstet Gynecol* 2003;188:1383–1392.

79. **Goldie SJ, Kim JJ, Wright TC.** Cost-effectiveness of human papillomavirus DNA testing for cervical cancer screening in women aged 30 years or more. *Obstet Gynecol* 2004;103:619–631.

80. **ASCUS-LSIL Triage Study (ALTS) Group.** A randomized trial on the management of low-grade squamous intraepithelial lesion cytology interpretations. *Am J Obstet Gynecol* 2003;188:1393–1400.

81. **Wright TC Jr, Cox JT, Massad LS, et al.** 2001 consensus guidelines for the management of women with cervical cytological abnormalities. *JAMA* 2002;287:2120–2129.

82. **Wright YC Jr, Cox JT, Massad LS, et al.** 2001 consensus guidelines for the management of women with cervical intraepithelial neoplasia. *Am J Obstet Gynecol* 2003;189:295–304.

83. **Wright TC, Massad LS, Dunton CJ, et al.** 2006 American Society for Colposcopy and Cervical Pathology-sponsored Consensus Conference. 2006 consensus guidelines for the management of women with cervical intraepithelial neoplasia or adenocarcinoma-in-situ. *Am J Obstet Gynecol* 2007;197:340–345.

84. **American Society for Colposcopy and Cervical Pathology (ASCCP) Consensus Guidelines. 2006.** (www.asccp.org).

85. **Guido R, Schiffman M, Solomon D, et al.** Postcolposcopy management strategies for women referred with low-grade squamous intraepithelial lesions or human papillomavirus DNA-positive atypical squamous cells of undetermined significance: a two-year prospective study. *Am J Obstet Gynecol* 2003;188:1401–1405.

86. **Cox JT, Schiffman M, Solomon D.** Prospective follow-up suggests similar risk of subsequent cervical intraepithelial neoplasia grade 2 or 3 among women with cervical intraepithelial neoplasia grade 1 or negative colposcopy and directed biopsy. *Am J Obstet Gynecol* 2003;188:1406–1412.

87. **Lee SSN, Collins RJ, Pun TC, et al.** Conservative treatment of low grade squamous intraepithelial lesions (LSIL) of the cervix. *Int J Gynaecol Obstet* 1998;60:35–40.

88. **Falls RK.** Spontaneous resolution rate of grade 1 cervical intraepithelial neoplasia in a private practice population. *Am J Obstet Gynecol* 1999;181:278–282.

89. **Holowaty P, Miller AB, Rohan T, et al.** Natural history of dysplasia of the uterine cervix. *J Natl Cancer Inst* 1999;91:252–258.

90. **Ostor AG.** Natural history of cervical intraepithelial neoplasia: a critical review. *Int J Gynecol Pathol* 1993;12:186–192.

91. **Mitchell MF, Tortolero-Luna G, Cook E, et al.** A randomized clinical trial of cryotherapy, laser vaporization, and loop electrosurgical excision for treatment of squamous intraepithelial lesions of the cervix. *Obstet Gynecol* 1998;92:737–744.

92. **Alvarez RD, Helm CW, Edwards RP, et al.** Prospective randomized trial of LLETZ versus laser ablation in patients with cervical intraepithelial neoplasia. *Gynecol Oncol* 1994;52:175–179.

93. **Campion M.** Preinvasive disease. In **Berek JS, Hacker NF.** *Berek & Hacker's gynecologic oncology*, 5th ed. Philadelphia: Lippincott Williams & Wilkins; 2010:268–340.

94. **Andersen ES, Thorup K, Larsen G.** The results of cryosurgery for cervical intraepithelial neoplasia. *Gynecol Oncol* 1988;30:21–25.

95. **Ostergard DR.** Cryosurgical treatment of cervical intraepithelial neoplasia. *Obstet Gynecol* 1980;56:231–233.

96. Creasman WT, Weed JC, Curry SL, et al. Efficacy of cryosurgical treatment of severe cervical intraepithelial neoplasia. *Obstet Gynecol* 1973;41:501–506.

97. Benedet JL, Miller DM, Nickerson KG, et al. The results of cryosurgical treatment of cervical intraepithelial neoplasia at one, five, and ten years. *Am J Obstet Gynecol* 1987;157:268–273.

98. Anderson MC, Hartley RB. Cervical crypt involvement by intraepithelial neoplasia. *Obstet Gynecol Surv* 1979;34:852–853.

99. Townsend DE. Cryosurgery for CIN. *Obstet Gynecol Surv* 1979;34:828.

100. Burke L. The use of the carbon dioxide laser in the therapy of cervical intraepithelial neoplasia. *Am J Obstet Gynecol* 1982;144:337–340.

101. Wright VC, Riopelle MA, Rubinstein E, et al. CO_2 laser and cervical intraepithelial neoplasia. *Acta Obstet Gynecol Scand Suppl* 1984;125:1–36.

102. Rylander E, Isberg A, Joelsson I. Laser vaporization of cervical intraepithelial neoplasia: a five-year follow-up. *Acta Obstet Gynecol Scand Suppl* 1984;125:33–36.

103. Jordan JA, Mylotte MJ, Williams DR. The treatment of cervical intraepithelial neoplasia by laser vaporization. *Br J Obstet Gynaecol* 1985;92:394–398.

104. Benedet JL, Miller DM, Nickerson KG. Results of conservative management of cervical intraepithelial neoplasia. *Obstet Gynecol* 1992;79:105–110.

105. Baggish MS, Dorsey JH, Adelson M. A ten-year experience treating cervical intraepithelial neoplasia with the CO_2 laser. *Am J Obstet Gynecol* 1989;161:60–68.

106. Prendiville W, Cullimore J, Norman S. Large loop excision of the transformation zone (LLETZ). A new method of management for women with cervical intraepithelial neoplasia. *Br J Obstet Gynaecol* 1989;96:1054–1060.

107. Whiteley PF, Olah KS. Treatment of cervical intraepithelial neoplasia: experience with the low-voltage diathermy loop. *Am J Obstet Gynecol* 1990;162:1272–1277.

108. Mor-Yosef S, Lopes A, Pearson S, et al. Loop diathermy cone biopsy. *Obstet Gynecol* 1990;75:884–886.

109. Bigrigg MA, Codling BW, Perason P, et al. Colposcopic diagnosis and treatment of cervical dysplasia at a single clinic visit: experience of low-voltage diathermy loop in 1000 patients. *Lancet* 1990;336:229–231.

110. Gunasekera PC, Phipps JH, Lewis BV. Large loop excision of the transformation zone (LLETZ) compared to carbon dioxide laser in the treatment of CIN: a superior mode of treatment. *Br J Obstet Gynaecol* 1990;97:995–998.

111. Howe DT, Vincenti AC. Is large loop excision of the transformation zone (LLETZ) more accurate than colposcopically directed punch biopsy in the diagnosis of cervical intraepithelial neoplasia? *Br J Obstet Gynaecol* 1991;98:588–591.

112. Minucci D, Cinel A, Insacco E. Diathermic loop treatment for CIN and HPV lesions: a follow-up of 130 cases. *Eur J Gynaecol Oncol* 1991;12:385–393.

113. Wright TC, Gagnon S, Richart RM, et al. Treatment of cervical intraepithelial neoplasia using the loop electrosurgical excision procedure. *Obstet Gynecol* 1992;79:173–178.

114. Luesley DM, Cullimore J, Redman CWE, et al. Loop diathermy excision of the cervical transformation zone in patients with abnormal cervical smears. *BMJ* 1990;300:1690–1693.

115. Murdoch JB, Grimshaw RN, Morgan PR, et al. The impact of loop diathermy on management of early invasive cervical cancer. *Int J Gynecol Cancer* 1992;2:129–133.

116. Chappatte OA, Bryne DL, Raju KS, et al. Histological differences between colposcopic-directed biopsy and loop excision of the transformation zone (LETZ): a cause for concern. *Gynecol Oncol* 1991;43:46–50.

117. Baggish MS. A comparison between laser excisional conization and laser vaporization for the treatment of cervical intraepithelial neoplasia. *Am J Obstet Gynecol* 1986;155:39–44.

118. Larsson G, Gullberg B, Grundsell H. A comparison of complications of laser and cold knife conization. *Obstet Gynecol* 1983;62:213–217.

119. Bostofte E, Berget A, Falck LJ, et al. Conization by carbon dioxide laser or cold knife in the treatment of cervical intra-epithelial neoplasia. *Acta Obstet Gynecol Scand* 1986;65:199–202.

120. Bjerre B, Eliasson G, Linell F, et al. Conization as only treatment of carcinoma in situ of the uterine cervix. *Am J Obstet Gynecol* 1976;125:143–152.

121. Kolstad P, Klem V. Long-term followup of 1121 cases of carcinoma in situ. *Obstet Gynecol* 1976;48:125–129.

122. Jones HW 3rd. Treatment of cervical intraepithelial neoplasia. *Clin Obstet Gynecol* 1990;33:826–836.

123. Samson SL, Bentley JR, Fahey TJ, et al. The effect of loop electrosurgical excision procedure on future pregnancy outcome. *Obstet Gynecol* 2005;105:325–332.

124. Luesley DM, McCrum A, Terry PB, et al. Complications of cone biopsy related to the dimensions of the cone and the influence of prior colposcopic assessment. *Br J Obstet Gynaecol* 1985;92:158–164.

125. Demopoulos RI, Horowitz LF, Vamvakas EC. Endocervical gland involvement by cervical intraepithelial neoplasia grade III: predictive value for residual and/or recurrent disease. *Cancer* 1991;68:1932–1936.

126. Duggan BD, Felix JC, Muderspach LI, et al. Cold-knife conization versus conization by the loop electrosurgical excision procedure: a randomized, prospective study. *Am J Obstet Gynecol* 1999;180:276–282.

127. Mathevet P, Chemali E, Roy M, et al. Long-term outcome of a randomized study comparing three techniques of conization: cold knife, laser, and LEEP. *Eur J Obstet Gynecol Reprod Biol* 2003;106:214–218.

128. Mahmoud I Shafi. The management of cervical intraepithelial neoplasia. In Jordan J, Singer A. *The Cervix*. Blackwell; 2006.

129. Goff BA, Atanasoff P, Brown E, et al. Endocervical glandular atypia in Papanicolaou smears. *Obstet Gynecol* 1992;79:101–104.

130. Boone ME, Baak JPA, Kurver JPH, et al. Adenocarcinoma in situ of the cervix: an underdiagnosed lesion. *Cancer* 1981;48:768–773.

131. Bertrand M, Lickrish GM, Colgan TJ. The anatomic distribution of cervical adenocarcinoma in situ: implications for treatment. *Am J Obstet Gynecol* 1987;157:21–25.

132. Muntz HG, Bell DA, Lage JM, et al. Adenocarcinoma in situ of the uterine cervix. *Obstet Gynecol* 1992;80:935–939.

133. Poynor EA, Barakat RR, Hoskins WJ. Management and follow-up of patients with adenocarcinoma in situ of the uterine cervix. *Gynecol Oncol* 1995;57:158–164.

134. Benedet JL, Sanders BH. Carcinoma in situ of the vagina. *Am J Obstet Gynecol* 1984;148:695–700.

135. Hoffman MS, DeCesare SL, Roberts WS, et al. Upper vaginectomy for in situ and occult, superficially invasive carcinoma of the vagina. *Am J Obstet Gynecol* 1992;166:30–33.

136. Gardner HL, Friedrich EG, Kaufman RH. The vulvar dystrophies, atypias, and carcinoma in situ: an invitational symposium. *J Reprod Med* 1976;17:131–137.

137. Jeffcoate TN. Chronic vulval dystrophies. *Am J Obstet Gynecol* 1966;95:61–74.

138. Committee on Terminology, International Society for the Study of Vulvar Disease. New nomenclature for vulvar disease. *Int J Gynecol Pathol* 1989;8:83.

139. Rodke G, Friedrich EG Jr, Wilkinson EJ. Malignant potential of mixed vulvar dystrophy (lichen sclerosus associated with squamous cell hyperplasia. *J Reprod Med* 1988;33:545–550.

140. Rusk D, Sutton GP, Look KY, et al. Analysis of invasive squamous cell carcinoma of the vulva and vulvar intraepithelial neoplasia for the presence of human papillomavirus DNA. *Obstet Gynecol* 1991;77:918–922.

141. Dubreuilh W. Pigmentation of the skin due to demodex folliculorum. *Br J Dermatol* 1901;13:403.

142. Lee RA, Dahlin DC. Paget's disease of the vulva with extension into the urethra, bladder, and ureters: a case report. *Am J Obstet Gynecol* 1981;140:834–836.

143. Hart WR, Millman JB. Progression of intraepithelial Paget's disease of the vulva to invasive carcinoma. *Cancer* 1977;40:2333–2337.

144. Buscema J, Woodruff JD, Parmley T, et al. Carcinoma in situ of the vulva. *Obstet Gynecol* 1980;55:225–230.

145. Friedrich EG Jr, Wilkinson EJ, Fu YS. Carcinoma in situ of the vulva: a continuing challenge. *Am J Obstet Gynecol* 1980;136:830–843.

146. Rutledge F, Sinclair M. Treatment of intraepithelial carcinoma of the vulva by skin excision and graft. *Am J Obstet Gynecol* 1968;102:807–818.

147. **Chafee W, Ferguson K, Wilkinson EJ.** Vulvar intraepithelial neaoplasia (VIN): principles of surgical therapy. *Colpo Gynecol Surg* 1988;4:125–130.

148. **Reid R.** Superficial laser vulvectomy. III. A new surgical technique for appendage-conserving ablation of refractory condylomas and vulvar intraepithelial neoplasia. *Am J Obstet Gynecol* 1985;152:504–509.

149. **Berek JS, Hacker NF, Lagasse LD.** Reconstructive operations. In:

Knapp RC, Berkowitz RS, eds. *Gynecologic oncology*. Philadelphia, PA: Saunders, 1994:420–432.

150. **Gunn RA, Gallager HS.** Vulvar Paget's disease: a topographic study. *Cancer* 1980;46:590–594.

151. **Stacy D, Burrell MO, Franklin EW III.** Extramammary Paget's disease of the vulva and anus: use of intraoperative frozen-section margins. *Am J Obstet Gynecol* 1986;155:519–523.

20 Early Pregnancy Loss and Ectopic Pregnancy

Amy J. Voedisch
Carrie E. Frederick
Antonia F. Nicosia
Thomas G. Stovall

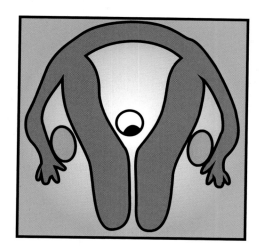

- **Spontaneous pregnancy loss is common, occurring in up to 20% of recognized conceptions.**

- **Following an ectopic pregnancy, approximately 15% of women will have a subsequent ectopic pregnancy.**

- **Single-dose *methotrexate* appears to be the treatment of choice if medical therapy is indicated and selected.**

- **Surgical management and medical therapy appear to be equivalent in a randomized comparison.**

An abnormal gestation can be either intrauterine or extrauterine. Extrauterine or ectopic pregnancy occurs when the fertilized ovum becomes implanted in tissue other than the endometrium. Although 70% of ectopic gestations are located in the ampullary segment of the fallopian tube, such pregnancies may also occur in other sites (Fig. 20.1) (1). Abnormal intrauterine pregnancy often results in pregnancy loss early in gestation. Such losses can be related to a number of factors such as age, previous pregnancy loss, and maternal smoking (Table 20.1). With both abnormal intrauterine and extrauterine gestation, early recognition is key to diagnosis and management.

Abnormal Intrauterine Pregnancy

Spontaneous Abortion

Spontaneous abortion is a pathologic process resulting in unintentional termination of the pregnancy prior to 20 weeks' gestation. **About 8% to 20% of known pregnancies terminate in spontaneous abortion** (2,3). **About 80% of spontaneous pregnancy losses occur in the first trimester; the incidence decreases with each gestational week** (4–6). In women who had one prior spontaneous abortion, the rate of spontaneous abortion in a subsequent pregnancy ranges from 13% to 20%; in women who had three consecutive losses, the rate is 33% (7). Patients should be reassured that, in most cases, spontaneous abortion does not recur. In women less than 36 years of age, when fetal cardiac activity is confirmed by ultrasound, the risk of spontaneous

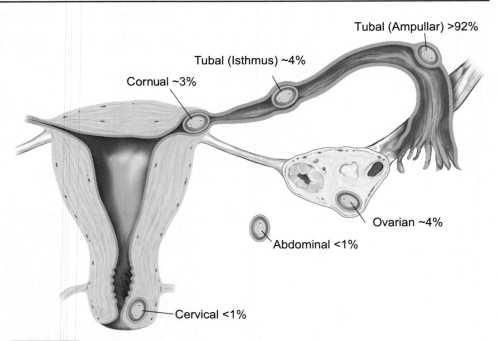

Tubal (Ampullar) >92%

Tubal (Isthmus) ~4%

Cornual ~3%

Ovarian ~4%

Abdominal <1%

Cervical <1%

Figure 20.1   Common sites of ectopic pregnancy.   (Adapted from **Seeber BE.** Suspected ectopic pregnancy. *Obstet Gynecol* 2006;107:399–413.)

abortion is less than 4.5%. For women older than 36, the risk of spontaneous abortion rises to 10%, and above 40 years may approach 30% (8). Risk factors for spontaneous abortion include increasing maternal age, closely spaced pregnancies (less than 3 to 6 months apart), history of previous spontaneous abortion, maternal diabetes, and maternal smoking during pregnancy (9–13).

With pelvic ultrasound, spontaneous abortion can be differentiated into various categories, based on examination findings and ultrasound findings. Missed abortion is defined as a nonviable intrauterine pregnancy in the presence of a closed cervix and little or no abdominal cramping or vaginal bleeding and can be subdivided into anembryonic gestation and embryonic demise. **Anembryonic gestation** is a pregnancy where the embryo failed to develop and is confirmed

Table 20.1 Potential Causes of Spontaneous Pregnancy Loss
Increased maternal age
Previous spontaneous abortion
Maternal smoking
Maternal systemic disease (diabetes mellitus, infection, thrombophilia, etc.)
Maternal alcohol consumption (moderate to high)
Increasing gravidity
Amphetamine use
Chromosomal or other embryologic abnormalities
Anembryonic gestation
Uterine anomalies
Intrauterine device in place
Placental anomalies
Severe maternal trauma
Extremes of maternal weight

when the mean gestational sac diameter measured by transvaginal ultrasound is greater than 20 mm and no embryonic pole is present. When an embryo is present with crown-rump length greater than 5 mm and no cardiac activity, this is classified as **embryonic demise,** and the pregnancy is nonviable (14).

Threatened Abortion

Threatened abortion **is defined as vaginal bleeding before 20 weeks of gestation. It occurs in at least 20% of all pregnancies** (15). **The distinction from missed or inevitable abortion requires ultrasound documentation of an intrauterine embryo or fetus with cardiac activity.** The bleeding is usually light and may be associated with mild lower abdominal or cramping pain. The differential diagnosis in these patients includes consideration of possible cervical polyps, vaginitis, cervical carcinoma, gestational trophoblastic disease, ectopic pregnancy, trauma, and foreign body. On physical examination, the abdomen usually is not tender, and the cervix is closed. Bleeding can be seen coming from the os, and usually there is no cervical motion or adnexal tenderness.

In the vast majority of cases, threatened abortion does not result in a pregnancy loss, but may be associated with poor outcomes later in pregnancy. In a study of 347 patients with a first-trimester pregnancy documented by ultrasonography, the overall rate of pregnancy loss was 6.1% to 4.2% in patients without bleeding and 12.4% in patients with bleeding (4). In a review of over 800 women presenting with first trimester vaginal bleeding or abdominal pain, nearly 14% with bleeding had spontaneous abortion compared with 2.5% in patients without bleeding (5). There is no effective therapy for a threatened intrauterine pregnancy. Bed rest and progesterone treatment, although often advocated, are not effective (16–18). Women with first trimester vaginal bleeding who do go on to have continuing pregnancies have nearly three times the risk of preterm birth between 28 and 31 weeks as women without bleeding, and a 50% higher likelihood of preterm birth between 32 to 36 weeks (19). First trimester bleeding may predict higher risk for intrauterine growth restriction, preterm premature rupture of membranes, and placental abruption (20). Bacterial vaginosis, if present, should be treated, as this is associated with increased risk for spontaneous abortion (21).

Inevitable Abortion

With an *inevitable abortion,* **the volume of bleeding is often greater than with other types of abortion, and the cervical os is open and effaced, but no tissue has passed.** Most patients have crampy lower abdominal pain, and some have cervical motion or adnexal tenderness. When it is certain that the pregnancy is not viable because the cervical os is dilated or excessive bleeding is present, the patient should be offered medical or surgical management. Blood type and Rh determination and a complete blood count should be obtained if there is any concern about the amount of bleeding. **Rh$_0$(D) immune globulin (*RhoGAM*) should be given if the patient's blood is Rh negative** (22). **It is acceptable to give a dose of 50 μg until 12 completed weeks; if this dose is not available, the standard 300 μg dose may be given.**

Incomplete Abortion

An incomplete abortion is a partial expulsion of the pregnancy tissue. Although most patients have vaginal bleeding, only some have passed tissue. Lower abdominal cramping is invariably present, and the pain may be described as resembling labor. On physical examination, the cervix is dilated and effaced, and bleeding is present. Often, clots are admixed with products of conception. If the bleeding is profuse, the patient should be examined promptly for tissue protruding from the cervical os; removal of this tissue with a ring forceps may reduce the bleeding. A vasovagal bradycardia may occur and responds to removal of the tissue. A complete blood count, maternal blood type, and Rh determination should be obtained; **Rh-negative patients should receive *RhoGAM*. If the patient is febrile, broad-spectrum antibiotic therapy should be administered.**

Management of Spontaneous Abortion

In women with stable vital signs and mild vaginal bleeding, three management options exist: expectant management, medical treatment, and suction curettage. Despite a wide range (25% to 76%) of success cited in the literature, expectant management may remain a desirable option for a stable and carefully counseled patient (23,24). Medical management with 800 μg of *misoprostol* placed vaginally can be up to 84% effective in achieving complete abortion (25). For incomplete abortion, the *misoprostol* dose can be reduced to 600 μg orally or 400 μg sublingually, with efficacy greater than 90% (26). Suction curettage should be performed in women with excessive bleeding, unstable vital signs, or in whom reliable follow-up is a concern.

Ectopic Gestation

Incidence

The most comprehensive data available on ectopic pregnancy rates were collected by the **Centers for Disease Control and Prevention (CDC). The incidence of ectopic pregnancy increased significantly in the past century.** In 1992, the latest year for which statistics are published, there were an estimated 108,800 ectopic pregnancies at a rate of 19.7 ectopic pregnancies per 1,000 reported pregnancies. This represents a sixfold increase compared with 1970 rates. The observed increase may represent an increase in detection and diagnosis resulting from more sensitive ultrasound technology, and a rise in sexually transmitted illnesses and assisted reproductive technologies (27). As Figure 20.2 demonstrates, while the absolute number of ectopic pregnancies continues to rise, the number of hospitalizations declined since the late 1980s, likely because of increasing outpatient management of this condition. Precise estimation of the true incidence of ectopic pregnancy is difficult, but the most recent estimate by the CDC is 2% of reported pregnancies (28). The data on demographic trends indicate that the highest rates occurred in women aged 35 to 44 years (27.2 per 1,000 reported pregnancies). When the data are analyzed by race, the risk for ectopic pregnancy among African Americans and other minorities (20.8 per 1,000) is 1.6 times greater than the risk among whites (13.4 per 1,000) (29). In 1992, 9% of all maternal deaths were attributable to ectopic pregnancy, down from 15% in 1988. The risk for death is higher for African Americans and other minorities than for whites. For all races, teenagers have the highest mortality rates, but the rate for African American and other minority teenagers is almost five times that of white teenagers (28,29). **After an ectopic pregnancy, there is an 8% to 15% chance of recurrent ectopic pregnancy, with single-dose *methotrexate* conferring the lowest risk, while linear salpingostomy is associated with the highest risk** (30). Many variables make accurate assessment of risk difficult (e.g., size and location of the ectopic pregnancy, status of the contralateral adnexa, treatment method, and history of infertility).

Etiology and Risk Factors

Ectopic pregnancy results from various factors that interrupt the successful migration of the conceptus to the endometrium. **The most important risk factors for ectopic pregnancy are a history of tubal surgery, including tubal ligation, prior ectopic pregnancy, *in utero***

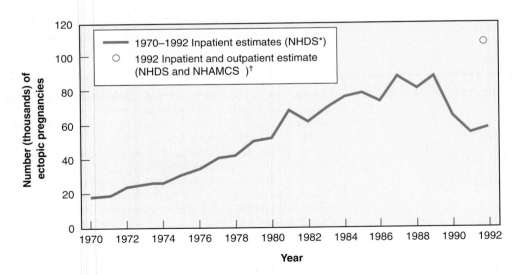

*National hospital discharge survey.
†National hospital ambulatory medical care survey.

Figure 20.2 **Estimation of the number of ectopic pregnancies (United States, 1970–1992).** (Adapted from *MMWR* 1995;44:46–48.)

diethylstilbestrol (**DES**) **exposure, and history of pelvic inflammatory disease** (31,32). Intrauterine device (IUD) use and infertility are associated with increased risk for ectopic gestation, but these relationships are complex. Up to half of women with ectopic pregnancy will have no identifiable risk factors (33–35). Many other risk factors, including smoking and multiple lifetime sexual partners, are weakly associated with ectopic pregnancy (32).

Myoelectrical activity is responsible for propulsive activity in the fallopian tube (36). This activity facilitates movement of the sperm and ova toward each other and propels the zygote toward the uterine cavity. Estrogen increases smooth muscle activity, and progesterone decreases muscle tone. Aging results in progressive loss of myoelectrical activity along the fallopian tube, which may explain the increased incidence of tubal pregnancy in perimenopausal women (36). Hormonal control of the muscular activity in the fallopian tube may explain the increased incidence of tubal pregnancy associated with failures of the morning-after pill, minipill, progesterone-containing IUDs, and ovulation induction. There is no increase in the incidence of chromosomal abnormalities in ectopic pregnancies (37).

Tubal Surgery

As would be expected, factors that disrupt normal tubal anatomy are the primary etiology for ectopic pregnancy. Women with prior tubal surgery have a more than 20-fold increased risk of subsequent ectopic pregnancy (32). Tubal repair or reconstruction may be performed to correct an obstruction, lyse adhesions, or evacuate an unruptured ectopic pregnancy. **Although it is clear that tubal surgery is associated with an increased risk for ectopic pregnancy, it is unclear whether the increased risk results from the surgical procedure or from the underlying problem.** A four- to fivefold increased risk is associated with salpingostomy, neosalpingostomy, fimbroplasty, anastomosis, and lysis of complex peritubal and periovarian adhesions (38). After tubal surgery, the overall rate of ectopic pregnancy is 2% to 7%, and the viable intrauterine pregnancy rate is 50% (38).

Though tubal sterilization remains one of the most effective forms of contraception, failures do occur; when they do, they are more likely to result in ectopic gestation. The 10-year cumulative incidence of pregnancy after any form of tubal sterilization is 18.5 per 1,000 woman-years and the likelihood of sterilization failure does not decrease with time since the procedure (39). Despite a greater proportion of poststerilization failures resulting in ectopic pregnancy, the absolute rate of ectopic pregnancy is decreased after sterilization (40). Calculating cumulative lifetime risk for ectopic pregnancy according to method of contraception, sterilized women have a lower cumulative risk for ectopic pregnancy than IUD users or nonusers of contraception, and women using barrier methods or oral contraceptives have the lowest risk (40).

The 10-year cumulative incidence of tubal pregnancy after any sterilization procedure is 7.3 per 1,000 procedures (41). The risk depends on the sterilization technique and the woman's age at the time of sterilization: postpartum partial salpingectomy and unipolar coagulation have the lowest rates of ectopic pregnancy (1.5 and 1.8 per 1,000 procedures), while bipolar coagulation techniques had the highest incidence (17.1 per 1,000 procedures). Spring clip and band application techniques have 10-year ectopic rates similar to the general incidence, 8.5 and 7.3 per 1,000 procedures, respectively (41). Women younger than 28 years at the time of sterilization are more likely to have a failure than women over 34 years.

Sterilization reversal increases risk for ectopic pregnancy. The exact risk depends on the method of sterilization, site of tubal occlusion, residual tube length, coexisting disease, and surgical technique. In general, the risk for reanastomosis of a cauterized tube is up to 17%, and it ranges from 6% to 9% for reversal of Pomeroy and 5% to 11% for reversal of ring procedures (42–47).

Prior Ectopic Pregnancy

A previous history of ectopic pregnancy is a risk factor for another occurrence. The likelihood of recurrence exists because of the factors that led to an initial ectopic implantation and may be affected by the type of treatment the patient received with the first episode. There is concern that conservation of the tube at the time of removal of an ectopic pregnancy would increase the risk for recurrent ectopic pregnancy (27,48). **The rates for intrauterine pregnancy (40%) and ectopic pregnancy (15%, range 4% to 28%) are similar after tubal removal or conservation** (49). In a series of 54 patients with conservative surgical procedures for management of ectopic pregnancy, the incidence of future ectopic pregnancy could be predicted by the status of the contralateral tube: normal (7%), abnormal (18%), or absent (25%) (50). In a later study of pregnancy outcomes of 200 patients treated with tubal conservation for ectopic pregnancy, preservation of the tube did not increase the incidence of repeat ectopic pregnancy, but it did improve overall fertility rates (51). The risk of recurrence after *methotrexate* treatment is similar to that encountered with salpingectomy (52,53). The risk of recurrent ectopic pregnancy after two prior episodes may be as high as 30% (54).

Pelvic Infection

The relationship of pelvic infection, tubal obstruction, and ectopic pregnancy is well documented. In a study of 2,500 women with suspected pelvic inflammatory disease (PID) who underwent diagnostic laparoscopy, the incidence of ectopic pregnancy in the subsequent pregnancy for those with laparoscopically confirmed disease was 9.1% compared with 1.4% in the women with normal laparoscopy (55). In a study of 415 women with laparoscopically proven PID, the incidence of tubal obstruction increased with successive episodes of PID: **13% after one episode, 35% after two, and 75% after three** (56).

Chlamydia is an important pathogen causing tubal damage and subsequent tubal pregnancy. Chlamydia was cultured from 7% to 30% of patients with tubal pregnancy (57,58). A strong association between chlamydia infection and tubal pregnancy was shown with serologic tests for chlamydia (59–62). Conception is three times as likely to be tubal in women with anti–*Chlamydia trachomatis* titers higher than 1:64 than in those women whose titers were negative (63). The number of episodes of chlamydia is directly associated with risk for ectopic pregnancy. In a retrospective cohort study of 11,000 women, those with two chlamydial infections were more than twice as likely to develop ectopic pregnancy as those with one, and women with three or more were at greater than four times higher risk (64). Women at risk for chlamydia infections should be diligently tested, treated when infection is present, and counseled about the risk of ectopic pregnancy.

Diethylstilbestrol   Women exposed to *DES in utero* who subsequently conceive are at increased risk for ectopic pregnancy. In a review by Goldberg and Falcone, the pooled risk of ectopic pregnancy in *DES*-exposed women was nine times that of nonexposed women (65). Structural tubal abnormalities were found in *DES*-exposed women, including foreshortening, constrictions, and distortions (66). The Collaborative *Diethylstilbestrol*-Adenosis Project, which monitored 327 *DES*-exposed women, found that about 50% had uterine cavity abnormalities. In *DES*-exposed women, the risk for ectopic pregnancy was 13% in those who had uterine abnormalities compared with 4% in those who had a normal uterus. No specific type of defect was related to the risk for ectopic pregnancy (67).

Contraceptive Use

It is not surprising that by reducing the overall likelihood of pregnancy, contraceptive use reduces the risk of ectopic pregnancy. There is concern that because of the various mechanisms of action of contraceptives, if a pregnancy were to occur, it might be more likely to be ectopic. In a meta-analysis of 13 studies examining the relationship between contraception and the risk of ectopic pregnancy, there was no increased risk in users of oral contraceptives or barrier methods compared with pregnant controls (40). There is no demonstrated increased risk in users of *depomedroxyprogesterone* injections, emergency contraceptive pills, or etonogestrel implants (68–70).

Hormonal and copper-containing IUDs are highly effective at preventing both intrauterine and extrauterine pregnancies. **Women who conceive with an IUD in place are more likely to have a tubal pregnancy than those not using contraceptives.** For women using the *levonorgestrel* intrauterine device, half of pregnancies will be ectopic, and 1 in 16 pregnancies in women with a copper IUD in place will be ectopic (71). The baseline risk of ectopic pregnancy in women not contracepting is 1 in 50. In a meta-analysis of studies investigating risk of ectopic pregnancy in IUD users compared with nonpregnant controls, IUD use had a protective effect with the exception of one study that showed no effect of IUD use (40). In the same meta-analysis, when IUD users were compared with pregnant controls, IUD use was associated with a significantly increased risk for ectopic pregnancy; the odds ratios ranged from 4.2 to 45. A common odds ratio could not be calculated because of heterogeneity between studies. The study with the most precise point estimate was a multinational case-control study conducted by the World Health Organization involving more than 2,200 women, which found an odds ratio of 4.2

(95% confidence interval, 2.5–6.9) (72). This suggests that while the intrauterine device decreases the risk of pregnancy overall, if a failure does occur, the device is more successful at preventing intrauterine pregnancy than tubal pregnancy. Past IUD use may slightly increase the risk of ectopic pregnancy. It should be noted that many of the studies that demonstrated this finding were conducted in the 1970s and 1980s, when women may have been using the *Dalkon Shield*, an IUD strongly associated with PID and ectopic pregnancy (73). The IUDs on the market in recent years are not associated with PID after the immediate insertion period (74).

Other Causes

Prior Abdominal Surgery   Many patients with ectopic pregnancies have a history of previous abdominal surgery. The role of abdominal surgery in ectopic pregnancy is unclear. In one study, there appeared to be no increased risk for cesarean delivery, ovarian surgery, or removal of an unruptured appendix (75). Other studies showed that ovarian cystectomy or wedge resection increases the risk for ectopic pregnancy, presumably because of peritubal scarring (76,77). Although there is agreement that an increased risk for ectopic pregnancy is associated with a ruptured appendix, one study did not confirm this finding (75).

Infertility   The incidence of ectopic pregnancy increases with age and parity, and there is a significant increase in nulliparous women undergoing infertility treatment (27,32,49). For nulliparous women, conceptions after at least 1 year of unprotected intercourse are 2.6 times more likely to be tubal (78). Additional risks for infertile women are associated with specific treatments, including reversal of sterilization, tuboplasty, ovulation induction, and *in vitro* fertilization (IVF). Various studies examining risk factors for ectopic pregnancy found that infertility increased the odds of tubal pregnancy at least 2.5 times and perhaps as much as 21 times (32).

Hormonal alterations characteristic of *clomiphene citrate* and gonadotropin ovulation-induction cycles may predispose to tubal implantation. About 1.1% to 4.6% of conceptions associated with ovulation induction are ectopic pregnancies (78–80). In many of these patients, the results of hysterosalpingography are normal, and there is no evidence of intraoperative tubal pathology. Hyperstimulation, with high estrogen levels, may play a role in tubal pregnancy; however, not all studies showed this relationship (81–83).

When the first pregnancy obtained with IVF was a tubal pregnancy; about 2% to 8% of the conceptions are tubal (84). Tubal factor infertility is associated with a further increased risk of 17% (85–88). Predisposing factors are unclear but may include placement of the embryo high in the uterine cavity, fluid reflux into the tube, and a predisposing tubal factor that prevents the refluxed embryo from returning to the uterine cavity.

Smoking   Cigarette smoking is associated with an increased risk for tubal pregnancy in a dose-dependent fashion. A case-control study showed a dose relationship: smokers of more than 20 cigarettes a day had a relative risk of 3.5 compared with nonsmokers, whereas smokers of up to 10 cigarettes had a risk of 2.3 (89). A case-control study in France found similar relative risk estimates (90). Alterations of tubal motility, ciliary activity, and blastocyst implantation are associated with nicotine intake.

Abortion   Multiple studies suggest an association between ectopic pregnancy and spontaneous abortion (79,91). With recurrent spontaneous abortion the risk may be increased up to four times (92). This may reflect a shared risk factor, such as with luteal phase defect. Substantial evidence found no increased risk with elective abortion; one study did find a slightly increased risk, particularly with multiple abortions (93–96).

Salpingitis Isthmica Nodosa   Salpingitis isthmica nodosa (SIN) is a noninflammatory patho-logic condition of the tube in which tubal epithelium extends into the myosalpinx and forms a true diverticulum. The incidence in healthy controls is 6% to 11%, but this condition is found more often in the tubes of women with an ectopic pregnancy than in nonpregnant women (97). In one study, 46% of women with isthmic tubal pregnancy were found to have SIN (98). Myome-trial electrical activity over the diverticula is abnormal. Whether tubal pregnancy is caused by SIN or whether the association is coincidental is unknown.

Endometriosis or Leiomyomas   Endometriosis or leiomyomas can cause tubal obstruction. Neither is commonly associated with ectopic pregnancy.

Histologic Characteristics

Chorionic villi, usually found in the lumen, are pathognomic findings of tubal pregnancy (99). **Gross or microscopic evidence of an embryo is seen in two-thirds of cases.** An unruptured tubal pregnancy is characterized by irregular dilation of the tube, with a blue discoloration caused by hematosalpinx. The ectopic pregnancy may not be readily apparent. Bleeding associated with tubal pregnancies is mainly extraluminal but may be luminal (hematosalpinx) and may extrude from the fimbriated end. A hematoma is frequently seen surrounding the distal segment of the tube. Patients who have tubal pregnancies that spontaneously resolved and those treated with *methotrexate* frequently have an enlargement of the ectopic mass associated with blood clots and extrusion of tissue from the fimbriated end. **Hemoperitoneum is nearly always present but is confined to the cul-de-sac unless tubal rupture occurred. The natural progression of tubal pregnancy is either expulsion from the fimbriated end (tubal abortion), involution of the conceptus, or rupture, usually around the eighth gestational week.** Some tubal pregnancies form a chronic inflammatory mass that is associated with involution and reestablishment of menses and thus is difficult to diagnose. Extensive histologic sampling may be required to disclose a few ghost villi.

Histologic findings associated with tubal gestation include evidence of chronic salpingitis and SIN. Inflammation associated with salpingitis causes adhesions as a result of fibrin deposition. Healing and cellular organization lead to permanent scarring between folds of tissue. This scarring may allow transport of sperm but not the passage of the larger blastocyst. About 45% of patients with tubal pregnancies have pathologic evidence of prior salpingitis (56).

The cause of SIN is unknown but is speculated to be an adenomyosis-like process or, less likely, inflammation (100). This condition is rare before puberty, indicating a noncongenital origin. Tubal diverticula are identified in about one-half of patients who have ectopic pregnancies, as opposed to 5% of women who do not have ectopic pregnancies (101).

Histologic findings include the Arias-Sella reaction, which is characterized by localized hyperplasia of endometrial glands that are hypersecretory. The cells have enlarged nuclei that are hyperchromatic and irregular (102). **The Arias-Sella reaction is a nonspecific finding that can be seen in patients with intrauterine pregnancies** (Fig. 20.3).

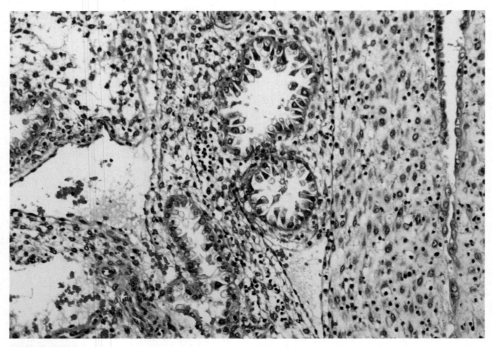

Figure 20.3   The Arias-Stella reaction of the endometrium. The glands are closely packed and hypersecretory with large, hyperchromatic nuclei suggesting malignancy.

Diagnosis

The diagnosis of ectopic pregnancy is complicated by the wide spectrum of clinical presentations, from asymptomatic cases to acute abdomen and hemodynamic shock. The diagnosis and management of a ruptured ectopic pregnancy is straightforward; the primary goal is achieving hemostasis. **If an ectopic pregnancy can be identified before rupture or irreparable tubal damage occurs, consideration may be given to optimizing future fertility.** With patients presenting earlier in the disease process, the number of those without symptoms or with minimal symptoms increased. There must be a high degree of suspicion of ectopic pregnancy, especially in areas of high prevalence. History and physical examination identify patients at risk, improving the probability of detection of ectopic pregnancy before rupture occurs.

History

Patients who have an ectopic pregnancy have an abnormal menstrual pattern or the perception of a spontaneous pregnancy loss. Pertinent points in the history include the menstrual history, previous pregnancy, infertility history, current contraceptive status, risk factor assessment, and current symptoms.

The classic symptom triad of ectopic pregnancy is pain, amenorrhea, and vaginal bleeding. This symptom group is present in about 50% of patients and is typical in patients with a ruptured ectopic pregnancy. Abdominal pain is the most common presenting symptom, but the severity and nature of the pain vary widely. There is no pathognomonic pain that is diagnostic of ectopic pregnancy. Pain may be unilateral or bilateral and may occur in the upper or lower abdomen. The pain may be dull, sharp, or crampy and either continuous or intermittent. With rupture, the patient may experience transient relief of the pain, as stretching of the tubal serosa ceases. Shoulder and back pain, thought to result from hemoperitoneal irritation of the diaphragm, may indicate intra-abdominal hemorrhage.

Physical Examination

The physical examination should include measurements of vital signs and examination of the abdomen and pelvis. Frequently, the findings before rupture and hemorrhage are nonspecific, and vital signs are normal. The abdomen may be nontender or mildly tender, with or without rebound. The uterus may be slightly enlarged, with findings similar to a normal pregnancy (103,104). Cervical motion tenderness may or may not be present. **An adnexal mass may be palpable in up to 50% of cases, but the mass varies markedly in size, consistency, and tenderness. A palpable mass may be the corpus luteum and not the ectopic pregnancy.** With rupture and intra-abdominal hemorrhage, the patient develops tachycardia followed by hypotension. Bowel sounds are decreased or absent. The abdomen is distended, with marked tenderness and rebound tenderness. Cervical motion tenderness is present. Frequently, the findings of the pelvic examination are inadequate because of pain and guarding.

History and physical examination may or may not provide useful diagnostic information. The accuracy of the initial clinical evaluation is less than 50% (105). Additional tests are frequently required to differentiate early viable intrauterine pregnancy or suspected ectopic or abnormal intrauterine pregnancy.

Laboratory Assessment

Quantitative β-human chorionic gonadotropin (β-hCG) measurements are the diagnostic cornerstone for ectopic pregnancy. **The hCG enzyme immunoassay, with a sensitivity of 25 mIU/mL, is an accurate screening test for detection of ectopic pregnancy. The assay is positive in virtually all documented ectopic pregnancies.**

Reference Standards

There are three reference standards for β-hCG measurement. The World Health Organization introduced the First International Standard (1st IS) in the 1930s. Testing for hCG and its subunits improved over the years. The Second International Standard (2nd IS), introduced in 1964, has varying amounts of β-hCG and β subunits. A purified preparation of β-hCG is now available. Originally referred to as the First International Reference Preparation (1st IRP), the test standard is now referred to as the Third International Standard (3rd IS). Although each standard has its own scale, the 2nd IS is about one-half of the 3rd IS. For example, if a level is reported as 500 mIU/mL (2nd IS), it is equivalent to a level of 1,000 mIU/mL (3rd IS). The assay standard used must be known to interpret hCG results correctly (106). In several recent articles, attention was drawn to a problem known as **phantom hCG, in which the presence of heterophile anti-**

bodies or proteolytic enzymes causes a false-positive hCG result. Because the antibodies are large glycoproteins, significant quantities of the antibody are not excreted in the urine. **In the patient with hCG levels less than 1,000 mIU/mL, a urine pregnancy test should be performed and confirmatory positive results obtained before instituting treatment** (107,108).

Doubling Time

The hCG level correlates somewhat with the gestational age (109). During the first 6 weeks of amenorrhea, serum hCG levels increase exponentially. During this period, the doubling time of hCG is relatively constant, regardless of the initial level. After the sixth week of gestation, when hCG levels are higher than 6,000 to 10,000 mIU/mL, the hCG rise is slower and not constant (110).

The hCG doubling time can help to differentiate an ectopic pregnancy from an intrauterine pregnancy—a 66% rise in the hCG level over 48 hours (85% confidence level) represents the lower limit of normal values for viable intrauterine pregnancies (111). **About 15% of patients with viable intrauterine pregnancies have less than a 66% rise in hCG level over 48 hours, and a similar percentage with an ectopic pregnancy have more than a 66% rise.** If the sampling interval is reduced to 24 hours, the overlap between normal and abnormal pregnancies is even greater. Patients with normal intrauterine pregnancies usually have more than a 50% rise in their hCG levels over 48 hours when the starting level is less than 2,000 mIU/mL. **The hCG pattern that is most predictive of an ectopic pregnancy is one that has reached a plateau (a doubling time of more than 7 days). For falling levels, a half-life of less than 1.4 days is rarely associated with an ectopic pregnancy, whereas a half-life of more than 7 days is most predictive of ectopic pregnancy.**

Serial hCG levels are usually required when the results of the initial ultrasonography examination are indeterminate (i.e., when there is no evidence of an intrauterine gestation or extrauterine cardiac activity consistent with an ectopic pregnancy). When the hCG level is less than 2,000, doubling time helps to predict viable intrauterine gestation (normal rise) versus nonviability (subnormal rise). With normally rising levels, a second ultrasonography examination is performed when the level is expected (by extrapolation) to reach 2,000 mIU/mL. Abnormally rising levels (less than 2,000 mIU/mL and less than 50% rise over 48 hours) indicate a nonviable pregnancy. The location (i.e., intrauterine versus. extrauterine) must be determined surgically, either by laparoscopy or dilation and curettage. Indeterminate ultrasonography results and an hCG level of less than 2,000 mIU/mL is diagnostic of nonviable gestation, either ectopic pregnancy or a complete abortion. Rapidly falling hCG levels (50% over 48 hours) occur with a completed abortion, whereas with an ectopic pregnancy levels rise or plateau.

Single Human Chorionic Gonadotropin Level

A single hCG measurement has limited usefulness because there is considerable overlap of values between normal and abnormal pregnancies at a given gestational age. The ectopic pregnancy site and hCG level do not correlate (112). Many patients in whom the diagnosis of ectopic pregnancy is being considered are uncertain about their menstrual dates. A single hCG level may be useful when measured by sensitive enzyme immunoassays that, if negative, exclude a diagnosis of ectopic pregnancy. Measurement of a single level may be helpful in predicting pregnancy outcome after timed conceptions using advanced reproductive technology. If the hCG level is more than 300 mIU/mL on day 16 to 18 after artificial insemination, there is an 88% chance of a live birth (113). If the hCG level is less than 300 mIU/mL, the chance of a live birth is only 22%. A single hCG level may facilitate the interpretation of ultrasonography when an intrauterine gestation is not visualized. **An hCG level greater than the ultrasound discriminatory zone indicates a possible extrauterine pregnancy.** Determination of serial hCG levels may be needed to differentiate an ectopic pregnancy from a completed abortion. Further tests are required for patients in whom ultrasonography examination results are inconclusive and hCG levels are below the discriminatory zone.

Serum Progesterone

The mean serum progesterone level in patients with ectopic pregnancies is lower than that in patients with normal intrauterine pregnancies (114,115). However, in studies of more than 5,000 patients with first-trimester pregnancies, a spectrum of progesterone levels was found in patients with both normal and abnormal pregnancies (35,116,117). About 70% of patients with a viable intrauterine pregnancy have serum progesterone levels higher than 25 ng/mL, whereas only 1.5% of patients with ectopic pregnancies have serum progesterone levels higher than 25 ng/mL, and most of these pregnancies exhibit cardiac activity (35,116,117).

A serum progesterone level can be used as an ectopic pregnancy screening test for both normal and abnormal pregnancy, particularly in settings in which hCG levels and ultrasonography are not readily available. A serum progesterone level of less than 5 ng/mL is highly suggestive of an abnormal pregnancy, but it is not 100% predictive. The risk of a normal pregnancy with a serum progesterone level of less than 5 ng/mL is about 1 in 1,500 (118). Serum progesterone measurements alone cannot be used to predict pregnancy nonviability.

Other Endocrinologic Markers

In an effort to improve early detection of ectopic pregnancy, various endocrinologic and protein markers were studied. Estradiol levels increase slowly from conception until 6 weeks of gestation and then rise rapidly as placental production of estradiol increases (119). Estradiol levels are significantly lower in ectopic pregnancies when compared with viable pregnancies. However, there is considerable overlap between normal and abnormal pregnancies and between intrauterine and extrauterine pregnancies (120,121).

Maternal serum creatinine kinase was studied as a marker for ectopic pregnancy diagnosis (122). Maternal serum creatine kinase levels were significantly higher in all patients with tubal pregnancy when compared with those in patients who had missed abortions or normal intrauterine pregnancies. No correlation was found between the creatine kinase level and the clinical presentation of the patient, and there was no correlation with the hCG levels. *Schwangerschafts protein 1* (SP$_1$), also known as pregnancy-associated plasma protein C (PAPP-C) or pregnancy-specific β-glycoprotein (PSBS), is produced by the syncytiotrophoblast (120). The main advantage of SP$_1$ level assessment may be in the diagnosis of conception after recent hCG administration. A level of 2 ng/L might be used for the diagnosis of pregnancy; however, it is doubtful that a diagnosis can be established before delay of menses. Although the level of SP$_1$ increases late in all patients with a nonviable pregnancy, a single SP$_1$ level assessment does not have prognostic value (123).

Relaxin is a protein hormone produced solely by the corpus luteum of pregnancy. It appears in the maternal serum at 4 to 5 weeks of gestation, peaks at about 10 weeks of gestation, and decreases until term (124). Relaxin levels are significantly lower in ectopic pregnancies and spontaneous abortions than in normal intrauterine pregnancies. Prorenin and active renin levels are significantly higher in viable intrauterine pregnancies than in either ectopic pregnancies or spontaneous abortions, with a single level of more than 33 pg/mL excluding the diagnosis of ectopic pregnancy (125). The clinical utility of relaxin, prorenin, and renin levels in diagnosing ectopic pregnancy is not yet determined.

CA125 is a glycoprotein, the origin of which is uncertain during pregnancy. Levels of CA125 rise during the first trimester and return to a nonpregnancy range during the second and third trimesters. After delivery, maternal serum concentrations increase (126,127). Levels of CA125 were studied in an effort to predict spontaneous abortion. Although a positive correlation was found between elevated CA125 levels 18 to 22 days after conception and spontaneous abortion, repeat measurements at 6 weeks of gestation did not correlate with outcome (128). Conflicting results were reported—one study showed a higher serum CA125 level in normal pregnancies than in ectopic pregnancies 2 to 4 weeks after a missed menses, whereas another study found higher CA125 levels for ectopic pregnancies compared with normal pregnancies (129,130).

Maternal serum α-fetoprotein (AFP) levels are elevated in ectopic pregnancies; however, the use of AFP measurements as a screening technique for ectopic pregnancy was not studied (131,132). A combination of AFP with three other markers—β-hCG, progesterone, and estradiol—has 98.5% specificity and 94.5% accuracy for the prediction of ectopic pregnancy (133,134). **Serum placental growth factor may prove to be a diagnostic biomarker for ectopic pregnancy because it was shown to be undetectable in ectopic and nonviable pregnancies.**

C-reactive protein is an acute-phase reactant that increases with trauma or infection. Levels of this protein are lower in patients with ectopic pregnancy than in patients with an acute infectious process. When an infectious process is part of the differential diagnosis, measurement of C-reactive protein may be beneficial (135).

Ultrasonography

Improvements in ultrasonography resulted in the earlier diagnosis of intrauterine and ectopic gestations (136). **The sensitivity of the β-hCG assay allows the diagnosis of pregnancy before direct visualization by ultrasonography.**

The complete examination should include both transvaginal and transabdominal ultrasonography. **Transvaginal ultrasonography is superior to transabdominal ultrasonography in evaluating intrapelvic structures.** The closeness of the vaginal probe to the pelvic organs allows use of higher frequencies (5–7 mHz), which improves resolution. **Intrauterine pregnancy can be diagnosed 1 week earlier with transvaginal than with transabdominal ultrasonography.** Evidence of an empty uterus, detection of adnexal masses and free peritoneal fluid, and direct signs of ectopic pregnancy are more reliably established with a transvaginal procedure (137–142). Transabdominal ultrasonography permits visualization of both the pelvis and abdominal cavity and should be included as part of the complete ectopic pregnancy evaluation to detect adnexal masses and hemoperitoneum.

The earliest ultrasonographic finding of an intrauterine pregnancy is a small fluid space and the gestational sac, surrounded by a thick echogenic ring, located eccentrically within the endometrial cavity. The earliest normal gestational sac is seen at 5 weeks of gestation with transabdominal ultrasonography and at 4 weeks of gestation with transvaginal ultrasonography (143,144). **As the gestational sac grows, a yolk sac is seen within it, followed by an embryo with cardiac activity.**

The appearance of a normal gestational sac may be simulated by intrauterine fluid collection, the pseudogestational sac, which occurs in 8% to 29% of patients with ectopic pregnancy (145–147). This ultrasonographic lucency, centrally located, probably represents bleeding into the endometrial cavity by the decidual cast. Clots within this lucency may mimic a fetal pole.

Morphologically, identification of the double decidual sac sign (DDSS) is the best method of ultrasonographically differentiating true sacs from pseudosacs (148). The double sac, believed to be the decidua capsularis and parietalis, is seen as two concentric echogenic rings separated by a hypoechogenic space. Although useful, this approach has some limitations in sensitivity and specificity—the DDSS sensitivity ranges from 64% to 95% (147). Pseudosacs may occasionally appear as the DDSS; intrauterine sacs of failed pregnancies may appear as pseudosacs.

The appearance of a yolk sac within the gestational sac is superior to the DDSS in confirming intrauterine pregnancy (149). The yolk sac is consistently visible on transabdominal ultrasonography with a gestational sac size of 2 cm and on transvaginal ultrasonography with a gestational sac size of 0.6 to 0.8 cm (150,151). Intrauterine sacs smaller than 1 cm on transabdominal ultrasonography and smaller than 0.6 cm on transvaginal ultrasonography are considered indeterminate. Larger sacs without DDSS or yolk sac represent either a failed intrauterine or ectopic pregnancy.

The presence of cardiac activity within the uterine cavity is definitive evidence of an intrauterine pregnancy. This finding essentially eliminates the diagnosis of ectopic pregnancy because the incidence of combined intrauterine and extrauterine pregnancy is 1 in 30,000.

The presence of an adnexal gestational sac with a fetal pole and cardiac activity is the most specific but least sensitive sign of ectopic pregnancy, occurring in only 10% to 17% of cases (135,152,153). The recognition of other characteristics of ectopic pregnancy improves ultrasonographic sensitivity. Adnexal rings (fluid sacs with thick echogenic rings) that have a yolk sac or nonliving embryo are accepted as specific ultrasonographic signs of ectopic pregnancy (154). Adnexal rings are visualized in 22% of ectopic pregnancies using transabdominal ultrasonography and in 38% using transvaginal ultrasonography (137). Other studies identified adnexal rings in 33% to 50% of ectopic pregnancies (135,153). The adnexal ring may not always be apparent because bleeding around the sac results in the appearance of a nonspecific adnexal mass.

Complex or solid adnexal masses are frequently associated with ectopic pregnancy; however, the mass may represent a corpus luteum, endometrioma, hydrosalpinx, ovarian neoplasm (e.g., dermoid cyst), or pedunculated fibroid (4,155–157). The presence of free cul-de-sac fluid is frequently associated with ectopic pregnancy and is no longer considered evidence of rupture. The presence of intra-abdominal free fluid should raise concern about tubal rupture (158,159).

Accurate interpretation of ultrasonography findings requires correlation with the hCG level (discriminatory zone) (146,151,154,160). **All viable intrauterine pregnancies can be visualized by transabdominal ultrasonography for serum hCG levels higher than 6,500 mIU/mL; none can be seen at 6,000 mIU/mL. The inability to detect an intrauterine gestation with serum hCG levels higher than 6,500 mIU/mL indicates the presence of an abnormal (failed intrauterine or ectopic) pregnancy. Intrauterine sacs seen at hCG levels below the discriminatory zone are abnormal and represent either failed intrauterine pregnancies or the pseudogestational sacs of ectopic pregnancy. If there is no definite sign of an intrauterine gestation (the empty uterus sign) and the hCG level is below the discriminatory zone, the differential diagnosis includes the following considerations:**

1. **Normal intrauterine pregnancy too early for visualization**
2. **Abnormal intrauterine gestation**
3. **Recent abortion**
4. **Ectopic pregnancy**
5. **Nonpregnant patient**

The discriminatory zone is lowered progressively with improvements in ultrasonography resolution. **Discriminatory zones for transvaginal ultrasonography are reported at levels from 1,000 to 2,000 mIU/mL** (146,151,154,160). Discriminatory zones vary according to the expertise of the examiner and capability of the equipment.

Although the discriminatory zone for intrauterine pregnancy is well established, there is no such zone for ectopic pregnancy. Levels of hCG do not correlate with the size of ectopic pregnancy. Regardless of how high the hCG level may be, nonvisualization does not exclude ectopic pregnancy. An ectopic pregnancy may be present anywhere in the abdominal cavity, making ultrasonographic visualization difficult.

Doppler Ultrasonography

A Doppler shift occurs whenever the source of an ultrasound beam is moving. The usual sources of Doppler-shifted frequencies are red blood cells. The presence of intravascular blood flow, flow direction, and flow velocity can be determined (161). Pulsed Doppler provides ultrasonographic control over which vessels are sampled. The vascular information is provided both by the shape of the time-velocity waveform (high- or low-resistance flow) and by its systolic, diastolic, and mean velocities (or Doppler frequency shifts) (162). Color flow Doppler ultrasonography analyzes very low amplitude signals from an entire ultrasound tomogram; the Doppler shift is then modulated into color. This information is used to gauge generalized tissue vascularity and to guide pulsed Doppler vascular sampling of specific vessels.

The waveform in the uterine arteries in the nongravid state and in the first trimester of pregnancy shows a high-resistance (little or no diastolic flow), low-velocity pattern. Conversely, a high-velocity, low-resistance signal is localized to the area of developing placentation (163–165). This pattern, seen near the endometrium, is associated with normal and abnormal intrauterine pregnancies and is termed *peritrophoblastic flow*. Whereas transvaginal ultrasonography requires a well-developed double decidual sac (or possibly cardiac activity) to localize an intrauterine gestation, the use of Doppler techniques allows detection of an intrauterine pregnancy at an earlier date. The combined use of Doppler and two-dimensional imaging allows the differentiation of pseudogestational sacs and true intrauterine gestational sacs and the differentiation of the empty uterus sign as either the presence of an intrauterine pregnancy (normal and abnormal) or absence of an intrauterine pregnancy (with an increased risk for ectopic pregnancy) (158,166).

A similar high-velocity, low-impedance flow characterizes ectopic pregnancies. The addition of Doppler to the ultrasonographic evaluation of suspected ectopic pregnancy improves diagnostic sensitivity for individual diagnoses: from 71% to 87% for ectopic pregnancy, from 24% to 59% for failed intrauterine pregnancy, and from 90% to 99% for normal intrauterine pregnancy (154,158,166). **Transvaginal color Doppler ultrasonography did not increase overall detection rates (167). Magnetic resonance imaging (MRI) was studied for its possible uses in the diagnosis of ectopic pregnancy. The role of MRI in the detection of ectopic pregnancy is inconclusive. It was 96% accurate in detecting fresh hematoma associated with ectopic pregnancy. Further studies need to be done to assess its predictive value (168).**

Dilation and Curettage

Uterine curettage is performed when the pregnancy is confirmed to be nonviable and the location of the pregnancy cannot be determined by ultrasonography. The decision to evacuate the uterus in the presence of a positive pregnancy test must be made with caution to avoid the unintentional disruption of a viable intrauterine pregnancy. Although suction curettage traditionally was performed in the operating room, it can be accomplished under local anesthesia on an outpatient basis. Endometrial sampling methods (e.g., a Novak curettage or Pipelle endometrial sampling device) are accurate in diagnosing abnormal uterine bleeding, but their reliability for intrauterine pregnancy evacuation was not studied. These devices might miss intrauterine villi and falsely suggest the diagnosis of ectopic pregnancy.

It is essential to confirm the presence of trophoblastic tissue as rapidly as possible so that therapy may be instituted. After tissue is obtained by curettage, it can be added to saline, in which it will float (Fig. 20.4). Decidual tissue does not float. Chorionic villi are usually identified by their characteristic lacy frond appearance. The sensitivity and specificity of this technique are 95% when the tissue is examined with the aid of a dissecting microscope. Because flotation of curettage sample tissue is not 100% accurate in differentiating an intrauterine from extrauterine gestation, histologic confirmation or serial β-hCG level measurement is required. The presence of chorionic villi may be assessed rapidly with frozen section analysis, which avoids the waiting period of at least 48 hours for permanent histologic evaluation. Immunocytochemical staining techniques are used to identify intermediate trophoblasts that are not normally identified by light microscopy (169).

When frozen section analysis is not available, serial assessment of hCG levels permits rapid diagnosis. After evacuation of an abnormal intrauterine pregnancy, the hCG level decreases by greater than 15% within 12 to 24 hours. A borderline fall may represent interassay variability. A repeat level should be obtained in 24 to 48 hours to confirm the decline. If the uterus is evacuated

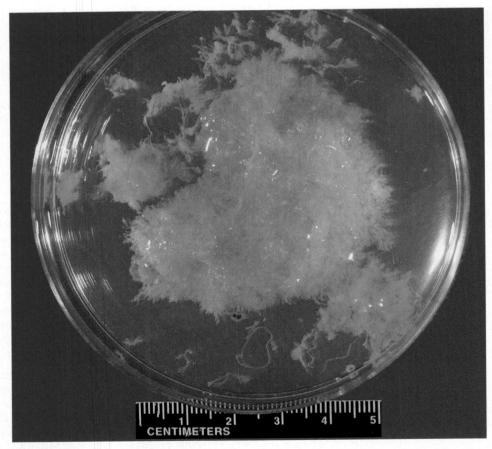

Figure 20.4   **When floated in saline, chorionic villi are often readily distinguishable as lacy fronds of tissue.**   (From **Stovall TG, Ling FW.** *Extrauterine pregnancy: clinical diagnosis and management.* New York: McGraw-Hill, 1993:186, with permission.)

and the pregnancy is extrauterine, the hCG level will plateau or continue to increase, indicating the presence of extrauterine trophoblastic tissue.

Culdocentesis

Culdocentesis was used widely as a diagnostic technique for ectopic pregnancy. With the use of hCG testing and transvaginal ultrasonography, culdocentesis is rarely indicated. The purpose of the procedure is to determine the presence of nonclotting blood, which increases the likelihood of ruptured ectopic pregnancy. After exposing the posterior vaginal fornix with a bivalve vaginal speculum, the posterior lip of the cervix is grasped with a tenaculum. The cul-de-sac is entered through the posterior vaginal wall with an 18- to 20-gauge spinal needle with a syringe attached. As the cul-de-sac is entered, suction is applied, and the intraperitoneal contents are aspirated. If nonclotting blood is obtained, the results are positive. If serous fluid is present, results are negative. A lack of fluid return or clotted blood is nondiagnostic.

Historically, if the culdocentesis results were positive, laparotomy was performed for a presumed diagnosis of ruptured tubal pregnancy. **The results of culdocentesis do not always correlate with the status of the pregnancy.** Although about 70% to 90% of patients with ectopic pregnancy have a hemoperitoneum demonstrated by culdocentesis, only 50% of patients have a ruptured tube (170). About 6% of women with positive culdocentesis results do not have an ectopic gestation at the time of laparotomy. Nondiagnostic taps occur in 10% to 20% of patients with ectopic pregnancy and are not definitive of the diagnosis. **A study concludes that culdocentesis is an obsolete tool in the diagnosis of suspected ectopic pregnancy** (171).

Laparoscopy

Laparoscopy is the gold standard for the diagnosis of ectopic pregnancy. The fallopian tubes are easily visualized and evaluated, but the diagnosis of ectopic pregnancy is missed in 3% to 4% of patients who have very small ectopic gestations. The ectopic gestation is seen distorting the normal tubal architecture. With earlier diagnosis, the possibility increases that a small ectopic pregnancy may not be visualized. Pelvic adhesions or previous tubal damage may compromise assessment of the tube. False-positive results occur when tubal dilation or discoloration is misinterpreted as an ectopic pregnancy, in which case the tube can be incised unnecessarily and damaged.

Diagnostic Algorithm

The presenting symptoms and physical findings of patients with unruptured ectopic pregnancies are similar to those of patients with normal intrauterine pregnancies (35). History, risk-factor assessment, and physical examination are the initial steps in the management of suspected ectopic pregnancy. Patients in a hemodynamically unstable condition should undergo immediate surgical intervention. Patients with a stable, relatively asymptomatic condition may be assessed as outpatients.

If the diagnosis of ectopic pregnancy can be confirmed without laparoscopy, several potential benefits result. First, both the anesthetic and surgical risks of laparoscopy are avoided; second, medical therapy becomes a treatment option. Because many ectopic pregnancies occur in histologically normal tubes, resolution without surgery may spare the tube from additional trauma and improve subsequent fertility. **An algorithm for the diagnosis of ectopic pregnancy without laparoscopy proved to be 100% accurate in a randomized clinical trial** (172,173) (Fig. 20.5). This screening algorithm shows the combined use of history and physical examination, serial hCG levels, serum progesterone levels, vaginal ultrasonography, and dilation and curettage. When hCG levels and transvaginal ultrasonography are available in a timely fashion, serum progesterone screening is not required. Serial hCG levels are used to assess pregnancy viability, correlated with transvaginal ultrasonography findings, and measured serially after a suction curettage. For patients in a stable condition, a treatment decision is never based on a single hCG level. After the initial evaluation, the patient is seen again at 24 to 48 hours for a repeat hCG level. At this time, transvaginal ultrasonography often is repeated so the findings can be correlated with the two hCG levels.

In this algorithm, **transvaginal ultrasonography is used as follows:**

1. **The identification of an intrauterine gestational sac or pregnancy effectively excludes the presence of an extrauterine pregnancy. If the patient has a rising hCG level of more than 2,000 mIU/mL, and no intrauterine gestational sac is**

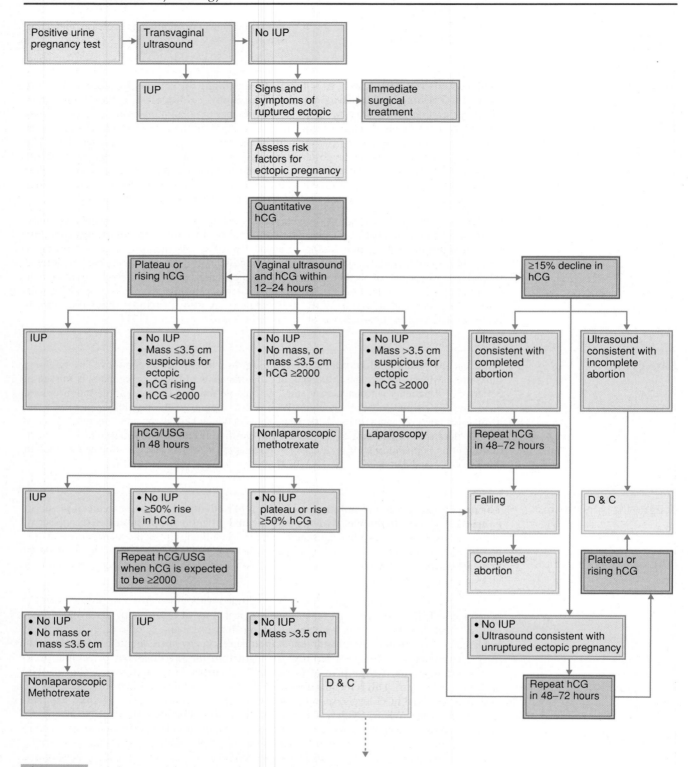

Figure 20.5   Nonlaparoscopic algorithm for diagnosis of ectopic pregnancy.

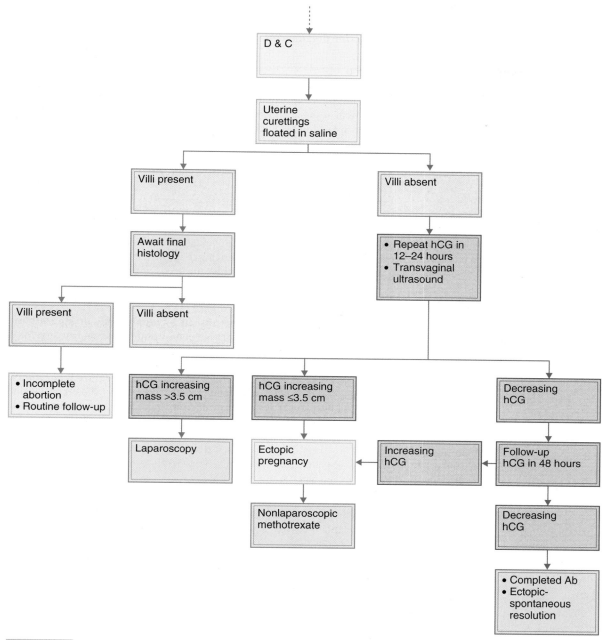

Figure 20.5 (*continued*) hCG, human chorionic gonadotropin; IUP, intrauterine pregnancy; USG, urine specific gravity; D&C, dilation and curettage.

identified, the patient is considered to have an extrauterine pregnancy and can be treated without further testing.

2. **Adnexal cardiac activity, when seen, definitively confirms the diagnosis of ectopic pregnancy.**

3. **A tubal mass as small as 1 cm can be identified and characterized. Masses greater than 3.5 cm with cardiac activity or larger than 4 cm without cardiac activity should not be treated with medical therapy.**

Suction curettage is used to differentiate nonviable intrauterine pregnancies from ectopic gestations (less than 50% rise in hCG level over 48 hours, an hCG level of less than 2,000 mIU/mL, and indeterminate ultrasonography findings). Performance of this procedure avoids unnecessary use of *methotrexate* in patients with abnormal intrauterine pregnancy that can be diagnosed only by evacuating the uterus. An unlikely potential problem with suction curettage is missing either an early nonviable intrauterine pregnancy or combined intrauterine and extrauterine pregnancies.

Treatment

Ectopic pregnancy can be effectively treated medically or surgically. Traditionally, exploratory laparotomy with unilateral salpingectomy was used for diagnosis and treatment for ectopic pregnancies. With techniques available that allow for early detection, including serum quantitative hCG levels and ultrasound, more conservative treatment options are available. Minimally invasive surgical techniques and medical management with *methotrexate* are the commonly used treatment options for ectopic pregnancies. **The treatment approach depends on the clinical circumstances, the site of the ectopic pregnancy, and the available resources.**

Surgical Treatment

Operative management is the most widely used treatment for ectopic pregnancy. The surgical approach (laparotomy versus. laparoscopy) and procedure (salpingectomy versus. salpingostomy) used to treat ectopic pregnancies depend on the clinical circumstances, available resources, and provider skill level. Each approach and procedure has associated risks and benefits, and the treatment employed must be individualized to best meet the needs of the patient and provider.

Laparotomy versus Laparoscopy

Treatment of an ectopic pregnancy can be accomplished by laparoscopy or laparotomy. The hemodynamic stability of the patient, size and location of the ectopic mass, and the surgeon's expertise all contribute to determining the appropriate surgical approach. **Laparotomy is indicated when the patient becomes hemodynamically unstable and an expedited abdominal entry is required. A ruptured ectopic pregnancy does not necessarily require laparotomy.** If the hemoperitoneum cannot be evacuated in a timely manner, laparotomy should be considered. Surgeon's experience with laparoscopy and the availability of laparoscopic equipment will determine the surgical approach. Cornual or interstitial pregnancies traditionally were treated with laparotomy, although laparoscopic management was described and is becoming common among skilled surgeons (174). Laparotomy is chosen for the management of most abdominal pregnancies. In some cases, the patient may have extensive abdominal or pelvic adhesive disease, making laparoscopy difficult and laparotomy more feasible.

Laparoscopy has advantages over laparotomy for management of ectopic pregnancy. In a case-control study of 50 patients comparing the use of laparoscopy and laparotomy for ectopic pregnancy management, hospital stay was significantly shorter (1.3 $\pm$ 0.8 versus. 3.0 $\pm$ 1.1 days), operative time was shorter (78 $\pm$ 26 versus. 104 $\pm$ 27 minutes), and convalescence was shorter (9 $\pm$ 8 versus. 26 $\pm$ 16 days) in the laparoscopy group (175). **Laparoscopic management was associated with significant cost savings when compared with laparotomy** ($4,368 $\pm$ $277 versus 5090 $\pm$ 168). Using a prospective analysis, 105 patients with tubal pregnancy were stratified with regard to age and risk factors and randomized to undergo either laparoscopic management or laparotomy (176). Subsequently, 73 patients underwent second-look laparoscopy to assess the degree of adhesion formation. Patients treated by laparotomy had significantly more adhesions at the surgical site than those treated by laparoscopy, but tubal patency rates were similar. A recent Cochrane review confirmed these findings and laparoscopic salpingostomy was associated with decreased cost, operative time, blood loss, and hospital stay when compared to salpingostomy at the time of a laparotomy (177).

An alternative to laparoscopy is the use of a minilaparotomy incision. This approach has the advantage of not requiring laparoscopic equipment and utilizes a smaller incision that should result in decreased postoperative pain and shorter recovery times for patients. A randomized control trial comparing minilaparotomy to laparotomy showed decreased complication rates and reduced costs associated with the minilaparotomy incision with similar success rates in the treatment of the ectopic pregnancy (177,178).

Salpingectomy versus Salpingostomy

There is debate about which surgical procedure is best. Salpingo-oophorectomy was once considered appropriate because it was theorized that this technique would eliminate transperitoneal migration of the ovum or zygote, which was thought to predispose to recurrent ectopic pregnancy

(179). Ovarian removal results in all ovulations occurring on the side with the remaining normal fallopian tube. Subsequent studies have not confirmed that ipsilateral oophorectomy increases the likelihood of conceiving an intrauterine pregnancy; therefore, this practice is not recommended (180). Whether to treat the ectopic pregnancy with a salpingostomy or salpingectomy is strongly debated and multiple studies investigated this issue. If one surgical technique resulted in higher treatment efficacy, lower rates of recurrent ectopic pregnancies, and higher rates of future intrauterine pregnancies, the decision would be clear. Studies have not demonstrated a clear advantage of either salpingectomy or salpingostomy. The decision to chose one technique over the other depends on the condition of the affected and contralateral fallopian tubes, history of a previous ectopic pregnancy in the affected tube, and the patient's desire for future fertility.

Linear salpingostomy can be considered when the patient has an unruptured ectopic pregnancy, wishes to retain her potential for future fertility, and the affected fallopian tube appears otherwise normal. If the contralateral tube appears damaged, a salpingostomy should be considered.

In a salpingostomy, the products of conception are removed through an incision made into the tube on its antimesenteric border. The procedure can be accomplished with needle-tip cautery, laser, scalpel, or scissors. It can be done with operative laparoscopic techniques or via a laparotomy. Contraindications to a salpingostomy include ruptured fallopian tube, use of extensive cautery to obtain hemostasis, severely damaged tube, and a recurrent ectopic pregnancy in the same tube. The main risk factor of salpingostomy is a persistent ectopic pregnancy resulting from failure to remove the entire pregnancy from the fallopian tube. This was reported in 5% to 20% of cases, and the rate appears to be higher in laparoscopic cases as compared to salpingostomies at the time of a laparotomy (181–184). Patients with high starting β-hCG levels, early gestations, and small ectopic pregnancies (<2 cm) are at greater risk of having a persistent pregnancy after a salpingostomy (185). Because of this risk, it is recommended to follow weekly β-hCG levels to ensure complete resolution of the ectopic pregnancy. β-hCG levels that persist or plateau can usually be treated successfully with a single dose of *methotrexate,* as described below (26).

Milking the tube to effect a tubal abortion was advocated; if the pregnancy is fimbrial, this technique may be effective. When milking was compared with linear salpingostomy for ampullary ectopic pregnancies, milking was associated with a twofold increase in the recurrent ectopic pregnancy rate (186).

Reproductive Outcome

Reproductive outcome after ectopic pregnancy is evaluated by determining tubal patency by hysterosalpingography, the subsequent intrauterine pregnancy rate, and the recurrent ectopic pregnancy rate. **Pregnancy rates are similar in patients treated by either laparoscopy or laparotomy. Tubal patency on the ipsilateral side after conservative laparoscopic management is about 84%** (187).

In a study of 143 patients followed after undergoing laparoscopic procedures for ectopic pregnancy, the overall intrauterine pregnancy rates for laparoscopic salpingostomy (60%) and laparoscopic salpingectomy (54%) were not significantly different (188). If the patient had evidence of tubal damage, pregnancy rates (42%) were significantly lower than in those women who did not have tubal damage (79%). In another study, the reproductive outcome of 188 patients followed for a mean of 7.2 years (range 3–15 years) was reported after conservation by laparotomy for ectopic pregnancy (189). An intrauterine pregnancy occurred in 83 (70%) patients, with a recurrent ectopic pregnancy rate of 13%, suggesting that reproductive outcome after an ectopic pregnancy treated by laparotomy is similar to that of patients undergoing laparoscopic or medical management. A recent Cochrane review showed no difference in tubal patency rate, future intrauterine pregnancy rates, and recurrent ectopic pregnancy rates in those patients treated with salpingostomy by either laparoscopy or laparotomy approach (177).

Medical Treatment	**The drug most frequently used for medical management of ectopic pregnancy is *methotrexate,*** although other agents were studied, including potassium chloride (KCl), hyperosmolar glucose, prostaglandins, and *RU-486.* These agents may be given systemically (intravenously, intramuscularly, or orally) or locally (laparoscopic direct injection, transvaginal ultrasonographically directed injection, or retrograde salpingography). Other agents besides *methotrexate* are not recommended for the treatment of ectopic pregnancy because their safety and efficacy are not well documented.

Table 20.2 Contraindications to Medical Therapy
Absolute Contraindications
Hemodynamically unstable
Ruptured ectopic pregnancy
Unable to comply with medical management follow-up
Breastfeeding
Immunodeficiency
Alcoholism, alcoholic liver disease or chronic liver disease
Preexisting blood dyscrasias
Known sensitivity to *methotrexate*
Active pulmonary disease
Peptic ulcer disease
Hepatic, renal, or hematologic disorder
Relative Contraindications
Gestational sac larger than 3.5 cm
Embryonic cardiac motion

Adapted from ACOG Practice Bulletin Medical Management of Ectopic Pregnancy, 2008.

Methotrexate

Methotrexate is a folic acid analogue that inhibits dehydrofolate reductase and thereby prevents synthesis of DNA. *Methotrexate* affects actively growing cells including trophoblastic tissues, malignant cells, bone marrow, intestinal mucosa, and respiratory epithelium (190). It is used extensively in the treatment of gestational trophoblastic disease (see Chapter 39). Initially, *methotrexate* was used for the treatment of trophoblastic tissue left *in situ* after exploration for an abdominal pregnancy (191). In 1982, Tanaka et al. treated an unruptured interstitial gestation with a 15-day course of intramuscular *methotrexate* (192). Multiple studies documented the safety and efficacy of *methotrexate* therapy for the management of ectopic pregnancies, and this is the first-line treatment for many providers. Approximately 35% of patients with ectopic pregnancies are candidates for primary therapy with *methotrexate* (193). *Methotrexate* is appropriate for primary treatment and may be given for the treatment of persistent ectopic pregnancies that failed surgical management.

Candidates for Methotrexate   Medical management of ectopic pregnancies with *methotrexate* is safe and effective, however, not all patients are candidates for this medical therapy. According to American College of Obstetricians and Gynecologists (ACOG) guidelines, *methotrexate* therapy can be considered for those patients with confirmed, or high suspicion for, ectopic pregnancy who are hemodynamically stable with no evidence of rupture. Table 20.2 documents the absolute contraindications to *methotrexate* therapy including breastfeeding, hepatic, renal, or hematologic disorders and known sensitivity to *methotrexate*. A patient who is unable to comply with the follow-up protocol should not be offered medical management. Relative contraindications to *methotrexate* therapy include gestational sac greater than or equal to 3.5 cm and embryonic cardiac motion (Table 20.2). Prior to the administration of *methotrexate*, a patient should have a complete blood count, blood type, liver function tests, electrolyte panel including creatinine, and a chest x-ray if there is any history of pulmonary disease. These studies are usually repeated 1 week after administration of *methotrexate* to evaluate for any potential complications from the therapy (190).

Methotrexate Dosing Regimens   *Methotrexate* is usually given via intramuscular injection but can be administered orally or by intravenous infusion. *Methotrexate* traditionally was administered using a multidose regimen, but single dosing protocols were developed that are easier for patient compliance (194).

Table 20.3 *Methotrexate* Treatment Regimens
Multidose Regimen
Administer *MTX* 1 mg/kg IM days 1, 3, 5, 7
Administer *leucovorin* 0.1 mg/kg days 2, 4, 6, 8
Measure β-hCG levels on days 1, 3, 5, 7 until 15% decrease between two measurements.
Once β-hCG levels drop 15%, stop *MTX* and monitor β-hCG weekly until nonpregnant level
Single-Dose Regimen
Administer *MTX* 50 mg/m^2 on day 0
Measure β-hCG level on days 4 and 7
If levels drop by 15%, monitor β-hCG weekly until nonpregnant level
If levels do not drop by 15%, repeat dose of *MTX* and measure β-hCG on days 4 and 7
Two-Dose Regimen
Administer *MTX* 50 mg/m^2 on days 0 and 4
Measure β-hCG level on days 4 and 7
If levels drop by 15%, monitor β-hCG weekly until nonpregnant level
If levels do not drop by 15%, repeat dose of *MTX* on days 7 and 11 and measure β-hCG on days 7 and 11. If levels drop 15%, monitor β-hCG weekly until nonpregnant level

MTX, methotrexate; IM, intramuscular; β-hCG, β-human chorionic gonadotropin;
Adapted from ACOG Practice Bulletin Medical Management of Ectopic Pregnancy, 2008.

The multidose regimen is outlined in Table 20.3. Patients receive 1 mg/kg of *methotrexate* intramuscularly on days 1, 3, 5, and 7 with leucovorin 0.1 mg/kg intramuscular administered on days 2, 4, 6, and 8. As a result of the repeat dosing of *methotrexate*, side effects are more common. The leucovorin helps reduce these side effects and increases patients' tolerance of the treatment. A patient may not require all four doses of *methotrexate* and her β-hCG levels should be monitored on days 1, 3, 5, and 7. If the β-hCG level drops 15% between two measurements, the regimen can be stopped and weekly β-hCG monitoring initiated. If the *methotrexate* is discontinued early, the patient should receive leucovorin after her final dose of *methotrexate* to help reduce potential side effects. If a patient's β-hCG level plateaus or increases, a second round of *methotrexate* and leucovorin can be given 1 week later. Earlier studies indicated approximately 19% will require all four doses, and 17% of women will require only one dose with this regimen (195,196). **A more recent meta-analysis showed 10% of women require only one dose, while nearly 54% will require all four doses.**

Methotrexate Single-Dose Regimens   Single-dose regimens were designed to increase patient compliance and simplify the administration of *methotrexate*. This regimen is well studied and safe and effective in the treatment of ectopic pregnancies. The single-dose regimen is detailed in Table 20.3.

Approximately 15% to 20% of patients in the single-dose regimen will require a second dose of *methotrexate* due to persistent β-hCG levels (194,197). The β-hCG level at the time of treatment appears to predict the subsequent success rate of single-dose therapy. Patients with β-hCG levels greater than 5,000 mIU/mL have a 14.3% chance of treatment failure compared to only 3.7% for women with levels less than 5,000 mIU/mL (198).

Compared with the multidose protocol, single-dose *methotrexate* is less expensive, patient acceptance is greater because less monitoring is required during treatment, and the treatment results and prospects for future fertility are comparable (194).

Methotrexate Two-Dose Regimen   The two-dose regimen was described as a cross between the single and multidose regimens. Because only 54% require all four doses of the multidose regimen, and 15% to 20% will require a second dose in the single-dose regimen, it is reasonable to consider a two-dose regimen of *methotrexate*. The protocol is outlined in Table 20.3 and involves

Table 20.4 Initiation of *Methotrexate*: Physician Checklist and Patient Instructions

Physician Checklist

Obtain hCG level.
Check CBC, liver function tests, creatinine, and blood type
Administer *RhoGAM* if patient is Rh-negative.
Identify unruptured ectopic pregnancy smaller than 3.5 cm (relative contraindication)
Obtain informed consent
Prescribe $FeSO_4$ 325 mg PO bid if hematocrit is less than 30%.
Schedule follow-up appointment on days 4 and 7.

Patient Instructions

Refrain from alcohol use, multivitamins containing folic acid, NSAID use, and sexual intercourse until hCG level is negative.
Call your physician if:
You experience prolonged or heavy vaginal bleeding.
The pain is prolonged or severe (lower abdomen and pelvic pain is normal during the first 10–14 days of treatment).
You use oral contraception or barrier contraceptive methods.

About 4%–5% of women experience unsuccessful *methotrexate* treatment and require surgery. hCG, human chorionic gonadotropin; SGOT, serum glutamic-oxaloacetic transaminase; BUN, blood urea nitrogen; CBC, complete blood count; *Rho-GAM*, $Rho_0(D)$ immune globulin; NSAIDs, nonsteroidal anti-inflammatory drugs; WBC, white blood cell; PO, by mouth; bid, twice daily.

the administration of *methotrexate* on day 0 and day 4 with monitoring of β-hCG levels on days 4 and 7. If there is less than a 15% drop between the two measures, a repeat administration of *methotrexate* is given on days 7 and 11 and β-hCG levels drawn accordingly. A single study showed an 87% success rate with low complication rates and high patient satisfaction (199).

Effectiveness of *Methotrexate*

The overall effectiveness of *methotrexate* therapy ranges from 78% to 96% (200). A meta-analysis in 2003 of 26 observational studies including 1,300 women revealed a significantly higher rate (93% versus. 88%) of successful treatment with multidose therapy (194). A meta-analysis comparing two randomized controlled trials showed no difference in success rates between the two regimens; however, the β-hCG levels in both of these studies were less than 3,000 mIU/mL (184,201,202).

When comparing *methotrexate* to laparoscopic salpingostomy, the multidose regimen has similar success rates. The single-dose regimen has lower initial success rates. After women receive additional doses as needed, the success rates are comparable between laparoscopic salpingostomy and single-dose *methotrexate* protocols (184).

Initiating Methotrexate   Outlined in Table 20.4 is a checklist that should be followed by the physician before initiating *methotrexate*. It includes instructions that are helpful to the patient.

Patient Follow-Up   **After intramuscular administration of *methotrexate*, regardless of the dose regimen used, patients are monitored on an outpatient basis with weekly β-hCG levels. These levels need to be monitored until the β-hCG reaches nonpregnant levels.** It is possible that tubal rupture may occur even if β-hCG levels are falling. Signs of a tubal rupture include severe pain, hemodynamic instability, and a drop in hematocrit. Patients who report severe or prolonged pain should be evaluated by measuring hematocrit levels and performing transvaginal ultrasonography. The ultrasonography findings during follow-up, although usually not helpful, can be used to provide reassurance that the tube is not ruptured (203). Cul-de-sac fluid is a common finding, and the amount of fluid may increase if a tubal abortion occurs. It is not necessary to intervene surgically, unless the patient has a precipitous drop in hematocrit levels or she becomes hemodynamically unstable.

Side Effects   **Side effects of *methotrexate* therapy are dose and frequency dependent. The most commonly reported side effects are the gastrointestinal symptoms of nausea, vomiting, stomatitis, and abdominal pain.** Because of these potential effects, women are cautioned against using alcohol and nonsteroidal anti-inflammatory medications while being treated with *methotrexate* (190). Other side effects include bone marrow suppression, hemorrhagic enteritis, alopecia, dermatitis, elevated liver enzyme levels, and pneumonitis (204). These side effects are usually mild and self-limited; few life-threatening side effects are reported with *methotrexate* treatment for ectopic pregnancy. The risk of these side effects does not appear to differ between single-dose and multidose regimens when adjusting for starting level of β-hCG at initiation of treatment. The frequency of reported side effects ranges from 30% to 40% (194). For those patients on prolonged therapy, *leucovorin* can reduce the incidence of these side effects and is included in the "multidose" regimen. Long-term follow-up of women treated with *methotrexate* for gestational trophoblastic disease shows no increase in congenital malformations, spontaneous abortions, or tumors recurring after chemotherapy (205). Treatment of ectopic pregnancy differs from that of gestational trophoblastic disease in that a smaller total dose of *methotrexate* is required and shorter treatment duration is used.

Although surgical management of ectopic pregnancy remains the mainstay of treatment worldwide, *methotrexate* treatment is appropriate in those patients who meet the treatment criteria previously detailed.

Reproductive Outcome   Reproductive function after *methotrexate* treatment can be assessed on the basis of repeat ectopic pregnancy rates, tubal patency, and pregnancy outcome. The risk of subsequent ectopic pregnancy is approximately 10% following either *methotrexate* or salpingostomy (52,53). The tubal patency rates are reported to be higher than 80% in those patients treated with either single-dose or multidose regimens with no difference in rates compared with women treated with salpingostomy (52,53). A randomized trial comparing *methotrexate* to laparoscopic salpingostomy showed no difference in tubal patency rates among the two groups, although in this trial patency rates were lower than previously reported at 66% in the salpingostomy group (206).

Subsequent spontaneous intrauterine pregnancy rates are similar between those women treated with *methotrexate* versus salpingostomy, with rates ranging from 36% to 64% (207,208). **Comparison of laparoscopically treated patients with *methotrexate*-treated patients indicates that the two methods have similar reproductive outcomes.**

Other Drugs and Techniques

Salpingocentesis is a technique in which agents such as KCl, *methotrexate,* prostaglandins, and hyperosmolar glucose are injected into the ectopic pregnancy transvaginally using ultrasonographic guidance, transcervical tubal cannulization, or laparoscopy. Agents injected under ultrasonographic guidance included *methotrexate,* KCl, combined *methotrexate* and KCl, and *prostaglandin* E_2 (162,209–215). The potential advantages of salpingocentesis include a one-time injection with the potential avoidance of systemic side effects. Reproductive function after this form of treatment was not reported. Because of the limited experience, this treatment cannot be recommended until there is further study.

Agents injected into the amniotic sac at laparoscopy included *prostaglandin* F_{2a}, hyperosmolar glucose, and *methotrexate* (216–218). This method has the obvious disadvantage of requiring laparoscopy, but it can be used if laparoscopy is performed for diagnosis. Other agents reported for the treatment of ectopic pregnancy include *RU-486* and anti-hCG antibody (219,220).

Types of Ectopic Pregnancy

Spontaneous Resolution   **Some ectopic pregnancies resolve by resorption or by tubal abortion, obviating the need for medical or surgical therapy** (221–225). The proportion of ectopic pregnancies that resolve spontaneously and the reason they do so while others do not are unknown. There are no specific criteria for patient selection that predict successful outcome after spontaneous resolution. A falling hCG level is the most common indicator used, but tubal rupture can occur even with falling hCG levels. Patients with low initial levels of β-hCG are generally the best candidates for expectant management, and there is a reported 88% success rate of spontaneous remission with an initial β-hCG level less than 200 mU/mL (226). These patients should be followed with serial β-hCG levels and active management initiated if these levels plateau or rise or the patient develops abdominal pain or signs of tubal rupture (190).

Persistent Trophoblastic Tissue

Persistent ectopic pregnancy occurs when a patient underwent conservative surgery (e.g., salpingostomy, fimbrial expression) and viable trophoblastic tissue remains. Histologically, there is no identifiable embryo, the implantation usually is medial to the previous tubal incision, and residual chorionic villi are confined to the tubal muscularis. Peritoneal trophoblastic tissue implants may be responsible for persistence (182,183,227–230).

The incidence of persistent ectopic pregnancy increased with the increased use of surgery that conserves the tubes. Persistence is diagnosed when the β-hCG levels plateau after conservative surgery. Risk factors for persistent ectopic pregnancy are based on the type of surgical procedure, the initial β-hCG level, the duration of amenorrhea, and the size of the ectopic pregnancy. Patients treated with laparoscopic salpingostomy have a higher rate of persistent ectopic pregnancies compared to those treated with salpingostomy at the time of a laparotomy, with an incidence of **persistence after laparoscopic linear salpingostomy ranging from 4% to 15%** (49,177). Other risk factors for persistent ectopic pregnancies include very early gestations (amenorrhea less than 7 weeks' duration), ectopic pregnancies less than 2 cm, and those with high starting β-hCG levels (183,185,229).

Persistent ectopic pregnancy can be treated surgically or medically; surgical therapy consists of either repeat salpingostomy or, more commonly, salpingectomy. *Methotrexate offers an alternative to patients who are hemodynamically stable at the time of diagnosis. Methotrexate may be the treatment of choice because the persistent trophoblastic tissue may not be confined to the tube and, therefore, not readily identifiable during repeat surgical exploration* (231–233).

Chronic Ectopic Pregnancy

Chronic ectopic pregnancy is a condition in which the pregnancy does not completely resorb during expectant management. The condition arises when there is persistence of the chorionic villi with bleeding into the tubal wall, which is distended slowly and does not rupture. It may arise from chronic bleeding from the fimbriated end of the fallopian tube with subsequent tamponade. In a series of 50 patients with a chronic ectopic pregnancy, pain was present in 86%, vaginal bleeding was present in 68%, and both symptoms were present in 58% (234). Ninety percent of the patients had amenorrhea ranging from 5 to 16 weeks (mean, 9.6 weeks). Most patients develop a pelvic mass that usually is symptomatic. The β-hCG level usually is low but may be absent; ultrasonography may be helpful in the diagnosis; rarely, bowel involvement or ureteral compression or obstruction exists (234,235).

This condition is treated surgically with removal of the affected tube. Often, the ovary must be removed because there is inflammation with subsequent adhesion development. A hematoma may be present secondary to chronic bleeding.

Nontubal Ectopic Pregnancy

Cervical Pregnancy   **The incidence of cervical pregnancy in the United States ranges from 1 in 2,400 to 1 in 50,000 pregnancies** and accounts for less than 1% of ectopic pregnancies (236,237). The cause of cervical ectopic pregnancies is unknown and the rare occurrence prevents identification of known risk factors. The incidence does appear to be higher with *in vitro* fertilization procedures, accounting for 3.7% of IVF-related ectopic pregnancies (238).

The clinical criteria for diagnosing a cervical pregnancy include the following findings (239):

1. Uterus is smaller than the surrounding distended cervix;
2. External os may be open;
3. Visible cervical lesion often blue or purple in color;
4. Profuse bleeding on manipulation of cervix.

Patients classically present with painless vaginal bleeding, but reports of associated cramping and pain are published (240).

Table 20.5 Ultrasound Criteria for Cervical Pregnancy

1. Gestational sac or placental tissue visualized within the cervix

2. Cardiac motion noted below the level of the internal os

3. No intrauterine pregnancy

4. Hourglass uterine shape with ballooned cervical canal

5. No movement of the sac with pressure from transvaginal probe (i.e., no "sliding sign" that is typically seen with incomplete abortions)

6. Closed internal os

Adapted from **Kung FT, Lin H, Hsu TY, et al.** Differential diagnosis of cervical ectopic pregnancy and conservative treatment with the combination of laparoscopy-assisted uterine artery ligation and hysteroscopic endocervical resection. *Fertil Steril* 2004;81:1642–1649.

When a cervical pregnancy is suspected, imaging studies are useful in confirming the diagnosis. Ultrasonographic diagnostic criteria are described that are helpful in differentiating a true cervical pregnancy from an ongoing spontaneous abortion (Table 20.5). MRI of the pelvis is used in this situation (241). Other potential diagnoses that must be differentiated from cervical pregnancy include cervical carcinoma, cervical or prolapsed submucousal leiomyomas, trophoblastic tumor, placenta previa, and low-lying placenta.

Management of cervical ectopic pregnancies includes medical treatment with *methotrexate* and surgical dilation and curettage. The ideal regimen for medical management is unknown and success is reported with both the single- and multidose regimens, as previously described. More advanced gestations, especially with fetal cardiac activity, may require a combination of multidose *methotrexate* and intra-amniotic/intrafetal injection of PCl. These injections require skill to avoid rupture of membranes during the procedure (240). As with tubal ectopic pregnancies, medical management is appropriate only for those patients who are hemodynamically stable.

If the patient and physician elect to proceed with surgical management, the preoperative preparation should include blood typing and cross-matching, establishment of intravenous access, and detailed informed consent. This consent should include the possibility of hemorrhage that may require transfusion or hysterectomy.

The diagnosis may not be suspected until the patient is undergoing suction curettage for a presumed incomplete abortion and hemorrhage occurs. In some cases, bleeding is light, whereas in others, there is hemorrhage. **Various techniques that can be used to control bleeding include uterine packing, lateral cervical suture placement to ligate the lateral cervical vessels, placement of a cerclage, and insertion of an intracervical 30-mL Foley catheter in an attempt to tamponade the bleeding. Alternatively, angiographic artery embolization can be used. If laparotomy is required, an attempt can be made to ligate the uterine or internal iliac arteries (242–244). When none of these methods is successful, hysterectomy is required.**

Ovarian Pregnancy   **A pregnancy confined to the ovary accounts for up to 3% of all ectopic pregnancies and is the most common type of nontubal ectopic pregnancy** (1). The incidence ranges from 1 in 40,000 to 1 in 7,000 deliveries (245,246). The diagnostic criteria were described in 1878 by Spiegelberg (Table 20.6) (247). Unlike tubal gestation, ovarian pregnancy is associated with neither PID nor infertility. The risk of ovarian ectopic pregnancies in patients using IUDs is controversial.

Patients have symptoms similar to those of ectopic pregnancies in other sites. Misdiagnosis is common because it is confused with a ruptured corpus luteum in up to 75% of cases (245). As with other types of ectopic pregnancy, an ovarian pregnancy was reported after hysterectomy (248). Ultrasonography makes preoperative diagnosis possible in some cases (249).

The treatment of ovarian pregnancy has changed. Whereas oophorectomy was advocated in the past, **ovarian cystectomy and/or wedge resection is now utilized with success** (250–252). Successful treatment with *methotrexate* is reported (253–255).

Table 20.6 Criteria for Ovarian Pregnancy Diagnosis
1. The fallopian tube on the affected side must be intact.
2. The fetal sac must occupy the position of the ovary.
3. The ovary must be connected to the uterus by the ovarian ligament.
4. Ovarian tissue must be located in the sac wall.

From **Spiegelberg O.** Casusistik der ovarialschwangerschaft. *Arch Gynaecol* 1878;13:73.

Abdominal Pregnancy   Abdominal pregnancies are classified as primary and secondary. Listed in Table 20.7 are criteria for classifying a primary abdominal pregnancy. Secondary abdominal pregnancies are the most common and result from tubal abortion or rupture or, less often, from subsequent implantation within the abdomen after uterine rupture. The incidence of abdominal pregnancy varies from 1 in 372 to 1 in 9,714 live births and accounts for 1.4% of ectopic pregnancies (1,256). Risk factors for abdominal pregnancy include PID, multiparity, endometriosis, assisted reproductive techniques, and tubal damage (257,258). **Abdominal pregnancy is associated with high morbidity and mortality, with the risk for death seven to eight times greater than from tubal ectopic pregnancy and 50 times greater than from intrauterine pregnancy** (256). There are scattered reports of term abdominal pregnancies. When this occurs, perinatal morbidity and mortality are high, usually as a result of growth restriction and congenital anomalies such as fetal pulmonary hypoplasia, pressure deformities, and facial and limb asymmetry. The incidence of congenital anomalies ranges from 20% to 40% (259,260).

The presentation of patients with an abdominal pregnancy varies and depends on the gestational age. In the first and early second trimesters, the symptoms may be the same as with tubal ectopic gestation; in advanced abdominal pregnancy, the clinical presentation is more variable. The patient may report painful fetal movement, fetal movements high in the abdomen, or sudden cessation of movements. Physical examination may disclose persistent abnormal fetal positioning, abdominal tenderness, a displaced uterine cervix, easy palpation of fetal parts, and palpation of the uterus separate from the gestation. The diagnosis may be suspected when there are no uterine contractions after *oxytocin* infusion. Other diagnostic aids include abdominal radiography, abdominal ultrasonography, CT, and MRI (261–263).

Because the pregnancy can continue to term, the potential maternal morbidity and mortality are very high. As a result, **surgical intervention is recommended when an abdominal pregnancy is diagnosed.** At surgery, the placenta can be removed if its vascular supply can be identified and ligated, but hemorrhage can occur, requiring abdominal packing that is left in place and removed after 24 to 48 hours. Angiographic arterial embolization was described (264). If the vascular supply cannot be identified, the cord is ligated near the placental base, and the placenta is left in place. Placental involution can be monitored using serial ultrasonography and assessment of β-hCG levels. Potential complications of leaving the placenta in place include bowel obstruction, fistula formation, and sepsis as the tissue degenerates. There are concerns regarding the use of *methotrexate* treatment in abdominal pregnancies. Specifically, there is

Table 20.7 Studdiford's Criteria for Diagnosis of Primary Abdominal Pregnancy
1. Presence of normal tubes and ovaries with no evidence of recent or past pregnancy.
2. No evidence of uteroplacental fistula.
3. The presence of a pregnancy related exclusively to the peritoneal surface and early enough to eliminate the possibility of secondary implantation after primary tubal nidation.

Adapted from **Anderson PM, Opfer EK, Busch JM, et al.** An early abdominal wall ectopic pregancy successfully treated with ultrasound guided intralesional methotrexate: a case report. *Obstet Gynecol Int* 2009; Article ID 247452

theoretically an increased risk of infection and sepsis resulting from the rapid tissue necrosis that occurs following *methotrexate* administration (265). There are reports of successful treatment of abdominal pregnancies with *methotrexate* in patients not considered to be optimal surgical candidates (266).

Interstitial Pregnancy **Interstitial pregnancies represent about 2.4% of ectopic pregnancies** (1). This section of the fallopian tube is relatively thick with an increased capacity to expand prior to rupture. This ability may allow these types of ectopic pregnancies to remain asymptomatic for 7 to 16 weeks of gestation (267). Late presentations are rare and these patients typically present between 6 to 8 weeks of gestation, similar to other types of ectopic pregnancies (268,269). The diagnosis of an interstitial ectopic pregnancy can be difficult, because this area has a relatively high level of vascular supply. Interstitial pregnancies represent a disproportionately large percentage of fatalities from ectopic pregnancy with a 2.5% mortality rate (268,270).

Treatment classically was a cornual resection by laparotomy, but early detection allows for a more conservative management approach in hemodynamically stable patients without evidence of rupture. Medical management with *methotrexate* is well described, with both the single- and multidose regimens. Approximately 10% to 20% of patients treated medically will ultimately require surgery and close follow-up, as is warranted with all medically managed ectopic pregnancies (271).

Although cornual wedge resection by laparotomy is an acceptable surgical option, minimally invasive techniques were described, including cornual excision, minicornual excision, and cornuostomy. Laparoscopic approaches are more widely used and are dependent on surgical skill. Transcervical suction evacuation under laparoscopic or ultrasound guidance is reported (271). The appropriate surgical technique and approach depends on the individual patient presentation and the surgeon's expertise.

Interligamentous Pregnancy **Interligamentous pregnancy is a rare form of ectopic pregnancy that occurs in about 1 of 300 ectopic pregnancies** (272). An interligamentous pregnancy usually results from trophoblastic penetration of a tubal pregnancy through the tubal serosa and into the mesosalpinx, with secondary implantation between the leaves of the broad ligament. It can occur if a uterine fistula develops between the endometrial cavity and the retroperitoneal space. As in abdominal pregnancy, with interligamentous pregnancy the placenta may be adherent to the uterus, bladder, and pelvic side walls. If possible, the placenta should be removed; when this is not possible, it can be left *in situ* and allowed to resorb. Cases of live birth are reported with this type ectopic gestation (272).

Heterotropic Pregnancy **Heterotropic pregnancy occurs when intrauterine and ectopic pregnancies coexist. The reported incidence varies widely from 1 in 100 to 1 in 30,000 pregnancies** (273). Patients who underwent assisted reproduction have a much higher incidence of heterotropic pregnancy than those who have a spontaneous conception (274,275). An intrauterine pregnancy is seen during ultrasonography examination, and an extrauterine pregnancy may be overlooked, delaying diagnosis. Serial β-hCG levels are not helpful because the intrauterine pregnancy causes the β-hCG level to rise appropriately.

The ectopic pregnancy is treated surgically if the intrauterine pregnancy is desired. When the ectopic pregnancy is removed, the intrauterine pregnancy continues in most patients. The rate of spontaneous abortion is higher with approximately one in three ending in miscarriage (276,277). It may be possible to treat the ectopic pregnancy using nonchemotherapeutic medical treatment, such as KCl, by transvaginal or laparoscopically directed injection; however, a reported 55% may require additional surgical treatment (278).

Multiple Ectopic Pregnancies **Twin or multiple ectopic gestations occur less frequently than heterotropic gestations and may appear in a variety of locations and combinations. Multiple ectopic pregnancies are thought to be rare, but with the advent of assisted reproductive technologies the incidence appears to be rising.** A recent review of bilateral tubal pregnancies reported 242 cases between 1918 and 2007, with 42 cases in the past 10 years alone. Fifty percent of these twin tubal pregnancies were associated with assisted reproductive technologies (279). Another review of 163 cases of tubal ectopic pregnancies had a reported rate of twin tubal pregnancies of 2.4% (280). Although most reports are confined to twin tubal gestations, ovarian, interstitial, and abdominal twin pregnancies were reported. Twin and triplet gestations were reported following partial salpingectomy and IVF (281,282). Management is similar to that of other types of ectopic pregnancy and is somewhat dependent on the location of the pregnancy.

Pregnancy after Hysterectomy The most unusual form of ectopic pregnancy is one that occurs after vaginal or abdominal hysterectomy (283,284). Such a pregnancy may occur after supracervical hysterectomy because the patient has a cervical canal that may provide intraperitoneal access. Pregnancy may occur in the perioperative period with implantation of the already fertilized ovum in the fallopian tube. Pregnancy after total hysterectomy probably occurs secondary to a vaginal mucosal defect that allows sperm into the abdominal cavity.

References

1. **Bouyer J, Coste J, Fernandez H, et al.** Sites of ectopic pregnancy: a 10 year population-based study of 1800 cases. *Hum Reprod* 2002;17:3224–3230.
2. **Wilcox AJ, Weinberg CR, O'Connor JF, et al.** Incidence of early loss of pregnancy. *N Engl J Med* 1988;319:189–194.
3. **Wang X, Chen C, Wang L, et al.** Conception, early pregnancy loss, and time to clinical pregnancy: a population-based prospective study. *Fertil Steril* 2003;79:577–584.
4. **Hill LM, Guzick D, Fries J, et al.** Fetal loss rate after ultrasonically documented cardiac activity between 6 and 14 weeks, menstrual age. *J Clin Ultrasound* 1991;19:221–223.
5. **Juliano M, Dabulis S, Heffner A.** Characteristics of women with fetal loss in symptomatic first trimester pregnancies with documented fetal cardiac activity. *Ann Emerg Med* 2008;52:143–147.
6. **Wyatt PR, Owolabi T, Meier C, et al.** Age-specific risk of fetal loss observed in a second trimester serum screening population. *Am J Obstet Gynecol* 2005;192:240–246.
7. **Stirrat GM.** Recurrent miscarriage. *Lancet* 1990;336:673–675.
8. **Deaton JL, Honore GM, Huffman CS, et al.** Early transvaginal ultrasound following an accurately dated pregnancy: the importance of finding a yolk sac or fetal heart motion. *Hum Reprod* 1997;12:2820–2823.
9. **Nybo Andersen AM, Wohlfahrt J, Christens P, et al.** Maternal age and fetal loss: population based register linkage study. *BMJ* 2000;320:1708–1712.
10. **Kleinhaus K, Perrin M, Friedlander Y, et al.** Paternal age and spontaneous abortion. *Obstet Gynecol* 2006;108:369–377.
11. **Buss L, Tolstrup J, Munk C, et al.** Spontaneous abortion: a prospective cohort study of younger women from the general population in Denmark. Validation, occurrence and risk determinants. *Acta Obstet Gynecol Scand* 2006;85:467–475.
12. **Chatenoud L, Parazzini F, di Cintio E, et al.** Paternal and maternal smoking habits before conception and during the first trimester: relation to spontaneous abortion. *Ann Epidemiol* 1998;8:520–526.
13. **Nielsen A, Hannibal CG, Lindekilde BE, et al.** Maternal smoking predicts the risk of spontaneous abortion. *Acta Obstet Gynecol Scand* 2006;85:1057–1065.
14. **Perriera L, Reeves MF.** Ultrasound criteria for diagnosis of early pregnancy failure and ectopic pregnancy. *Semin Reprod Med* 2008;26:373–382.
15. **Makrydimas G, Sebire NJ, Lolis D, et al.** Fetal loss following ultrasound diagnosis of a live fetus at 6–10 weeks of gestation. *Ultrasound Obstet Gynecol* 2003;22:368–372.
16. **Sotiriadis A, Papatheodorou S, Makrydimas G.** Threatened miscarriage: evaluation and management. *BMJ* 2004;329:152–155.
17. **Gerhard I, Gwinner B, Eggert-Kruse W, et al.** Double-blind controlled trial of progesterone substitution in threatened abortion. *Biol Res Pregnancy Perinatol* 1987;8:26–34.
18. **Harrison RF.** A comparative study of human chorionic gonadotropin, placebo, and bed rest for women with early threatened abortion. *Int J Fertil Menopausal Stud* 1993;38:160–165.
19. **Lykke JA, Dideriksen KL, Lidegaard O, et al.** First-trimester vaginal bleeding and complications later in pregnancy. *Obstet Gynecol* 2010;115:935–944.
20. **Weiss JL, Malone FD, Vidaver J, et al.** Threatened abortion: a risk factor for poor pregnancy outcome, a population-based screening study. *Am J Obstet Gynecol* 2004;190:745–750.
21. **Leitich H, Bodner-Adler B, Brunbauer M, et al.** Bacterial vaginosis as a risk factor for preterm delivery: a meta-analysis. *Am J Obstet Gynecol* 2003;189:139–147.
22. **American College of Obstetrics and Gynecology.** ACOG Practice Bulletin. Prevention of Rh D alloimmunization. Number 4, May 1999 (replaces educational bulletin Number 147, October 1990). Clinical management guidelines for obstetrician-gynecologists. *Int J Gynaecol Obstet* 1999;66:63–70.
23. **Ballagh SA, Harris HA, Demasio K.** Is curettage needed for uncomplicated incomplete spontaneous abortion? *Am J Obstet Gynecol* 1998;179:1279–1282.
24. **Jurkovic D, Ross JA, Nicolaides KH.** Expectant management of missed miscarriage. *Br J Obstet Gynaecol* 1998;105:670–671.
25. **Zhang J, Gilles JM, Barnhart K, et al.** A comparison of medical management with misoprostol and surgical management for early pregnancy failure. *N Engl J Med* 2005;353:761–769.
26. **Blum J, Winikoff B, Gemzell-Danielsson K, et al.** Treatment of incomplete abortion and miscarriage with misoprostol. *Int J Gynaecol Obstet* 2007;99(Suppl 2):S186–S189.
27. **Seeber BE, Barnhart KT.** Suspected ectopic pregnancy. *Obstet Gynecol* 2006;107:399–413.
28. **Anonymous.** Ectopic pregnancy—United States, 1990–1992. *MMWR Morb Mortal Wkly Rep* 1995;44:46–48.
29. **Anonymous.** Ectopic pregnancy—United States, 1988–1989. *MMWR Morb Mortal Wkly Rep* 1992;41:591–594.
30. **Yao M, Tulandi T.** Current status of surgical and nonsurgical management of ectopic pregnancy. *Fertil Steril* 1997;67:421–433.
31. **Murray H, Baakdah H, Bardell T, et al.** Diagnosis and treatment of ectopic pregnancy. *CMAJ* 2005;173:905–912.
32. **Ankum WM, Mol BW, Van der Veen F, et al.** Risk factors for ectopic pregnancy: a meta-analysis. *Fertil Steril* 1996;65:1093–1099.
33. **Buckley RG, King KJ, Disney JD, et al.** History and physical examination to estimate the risk of ectopic pregnancy: validation of a clinical prediction model. *Ann Emerg Med* 1999;34:589–594.
34. **Dart RG, Kaplan B, Varaklis K.** Predictive value of history and physical examination in patients with suspected ectopic pregnancy. *Ann Emerg Med* 1999;33:283–290.
35. **Stovall TG, Kellerman AL, Ling FW, et al.** Emergency department diagnosis of ectopic pregnancy. *Ann Emerg Med* 1990;19:1098–1103.
36. **Pulkkinen MO, Talo A.** Tubal physiologic consideration in ectopic pregnancy. *Clin Obstet Gynecol* 1987;30:164–172.
37. **Coste J, Fernandez H, Joye N, et al.** Role of chromosome abnormalities in ectopic pregnancy. *Fertil Steril* 2000;74:1259–1260.
38. **Lavy G, Diamond MP, DeCherney AH.** Ectopic pregnancy: its relationship to tubal reconstructive surgery. *Fertil Steril* 1987;47:543–556.
39. **Peterson HB, Xia Z, Hughes JM, et al.** The risk of pregnancy after tubal sterilization: findings from the U.S. Collaborative Review of Sterilization. *Am J Obstet Gynecol* 1996;174:1161–1170.
40. **Mol BW, Ankum WM, Bossuyt PM, et al.** Contraception and the risk of ectopic pregnancy: a meta-analysis. *Contraception* 1995;52:337–341.
41. **Peterson HB, Xia Z, Hughes JM, et al.** The risk of ectopic pregnancy after tubal sterilization. U.S. Collaborative Review of Sterilization Working Group. *N Engl J Med* 1997;336:762–767.

42. **Rock JA, Guzick DS, Katz E, et al.** Tubal anastomosis: pregnancy success following reversal of Falope ring or monopolar cautery sterilization. *Fertil Steril* 1987;48:13–17.

43. **Henderson SR.** The reversibility of female sterilization with the use of microsurgery: a report on 102 patients with more than one year of follow-up. *Am J Obstet Gynecol* 1984;149:57–65.

44. **Spivak MM, Librach CL, Rosenthal DM.** Microsurgical reversal of sterilization: a six-year study. *Am J Obstet Gynecol* 1986;154:355–361.

45. **DeCherney AH, Mezer HC, Naftolin F.** Analysis of failure of microsurgical anastomosis after midsegment, non-coagulation tubal ligation. *Fertil Steril* 1983;39:618–622.

46. **Hulka JF.** Spring clip technique for sterilization. *Obstet Gynecol* 1982;60:760.

47. **Vasquez G, Winston RM, Boeckx W, et al.** Tubal lesions subsequent to sterilization and their relation to fertility after attempts at reversal. *Am J Obstet Gynecol* 1980;138:86–92.

48. **Hajenius PJ, Mol BW, Ankum WM, et al.** Suspected ectopic pregnancy: expectant management in patients with negative sonographic findings and low serum hCG concentrations. *Early Pregnancy* 1995;1:258–262.

49. **Farquhar CM.** Ectopic pregnancy. *Lancet* 2005;366:583–591.

50. **Langer R, Bukovsky I, Herman A, et al.** Conservative surgery for tubal pregnancy. *Fertil Steril* 1982;38:427–430.

51. **Hallatt JG.** Tubal conservation in ectopic pregnancy: a study of 200 cases. *Am J Obstet Gynecol* 1986;154:1216–1221.

52. **Stovall TG, Ling FW, Buster JE.** Reproductive performance after methotrexate treatment of ectopic pregnancy. *Am J Obstet Gynecol* 1990;162:1620–1624.

53. **Stovall TG.** Medical management should be routinely used as primary therapy for ectopic pregnancy. *Clin Obstet Gynecol* 1995;38:346–352.

54. **Tulandi T.** Reproductive performance of women after two tubal ectopic pregnancies. *Fertil Steril* 1988;50:164–166.

55. **Westrom L, Joesoef R, Reynolds G, et al.** Pelvic inflammatory disease and fertility. A cohort study of 1,844 women with laparoscopically verified disease and 657 control women with normal laparoscopic results. *Sex Transm Dis* 1992;19:185–192.

56. **Westrom L.** Effect of acute pelvic inflammatory disease on fertility. *Am J Obstet Gynecol* 1975;121:707–713.

57. **Diquelou JY, Pia P, Tesquier L, et al.** [The role of *Chlamydia trachomatis* in the infectious etiology of extra-uterine pregnancy]. *J Gynecol Obstet Biol Reprod (Paris)* 1988;17:325–332.

58. **Berenson A, Hammill H, Martens M, et al.** Bacteriologic findings with ectopic pregnancy. *J Reprod Med* 1991;36:118–120.

59. **Coste J, Job-Spira N, Fernandez H, et al.** Risk factors for ectopic pregnancy: a case-control study in France, with special focus on infectious factors. *Am J Epidemiol* 1991;133:839–849.

60. **Svensson L, Mardh PA, Ahlgren M, et al.** Ectopic pregnancy and antibodies to *Chlamydia trachomatis*. *Fertil Steril* 1985;44:313–317.

61. **Brunham RC, Binns B, McDowell J, et al.** *Chlamydia trachomatis* infection in women with ectopic pregnancy. *Obstet Gynecol* 1986;67:722–726.

62. **Miettinen A, Heinonen PK, Teisala K, et al.** Serologic evidence for the role of *Chlamydia trachomatis*, *Neisseria gonorrhoeae*, and *Mycoplasma hominis* in the etiology of tubal factor infertility and ectopic pregnancy. *Sex Transm Dis* 1990;17:10–14.

63. **Chow JM, Yonekura ML, Richwald GA, et al.** The association between *Chlamydia trachomatis* and ectopic pregnancy. A matched-pair, case-control study. *JAMA* 1990;263:3164–3167.

64. **Hillis SD, Owens LM, Marchbanks PA, et al.** Recurrent chlamydial infections increase the risks of hospitalization for ectopic pregnancy and pelvic inflammatory disease. *Am J Obstet Gynecol* 1997;176:103–107.

65. **Goldberg JM, Falcone T.** Effect of diethylstilbestrol on reproductive function. *Fertil Steril* 1999;72:1–7.

66. **DeCherney AH, Cholst I, Naftolin F.** Structure and function of the fallopian tubes following exposure to diethylstilbestrol (DES) during gestation. *Fertil Steril* 1981;36:741–745.

67. **Barnes AB, Colton T, Gundersen J, et al.** Fertility and outcome of pregnancy in women exposed *in utero* to diethylstilbestrol. *N Engl J Med* 1980;302:609–613.

68. **Borgatta L, Murthy A, Chuang C, et al.** Pregnancies diagnosed during Depo-Provera use. *Contraception* 2002;66:169–172.

69. **Trussell J, Hedley A, Raymond E.** Ectopic pregnancy following use of progestin-only ECPs. *J Fam Plann Reprod Health Care* 2003;29:249.

70. **Sivin I.** Risks and benefits, advantages and disadvantages of levonorgestrel-releasing contraceptive implants. *Drug Saf* 2003;26:303–335.

71. **Furlong LA.** Ectopic pregnancy risk when contraception fails. A review. *J Reprod Med* 2002;47:881–885.

72. **Anonymous.** A multinational case-control study of ectopic pregnancy. The World Health Organization's Special Programme of Research, Development and Research Training in Human Reproduction: Task Force on Intrauterine Devices for Fertility Regulation. *Clin Reprod Fertil* 1985;3:131–143.

73. **Xiong X, Buekens P, Wollast E.** IUD use and the risk of ectopic pregnancy: a meta-analysis of case-control studies. *Contraception* 1995;52:23–34.

74. **Farley TM, Rosenberg MJ, Rowe PJ, et al.** Intrauterine devices and pelvic inflammatory disease: an international perspective. *Lancet* 1992;339:785–788.

75. **Ni HY, Daling JR, Chu J, et al.** Previous abdominal surgery and tubal pregnancy. *Obstet Gynecol* 1990;75:919–922.

76. **Trimbos-Kemper T, Trimbos B, van Hall E.** Etiological factors in tubal infertility. *Fertil Steril* 1982;37:384–388.

77. **Weinstein D, Polishuk WZ.** The role of wedge resection of the ovary as a cause for mechanical sterility. *Surg Gynecol Obstet* 1975;141:417–418.

78. **Marchbanks PA, Coulam CB, Annegers JF.** An association between clomiphene citrate and ectopic pregnancy: a preliminary report. *Fertil Steril* 1985;44:268–270.

79. **Chow WH, Daling JR, Cates W Jr, et al.** Epidemiology of ectopic pregnancy. *Epidemiol Rev* 1987;9:70–94.

80. **Cohen J, Mayaux MJ, Guihard-Moscato ML, et al.** *In-vitro* fertilization and embryo transfer: a collaborative study of 1163 pregnancies on the incidence and risk factors of ectopic pregnancies. *Hum Reprod* 1986;1:255–258.

81. **McBain JC, Evans JH, Pepperell RJ, et al.** An unexpectedly high rate of ectopic pregnancy following the induction of ovulation with human pituitary and chorionic gonadotrophin. *Br J Obstet Gynaecol* 1980;87:5–9.

82. **Gemzell C, Guillome J, Wang CF.** Ectopic pregnancy following treatment with human gonadotropins. *Am J Obstet Gynecol* 1982;143:761–765.

83. **Oelsner G, Menashe Y, Tur-Kaspa I, et al.** The role of gonadotropins in the etiology of ectopic pregnancy. *Fertil Steril* 1989;52:514–516.

84. **Steptoe PC, Edwards RG.** Reimplantation of a human embryo with subsequent tubal pregnancy. *Lancet* 1976;1:880–882.

85. **Corson SL, Dickey RP, Gocial B, et al.** Outcome in 242 *in vitro* fertilization-embryo replacement or gamete intrafallopian transfer-induced pregnancies. *Fertil Steril* 1989;51:644–650.

86. **Herman A, Ron-El R, Golan A, et al.** The role of tubal pathology and other parameters in ectopic pregnancies occurring in *in vitro* fertilization and embryo transfer. *Fertil Steril* 1990;54:864–868.

87. **Dor J, Seidman DS, Levran D, et al.** The incidence of combined intrauterine and extrauterine pregnancy after in vitro fertilization and embryo transfer. *Fertil Steril* 1991;55:833–834.

88. **Strandell A, Thorburn J, Hamberger L.** Risk factors for ectopic pregnancy in assisted reproduction. *Fertil Steril* 1999;71:282–286.

89. **Saraiya M, Berg CJ, Kendrick JS, et al.** Cigarette smoking as a risk factor for ectopic pregnancy. *Am J Obstet Gynecol* 1998;178:493–498.

90. **Bouyer J, Coste J, Shojaei T, et al.** Risk factors for ectopic pregnancy: a comprehensive analysis based on a large case-control, population-based study in France. *Am J Epidemiol* 2003;157:185–194.

91. **Honore LH.** A significant association between spontaneous abortion and tubal ectopic pregnancy. *Fertil Steril* 1979;32:401–402.

92. **Fedele L, Acaia B, Parazzini F, et al.** Ectopic pregnancy and recurrent spontaneous abortion: two associated reproductive failures. *Obstet Gynecol* 1989;73:206–208.

93. **Thorp JM Jr, Hartmann KE, Shadigian E.** Long-term physical and psychological health consequences of induced abortion: review of the evidence. *Obstet Gynecol Surv* 2003;58:67–79.

94. **Atrash HK, Strauss LT, Kendrick JS, et al.** The relation between induced abortion and ectopic pregnancy. *Obstet Gynecol* 1997;89:512–518.

95. **Skjeldestad FE, Atrash HK.** Evaluation of induced abortion as a risk factor for ectopic pregnancy. A case-control study. *Acta Obstet Gynecol Scand* 1997;76:151–158.

96. **Tharaux-Deneux C, Bouyer J, Job-Spira N, et al.** Risk of ectopic pregnancy and previous induced abortion. *Am J Public Health* 1998;88:401–405.

97. **Jenkins CS, Williams SR, Schmidt GE.** Salpingitis isthmica nodosa: a review of the literature, discussion of clinical significance, and consideration of patient management. *Fertil Steril* 1993;60:599–607.

98. **Homm RJ, Holtz G, Garvin AJ.** Isthmic ectopic pregnancy and salpingitis isthmica nodosa. *Fertil Steril* 1987;48:756–760.

99. **Niles, Clark JF.** Pathogenesis of tubal pregnancy. *Am J Obstet Gynecol* 1969;105:1230–1234.

100. **Benjamin CL, Beaver DC.** Pathogenesis of salpingitis isthmica nodosa. *Am J Clin Pathol* 1951;21:212–222.

101. **Persaud V.** Etiology of tubal ectopic pregnancy. Radiologic and pathologic studies. *Obstet Gynecol* 1970;36:257–263.

102. **Arias-Stella J.** The Arias-Stella reaction: facts and fancies four decades after. *Adv Anat Pathol* 2002;9:12–23.

103. **Stabile I, Grudzinskas JG.** Ectopic pregnancy: a review of incidence, etiology, and diagnostic aspects. *Obstet Gynecol Surv* 1990;45:335–347.

104. **Seeber B.** Endometrial stripe thickness and pregnancy outcome in first trimester pregnancies with pain bleeding or both. *J Reprod Med* Sep 2007;52:757.

105. **Tuomivaara L, Kauppila A, Puolakka J.** Ectopic pregnancy—an analysis of the etiology, diagnosis and treatment in 552 cases. *Arch Gynecol* 1986;237:135–147.

106. **Storring PL, Gaines-Das RE, Bangham DR.** International reference preparation of human chorionic gonadotrophin for immunoassay; potency estimates in various bioassays and protein binding assay systems; and international reference preparations of the alpha and beta subunits of human chorionic gonadotrophin for immunoassay. *J Endocrinol* 1980;84:295–310.

107. **Cole LA.** Phantom hCG and phantom choriocarcinoma. *Gynecol Oncol* 1998;71:325–329.

108. **Rotmensch S, Cole LA.** False diagnosis and needless therapy of presumed malignant disease in women with false-positive human chorionic gonadotropic concentration. *Lancet* 2000;35:712–715.

109. **Marshall JR, Hammond CB, Ross GT, et al.** Plasma and urinary chorionic gonadotropin during early human pregnancy. *Obstet Gynecol* 1968;32:760–764.

110. **Daus K, Mundy D, Graves W, et al.** Ectopic pregnancy: what to do during the 20-day window. *J Reprod Med* 1989;34:162–166.

111. **Kadar N, Caldwell BV, Romero R.** A method of screening for ectopic pregnancy and its indications. *Obstet Gynecol* 1981;58:162–165.

112. **Cartwright PS, Moore RA, Dao AH, et al.** Serum beta-human chorionic gonadotropin levels relate poorly with the size of a tubal pregnancy. *Fertil Steril* 1987;48:679–680.

113. **Pearlstone AC, Oei ML, Wu TCJ.** The predictive value of a single, early human chorionic gonadotropin measurement and the influence of maternal age on pregnancy outcome in an infertile population. *Fertil Steril* 1992;57:302–304.

114. **Milwidsky A, Adoni A, Segal S, et al.** Chorionic gonadotropin and progesterone levels in ectopic pregnancy. *Obstet Gynecol* 1977;50:145–147.

115. **Radwanska E, Frankenberg J, Allen EI.** Plasma progesterone levels in normal and abnormal early human pregnancy. *Fertil Steril* 1978;30:398–402.

116. **Stovall TG, Ling FW, Andersen RN, et al.** Improved sensitivity and specificity of a single measurement of serum progesterone over serial quantitative beta-human chorionic gonadotrophin in screening for ectopic pregnancy. *Hum Reprod* 1992;7:723–725.

117. **Stovall TG, Ling FW, Cope BJ, et al.** Preventing ruptured ectopic pregnancy with a single serum progesterone. *Am J Obstet Gynecol* 1989;160:1425–1431.

118. **Cowan BD, Vandermolen DT, Long CA, et al.** Receiver operator characteristics, efficiency analysis, and predictive value of serum progesterone concentration as a test for abnormal gestations. *Am J Obstet Gynecol* 1992;166:1729–1734.

119. **Barnes ER, Oelsner G, Benveniste R, et al.** Progesterone, estradiol, and alpha-human chorionic gonadotropin secretion in patients with ectopic pregnancy. *J Clin Endocrinol Metab* 1986;62:529–531.

120. **Witt BR, Wolf GC, Wainwright CJ, et al.** Relaxin, CA125, progesterone, estradiol, Schwangerschaft protein, and human chorionic gonadotropin as predictors of outcome in threatened and non-threatened pregnancies. *Fertil Steril* 1990;53:1029–1036.

121. **Guillaume J, Benjamin F, Sicuranza BJ, et al.** Serum estradiol as an aid in the diagnosis of ectopic pregnancy. *Obstet Gynecol* 1990;76:1126–1129.

122. **Lavie O, Beller U, Neuman M, et al.** Maternal serum creatine kinase: a possible predictor of tubal pregnancy. *Am J Obstet Gynecol* 1993;169:1149–1150.

123. **Ho PC, Chan SYW, Tang GWK.** Diagnosis of early pregnancy by enzyme immunoassay of Schwangerschafts-protein 1. *Fertil Steril* 1988;49:76–80.

124. **Bell RJ, Eddie LW, Lester AR, et al.** Relaxin in human pregnancy serum measured with an homologous radioimmunoassay. *Obstet Gynecol* 1987;69:585–589.

125. **Meunier K, Mignot TM, Maria B, et al.** Predictive value of the active renin assay for the diagnosis of ectopic pregnancy. *Fertil Steril* 1991;55:432–435.

126. **Niloff JM, Knapp RC, Schaetzl E, et al.** CA125 antigen levels in obstetric and gynecologic patients. *Obstet Gynecol* 1984;64:703–707.

127. **Kobayashi F, Sagawa N, Nakamura K, et al.** Mechanism and clinical significance of elevated CA125 levels in the sera of pregnant women. *Am J Obstet Gynecol* 1989;160:563–566.

128. **Check JH, Nowroozi K, Winkel CA, et al.** Serum CA125 levels in early pregnancy and subsequent spontaneous abortion. *Obstet Gynecol* 1990;75:742–744.

129. **Brumsted JR, Nakajima ST, Badger G, et al.** Serum concentration of CA125 during the first trimester of normal and abnormal pregnancies. *J Reprod Med* 1990;35:499–502.

130. **Sadovsky Y, Pineda J, Collins JL.** Serum CA125 levels in women with ectopic and intrauterine pregnancies. *J Reprod Med* 1991;36:875–878.

131. **Cederqvist LL, Killackey MA, Abdel-Latif N, et al.** Alpha-fetoprotein and ectopic pregnancy. *BMJ* 1983;286:1247–1248.

132. **Grosskinsky CM, Hage ML, Tyrey L, et al.** hCG, progesterone, alpha-fetoprotein, and estradiol in the identification of ectopic pregnancy. *Obstet Gynecol* 1993;81:705–709.

133. **Horne A, Shaw JL, Murdoch A, et al.** Placental growth factor: a promising diagnostic biomarker for tubal ectopic pregnancy. *J Clin Endocrinol Metab* 2010;96:E104–108.

134. **Cartwright J, Duncan WC, Critchley HO, et al.** Serum biomarkers of tubal ectopic pregnancy: current candidates and future possibilities. *Reproduction* 2009;138:9–22.

135. **Theron GB, Shepherd EGS, Strachan AF.** C-reactive protein levels in ectopic pregnancy, pelvic infection and carcinoma of the cervix. *S Afr Med J* 1986;69:681–682.

136. **Cacciatore B.** Can the status of tubal pregnancy be predicted with transvaginal sonography? A prospective comparison of sonographic, surgical, and serum hCG findings. *Radiology* 1990;177:481–484.

137. **Thorsen MK, Lawson TL, Aiman EJ, et al.** Diagnosis of ectopic pregnancy: endovaginal vs transabdominal sonography. *Am J Roentgenol* 1990;155:307–310.

138. **Bateman BG, Nunley WC Jr, Kolp LA, et al.** Vaginal sonography findings and hCG dynamics of early intrauterine and tubal pregnancies. *Obstet Gynecol* 1990;75:421–427.

139. **Cacciatore B, Stenman UH, Ylostalo P.** Comparison of abdominal and vaginal sonography in suspected ectopic pregnancy. *Obstet Gynecol* 1989;73:770–774.

140. **Condous G.** The accuracy of transvaginal ultrasonography for the diagnosis of ectopic pregnancy prior to surgery. *Hum Reprod* 2005;20:1404–1409.

141. **Fleischer AC, Pennell RG, McKee MS, et al.** Ectopic pregnancy: features at transvaginal sonography. *Radiology* 1990;174:375–378.

142. **Timor-Tritsch IE, Yeh MN, Peisner DB, et al.** The use of transvaginal ultrasonography in the diagnosis of ectopic pregnancy. *Am J Obstet Gynecol* 1989;161:157–161.

143. Bree RL, Marn CS. Transvaginal sonography in the first trimester: embryology, anatomy, and hCG correlation. *Semin Ultrasound CT MR* 1990;11:12–21.

144. Bottomley C. The optimal timing of an ultrasound scan to assess the location and viability of an early pregnancy. *Hum Reprod* 2009;24:1811–1817.

145. Cacciatore B, Ylostalo P, Stenman UH, et al. Suspected ectopic pregnancy: ultrasound findings and hCG levels assessed by an immunofluorometric assay. *BJOG* 1988;95:497–502.

146. Abramovici H, Auslender R, Lewin A, et al. Gestational-pseudogestational sac: a new ultrasonic criterion for differential diagnosis. *Am J Obstet Gynecol* 1983;145:377–379.

147. Nyberg DA, Filly RA, Laing FC, et al. Ectopic pregnancy, diagnosis by sonography correlated with quantitative hCG levels. *J Ultrasound Med* 1987;6:145–150.

148. Bradley WG, Fiske CE, Filly RA. The double sac sign of early intrauterine pregnancy: use in exclusion of ectopic pregnancy. *Radiology* 1982;143:223–226.

149. Nyberg DA, Mack LA, Harvey D, et al. Value of the yolk sac in evaluating early pregnancies. *J Ultrasound Med* 1988;7:129–135.

150. Jain KA, Hamper UM, Sanders RC. Comparison of transvaginal and transabdominal sonography in the detection of early pregnancy and its complications. *AJR Am J Roentgenol* 1988;151:1139–1143.

151. Bree RL, Edwards M, Bohm VM, et al. Transvaginal sonography in the evaluation of normal early pregnancy: correlation with hCG level. *AJR Am J Roentgenol* 1989;53:75–79.

152. Nyberg DA, Hughes MP, Mack LA, et al. Extrauterine findings of ectopic pregnancy at transvaginal US: importance of echogenic fluid. *Radiology* 1991;178:823–826.

153. Rottem S, Thaler I, Levron J, et al. Criteria for transvaginal sonographic diagnosis of ectopic pregnancy. *J Clin Ultrasound* 1990;18:274–279.

154. Nyberg DA, Mack LA, Laing FC, et al. Early pregnancy complications: endovaginal sonographic findings correlated with human chorionic gonadotropin levels. *Radiology* 1988;167:619–622.

155. Goldstein SR. Embryonic death in early pregnancy: a new look at the first trimester. *Obstet Gynecol* 1994;84:294–297.

156. Westrom L, Bengtsson LPH, Mardh P-A. Incidence, trends, and risks of ectopic pregnancy in a population of women. *BMJ* 1981;282:15–18.

157. Brown DL. Transvaginal sonography for diagnosing ectopic pregnancy: positivity criteria and performance characteristics. *J Ultrasound Med* 1994;13:259–266.

158. Emerson DS, Cartier MS, Altieri LA, et al. Diagnostic efficacy of endovaginal color Doppler flow imaging in an ectopic pregnancy screening program. *Radiology* 1992;183:413–420.

159. Dart R. Isolated fluid in the cul-de-sac how well does it predict ectopic pregnancy? *Am J Emerg Med* 2002;20:1–4.

160. Bernaschek G, Rudelstorfer R, Csaicsich P. Vaginal sonography versus serum human chorionic gonadotropin in early detection of pregnancy. *Am J Obstet Gynecol* 1988;158:608–612.

161. Diamond MP, DeCherney AH. Ectopic pregnancy. Philadelphia, PA: WB Saunders, 1991:1–163.

162. Menard A, Crequat J, Mandelbrot L, et al. Treatment of unruptured tubal pregnancy by local injection of methotrexate under transvaginal sonographic control. *Fertil Steril* 1990;54:47–50.

163. Campbell S, Pearce JM, Hackett G, et al. Qualitative assessment of uteroplacental blood flow: early screening test for high-risk pregnancies. *Obstet Gynecol* 1986;68:649–653.

164. McCowan LM, Ritchie K, Mo LY, et al. Uterine artery flow velocity waveforms in normal and growth-retarded pregnancies. *Am J Obstet Gynecol* 1988;158:499–504.

165. Taylor KJ, Ramos IM, Feyock AL, et al. Ectopic pregnancy: duplex Doppler evaluation. *Radiology* 1989;173:93–97.

166. Dillon EH, Feyock AL, Taylor KJW. Pseudogestational sacs: Doppler US differentiation from normal or abnormal intrauterine pregnancies. *Radiology* 1990;176:359–364.

167. Chew S. The role of TVUS and colour Doppler imaging in the detection of ectopic pregnancy. *J Obstetrics Gynaecol Res* 1996;22:455–460.

168. Condous G. The conservative management of early pregnancy complication: a review of the literature. *Ultrasound Obstet Gynecol* 2003;22:420–430.

169. Kurman RJ, Main CS, Chen HC. Intermediate trophoblast: a distinctive form of trophoblast with specific morphological, biochemical, and functional features. *Placenta* 1984;5:349–369.

170. Vermesh M, Graczykowski JW, Sauer MV. Reevaluation of the role of culdocentesis in the management of ectopic pregnancy. *Am J Obstet Gynecol* 1990;162:411–413.

171. Glezerman M, Press F, Carpman M. Culdocentesis is an obsolete diagnostic tool in suspected ectopic pregnancy. *Arch Obst Gynecol* 1992;252:5–9.

172. Stovall TG, Ling FW, Carson SA, et al. Serum progesterone and uterine curettage in the differential diagnosis of ectopic pregnancy. *Fertil Steril* 1992;57:456–458.

173. Stovall TG, Ling FW. Ectopic pregnancy: diagnostic and therapeutic algorithms minimizing surgical intervention. *J Reprod Med* 1993;38:807–812.

174. Hill GA, Segars JH Jr, Herbert CM III. Laparoscopic management of interstitial pregnancy. *J Gynecol Surg* 1989;5:209–212.

175. Gray DT, Thorburn J, Lundorff P, et al. A cost-effectiveness study of a randomised trial of laparoscopy versus laparotomy for ectopic pregnancy. *Lancet* 1995;345:1139–1143.

176. Lundorff P, Hahlin M, Kallfelt B, et al. Adhesion formation after laparoscopic surgery in tubal pregnancy: a randomized trial versus laparotomy. *Fertil Steril* 1991;55:911–915.

177. Hajenius PJ, Mol F, Mol BW, et al. Interventions for tubal ectopic pregnancy. *Cochrane Database Syst Rev* 2007;1:CD000324.

178. Sharma JB, Gupta S, Malhotra M, et al. A randomized controlled comparison of minilaparotomy and laparotomy in ectopic pregnancy cases. *Indian J Med Sci* 2003;57:493–500.

179. Jeffcoate TN. Salpingectomy or salpingo-oophorectomy. *J Obstet Gynaecol Br Emp* 1955;62:214–215.

180. Schenker JG, Eyal F, Polishuk WZ. Fertility after tubal surgery. *Surg Gynecol Obstet* 1972;135:74–76.

181. Dimarchi JM, Kosasa TS, Kobara TY, et al. Persistent ectopic pregnancy. *Obstet Gynecol* 1987;70:555–560.

182. Vermesh M, Silva PD, Sauer MV, et al. Persistent tubal ectopic gestation: patterns of circulating beta-human chorionic gonadotropin and progesterone, and management options. *Fertil Steril* 1988;50:584–588.

183. Seifer DB, Gutmann JN, Grant WD, et al. Comparison of persistent ectopic pregnancy after laparoscopic salpingostomy versus salpingectomy at laparotomy for ectopic pregnancy. *Obstet Gynecol* 1993;81:378–382.

184. Mol F, Mol BW, Ankum WM. Current evidence on surgery, systemic methotrexate and expectant management in the treatment of tubal ectopic pregnancy: a systematic review and meta-analysis. *Hum Reprod Update* 2008;14:309–319.

185. Gracia CR, Brown HA, Barnhart KT. Prophylactic methotrexate after linear salpingostomy: a decision analysis. *Fertil Steril* 2001;76:1191–1195.

186. Smith HO, Toledo AA, Thompson JD. Conservative surgical management of isthmic ectopic pregnancies. *Am J Obstet Gynecol* 1987;157:604–610.

187. Vermesh M, Silva PD, Rosen GF, et al. Management of unruptured ectopic gestation by linear salpingostomy: a prospective, randomized clinical trial of laparoscopy versus laparotomy. *Obstet Gynecol* 1989;73:400–404.

188. Silva PD, Schaper AM, Rooney B. Reproductive outcome after 143 laparoscopic procedures for ectopic pregnancy. *Obstet Gynecol* 1993;81:710–715.

189. Langer R, Raziel A, Ron-El R, et al. Reproductive outcome after conservative surgery for unruptured tubal pregnancies—a 15-year experience. *Fertil Steril* 1990;53:227–231.

190. American College of Obstetricians and Gynecologists. Medical management of ectopic pregnancy. ACOG Practice Bulletin No. 94. *Obstet Gynecol* 2008;111:479–485.

191. St. Clair JT, Whealer DA, Fish SA. Methotrexate in abdominal pregnancy. *JAMA* 1969;208:529–531.

192. Tanaka T, Hayashi H, Kutsuzawa T, et al. Treatment of interstitial ectopic pregnancy with methotrexate: report of a successful case. *Fertil Steril* 1982;37:851–852.

193. Van Den, Eeden SK, Shan J, et al. Ectopic pregnancy rate and treatment utilization in a large managed care organization. *Obstet Gynecol* 2005;105:1052.

194. **Barnhart KT, Gosman G, Asnby R, et al.** The medical management of ectopic pregnancy: a meta-analysis comparing "single dose" and multidose regimens. *Obstet Gynecol* 2003;101:778–784.

195. **Stovall TG, Ling FW, Buster JE.** Outpatient chemotherapy of unruptured ectopic pregnancy. *Fertil Steril* 1989;51:435–438.

196. **Stovall TG, Ling FW, Gray LA.** Single-dose methotrexate for treatment of ectopic pregnancy. *Obstet Gynecol* 1991;77:754–757.

197. **Lipscomb GH, Bran D, McCord ML, et al.** Analysis of three hundred fifteen women with tubal ectopic pregnancies treated with single-dose methotrexate. *Am J Obstet Gynecol* 1998;178:1354–1358.

198. **Menon S, Colins J, Barnhart KT.** Establishing a human chorionic gonadotropin cutoff to guide methotrexate treatment of ectopic pregnancy: a systematic review. *Fertil Steril* 2007;87:481–484.

199. **Barnhart KT, Hummel AC, Sammel MD, et al.** Use of "2-dose" regimen of methotrexate to treat ectopic pregnancy. *Fertil Steril* 2007;87:250–256.

200. **Pisarka MD, Carson SA, Buster JE.** Ectopic pregnancy. *Lancet* 1998;351:1115–1120.

201. **Klauser CK, May WL, Johnson VK, et al.** Methotrexate for ectopic pregnancy: a randomized single dose compared with multiple dose. *Obstet Gynecol* 2005;105:64S.

202. **Alleyassin A, Khademi A, Aghahosseini M, et al.** Comparison of success rates in the medical management of ectopic pregnancy with single-dose and multiple dose administration of methotrexate: a prospective, randomized clinical trial. *Fertil Steril* 2006;85:1661–1666.

203. **Brown DL, Felker RE, Stovall TG, et al.** Serial endovaginal sonography of ectopic pregnancies treated with methotrexate. *Obstet Gynecol* 1991;77:406–409.

204. **Berkowitz RS, Goldstein DP, Jones MA, et al.** Methotrexate with citrovorum factor rescue: reduced chemotherapy toxicity in the management of gestational trophoblastic neoplasms. *Cancer* 1980;45:423–426.

205. **Rustin GJS, Rustin F, Dent J, et al.** No increase in second tumors after cytotoxic chemotherapy for gestational trophoblastic tumors. *N Engl J Med* 1983;308:473–476.

206. **Hajenius PJ, Engelsbel S, Mol BW, et al.** Randomized trial of systemic methotrexate versus laparoscopic salpingostomy in tubal pregnancy. *Lancet* 1997;350:774–779.

207. **Olofsson JI, Poromaa IS, Ottander U, et al.** Clinical and pregnancy outcome following ectopic pregnancy; a prospective study comparing expectancy, surgery and systemic methotrexate treatment. *Acta Obstet Gynecol Scand* 2001;80:744–749.

208. **Dias Pereira G, Hajenius PJ, Mol BW, et al.** Fertility outcome after systemic methotrexate and laparoscopic salpingostomy for tubal pregnancy. *Lancet* 1999;353:724–745.

209. **Shalev E, Peleg D, Bustan M, et al.** Limited role for intratubal methotrexate treatment of ectopic pregnancy. *Fertil Steril* 1995;63:20–24.

210. **Tulandi T, Atri M, Bret P, et al.** Transvaginal intratubal methotrexate treatment of ectopic pregnancy. *Fertil Steril* 1992;58:98–100.

211. **Fernandez H, Benifla JL, Lelaidier C, et al.** Methotrexate treatment of ectopic pregnancy: 100 cases treated by primary transvaginal injection under sonographic control. *Fertil Steril* 1993;59:773–777.

212. **Fernandez H, Pauthier S, Daimerc S, et al.** Ultrasound-guided injection of methotrexate versus laparoscopic salpingotomy in ectopic pregnancy. *Fertil Steril* 1995;63:25–29.

213. **Oelsner G, Admon D, Shalev E, et al.** A new approach for the treatment of interstitial pregnancy. *Fertil Steril* 1993;59:924–925.

214. **Aboulghar MA, Mansour RT, Serour GI.** Transvaginal injection of potassium chloride and methotrexate for the treatment of tubal pregnancy with a live fetus. *Hum Reprod* 1990;5:887–888.

215. **Feichtinger W, Kemeter P.** Treatment of unruptured ectopic pregnancy by needling of sac and injection of methotrexate or PGE$_2$ under transvaginal sonography control. *Arch Gynecol Obstet* 1989;246:85–89.

216. **Hagstrom HG, Hahlin M, Sjöblom P, et al.** Prediction of persistent trophoblastic activity after local prostaglandin F_{2a} injection for ectopic pregnancy. *Hum Reprod* 1994;9:1170–1174.

217. **Laatikainen T, Tuomivaara L, Kauppila K.** Comparison of a local injection of hyperosmolar glucose solution with salpingostomy for the conservative treatment of tubal pregnancy. *Fertil Steril* 1993;60:80–84.

218. **Kojima E, Abe Y, Morita M, et al.** The treatment of unruptured tubal pregnancy with intratubal methotrexate injection under laparoscopic control. *Obstet Gynecol* 1990;75:723–725.

219. **Kenigsberg D, Porte J, Hull M, et al.** Medical treatment of residual ectopic pregnancy: RU 486 and methotrexate. *Fertil Steril* 1987;47:702–703.

220. **Frydman R, Fernandez H, Troalen F, et al.** Phase I clinical trial of monoclonal anti-human chorionic gonadotropin antibody in women with an ectopic pregnancy. *Fertil Steril* 1989;52:734–738.

221. **Garcia AJ, Aubert JM, Sama J, et al.** Expectant management of presumed ectopic pregnancies. *Fertil Steril* 1987;48:395–400.

222. **Carson SA, Stovall TG, Ling FW, et al.** Low human chorionic somatomammotropin fails to predict spontaneous resolution of unruptured ectopic pregnancies. *Fertil Steril* 1991;55:629–630.

223. **Fernandez H, Rainhorn JD, Papiernik E, et al.** Spontaneous resolution of ectopic pregnancy. *Obstet Gynecol* 1988;71:171–174.

224. **Gretz E, Quagliarello J.** Declining serum concentrations of the beta-subunit of human chorionic gonadotropin and ruptured ectopic pregnancy. *Am J Obstet Gynecol* 1987;156:940–941.

225. **Makinen JI, Kivijarvi AK, Irjala KMA.** Success of non-surgical management of ectopic pregnancy. *Lancet* 1990;335:1099.

226. **Korhonen J, Stenman UH, Ylotalo P.** Serum human chorionic gonadotropin dynamics during spontaneous resolution of ectopic pregnancy. *Fertil Steril* 1994;61:632–636.

227. **Seifer DB, Gutmann JN, Doyle MB, et al.** Persistent ectopic pregnancy following laparoscopic linear salpingostomy. *Obstet Gynecol* 1990;76:1121–1125.

228. **Pouly JL, Mahnes H, Mage G, et al.** Conservative laparoscopic treatment of 321 ectopic pregnancies. *Fertil Steril* 1986;46:1093–1097.

229. **Lundorff P, Hahlin M, Sjoblom P, et al.** Persistent trophoblast after conservative treatment of tubal pregnancy: prediction and detection. *Obstet Gynecol* 1991;77:129–133.

230. **Cartwright PS.** Peritoneal trophoblastic implants after surgical management of tubal pregnancy. *J Reprod Med* 1991;36:523–524.

231. **Higgins KA, Schwartz MB.** Treatment of persistent trophoblastic tissue after salpingostomy with methotrexate. *Fertil Steril* 1986;45:427–428.

232. **Rose PG, Cohen SM.** Methotrexate therapy for persistent ectopic pregnancy after conservative laparoscopic management. *Obstet Gynecol* 1990;76:947–949.

233. **Bengtsson G, Bryman I, Thorburn J, et al.** Low-dose oral methotrexate as second-line therapy for persistent trophoblast after conservative treatment of ectopic pregnancy. *Obstet Gynecol* 1992;79:589–591.

234. **Cole T, Corlett RC Jr.** Chronic ectopic pregnancy. *Obstet Gynecol* 1982;59:63–68.

235. **Rogers WF, Shaub M, Wilson R.** Chronic ectopic pregnancy: ultrasonic diagnosis. *J Clin Ultrasound* 1977;5:257–260.

236. **Parente JT, Ou CS, Levy J, et al.** Cervical pregnancy analysis: a review and report of five cases. *Obstet Gynecol* 1983;62:79–82.

237. **Marcovici I, Rosenzweig BA, Brill AI, et al.** Cervical pregnancy. *Obstet Gynecol Surv* 1994;49:49–55.

238. **Karande VC, Flood JT, Heard N, et al.** Analysis of ectopic pregnancies resulting from *in-vitro* fertilization and embryo transfer. *Hum Reprod* 1991;6:446.

239. **Hofmann HMH, Urdl W, Hofler H, et al.** Cervical pregnancy: case reports and current concepts in diagnosis and treatment. *Arch Gynecol Obstet* 1987;241:63–69.

240. **Leeman LM, Wendland CL.** Cervical ectopic pregnancy: diagnosis with endovaginal ultrasound examination and successful treatment with methotrexate. *Arch Fam Med* 2000;9:72–77.

241. **Bader-Armstrong B, Shah Y, Rubens D.** Use of ultrasound and magnetic resonance imaging in the diagnosis of cervical pregnancy. *J Clin Ultrasound* 1989;17:283–286.

242. **Bernstein D, Holzinger M, Ovadia J, et al.** Conservative treatment of cervical pregnancy. *Obstet Gynecol* 1981;58:741–742.

243. **Wharton KR, Gore B.** Cervical pregnancy managed by placement of a Shirodkar cerclage before evacuation: a case report. *J Reprod Med* 1988;33:227–229.

244. **Nolan TE, Chandler PE, Hess LW, et al.** Cervical pregnancy managed without hysterectomy: a case report. *J Reprod Med* 1989;34:241–243.

245. **Hallatt JG.** Primary ovarian pregnancy: a report of twenty-five cases. *Am J Obstet Gynecol* 1982;143:55–60.

246. **Grimes HG, Nosal RA, Gallagher JC.** Ovarian pregnancy: a series of 24 cases. *Obstet Gynecol* 1983;61:174–180.

247. **Spiegelberg O.** Casusistik der ovarialschwangerschaft. *Arch Gynaecol* 1878;13:73.

248. **Malinger G, Achiron R, Treschan O, et al.** Case report: ovarian pregnancy-ultrasonographic diagnosis. *Acta Obstet Gynecol Scand* 1988;67:561–563.

249. **DeVries K, Atad J, Arodi J, et al.** Primary ovarian pregnancy: a conservative surgical approach by wedge resection. *Int J Fertil* 1981;26:293–294.

250. **Van Coevering RJ, Fisher JE.** Laparoscopic management of ovarian pregnancy: a case report. *J Reprod Med* 1988;33:774–776.

251. **Russell JB, Cutler LR.** Transvaginal ultrasonographic detection of primary ovarian pregnancy with laparoscopic removal: a case report. *Fertil Steril* 1989;51:1055–1056.

252. **Tinelli A, Hudelist G, Malvasi A, et al.** Laparoscopic management of ovarian pregnancy. *J Soc Laparosc Surg* 2008;12:169–172.

253. **Habbu J, Read MD.** Ovarian pregnancy successfully treated with methotrexate. *J Obstet Gynaecol* 2006; 26:587–588.

254. **Raziel A, Golan A.** Primary ovarian pregnancy successfully treated with methotrexate. *Am J Obstet Gynecol* 1993;169:1362–1363.

255. **Shamma FN, Schwartz LB.** Primary ovarian pregnancy successfully treated with methotrexate. *Am J Obstet Gynecol* 1992;167:1307–1308.

256. **Atrash HK, Friede A, Hogue CJR.** Abdominal pregnancy in the United States: frequency and maternal mortality. *Obstet Gynecol* 1987;69:333–337.

257. **Ludwig M, Kaisi M, Bauer O, et al.** The forgotten chid—a case of heterotopic, intraabdominal and intrauterine pregnancy carried to term. *Hum Reprod* 1999;14:1372–1374.

258. **Tsudo T, Harada T, Yoshioka H, et al.** Laparoscopic management of early primary abdominal pregnancy. *Obstet Gynecol* 1997;90:687–688.

259. **Rahman MS, Al-Suleiman SA, Rahman J, et al.** Advanced abdominal pregnancy—observations in 10 cases. *Obstet Gynecol* 1982;59:366–372.

260. **Stevens CA.** Malformations and deformations in abdominal pregnancy. *Am J Med Genetics* 1993;47:1189–1195.

261. **Stanley JH, Horger EO III, Fagan CJ, et al.** Sonographic findings in abdominal pregnancy. *AJR Am J Roentgenol* 1986;147:1043–1046.

262. **Harris MB, Angtuaco T, Frazer CN, et al.** Diagnosis of a viable abdominal pregnancy by magnetic resonance imaging. *Am J Obstet Gynecol* 1988;159:150–151.

263. **Lockhat F, Corr P, Ramphal S, et al.** The value of magnetic resonance imaging in the diagnosis and management of extra-uterine abdominal pregnancy. *Clin Radiol* 2006;61:264–269.

264. **Martin JN Jr, Ridgway LE III, Connors JJ, et al.** Angiographic arterial embolization and computed tomography-directed drainage for the management of hemorrhage and infection with abdominal pregnancy. *Obstet Gynecol* 1990;76:941–945.

265. **Martin JN Jr, Sessums JK, Martin RW, et al.** Abdominal pregnancy: current concepts of management. *Obstet Gynecol* 1988;71:549–557.

266. **Moores KL, Keriakos RH, Anumba DO, et al.** Management challenges of a live 12-week sub-hepatic intra-abdominal pregnancy. *BJOG* 2010;117:365–368.

267. **Lau S, Tulandi T.** Conservative medical and surgical management of interstitial ectopic pregnancy. *Fertil Steril* 1999;72:207–215.

268. **MacRae R, Olowu O, Rizzuto MI, et al.** Diagnosis and laparoscopic management of 11 consecutive cases of cornual ectopic pregnancy. *Arch Gynecol Obstet* 2009;280:59–64.

269. **Elito J, Camano L.** Unruptured tubal pregnancy: different treatments for early and late diagnosis. *Sao Paulo Med J* 2006;124:321–324.

270. **Walker JJ.** Ectopic pregnancy. *Clin Obstet Gynecol* 2007;50:89–99.

271. **Moawad NS, Mahajan ST, Moniz MH, et al.** Current diagnosis and treatment of interstitial pregnancy. *Am J Obstet Gynecol* 2010;202:15–29.

272. **Vierhout ME, Wallenburg HCS.** Intraligamentary pregnancy resulting in a live infant. *Am J Obstet Gynecol* 1985;152:878–879.

273. **Reece EA, Petrie RH, Sirmans MF, et al.** Combined intrauterine and extrauterine gestations: a review. *Am J Obstet Gynecol* 1983;146:323–330.

274. **Tal J, Haddad S, Gordon N, et al.** Heterotopic pregnancy after ovulation induction and assisted reproductive technologies: a literature review from 1971 to 1993. *Fertil Steril* 1996;66:1–12.

275. **Cheng PJ, Chueh HY, Qiu JT.** Heterotopic pregnancy in a natural conception cycle presenting as hematometra. *Obstet Gynecol* 2004;104:1195–1198.

276. **Clayton HB, Schieve LA, Peterson HB, et al.** A comparison of heterotopic and intrauterine-only pregnancy outcomes after assisted reproductive technologies in the United States from 1999 to 2002. *Fertil Steril* 2007;87:303–309.

277. **Goldberg JM, Bedaiwy MA.** Transvaginal local injection of hyperosmolar glucose for the treatment of heterotopic pregnancies. *Obstet Gynecol* 2006;107:509–510.

278. **Goldstein JS, Ratts VS, Philpott T, et al.** Risk of surgery after use of potassium chloride for treatment of tubal heterotopic pregnancy. *Obstet Gynecol* 2006;107:506–508.

279. **De Los Rios JF.** Bilateral ectopic pregnancy. *J Minim Invasive Gynecol* 2007;14:419–427.

280. **Svirsky R, Maymon R, Vaknin Z, et al.** Twin tubal pregnancy: a rising complication? *Fertil Steril* 2010;94:1910.e13–e16.

281. **Adair CD, Benrubi GI, Sanchez-Ramos L, et al.** Bilateral tubal ectopic pregnancies after bilateral partial salpingectomy: a case report. *J Reprod Med* 1994;39:131–133.

282. **Goffner L, Bluth MJ, Fruauff A, et al.** Ectopic gestation associated with intrauterine triplet pregnancy after in vitro fertilization. *J Ultrasound Med* 1993;12:63–64.

283. **Jackson P, Barrowclough IW, France JT, et al.** A successful pregnancy following total hysterectomy. *Br J Obstet Gynaecol* 1980;87:353–355.

284. **Nehra PC, Loginsky SJ.** Pregnancy after vaginal hysterectomy. *Obstet Gynecol* 1984;64:735–737.

21 Benign Breast Disease

Camelia A. Lawrence
Baiba J. Grube
Armando E. Giuliano

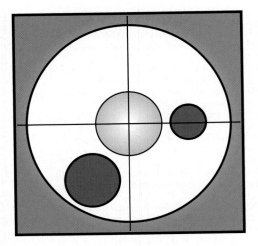

- **Early detection of breast cancer is improved by risk assessment, clinical breast examination, screening mammography, and magnetic resonance imaging in selected patients.**

- **Triple-test concordance requires agreement between results of clinical breast examination, breast imaging, and tissue diagnosis. In the absence of concordance, further diagnostic intervention is required.**

- **The most common benign breast problems include fibrocystic changes and mastalgia. These problems are usually best treated by reassurance. Pharmaceutic agents are available but have side effects that usually are not well tolerated.**

- **Histologic differences exist between fibroadenomas and phyllodes tumors; phyllodes tumors require excision, whereas small asymptomatic fibroadenomas can be observed if the diagnosis is confirmed by histologic or cytologic assessment and there is no evidence of growth.**

- **Spontaneous, unilateral, bloody discharge requires histologic evaluation to exclude malignancy, but symptoms usually are caused by a benign process such as intraductal papilloma or duct ectasia.**

- **Breast abscesses are managed with fine needle aspiration and antibiotics; the use of incision and drainage is reserved for recurrence.**

Benign breast diseases are among the most common diagnoses that the busy obstetrician-gynecologist will see in practice. An ability to accurately and promptly diagnose both benign and malignant breast diseases is within the purview of the practicing gynecologist (1). Benign breast disease is a complex entity with a range of physiologic changes and clinical manifestations that have an impact on a woman's health independent of breast cancer risk (2).

Detection

Evaluation of a new breast symptom begins with assessment of symptoms based on a thorough clinical history (3). The history should include questions regarding current symptoms, duration of the condition, fluctuation of the signs and symptoms, and factors that aggravate or relieve the symptom. **Assessment of breast problems should focus on the following points:**

- **Nipple discharge**

- **Characteristics of discharge (spontaneous or nonspontaneous, appearance, unilateral or bilateral, single or multiple duct involvement)**

- **Breast mass (size and change in size, density, or texture)**

- **Breast pain (cyclic versus continuous)**

- **Association of symptoms with menstrual cycle**

- **Change in breast shape, size, or texture**

- **Previous breast biopsies**

- **History of breast trauma**

The patient should be questioned about the following risk factors for breast cancer (see Chapter 40 for more details):

- **Sex**

- **Increasing age (approximately 50% of breast cancers occur *after* age 65)**

- **Age of menarche less than 12 years**

- **Nulliparity or first pregnancy at greater than 30 years of age**

- **Late menopause (older than 55 years of age)**

- **Family history of breast cancer (especially premenopausal or bilateral disease)**

- **Number of first-degree relatives with breast cancer and their ages when diagnosed**

- **Family history of male breast cancer**

- **Inherited conditions associated with a high risk for breast cancer, including *BRCA1* and *BRCA2* genes, Li-Fraumeni syndrome, Cowden's disease, ataxia telangiectasia syndrome, and Peutz-Jeghers syndrome**

- **Other malignancies (ovary, colon, and prostate)**

- **Pathology of previous breast biopsy showing atypia or lobular or ductal carcinoma *in situ***

- **Hormone therapy**

- **Alcohol consumption**

- **Postmenopausal weight gain**

- **Personal history of breast cancer**

Breast cancer risk can be determined by the **Gail Risk assessment model,** which is available electronically (4). **The Gail Risk assessment model calculates risk based on patient race, age, age of menarche, age of first live birth, number of first-degree relatives with breast cancer, number of previous breast biopsies, and presence of atypia on the biopsy.**

It is important to obtain a current list of medications used, including hormone therapy and herbal medications such as phytoestrogens. The gestational history should take into consideration the possibility that the patient may be pregnant or has a prior history of miscarriage or abortion. A personal history of exposure to radiation, especially in the treatment of childhood malignancies, is associated with a higher incidence of developing breast cancer (5). The goal of breast evaluation is to determine clearly whether the symptom represents a benign breast condition or may be indicative of a neoplastic process.

Physical Examination

Breast tumors, particularly cancerous ones, usually are asymptomatic and are discovered by the patient or through physical examination or screening mammography. Typically, the breast changes slightly during the menstrual cycle. During the premenstrual phase, most women have increased innocuous nodularity and mild engorgement of the breast. Rarely these characteristics can obscure an underlying lesion and make examination difficult. Findings should be carefully documented in the medical record to serve as a baseline for future reference.

Inspection

Inspection is performed initially while the patient is seated comfortably with her arms relaxed at her sides. The breasts are compared for symmetry, contour, and skin appearance. Edema or erythema is identified easily, and skin dimpling or nipple retraction is shown by having the patient raise her arms above her head and then press her hands on her hips, thereby contracting the pectoralis muscles (Fig. 21.1). Palpable and even nonpalpable tumors that distort Cooper's ligaments may lead to skin dimpling with these maneuvers.

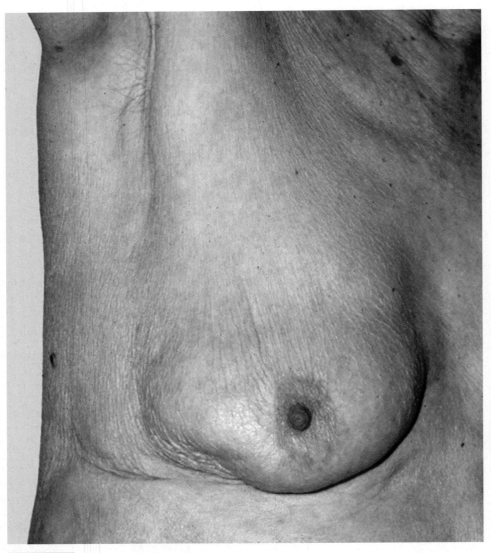

Figure 21.1 **Raising the arm reveals retraction of the skin of the lower outer quadrant caused by a small palpable carcinoma.** (From **Kruper L, Giuliano AE.** Breast disease. In: **Berek JS, Hacker NF, eds.** *Berek & Hacker's Gynecologic Oncology,* 5th ed. Philadelphia: Lippincott Williams & Wilkins, 2010:615, with permission.)

Palpation

While the patient is seated, each breast should be palpated methodically. Some physicians recommend palpating the breast in long strips, but the exact palpation technique used is probably not as important as the thoroughness of its application over the entire breast. One very effective method is to palpate the breast in enlarging concentric circles until the entire breast is covered. A pendulous breast can be palpated by placing one hand between the breast and the chest wall and gently palpating the breast between both examining hands. The axillary and supraclavicular areas should be palpated for enlarged lymph nodes. The entire axilla, the upper outer quadrant of the breast, and the axillary tail of Spence are palpated for possible masses. **While the patient is supine with one arm over her head, the ipsilateral breast is again methodically palpated from the clavicle to the costal margin and from the sternum to the latissimus dorsi laterally.** If the breast is large, a pillow or towel may be placed beneath the scapula to elevate the side being examined; otherwise, the breast tends to fall to the side, making palpation of the lateral hemisphere more difficult. The major features to be identified on palpation of the breast are temperature, texture and thickness of skin, generalized or focal tenderness, nodularity, density, asymmetry, dominant masses, and nipple discharge. Most premenopausal patients have normally nodular breast parenchyma. The nodularity is diffuse but predominantly in the upper outer quadrants, where there is more breast tissue. These benign parenchymal nodules are small, similar in size, and indistinct. By comparison, breast cancer usually occurs in the form of a nontender, firm mass with irregular margins. A cancerous mass feels distinctly different from the surrounding nodularity. A malignant mass may be fixed to the skin or to the underlying fascia. A suspicious mass is usually unilateral. Similar findings in both breasts are unlikely to represent malignant disease (6).

Breast Self-Examination

There is controversy about recommending breast self-examination (BSE). There is no evidence that doing BSE improves survival rates from breast cancer (7). Staunch opponents of BSE argue that it doubles a woman's risk of undergoing a breast biopsy for benign pathology (8). BSE increases breast health awareness and helps promote early detection of cancer (9–11). Most breast cancers are detected by women themselves (48%), followed by breast imaging (41%), and by physician clinical examination in only 11% (12). Although young women have a low incidence of breast cancer, it is important to teach BSE early so it becomes habitual. Organizations such as the American Cancer Society sponsor courses in BSE. Reassurance, support, and patient education may encourage women to overcome psychological barriers to routine BSE (13). Such instruction is available through electronic resources (14).

The following seven "P"s represent the essential components of breast examination:

- **Positions**
- **Palpation**
- **Pads of fingers for palpation**
- **Pressure**
- **Perimeter**
- **Pattern of search**
- **Patient education**

The woman should inspect her breasts while standing or sitting before a mirror, looking for any asymmetry, skin dimpling, or nipple retraction. Elevating her arms over her head or pressing her hands against her hips to contract the pectoralis muscles will highlight any skin dimpling. Finally, the woman should examine her breasts while bending over and leaning forward. While standing or sitting, she should carefully palpate her breasts with the fingers of the opposite hand. She should lie down and again palpate each quadrant of the breast as well as the axilla using the pads of the three middle fingers with three pressures—light, medium, and deep—covering the entire breast from the clavicle to the inframammary fold, from sternum to latissimus dorsi laterally. The area within the perimeter of the breast should be palpated, preferably using an up-and-down method called vertical stripe, rather than the concentric circular or radial methods, in which the edges of the breast tissue often are omitted. Many women feel anxious about performing breast examination. The examination may be performed while showering; soap and water may increase the sensitivity of palpation, and the privacy of the shower may provide a less anxiety-provoking environment.

It is helpful for all women to examine their breasts at the same time each month to develop a routine. Premenopausal women should examine their breasts monthly 7 to 10 days after the onset of the menstrual cycle. For postmenopausal women, selection of a specific calendar date is a helpful way to remember to perform a monthly BSE. Women should be instructed to report any abnormalities or changes to their physicians. If the physician cannot confirm the patient's findings, the examination should be repeated in 1 month or after her next menstrual period.

Breast Imaging

Mammography

Screen-film mammography was considered the best method for imaging the breast (15). Full-field digital mammography, which records mammographic images on a computer, is a modification of screen-film mammography (16). Some advantages of digital mammography include lower radiation exposure, ability to manipulate a computerized image for optimal viewing, and access to distance consultations through telemammography (17). Studies comparing the sensitivity of full-field digital mammography with screen-film mammography in detecting cancer had mixed results. The Digital Mammographic Imaging Screening Trial (DMIST) consisted of 49,528 asymptomatic women presenting for screening mammography, who underwent both digital and film mammography. Results suggested that while the overall accuracy of digital and film mammography for screening breast cancer is similar, digital mammography may be more accurate in women under the age of 50 years, women with radiographically dense breast, and premenopausal or perimenopausal women (18).

Slow-growing breast cancers can be identified by mammography at least 2 years before the mass reaches a size detectable by palpation. These tumors have a less aggressive biologic behavior than interval breast cancers (19–21). Mammography is the only reproducible method of detecting nonpalpable breast cancer, but its use depends on the availability of state-of-the-art equipment and a dedicated breast radiologist.

Compression of the breast is necessary to obtain good images, and patients should be forewarned that breast compression is uncomfortable. With good technique and well-maintained modern equipment, exposure to radiation can be limited. Full-field digital mammography (FFDM) has a 22% lower mean glandular radiation dose than film-screen mammography per acquired view. FFDM delivers 1.86 mGy average breast radiation dose per view compared to 2.37 mGy for film screen (22).

Indications for Mammography

The indications for mammography are as follows:

1. **To screen, at regular intervals, women who are at high risk for developing breast cancer.** About one-third of the abnormalities detected on screening mammography prove malignant when biopsy is performed (23).

2. **To evaluate a questionable or ill-defined breast mass or other suspicious change in the breast that is detected by clinical breast examination.**

3. **To establish a baseline breast mammogram and reevaluate patients at yearly intervals to diagnose a potentially curable breast cancer before it has been diagnosed clinically.**

4. **To search for occult breast cancer in a patient with metastatic disease in axillary nodes or elsewhere from an unknown primary origin.**

5. **To screen for unsuspected cancer before cosmetic operations or biopsy of a mass.**

6. **To monitor breast cancer patients who were treated with a breast-conserving surgery and radiation.**

Screening

Screening programs to evaluate asymptomatic, healthy women combine physical examination with mammographic screening to identify breast abnormalities. During the past 30 years, there was an increase in the use of mammography, mammographic screening, and public awareness of breast health care. The cancer detection rate for screening mammography is 5 per 1,000 screening examinations (24). The cancer detection rate is 11-fold higher, at 55 per 1,000 examinations, when breast imaging is performed for a specific finding (i.e., diagnostic imaging) (24). Of seven randomized mammographic screening trials performed, five demonstrated a reduction in overall mortality from breast cancer screening programs (25–32). A study from the Rhode Island Cancer Registry indicates that the institution of population-based breast cancer screening programs can result in the reduction in the median tumor size at initial detection from 2.0 to 1.5 cm, which is associated with a 25% reduction in mortality (33). A study from the Norwegian breast-cancer screening program was associated with a reduction in the rate of death from breast cancer, but the screening itself accounted for only about a third of total reduction (30). Detecting breast cancer before it spreads to the axillary nodes greatly increases the chance of survival; about 85% of women with such cancer will survive at least 5 years (31,34). Because breast cancer presents first as local disease, screening mammography for breast cancer in asymptomatic women can detect small tumors and offer a better prognosis. These tumors had less opportunity to metastasize regionally or systemically; thus women have more options for treatment with reduced toxicity.

The American Cancer Society published an extensive review of the benefits, limitations, and potential harms of screening mammography (35). It addresses the role of physical examination, discusses screening in older and high-risk women, and reviews the role of newer technologies. **A summary of the guidelines recommends that women of average risk for breast cancer begin mammographic screening at age 40. The rationale for beginning mammographic screening at age 40 is a 24% reduction in mortality in screened populations** (28). For women in their 20s and 30s, a clinical breast examination is suggested at least every 3 years, and preferably annually, as part of a well-woman examination. For women older than age 40 years, annual clinical breast examination and mammography are recommended. For older women, recommendations for mammographic screening may be individualized based on the presence of any comorbidities. Chronologic age alone should not be considered a contraindication to mammographic screening as long as a woman is in reasonable health and would be a candidate for breast cancer surgery (35). **The American Geriatrics Society recommends annual or at least biennial mammography for women up to age 75 years, and after that age, every 2 to 3 years if the woman has a life expectancy of more than 4 years** (36). The reasons for liberalization of the screening interval recommendations for older women include improved biology profile, slower growth rate, and lower risk for recurrence (37–41). The natural history of the disease in older women must be balanced against life expectancy as a function of overall health (42). **For high-risk women, consideration can be given to earlier initiation of screening (5 to 10 years earlier than the age of the index case) and shorter intervals between screening,** and the use of additional imaging modalities such as breast ultrasonography and magnetic resonance imaging (MRI) with dedicated breast coils. No screening test is perfect, and false-negative imaging studies or benign clinical examinations may lead the patient to an erroneous sense of well-being only to be confronted later with a subsequent cancer. Likewise, a false-positive result can lead to significant anxiety and unnecessary biopsy.

Mammographic Abnormalities

A mammographic abnormality includes a mass (solid versus cystic), microcalcifications (benign, indeterminate, suspicious), asymmetric density, architectural distortion, and appearance of a new density. There are eight morphologic categories of mammographic abnormalities (43,44):

1. **Calcification distribution**
2. **Number of calcifications**
3. **Description of calcifications**
4. **Mass margin**
5. **Shape of mass**
6. **Density of mass**
7. **Associated findings**
8. **Special cases**

Mammographic abnormalities should be visible on two views, usually craniocaudal (CC) and mediolateral oblique (MLO). The lesion should triangulate to the same location on those two views. Calcifications can be macrocalcifications, which are coarse and usually represent benign degenerative breast conditions. Calcifications associated with breast cancer are clustered pleomorphic microcalcifications; typically five to eight or more calcifications are aggregated in one part of the breast (45). These calcifications may be associated with a mammographic mass density. A mass density may appear without evidence of calcifications. It can represent a cyst, benign tumor, or a malignancy. A malignant density usually has irregular or ill-defined borders and may lead to architectural distortion, which may be subtle and difficult to detect in a dense breast. Other mammographic findings suggesting breast cancer are architectural distortion, asymmetric density, skin thickening or retraction, or nipple retraction. Examples of mammographic abnormalities can be found in several electronic sources (46).

Mammographic Reports

The American College of Radiology recommended the **Breast Imaging Reporting and Data System (BI-RADS)** as a standardized scheme for describing mammographic lesions (47). In the BI-RADS system, there are six categories for mammographic findings (other than incomplete) (43,44).

0. **Incomplete, needs further imaging**
1. **Negative**
2. **Benign finding**
3. **Probably benign, short-interval follow-up recommended**
4. **Suspicious finding and biopsy should be considered**
5. **Highly suggestive of malignancy and appropriate action should be undertaken**
6. **Known malignancy (a category that is often used for follow-up of a lesion that is undergoing neoadjuvant treatment)**

The patient should be referred for tissue diagnosis if the report identifies a lesion as a category 4 or 5 (47). A category 0 indicates incomplete evaluation, and further diagnostic studies are required. Category 3 connotes a finding that is most likely benign; a short-interval follow-up is recommended, and breast examination by an expert should be considered.

Correlation of Findings

Biopsy must be performed on patients with a dominant or suspicious mass despite absence of mammographic findings (48). Mammography should be performed before biopsy so other suspicious areas can be noted and the contralateral breast can be checked (Fig. 21.2). **Mammography is never a substitute for biopsy because it may not reveal clinical cancer,** especially when it occurs in the dense breast tissue of young women with fibrocystic changes. The sensitivity of mammography is 75%, with a specificity of 92.3% depending on the patient's age; breast density; use of hormone therapy; and the size, location, and mammographic appearance of the tumor (49). Mammography is less sensitive in young women with dense breast tissue than in older women, who tend to have fatty breasts, in which mammography can detect at least 90% of malignancies (50). Small tumors, particularly those without calcifications, are more difficult to detect, especially in women with dense breasts.

Ultrasonography

Breast ultrasonography is used for focused scanning of a questionable finding or for evaluation of a mammographic finding (51). Reliable, portable, computer-enhanced ultrasonography with high-frequency transducers and improved imaging is available to evaluate and treat problems of the breast (52). It is a sensitive, minimally invasive technique that is used frequently to evaluate some breast symptoms, especially in younger women with dense breast tissue, but is dependent on the availability of a skilled ultrasonographer (53). Some lesions can be detected only with ultrasonography (54). It is the preferred modality to distinguish a solid from a cystic mass (51). Breast ultrasonography is not recommended for routine screening, but is being studied as a means to screen women with dense breast tissue (54). Ultrasonography has a higher false-positive rate than mammography (51,53–55).

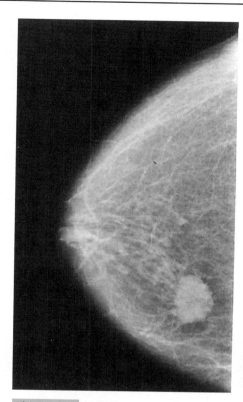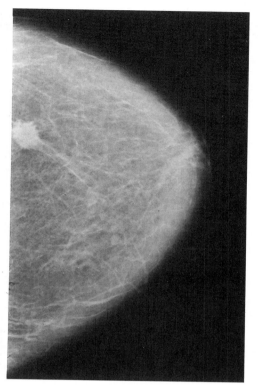

Figure 21.2   Bilateral mammography shows the extent of breast carcinoma, illustrating the importance of bilateral mammography in the workup of a clinically apparent mass. (From **Kruper L, Giuliano AE.** Breast disease. In: **Berek JS, Hacker NF, eds.** *Berek & Hacker's Gynecologic Oncology,* 5th ed. Philadelphia: Lippincott Williams & Wilkins, 2010:617, with permission.)

Following are indications for breast ultrasonography:

- **Characterization:**
  Palpable abnormality
  Ambiguous mammographic findings
  Silicone leak
  Mass in woman younger than 30 years, lactating, or pregnant

- **Guidance for interventional procedures**

- **Possible role for additional imaging in high-risk individuals**

Ultrasonography is useful in distinguishing benign from malignant lesions identified by mammography (56). Ultrasonography may be especially useful if the patient feels a mass, but the physician cannot detect an abnormality and the mammogram does not disclose one. It may identify cancers in the dense breast tissue of premenopausal women, but it is usually used to distinguish a benign cyst from a solid tumor. Ultrasonography cannot reliably detect microcalcifications, and it is not as useful as mammography in assessing women with fatty breasts.

Handheld or real-time ultrasonography is 95% to 100% accurate in differentiating solid masses from cysts (57). This finding is of limited clinical value because a dominant mass should be evaluated by biopsy, and a cystic mass can be studied by needle aspiration, which is far less expensive than ultrasonography. If a lesion proves to be a simple cyst, no further evaluation is necessary. Rarely ultrasonography may identify a small cancer within a cyst, an intracystic carcinoma. These complex cysts warrant surgical biopsy.

Magnetic Resonance Imaging

Magnetic resonance imaging may be of value in assessing breast lesions of an indeterminate nature detected by clinical and mammographic examination or occurring in patients who have implants (58). Both MRI and positron emission tomography (PET) are used to identify occult lesions, and MRI is increasing in popularity as a means of imaging the breast (58–60). It tends to be highly sensitive but not specific, leading to biopsies of benign lesions. Image enhancement with gadolinium discriminates between benign and malignant lesions with varying degrees of accuracy.

Several roles are proposed for breast MRI. The lack of radiation exposure makes MRI theoretically an ideal method for screening of healthy women, but widespread use is not cost-effective. Focal asymmetry is usually benign but can represent a malignancy. MRI may help identify those patients with focal asymmetric areas who should undergo biopsy. A scar can easily be distinguished from recurrent tumor based on the evaluation and diminution of the scar over time. Some scars do not resolve rapidly and are confused with cancer or, more commonly, with recurrent cancer after breast-conserving surgery and whole breast irradiation. Ideally, such cases are evaluated with MRI, sometimes obviating the need for biopsy. MRI is extremely useful in identifying silicone released by ruptured breast implants in patients with augmented breasts (Fig. 21.3). In patients with implants, MRI with gadolinium may be performed to detect breast cancer even if silicone release is not suspected. There may be a role for **MRI in evaluation of specific conditions. It is used for the following indications:**

- **Stage tumor to rule out multicentric disease.**

- **Differentiate postoperative scar from recurrence after breast-conserving surgery.**

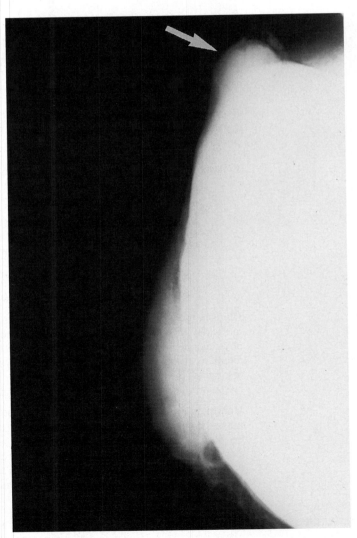

Figure 21.3 **Mammography shows implant and extracapsular free silicone** (*arrow*).

- **Find a lesion seen in only one view of mammogram.**

- **Evaluate positive axillary nodes in the presence of negative mammogram and clinical breast examination results.**

- **Rule out silicone implant rupture.**

- **Assess focal asymmetry.**

- **Detect additional ipsilateral and contralateral cancers.**

- **Evaluate the effect of neoadjuvant chemotherapy.**

The American Cancer Society recommends annual MRI screening for women who are high risk (greater than 20% lifetime risk) and consideration given to women with moderate risk (15% to 20% lifetime risk) (61). A study from the Netherlands in high-risk women reported 71% sensitivity for MRI compared with 17.9% for clinical breast examination and 40% for mammography (62). The International Cooperative Magnetic Resonance Mammography Study will help identify the advantages and limitations of MRI. At present, MRI should be considered only after conventional imaging is performed; it should not be used as a screening tool or a substitute for mammography or biopsy. Centers that perform MRI should have the ability to perform MRI-guided biopsies of lesions detected with MRI only and that are not visible with mammogram or ultrasound.

Positron Emission Tomography Scan

PET scanning is a diagnostic modality that assesses the metabolic activity of tumors. Radioactive fluorodeoxyglucose (FDG) is an analogue of glucose that is metabolized by tissues of high metabolic activity. Although not specifically approved for the initial diagnosis of breast cancer or for staging the axilla, it can be useful in patients with advanced disease (59,63). This technique is used to identify occult breast lesions with positive axillary lymph nodes (59).

Breast Tissue Evaluation: Histology and Cytology

The safest course is tissue or cytologic biopsy evaluation of all dominant masses found on physical examination and, in the absence of a mass, evaluation of suspicious lesions shown by breast imaging. Over 1 million women have breast biopsies each year in the United States. Between 70% and 80% of these biopsies yield a benign lesion (64). The diagnosis of a benign breast lesion versus breast cancer is often difficult to determine based on clinical examination and requires evaluation of tissue by fine needle aspiration cytology (FNAC), core needle biopsy (CNB), or excisional biopsy (EB). Both FNAC and CNB are reasonable techniques for the evaluation of a palpable or image-identified lesion. CNB evolved as the diagnostic procedure of choice. More than half of all breast biopsies use a core-needle technique. The sensitivity of CNBs performed using either stereotactic or ultrasound guidance is 97% to 99% (65). CNB is used increasingly to diagnose breast cancer and to determine tumor histology, grade, and marker expression; select neoadjuvant therapy; and predict sentinel lymph node status (66). CNB and fine needle aspiration (FNA) are less invasive and achieve better cosmesis than excisional or even incisional biopsy. The main limitations of FNA are high rate of insufficient sampling and inability to distinguish invasive from noninvasive cancers. CNB is a well-accepted alternative to surgical biopsy and can avoid surgical biopsies in most patients (67). Investigators of the Fifth Radiologic Diagnostic Oncology Group demonstrated that image-guided biopsy of breast lesions provides high diagnostic accuracy. The sensitivity, specificity, and accuracy of CNB were 0.91, 1.00, and 0.98, respectively (68).

About 30% of lesions suspected to be cancer prove on biopsy to be benign, and about 15% of lesions believed to be benign prove to be malignant (23). Dominant masses or suspicious nonpalpable breast lesions require histopathological examination. Histologic or cytologic diagnosis should be obtained before the decision is made to monitor a breast mass (69). An exception may be a premenopausal woman with a nonsuspicious mass presumed to be fibrocystic disease. **An apparently fibrocystic lesion that does not completely resolve within several menstrual cycles should be sampled for biopsy. Any mass in a postmenopausal woman who is not taking estrogen therapy should be presumed to be malignant.** Some clinicians will monitor a mass when results of the clinical diagnosis, breast imaging studies, and cytologic studies are all in agreement, such as with fibroadenoma. Many clinicians will not leave a dominant mass in the breast even when FNAC or CNB results are negative, unless the FNA or CNB shows fibroadenoma. Such cases require periodic follow-up. Some surgeons excise lesions when the sampling technique shows only fibrocystic disease. Figures 21.4 and 21.5 present algorithms for management of breast masses in premenopausal and postmenopausal patients. Simultaneous evaluation of a breast mass using clinical breast examination, radiography, and needle biopsy can lower the risk of missing cancer to only 1%, effectively reducing the rate of diagnostic failure and increasing the quality of patient care (70).

If the presence of breast cancer is strongly suggested by physical examination, the diagnosis can be confirmed by FNAC or CNB, and the patient may be counseled regarding treatment. Treatment should not be determined based on results of physical examination and mammography alone, in the absence of biopsy results. The most reasonable approach to the diagnosis and treatment of breast cancer is outpatient biopsy (either FNAC, CNB, or EB), followed by definitive surgery at a later date if needed. **This two-step approach allows patients to adjust to the diagnosis of cancer, carefully consider alternative forms of therapy, and seek a second opinion. Studies show no adverse effect from the 1- to 2-week delay associated with the two-step procedure (71). Because cancer is found in the minority of patients who require biopsy for diagnosis of a breast mass, definitive treatment should not be undertaken without an unequivocal histologic diagnosis of cancer.**

Fine-Needle Aspiration

With FNAC, cells from a breast tumor are aspirated with a small (usually 22-gauge) needle and examined by a pathologist. Precise guidelines for this technique are available (72). It can be performed easily, with no morbidity, and is much less expensive than excisional or open biopsy. It requires the availability of a pathologist skilled in the cytologic diagnosis of breast cancer to interpret the results, and it is subject to sampling problems, particularly when lesions are deep. Cytologic diagnoses must be correlated with clinical and imaging findings to achieve triple-test concordance and to decrease the false-negative rate (73). **The triple-test concordance (i.e., concordance between fine-needle aspiration, physical examination, and mammography) is the foundation of breast evaluation. The triple-test results are more powerful than each modality alone** (74). The incidence of false-positive diagnoses was 0% to 0.3%, and the rate of false-negative diagnoses was 1.4% to 2.3% in several recent studies (74,75).

Core Needle Biopsy

A core of tissue can be obtained from palpable lesions using a large cutting needle (76). Image-guided large-core needle biopsy is a reliable diagnostic alternative to surgical excision of suspicious nonpalpable breast lesions (77). As in the case of any needle biopsy, the main drawback is false-negative findings caused by improper positioning of the needle. False-negative findings may be reduced if core biopsy is performed with ultrasonographic guidance. **The interpretation of results from CNB is classified by categories B1 to B5** (78):

B1: Normal tissue
B2: Benign lesions: fibroadenomas, fibrocystic change, sclerosing adenosis, duct ectasia, fat necrosis, abscess
B3: Uncertain malignant potential: atypical epithelial hyperplasia, lobular neoplasia, phyllodes tumor, papillary lesions, radial scar, complex sclerosing lesions
B4: Suspicious
B5: Malignant

Open Excisional Biopsy

Open biopsy with local anesthesia as a separate procedure before deciding on definitive treatment is the most reliable means of diagnosis. Its utility is reserved for when the results of needle biopsy are nondiagnostic or equivocal.

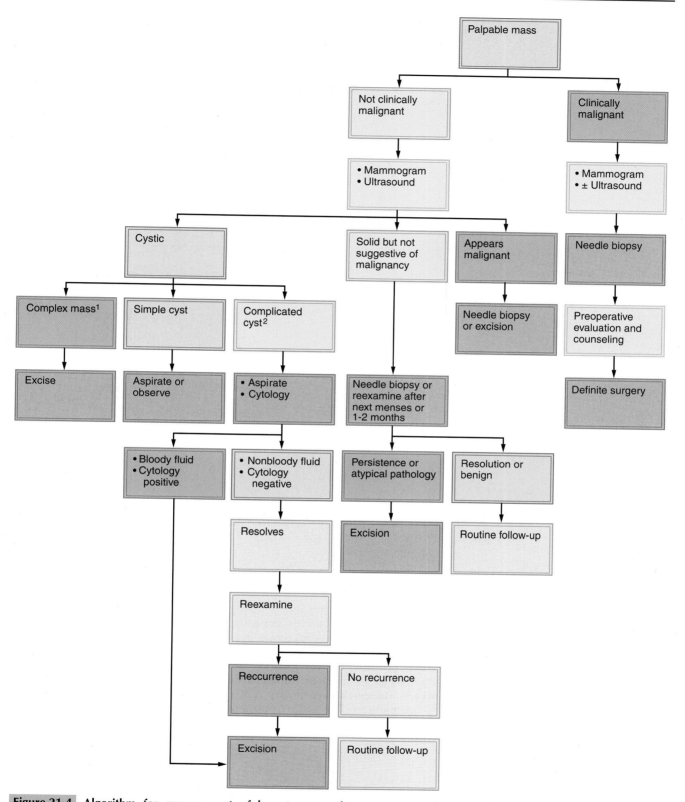

Figure 21.4 Algorithm for management of breast masses in premenopausal women.
(Revised and updated from **Kruper L, Giuliano AE.** Breast disease. In: **Berek JS, Hacker NF, eds.** *Berek & Hacker's Gynecologic Oncology*, 5th ed. Philadelphia: Lippincott Williams & Wilkins, 2010:628, with permission.)

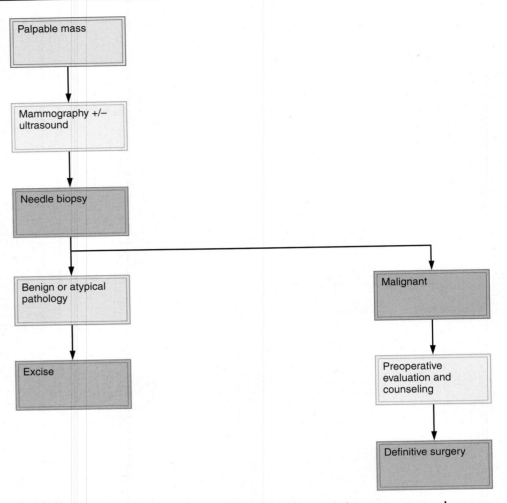

Figure 21.5 **Algorithm for management of breast masses in postmenopausal women.** (Revised and updated from **Kruper L, Giuliano AE.** Breast disease. In: **Berek JS, Hacker NF, eds.** *Berek & Hacker's Gynecologic Oncology,* 5th ed. Philadelphia: Lippincott Williams & Wilkins, 2010:629, with permission.)

Histologic Analysis

Histologic evaluation with hematoxylin and eosin (H&E) staining confirms benign or malignant disease. Images of benign and malignant breast lesions can be viewed through the Internet Pathology Laboratory for Medical Education (79). **Assessment of prognostic factors, tumor grade; estrogen, progesterone, her-2/*neu* receptor status; and proliferative indices is performed on paraffin-fixed tissue by immunohistochemistry (78). Her-2/*neu* assessment in breast cancer by immunohistochemistry (IHC) is appropriate for patients with tumors that score 3+. Fluorescence *in situ* hybridization (FISH) is recommended for 2+ IHC to more accurately assess her-2/*neu* amplification and provide better prognostic information** (80).

Ductal Lavage Cytology

Ductal lavage using a microcatheter is a modality that was investigated in high-risk women (81). Patients undergo gentle nipple suction to elicit nipple fluid. A duct that yields fluid is cannulated with a microcatheter, and 10 to 20 mL of saline are introduced in 2- to 4-mL increments. **The cytologic assessment of a sample obtained by ductal lavage is more sensitive than that of nipple aspiration. Ductal lavage performed to identify abnormal cells is not an effective tool in detecting breast cancer and is rarely performed** (81).

Benign Breast Conditions

Benign breast disorders account for most breast problems. These conditions are frequently considered in the context of excluding breast cancer and often are unrecognized for their own associated morbidity (82). To provide appropriate management, it is important to consider benign breast disorders from four aspects: (i) clinical picture, (ii) medical significance, (iii) treatment intervention, and (iv) pathologic etiology (83). A framework for understanding benign breast problems is called Aberrations of Normal Development and Involution (ANDI) (2,82,83). It includes symptoms, histology, endocrine state, and pathogenesis in a progression from a normal to a disease state. Most benign breast conditions arise from normal changes in breast development, hormone cycling, and reproductive evolution (82).

Three life cycles reflect different reproductive phases in a woman's life and are associated with unique breast manifestations.

1. **During the early reproductive period (15–25 years), lobule and stromal formation occurs.** The ANDI conditions associated with this period are fibroadenoma (mass) and juvenile hypertrophy (excessive breast development). In this first stage, the progression from ANDI to a disease state results in the formation of giant fibroadenomas and multiple fibroadenomas.

2. **During the mature reproductive period (25 to 40 years), cyclic hormonal changes affect glandular tissue and stroma.** In this second period, the ANDI is an exaggeration of these cyclic effects, such as cyclic mastalgia and generalized nodularity.

3. **The third phase is involution of lobules and ducts or turnover of epithelia, which occurs during ages 35 to 55 years.** The ANDI associated with lobular involution are macrocysts (lumps) and sclerosing lesions (mammographic abnormalities). Those associated with ductal involution are duct dilation (nipple discharge) and periductal fibrosis (nipple retraction), and those with epithelial turnover are mild hyperplasia (pathologic description).

Disease conditions with increased epithelial turnover are epithelial hyperplasias with atypia. Breasts are under endocrine control and show a wide range of appearances during reproductive life. ANDI classification allows the clinician to understand the pathogenesis of these conditions and to understand that these disorders are aberrations of a normal process that does not usually require any specific treatment (82).

Fibrocystic Change

Fibrocystic change, the most common lesion of the breast, is an imprecise term that covers a spectrum of clinical signs, symptoms, and histologic changes (76). The term refers to a histologic picture of fibrosis, cyst formation, and epithelial hyperplasia (83). Cysts arise from the breast lobules and are an aberration of normal breast involution (82). Macroscopic cysts occur in approximately 7% of women, and microscopic, nonpalpable cysts occur in about 40% of women (84). It is common in women 35 to 55 years of age, but rare in postmenopausal women not taking hormone therapy. The presence of estrogen seems necessary for the clinical symptoms to occur. This finding is supported by the observation that it is present bilaterally, increased in the perimenopausal age group, and responsive to endocrine therapy (85). In essence, a diagnosis of fibrocystic change can lead to significant patient anxiety but is of little clinical significance as long as malignancy is excluded (86). These lesions are associated with benign changes in the breast epithelium.

Cyst Fluid Analysis

Investigators examined the electrolyte and protein content of cyst fluid, but this is of little significance in the clinical management of fibrocystic disease. The potassium-to-sodium ratio is a marker that may be used to distinguish cyst subtypes (87). Cysts are either lined by apocrine epithelium with a high potassium-to-sodium ratio and a higher hormone or steroid concentration (type I); or by flattened lobule epithelium with a low potassium-to-sodium ratio and a higher concentration of albumin, carcinoembryonic antigen, CA125, and steroid hormone–binding globulin (type II) (87). Apocrine cysts produce and secrete large amounts of prostate-specific antigen (PSA) (88). The role of this serine protease in proliferative breast disease is not fully understood.

Clinical Findings in Fibrocystic Disease

Fibrocystic changes may produce an asymptomatic mass that is smooth, mobile, and potentially compressible. Fibrocystic change is more often accompanied by pain or tenderness and sometimes nipple discharge. In many cases, discomfort coincides with the premenstrual phase of the cycle, when the cysts tend to enlarge. Fluctuations in size and rapid appearance or disappearance of a breast mass are common. Multiple or bilateral masses appear frequently, and many patients have a history of a transient mass in the breast or cyclic breast pain. Cyclic breast pain is the most commonly associated symptom of fibrocystic changes.

Differential Diagnosis

Pain, fluctuation in size, multiplicity of lesions, and bilaterality are the features most helpful to differentiate fibrocystic disease from carcinoma. If a dominant mass is present, the diagnosis of cancer should be suspected until it is disproved by complete aspiration of a cyst, or histopathologic analysis if a mass is present after aspiration, or by breast imaging. Microscopic findings associated with fibrocystic disease include cysts (gross and microscopic), papillomatosis, adenosis, fibrosis, and ductal epithelial hyperplasia (89).

Diagnostic Tests

Patients with cystic disease may have a discrete fibrocystic mass that is frequently indistinguishable from carcinoma, based on clinical findings. Mammography may be helpful, but there are no mammographic signs diagnostic of fibrocystic change. Ultrasonography is useful in differentiating a cystic from a solid mass. **Characteristic findings on ultrasonography that confirm a simple cyst include the following:**

- **Mass with thin walls**
- **Smooth round shape**
- **Absence of internal echoes**
- **Posterior acoustic enhancement**

If these imaging criteria are not met, a tissue diagnosis of the mass usually requires a FNA, FNAC, or EB. The finding of a simple cyst by ultrasonography rules out carcinoma. **Any lesion that is suspicious by mammography or ultrasonography should be biopsied.**

When the diagnosis of fibrocystic change is established by ultrasonography or is practically certain because the history is classic, aspiration of a discrete mass, suggestive of a cyst, is indicated if the patient is symptomatic, the cyst obscures visualization of breast tissue on mammography and prevents adequate imaging, or if the ultrasonographic criteria are not met. In one study of a screened population, 1% of individuals developed a new cyst that resolved in more than 50% of cases (90). Aspiration may be performed with ultrasonographic guidance, but image guidance is usually not necessary if the cyst is palpable (91). FNA of a cyst is a minimally invasive procedure performed with a 21- or 22-gauge needle without local anesthesia and is not associated with significant risks or complications. There is minimal pain and little risk for infection or bleeding. Benign cyst fluid is straw colored to dark green to brownish and does not need to be submitted for cytologic evaluation (6). Injection of air into the cyst cavity is reported to reduce the likelihood of cyst recurrence but generally is not performed. The patient should be reexamined at a short interval thereafter for cyst recurrence. Cysts will reoccur in 30% of patients, cause anxiety, and require repeated evaluations (84). **Tissue biopsy should be performed in the presence of the following findings:**

- **No cyst fluid is obtained.**
- **The fluid is bloody.**
- **The fluid is thick.**
- **The cyst is complex.**
- **There is an intracystic mass.**
- **A mass persists after aspiration.**
- **A persistent mass is noted at any time during follow-up.**

If a needle biopsy is performed and results are negative for malignancy, a suspicious mass that does not resolve over several months should be excised. Surgery should be conservative, because the primary objective is to exclude cancer. Simple mastectomy or extensive removal of breast tissue is not indicated for fibrocystic disease. Most patients do not require treatment for fibrocystic changes, just reassurance that fibrocystic change is a transient phenomenon of aging that is associated with hormonal effects on the breast glandular tissue that eventually subsides.

Fibrocystic Change and Risk for Breast Cancer

Fibrocystic change is not associated with an increased risk of breast cancer unless there is histologic evidence of epithelial proliferative changes, with or without atypia (92–97). The common coincidence of fibrocystic disease and malignancy in the same breast reflects the fact that both processes are common events. Approximately 80% of biopsies show fibrocystic changes. In an evaluation of the relationship between fibrocystic change and breast cancer in 10,366 women who underwent biopsy between 1950 and 1968 and were followed for a median of 17 years, approximately 70% of the biopsies showed nonproliferative breast disease, whereas 30% showed proliferative breast disease (95). Cytologic atypia were present in 3.6% of cases. Women with nonproliferative disease had no increased risk of breast cancer, whereas women with proliferative breast disease and no atypical hyperplasia had a twofold higher risk of breast cancer. **Patients whose biopsy results showed atypical ductal or lobular hyperplasia had an approximately fivefold higher risk than women with nonproliferative disease to develop invasive breast cancer in either breast.** Patients with carcinoma *in situ* have an eight- to tenfold risk of developing breast cancer. This risk is bilateral for lobular lesions and ipsilateral for ductal lesions. A family history of breast cancer added little risk for women with nonproliferative disease, but family history plus atypia increased breast cancer risk 11-fold. The presence of cysts alone did not increase the risk of breast cancer, but cysts combined with a family history of breast cancer increased the risk about threefold (76,92–97). Women with these risk factors (family history of breast cancer and proliferative breast disease) should be followed carefully with physical examination and mammography. For such women, age-specific probability of developing invasive breast carcinoma in the next 10 years is 1 in 2,000 (age 20), 1 in 256 (age 30), 1 in 67 (age 40), 1 in 39 (age 50), and 1 in 29 (age 60) (93). The relative risk for developing breast cancer depends on the type of proliferative lesion diagnosed.

Management of Fibrocystic Change

Fibrocystic change is a normal evolutionary change in breast development and involution and does not require a specific treatment other than a good clinical breast examination and age-appropriate mammographic screening or imaging studies directed to signs and symptoms. A number of nutritional and dietary supplements were investigated to relieve symptoms. The role of caffeine consumption in the aggravation of fibrocystic change is controversial (98–101). Results of some studies suggest that eliminating caffeine from the diet is associated with improvement of symptoms (100,101). Many patients are aware of these studies and report relief of symptoms after discontinuing intake of coffee, tea, and chocolate. Similarly, many women find vitamin E (150 to 600 IU daily) or B$_6$ (200 to 800 mg per day) helpful (102,103). Observations about these effects are difficult to confirm and are anecdotal (104–106). A recent review of nutritional interventions for fibrocystic breast conditions that evaluated evening primrose oil, vitamin E, or pyridoxine suggested that there are insufficient data to draw clear conclusions about their effectiveness (107). Exacerbations of pain, tenderness, and cyst formation may occur at any time until menopause, when symptoms usually subside unless patients are taking *estrogen*. **A patient with fibrocystic changes should be advised to examine her own breasts each month just after menstruation and to inform her physician if a mass appears.**

Mastalgia

Mastalgia is a recognized organic condition that is studied less thoroughly than other breast problems (108,109). Inflammatory cytokines were implicated in the etiology of breast pain. A study evaluating expression of interleukin-6 and tumor necrosis factor-α in painful and non-painful breast tissue showed lower levels of these cytokines in painful breast tissue during the luteal phase; however, these levels did not reach statistical significance (110). Elevated estrogen, low progesterone, or an imbalance in the ratio of estrogen and progesterone were suggested as a possible cause for the symptoms (111).

Natural History of Mastalgia

Approximately 70% to 80% of women experience severe breast pain at some time in their lives (112,113). Mastalgia accounts for 30% to 47% of breast clinical evaluations (111,114). In 15% of the patients, the mastalgia is so severe that it alters lifestyle and requires repeated investigations and treatment (112). Mastalgia interferes with sexual (48%), physical (37%), social (12%), and work or school activities (8%) (115).

Types of Mastalgia

Breast pain is a distressing constellation of symptoms that is classified as cyclic, noncyclic, or extramammary (116). Cyclic mastalgia is related to exaggerated premenstrual symptoms beginning in the luteal phase of the menstrual cycle, associated with breast engorgement, pain, ache, heaviness, and tenderness that is bilateral and can last for more than 7 days in 11% of women (116–118). Cyclical mastalgia is more prevalent in women in their third and fourth decades of life and accounts for two-thirds of all breast pain symptoms (119). **Noncyclic mastalgia** is independent of menstrual cycles and is described as achy, burning soreness. It may be intermittent or constant, is usually unilateral, occurs in the fourth and fifth decades, and is more difficult to treat than cyclic mastalgia (116). **Extramammary pain** is perceived to be located in the breast but is related to an extramammary site. Chest wall muscular pain, costal cartilage symptoms, herpes zoster, radiculopathies, and rib fractures are among some of the more common causes of extramammary pain. Costochondritis (Tietze syndrome) is a manifestation of chest wall pain that is frequently interpreted as breast pain.

Management of Mastalgia

Breast pain is an unlikely symptom of malignancy, and when malignancy is excluded by a clinical breast examination and age-appropriate breast imaging for focal breast pain, the most important treatment is reassurance. Treatments include medications, such as anesthetics, diuretics, *bromocriptine,* and *tamoxifen;* vitamins and supplements, such as evening primrose oil; mechanical support with a well-fitting bra; local excision; and decreased fat intake and reduction in methylxanthines from caffeine, tea, and chocolate (108,116). **Discontinuation of hormone therapy may be effective in some women. Maintenance of a pain score diary is important to understand the relationship of pain to factors such as the menstrual cycle, activities of daily living, and stress.** External support may be effective for breast pain associated with generalized fibrocystic changes and is best treated by avoiding trauma and by wearing (night and day) a brassiere that gives good support and protection (120). One study evaluated resolution of symptoms in 200 women randomized either to a regimen of *danazol* (200 mg per day) or to mechanical support with a sports brassiere worn for regular activities for 12 weeks. The group using mechanical support had 85% relief of symptoms compared with 58% improvement in the *danazol* group. Symptoms recurred after discontinuance of treatment with *danazol* (113). The *danazol* group experienced drug-related side effects in 42%, which led to discontinuance of the medication in 15%. The breast has minimal structural support and is at significant risk for motion-related displacement resulting in mastalgia. The use of external support to minimize breast motion appears to be effective in reducing breast pain. The application of heat packs or cold packs and light breast massage may reduce symptoms in some individuals (116).

Hormone-modulating drugs, including *danazol, bromocriptine, tamoxifen,* and *Depo-Provera,* are recognized drug treatments for mastalgia, although *tamoxifen* is not approved for this use in the United States (116,121–124). These drugs are associated with significant side effects that limit their general use (116). **Withdrawal of birth control pills or hormone therapy may be all that is required to alleviate symptoms** (116).

Danazol is a synthetic androgen that suppresses release of pituitary gonadotropin, prevents luteinizing hormone surge, and inhibits ovarian steroid formation. It is the only medication approved by the U.S. Food and Drug Administration for mastalgia (116). The androgenic effects—acne, edema, change in voice, weight gain, headaches, depression, and hirsutism—often are intolerable, and many patients stop taking *danazol* even when symptoms are improved (122). It can be initiated at doses of 100 to 200 mg twice daily orally for patients with severe pain and then tapered to a lower dose of 100 mg per day (122). A survey of surgeons in Great Britain revealed that 75% prescribed *danazol* as first-line therapy (108). A study conducted to evaluate the response to administration of *danazol* revealed a 79% amelioration of symptoms (125). This approach reduced the premenstrual mastalgia and resulted in virtually no side effects.

The use of oral progesterone agents reduces cyclical breast pain (111). Further studies may be warranted to see whether *medroxyprogesterone acetate* suppresses cyclic mastalgia in reproductive-age women.

Breast pain is increased in some individuals who have elevated prolactin (PRL) levels induced by thyrotropin-releasing hormone (TRH) (116). *Bromocriptine* is a dopamine antagonist that inhibits the release of PRL. *Bromocriptine* (2.5 mg twice daily) given for 3 to 6 months is effective in reducing mastalgia in women who have TRH-induced elevation of PRL (123). Patients who have normal TRH levels, are resistant to *bromocriptine*, or do not tolerate the side effects of nausea, vomiting, and headache respond favorably to progesterone and systemic nonsteroidal anti-inflammatory drugs (NSAIDs).

Prolactin induces active transport of iodine in breast tissue (126,127). Iodine deficiency in rats causes hyperplasia and atypia (128). Iodine replacement is associated with improvement in subjective pain (129). A randomized, double-blind study with supraphysiologic levels of iodine in women with documented cyclic mastalgia demonstrated dose-dependent reduction in physician-assessed and self-reported pain at 3 and 6 months of treatment (130).

Goserelin is a potent synthetic analogue of luteinizing hormone-releasing hormone (LHRH) that causes reversible reduction in serum estrogen level and decrease in breast pain (131). Side effects of *goserelin* include vaginal dryness, hot flushes, decreased libido, oily skin and hair, and decreased breast size. A recent clinical trial randomized 147 women into *goserelin* versus placebo groups. The study had a 49% drop-out rate. The mean breast pain score decreased by 67% in the *goserelin* arm and 35% in the placebo arm. The authors concluded that *goserelin* is an effective treatment for mastalgia with significant side effects and should be kept as second-line therapy. Hormonal blockade of the estrogen receptor is another approach to minimizing the effects of circulating estrogen on breast pain. Treatment with the selective estrogen receptor modulator *tamoxifen* demonstrated reduction in breast pain at 10 and 20 mg per day, with equivalent effects compared with *danazol* and *bromocriptine* in most studies (124,132–134). Topical nonsteroidal therapy is another option for women with mastalgia (135). Gel forms of NSAIDs often are used for relief of pain. Patients were stratified by cyclic versus noncyclic pain and then randomized to treatment with NSAIDs versus placebo. There was a significant reduction in cyclic and noncyclic pain in all groups, but the magnitude of change was greater in the treatment arms and similar for cyclic and noncyclic pain. Use of NSAIDs appears to be a less toxic treatment and may be considered as an option for both cyclic and noncyclic breast pain.

Nonhormonal therapies such as dietary restrictions, vitamins and supplements, and restriction of methylxantines were investigated as possible treatments for mastalgia because they are less likely to be associated with adverse drug-related side effects (116). Because mastalgia is one of the symptoms associated with fibrocystic disease, the treatments described for fibrocystic disease are relevant to mastalgia. A low-fat diet was effective in one randomized trial (136). Ninety percent of patients taking in 15% dietary fat experienced resolution of pain symptoms after 6 months compared with only 22% of those on a diet containing 36% fat ($p = .0023$). Evening primrose oil containing essential fatty acids (γ-linolenic acid [GLA]) was studied because of its affect on prostaglandin synthesis (137). It was used as first-line therapy, reserving *danazol* and *bromocriptine* for treatment of more severe symptoms (112). In a small prospective mastalgia trial, women were given eight capsules of evening primrose oil daily for 4 months (320 mg GLA) (138). Those who responded had a lower level of essential fatty acids at the time of initiation when compared with poor responders, suggesting that evening primrose oil increases essential fatty acids and that this increase may be associated with the improvement in symptoms in the responders. Two other trials failed to demonstrate efficacy of evening primrose oil capsules over placebo (139,140). In a Dutch trial, 124 women with cyclic or noncyclic pain lasting on average 7 or more days (minimum 5 days) were randomized to receive the following regimens: (i) fish oil and control oil, (ii) evening primrose oil and control oil, (iii) fish and evening primrose oil, or (iv) both control oils for 6 months (139). There was a statistically significant reduction in the number of days per month with pain but not in the pain score in the entire study population. There was a greater reduction in cyclic than noncyclic pain symptoms, and this finding was true for both the test oils and for the control oils. The authors concluded that neither fish oil nor evening primrose oil had a better effect than the less expensive wheat germ and corn oils. A second large double-blind randomized prospective trial was conducted in 555 women with cyclic mastalgia of moderate to severe degree present for at least 7 days of a menstrual cycle (140). The four groups were (i) GLA and placebo antioxidants, (ii) placebo fatty acids and antioxidants, (iii) GLA and placebo antioxidants, and (iv) placebo fatty acids and placebo antioxidants. The treatments were given in a blinded fashion for 4 months. All groups had a similar 35% reduction in symptoms. This treatment was followed by open treatment with GLA in all groups and blinded treatment with antioxidants. There was continued improvement of symptoms in all groups with a reduction in mastalgia by 50% over the next 12 months. This is the largest and best-controlled study to date evaluating GLA for relief of mastalgia, and GLA was not found to be superior to placebo. The results of this study were not consistent with those from previous smaller studies. The authors cannot exclude a significant psychologic impact that may confound the effect of GLA. GLA use was found to be safe, without any significant side effects, and was prescribed as therapy for mastalgia because of its lack of side effects. The randomized trials, however, bring into serious question the efficacy of these options.

Fibroepithelial Lesions

Fibroadenoma

Fibroadenomas are the most common benign tumors of the breast. In one series, they accounted for 50% of all breast biopsies (141). They usually occur in young women (age 20 to 35 years) and may occur in teenagers (142). In women younger than 25 years, fibroadenomas are more common than cysts. They rarely occur after menopause, although occasionally they are found, often calcified, in postmenopausal women. For this reason, it is postulated that fibroadenomas are responsive to estrogen stimulation. A study reports the *de novo* occurrence of fibroadenoma in 51 women older than age 35 years who had no evidence of a palpable or mammographic visualized lesion in well-documented prior visits (143). Fibroadenomas may appear as single masses or as multiple lesions.

Clinically, a young woman usually notices a mass while showering or dressing. Most masses are 2 to 3 cm in diameter when detected, but they can become extremely large (i.e., the giant fibroadenoma). On physical examination, they are firm, smooth, and rubbery. They do not elicit an inflammatory reaction, are freely mobile, and cause no dimpling of the skin or nipple retraction. They are often bilobed, and a groove can be palpated on examination. On mammographic and ultrasonographic imaging, the typical features are of a well-defined, smooth, solid mass with clearly defined margins and dimensions that are longer than wide and craniocaudad dimensions that are less than the length.

Fibroadenoma is not associated with an increased risk for breast cancer (144). The natural history of fibroadenoma can be regression, growth, or no change in size. Most fibroadenomas are static or cease growth at approximately 2 to 3 cm, about 15% of tumors regress spontaneously, and only 5% to 10% progress (145). Because transformation of a fibroadenoma into cancer is rare and regression is frequent, current management recommendations are conservative unless there is evidence of growth (141). A suspected fibroadenoma should be confirmed by FNAC or CNB and observed for increase in size or excised based on patient preference. Rarely will the fibroadenoma increase to more than 2 to 3 cm in size. Large or growing fibroadenomas must be excised. Complete excision of a fibroadenoma with local anesthesia can be performed to treat the lesion and confirm the absence of malignancy. Less invasive local treatment of a fibroadenoma is advocated by some and can be performed with either ultrasonographically guided percutaneous vacuum-assisted biopsy devices or percutaneous cryoablation (146,147). A young woman with a clinical fibroadenoma can undergo needle cytology and observation of the mass (148). Acceptance of observation varies, and many women choose to have the fibroadenoma excised (149).

On gross examination of an excised mass, the fibroadenoma appears encapsulated and sharply delineated from the surrounding breast parenchyma. Microscopically, there is proliferation of both the epithelial and stromal component. In longstanding lesions and in postmenopausal patients, calcifications may be observed within the stroma.

Multiple Fibroadenomas

Multiple fibroadenomas occur in some women and were reported to occur more frequently in premenopausal women undergoing immunosuppression for transplant (150–152). Excision of all lesions through separate incisions could leave significant scarring and deformity. Excision of these mobile lesions through a single periareolar incision was suggested, but this approach can lead to significant ductal disruption (153). Another approach is through an incision in the inframammary crease. Alternatively, these lesions can be treated with observation based on triple-test concordance of results of a classic clinical examination with histologic corroboration with FNAC and ultrasonographic diagnostic criteria consistent with a fibroadenoma (151).

Phyllodes Tumor

Phyllodes tumors are rare fibroepithelial tumors that display a spectrum of clinical and pathologic behaviors that are benign, borderline, and malignant (154,155). The distribution of phyllodes tumors demonstrates that **most tumors are benign (70%) compared with malignant (23%) and borderline lesions (7%)** (156). This distribution is similar to a larger, older study that reported an incidence of 64% benign, 21% malignant, and 14% borderline phyllodes tumors (157). The incidence in some studies should be viewed with caution because of variation in histologic interpretation (156). Phyllodes tumors may occur at any age but tend to be more common in women who are in their late 30s, 40s, and 50s (156,158–162). **These lesions are rarely bilateral and usually appear as isolated masses that are difficult to distinguish clinically from a fibroadenoma.** Patients often relate a long history of a previously stable nodule that suddenly increases in size. Reported sizes range from 1.0 to 50 cm (154,163,164). Size is not a dependable diagnostic criterion, although phyllodes tumors tend to be larger than fibroadenomas, probably because of their rapid growth. There are no good clinical criteria by which to distinguish a phyllodes tumor from a fibroadenoma. Whereas observation of a fibroadenoma is acceptable, excision of a phyllodes tumor is necessary for local control and for determination of benign or malignant features. To avoid unnecessary excision of benign fibroadenomas that are indistinguishable from phyllodes tumors on clinical examination, imaging criteria were sought to aid in identifying patients who require EB for complete histopathologic evaluation and local control. Mammography may show a halo around a phyllodes tumor mass but cannot reliably distinguish a fibroadenoma from a phyllodes tumor (165–167). Ultrasonography evaluation has limitations even when color and pulse Doppler ultrasonography are used in conjunction with it (163).

Microscopic evaluation of a lesion is important to determine the diagnosis. The histologic distinction between fibroadenoma, benign, borderline, and malignant phyllodes tumor can be very difficult on minimal tissue sampling with FNAC or CNB (168,169). It may be easier to distinguish benign phyllodes from malignant phyllodes tumors than benign phyllodes tumors from fibroadenomas (170). Histologic features that stratify lesions include number of mitoses per high power field, stromal cellularity, pushing or infiltrating tumor margin, cellular atypia, tumor necrosis, and stromal overgrowth (171).

If a lesion cannot be clearly characterized as a fibroadenoma, excision may be necessary. Factors that are considered in recommending excision include older age, new mass in a well-screened individual, rapid growth, size greater than 2.5 to 3 cm, suspicious FNAC or CB, and mammographic or ultrasonographic features that demonstrate lobulation and intramural cysts. If observation is elected, repeat clinical examination and imaging in a short interval is essential to evaluate change in size.

Treatment of biopsy-proven phyllodes tumor is wide local excision, attempting to obtain a 1- to 2-cm margin (156–161). Massive tumors, or large tumors in relatively small breasts, may require mastectomy; otherwise, mastectomy should be avoided, and axillary lymph node dissection is not indicated. Often, however, a patient will undergo excisional biopsy of a mass believed to be fibroadenoma, and final histologic examination reveals a phyllodes tumor. Reexcision with normal breast margins is recommended for borderline and malignant phyllodes tumors (159). An expectant approach is an option for unanticipated diagnosis of benign phyllodes tumors (157).

The prognosis of benign and malignant phyllodes tumors is variable (154,155,157,162,172). **Tumors judged to be benign phyllodes tumors can recur locally in up to 10% of patients** (159–161). Recurrence is associated with margin involvement, whereas mortality correlates with size and grade (173). In a series reviewing only high-grade malignant phyllodes tumors, size and excision margins were associated with local recurrence and metastatic spread, and mastectomy may be required to achieve complete surgical excision (174). **Malignant phyllodes tumors tend to recur locally and occasionally may metastasize to the lung, although brain, pelvic, and bone metastases also may occur** (160–162). The stromal component of the tumor is malignant and metastasizes, behaving like a sarcoma. Axillary involvement is extremely unusual. Often, the appearance of metastasis is the first sign that a phyllodes tumor is malignant.

Chemotherapy for metastatic phyllodes tumors should be based on regimens for sarcoma, not adenocarcinoma (159). Radiation therapy generally is not used in the treatment of phyllodes tumors. In the presence of a bulky tumor, positive margins, recurrence, or malignant histology, radiation therapy may be of some benefit (175).

Breast Conditions Requiring Evaluation

Nipple Discharge

Nipple discharge is a presenting breast symptom in 4.5% of patients seeking evaluation of a breast symptom, with 48% spontaneous and 52% provoked (176). Nipple discharge that does not occur spontaneously has no pathologic significance. Provoked or self-induced nipple discharge should be managed by reassurance and instruction to discontinue manipulation. Spontaneous nipple discharge is more likely to be associated with an underlying pathologic problem than provoked discharge. **Although it is a distressing finding, spontaneous nipple discharge is infrequently found to be associated with carcinoma, ranging from 4% to 10%** (176–178). Nipple discharge can be caused by neoplastic or nonneoplastic processes (179). Nonneoplastic processes include galactorrhea, physiologic changes resulting from mechanical manipulation, parous condition, periductal mastitis, subareolar abscess, fibrocystic change, and mammary duct ectasia. Neoplastic causes of nipple discharge in nonlactating women are solitary intraductal papilloma, carcinoma, papillomatosis, squamous metaplasia, and adenosis (176,179,180). Extramammary causes are related to hormones and drugs (179). **Following are the important characteristics of the discharge and other factors to be evaluated by history and physical examination** (180):

1. **Nature of discharge (serous, bloody, or milky)**
2. **Association with a mass**
3. **Unilateral or bilateral**
4. **Single or multiple ducts**
5. **Discharge that is spontaneous (persistent or intermittent) or expressed by pressure at a single site or on entire breast**
6. **Relation to menses**
7. **Premenopausal or postmenopausal**
8. **Hormonal medication (contraceptive pills or estrogen)**

Unilateral, spontaneous, bloody, or serosanguinous discharge from a single duct is usually caused by an intraductal papilloma or, rarely, by an intraductal cancer. In either case, a mass may not be palpable. The involved duct may be identified by pressure at different sites around the nipple and at the margin of the areola. Bloody discharge is more suggestive of cancer but usually is caused by a benign papilloma in the duct. In premenopausal women, spontaneous multiple-duct discharge, unilateral or bilateral, is most marked just before menstruation. It often is caused by fibrocystic change. Discharge may be green or brownish. Papillomatosis and ductal ectasia are usually seen on biopsy. If a mass is present, it should be removed. Milky discharge from multiple ducts in nonlactating women presumably reflects increased secretion of pituitary prolactin; serum prolactin and thyroid-stimulating hormone levels should be evaluated to detect a pituitary tumor or hypothyroidism. Hypothyroidism may cause galactorrhea. Alternatively, *phenothiazines* may cause milky discharge that disappears when the medication is discontinued. Oral contraceptive agents may cause clear, serous, or milky discharge from multiple ducts or, less often, from a single duct. The discharge is more evident just before menstruation and disappears when the medication is stopped.

Chronic unilateral nipple discharge, especially if it is bloody, is an indication for resection of the involved ducts. Mammography and ultrasonography are performed to rule out an associated mass. On occasion, ductography may be performed to identify a filling defect before excision of the duct system, but usually this technique is of little value (178). Ductography is not a substitute for excision because it misses multiple lesions and cannot visualize the periphery (181).

Fiberoptic ductoscopy is a technology used to evaluate patients with nipple discharge (182). In 259 patients with nipple discharge, fiberoptic ductoscopy successfully detected intraductal papillary lesions in 92 patients (36%). Office-based, minimally invasive breast ductoscopy with intraductal biopsy is available in some centers (183,184). It was performed for diagnosis in 83 patients with nipple discharge (183). A diagnosis of severe or malignant atypia was established in 21% of patients.

Cytologic examination of nipple discharge or cyst fluid rarely is performed. **Cytologic examination usually is of no value but may identify malignant cells** (178). Negative findings do not rule out cancer, which is more likely in women older than 50 years of age. In any case, the involved duct—and a mass, if present—should be excised (177,178,180,185). Complete histopathologic evaluation of the involved ductal system is the preferred method of diagnosis, and cytologic assessment should not be relied on for diagnosis.

The usual approach for nipple discharge is surgical excision through a periareolar incision adjacent to the trigger point, the pressure point that elicits nipple discharge (179). A microdochetomy of a single duct or a central duct excision of the major subareolar ducts can be performed under local or general anesthesia. The putative duct can be cannulated, methylene blue can be injected, or a lacrimal probe can be inserted into the duct for localization. A resection of breast tissue for 3 to 5 cm, or until no bloody fluid can be identified in the ductal system, is performed. The patient must be warned of possible skin and nipple loss as a result of compromised vascularity, change in nipple sensation, deformity, inability to breastfeed, and recurrence if only a single duct if removed.

When there is a history of unilateral nipple discharge, localization is not possible, and no mass is palpable, the patient should be reexamined every week for 1 month. When unilateral discharge persists, even without definite localization or tumor, surgical exploration should be considered. The alternative is careful follow-up at intervals of 1 to 3 months. Mammography should be performed. Purulent discharge may originate in a subareolar abscess and requires excision of the related lactiferous sinus (186).

Erosive Adenomatosis of the Nipple

Erosive adenomatosis is a rare benign condition of the nipple that mimics Paget's disease (187). Patients seek treatment for pruritus, burning, and pain. On clinical examination, the nipple can appear ulcerated, crusting, scaling, indurated, and erythematous. The nipple can be enlarged and more prominent during menstrual cycles (188). The differential diagnosis includes squamous cell carcinoma, psoriasis, contact dermatitis, seborrheic keratosis, adenocarcinoma metastatic to the skin, and unusual primary tumors of the nipple (187). Biopsy should be performed to diagnose the lesion. Local excision is curative (187).

Fat Necrosis

Fat necrosis of the breast is rare but clinically important because it produces a mass, often accompanied by skin or nipple retraction, which is indistinguishable from carcinoma. Fat necrosis often presents as a confusing clinical finding. Trauma is presumed to be the cause, although only about one-half of patients have a history of injury to the breast. Ecchymosis is occasionally seen near the tumor. Tenderness may or may not be present. If untreated, the mass associated with fat necrosis gradually disappears. Diagnostic imaging studies are usually insufficient (189). As a rule, the safest course is needle-core or excisional biopsy of the entire mass to rule out carcinoma (189). Fat necrosis is common after segmental resection and radiation therapy or transverse rectus abdominis musculocutaneous (TRAM) flap (190).

Breast Abscess

Lactational Abscesses

Infection in the breast is rare unless the patient is lactating. Lactational mastitis must be distinguished from lactational abscess (191). During lactation, an area of redness, tenderness, and induration frequently develops in the breast. **Lactational mastitis is caused by transmission of bacteria during nursing and poor hygiene. The organism most commonly found in lactational mastitis and abscesses is *Staphylococcus aureus*** (192). If mastitis is diagnosed, manual pressure, antibiotics, and continued breastfeeding are recommended. In its early stages, the infection often can be treated while breastfeeding is continued by administering an antibiotic such as *dicloxacillin* 250 mg four times daily, or *oxacillin* 500 mg four times daily, for 7 to

10 days. **If the lesion progresses to a localized mass with local and systemic signs of infection, an abscess is present. It should be drained, and breastfeeding should be discontinued.**

Nonlactational Abscess

Rarely, infections or abscesses may develop in young or middle-aged women who are not lactating (193). The approach to nonlactational abscess is conservative (194,195). A suspected abscess should be evaluated with preliminary ultrasonography to detect the presence of an inflammatory mass, frank pus, solitary cavity, or a multiloculated abscess (196). Aspiration of pus, if present, and antibiotic therapy is instituted with reaspiration, if necessary (196). When the fluid collection is greater than 3 mL, percutaneous drain placement is an option (194). A single aspiration is sufficient in about one-half of patients (194). Recurrent abscess formation is low (10%) (194). Bacteriologic analysis of 190 abscesses in nonlactating and lactating women showed a preponderance of gram-positive cocci. *S. aureus* was the most common organism isolated (51.3%). Of these, 8.6% were methicillin-resistant *S. aureus*. Other common organisms included mixed anaerobes (13.7%) and anaerobic cocci (6.3%) (196). **If these infections recur after multiple aspirations, incision and drainage followed by excision of the involved lactiferous duct or ducts at the base of the nipple may be necessary during a quiescent interval.** In virtually all cases, mammillary sinus (lactiferous duct fistula) can be confirmed as the cause of reinfection or persistent infection (197). Inflammatory carcinoma is a consideration when erythema of the breast is present. Patients should not undergo prolonged treatment for an apparent infection unless biopsy eliminated the possibility of inflammatory carcinoma.

Subareolar Abscess and Lactiferous Duct Fistula

Subareolar abscess and fistula of the lactiferous ducts secondary to squamous metaplasia can occur (198). The distal duct can be occluded with inspissated debris. Two large reviews report a high association of lactiferous duct fistulae in women who smoke (199,200). The definitive treatment for lactiferous duct sinus is excision of the lactiferous duct and drainage of the abscess cavity. In both studies, **the recurrence rate was greater when only incision and drainage were performed.** The most common organism occurring in primary subareolar abscess was *S. aureus,* but anaerobic organisms occurred more frequently in chronic recurring abscesses (200).

Disorders of Breast Augmentation

Estimates indicate that nearly 4 million women in the United States have undergone augmentation mammoplasty. Breast implants are usually placed under the pectoralis muscle or, less desirably, in the subcutaneous tissue of the breast. Most implants are made of an outer silicone shell filled with a silicone gel or saline.

The complications of breast implantation are significant. Rates of contracture vary in the literature from less than 10% to over 60%. Capsular contraction or scarring around the implant, leading to firmness and distortion of the breast, can be painful and sometimes requires removal of the implant and capsule. Implant rupture may occur in as many as 5% to 10% of women, and bleeding of gel through the capsule is even more common (201). In 2006, the U.S. Food and Drug Administration approved silicone gel filled implants for use in women 22 years or older for cosmetic purposes and for reconstruction after breast surgery or in women with traumatic or congenital breast defects (202). The agency recommends MRI scanning 3 years after the first implant surgery and then every 2 years for the detection of implant rupture.

The agency advised symptomatic women with ruptured implants to discuss the need for surgical removal with their physicians. When there is no evidence of associated symptoms or rupture, implant removal is generally not indicated because the risks of removal are probably greater than the risk of retention. If screening ultrasonography shows no rupture, the probability of rupture is 2.2% (203). If ultrasonography shows rupture, true rupture is present in 37.8%. In this setting, a large number of women would have normal implants removed. When MRI is used in addition to ultrasonography, the probability of rupture increases to 86%.

The suggested association between silicone gel and autoimmune disease is poorly documented (204,205). Among the multiple meta-analyses conducted thus far, none have identified a significant association between breast implants and connective-tissue disease (206). Subsequent studies demonstrated no clinical data proving an increased incidence of connective tissue disorders in patients with silicone gel breast implants (207–209). The data continue to reaffirm previous observations that there is no evidence of an association between breast implants and connective tissue diseases (210). In a study of Danish women undergoing reduction mammoplasty compared with silicone implant augmentation, there was no increased incidence of antinuclear antibodies or other autoantibodies between the groups (211). The augmentation group experienced capsular contraction and more pain than the group undergoing reduction mammoplasty. Any association between implants and an increased incidence of breast cancer is unlikely (212). Breast cancer may develop in any patient with a silicone gel prosthesis.

References

1. **Pearlman, MD, Giffin JL.** Benign breast disease. *Obstet Gynecol* 2010;116:747–747.
2. **Harris J, Morrow M, Lippman M, et al.** *Diseases of the breast.* Philadelphia: Lippincott Williams & Wilkins, 2009.
3. **Miltenburg DM, Speights VO Jr.** Benign breast disease. *Obstet Gynecol Clin North Am* 2008;35:285–300.
4. **Gail Risk Assessment.** Breast cancer risk assessment tool. Available online at: http://www.cancer.gov/bcrisktool
5. **O'Brien MM, Donaldson SS, Balise RR, et al.** Second malignant neoplasms in survivors pediatric Hodgkin's lymphoma treated with low-dose radiation and chemotherapy. *J Clin Oncol* 2010;28:1232–1239.
6. **Rodden AM.** Common breast concerns. *Prim Care* 2009;36:103–113.
7. **Smith RA, Cokkinides V, Brawley OW.** Cancer screening in the United States, 2008: a review of current American Cancer Society guidelines and cancer screening issues. *CA Cancer J Clin.* 2008;58:161–179.
8. **Kosters JP, Gotzsche PC.** Regular self-examination or clinical examination for early detection of breast cancer. *Cochrane Database Syst Rev* 2003;2:CD003373.
9. **Austoker J.** Breast self examination. *BMJ* 2003;326:1–2.
10. **Weiss NS.** Breast cancer mortality in relation to clinical breast examination and breast self-examination. *Breast J* 2003;9:86–89.
11. **Nelson HD, Tyne K, Naik A, et al.** Screening for breast cancer: systematic evidence review update for the US Preventative Services Task Force. *Rockville (MD) Agency Healthcare Res Qual (US);* 2009;10-05142-EF-1.
12. **Newcomer L, Newcomb P, Trentham-Dietz A, et al.** Detection method and breast carcinoma histology. *Cancer* 2002;95:470–477.
13. **van Dooren S, Rijnsburger AJ.** Psychological distress and breast self-examination frequency in women at increased risk for hereditary or familial breast cancer. *Community Genet* 2003;6:235–241.
14. **Breast self-examination tutorial.** Available online at: http://www.komen.org/bse http://ww5.komen.org/BreastCancer/BreastSelfAwareness.html?ecid=vanityurl:28
15. **Committee on Technologies for the Early Detection of Breast Cancer.** *Mammography and beyond: developing technologies for the early detection of breast cancer.* Washington, DC: National Academy Press, 2005.
16. **Lewin J, Hendrick RE, D'Orsi CJ, et al.** Comparison of full-field digital mammography with screen-film mammography for cancer detection: results of 4,945 paired examinations. *Radiology* 2001;218:873–880.
17. **Nees AV.** Digital mammography: are there advantages in screening for breast cancer? *Acad Radiol* 2008;15:401–407.
18. **Pisano E, Gatsonis C, Hendrick E, et al.** Diagnostic performance of digital versus film mammography for breast cancer screening. *N Engl J Med* 2005;353:1773–1783.
19. **Paquelet JR, Hendrick RE.** Lesion size inaccuracies in digital mammography. *AJR Am J Roentgenol* 2010;194:115–118.
20. **Buist DS, Porter PL, et al.** Factors contributing to mammography failure in women age 40–49 years. *J Natl Cancer Inst* 2004;96:1432–1440.
21. **Palka I, Kelemen G, Ormandi K, et al.** Tumor characteristics in screen-detected and symptomatic breast cancers. *Pathol Oncol Res* 2008;14:161–167.
22. **Hendrick RE, Pisano ED, Averbukh A, et al.** Comparison of acquisition parameters and breast dose in digital mammography and screen-film mammography in the American College of Radiology Imaging Network digital mammographic imaging screening trial. *AJR Am J Roentgenol* 2010;194:362–369.
23. **Bassett L, Liu TH, Giuliano AE, et al.** The prevalence of carcinoma in palpable vs. impalpable, mammographically detected lesions. *Am J Roentgenol* 1991;157:21–24.
24. **Tice JA, Kerlikowse K.** Screening and prevention of breast cancer in primary care. *Prim Care* 2009;36:533–558.
25. **Nystrom L, Anderson T, Bjurstam N, et al.** Long-term effects of mammography screening: updated overview of the Swedish randomised trials. *Lancet* 2002;359:909–919.
26. **Miller A, To T, Baines CJ, et al.** National breast screening study-1: breast cancer mortality after 11 to 16 years of follow-up: a randomized screening trial of mammography in women age 40–49 years. *Ann Intern Med* 2002;137:305–312.
27. **Miller A, To T, Baines CJ, et al.** Canadian national breast screening study-2: 13-year results of a randomized trial in women aged 50–59 years. *J Natl Cancer Inst* 2000;92:1490–1499.
28. **Duffy S, Tabar L, Smith R.** The mammographic screening trials: commentary on the recent work of Olsen Gotzsche. *CA Cancer J Clin* 2002;52:68–71.
29. **Alexander F, Anderson T, Brown HK, et al.** 14 years of follow-up from the Edinburgh randomised trial of breast-cancer screening. *Lancet* 1999;353:1903–1908.
30. **Kalager M, Zelen M, Langmark F, et al.** Effect of screening mammography on breast-cancer specific mortality in Norway. *N Engl J Med* 2010;363:1203–1210.
31. **Tabar L, Vitak B, Chen, HH, et al.** Two-county trial twenty years later: updated mortality results and new insights from long-term follow-up. *Radiol Clin North Am* 2000;38:625–651.
32. **UKDG, UK Trials of Early Detection of Breast Cancer Group.** 16-year mortality from breast cancer in the UK trial of early detection of breast cancer. *Lancet* 1999;353:1909–1914.
33. **Coburn NG, Chung MA, Fulton J, et al.** Decreased breast cancer tumor size, stage, and mortality in Rhode Island: an example of a well-screened population. *Cancer Control* 2004;11:222–230.
34. **Botteri E, Bagnardi V, Goldhirsch A, et al.** Axillary lymph nodes involvement in women with breast cancer: does it depend on age? *Clin Breast Cancer* 2010; 4:318–321.
35. **Smith R, Cokkinides V, Brawley OW.** Cancer screening in the United States, 2009: a review of current American Cancer Society guidelines and issues in cancer screening. *CA Cancer J Clin* 2009;59:27–41.
36. **American Geriatrics Society Clinical Practice Committee.** AGS position statement: breast cancer screening in older women. *J Am Geriatr Soc* 2000;48:842–844.
37. **Mandelblatt JS, Schechter CB, Yabroff KR, et al.** Toward optimal screening strategies for older women. Costs, benefits and harms of breast cancer screening by age, biology and health status. *J Gen Intern Med* 2005;20:487–496.
38. **Schonberg MA, Silliman RA, Marcantonio ER.** Weighing the benefits and burdens of mammography screening among women age 80 years or older. *J Clin Oncol* 2009;27:1774–1780.
39. **Badgwell BD, Giordano SH, Duan ZZ, et al.** Mammography before diagnosis among women age 80 years and older with breast cancer. *J Clin Oncol* 2008;26:2482–2488.
40. **U.S. Preventative Services Task Force.** Screening for breast cancer: U.S. Preventive Services Task Force recommendation statement. *Ann Intern Med* 2009;151:716–726.
41. **Smith RA, Cokkinides V, Brooks D, et al.** Cancer screening in the United States, 2010: a review of current American Cancer

Society guidelines and issues in cancer screening. *CA Cancer J Clin* 2010;60:99–119.

42. **Albert RH, Clark MM.** Cancer screening in the older patient. *Am Fam Phys* 2008;78:1369–1374.

43. **American College of Radiology.** *Breast imaging reporting and data system (BI-RADS).* 4th ed. Reston, VA: American College of Radiology, 2003.

44. **Elmore J, Armstrong K, Lehman C, et al.** Screening for breast cancer. *JAMA* 2005;293:1245–1256.

45. **Weigel S, Decker T, Korsching E, et al.** Calcifications in digital mammographic screening; improvement of early detection of invasive breast cancer? *Radiology* 2010;255:738–745.

46. **Lanzieri CF, Molter JP, Legan GJ.** University Hospitals of Cleveland. Available online at: uhrad.com//mamarc.htm

47. **Lazarus E, Mainiero MB, Schepps B, et al.** BI-RADS lexicon for UD and mammography interobserver variability and PPV. *Radiology* 2006;239:385–391.

48. **Parikh JR.** ACR appropriateness criteria on palpable breast masses. *J Am Coll Radiol* 2007;285–288.

49. **Carney P, Miglioretti D, Yankaskas BC, et al.** Individual and combined effects of age, breast density, and hormone replacement therapy use on the accuracy of screening mammography. *Ann Intern Med* 2003;138:168–175.

50. **Stone J, Warren RM, Pinney E, et al.** Determinants of percentage and area measures of mammographic density. *Am J Epidemiol* 2009;170:1571–1578.

51. **Madjar H.** Role of breast ultrasound for the detection and differentiation of breast lesions. *Breast Care* 2010;5:109–114.

52. **Dillion MF, Hill AD, Quinn CM, et al.** The accuracy of ultrasound, stereotactic and clinical core biopsies in the diagnosis of breast cancer with an analysis of false negative cases. *Ann Surg* 2005;242:701–707.

53. **Kelly KM, Dean J, Columada WS, et al.** Breast cancer detection using automated whole breast ultrasound and mammography in radiologically dense breasts. *Eur Radiol* 2010;20:734–742.

54. **Nothacker M, Duda V, Hahn M, et al.** Early detection of breast cancer: benefits and risk of supplemental breast ultrasound in asymptomatic women with mammographically dense breast tissue. A systematic review. *BMC Cancer* 2009;9:335–344.

55. **Irwig L, Houssami N, van Vliet C.** New technologies in screening for breast cancer: a systematic review of their accuracy. *Br J Cancer* 2004;90:2118–2122.

56. **Hong AS, Rosen E, Soo MS, et al.** BI-RADS for sonography: positive and negative predictive values of sonographic features. *AJR Am J Roentgenol* 2005;184:1260–1265.

57. **Chang YW, Kwon KH, Goo DE, et al.** Sonographic differentiation of benign and malignant cystic lesions of the breast. *J Ultrasound Med* 2007;26:47–53.

58. **Weinstein S, Rosen M.** Breast MR imaging: current indications and advanced imaging techniques. *Radiol Clin North Am* 2010;48:1013–1042.

59. **Veronesi U, De Cicco C, Galimberti VE, et al.** A comparative study on the value of FDG-PET and sentinel node biopsy to identify occult axillary metastases. *Ann Oncol* 2007;18:473–478.

60. **Buchanan Cl, Morris EA, Dorn PL, et al.** Utility of breast magnetic resonance imaging in patients with occult primary breast cancer. *Ann Surg Oncol* 2005;12:1045–1053.

61. **Saslow D, Boetes C, Burke W, et al.** American Cancer Society guidelines for breast screening and MRI as an adjunct to mammography. *CA Cancer J Clin* 2007;57:75–89.

62. **Kriege M, Brekelmans C, Coetes C, et al.** Efficacy of MRI and mammography for breast-cancer screening in women with a familial or genetic predisposition. *N Engl J Med* 2004;351:427–437.

63. **Tafra L.** Positron emission tomography (PET) and mammography (PEM) for breast cancer: importance to surgeons. *Ann Surg Oncol* 2007;14:3–13.

64. **Berner A, Davidson B, Sigstad E, et al.** Fine-needle aspiration cytology vs. core biopsy in the diagnosis of breast lesions. *Diagn Cytopathol* 2003;29:344–348.

65. **Bruening W, Schoelles K, Treadwell J, et al.** Comparative effectiveness of core-needle and open surgical biopsy for the diagnosis of breast lesions. Agency for Healthcare Research and Quality. Dec. 2009. Report NO. 10-EHC007-EF.

66. **Ough M, Velasco J, Hieken T.** A comparative analysis of core needle biopsy and final excision for breast cancer: histology and marker expression. *Am J Surg* 2010;201:685–687.

67. **Usami S, Moriya T.** Pathological aspects of core needle biopsy for non-palpable breast lesions. *Breast Cancer* 2005;12:272–278.

68. **Fajardo LL, Pisano ED.** Radiologist investigators of the radiologic diagnostic oncology group V: stereotactic and sonographic large-core biopsy of nonpalpable breast lesions. *Acad Radiol* 2004;11:293–308.

69. **Bevers T, Anderson B, Borgen P, et al.** Breast cancer screening and diagnosis. *NCCN Practice Guidelines in Oncology* 2004;1:1–74.

70. **Kerlikowske K, Smith-Bindman, Ljung BM, et al.** Evaluation of abnormal mammography results and palpable breast abnormalities. *Ann Intern Med* 2003;139:274–284.

71. **Brazda A, Estroff J.** Delays in time to treatment and survival impact in breast cancer. *Ann Surg Oncol* 2010;17:291–296.

72. **Abati A, Simsir A.** Breast fine needle aspiration biopsy: prevailing recommendations and **contemporary practices**. *Clin Lab Med* 2005;25:631–654.

73. **Morris AM, Flowers CR.** Comparing the cost effectiveness of the triple test score to traditional methods for evaluating palpable breast masses. *Med Care* 2003;41:962–971.

74. **Ahmed I, Nazir R, Chaudhary MY, et al.** Triple assessment of breast lump. *J Coll Physician Surg* 2007;17:535–538.

75. **Ciatto S, Houssami N.** Breast imaging and needle biopsy in women with clinically evident breast cancer: does combined imaging change overall diagnostic sensitivity? *Breast* 2007;16:382–386.

76. **Vimpeli SM, Saarenmaa I, Huhtula H, et al.** Large-core needle biopsy versus fine needle aspiration biopsy in solid breast lesions: comparison of cost and diagnostic value. *Acta Radiol* 2008;49:863–869.

77. **Kuo YL, Chang TW.** Can concurrent core biopsy and fine needle aspiration biopsy improve the false negative rate of sonographically detectable breast lesions? *BMC Cancer* 2010;10:371–377.

78. **Ellis I, Humphreys M, Michell M, et al.** Best Practice No. 179: guidelines for breast needle core biopsy handling and reporting in breast screening assessment. *J Clin Pathol* 2005;57:897–902.

79. **Blaylock RC, Byrne JLB, Clayton F, et al.** The Internet pathology laboratory for medical education. Available online at: http://202.193.198.50/glblnet/severbj1/bl/WEBPATH.HTM

80. **Ciampa A, Xu B, Bayiee D, et al.** HER-2 status in breast cancer; correlation of gene amplification by FISH with immunohistochemistry expression using advanced cellular imaging system. *Appl Immunohistochem Mol Morphol* 2006;14:132–137.

81. **Vaugh A, Crowe JP.** Mammary ductoscopy and ductal washings for the evaluation of patients with pathologic nipple discharge. *Breast* 2009;15:254–260.

82. **Courtillot C, Plu-Bureau, Binart N, et al.** Benign breast diseases. *J Mammary Gland Bio Neoplasia* 2005;10:325–335.

83. **Santen RJ, Mansel R.** Benign breast disorder. *N Engl J Med* 2005;353:275–285.

84. **Berg Wa, Sechin AG, Marques H, et al.** Cystic breast masses and the ACRIN 6666 experience. *Radiol Clin North Am* 2010;48:931–987.

85. **Schindler AE.** Non-contraceptive benefits of hormonal contraceptives. *Minerva Ginecol* 2010;62:319–329.

86. **Iwanitsu Y, Shimoda K, Abe H, et al.** Anxiety, emotional suppression, and psychological distress before and after breast cancer diagnosis. *Psychosomatics* 2005;46:19–24.

87. **Mannello F, Tonti GA, Papa S.** Human gross cyst breast disease and cystic fluid: bio-molecular, morphological and clinical studies. *Breast Cancer Res Treat* 2006;97:115–129.

88. **Radowicki S, Kunicki M, Bandurska-Stankiewicz E.** Prostate-specific antigen in the serum of women with benign breast disease. *Eur J Obstet Gynecol Reprod Bio* 2008;138:212–216.

89. **Katz VL, Lentz G, Lobo RA, et al.** *Comprehensive gynecology: fibrocystic changes.* Philadelphia, PA: Mosby, 2007.

90. **Daly CP, Bailey JE, Klein KA, et al.** Complicated breast cyst on sonography: is aspiration necessary to exclude malignancy? *Acad Radiol* 2008;15:610–617.

91. **Vargas H, Vargas M, Gonzalez KD, et al.** Outcomes of sonography-based management of breast cysts. *Am J Surg* 2004;188:443–447.

92. **Kabat GC, Jones JG, Olson N, et al.** A multi-center prospective cohort study of benign breast and risk of subsequent breast cancer. *Cancer Causes Control* 2010;26:82–826.

93. **Fitzgibbons P, Henson DE, Hutter RV, et al.** Benign breast changes and the risk of subsequent breast cancer: an update of the 1985 consensus statement. *Arch Pathol Lab Med* 1998;122:1053–1055.

94. **Chun J, El-Tamer M, Joseph KA, et al.** Predictors of breast cancer development in a high-risk population. *Am J Surg* 2006;192:474–477.

95. **Page D, Dupont WD.** Anatomic markers of human premalignancy and risk of breast cancer. *Cancer* 1990;66:1326–1335.

96. **Hartmann LC, Sellers TA, Frost MN, et al.** Benign breast disease and the risk of breast cancer. *N Engl J Med* 2005;352:229–237.

97. **Worsham MJ, Raju U, Lu M, et al.** Risk factors for breast cancer from benign breast diseases in a diverse population. *Breast Cancer Res Treat* 2009;118:1–7.

98. **Webb Pm, Bryne C, Schnitt SJ, et al.** A prospective study of diet and benign breast disease. *Cancer Epidemiol Biomarkers Prev* 2004;13:1106–1113.

99. **Ishitani K, Lin T, Manson JE, et al.** Caffeine consumption and risk of breast cancer in a large cohort of women. *Arch Intern Med* 2008;168:2022–2031.

100. **Ganmaa D, Willett W, Fiskanich D, et al.** Coffee, tea, caffeine and risk breast cancer: a 22-year follow-up. *Int J Cancer* 2008;122:2071–2076.

101. **Holmes MD, Willett WC.** Does diet affect breast cancer risk? *Breast Cancer Res* 2004;6:170–178.

102. **Parsay S, Olfati F, Nahidi S, et al.** Therapeutic effects of vitamin E on cyclic mastalgia. *Breast J* 2009;15:510–514.

103. **Kashanian M, Manzinami R, Jalalmanesh S.** Pyridoxine (vitamin B$_6$) therapy for premenstrual syndrome. *Int J Gynaecol Obstet* 2007;96:43–44.

104. **Pruthis S, Wahner-Roedler DL, Torkelson CJ, et al.** Vitamin E and evening primrose oil for management of cyclical mastalgia: a randomized pilot study. *Altern Med Rev* 2010;15:59–67.

105. **Smallwood J, A-Kye D, Taylor I.** Vitamin B6 in the treatment of premenstrual mastalgia. *Br J Clin Pract* 1986;40:532–533.

106. **Ernster V, Goodson W 3rd, Hunt T, et al.** Vitamin E and benign breast "disease": a double-blind, randomized clinical trial. *Surgery* 1985;97:490–494.

107. **Horner N, Lampe J.** Potential mechanisms of diet therapy for fibrocystic breast conditions show inadequate evidence of effectiveness. *J Am Diet Assoc* 2000;100:1368–1380.

108. **Kaviani A, Mehrdad N, Najafi M, et al.** Comparison of naproxen with placebo for the management of noncyclical breast pain: a randomized, double blind, controlled trial. *World J Surg* 2008;32:2464–2470.

109. **Bundred NJ.** Breast pain. *Clin Evid (Online)*. 2007;2007:pii0812.

110. **Ramakrishnan R, Werbeck J, Khurana K, et al.** Expression of interleukin-6, and tumor necrosis factor a and histopathologic findings in painful and nonpainful breast tissue. *Breast J* 2003;9:91–97.

111. **Ford O, Lethaby A, Roberts H, et al.** Progesterone for premenstrual syndrome. *Cochrane Database Syst Rev* 2009;2:CD003415.

112. **Olawaiye A, Witham-Leitch M, Danakas G, et al.** Mastalgia: a review of management. *Reprod Med* 2005;50:933–939.

113. **Hadi M.** Sports brassiere: is it a solution for mastalgia? *Breast J* 2000;6:407–409.

114. **Eberl MM, Phillips RL Jr, Lamberts H, et al.** Characterizing breast symptoms in family practice. *Ann Fam Med* 2008;6:528–533.

115. **Browne M.** Prevalence and impact of cyclic mastalgia in a United Stated clinic-based sample. *Am J Obstet Gynecol* 1997;177:126–132.

116. **Smith R, Pruthi S, Fitzpatrick L.** Evaluation and management of breast pain. *Mayo Clin Proc* 2004;79:353–372.

117. **Rosolowich V, Saettler E, Szuck B, et al.** Mastalgia. Society of Obstetricians and Gynecologists of Canada (SOGC). *J Obstet Gynaecol Can* 2006;28:49–71.

118. **Dennerstein L, Lehert P, Bäckström TC, Heinemann K.** Premenstrual symptoms—severity, duration and typology: an international cross-sectional study. *Menopause Int* 2009;15:120–126.

119. **Davies E, Gateley C, Miers M, et al.** The long-term course of mastalgia. *J R Soc Med* 1998;91:462–464.

120. **Gumm R, Cunnick GH, Mokbel K.** Evidence for the management of mastalgia [review]. *Curr Med Res Opin* 2004;20:681–684.

121. **Ortíz-Mendoza CM, Lucas Flores MA, et al.** Mastalgia treatment with *tamoxifen*. *Ginecol Obstet Mex* 2003;71:502–507.

122. **Ortiz-Mendoza CM, Olvera-Mancilla M.** Danazol effectivity in control of moderate to severe mastalgia. *Cir Cir* 2004;72:479–482.

123. **Srivastava A, Mansel RE, Arvind N, et al.** Evidence-based management of mastalgia: a meta-analysis of randomised trials. *Breast* 2007;16:503–512.

124. **Oksa S, Luukkaala T, Mäenpää J.** *Toremifene* for premenstrual mastalgia: a randomised, placebo-controlled crossover study. *BJOG* 2006;113:713–718.

125. **Ortiz-Mendoza CM, Olvera-Mancilla M.** *Danazol* effectivity in control of moderate to severe mastalgia. *Cir Cir* 2004;72:479–482.

126. **Kilbane M, Ajjan R, Weetman A, et al.** Tissue iodine content and serum-mediated 125I uptake-blocking activity in breast cancer. *J Clin Endocrinol Metab* 2000;85:1245–1250.

127. **Rillema J, Collins S, Williams C.** Prolactin stimulation of iodine uptake and incorporation into protein is polyamine-dependent in mouse mammary gland explants. *Proc Soc Exp Biol Med* 2000;224:41–44.

128. **Eskin B, Bartusda D, Dunn M, et al.** Mammary gland dysplasia in iodine deficiency. *JAMA* 1967;200:115–119.

129. **Patrick L.** Iodine: deficiency and therapeutic considerations. *Altern Med Rev* 2008;13:116–127.

130. **Kessler J.** The effect of supraphysiologic levels of iodine on patients with cyclic mastalgia. *Breast J* 2004;10:328–336.

131. **Mansel R, Goyal A, Preece P, et al.** European randomized, multicenter study of *goserelin* (*Zoladex*) in the management of mastalgia. *Am J Obstet Gynecol* 2004;191:1942–1949.

132. **Sandrucci S, Mussa A, Festa V.** Comparison of *tamoxifen* and *bromocriptine* in management of fibrocystic breast disease: a randomized blind study. *Ann N Y Acad Sci* 1990;586:626–628.

133. **GEMB.** *Tamoxifen* therapy for cyclical mastalgia: dose randomized trial. *Breast* 1997;11:212–213.

134. **Olawaiye A, Witham-Leiteh M, Danaka S, et al.** Mastalgia: a review of management. *J Reprod Med* 2005;50:933–939.

135. **Colak T, Ipek T, Kanik A, et al.** Efficacy of topical nonsteroidal antiinflammatory drugs in mastalgia treatment. *J Am Coll Surg* 2003;196:525–530.

136. **Boyd N, McGuire V, Shannon P, et al.** Effect of a low-fat high-carbohydrate diet on symptoms of cyclical mastopathy. *Lancet* 1988;2:128–132.

137. **Stonemetz D.** A review of the clinical efficacy of evening primrose. *Holist Nurs Pract* 2008;22:171–174.

138. **Gateley C, Maddox P, Pritchard G, et al.** Plasma fatty acid profiles in benign breast disorders. *Br J Surg* 1992;79:407–409.

139. **Blommers J, Lange-de Klerk E, Kuik D, et al.** Evening primrose oil and fish oil for severe chronic mastalgia: a randomized, double-blind, controlled trial. *Am J Obstet Gynecol* 2002;187:1389–1394.

140. **Goyal A, Mansel R, Group ES.** A randomized multicenter study of *gamolenic acid* (*Efamast*) with and without antioxidant vitamins and minerals in the management of mastalgia. *Breast J* 2005;11:41–47.

141. **Smith GE, Burrows P.** Ultrasound diagnosis of fibroadenoma—is biopsy always necessary? *Clin Radiol* 2008;63:511–515.

142. **Jayasinghe Y, Simmons PS.** Fibroadenomas in adolescence [review]. *Curr Opin Obstet Gynecol* 2009;21:402–406.

143. **Foxcroft L, Evans E, Hirst C.** Newly arising fibroadenomas in women aged 35 and over. *Aust N Z J Surg* 1998;68:419–422.

144. **Manfrin E, Mariotto R, Remo A, et al.** Benign breast lesions at risk of developing cancer—a challenging problem in breast cancer screening programs. *Cancer* 2009;115:499–507.

145. **Sperber F, Blank A, Metser U, et al.** Diagnosis and treatment of breast fibroadenoma by ultrasound-guided vacuum-assisted biopsy. *Arch Surg* 2003;138:796–800.

146. **Fine R, Whitworth P, Kim J, et al.** Low-risk palpable breast masses removed using a vacuum-assisted handheld device. *Am J Surg* 2003;186:362–367.

147. **Edwards M, Broadwater R, Tafra L, et al.** Progressive adoption of cryoablative therapy for breast fibroadenoma in community practice. *Am J Surg* 2004;188:221–224.

148. **Park Y-M, Kim E, Lee JH, et al.** Palpable breast masses with probably benign morphology at sonography: can biopsy be deferred? *Acta Radiol* 2008;48:1104–1111.

149. **Ranieri E, Ersilia S, Barberi G, et al.** Diagnosis and treatment of fibroadenoma of the breast: 20 years' experience. *Chir Ital* 2006;58:295–297.

150. **Alkhunaizi AM, Ismail A, Yousif BM.** Breast fibroadenomas in renal transplant recipients. *Transplant Proc* 2004;36:1839–1840.

151. **Seo YL, Choi CS, Yoon DY, et al.** Benign breast diseases associated with cyclosporine therapy in renal transplant recipients. *Transplant Proc* 2005;37:4315–4319.

152. **Darwish A, Nasr AO, El Hassan LA, et al.** Cyclosporine—a therapy-induced multiple bilateral breast and accessory axillary breast fibroadenomas: a case report. *J Med Case Rep* 2010;4:267.

153. **Jayasinghe Y, Simmons PS.** Fibroadenomas in adolescence. *Curr Opin Obstet Gynecol* 2009;21:402–406.

154. **Tse GM, Niu Y, Shi HJ.** Phyllodes tumor of the breast: an update. *Breast Cancer* 2010;17:29–34.

155. **Guerrero M, Ballard B, Grau A.** Malignant phyllodes tumor of the breast: review of the literature and case report of stromal overgrowth. *Surg Oncol* 2003;12:27–37.

156. **Chen WH, Cheng Sp, Tzen Cy, et al.** Surgical treatment of phyllodes tumors of the breast: retrospective review of 172 cases. *J Surg Oncol* 2005;91:185–194.

157. **Zurrida S, Bartoli C, Galimberti V, et al.** Which therapy for unexpected phyllode tumour of the breast? *Eur J Cancer* 1992;28:654–657.

158. **Karim RZ, Gerega SK, Ynag YH, et al.** Phyllodes tumor of the breast: a clinicopathological analysis of 65 cases from a single institution. *Breast* 2009;18:165–170.

159. **Grabowski J, Salztein SL, Sadler GR, et al.** Malignant phyllodes tumors: a review of 752 cases. *Am Surg* 2007;73:967–969.

160. **Ben Hassouna J, Damak T, Gamoudi A, et al.** Phyllodes tumors of the breast: a case series of 106 patients. *Am J Surg* 2006;192:141–147.

161. **Belkacemi Y, Bousquet G, Marsiglia H, et al.** Phyllodes tumor of the breast. *Int J Radiat Oncol Biol Phys* 2008;70:492–500.

162. **Barrio AV, Clark BD, Goldberg JI, et al.** Clinicopathologic features and long-term outcomes of 292 phyllodes tumors of the breast. *Ann Surg Oncol* 2007;14:2961–2970.

163. **Chao T-C, Lo Y-F, Chen M-F.** Phyllodes tumors of the breast. *Eur Radiol* 2003;13:88–93.

164. **Kurt A, Tatlidede S, Sade C, et al.** A giant cystosarcoma phyllodes. *Breast J* 2004;10:546–547.

165. **Foxcroft LM, Evans EB, Porter AJ.** Difficulties in the pre-operative diagnosis of phyllodes tumors of the breast: a study of 84 cases. *Breast* 2007;16:27–37.

166. **Franceschini G, Masetti R, Brescia A, et al.** Phyllodes tumor of the breast: magnetic resonance imaging findings and surgical treatment. *Breast J* 2005;11:44–45.

167. **Kraemer B, Hoffmann J, Roehm C, et al.** Cystosarcoma of the breast: a rare diagnosis: case studies and review of literature. *Arch Gynecol Obstet* 2007;276:649–653.

168. **Giri D.** Recurrent challenges in the evaluation of fibroepithelial lesions. *Arch Pathol Lab Med* 2009;133:713–721.

169. **Bode MK, Rissanen T, Apaja-Sarkkinen M.** Ultrasonography and core needle biopsy in the differential diagnosis of fibroadenoma and phyllodes tumor. *Acta Radiol* 2007;48:708–713.

170. **Tomimaru Y, Komoike Y, Egawa C, et al.** A case of phyllodes tumor of the breast with a lesion mimicking fibroadenoma. *Breast Cancer* 2005;12:322–326.

171. **Roa JC, Tapia O, Carrasco P, et al.** Prognostic factors of phyllodes tumor of the breast. *Pathol Int* 2006;56:309–314.

172. **Macdonald OK, Lee CM, Tward JD, et al.** Malignant phyllodes tumor of the female breast: association of primary therapy with cause-specific survival from the Surveillance, Epidemiology, and End Results (SEER) program. *Cancer* 2006;107:2127–2133.

173. **Cheng SP, Chang YC, Liu TP, et al.** Phyllodes tumor of the breast: the challenge persists. *World J Surg* 2006;30:1414–1421.

174. **Asoglu O, Ugurlu MM, Blanchard K, et al.** Risk factors for recurrence and death after primary surgical treatment of malignant phyllodes tumors. *Ann Surg Oncol* 2004;11:1011–1017.

175. **Barth RJ Jr, Wells WA, Mitchell SE, et al.** A prospective, multi-institutional study of adjuvant radiotherapy after resection of malignant phyllodes tumors. *Ann Surg Oncol* 2009;16:2288–2294.

176. **Goksel H, Yagmurdur M, Demirhan B, et al.** Management strategies for patients with nipple discharge. *Langenbecks Arch Surg* 2005;390:52–58.

177. **Montroni I, Santini D, Zucchini G, et al.** Nipple discharge: is its significance as a risk factor for breast cancer fully understood? Observational study including 915 consecutive patients who underwent selective duct excision. *Breast Cancer Res Treat* 2010;123:895–900.

178. **Lang JE, Kuerer HM.** Breast ductal secretions: clinical features, potential uses, and possible applications. *Cancer Control* 2007;14:350–359.

179. **Alcock C, Layer GT.** Predicting occult malignancy in nipple discharge. *ANZ J Surg* 2010;80:646–649.

180. **Hussain AN, Policarpio C, Vincent MT.** Evaluating nipple discharge. *Obstet Gynecol Surv* 2006;61:278–283.

181. **Morrogh M, Park A, Elkin EB, et al.** Lessons learned from 416 cases of nipple discharge of the breast. *Am J Surg.* 2010;200:73–80.

182. **Ling H, Liu GY, Lu JS, et al.** Fiberoptic ductoscopy-guided intraductal biopsy improve the diagnosis of nipple discharge. *Breast J* 2009;15:168–175.

183. **Dooley W, Francescatti D, Clark L, et al.** Office-based breast ductoscopy for diagnosis. *Am J Surg* 2004;188:415–418.

184. **Beechy-Newman N, Kulkarni D, Kothari A, et al.** Throwing light on nipple discharge. *Breast J* 2005;11:138–139.

185. **Wahner-Roedler D, Reynolds C, Morton M.** Spontaneous unilateral nipple discharge: when screening tests are negative—a case report and review of current diagnostic management of a pathologic nipple discharge. *Breast J* 2003;9:49–52.

186. **Mandal S, Jain S.** Purulent nipple discharge—a presenting manifestation in tuberculous mastitis. *Breast J* 2007;13:205.

187. **El Idrissi F, Fadii A.** Erosive adenomatosis of the nipple. *J Gynecol Obstet Biol Reprod* 2005;34:813–814.

188. **Ku BS, Kwon OE, Kim DC, et al.** A case of erosive adenomatosis of nipple treated with total excision using purse-string suture. *Dermatol Surg* 2006;32:1093–1096.

189. **Haj M, Loberant N, Salamon V, et al.** Membranous fat necrosis of the breast: diagnosis by minimally invasive technique. *Breast J* 2004;10:504–508.

190. **Tan PH, Lai LM, Carrington EV, et al.** Fat necrosis of the breast—a review. *Breast* 2006;15:313–318.

191. **Dener C, Inan A.** Breast abscesses in lactating women. *World J Surg* 2003;27:130–133.

192. **Moazzez A, Kelso RL, Towfigh S, et al.** Breast abscess bacteriologic features in the era of community-acquired methicillin-resistant *Staphylococcus aureus* epidemics. *Arch Surg* 2007;142:881–884.

193. **Rizzo M, Gabram S.** Management of breast abscesses in nonlactating women. *Am Surg* 2010;76:292–295.

194. **Berna-Serna J, Madrigal M, Berna-Serna J.** Percutaneous management of breast abscesses: an experience of 39 cases. *Ultrasound Med Biol* 2004;30:1–6.

195. **Christensen AF, Al-Suliman, Nielsen KR, et al.** Ultrasound-guided drainage of breast abscess: results in 151 patients. *Br J Radiol* 2005;78:186–188.

196. **Dabbas N, Chand M, Pallett A, et al.** Have the organisms that cause breast abscess changed with time? Implications for appropriate antibiotic usage in primary and secondary care. *Breast J* 2010;16:412–415.

197. **Bharat A, Gao F, Aft RL, et al.** Predictors of primary breast abscesses and recurrence. *World J Surg* 2009;33:2582–2586.

198. **Li S, Grant C, Degnim A, et al.** Surgical management of recurrent subareolar breast abscesses: Mayo clinical experience. *Am J Surg* 2006;192:528–529.

199. **Lannin D.** Twenty-two-year experience with recurring subareolar abscess and lactiferous duct fistula treated by a single breast surgeon. *Am J Surg* 2004;188:407–410.

200. **Versluijs-Ossewaarde F, Roumen R, Goris R.** Subareolar breast abscesses: characteristics and results of surgical treatment. *Breast J* 2005;11:179–182.

201. **Gorczyca DP, Gorczyca SM, Gorczyca KL.** The diagnosis of silicone breast implant rupture. *Plast Reconstr Surg* 2007;120:49–61.

202. **Tanne J.** FDA approves silicone implants 14 years after their withdrawal. *BMJ* 2006;333:1139.

203. **Chung K, Greenfield ML, Walters M.** Decision-analysis methodology in the work-up of women with suspected silicone breast implant rupture. *Plast Reconstr Surg* 1998;102:689–695.

204. **Lipworth L, Tarone RE, McLaughlin JK.** Silicone breast implants and connective tissue disease: an updated review of the epidemiologic evidence. *Ann Plast Surg* 2004;52:598–601.

205. **Fryzek JP, Holmich L, McLaughlin JK, et al.** A nationwide study

of connective tissue disease and other rheumatic conditions among Danish women with long-term cosmetic breast implantation. *Ann Epidemiol* 2007;17:374–379.

206. **Janowsky E, Lawrence L, Hulka BS.** Meta-analyses of relationship between silicone breast implants and the risk of connective-tissue diseases. *N Engl J Med* 2000;342:781–790.

207. **Holmich LR, Lipworth L, McLaughlin JK, et al.** Breast implant rupture and connective tissue disease: a review of the literature. *Plast Reconstr Surg* 2007;120:62–69.

208. **Bar-Meir E, Eherenfeld M, Shoenfeld Y.** Silicone gel breast implants and connective tissue disease—a comprehensive review. *Autoimmunity* 2003;36:193–197.

209. **McLaughlin JK, Lipworth L, Murphy DK, et al.** The safety of silicone gel-filled breast implants: a review of the epidemiologic evidence. *Ann Plastic Surg* 2007;59:569–580.

210. **Lipworth L, Tarone R, McLaughlin J.** Silicone breast implants and connective tissue disease: an update review of the epidemiologic evidence. *Ann Plast Surg* 2004;52:598–601.

211. **Breiting V, Holmich L, Brandt B, et al.** Long-term health status of Danish women with silicone breast implants. *Plast Reconstr Surg* 2004;114:217–226.

212. **Friis S, Holmich LR, McLaughlin JK, et al.** Cancer risk among Danish women with cosmetic breast implants. *Int J Cancer* 2006;118:998–1003.

OPERATIVE GYNECOLOGY

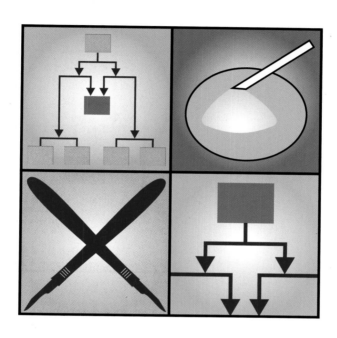

22 Preoperative Evaluation and Postoperative Management

Daniel L. Clarke-Pearson
Emily Ko
Lisa Abaid
Kevin Schuler

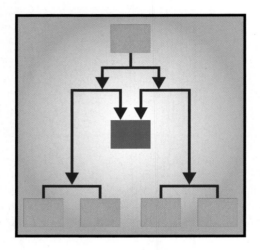

- The preoperative evaluation should be complete and thorough, taking into account the essential aspects of the patient's general medical condition and prior surgical history. The risks, benefits, and potential complications of the surgical procedure should be discussed with the patient, including the most frequent complications of the particular surgical procedure. Alternative management, if any, should be presented.

- A calculated body mass index (BMI) can be used as a surrogate marker for nutritional status.

- Careful and meticulous fluid and electrolyte management is essential for all patients undergoing major surgical procedures.

- Although satisfactory analgesia is easily achievable with available methods, patients continue to suffer unnecessarily from postoperative pain.

- Prophylactic antibiotics should be employed judiciously. Prompt identification of perioperative infections and their specific treatments are critical to minimize the impact of this common morbidity.

- Early in the clinical course, a postoperative small bowel obstruction may exhibit signs and symptoms identical to those of ileus. Initial conservative management as outlined for the treatment of ileus is appropriate.

- Because pulmonary embolism is the leading cause of death following gynecologic surgical procedures, the use of prophylactic venous thromboembolism regimens is an essential part of management. In patients at moderate risk, intermittent pneumatic compression (IPC) during and after gynecologic surgery reduces the incidence of deep venous thrombosis on a level similar to that of low-dose or low molecular weight *heparin*. A combination of mechanical (IPC) and pharmacologic prophylaxis is recommended for high-risk patients.

- **Patients who are predisposed to cardiovascular, respiratory, and endocrine illnesses must be thoroughly evaluated preoperatively. Coronary artery disease and chronic obstructive pulmonary disease (COPD) are major risk factors for patients undergoing abdominal surgery. Patients with hypertension should receive medication to control their blood pressure before surgery. Perioperative management of medical complications must be prompt and meticulous.**

The successful outcome of gynecologic surgery is based on thorough evaluation, careful preoperative preparation, and attentive postoperative care. This chapter discusses approaches to the general perioperative management of patients undergoing major gynecologic surgery with specific medical problems that could complicate the surgical outcome.

Medical History and Physical Examination

Gynecologic surgery should be undertaken only after gaining a thorough understanding of a patient's medical history and performing a complete physical examination.

1. **The medical history should include detailed questions to identify any medical illnesses that might be aggravated by surgery or anesthesia.** Coronary artery disease, pulmonary diseases, and obesity are the most common causes of postoperative complications.

2. **Medications currently being taken (including nonprescription drugs) and those discontinued within the month before surgery should be recorded.** Information about the use of "alternative therapies," herbs, and vitamins should be elicited (1,2). Specific instructions must be given to the patient regarding the need to discontinue any medications before surgery (e.g., *aspirin*, antiplatelet agents, diuretics, hormone replacement, or oral contraceptives), and those medications that should be continued (e.g., beta-blockers, α-2 agonists, statins, H_2 blockers, and proton pump inhibitors). Collaboration with the anesthesiologist in making decisions about continuing preoperative medications is essential. In the case of herbal medications, there is no evidence that herbal medications improve surgical outcomes and many may increase complications (Table 22.1). It is recommended that all herbal medications be discontinued at least a week before surgery.

3. **The patient should be questioned regarding known allergies to medications (e.g., sulfa and *penicillin*), foods, or environmental agents.** A history of sensitivity to shellfish may be the only clue of iodine sensitivity, which could be fatal if intravenous contrast is administered without corticosteroid preparation.

4. **Previous surgical procedures, and the patient's course following those surgical procedures, should be reviewed to identify and protect against potential complications.** The patient should be asked about specific complications, such as excessive bleeding, wound infection, venous thromboembolism, peritonitis, or bowel obstruction. Prior pelvic surgery should alert the gynecologist to the possibility of distorted surgical anatomy such as adhesions or ureteral stricture from previous periureteral scarring. In such cases, it may be prudent to identify any preexisting abnormality by performing computed tomography (CT) or other imaging. Many patients may not be entirely clear about the extent of the previous surgical procedure or the details of intraoperative findings. Therefore, operative notes from previous procedures should be obtained and reviewed.

5. **Family history may identify familial traits that might complicate planned surgery.** A family history of excessive intraoperative or postoperative bleeding, venous thromboembolism, malignant hyperthermia, and other potentially inherited conditions should be sought.

6. **The review of systems should be detailed to identify any coexisting medical or surgical conditions.** Inquiry about gastrointestinal and urologic function is particularly important before undertaking pelvic surgery because many gynecologic diseases involve adjacent nongynecologic viscera. The patient may have less serious symptoms, which could be corrected along with performing the primary surgery (e.g., stress urinary incontinence, fecal soiling, symptomatic cystocele).

Table 22.1 Potential Effects of Common Herbal and Dietary Supplements

Herb/Dietary Supplement	Potential Perioperative Effect
Aconite	Potential ventricular arrhythmias
Aloe	May potentiate thiazides
Black cohosh	May potentiate hypotensive effects
Danshen	May cause bleeding
Dong quai	May cause bleeding
Echinacea	Allergic reactions; decreased effectiveness of immunosuppressants
Ephedra/ma huang	Risk of myocardial ischemia and stroke from tachycardia and hypertension; ventricular arrhythmias with halothane; long-term use may cause intraoperative hemodynamic instability; life-threatening interaction with monoamine oxidase inhibitors, anesthesia, potential for withdrawal
Licorice	May cause hypertension and hypokalemia
Senna	May cause electrolyte imbalance
St. John's wort	Induction of cytochrome p450 enzyme; excessive sedation and delayed emergence from general anesthesia; potential serotonin syndrome if used in combination with other serotoneregic agents
Valerian	Excessive sedation and delayed emergence from general anesthesia; benzodiazepine-like acute withdrawal
Yerba mate	May cause hypertension or hypotension and excess sympathetic nervous system stimulation

7. **Although many women undergoing gynecologic surgical procedures are otherwise healthy, with pathology identified only on pelvic examination, other major organ systems should not be neglected in the physical examination.** Identification of abnormalities, such as a heart murmur, pulmonary compromise, hernia, or osteoarthritis of hips or knees should lead the surgeon to obtain additional testing and consultation to minimize intraoperative and postoperative complications.

Laboratory Evaluation

"Routine" preoperative laboratory testing of healthy women is to be discouraged as abnormal results are infrequent and are rarely of consequence in the surgical or anesthetic management of the patient (3). Despite well-established guidelines, approximately 90% of patients undergo unnecessary testing in a major university medical center (4). The selection of appropriate preoperative laboratory studies should depend on the type of the anticipated surgical procedure and the patient's medical status.

Chest x-ray:
Over age 60 years undergoing major surgery
American Society of Anesthesiologists (ASA) 3 or greater
Cardiovascular disease
Electrocardiogram (5):
Over age 60 years undergoing major surgery
Any cardiovascular disease or diabetes
Complete blood count:
Major surgery
ASA 3 or greater

Renal function:
   Recognized renal or cardiovascular disease
Coagulation studies (activated partial thromboplastin time [APTT], prothrombin time [PT], platelet count):
   Not recommended unless patient has history of bleeding or liver disease (6)
Urinalysis:
   Not recommended; may be considered given symptoms or history

Imaging of adjacent organ systems should be undertaken in individual cases as follows:

1. CT urography is helpful to delineate ureteral patency and course, especially in the presence of a pelvic mass, gynecologic cancer, or congenital müllerian anomaly. A CT urogram is not of value in the evaluation of most patients undergoing pelvic surgery (7).

2. Upper endoscopy, colonoscopy, barium enema, or upper gastrointestinal studies with small bowel assessment may be of value in evaluating some patients before undergoing pelvic surgery. Because of the proximity of the female genital tract to the lower gastrointestinal tract, the rectum and sigmoid colon may be involved with benign (endometriosis or pelvic inflammatory disease) or malignant gynecologic conditions. Conversely, a pelvic mass could have a gastrointestinal origin such as a diverticular abscess or a mass of inflamed small intestines (Crohn disease) or, rarely, a gastric or pancreatic carcinoma. Any patient with gastrointestinal symptoms should be further evaluated.

3. Other imaging studies, including ultrasonography, CT scanning, or magnetic resonance imaging (MRI), may be useful in selected patients such as in the evaluation of a pelvic mass.

Preoperative Discussion and Informed Consent

The preoperative discussion should include a description of the surgical procedure, its expected outcome and risks and is the basis for obtaining signed informed consent (8,9). Informed consent is an educational process for the patient and her family and fulfills the physician's need to convey information in understandable terms. The items listed in Table 22.2 should be discussed, and, after each item, the patient and family should be invited to ask questions. Documentation of the discussion is an important component of the patient's record that the physician should always include with the preprinted consent form.

Following are components of the informed consent process:

1. **A discussion of the nature and the extent of the disease process should include an explanation in lay terms of the significance of the disease or condition.** Printed materials, computer-based learning programs, and videotapes may assist in this process. The patient's competency to understand the discussion and written consent should be assessed. If the patient speaks a different language, a qualified interpreter should be present and the presence of the interpreter documented.

Table 22.2 Outline of Key Points of the Preoperative Informed Consent Discussion
1. The nature and extent of the disease process
2. The extent of the actual operation proposed and the potential modifications of the operation, depending on intraoperative findings
3. The anticipated benefits of the operation, with a conservative estimate of successful outcome
4. The risks and potential complications of the surgery
5. Alternative methods of therapy and the risks and results of those alternative methods of therapy
6. The results likely if the patient is not treated

2. **The goals of surgery should be discussed in detail.** Some gynecologic surgical procedures are performed purely for diagnostic purposes (e.g., dilation and curettage, cold knife conization, diagnostic laparoscopy), whereas most are aimed at correcting a specific problem. The extent of the surgery should be outlined, including which organs will be removed. Most patients like to be informed regarding the type of surgical incision and the estimated duration of anesthesia.

3. **The expected outcome of the surgical procedure should be explained.** If the procedure is being performed for diagnostic purposes, the outcome will depend on surgical or pathologic findings that are not known before surgery. When treating an anatomic deformity or disease, the expected success of the operation should be discussed, and the potential for failure of the operation (e.g., failure of tubal sterilization or the possibility that stress urinary incontinence may not be alleviated). When treating cancer, the possibility of finding more advanced disease and the potential need for adjunctive therapy (e.g., postoperative radiation therapy or chemotherapy) should be mentioned. Other issues of importance to the patient include discussion of loss of fertility or loss of ovarian function. These issues should be raised by the physician to ensure that the patient adequately understands the pathophysiology that may result from the surgery and to allow her to express her feelings regarding these emotionally charged issues. Unanticipated findings at the time of surgery should be mentioned. For example, if the ovaries are unexpectedly found to be diseased, the best surgical judgment may be that they should be removed.

4. **The risks and potential complications of the surgical procedure should be discussed, including the most frequent complications of the particular surgical procedure.** For most major gynecologic surgery, the risks include intraoperative and postoperative hemorrhage, postoperative infection, venous thromboembolism, injury to adjacent viscera, and wound complications. The patient should understand that minimally invasive surgery may have many of the same risks of injury or complications as does "open" surgery. Given the potential for transfusion of blood products, it should be clarified whether the patient would object to receiving a transfusion. Preexisting medical problems (e.g., diabetes, obesity, chronic obstructive pulmonary disease [COPD], coronary artery disease) result in additional risks and should be reviewed with the patient. Measures that will be taken to reduce the risk of complications should be described (e.g., prophylactic antibiotics, bowel preparation, venous thromboembolism prophylaxis).

5. **The usual postoperative course should be discussed in enough detail to allow the patient to understand what to expect in the days following surgery.** Information regarding the need for a suprapubic catheter, prolonged central venous monitoring, or an intensive care stay helps the patient accept her postoperative course and avoids surprises to the patient and her family that may be disconcerting. The expected duration of the recovery period, both in and out of the hospital, should be outlined.

6. **Alternative methods of therapy should be discussed, including medical management or other surgical approaches.** The patient should have an understanding of the outcome of the disease if nothing is done.

General Considerations

Nutrition

Young patients undergoing elective gynecologic surgery have adequate nutritional stores and, for the most part, do not require nutritional support. **All patients should have a nutritional assessment, especially elderly patients and those undergoing gynecologic cancer surgery or other major gynecologic procedures in which a prolonged postoperative recovery is expected.** Nutritional status should be reassessed at regular intervals postoperatively until the patient successfully returns to a regular diet.

A nutritional assessment includes a careful history and physical examination, which are the most useful, reliable, and cost-effective methods of determining a patient's nutritional status. In particular, information about recent weight loss, dietary history, fad diets, extreme exercise, or anorexia or bulimia should be elucidated. Physical evidence of malnutrition includes temporal wasting, muscle wasting, ascites, and edema. Accurate height and weight measurements should be obtained and an ideal body weight, percentage ideal body weight, and percentage usual body weight may be calculated. Many Internet-based body weight calculators are available. A variety of techniques were developed to determine a patient's nutritional state; however, many methods lack clinical utility outside of a research setting. Anthropometric measurements of skin-fold thickness and arm-muscle circumference provide an estimate of total body fat and lean muscle mass.

The calculated body mass index (BMI) can be used as a surrogate marker for nutritional status. **The BMI is calculated as body weight in kilograms divided by the height in square centimeters. A BMI less than 22 increases the risk of malnutrition, and a BMI less than 19 gives clear evidence of malnutrition** (10).

Patients who have lost less than 6% of their ideal body weight do not need preoperative nutritional intervention. However, **patients who have lost more than 10% of their ideal body weight in 6 months meet the definition of severely malnourished and should be considered for preoperative intervention** (11). Patients who have lost between 6% and 10% should undergo further studies to determine if preoperative intervention is needed. Laboratory assessments of albumin, transferrin, and prealbumin may be obtained in addition to the routine preoperative tests. The degree of malnutrition can in part be determined by serum concentrations of albumin, transferrin, and prealbumin. The levels of these serum proteins are greatly influenced by the patient's level of hydration. Prealbumin has the shortest half-life, at 2 to 3 days, and levels of this protein are depressed very early in comparison with serum transferrin and albumin, which have half-lives of 8 and 20 days, respectively (12). Serum albumin is a substitute for the Prognostic Nutritional Index, which is a time-consuming calculation, in assessing malnutrition in women with gynecologic malignancies (13). **A serum albumin level of 3.5 to 5.0 is in the normal range, 2.8 to 3.4 is considered to indicate mild malnutrition, 2.1 to 2.7 moderate malnutrition, and less than 2.1 severe malnutrition** (14). **Hypoalbuminemia is correlated with morbidity, mortality, and increased postoperative complication rates in data from the National Surgical Quality Improvement Program** (15). Decisions regarding the need for nutritional support should be based on several individualized factors. These factors include the patient's prior nutritional state, the anticipated length of time in which the patient will not be able to eat, the severity of surgery, and the likelihood of complications. The nutritional assessment should determine whether the cause of the malnutrition is increased enteral loss (malabsorption, intestinal fistula), decreased oral intake, increased nutritional requirements as a result of hypermetabolism (sepsis, malignancy), or a combination of these factors. Severe malnutrition, if not corrected, can further complicate the postoperative problem by causing altered immune function, chronic anemia, impaired wound healing, and eventually multiple organ system failure and death.

The patient's nutritional requirements are increased by surgery for several reasons. First, there is a period following surgery during which oral intake is not allowed or is very limited. In addition, the operation itself causes increased protein catabolism, increased energy requirements, and a negative nitrogen balance. If the surgery is uncomplicated and the patient is without food for less than 7 days, this response is limited and patients usually recover without the need for nutritional support. An adequate diet is defined as providing 75% of estimated caloric and protein needs. Therefore, **if an adequate oral diet is not expected for 7 to 10 days, perioperative nutritional support may be required to avoid progressive malnutrition and associated complications** (14). Perioperative nutritional support reduces operative morbidity and decreases the length of hospitalization when commenced early in the postoperative course. Patients with either normal nutritional indices or mild or moderate malnutrition, who will be undergoing surgical procedures likely to require a prolonged catabolic period of more than 7 to 10 days, should have enteral or parenteral nutrition instituted in the early postoperative period as soon as the patient is hemodynamically stable. This type of management should be strongly considered in patients undergoing pelvic exenterations, urinary diversions, or multiple enterectomies (16). Preoperative nutritional support is indicated for patients who have significant preexisting malnutrition or require major elective surgery. **According to the American Society for Parenteral and Enteral Nutrition (ASPEN) guidelines, evidence-based medicine supports the use of preoperative nutritional support for 7 to 14 days in moderately to severely malnourished patients undergoing major nonemergent gastrointestinal surgery** (12). A Veterans Affairs Total Parenteral Nutrition Cooperative Study found that severely malnourished patients preconditioned with total parenteral nutrition (TPN) had fewer complications than did control patients, excluding infectious complications (17). In a meta-analysis review of 22 studies of preoperative TPN use, a 10% decrease in postoperative complications occurred in TPN-supported patients (18). In a prospective trial including 108 women with ovarian cancer who underwent surgical cytoreduction, 88 patients had prealbumin levels less than 18 mg/dL and 24 had prealbumin levels less than 10 mg/dL (19). All postoperative mortality (23%) and 61.5% of all complications occurred in women with prealbumin less than 10 mg/dL. Women who received preoperative TPN and had prealbumin levels that increased to greater than 10 mg/dL did not have significantly increased complications. These findings lend support to consideration of preoperative TPN or neoadjuvant chemotherapy with interval cytoreduction when the nutritional status improves. These findings are encouraging but not supported by all studies or meta-analyses (20). If preoperative TPN is prescribed, it should be tapered and stopped at midnight before surgery, restarted 24 to 72 hours after the procedure, and continued until the patient is able to meet nutritional requirements.

ASPEN guidelines do not support the routine use of nutritional support in the immediate postoperative period for patients undergoing major gastrointestinal surgery; however, the guidelines do indicate a role for nutritional support postoperatively in patients in whom oral intake will be inadequate for 7 to 10 days (12). Clinical trials demonstrate that TPN can improve nutritional status as measured by biochemical assays, immune function, and nitrogen balance. The effect of TPN on clinical outcome is less well established. **Despite what seems reasonable, based on common sense and preoperative nutritional parameters, the data do not support TPN for mild to moderately malnourished patients. With severe malnutrition, preoperative TPN seems to be beneficial and should be instituted.**

Route of Administration

After the decision is made that nutritional support is required, the appropriate route of administration must be determined. ***Enteral nutrition* should be considered primarily because it is easy to deliver, associated with the fewest complications, linked to enhanced wound healing, and relatively inexpensive** (21). Contraindications to this route of delivery include intestinal obstruction, gastrointestinal bleeding, and diarrhea. Many types of preparations are commercially available and can be chosen based on their caloric content, fat content, protein content, osmolality, viscosity, and price. Depending on the patient's problem, the route of delivery may be through a Dobhoff feeding tube, a gastrostomy tube, or a feeding jejunostomy tube (22). If the gastrointestinal tract is unusable for more than 7 days postoperatively, TPN should be implemented.

Total parenteral nutrition must be delivered through a central vein and has wide acceptance as a means of providing nutritional support for surgically ill patients. It must be delivered through a subclavian or internal jugular vein, and the catheter must be placed using meticulous sterile surgical technique. Only intravenous access lines in the right atrium, superior vena cava, or inferior vena cava can be truly deemed central lines (23). Proper daily care is required to avoid infectious complications. When managed by an experienced team, the most frequent complication, infection, can be minimized (24).

Composition of Total Parenteral Nutrition Solutions

1. **Calories. The daily caloric requirements can be met by providing 1,000 calories more than the patient's basal energy expenditure.** Caloric requirements can be calculated based on **Long's modification of the Harrison-Benedict formula** for actual energy expenditure (AEE) (25). This is the most accurate available method to calculate an individual's AEE:

$$\textbf{AEE (women)} = [\textbf{655.10} + \textbf{9.56 Weight (kg)} + \textbf{1.85 Height (cm)} - \textbf{4.68 Age (yrs)}]$$
$$\times \textbf{(activity factor)} \times \textbf{(injury factor)}$$

   Activity factor: confined to bed (1.2), out of bed (1.3).
   Injury factor: minor surgery (1.2), skeletal trauma (1.3), major sepsis (1.6), severe burn (2.1).
   Alternatively, daily caloric requirements can be met by giving the patient 35 kcal/kg/day for maintenance and 45 kcal/kg/day for anabolic states.

2. **Protein. Daily nitrogen requirements may be met by providing 1 g of nitrogen (6.25 g of protein) for every 130 to 150 calories.** Protein is provided by synthetic amino acids. **The amino acids provide 15% to 20% of total calories** (24).

3. **Carbohydrates.** The carbohydrate base of TPN is dextrose (glucose) in approximately 25% solution. Adults need approximately 100 g of dextrose per day at baseline. The

maximal rate of glucose oxygenation in adults is approximately 7 g/kg/day, and glucose administration in excess of the caloric requirements can lead to fatty infiltration of the liver and other metabolic complications. When given by TPN infusion, the dextrose tolerance in critically ill patients is 5 mg/kg/min (24). Insulin should be used to maintain serum glucose concentration between 150 and 250 mg/dL, and it may be added directly to the TPN solution.

4. **Fats.** Lipids in a 10% to 20% emulsion can be given as further caloric supplement and supply the essential fatty acids, linoleic acid, and α-linoleic acids. More calories can be given in the form of free fatty acids, which are the major source of energy for most peripheral tissues. When lipids are used as a major source of calories, a minimum of 50 to 150 g per day of glucose should also be given to provide a substrate for the central nervous system. Most patients can tolerate up to 2 g of fat per kilogram of weight per day, and daily dosages should not exceed 4 g of fat per kilogram of weight per day. In critically ill patients, the lipid content should not exceed 1 g/kg/day. These lipid emulsions are isotonic and can be delivered simultaneously with the protein and carbohydrate mixture in a 3-L bag over a 24-hour infusion. **In general, 30% to 50% of nonprotein calories should be supplied in lipid form.** Serum triglyceride levels should be monitored to ensure that the patient can metabolize the fat.

5. **Electrolytes, vitamins, and minerals.** In addition to calories and protein, nutritional support should be maintained in terms of electrolytes, vitamins, and trace elements. Daily maintenance requirements for electrolytes are as follows: sodium, 40 to 50 mEq; potassium, 30 to 40 mEq; magnesium, 8 to 10 mEq; calcium, 2 to 5 mEq; and phosphate, 13 to 25 mmol (24). A number of vitamins and trace elements must also be supplied to ensure that the patient is eumetabolic.

Fluid and Electrolytes

Water constitutes approximately 50% to 55% of the body weight of the average woman. Two-thirds of this water is contained in the intracellular compartment. One-third is contained in the extracellular compartment, of which one-fourth is contained in plasma, and the remaining three-fourths is in the interstitium.

Osmolarity, or tonicity, is a property derived from the number of particles in a solution. Sodium and chloride are the primary electrolytes contributing to the osmolarity of the extracellular compartment. Potassium and, to a lesser extent, magnesium and phosphate are the major intracellular electrolytes. Water flows freely between the intracellular and the extracellular spaces to maintain osmotic neutrality throughout the body. Any shifts in osmolarity in any fluid spaces within the body are accompanied by corresponding shifts in free water from spaces of lower to higher osmolarity, thus maintaining equilibrium.

The average adult daily fluid maintenance requirement is approximately 30 mL/kg/day, or 2,000 to 3,000 mL per day (26). **This level is offset partially by insensible losses of 1,200 mL per day, which include losses from the lungs (600 mL), skin (400 mL), and gastrointestinal tract (200 mL).** Urinary output from the kidney accounts for the remainder of the fluid loss, and this output will vary depending on total body intake of water and sodium. Approximately 600 to 800 mOsm of solute are excreted by the kidneys daily. Healthy kidneys can concentrate urine up to approximately 1,200 mOsm and, therefore, the minimum output can range between 500 and 700 mL per day. The maximal urine output of the kidney can be as high as 20 L per day, as seen in patients with diabetes insipidus. In healthy individuals, the kidney adjusts output commensurate with daily fluid intake.

The major extracellular buffer used in the acid-base balance is the bicarbonate-carbonic acid system: $CO_2 + H_2O \leftrightarrow H_2CO_3 \leftrightarrow H^+ + HCO_3^+$ (27). Typically, the body will maintain a bicarbonate-to-carbonic acid ratio of 20:1 to maintain an extracellular pH of 7.4. Both the lung and the kidney play integral roles in the maintenance of normal extracellular pH via retention or excretion of carbon dioxide and bicarbonate. Under conditions of alkalosis, minute ventilation decreases and renal excretion of bicarbonate increases to restore the normal ratio of bicarbonate to carbonic acid; the opposite occurs with acidosis.

Ultimately, the kidney plays the most important role in fluid and electrolyte balance through excretion and retention of water and solute. Circulating antidiuretic hormone and aldosterone help modulate the process. Serum osmolarity affects hypothalamic release of antidiuretic hormone and aldosterone secretion in response to renal perfusion. Under states of dehydration or hypovolemia, serum antidiuretic hormone levels increase, leading to increased resorption of water in the distal tubule of the kidney. Increased aldosterone release promotes increased sodium and water retention. The opposite occurs in states of fluid excess. Individuals with normal renal function and circulating antidiuretic hormone and aldosterone levels maintain normal serum osmolarity and electrolyte composition, despite daily fluctuations of fluid and electrolyte intake.

Various disease states can alter the normal fluid and electrolyte homeostatic mechanisms, making perioperative fluid and electrolyte management more difficult. Patients with intrinsic renal disease are unable to excrete solute and to maintain acid-base balance. In patients undergoing the stress of chronic starvation or severe illness, there may be an inappropriately high level of circulating antidiuretic hormone and aldosterone, resulting in fluid and sodium retention. With severe cardiac disease, secondary renal hypoperfusion can lead to increased aldosterone synthesis and increased sodium and water retention by the kidney. Patients with severe diabetes can have significant osmotic diuresis as well as acid-base dysfunction secondary to circulating keto acids. Treatment of renal, cardiac, or endocrine disorders preoperatively is imperative and often will rectify fluid and electrolyte abnormalities.

Special attention is warranted in the elderly patient undergoing surgery. Normal physiological changes associated with aging can increase the likelihood of fluid and electrolyte disorders. These changes include decreased glomerular filtration rate, decreased urinary concentrating ability, and narrowed limits for excretion of water and electrolytes (28). Fluid and electrolyte management in the perioperative period requires knowledge of the daily fluid and electrolyte requirements for maintenance, replacement of ongoing fluid and electrolyte losses, as well as correction of any existing abnormalities.

Fluid and Electrolyte Maintenance Requirements

The body adjusts to higher and lower volumes of intake by changes in plasma tonicity. Alterations in plasma tonicity induce adjustments in circulating antidiuretic hormone levels, which ultimately regulate the amount of water retained in the distal tubule of the kidney. In the preoperative and the early postoperative periods, it is usually necessary to replace only sodium and potassium. Chloride is automatically replaced, concomitant with sodium and potassium, because chloride is the usual anion used to balance sodium and potassium in electrolyte solutions. There are various commercially available solutions containing 40 mmol of sodium chloride, with smaller amounts of potassium, calcium, and magnesium, designed to meet the requirements of a patient who is receiving 3 L of intravenous fluids per day. **The daily requirement can be met by any combination of intravenous fluids. For example, 2 L of D5 (5% dextrose)/0.45 normal saline (7 mEq sodium chloride each), supplemented with 20 mEq of potassium chloride, followed by 1 L of D5W (5% dextrose in water) with 20 mEq of potassium chloride, would suffice.**

Fluid and Electrolyte Replacement

Fluid and electrolyte losses beyond the daily average must be replaced by appropriate solutions. The choice of solutions for replacement depends on the composition of the fluids lost. Often, it is difficult to measure free water loss, particularly in patients who have high losses from the lungs, skin, or the gastrointestinal tract. Weighing these patients daily can be very useful. Up to 300 g of weight loss daily can be attributable to weight loss from catabolism of protein and fat in the patient who is taking nothing by mouth (26). Any loss beyond this level represents fluid loss, which should be replaced accordingly.

Patients with a high fever can have increased pulmonary and skin loss of free water, sometimes in excess of 2 to 3 L per day. These losses should be replaced with free water in the form of D5W. Perspiration typically has one-third the osmolarity of plasma and can be replaced with D5W or, if the loss is excessive, with D5/0.25 normal saline.

Patients with acute blood loss need replacement with appropriate isotonic fluid or blood or both. There is a wide range of plasma volume expanders, including albumin, dextran, and hetastarch solutions, that contain large molecular weight particles (<50 kDa molecular weight). These particles are slow to exit the intravascular space, and about one-half of the particles remain after 24 hours. Controversy exists over the ideal strategy for intravascular volume replacement (29). A systematic review of 25 randomized clinical trials demonstrated preserved renal function and reduced intestinal edema in surgical patients receiving hyperoncotic albumin solutions, as compared with control fluids (30). Meta-analyses on the use of human albumin and crystalloids versus colloids in fluid resuscitation did not show a benefit in mortality rates (31,32). Caution is required in interpreting results from these pooled controlled trials because mortality outcome was not the end point of most of the studies, and publication bias is a limitation. Possible side effects with synthetic colloid solutions include adverse affects on hemostasis, severe anaphylactic reactions, and impairment of renal function (29). These solutions are expensive and **for most cases, simple replacement with 0.9 normal saline or lactated Ringer's solution will suffice.** One-third of the volume of lactated Ringer's solution or normal saline typically will remain in the intravascular space and the remainder goes to the interstitium.

Appropriate replacement of gastrointestinal fluid loss depends on the source of fluid loss in the gastrointestinal tract. Gastrointestinal secretions beyond the stomach and up to the colon are typically isotonic with plasma, with similar amounts of sodium, slightly lower amounts of chloride, slightly alkaline pH, and more potassium (in the range of 10 to 20 mEq/L). Under normal conditions, stool is hypotonic. However, under conditions of increased flow (i.e., severe diarrhea), stool contents are isotonic with a composition similar to that of the small bowel contents. Gastric contents are typically hypotonic, with one-third the sodium of plasma, increased amounts of hydrogen ion, and low pH.

In patients who have gastric outlet obstruction, nausea, and vomiting, or who undergo nasogastric suction, appropriate replacement of gastric secretions can be provided with a solution such as D5/0.45 normal saline with 20 mEq/L of potassium. Potassium supplementation is particularly important to prevent hypokalemia in these patients, whose kidneys attempt to conserve hydrogen ions in the distal tubule of the kidney in exchange for potassium ions.

In patients with bowel obstruction, 1 to 3 L of fluid can be sequestered daily in the gastrointestinal tract. This fluid should be replaced with isotonic saline or lactated Ringer's solution. Similarly, patients with enterocutaneous fistulas or new ileostomies should receive replacement with isotonic fluids.

Correction of Existing Fluid and Electrolyte Abnormalities

Patients who have fluid or electrolyte abnormalities preoperatively can pose a diagnostic challenge. The correct diagnosis and therapy is contingent on a correct assessment of total body fluid and electrolyte status. The management of hyponatremia, for example, may be either fluid restriction or fluid replacement. The choice of treatment depends on whether there is overall extracellular fluid excess and normal body sodium stores or decreased overall total body sodium stores and extracellular fluid. A detailed history is necessary to disclose any underlying medical illness and to assess the amount and duration of any abnormal fluid losses or intake. Initial evaluation should include an assessment of hemodynamic, clinical, and urinary parameters to determine the overall level of hydration as well as the fluid status of the extracellular fluid compartment. The patient who has good skin turgor, moist mucosa, stable vital signs, and good urinary output is well hydrated. Nonpitting edema is indicative of extracellular fluid excess, whereas patients with orthostasis, sunken eyes, parched mouth, and decreased skin turgor have extracellular volume contraction. A patient's overall extracellular fluid status does not always reflect the hydration status of the intravascular compartment. A patient can have increased interstitial fluid and yet be intravascularly dry, requiring replacement with isotonic fluid.

The laboratory workup for patients who may have preexisting fluid problems should include assessment of blood hematocrit, serum chemistry, glucose, blood urea nitrogen (BUN) and creatinine, urine osmolarity, and urine electrolyte levels. Serum osmolarity is mainly a function of the concentration of sodium and is given by the following equation:

$$2[Na^+] + glucose\,(mg/dL)/18 + BUN\,(mg/dL)/2.8$$

Normal serum osmolarity is typically 290 to 300 mOsm. Blood hematocrit will rise or fall inversely at a rate of 1% per 500-mL alteration of extracellular fluid volume. The BUN:creatinine ratio is typically 10:1 but will rise to a ratio of greater than 20:1 under conditions of extracellular fluid contraction. Under conditions of extracellular fluid deficit, urine osmolarity will typically be high (>400 mOsm), whereas urine sodium concentration is low (<15 mEq/L), indicative of an attempt by the kidney to conserve sodium. Under conditions of extracellular fluid excess or in cases of renal disease in which the kidney has impaired ability to retain sodium and water, urine osmolarity will be low and urine sodium will be high (>30 mEq/L). Changes in sodium can give insight into the degree of extracellular fluid excess or deficit. In the average person, the serum sodium rises by 3 mmol/L for every liter of water deficit and falls by 3 mmol/L for each liter of water excess. One must be careful in making these estimates because patients with prolonged water and electrolyte loss can have low serum sodium levels and marked water deficits.

Specific Electrolyte Disorders

Hyponatremia

Because sodium is the major extracellular cation, shifts in serum sodium levels are usually inversely correlated with the hydration state of the extracellular fluid compartment. The pathophysiology of hyponatremia is usually expansion of body fluids leading to excess total body water (27,33). Symptomatic hyponatremia usually does not occur until the serum sodium is below 120 to 125 mEq/L. The severity of the symptoms (nausea, vomiting, lethargy, seizures) is related more to the rate of change of serum sodium than to the actual serum sodium level.

Hyponatremia in the form of extracellular fluid excess can be seen in patients with renal or cardiac failure and in conditions such as nephrotic syndrome, in which total body salt and water are increased, with a relatively greater increase in the latter. Administration of hypertonic saline to correct the hyponatremia would be inappropriate in this setting. The treatment should include, in addition to correcting the underlying disease process, water restriction with diuretic therapy. Inappropriate secretion of antidiuretic hormone (ADH) can occur with head trauma, pulmonary or cerebral tumors, and states of stress. The abnormally elevated ADH results in excess water retention. Treatment includes water restriction and, if possible, correction of the underlying cause. *Demeclocycline,* a *tetracycline* antibiotic, is effective in this disorder via its action in the kidney. The introduction of vasopressin receptor antagonists, such as *tolvaptan,* may replace *demeclocycline* as the drug of choice for the syndrome of inappropriate ADH secretion (34).

Inappropriate replacement of body salt losses with water alone will result in hyponatremia. This situation will typically occur in patients who lose large amounts of electrolytes secondary to vomiting, nasogastric suction, diarrhea, or gastrointestinal fistulas, and who received replacement with hypotonic solutions. Simple replacement with isotonic fluids and potassium will usually correct the abnormality. Rarely, rapid correction of the hyponatremia is necessary, in which case hypertonic saline (3%) can be administered. Hypertonic saline should be administered very cautiously to avoid a rapid shift in serum sodium, which will induce central nervous system dysfunction.

Hypernatremia

Hypernatremia is an uncommon condition that can be life-threatening if severe (serum sodium greater than 160 mEq/L). The pathophysiology is extracellular fluid deficit. The resultant hyperosmolar state leads to decreased water volume in cells in the central nervous system, which, if severe, can cause disorientation, seizures, intracranial bleeding, and death. The causes include excessive extrarenal water loss, which can occur in patients who have a high fever, have undergone tracheostomy in a dry environment, or have extensive thermal injuries; who have diabetes insipidus, either central or nephrogenic; and who have iatrogenic salt loading. The treatment involves correction of the underlying cause (correction of fever, humidification of the tracheostomy, administration of desmopressin for control of central diabetes insipidus) and replacement with free water either by the oral route or intravenously with D5W. As with severe hyponatremia, marked hypernatremia should be corrected slowly, no faster than 10 mEq per day, unless the patient is symptomatic from severe acute hypernatremia (35).

Hypokalemia

Hypokalemia may be encountered preoperatively in patients with significant gastrointestinal fluid loss (prolonged emesis, diarrhea, nasogastric suction, intestinal fistulas) and marked urinary potassium loss secondary to renal tubular disorders (renal tubular acidosis, acute tubular necrosis, hyperaldosteronism, prolonged diuretic use). It can arise from prolonged administration of potassium-free parenteral fluids in patients who are restricted from ingesting anything by mouth. The symptoms associated with hypokalemia include neuromuscular disturbances, ranging from muscle weakness to flaccid paralysis, and cardiovascular abnormalities, including hypotension, bradycardia, arrhythmias, and enhancement of digitalis toxicity. These symptoms rarely occur unless the serum potassium level is less than 3 mEq/L. The treatment is potassium replacement. Oral therapy is preferable in patients who are on an oral diet.

If necessary, potassium replacement can be given intravenously in doses that should not exceed 10 mEq per hour.

Hyperkalemia

Hyperkalemia is encountered infrequently in preoperative patients. It is usually associated with renal impairment but can be seen in patients who have adrenal insufficiency, are taking potassium-sparing diuretics, and have marked tissue breakdown such as that occurring with crush injuries, massive gastrointestinal bleeding, or hemolysis. The clinical manifestations are mainly cardiovascular. Marked hyperkalemia (potassium >7 mEq/L) can result in bradycardia, ventricular fibrillation, and cardiac arrest. The treatment chosen depends on the severity of the hyperkalemia and whether there are associated cardiac abnormalities detected with electrocardiography. *Calcium gluconate* (10 mL of a 10% solution), given intravenously, can offset the toxic effects of hyperkalemia on the heart. One ampule each of sodium bicarbonate and D5W, with or without insulin, will cause a rapid shift of potassium into cells. Over the longer term, cation exchange resins such as *sodium polystyrene sulfate* (*Kayexalate*), taken orally or by enema, will bind and decrease total body potassium. Hemodialysis is reserved for emergent conditions in which other measures are not sufficient or have failed (35).

Postoperative Fluid and Electrolyte Management

Several hormonal and physiologic alterations in the postoperative period may complicate fluid and electrolyte management. The stress of surgery induces an inappropriately high level of circulating ADH. Circulating aldosterone levels are increased, especially if sustained episodes of hypotension occurred either intraoperatively or postoperatively. The elevated levels of circulating ADH and aldosterone make postoperative patients prone to sodium and water retention.

Total body fluid postoperative volume may be altered significantly. First, 1 mL of free water is released for each gram of fat or tissue that is catabolized and, in the postoperative period, several hundred milliliters of free water are released daily from tissue breakdown, particularly in the patient who has undergone extensive intra-abdominal dissection and who is restricted from ingesting food and fluids by mouth. This free water is often retained in response to the altered levels of ADH and aldosterone. Second, fluid retention is further enhanced by third spacing, or sequestration of fluid in the surgical field. **The development of an ileus may result in an additional 1 to 3 L of fluid per day being sequestered in the bowel lumen, bowel wall, and peritoneal cavity.**

In contrast to renal sodium homeostasis, the kidney lacks the capacity for retention of potassium. **In the postoperative period, the kidneys continue to excrete a minimum of 30 to 60 mEq/L of potassium daily, irrespective of the serum potassium level and total body potassium stores** (27). If this potassium is not replaced, hypokalemia may develop. Tissue damage and catabolism during the first postoperative day usually result in the release of sufficient intracellular potassium to meet the daily requirements. Beyond the first postoperative day, potassium supplementation is necessary.

Correct maintenance of fluid and electrolyte balance in the postoperative period starts with the preoperative assessment, with emphasis on establishing normal fluid and electrolyte parameters before surgery. Postoperatively, close monitoring of daily weight, urine output, serum hematocrit, serum electrolytes, and hemodynamic parameters will yield the necessary information to make correct adjustments in crystalloid replacement. The normal daily fluid and electrolyte requirements must be met and any unusual fluid and electrolyte losses, including those from the gastrointestinal tract, lungs, or skin, must be compensated. After the first few postoperative days, third-space fluid begins to return to the intravascular space, and ADH and aldosterone levels revert to normal. The excess fluid retained perioperatively is mobilized and excreted through the kidneys, and exogenous fluid requirements decrease. Patients with inadequate cardiovascular or renal reserve are prone to fluid overload during this time of third-space reabsorption, especially if intravenous fluids are not appropriately reduced.

The most common fluid and electrolyte disorder in the postoperative period is fluid overload. Fluid excess can occur concomitantly with normal or decreased serum sodium. Large amounts of isotonic fluids are usually infused intraoperatively and postoperatively to maintain blood pressure and urine output. Because the infused fluid is often isotonic with plasma, it will remain in the extracellular space. Under such conditions, serum sodium will remain within normal levels. Fluid excess with hypotonicity (decreased serum sodium) can occur if large amounts of isotonic fluid losses (e.g., blood and gastrointestinal tract) are inappropriately replaced with hypotonic fluids. The predisposition toward retention of free water in the immediate postoperative period compounds the problem. An increase in body weight occurs concomitantly with the fluid expansion. In the patient who is not allowed anything by mouth, catabolism should induce a daily weight loss as great as 300 g per day. The patient who is gaining weight in excess of 150 g per day is in a state of fluid expansion. Simple fluid restriction will correct the abnormality. When necessary, diuretics can be used to increase urinary excretion.

States of fluid dehydration are uncommon but will occur in patients who have large daily losses of fluid that are not replaced. **Gastrointestinal losses should be replaced with the appropriate fluids. Patients with high fevers should be given appropriate free water replacement, because up to 2 L per day of free water can be lost through perspiration and hyperventilation.** Although these increased losses are difficult to monitor, a reliable estimate can be obtained by monitoring body weight.

Postoperative Acid-Base Disorders

A variety of metabolic, respiratory, and electrolyte abnormalities in the postoperative period can result in an imbalance in normal acid-base homeostasis, leading to alkalosis or acidosis. Changes in the respiratory rate directly affect the amount of carbon dioxide that is exhaled. ***Respiratory acidosis* will result from carbon dioxide retention in patients who have hypoventilation from central nervous system depression.** This condition can result from oversedation with narcotics, particularly in the presence of concurrent severe chronic obstructive pulmonary disease. ***Respiratory alkalosis* can result from hyperventilation caused by excitation of the central nervous system by drugs, pain, or excess ventilator support.** Numerous metabolic derangements can result in metabolic *alkalosis* or *acidosis*. Proper fluid and electrolyte replacement as well as maintenance of adequate tissue perfusion will help prevent most acid-base disorders that occur during the postoperative period.

Alkalosis

The most common acid-base disorder encountered in the postoperative period is alkalosis (27). Alkalosis is usually of no clinical significance and resolves spontaneously. Several etiologic factors may include hyperventilation associated with pain; posttraumatic transient hyperaldosteronism, which results in decreased renal bicarbonate excretion; nasogastric suction, which removes hydrogen ions; infusion of bicarbonate during blood transfusions in the form of citrate, which is converted to bicarbonates; administration of exogenous alkali; and use of diuretics. Alkalosis can be corrected with removal of the inciting cause and the correction of extracellular fluid and potassium deficits (Table 22.3). Full correction usually can be safely achieved over 1 to 2 days.

Marked alkalosis, with serum pH higher than 7.55, can result in serious cardiac arrhythmias or central nervous system seizures. Myocardial excitability is particularly pronounced with concurrent hypokalemia. Under such conditions, fluid and electrolyte replacement may not

Table 22.3 Causes of Metabolic Alkalosis		
Disorder	*Source of Alkali*	*Cause of Renal HCO Retention*
Gastric alkalosis		
Nasogastric suction	Gastric mucosa	$\downarrow\downarrow$ECF, $\downarrow$K
Vomiting		
Renal alkalosis		
Diuretics	Renal epithelium	$\downarrow$ECF, $\downarrow$K
Respiratory acidosis and diuretics		$\downarrow$ECF, $\downarrow$K, $\uparrow$PCO$_2$
Exogenous base	NaHCO$_3$, Na citrate, Na lactate	Coexisting disorder of ECF, K, PaCO$_2$

$\downarrow$ECF, extracellular fluid depletion; $\downarrow$K, potassium depletion; $\uparrow\uparrow$PCO$_2$, carbon dioxide retention; NaHCO$_3$, sodium bicarbonate; PaCO$_2$, partial pressure of carbon dioxide, arterial.

be sufficient to correct the alkalosis rapidly. *Acetazolamide* (250 to 500 mg) can be given orally or intravenously two to four times daily to induce renal bicarbonate diuresis. Treatment with an acidifying agent rarely is necessary and should be reserved for acutely symptomatic patients (i.e., those with cardiac or central nervous system dysfunction) or for patients with advanced renal disease. Under such conditions, *hydrogen chloride* (5 to 10 mEq per hour of a 100-mmol solution) can be given via a central intravenous line. *Ammonium chloride* can be given orally or intravenously but should not be given to patients with hepatic disease.

Acidosis

Metabolic acidosis **is less common than alkalosis during the postoperative period, but acidosis can be serious because of its effect on the cardiovascular system.** Under conditions of acidosis, there are decreased myocardial contractility, a propensity for vasodilation of the peripheral vasculature leading to hypotension, and refractoriness of the fibrillating heart to defibrillation (27). These effects promote decompensation of the cardiovascular system and can hinder attempts at resuscitation.

Metabolic acidosis results from a decrease in serum bicarbonate levels caused by the consumption and replacement of bicarbonate by circulating acids or the replacement by other anions such as chloride. The proper workup includes a measurement of the anion gap:

$$\text{Anion gap} = (Na^+ + K^+) - (Cl^- + HCO_3{}^-) = 10 \text{ to } 14 \text{ mEq/L (normal)}$$

The anion gap is composed of circulating protein, sulfate, phosphate, citrate, and lactate (36).

With metabolic acidosis, the anion gap can be increased or normal. An increase in circulating acids will consume and replace bicarbonate ion, increasing the anion gap. The causes include an increase in circulating lactic acid secondary to anaerobic glycolysis, such as that seen under conditions of poor tissue perfusion; increased ketoacids, as with cases of severe diabetes or starvation; exogenous toxins; and renal dysfunction, which leads to increased circulating sulfates and phosphates (37). The diagnosis can be established via a thorough history and measurement of serum lactate (normal <2 mmol/L), serum glucose, and renal function parameters. Metabolic acidosis in the face of a normal anion gap is usually the result of an imbalance of the ions chloride and bicarbonate, which occurs under conditions leading to excess chloride and decreased bicarbonate. Hyperchloremic acidosis can be seen in patients who underwent saline loading. Bicarbonate loss will be seen in patients with small bowel fistulas, new ileostomies, severe diarrhea, or renal tubular acidosis. In patients with marked extracellular volume expansion, which often occurs postoperatively, the relative decrease in serum sodium and bicarbonate will result in a mild acidosis. A summary of the various causes of metabolic acidosis is shown in Table 22.4.

The treatment of metabolic acidosis depends on the cause. In patients with lactic acidosis, restoration of tissue perfusion is imperative. This state can be accomplished through cardiovascular and pulmonary support as needed, oxygen therapy, and aggressive treatment of systemic

Table 22.4 Causes of Metabolic Acidosis

High Anion Gap	Normal Anion Gap	
	Hyperkalemic	*Hypokalemic*
Uremia	Hyporeninism	Diarrhea
Ketoacidosis	Primary adrenal failure	Renal tubular acidosis
Lactic acidosis	NH_2Cl	Ileal and sigmoid bladders
Aspirin	Sulfur poisoning	Hyperalimentation
Paraldehyde	Early chronic renal failure	
Methanol	Obstructive uropathy	
Ethylene glycol		
Methyl malonic aciduria		
NH_2Cl (chloramine)		

Adapted from **Narins RG, Lazarus MJ.** Renal system. In: **Vandam LD, ed.** *To make the patient ready for anesthesia: medical care of the surgical patient,* 2nd ed. Menlo Park, CA: Addison Wesley, 1984:67–114.

Table 22.5 Acid-Base Disorders and Their Treatment				
Primary Disorder	*Defect*	*Common Causes*	*Compensation*	*Treatment*
Respiratory acidosis	Carbon dioxide (hypoventilation)	Central nervous system depression Airway and lung impairment	Renal excretion of acid salts Bicarbonate retention Chloride shift into red blood cells	Restoration ventilation Control of excess dioxide production
Respiratory alkalosis	Hyperventilation	Central nervous excitation system Excess ventilator support	Renal excretion of sodium, potassium bicarbonate Absorption of hydrogen and chloride ions Lactate release from red blood cells	Correction hyperventilation
Metabolic acidosis	Excess loss of base Increased nonvolatile acids	Excess chloride versus sodium Increased bicarbonate loss Lactic, ketoacidosis Uremia Dilution acidosis	Respiratory alkalosis Renal excretion of hydrogen and chloride ions Resorption of potassium bicarbonate	Increase sodium load Give bicarbonate for pH <7.2 Restore buffers, protein, hemoglobin
Metabolic alkalosis	Excess loss of chloride and potassium Increased bicarbonate	Gastrointestinal losses of chloride Excess intake of bicarbonate Diuretics Hypokalemia Extracellular fluid volume contraction	Respiratory acidosis May be hypoxia Renal excretion of bicarbonate and potassium Absorption of hydrogen and chloride ions	Increased chloride content Potassium replacement *Acetazolamide* (*Diamox*) to waste bicarbonate Vigorous volume replacement Occasional 0.1 NaHCl as needed

NaHCl, sodium hydrochloride.

infection wherever appropriate. Ketosis from diabetes can be corrected gradually with *insulin* therapy. Ketosis resulting from chronic starvation or from lack of caloric support postoperatively can be corrected with nutrition. In patients with normal anion gap acidosis, bicarbonate lost from the gastrointestinal tract should be replaced, excess chloride administration can be curtailed, and, where necessary, a loop diuretic can be used to induce renal clearance of chloride. Dilutional acidosis can be corrected with mild fluid restriction.

Bicarbonates should not be given unless serum pH is lower than 7.2 or severe cardiac complications secondary to acidosis are present. Close monitoring of serum potassium levels is mandatory. Under states of acidosis, potassium will exit the cell and enter the circulation. The patient with a normal potassium concentration and metabolic acidosis is actually depleted of intracellular potassium. Treatment of the acidosis without potassium replacement will result in severe hypokalemia with its associated risks. A summary of the various acid-base abnormalities and associated therapies is shown in Table 22.5.

Perioperative Pain Management

Although satisfactory analgesia is easily achievable with available methods, patients continue to suffer unnecessarily from postoperative pain. Studies consistently show that 25% to 50% of patients suffer moderate to severe pain in the postoperative period (38,39). There are several reasons for the existing inadequacies in pain management. First, patient expectations of pain relief are low and they are not aware of the extent of analgesia that they should expect. In a study of the perception of pain relief after surgery, 86% of patients had moderate to severe pain after surgery, but 70% felt that the pain was as severe as they expected (40). Second, there is a lack of formal physician training in pain management. This lack is epitomized by the commonly written order prescribing a range of narcotic to be given intramuscularly every 3 to 4 hours as needed, leaving pain management decisions to the nursing staff, with no attempt made to titrate the dose of the prescribed narcotic commensurate with individual patient requirements. Third, attitudes continue to be influenced by the common misconception that the use of narcotics in the postoperative period results in opioid dependence. In one review, 20% of nurses responding to a staff questionnaire expressed concern that the use of opioid analgesics during the postoperative period could cause addiction (40). Studies confirm that nurses administer less than one-fourth of the total dose of narcotic that is prescribed on an as-needed basis. To facilitate acute pain management and reduce the number of adverse outcomes, the American Society of Anesthesiologists established practice guidelines for acute pain management in the perioperative setting (41).

The *minimal effective analgesic concentration* (MEAC) refers to the serum concentration of a drug below which very little analgesia is achieved. At the MEAC, receptor and plasma concentrations of a drug are in equilibrium. Steady-state drug concentrations above the MEAC are difficult to achieve with intramuscular depot injection (42). In one study, patients receiving intramuscular injections with *meperidine hydrochloride (Demerol)* every 4 hours experienced marked intrapatient and interpatient variations in narcotic drug peak concentrations and in the time required to reach these peaks. As a result, serum concentrations of drug were above the MEAC an average of only 35% of each 4-hour dosing interval (43). Variable pain control following intermittent intramuscular injections is the result of inadequate, highly variable, and unpredictable blood concentrations (44). Adequate analgesia can be achieved through intramuscular or subcutaneous modes of administration, but unpredictable absorption can make titration difficult. Small intravenous boluses can be more easily titrated but may be shorter acting, requiring more frequent injections and thus intensive nursing care, whereas larger intravenous boluses may be associated with a higher incidence of central nervous system and respiratory depression. **The *patient-controlled analgesia* (PCA) technique, which allows patients to self-administer small doses of narcotic on demand, allows titration of measured boluses of narcotic as needed to relieve pain. This technique can provide a more thorough analgesia with maintenance of steady-state drug concentrations above the MEAC.**

Irrespective of the route of administration, analgesics must be front loaded to provide prompt analgesia from the start. Without front loading, attainment of the MEAC will not occur for at least three elimination half-lives of the narcotic agent that is used. After front loading, additional small boluses of narcotic can be administered until analgesia is achieved. From the total dose of drug required to achieve analgesia, maintenance drug dosages can then be determined and administered either as a continuous infusion or on a scheduled basis, so that the dose of drug administered offsets the amount that is cleared. Thereafter, prescribed doses of narcotic can be adjusted as needed.

Patient-Controlled Analgesia

Devices for administering PCA are electronically controlled infusion pumps that deliver a preset dose of narcotic into a patient's indwelling intravenous catheter upon patient request. The devices all contain delay intervals or lockout times during which patient demands for more narcotic are not met. **These devices eliminate the delay between the onset of pain and the administration of analgesic agents, a common problem inherent with on-demand analgesic orders in busy hospital wards.** Patient-controlled analgesia has excellent patient acceptance. Compared with conventional intramuscular injections, serum narcotic levels have significantly lower variability in patients using PCA (42). Patients using PCA have improved analgesia, a lower incidence of postoperative pulmonary complications, and less confusion than those given intramuscular narcotics (45). The total dose of narcotic used is lower with PCA than with conventional intramuscular depot injection.

The use of PCA does not eliminate the adverse side effects of narcotics. Potentially life-threatening respiratory depression is seen in as many as 0.5% of patients using PCA. The use of a continuous narcotic infusion in addition to demand dosing is associated with a fourfold increase in respiratory depression. Elderly patients and those with preexisting respiratory compromise are at risk for respiratory depression (42).

Carefully supervised regimens using continuous infusions, on-demand intramuscular therapy, or fixed dosage schedules (every 4-hour dosing) with on-demand supplementation can have analgesic efficacy comparable with PCA. The type of close supervision required to achieve adequate on-demand analgesia without PCA is difficult to maintain. **Use of PCA shortens the time between the onset of pain and the administration of pain medication, provides more continuous access to analgesics, and allows for an overall steadier state of pain control.**

Epidural and Spinal Analgesia

Anesthetics and narcotics administered either in the epidural space or intrathecally are among the most potent analgesic agents available; the efficacy of these agents is greater than that provided by intravenous PCA techniques. These drugs can be administered in several ways, including a single-shot dose given by epidural or intrathecal injection, intermittent injection given either on schedule or on demand, and continuous infusion.

Because of the risk of central nervous system infections and headaches, intrathecal administration is usually limited to a single dose of narcotic, local anesthetic, or both. In comparison with epidural administration, duration of action for a single dose is increased via the intrathecal route as a result of the high concentrations of drug attained in the cerebrospinal fluid. The risk of central nervous system and respiratory depression, and systemic hypotension, is increased. The low doses of opioids required for intrathecal analgesia are sufficient to be associated with an increased risk of respiratory depression (46). Some investigators warn against the use of intrathecal spinal analgesia outside the intensive care setting.

Epidural administration is the preferred approach and provides extended (>24 hours) pain control during the postoperative period. Relative contraindications are the presence of coagulopathy, sepsis, and hypotension. Both anesthetic and narcotic agents are used with excellent efficacy. Among the anesthetic agents, *bupivacaine* is the most popular, providing excellent analgesia with minimal toxicity. Epidural analgesia is most suited for pain control in the lower abdomen and extremities. Potential adverse effects of epidural anesthetic agents include urinary retention, motor weakness, hypotension, and central nervous system and cardiac depression. In contrast to anesthetic agents, opioids offer excellent analgesia without accompanying sympathetic blockade. Epidural opioids tend to have a much longer duration of action, and hypotension is a rare complication. Compared with epidural anesthetics, there is a higher incidence of nausea and vomiting, respiratory depression, and pruritus (47).

Compared with analgesics administered intramuscularly or intravenously, epidural analgesia is associated with improved pulmonary function postoperatively, a lower incidence of pulmonary complications, a decrease in postoperative venous thromboembolic complications (most likely secondary to earlier ambulation), fewer gastrointestinal side effects, a lower incidence of central nervous system depression, and shorter convalescence (47). **A systematic review concluded that continuous epidural anesthesia is more effective than intravenous opioid PCA in reducing postoperative pain for up to 72 hours after abdominal surgery** (48). Severe respiratory depression, which occurs in less than 1% of patients, is the most serious potential complication. A lower incidence of respiratory depression occurs with the more lipophilic drugs such as *fentanyl,* which is quickly absorbed within the spinal cord and is less likely to diffuse to the central nervous system respiratory control centers. Pruritus, nausea, and urinary retention are common but can be managed easily and usually are of little clinical significance. Cost is perhaps the main and most limiting drawback of epidural analgesia.

Close monitoring by nursing staff is required for safe administration of epidural analgesia. An intensive care setting is not necessary. Epidural analgesics can be administered safely in a hospital ward setting under close nursing supervision, using respiratory monitoring with hourly ventilatory checks during the first 8 hours of epidural analgesia.

Nonsteroidal Anti-inflammatory Drugs

Current therapeutic strategies for perioperative pain control are largely dependent on multimodal therapy with opioid analgesics and nonsteroidal anti-inflammatory drugs (NSAIDs). The nonselective NSAID *ketorolac* is a potent drug that can be given orally or parenterally. **Ketorolac has a slightly slower onset of activity than *fentanyl* but has an analgesic potency comparable to *morphine*.** The theoretical advantages of NSAIDs over opioids include absence of respiratory depression, lack of abuse potential, decreased sedative effects, decreased nausea, early return of bowel function, and faster recovery. In clinical studies, *ketorolac* is found to have analgesic effects similar to those of morphine in postoperative orthopedic patients and, when used in conjunction with PCA, significantly reduced opioid requirements (49,50). Depending on the type of surgery, *ketorolac* has an opioid dose-sparing effect of a mean of 36% and improves analgesic control of moderate to severe pain 24 hours postoperatively (51). In the obstetric population, intravenous *ketorolac* is effective in reducing postoperative narcotic use after cesarean delivery (52). Although the U.S. Food and Drug Administration has not approved *ketorolac* for use during lactation, it was quantified in breast milk and has lower levels than *ibuprofen* (53).

Potential adverse effects associated with the use of NSAIDs include an increased risk of renal compromise (particularly in patients suffering from acute hypovolemia), gastrointestinal side effects, hypersensitivity reactions, and bleeding. The effects of *ketorolac* on bleeding are inconsistent. Studies of *ketorolac* on healthy volunteers showed transient increases in bleeding time and decreases in platelet aggregation, but these changes were not clinically significant (54). A retrospective cohort study showed increased risk of gastrointestinal and operative site bleeding in elderly patients receiving high doses of *ketorolac,* between 105 and 120 mg per day. Increased risk for all gastrointestinal bleeding was associated with use of *ketorolac* for more than 5 days (55). Controlled prospective studies did not show a significant increase in blood loss in patients who receive NSAIDs perioperatively. *Ketorolac* may be associated with elevated rates of acute renal failure when therapy exceeds 5 days (56). A meta-analyses of the use of postoperative NSAIDs in patients with normal preoperative renal function showed a clinically insignificant reduction in renal function (57). These agents should be used with extreme care, if at all, in patients with asthma, because 5% to 10% of adult patients with asthma are sensitive to *aspirin* and other NSAID preparations.

With the advantages of less gastrointestinal toxicity and a lack of antiplatelet effects, selective cyclooxygenase-2 (COX-2) inhibitors are a valuable option in perioperative pain management (58). Although evidence exists showing an increased risk of serious cardiovascular events associated with COX-2 inhibitors, short-term use of these agents in the perioperative setting can be considered in low-risk patients without existing cardiovascular disease (59–64).

In addition to NSAIDs, other adjuvant analgesics are being explored to minimize opioid use and the accompanying side effects, which can delay recovery. *Capsaicin* is a nonnarcotic that promotes release of substance P, a neurotransmitter for pain and heat, which initially results in a burning sensation, but eventually leads to substance P depletion and a reduction in pain. It is available in both topical and injectable preparations. *Ketamine* blocks centrally located *N*-methyl-D-aspartate pain receptors, and at low subanesthetic doses can reduce central sensitization caused by surgery and prevent opioid-induced hyperalgesia. At higher doses, *ketamine* is associated with hallucinations, dizziness, nausea, and vomiting. *Gabapentin* and *pregabalin* are nonnarcotics that prevent the release of excitatory neurotransmitters that relay pain signals. They reduce opioid requirements and are effective antihyperalgesic agents (64).

Antimicrobial Prophylaxis in Gynecologic Surgery

Gynecologic procedures often involve breaching the reproductive and gastrointestinal tracts, which harbor endogenous bacteria capable of causing polymicrobial infections in the postoperative period (Table 22.6). **Despite great advances in aseptic technique and drug development, bacterial contamination of the operative site and postoperative infections are an inevitable part of the practice of gynecologic surgery.** Prevention of these surgical complications includes

Table 22.6 Bacteria Indigenous to the Lower Genital Tract

Lactobacillus	*Enterobacter agglomerans*
Diphtheroids	*Klebsiella pneumoniae*
Staphylococcus aureus	*Proteus mirabilis*
Staphylococcus epidermidis	*Proteus vulgaris*
Streptococcus agalactiae	*Morganella morganii*
Streptococcus faecalis	*Citrobacter diversus*
α-Hemolytic streptococci	*Bacteroides* species
Group D streptococci	*B. disiens*
Peptostreptococci	*B. fragilis*
Peptococcus	*B. melaninogenicus*
Clostridium	
Gaffky anaerobia	
Escherichia coli	
Fusobacterium	
Enterobacter cloacae	

Table 22.7 Antibiotic Prophylaxis Regimens by Procedure		
Procedure	*Antibiotic*	*Dose*
Hysterectomy	*Cefazolin[a]*	1 g or 2 g IV[b]
Urogynecology	*Clindamycin[c]* plus	600 mg IV
procedures, including	gentamicin or	1.5 mg/kg IV
those involving mesh	quinolone[d] or	400 mg IV
	aztreonam	1 g IV
	Metronidazole[c] plus	500 mg IV
	gentamycin or	1.5 mg/kg IV
	quinolone[d]	400 mg IV
		1 g IV
Hysterosalpingogram or Chromotubation	*Doxycycline[e]*	100 mg orally, twice daily for 5 days
Induced abortion/dilation and evacuation	Doxycycline Metronidazole	100 mg orally 1 hour before procedure and 200 mg orally after procedure 500 mg orally twice daily for 5 days

[a]Alternatives include *cefotetan, cefoxitin, cefuroxime,* or *ampicillin-sulbactam.*
[b]A 2-g dose is recommended in women with a body mass index greater than 35 or weight greater than 100 kg or 220 lb.
[c]Antimicrobial agents of choice in women with a history of immediate hypersensitivity to *penicillin.*
[d]*Ciprofloxacin* or *levofloxacin* or *moxifloxacin.*
[e]If patient has a history of pelvic inflammatory disease or procedure demonstrates dilated fallopian tubes. No prophylaxis is indicated for a study without dilated tubes.
Adapted from Antibiotic prophylaxis for gynecologic procedures. *American College of Obstetricians and Gynecologists Practice Bulletin* No. 104, May 2009.

using proper aseptic technique, minimizing tissue trauma, minimizing the amount foreign material in the surgical site, controlling diabetes, avoiding immunologic suppression, maximizing tissue oxygenation, draining blood and serum from the surgical site, and using prophylactic antibiotics. Antibiotic prophylaxis is given with the belief that antibiotics enhance the immune mechanisms in host tissues that resist infections by killing the bacteria that inoculate the surgical site during surgery (65).

Infections in the skin or pelvis that result from gynecologic surgery (e.g., parametritis, cuff cellulitis, pelvic abscess) typically are polymicrobial in nature. These infections are complex and often involve gram-negative rods, gram-positive cocci, and anaerobes. Antibiotic prophylaxis should be sufficiently broad to cover these potential pathogens (66) (Table 22.7).

The timing of antimicrobial prophylaxis is important. There is a relatively narrow window of opportunity for affecting outcomes (67). In the United States, it is customary to give antimicrobial prophylaxis shortly before or during the induction of anesthesia. **Data revealed that a delay of 3 hours or more between the time of bacterial inoculation (i.e., skin incision) and administration of antibiotics may result in ineffective prophylaxis. Evidence indicates that for prophylaxis, one dose of antibiotic is appropriate. When the surgical procedure proceeds longer than 1 to 2 times the half-life of the drug or blood loss is greater than 1.5 L, additional intraoperative doses of antibiotics should be administered to maintain adequate levels of medication in serum and tissues** (68,69). There are no data to support the continuation of prophylactic antimicrobial agents into the postoperative period for routine gynecologic procedures. For cases involving colorectal resection, a reduction in surgical site infections (SSI) was seen when antibiotics were continued for up to 24 hours. Other measures to reduce SSI incidence were taken, including tight glycemic control, maintenance of intraoperative normothermia, and placement of subcutaneous drains in obese patients (70).

Cephalosporins emerged as the most important class of antimicrobial agents for prophylaxis. These drugs have a broad spectrum and relatively low incidence of adverse reactions. *Cefazolin* (1 g) appears to be widely used in the United States by gynecologic surgeons because of its relatively low cost and long half-life (1.8 hours). Other cephalosporins such as *cefoxitin, cefotaxime,* and *cefotetan* commonly are used for prophylaxis. These agents appear to have a broader spectrum of activity against anaerobic bacteria and are appropriate selections when colorectal resections are possible, such as during a debulking surgery for ovarian cancer. For the majority of gynecologic procedures, there is little evidence that a clinically relevant distinction exists between *cefazolin* and the other agents. Morbidly obese patients, defined as having a BMI greater than 35 or weight greater than 100kg, should receive 2 g of *cefazolin* to achieve appropriate blood and tissue antibiotic concentrations (71).

Antimicrobial prophylaxis, although usually beneficial, is not without risk. Anaphylaxis is the most life-threatening complication from antibiotic use. Anaphylactic reactions to penicillins are reported in 0.2% courses of treatment. The fatality rate is 0.0001%. Data indicate that it is safe to administer *cephalosporins* to women who report a history of adverse reactions to *penicillins*. The incidence of adverse reactions (e.g., skin flushing, itching) in women with a history of *penicillin* allergy who are given *cephalosporins* is 1% to 10%. The incidence of anaphylaxis in this setting is less than 0.02% (72).

A single dose of broad-spectrum antibiotics can result in pseudomembranous colitis, caused by *Clostridium difficile*. Diarrhea may develop in as many as 15% of hospitalized patients treated with beta-lactam antibiotics (73). In patients receiving *clindamycin*, the rate of diarrhea is nearly 10% to 25% (74). These gastrointestinal complications from antibiotics may cause serious morbidity in the surgical patient, and the surgeon should be able to recognize and manage these problems.

Not all gynecologic surgery patients need to receive prophylactic antibiotics. The surgeon should choose agents to cover procedures based on available data, thereby avoiding the potential for adverse reactions and minimizing the unnecessary use of antibiotics, which may contribute to increased rates of antimicrobial resistance. In patients with *cephalosporin* allergies or anaphylaxis to *penicillin*, other drugs or combinations should be chosen to provide adequate prophylactic coverage. Antimicrobial prophylaxis options for common gynecologic procedures are presented in Table 22.6. Antibiotic prophylaxis is not indicated for diagnostic or operative laparoscopy, exploratory laparotomy, or diagnostic or operative hysteroscopy, including endometrial ablation, intrauterine device insertions, endometrial biopsy, or urodynamics (75).

Subacute Bacterial Endocarditis Prophylaxis

It was thought that women who had severe valvular disease or other cardiac conditions required antibiotic prophylaxis prior to genitourinary (GU) or gastrointestinal (GI) procedures in order to prevent bacterial endocarditis as a result of the transient bacteremia provoked by the surgery. After reviewing the pertinent evidence-based literature, the American Heart Association issued revised guidelines in 2007 stating that antibiotic prophylaxis was not necessary solely to prevent endocarditis in patients undergoing GI or GU procedures, including hysterectomy (Table 22.8) (76).

Table 22.8 Recommendations for Prophylaxis of Bacterial Endocarditis

Highest-Risk Patients	Agents	Regimen (within 30 – 60 min of starting procedure)
Standard regimen	Amoxicillin	2 g PO
	Ampicillin	2.0 g IM or IV
	or	
	Cefazolin or ceftriaxone	1 g IM or IV
	Cephalexin	2 g
Penicillin-allergic (oral)	Cephalexin	2 g
	Clindamycin	600 mg
	Azithromycin or clarithromycin	500 mg
Penicillin-allergic (non-oral)	Cefazolin or ceftriaxone	1 g IM or IV
	Clindamycin	600 mg IM or IV

IM, intramuscularly; IV, intravenously.
Derived from Wilson W, Taubert KA, Gewitz M, et al. Prevention of infective endocarditis: guidelines from the American Heart Association: a guideline from the American Heart Association Rheumatic Fever, Endocarditis, and Kawasaki Disease Committee, Council on Cardiovascular Disease in the Young, and the Council on Clinical Cardiology, Council on Cardiovascular Surgery and Anesthesia, and the Quality of Care and Outcomes Research Interdisciplinary Working Group. *Circulation* 2007;116:1736–1754.

Postoperative Infections

Infections are a major source of morbidity in the postoperative period. Risk factors for infectious morbidity include the absence of perioperative antibiotic prophylaxis, contamination of the surgical field from infected tissues or from spillage of large bowel contents, an immunocompromised host, poor nutrition, chronic and debilitating severe illness, poor surgical technique, and preexisting focal or systemic infection. Sources of postoperative infection can include the lung, urinary tract, surgical site, pelvic sidewall, vaginal cuff, abdominal wound, and sites of indwelling intravenous catheters. Early identification and treatment of infection will result in the best outcome for these potentially serious complications.

Although infectious morbidity is an inevitable complication of surgery, the incidence of infections can be decreased by the appropriate use of simple preventive measures. In cases that involve transection of the large bowel, spillage of fecal contents inevitably occurs. A thorough preoperative mechanical and antibiotic bowel preparation in combination with systemic antibiotic prophylaxis will help decrease the incidence of postoperative pelvic and abdominal infections in these patients. The surgeon can further decrease the risk of postoperative infections by using meticulous surgical technique. Blood and necrotic tissue are excellent media for the growth of aerobic and anaerobic organisms. In cases in which there is higher-than-usual potential for serum and blood to collect in spaces that were contaminated by bacterial spill, closed-suction drainage may reduce the risk of infection. Antibiotic therapy, rather than prophylaxis, should be initiated during surgery in patients who have frank intra-abdominal infection or pus. Elective surgical procedures should be postponed in patients who have preoperative infections. In an epidemiologic study conducted by the Centers for Disease Control and Prevention (CDC), the incidence of nosocomial surgical infections ranged from 4.3% in community hospitals to 7% in municipal hospitals (77). Data confirmed this, with an incidence of 2% to 5% (78). Urinary tract infections accounted for approximately 40% of these nosocomial infections. Infections of the skin and wound accounted for approximately one-third of the infections, and respiratory tract infections accounted for approximately 16%. In patients who had any type of infection before surgery, the risk of infection at the surgical wound site increased fourfold. Rates of infection were higher in older patients, in patients with increased length of surgery, and in those with increased length of hospital stay before surgery. The relative risk was three times higher in patients with a community-acquired infection before surgery. These community-acquired infections included infections of the urinary and respiratory tracts.

Historically, the standard definition of febrile morbidity for surgical patients was the presence of a temperature higher than or equal to 100.4°F (38°C) on two occasions at least 4 hours apart during the postoperative period, excluding the first 24 hours. Other sources defined fever as two consecutive temperature elevations greater than 101.0°F (38.3°C) (79,80). Febrile morbidity is estimated to occur in as many as one-half of patients; it is often self-limited, resolves without therapy, and is usually noninfectious in origin (81). Overzealous evaluations of postoperative fever, especially during the early postoperative period, are time consuming, expensive, and sometimes uncomfortable for the patient (81). **The value of 101.0°F is more useful than 100.4°F to distinguish an infectious cause from an inconsequential postoperative fever.**

The assessment of a febrile surgical patient should include a review of the patient's history with regard to risk factors. Both the history and the physical examination should focus on the potential sites of infection (Table 22.9). The examination should include inspection of the pharynx, a thorough pulmonary examination, percussion of the kidneys to assess for costovertebral angle tenderness, inspection and palpation of the abdominal incision, examination of sites of intravenous catheters, and an examination of the extremities for evidence of deep venous thrombosis or thrombophlebitis. In gynecologic patients, an appropriate workup may include inspection and palpation of the vaginal cuff for signs of induration, tenderness, or purulent drainage. A pelvic examination should be performed to identify a mass consistent with a pelvic hematoma or abscess and to look for signs of pelvic cellulitis.

Patients with fever in the early postoperative period should have an aggressive pulmonary toilet, including incentive spirometry (80). If the fever persists beyond 72 hours postoperatively, additional laboratory and radiologic data may be obtained. The evaluation may include complete and differential white blood cell counts and a urinalysis. In one study, results from fever workups included positive blood cultures in 9.7% of patients, a positive urine culture in 18.8%, and a positive chest x-ray in 14%. These data support the need for a tailored workup based on the

Table 22.9 Posthysterectomy Infections	
Operative Site	*Nonoperative Site*
Vaginal cuff	Urinary tract
Pelvic cellulitis	Asymptomatic bacteriuria
Pelvic abscess	Cystitis
Supervaginal, extraperitoneal	Pyelonephritis
Intraperitoneal	Respiratory
Adnexa	Atelectasis
Cellulitis	Pneumonia
Abscess	Vascular
Abdominal incision	Phlebitis
Cellulitis	Septic pelvic thrombophlebitis
Simple	
Progressive bacterial synergistic	
Necrotizing fasciitis	
Myonecrosis	

patient's clinical picture (82). Blood cultures can be obtained but will most likely be of little yield unless the patient has a high fever (102°F). In patients with costovertebral angle tenderness, intravenous pyelogram may be indicated to rule out the presence of ureteral damage or obstruction from surgery, particularly in the absence of laboratory evidence of urinary tract infection. Patients who have persistent fevers without a clear localizing source should undergo CT scanning of the abdomen and pelvis to rule out the presence of an intra-abdominal abscess. If fever persists in patients who had gastrointestinal surgery, a barium enema or upper gastrointestinal studies with small bowel assessment may be indicated late in the course of the first postoperative week to rule out an anastomotic leak or fistula.

Urinary Tract Infections

Historically, the urinary tract was the most common site of infection in surgical patients (83). The incidence reported in the gynecologic literature is less than 4% (84,85). This decrease in urinary tract infections is most likely the result of increased perioperative use of prophylactic antibiotics. The incidence of postoperative urinary tract infection in gynecologic surgical patients not receiving prophylactic antibiotics is confirmed to be as high as 40%, and **even a single dose of perioperative prophylactic antibiotic decreases the incidence of postoperative urinary tract infection to as low as 4%** (86,87).

Symptoms of a urinary tract infection may include urinary frequency, urgency, and dysuria. In patients with pyelonephritis, other symptoms include headache, malaise, nausea, and vomiting. A urinary tract infection is diagnosed on the basis of microbiology and is defined as the growth of 10^5 organisms per milliliter of urine cultured. Most infections are caused by coliform bacteria, with *Escherichia coli* being the most frequent pathogen. Other pathogens include *Klebsiella, Proteus,* and *Enterobacter* species. *Staphylococcus* organisms are the causative bacteria in fewer than 10% of cases.

Despite the high incidence of urinary tract infections in the postoperative period, few of these infections are serious. Most are confined to the lower urinary tract, and pyelonephritis is a rare complication (88). Catheterization of the urinary tract, either intermittently or continuously with the use of an indwelling catheter, is implicated as a main cause of urinary tract contamination (89). More than 1 million catheter-associated urinary tract infections occur yearly in the United States, and **catheter-associated bacteria remains the most common etiology of gram-negative bacteremia in hospitalized patients.** Bacteria adhere to the surface of urinary catheters and grow within bile films, which appear to protect embedded bacteria from antibiotics, making treatment less effective. The use of urinary tract catheters should be minimized. An indwelling catheter should be removed or replaced in a patient undergoing treatment for catheter-related infections.

The treatment of urinary tract infection includes hydration and antibiotic therapy. Commonly prescribed and effective antibiotics include *penicillin, sulfonamides, cephalosporins, fluoroquinolones,* and *nitrofurantoin*. The choice of antibiotic should be based on knowledge of the susceptibility of organisms cultured at a particular institution. In some institutions, for example, more than 40% of *E. coli* strains are resistant to *ampicillin*. For uncomplicated urinary tract infections, an antibiotic that has good activity against *E. coli* should be given in the interim while awaiting results of the urine culture and sensitivity data.

Patients who have a history of recurrent urinary tract infections, those with chronic indwelling catheters (Foley catheters or ureteral stents), and those who have urinary conduits should be treated with antibiotics that will be effective against the less common urinary pathogens such as *Klebsiella* and *Pseudomonas*. Chronic use of *fluoroquinolones* for prophylaxis is not advised because these agents are notorious for inducing antibiotic-resistant strains of bacteria.

Pulmonary Infections

The respiratory tract is an uncommon site for infectious complications in gynecologic surgical patients. In one study only six cases of pneumonia occurred in more than 4,000 women who underwent elective hysterectomy (85). This low incidence is probably a reflection of the young age and good health status of gynecologic patients in general. In acute care facilities, pneumonia is a frequent hospital-acquired infection, particularly in elderly patients (90). Risk factors include extensive or prolonged atelectasis, preexistent COPD, severe or debilitating illness, central neurologic disease causing an inability to clear oropharyngeal secretions effectively, nasogastric suction, and a prior history of pneumonia (90,91). In surgical patients, early ambulation and aggressive management of atelectasis are the most important preventive measures. The role of prophylactic antibiotics remains unclear.

A significant percentage (40% to 50%) of cases of hospital-acquired pneumonia is caused by gram-negative organisms (83). These organisms gain access to the respiratory tract from the oral pharynx. Gram-negative colonization of the oral pharynx is increased in patients in acute care facilities and is associated with the presence of nasogastric tubes, preexisting respiratory disease, mechanical ventilation, and tracheal intubation (92). The use of antimicrobial drugs seems to significantly increase the frequency of colonization of the oral pharynx with gram-negative bacteria.

A thorough lung examination should be included in the assessment of all febrile surgical patients. In the absence of significant lung findings, chest radiography is probably of little benefit in patients at low risk for postoperative pulmonary complications. In patients with pulmonary findings or with risk factors for pulmonary complications, chest radiography should be performed. A sputum sample should be obtained for Gram stain and culture. The treatment should include postural drainage, aggressive pulmonary toilet, and antibiotics. The antibiotic chosen should be effective against both gram-positive and gram-negative organisms. In patients who are receiving assisted ventilation, the antibiotic spectrum should include drugs that are active against *Pseudomonas* organisms.

Phlebitis

Historically, intravenous catheter–related infections were common; the reported incidence is 25% to 35% in the 1980s (93). Because the incidence of catheter-related phlebitis increases significantly after 72 hours, intravenous catheters should be changed at least every 3 days according to the CDC (94). The institution of intravenous therapy teams decreased the incidence of phlebitis by as much as 50% in one study (95). In combination, these measures led to a dramatic decrease in peripheral catheter site infection.

The intravenous site should be inspected daily, and the catheter should be removed if there is any associated pain, redness, or induration. Phlebitis can occur even with close surveillance of the intravenous site. In one study, more than 50% of the cases of phlebitis became evident more than 12 hours after discontinuation of intravenous catheters (96). Less than one-third of patients had symptoms related to the intravenous catheter site 24 hours before the diagnosis of phlebitis.

Phlebitis can be diagnosed based on the presence of fever, pain, redness, induration, or a palpable venous cord. Occasionally, suppuration will be present. Phlebitis is usually self-limited and resolves within 3 to 4 days. The treatment includes application of warm, moist compresses and prompt removal of any catheters from the infected vein. Antibiotic therapy with antistaphylococcal agents should be instituted for catheter-related sepsis. Excision or drainage of an infected vein rarely is necessary.

Wound Infections

The results of a prospective study of more than 62,000 wounds were revealing in regard to the epidemiology of wound infections (97). The wound infection rate varied markedly, depending on the extent of contamination of the surgical field. The wound infection rate for clean surgical cases (infection not present in the surgical field, no break in aseptic technique, no viscus entered) was lower than 2%, whereas the incidence of wound infections with dirty, infected cases was 40% or higher. Preoperative showers with *hexachlorophene* slightly lowered the infection rate for clean wounds, whereas preoperative shaving of the wound site with a razor increased the infection rate. A 5-minute wound preparation immediately before surgery was as effective as preparation for 10 minutes. The wound infection rate increased with the duration of preoperative hospital stay and with the duration of surgery. Incidental appendectomy increased the risk of wound infection in patients undergoing clean surgical procedures. The study concluded that the **incidence of wound infections could be decreased by short preoperative hospital stays, hexachlorophene showers before surgery, minimizing shaving of the wound site, use of meticulous surgical technique, decreasing operative time as much as possible, bringing drains out through sites other than the wound, and dissemination of information to surgeons regarding their wound infection rates.** A program instituting these conclusions led to a decrease in the clean wound infection rate from 2.5% to 0.6% over an 8-year period. The wound infection rate in most gynecologic services is lower than 5%, reflective of the clean nature of most gynecologic operations.

The symptoms of wound infection often occur late in the postoperative period, usually after the fourth postoperative day, and may include fever, erythema, tenderness, induration, and purulent drainage. Wound infections that occur on postoperative days 1 through 3 are generally caused by streptococcal and *Clostridia* infections. The management of wound infections is mostly mechanical and involves opening the infected portion of the wound above the fascia, with cleansing and debridement of the wound edges as necessary. Wound care, consisting of debridement and dressing changes two to three times daily with mesh gauze, will promote growth of granulation tissue, with gradual filling in of the wound defect by secondary intention. Clean, granulating wounds can often be secondarily closed with good success, shortening the time required for complete wound healing.

The technique of delayed primary wound closure can be used in contaminated surgical cases to lower the incidence of wound infection. This technique involves leaving the wound open above the fascia at the time of the initial surgical procedure. Vertical interrupted mattress sutures through the skin and subcutaneous layers are placed 3 cm apart but are not tied. Wound care is instituted immediately after surgery and continued until the wound is noted to be granulating well. Sutures may then be tied and the skin edges further approximated using sutures or staples. **Using this technique of delayed primary wound closure, the overall wound infection rate is decreased from 23% to 2.1% in high-risk patients (98).**

Pelvic Cellulitis

Vaginal cuff cellulitis is present in most patients who underwent hysterectomy. It is characterized by erythema, induration, and tenderness at the vaginal cuff. A purulent discharge from the apex of the vagina may be present. The cellulitis is often self-limited and does not require any treatment. Fever, leukocytosis, and pain localized to the pelvis may accompany severe cuff cellulitis and most often signifies extension of the cellulitis to adjacent pelvic tissues. In such cases, broad-spectrum antibiotic therapy should be instituted with coverage for gram-negative, gram-positive, and anaerobic organisms. If purulence at the vaginal cuff is excessive or if there is a fluctuant mass noted at the vaginal cuff, the vaginal cuff should be gently probed and opened with a blunt instrument. The cuff can be left open for dependent drainage or, alternatively, a drain can be placed into the lower pelvis through the cuff and removed when drainage, fever, and symptoms in the lower pelvic region have resolved.

Intra-abdominal and Pelvic Abscess

The development of an abscess in the surgical field or elsewhere in the abdominal cavity is an uncommon complication after a gynecologic surgery. It is likely to occur in contaminated cases in which the surgical site is not adequately drained or as a secondary complication of hematomas. **The causative pathogens in patients who have intra-abdominal abscesses are usually polymicrobial in nature.** The aerobes most commonly identified include *E. coli, Klebsiella, Streptococcus, Proteus,* and *Enterobacter.* Anaerobic isolates are common, usually from the *Bacteroides* group. These pathogens arise mainly from the vaginal tract but can be derived from the gastrointestinal tract, particularly when the colon was entered at the time of surgery.

Intra-abdominal abscess is sometimes difficult to diagnose. The evolving clinical picture is often one of persistent febrile episodes with a rising white blood cell count. Findings on abdominal examination may be equivocal. If an abscess is located deep in the pelvis, it may be palpable by pelvic or rectal examination. For abscesses above the pelvis, the diagnosis will depend on radiologic confirmation.

Ultrasonography can occasionally delineate fluid collections in the upper abdomen and in the pelvis. Bowel gas interference makes visualization of fluid collections or abscesses in the midabdomen difficult to distinguish. **Computed tomography scanning is more sensitive and specific for diagnosing intra-abdominal abscesses and often is the radiologic procedure of choice.** Occasionally, if conventional radiologic methods fail to identify an abscess and the index of suspicion for an abscess remains high, labeled leukocyte scanning may be useful for locating the infected focus.

Standard therapy for intra-abdominal abscess is evacuation and drainage combined with appropriate parenteral administration of antibiotics. Abscesses located low in the pelvis, particularly in the area of the vaginal cuff, can be reached through a vaginal approach. In many patients, the ability to drain an abscess by placement of a drain percutaneously under CT guidance obviated the need for surgical exploration. With CT guidance, a pigtail catheter is placed into an abscess cavity via transperineal, transrectal, or transvaginal approaches. The catheter is left in place until drainage decreases. Transperineal and transrectal drainage of deep pelvic abscesses is successful in 90% to 93% of patients, obviating the need for surgical management (99,100). **For those patients in whom radiologic drainage is not successful, surgical exploration and evacuation are indicated.** The standard approach to initial antibiotic therapy is the combination of *ampicillin, gentamicin,* and *clindamycin.* Adequate treatment can be achieved with available broad-spectrum single agents (including the broad-spectrum *penicillin*), second- and third-generation cephalosporins, *levofloxacin* and *metronidazole,* and the *sulbactam-clavulanic acid*–containing preparations (101).

Necrotizing Fasciitis

Necrotizing fasciitis is an uncommon infectious disorder, affecting roughly 1,000 patients per year (102). This disease process is characterized by a rapidly progressive bacterial infection that involves the subcutaneous tissues and fascia while characteristically sparing underlying muscle. Systemic toxicity is a frequent feature of this disease, as manifested by the presence of dehydration, septic shock, disseminated intravascular coagulation, and multiple organ system failure.

The pathogenesis of necrotizing fasciitis involves a polymicrobial infection of the dermis and subcutaneous tissue. Hemolytic *streptococcus* was initially believed to be the primary pathogen responsible for the infection in necrotizing fasciitis (103). Other organisms are often cultured in addition to *streptococcus,* including other gram-positive organisms, coliforms, and anaerobes (104). Bacterial enzymes such as hyaluronidase and lipase released in the subcutaneous space destroy the fascia and adipose tissue and induce a liquefactive necrosis. Noninflammatory intravascular coagulation or thrombosis subsequently occurs. Intravascular coagulation results in ischemia and necrosis of the subcutaneous tissues and skin. Subcutaneous spread of up to 1 inch per hour can be seen, often with little effect on the overlying skin (104). Late in the course of the infection, destruction of the superficial nerves produces anesthesia in the involved skin. The release of bacteria and bacterial toxins into the systemic circulation can cause septic shock, acid-base disturbances, and multiple organ impairment.

The diagnosis is often difficult to make early in the disease course. **Most patients with necrotizing fasciitis develop erythema, edema, and pain, which in the early stages of the disease is disproportionately greater than that expected from the degree of cellulitis present and characteristically extends beyond the border of erythema** (105). Late in the course of the infection, the involved skin may be anesthetized secondary to necrosis of superficial nerves. Temperature abnormalities, both hyperthermia and hypothermia, are concomitant with the release of bacterial toxins and with bacterial sepsis (104). The involved skin is initially tender, erythematous, and warm. Edema develops, and the erythema spreads diffusely, fading into normal skin, characteristically without distinct margins or induration. Subcutaneous microvascular thrombosis induces ischemia in the skin, which becomes cyanotic and blistered. As necrosis develops, the skin becomes gangrenous and may slough spontaneously (104). Most patients will have leukocytosis and acid-base abnormalities. Subcutaneous gas may develop, which can be identified by palpation and by radiography. The finding of subcutaneous gas by radiography is often indicative of clostridial infection, although it is not a specific finding and may be caused by other organisms. These organisms include *Enterobacter, Pseudomonas,* anaerobic streptococci, and *Bacteroides,* which, unlike clostridial infections, spare the muscles underlying the affected area. A tissue biopsy specimen for Gram stain and aerobic and anaerobic culture should be obtained from the necrotic center of the lesion to identify the etiologic organisms (105). Although necrotizing fasciitis often is diagnosed during surgery, a high index of suspicion and liberal use of frozen-section biopsy can provide an early life-saving diagnosis and minimize morbidity (104).

Predisposing risk factors for necrotizing fasciitis include diabetes mellitus, alcoholism, an immunocompromised state, hypertension, peripheral vascular disease, intravenous drug abuse, and obesity (104). The most frequent site of infection is in the extremities, but the infection can occur anywhere in the subcutaneous tissues, including the head and neck, trunk, and perineum. Necrotizing fasciitis occurs after trauma, surgery, burns, and lacerations; as a secondary complication in perirectal infections or Bartholin duct abscesses; and *de novo* (103,106–109). Increased age, delay in diagnosis, inadequate debridement during initial surgery, extensive disease at the time of diagnosis, and the presence of diabetes mellitus are all factors that are associated with an increased likelihood of mortality from necrotizing fasciitis (104–106). Early diagnosis and aggressive management of this lethal disease contribute to improved survival.

Successful management of necrotizing fasciitis involves early recognition, immediate initiation of resuscitative measures (including correction of fluid, acid-base, electrolyte, and hematologic abnormalities), aggressive surgical debridement and redebridement as necessary, and broad-spectrum intravenous antibiotic therapy (104). During surgery, the incision should be made through the infected tissue down to the fascia. An ability to undermine the skin and subcutaneous tissues with digital palpation often will confirm the diagnosis. Multiple incisions can be made sequentially toward the periphery of the affected tissue until well-vascularized, healthy, resistant tissue is reached at all margins. The remaining affected tissue must be excised. The wound can be packed and sequentially debrided on a daily basis as necessary until healthy tissue is displayed at all margins. **Hyperbaric oxygen therapy may be of some benefit, particularly in patients for whom culture results are positive for anaerobic organisms** (110). Retrospective nonrandomized studies demonstrated that the addition of hyperbaric oxygen therapy to surgical debridement and antimicrobial therapy appears to significantly decrease both wound morbidity and overall mortality in patients with necrotizing fasciitis (110). The benefit of hyperbaric therapy demonstrated in one study was remarkable, given that patients receiving hyperbaric oxygen were sicker and had a higher incidence of diabetes mellitus, leukocytosis, and shock (106).

After the initial resuscitative efforts and surgical debridement, the primary concern is the management of the open wound. Allograft and xenograft skin can be used to cover open wounds, thus decreasing heat and evaporative water loss. Temporary biologic closure of open wounds seems to decrease bacterial growth (111). Amniotic membranes were effective wound covering in patients with necrotizing fasciitis (112).

A new technology demonstrated to significantly improve wound healing in laboratory and clinical studies is a vacuum-assisted closure (VAC) method that uses a subatmospheric pressure technique (113–115). In situations in which spontaneous closure is not likely, the VAC device may allow for the development of a suitable granulation bed and prepare the tissue for graft placement, thereby increasing the probability of graft survival. Skin flaps can be mobilized to help cover open wounds when the infections resolve and granulation begins.

Gastrointestinal Preparation

Traditionally, mechanical bowel preparation was advised before abdominal surgery, especially if colonic surgery was anticipated. Despite the infrequent need for colonic surgery (or injury) when performing gynecologic surgery, bowel preparation is part of the standard practice for many gynecologists. Advantages of mechanical bowel preparation include reduction of gastrointestinal contents, which facilitates the surgical procedure by allowing more room in the abdomen and pelvis. If a rectosigmoid colon enterotomy occurs, the mechanical bowel preparation eliminates formed stool and reduces the risk of bacterial contamination, thus reducing infectious complications.

Randomized clinical trials questioned the need for mechanical bowel preparation in colonic surgery (116). Although somewhat controversial, a meta-analyses including almost 5,000 patients showed no statistical difference between the groups for anastomotic leakage ($p = 0.46$), pelvic or abdominal abscess ($p = 0.75$), and wound sepsis ($p = 0.11$). The use of different mechanical regimes did not influence primary and secondary outcomes. The authors concluded that this **analysis demonstrates that any kind of mechanical bowel preparation should be omitted before colonic surgery.** The main limitation concerned rectal surgery for which the limited data preclude any interpretation.

A randomized trial of mechanical bowel preparation versus no bowel preparation with rectal surgery found that the overall and site-specific infectious morbidity rates were significantly higher in no preparation versus the mechanical preparation group. Regarding anastomotic leakage, length of hospital stay, major morbidity and mortality rates, there was no significant difference between the no preparation and mechanical bowel preparation groups. This was the first randomized trial to demonstrate that rectal cancer surgery without mechanical preparation is associated with higher risk of overall and infectious morbidity rates without any significant increase of anastomotic leakage rate. It suggests continuing to perform mechanical preparation before elective rectal resection for cancer (117).

Despite evidence of the infectious complications associated with mechanical preparation or no preparation, many gynecologic surgeons prefer a mechanical preparation to aid with exposure in the pelvic operative field. This may be particularly relevant to the surgeon performing minimally invasive surgery.

Mechanical bowel preparation may be accomplished as presented in (Table 22.10). The traditional use of laxatives and enemas requires at least 12 to 24 hours and causes moderate abdominal distention and crampy pain. Randomized trials comparing traditional mechanical bowel preparation (magnesium citrate and enemas) with oral gut lavage (*PEG electrolyte solution, GoLYTELY*) found that the use of approximately 4 L of *GoLYTELY* (administered until the rectal effluent is clear) provides more complete, faster, and more comfortable bowel preparation (118). **However, the ingestion of 4 L of fluid is problematic for many patients, so magnesium citrate may be preferable when mechanical preparation is to be used.**

An alternative mechanical preparation method is the use of oral *sodium phosphate* (*Phospho-Soda*). When evaluated in a randomized trial comparing the 4 L of *GoLYTELY* with oral *sodium phosphate*, colonoscopic examination disclosed that both methods were equally effective in colonic cleansing, and more patients preferred the *sodium phosphate* method (119). Some patients are at higher risk to develop acute phosphate nephropathy, leading to acute renal failure or worsening of chronic renal disease after the use of *sodium phosphate*. Although the pathophysiology is not fully understood, it may be secondary to substantial fluid shifts and electrolyte changes. It is speculated that potential etiologic factors included inadequate hydration, increased patient age, a history of hypertension, and current use of an angiotensin receptor

Table 22.10 Mechanical Bowel Preparation

Preoperative Day 1 Clear liquid diet

Mechanical Prep

4 L of GoLYTELY
OR
Fleet Phospho-Soda Saline laxative (3 oz. bottle)[a]
(one bottle of laxative 1 p.m. and another at 7 p.m.)
Fleet enemas until no solid stool in p.m. (optional)

Antibiotic Prep (Optional)

Neomycin (oral), 1 g every 4 h for three doses (4, 8, 12 p.m.)
Erythromycin (oral), 1 g every 4 h for three doses or *metronidazole* 500 mgm every 4 h
 for three doses

[a]Be aware of acute phosphate nephropathy. Avoid use of phospho-soda in patients with inadequate hydration, increased age, a history of hypertension, current use of an angiotensin receptor blocker, or angiotensin-conversing enzyme (ACE) inhibitors; renal disease or chronic heart failure and those taking nonsteroidal anti-inflammatory drugs (NSAIDs) or diuretics.

blocker or angiotension-converting enzyme (ACE) inhibitors. Patients with chronic renal disease or chronic heart failure and those taking NSAIDs or diuretics appear to be at higher risk of acute phosphate nephropathy (120). For these patients, the guidelines recommend an alternative bowel preparation agent, *polyethylene glycol,* which is not associated with volume shifts and electrolyte abnormalities (121,122).

Oral antibiotic prophylaxis was advised over the past three decades to reduce the infectious complications following colonic surgery. The usual regimen was a combination of oral *erythromycin* and *neomycin* taken the day before surgery. Many surgeons would substitute oral *metronidazole* for *erythromycin* because patients tolerate it better. **With the use of perioperative parental antibiotics, the benefit of oral antibiotics is questioned and most surgeons abandoned the use of oral antibiotics in favor of perioperative parenteral antibiotics.**

Postoperative Gastrointestinal Complications

Ileus

Following open abdominal or pelvic surgery, most patients experience some degree of intestinal ileus. The exact mechanism by which this arrest and disorganization of gastrointestinal motility occurs is unknown, but it appears to be associated with the opening of the peritoneal cavity and is aggravated by manipulation of the intestinal tract and prolonged surgical procedures. Infection, peritonitis, and electrolyte disturbances may result in ileus. For most patients undergoing common gynecologic operations, the degree of ileus is minimal, and gastrointestinal function returns relatively rapidly, allowing the resumption of oral intake within a few days of surgery. Patients who have persistently diminished bowel sounds, abdominal distention, and nausea and vomiting require further evaluation and more aggressive management. **Patients with symptoms of ileus or small bowel obstruction who underwent minimally invasive surgery are a different matter. Minimally invasive surgery should result in a daily improvement in GI function. An "ileus" in the case of minimally invasive surgery more likely represents GI injury, which should be evaluated immediately with a CT scan using GI contrast.**

Ileus is usually manifested by abdominal distention and should be evaluated by physical examination. Pertinent points of the abdominal examination include assessment of the quality of bowel sounds and palpation in search of distension, masses, tenderness, or rebound. The possibility that the patient's signs and symptoms may be associated with a more serious intestinal obstruction or intestinal complication (such as a perforation) must be considered. Pelvic examination should be performed to evaluate the possibility of a pelvic abscess or hematoma that may contribute to the ileus. **Abdominal radiography to evaluate the abdomen in the flat (supine) position and in the upright position will aid in the diagnosis of an ileus. The most common radiographic findings include dilated loops of small and large bowel and air-fluid levels while the patient is in the upright position.** Sometimes, massive dilation of the colon or stomach may be noted. The remote possibility of distal colonic obstruction suggested by a dilated cecum should be excluded by rectal examination, proctosigmoidoscopy, colonoscopy, or barium enema. In the postoperative gynecology patient, especially in the upright position, the abdominal x-ray may show free air. This common finding following surgery lasts 7 to 10 days in some instances and is not indicative of a perforated viscus in most patients.

The initial management of a postoperative ileus is aimed at gastrointestinal tract decompression and maintenance of appropriate intravenous replacement fluids and electrolytes.

1. **The patient should be made NPO status (nothing by mouth) with intravenous (IV) fluids and electrolytes.** If nausea and vomiting persist, **a nasogastric tube should be used to evacuate the stomach of its fluid and gaseous contents.** Continued nasogastric suction removes swallowed air, which is the most common source of gas in the small bowel.

2. **Fluid and electrolyte replacement must be adequate to keep the patient well hydrated and in metabolic balance.** Significant amounts of third-space fluid loss occur in the bowel wall, the bowel lumen, and the peritoneal cavity during the acute episode. Gastrointestinal fluid losses from the stomach may lead to metabolic alkalosis and depletion of other electrolytes as well. Careful monitoring of serum chemistry levels and appropriate replacement are necessary.

3. **Most cases of severe ileus begin to improve over a period of several days.** This improvement is recognizable by a reduction in the abdominal distention, return of normal bowel sounds, and passage of flatus or stool. Repeat abdominal radiographs should be obtained as necessary for further monitoring.

4. **When the gastrointestinal tract function appears to have returned to normal, the nasogastric tube may be removed and a liquid diet instituted.**

5. **If a patient shows no evidence of improvement during the first 48 to 72 hours of medical management, other causes of ileus should be sought.** Such cases may include ureteral injury, peritonitis from pelvic infection, unrecognized gastrointestinal tract injury with peritoneal spill, or fluid and electrolyte abnormalities such as hypokalemia. With persistent ileus, the use of water-soluble upper gastrointestinal contrast studies (CT scan with oral contrast) may assist in the resolution, but prospective randomized data regarding this maneuver are lacking.

Small Bowel Obstruction

Obstruction of the small bowel following major gynecologic surgery occurs in approximately 1% to 2% of patients (123). The most common cause of small bowel obstruction is adhesions to the operative site. If the small bowel becomes adherent in a twisted position, partial or complete obstruction may result from distention, ileus, or bowel wall edema. Less common causes of postoperative small bowel obstruction include entrapment of the small bowel into an incisional hernia and an unrecognized defect in the small bowel or large bowel mesentery. **Early in its clinical course, a postoperative small bowel obstruction may exhibit signs and symptoms identical to those of ileus. Initial conservative management as outlined for the treatment of ileus is appropriate.** Because of the potential for mesenteric vascular occlusion and resulting ischemia or perforation, worsening symptoms of abdominal pain, progressive distention, fever, leukocytosis, or acidosis should be evaluated carefully because immediate surgery may be required.

In most cases of small bowel obstruction following gynecologic surgery, the obstruction is only partial and the symptoms usually resolve with conservative management.

1. **Further evaluation after several days of conservative management may be necessary.** Evaluation of the gastrointestinal tract with barium enema, an upper gastrointestinal study, or a CT scan with small bowel assessment is appropriate. In most cases, complete obstruction is not documented, although a narrowing ("transition point") or tethering of the segment of small bowel may indicate the site of the problem.

2. **Further conservative management with nasogastric decompression and intravenous fluid replacement may allow time for bowel wall edema or torsion of the mesentery to resolve.**

3. **If resolution is prolonged and the patient's nutritional status is marginal, the use of TPN may be necessary.**

4. **Conservative medical management of postoperative small bowel obstruction usually results in complete resolution.** If persistent evidence of small bowel obstruction remains after full evaluation and an adequate trial of medical management, exploratory laparotomy may be necessary to manage the obstruction. In most cases, lysis of adhesions is all that is required, although a segment of small bowel that is badly damaged or extensively sclerosed from adhesions may require resection and reanastomosis.

Colonic Obstruction

Postoperative colonic obstruction following surgery for most gynecologic conditions is exceedingly rare. It is associated with a pelvic malignancy, which in most cases was known at the time of the initial operation. Advanced ovarian carcinoma is the most common cause of colonic obstruction in postoperative gynecologic surgery patients, and it is caused by extrinsic impingement on the colon by the pelvic malignancy. Intrinsic colonic lesions may be undetected, especially in a patient with some other benign gynecologic condition. When colonic obstruction is manifested by abdominal distention and abdominal radiography reveals a dilated colon and enlarging cecum, further evaluation of the large bowel is required by barium enema or colonoscopy. **Dilation of the cecum to more than 10 to 12 cm in diameter as viewed by abdominal radiography requires immediate evaluation and surgical decompression by performing colectomy or colostomy.** Surgery should be performed as soon as the obstruction is documented. Conservative management of colonic obstruction is not appropriate because the complication of colonic perforation has an exceedingly high mortality rate. In patients who are too ill to undergo surgery, the interventional radiologist may be able to place a cecostomy tube or the gastroenterologist may place a colonic stent (124).

Diarrhea

Episodes of diarrhea often occur following abdominal and pelvic surgery as the gastrointestinal tract returns to its normal function and motility. Prolonged and multiple episodes may represent a pathologic process such as impending small bowel obstruction, colonic obstruction, or pseudomembranous colitis. Excessive amounts of diarrhea should be evaluated by abdominal radiography and stool samples tested for the presence of ova and parasites, bacterial culture, and *Clostridium difficile* toxin. Proctoscopy and colonoscopy may be advisable in severe cases. Evidence of intestinal obstruction should be managed as outlined previously. Infectious causes of diarrhea should be managed with the appropriate antibiotics and fluid and electrolyte replacement. **C. difficile–associated pseudomembranous colitis may result from exposure to any antibiotic. Discontinuation of these antibiotics (unless they are needed to treat another severe infection) is advisable, along with the institution of appropriate therapy.** Oral *metronidazole* is a suitable agent for instituting therapy and is less expensive than *vancomycin*. Therapy should be continued until the diarrhea abates, and several weeks of oral therapy may be required to obtain complete resolution of the pseudomembranous colitis.

Fistula

Gastrointestinal fistulas are relatively rare following gynecologic surgery. They are most often associated with malignancy, prior radiation therapy, intestinal resection with anastomosis, or surgical injury to the large or small bowel that was improperly repaired or unrecognized. Signs and symptoms of gastrointestinal fistula are often similar to those of small bowel obstruction or ileus, except that fever is usually a more prominent component of the patient's symptoms. When fever is associated with gastrointestinal dysfunction postoperatively, evaluation should include early assessment of the gastrointestinal tract to confirm its continuity. **When fistula is suspected, the use of water-soluble gastrointestinal contrast material is advised to avoid the complication of barium peritonitis.** Evaluation with abdominal pelvic CT scan may assist in identification of a fistula and associated abscess. **Recognition of an intraperitoneal gastrointestinal leak or fistula formation usually requires immediate surgery, unless the fistula drained spontaneously through the abdominal wall or vaginal cuff.**

An *enterocutaneous fistula* arising from the small bowel and draining spontaneously **through the abdominal incision may be managed successfully with medical therapy.** Therapy should include nasogastric decompression, replacement of intravenous fluids as well as TPN, and appropriate antibiotics to treat an associated mixed bacterial infection. If the infection is under control and there are no other signs of peritonitis, the surgeon may consider allowing potential resolution of the fistula over a period of up to 2 weeks. Some authors suggested the use of *somatostatin* to decrease intestinal tract secretion and allow earlier healing of the fistula. In some cases, the fistula will close spontaneously with this mode of management. If the enterocutaneous fistula does not close with conservative medical management, surgical correction with resection, bypass, or reanastomosis will be necessary.

A *rectovaginal fistula* that occurs following gynecologic surgery is usually the result of surgical trauma that may have been aggravated by the presence of extensive adhesions and scarring in the rectovaginal septum associated with endometriosis, pelvic inflammatory disease, or pelvic malignancy. **A small rectovaginal fistula may be managed with a conservative medical approach, in the hope that decreasing the fecal stream will allow closure of the fistula.** A small fistula that allows continence except for an occasional leak of flatus may be managed conservatively until the inflammatory process in the pelvis resolves. At that point, usually several months later, correction of the fistula is appropriate. Large rectovaginal fistulas for which there is no hope of spontaneous closure are best managed by performing an initial diverting colostomy followed by repair of the fistula after inflammation resolves. After the fistula closure is healed and deemed successful, the colostomy can be reversed.

Thromboembolism

Risk Factors

Deep venous thrombosis and pulmonary embolism are largely preventable, yet significant complications in postoperative patients. The magnitude of this problem is relevant to the

Table 22.11 Thromboembolism Risk Stratification

Low Risk

Minor surgery

No other risk factors[a]

Moderate Risk

Age >40 years and major surgery

Age <40 years with other risk factors[a] and major surgery

High Risk

Age >60 years and major surgery

Cancer

History of deep venous thrombosis or pulmonary embolism

Thrombophilias

Highest Risk

Age >60 and cancer or history of venous thromboembolism

[a]Risk factors: obesity, varicose veins, history of deep venous thrombosis or pulmonary embolism, current estrogen, *tamoxifen,* or oral contraceptive use.

gynecologist, because **40% of all deaths following gynecologic surgery are directly attributed to pulmonary emboli,** and it is the most frequent cause of postoperative death in patients with uterine or cervical carcinoma (125,126).

The causal factors of venous thrombosis were first proposed by Virchow in 1858 and include a hypercoagulable state, venous stasis, and vessel endothelial injury. Risk factors include major surgery; advanced age; nonwhite race; malignancy; history of deep venous thrombosis, lower extremity edema, or venous stasis changes; presence of varicose veins; being overweight; a history of radiation therapy; and hypercoagulable states, such as factor V Lieden, pregnancy, and use of oral contraceptives, estrogens, or *tamoxifen.* Intraoperative factors associated with postoperative deep venous thrombosis include increased anesthesia time, increased blood loss, and the need for transfusion in the operating room. It is important to recognize these risk factors and to provide the appropriate level of venous thrombosis prophylaxis (127,128). The levels of thromboembolism risk are listed in Table 22.11.

Prophylactic Methods

A number of prophylactic methods significantly reduced the incidence of deep venous thrombosis, and a few studies included a large enough patient population to show a reduction in fatal pulmonary emboli (129). The ideal prophylactic method would be effective, free of significant side effects, well accepted by the patient and nursing staff, widely applicable to most patients, and inexpensive.

Low-Dose Heparin

The use of small doses of subcutaneously administered *heparin* for the prevention of deep venous thrombosis and pulmonary embolism is the most widely studied of all prophylactic methods. **More than 25 controlled trials demonstrated that *heparin* given subcutaneously 2 hours preoperatively and every 8 to 12 hours postoperatively is effective in reducing the incidence of deep venous thrombosis. The value of low-dose *heparin* in preventing fatal pulmonary emboli was established by a randomized, controlled multicenter international trial, which demonstrated a significant reduction in fatal postoperative pulmonary emboli in general surgery patients receiving low-dose *heparin* every 8 hours postoperatively** (129). Trials of low-dose *heparin* in gynecologic surgery patients showed a significant reduction in postoperative deep venous thrombosis.

Although low-dose *heparin* is considered to have no measurable effect on coagulation, most large series noted an increase in the bleeding complication rate, especially a higher incidence of wound hematoma (130). Although relatively rare, thrombocytopenia is associated with low-dose *heparin* use and was found in 6% of patients after gynecologic surgery (130). If patients remain on low-dose *heparin* for more than 4 days, it is reasonable to check their platelet count to assess the possibility of *heparin*-induced thrombocytopenia.

Low-Molecular-Weight Heparin

Low-molecular-weight heparins (LMWH) are fragments of *heparin* that vary in size from 4,500 to 6,500 Da. When compared with unfractionated *heparin*, *LMWH* have more anti-Xa and less antithrombin activity, leading to less effect on partial thromboplastin time and possibly leading to fewer bleeding complications (131). An increased half-life of 4 hours results in increased bioavailability when compared with unfractionated *heparin*. The increase in half-life of *LMWH* allows the convenience of once-a-day dosing.

Randomized controlled trials compared *LMWH* with *unfractionated heparin* in patients undergoing gynecologic surgery. In all studies, there was a similar incidence of deep venous thrombosis (DVT). Bleeding complications were similar between the *unfractionated heparin* and *LMWH* groups (132). A meta-analysis of general surgery and gynecological surgery patients from 32 trials indicated that daily *LMWH* administration is as effective as *unfractionated heparin* in DVT prophylaxis without any difference in hemorrhagic complications (133).

Mechanical Methods

Stasis in the veins of the legs occurs while the patient is undergoing surgery and continues postoperatively for varying lengths of time. Stasis occurring in the capacitance veins of the calf during surgery, plus the hypercoagulable state induced by surgery, are the prime factors contributing to the development of acute postoperative DVT. Prospective studies of the natural history of postoperative DVT showed that the calf veins are the predominant site of thrombi and that most thrombi develop within 24 hours of surgery (134).

Although probably of only modest benefit, reduction of stasis by short preoperative hospital stays and early postoperative ambulation should be encouraged for all patients. Elevation of the foot of the bed, raising the calf above heart level, allows gravity to drain the calf veins and should further reduce stasis.

Graduated Compression Stockings   Controlled studies of graduated compression stockings are limited but do suggest modest benefit when they are carefully fitted (135). Poorly fitted stockings may be hazardous to some patients who develop a tourniquet effect at the knee or midthigh (126). Variations in human anatomy do not allow perfect fit of all patients to available stocking sizes. The simplicity of graduated compression stockings and the absence of significant side effects are probably the two most important reasons that they are included in routine postoperative care. Compared to thigh length stockings, calf-high stockings appear to offer the same degree of venous thromboembolism protection.

Intermittent Pneumatic Compression   The largest body of literature dealing with the reduction of postoperative venous stasis deals with intermittent compression of the leg by pneumatically inflated sleeves placed around the calf or leg during intraoperative and postoperative periods. Various pneumatic compression devices and leg sleeve designs are available, and the literature has not demonstrated superiority of one system over another. **Calf compression during and after gynecologic surgery significantly reduces the incidence of DVT on a level similar to that of low-dose *heparin*.** In addition to increasing venous flow and pulsatile emptying of the calf veins, intermittent pneumatic compression appears to augment endogenous fibrinolysis, which may result in lysis of very early thrombi before they become clinically significant (136).

The duration of postoperative external pneumatic compression differed in various trials. External pneumatic compression may be effective when used in the operating room and for the first 24 hours postoperatively in patients with benign conditions who will ambulate on the first postoperative day (136,137).

External pneumatic compression used in patients undergoing major surgery for gynecologic malignancy reduced the incidence of postoperative venous thromboembolic complications by nearly threefold, but only if calf compression was applied intraoperatively and for the first 5 postoperative days (138,139). Patients with gynecologic malignancies may remain at risk for a longer period than general surgical patients because of stasis and hypercoagulable states; therefore, these patients appear to benefit from longer use of intermittent pneumatic compression.

Intermittent pneumatic leg compression has no significant side effects or risks and is considered slightly more cost-effective when compared with pharmacologic methods of prophylaxis (140). Compliance in wearing the leg compression while in bed is of utmost importance, and the patient and nursing staff should be educated to the proper regimen for maximum benefit.

The use of low-dose *heparin* or *LMWH* or intermittent pneumatic compression is a reasonable strategy in the care of women at moderate risk for postoperative venous thromboembolism. In high-risk patients, consideration should be given to using a pharmacologic method along with intermittent pneumatic compression.

Management of Postoperative Deep Venous Thrombosis and Pulmonary Embolism

Because pulmonary embolism is the leading cause of death following gynecologic surgical procedures, identification of high-risk patients and the use of prophylactic venous thromboembolism regimens are essential parts of management (125,126,141).

The early recognition of DVT and pulmonary embolism and immediate treatment are critical. Most pulmonary emboli arise from the deep venous system of the leg following gynecologic surgery; the pelvic veins are a known source of fatal pulmonary emboli.

The signs and symptoms of DVT of the lower extremities include pain, edema, erythema, and prominent vascular pattern of the superficial veins. These signs and symptoms are relatively nonspecific; 50% to 80% of patients with these symptoms will not have DVT (142). Conversely, approximately 80% of patients with symptomatic pulmonary emboli have no signs or symptoms of thrombosis in the lower extremities (143). Because of the lack of specificity when signs and symptoms are recognized, additional tests should be performed to establish the diagnosis of DVT.

Diagnosis

Doppler Ultrasound   **B-mode duplex Doppler imaging is the most common technique for the diagnosis of symptomatic venous thrombosis, especially when it arises in the proximal lower extremity.** With duplex Doppler imaging, the femoral vein can be visualized and clots may be seen directly (144). Compression of the vein with the ultrasound probe tip allows assessment of venous collapsibility; the presence of a thrombus diminishes vein wall collapsibility. Doppler imaging is less accurate when evaluating the calf and the pelvic veins.

Venography   Although venography is the standard technique for diagnosis of DVT, other diagnostic studies are accurate when performed by a skilled technologist and, in nearly all patients, may replace the need for contrast venography. Venography is moderately uncomfortable, requires the injection of a contrast material that may cause allergic reaction or renal injury, and may result in phlebitis in approximately 5% of patients (145). If the results of noninvasive imaging are normal or inconclusive and the clinician remains concerned given clinical symptoms, venography should be performed to obtain a definitive answer.

Magnetic Resonance Venography   In addition to having a sensitivity and specificity comparable to venography, magnetic resonance venography (MRV) may detect thrombi in pelvic veins that are not imaged by venography (146). The primary drawback to MRV is the time involved in examining the lower extremity and pelvis and the expense of this technology.

Treatment

Deep Venous Thrombosis

The treatment of postoperative DVT requires the immediate institution of anticoagulant therapy. Treatment may be with either *unfractionated heparin* or *LMWH*, followed by 6 months of oral anticoagulant therapy with *warfarin (Coumadin)*.

Unfractionated Heparin   After venous thromboembolism is diagnosed, *unfractionated heparin* should be initiated to prevent proximal propagation of the thrombus and allow physiological thrombolytic pathways to dissolve the clot. An initial bolus of 80 U per kilogram is given intravenously, followed by a continuous infusion of 1,000 to 2,000 U per hour (18 U/kg/hour).

Table 22.12 Heparin Administration for Treatment of Deep Venous Thrombosis or Pulmonary Embolism: Weight-Based Nomogram

Time of Administration	Dose
Initial dose	80-U/kg bolus, then 18 U/kg/h
The APTT should be measured every 6 h and the heparin dose adjusted as follows:	
APTT <35 seconds (<1.2 × control)	80-U/kg bolus, then 4 U/kg/h
APTT 35–45 seconds (1.2–1.5 × control)	40-U/kg bolus, then 2 U/kg/h
APTT 46–70 seconds (1.5–2.3 × control)	No change
APTT 71–90 seconds (2.3–3 × control)	Decrease infusion rate by 2 U/kg/h
APTT >90 seconds (>3 × control)	Hold infusion for 1 h, then decrease infusion rate by 3 U/kg/h

APTT, activated partial thromboplastin time.
Reprinted from **Raschke RA, Reilly BM, Guidry JR, et al.** The weight-based heparin dosing nomogram compared with a "standard care" nomogram. *Ann Intern Med* 1993;119:874–881, with permission.

Heparin dosage is adjusted to maintain activated partial thromboplastin time (APTT) levels at a therapeutic level 1.5 to 2.5 times the control value. Initial APTT should be measured after 6 hours of *heparin* administration and the dose adjusted as necessary. Patients having subtherapeutic APTT levels in the first 24 hours have a 15-fold increased risk of recurrent VTE when compared to patients who are adequately anticoagulated. Patients should be managed aggressively using intravenous *heparin* to achieve prompt anticoagulation. A weight-based nomogram is helpful in achieving a therapeutic APTT level (Table 22.12) (147). **Oral anticoagulant (*warfarin*) administration may be started on the first day of *heparin* infusion. The international normalized ration (INR) should be monitored daily until a therapeutic level is achieved (2.0 to 3.0 times normal value).** The change in the INR resulting from *warfarin* administration often precedes the anticoagulant effect by approximately 2 days, during which time low protein C levels are associated with a transient hypercoagulable state. Therefore, *heparin* should be administered until the INR was maintained in a therapeutic range for at least 2 days, confirming proper *warfarin* dose. Intravenous *heparin* may be discontinued in 5 days if an adequate IRN level is established.

Low-Molecular-Weight Heparin   Two *LMWH* preparations (*enoxaparin* and *dalteparin*) **were effective in the treatment of venous thromboembolism and have a cost-effective advantage over intravenous *heparin* in that they may be administered in the outpatient setting.** The dosages used in treatment of thromboembolism are unique and weight adjusted according to each *LMWH* preparation. Because *LMWH* has a minimal effect on APPT, serial laboratory monitoring of these levels is not necessary. Similarly, monitoring of anti-Xa activity (except in difficult cases or those with renal impairment) is not of significant benefit in a dose adjustment of *LMWH*. The increased bioavailability associated with *LMWH* allows for twice-a-day dosing, potentially making outpatient management an option for a subset of patients. **A meta-analysis involving more than 4,000 patients from 22 trials suggests that *LMWH* is more effective, safer, and less costly when compared with *unfractionated heparin* in preventing recurrent thromboembolism** (148).

Pulmonary Embolism

Many of the signs and symptoms of pulmonary embolism are associated with other, more commonly occurring pulmonary complications following surgery. **The classic findings of pleuritic chest pain, hemoptysis, shortness of breath, tachycardia, and tachypnea should alert the physician to the possibility of a pulmonary embolism.** Many times the signs are subtle and may be demonstrated only by a persistent tachycardia or a slight elevation in the respiratory rate. Patients suspected of pulmonary embolism should be evaluated initially by chest x-ray, electrocardiography, and arterial blood gas assessment. Any evidence of abnormality should be further evaluated by a spiral CT scan of the chest or a ventilation-perfusion lung scan. A high percentage of lung scans may be interpreted as "indeterminate." In this setting, careful clinical evaluation and judgment are required to decide whether pulmonary arteriography should be performed to document or exclude the presence of a pulmonary embolism.

The treatment of pulmonary embolism is as follows:

1. Immediate anticoagulant therapy, identical to that outlined for the treatment of DVT, should be initiated.

2. Respiratory support, including oxygen and bronchodilators and an intensive care setting, if necessary.

3. Although massive pulmonary emboli are usually quickly fatal, rarely pulmonary embolectomy is successful.

4. Pulmonary artery catheterization with the administration of thrombolytic agents bears further evaluation and may be important in patients with massive pulmonary embolism.

5. Vena cava interruption may be necessary in situations in which anticoagulant therapy is ineffective in the prevention of rethrombosis and repeated embolization from the lower extremities or pelvis. A vena cava filter may be inserted percutaneously above the level of the thrombosis and caudad to the renal veins. In most cases, anticoagulant therapy is sufficient to prevent repeat thrombosis and embolism and to allow the patient's own endogenous thrombolytic mechanisms to lyse the pulmonary embolus.

Management of Medical Problems

Endocrine Disease

The three most frequent endocrine disorders that occur in patients undergoing gynecologic surgery are diabetes mellitus, thyroid disease, and adrenal abnormalities. The pathophysiology of these disorders aids in understanding the effects of surgery on patients with these problems.

Diabetes Mellitus

According to the American Diabetes Association, 9.3 million American women, or 10.2% of all women older than 20 years, suffer from diabetes (149). Approximately 50% of individuals with diabetes mellitus (DM) will require surgery during their lives (150). Many of these procedures are a direct result of the complications of DM: retinopathy, nephropathy, large- and small-vessel occlusive disease, and coronary artery disease. It is the direct effect of DM on the end organs that determines the risk of surgery, rather than the type or duration of surgery, or the management of the condition itself. Diabetes mellitus is a complicated medical disorder of glucose metabolism that is related to a lack of production of, or resistance to, insulin.

Patients with DM experience exaggerated hyperglycemia during surgery. This hyperglycemia is multifactorial in origin and is secondary to increased catecholamine production, which inhibits pancreatic release of insulin and causes increased insulin resistance at the end organs. Elevations in instrumental hormones, such as cortisol, growth hormone, and glucagon, enhance gluconeogenesis and glycogenolysis (151). Goals of the preoperative assessment and perioperative management are to ensure metabolic homeostasis and to anticipate problems arising from preexisting complications.

Preoperative Risk Assessment

Preoperative risk assessment for diabetes should begin with a review of systems. Nocturia, polyuria, polydipsia, glucosuria, obesity, previous gestational diabetes, ethnicity, and family history are relevant aspects of the history. The current criteria for diagnosis of diabetes include (152):

1. Polyuria, polydipsia, or unexplained weight loss with a random nonfasting glucose of ≥ 200 mg/dL, *or*

2. Fasting glucose ≥ 126 mg/dL (in which fasting is defined as no food intake for 8 hours), *or*

3. Two-hour oral glucose tolerance test of 75 g, with serum glucose ≥ 200 mg/dL, *or*

4. Hemoglobin A1$_c$ $\geq 6.5\%$.

Confirmation of the diagnosis requires repeating the same test on a different day or concordant results of two different tests simultaneously.

Preoperative risk assessment in the previously diagnosed individual with diabetes should begin with the knowledge of the type of diabetes. Type 1 (insulin dependent) diabetes, or type 2 diabetes (noninsulin dependent), should be established because the perioperative management of each differs. The patient's routine glucose management strategies, glucose levels, medications, and baseline hemoglobin $A1_c$ should be assessed (153). The presence of end-organ complications of diabetes should be documented.

Large- and small-vessel arterial occlusive disease is the single most important risk factor in the preoperative setting. A careful history and physical examination should be performed to determine the presence or absence of coronary artery or cerebral vascular disease (150). When extended surgery is possible, as with surgery for gynecologic cancer, exercise stress testing or dipyridamole-thallium imaging should be considered to rule out occult coronary artery disease. Perioperative beta-blockade should be continued for patients already on beta-blockers at baseline. For patients with inducible ischemia, coronary artery disease, or multiple clinical risk factors for heart disease, perioperative beta-blockade should be considered, with initiation and careful titration of medication several weeks prior to surgery (154,155). Assessment of end-organ disease in the retina, kidney, and carotid arteries or evidence of peripheral vascular disease by the presence of foot ulcers should alert the clinician to the presence of small- or large-vessel disease. Diabetic nephropathy should be documented carefully preoperatively. Imaging studies using contrast dye should be avoided, and alternative testing should be performed to reduce the incidence of acute tubular necrosis. If a contrast study must be performed, adequate hydration both before and after the procedure is essential, and oral *metformin* should be withheld for 24 to 48 hours after the procedure.

Diabetes is associated with increased perioperative infections (156). Preoperative evaluation should include examination of the skin and urine sediment to detect asymptomatic infection. Wound infections, skin infections, pneumonia, and urinary tract infections account for two-thirds of the postoperative complications in patients with diabetes (151). There is a known predisposition for patients with DM to have increased colonization by *methicillin*-resistant *Staphylococcus aureus,* increased infections by gram-negative and staphylococcal bacteria, and an increased incidence of gram-negative and group B streptococcal sepsis (157–159). Seven percent of individuals with diabetes will have postoperative gram-negative sepsis, a rate approximately seven times higher than that of the nondiabetic population. These complications occur more often in patients with poor glucose control, probably caused by impaired leukocyte function in the presence of hyperglycemia (160,161). Individuals with DM have an increased risk of wound dehiscence and wound infection, possibly related to an impaired immune function, with changes in phagocytosis, cell-mediated immunity, and intracellular bactericidal activity (162). Autonomic neuropathy was documented in patients with DM, and these autonomic impairments can lead to intraoperative hypotension, cardiac arrhythmias, sudden death and abnormal motility of the esophagus, stomach, and small intestine (151). Peripheral sensory and motor neuropathies may or may not be present. The presence of any manifestations of autonomic neuropathy intra-operatively should prompt close monitoring of the affected organ system in the postoperative period.

The traditional goal for glucose control perioperatively is to maintain the glucose level below 200 mg/dL (151,153). **Significant debate continues regarding whether strict glycemic control below 110 mg/dL may be beneficial in critically ill patients** (163,164). **Perioperative hyperglycemia (>250 mg/dL) is associated with increased susceptibility to infection and poor wound healing.** Extreme hyperglycemia predisposes type 1 DM patients to metabolic acidosis, and surgery should be canceled until normal acid-base balance is documented. Hyperosmolar hyperglycemic nonketotic states must be recognized before surgery. Electrolyte disturbances, especially those related to sodium and potassium, should be corrected preoperatively. Hypoglycemia should be avoided during the perioperative period.

The history and type of DM are important factors to consider when devising a perioperative management plan. Patients with non*insulin*-dependent diabetes (type 2) whose condition is controlled with oral hypoglycemic agents or diet are best treated with intravenous fluids containing no dextrose and should not be given *insulin* intraoperatively. Oral administration of hypoglycemic agents should be discontinued when the patient ceases oral intake of food, and hyperglycemic episodes in the perioperative period are treated with sliding-scale regular *insulin* if blood sugar levels exceed 200 mg/dL (151,153).

Insulin-dependent or type 1 diabetes poses a more difficult problem. These patients are insulin deficient and therefore require a basal rate of insulin at all times. Likewise, they require a baseline intake of glucose. They risk developing diabetic ketoacidosis whether

or not they are eating (153). **Preoperatively, the goals include avoiding ketoacidosis and hypoglycemia, and, to a lesser extent, hyperglycemia. Traditionally, approximately one-third to one-half of the patient's usual daily dose of *NPH insulin* (intermediate acting) is given subcutaneously the morning of surgery. Omit any short-acting *insulin* without oral intake. An infusion of 5% dextrose should be given while being restricted from oral intake. Additional regular *insulin* can be administered in the operating room as needed** (150,153). If patients are normally on a continuous *insulin* infusion, they may continue at their usual infusion rate. There is no single regimen that is superior for the intraoperative management of type 1 diabetic patients. A continuous intravenous *insulin* infusion is indicated for patients with unstable type 1 diabetes, those who require emergency surgery while in ketoacidosis, and those undergoing long, complex procedures (161). Consultation with endocrine and anesthesia colleagues can be helpful in managing these complex regimens.

Postoperative Management   Postoperative monitoring of patients with DM includes careful monitoring of serum glucose levels. **If an intravenous *insulin* regimen is used, blood glucose levels must be checked every 1 to 2 hours. If a sliding-scale *insulin* administration is used, blood glucose should be checked and documented approximately every 6 hours until the patient is eating and stable on her preoperative regimen. The serum glucose level should be maintained at less than 250 mg/dL, and ideally below 140 mg/dL when fasting and below 180 mg/dL with random draws** (165,166). For type 2 diabetics, oral hypoglycemics can be restarted when the patient resumes eating, except with *metformin,* which requires normal renal and liver function (153).

It is essential to prevent the development of severe hypoglycemia or hyperglycemia and the associated complications of diabetic ketoacidosis or a hyperosmolar state. Rigorous perioperative management may obviate some of the infectious and wound-healing complications that are more common in these patients (167).

Thyroid Syndromes

Thyroid dysfunction should be suspected in any patient with a history of hyperthyroidism, use of thyroid replacement medication or antithyroid medication, prior thyroid surgery, or radioactive iodine therapy.

Hyperthyroidism

Diffuse toxic goiter (Grave's disease) is the most common cause of hyperthyroidism and results from abnormal stimulation of the thyroid gland by antithyroid antibodies. Other causes of hyperthyroidism include multinodular goiter, excess thyroid hormone, or thyroiditis. Any signs or symptoms suggestive of weight loss, tachycardia, atrial fibrillation, goiter, or proptosis should initiate a more extensive laboratory evaluation of thyroid function. Total thyroxin, free tri-iodothyronine (T_3), free thyroxin (T_4), and thyroid-stimulating hormone (TSH) tests are useful in diagnosis. **In hyperthyroidism, the free T_4 level will be elevated, and the TSH level will be suppressed** (154). A new diagnosis of hyperthyroidism necessitates postponement of elective surgery until adequate treatment with antithyroid medication is received because of the risk of thyroid storm. Thyroid storm is associated with mortality of up to 40% (168). Stable thyroid conditions do not require any special preoperative treatments or tests. **Ideally, an euthyroid state should be maintained for 3 months before elective surgery.** In emergent situations, beta-blockers can be used to counter sympathomimetic drive such as palpitations, diaphoresis, and anxiety. Antithyroid medications such as *propylthiouracil (PTU)* or *radioactive iodine* do not render patients euthyroid quickly enough for urgent surgery. *Radioactive iodine* requires 6 to 18 weeks to establish a euthyroid state (154). When thyroid dysfunction is corrected and maintained for several months, elective surgery can proceed without additional perioperative monitoring. Antithyroid medications should be resumed with return of bowel function. If a prolonged delay in resumption of oral intake is encountered, *PTU* and *methimazole* can be administered rectally (169). **When time does not permit establishment of a euthyroid state preoperatively, oral administration of *PTU* and a *beta-blocker* can be implemented for 2 weeks before surgery, and with careful monitoring, optimal results can be achieved** (170). Alternatively, oral *beta-blockers, glucocorticoids,* and *sodium iopanoate* can be used for 5 days, followed by surgery on day 6 (169). In the emergent setting, close monitoring of the patient for tachycardia, arrhythmias, and hypertension is necessary. *Beta-blockers* can control these symptoms until definitive therapy can be initiated after recovery from surgery.

Any signs suggestive of the development of thyroid storm—including hemodynamic instability, tachycardia, arrhythmias, hyperreflexia, diarrhea, fever, delirium, or congestive heart failure—mandate transfer to an intensive care setting for optimal monitoring and management in consultation with a medical endocrinologist. Such thyroid instability can be triggered by underlying infection, which requires diagnosis and treatment to facilitate management of this medical emergency. The mortality rate from thyroid storm is reportedly between 10% and 75% (169). Treatment of thyroid storm consists of *beta-blockers, thioamides, iodine, iodinated contrast agents,* and *corticosteroids* (151). *Aspirin* should not be given for fever in the patient with thyroid storm because it may interfere with the protein binding of T_4 and T_3, resulting in increased free serum concentrations (151).

Hypothyroidism

The incidence of hypothyroidism is approximately 1% in the adult population, and 5% in adults older than 50 years (154). **In women older than 60 years, the incidence of hypothyroidism may approach 6%** (168). **Hypothyroidism is 10 times more common in women than in men** (154). Many such cases are secondary to previous antithyroid therapy (*radioactive iodine* or *thyroidectomy*) for hyperthyroidism. The most common primary cause of hypothyroidism is Hashimoto's thyroiditis, an autoimmune condition (154). A history of lethargy, cold intolerance, lassitude, weight gain, fluid retention, constipation, dry skin, hoarseness, periorbital edema, and brittle hair can be indicative of inadequate thyroid function. In this setting, physical findings of increased relaxation phase of deep tendon reflexes, cardiomegaly, pleural or pericardial effusions, or peripheral edema should stimulate further investigation of thyroid function by assessment of TSH and free T_4 levels. Hypothyroidism decreases cardiac output by 30% to 50% as a result of decreased stroke volume and heart rate (171). Hyponatremia may be associated with hypothyroidism because of the inability of the kidneys to excrete water (171). When elective surgery is planned for severely hypothyroid patients, surgery should be postponed until thyroid replacement therapy is initiated (154). In patients with mild or moderate hypothyroidism, the delay of surgery is controversial (154).

For young patients with mild to moderate hypothyroidism, a starting dose of 1.6 μg/kg of thyroid hormone replacement can be given. In elderly patients, *thyroxin* dosage (0.025 mg once a day) should be given with interval dose increases every 4 to 6 weeks until the patient is euthyroid (168). **Dosage levels can ultimately be titrated against TSH levels.** In severely hypothyroid patients requiring urgent or emergent surgery, intravenous T_3 or T_4 may be given, along with intravenous *corticosteroids* to avoid consequences of unrecognized adrenal insufficiency (151,154).

In the immediate postoperative setting, T_4 therapy can be held for 5 to 7 days while waiting for return of bowel function because the half-life of circulating T_4 is approximately 5 to 9 days (170). If more than 5 to 7 days of decreased bowel function are expected, T_4 can be given by the intramuscular or intravenous route at approximately 80% of the oral dose (171,172).

Adrenal Insufficiency

Adrenal insufficiency may result in catastrophic postoperative complications, including death. The most common cause of adrenal insufficiency in the surgical patient is secondary to the exogenous use of *corticosteroids*. The physician should ascertain whether a patient used exogenous steroids for asthma (including inhaled steroids), malignant conditions, arthritis, or irritable bowel syndrome. The type of steroid use, the route, the dose, the duration, and the temporal relationship to the timing of the surgical procedure must be determined. The type of surgical procedure and its associated stress should be taken into consideration. The use of high doses of exogenous steroids for prolonged periods can cause circulatory collapse, and they have adverse effects on wound healing and immunocompetence.

The daily replacement dose of cortisol is approximately 5 to 7.5 mg of *prednisone.* **Suppression of the hypothalamic–pituitary–adrenal (HPA) axis by exogenous steroids for more than a few weeks may produce relative adrenal insufficiency.** When systemic steroids are used for longer periods, adrenal insufficiency may persist for up to 1 year. Short courses of low-dose oral steroids (<5 mg of *prednisone* in a single morning dose for any duration of time, alternate-day dosing of short-acting glucocorticoids, and any dose of corticosteroids given for less than 3 weeks) are not thought to cause clinically significant suppression of the HPA axis (151,172). Use of inhaled corticosteroids of over 0.8 mg per day or class I topical glucocorticoids of 2 g per day or more may cause suppression (172).

Table 22.13 Guidelines for Adrenal Supplementation Therapy[a]

Medical or Surgical Stress	Corticosteroid Dosage
Minor Inguinal hernia repair Colonoscopy Mild febrile illness Mild-moderate nausea/vomiting Gastroenteritis	25 mg of *hydrocortisone* or 5 mg of *methylprednisolone* IV on day of procedure only
Moderate Open cholecystectomy Hemicolectomy Significant febrile illness Pneumonia Severe gastroenteritis	50–75 mg of *hydrocortisone* or 10–15 mg of *methylprednisolone* IV on day of procedure Taper quickly over 1–2 days to usual dose
Severe Major cardiothoracic surgery Whipple procedure Liver resection Pancreatitis	100–150 mg of *hydrocortisone* or 20–30 mg of *methylprednisolone* IV on day of procedure Rapid taper to usual dose over next 1–2 days
Critically Ill Sepsis-induced hypotension or shock	50–100 mg of *hydrocortisone* IV every 6–8 h or 0.18 mg/kg/h as a continuous infusion + 50 μg/d of *fludrocortisone* until shock resolved. May take several days to a week or more, then gradually taper, following vital signs and serum sodium.

IV, intravenously.

[a]Patients receiving 5 mg/d or less of *prednisone* should receive their normal daily replacement but do not require supplementation. Patients who receive greater than 5 mg/d of *prednisone* should receive the above therapy in addition to their maintenance therapy.

Reprinted from **Coursin DB, Wood KE.** Corticosteroid supplementation for adrenal insufficiency. *JAMA* 2002;287:236–240, with permission.

If either the dose or duration of glucocorticoid administration exceeds the preceding regimen, biochemical tests are recommended to preoperatively evaluate the function of the adrenal gland. The easiest and safest test to assess HPA function is the *cosyntropin* stimulation test. *Cosyntropin*, a synthetic analogue of adrenocorticotropic hormone, is given in a dose of 250 μg intravenously, and a blood sample is collected 30 minutes after the injection and assayed for plasma cortisol. A plasma cortisol value of greater than 18 to 20 μg/dL indicates adequate adrenal function (151,154). If the history regarding exogenous steroid use is unclear, the *cosyntropin* stimulation test should be considered as a preoperative test to determine whether the patient will need perioperative glucocorticoid coverage. The amount of glucocorticoid replacement should be equivalent to the normal physiologic response to surgical stress (Table 22.13) (173).

For minor surgical stress, such as colonoscopy, the glucocorticoid target is approximately 25 mg of *hydrocortisone* equivalent on the day of the procedure (173). For moderate surgical stress, for example, open cholecystectomy, the glucocorticoid target is 50 to 75 mg of *hydrocortisone* equivalent on the day of the procedure and tapered quickly for 1 to 2 days (173). The patient should receive her normal daily dose preoperatively, followed by 50 mg of *hydrocortisone* intravenously administered intraoperatively. For major surgical stress, such as liver resection, the glucocorticoid target range is 100 to 150 mg *hydrocortisone* equivalent on the day of the procedure, tapering rapidly over the next 1 to 2 days to the usual dosage (173). The patient should receive her normal daily dose preoperatively.

Administration of high-dose steroids should be stopped as soon as possible postoperatively because they can inhibit wound healing and promote infection. Hypertension and glucose intolerance can develop. When a prolonged or involved procedure is performed and longer steroid use is necessary, careful tapering may be required. The previously recommended approach was to halve the dose of *hydrocortisone* on a daily basis until a dose of 25 mg is reached. Eliminating one daily dose each day until the drug is stopped was considered the safest method of withdrawal; no consensus on the timing or duration of steroid tapering exists. Addison's disease is uncommon but should be considered in the differential diagnosis if the patient develops perioperative hypotension after steroids are withdrawn. In addition to blood and isotonic fluid replacement, a "stress" dose of steroids should be given if adrenal insufficiency is suspected and sepsis and hypovolemia are excluded.

Cardiovascular Diseases

The incidence of perioperative cardiovascular complications decreased markedly as a result of improvements in preoperative detection of high-risk patients, preoperative preparation, and surgical and anesthetic techniques (174).

Preoperative Evaluation

The goal of a preoperative cardiac evaluation is to determine the presence of heart disease, its severity, and the potential risk to the patient during the perioperative period. Every patient should be questioned about symptoms of cardiac disease including chest pain, dyspnea on exertion, peripheral edema, wheezing, syncope, claudication, or palpitations. Patients with a history of cardiac disease should be evaluated for worsening of symptoms, which indicates progressive or poorly controlled disease. Records of previous treatment should be obtained. Prescriptions for antihypertensive, anticoagulant, antiarrhythmic, antilipid, or antianginal medications may be the only indication of cardiac problems. In patients without known heart disease, the presence of DM, hyperlipidemia, hypertension, tobacco use, or a family history of heart disease identifies patients at higher risk for heart disease who should be more carefully screened.

On physical examination, the presence of findings such as hypertension, jugular venous distention, laterally displaced point of maximum impulse, irregular pulse, third heart sound, pulmonary rales, heart murmurs, peripheral edema, or vascular bruits should prompt a more complete evaluation. Laboratory evaluation of patients with known or suspected heart disease should include a blood count and serum chemistry analysis. Patients with heart disease tolerate anemia poorly. Serum sodium and potassium levels are particularly important in patients taking diuretics and digitalis. Blood urea nitrogen and creatinine values provide information on renal function and hydration status. Assessment of blood glucose levels may detect undiagnosed DM. Chest radiography and electrocardiography are mandatory as part of the preoperative evaluation, and the results may be particularly helpful when compared with those of previous studies.

Coronary Artery Disease

Coronary artery disease is a major risk factor for patients undergoing abdominal surgery. In an adult population without a prior history of myocardial infarction, the incidence of myocardial infarction following surgery is 0.1% to 0.7% (175). **In patients who had a prior myocardial infarction, the reinfarction rate is 2.8% to 7%** (176). The risk of reinfarction is inversely proportional to the length of time between infarction and surgery. At 3 months or less, the risk of reinfarction is 5.7%, and from 3 to 6 months, the rate falls to 2.3%. Six months after myocardial infarction, the reinfarction rate is 1.5% (175). Careful perioperative management can lower the reinfarction rate in patients who had recent infarctions. Perioperative myocardial infarction is associated with a mortality rate of 26% to 70% (177).

Because of the high mortality and morbidity associated with perioperative myocardial infarction, considerable effort is made to predict perioperative cardiac risk. **A prospective evaluation of preoperative cardiac risk factors using a multivariate analysis identified independent cardiac risk factors for patients undergoing noncardiac surgery** (177). Using these factors, a cardiac risk index was created that placed a patient in one of four risk classes. This cardiac risk index was further modified and validated prospectively, resulting in a tool for clinical risk assessment in nonemergent major noncardiac surgery, the Revised Cardiac Risk Index (178). Risk factors include high-risk surgical procedures, history of ischemic heart disease, history of congestive heart failure, history of transient ischemic attack or stroke, preoperative insulin therapy, and preoperative serum creatinine levels greater than 2.0 mg/dL. Depending on the number of risk factors, the risk of major cardiac events (myocardial infarction, cardiac arrest, pulmonary edema, and complete heart block) range from 0.5% to 9.1% (Table 22.14).

Risk assessment is stratified into three major categories: (i) clinical predictors, (ii) functional capacity, and (iii) surgery-specific risk (179). Clinical predictors of increased perioperative

Table 22.14 Major Cardiac Event Rates by the Revised Cardiac Risk Index			
Class	*(number of risk factors)*	*Events/Patient*	*Event Rate% (95% CI)*
I	(0)	2/488	0.4 (0.05, 1.5)
II	(1)	5/567	0.9 (0.3, 2.1)
III	(2)	17/258	6.6 (3.9, 10.3)
IV	(3)	12/109	11.0 (5.8, 18.4)

CI, confidence interval.
Adapted from **Lee TH, Marcantonio ER, Mangione CM, et al.** Derivation and prospective validation of a simple index for prediction of cardiac risk of major noncardiac surgery. *Circulation* 1999;100: 1043–1049.

cardiac risk were formerly divided into major, intermediate, and minor factors. The intermediate category was replaced by clinical risk factors from the revised cardiac risk index (Table 22.15). The patient's functional status is assessed by a thorough history (Table 22.16), and self-reported exercise tolerance can be used to predict perioperative risk, based on a system of metabolic equivalents (METS) (180). **Surgery-specific risk is subdivided into high-risk procedures (emergent major operations, aortic and vascular procedures, and prolonged surgical procedures associated with large fluid shifts or blood loss), intermediate-risk procedures (intraperitoneal and intrathoracic), and low-risk procedures (endoscopic, breast surgery, and ambulatory procedures). Patients with poor functional capacity and any clinical risk factor undergoing more than low-risk nonemergent surgery should undergo preoperative testing, based on American Heart Association (AHA) guidelines** (179).

In an effort to quantify preoperative cardiac risk, several tests are used to assess cardiovascular function. Electrocardiogram should be considered for anyone other than asymptomatic persons undergoing low risk procedures. Echocardiography may be used to evaluate left ventricular function (179). Patients who have dyspnea of unknown origin, current or past heart failure,

Table 22.15 Clinical Predictors of Increased Perioperative Cardiovascular Risk
Major
Unstable coronary syndromes: acute ($\leq$7 days) or recent (7 < days $\leq$ 1 month) MI, unstable or severe angina Decompensated congestive heart failure Significant arrhythmias (high-grade AV block, symptomatic ventricular arrhythmias, supraventricular arrhythmias with uncontrolled ventricular rate) Severe valvular disease
Intermediate
History of cerebrovascular disease Prior ischemic cardiac disease Compensated or prior congestive heart failure Diabetes mellitus Renal insufficiency
Minor
Advanced age Abnormal ECG (LVH, LBBB, ST-T abnormalities) Rhythm other than sinus Uncontrolled systemic hypertension

MI, myocardial infarction; AV, atrioventricular; ECG, electrocardiogram; LVH, left ventricular hypertrophy; LBBB, left bundle branch block.
Adapted from **Fleisher LA, Beckman JA, Brown KA, et al.** 2009 ACCF/AHA focused update on perioperative beta blockade incorporated into the ACC/AHA 2007 guidelines on perioperative cardiovascular evaluation and care for noncardiac surgery: a report of the American College of Cardiology Foundation/American Heart Association Task Force on Practice Guidelines. *Circulation* 2009;120:e169–e276.

Table 22.16 Functional Capacity Assessment from Clinical History
Excellent
Carry 24 lb up eight steps
Carry objects that weigh 80 lb
Outdoor work (shovel snow, spade soil)
Recreation (ski, basketball, squash, handball, jog, or walk 5 mph)
Moderate
Have sexual intercourse without stopping
Walk at 4 mph on ground level
Outdoor work (garden, rake, weed)
Recreation (roller-skate, dance)
Poor
Shower and dress without stopping
Basic housework
Walk 2.5 mph on level ground
Recreation (golf, bowl)

Adapted from **Mehta RH, Bossone E, Eagle KA.** Perioperative cardiac risk assessment for noncardiac surgery. *Cardiologia* 1999;44:409–418.

prior cardiomyopathy, or with any of the above factors and no cardiac assessment in the past 12 months should consider echocardiogram testing preoperatively (179). ***Exercise stress testing before surgery can identify patients who have ischemic heart disease not apparent at rest.*** AHA guidelines recommend noninvasive stress testing for patients with one to two clinical risk factors, undergoing intermediate risk surgery with poor functional capacity of METS less than 4. Likewise, it is recommended for patients with greater clinical risk factors or those undergoing high-risk surgery (179). These patients are at increased risk of developing cardiac complications in the perioperative period. In a study of patients undergoing peripheral vascular surgery, a high-risk group of patients was identified who had ischemic electrocardiographic changes when they exercised to less than 75% of their maximal predicted heart rate. In this group, the incidence of perioperative myocardial infarction was 25% and the overall cardiac mortality rate was 18.5%. Conversely, no perioperative infarctions occurred in patients who were able to exercise to more than 75% of their maximal predicted heart rate and who had no electrocardiographic evidence of ischemia (181). The prognostic value of stress testing was not supported in another prospective study that found that only an abnormal preoperative resting electrocardiography result was an independent risk factor (182). The exercise stress test must be selectively applied to a high-risk population because its predictive value depends on the prevalence of the disease. It is not prudent to screen all patients preoperatively; it is preferable to rely on a careful history to identify patients with symptoms of cardiac disease for whom the test would be most predictive.

Exercise stress testing is limited in some patients who cannot exercise because of musculoskeletal disease, pulmonary disease, or severe cardiac disease. *Dipyridamole-thallium scanning* may be used to overcome the limitations of exercise stress testing. This study has a high degree of sensitivity and specificity but a low positive predictive value (179,183). It relies on the ability of *dipyridamole* to dilate normal coronary arteries but not stenotic vessels. Normally perfused myocardium readily takes up *thallium* when it is given intravenously. Conversely, hypoperfused myocardium does not show good uptake of *thallium* when scanned 5 minutes after injection. Reperfusion and uptake of *thallium* 3 hours after injection identify viable but high-risk myocardium. Old infarctions are identified as areas without uptake. Several studies show an increasing risk of perioperative myocardial infarction dependent on the extent of reperfusion of *thallium*, or reversible defect, ranging from 3% to 49% (184,185). The *dipyridamole-thallium* scan is applicable to clinically high-risk patients who are unable to exercise because it uses a medically induced "stress."

Dobutamine stress echocardiography is another test to evaluate cardiac risk in patients who are unable to exercise. This method identifies regional cardiac wall motion abnormalities after *dobutamine* infusion to identify patients at high risk for cardiac events. Positive and negative predictive values are similar to those of *dipyridamole-thallium* testing for a perioperative event

(186,187). *Dipyridamole-thallium* testing is preferred for patients with known cardiac arrhythmias, and *dobutamine* is preferred for patients with bronchospastic lung disease and in those with severe cardiac stenosis (188). Coronary angiography should be considered only in patients who have an indication for angiography independent of the planned surgery, such as patients with acute coronary syndromes, unstable angina, angina refractory to medical therapy, or high-risk results on noninvasive testing.

Preoperative testing should be used discriminately in intermediate-risk patients. Controversy exists regarding the accuracy of these tests to provide prognostic information beyond what is obtained from clinical risk stratification for nonvascular procedures. Diagnostic testing should not lead to unnecessary additional testing or harmful delays in surgery. **The American College of Cardiology and the American Heart Association present an updated detailed algorithm that incorporates risk-factor stratification to guide clinicians to proceed directly to surgery, to delay surgery and obtain preoperative noninvasive testing, or to attempt risk factor modification** (179).

It is rare for patients who are younger than 50 years and who do not have diabetes, hypertension, hypercholesterolemia, or coronary artery disease to suffer a perioperative myocardial infarction. In contrast, patients with coronary artery disease are at increased risk of myocardial infarction in the postoperative period. Prevention, early recognition, and treatment are important because myocardial infarctions that occur in the postoperative period have mortality rates of up to 25% and are associated with increased rates of cardiovascular death in the 6 months following surgery (189).

Nearly two-thirds of postoperative myocardial infarctions occur during the first 3 days postoperatively (189). Although the pathophysiologic factors are complex, the causes of postoperative myocardial ischemia and infarction are related to decreased myocardial oxygen supply coupled with increased myocardial oxygen requirements. In postoperative patients, conditions that decrease oxygen supply to the myocardium include tachycardia, increased preload, hypotension, anemia, and hypoxia (190). Conditions that increase myocardial oxygen consumption are tachycardia, increased preload, increased afterload, and increased contractility. Tachycardia and increased preload are the most important causes of ischemia, because both conditions decrease oxygen supply to the myocardium while simultaneously increasing myocardial oxygen demand. Tachycardia decreases the diastolic time, which, when the coronary arteries are perfused, decreases the volume of oxygen available to the myocardium. Increased preload increases the pressure exerted by the myocardial wall on the arterioles within it, thus decreasing myocardial blood flow.

Other factors associated with perioperative myocardial ischemia include physiologic responses to the stress of intubation, intravenous or arterial line placement, emergence from anesthesia, pain, and anxiety. These stresses result in catecholamine stimulation of the cardiovascular system, resulting in increased heart rate, blood pressure, and contractility, which may induce or worsen myocardial ischemia. Loss of intravascular volume because of third spacing of fluids or postoperative hemorrhage can induce ischemia.

Postoperative myocardial infarction is often difficult to diagnose. Chest pain, which is present in 90% of nonsurgical patients with myocardial infarction, may be present in only 50% of patients with postoperative infarction because myocardial pain may be masked by coexisting surgical pain and the use of analgesics (175). It is important to maintain a high level of suspicion for postoperative infarction in patients with coronary artery disease. The presence of arrhythmia, congestive heart failure, hypotension, dyspnea, or elevations of pulmonary artery pressure may indicate infarction and should prompt a thorough cardiac investigation and electrocardiographic monitoring. **Measurement of creatinine phosphokinase myocardial band (CPK-MB) isoenzyme and troponin T levels are the most sensitive and specific indicators of myocardial infarction, and assessments should be obtained for all patients suspected of myocardial infarction** (189).

Despite the high incidence of silent myocardial infarction, routine use of postoperative electrocardiography (ECG) for all patients with cardiovascular disease is controversial. Many patients will exhibit P-wave changes that spontaneously resolve and do not represent ischemia or infarction. Conversely, patients with proven myocardial infarctions may show few, if any, ECG abnormalities. The American College of Cardiology and American Heart Association advise consideration of postoperative surveillance via ST-segment monitoring for myocardial infarction in patients with known or suspected coronary artery disease (191). In a review of over 2,400 patients, the sensitivity of predicting postoperative cardiac events was 55% to 100%, specificity 37% to 85%, positive predictive value 7% to 57%, and negative predictive value 89% to 100% (192). If routine screening of asymptomatic patients is desired, ECG should be performed 24 hours following surgery because significant ECG changes that occur immediately postoperatively will persist for 24 hours. It is prudent to continue serial ECG assessments for at least 3 days postoperatively.

Postoperative management of patients with coronary artery disease is based on maximizing delivery of oxygen to the myocardium and decreasing myocardial oxygen utilization. Most patients benefit from supplemental oxygen in the postoperative period, although special care should be exercised in patients with COPD. Oxygenation can easily be monitored by pulse oximetry. Anemia is detrimental because of loss of oxygen-carrying capacity and resultant tachycardia and should, therefore, be carefully corrected in high-risk patients. Although transfusion criteria are not absolute, all patients with a hemoglobin less than 6 mg/dL, and hemoglobin of 6 to 10 mg/dL with significant cardiac risk factors should be offered blood transfusion (193).

Patients with coronary artery disease may benefit from pharmacologic control of hyperadrenergic states that result from increased postoperative catecholamine production. Beta-blockers decrease heart rate, myocardial contractility, and systemic blood pressure, all of which are increased by adrenergic stimulation. Perioperative use of β_1 selective beta-blocker is shown to significantly reduce perioperative ischemia, myocardial infarction, and overall mortality caused by cardiac death and congestive heart failure in the perioperative period (194–196). The POISE (Perioperative Ischemic Evaluation) trial, a randomized controlled trial of *metoprolol,* enrolling 8,000 patients undergoing noncardiac surgery, revealed a reduction in cardiovascular death, myocardial infarction, and cardiac arrest. There was an increased risk of stroke and total mortality (197). The AHA provides the following guidelines: Continue beta-blocker therapy in patients on baseline beta-blockers for treatment of cardiac disease. Consider initiating and titrating beta-blockers in patients with coronary artery disease or high cardiac risk (as defined by the presence of more than one clinical risk factor) who are undergoing intermediate-risk surgery (155). Therapy should be initiated at least 1 week before surgery to allow for proper titration. The timing and optimal duration of beta-blocker therapy remains an area of uncertainty. Nevertheless, for patients already on beta-blocker therapy, they should continue it perioperatively because abrupt withdrawal results in a rebound hyperadrenergic state.

Prophylactic use of other agents such as *nitroglycerin* and calcium-channel blockers remains controversial, as data did not show a consistent benefit toward reducing risk of ischemic cardiac events. *Nitroglycerin* may cause hypotension, which may worsen cardiac status (155).

Congestive Heart Failure

Patients with congestive heart failure (CHF) face a substantially increased risk of myocardial infarction during and after surgery (177). The postoperative development of pulmonary edema may be associated with a high mortality rate, especially if it occurs in the setting of cardiac ischemia (198,199). Because patients with heart failure at the time of surgery are significantly more likely to develop complications, every effort should be made to diagnose and treat CHF before surgery (178,200). The signs and symptoms of CHF are listed in Table 22.17 and should be assessed based on preoperative history and physical examination. Patients who are able to

Table 22.17 Signs and Symptoms of Congestive Heart Failure
1. Presence of an S_3 gallop
2. Jugular venous distention
3. Lateral shift of the point of maximal impulse
4. Lower-extremity edema
5. Basilar rales
6. Increased voltage on electrocardiogram
7. Evidence of pulmonary edema or cardiac enlargement on chest radiograph
8. Tachycardia

perform usual daily activities without developing CHF are at limited risk of perioperative heart failure.

To prevent severe postoperative complications, CHF must be corrected preoperatively. Treatment usually relies on aggressive diuretic therapy, although care must be taken to avoid dehydration, which may result in hypotension during the induction of anesthesia. Hypokalemia can result from diuretic therapy and is especially deleterious to patients who are taking *digitalis.* In addition to diuretics and *digitali*s, treatment often includes the use of preload- and afterload-reducing agents. Optimal use of these drugs and correction of CHF may be aided by consultation with a cardiologist. It is preferable to continue the usual regimen of cardioactive drugs throughout the perioperative period.

Postoperative CHF frequently results from excessive administration of intravenous fluids and blood products. Other common postoperative causes are myocardial infarction, systemic infection, pulmonary embolism, and cardiac arrhythmias. The cause of postoperative heart failure must be diagnosed because, to be successful, treatment should be directed simultaneously to the underlying cause. Postoperative diagnosis of CHF is more difficult than preoperative diagnosis because the signs and symptoms of CHF are not specific and may result from other causes. The most reliable method of detecting CHF is chest radiography, in which the presence of cardiomegaly or evidence of pulmonary edema is a helpful diagnostic feature.

Acute postoperative CHF frequently manifests as pulmonary edema. Treatment of pulmonary edema may include the use of intravenous *furosemide,* supplemental oxygen, *morphine sulfate,* and elevation of the head of the bed. Intravenous *aminophylline* may be useful if cardiogenic asthma is present. Electrocardiography, in addition to laboratory evaluation, including arterial blood gas, serum electrolyte, and renal function chemistry measurements, should be obtained expediently. If the patient's condition does not improve rapidly, she should be transferred to an intensive care unit.

Arrhythmias

Nearly all arrhythmias found in otherwise healthy patients are asymptomatic and of limited consequence. In patients with underlying cardiac disease, however, even brief episodes of arrhythmias may result in significant cardiac morbidity and mortality.

Preoperative evaluation of arrhythmias by a cardiologist and anesthesiologist is important because many anesthetic agents and surgical stress contribute to the development or worsening of arrhythmias. In patients undergoing continuous electrocardiographic monitoring during surgery, a 60% incidence of arrhythmias, excluding sinus tachycardia, are reported (201). **Patients with heart disease have an increased risk of arrhythmias, most commonly ventricular arrhythmias** (201). Patients without cardiac disease are more likely to develop supraventricular arrhythmias during surgery. Patients taking antiarrhythmic medications before surgery should continue taking those drugs during the perioperative period. Initiation of antiarrhythmic medications is rarely indicated preoperatively, but consultation with a cardiologist is recommended for patients in whom arrhythmias are detected before surgery.

Patients with first-degree atrioventricular (AV) block or asymptomatic Mobitz I (Wenckebach) second-degree AV block require no preoperative therapy. A pacemaker is appropriate in patients with symptomatic Mobitz II second- or third-degree AV block before elective surgery (202). In emergency situations, a pacing pulmonary artery catheter can be used. Before performing surgery on patients with a permanent pacemaker, the type and location of the pacemaker should be determined because electrocautery units may interfere with demand-type pacemakers (203). **When performing gynecologic surgery on patients with pacemakers, it is preferable to place the electrocautery unit ground plate on the leg to minimize interference by preventing the pacemaker generator from sitting within the electrocautery circuit and to maximize distance from the pacemaker device. If possible, use of bipolar cautery devices are recommended rather than monopolar devices. In patients with a demand pacemaker in place, the pacemaker should be converted preoperatively to the fixed-rate (or asynchronous) mode. Although this can be accomplished oftentimes by placing a magnet over the pacemaker, it may be better to reprogram the pacemaker preoperatively and then again postoperatively. Patients should be monitored continuously intraoperatively with both telemetry and continuous pulse oximeter. Close coordination with anesthesia and cardiology is imperative. Patients with an implantable cardioverter defibrillator device should have their device programmed off prior to surgery and reprogrammed postoperatively (155).**

Surgery is not contraindicated in patients with bundle branch blocks or hemiblocks (204). Perioperative mortality rates are not increased by bundle-branch block. Complete heart block rarely develops during noncardiac surgical procedures in patients with conduction system disease. The presence of a left bundle-branch block may indicate the presence of aortic stenosis, which can increase surgical mortality if it is severe.

Valvular Heart Disease

Although there are many forms of valvular heart disease, two types—aortic and mitral stenosis—primarily are associated with significantly increased operative risk (205). Patients with significant aortic stenosis appear to be at greatest risk, which is increased in the presence of atrial fibrillation, congestive heart failure, or coronary artery disease. Significant stenosis of aortic or mitral valves should be repaired before elective gynecologic surgery (176).

Severe valvular heart disease usually is evident during physical exertion. Common findings in such patients are listed in Table 22.18. The classic history presented by patients with severe aortic stenosis includes exercise dyspnea, angina, and syncope, whereas symptoms of mitral stenosis are paroxysmal and effort dyspnea, hemoptysis, and orthopnea. Most patients have a remote history of rheumatic fever. Severe stenosis of either valve is considered to be a valvular area of less than 1 cm^2, and diagnosis can be confirmed by echocardiography or cardiac catheterization.

Patients with valvular abnormalities are subdivided by the American Heart Association into risk groups for the development of subacute bacterial endocarditis following surgery. **Patients in the highest risk groups should receive prophylactic antibiotics immediately preoperatively to prevent subacute bacterial endocarditis** (Table 22.8). As defined by the American Heart Association, only patients with prosthetic cardiac valves, congenital heart disease, and cardiac transplantation who develop cardiac valvulopathy should receive perioperative endocarditis prophylaxis (76). All other patients do not require antibiotics for subacute bacterial endocarditis prophylaxis. Routine prophylaxis for GI or GU procedures is not recommended. Only in cases of a known infection of the GI or GU tract should antibiotics coverage for enterococcus with *amoxicillin* or *ampicillin* or *vancomycin* be provided.

Patients with aortic and mitral stenosis tolerate sinus tachycardia and other tachyarrhythmias poorly. In patients with aortic stenosis, sufficient levels of *digitalis* should be provided to correct preoperative tachyarrhythmias, and *propranolol* may be used to control sinus tachycardia. Patients with mitral valve stenosis often have atrial fibrillation and, if present, *digitalis* should be used to reduce rapid ventricular response.

Patients with mechanical heart valves usually tolerate surgery well (206). These patients should receive antibiotic prophylaxis (Table 22.8). If the patient is taking *aspirin* therapy, it should be discontinued 1 week before the procedure and restarted as soon as it is considered safe by the

Table 22.18 Signs and Symptoms of Valvular Heart Disease
Aortic stenosis
1. Systolic murmur at right sternal border, which radiates into carotids
2. Decreased systolic blood pressure
3. Apical heave
4. Chest radiograph with calcified aortic ring, left ventricular enlargement
5. Electrocardiogram with high R waves, depressed T waves in lead I, and precordial leads
Mitral stenosis
1. Precordial heave
2. Diastolic murmur at apex
3. Mitral opening snap
4. Suffused face and lips
5. Chest radiograph with left atrial dilation
6. Electrocardiogram with large P waves and right axis deviation

surgeon. Patients with a bileaflet aortic valve with no risk factors (atrial fibrillation, previous thromboembolism, left ventricular dysfunction, a hypercoagulable state, older generation thrombogenic valve) generally do not require anticoagulation bridging. *Warfarin* should be stopped 72 hours prior to the procedure and resumed 24 hours after the procedure. In contrast, patients with a mechanical aortic valve and any above mentioned risk factor, or a mechanical mitral valve, should be bridged with intravenous unfractionated *heparin* when the INR falls below 2. The *heparin* drip should be stopped approximately 6 to 8 hours before the procedure and restarted as soon as possible after surgery when the patient is deemed stable from postoperative bleeding risk. The *heparin* bridge can be stopped when the INR reaches therapeutic levels (207).

In the postoperative period, patients with mitral stenosis should be carefully monitored for pulmonary edema because they may not be able to compensate for the amount of intravenous fluid administered during surgery. Prevention of tachycardia is important, as it may lead to pulmonary edema. Patients with mitral stenosis frequently have pulmonary hypertension and decreased airway compliance. They may require more pulmonary support and therapy postoperatively, including prolonged mechanical ventilation.

For patients with significant aortic stenosis, it is imperative that a sinus rhythm be maintained during the postoperative period. Even sinus tachycardia can be deleterious because it shortens the diastolic time. Bradycardia less than 45 beats per minute should be treated with *atropine*. Supraventricular dysrhythmias may be controlled with *verapamil* or direct-current cardioversion. Particular attention should be provided to the maintenance of proper fluid status, digoxin levels, electrolyte levels, and blood replacement.

Hypertension

Patients with controlled essential hypertension have no increased risk of perioperative cardiac morbidity or mortality (208). Patients with concomitant heart disease are at elevated risk and should be completely evaluated by a cardiologist preoperatively. Laboratory studies should include an ECG, chest radiography, blood count, urinalysis, and serum electrolytes and creatinine measurement. Antihypertensive medications should be continued perioperatively. Beta-blockers should be continued, parenterally if necessary, to avoid rebound tachycardia, hypercontractility, and hypertension. *Clonidine* may cause significant rebound hypertension if withdrawn acutely. Angiotensin converting enzyme inhibitor agents and angiotensin II receptor antagonists are associated with increased intraoperative hypotension and perioperative renal dysfunction possibly resulting from a hypovolumic state. It may be prudent to withhold these agents on the morning of surgery and resume them postoperatively when good renal function and euvolumia is confirmed (155).

Patients with diastolic pressures higher than 110 mm Hg or systolic pressures higher than 180 mm Hg should receive medication to control their hypertension before surgery. Beta-blockers may be particularly effective agents for treatment of preoperative hypertension (179). Chronically hypertensive patients are very susceptible to intraoperative hypotension because of impaired autoregulation of blood flow to the brain and require a higher mean arterial pressure to maintain adequate perfusion (209). During induction of anesthesia, episodes of hypertension occur, and such episodes are seen more frequently in patients with baseline hypertension.

Postoperative hypertension is usually treated parenterally because gastrointestinal absorption may be diminished, and transdermal absorption can be erratic in patients who are cold and rewarming. Commonly used parenteral antihypertensives are listed in Table 22.19.

Perioperative Antiplatelet Agents

Increasing numbers of patients undergo coronary revascularization procedures, otherwise known as coronary artery bypass grafting, or percutaneous coronary intervention, typically stent placement. With the evolution of bare metal and drug-eluting stents, perioperative management of cardiovascular thrombotic risk versus perioperative bleeding and mortality is challenged. Given that drug-eluting stents generally require 12 months' treatment with dual agent *aspirin* and thienopyridine (i.e., clopidogrel), the American College of Cardiology and American Heart Association (ACC/AHA) guidelines recommend avoiding elective surgery within 12 months of drug-eluting stent placement. When surgery cannot wait, the ACC/AHA recommends continuation of *aspirin* perioperatively, discontinuation of *thienopyridine* 5 days prior to surgery, and resuming it as soon as possible postoperatively. Ultimately the risk of perioperative morbidity secondary to bleeding must be weighed against the risk of repeat thrombosis and cardiovascular morbidity and mortality. If a patient requires new placement of a cardiac stent and requires a

Table 22.19 Common Parenteral Antihypertensives

Drug	Route	Initial Dose	Onset	Duration	Side Effects
Nitroprusside	IV infusion	0.5 μg/min	Immediate	2–5 min	Tachycardia, nausea
Labetalol	IV infusion	20 mg	5–10 min	4 h	Bronchospasm, dizziness, nausea
Esmolol	IV infusion	50 μg/min	2 h	9 min	Headache, somnolence, dizziness, hypotension
Nifedipine	Sublingual	10 mg	5 min	2 min	Hypotension, headache, dizziness, nausea, peripheral edema
Verapamil	IV infusion	5–10 mg	3–5 min	2–5 h	Nausea, headache, hypotension, dizziness, pulmonary edema

IV, intravenous.

noncardiac surgery in the following 12 months, placement of a bare metal stent is recommended rather than a drug-eluting stent, as these require only 4 to 6 weeks of dual-antiplatelet therapy. Again, *aspirin* should be continued perioperatively. Following a newly placed bare metal stent, noncardiac surgery should be scheduled at least 30 to 45 days after the stent placement to decrease cardiac morbidity (179).

Hemodynamic Monitoring

Hemodynamic monitoring is integral to the perioperative management of patients with cardiovascular and pulmonary diseases. The major impetus for this advancement resides in the need for the quantitative estimate of cardiac function, resulting in the development of bedside pulmonary artery catheterization. The impact of monitoring cardiac function is demonstrated by the significant reduction of myocardial infarctions in high-risk patients who are aggressively monitored for 72 to 96 hours postoperatively (175).

Before the development of the pulmonary artery catheter, central venous pressure (CVP) measurement was used to assess intravascular volume status and cardiac function. To measure the CVP, a catheter is placed in the central venous system, most frequently the superior vena cava. A water manometer or a calibrated pressure transducer is connected to the CVP line, allowing an estimation of right atrial pressure. Right atrial pressure is determined by the balance between cardiac output and venous return. Cardiac output is determined by heart rate, myocardial contractility, preload, and afterload. If the pulmonary vascularity and left ventricular function are normal, the CVP accurately reflects the left ventricular end-diastolic pressure (LVEDP). The LVEDP reflects cardiac output or systemic perfusion and was considered the standard estimator of left ventricular pump function. Venous return is determined primarily by the mean systemic pressure, which propels blood toward the heart, balanced against resistance to venous return, which acts in the opposite direction. If right ventricular function is normal, the CVP accurately reflects intravascular volume.

Left and right ventricular function is frequently abnormal or discordant; therefore, the relationship of CVP to cardiac function and to intravascular volume is not maintained. When this occurs, measurement of pulmonary artery occlusion pressure can be used to accurately assess volume status and cardiovascular function. The use of a pulmonary artery catheter allows detection of changes in cardiovascular function with more sensitivity and rapidity than clinical observation.

The balloon-tipped pulmonary artery catheter (Swan-Ganz catheter) can measure pulmonary artery and pulmonary artery occlusion pressures (210). The catheter can measure cardiac output, be used to perform intracavitary electrocardiography, and provide temporary cardiac pacing. The standard pulmonary artery occlusion catheter is a 7-French, radiopaque, flexible, polyvinyl chloride, 4-lumen catheter with a 1.5-mL latex balloon at its distal tip. Most often, a right internal jugular cannulation is used for placement of the catheter, because this site provides the most direct access into the right atrium and has fewer complications when compared with a subclavian route of placement. After the catheter is placed into the right atrium, the balloon is inflated, and the catheter is pulled by blood flow through the right ventricle into the pulmonary artery. The position of the catheter can be identified and followed by the various pressure waveforms generated by the right atrium, right ventricle, and pulmonary artery. As the catheter passes through increasingly smaller branches of the pulmonary artery, the inflated balloon eventually occludes the pulmonary artery.

The distal lumen of the catheter, which is beyond the balloon, measures left atrial pressure (LAP) and, in the absence of mitral valvular disease, LAP approximates LVEDP. Pulmonary–capillary wedge pressure (PCWP) equals the LAP, which equals LVEDP and is normal at 8 to 12 mm Hg. Because the standard pulmonary artery catheter has an incorporated thermistor, thermodilution studies can be performed to determine cardiac output. This thermodilution method is performed by injecting cold 5% dextrose in water through the proximal port of the catheter, which cools the blood entering the right atrium. The change in temperature measured at the more distal thermistor (4 cm from the catheter tip) generates a curve proportional to cardiac output. Knowledge of the cardiac output is helpful in establishing cardiovascular diagnoses. For example, a patient with hypotension, low-to-normal wedge pressure, and a cardiac output of 3 L per minute is most likely hypovolemic. The same patient with a cardiac output of 8 L per minute is probably septic with resultant low systemic vascular resistance.

Pulmonary artery catheters are associated with a small but significant complication rate. The complications can be grouped into those occurring during venous cannulation or insertion, during maintenance and use, and those related to interpretation of hemodynamic data (210). The most common problems encountered during venous access are cannulation of the carotid or subclavian artery and introduction of a pneumothorax. Problems resulting from the catheter itself include dysrhythmias, sepsis, and disruption of the pulmonary artery. Pulmonary artery catheters (PAC) should be placed under the supervision of experienced personnel in a setting in which complications can be rapidly diagnosed and treated. Accessory equipment such as resuscitation equipment and an external pacing device must be immediately available. Ultrasound and fluoroscopic equipment if available may aid in PAC placement (211).

The effect of PAC use on patient outcome is controversial. Several large trials did not confer a definite benefit to PAC use. One multi-institutional study examined the association of PAC placement within the first 24 hours of hospital stay and its associated outcomes. They found a higher mortality rate in patients who received a PAC than those who did not have a PAC (212). The study was limited because it was retrospective and not randomized. A randomized controlled trial of 1,994 high-risk (American Society of Anesthesiologists class III or IV risk) patients age 60 or older undergoing urgent or elective major noncardiac surgery compared outcomes of those who underwent PAC placement versus standard care. Results analyzed by a blinded assessor revealed no benefit of PAC over standard care with central venous catheters (213). Another randomized controlled trial enrolling 65 intensive care units in the United Kingdom found no difference in mortality among critically ill patients managed with or without a PAC (214). A meta-analysis of 13 randomized controlled trials of PAC use found no significant difference in mortality rates and an increased use of ionotropes and intravenous vasodilators (215). **Routine preoperative use of PAC in noncardiac surgery patients is no longer indicated. Use of PAC in critically ill patients postoperatively remains controversial.**

Hematologic Disorders

The presence of hematologic disorders, although uncommon in gynecologic patients, significantly affects operative morbidity and mortality and should be considered routinely in preoperative evaluation. Preoperative assessment should include consideration of anemia, platelet and coagulation disorders, white blood cell function, and immunity.

Anemia

Moderate anemia is not in itself a contraindication to surgery because it can be corrected by transfusion. If possible, surgery should be postponed until the cause of the anemia can be identified and the anemia corrected without resorting to transfusion. By tradition, anesthetic and surgical practice recommended a hemoglobin level of greater than 10 g/dL or a hematocrit of greater than 30%. Data suggest a lower tolerance for pre- and intraoperative transfusion threshold to improve intra- and postoperative morbidity and mortality (216–219). It remains that no universal "transfusion threshold" is agreed upon, but that a hematocrit of less than 24% should prompt strong consideration (219). The circulating blood volume provides oxygen-carrying capacity and tissue oxygenation. Usually this capacity is reflected by the hemoglobin level and hematocrit. Under certain circumstances this is not the case. After an acute blood loss or before plasma expansion by extracellular fluid occurs, hematocrit measurements may be normal despite a low circulating blood volume. Conversely, overhydration may result in low hematocrit and hemoglobin levels despite adequate red blood cell mass.

Individual tolerance of anemia depends on overall physical fitness and cardiovascular reserve. The effects of anemia depend on its magnitude, the rate at which it occurs, the oxygen requirement of the patient, and the ability of physiologic mechanisms to compensate (220). Maintenance of adequate tissue perfusion requires an increase in cardiac output as hemoglobin concentration falls (193). In the healthy patient, oxygen delivery is unchanged when it falls below 7 g/dL (221). In contrast, a patient with ischemic heart disease will not tolerate anemia as well (222). The presence of cardiac, pulmonary, or other serious illness justifies a more conservative approach to the management of anemia. Patients with longstanding anemia may have normal blood volume levels and tolerate surgical procedures well. There is no evidence that mild to moderate anemia increases perioperative morbidity or mortality (222).

Autologous blood transfusion may be an acceptable option for patients. Patients with normal hematocrit levels may store autologous blood preoperatively to reduce the need for allogenic blood transfusion and minimize the risk of infections and immunologic problems (193). *Recombinant human erythropoietin* may increase collection and reduce preoperative anemia in these patients (223,224). Intraoperative blood collection and homologous transfusion can be employed to limit the need for allogenic blood transfusion.

Autologous blood donation is advocated as a safer alternative for the patient; however, the use of preoperative autologous blood donation has come under scrutiny (225,226). **Preoperative autologous blood may lead to more liberal blood transfusion, iatrogenic anemia, volume overload, and bacterial contamination** (227). Preoperative autologous blood donation is poorly cost-effective (228). The National Heart, Lung, and Blood Institute does not recommend collection of autologous blood for procedures with a likelihood of transfusion less than 10%, such as uncomplicated abdominal and vaginal hysterectomies (229).

Platelet and Coagulation Disorders

Surgical hemostasis is provided by platelet adhesion to injured vessels, which plugs the opening as the coagulation cascade is activated, resulting in the formation of fibrin clots. Functional platelets and coagulation pathways are necessary to prevent excessive surgical bleeding. Platelet dysfunction is encountered preoperatively more frequently than coagulation disorders.

Platelets may be deficient in both number and function. The normal peripheral blood count is 150,000 to 400,000 per mm^3, and the normal lifespan of a platelet is approximately 10 days. Although there is no clear-cut correlation between the degree of thrombocytopenia and the presence or amount of bleeding, several generalizations can be made. If the platelet count is higher than 100,000/mm^3 and the platelets are functioning normally, there is little chance of excessive bleeding during surgical procedures. Patients with a platelet count higher than 75,000/mm^3 almost always have normal bleeding times, and a platelet count higher than 50,000/mm^3 is probably adequate. **A platelet count lower than 20,000/mm^3 often will be associated with severe and spontaneous bleeding.** Platelet counts higher than 1,000,000/mm^3 are often, paradoxically, associated with bleeding.

If the patient's platelet count is lower than 100,000/mm^3, an assessment of bleeding time should be obtained. If the bleeding time is abnormal and surgery must be performed, an attempt should be made to raise the platelet count by administering platelet transfusions immediately before surgery. In patients with immune destruction of platelets, human leukocyte antigen (HLA)–matched donor-specific platelets may be required to prevent rapid destruction of transfused platelets. If surgery can be postponed, a hematology consultation should be obtained to identify and treat the cause of the platelet abnormality.

Abnormally low platelet counts result from either decreased production or increased consumption of platelets. Although there are numerous causes of thrombocytopenia, most are exceedingly uncommon. Decreased platelet production may be drug induced and is associated with the use of sulfonamides, cinchona alkaloids, *thiazide* diuretics, NSAIDs, gold salts, *penicillamine,* anticonvulsants, and *heparins* (230). Decreased platelet count is a feature of several diseases, including vitamin B$_{12}$ and folate deficiency, aplastic anemia, myeloproliferative disorders, renal failure, and viral infections. Inherited congenital thrombocytopenia is extremely rare. More commonly, thrombocytopenia results from immune destruction of platelets by diseases such as idiopathic thrombocytopenia purpura and collagen vascular disorders. **Consumptive thrombocytopenia is a feature of disseminated intravascular coagulation, which is**

encountered most frequently in conjunction with sepsis or malignancy in the preoperative population.

Platelet dysfunction most often is acquired, but may be inherited. Occasionally, a patient with von Willebrand disease, the second most common inherited disorder of coagulation, may be encountered in the preoperative setting. More commonly, platelet dysfunction results from the use of drugs (e.g., *aspirin* and *amitriptyline*), and in patients with resulting prolonged bleeding time, the drug should be withheld for 7 to 10 days before surgery. Uremia and hepatic diseases can affect platelet function.

Platelet dysfunction is more difficult to diagnose than abnormalities of platelet count. A history of easy bruising, petechiae, bleeding from mucous membranes, or prolonged bleeding from minor wounds may signify an underlying abnormality of platelet function. Such dysfunction can be identified with the help of a bleeding time, but full characterization of the underlying etiology should be carried out with hematologic consultation. If at all possible, surgery should be postponed until therapy is instituted.

Disorders of the coagulation cascade often are diagnosed through a personal or family history of excessive bleeding during minor surgery, childbirth, or menses. Many women with menorrhagia are referred for surgical intervention and require a thorough preoperative evaluation for possible inherited disorders of hemostasis, such as factor VIII (hemophilia), factor IX (Christmas disease), factor XI deficiencies, and von Willebrand disease. Von Willebrand disease is the most common hereditary bleeding disorder, with prevalence in the general population of roughly 1% (231). Seventy percent to 90% of patients with von Willebrand disease have menorrhagia (231). Identified women can be treated effectively with *desmopressin* nasal spray, avoiding unanticipated or excessive bleeding during surgery (232). In the absence of a genetic diagnosis, the diagnosis of von Willebrand disease is difficult and involves a combination of clinical and laboratory assessments, including von Willebrand factor antigen and von Willebrand factor functional activity or ristocetin cofactor assay (232). Physiologic fluctuations occur with von Willebrand factor levels, requiring repeat testing and consultation or referral to a hematologist. It is recommended that women presenting with menorrhagia without obvious pelvic abnormalities should be routinely screened for inherited bleeding disorders before undergoing invasive procedures.

There are few commonly prescribed drugs that affect coagulation factors, the exceptions being *warfarin* and *heparin*. Disease states that may be associated with decreased coagulation factor levels are primarily liver disease, vitamin K deficiency (secondary to obstructive biliary disease, intestinal malabsorption, or antibiotic reduction of bowel flora), and disseminated intravascular coagulation.

Preoperative laboratory screening for coagulation deficiencies is controversial. Routine screening is not warranted in patients who do not have historical evidence of a bleeding problem (233). Patients who are seriously ill or who will be undergoing extensive surgical procedures should undergo testing preoperatively to determine prothrombin time, partial thromboplastin time, fibrinogen level, and platelet count.

White Blood Cells and Immune Function

Abnormally high or low white blood cell counts are not an absolute contraindication to surgery; they should be considered relative to the need for surgery. Evaluation of an elevated or decreased white blood cell count should be undertaken before elective surgery. **Patients with absolute granulocyte counts lower than 1,000/mm^3 are at increased risk of severe infection and perioperative morbidity and mortality and should undergo surgery only for life-threatening indications** (234).

Blood Component Replacement

Packed red blood cells, which may be stored for several weeks, are used for most postoperative transfusions. Most clotting factors are stable for long periods. The exceptions are factors V and VIII, which decrease to 15% and 50% of normal, respectively. Most hematologic problems observed in the postoperative period are related to perioperative bleeding and blood component replacement. Although the primary cause of the bleeding is usually lack of surgical hemostasis, other factors, including deranged coagulation, may compound the problem. Such coagulopathy can result from massive transfusion (less than one blood volume) and is thought to be caused by dilution of platelets and labile coagulation factors by platelet- and factor-poor packed red blood cells (PRBCs), fibrinolysis, and disseminated intravascular coagulation.

A review in *Transfusion* questioned the traditional practice of limiting blood component replacement in massive transfusion. Summarizing 14 articles and encompassing nearly 4,600 patients, the conclusions note a decrease in all-cause mortality with more liberal transfusion of platelets and fresh frozen plasma (FFP) (235).

A task force for the American Society of Anesthesiologists **recommended critical values for replacement in patients with massive transfusion and microvascular bleeding** (193):

1. **Platelet transfusion usually is indicated for counts less than 50,000/mm³ (with intermediate platelet counts, i.e., 50,000/mm³ to 100,000/mm³, the transfusion of platelet concentrates should be based on the risk of more significant bleeding).**

2. **Fresh frozen plasma therapy is indicated if the prothrombin or activated partial thromboplastin time values exceed 1.5 times the normal value.**

3. **Cryoprecipitate transfusion is indicated if fibrinogen concentrations decrease to less than 80 to 100 mg/dL.**

Cryoprecipitate transfusions are recommended for prophylaxis in nonbleeding perioperative patients with fibrinogen deficiencies or von Willebrand disease refractory to *desmopressin acetate* and bleeding patients with von Willebrand disease (232).

Donor blood is stored in the presence of citrate, which chelates calcium to prevent clotting, increasing the theoretical risk of hypocalcemia following massive transfusion. Citrate is metabolized at a rate equivalent to 20 U of blood transfused per hour; thus, routine supplementation of calcium is unnecessary. Close monitoring of calcium levels is required in patients with hypothermia, liver disease, or hyperventilation because citrate metabolism may be slowed. Hepatic metabolism of citrate to bicarbonate can result in metabolic alkalosis following transfusion, resulting in subsequent hypokalemia, despite the high level of extracellular potassium in stored blood.

Pulmonary Disease

In patients undergoing abdominal surgery, several pulmonary physiologic changes manifest secondary to immobilization, anesthetic irritation of the airways, and the splinting of breathing that inevitably occurs secondary to incisional pain. Pulmonary physiologic changes include a decrease in the functional residual capacity (FRC), an increase in ventilation perfusion mismatching, and impaired mucociliary clearance of secretions from the tracheobronchial tree (236). **Risk factors for postoperative pulmonary complications include the following** (237,238) (Table 22.20):

- **Upper abdominal or thoracic, or abdominal aortic aneurysm surgery**

- **Surgical procedure time longer than 3 hours**

- **COPD**

- **Smoking within 2 months of surgery**

- **Use of *pancuronium* for general anesthesia**

Table 22.20 Predictors of Postoperative Pulmonary Complications[a]	
Parameter	*Value*
Maximal breathing capacity	<50% predicted
FEV_1	<1 L
FVC	<70% predicted
FEV_1/FVC	<65% predicted
PaO_2	<60 mm Hg
$PaCO_2$	>45 mm Hg

FEV, forced expiration volume; FVC, forced vital capacity; PaO_2, partial pressure of oxygen, arterial; $PaCO_2$, partial pressure of carbon dioxide, arterial.
[a]*Complication* defined as atelectasis or pneumonia.
Adapted from **Blosser SA, Rock P.** Asthma and chronic obstructive lung disease. In: **Breslow MJ, Miller CJ, Rogers MC, eds.** *Perioperative management.* St. Louis, MO: Mosby, 1990:259–280.

- **New York Heart Association Class II pulmonary hypertension**
- **General anesthesia**
- **Pancuronium**
- **Emergency surgery**
- **Poor nutrition (serum albumin <3.5mg/dL or BUN <8).**

Probable risk factors include general anesthesia, preoperative partial pressure of carbon dioxide, arterial ($PaCO_2$) greater than 45 mm Hg, and emergency surgery. Risk factors that could increase the postoperative risk are upper respiratory infection, abnormal chest x-ray, and age. Preoperative pulmonary function testing is of unproven value in patients not undergoing thoracic surgery (237). This is based on multiple reasons: first, a lower limit of forced expiration volume (FEV_1) did not correlate with pulmonary complications; second, pulmonary complications can occur in the context of a normal FEV_1; and third, if an FEV_1 were able to predict a pulmonary complication putting the patient at increased risk, it would not change the need for aggressive postoperative prophylactic measures (237). The routine performance of preoperative arterial blood gas measurements does not improve assessment of risk (236). Non-invasive pulse-oximetry measurements can detect patients with hypoxemia (236). The presence of hypercarbia on arterial blood gas measurements does not predict postoperative pulmonary complications (236).

Young, healthy patients rarely have abnormal chest x-rays. Chest x-rays should not be performed routinely in these patients. Most patients with abnormal chest x-rays have history or physical examination findings suggestive of pulmonary disease. Chest x-rays should be limited to patients older than 50 years of age, with a history of smoking or of pulmonary disease, who have evidence of cardiopulmonary disease and in whom a metastatic malignancy is suspected. Although they have limited usefulness in predicting postoperative pulmonary complications, chest x-rays provide a valuable baseline in elderly patients, patients with chronic pulmonary diseases, and those with known lung metastases (236–238).

Asthma

Asthma affects approximately 22 million individuals in the United States, including 6% of children (239). It is characterized by a history of episodic wheezing, physiologic evidence of reversible obstruction of the airways either spontaneously or following bronchodilator therapy, and pathologic evidence of chronic inflammatory changes in the bronchial submucosa. Asthma is not a disease of airway physiology in which hypertrophy and increased contractility of bronchial smooth muscle is the dominant lesion; rather, it is an inflammatory disease affecting the airways that secondarily results in epithelial damage, leukocytic infiltration, and increased sensitivity of the airways to a number of stimuli. The treatment of asthma is directed toward relaxing the airways and alleviating inflammation (239).

Multiple stimuli are noted to precipitate or exacerbate asthma, including environmental allergens or pollutants, respiratory tract infections, exercise, cold air, emotional stress, nonselective beta-adrenergic blockers, and NSAIDs (239). Management of asthma includes removal of the inciting stimuli as well as use of appropriate pharmacologic therapy. The optimal therapy for asthma involves managing the acute symptoms and long-term management of the inflammatory component of the disease.

Pharmacotherapy of Asthma

The treatment of asthma is divided into long-term control modalities and short-term modalities. **Recognizing the underlying pathophysiology in asthma as an inflammatory condition, inhaled corticosteroids are the cornerstone for maintenance therapy.** Onset of action is slow (several hours), and up to 3 months of steroid therapy may be required for optimal improvement of bronchial hyperresponsiveness. Even with acute bronchospasm, steroid treatment can enhance the beneficial effect of beta-adrenergic treatment. During acute exacerbations of asthma, a short course of oral steroids, in addition to inhaled steroids, may be necessary. For adults with chronic asthma, only a minority will require chronic oral steroid therapy. Patients taking oral steroids should receive intravenous steroid support in the form of 100 mg of hydrocortisone IV every 8 hours perioperatively, sharply tapering within 24 hours of surgery to avoid adrenal insufficiency. Other long-term control therapies include (239):

1. Leukotriene modifiers (i.e., *montelukast*): These agents interfere with leukotrienes, substances released from mast cells, eosinophils, and basophils important in the inflammatory response.

2. *Cromolyn sodium:* Highly active in the treatment of seasonal allergic asthma in children and young adults. It is usually not as effective in older patients or in patients in whom asthma is not allergic in nature.

3. Immunomodulators: *Omalizumab,* a monoclonal antibody to immunoglobulin E (IgE), has gained support for prevention and may be an important adjunct in symptomatic suppression.

4. Long term beta$_2$-adrenergic agonists (i.e., *salmeterol*): Although not appropriate for single agent management or use in mild disease, they are an important adjunct in the suppression of symptoms in patients with significant disease.

5. Methylxanthines (i.e., *theophylline*): These were relegated to third-line status in the management of asthma. *Theophylline* toxicity can develop when other drugs such as *ciprofloxacin, erythromycin, allopurinol, Inderal,* or *cimetidine* are concomitantly administered. Therapeutic serum levels must be monitored closely.

β_2-adrenergic agonists remain the first-line drugs for acute asthma attacks. These drugs, inhaled four to six times daily, rapidly relax smooth muscle in the airways and are effective for up to 6 hours. Studies of beta$_2$ agonists in chronic asthma failed to show any influence of these agents on the inflammatory component of asthma. β_2 agonists are recommended for short-term relief of bronchospasm ("rescue inhalers") or as first-line treatment for patients with very infrequent symptoms or symptoms provoked solely by exercise (239).

Anticholinergic agents are weak bronchodilators that work via inhibition of muscarinic receptors in the smooth muscle of the airways. The quaternary derivatives such as *ipratropium bromide* (*Atrovent*) are available in an inhaled form that is not absorbed systemically. Anticholinergic drugs may provide additional benefit in conjunction with standard steroid and bronchodilator therapy but should not be used as single-agent therapy because they do not inhibit mast cell degranulation, do not have any effect on the late response to allergens, and do not have an anti-inflammatory effect (239).

Perioperative Management of Asthma

In patients with asthma, elective surgery should be postponed whenever possible until pulmonary function and pharmacotherapeutic management are optimized. The most recent guidelines of the American Academy of Allergy, Asthma and Immunology's recommend three interventions to reduce perioperative pulmonary complications related to asthma (239):

1. Review the patient's asthmatic control, including the need for oral steroids.

2. Optimize the patient's symptomatic control through the use of long-acting pharmacotherapy, including oral steroids if needed.

3. For patients on oral steroid therapy within 6 months of therapy or for patients using large doses of inhaled corticosteroids, consider perioperative stress dose steroids.

For mild asthma, the use of inhaled beta-adrenergic agonists preoperatively may be all that is required. For chronic asthma, optimization of steroid therapy will greatly decrease alveolar inflammation and bronchiolar hyperresponsiveness. Inhaled beta$_2$-agonists should be added to therapy as needed for further control of asthma. Each drug prescribed should be used in maximal dosage before adding an additional agent. Preoperative treatment with combined corticosteroids and an inhaled beta$_2$-adrenergic agonist for a 5-day period may decrease the risk of postoperative bronchospasm in patients with asthma (240). For patients undergoing emergent surgery who have significant bronchoconstriction, a multimodal approach should be instituted, including aggressive bronchodilator inhalation therapy and intravenous steroid therapy. The role of spirometry, outside of cardiothoracic procedures, has limited value in predicting postoperative pulmonary complications and should be limited to the confirmation of undiagnosed obstructive pulmonary disease (241).

Chronic Obstructive Pulmonary Disease

COPD is the greatest risk factor for the development of postoperative pulmonary complications. COPD encompasses both chronic bronchitis and emphysema, disease entities that often occur in tandem. Cigarette smoke is implicated in the pathogenesis of both, and any treatment plan must include cessation of smoking (242). Chronic bronchitis is defined as the presence of productive cough on most days for at least 3 months per year and for at least 2 successive years (243). It is characterized by chronic airway inflammation and excessive mucus production. The histologic changes of emphysema include destruction of alveolar septa and distension of airspaces distal to terminal alveoli. The destruction of alveoli results in air trapping, loss of pulmonary elastic recoil, collapse of the airways in expiration, increased work of breathing, and significant ventilation-perfusion mismatching (243). The impaired ability to cough effectively and clear secretions predisposes patients with COPD to atelectasis and pneumonia in the postoperative period.

Patients with COPD and a history of heavy smoking account for most postoperative pulmonary complications in gynecologic surgical patients. The severity of COPD can be determined preoperatively via a thorough history and physical examination. According to recommendations regarding the use of preoperative pulmonary function tests by the American College of Physicians, these should be reserved for individuals in whom COPD is suspected, but unconfirmed (237,241). Typically, patients with COPD demonstrate impaired expiratory air flow, manifested by diminished FEV_1, forced vital capacity (FVC).

Data suggest that arterial blood gas measurements may show varying degrees of hypoxemia and hypercapnia: routine use of preoperative arterial blood gas measurement does not stratify patients into a higher risk subset for postoperative complications (236).

The preoperative preparation of the patient at risk for postoperative pulmonary complications should include cessation of smoking for as long as possible preoperatively; whereas 2 to 3 days of smoking abstinence are sufficient for carboxyhemoglobin levels to return to normal. One to 2 weeks of cessation decreases sputum volume. Two months of smoking abstinence is required to significantly lower the risk of postoperative pulmonary complications (236). Longer periods of abstinence can be counseled in patients undergoing elective surgery.

In patients with severe COPD, maximum improvement in airflow limitation can be achieved with a therapeutic trial of high-dose oral corticosteroids followed by a 2-week trial of high-dose inhaled steroid (*beclomethasone* 1.5 mg per day or the equivalent) in addition to inhaled bronchodilator therapy. Ideally, oral and inhaled steroid therapy should be initiated 1 to 2 weeks preoperatively. Inhaled steroids, in particular, address the inflammatory component of COPD. Oral steroid therapy initiated preoperatively should be maintained throughout the perioperative period and then tapered postoperatively. Beta-adrenergic agonist therapy can be initiated at least 72 hours preoperatively and is beneficial in patients who demonstrate either clinical or spirometric improvement on bronchodilators.

Patients with COPD and an active bacterial infection suggested by purulent sputum should undergo a full course of antibiotic therapy before surgery. The antibiotic used should cover the most likely etiologic organisms, *Streptococcus pneumoniae* and *Haemophilus influenzae*. In any patient with acute upper respiratory infection, surgery should be delayed if possible. The use of antibiotics to sterilize the sputum in the absence of evidence of an acute infection should be avoided because this practice may lead to bacterial resistance.

Aggressive pulmonary toilet, including incentive spirometry, chest physical therapy, and continuous positive airway pressure devices, reduced the risk of perioperative pulmonary complications in patients undergoing upper abdominal surgery, many of which can be instituted preoperatively (237).

Postoperative Pulmonary Management

Atelectasis

Atelectasis accounts for more than 90% of all postoperative pulmonary complications. The pathophysiology involves a collapse of the alveoli, resulting in ventilation-perfusion mismatching, intrapulmonary venous shunting, and a subsequent drop in the PaO_2. Collapsed alveoli are susceptible to superimposed infection, and if managed improperly, atelectasis will progress to pneumonia. Patients with atelectasis have a decreased FRC as well as decreased lung compliance, resulting in increased work during breathing. Despite the decrease in PaO_2, the partial pressure of carbon dioxide (PCO_2) remains unaffected unless atelectatic changes progress to large volumes of the lung or preexisting lung disease is present.

Physical findings associated with atelectasis may include a low-grade fever. Auscultation of the chest may reveal decreased breath sounds at the bases or dry rales upon inspiration. Percussion of the posterior thorax may suggest elevation of the diaphragm. Radiologic findings include the presence of horizontal lines or plates on posteroanterior chest x-rays, occasionally with adjacent areas containing hyperinflation. These changes are most pronounced during the first 3 postoperative days.

Therapy for atelectasis should be aimed at expanding the alveoli and increasing the FRC. The most important maneuvers are those that promote maximal inspiratory pressure, which is maintained for as long as possible. This exercise promotes an expansion of the alveoli and secretion of surfactant, which stabilizes alveoli. It can be achieved with aggressive supervised use of incentive spirometry, deep breathing exercises, coughing, and in some cases, the use of positive expiratory pressure with a mask (continuous positive airway pressure). Oversedation should be avoided, and patients should be encouraged to ambulate and change positions frequently. Fiberoptic bronchoscopy for removal of mucopurulent plugs should be reserved for patients who fail to improve with the usual measures.

Cardiogenic (High-Pressure) Pulmonary Edema

Cardiogenic pulmonary edema can result from myocardial ischemia, myocardial infarction, or from intravascular volume overload, particularly in patients who have low cardiac reserve or renal failure. The process usually begins with an increase in the fluid in the alveolar septa and bronchial vascular cuffs, ultimately seeping into the alveoli. Complete filling of the alveoli impairs secretion and production of surfactant. Concomitant with alveolar flooding, there is a decrease in lung compliance, impairment of the oxygen diffusion capacity, and an increase in the arteriolar–alveolar oxygen gradient. Ventilation-perfusion mismatching in the lung results in a decrease in the PaO_2, resulting eventually in decreased oxygenation of the tissues and impairment of cardiac contractility.

Symptoms may include tachypnea, dyspnea, wheezing, and use of the accessory muscles of respiration. Clinical signs may include distention of the jugular veins, peripheral edema, rales upon auscultation of the lungs, and an enlarged heart. Radiographic findings may include the presence of bronchiolar cuffing and increased interstitial fluid markings extending to the periphery of the lung. The diagnosis can be confirmed with the use of central hemodynamic monitoring, which will denote an elevated central venous pressure and, more specifically, an elevation in the pulmonary capillary wedge pressure.

The patient's volume status should be evaluated thoroughly. In addition, myocardial ischemia or infarction should be ruled out by performing ECG and analyzing cardiac enzyme levels. The management of cardiogenic pulmonary edema includes oxygen support, aggressive diuresis, and afterload reduction to increase the cardiac output. In the absence of myocardial infarction, an inotropic agent may be used. Mechanical ventilation should be reserved for cases of acute respiratory failure.

Noncardiogenic Pulmonary Edema (Adult Respiratory Distress Syndrome)

In contrast with cardiogenic pulmonary edema, in which alveolar flooding is a result of an increase in the hydrostatic pressure of the pulmonary capillaries, alveolar flooding in patients with adult respiratory distress syndrome (ARDS) is the result of an increase in pulmonary capillary permeability. The primary pathophysiologic process is one of damage to the capillary side of the alveolar–capillary membrane. This damage results in rapid movement of fluid containing high concentrations of protein from the capillaries to the pulmonary parenchyma and alveoli. Lung compliance decreases and oxygen diffusion capacity is impaired, resulting in hypoxemia. If not managed aggressively, respiratory failure may result; when managed aggressively, the mortality rate associated with ARDS is high. There are a number of causes and several distinct states of ARDS. **The causes of ARDS include shock, sepsis, multiple red blood cell transfusions, aspiration injury, inhalation injury, pneumonia, pancreatitis, disseminated intravascular coagulation, and fat emboli** (244). Twenty-eight-day mortality is reported between 25% to 40%, with overall mortality as high as 70% (244,245). Irrespective of the cause, which should be identified and treated if possible, the evolving clinical picture and management are very similar.

Clinically, ARDS passes through several stages. Initially, patients develop tachypnea and dyspnea with no remarkable findings on clinical evaluation or on chest x-ray. Chest x-rays eventually reveal bilateral diffuse pulmonary infiltrates. As lung compliance becomes impaired, functional residual capacity, tidal volume, and vital capacity decrease. The PaO_2 decreases and, characteristically, increases only marginally with oxygen supplementation. An attempt should be made to maintain the arterial oxygen level above 90%. This may be achievable initially by administering oxygen by mask. For patients with severe hypoxemia, endotracheal intubation with positive-pressure ventilation should be instituted. Traditionally, the goal was to maintain normal arterial gases, with increased minute ventilation and pressure as needed to maintain these, with little insight into the long-term repercussions that this modality employs. Data over the past 5 to 10 years show that "normal" or increased tidal volumes and pressures are linked to significant barotrauma and injury to alveoli. Elevated positive end-expiratory pressure (PEEP) increasingly was used to recruit alveoli, with decreases in the amount of fraction of inspired oxygen (FIO_2) and minute ventilation required to maintain oxygenation in this setting, with limited success when compared to lower PEEP levels, controlling for tidal volume and end-inspiratory pressures (246).

Attempts to manage and treat the cause of ARDS must include aggressive efforts toward hemodynamic and circulatory resuscitation in patients with shock. Nosocomial pneumonia is present in 50% of patients with ARDS, and broad-spectrum antibiotic therapy should be administered appropriately for patients with suspected pneumonia or sepsis. Patients who have disseminated intravascular coagulopathy may require replacement with cryoprecipitate or FFP. Other measures for general care should include the placement of a nasogastric tube, gastric acid suppression with H_2 blockers, and administration of steroids in patients with the fat emboli syndrome.

Hemodynamic monitoring is invaluable and should be initiated early in the course of the disease process in the appropriate intensive care unit setting. Patients with any evidence of fluid overload should receive aggressive diuresis, whereas others may require fluid resuscitation for maintenance of tissue perfusion while the pulmonary–capillary wedge pressure is maintained below 15 mm Hg. Pulmonary wedge pressure may be falsely elevated when PEEP is being applied. **The goal of management is to maintain the lowest pulmonary–capillary wedge pressure, with acceptable cardiac output and blood pressure.** In the setting of hypotension and oliguria, inotropic support with *dopamine* or *dobutamine* or both is helpful.

With aggressive management, particularly if the inciting cause is identified and treated, ARDS can be reversed during the first 48 hours with few sequelae. After the first 48 hours, progression of the ARDS will cause lung damage that may leave residual pulmonary fibrosis. The long-term outcome is usually apparent within the first 10 days, at which time approximately half of patients are weaned from ventilatory support or they die (244).

Renal Disease

The need for surgical intervention in patients with renal impairment resulted in the development of a very specialized medical approach to their care. Precautions are necessary to compensate for the kidneys' impaired ability to regulate fluids and electrolytes and excrete metabolic waste products. Equally important are the unique problems that develop in patients with chronic renal impairment, including an increased risk of sepsis, coagulation defects, impaired immune function and wound healing, and a propensity to develop specific acid-base abnormalities. Special consideration must be given to a variety of different medications, anesthetic agents, and numerous hematologic and nutritional factors that are important in the successful surgical care of patients with renal insufficiency.

Management of fluid levels and cardiovascular hemodynamics in patients with acute or chronic renal impairment is paramount. Intravascular fluid volume changes that lead to hypertension or hypotension are very common in these patients and often are difficult to manage secondary to autonomic dysfunction, acidosis, and other problems that are inherent to the underlying kidney disease. Patients undergoing dialysis in whom major abdominal or pelvic surgery is contemplated should be treated using invasive monitoring, both intra- and postoperatively. The results of physical examination and CVP monitoring correlate poorly with left cardiac filling pressures. Swan-Ganz catheter measurements will help guide fluid replacement and avoid volume overload. Invasive hemodynamic monitoring should be continued as needed throughout the first postoperative week because third spacing will occur during this period.

Postoperative dialysis usually is necessary to avoid problems associated with fluid overload and hyperkalemia. Dialysis-dependent patients should undergo dialysis approximately 24 hours following surgery. A short-lived but rather significant fall in the number of platelets occurs during dialysis; in addition, *heparin* is used in hemodialysis equipment to prevent clotting. Because of these factors and concerns about postoperative bleeding, dialysis is usually avoided during the first 12 to 24 hours following surgery. Although ischemic heart disease is the most common cause of death in patients with renal insufficiency, it is not a major cause of perioperative mortality (247). A large percentage of perioperative deaths of patients with renal insufficiency are associated with hyperkalemia that is controlled most effectively by dialysis (248).

Patients with chronic renal failure are at an increased risk for postoperative infections resulting from abnormalities in neutrophil and monocyte function (249). Appropriate preoperative antibiotic prophylaxis and accurate assessment of nutritional status help lower the incidence of postoperative infectious complications.

The major hematologic concern in patients with chronic renal insufficiency is the increased incidence of bleeding. These bleeding problems are secondary to abnormal bleeding times and, in particular, disorders of platelet function related to a decreased amount of factor VIII and von Willebrand antigen in the serum of uremic patients. Anemia, which is common in patients with renal insufficiency, can contribute to prolonged bleeding times (250). Abnormalities in arachidonic acid metabolism, acquired platelet storage pool deficiency, and disturbed regulation of platelet calcium content all contribute to an increased tendency for uremic patients to have significant bleeding during surgery (251). The bleeding time should be routinely checked preoperatively in these patients, and abnormalities should be corrected before surgery. Options for the correction of bleeding time in uremic patients include infusion of *desmopressin* or *cryoprecipitate,* both of which act to increase plasma levels of factor VIII and von Willebrand antigen (252,253).

Normal renal function is essential for maintenance of acid-base balance in the body. Patients with renal insufficiency can have a normal anion gap or an elevated anion gap acidosis. When mild renal insufficiency develops, a normal anion gap is present, whereas in more significant and severe renal dysfunction, an elevated anion gap acidosis occurs. Hemodialysis corrects metabolic acidosis. If a patient is severely acidotic (pH <7.15) and emergency surgery is planned, correction of the blood pH to 7.25 using intravenous *sodium bicarbonate* is indicated. However, correction of metabolic acidosis should be carried out slowly, because in patients with hypocalcemia, seizures may be precipitated (254). It is important to exclude other causes of elevated anion gap acidosis, such as ketoacidosis secondary to diabetes, lactic acidosis secondary to infection, or in rare instances, poisoning with *ethylene glycol, methanol,* or *aspirin.*

Impaired kidney function causes phosphate retention by the kidney and impaired vitamin D metabolism. Therefore, hypocalcemia is common in patients with renal insufficiency, but tetany and other signs of hypocalcemia are relatively uncommon because metabolic acidosis increases the level of ionized calcium. Oral phosphate binders, such as *aluminum hydroxide* (1 to 2 g per meal), and dietary phosphate restriction (1 g per day) is the usual treatment for hypocalcemia–hyperphosphatemia in patients with renal insufficiency. In chronic situations, because of central nervous system toxicity associated with elevated aluminum levels, it is preferable to treat hypocalcemia–hyperphosphatemia with large doses of *calcium carbonate* (6 to 12 g per day) rather than with the standard aluminum-containing antacids (255).

Approximately 20% of patients with renal insufficiency exhibit clinical evidence of protein calorie malnutrition. Vitamin deficiencies, most notably with water-soluble vitamins, occur with dialysis. Nutritional disturbances in patients with chronic renal insufficiency arise secondary to deficiencies in protein intake, and studies show that, in patients with chronic renal insufficiency, their kidneys are hyperfiltrating (256). Postoperatively, both protein and caloric intake may need to be increased dramatically to meet catabolic demands in surgical patients. As much as 1.5 g/kg of protein and 45 kcal/kg of calories may be needed (256).

Wound healing is impaired in patients with chronic renal failure, and wound dehiscence and evisceration are potential problems. Wound healing is most appropriately aided by nutritional assessment preoperatively and maintenance of adequate caloric and protein intake in the perioperative setting. Antibiotic prophylaxis should be used in these patients, and uremia should be treated with dialysis as indicated. A running mass closure of the midline vertical incision with continuous monofilament sutures should be used to decrease the risk of wound dehiscence and evisceration (256).

Patients with chronic renal disease have an altered ability to excrete drugs and are prone to significant metabolic derangements secondary to the altered bioavailability of many commonly used medications. Because of this, and the effect of dialysis on drug pharmacokinetics, the gynecologic surgeon and nephrologist must be aware of the lowered metabolism and bioavailability of narcotics, barbiturates, muscle relaxants, antibiotics, and other drugs that require renal clearance. Of particular note is the inability of patients with renal insufficiency to clear the neuromuscular blockade caused by *pancuronium* (257). Care must be taken with *D-tubocurarine,* especially if repeated doses are given (258). *Midazolam, propofol, vecuronium,* and *atracurium* are used safely in patients with renal failure (254). *Succinylcholine* is reported to cause significant hyperkalemic responses in patients with renal failure (259). When *succinylcholine* is used in patients with chronic renal insufficiency, careful monitoring of the serum potassium level is necessary (260).

Perioperative acute renal failure in previously normal patients may be caused by decreased renal perfusion, nephrotoxins, or both. Patients with impaired cardiac function, intravascular volume depletion, sepsis, or hypotension fall under the first category. Nephrotoxic medications such as *aminoglycosides,* chemotherapeutic agents such as *cisplatin,* or iodinated contrast agents fall under the second category (261–263). The risk of renal impairment becomes cumulative if more than one of these factors exist at the same time, and especially if a variety of factors are associated with intervascular volume depletion (264). Several measurements should be used to avoid acute renal failure. All nephrotoxic drugs should be discontinued when possible. When it is not practical to withdraw medication, strict attention should be paid to the pharmacokinetic characteristics of each drug and to the regular measurements of serum creatinine levels. Patients with diabetes should be given reduced doses of radiocontrast agents and should be well hydrated because they are particularly susceptible to renal injury from these materials (265). Volume repletion is essential to lower the incidence of renal impairment (266).

Liver Disease

Management of perioperative problems in gynecologic patients with liver disease requires a comprehensive understanding of normal liver physiology and the pathophysiology underlying diseases of the liver that may complicate surgery or recovery. **Patients with liver disease often have numerous complicated problems involving nutrition, coagulation, wound healing, encephalopathy, and infection.**

History and Physical Examination

Patients with a history of alcohol abuse, drug use, hepatitis, jaundice, blood product exposure, or a family member with liver disease should undergo biochemical evaluation. During the physical examination, note should be made of any jaundice, signs of muscle wastage, ascites, right upper quadrant tenderness, palmar erythema, or hepatomegaly.

Laboratory Testing

The biochemical profile (alkaline phosphatase, calcium, lactate dehydrogenase, bilirubin, serum glutamic–oxaloacetic transaminase, cholesterol, uric acid, phosphorous, albumin, total protein, and glucose) is not useful for routine preoperative evaluation (267). Mild abnormalities can result in further extensive testing that requires consultation, delays in surgery, and increased cost without net benefit. A possible exception is selected use of biochemical testing when the history or physical examination reveals abnormalities. Patients with known liver disease should undergo albumin and bilirubin testing using the Child's risk classification (Table 22.21). This system

	Table 22.21 Child's Classification of Liver Dysfunction		
	Child Classification		
Parameter	*A*	*B*	*C*
Bilirubin	<2.0	2.0–3.0	>3.0
Albumin	>3.5	3.0–3.5	<3.0
Ascites	None	Easily controlled	Poor controlled
Encephalopathy	None	Mild	Advanced
Nutritional status	Excellent	Good	Poor

was originally designed to predict mortality following portosystemic shunt surgery. It divides patients into three classes of severity based on five easily assessed clinical parameters. Measurement of prothrombin time may be helpful in patients with significant histories of liver disease. If a history of hepatitis is ascertained, the patient should be tested for serum aminotransferase, alkaline phosphatase, bilirubin, albumin levels, and prothrombin time. Serologic documentation of hepatitis is important. If a patient has a known malignancy, biochemical testing of the liver may be of some benefit as a screen for metastatic disease, although this was not proven conclusively.

Anesthesia

With few exceptions, most anesthetic agents, including those administered by epidural or spinal routes, reduce hepatic blood flow and decrease oxygenation of the liver. Other perioperative factors—hemorrhage, intraoperative hypotension, hypercarbia, congestive heart failure, and intermittent positive pressure ventilation, especially in critically ill patients—lead to decreased hepatic perfusion and hypoxia (268).

Drug Metabolism

Patients with altered liver function should be carefully monitored because of the prolonged action of many medications used during surgery. In addition to impaired metabolism, hypoalbuminemia decreases drug binding, which alters serum levels and biliary clearance rates. The degree of hepatic metabolism varies greatly, depending on the type of medication considered. For inhalation anesthetics, *isoflurane* is preferred because it undergoes minimal hepatic metabolism in comparison with *halothane* or *enflurane*. Narcotics, induction agents, sedatives, and neuromuscular blocking agents all undergo abnormal metabolism in patients with decompensated liver disease. *Diazepam, meperidine,* and *phenobarbital* cause prolonged depression of consciousness and may precipitate hepatic encephalopathy because of their altered rates of clearance. *Sufentanil* and *fentanyl* are the preferred narcotics. *Oxazepam,* a benzodiazepine that does not undergo hepatic metabolism, is considered safe. Muscle relaxants, such as *D-tubocurarine, pancuronium,* and *vecuronium,* cause prolonged neuromuscular blockade in patients with impaired liver function and are not ideal drugs to use in this situation. *Atracurium* is not metabolized by the liver and is the preferred muscle relaxant for patients with abnormal hepatic function. *Succinylcholine* metabolism is prolonged in patients with hepatic dysfunction and must be used with great caution (269).

Determination of Operative Risk

Although it is well known that acute hepatobiliary damage results in increased morbidity and mortality in the surgical patient, estimating the operative risk in patients with hepatic dysfunction is difficult based on the history and physical examination. **The most accurate method for risk assessment of surgery in patients with hepatic dysfunction is Child's classification** (Table 22.21). Using this system, accurate assessment of morbidity and mortality can be directly related to the degree of liver dysfunction (270). The Child's classification is useful for patients undergoing a variety of different types of abdominal surgery. Data show operative mortalities of 10%, 30%, and 82% for each of the three Child's classifications, respectively, while other data called this into question with operative mortality of 2%, 12%, and 12% (271,272). The major cause of perioperative death was often sepsis. This classification correlated significantly with postoperative complications such as bleeding, renal failure, wound dehiscence, and sepsis. Another method for determining operative risk in patients with cirrhosis is the Model for End-Stage Liver Disease (MELD), which takes into account the patient's prothrombin time, bilirubin, and creatinine with various iterations used to better predict perioperative morbidity and mortality (273,274). Originally designed to predict outcomes in cirrhotic patients undergoing the transjugular intrahepatic portosystemic shunt (TIPS) procedure, it was further studied to include patients undergoing other surgical procedures. In patients with a MELD score greater than 15, elective surgery should be deferred (275).

Acute Viral Hepatitis

Acute viral hepatitis poses an increased risk of operative complications and perioperative mortality and is a contraindication for elective surgery (276). Elective surgery should be delayed for approximately 1 month after the results of all biochemical tests have returned to normal (277). In patients with ectopic pregnancy, hemorrhage, or bowel obstruction secondary to malignancy, surgical intervention must take place before normalization of serum transaminase levels (276). In these situations, the perioperative morbidity (12%) and mortality (9.5%) rates are much higher than when they are performed under ideal situations (269).

Chronic Hepatitis

Chronic hepatitis is a group of disorders characterized by inflammation of the liver for at least 6 months. The disease is divided by morphologic and clinical criteria into chronic persistent hepatitis and chronic active hepatitis. A liver biopsy is usually required to establish the extent and type of injury. The surgical risk in these patients correlates most closely with the severity of disease. The risk of surgery in patients with asymptomatic or mild disease is minimal in contrast to a significant risk for those patients who have symptomatic chronic active hepatitis (278). Elective surgery is contraindicated in symptomatic patients, and nonelective surgery is associated with significant morbidity (277). In the nonelective situation, patients taking long-term *glucocorticoid* therapy should be given appropriate stress coverage with a higher dose of *glucocorticoids* during the perioperative period. Preoperatively, patients who are not taking steroids should receive *prednisone* and *azathioprine*, which are shown to reduce the perioperative risk of complications and may result in remission in as many as 80% of patients (279). **Asymptomatic carriers of the hepatitis B virus (HBV; individuals who test positive for the HBV surface antigen) are not at increased risk for postoperative complications in the absence of elevated aminotransferase levels and liver inflammation.** There is a significant risk to the health care professional operating on these individuals. In cases of needlestick in which the patient's hepatitis status is unknown, both the health care worker and the patient should be tested for hepatitis C virus (HCV) antibody and HBV serologic markers. If markers for HBV infection are present, *hepatitis B immune globulin* should be administered to unvaccinated medical personnel. A vaccination series should be initiated during the early postoperative period. If the health care worker is immune (surface antibody positive), no treatment is necessary (269). All medical personnel, and especially those in the surgical subspecialties, should receive a full course of recombinant hepatitis B vaccine as recommended by the CDC (280). Treatment for chronic hepatitis B in the 1990s centered around *interferon-α* with data in the 2000s showing increased benefit from the use of nucleoside analogues, including *lamivudine* and *tenofovir* (281,282). *Pegylated interferon* and *ribavirin* are used in the standard treatment of HCV (283). Consideration should be given to using these medications for patients in whom surgery cannot be avoided but is not emergent.

Alcoholic Liver Disease

Alcoholic liver disease encompasses a spectrum of diseases including fatty liver, acute alcoholic hepatitis, and cirrhosis. Elective surgery is not contraindicated in patients with fatty liver because liver function is preserved. **If nutritional deficiencies are discovered, they should be corrected before elective surgery.** Acute alcoholic hepatitis is characterized on biopsy by hepatocyte edema, polymorphonuclear leukocyte infiltration, necrosis, and the presence of Mallory bodies. Elective surgery in these patients is contraindicated (284). Abstinence from alcohol for approximately 6 to 12 weeks along with clinical resolution of the biochemical abnormalities are recommended before surgery is considered. Severe alcoholic hepatitis may persist for several months despite abstinence and, if any question of continued activity exists, a liver biopsy should be repeated (285). In cases of urgent or emergent surgery on patients with alcohol dependence, administration of tapered doses of *benzodiazepine* is appropriate as prophylaxis against alcohol withdrawal.

Cirrhosis

Cirrhosis is an irreversible liver lesion characterized histologically by parenchymal necrosis, nodular degeneration, fibrosis, and a disorganization of hepatic lobular architecture. The most serious complication of cirrhosis is portal venous hypertension, which ultimately leads to bleeding from esophageal varices, ascites, and hepatic encephalopathy. Conventional liver biochemical test results correlate poorly with the degree of liver impairment in patients with cirrhosis. Hepatic dysfunction may be somewhat quantified by low albumin levels and prolonged prothrombin times.

Surgical risk is increased in patients with advanced liver disease, although it is substantially greater in emergency surgery than in elective surgery. Perioperative mortality correlates with the severity of cirrhosis and can be estimated through the use of the Child's classification (Table 22.21). In patients with Child's class A cirrhosis, surgery can usually be performed without significant risk, whereas in patients with Child's class B or C, surgery poses a major risk and requires careful preoperative consideration. Preoperative preparation should include the following measures: (i) optimizing nutritional status by enteral and parenteral nutrition and supplementation with vitamin B_1, (ii) correcting coagulopathy with administration of FFP or cryoprecipitate or both, (iii) minimizing preexisting encephalopathy, (iv) preventing sepsis from spontaneous bacterial peritonitis by administering prophylactic antibiotic therapy, and (v) optimizing renal function and carefully correcting electrolyte abnormalities (286). Meticulous preoperative preparation focused on correcting abnormalities associated with advanced liver disease may improve surgical outcomes (287).

References

1. **Kaye AD, Kucera I, Sabar R.** Perioperative anesthesia clinical considerations of alternative medicines. *Anesthesiol Clin North Am* 2004;22:125–139.

2. **Philp R.** *Herbal-drug interactions and adverse effects: An evidence-based quick reference guide.* New York: McGraw-Hill Professional, 2003.

3. **Blery C, Charpak Y, Szatan M, et al.** Evaluation of a protocol for selective ordering of preoperative tests. *Lancet* 1986;1:139–141.

4. **St. Clair CM, Shah M, Diver EJ, et al.** Adherence to evidence-based guidelines for preoperative testing in women undergoing gynecologic surgery. *Obstet Gynecol* 2010;116:694–700.

5. **Lamers RJ, van Engelshoven JM, Pfaff A.** [Once again, the routine preoperative thorax photo]. *Ned Tijdschr Geneeskd* 1989;133:2288–2291.

6. **Rohrer MJ, Michelotti MC, Nahrwold DL.** A prospective evaluation of the efficacy of preoperative coagulation testing. *Ann Surg* 1988;208:554–557.

7. **Piscitelli JT, Simel DL, Addison WA.** Who should have intravenous pyelograms before hysterectomy for benign disease? *Obstet Gynecol* 1987;69:541–545.

8. **ACOG Committee.** Opinion No. 439: informed consent. *Obstet Gynecol* 2009;114(Pt 1):401–408.

9. **Abed H, Rogers R, Helitzer D, et al.** Informed consent in gynecologic surgery. *Am J Obstet Gynecol* 2007;197:674 e1–e5.

10. **Rosenthal RA.** Nutritional concerns in the older surgical patient. *J Am Coll Surg* 2004;199:785–791.

11. **Windsor JA, Hill GL.** Weight loss with physiologic impairment. A basic indicator of surgical risk. *Ann Surg* 1988;207:290–296.

12. **Huckleberry Y.** Nutritional support and the surgical patient. *Am J Health Syst Pharm* 2004;61:671–684.

13. **Santoso JT, Canada T, Latson B, et al.** Prognostic nutritional index in relation to hospital stay in women with gynecologic cancer. *Obstet Gynecol* 2000;95(Pt 1):844–846.

14. **Salvino RM, Dechicco RS, Seidner DL.** Perioperative nutrition support: who and how. *Cleve Clin J Med* 2004;71:345–351.

15. **Gibbs J, Cull W, Henderson W, et al.** Preoperative serum albumin level as a predictor of operative mortality and morbidity: results from the National VA Surgical Risk Study. *Arch Surg* 1999;134:36–42.

16. **Soper JT, Berchuck A, Creasman WT, et al.** Pelvic exenteration: factors associated with major surgical morbidity. *Gynecol Oncol* 1989;35:93–98.

17. **The Veterans Affairs Total Parenteral Nutrition Cooperative Study Group.** Perioperative total parenteral nutrition in surgical patients. *N Engl J Med* 1991;325:525–532.

18. **Klein S, Kinney J, Jeejeebhoy K, et al.** Nutrition support in clinical practice: review of published data and recommendations for future research directions. National Institutes of Health, American Society for Parenteral and Enteral Nutrition, and American Society for Clinical Nutrition. *JPEN J Parenter Enteral Nutr* 1997;21:133–156.

19. **Geisler JP, Linnemeier GC, Thomas AJ, et al.** Nutritional assessment using prealbumin as an objective criterion to determine whom should not undergo primary radical cytoreductive surgery for ovarian cancer. *Gynecol Oncol* 2007;106:128–131.

20. **Koretz RL, Lipman TO, Klein S.** AGA technical review on parenteral nutrition. *Gastroenterology* 2001;121:970–1001.

21. **Heuschekel R, Duggan C.** Enteral feeding: gastric versus post-pyloric. *UpToDate* 2010. Available online at: http://www.uptodate.com/contents/enteral-feeding-gastric-versus-post-pyloric

22. **Pearce CB, Duncan HD.** Enteral feeding. Nasogastric, nasojejunal, percutaneous endoscopic gastrostomy, or jejunostomy: its indications and limitations. *Postgrad Med J* 2002;78:198–204.

23. **Duro D, Collier S, Duggan C.** Overview of parenteral and enteral nutrition. *UpToDate* 2010. Available online at: http://www.uptodate.com/contents/overview-of-parenteral-and-enteral-nutrition

24. **Worthington P.** *Practical aspects of nutritional support: an advanced practice guide.* Philadelphia, PA: Saunders, 2004.

25. **Long CL, Schaffel N, Geiger JW, et al.** Metabolic response to injury and illness: estimation of energy and protein needs from indirect calorimetry and nitrogen balance. *JPEN J Parenter Enteral Nutr* 1979;3:452–456.

26. **Pestana C.** *Fluids and electrolytes in the surgical patient.* Baltimore, MD: Williams & Wilkins, 2000.

27. **Miller TA, Duke JH.** Fluid and electrolyte management. In: **Dudrick SJ, Baue AE, Aiseman B, eds.** *ACS manual of preoperative and postoperative care.* Philadelphia, PA: WB Saunders, 1983:38–67.

28. **Luckey AE, Parsa CJ.** Fluid and electrolytes in the aged. *Arch Surg* 2003;138:1055–1060.

29. **Boldt J.** Volume replacement in the surgical patient—does the type of solution make a difference? *Br J Anaesth* 2000;84:783–793.

30. **Jacob M, Chappell D, Conzen P, et al.** Small-volume resuscitation with hyperoncotic albumin: a systematic review of randomized clinical trials. *Crit Care* 2008;12:R34.

31. **Alderson P, Bunn F, Lefebvre C, et al.** Human albumin solution for resuscitation and volume expansion in critically ill patients. *Cochrane Database Syst Rev* 2004;4:CD001208.

32. **Roberts I, Alderson P, Bunn F, et al.** Colloids versus crystalloids for fluid resuscitation in critically ill patients. *Cochrane Database Syst Rev* 2004;4:CD000567.

33. **Cogan M.** *Fluid and electrolytes.* New Haven, CT: Appleton & Lange, 1991.

34. **Schrier RW, Gross P, Gheorghiade M, et al.** *Tolvaptan,* a selective oral vasopressin V2-receptor antagonist, for hyponatremia. *N Engl J Med* 2006;355:2099–2112.

35. **Mullins RJ.** Shock, electrolytes, and fluid. In: **Townsend CM, et al, eds.** *Sabiston textbook of surgery.* Philadelphia, PA: Elsevier Saunders, 2004:69–112.

36. **Narins RG.** Renal systems. In: **Vandem L, ed.** *To make the patient ready for anesthesia: medical care of the surgical patient.* Stoneham, MA: Butterworth, 1984:67–114.

37. **Wish JB, Cacho CP.** Acid/base and electrolyte disorders. In: Sivak ED, Higgins TL, Seiver A, eds. *The high risk patient: management of the critically ill.* Baltimore, MD: Williams & Wilkins, 1995:755–782.

38. **Apfelbaum JL, Chen C, Mehta SS, et al.** Postoperative pain experience: results from a national survey suggest postoperative pain continues to be undermanaged. *Anesth Analg* 2003;97:534–540.

39. **Huang N, Cunningham F, Laurito CE, et al.** Can we do better with postoperative pain management? *Am J Surg* 2001;182:440–448.

40. **Kuhn S, Cooke K, Collins M, et al.** Perceptions of pain relief after surgery. *BMJ* 1990;300:1687–1690.

41. **Anonymous.** Practice guidelines for acute pain management in the perioperative setting: an updated report by the American Society of Anesthesiologists Task Force on Acute Pain Management. *Anesthesiology* 2004;100:1573–1581.

42. **Etches RC.** Patient-controlled analgesia. *Surg Clin North Am* 1999; 79:297–312.

43. **Austin KL, Stapleton JV, Mather LE.** Multiple intramuscular injections: a major source of variability in analgesic response to meperidine. *Pain* 1980;8:47–62.

44. **Jain S, Datta S.** Postoperative pain management. *Chest Surg Clin North Am* 1997;7:773–799.

45. **Egbert AM, Parks LH, Short LM, et al.** Randomized trial of postoperative patient-controlled analgesia vs intramuscular narcotics in frail elderly men. *Arch Intern Med* 1990;150:1897–1903.

46. **Rawal N, Arnér S, Gustafsson LL, et al.** Present state of extradural and intrathecal opioid analgesia in Sweden. A nationwide follow-up survey. *Br J Anaesth* 1987;59:791–799.

47. **Rawal N.** Epidural and spinal agents for postoperative analgesia. *Surg Clin North Am* 1999;79:313–344.

48. **Werawatganon T, Charuluxanun S.** Patient controlled intravenous opioid analgesia versus continuous epidural analgesia for pain after intra-abdominal surgery. *Cochrane Database Syst Rev* 2005;1:CD004088.

49. **DeAndrade JR, Maslanka M, Maneatis T, et al.** The use of ketorolac in the management of postoperative pain. *Orthopedics* 1994;17:157–166.

50. **Etches RC, Warriner CB, Badner N, et al.** Continuous intravenous administration of ketorolac reduces pain and morphine consumption after total hip or knee arthroplasty. *Anesth Analg* 1995;81:1175–1180.

51. **Macario A, Lipman AG.** Ketorolac in the era of cyclo-oxygenase-2 selective nonsteroidal anti-inflammatory drugs: a systematic review of efficacy, side effects, and regulatory issues. *Pain Med* 2001;2:336–351.

52. **Lowder JL, Shackelford DP, Holbert D, et al.** A randomized, controlled trial to compare ketorolac tromethamine versus placebo after cesarean section to reduce pain and narcotic usage. *Am J Obstet Gynecol* 2003;189:1559–1562.

53. **Wischnik A, Manth SM, Lloyd J, et al.** The excretion of ketorolac tromethamine into breast milk after multiple oral dosing. *Eur J Clin Pharmacol* 1989;36:521–524.

54. **Greer IA.** Effects of ketorolac tromethamine on hemostasis. *Pharmacotherapy* 1990;10(Pt 2):71S–76S.

55. **Strom BL, Berlin JA, Kinman JL, et al.** Parenteral ketorolac and risk of gastrointestinal and operative site bleeding. A postmarketing surveillance study. *JAMA* 1996;275:376–382.

56. **Feldman HI, Kinman JL, Berlin JA, et al.** Parenteral ketorolac: the risk for acute renal failure. *Ann Intern Med* 1997;126:193–199.

57. **Lee A, Cooper MC, Craig JC, et al.** Effects of nonsteroidal anti-inflammatory drugs on postoperative renal function in adults with normal renal function. *Cochrane Database Syst Rev* 2004;2: CD002765.

58. **Gajraj NM, Joshi GP.** Role of cyclooxygenase-2 inhibitors in postoperative pain management. *Anesthesiol Clin North Am* 2005;23:49–72.

59. **Bresalier RS, Quan H, Bolognese JA, et al.** Cardiovascular events associated with rofecoxib in a colorectal adenoma chemoprevention trial. *N Engl J Med* 2005;352:1092–1102.

60. **Fitzgerald GA.** Coxibs and cardiovascular disease. *N Engl J Med* 2004;351:1709–1711.

61. **FitzGerald GA, Patrono C.** The coxibs, selective inhibitors of cyclooxygenase-2. *N Engl J Med* 2001;345:433–442.

62. **Nussmeier NA, Whelton AA, Brown MT, et al.** Complications of the COX-2 inhibitors parecoxib and valdecoxib after cardiac surgery. *N Engl J Med* 2005;352:1081–1091.

63. **Solomon SD, McMurray JJ, Pfeffer MA, et al.** Cardiovascular risk associated with *celecoxib* in a clinical trial for colorectal adenoma prevention. *N Engl J Med* 2005;352:1071–1080.

64. **Vadivelu N, Mitra S, Narayan D.** Recent advances in postoperative pain management. *Yale J Biol Med* 2010;83:11–25.

65. **Tanos V, Rojansky N.** Prophylactic antibiotics in abdominal hysterectomy. *J Am Coll Surg* 1994;179:593–600.

66. **Dellinger EP, Gross PA, Barrett TL, et al.** Quality standard for antimicrobial prophylaxis in surgical procedures. The Infectious Diseases Society of America. *Infect Control Hosp Epidemiol* 1994; 15:182–188.

67. **Burke JF.** The effective period of preventive antibiotic action in experimental incisions and dermal lesions. *Surgery* 1961;50:161–168.

68. **Dellinger EP, Gross PA, Barrett TL, et al.** Quality standard for antimicrobial prophylaxis in surgical procedures. Infectious Diseases Society of America. *Clin Infect Dis* 1994;18:422–427.

69. **Swoboda SM, Merz C, Kostuik J, et al.** Does intraoperative blood loss affect antibiotic serum and tissue concentrations? *Arch Surg* 1996;131:1165–11712.

70. **Hedrick TL, Heckman JA, Smith RL, et al.** Efficacy of protocol implementation on incidence of wound infection in colorectal operations. *J Am Coll Surg* 2007;205:432–438.

71. **Forse RA, Karam B, MacLean LD, et al.** Antibiotic prophylaxis for surgery in morbidly obese patients. *Surgery* 1989;106:750–757.

72. **Idsoe O, Guthe T, Wilcox RR, et al.** Nature and extent of penicillin side-reactions, with particular reference to fatalities from anaphylactic shock. *Bull World Health Organ* 1968;38:159–188.

73. **McFarland LV, Surawicz CM, Greenberg, RN, et al.** Prevention of beta-lactam-associated diarrhea by *Saccharomyces boulardii* compared with placebo. *Am J Gastroenterol* 1995;90:439–448.

74. **Bartlett JG.** Antibiotic-associated diarrhea. *Clin Infect Dis* 1992; 15:573–581.

75. **Antibiotic prophylaxis for gynecologic procedures.** ACOG Practice Bulletin No.104. *Obstet Gynecol* 2009;113:1180–1189.

76. **Wilson W, Taubert KA, Gewitz M, et al.** Prevention of infective endocarditis: guidelines from the American Heart Association: a guideline from the American Heart Association Rheumatic Fever, Endocarditis, and Kawasaki Disease Committee, Council on Cardiovascular Disease in the Young, and the Council on Clinical Cardiology, Council on Cardiovascular Surgery and Anesthesia, and the Quality of Care and Outcomes Research Interdisciplinary Working Group. *Circulation* 2007;116:1736–1754.

77. **Brachman PS, Dan BB, Haley RW, et al.** Nosocomial surgical infections: incidence and cost. *Surg Clin North Am* 1980;60:15–25.

78. **Anderson DJ, Sexton DJ, Kanafani ZA, et al.** Severe surgical site infection in community hospitals: epidemiology, key procedures, and the changing prevalence of methicillin-resistant *Staphylococcus aureus*. *Infect Control Hosp Epidemiol* 2007;28:1047–1053.

79. **Lyon DS, Jones JL, Sanchez A.** Postoperative febrile morbidity in the benign gynecologic patient. Identification and management. *J Reprod Med* 2000;45:305–309.

80. **O'Grady NP, Barie PS, Bartlett JG, et al.** Guidelines for evaluation of new fever in critically ill adult patients: 2008 update from the American College of Critical Care Medicine and the Infectious Diseases Society of America. *Crit Care Med* 2008;36:1330–1349.

81. **Schey D, Salom EM, Papadia A, et al.** Extensive fever workup produces low yield in determining infectious etiology. *Am J Obstet Gynecol* 2005;192:1729–1734.

82. **Schwandt A, Andrews SJ, Fanning J.** Prospective analysis of a fever evaluation algorithm after major gynecologic surgery. *Am J Obstet Gynecol* 2001;184:1066–1067.

83. **Wallace WC, Cinat ME, Nastanski F, et al.** New epidemiology for postoperative nosocomial infections. *Am Surg* 2000;66:874–878.

84. **Bartzen PJ, Hafferty FW.** Pelvic laparotomy without an indwelling catheter. A retrospective review of 949 cases. *Am J Obstet Gynecol* 1987;156:1426–1432.

85. **Hemsell DL.** Infections after gynecologic surgery. *Obstet Gynecol Clin North Am* 1989;16:381–400.

86. **Kingdom JC, Kitchener HC, MacLean AB.** Postoperative urinary tract infection in gynecology: implications for an antibiotic prophylaxis policy. *Obstet Gynecol* 1990;76:636–638.

87. **Cormio G, Vicino M, Loizzi V, et al.** Antimicrobial prophylaxis in vaginal gynecologic surgery: a prospective randomized study comparing *amoxicillin-clavulanic acid* with *cefazolin*. *J Chemother* 2007;19:193–197.

88. **Boyd ME.** Postoperative gynecologic infections. *Can J Surg* 1987; 30:7–9.

89. **Kunin CM.** Catheter-associated urinary tract infections: a syllogism compounded by a questionable dichotomy. *Clin Infect Dis* 2009;48:1189–1190.

90. **Harkness GA, Bentley DW, Roghmann KJ.** Risk factors for nosocomial pneumonia in the elderly. *Am J Med* 1990;89:457–463.

91. **Rothan-Tondeur M, Meaume S, Girard L, et al.** Risk factors for nosocomial pneumonia in a geriatric hospital: a control-case one-center study. *J Am Geriatr Soc* 2003;51:997–1001.

92. **Koeman M, van der Ven AJ, Ramsay G, et al.** Ventilator-associated pneumonia: recent issues on pathogenesis, prevention and diagnosis. *J Hosp Infect* 2001;49:155–162.

93. **Tomford JW, Hershey CO, McLaren CE, et al.** Intravenous therapy team and peripheral venous catheter-associated complications. A prospective controlled study. *Arch Intern Med* 1984;144:1191–1194.

94. **O'Grady NP, Alexander M, Dellinger EP, et al.** Guidelines for the prevention of intravascular catheter-related infections. Centers for Disease Control and Prevention. *MMWR Recomm Rep* 2002;51(RR-10):1–29.

95. **Soifer NE, Borzak S, Edlin BR, et al.** Prevention of peripheral venous catheter complications with an intravenous therapy team: a randomized controlled trial. *Arch Intern Med* 1998;158:473–477.

96. **Hershey CO, Tomford JW, McLaren CE, et al.** The natural history of intravenous catheter-associated phlebitis. *Arch Intern Med* 1984;144:1373–1375.

97. **Cruse PJ, Foord R.** The epidemiology of wound infection. A 10-year prospective study of 62,939 wounds. *Surg Clin North Am* 1980;60:27–40.

98. **Brown SE, Allen HH, Robins RN.** The use of delayed primary wound closure in preventing wound infections. *Am J Obstet Gynecol* 1977;127:713–717.

99. **Sperling DC, Needleman L, Eschelman DJ, et al.** Deep pelvic abscesses: transperineal US-guided drainage. *Radiology* 1998;208:111–115.

100. **Sudakoff GS, Lundeen SJ, Otterson MF.** Transrectal and transvaginal sonographic intervention of infected pelvic fluid collections: a complete approach. *Ultrasound Q* 2005;21:175–185.

101. **Larsen JW, Hager WD, Livengood CM, et al.** Guidelines for the diagnosis, treatment and prevention of postoperative infections. *Infect Dis Obstet Gynecol* 2003;11:65–70.

102. **Ellis Simonsen SM, van Orman ER, Hatch BE, et al.** Cellulitis incidence in a defined population. *Epidemiol Infect* 2006;134:293–299.

103. **Meleney R.** Hemolytic streptococcus gangrene. *Arch Surg* 1925;9:317–321.

104. **Sarani B, Strong M, Pascual J, et al.** Necrotizing fasciitis: current concepts and review of the literature. *J Am Coll Surg* 2009;208:279–288.

105. **Wong CH, Wang YS.** The diagnosis of necrotizing fasciitis. *Curr Opin Infect Dis* 2005;18:101–106.

106. **Riseman JA, Zamboni WA, Curtis A, et al.** Hyperbaric oxygen therapy for necrotizing fasciitis reduces mortality and the need for debridements. *Surgery* 1990;108:847–850.

107. **Stamenkovic I, Lew PD.** Early recognition of potentially fatal necrotizing fasciitis. The use of frozen-section biopsy. *N Engl J Med* 1984;310:1689–1693.

108. **Umbert IJ, Winkelmann RK, Oliver GF, et al.** Necrotizing fasciitis: a clinical, microbiologic, and histopathologic study of 14 patients. *J Am Acad Dermatol* 1989;20(Pt 1):774–781.

109. **Wilkerson R, Paull W, Coville FV.** Necrotizing fasciitis. Review of the literature and case report. *Clin Orthop Relat Res* 1987;216:187–192.

110. **Jallali N, Withey S, Butler PE.** Hyperbaric oxygen as adjuvant therapy in the management of necrotizing fasciitis. *Am J Surg* 2005;189:462–466.

111. **Robson MC, Krizek TJ, Koss N, et al.** Amniotic membranes as a temporary wound dressing. *Surg Gynecol Obstet* 1973;136:904–906.

112. **Rothman PA, Wiskind AK, Dudley AG.** Amniotic membranes in the treatment of necrotizing fasciitis complicating vulvar herpes virus infection. *Obstet Gynecol* 1990;76(Pt 2):534–536.

113. **Alvarez AA, Maxwell GL, Rodriguez GC.** Vacuum-assisted closure for cutaneous gastrointestinal fistula management. *Gynecol Oncol* 2001;80:413–416.

114. **Argenta PA, Rahaman J, Gretz HF, et al.** Vacuum-assisted closure in the treatment of complex gynecologic wound failures. *Obstet Gynecol* 2002;99:497–501.

115. **Schimp VL, Worley C, Brunello S, et al.** Vacuum-assisted closure in the treatment of gynecologic oncology wound failures. *Gynecol Oncol* 2004;92:586–591.

116. **Slim K, Vicaut E, Launay-Savary MV, et al.** Updated systematic review and meta-analysis of randomized clinical trials on the role of mechanical bowel preparation before colorectal surgery. *Ann Surg* 2009;249:203–209.

117. **Bretagnol F, Panis Y, Rullier E, et al.** Rectal cancer surgery with or without bowel preparation: the French GRECCAR III multicenter single-blinded randomized trial. *Ann Surg* 2010;252:863–868.

118. **Beck DE, Harford FJ, DiPalma JA.** Comparison of cleansing methods in preparation for colonic surgery. *Dis Colon Rectum* 1985;28:491–495.

119. **Cohen SM, Wexner SD, Binderow SR, et al.** Prospective, randomized, endoscopic-blinded trial comparing precolonoscopy bowel cleansing methods. *Dis Colon Rectum* 1994;37:689–696.

120. **Markowitz GS, Stokes MB, Radhakrisnan J, et al.** Acute phosphate nephropathy following oral sodium phosphate bowel purgative: an underrecognized cause of chronic renal failure. *J Am Soc Nephrol* 2005;16:3389–3396.

121. **Wexner SD, Beck DE, Baron TH, et al.** A consensus document on bowel preparation before colonoscopy: prepared by a task force from the American Society of Colon and Rectal Surgeons (ASCRS), the American Society for Gastrointestinal Endoscopy (ASGE), and the Society of American Gastrointestinal and Endoscopic Surgeons (SAGES). *Gastrointest Endosc* 2006;63:894–909.

122. **Enestvedt BK, Fennerty MB, Eisen GM.** Randomised clinical trial: *MiraLAX* vs. *GoLYTELY*—a controlled study of efficacy and patient tolerability in bowel preparation for colonoscopy. *Aliment Pharmacol Ther* 2011;33:33–40.

123. **Ratcliff JB, Kapernick P, Brooks GG, et al.** Small bowel obstruction and previous gynecologic surgery. *South Med J* 1983;76:1349–1350, 1360.

124. **Carter J, Valmadre S, Dalrymple C, et al.** Management of large bowel obstruction in advanced ovarian cancer with intraluminal stents. *Gynecol Oncol* 2002;84:176–179.

125. **Jeffcoate TN, Tindall VR.** Venous thrombosis and embolism in obstetrics and gynaecology. *Aust N Z J Obstet Gynaecol* 1965;5:119–130.

126. **Clarke-Pearson DL, Jelovsek FR, Creasman WT.** Thromboembolism complicating surgery for cervical and uterine malignancy: incidence, risk factors, and prophylaxis. *Obstet Gynecol* 1983;61:87–94.

127. **Clayton JK, Anderson JA, McNicol GP.** Preoperative prediction of postoperative deep vein thrombosis. *BMJ* 1976;2:910–912.

128. **Clarke-Pearson DL, DeLong ER, Synan IS, et al.** Variables associated with postoperative deep venous thrombosis: a prospective study of 411 gynecology patients and creation of a prognostic model. *Obstet Gynecol* 1987;69:146–150.

129. **Kakkar VV, Corrigan TP, Fossard DP, et al.** Prevention of fatal postoperative pulmonary embolism by low doses of heparin. Reappraisal of results of international multicentre trial. *Lancet* 1977;1:567–569.

130. **Clarke-Pearson DL, DeLong ER, Synan IS, et al.** Complications of low-dose *heparin* prophylaxis in gynecologic oncology surgery. *Obstet Gynecol* 1984;64:689–694.

131. **Tapson VF, Hull RD.** Management of venous thromboembolic disease. The impact of low-molecular-weight *heparin*. *Clin Chest Med* 1995;16:281–294.

132. **Borstad E, Urdal K, Handeland G, et al.** Comparison of low molecular weight *heparin* vs. unfractionated *heparin* in gynecological surgery. II: Reduced dose of low molecular weight *heparin*. *Acta Obstet Gynecol Scand* 1992;71:471–475.

133. **Jorgensen LN, Wille-Jorgensen P, Hauch O.** Prophylaxis of postoperative thromboembolism with low molecular weight *heparins*. *Br J Surg* 1993;80:689–704.

134. **Clarke-Pearson DL, Synan IS, Colemen RE, et al.** The natural history of postoperative venous thromboemboli in gynecologic oncology: a prospective study of 382 patients. *Am J Obstet Gynecol* 1984;148:1051–1054.

135. **Scurr JH, Ibrahim SZ, Faber RG, et al.** The efficacy of graduated compression stockings in the prevention of deep vein thrombosis. *Br J Surg* 1977;64:371–373.

136. **Salzman EW, Ploetz J, Bettmann M, et al.** Intraoperative external pneumatic calf compression to afford long-term prophylaxis against deep vein thrombosis in urological patients. *Surgery* 1980;87:239–242.

137. **Nicolaides AN, Fernandes J, Pollock AV.** Intermittent sequential pneumatic compression of the legs in the prevention of venous stasis and postoperative deep venous thrombosis. *Surgery* 1980;87:69–76.

138. **Clarke-Pearson DL, Synan IS, Hinshaw WM, et al.** Prevention of postoperative venous thromboembolism by external pneumatic calf compression in patients with gynecologic malignancy. *Obstet Gynecol* 1984;63:92–98.

139. **Clarke-Pearson DL, Creasman WT, Coleman RE, et al.** Perioperative external pneumatic calf compression as thromboembolism prophylaxis in gynecologic oncology: report of a randomized controlled trial. *Gynecol Oncol* 1984;18:226–232.

140. **Maxwell GL, Myers ER, Clarke-Pearson DL.** Cost-effectiveness of deep venous thrombosis prophylaxis in gynecologic oncology surgery. *Obstet Gynecol* 2000;95:206–214.

141. **Creasman WT, Weed JC Jr.** Complications of radical hysterectomy. In: Schaefer G, ed. *Complications in Obstetrics and Gynecologic Surgery*. Hagerstown, MD: Harper & Row, 1981:389–398.

142. **Haeger K.** Problems of acute deep venous thrombosis. I. The interpretation of signs and symptoms. *Angiology* 1969;20:219–223.

143. **Palko PD, Nanson EM, Fedoruk SO.** The early detection of deep venous thrombosis using I131-tagged human fibrinogen. *Can J Surg* 1964;7:215–226.

144. **Lensing AW, Prandoni P, Brandjes D, et al.** Detection of deep-vein thrombosis by real-time B-mode ultrasonography. *N Engl J Med* 1989;320:342–345.

145. **Athanasoulis C.** Phlebography for the diagnosis of deep leg vein thrombosis, prophylactic therapy of deep venous thrombosis and pulmonary embolism. In: *DHEW Publication (NIH). No. 76-866.* 1975:62–76.

146. **Montgomery KD, Potter HG, Helfet DL.** Magnetic resonance venography to evaluate the deep venous system of the pelvis in patients who have an acetabular fracture. *J Bone Joint Surg Am* 1995;77:1639–1649.

147. **Raschke RA, Reilly BM, Guidry JR, et al.** The weight-based heparin dosing nomogram compared with a "standard care" nomogram. A randomized controlled trial. *Ann Intern Med* 1993;119:874–881.

148. **van Dongen CJ, van den Belt AG, Prins MH, et al.** Fixed dose subcutaneous low molecular weight *heparins* versus adjusted dose unfractionated *heparin* for venous thromboembolism. *Cochrane Database Syst Rev* 2004;4:CD001100.

149. **National Estimates of Diabetes.** C.f.D.C.a.P. 2007 National Diabetes Fact Sheet Figures: General information and national estimates on diabetes in the United States, 2007. Available online at: http://www.cdc.gov/diabetes/pubs/factsheet07.htm

150. **Glister BC, Vigersky RA.** Perioperative management of type 1 diabetes mellitus. *Endocrinol Metab Clin North Am* 2003;32:411–436.

151. **Kohl BA, Schwartz S.** Surgery in the patient with endocrine dysfunction. *Med Clin North Am* 2009;93:1031–1047.

152. **McCullouch DK.** Diagnosis of diabetes mellitus. UpToDate 2011. Available online at: http://www.uptodate.com/contents/diagnosis-of-diabetes-mellitus

153. **Khan NA, Ghali WA, Cagliero E.** Perioperative management of diabetes mellitus. *UpToDate* 2011. Available online at: http://www.uptodate.com/contents/perioperative-management-of-diabetes-mellitus

154. **Connery LE, Coursin DB.** Assessment and therapy of selected endocrine disorders. *Anesthesiol Clin North Am* 2004;22:93–123.

155. **Fleischmann KE, Beckman JA, Buller CE, et al.** 2009 ACCF/AHA focused update on perioperative beta blockade: a report of the American College of Cardiology Foundation/American Heart Association Task Force on Practice Guidelines. *Circulation* 2009;120:2123–2151.

156. **Malone DL, Genuit T, Tracy JK, et al.** Surgical site infections: reanalysis of risk factors. *J Surg Res* 2002;103:89–95.

157. **Fabian TC.** Empiric therapy for pneumonia in the surgical intensive care unit. *Am J Surg* 2000;179(Suppl 1):18–23.

158. **Graham PL 3rd, Lin SX, Larson EL.** A U.S. population-based survey of *Staphylococcus aureus* colonization. *Ann Intern Med* 2006;144:318–325.

159. **Reynolds C.** Management of the diabetic surgical patient. A systematic but flexible plan is the key. *Postgrad Med* 1985;77:265–269, 272–276, 279.

160. **Hirsch IB, McGill JB.** Role of insulin in management of surgical patients with diabetes mellitus. *Diabetes Care* 1990;13:980–991.

161. **Jacober SJ, Sowers JR.** An update on perioperative management of diabetes. *Arch Intern Med* 1999;159:2405–2411.

162. **Weintrob AC, Sexton DJ.** Susceptibility to infections in persons with diabetes mellitus. *UpToDate* 2011. Available online at: http://www.uptodate.com/contents/susceptibility-to-infections-in-persons-with-diabetes-mellitus

163. **Stapleton RD, Heyland DK.** Glycemic control and intensive insulin therapy in critical illness. *UpToDate* 2011. Available online at: http://www.uptodate.com/contents/glycemic-control-and-intensive-insulin-therapy-in-critical-illness

164. **Van den Berghe G, Wilmer A, Milants I, et al.** Intensive insulin therapy in mixed medical/surgical intensive care units: benefit versus harm. *Diabetes* 2006;55:3151–3159.

165. **Moghissi ES, Korytkowski MT, DiNardo M, et al.** American Association of Clinical Endocrinologists and American Diabetes Association consensus statement on inpatient glycemic control. *Endocr Pract* 2009;15:353–369.

166. **Moghissi ES, Korytkowski MT, DiNardo M, et al.** American Association of Clinical Endocrinologists and American Diabetes Association consensus statement on inpatient glycemic control. *Diabetes Care* 2009;32:1119–1131.

167. **Galloway JA, Shuman CR.** Diabetes and surgery. A study of 667 cases. *Am J Med* 1963;34:177–191.

168. **Manzullo EF, Welsh GA, Ross DS.** Nonthyroid surgery in the patient with thyroid disease. *UpToDate* 2010. Available online at: http://www.uptodate.com/contents/nonthyroid-surgery-in-the-patient-with-thyroid-disease

169. **Langley RW, Burch HB.** Perioperative management of the thyrotoxic patient. *Endocrinol Metab Clin North Am* 2003;32:519–534.

170. **Goldmann DR.** Surgery in patients with endocrine dysfunction. *Med Clin North Am* 1987;71:499–509.

171. **Stathatos N, Wartofsky L.** Perioperative management of patients with hypothyroidism. *Endocrinol Metab Clin North Am* 2003;32:503–518.

172. **Welsh GA, Manzullo EF, Nieman LK.** The surgical patient taking glucocorticoids. *UpToDate* 2010. Available online at: http://www.uptodate.com/contents/the-surgical-patient-taking-glucocorticoids

173. **Coursin DB, Wood KE.** Corticosteroid supplementation for adrenal insufficiency. *JAMA* 2002;287:236–240.

174. **Becker RC, Underwood DA.** Myocardial infarction in patients undergoing noncardiac surgery. *Cleve Clin J Med* 1987;54:25–28.

175. **Rao TL, Jacobs KH, El-Etr AA.** Reinfarction following anesthesia in patients with myocardial infarction. *Anesthesiology* 1983;59:499–505.

176. **Mehta RH, Bossone E, Eagle KA.** Perioperative cardiac risk assessment for noncardiac surgery. *Cardiologia* 1999;44:409–418.

177. **Goldman L, Caldera DL, Nussbaum SR, et al.** Multifactorial index of cardiac risk in noncardiac surgical procedures. *N Engl J Med* 1977;297:845–850.

178. **Lee TH, Marcantonio ER, Mangione CM, et al.** Derivation and prospective validation of a simple index for prediction of cardiac risk of major noncardiac surgery. *Circulation* 1999;100:1043–1049.

179. **Fleisher LA, Beckman JA, Brown KA, et al.** 2009 ACCF/AHA focused update on perioperative beta blockade incorporated into the ACC/AHA 2007 guidelines on perioperative cardiovascular evaluation and care for noncardiac surgery: a report of the American College of Cardiology Foundation/American Heart Association Task Force on Practice Guidelines. *Circulation* 2009;120:e169–e276.

180. **Reilly DF, McNeely MJ, Doerner D, et al.** Self-reported exercise tolerance and the risk of serious perioperative complications. *Arch Intern Med* 1999;159:2185–2192.

181. **Cutler BS, Wheeler HB, Paraskos JA, et al.** Applicability and interpretation of electrocardiographic stress testing in patients with peripheral vascular disease. *Am J Surg* 1981;141:501–506.

182. **Carliner NH, Fisher ML, Plotnick GD, et al.** Routine preoperative exercise testing in patients undergoing major noncardiac surgery. *Am J Cardiol* 1985;56:51–58.

183. **Auerbach A, Goldman L.** Assessing and reducing the cardiac risk of noncardiac surgery. *Circulation* 2006;113:1361–1376.

184. **Etchells E, Meade M, Tomlinson G, et al.** Semiquantitative dipyridamole myocardial stress perfusion imaging for cardiac risk assessment before noncardiac vascular surgery: a meta-analysis. *J Vasc Surg* 2002;36:534–540.

185. **Younis L, Stratmann H, Takase B, et al.** Preoperative clinical assessment and dipyridamole thallium-201 scintigraphy for prediction and prevention of cardiac events in patients having major noncardiovascular surgery and known or suspected coronary artery disease. *Am J Cardiol* 1994;74:311–317.

186. **Davila-Roman VG, Waggoner AD, Sicard GA, et al.** Dobutamine stress echocardiography predicts surgical outcome in patients with an aortic aneurysm and peripheral vascular disease. *J Am Coll Cardiol* 1993;21:957–963.

187. **Lane RT, Sawada SG, Segar DS, et al.** Dobutamine stress echocardiography for assessment of cardiac risk before noncardiac surgery. *Am J Cardiol* 1991;68:976–977.

188. **Shammash JB, Kimmel SE, Morgan JP.** Estimation of cardiac risk prior to noncardiac surgery. *UpToDate* 2010. Available online at: http://www.uptodate.com/contents/estimation-of-cardiac-risk-prior-to-noncardiac-surgery

189. **Devereaux PJ, Goldman L, Cook DJ, et al.** Perioperative cardiac events in patients undergoing noncardiac surgery: a review of the

magnitude of the problem, the pathophysiology of the events and methods to estimate and communicate risk. *CMAJ* 2005;173:627–634.

190. **Kaplan J.** Hemodynamic monitoring. In: **Kaplan J, ed.** *Cardiac anesthesia.* New York: Grune & Stratton, 1987:179–226.

191. **Fleischmann KE, Beckman JA, Buller CE, et al.** 2009 ACCF/AHA focused update on perioperative beta blockade. *J Am Coll Cardiol* 2009;54:2102–2128.

192. **Landesberg G.** Monitoring for myocardial ischemia. *Best Pract Res Clin Anaesthesiol* 2005;19:77–95.

193. **Anonymous.** Practice guidelines for perioperative blood transfusion and adjuvant therapies: an updated report by the American Society of Anesthesiologists Task Force on Perioperative Blood Transfusion and Adjuvant Therapies. *Anesthesiology* 2006;105:198–208.

194. **Auerbach AD, Goldman L.** Beta-blockers and reduction of cardiac events in noncardiac surgery: clinical applications. *JAMA* 2002;287:1445–1457.

195. **Mangano DT, Layug EL, Wallace A, et al.** Effect of atenolol on mortality and cardiovascular morbidity after noncardiac surgery. Multicenter Study of Perioperative Ischemia Research Group. *N Engl J Med* 1996;335:1713–1720.

196. **Wallace A, Layug B, Tateo I, et al.** Prophylactic atenolol reduces postoperative myocardial ischemia. McSPI Research Group. *Anesthesiology* 1998;88:7–17.

197. **Devereaux PJ, Yang H, Yusuf S, et al.** Effects of extended-release metoprolol succinate in patients undergoing non-cardiac surgery (POISE trial): a randomised controlled trial. *Lancet* 2008;371:1839–1847.

198. **Arieff AI.** Fatal postoperative pulmonary edema: pathogenesis and literature review. *Chest* 1999;115:1371–1377.

199. **Mangano DT, Browner WS, Hooenberg M, et al.** Long-term cardiac prognosis following noncardiac surgery. The Study of Perioperative Ischemia Research Group. *JAMA* 1992;268:233–239.

200. **Ashton CM, Petersen NJ, Wray NP, et al.** The incidence of perioperative myocardial infarction in men undergoing noncardiac surgery. *Ann Intern Med* 1993;118:504–510.

201. **Kuner J, Enescu V, Utsu F, et al.** Cardiac arrhythmias during anesthesia. *Dis Chest* 1967;52:580–587.

202. **Blaustein AS.** Preoperative and perioperative management of cardiac patients undergoing noncardiac surgery. *Cardiol Clin* 1995;13:149–161.

203. **Lerner SM.** Suppression of a demand pacemaker by transurethral electrocautery. *Anesth Analg* 1973;52:703–706.

204. **Dorman T, Breslow MJ, Pronovost PJ, et al.** Bundle-branch block as a risk factor in noncardiac surgery. *Arch Intern Med* 2000;160:1149–1152.

205. **Skinner JF, Pearce ML.** Surgical risk in the cardiac patient. *J Chronic Dis* 1964;17:57–72.

206. **Maille JG, Dyrda I, Paiement B, et al.** Patients with cardiac valve prosthesis: subsequent anaesthetic management for non-cardiac surgical procedures. *Can Anaesth Soc J* 1973;20:207–216.

207. **Bonow RO, Carabello B, de Leon AC, et al.** ACC/AHA guidelines for the management of patients with valvular heart disease. executive summary. A report of the American College of Cardiology/American Heart Association Task Force on Practice Guidelines (Committee on Management of Patients with Valvular Heart Disease). *J Heart Valve Dis* 1998;7:672–707.

208. **Goldman L, Caldera DL, Southwick FS, et al.** Cardiac risk factors and complications in non-cardiac surgery. *Medicine (Baltimore)* 1978;57:357–370.

209. **Strandgaard S, Olesen J, Skinhoj E, et al.** Autoregulation of brain circulation in severe arterial hypertension. *BMJ* 1973;1:507–510.

210. **Weinhouse GL.** Pulmonary artery catheterization: indications and complications. *UpToDate* 2010. Available online at: http://www.uptodate.com/contents/pulmonary-artery-catheterization-indications-and-complications

211. **Weinhouse GL.** Insertion of pulmonary artery catheters. *UpToDate* 2010. Available online at: http://www.uptodate.com/contents/insertion-of-pulmonary-artery-catheters

212. **Connors AF Jr, Speroff T, Dawson NV, et al.** The effectiveness of right heart catheterization in the initial care of critically ill patients. SUPPORT investigators. *JAMA* 1996;276:889–897.

213. **Sandham JD, Hull RD, Brant RF, et al.** A randomized, controlled trial of the use of pulmonary-artery catheters in high-risk surgical patients. *N Engl J Med* 2003;348:5–14.

214. **Harvey S, Harrison DA, Singer M, et al.** Assessment of the clinical effectiveness of pulmonary artery catheters in management of patients in intensive care (PAC-Man): a randomised controlled trial. *Lancet* 2005;366:472–477.

215. **Shah MR, Hasselblad V, Stevenson LW, et al.** Impact of the pulmonary artery catheter in critically ill patients: meta-analysis of randomized clinical trials. *JAMA* 2005;294:1664–1670.

216. **Bernard AC, Davenport DL, Chang PK, et al.** Intraoperative transfusion of 1 U to 2 U packed red blood cells is associated with increased 30-day mortality, surgical-site infection, pneumonia, and sepsis in general surgery patients. *J Am Coll Surg* 2009;208:931–939.

217. **Corwin HL, Gettinger A, Pearl RG, et al.** The CRIT study: anemia and blood transfusion in the critically ill—current clinical practice in the United States. *Crit Care Med* 2004;32:39–52.

218. **Hebert PC, Yetisir E, Martin C, et al.** Is a low transfusion threshold safe in critically ill patients with cardiovascular diseases? *Crit Care Med* 2001;29:227–234.

219. **Wu WC, Smith TS, Henderson WG, et al.** Operative blood loss, blood transfusion, and 30-day mortality in older patients after major noncardiac surgery. *Ann Surg* 2010;252:11–17.

220. **Greenburg AG.** Benefits and risks of blood transfusion in surgical patients. *World J Surg* 1996;20:1189–1193.

221. **Weiskopf RB, Viele MK, Feiner J, et al.** Human cardiovascular and metabolic response to acute, severe isovolemic anemia. *JAMA* 1998;279:217–221.

222. **Madjdpour C, Spahn DR, Weiskopf RB.** Anemia and perioperative red blood cell transfusion: a matter of tolerance. *Crit Care Med* 2006;34(5 Suppl):S102–S108.

223. **Price TH, Goodnough LT, Vogler WR, et al.** The effect of recombinant human erythropoietin on the efficacy of autologous blood donation in patients with low hematocrits: a multicenter, randomized, double-blind, controlled trial. *Transfusion* 1996;36:29–36.

224. **Price TH, Goodnough LT, Vogler WR, et al.** Improving the efficacy of preoperative autologous blood donation in patients with low hematocrit: a randomized, double-blind, controlled trial of recombinant human erythropoietin. *Am J Med* 1996;101:22S–27S.

225. **Goodnough LT.** Autologous blood donation. *Anesthesiol Clin North Am* 2005;23:263–270.

226. **Goodnough LT, Brecher ME, Kanter MH, et al.** Transfusion medicine. Second of two parts—blood conservation. *N Engl J Med* 1999;340:525–533.

227. **Kanter MH, van Maanen D, Anders KH, et al.** Preoperative autologous blood donations before elective hysterectomy. *JAMA* 1996;276:798–801.

228. **Horowitz NS, Gibb RK, et al.** Utility and cost-effectiveness of preoperative autologous blood donation in gynecologic and gynecologic oncology patients. *Obstet Gynecol* 2002;99(Pt 1):771–776.

229. **Anonymous.** Transfusion alert: use of autologous blood. National Heart, Lung, and Blood Institute Expert Panel on the use of Autologous Blood. *Transfusion* 1995;35:703–711.

230. **Pedersen-Bjergaard U, Andersen M, Hansen PB.** Drug-specific characteristics of thrombocytopenia caused by non-cytotoxic drugs. *Eur J Clin Pharmacol* 1998;54:701–706.

231. **James AH.** Von Willebrand disease in women: awareness and diagnosis. *Thromb Res* 2009;124(Suppl 1):S7–S10.

232. **Federici AB, Mannucci PM.** Management of inherited von Willebrand disease in 2007. *Ann Med* 2007;39:346–358.

233. **Myers ER, Clarke-Pearson DL, Olt GJ, et al.** Preoperative coagulation testing on a gynecologic oncology service. *Obstet Gynecol* 1994;83:438–444.

234. **Bodey GP, Buckley M, Sathe YS, et al.** Quantitative relationships between circulating leukocytes and infection in patients with acute leukemia. *Ann Intern Med* 1966;64:328–340.

235. **Johansson PI, Stensballe J.** Hemostatic resuscitation for massive bleeding: the paradigm of plasma and platelets—a review of the current literature. *Transfusion* 2010;50:701–710.

236. **Rock P, Passannante A.** Preoperative assessment: pulmonary. *Anesthesiol Clin North Am* 2004;22:77–91.

237. **Bapoje SR, Whitaker JF, Schulz T, et al.** Preoperative evaluation of the patient with pulmonary disease. *Chest* 2007;132:1637–1645.

238. **Smetana GW.** Preoperative pulmonary evaluation. *N Engl J Med* 1999;340:937–944.

239. **Expert Panel Report 3 (EPR-3).** Guidelines for the diagnosis and management of asthma—Summary Report 2007. *J Allergy Clin Immunol* 2007;120(Suppl):S94–S138.

240. **Silvanus MT, Groeben H, Peters J.** Corticosteroids and inhaled *salbutamol* in patients with reversible airway obstruction markedly decrease the incidence of bronchospasm after tracheal intubation. *Anesthesiology* 2004;100:1052–1057.

241. **Qaseem A, Snow V, Fitterman N, et al.** Risk assessment for and strategies to reduce perioperative pulmonary complications for patients undergoing noncardiothoracic surgery: a guideline from the American College of Physicians. *Ann Intern Med* 2006;144:575–580.

242. **Sutherland ER, Cherniack RM.** Management of chronic obstructive pulmonary disease. *N Engl J Med* 2004;350:2689–2697.

243. **Barnes PJ.** Chronic obstructive pulmonary disease. *N Engl J Med* 2000;343:269–280.

244. **Wheeler AP, Bernard GR.** Acute lung injury and the acute respiratory distress syndrome: a clinical review. *Lancet* 2007;369:1553–1564.

245. **Weinacker AB, Vaszar LT.** Acute respiratory distress syndrome: physiology and new management strategies. *Annu Rev Med* 2001;52:221–237.

246. **Brower RG, Lanken PN, MacIntyre N, et al.** Higher versus lower positive end-expiratory pressures in patients with the acute respiratory distress syndrome. *N Engl J Med* 2004;351:327–336.

247. **Anonymous.** Demography of dialysis and transplantation in Europe, 1984. Report from the European Dialysis and Transplant Association Registry. *Nephrol Dial Transplant* 1986;1:1–8.

248. **Blumberg A, Weidmann P, Shaw S, et al.** Effect of various therapeutic approaches on plasma potassium and major regulating factors in terminal renal failure. *Am J Med* 1988;85:507–512.

249. **Lewis SL, Van Epps DE.** Neutrophil and monocyte alterations in chronic dialysis patients. *Am J Kidney Dis* 1987;9:381–395.

250. **Hellem AJ, Borchgrevink CF, Ames SB.** The role of red cells in haemostasis: the relation between haematocrit, bleeding time and platelet adhesiveness. *Br J Haematol* 1961;7:42–50.

251. **Remuzzi G.** Bleeding disorders in uremia: pathophysiology and treatment. *Adv Nephrol Necker Hosp* 1989;18:171–186.

252. **Janson PA, Jubelirer SJ, Weinstein MJ, et al.** Treatment of the bleeding tendency in uremia with cryoprecipitate. *N Engl J Med* 1980;303:1318–1322.

253. **Mannucci PM, Remuzzi G, Pusineri F, et al.** Deamino-8-D-arginine vasopressin shortens the bleeding time in uremia. *N Engl J Med* 1983;308:8–12.

254. **Stoelting R, Dierdorf S.** Renal disease. In: Stoelting R, Dierdorf E, eds. *Anesthesia and co-existing disease.* New York: Churchill Livingstone, 1993:289–312.

255. **Tonelli M, Pannu N, Manns B.** Oral phosphate binders in patients with kidney failure. *N Engl J Med* 2010;362:1312–1324.

256. **Hostetter TH, Olson JL, Rennke HG, et al.** Hyperfiltration in remnant nephrons: a potentially adverse response to renal ablation. *J Am Soc Nephrol* 2001;12:1315–1325.

257. **Miller R.** *Pharmacology of muscle relaxants and their antagonists.* New York: Churchill Livingstone, 1986.

258. **Mazze R.** *Anesthesia for patients with abnormal renal function and genitourinary problems.* New York: Churchill Livingstone, 1986.

259. **Roth F, Wuthrich H.** The clinical importance of hyperkalaemia following suxamethonium administration. *Br J Anaesth* 1969;41:311–316.

260. **Silberman H.** Renal failure and the surgeon. *Surg Gynecol Obstet* 1977;144:775–784.

261. **Bullock ML, Umen AJ, Finkelstein M, et al.** The assessment of risk factors in 462 patients with acute renal failure. *Am J Kidney Dis* 1985;5:97–103.

262. **Hou SH, Bushinsky DA, Wish JB, et al.** Hospital-acquired renal insufficiency: a prospective study. *Am J Med* 1983;74:243–248.

263. **Meyer RD.** Risk factors and comparisons of clinical nephrotoxicity of aminoglycosides. *Am J Med* 1986;80:119–125.

264. **Shusterman N, Strom BL, Murray TG, et al.** Risk factors and outcome of hospital-acquired acute renal failure. Clinical epidemiologic study. *Am J Med* 1987;83:65–71.

265. **Lameire NH.** Contrast-induced nephropathy—prevention and risk reduction. *Nephrol Dial Transplant* 2006;21:i11–i23.

266. **Bush HL Jr, Huse JB, Johnson WC, et al.** Prevention of renal insufficiency after abdominal aortic aneurysm resection by optimal volume loading. *Arch Surg* 1981;116:1517–1524.

267. **Cebul RD, Beck JR.** Biochemical profiles. Applications in ambulatory screening and preadmission testing of adults. *Ann Intern Med* 1987;106:403–413.

268. **Batchelder BM, Cooperman LH.** Effects of anesthetics on splanchnic circulation and metabolism. *Surg Clin North Am* 1975;55:787–794.

269. **Maze M, Bass NM.** *Anesthesia and the hepatobilliary system.* New York: Churchill Livingstone, 2000.

270. **Child C, Turcotte JG.** Surgery and portal hypertension. In: **Child C, ed.** *The liver and portal hypertension.* Philadelphia, PA: WB Saunders, 1964:1–85.

271. **Mansour A, Watson W, Sahyani V, et al.** Abdominal operations in patients with cirrhosis: still a major surgical challenge. *Surgery* 1997;122:730–736.

272. **Telem DA, Schiano T, Goldstone R, et al.** Factors that predict outcome of abdominal operations in patients with advanced cirrhosis. *Clin Gastroenterol Hepatol* 2010;8:451–458.

273. **Kamath PS, Wiesner RH, Malinchoc M, et al.** A model to predict survival in patients with end-stage liver disease. *Hepatology* 2001;33:464–470.

274. **Malinchoc M, Kamath PS, Gordon FD, et al.** A model to predict poor survival in patients undergoing transjugular intrahepatic portosystemic shunts. *Hepatology* 2000;31:864–871.

275. **Hanje AJ, Patel T.** Preoperative evaluation of patients with liver disease. *Nat Clin Pract Gastroenterol Hepatol* 2007;4:266–276.

276. **Terblanche J.** Sclerotherapy for prophylaxis of variceal bleeding. *Lancet* 1986;1:961–963.

277. **Lamont J.** The liver. In: **Vandam L, ed.** *To make the patient ready for anesthesia: medical care of the surgical patient.* Menlo Park, CA: Addison Wesley, 1984:47–66.

278. **Blamey SL, Fearpm KC, Gilmour WH, et al.** Prediction of risk in biliary surgery. *Br J Surg* 1983;70:535–538.

279. **Czaja AJ, Summerskill WH.** Chronic hepatitis. To treat or not to treat? *Med Clin North Am* 1978;62:71–85.

280. **Mast EE, Weinbaum CM, Fiore AE, et al.** A comprehensive immunization strategy to eliminate transmission of hepatitis B virus infection in the United States: recommendations of the Advisory Committee on Immunization Practices (ACIP) Part II: immunization of adults. *MMWR Recomm Rep* 2006;55(RR-16):1–33.

281. **Liaw YF, Sung JJ, Chow WC, et al.** *Lamivudine* for patients with chronic hepatitis B and advanced liver disease. *N Engl J Med* 2004;351:1521–1531.

282. **Marcellin P, Heathcote EJ, Buti M, et al.** *Tenofovir disoproxil fumarate* versus *adefovir dipivoxil* for chronic hepatitis B. *N Engl J Med* 2008;359:2442–2455.

283. **Keam SJ, Cvetkovic RS.** Peginterferon-alpha-2a (40 kD) plus ribavirin: a review of its use in the management of chronic hepatitis C mono-infection. *Drugs* 2008;68:1273–1317.

284. **Chiang PP.** Perioperative management of the alcohol-dependent patient. *Am Fam Physician* 1995;52:2267–2273.

285. **Matloff D, Kapkan MM.** Gastroenterology. In: **Molitch M, ed.** *Management of medical problems in surgical patients.* Philadelphia, PA: FA Davis, 1982:219–252.

286. **Wiklund RA.** Preoperative preparation of patients with advanced liver disease. *Crit Care Med* 2004;32(Suppl):S106–S115.

287. **O'Leary JG, Yachimski PS, Friedman LS.** Surgery in the patient with liver disease. *Clin Liver Dis* 2009;13:211–231.

23

Gynecologic Endoscopy

Malcolm G. Munro
Andrew I. Brill
William H. Parker

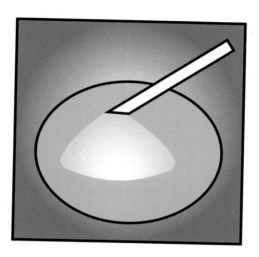

- **Positioning the insufflation needle and the primary cannula are best accomplished with the patient in an unaltered horizontal position.**

- **Proper patient selection is critical for laparoscopic management of ovarian cysts because of concerns about an adverse effect on prognosis with malignant tumors.**

- **Laparoscopic myomectomy often requires laparoscopic suturing; thus, more technical skills are needed than with many other endoscopic procedures.**

- **Laparoscopic hysterectomy comprises any removal of the uterus where at least part of the dissection is accomplished laparoscopically while the remainder, if any, is finished vaginally.**

- **Dehiscence and hernia risk appear to significantly increase when the fascial incision is larger than 10 mm in diameter.**

- **The incidence of unintended electrosurgical activation injuries can be reduced if the surgeon always remains in direct control of electrode activation and if all electrosurgical hand instruments are removed from the peritoneal cavity when not in use.**

- **Patients recovering from laparoscopic surgery usually experience daily improvement. Pain diminishes, gastrointestinal function returns rapidly, and fever is extremely unusual. Therefore, if a patient's condition is not improving, possible complications of anesthesia or surgery should be considered.**

Endoscopy is a procedure that uses a narrow telescope to view the interior of a viscus or preformed space. Although the first medical endoscopic procedures were performed more than 100 years ago, the potential of this method was realized only recently. Endoscopes are used to perform a variety of operations. **In gynecology, endoscopes are used most often to diagnose conditions by direct visualization of the peritoneal cavity (laparoscopy) or the inside of the uterus (hysteroscopy).**

When used appropriately, endoscopic surgery offers the benefits of reduced pain, improved cosmesis, lower cost, and faster recovery. The indications for endoscopic surgery are outlined here and described in more detail in the appropriate chapters. The technology, potential uses, and complications of laparoscopy and hysteroscopy are summarized here.

Laparoscopy

The past four decades have witnessed rapid progress and technologic advances in gynecologic laparoscopy. Operative laparoscopy was developed in the 1970s, and in the early 1980s, laparoscopy was first used to direct the application of electrical or laser energy for the treatment of advanced stages of endometriosis. The use of high-resolution, and, more recently, high-definition video cameras in operative laparoscopy made it easier to view the pelvis during the performance of complex procedures (1,2). Most procedures that previously were performed using traditional techniques are feasible with the laparoscope, including adnexal procedures such as ectopic pregnancy and ovarian cystectomy; uterine surgery, such as myomectomy and hysterectomy; and reconstruction of the pelvic floor, such as retropubic urethropexy and sacral colposuspension. The endoscopic approach may have drawbacks in some patients. Although many laparoscopic procedures appear to reduce the cost and morbidity associated with surgery, others were replaced by even less invasive procedures, and a few were not effective replacements for more traditional operations. The use of microprocessor-assisted laparoscopy allows the surgeon to operate remotely from the operative field, in a sitting position, with the "robot" allowing translation of natural hand manipulations to the peritoneal cavity with the specially designed instruments. The value of this and other techniques and indications for operative endoscopy are still under investigation and constantly in a state of evolution.

Diagnostic Laparoscopy

The lens of a laparoscope can be positioned to allow wide-angle or magnified views of the peritoneal cavity. The clarity and illumination of the optics allow a better appreciation of fine detail than is possible with the naked eye. Laparoscopy is the standard method for the diagnosis of endometriosis and adhesions because no other imaging technique provides the same degree of sensitivity and specificity.

There are limitations to laparoscopy. The view of the operative field may be restricted, and if tissue or fluid becomes attached to the lens, vision may be obscured. Soft tissues, intramural myomas, or the inside of a hollow viscus cannot be palpated. For assessment of these tissues, an imaging modality, such as ultrasonography, computed tomography (CT), or magnetic resonance imaging (MRI), is superior. **Because of its ability to view soft tissue, ultrasonography is more accurate than laparoscopy for the evaluation of the inside of adnexal masses. The intraluminal contour of the uterus can be shown only by hysteroscopy or contrast imaging such as saline infusion sonography, hysterosalpingography, or MRI. Ultrasonography, in combination with serum assays of β-human chorionic gonadotropin (β-hCG) and progesterone, can be used to diagnose ectopic pregnancy, usually allowing medical therapy to be given without laparoscopic confirmation** (3). As a result of the advances in blood tests and imaging technology, laparoscopy more often is used to confirm a clinical impression than for initial diagnosis.

Laparoscopy may disclose abnormalities that are not necessarily related to the patient's problem. Although endometriosis, adhesions, leiomyomas, and small cysts in the ovaries are common, they are frequently asymptomatic. Thus, **diagnostic laparoscopy must be performed prudently,** interpreting findings in the context of the clinical problem and other diagnoses.

Therapeutic (Operative) Laparoscopy

The role of laparoscopy in the operative management of gynecologic conditions is evolving. Many procedures previously performed as traditional abdominal and vaginal operations are feasible or even readily performed under laparoscopic direction. **Operative laparoscopy has the benefit of shorter hospital stays, less postoperative pain, and faster return to normal activity.** These general features of laparoscopic procedures contribute to a reduction in the "indirect costs" of surgical care, including less time away from work and a diminished need for postdischarge supportive care in the home (4). In addition to the other benefits of endoscopic procedures, adhesions are less likely to form with laparoscopic surgery than with laparotomy. Because sponges are not used, the amount of direct peritoneal trauma is reduced substantially, and contamination of the peritoneal cavity is minimized. The reduced exposure to the drying effect of room air allows the peritoneal surface to remain more moist and, therefore, less susceptible to injury and adhesion formation.

Despite these advantages, there are potential limitations: exposure of the operative field can be reduced; instruments are small and can be used only through fixed ports; and the ability to manipulate the pelvic viscera is limited. In some cases, the cost of hospitalization increases, despite a shortened stay, because of prolonged operating room time and the use of more expensive surgical equipment and supplies. Efficacy may be reduced if a surgeon cannot adequately replicate the abdominal operation. In some patients, there is an increased risk of complications, which can be attributed to the innate limitations of laparoscopy, the level of surgical expertise, or both. With an adequate combination of ability, training, and experience, however, operative time is comparable to those of traditional abdominal surgery and complications may be reduced.

Tubal Surgery

Sterilization   Laparoscopic sterilization has been used extensively since the late 1960s, and while it can be performed with local anesthetics, it is usually accomplished under general anesthesia. The fallopian tubes can be occluded by suture, clips, silastic rings, or with radiofrequency electrocoagulation, most commonly with a bipolar electrocoagulation instrument (see Chapter 10). When an "operative laparoscope" is used, only one incision is required because the sheath in such a system contains an instrument channel. Otherwise, a second port is needed for the introduction of the occluding instrument. Patients generally remain in the hospital only for a few hours; even when general anesthesia is used. Postoperative pain is usually minor and related to gas that remains in the peritoneal cavity (shoulder pain, dyspnea), and in the case of occlusive devices, pain at the surgical site. These effects normally disappear within a few days. The failure rate is about 5.4 per 1,000 woman-years (5,6). The use of laparoscopic tubal sterilization was impacted by the availability of office vasectomy, effective intrauterine contraception, and the development of office-based hysteroscopic sterilization techniques, discussed later in this chapter.

Ectopic Gestation   Medical therapy with *methotrexate* is considered first-line therapy for tubal pregnancies that meet criteria that may include the following: no cardiac activity, tubal mass smaller than 4 cm as determined by ultrasonography, and β-hCG level less than 10,000 (7,8). **When surgical therapy is required, ectopic gestation can usually be managed successfully by using laparoscopic salpingotomy, salpingectomy, or segmental resection of a portion of the oviduct** (see Chapter 20) (9,10). Salpingotomy is performed with scissors, a laser, or an electrosurgical electrode after carefully injecting the mesosalpinx with a dilute *vasopressin*-containing solution (20 U in 100 mL of normal saline). For salpingectomy, the vascular pedicles are usually secured with electrosurgical desiccation or coagulation, but it is possible using ligatures or clips. Tissue is usually removed from the peritoneal cavity through one of the laparoscopic cannulas.

When salpingotomy is performed, regardless of the route, there is about a 5% chance that trophoblastic tissue remains. In such instances, medical treatment with *methotrexate* is appropriate (see Chapter 20). Consequently, β-hCG levels should be measured weekly until there is confidence that complete excision occurred (11–13).

Ovarian Surgery

Ovarian Masses   **Laparoscopic removal of selected ovarian masses is a well-established technique supported by high quality evidence (14–16). Proper patient selection is critical for laparoscopic management of adnexal masses because of the possible adverse effect of laparoscopic approaches on prognosis with malignant tumors** (17,18). Preoperative ultrasonography is mandatory. Sonolucent lesions with thin walls and no solid components are at very low risk for malignancy and, therefore, are suitable for laparoscopic removal. For postmenopausal women, the measurement of CA125 levels is useful in identifying candidates for laparoscopic management (19,20). Combining age, menopausal status, an ultrasound score, and the serum CA125 level into a "risk of malignancy index" seems to offer an effective approach to the identification of cysts at high risk for epithelial malignancy (21–23). Lesions with ultrasonographic findings suggestive of mature teratoma (dermoid), endometrioma, or hemorrhagic or other cysts presenting with torsion or other causes of acute pain may be suitable for endoscopic management (24–27). **Ovarian tumors should be assessed by frozen histologic section, and any frank malignancy should be managed expeditiously by laparotomy (14,18,20).**

The technique for performing laparoscopy for oophorectomy and cystectomy is similar to that used for laparotomy (13). For cystectomy, scissors are used to incise the ovarian capsule, and blunt dissection or aqua dissection is used to separate the cyst from the ovary. If oophorectomy is performed, the vascular pedicles are occluded and transected, usually with radiofrequency electrosurgical coagulation and cutting systems, but in some instances with sutures, clips, or linear cutting and stapling devices. The ureter should be identified and should be clear of the pedicle to be transected. Cysts that appear to be benign may be drained before extraction through a laparoscopic cannula or, less commonly, a posterior culdotomy. If there is concern about the impact of spilled cyst contents, the specimen should be removed in a retrieval bag inserted into the peritoneal cavity through a laparoscopic port. Some authors describe a minilaparotomy technique, or enlarging one port site incision, to exteriorize the mass, drain it externally without intraperitoneal spill, remove the cyst or ovary, and then reintroduce the adnexa into the peritoneal cavity (28).

Although in the past the ovary routinely was closed after cystectomy, this practice may be unnecessary and could contribute to the formation of adhesions (29). There is controversy about this point as at least one randomized clinical trial (class 1) suggested that suture-based closure of the ovary is associated with fewer adhesions than using electrodesiccation alone (30).

Other Ovarian Surgery

Ovarian torsion, previously treated by laparotomy and oophorectomy, often can be managed laparoscopically (31,32). Even if there is apparent necrosis, the adnexa can be untwisted, usually with preservation of normal ovarian function (26,33). Performing a cystectomy at the same time that the ovary is untwisted greatly reduces the likelihood that ovarian function will be maintained. Rarely is adnexectomy indicated.

Polycystic ovarian syndrome can be treated laparoscopically using electrosurgery or laser vaporization to perform ovarian "drilling." This procedure reduces the volume of ovarian stromal tissue and may lead to a temporary return of normal ovulation (34–36). Although such procedures were successful in a number of randomized trials, postoperative adhesions form in 15% to 20% of patients, which underscores the need to first exhaust medical treatment (37–39).

Uterine Surgery

Myomectomy

Laparoscopic myomectomy, although feasible, may be difficult to perform because proper closure of the myometrium requires laparoscopically directed suturing and, thus, requires more technical skills than many other endoscopic procedures. While it is possible that microprocessor-assisted (robotic) laparoscopic myomectomy may allow more surgeons to suture effectively under laparoscopic guidance, in expert hands there appears to be no benefit to robotic surgery in any measurable perioperative outcome (40).

There remain some questions regarding the efficacy of laparoscopic myomectomy, especially as it relates to the treatment of infertility and heavy menstrual bleeding, each of which are thought to be secondary to submucous myomas. Although there are some well-designed randomized clinical trials evaluating infertility outcomes comparing laparoscopic myomectomy to that performed by laparotomy, the sample sizes are still relatively small, and the cases are highly selected, limiting the size and number of the lesions to be removed (41,42). In these trials, fertility outcomes were similar between the laparoscopic and the laparotomic approaches. These and other trials evaluating perioperative outcomes, such as duration of admission, surgical pain, and operative complications, found the laparoscopic approach to be superior (43).

Proper patient selection for myomectomy, regardless of route, is extremely important, particularly because, by age 50, the prevalence of leiomyomas may be as high as 70% in whites and 80% in women of African ancestry (44). It is relatively easy to mistakenly ascribe symptoms to the presence of leiomyomas. Unless the myoma involves the endometrial cavity, it is unlikely to contribute to heavy menstrual bleeding or infertility; the impact of intramural myomas on infertility is not well understood (45). Leiomyomas that cause pressure are often large and may be located near vital vascular structures that may preclude the laparoscopic approach even in expert hands. Many women will do well with expectant or medical management or with procedural alternatives such as uterine artery embolization. The surgeon should freely select a laparotomic approach, either at the outset or during the procedure, if technical limitations put the patient at risk or otherwise compromise the potential relevant clinical outcomes (46). **Patients who have pedunculated or subserosal leiomyomas that cause bothersome discomfort or pain in association with torsion are especially good candidates for laparoscopic excision** (13,47).

Hysterectomy

Laparoscopic hysterectomy encompasses a variety of procedures, including the facilitation of vaginal hysterectomy with variable extents of endoscopic dissection, supracervical hysterectomy by dissection, amputation and mechanical removal of the fundus, and the removal of the entire uterus under laparoscopic direction (48–50). In most environments, the procedure is performed with a combination of electrosurgical vessel sealing devices and mechanical cutting systems, often incorporated into a single instrument. In some instances sutures, clips, and linear cutting and stapling devices are employed in the process of dissecting or occluding vascular pedicles.

Compared to vaginal hysterectomy, there is a slightly higher risk of complications with laparoscopic hysterectomy, but this risk is probably lower than for abdominal hysterectomy (51). As experience is gained with laparoscopic hysterectomy, these outcomes may approach those of vaginal hysterectomy. The procedural costs of laparoscopic hysterectomy are greater than either vaginal or abdominal hysterectomy but can be dramatically reduced when reusable instruments are employed (4,52). Most studies show less postoperative pain, shorter hospital stays, and faster postoperative recovery with laparoscopic hysterectomy than with abdominal hysterectomy (51,53). There is evidence that pain scores and quality-of-life measures, including sexual activity and physical and mental functioning, were significantly better for women who underwent laparoscopic versus abdominal hysterectomy (54). These differences were present at 6 weeks following surgery and remained at the 12-month follow-up visit. When the societal benefits of faster return to work or family are considered, the cost of laparoscopic surgery is significantly less (4).

Selection of the route of hysterectomy must be done considering the anatomy, the disorder or disease state, the patient's wishes, and the training and experience of the surgeon. Laparoscopic hysterectomy offers no advantage for women in whom vaginal hysterectomy is possible because the endoscopic approach is more expensive and probably has a higher risk for perioperative morbidity (51). The ideal place for laparoscopic hysterectomy is as a replacement for abdominal hysterectomy.

Outside of physician training, there are relatively few remaining indications for abdominal hysterectomy, which should be reserved for the minority of women for whom a laparoscopic or vaginal approach is not appropriate, including (i) patients with medical conditions, such as cardiopulmonary disease, where the risks of either general anesthesia or the increased intraperitoneal pressure associated with laparoscopy are deemed unacceptable; or (ii) where morcellation is known or likely to be required and uterine malignancy is either known or suspected. For both laparoscopic and vaginal hysterectomy the reasons include: (i) hysterectomy is indicated but there is no access to the surgeons or facilities required for vaginal or laparoscopic hysterectomy and referral is not feasible; or (ii) circumstances where anatomy is so distorted by uterine disease or adhesions that a vaginal or laparoscopic approach is not deemed safe or reasonable by individuals with recognized expertise in either vaginal or laparoscopic hysterectomy techniques (52,54). For surgeons without the skill and training to perform minimally invasive hysterectomy (either vaginal or laparoscopic), for benign indications, consideration should be given for referral to a gynecologist with such training.

Infertility Operations

When infertility occurs secondary to disruption of the normal anatomy or anatomic relationships by an inflammatory process, laparoscopically directed operations used to restore anatomy include fimbrioplasty, adhesiolysis, and salpingostomy for distal obstruction (55). Fimbrioplasty is distinguished from salpingostomy because it is performed in the absence of preexisting complete distal obstruction. Endometriosis associated with adnexal distortion can be treated by laparoscopic adhesiolysis. Whereas there is no known additional benefit of medical treatment of coexistent active endometriosis, the evidence relating to ablation of minimal and mild endometriosis is mixed, although when subjected to meta-analytic technique, there is a slight fecundity benefit for those undergoing laparoscopic ablation (56–58). Laparoscopy is used for procedures in which gametes (gamete intrafallopian transfer) or zygotes (zygote intrafallopian transfer) are placed into the fallopian tube after oocytes are removed either via ultrasound- or laparoscopically guided technique.

Adhesiolysis may be accomplished by blunt or sharp dissection with scissors, ultrasonic shears, or an electrosurgical electrode. There is no evidence that laser-based instruments provide any additional value over less expensive techniques such as electrosurgery (59–61). The dissecting instruments are usually passed through an ancillary port; when laser energy is used, the channel of the operating laparoscope may be used for this purpose. Although there is controversy regarding the most appropriate modality for adhesiolysis, these methods are probably equally effective in appropriately trained hands.

Laparoscopic operations for the treatment of mechanical infertility are probably equally effective to similar procedures performed by laparotomy. In patients with extensive adhesions, successful outcomes are unlikely regardless of the approach. Consequently, assisted reproductive technologies such as *in vitro* **fertilization and embryo transfer are necessary in these situations** (see Chapter 32) (13,55).

Endometriosis

The laparoscopic management of endometriomas parallels that of adnexal masses, although the ultrasonographic complexity of endometriomas sometimes makes it difficult to distinguish them preoperatively from a neoplasm (62). The close attachment of the endometrioma to the ovarian cortex and stroma may make it difficult to find surgical dissection planes, and incomplete removal increases the risk of recurrence. In such instances there may be a tendency either to compromise the function of the remaining ovary by attempting complete removal or to risk recurrence by leaving part of the endometrioma in place. A Cochrane review found good evidence that excisional surgery for endometriomas decreases the recurrence of the endometrioma, decreases the recurrence of pain symptoms, and in women who were previously subfertile, increases subsequent spontaneous pregnancy (63). Consequently, where possible the excisional approach should be the goal. Multifocal endometriosis may be treated by mechanical excision or ablation, the latter using coagulation or vaporization with either electrical or laser energy. With proper use, each energy source creates about the same amount of thermal injury (59–61). Endometriosis frequently is deeper than appreciated initially, making excisional techniques valuable in many instances (64,65).

Pelvic Floor Disorders

Laparoscopy can be used to guide procedures to treat pelvic support defects, including culdoplasty, enterocele repair, vaginal vault suspension, paravaginal repair, and retropubic cystourethropexy for urinary stress incontinence. Although these conditions can be treated vaginally, the laparoscopic approach may offer benefits, particularly with retropubic urethropexy. There is some evidence that the laparoscopic approach is effective when compared with the traditional methods, but, in most instances, vaginal or laparoscopic mesh-based techniques seem to be the most frequently used approaches (66,67). Using the same surgical principles applied during traditional pelvic floor repair, laparoscopy promises better access to key anatomical landmarks and potentially more accurate suture placement (68). Whereas apical and anterior compartment defects can be successfully corrected via laparoscopy, posterior and perineal defects are best visualized and repaired using vaginal techniques. The laparoscopic treatment of enterocele and vault prolapse may be useful in patients who require abdominal approaches after failure of a previous vaginal procedure. Because of the anatomical proximity of the pelvic ureter to the uterosacral ligament and anterolateral vagina, bilateral ureteral patency should be confirmed cystoscopically after laparoscopic vaginal vault suspension, enterocele repair, culdoplasty, cystourethropexy, or paravaginal repair.

Gynecologic Malignancies

The role of laparoscopy in the management of gynecologic malignancy is not clearly established (69–71). A study performed by the Gynecology Oncologic Group showed that laparoscopic management of presumed stage I endometrial cancer was feasible (72). Larger-scale studies suggest that women treated with a laparoscopic approach do not fare worse than those treated via laparotomy (73,74). The potential for laparoscopic lymphadenectomy fostered a resurgence of interest in vaginal radical hysterectomy for stage I carcinoma of the cervix. Laparoscopy is being investigated for the staging of early ovarian malignancy and for second-look surgery (75,76).

Patient Preparation and Communication

The rationale, alternatives, risks, and potential benefits of the selected approach should be explained to the prospective patient. She should be advised concerning the likely outcome of expectant management if the procedure was not performed.

The expectations and risks of diagnostic laparoscopy, and those of any other procedures that may be needed, must be explained. It may be helpful to compare risks and recovery with the same procedure performed via abdominal surgery. The risks of laparoscopy include those associated with anesthesia, infection, bleeding, and injury to the abdominal and pelvic viscera. The possibility of conversion to laparotomy if a complication should occur or if the procedure cannot be completed via laparoscopic surgery should also be discussed. Infection is uncommon with laparoscopic surgery. For procedures involving extensive dissection, there is a higher risk for visceral injury. These risks should be clearly presented in a fashion that includes both the possibilities of immediate and delayed recognition. The patient should be given realistic expectations regarding postoperative disability. **Because pain and visceral dysfunction normally continue to improve after uncomplicated laparoscopy, the patient should be instructed to communicate immediately any regression in her recovery.** After diagnostic or brief operative procedures, patients can be discharged on the day of surgery and usually require 24 to 72 hours off work or school. If extensive dissection—a major surgical procedure performed laparoscopically—is necessary or if the surgery lasts longer than 4 hours, hospital admission may be necessary, and the period of disability may then be as long as 10 to 14 days.

Preoperative mechanical bowel preparation was perceived as reducing the morbidity of colonic surgery should an injury occur and improving visualization and exposure of the operative field at laparoscopy. There is an abundance of high-quality evidence demonstrating that preoperative mechanical bowel preparation does not reduce the morbidity of colonic surgery (77). There is one high-quality trial that shows that mechanical bowel preparation may not improve visualization at gynecologic laparoscopy (78). It is premature to abandon preoperative bowel preparation to improve visualization, because, in a small subset of patients, it may facilitate surgery. Mechanical bowel preparation should be considered to help improve visualization in selected instances where stool in the colon might compromise visualization of the operative field.

Communication with the family or other designated individuals should be arranged prior to the procedure. The patient should arrange for a friend or family member to be present to discuss the results of the procedure with the physician and to drive her home if she is discharged the same day.

Equipment and Technique

To facilitate the discussion of laparoscopic equipment, supplies, and techniques, it is useful to divide procedures into "core competencies," which are as follows:

1. Patient positioning
2. Operating room organization
3. Peritoneal access
4. Visualization
5. Manipulation of tissue and fluid
6. Cutting, hemostasis, and tissue fastening
7. Tissue extraction
8. Incision management

Patient Positioning

Proper positioning of the patient is essential for patient safety, comfort of the operator, and optimal visualization of the pelvic organs. There may be advantages to positioning the patient while awake to reduce the frequency of positioning-related complications. Laparoscopy is performed on an operating table that can be tipped to create a steep, head-down (Trendelenburg) position that allows the bowel to move out of the pelvis to facilitate visualization after the cannulas is placed. The footrest can be dropped to allow access to the perineum. The patient is placed in the low lithotomy position, with the legs appropriately supported in stirrups and the buttocks protruding slightly from the lower edge of the table (Fig. 23.1). The thighs are usually kept in the neutral position to preserve the sacroiliac angle, reducing the tendency of

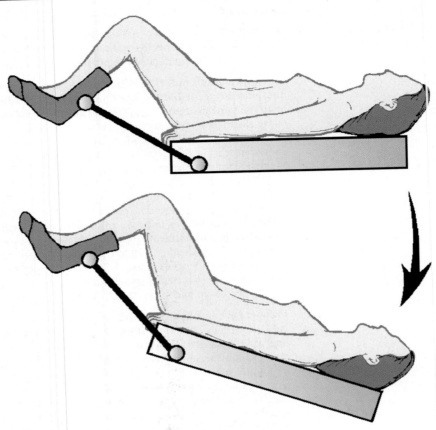

Figure 23.1   **Patient positioning: the low lithotomy position.** The patient's buttocks are positioned so that the perineum is at the edge of the table. The legs are well supported with stirrups, with the thighs in slight flexion. Too much flexion may impede the manipulation of laparoscopic instruments while in the Trendelenburg (head-down) position.

bowel to slide into the peritoneal cavity. **The feet should rest flat, and the lateral aspect of the knee should be protected with padding or a special stirrup to avoid peroneal nerve injury.** The knees should be kept in at least slight flexion to minimize stretching of the sciatic nerve and to provide more stability in the Trendelenburg position. **The arms are positioned at the patient's side by adduction and pronation to allow freedom of movement for the surgeon and to lower the risk for brachial plexus injury** (Fig. 23.2). Care must be exercised to protect the patient's fingers and hands from injury when the foot of the table is raised or lowered. After the patient is properly positioned, the bladder should be emptied with a catheter and a uterine manipulator positioned in the endometrial cavity and secured either by an intracavitary balloon or attached to the cervix as appropriate.

Operating Room Organization

The arrangement of instruments and equipment is important for safety and efficiency. The orientation depends on the operation, the instruments used, and whether the surgeon is right- or left-handed. An orientation for a right-handed operator is shown in Figure 23.2.

For pelvic surgery, the television monitor is typically placed at or over the foot of the table within the angle formed by the patient's legs. If two monitors are available, one may be positioned at each foot of the patient allowing both the surgeon and the assistant the opportunity to view the surgical field without having to turn the head.

The surgeon usually stands by the patient's left side, at an angle facing the patient's contralateral foot. The nurse or technician and instrument table are positioned near the foot of the operating table to avoid obscuring the video monitor. The insufflator may be placed on the patient's right side, in front of the surgeon, to allow continuous monitoring of the inflation rate and

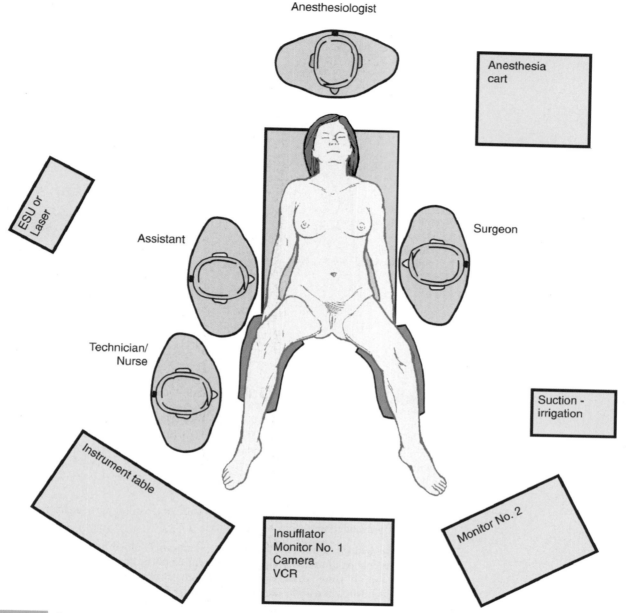

Figure 23.2 **Operating room organization.** The patient's arms are at the sides. The right-handed surgeon stands on the patient's left. Instruments and equipment are distributed around the patient within view of the surgeon. For pelvic surgery, the monitor should be located between the patient's legs.

intra-abdominal pressure. The energy source (e.g., electrosurgical or ultrasonic generator) may be positioned on the patient's right side to permit visualization of the power output.

Peritoneal Access

Before inserting the laparoscope, a primary cannula (or port) must be positioned in the abdominal wall to establish access to the peritoneal cavity. **The *closed technique* is a blind approach in which the cannula is introduced with an obturator designed to penetrate the abdominal layers. In *open laparoscopy,* initial entry into the peritoneal cavity is achieved with minilaparotomy using either a transverse subumbilical or midline infraumbilical incision down to the rectus fascia, to which the cannula is fixed into position with sutures or other suitable techniques.** Gynecologists generally favor a closed technique, preinflating the peritoneal cavity with CO_2 through a hollow insufflation needle. In either case, additional cannulas are

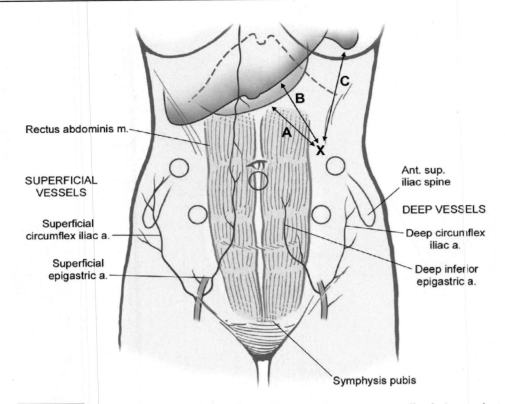

Rectus abdominis m.

SUPERFICIAL
VESSELS

Superficial
circumflex iliac a.

Superficial
epigastric a.

Ant. sup.
iliac spine

DEEP VESSELS

Deep circumflex
iliac a.

Deep inferior
epigastric a.

Symphysis pubis

Figure 23.3   **Vascular anatomy of the anterior abdominal Figure 23.3 wall relative to the sites of port insertion.** The location of the vessels that can be traumatized when inserting trocars into the anterior abdominal wall is indicated. The lateral trocars should be placed lateral to the inferior epigastric vessels that course medially to lie under the rectus muscle anterior to the posterior rectus sheath. The relative anatomy of the left upper quadrant port site is shown: the closest structure is the stomach **(A)** (approximately 4 cm away) and the left lobe of the liver **(B)** approximately (4 cm away). The spleen **(C)** is approximately 12 cm away.

subsequently inserted under direct vision to allow the use of laparoscopic hand instruments such as scissors, probes, and other manipulating devices.

Insertion of the insufflation needle and primary cannula is aided by an understanding of the normal underlying anatomy, especially the location of the larger retroperitoneal vessels (Fig. 23.3). A "safety zone" exists inferior to the sacral promontory in the area bounded cephalad by the bifurcation of the aorta, posteriorly by the sacrum, and laterally by the iliac vessels (79). In women placed in the Trendelenburg position, the great vessels are oriented more cephalad and anterior, making them more vulnerable to injury unless appropriate adjustments are made in the angle of insertion (Fig. 23.4) (80). Therefore, positioning of the insufflation needle and the primary cannula is best accomplished with the patient in an unaltered supine (horizontal) position. This approach facilitates the evaluation of the upper abdomen, which is limited if the intraperitoneal contents are shifted cephalad by the head-down (Trendelenburg) position.

Insufflation Needles

Virtually all insufflation needles are modifications of the hollow needle designed by Verres (Fig. 23.5). In cases uncomplicated by previous pelvic surgery, the preferred site for insertion is the base of the umbilicus, where the abdominal wall is the thinnest and usually avascular.

1. **A midline infraumbilical incision adequate for the needle is made at the base of the umbilicus with a small scalpel, and the abdominal wall is maximally lifted, either manually or with instruments.** Elevation is accomplished manually after affixing towel clips to the abdominal wall on either side lateral to the umbilicus or opposite one another within the edge of the umbilical incision itself (81).

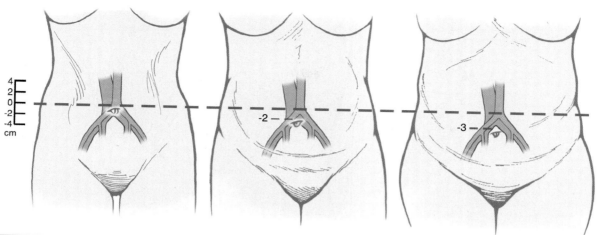

Figure 23.4 **Vascular anatomy.** Location of the great vessels and their changing relationship to the umbilicus with increasing patient weight (from left to right).

Safe insertion of the insufflation needle mandates that the instrument be maintained in a midline, sagittal plane while the operator directs the tip between the iliac vessels, anterior to the sacrum but inferior to the bifurcation of the aorta and the proximal aspect of the vena cava. Because the sacral promontory is commonly covered in part by the left common iliac vein, vascular injury may occur in the midline below the bifurcation (82).

To reduce the risk of retroperitoneal vascular injury while minimizing the chance of inadvertent preperitoneal insufflation, in women of average weight, **the insufflation needle is directed to the patient's spine at a 45-degree angle.** In heavy to obese individuals, this angle may be increased incrementally to nearly 90 degrees, accounting for the increasing thickness of the abdominal wall and the tendency of the umbilicus to gravitate caudad with increasing abdominal girth (79,83). The needle's shaft is held by the tips of the fingers and steadily but purposefully guided into position only far enough to allow the tip's entry into the peritoneal cavity. The tactile and visual feedback created when the needle passes through the facial and peritoneal layers of the abdominal wall may provide guidance and help prevent overaggressive insertion attempts. This proprioceptive feedback is less apparent with disposable needles than with the classic Verres needle. With the former, the surgeon must listen to the "clicks" as the needle obturator retracts when it passes through the rectus fascia and the peritoneum. The

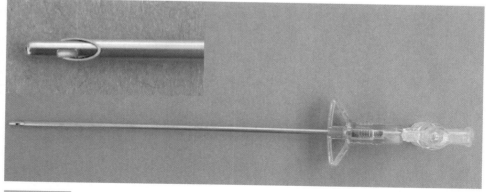

Figure 23.5 **Insufflation needle.** When pressed against tissue such as fascia or peritoneum, the spring-loaded blunt obturator (*inset*) is pushed back into the hollow needle, revealing its sharpened end. When the needle enters the peritoneal cavity, the obturator springs back into position, protecting the intraabdominal contents from injury. The handle of the hollow needle allows the attachment of a syringe or tubing for insufflation of the distention gas.

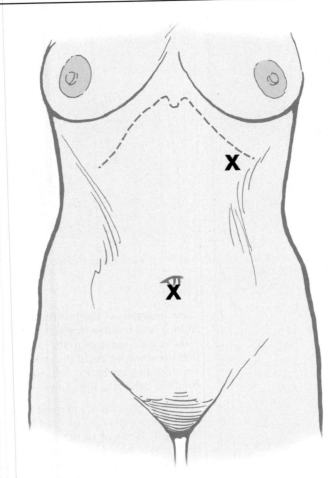

Figure 23.6 **Insufflation needle and cannula insertion sites.** In most instances, both the insufflation needle, if used, and the primary cannula are inserted through the umbilicus. When subumbilical adhesions are known or suspected, the insufflation needle may be placed through the pouch of Douglas or in the left upper quadrant after evacuation of the gastric contents with an orogastric tube.

needle should never be forced. Regardless of technique, the underlying retroperitoneal vessels are protected ultimately by limiting the insertion depth of the insufflation needle.

2. **In instances where known or suspected intra-abdominal adhesions surround the umbilicus, alternative sites should be used for insufflation needle insertion.** These sites include the left upper quadrant, most often at the left costal margin, the pouch of Douglas, and the fundus of the uterus (Fig. 23.6). The left upper quadrant is preferred if hepatosplenomegaly is not present and the patient has not previously had surgery in this area. In such patients, the stomach must be decompressed with a nasogastric or orogastric tube before the needle is inserted (84). While at this location the distance between the skin and the posterior peritoneum is generally more than 11 cm, in thin individuals, it may be as little as 7 cm, so the angle of insertion should take this into account. The needle should be directed medially, about 10 to 15 degrees to avoid the kidney and renal artery; in women of relatively high body mass index it can be placed at a 90-degree angle to the skin, and in thin women, this angle should be reduced to about 45 degrees (84,85).

3. **Before insufflation, the operator should try to detect whether the insufflation needle was malpositioned in the omentum, mesentery, blood vessels, or hollow organs such as the stomach or bowel.** The most direct approach is to use a specially designed insufflation needle that has an integrated cannula through which a small diameter (2 mm) laparoscope can be passed to visualize the point of entry. Otherwise, indirect methods are

necessary. Using a syringe attached to the insufflation needle, blood or gastrointestinal contents may be aspirated. To facilitate this examination, a small amount of saline may be injected into the syringe. If the needle is appropriately positioned, negative intra-abdominal pressure is created by lifting the abdominal wall. This negative pressure may be demonstrated by aspiration of a drop of saline placed over the open, proximal end of the needle or, preferably, by using the digital pressure gauge on the insufflator.

4. **Additional signs of proper placement may be sought after starting insufflation. The intra-abdominal pressure reading should be low, reflecting only systemic resistance to the flow of CO_2.** Consequently, there should be little deviation from a baseline measurement, generally less than 10 mm Hg. The pressure varies with respiration and is slightly higher in obese patients. The earliest reassuring sign is the loss of liver "dullness" over the lateral aspect of the right costal margin. This sign may be absent if there are dense adhesions in the area, usually the result of previous surgery. Symmetric distention is unlikely to occur when the needle is positioned extraperitoneally. Proper positioning can be shown by lightly compressing the xiphoid process, which increases the pressure measured by the insufflator.

5. **The amount of gas transmitted into the peritoneal cavity should depend on the measured intraperitoneal pressure, not the volume of gas inflated.** Intraperitoneal volume capacity varies significantly between individuals. Many surgeons prefer to insufflate to 25 to 30 mm Hg for positioning the cannulas, and a body of evidence exists supporting this approach (86). This level usually provides extra volume and enough counter pressure against the peritoneum, facilitating introduction of the cannula and potentially reducing the chance of bowel or posterior abdominal wall and vessel trauma. After placement of the cannulas, the pressure should be dropped to 10 to 15 mm Hg, which reduces the risk of subcutaneous insufflation leading to crepitus and essentially eliminates hypercarbia or decreased venous return of blood to the heart (84,86,87).

Primary Access Cannulas

Laparoscopic cannulas (or ports) allow the insertion of laparoscopic instruments into the peritoneal cavity while maintaining the pressure created by the distending gas (Figs. 23.7 and 23.8). Cannulas are hollow tubes with a valve or sealing mechanism at or near the proximal end. The cannula may be fitted with a Luer-type port that allows attachment to tubing connected with the CO_2 insufflator. Larger-diameter cannulas (8 to 15 mm) may be fitted with adapters or specialized valves that allow the insertion of smaller-diameter instruments without loss of intraperitoneal pressure.

The obturator is a longer instrument of slightly smaller diameter that is passed through the cannula, exposing its tip. Most obturators are called *trocars* because their tip is designed to penetrate the abdominal wall after the creation of an appropriately sized skin incision. Many disposable trocar-cannula systems are designed with a safety mechanism—usually a pressure-sensitive spring that either retracts the trocar or deploys a protective sheath around its tip after passage through the abdominal wall. None of these protective devices makes insertion safer, and they all increase the cost of the equipment.

In the "closed" laparoscopic access technique, cannulas can be inserted either after the successful creation of a pneumoperitoneum or without previously instilling intraperitoneal gas, also referred to as *direct insertion*. With open laparoscopy, there may be less risk of injury to the major blood vessels such as the aorta, inferior vena cava, and common iliacs. Open laparoscopy cannot prevent all insertion accidents because intestine can be entered inadvertently no matter how small the incision. There is little evidence that a pneumoperitoneum is necessary, at least in the absence of preexisting abdominal wall adhesions. **In women with no previous surgery, the primary puncture can be performed with a trocar-cannula system, which reduces operating time. The first, or primary, cannula must be of sufficient caliber to permit passage of the laparoscope and usually is inserted in or at the lower border of the umbilicus.** The incision should be extended only enough to allow insertion of the cannula; otherwise, leakage of gas may occur around the sheath. The patient should be in an unaltered supine position during placement of the primary cannula. For the primary puncture, either the surgeon or the assistant should elevate the abdominal wall as described previously. Both hands can be positioned on the device, using one to provide counter pressure and control to

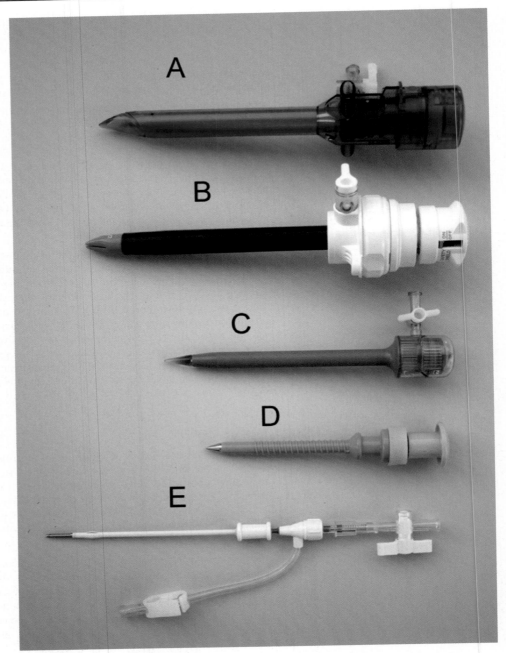

Figure 23.7   Disposable access systems. These instruments are designed for single use. A 12-mm internal diameter blunt access system is shown in (**A**). The next device (**B**) has a 12 mm internal diameter, but has a deployable blade that is used to cut through the abdominal wall. A smaller diameter blunt conical device is shown in (**C**) while a sharp conical access system is presented in (**D**). Both (**C**) and (**D**) have a 5-mm inside diameter. A narrow, 2.7-mm diameter cannula is shown in (**E**). The trocar for this system is a long insufflation needle with a spring deployable obturator.

prevent "overshoot" and resultant injury to bowel or vessels. **The angle of insertion is the same as for the insufflation needle; adjustments are made according to the patient's weight and body habitus** (79). The laparoscope should be inserted to confirm proper intraperitoneal placement before the insufflation gas is allowed to flow. **Previous abdominal surgery increases the incidence of adhesions of the bowel to the anterior abdominal wall, frequently near the umbilicus and in the path of the primary trocar-cannula system** (88,89). In such patients,

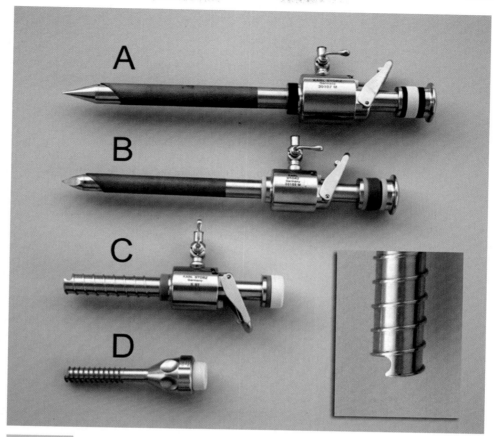

Figure 23.8 **Reusable access systems.** **A:** A sharp conical device, while (**B**) represents a pyramidal-tipped design. **C** and **D** (and *inset*): Images of the so-called EndoTip device that can be positioned in the abdominal wall by simply twisting or screwing it in without the requirement of a trocar.

another primary insertion site, such as the left upper quadrant, should be selected, even if it is used solely for conveying a narrow "scout" laparoscope, some types of which can be inserted through a trocar cannula system with a design similar to that of an insufflation needle (Fig. 23.9). Using such a laparoscope, the presence of adhesions under the incision can be identified and the umbilical cannula can be inserted under direct vision. If adhesions are noted under the incision, appropriate placement of secondary cannulas may be used to introduce instruments for adhesiolysis. Alternate insertion sites for primary cannulas are shown in Figure 23.6.

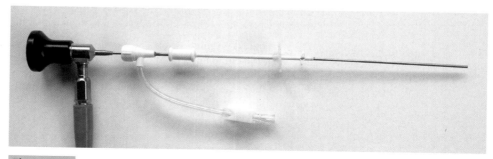

Figure 23.9 **"Scout" laparoscope.** The 2-mm laparoscope from Figure 23.8 and the 2.7-mm access system from Figure 23.7 are shown here assembled. The tubing is connected to inflow gas, usually carbon dioxide.

Ancillary Cannulas

Ancillary cannulas are necessary to perform most diagnostic and operative laparoscopic procedures. Most currently available disposable ancillary cannulas are identical to those designed for insertion of the primary cannula; however, simple cannulas without the so-called safety mechanisms and insufflation ports are generally sufficient (Figs. 23.7D and 23.8D). Some investigators are evaluating the value of systems that allow the insertion of multiple cannulas through a single port, an approach that has the potential to improve surgical cosmesis by reducing the number of incisions created (90–92).

Proper positioning of these ancillary cannulas depends on a sound knowledge of the abdominal wall vascular anatomy. **For the secondary puncture, the patient may be tipped head down (Trendelenburg), allowing the abdominal contents to shift from beneath the incision sites, and thus making it unnecessary to lift the abdominal wall during secondary cannula insertion.** Alternatively, the intraperitoneal pressure may be maintained at 25 to 30 mm Hg to allow insertion of the secondary cannulas prior to placing the patient in the Trendelenburg position.

Ancillary cannulas should always be inserted under direct vision because injury to bowel or major vessels can occur. Before insertion, the bladder should be drained with a urethral catheter. The insertion sites depend on the procedure, the disease, the patient's body habitus, and the surgeon's preference. For diagnostic laparoscopy, the most useful and cosmetically acceptable site for insertion of an ancillary cannula is in the midline of the lower abdomen, about 2 to 4 cm above the symphysis. The ancillary cannula should not be inserted too close to the symphysis because it limits the mobility of the ancillary instruments and access to the cul-de-sac. Laparoscopic cannulas can become dislodged and slip out of the incision during a procedure. There are a variety of cannula designs designed to reduce slippage, which include those with threaded exteriors and anchoring systems with balloon tips.

Lateral placement of lower-quadrant cannulas is useful for operative laparoscopy, but the superficial and inferior epigastric vessels must be located to avoid injury (Fig. 23.3). Transillumination of the abdominal wall from within permits the identification of the superficial inferior epigastric vessels in most thin women. The deep inferior epigastric vessels cannot be identified by this mechanism because of their location deep to the rectus sheath. **The most consistent landmarks are the medial umbilical ligaments (obliterated umbilical arteries) and the exit point of the round ligament into the inguinal canal.** At the pubic crest, the deep inferior epigastric vessels can often be visualized between the medially located umbilical ligament and the laterally positioned exit point of the round ligament. The cannula should be inserted medial or lateral to the vessels if they are visualized. **If the vessels cannot be seen and it is necessary to position the cannula laterally, the device should be placed 3 to 4 cm lateral to the medial umbilical ligament or lateral to the lateral margin of the rectus abdominis muscle.** If the incision is placed too far laterally, it will endanger the deep circumflex epigastric artery. The risk of injury can be minimized by placing a 22-gauge spinal needle through the skin at the desired location, in order to directly observe the entry through the laparoscope. This provides reassurance that a safe location is identified and allows visualization of the peritoneal needle hole, which provides a precise target for inserting the cannula.

Even after a properly positioned incision, the abdominal wall vessels can be injured if a trocar slides medially during placement. Large-diameter devices are more likely to cause injury; therefore, the smallest cannulas necessary to perform the procedure should be used. Ancillary cannulas should not be placed too close together because this results in hindrance of the hand instruments, which compromises access and maneuverability.

The incision made must be of adequate length to allow easy insertion of the device through the skin—a 1-cm long incision is inadequate to allow passage of a 1-cm diameter device. It is important to know that the outside diameter of a cannula is larger than the inside diameter, to allow for the thickness of the material used to create the port. In some instances, this can add two or more millimeters to the device diameter, and, therefore, increase the length of the required incision.

Endoscopes

During endoscopy, the image must be transferred through an optical system. Although direct optical viewing is feasible and often used for diagnostic purposes, virtually all operative laparoscopy is performed using video guidance.

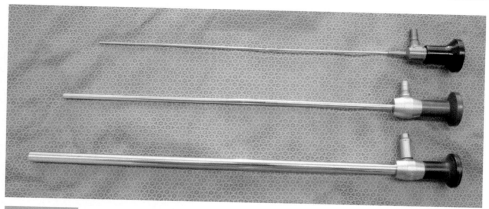

Figure 23.10 **Laparoscopes.** Three 0-degree laparoscopes are shown. From top to bottom, 2-mm, 5-mm and 10-mm diameter.

Laparoscopes are more than simple telescopes; they serve a dual purpose—transmission of light into a dark and closed cavity and provision of an image of the operative field. The light is generally transmitted from a cold light source via a fiberoptic cable to an attachment on the endoscope that passes the light to the distal end of the telescope via a peripherally arranged array of fiberoptic bundles. The image is obtained by a distally positioned lens and transmitted to the eyepiece via a series of rod shaped lenses. The eyepiece can be used to view the peritoneal contents directly or can serve as a point of attachment for a digital video camera. Some endoscopes transmit the image through a collection of densely packed fiberoptic bundles—an approach that diminishes resolution, but allows flexibility of the endoscope, and that is of great value for small-caliber telescopes or when the device is designed to be steerable with an articulated distal end. Another option is to position a digital chip on the end of the system, which then functions as a camera, obviating the need to have any lenses or fibers to transmit the image, a design that is colloquially called "chip-on-a-stick."

A laparoscope with an integrated straight channel, parallel to the optical axis, is called an operating laparoscope because the channel allows for the introduction of operating instruments. Operative endoscopes are of relatively larger caliber than standard laparoscopes, may have smaller fields of view, and may present increased risks associated with the use of monopolar electrosurgical instruments. Standard, viewing-only laparoscopes permit better visualization at a given diameter.

In general, the wider the diameter of the laparoscope, the brighter the image, resulting from either more light or wider lenses, which improve the viewing experience for the surgeon. Narrow-diameter laparoscopes generally allow reduced transfer of light both into and out of the peritoneal cavity; therefore, they require a more sensitive camera or a more powerful light source for adequate illumination. In the past, ideal illumination was provided by 10-mm diagnostic laparoscopes, but improvements in optics allowed the 5-mm diameter laparoscope to become the standard in many operating rooms (Fig. 23.10).

The viewing angle depicts the relationship of the visual field to the axis of the endoscope and typically ranges from 0 to 45 degrees to the horizontal. The 0-degree scope is the standard for gynecologic surgery. The 30-degree angle scope is invaluable in difficult situations, such as the performance of laparoscopic sacrocolpopexy, some myomectomies, and hysterectomy in the presence of large myomas.

Image Visualization Systems

The video camera is usually attached to the eyepiece of the endoscope where it captures the image and transmits it to the body of the camera located outside the operative field, where it is processed and sent to a monitor and, if desired, a recording device (Fig. 23.11). Laparoscopes without an optical path were introduced, with the sensor located on the distal tip of the endoscope, a design that requires a remote camera location. The resolution capability of the monitor should be at least equal to that provided by the camera. Most monitors have the potential to display about 800 horizontal lines of resolution while high definition (HD) systems generally possess 1,080 lines. The more light transmitted through the endoscope, the better the video visualization. The best

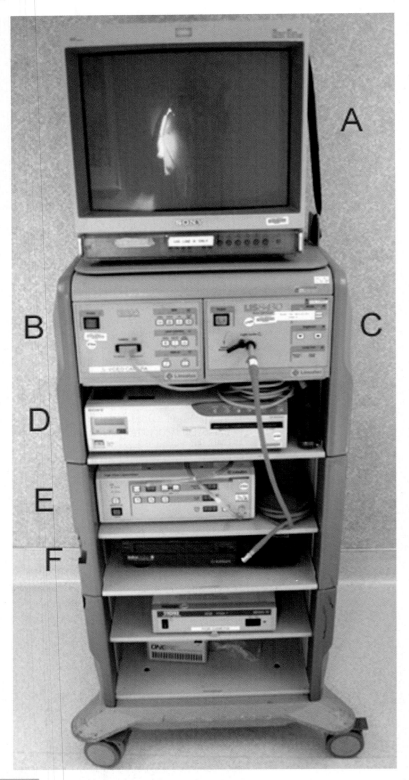

Figure 23.11   Laparoscopic tower. This tower comprises a monitor (**A**), a camera body or base unit (**B**) attached to a camera sensor; a light source (**C**) attached to a cable, which in turn will be connected with the endoscope; a still-image printer (**D**), and an insufflation machine (**E**). A video recorder is shown in (**F**).

available output is achieved from 250 to 300 watts, usually using xenon or metal halide bulbs. Most camera systems are integrated with the light source to vary light output automatically, depending on the amount of exposure required. Light guides or cables transmit light from the source to the endoscope via a bundle of densely packed optical fibers (fiberoptic). Fiberoptic cables lose function over time, generally secondary to breakage of the fiber bundles, especially if they are mishandled.

Creation of a Working Space

The peritoneal cavity is only a potential space, so it is necessary to fill it with a gas, typically CO_2, to create a working environment. Other approaches are being explored that use mechanical lifting systems that allow room air into the peritoneal cavity.

Carbon dioxide is injected into the peritoneal cavity under pressure by a machine called an insufflator. The insufflator delivers the CO_2 from a gas cylinder to the patient through tubing connected to a Luer adaptor on one of the laparoscopic cannulas. Most insufflators can be set to maintain a predetermined intra-abdominal pressure. High flow rates (9 to 20 L per minute) are especially useful for maintaining exposure when suction of smoke or fluid depletes the volume of intraperitoneal gas.

Intraperitoneal retractors attached to a pneumatic or mechanical lifting system can be used to create an intraperitoneal space much like a tent (93). This gasless or isobaric technique may have some advantages over pneumoperitoneum, particularly in patients with cardiopulmonary disease. Airtight cannulas are not necessary, and instruments do not need to have a uniform, narrow, cylindrical shape. Consequently, some conventional instruments may be used directly through the incisions.

Manipulation of Tissue and Fluid

Fluid Management

Fluid may be disseminated into the peritoneal cavity through wide-caliber arthroscopy or cystoscopy tubing using gravity pressure and an infusion cuff or a high-pressure mechanical pump. The pumps deliver fluid faster than the other techniques, and the highly pressurized stream of fluid may facilitate blunt dissection (hydro- or aqua dissection). Small volumes of fluid can be removed with a syringe attached to a cannula; for large volumes, it is necessary to use suction generated by a machine or a wall source.

The type of cannulas used for suction and irrigation depends on the irrigation fluid used and the fluid being removed. For ruptured ectopic gestations or other procedures in which there is a large amount of blood and clots, large-diameter cannulas (7 to 10 mm) are preferred. Cannulas with narrow tips are more effective in generating the high pressure needed for hydrodissection.

If large volumes of fluid are required, isotonic fluids should be used to avoid fluid overload and electrolyte imbalance. **If electrosurgery is to be performed, small volumes of a nonelectrolyte-containing solution such as glycine or sorbitol can be used for hemostasis and irrigation.** *Heparin* **(1,000 to 5,000 U/L) can be added to irrigating solution to prevent blood from clotting and facilitate fluid removal.**

Uterine Manipulators

Uterine manipulation is an important component of the strategy to maximize visualization for most pelvic procedures, especially for myomectomy and hysterectomy. A properly designed uterine manipulator should have an intrauterine component, or obturator, and a method for attaching the device to the uterus. Articulation of the instrument permits acute anteversion or retroversion, both of which are extremely useful procedural maneuvers. If the uterus is large, longer and wider obturators can be used for more effective control. Two types of uterine manipulators are shown in Figure 23.12. A hollow channel attached to a port allows intraoperative instillation of liquid dye to aid in the identification of the endometrial cavity (during myomectomy) or to demonstrate tubal patency.

Grasping Forceps

The forceps used during laparoscopy should, to the extent possible, replicate those used in open surgery. Disposable instruments generally do not have the quality, strength, or precision

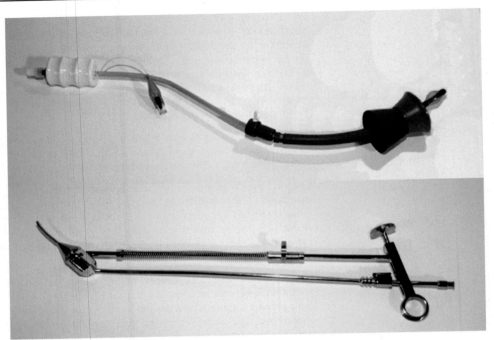

Figure 23.12 **Uterine manipulators. Top:** The disposable "V-Care" device. At the tip is a balloon inflated to maintain the device in the endometrial cavity. Next to the tip is a cervical collar that serves to facilitate identification of the vaginal fornices and cutting of the vagina in laparoscopic total hysterectomy. The blue truncated cone maintains a seal so that gas will not leak out when culdotomy is performed. **Bottom:** The reusable Valtchev manipulator. The ring handle allows the surgeon to antevert the uterus.

of nondisposable forceps (Fig. 23.13). Instruments with teeth (toothed forceps) are necessary to securely grasp the peritoneum or the edge of an ovary for the removal of an ovarian cyst. Instruments designed to be minimally traumatic, like Babcock clamps, are needed to retract the fallopian tube safely. Tenaculum-like instruments are desirable to retract leiomyomas or the uterus. A ratchet is useful for holding tissue without arduous hand pressure. Graspers should be insulated if unipolar radiofrequency instruments are being used to attain hemostasis.

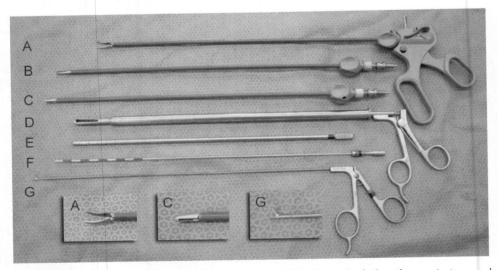

Figure 23.13 **Laparoscopic instruments for grasping and manipulating tissue. A:** (*top* and *inset*) are 5-mm diameter graspers with a curved tip, often called "Maryland" graspers. Other reusable tips (**B**) and (**C**) may be positioned in the same handle as is shown for (**A**). **D:** A 10-mm claw grasper, while (**E**) and (**F**) are 5- and 2-mm manipulating probes respectively. **G:** A 2-mm grasping forceps.

Cutting, Hemostasis, and Tissue Fixation

Cutting can be achieved by mechanical means or by using laser, radiofrequency electrical, or ultrasonic energy. The methods for maintaining or securing hemostasis include sutures, clips, linear staplers, energy sources, and topical or injectable substances. Secure apposition or tissue fixation may be accomplished with sutures, clips, or staples. With appropriate training, a skilled surgeon can obtain good results with any combination of these techniques for cutting, hemostasis, and tissue fixation. Studies in animals have not demonstrated any difference in injury characteristics when cutting is performed with either laser or radiofrequency energy and randomized controlled studies have shown no differences in fertility outcomes (59–61,94). Therefore, differences in results are likely to be caused by other factors, such as patient selection, extent of disease, and degree of surgical expertise.

Cutting

The most useful cutting instruments are scissors (Fig. 23.14, bottom). Because it is difficult to sharpen laparoscopic scissors, most surgeons prefer disposable instruments that can be used until dull and then discarded. Another mechanical cutting tool is the linear stapler–cutter that can simultaneously cut and hemostatically staple the edges of the incision. The cost and large dimensions of the instruments limit their practical use to only a few highly selected situations, such as separation of the uterus from the ovary and fallopian tube during laparoscopic hysterectomy. Devices that coagulate tissue and mechanically transect it are designed to be narrow enough to be practical and effective enough to become the dominant devices for laparoscopic cutting, when concomitant sealing of vessels is a requirement.

Laser and electrical sources of energy manifest their effect by conversion of electromagnetic energy (Fig. 23.14) **to mechanical energy, which is then transformed into thermal energy. Highly focused radiofrequency electrical current (high-power or current density), generated by a specially designed electrosurgical generator produces vaporization or cutting by raising the intracellular temperature above 100°C, which rapidly converts water to**

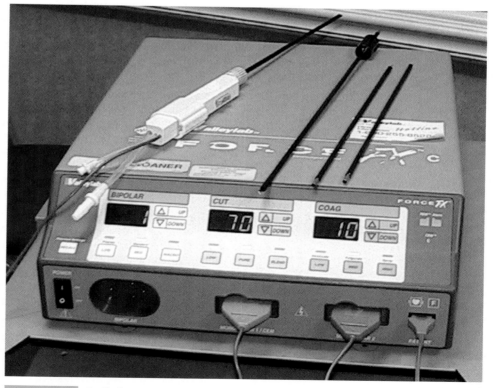

Figure 23.14 **Radiofrequency electrosurgical generator.** Displayed is the Force FX generator with unipolar laparoscopic electrodes. The device is capable of outputting high-voltage ("coagulation") and low-voltage ("cut") waveforms for unipolar instruments and a low-voltage bipolar circuit for bipolar instruments.

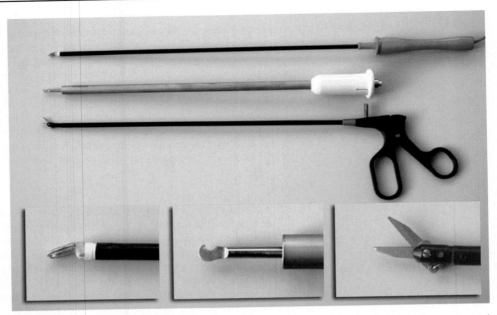

Figure 23.15 **Laparoscopic cutting devices.** *Top* and *inset left* is a bipolar electrosurgical spatula. *Middle* and *center inset* is a harmonic scalpel. This device oscillates at 55,000 Hz to cut tissue. Bottom and inset right are laparoscopic scissors. They may be connected to an electrosurgical generator to act as a unipolar electrosurgical instrument.

steam with a massive increase in intracellular volume. This expansion ruptures the already damaged cell membrane, resulting in cellular and tissue vaporization into a cloud of steam, ions, and protein particles. If the instrument used to focus this energy is moved in a linear fashion, tissue transection or cutting will result. Less focused radiofrequency energy (moderate current density) elevates intracellular temperature, causing desiccation, rupture of hydrogen bonds, and tissue coagulation, but vaporization does not occur.

Monopolar electrosurgical instruments that are narrow or pointed are capable of generating the high-power densities necessary to vaporize or cut tissue. Continuous or modulated and relatively low voltage outputs tend to be the most effective. For optimal results, the instrument should be used in a noncontact fashion, following (not leading) the energy through the tissue. Specially designed bipolar cutting probes that contain both the active and dispersive electrode are available. The active electrode is shaped as a needle, or even a blade, while the other larger-surface-area electrodes are designed to be dispersive (Fig. 23.15, top). Laparoscopic scissors are generally of unipolar design and are intended to cut mechanically; energy may be applied simultaneously for desiccation and hemostasis when cutting tissue that contains small blood vessels (Fig. 23.15, bottom).

Laser energy can be focused to vaporize and cut tissue. The most efficient laser-based cutting instrument is the CO_2 laser, which has the drawback of requiring linear transmission because light cannot be conducted effectively along bendable fibers. The potassium-titanyl-phosphate (KTP) and neodymium:yttrium, aluminum, garnet (Nd:YAG) lasers are effective cutting tools. They are capable of propagating energy along bendable quartz fibers but have a slightly greater degree of collateral thermal injury than radiofrequency electrical or CO_2 laser energy. These limitations and their additional expense constrict the value of these lasers.

Ultrasonic cutting is accomplished mechanically using a blade that oscillates back and forth in a linear fashion (Fig. 23.15, center). The oscillation is achieved using an element located in a handle that vibrates the blade, hook, or one arm of the clamp 55,000 times per second (55 kHz). The distance of the oscillation can be varied and determines the efficiency of the cutting process. The tip of the device cuts mechanically, but there is a degree of collateral thermal tissue coagulation injury that can be used for hemostasis. In low-density tissue, the process of mechanical cutting is augmented by the process of cavitation, in which reduction of local atmospheric pressure allows vaporization of intracellular water at lower temperatures than those required for laser or electrosurgical vaporization.

Hemostasis

Because of the visual, tactile, and mechanical limitations of laparoscopy, prevention of bleeding is important for efficient, effective, and safe procedures. Radiofrequency electricity is the least expensive and most versatile method for achieving hemostasis during laparoscopy and can be applied with either monopolar or bipolar instruments. Regardless of the type of system, the process of electrical desiccation and coagulation is best achieved by contacting the tissue with the activated electrode using continuous low-voltage or "cutting" current. With adequate power, typically 20 to 30 watts (depending, in part, on the surface area of the electrodes), tissue will be heated, desiccated, and coagulated. Blood vessels should be compressed with the blades of the forceps before the electrode is activated so that the "heat sink" effect of flowing blood is eliminated. This allows the opposing walls of the vessel to bond, forming a strong tissue seal in a process called *coaptive coagulation*. Bipolar devices can be fitted with a serial ammeter that measures the current flowing through the system. When the tissue between the blades of the forceps is completely desiccated, the device is no longer able to conduct electricity, which can trigger a visual or auditory cue for the surgeon. Alternatively, the generator can be designed to stop automatically when current is no longer being conducted by the tissue between the blades of the forceps. The surgeon can reduce lateral thermal spread of radiofrequency energy by manually pulsing delivery or by simultaneously running irrigation fluid over the pedicle. Automated generators that pulse energy automatically are available, and such bipolar systems can include mechanical blades to cut tissues following coagulation of the tissue (Fig. 23.16).

Control of superficial bleeding can be achieved with *fulguration*, the near-contact spraying of tissue with a unipolar instrument using modulated, high-voltage radiofrequency waveforms from the "coagulation" side of the electrosurgical generator. Care must be taken to safely perform laparoscopic fulguration, ensuring that the entire shaft of the laparoscopic instrument is well away from the bowel.

Ultrasonic instruments can be used for hemostasis as well. Those with a forceps-like end effector disperse the mechanical energy in a way that allows the tissue to be heated and coagulated. These

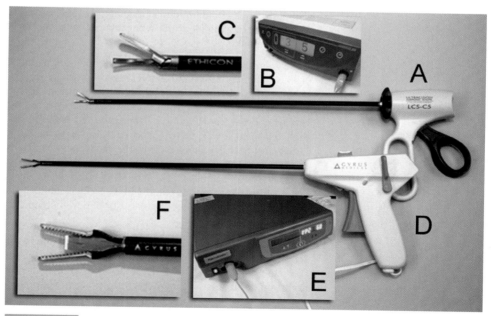

Figure 23.16   Displayed are two devices that cut and coagulate or seal tissue. *Top* (**A–C**) are the ligating cutting shears (LCS) that are based on the same technology as the harmonic scalpel displayed in Figure 23.13. The bottom blade oscillates (**C**), while the top blade is opened to grasp the tissue and used by the surgeon to slowly transect and seal the blood vessels in the tissue being transected. The PlasmaKinetic (**D–F**) is a bipolar radiofrequency device that, using electrical impedance, tells the surgeon when the tissue is coagulated. Then the orange trigger (*top*) is pushed deploying the blade (**F**), thereby cutting the coagulated tissue.

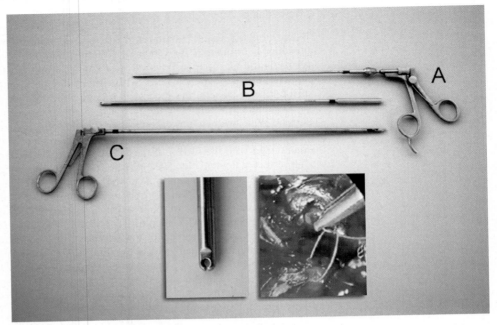

Figure 23.17 **Laparoscopic suturing instruments.** The 3-mm and 5-mm diameter laparoscopic needle drivers are displayed in (**A**) and (**C**), while a knot manipulator is shown in (**B**) and *inset left*. The device is shown transferring a knot into the peritoneal cavity (*inset right*).

so-called ligating-cutting shears cut when high pressure is exerted in the handle by the surgeon (Fig. 23.16A–C).

Hemostatic clips may be applied with specially designed laparoscopic instruments. Nonabsorbable clips made of titanium are useful for relatively narrow vessels, and longer, delayed absorbable, self-retaining clips are generally preferred for larger vessels, 3 or 4 mm or more. Clips may be of particular value when securing relatively large vessels near an important structure such as the ureter.

Laparoscopic suturing is a method for maintaining hemostasis (95–97). Compared with clips or linear staplers, suturing has a relatively low materials cost, although operating time may be longer and more expensive. **The two basic methods for securing a ligature around a blood vessel depend on where the knot is tied; ligatures are intracorporeal and extracorporeal. Intracorporeal knots replicate the standard instrument-tied knot and are formed within the peritoneal cavity. Extracorporeal knots are created outside the abdomen under direct vision and then transferred into the peritoneal cavity by knot manipulators** (Fig. 23.17). Pretied knotted suture loops attached to long introducers, called Endoloops®, may be used to secure vascular pedicles. Care should be taken to make sure that they are tightly secured and that no other tissue is incorporated in the loop. A number of devices that facilitate the formation and tying of knots are either available or in development.

Small areas of low volume bleeding can be treated with topical hemostatic agents. **Topical agents such as microfibrillar collagen are available in 5-mm and 10-mm diameter laparoscopic applicators** (Fig. 23.13). Fibrin sealants (e.g., Tisseel®) and bovine thrombin and gelatin (Floseal®)can also be used. **A solution of dilute vasopressin may be injected locally to maintain hemostasis for myomectomy or removal of ectopic pregnancy.**

Tissue Extraction

After excising tissue, it is usually necessary to remove it from the peritoneal cavity. Small samples can be pulled through an appropriate-sized cannula with grasping forceps; however, larger specimens may not fit. If the specimen is cystic, it may be drained by a needle or incised, shrinking it to a size suitable for removal through the cannula or one of the small laparoscopic incisions. **If there is concern for malignancy, an alternative is to place the specimen in an endoscopic retrieval bag before drainage to prevent spillage** (Fig. 23.18). More solid tissue may be morcellated with scissors, ultrasonic equipment, electrosurgery or electromechanical

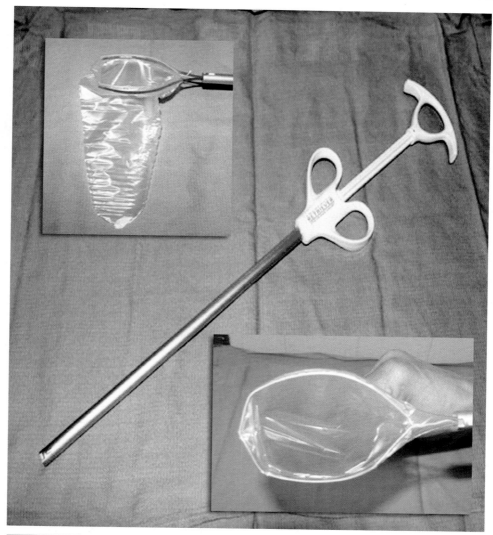

Figure 23.18   Specimen removal bag. This 10-mm diameter bag is positioned in the peritoneal cavity. Then the bag is deployed (*insets*), allowing the surgeon to place specimens for removal.

morcellators. If monopolar radiofrequency instruments are used for electrosurgical morcellation, the specimen must remain attached to the patient to preserve the integrity of the electrical circuit. Alternatively, special bipolar needles are available that do not require a dispersive electrode.

Larger specimens may be removed by inserting a larger cannula through an incision in the cul-de-sac (posterior culdotomy) or by extending one of the laparoscopy incisions. With the exception of culdotomy (colpotomy), extension of the umbilical incision may be the most cosmetic approach because incisions up to 3 cm in length can be concealed successfully. When the umbilical location is selected, removal of the tissue can be directed from an endoscope positioned in one of the ancillary ports. Electronic morcellators are available to remove large tissue specimens by reducing them to smaller sections (Fig. 23.19). These are especially useful for laparoscopic myomectomy and laparoscopic supracervical hysterectomy.

Incision Management

Dehiscence and hernia risk appear to significantly increase when the fascial incision is larger than 10 mm in diameter (98,99). Closure of the fascia should take place under direct laparoscopic vision to prevent the accidental incorporation of bowel into the incisions, and the peritoneum should be included to reduce the risk of Richter's hernia. A small-caliber laparoscope passed through one of the narrow cannulas can be used to direct the fascial closure using curved needles or a ligature carrier especially designed for this purpose.

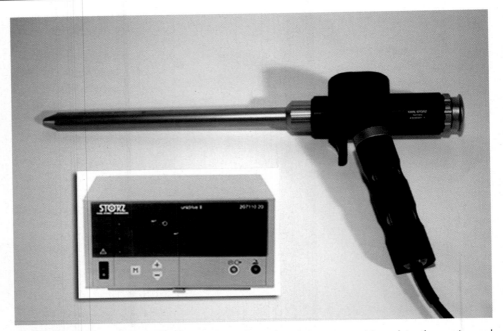

Figure 23.19 **Electromechanical morcellator.** This device is positioned in the peritoneal cavity and attached to the power generator (*inset*). The blunt obturator is removed; a grasping instrument inserted through the lumen is used to withdraw the tissue, which is cut by a cylindrical blade. The motor is activated by a foot pedal.

Complications

After laparoscopic surgery patients usually experience a rapid recovery. Pain diminishes, gastrointestinal function improves quickly, and fever is extremely unusual. Therefore, if a patient's condition is not improving, possible complications of anesthesia or surgery should be considered. Laparoscopic procedures can be complicated by infections, trauma, or hemorrhage, and by problems associated with anesthetic use. The incidence of infection is lower than with procedures performed by laparotomy. Problems associated with visualization in conjunction with the change in anatomic perspective may increase the risk of damage to blood vessels or vital structures such as the bowel, ureter, or bladder.

Anesthetic and Cardiopulmonary Complications

A review of laparoscopic tubal sterilization in 9,475 women found no deaths from complications of anesthesia (100,101). The potential risks of general anesthesia include hypoventilation, esophageal intubation, gastroesophageal reflux, bronchospasm, hypotension, narcotic overdose, cardiac arrhythmias, and cardiac arrest. These risks can be exacerbated by some of the inherent features of gynecologic laparoscopy. For example, the Trendelenburg position, in combination with the increased intraperitoneal pressure provided by pneumoperitoneum, places greater compression on the diaphragm, increasing the risk of hypoventilation, hypercarbia, and metabolic acidosis. This position, combined with anesthetic agents that relax the esophageal sphincter, promotes regurgitation of gastric content, which in turn can lead to aspiration, bronchospasm, pneumonitis, and pneumonia. Parameters of cardiopulmonary function associated with both CO_2 and N_2O insufflation include reduced PO_2, O_2 saturation, tidal volume, and minute ventilation and increased respiratory rate. The use of intraperitoneal CO_2 as a distention medium is associated with an increase in PCO_2 and a decrease in pH. Elevation of the diaphragm may be associated with basilar atelectasis, resulting in right-to-left shunt and ventilation–perfusion mismatch (102).

Carbon Dioxide Embolus

Carbon dioxide is the most widely used peritoneal distention medium, largely because the rapid absorption of CO_2 in blood reduces the significance of gas emboli. If large amounts of CO_2 gain access to the central venous circulation, if peripheral vasoconstriction occurs, or if the splanchnic blood flow is decreased by excessively high intraperitoneal pressure, severe cardiorespiratory compromise may result.

The signs of CO_2 embolus include sudden and otherwise unexplained hypotension, cardiac arrhythmia, cyanosis, and heart murmurs. The end-tidal CO_2 level may increase, and findings consistent with pulmonary edema may manifest (103). Accelerating pulmonary hypertension may occur, resulting in right-sided heart failure.

Because gas embolism may result from direct intravascular injection through an insufflation needle, the proper placement of the insufflation needle must be ensured. Although the initial intraperitoneal pressure may be set at 20 to 30 mm Hg for port placement, it should be maintained at 8 to 12 mm for the rest of the case (104). The risk of CO_2 embolus is reduced by careful hemostasis because open venous channels are the portal of entry for gas into the systemic circulation. The anesthesiologist should continuously monitor the patient's color, blood pressure, heart sounds, heartbeat, and end-tidal CO_2 to allow early recognition of the signs of CO_2 embolus.

If CO_2 embolus is suspected or diagnosed, the surgeon must evacuate the CO_2 from the peritoneal cavity and place the patient in the left lateral decubitus position, with the head below the level of the right atrium. A large-bore central venous line should be inserted immediately to allow aspiration of gas from the heart. Because the findings are nonspecific, the patient should be evaluated for other causes of cardiovascular collapse.

Cardiovascular Complications

Cardiac arrhythmias occur relatively frequently during laparoscopic surgery and are related to a number of factors, the most significant of which are hypercarbia and acidemia. Early reports of laparoscopy-associated arrhythmia were associated with spontaneous respiration; therefore, most anesthesiologists adopted the practice of mechanical ventilation during laparoscopic surgery. The incidence of hypercarbia is reduced by operating with intraperitoneal pressures at levels less than 12 mm Hg (105).

The risk of cardiac arrhythmia may be reduced by using NO_2 as a distending medium (see the preceding discussion in "Peritoneal Access"). Although NO_2 is associated with a decreased incidence of arrhythmia, it is insoluble in blood and, therefore, its use may increase the risk of gas embolus. External lifting systems avoid the complication of hypercarbia and can provide protection against cardiac arrhythmia (106).

Hypotension can occur because of decreased venous return secondary to very high intraperitoneal pressure, and this condition may be potentiated by volume depletion. Vagal discharge may occur in response to increased intraperitoneal pressure, which can cause hypotension secondary to cardiac arrhythmias (106). These side effects should be considered when performing surgery on patients with preexisting cardiovascular disease.

Gastric Reflux

Gastric regurgitation and aspiration can occur during laparoscopic surgery, especially in patients with obesity, gastroparesis, hiatal hernia, or gastric outlet obstruction. In these patients, the airway must be maintained with a cuffed endotracheal tube, and the stomach must be decompressed (e.g., with a nasogastric tube). The lowest necessary intraperitoneal pressure should be used to minimize the risk of aspiration. Patients should be moved out of the Trendelenburg position before being extubated. Routine preoperative administration of *metoclopramide,* H2-blocking agents, and nonparticulate antacids reduces the risk of aspiration.

Extraperitoneal Insufflation

The most common causes of extraperitoneal insufflation are preperitoneal placement of the insufflating needle and leakage of CO_2 around the cannula sites. Although this condition is usually mild and limited to the abdominal wall, subcutaneous emphysema can become extensive, involving the extremities, the neck, and the mediastinum. Another relatively common site for emphysema is the omentum or mesentery, a circumstance that may be mistaken for preperitoneal insufflation.

Subcutaneous emphysema may be identified by the palpation of crepitus, usually in the abdominal wall. Emphysema can extend along contiguous fascial plains to the neck, where it can be visualized directly. This finding may reflect mediastinal emphysema, which may indicate impending cardiovascular collapse (107–110).

The risk of subcutaneous emphysema is reduced by the proper positioning of the insufflation needle and by maintaining a low intraperitoneal pressure after placement of the desired cannulas. Other approaches that reduce the chance of subcutaneous emphysema include open laparoscopy and the use of abdominal wall lifting systems that make gas unnecessary.

If the insufflation occurred extraperitoneally, the laparoscope can be removed and the procedure can be repeated. Difficulty may ensue because of the altered anterior peritoneum. Open laparoscopy or the use of an alternate site, such as the left upper quadrant, should be considered. One approach is to leave the laparoscope in the expanded preperitoneal space while the insufflation needle is reinserted under direct vision through the peritoneal membrane caudad to the tip of the laparoscope (111).

In mild cases of subcutaneous emphysema, the findings quickly resolve after evacuation of the pneumoperitoneum, and no specific intraoperative or postoperative therapy is required. When the extravasation extends to the neck, it is usually preferable to terminate the procedure because pneumomediastinum, pneumothorax, hypercarbia, and cardiovascular collapse may result. Following termination of the procedure, it is prudent to obtain a chest x-ray. The patient's condition should be managed expectantly unless a tension pneumothorax results, in which case immediate evacuation must be performed using a chest tube or a wide-bore needle (14 to 16 gauge) inserted in the second intercostal space in the midclavicular line.

Electrosurgical Complications

Complications of electrosurgery occur secondary to thermal injury from unintended or inappropriate use of the active electrode, current diversion to an undesirable path, or injury at the site of the dispersive electrode. Such complications may occur with the use of these instruments during laparoscopic, abdominal, or vaginal surgery. Active electrode injury can occur with either unipolar or bipolar instruments, whereas trauma secondary to current diversion and dispersive electrode accidents occurs only with unipolar devices. Complications of electrosurgery are reduced by adherence to safety protocols coupled with a sound understanding of the principles of electrosurgery and the circumstances that can lead to injury (112).

Active Electrode Trauma

If the foot pedal is accidentally depressed, tissue adjacent to the electrode will be traumatized. Potential sites of injury include the bowel, ureter, and other intraperitoneal structures, or, if the electrode lies on the abdomen, the skin. Injury from direct extension of thermal effect can occur when the zone of vaporization or coagulation extends to large blood vessels or vital structures such as the bladder, ureter, or bowel. Bipolar instruments may reduce but do not eliminate the risk of thermal injury to adjacent tissue (113). Blood vessels should be isolated before electrosurgical coagulation, especially when they are near vital structures, and appropriate amounts of energy must be applied to allow an adequate margin of noncoagulated tissue.

The diagnosis of direct thermal visceral injury may be difficult. If unintended activation of the electrode occurs, nearby intraperitoneal structures should be evaluated carefully. The appearance can be affected by several factors, including the output of the generator, the type of electrode, its proximity to tissue, and the duration of activation. The diagnosis of visceral thermal injury is often delayed until signs and symptoms of fistula or peritonitis secondary to perforation appear. Because these complications may not manifest until 2 to 10 days after surgery, patients should be advised to report any postoperative fever or increasing abdominal pain.

Thermal injury to the bowel, bladder, or ureter that is recognized at the time of laparoscopy should be managed immediately, taking into consideration the potential extent of the zone of coagulative necrosis (114). Incisions made with the focused energy from a pointed electrode are associated with a minimal amount of surrounding thermal injury. Prolonged or even transient contact with a relatively large-caliber electrode may produce a zone of thermal necrosis that may be much larger than visually apparent. In such cases, wide excision or resection of up to several centimeters of bowel may be necessary. The choice of route of access for any required surgical repairs depends in part on the nature of the injury and on the skills and training of the surgeon.

The incidence of unintended activation injuries can be reduced if the surgeon is always in direct control of electrode activation and if all electrosurgical hand instruments are

removed from the peritoneal cavity when not in use. When removed from the peritoneal cavity, the instruments should be detached from the electrosurgical generator, or they should be stored in an insulated pouch near the operative field. These measures prevent damage to the patient's skin if the electrode is accidentally activated.

Current Diversion

Current diversion occurs when the radiofrequency circuit follows an unintended path between the active electrode and the electrosurgical generator. This may occur with insulation defects, direct coupling, or capacitative coupling. In older, grounded systems, unlikely to be in use, current can be diverted if any part of the patient's body touches a conductive and grounded object. In any of these situations, if the power density becomes high enough, unintended and severe thermal injury can result.

Insulation Defects

If the insulation coating the shaft of a monopolar electrosurgical instrument becomes defective, it can allow current diversion to adjacent tissue, most often bowel, potentially resulting in significant injury. This happens in part because such defects create a zone of high current density (Fig. 23.20A). Therefore, the instruments should be examined before each procedure to detect worn or obviously defective insulation. **When using monopolar laparoscopic instruments, the shaft of the device should be kept away from vital structures and, if possible, totally visible in the operative field.**

Direct Coupling

Direct coupling occurs when an activated electrode touches and energizes another uninsulated metal conductor such as a laparoscope, cannula, or other instrument. Direct coupling is often used for hemostasis when a grasping instrument is used to occlude a blood vessel while a separate activated electrode is used to provide the energy for desiccation and coagulation. If this occurs while the noninsulated device rests against structures such as bowel or the urinary tract, injury may occur (Fig. 23.20B). The risk of direct coupling can be reduced by eliminating the simultaneous use of noninsulated and monopolar instruments. The surgeon should visually confirm that there is no contact with other conductive instruments before activating a monopolar instrument.

Capacitive Coupling

Capacitance is the ability of a conductor to establish an electrical current in an unconnected nearby circuit. An electrical field is established around the shaft of any activated unipolar instrument (including the cord), a circumstance that creates a potential capacitor. This field is harmless if the circuit is completed through a dispersive, low-power density pathway (Fig. 23.21). For example, if capacitative coupling occurs between a monopolar laparoscopic instrument and a metal cannula positioned in the abdominal wall, the current is harmlessly dispersed in the abdominal wall at the point where it connects with the dispersive electrode (Fig. 23.21A). However, if the metal cannula is anchored to the skin by a nonconductive plastic retaining sleeve or "gripper" (a hybrid system), the current cannot access the abdominal wall because the sleeve acts as an insulator (Fig. 23.21B). Instead, the capacitor will have to "look" elsewhere to complete the circuit. The bowel or any other nearby conductor can become the target of a relatively high-power density discharge (Fig. 23.21C). This situation can occur when a unipolar instrument is inserted through an operating laparoscope that, in turn, is passed through a nonconductive plastic laparoscopic cannula. In this configuration, the plastic port acts as the insulator. If the electrode capacitively couples with the metal laparoscope, nearby bowel will be at risk for significant thermal injury (115). The circumstance occurs with the relatively new "single port" systems where the laparoscope and hand instruments, including monopolar instruments, are passed through the same concentrated array of ports. This situation is identical to that of the "operating" laparoscope with an increased risk that the laparoscope or other instruments function as capacitors.

The risk of capacitive coupling-related complications can be reduced in a number of ways. First, it is important to avoid the use of hybrid laparoscope-cannula systems that contain a mixture of conductive and nonconductive elements. Instead, the use of all-plastic or all-metal cannula systems is preferred. It may be best to avoid or at least minimize the use of monopolar instruments

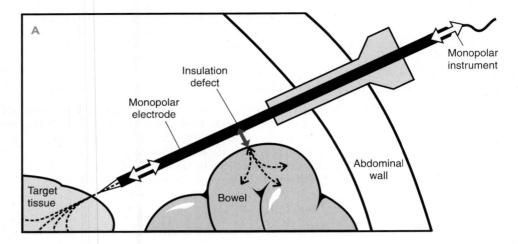

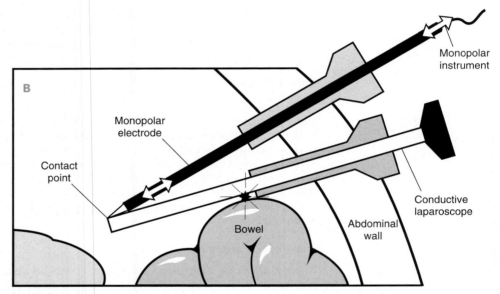

Figure 23.20   **Current diversion secondary to insulation defects and direct coupling.** These events may occur with the use of monopolar instrumentation when there is a defect in the insulation **(A)** or, classically, to contact a conductive instrument that, in turn, touches other intraperitoneal structures. In the example depicted **(B)**, the active electrode is touching the laparoscope, and current is transferred to bowel through a small enough contact point that thermal injury results. Another common target of such coupling is to noninsulated hand instruments.

using operating laparoscopes or multiport, single site access systems. If an operating laparoscope is to be used, all-metal cannula systems should be the rule unless there is no intent to use unipolar electrosurgical instruments through the operating channel. Finally, minimizing the use of high voltage, modulated current ("coagulation" current) will reduce the risk of capacitative coupling.

Dispersive Electrode Burns

Modern electrosurgical units are designed with isolated circuits and impedance monitoring systems that shut down the machine if dispersive electrode ("patient pad") detachment occurs. The use of isolated-circuit electrosurgical generators with dispersive electrode monitors has virtually eliminated dispersive electrode–related thermal injury. Dispersive electrode monitoring is accomplished by measuring the impedance in the dispersive electrode, which should always be low because of the large surface area. Without such devices, partial detachment of the dispersive

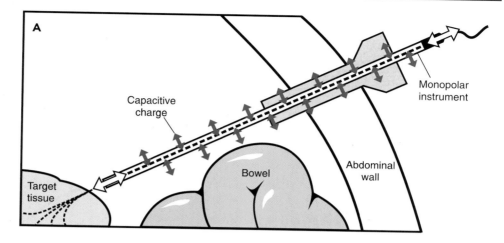

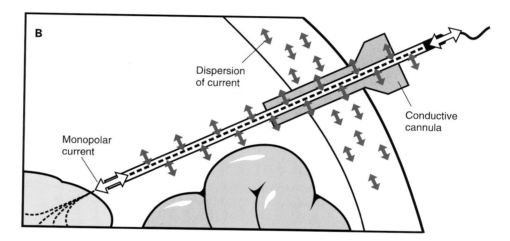

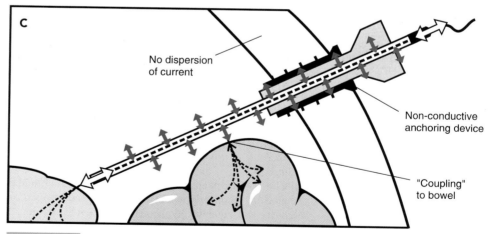

Figure 23.21 **Capacitative coupling.** **A:** All activated monopolar electrodes emit a surrounding charge, proportional to the voltage of the current. This makes the electrode a potential capacitor. **B:** Generally, as long as the charge is allowed to disperse through the abdominal wall, no sequelae result. However, if the "return" to the dispersive electrode is blocked by insulation, such as a plastic anchor (**C**), the current can couple to a conductive cannula or directly to bowel.

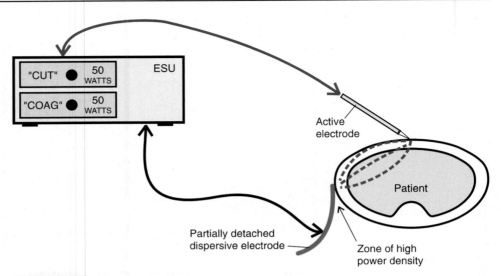

Figure 23.22 **Dispersive electrode burns.** If the dispersive electrode becomes partially detached, the current density may increase to the point that a skin burn results.

electrode could result in a thermal injury because reducing the surface area of the electrode in contact with the skin raises the current density (Fig. 23.22).

Because a few ground-referenced machines without such safeguards may still be in use, it is important to know the type of electrosurgical unit used in the operating room. If the electrosurgical generator is ground referenced and if the dispersive electrode becomes detached, unplugged, or otherwise ineffective, the current seeks any grounded conductor, such as electrocardiograph patch electrodes or the conductive metal components of the operating table (Fig. 23.23). If the conductor has a small surface area, the current or power density may become high enough to cause thermal injury (Fig. 23.24).

Hemorrhagic Complications

Great Vessel Injury

The most dangerous hemorrhagic complications are injuries to the great vessels, including the aorta and the vena cava, the common iliac vessels and their branches, and the internal and external iliac arteries and veins. The most catastrophic injuries occur secondary to insertion of an insufflation needle or the tip of the obturator (trocar) used to position the primary or ancillary cannulas. The vessels most frequently damaged are the aorta and the right common iliac artery as it branches from the aorta in the midline. The anatomically more posterior location of the vena cava and the iliac veins provides relative protection, but not immunity, from injury (116). After vascular injury, patients usually develop profound hypotension with or without hemoperitoneum. In some instances, blood is aspirated through the insufflation needle before the introduction of the distending gas. **In such instances, the needle should be left in place while immediate preparations are made to obtain blood products and perform laparotomy.** The bleeding frequently will be contained in the retroperitoneal space, which usually delays the diagnosis; consequently, hypovolemic shock may develop. To avoid late recognition, the course of each great vessel must be identified before completing the procedure. Because it is difficult to assess the volume of blood filling the retroperitoneal space, immediate laparotomy is indicated if retroperitoneal bleeding is suspected. A midline incision should be made to allow access to the great vessels. Upon entry into the peritoneal cavity, the aorta and vena cava should immediately be compressed just below the level of the renal vessels to gain at least temporary control of blood loss. The most appropriate course of action depends on the site and extent of injury. Vascular or general surgery consultation may be necessary to evaluate and repair significant vascular injuries. Although most of these injuries are small and amenable to repair with suture, some are larger and require the insertion of a vascular graft. Deaths have occurred as a result of these injuries.

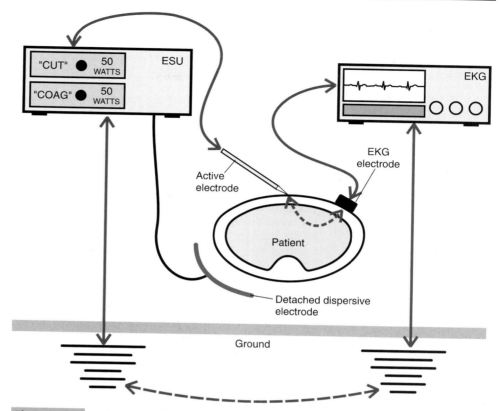

Figure 23.23 **Risk of ground-referenced generators.** Current diversion along alternate pathways is a risk associated with ground-referenced electrosurgical generators, particularly if the dispersive electrode is detached. In the example depicted, the relatively high current density at the electrocardiogram electrode site may result in a skin burn.

Abdominal Wall Vessel Injury

The abdominal wall vessels most commonly injured during laparoscopy are the superficial inferior epigastric vessels as they branch from the femoral artery and vein and course cephalad in each lower quadrant. They are invariably damaged by the initial passage of an ancillary trocar-cannula system or by the introduction of a wider device later in the procedure. The problem may be recognized immediately by the observation of blood dripping along the cannula or out through the incision. However, the bleeding may be obstructed by the cannula until it is withdrawn at the end of the operation.

The more serious injuries are those to the deep inferior epigastric vessels, which are branches of the external iliac artery and vein that course cephalad but are deep to the rectus fascia and often deep to the muscles (Fig. 23.3). More laterally located are the deep circumflex iliac vessels, which are not often encountered in laparoscopic surgery. Laceration of these vessels may cause profound blood loss, particularly when the trauma is unrecognized and causes extraperitoneal bleeding.

Signs of injury, in addition to blood dripping down the cannula, include the postoperative appearance of shock and abdominal wall discolorization or hematoma located near the incision. In some instances, the blood may track to a more distant site, presenting as a pararectal or vulvar mass. Delayed diagnosis may be prevented by laparoscopic evaluation of each peritoneal incision after removal of the cannula.

Superficial inferior epigastric vessel trauma usually stops bleeding spontaneously; therefore, expectant management is appropriate. A straight ligature carrier can be used to repair lacerated deep inferior epigastric vessels. Alternatively, a Foley catheter may be inserted through the cannula, inflated, put on traction, and held in place with a clamp for up to 24 hours. If a postoperative hematoma develops, local compression should be used

initially. **Open removal or aspiration of the hematoma should not be undertaken because it may inhibit the tamponade effect and increase the risk of abscess. If the mass continues to enlarge or if signs of hypovolemia develop, the wound must be explored.**

Intraperitoneal Vessel Injury

Hemorrhage may result from inadvertent entry into a vessel or failure of a specific occlusive technique. In addition to delayed hemorrhage, there may be a further delay in diagnosis at laparoscopy as a result of the restricted visual field and the temporary occlusive pressure exerted by CO_2 in the peritoneal cavity.

Inadvertent division of an artery or vein is usually evident immediately. **Transected arteries may go into spasm and bleed minutes to hours later, going unnoticed temporarily because of the limited visual field of the laparoscope. Therefore, at the end of the procedure, all areas of dissection must be carefully examined.** Carbon dioxide should be vented, which decreases the intraperitoneal pressure so that blood vessels temporarily occluded by higher pressure can be recognized.

Gastrointestinal Complications

The stomach, the small bowel, and the colon can be injured during laparoscopy. Mechanical entry into the large or small bowel can occur 10 times more often when laparoscopy is performed in patients who have had prior intraperitoneal inflammation or abdominal surgery. Loops of intestine can adhere to the abdominal wall under the insertion site and be injured (117,118).

Insufflation Needle Injuries

Needle entry into the gastrointestinal tract may be more common than reported because it may go unnoticed and without further complication. Gastric entry may be identified by the increased filling pressure, asymmetric distention of the peritoneal cavity, or aspiration of gastric particulate matter through the lumen of the needle. Initially, the hollow, capacious stomach may allow the insufflation pressure to remain normal. Signs of bowel entry are the same as those for gastric injury, with the addition of feculent odor.

If particulate debris is identified, the needle should be left in place, and an alternate insertion site should be identified, such as the left upper quadrant. Immediately after successful entry into the peritoneal cavity, the site of injury can be identified. Defects must be repaired immediately by laparoscopy or laparotomy.

Trocar or Obturator Injuries

Damage caused by a sharp tipped obturator or trocar is usually more serious than needle injury. Inadvertent gastric entry usually is associated with stomach distention because of aerophagia, difficult or improper intubation, or mask induction with inhalation anesthetic. Most often the injury is created by the trocar-cannula system used for primary access. Ancillary cannulas may result in visceral injury, although placement of these cannulas under direct vision helps reduce the risk of injury. **The risk of gastric perforation can be minimized with the selective use of preoperative nasogastric or oral gastric suction when left upper-quadrant entries are used or when the intubation was difficult.** Open laparoscopy likely has little impact on the risk for gastrointestinal complications, particularly those related to adhesions to the anterior abdominal wall from previous surgery. For high-risk patients, left upper quadrant needle and trocar-cannula insertion with a properly decompressed stomach may be preferable (119–122).

If the trocar of a primary cannula penetrates the bowel, the condition is usually diagnosed when the mucosal lining of the gastrointestinal tract is visualized. If the large bowel is entered, a feculent odor may be noted. However, the injury may not be recognized immediately because the cannula may not stay within the bowel or may pass through the lumen. Such injuries usually occur when a single loop of bowel is adherent to the anterior abdominal wall. The injury may not be recognized until peritonitis, abscess, enterocutaneous fistula, or death occurs (123,124). Therefore, at the end of the procedure, the removal of the primary cannula must be viewed either through the cannula or an ancillary port, a process facilitated by routine direct visualization of closure of the incision of the primary port.

Trocar-related injuries to the stomach and bowel require repair as soon as they are recognized. If the injury is small, a trained operator can repair the defect under laparoscopic direction using a double layer of running 2-0 or 3-0 absorbable sutures. Extensive lesions may require resection and reanastomosis, which in most instances requires at least a small laparotomy. The preoperative use of mechanical bowel preparation in selected high-risk cases minimizes the need for laparotomy or colostomy, but recent evidence suggests that bowel surgery, if necessary, may be safely performed in unprepared bowel (125).

Dissection and Thermal Injury

When mechanical bowel trauma is recognized during the dissection, treatment is the same as that described for trocar injury. **Should the injury involve radiofrequency electrical energy, it is important to recognize that the zone of desiccation and coagulation may exceed the area of visual damage.** This is especially true if the exact mechanism of the thermal injury is unknown or if injury results from contact with a relatively large surface area electrode that would be more likely to create a large coagulation injury. Conversely, **bowel injury created under direct vision with a radiofrequency needle or blade electrode is associated with little collateral coagulation effect and can be managed similar to a mechanically induced lesion.** Consequently, surgical repair should be implemented considering these factors, and should include, if necessary, resection of ample margins around the injury. **Thermal injury may be handled expectantly if the lesion seems superficial and confined,** such as when fulguration (noncontact arcing of modulated high-voltage current) involves bowel. In such instances, the depth of injury is generally less than half a millimeter. In a study of 33 women with such injuries who were managed expectantly in the hospital, only 2 required laparotomy for repair of perforation (126).

Urologic Injury

Damage to the bladder or ureter may occur secondary to mechanical or thermal trauma incurred during laparoscopic procedures. Ideally, such injury should be prevented; otherwise, as is the case for most complications, it is preferable to identify the trauma intraoperatively.

Bladder Injury

Bladder injury can result from the perforation of the undrained bladder by an insufflation needle or trocar, or it may occur while the bladder is being dissected from adherent structures or from the anterior uterus (127,128). The frequency of injury is difficult to estimate and varies with the procedure. Estimates of the frequency of unintentional cystotomy associated with laparoscopic hysterectomy range from 0.4% to 3.2% and appear to be more frequent in the context of a previous cesarean section (129,130). The injury may be readily apparent by direct visualization. If an indwelling catheter is in place, hematuria or pneumaturia (CO_2 in the catheter drainage system) may be noticed. A bladder laceration can be confirmed by injecting sterile milk or a diluted methylene blue solution through a transurethral catheter. Thermal injury to the bladder, however, may not be apparent initially and, if missed, can present as peritonitis or a fistula.

Routine preoperative bladder drainage usually prevents trocar-related cystotomies. Separation of the bladder from the uterus or other adherent structures requires good visualization, appropriate retraction, and excellent surgical technique. Sharp mechanical dissection is preferred, particularly when relatively dense adhesions are present.

Very small-caliber injuries to the bladder (1 to 2 mm) may be treated with bladder catheterization for 3 to 7 days. If repair is undertaken immediately, catheterization is unnecessary. **When a larger injury is identified, it can be repaired laparoscopically** (127,128,131). **If the laceration is near to or involves the trigone, an open procedure should be used.** The mechanism of injury should be taken into consideration in making this evaluation because electrical injuries often extend beyond the visible limits of the apparent defect. If a coagulation-induced thermal injury occurred, the coagulated portion should be excised.

For small lesions, closure may be performed with layers of absorbable 2-0 to 3-0 sutures. Postoperative catheterization with either a transurethral or suprapubic catheter should be maintained for 2 to 5 days for small fundal lacerations and for 10 to 14 days for injuries to the trigone. Cystography should be considered before the urinary catheter is removed.

Ureteral Injury

One of the most common causes of ureteral injury during laparoscopy is electrosurgical trauma (113,132,133). Ureteral injury can occur after mechanical dissection, including linear cutting and stapling devices (133–135). **Although intraoperative recognition of ureteral injury is possible, the diagnosis is usually delayed** (132,133). Ureteral lacerations may be confirmed intraoperatively, visually, or following the intravenous injection of indigo carmine. Thermal injury presents up to 14 days after surgery with fever, abdominal or flank pain, and peritonitis. Leukocytosis may be present, and intravenous pyelography shows extravasation of urine or urinoma. Mechanical obstruction from staples or a suture may be recognized intraoperatively by direct visualization. **Cystoscopy following the intravenous injection of indigo carmine may be used to confirm failure of the dye to pass through the ureter.** Abdominal ultrasound may be helpful, but a CT urogram can more precisely identify the site and degree of the obstruction. Unrecognized ureteral obstruction may present a few days to 1 week after surgery with flank pain and often fever (136).

Discharge or continuous incontinence is a delayed sign of ureterovaginal or vesicovaginal fistula. **A vesicovaginal fistula can be confirmed by filling the bladder with methylene blue and then detecting dye on a tampon previously placed in the vagina. With a ureterovaginal fistula, the methylene blue will not pass into the vagina, but it can be detected with the intravenous injection of indigo carmine.**

Knowledge of the course of the ureter through the pelvis is a prerequisite to reducing the risk of injury. The ureter can usually be seen through the peritoneum of the pelvic sidewall between the pelvic brim and the attachment of the broad ligament. Because of variation from one patient to another or the presence of disease, the location of the ureter can become obscured, making it necessary to enter the retroperitoneal space. The techniques used for retroperitoneal dissection are important factors in reducing the risk of ureteric injury. Blunt and sharp dissection with scissors is preferred, although hydrodissection can be used (137). The selective placement of ureteral stents may be helpful in preventing injury.

Ureteral injury can be treated immediately if it is diagnosed intraoperatively. Although limited damage may heal over a ureteral stent left in place for 10 to 21 days, repair is indicated in most patients. Laparoscopic repair of ureteric lacerations and transections is performed, but most injuries require laparotomy (132,138).

Incomplete or small obstructions and lacerations may be treated successfully with either a retrograde or anterograde ureteral stent. Urinomas may be drained percutaneously. If a stent cannot be placed successfully, a percutaneous nephrostomy should be performed before operative repair is undertaken. Repair may be accomplished by excision and reanastamosis, or, more commonly, ureteric reimplantation with or without facilitating procedures such as a psoas hitch or a Boarie flap.

Neurologic Injury

Peripheral nerve injury is usually related either to poor positioning of the patient or to excessive pressure exerted by the surgeons. Placing the patient in the modified lithotomy position while she is awake may decrease this risk because the patient can determine whether any undue pressure or discomfort is felt (139). **Nerve injury may also occur as a result of the surgical dissection.**

In the extremities, the trauma may be direct, such as when the common peroneal nerve is compressed against a stirrup. **The femoral nerve or the sciatic nerve or its branches may be overstretched and damaged by excessive flexion or external rotation of the hips. The peroneal nerve may be injured by compression if the lateral head of the fibula rests against the stirrup** (139–141). **Brachial plexus injuries may occur secondary to the surgeon or assistants leaning against an abducted arm during the procedure.** If the patient is placed in a steep Trendelenburg position, the brachial plexus may be damaged because of the pressure exerted on the shoulder joint. In most cases, sensory or motor deficits are found as the patient emerges from anesthesia. The likelihood of brachial plexus injury can be reduced with adequate padding and support of the arms and shoulders or by placing the patient's arms in an adducted position.

Most injuries to peripheral nerves resolve spontaneously. The time to recovery depends on the site and severity of the lesion. For most peripheral injuries, full sensory nerve recovery occurs in 3 to 6 months. Recovery may be hastened by the use of physical therapy, appropriate braces, and electrical stimulation of the affected muscles. Open microsurgery should be performed for transection of major intrapelvic nerves.

Incisional Hernia and Wound Dehiscence	Incisional hernia after laparoscopy was reported in more than 900 cases (98,99). The most common defect is dehiscence that develops in the immediate postoperative period. Hernias may be asymptomatic or may cause pain, fever, periumbilical mass, obvious evisceration, and the symptoms and signs of mechanical bowel obstruction. **Although no incision is immune to the risk, defects that are larger than 10 mm in diameter are particularly vulnerable** (99,142,143).

Richter's hernias contain only a portion of the intestine in the defect, and the diagnosis is often delayed because the typical symptoms and findings of mechanical bowel obstruction may be absent. The initial symptom is usually pain. These hernias most often occur in incisions that are lateral to the midline where there is a greater amount of preperitoneal fat creating a potential space for incarceration. Fever can be present if incarceration occurs, and peritonitis may result from subsequent perforation. The condition is difficult to diagnose, requires a high index of suspicion, and may be confirmed with ultrasonography or CT (144).

In most cases, these occurrences can be prevented by using small-caliber cannulas, when possible, and with routine fascial and peritoneal closure of defects made by peritoneal access. The risk of inadvertent incorporation of the intestine into the wound can be reduced by viewing the closure with a smaller-caliber laparoscope passed through a narrow caliber ancillary port. All ancillary cannulas should be removed under direct vision to ensure that bowel is not drawn into the incision and that there is an absence of active incisional bleeding.

The management of laparoscopic incisional defects depends on the time of presentation and the presence and condition of entrapped bowel. Evisceration always requires surgical intervention. If the condition is diagnosed immediately, the intestine is replaced in the peritoneal cavity (if there is no evidence of necrosis or intestinal defect), and the incision is repaired, usually with laparoscopic guidance. If the diagnosis is delayed or the bowel is incarcerated or at risk of perforation, laparotomy is necessary to repair or resect the intestine.

Infection

Wound infections after laparoscopy are uncommon; most are minor skin infections that can be treated successfully with expectant management, drainage, or antibiotics (145). Severe necrotizing fasciitis rarely occurs. Bladder infection, pelvic cellulitis, and pelvic abscess were reported (146).

Laparoscopy is associated with a much lower risk of infection than open abdominal or vaginal surgery. Prophylactic antibiotics should be offered to selected patients (e.g., those with enhanced risk for bacterial endocarditis and those for whom total hysterectomy is planned). Patients should be instructed to monitor their body temperature after discharge and to report immediately a temperature higher than 38°C.

Hysteroscopy

The hysteroscope is an endoluminal endoscope, adapted from the urological cystoscope that can be used to aid diagnosis or to direct the performance of a variety of intrauterine procedures. Hysteroscopic lysis of intrauterine adhesions was first described in 1973 (147). The technique of endoscopically guided electrosurgical resection was adapted from urology to gynecology for the removal of uterine leiomyomas (148). Hysteroscopic division of uterine septa was originally developed using a mechanical technique with specially designed scissors (149). Hysteroscopic destruction of the endometrium, generally termed endometrial ablation (EA), was originally reported using Nd:YAG laser vaporization, but subsequent innovators used the urological resectoscope to ablate the endometrium using electrosurgical coagulation, resection, or vaporization (150–152). Hysteroscopically guided thermal ablation with heated fluid was described, as the only endoscopically guided technique for nonresectoscopic EA. Developments in the design of endoscopes resulted in smaller-diameter instruments that retain the ability to provide a high-quality image and facilitate the use of hysteroscopy in an office or procedure room setting.

Diagnostic Hysteroscopy   The goal for evaluation of the uterine cavity is to obtain either a sample of the endometrium, usually for the detection of hyperplasia or neoplasia, or to identify structural abnormalities, typically a uterine septum or focal lesions, such as adhesions, polyps, or myomas. Blind endometrial sampling is the diagnostic mainstay for the detection of endometrial hyperplasia, whereas transvaginal ultrasonography, hysterography, MRI and hysteroscopy are options for the detection and characterization of structural anomalies. **Hysteroscopic examination is superior to hysterography for evaluation of the endometrial cavity, but the diagnostic accuracy of transvaginal ultrasonography is comparable, when intrauterine saline or gel is used as a contrast medium, a procedure called sonohysterography or saline infusion sonography (SIS)** (153–156). MRI and ultrasound-based techniques have the advantage of allowing evaluation of the myometrium, whereas office-based hysteroscopy allows simultaneous removal of small polyps and even some myomas. Diagnostic hysteroscopy provides information not obtained by blind endometrial sampling, such as detection of endometrial polyps or submucous leiomyomas (157–163). Malignant or hyperplastic polyps or other localized lesions can be identified with hysteroscopy and removed via directed biopsy (160). Blind curettage remains an effective approach for the identification of global endometrial histopathology (157,162,164). **Following are potential indications for diagnostic hysteroscopy:**

1. Unexplained abnormal uterine bleeding
   - Premenopausal
   - Postmenopausal
2. Selected infertility cases
   - Abnormal hysterography or transvaginal ultrasonography
   - Unexplained infertility
3. **3.** Recurrent spontaneous abortion

For most patients, diagnostic hysteroscopy can be performed in an office or procedure room setting with minimal discomfort and at a much lower cost than in a surgical center or a traditional operating room. For some, concerns about patient comfort or a preexisting medical condition may preclude office hysteroscopy. In many patients hysteroscopy can provide more information than blind curettage, but it should be used prudently. For most patients, other diagnostic or therapeutic measures can be undertaken before, or instead of, diagnostic hysteroscopy. For example, for women in the late reproductive years who have abnormal uterine bleeding (AUB) or for those with postmenopausal bleeding, transvaginal sonography or office endometrial biopsy or curettage is typically adequate to evaluate for neoplasia and provide enough information to support an initial management strategy. In the absence of a satisfactory diagnosis or if unexplained bleeding continues without response to treatment, further investigation is appropriate, using one or a combination of ultrasound, endometrial sampling, SIS, or office hysteroscopy. For women in their earlier reproductive years who have AUB, medical or expectant management may be used initially, depending on the severity and inconvenience of the bleeding. For those who do not respond to medical treatments such as oral contraceptives, further diagnostic procedures such as transvaginal ultrasonography, SIS, or hysteroscopy with biopsy can be performed (165).

For women with infertility, hysterosalpingography is the best initial imaging step because it provides information about the patency of the oviducts. In the presence of a suspicious or identified abnormality in the endometrial cavity, hysteroscopy or sonohysterography can be performed to confirm the diagnosis, to better define the abnormality, and perhaps to direct the removal of a lesion. Some experts consider hysteroscopy or MRI mandatory for such patients because of the high occurrence of false-negative radiologic images in those with intrauterine anomalies (166). In women with previous *in vitro* fertilization failure, there is evidence that hysteroscopic identification and treatment of these "missed" anomalies improves pregnancy rates (167). Confirmation of patency of the oviduct is unnecessary in women who have recurrent abortions; therefore, these patients can be evaluated primarily with hysteroscopy.

Operative Hysteroscopy   A number of intrauterine procedures can be performed under endoscopic direction, including adhesiolysis, sterilization, division of a uterine septum, resection of myomas and polyps, removal of retained products of conception, and endometrial destruction through Nd:YAG laser vaporization or radiofrequency resection, desiccation, or vaporization. Hysteroscopy may be used to direct the removal of foreign bodies, including imbedded intrauterine contraceptive devices (IUDs).

Foreign Body

If the string of an IUD is absent, the device usually can be removed with a specially designed hook or a toothed curette (e.g., Novak). When removal is difficult or impossible, the location of the device may be confirmed by hysteroscopy, allowing removal with a grasping forceps. If the device is not seen or if only a portion is visible hysteroscopically and the remainder is imbedded in the myometrium, then individualized management is recommended, usually following appropriate imaging studies to identify the more precise location of the device.

Septum

When recurrent pregnancy loss is associated with a single corpus containing a uterine septum, hysteroscopic division of the septum improves pregnancy outcome (the frequency of spontaneous abortion) at a rate comparable to abdominal metroplasty, with reduced morbidity and cost (see Chapter 33) (168–173). There are fewer data regarding infertility but there is some evidence that metroplasty does improve fecundity (174). Confirmation of the external architecture of the corpus is important and can be achieved using either MRI or three-dimensional ultrasound. One group described an office method of "see and treat" where dissection is continued until attaining two of three criteria (pain, bleeding, the visualization of myometrial fibers) to determine the end point of septal transection (175). This procedure can be successfully performed in the office setting using local anesthesia protocols, with additional 0.05% *lidocaine* with 1/200,000 *epinephrine* directly injected into the septum. The procedure may be performed mechanically with scissors or with energy-based techniques such as the Nd:YAG laser or an electrosurgical knife, needle, or loop. Because most septa have few vessels, scissors can be used to avoid the minimal risk for thermal damage.

Endometrial Polyps

Endometrial polyps are frequently associated with abnormal uterine bleeding and infertility. Although such polyps can be removed with blind curettage, many are missed (157,159,162,163). Therefore, known or suspected endometrial polyps are treated more successfully with hysteroscopic guidance, which usually can be performed as an office procedure. Hysteroscopy may be used either to evaluate the result of blind curettage, to determine if the polyp is avulsed, or to direct the use of grasping forceps or small caliber scissors. Alternatively, for larger polyps, special polyp snares, electrosurgical needles, mechanical morcellators, or a uterine resectoscope may be used to sever the stalk or morcellate the lesion. For patients with infertility and endometrial polyps, it is not clear whether or not polyp number and size are related to outcome (176). Consequently, removal of all accessible polyps should be attempted if the process can be completed with minimal trauma.

Leiomyomas

Hysteroscopy may be used to remove selected leiomyomas that involve the uterine cavity in women with heavy menstrual bleeding, infertility, or recurrent first trimester spontaneous pregnancy loss (155,177–183). This approach is limited based on the location, size, and number of the lesions. Preoperative administration of gonadotropin-releasing hormone (GnRH) agonists may help shrink submucous myomas, facilitating their complete removal, and more importantly, reduce operating time and systemic absorption of distension media (184–186).

To help document and evaluate the results of hysteroscopically directed myoma surgery, a classification system was developed that is based on the proportion of the myoma that is in the uterine cavity. **In patients with myomas that are entirely intracavitary (type 0), excision is feasible and in many instances relatively easy, depending in part on the diameter; whereas in larger type II lesions an abdominal approach with laparoscopy or laparotomy is frequently necessary.** Small type 0 leiomyomas may be removed following transection of the stalk with scissors or an electrode attached to a uterine resectoscope. For larger type 0 lesions, or for type I myomas, mechanical or electrosurgical morcellation with a resectoscope is necessary before removal. For a limited number of type II myomas, careful dissection into the avascular plane interposed between the tumor and the myometrial pseudocapsule may be attempted, provided that satisfactory ultrasonography or MRI demonstrated an adequate margin of myometrium between the deepest aspect of the lesion and the uterine serosa. It may be preferable to undertake such procedures with laparoscopic monitoring to verify that bowel is not adjacent to the zone of dissection. Patients should be counseled that for some type I and many type II myomas, more than one procedure might be required to complete excision (178,187). The use of intrauterine prostaglandin $F_{2\alpha}$ was described to facilitate extrusion of type II myomas (188).

Endometrial Ablation

Heavy menstrual bleeding that does not respond to oral medical therapy may be managed by EA using coagulation, resection, or vaporization, provided the patient is willing to forgo future fertility (51). Alternatively, or if future fertility is desired, a *levonorgestrel*-releasing intrauterine contraceptive device can provide virtually equal clinical outcomes (189,190). Ablation may be performed with the laser, radiofrequency electrosurgical desiccation, resection, or vaporization using a uterine resectoscope, or by any of a number of nonresectoscopic techniques, including those employing thermal balloons, cryotherapy, heated free fluid, or microwave or bipolar radiofrequency systems (151,152,187,191–195). Many of these endometrial ablation devices can be used in an office setting using local anesthetic protocols.

Endometrial resection is an EA technique performed with an electrosurgical loop electrode to shave the endometrium and superficial myometrium (109,142,143,150,196,197). Vaporization utilizes specially designed electrodes that are attached to standard resectoscopes but which are capable of destroying large volumes of tissue without morcellation (187). Ablation is achieved using ball or barrel-shaped electrodes that coagulate the endometrial surface (51,152). Complications of these procedures include fluid overload, electrolyte imbalances (if nonelectrolytic or even isosmotic media are used), uterine perforation, bleeding, and intestinal and urinary tract injury (198,199). The risk of uterine perforation may be reduced by using a combination of resection or vaporization and electrosurgical ablation; the latter is most suitable for the thinner areas of the myometrium in the cornu (177). The preoperative use of GnRH analogues or *danazol* may reduce operating time. GnRH may reduce bleeding and the amount of fluid absorbed into the systemic circulation (186).

For many women, these procedures succeed in reducing or eliminating menses without hysterectomy or long-term medical therapy (51,200). Success rates vary and depend on the duration of follow-up and the definition of success. For many patients, amenorrhea is the goal, whereas for others, it is normalization of menses. About 75% to 95% of patients are satisfied with the surgical procedure after 1 year. Amenorrhea rates range from about 30% to 90% (depending in part upon the technique), but 40% to 50% of patients have amenorrhea, is a useful number to quote to patients considering the procedure. In comparative studies, there is no advantage of laser over electrosurgical techniques (198,201). The nonresectoscopic techniques have similar clinical outcomes, thus reducing the need for resectoscopic ablation. However, the nonresectoscopic approaches all have limitations defined by the size or configuration of the endometrial cavity. Consequently, for those women with heavy menstrual bleeding who are not suitable for nonresectoscopic techniques because of large uteri (>12 cm sounded length), resectoscopic endometrial ablation remains a viable option (161,202).

The long-term efficacy and impact of ablation or resection on women with adenomyosis is unknown. Because some endometrium inevitably cannot be ablated, there is the potential for endometrial cancer; therefore, postmenopausal women who underwent ablation or resection should take *progestin* as a part of hormonal therapy (203).

Sterilization

Sterilization can be performed under hysteroscopic guidance, an approach that eliminates the disadvantages and risks associated with abdominal or laparoscopic techniques (204). Two such techniques are available and others are under development. The Essure® system comprises a nickel-titanium coil with a Dacron filament that can be inserted relatively quickly in an office or procedure room setting (see Chapter 10). The Adiana® device uses a rice grain–sized porous silicon plug that is positioned in the proximal tube following the application of an aliquot of RF radiofrequency current. It is designed for office use under local anesthesia. North American protocols require that hysterosalpingography be performed 3 months after the procedure to ensure that bilateral tubal occlusion took place.

Synechiae

Asherman syndrome is the presence of adhesions in the endometrial cavity that can result in infertility or recurrent spontaneous abortion with or without amenorrhea. These synechiae may be detected on a hysterogram or sonohysterogram, but are best shown with diagnostic hysteroscopy. Relatively thin, fragile synechiae may be divided with the tip of a rigid diagnostic hysteroscope (205). Thicker lesions may require division by semirigid or rigid scissors or energy-based instruments such as a resectoscope or an operative hysteroscope with either a radiofrequency electrode or an Nd:YAG laser. Reproductive outcome depends on the extent of the preoperative endometrial damage (206,207). This is another hysteroscopic procedure that is amenable to performance in the office, at least in selected cases without complete obliteration, but the surgeon must be careful to maintain orientation within the endometrial cavity.

Patient Preparation and Communication

Diagnostic hysteroscopy procedures traditionally were performed in the office or clinic settings, and operative hysteroscopy usually was performed in an operating room or hospital surgical center. Much is changing; in a number of centers, 90% of the operative hysteroscopies are performed in an office procedure room setting using local and verbal anesthesia. The patient should understand the rationale for the procedure, and the anticipated discomfort, the potential risks, and the expectant, medical, and surgical alternatives. The nature of the procedure and the chance of therapeutic success should be explained, and she should be given a realistic estimate of success based on the operator's experience.

Diagnostic Hysteroscopy: Risks

The risks of diagnostic hysteroscopy are few, and those complications that occur rarely have severe consequences (199). The uncommon adverse events that should be discussed with the patient include perforation, bleeding, and those related to anesthesia and the distention media. After diagnostic hysteroscopy, most patients have slight vaginal bleeding and occasionally, lower abdominal cramps. Severe cramps, dyspnea, and upper abdominal and right shoulder pain can develop if CO_2 is used as the distension media and it passes through the fallopian tubes into the peritoneal cavity. Consequently, even in an office environment, the patient should be encouraged to have a friend or relative escort her home.

Operative Hysteroscopy: Risks

Counseling before operative hysteroscopy varies depending on the planned procedure, the type of anesthesia, and the procedure location—office or operating room. Overall, **the risks of operative hysteroscopy are higher than those of diagnostic hysteroscopy, but these increased risks are largely confined to procedures such as adhesiolysis of severe intrauterine synechiae or resection of leiomyomas that are either large or that extend deeply into the myometrium.** These risks include those associated with anesthesia, which are intrinsic to all hysteroscopic procedures, and are related to the specific surgical procedure to be performed. **With any hysteroscopic procedure, air embolus is a possibility, as are complications associated with the gaseous or fluid distention media used.** Hypotonic distension media may not be tolerated in some patients if there is significant intravascular absorption, especially in patients with underlying cardiovascular disease. The patient must be aware of the risks associated with uterine perforation, which range from failure to complete the procedure, to hemorrhage, or damage to the intestines or the urinary tract. If such complications occur, laparotomy may be necessary to repair the injury.

Equipment and Technique

The equipment required for hysteroscopy depends on the reason for the procedure. The surgeon must be knowledgeable about the equipment, its mechanisms, and the technical specifications to facilitate efficiency, optimal clinical outcome, and a decreased probability of complications. A typical hysteroscopy setup for diagnostic and minor operative procedures is shown in Figures 23.24 and 23.25. Core competencies required for hysteroscopy are as follows:

1. Patient positioning and cervical exposure
2. Anesthesia
3. Cervical dilation
4. Uterine distention
5. Visualization and imaging
6. Intrauterine cutting and hemostasis
7. Other instrumentation

Patient Positioning and Cervical Exposure

Hysteroscopy is performed in a modified dorsal lithotomy position; the patient is supine, and the legs are held in stirrups. For hysteroscopic procedures performed while the patient is conscious, comfort must be considered in conjunction with the need to gain good exposure of the perineum.

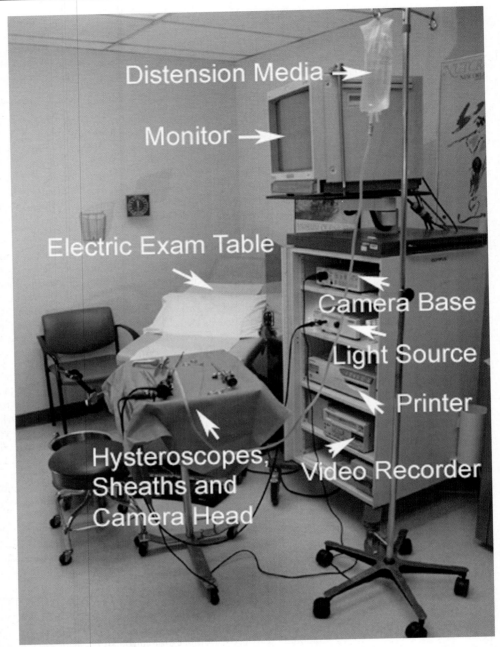

Figure 23.24   Office hysteroscopy setup. Hysteroscopic procedures are facilitated with an electric examination table. Distension media may be positioned on an intravenous pole, but wide, cystoscopy tubing allows maintenance of higher intrauterine pressures suitable for viewing and performing simple procedures such as polypectomy or transcervical sterilization. A light source is necessary and a camera desirable. The camera is attached to the monitor and may be connected to a printer and/or video recorder. The camera head is attached to a flexible hysteroscope.

Stirrups that hold and support the knees, calves, and ankles permit prolonged procedures. "Candy cane" stirrups are inappropriate for hysteroscopic surgery and for conscious patients.

The smallest speculum possible should be used to expose the cervix. A bivalve speculum hinged on only one side allows its removal without disturbing the position of the tenaculum and hysteroscope. The use of weighted specula should be avoided in conscious patients because of the discomfort involved.

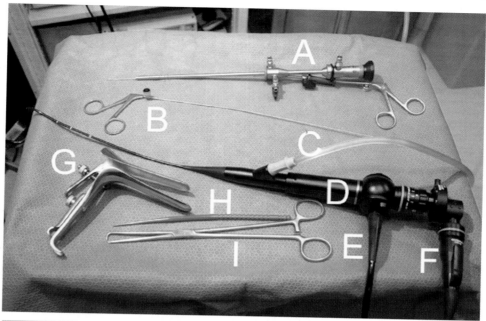

Figure 23.25 Office hysteroscopy instruments. An assembled continuous flow operating hysteroscope with a 5.5-mm diameter external sheath is shown in (**A**). A 5-French semirigid scissors occupies the working channel. An additional biopsy forceps is shown in (**B**). Tubing transporting media to the system is shown in (**C**) going into a 3-mm external diameter flexible and steerable hysteroscope (**D**). A medical video camera is attached to the hysteroscope (**F**) and the light source is attached at (**E**). An open speculum (**G**) facilitates removal with instruments in place. A small dilator (**H**) or series of dilators will be necessary for a large number of patients. A tenaculum (**I**) attached to the cervix frequently facilitates both dilation and entry of the hysteroscope into the endometrial cavity.

Anesthesia

The anesthetic requirements for hysteroscopy vary greatly, depending on the patient's level of anxiety, the status of her cervical canal, the procedure, and the outside diameter of the hysteroscope or sheath. **In some patients, diagnostic hysteroscopy is possible without anesthesia, especially if the patient is parous or if narrow-caliber (<3 mm in outside diameter) hysteroscopes and sheaths are used (208). In many instances the pain of cervical dilation can be avoided or minimized with the preprocedural use of oral or vaginal misoprostol (see below) or by inserting a laminaria "tent" in the cervix 3 to 8 hours before the procedure.** Laminaria are thin rods of natural (slippery elm) or synthetic construction that, when passed through the internal os, expand over several hours thereby dilating the cervix. However, if laminaria are left in place too long (e.g., longer than 24 hours), the cervix may overdilate, which is can be counterproductive for CO_2 insufflation.

For most diagnostic and many operative procedures, effective cervical anesthesia is obtained using local anesthesia, allowing the hysteroscopy to be done in an office procedure room. Evidence suggests that the paracervical block may be the most effective (208,209). Following exposure of the cervix with a vaginal speculum, a spinal needle can be used to instill about 3 mL of 0.5% to 1% _lidocaine_ into the anterior lip of the cervix to allow attachment of a tenaculum and manipulation of the exocervix. While the exact location and depth of the injection varies with providers and studies, the uterosacral ligament location (about 4 mm deep at approximately at the 4- and 8-o'clock positions as one looks at the cervix) was demonstrated successful (210). Care must be taken to avoid intravascular injection. An alternative technique is the use of an intracervical block where the anesthetic agent is injected evenly around the circumference of the cervix, attempting to reach the level of the internal os. The efficacy of this approach is unclear based on published studies (208). Recognizing the complex innervation of the uterus, alternative or additional topical anesthesia may be applied to the cervical canal or to the endometrium, or both, using anesthetic spray, gel, or cream. It is unclear how effective these approaches are because many of the study protocols seemed to allow inadequate time between application and initiation of the procedure (211). A number of options were presented, including instillation of 5 mL of 2% *mepivacaine* into the endometrial cavity with a syringe, or the application of similar amounts of 2% *lidocaine* gel. Many operative procedures can be performed with these techniques combined, if deemed necessary, with the oral or intravenous use of anxiolytics or analgesics, although the use of such systemic agents mandates continuous monitoring of blood pressure and oxygenation and the availability of appropriate resuscitative staff and equipment. An important component of the optimal use of local anesthesia is allowing sufficient time from the injection or application of the agents before the commencement of the procedure. While injectable local anesthetic agents such as *lidocaine* and *mepivacaine* may have an onset of action in 2 to 3 minutes, it may take up to 15 to 20 minutes to obtain a maximal effect. If local anesthesia is not deemed appropriate, regional or general anesthesia may be used in the context of a surgical center or operating room.

Cervical Dilation

In many instances, and particularly in vaginally parous women, dilation of the cervix will be unnecessary, especially if narrow caliber hysteroscopic systems are used. Dilation will be necessary some of the time, and, although seemingly simple, cervical stenosis or suboptimal technique can result in perforation that compromises the entire procedure. If the objective lens of the endoscope cannot be placed in the endometrial cavity the hysteroscopy cannot be done. The process of dilation should be undertaken carefully, respecting the orientation of the cervix to the axis of the vaginal canal (version) and that of the corpus to the cervix (flexion). In difficult circumstances, simultaneous ultrasound may be valuable, and difficult dilation may be facilitated directly with the hysteroscope.

There are a number of options available to facilitate cervical dilation. There is evidence that *prostaglandin E$_1$ (misoprostol)* administered 400 μg orally or 200 to 400 μg vaginally, approximately 12 to 24 hours before the procedure facilitates cervical dilation (212–215). *Misoprostol* alone may not be effective in postmenopausal women, but one well-designed randomized trial demonstrated that vaginal *estrogen,* administered daily for 2 weeks before the procedure facilitates the effect of the prostaglandin in this group of patients (215). Alternatively, there is evidence that intraoperatively administered intracervical *vasopressin* (0.05 U/mL, 4 cc at 4 and 8 o'clock) substantially reduces the force required for cervical dilation (216). Regardless of the circumstance, the cervix should be dilated as atraumatically as possible. It is best to avoid using a uterine sound because it can traumatize the canal or the endometrium, causing unnecessary bleeding and uterine perforation.

Uterine Distention

Distention of the endometrial cavity is necessary to create a viewing space. The choices include CO_2 gas, high-viscosity 32% *dextran* 70, and a number of low-viscosity fluids, including glycine, sorbitol, saline, and dextrose in water. **A pressure of 45 mm Hg or higher is generally required for adequate distention of the uterine cavity and to visualize the tubal ostia. To minimize extravasation, this pressure should not exceed the mean arterial pressure.** For each of the fluids, there are several methods used to create this pressure by infusion into the endometrial cavity.

Sheaths

A rigid hysteroscope is passed into the endometrial cavity through an external sheath. The design and diameter of the sheath reflect both the dimensions of the endoscope and the purpose of the instrument. Typical diagnostic hysteroscopes have a sheath slightly wider than the telescope, allowing infusion of the distention media. Operative sheaths have additional channels to permit the passage or efflux of distention media and the insertion of laser fibers, electrosurgical instruments or semirigid scissors, biopsy devices, or grasping forceps. These sheaths are usually 5 to 8 mm in diameter, and some allow continuous flow of distention media in and out of the endometrial cavity (Figs. 23.25 and 23.26).

Media

CO_2 **provides an excellent view for diagnostic purposes, but it is unsuitable for operative hysteroscopy and for diagnostic procedures when the patient is bleeding because there is no effective way to remove blood and other debris from the endometrial cavity. To prevent** CO_2 **embolus, the gas must be instilled by an insufflator that is specially designed for**

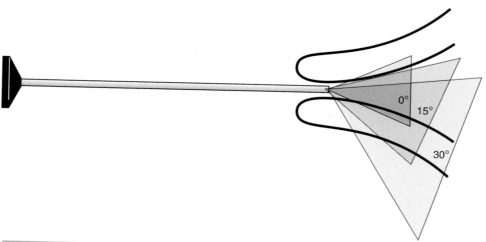

Figure 23.26 **Hysteroscope optics.** Panoramic (0°) and oblique (15° and 30°) viewing angles.

the procedure—the intrauterine pressure is kept below 100 mm Hg and the flow rate is maintained at less than 100 mL per minute.

Normal saline is a useful and safe medium for procedures that do not require radiofrequency electricity from standard monopolar resectoscopes. Even if there is absorption of a substantial volume of solution, saline typically does not cause electrolyte imbalance. Therefore, saline is a good fluid for minor procedures performed in the office. The development of bipolar radiofrequency instrumentation for hysteroscopic surgery allowed the application of saline as a distending medium in even more advanced and complex procedures.

Dextran 70 **is useful for patients who are bleeding because it does not mix with blood.** However, it is expensive and tends to "caramelize" on instruments, which must be disassembled and thoroughly cleaned in warm water immediately after each use. Anaphylactic reactions, fluid overload, and electrolyte disturbances can occur.

For standard operative hysteroscopy with monopolar radiofrequency resectoscopes, low-viscosity, nonconductive fluids such as 1.5% glycine, 3% sorbitol, and 5.0% mannitol are used most often. These solutions can be used with standard, monopolar radiofrequency instrumentation because there are no electrolytes to disperse the current and impede the electrosurgical effect. Each of these media is inexpensive and readily available, usually in 3-L bags suitable for continuous-flow hysteroscopy. Because each fluid is electrolyte-free, extravasation into the systemic circulation can be associated with electrolyte disturbances. Compared with 1.5% glycine or 3.0% sorbitol, 5% mannitol is isomolar and it functions as a diuretic, both advantages when performing resectoscopic surgery. **Regardless of the electrolyte content of the fluid distending media, systemic "absorption" must be monitored continuously or at least frequently (every 5 minutes) by collecting outflow from the sheath and subtracting it from the total infused volume.** The fact that the manufacturer frequently fills the bags with more than the indicated 3 L makes accurate calculation of absorbed volume even more difficult (217). There are a number of machines designed to provide continuous feedback to the surgeon regarding the degree of negative fluid balance. Absorbed volumes greater than 1 L mandate the measurement of electrolyte levels. The risk of fluid overload is reduced by the judicious restriction of intravenous fluid by the anesthesiologist. The administration of an appropriate dose of *furosemide* should be considered, and the surgeon should plan for the expeditious completion of the procedure. If there is more than a preset limit (1.5 to 2 L of extravasated fluid), the procedure should be stopped. Excessive circulating sorbitol may cause hyperglycemia, and large volumes of glycine may elevate levels of ammonia in the blood (218).

Media Delivery Systems

Syringes can be used for office diagnostic procedures and are especially good for infusing *dextran* solution. The syringe can be operated by the surgeon and is either connected directly to the sheath or attached by connecting tubing. Because this technique is so tedious, it is suited only for simple operations.

Continuous hydrostatic pressure is effectively achieved by elevating the vehicle containing the distention media above the level of the patient's uterus. The achieved pressure is the product of the width of the connecting tubing and the elevation—for operative hysteroscopy with 10-mm tubing, intrauterine pressure ranges from 70 to 100 mm Hg when the bag is between 1 to 1.5 m above the uterine cavity.

A pressure cuff may be placed around the infusion bag to elevate the pressure in the system. Caution must be exercised because this technique causes increasing extravasation if intrauterine pressure rises above the mean arterial pressure.

A variety of infusion pumps is available, ranging from simple devices to instruments that maintain a preset intrauterine pressure. Simple pump devices continue to press fluid into the uterine cavity regardless of resistance, whereas the pressure-sensitive pumps reduce the flow rate when the preset level is reached, thereby impeding the efflux of blood and debris and compromising the view.

Imaging

Endoscopes

Hysteroscopes are available in two basic types—flexible and rigid. Flexible hysteroscopes are self-contained in that they do not require a sheath; the single integrated channel is used to transmit gas or fluid to the endometrial cavity for distention. As a result, these instruments are generally of smaller diameter than rigid systems. In addition, they can be designed to be "steerable," allowing angled viewing. Flexible hysteroscopes utilize fiberoptic bundles rather than lenses to transmit the image to the observer and, consequently, have lower resolution than rigid instruments of a similar diameter and typically do not have a channel with a caliber suitable for most hand instruments. Rigid hysteroscopes are more durable and provide a superior image. The most commonly used hysteroscopes are 3 to 4 mm in diameter, although those using fibers can be smaller than 2 mm in diameter.

Rigid endoscopes require an angled (fore-oblique) lens to provide the angled view useful for operative hysteroscopy and are available in 0-degree, 12- to 15-degree, and 25- to 30-degree models (Fig. 23.26). The 0-degree telescope provides a panoramic view and is best for diagnostic procedures. Hysteroscopes with 25- to 30-degree angles are most often used for cannulation of the fallopian tubes or placement of sterilization devices, whereas 12- to 15-degree designs are a suitable compromise useful for diagnosis and ablation or resection. The utility of endoscopes with larger fore-oblique views may be offset by the tendency of resectoscopic electrodes to leave the visual field on full extension.

Light Sources and Cables

Adequate illumination of the endometrial cavity is essential. Because it runs from a standard 110- or 220-volt wall outlet, the light source requires no special electrical connections. For most cameras and endoscopes, the element must have at least 150 watts of power for direct viewing and preferably 250 watts or more for video and operative procedures (219).

Video Imaging

Although diagnostic hysteroscopy may be performed with direct visualization, it is best to use video guidance for prolonged operations. Video imaging is important for teaching and recording pathology and procedures. The camera must be sensitive because of the narrow diameter of the endoscope and the frequently dark background of the endometrial cavity, particularly when it is enlarged or when blood is in the field. (Fig. 23.25).

Image Documentation

A small video camera can be used to teach and to coordinate the procedure with the operating room team. It allows the acquisition of still or video images for future reference or teaching. When a video recorder is used, the camera should be attached directly to the recorder to preserve the image quality. A number of video recording formats are available, each with inherent advantages and disadvantages. Some video printers provide images suitable for a medical record. Newer high-definition digital cameras provide high-quality video still images as well as high-resolution digital video, suitable for publication or teaching.

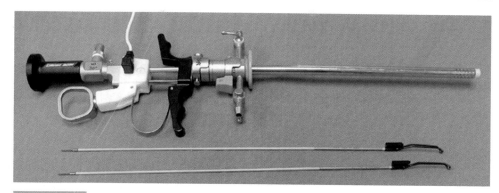

Figure 23.27   Resectoscope. The assembled resectoscope is shown, with two electrodes in the foreground. Manipulation of the electrode is via the white handle in the proximal portion of the device.

Intrauterine Cutting and Hemostasis

The instruments available for use through operative hysteroscopes include biopsy, grasping, cutting, and punch-biopsy devices. These tools are narrow and flexible enough to navigate the 1- to 2-mm diameter operating channel (Fig. 23.25). Although their value is limited by their small size and flimsy construction; the scissors can divide adhesions, the biopsy forceps can sample targeted lesions, and the grasping forceps can remove small polyps or intrauterine devices. Some operative hysteroscopes are designed to allow passage of fibers for the conduction of Nd:YAG laser energy, although this modality is generally superseded by electrosurgical electrodes.

The uterine resectoscope is similar to the one used in urology and is designed to apply radiofrequency electrical current to the endometrial cavity (Fig. 23.27). An understanding of the principles of electrosurgery is mandatory for safe and effective use of this instrument. By sliding the "working element," one of a variety of electrode tips can be manipulated back and forth within the cavity. Tissue can be divided with a pointed electrode, excised with a loop, or desiccated with a rolling ball or bar. An electrode with multiple tips or edges can vaporize tissue, provided higher wattage generator outputs are used. A clear operative field is maintained by the continuous flow of nonconductive distending media in and out of the cavity. Although basic design modifications made the resectoscope more useful in gynecology, extraction of resected fragments is time consuming. The most effective approach is the periodic use of a uterine curette or specially designed polyp or myoma forceps inserted after removal of the hysteroscope. Alternatively, much of the myoma or endometrium can be vaporized, thereby minimizing the need for periodic but time-consuming removal of tissue "chips." If vaporization is used, it is important to obtain representative samples of the endometrium or myoma for pathological analysis.

Other Instrumentation

For any hysteroscopic procedure, it is necessary to have available a cervical tenaculum, dilators, uterine curette, and appropriate-sized vaginal specula. When using the resectoscope, it is helpful to have a solid-state, isolated circuit electrosurgical generator capable of delivering both modulated and nonmodulated radiofrequency current. Laparoscopy or laparotomy may be necessary for emergencies secondary to uterine perforation.

Complications

The potential risks of positioning a hysteroscopic system in the endometrial cavity solely for viewing ("diagnostic hysteroscopy") are largely limited to cervical trauma and uterine perforation. Other adverse events such as infection, excessive bleeding, and complications related to the distention media are extremely uncommon when the procedure is short and does not involve instrumentation of the myometrium (0% to 1%) (199). **The risks of operative hysteroscopy are related to one of five aspects of the procedure performed: (i) anesthesia, (ii) the distention media, (iii) perforation, (iv) bleeding, and (v) thermal trauma (198,199).**

Anesthesia

Local anesthetic protocols typically include the intracervical or paracervical injection of 0.5% to 2% *lidocaine* or *mepivacaine* solution, with or without a local vasoconstrictor such as adrenaline. Overdosage is prevented by ensuring that intravascular injection is avoided and by not exceeding the maximum recommended doses (*lidocaine*, 4 mg/kg; *mepivacaine*, 3 mg/kg). The use of a dilute vasoconstrictor such as *epinephrine* 1/200,000 reduces the amount of systemic absorption of the agent, virtually doubling the maximum dose that can be used and facilitates the onset of action of local anesthetic agents (220).

Complications of intravascular injection or anesthetic overdose include allergy, neurologic effects, and impaired myocardial conduction. Allergy is characterized by the typical symptoms of agitation, palpitations, pruritus, coughing, shortness of breath, urticaria, bronchospasm, shock, and convulsions. Treatment measures include administration of oxygen, isotonic intravenous fluids, intramuscular or subcutaneous adrenaline, and intravenous prednisolone and aminophylline. Cardiac effects related to impaired myocardial conduction include bradycardia, cardiac arrest, shock, and convulsions. Emergency treatment measures include the administration of oxygen, intravenous *atropine* (0.5 mg), and intravenous *adrenaline* and the initiation of appropriate cardiac resuscitation. The most common central nervous system manifestations are paresthesia of the tongue, drowsiness, tremor, and convulsions. Options for therapy include intravenous *diazepam* and respiratory support.

Distention Media	### Carbon Dioxide

Carbon dioxide is highly soluble in blood; consequently such emboli as occur are usually clinically insignificant; however, in rare instances, CO_2 emboli may result in serious intraoperative morbidity and even death (221–223). These risks can be eliminated by avoiding the use of CO_2 with operative procedures, by ensuring that the insufflation pressure is always lower than 100 mm Hg, and that the flow rate is lower than 100 mL per minute. The insufflator used must be especially designed for hysteroscopy; it is difficult to set laparoscopic insufflator flow rates below 1,000 mL per minute.

Dextran 70

Dextran 70 is a hyperosmolar medium that, rarely, can induce an allergic response or coagulopathy (224,225). Similar to other types of distention media, if sufficient volumes are infused, vascular overload and heart failure can occur (226,227). Because *dextran* is hydrophilic, it can draw six times its own volume into the systemic circulation. Consequently, the volume of this agent should be limited to less than 300 mL.

Low-Viscosity Fluids

The low-viscosity fluids—1.5% glycine, 3% sorbitol, and 5.0% mannitol—are used commonly because of their low cost, compatibility with standard electrosurgery, and availability in large-volume bags. However, should these electrolyte free and usually hypotonic media be absorbed to excess in the systemic circulation, they can create serious fluid and electrolyte disturbances, a potentially dangerous complication that can result in pulmonary edema, hyponatremia, heart failure, cerebral edema, and even death. There are a number of published guidelines describing the steps required to reduce the risk of fluid overload at the time of hysteroscopy (228).

1. **Before undertaking anything but simple operative procedures using these agents, baseline serum electrolyte levels should be measured.** Women with cardiopulmonary disease should be evaluated carefully. The selective preoperative use of agents such as GnRH agonists may reduce operating time and media absorption. Intracervical injection of 8 mL of a dilute *vasopressin* solution (0.01 U/mL) immediately prior to surgery is effective at reducing the amount of systemic absorption of distending media (229). The duration of this effect may be limited to approximately 20 to 30 minutes, so repeat dosing may be useful for optimal effect.

2. **In the operating room, media infusion and collection should take place in a closed system to allow accurate measurement of the "absorbed" volume.** The volume should be measured continuously with a device specifically designed for the purpose or, if such a system is not available, calculated every 5 minutes by support staff who are trained in these calculations and unencumbered by duties that may interfere with this task.

3. **The lowest intrauterine pressure necessary for adequate distention should be used to complete the operation, preferably at a level that is below the mean arterial**

pressure. A good range for operative procedures is 70 to 80 mm Hg, which can be achieved with a specially designed pump or by maintaining the meniscus of the infusion bag 1 m above the level of the patient's uterus. If greater intrauterine pressure is needed for adequate distention, the anesthesiologist may temporarily raise the mean arterial pressure by administration of a vasoactive agent such as *phenylephrine.*

4. **Deficits of more than 1 L require repeat measurement of serum electrolyte levels and consideration of intravenous *furosemide* in a dose appropriate to the patient's renal function.** When such a deficit exists, the procedure should be completed expeditiously. If the deficit reaches a preset limit (1.5 to 2 L), the procedure should be terminated, and a diuretic such as mannitol or *furosemide* should be used as needed. Patients with cardiovascular compromise will typically have a lower tolerance for fluid deficits, a circumstance that mandates setting a lower limit for systemic absorption and consequent termination of the procedure (230).

Perforation

Perforation may occur during dilation of the cervix, positioning of the hysteroscope, or as a consequence of the intrauterine procedure. With complete perforation, the endometrial cavity typically does not distend, and the visual field is generally lost. **When perforation occurs during dilation of the cervix, the procedure must be terminated, but, because of the blunt nature of the dilators, usually there are no other injuries.** If the uterus is perforated by the activated tip of a laser, or electrode, there is a risk for bleeding or injury to the adjacent viscera. Therefore, the operation must be stopped and **laparoscopy or laparotomy should be performed.** Injury to the uterus is relatively easy to detect with a laparoscope. However, mechanical or thermal injury to the bowel, ureter, or bladder is more difficult to detect and laparoscopy is frequently inadequate to make a complete evaluation. If the patient's condition is managed expectantly, she should be advised of the situation and asked to report any symptoms of bleeding or visceral trauma such as fever, increasing pain, nausea, and vomiting.

Bleeding

Bleeding that occurs during or after hysteroscopy generally results from trauma to the vessels in the myometrium or injury to other vessels in the pelvis. Myometrial vessels are more susceptible to laceration with resectoscopic techniques that require myometrial dissection for procedures such as endometrial resection or type II myomectomy.

In planning operations that involve deep resection, autologous blood can be obtained before surgery. The risk for bleeding may be reduced by the preoperative injection of diluted vasopressin into the cervical stroma (229). The risk of injury to branches of the uterine artery can be lowered by limiting the depth of resection in the lateral endometrial cavity near the uterine isthmus, where ablative techniques should be considered. When bleeding is encountered during resectoscopic procedures, the ball electrode can be used to desiccate the vessel electrosurgically. Intractable bleeding may respond to the injection of diluted vasopressin or to the inflation of a 30-mL Foley catheter balloon or similar device in the endometrial cavity (177).

Thermal Trauma

Thermal injury to the intestine or ureter may be difficult to diagnose, and symptoms may not occur for several days to 2 weeks. Therefore, the patient should be advised of the symptoms that could indicate peritonitis.

References

1. **Nezhat C, Hood J, Winer W, et al.** Video laseroscopy and laser laparoscopy in gynaecology. *Br J Hosp Med* 1987;38:219–224.
2. **Pierre SA, Ferrandino MN, Simmons WN, et al.** High definition laparoscopy: objective assessment of performance characteristics and comparison with standard laparoscopy. *J Endourol* 2009;23:523–528.
3. **Stovall TG, Ling FW, Gray LA.** Single-dose *methotrexate* for treatment of ectopic pregnancy. *Obstet Gynecol* 1991;77:754–757.
4. **Ellstrom M, Ferraz-Nunes J, Hahlin M, et al.** A randomized trial with a cost-consequence analysis after laparoscopic and abdominal hysterectomy. *Obstet Gynecol* 1998;91:30–34.
5. **Bhiwandiwala PP, Mumford SD, Feldblum PJ.** A comparison of different laparoscopic sterilization occlusion techniques in 24,439 procedures. *Am J Obstet Gynecol* 1982;144:319–331.
6. **Ryder RM, Vaughan MC.** Laparoscopic tubal sterilization. Methods, effectiveness, and sequelae. *Obstet Gynecol Clin North Am* 1999;26:83–97.
7. **Lipscomb GH, Gomez IG, Givens VM, et al.** Yolk sac on transvaginal ultrasound as a prognostic indicator in the treatment of ectopic pregnancy with single-dose methotrexate. *Am J Obstet Gynecol* 2009;200:338 e1–e4.
8. **Potter MB, Lepine LA, Jamieson DJ.** Predictors of success with methotrexate treatment of tubal ectopic pregnancy at Grady Memorial Hospital. *Am J Obstet Gynecol* 2003;188:1192–1194.

9. **Hajenius PJ, Mol F, Mol BW, et al.** Interventions for tubal ectopic pregnancy. *Cochrane Database Syst Rev* 2007;1:CD000324.

10. **Maruri F, Azziz R.** Laparoscopic surgery for ectopic pregnancies: technology assessment and public health implications. *Fertil Steril* 1993;59:487–498.

11. **American College of Obstetricians and Gynecologists.** ACOG Practice Bulletin No. 94: medical management of ectopic pregnancy. *Obstet Gynecol* 2008;111:1479–1185.

12. **Gomel V.** Management of ectopic gestation: surgical treatment is usually best. *Clin Obstet Gynecol* 1995;38:353–361.

13. **Gomel V, Taylor PJ.** Diagnostic and operative laparoscopy. St. Louis: CV Mosby; 1995.

14. **Canis M, Mage G, Pouly JL, et al.** Laparoscopic diagnosis of adnexal cystic masses: a 12-year experience with long-term follow-up. *Obstet Gynecol* 1994;83:707–712.

15. **Mecke H, Lehmann-Willenbrock E, Ibrahim M, et al.** Pelviscopic treatment of ovarian cysts in premenopausal women. *Gynecol Obstet Invest* 1992;34:36–42.

16. **Medeiros LR, Rosa DD, Bozzetti MC, et al.** Laparoscopy versus laparotomy for benign ovarian tumour. *Cochrane Database Syst Rev* 2009;2:CD004751.

17. **Lehner R, Wenzl R, Heinzl H, et al.** Influence of delayed staging laparotomy after laparoscopic removal of ovarian masses later found malignant. *Obstet Gynecol* 1998;92:967–971.

18. **Vergote I.** Role of surgery in ovarian cancer: an update. *Acta Chir Belg* 2004;104:246–256.

19. **Parker WH, Berek JS.** Management of selected cystic adnexal masses in postmenopausal women by operative laparoscopy: a pilot study. *Am J Obstet Gynecol* 1990;163:1574–1577.

20. **Parker WH, Levine RL, Howard FM, et al.** A multicenter study of laparoscopic management of selected cystic adnexal masses in postmenopausal women. *J Am Coll Surg* 1994;179:733–737.

21. **Jacobs I, Oram D, Fairbanks J, et al.** A risk of malignancy index incorporating CA125, ultrasound and menopausal status for the accurate preoperative diagnosis of ovarian cancer. *Br J Obstet Gynaecol* 1990;97:922–929.

22. **Harry VN, Narayansingh GV, Parkin DE.** The risk of malignancy index for ovarian tumours in northeast Scotland—a population based study. *Scott Med J* 2009;54:21–23.

23. **van den Akker PA, Aalders AL, Snijders MP, et al.** Evaluation of the Risk of Malignancy Index in daily clinical management of adnexal masses. *Gynecol Oncol* 2010;116:384–388.

24. **Howard FM.** Surgical management of benign cystic teratoma. Laparoscopy vs. laparotomy. *J Reprod Med* 1995;40:495–499.

25. **Savasi I, Lacy JA, Gerstle JT, et al.** Management of ovarian dermoid cysts in the pediatric and adolescent population. *J Pediatr Adolesc Gynecol* 2009;22:360–364.

26. **Galinier P, Carfagna L, Delsol M, et al.** Ovarian torsion. Management and ovarian prognosis: a report of 45 cases. *J Pediatr Surg* 2009;44:1759–1765.

27. **Kavallaris A, Mytas S, Chalvatzas N, et al.** Seven years' experience in laparoscopic dissection of intact ovarian dermoid cysts. *Acta Obstet Gynecol Scand* 2010;89:390–392.

28. **Rhode JM, Advincula AP, Reynolds RK, et al.** A minimally invasive technique for management of the large adnexal mass. *J Minim Invasive Gynecol* 2006;13:476–479.

29. **Anonymous.** Postoperative adhesion development after operative laparoscopy: evaluation at early second-look procedures. Operative Laparoscopy Study Group. *Fertil Steril* 1991;55:700–704.

30. **Pellicano M, Bramante S, Guida M, et al.** Ovarian endometrioma: postoperative adhesions following bipolar coagulation and suture. *Fertil Steril* 2008;89:796–799.

31. **Mage G, Canis M, Manhes H, et al.** Laparoscopic management of adnexal torsion. A review of 35 cases. *J Reprod Med* 1989;34:520–524.

32. **Vancaillie T, Schmidt EH.** Recovery of ovarian function after laparoscopic treatment of acute adnexal torsion. A case report. *J Reprod Med* 1987;32:561–562.

33. **Cohen SB, Oelsner G, Seidman DS, et al.** Laparoscopic detorsion allows sparing of the twisted ischemic adnexa. *J Am Assoc Gynecol Laparosc* 1999;6:139–143.

34. **Gjonnaess H.** Polycystic ovarian syndrome treated by ovarian electrocautery through the laparoscope. *Fertil Steril* 1984;41:20–25.

35. **Huber J, Hosmann J, Spona J.** Polycystic ovarian syndrome treated by laser through the laparoscope. *Lancet* 1988;2:215.

36. **Kovacs G, Buckler H, Bangah M, et al.** Treatment of anovulation due to polycystic ovarian syndrome by laparoscopic ovarian electrocautery. *Br J Obstet Gynaecol* 1991;98:30–35.

37. **Farquhar C, Lilford RJ, Marjoribanks J, et al.** Laparoscopic "drilling" by diathermy or laser for ovulation induction in anovulatory polycystic ovary syndrome. *Cochrane Database Syst Rev* 2007;3:CD001122.

38. **Gurgan T, Kisnisci H, Yarali H, et al.** Evaluation of adhesion formation after laparoscopic treatment of polycystic ovarian disease. *Fertil Steril* 1991;56:1176–1178.

39. **Naether OG, Fischer R.** Adhesion formation after laparoscopic electrocoagulation of the ovarian surface in polycystic ovary patients. *Fertil Steril* 1993;60:95–98.

40. **Bedient CE, Magrina JF, Noble BN, et al.** Comparison of robotic and laparoscopic myomectomy. *Am J Obstet Gynecol* 2009;201:566 e1–e5.

41. **Palomba S, Zupi E, Falbo A, et al.** A multicenter randomized, controlled study comparing laparoscopic versus minilaparotomic myomectomy: reproductive outcomes. *Fertil Steril* 2007;88:933–941.

42. **Seracchioli R, Rossi S, Govoni F, et al.** Fertility and obstetric outcome after laparoscopic myomectomy of large myomata: a randomized comparison with abdominal myomectomy. *Hum Reprod* 2000;15:2663–2668.

43. **Jin C, Hu Y, Chen XC, et al.** Laparoscopic versus open myomectomy—a meta-analysis of randomized controlled trials. *Eur J Obstet Gynecol Reprod Biol* 2009;145:14–21.

44. **Day Baird D, Dunson DB, Hill MC, et al.** High cumulative incidence of uterine leiomyoma in black and white women: ultrasound evidence. *Am J Obstet Gynecol* 2003;188:100–107.

45. **Pritts EA, Parker WH, Olive DL.** Fibroids and infertility: an updated systematic review of the evidence. *Fertil Steril* 2009;91:1215–1223.

46. **Luciano AA.** Myomectomy. *Clin Obstet Gynecol* 2009;52:362–371.

47. **Sutton C, Diamond MP.** Endoscopic surgery for gynecologists. St. Louis: CV Mosby, 1993.

48. **Munro MG, Deprest J.** Laparoscopic hysterectomy: does it work? A bicontinental review of the literature and clinical commentary. *Clin Obstet Gynecol* 1995;38:401–425.

49. **Summitt RLJ, Stovall TG, Lipscomb GH, et al.** Randomized comparison of laparoscopy-assisted vaginal hysterectomy with standard vaginal hysterectomy in an outpatient setting. *Obstet Gynecol* 1992;80:895–901.

50. **Munro MG, Parker WH.** A classification system for laparoscopic hysterectomy. *Obstet Gynecol* 1993;82:624–629.

51. **Nieboer TE, Johnson N, Lethaby A, et al.** Surgical approach to hysterectomy for benign gynaecological disease. *Cochrane Database Syst Rev* 2009;3:CD003677.

52. **Johns DA, Carrera B, Jones J, et al.** The medical and economic impact of laparoscopically assisted vaginal hysterectomy in a large, metropolitan, not-for-profit hospital. *Am J Obstet Gynecol* 1995;172:1709–1715; discussion 15–19.

53. **Walsh CA, Walsh SR, Tang TY, et al.** Total abdominal hysterectomy versus total laparoscopic hysterectomy for benign disease: a meta-analysis. *Eur J Obstet Gynecol Reprod Biol* 2009;144:3–7.

54. **Marana R, Busacca M, Zupi E, et al.** Laparoscopically assisted vaginal hysterectomy versus total abdominal hysterectomy: a prospective, randomized, multicenter study. *Am J Obstet Gynecol* 1999;180:270–275.

55. **Munro M, Gomel V.** Fertility-promoting laparoscopically-directed procedures. *Reprod Med Rev* 1994;3:29–42.

56. **Marcoux S, Maheux R, Berube S.** Laparoscopic surgery in infertile women with minimal or mild endometriosis. Canadian Collaborative Group on Endometriosis. *N Engl J Med* 1997;337:217–222.

57. **Parazzini F.** Ablation of lesions or no treatment in minimal-mild endometriosis in infertile women: a randomized trial. Gruppo Italiano per lo Studio dell'Endometriosi. *Hum Reprod* 1999;14:1332–1334.

58. **Jacobson TZ, Duffy JM, Barlow D, et al.** Laparoscopic surgery for subfertility associated with endometriosis. *Cochrane Database Syst Rev* 2010;1:CD001398.

59. **Filmar S, Jetha N, McComb P, et al.** A comparative histologic study on the healing process after tissue transection. I. Carbon dioxide

laser and electromicrosurgery. *Am J Obstet Gynecol* 1989;160:1062–1067.

60. **Filmar S, Jetha N, McComb P, et al.** A comparative histologic study on the healing process after tissue transection. II. Carbon dioxide laser and surgical microscissors. *Am J Obstet Gynecol* 1989;160:1068–1072.

61. **Munro MG, Fu YS.** Loop electrosurgical excision with a laparoscopic electrode and carbon dioxide laser vaporization: comparison of thermal injury characteristics in the rat uterine horn. *Am J Obstet Gynecol* 1995;172:1257–1262.

62. **Van Holsbeke C,** Van **Calster B, Guerriero S, et al.** Endometriomas: their ultrasound characteristics. *Ultrasound Obstet Gynecol* 2010;35:730–740.

63. **Hart RJ, Hickey M, Maouris P, et al.** Excisional surgery versus ablative surgery for ovarian endometriomata. *Cochrane Database Syst Rev* 2008;2:CD004992.

64. **Chapron C, Dubuisson JB.** Management of deep endometriosis. *Ann N Y Acad Sci* 2001;943:276–280.

65. **Chapron C, Jacob S, Dubuisson JB, et al.** Laparoscopically assisted vaginal management of deep endometriosis infiltrating the rectovaginal septum. *Acta Obstet Gynecol Scand* 2001;80:349–354.

66. **Miklos JR, Kohli N.** Laparoscopic paravaginal repair plus Burch colposuspension: review and descriptive technique. *Urology* 2000;56:64–69.

67. **Ross JW.** Multichannel urodynamic evaluation of laparoscopic Burch colposuspension for genuine stress incontinence. *Obstet Gynecol* 1998;91:55–59.

68. **Paraiso MF, Walters MD.** Laparoscopic pelvic reconstructive surgery. *Clin Obstet Gynecol* 2000;43:594–603.

69. **Canis M, Pouly JL, Wattiez A, et al.** Laparoscopic management of adnexal masses suspicious at ultrasound. *Obstet Gynecol* 1997;89:679–683.

70. **Fowler JM, Carter JR.** Laparoscopic management of the adnexal mass in postmenopausal. *J Gynecol Tech* 1995;1:7–10.

71. **Possover M, Krause N, Plaul K, et al.** Laparoscopic para-aortic and pelvic lymphadenectomy: experience with 150 patients and review of the literature. *Gynecol Oncol* 1998;71:19–28.

72. **Homesley HD, Boike G, Spiegel GW.** Feasibility of laparoscopic management of presumed stage I endometrial carcinoma and assessment of accuracy of myoinvasion estimates by frozen section: a gynecologic oncology group study. *Int J Gynecol Cancer* 2004;14:341–347.

73. **Tozzi R, Malur S, Koehler C, et al.** Analysis of morbidity in patients with endometrial cancer: is there a commitment to offer laparoscopy? *Gynecol Oncol* 2005;97:4–9.

74. **Ghezzi F, Cromi A, Uccella S, et al.** Laparoscopic versus open surgery for endometrial cancer: a minimum 3-year follow-up study. *Ann Surg Oncol* 2010;17:271–278.

75. **Nezhat FR, Ezzati M, Chuang L, et al.** Laparoscopic management of early ovarian and fallopian tube cancers: surgical and survival outcome. *Am J Obstet Gynecol* 2009;200:83 e1–e6.

76. **Ghezzi F, Cromi A, Siesto G, et al.** Laparoscopy staging of early ovarian cancer: our experience and review of the literature. *Int J Gynecol Cancer* 2009;19(Suppl 2):S7–S13.

77. **Slim K, Vicaut E, Launay-Savary MV, et al.** Updated systematic review and meta-analysis of randomized clinical trials on the role of mechanical bowel preparation before colorectal surgery. *Ann Surg* 2009;249:203–209.

78. **Muzii L, Bellati F, Zullo MA, et al.** Mechanical bowel preparation before gynecologic laparoscopy: a randomized, single-blind, controlled trial. *Fertil Steril* 2006;85:689–693.

79. **Pickett SD, Rodewald KJ, Billow MR, et al.** Avoiding major vessel injury during laparoscopic instrument insertion. *Obstet Gynecol Clin North Am* 2010;37:387–397.

80. **Nezhat F, Brill AI, Nezhat CH, et al.** Laparoscopic appraisal of the anatomic relationship of the umbilicus to the aortic bifurcation. *J Am Assoc Gynecol Laparosc* 1998;5:135–140.

81. **Roy GM, Bazzurini L, Solima E, et al.** Safe technique for laparoscopic entry into the abdominal cavity. *J Am Assoc Gynecol Laparosc* 2001;8:519–528.

82. **Nezhat CH, Nezhat F, Brill AI, et al.** Normal variations of abdominal and pelvic anatomy evaluated at laparoscopy. *Obstet Gynecol* 1999;94:238–242.

83. **Hurd WW, Bude RO, DeLancey JO, et al.** The relationship of the umbilicus to the aortic bifurcation: implications for laparoscopic technique. *Obstet Gynecol* 1992;80:48–51.

84. **Brill AI, Cohen BM.** Fundamentals of peritoneal access. *J Am Assoc Gynecol Laparosc* 2003;10:286–298.

85. **Giannios NM, Gulani V, Rohlck K, et al.** Left upper quadrant laparoscopic placement: effects of insertion angle and body mass index on distance to posterior peritoneum by magnetic resonance imaging. *Am J Obstet Gynecol* 2009;201:522 e1–e5.

86. **Vilos GA, Ternamian A, Dempster J, et al.** Laparoscopic entry: a review of techniques, technologies, and complications. *J Obstet Gynaecol Can* 2007;29:433–465.

87. **Vilos GA, Vilos AG.** Safe laparoscopic entry guided by Veress needle CO2 insufflation pressure. *J Am Assoc Gynecol Laparosc* 2003;10:415–420.

88. **Audebert AJ, Gomel V.** Role of microlaparoscopy in the diagnosis of peritoneal and visceral adhesions and in the prevention of bowel injury associated with blind trocar insertion. *Fertil Steril* 2000;73:631–635.

89. **Brill AI, Nezhat F, Nezhat CH, et al.** The incidence of adhesions after prior laparotomy: a laparoscopic appraisal. *Obstet Gynecol* 1995;85:269–272.

90. **Fader AN, Rojas-Espaillat L, Ibeanu O, et al.** Laparoendoscopic single-site surgery (LESS) in gynecology: a multi-institutional evaluation. *Am J Obstet Gynecol* 2010;203:501e1–e6.

91. **Fader AN, Cohen S, Escobar PF, et al.** Laparoendoscopic single-site surgery in gynecology. *Curr Opin Obstet Gynecol* 2010;22:331–338.

92. **Escobar PF, Bedaiwy MA, Fader AN, et al.** Laparoendoscopic single-site (LESS) surgery in patients with benign adnexal disease. *Fertil Steril* 2010;93:2074e7–e10.

93. **Palomba S, Zupi E, Falbo A, et al.** New tool (Laparotenser) for gasless laparoscopic myomectomy: a multicenter-controlled study. *Fertil Steril.* 2010;94:1090–1096.

94. **Tulandi T.** Salpingo-ovariolysis: a comparison between laser surgery and electrosurgery. *Fertil Steril* 1986;45:489–491.

95. **Munro MG.** Principles of laparoscopic suturing. In: Stoval TJ, Sammarco MJ, Steege JF, eds. Gynecological endoscopy: principles in practice. Baltimore: Williams & Wilkins, 1996:193–244.

96. **Munro MG.** Laparoscopic suturing. In: Jain N, ed. Atlas of gynecologic endoscopy. New Delhi: Jaype, 2004. pp 64-84.

97. **Kho CH.** Laparoscopic suturing in the vertical zone. Endo Press, Tuttlingen, Germany 2006.

98. **Boike GM, Miller CE, Spirtos NM, et al.** Incisional bowel herniations after operative laparoscopy: a series of nineteen cases and review of the literature. *Am J Obstet Gynecol* 1995;172:1726–1733.

99. **Montz FJ, Holschneider CH, Munro MG.** Incisional hernia following laparoscopy: a survey of the American Association of Gynecologic Laparoscopists. *Obstet Gynecol* 1994;84:881–884.

100. **Peterson HB, DeStefano F, Rubin GL, et al.** Deaths attributable to tubal sterilization in the United States, 1977 to 1981. *Am J Obstet Gynecol* 1983;146:131–136.

101. **Jamieson DJ, Hillis SD, Duerr A, et al.** Complications of interval laparoscopic tubal sterilization: findings from the United States Collaborative Review of Sterilization. *Obstet Gynecol* 2000;96:997–1002.

102. **Hirvonen EA, Nuutinen LS, Kauko M.** Ventilatory effects, blood gas changes, and oxygen consumption during laparoscopic hysterectomy. *Anesth Analg* 1995;80:961–966.

103. **Lee Y, Kim ES, Lee HJ.** Pulmonary edema after catastrophic carbon dioxide embolism during laparoscopic ovarian cystectomy. *Yonsei Med J* 2008;49:676–679.

104. **Gutt CN, Oniu T, Mehrabi A, et al.** Circulatory and respiratory complications of carbon dioxide insufflation. *Dig Surg* 2004;21:95–105.

105. **Ishizaki Y, Bandai Y, Shimomura K, et al.** Safe intraabdominal pressure of carbon dioxide pneumoperitoneum during laparoscopic surgery. *Surgery* 1993;114:549–554.

106. **Myles PS.** Bradyarrhythmias and laparoscopy: a prospective study of heart rate changes with laparoscopy. *Aust N Z J Obstet Gynaecol* 1991;31:171–173.

107. **Bard PA, Chen L.** Subcutaneous emphysema associated with laparoscopy. *Anesth Analg* 1990;71:101–102.

108. **Kalhan SB, Reaney JA, Collins RL.** Pneumomediastinum and subcutaneous emphysema during laparoscopy. *Cleve Clin J Med* 1990;57:639–642.

109. **Kent RB.** Subcutaneous emphysema and hypercarbia following laparoscopic cholecystectomy. *Arch Surg* 1991;126:1154–1156.

110. **Ko ML.** Pneumopericardium and severe subcutaneous emphysema after laparoscopic surgery. *J Minim Invasive Gynecol* 2010;17:531–533.

111. **Kabukoba JJ, Skillern LH.** Coping with extraperitoneal insufflation during laparoscopy: a new technique. *Obstet Gynecol* 1992;80:144–145.

112. **Brill AI.** Energy systems for operative laparoscopy. *J Am Assoc Gynecol Laparosc* 1998;5:333–345; quiz 47–49.

113. **Grainger DA, Soderstrom RM, Schiff SF, et al.** Ureteral injuries at laparoscopy: insights into diagnosis, management, and prevention. *Obstet Gynecol* 1990;75:839–843.

114. **Soderstrom RM.** Electrosurgical injuries during laparoscopy: prevention and management. *Curr Opin Obstet Gynecol* 1994;6:248–250.

115. **Engel T, Harris FW.** The electrical dynamics of laparoscopic sterilization. *J Reprod Med* 1975;15:33–42.

116. **Baadsgaard SE, Bille S, Egeblad K.** Major vascular injury during gynecologic laparoscopy. Report of a case and review of published cases. *Acta Obstet Gynecol Scand* 1989;68:283–285.

117. **Chi I, Feldblum PJ, Balogh SA.** Previous abdominal surgery as a risk factor in interval laparoscopic sterilization. *Am J Obstet Gynecol* 1983;145:841–846.

118. **Franks AL, Kendrick JS, Peterson HB.** Unintended laparotomy associated with laparoscopic tubal sterilization. *Am J Obstet Gynecol* 1987;157:1102–1105.

119. **Childers JM, Brzechffa PR, Surwit EA.** Laparoscopy using the left upper quadrant as the primary trocar site. *Gynecol Oncol* 1993;50:221–225.

120. **Penfield AJ.** How to prevent complications of open laparoscopy. *J Reprod Med* 1985;30:660–663.

121. **Reich H.** Laparoscopic bowel injury. *Surg Laparosc Endosc* 1992;2:74–78.

122. **Agarwala N, Liu CY.** Safe entry techniques during laparoscopy: left upper quadrant entry using the ninth intercostal space—a review of 918 procedures. *J Minim Invasive Gynecol* 2005;12:55–61.

123. **Deziel DJ, Millikan KW, Economou SG, et al.** Complications of laparoscopic cholecystectomy: a national survey of 4,292 hospitals and an analysis of 77,604 cases. *Am J Surg* 1993;165:9–14.

124. **Wolfe BM, Gardiner BN, Leary BF, et al.** Endoscopic cholecystectomy. An analysis of complications. *Arch Surg* 1991;126:1192–1198.

125. **Zmora O, Mahajna A, Bar-Zakai B, et al.** Colon and rectal surgery without mechanical bowel preparation: a randomized prospective trial. *Ann Surg* 2003;237:363–367.

126. **Mirhashemi R, Harlow BL, Ginsburg ES, et al.** Predicting risk of complications with gynecologic laparoscopic surgery. *Obstet Gynecol* 1998;92:327–331.

127. **Font GE, Brill AI, Stuhldreher PV, et al.** Endoscopic management of incidental cystotomy during operative laparoscopy. *J Urol* 1993;149:1130–1131.

128. **Ostrzenski A, Ostrzenska KM.** Bladder injury during laparoscopic surgery. *Obstet Gynecol Surv* 1998;53:175–180.

129. **Soong YK, Yu HT, Wang CJ, et al.** Urinary tract injury in laparoscopic-assisted vaginal hysterectomy. *J Minim Invasive Gynecol* 2007;14:600–605.

130. **Jelovsek JE, Chiung C, Chen G, et al.** Incidence of lower urinary tract injury at the time of total laparoscopic hysterectomy. *JSLS* 2007;11:422–427.

131. **Reich H, McGlynn F.** Laparoscopic repair of bladder injury. *Obstet Gynecol* 1990;76:909–910.

132. **Gomel V, James C.** Intraoperative management of ureteral injury during operative laparoscopy. *Fertil Steril* 1991;55:416–419.

133. **Ostrzenski A, Radolinski B, Ostrzenska KM.** A review of laparoscopic ureteral injury in pelvic surgery. *Obstet Gynecol Surv* 2003;58:794–799.

134. **Steckel J, Badillo F, Waldbaum RS.** Uretero-fallopian tube fistula secondary to laparoscopic fulguration of pelvic endometriosis. *J Urol* 1993;149:1128–1129.

135. **Woodland MB.** Ureter injury during laparoscopy-assisted vaginal hysterectomy with the endoscopic linear stapler. *Am J Obstet Gynecol* 1992;167:756–757.

136. **Parpala-Sparman T, Paananen I, Santala M, et al.** Increasing numbers of ureteric injuries after the introduction of laparoscopic surgery. *Scand J Urol Nephrol* 2008;42:422–427.

137. **Nezhat C, Nezhat FR.** Safe laser endoscopic excision or vaporization of peritoneal endometriosis. *Fertil Steril* 1989;52:149–151.

138. **Nezhat C, Nezhat F.** Laparoscopic repair of ureter resected during operative laparoscopy. *Obstet Gynecol* 1992;80:543–544.

139. **Irvin W, Andersen W, Taylor P, et al.** Minimizing the risk of neurologic injury in gynecologic surgery. *Obstet Gynecol* 2004;103:374–382.

140. **Gombar KK, Gombar S, Singh B, et al.** Femoral neuropathy: a complication of the lithotomy position. *Reg Anesth* 1992;17:306–308.

141. **Loffer FD, Pent D, Goodkin R.** Sciatic nerve injury in a patient undergoing laparoscopy. *J Reprod Med* 1978;21:371–372.

142. **Bloom DA, Ehrlich RM.** Omental evisceration through small laparoscopy port sites. *J Endourol* 1993;7:31–33.

143. **Plaus WJ.** Laparoscopic trocar site hernias. *J Laparoendosc Surg* 1993;3:567–570.

144. **Ozcakir T, Tavmergen E, Goker EN, et al.** CT scanning to diagnose incisional hernias after laparoscopy. *J Am Assoc Gynecol Laparosc* 2000;7:595–597.

145. **Gynaecological Laparoscopy:** The report of the working party of the confidential inquiry into gynaecological laparoscopy. London: Royal College of Obstetricians and Gynaecologists, 1978.

146. **Glew RH, Pokoly TB.** Tuboovarian abscess following laparoscopic sterilization with silicone rubber bands. *Obstet Gynecol* 1980;55:760–762.

147. **Levine RU, Neuwirth RS.** Simultaneous laparoscopy and hysteroscopy for intrauterine adhesions. *Obstet Gynecol* 1973;42:441–445.

148. **Neuwirth RS, Amin HK.** Excision of submucus fibroids with hysteroscopic control. *Am J Obstet Gynecol* 1976;126:95–99.

149. **Chervenak FA, Neuwirth RS.** Hysteroscopic resection of the uterine septum. *Am J Obstet Gynecol* 1981;141:351–353.

150. **DeCherney A, Polan ML.** Hysteroscopic management of intrauterine lesions and intractable uterine bleeding. *Obstet Gynecol* 1983;61:392–397.

151. **Goldrath MH, Fuller TA, Segal S.** Laser photovaporization of endometrium for the treatment of menorrhagia. *Am J Obstet Gynecol* 1981;140:14–19.

152. **Vancaillie TG.** Electrocoagulation of the endometrium with the ball-end resectoscope. *Obstet Gynecol* 1989;74:425–427.

153. **Golan A, Ron-El R, Herman A, et al.** Diagnostic hysteroscopy: its value in an in-vitro fertilization/embryo transfer unit. *Hum Reprod* 1992;7:1433–1434.

154. **Valle RF.** Hysteroscopy in the evaluation of female infertility. *Am J Obstet Gynecol* 1980;137:425–431.

155. **Cicinelli E, Romano F, Anastasio PS, et al.** Transabdominal sonohysterography, transvaginal sonography, and hysteroscopy in the evaluation of submucous myomas. *Obstet Gynecol* 1995;85:42–47.

156. **Dueholm M, Lundorf E, Hansen ES, et al.** Evaluation of the uterine cavity with magnetic resonance imaging, transvaginal sonography, hysterosonographic examination, and diagnostic hysteroscopy. *Fertil Steril* 2001;76:350–357.

157. **Crescini C, Artuso A, Repetti F, et al.** [Hysteroscopic diagnosis in patients with abnormal uterine hemorrhage and previous endometrial curettage]. *Minerva Ginecol* 1992;44:233–235.

158. **Gimpelson RJ.** Office hysteroscopy. *Clin Obstet Gynecol* 1992;35:270–281.

159. **Gimpelson RJ, Rappold HO.** A comparative study between panoramic hysteroscopy with directed biopsies and dilatation and curettage. A review of 276 cases. *Am J Obstet Gynecol* 1988;158:489–492.

160. **Iossa A, Cianferoni L, Ciatto S, et al.** Hysteroscopy and endometrial cancer diagnosis: a review of 2007 consecutive examinations in self-referred patients. *Tumori* 1991;77:479–483.

161. **Itzkowic DJ, Laverty CR.** Office hysteroscopy and curettage—a safe diagnostic procedure. *Aust N Z J Obstet Gynaecol* 1990;30:150–153.

162. **Loffer FD.** Hysteroscopy with selective endometrial sampling compared with D&C for abnormal uterine bleeding: the value of a negative hysteroscopic view. *Obstet Gynecol* 1989;73:16–20.

163. **Brooks PG, Serden SP.** Hysteroscopic findings after unsuccessful dilatation and curettage for abnormal uterine bleeding. *Am J Obstet Gynecol* 1988;158:1354–1357.

164. **Marty R, Amouroux J, Haouet S, et al.** The reliability of endometrial biopsy performed during hysteroscopy. *Int J Gynaecol Obstet* 1991;34:151–155.

165. **Chambers JT, Chambers SK.** Endometrial sampling: When? Where? Why? With what? *Clin Obstet Gynecol* 1992;35:28–39.

166. **El-Mazny A, Abou-Salem N, El-Sherbiny W, et al.** Outpatient hysteroscopy: a routine investigation before assisted reproductive techniques? *Fertil Steril* 2010;95:272–276.

167. **Makrakis E, Hassiakos D, Stathis D, et al.** Hysteroscopy in women with implantation failures after *in vitro* fertilization: findings and effect on subsequent pregnancy rates. *J Minim Invasive Gynecol* 2009;16:181–187.

168. **Daly DC, Maier D, Soto-Albors C.** Hysteroscopic metroplasty: six years' experience. *Obstet Gynecol* 1989;73:201–205.

169. **DeCherney AH, Russell JB, Graebe RA, et al.** Resectoscopic management of mullerian fusion defects. *Fertil Steril* 1986;45:726–728.

170. **March CM, Israel R.** Hysteroscopic management of recurrent abortion caused by septate uterus. *Am J Obstet Gynecol* 1987;156:834–842.

171. **Valle RF, Sciarra JJ.** Hysteroscopic treatment of the septate uterus. *Obstet Gynecol* 1986;67:253–257.

172. **Valli E, Vaquero E, Lazzarin N, et al.** Hysteroscopic metroplasty improves gestational outcome in women with recurrent spontaneous abortion. *J Am Assoc Gynecol Laparosc* 2004;11:240–244.

173. **Zlopasa G, Skrablin S, Kalafatic D, et al.** Uterine anomalies and pregnancy outcome following resectoscope metroplasty. *Int J Gynaecol Obstet* 2007;98:129–133.

174. **Mollo A, De Franciscis P, Colacurci N, et al.** Hysteroscopic resection of the septum improves the pregnancy rate of women with unexplained infertility: a prospective controlled trial. *Fertil Steril* 2009;91:2628–2831.

175. **Di Spiezio Sardo A, Bettocchi S, Bramante S, et al.** Office vaginoscopic treatment of an isolated longitudinal vaginal septum: a case report. *J Minim Invasive Gynecol* 2007;14:512–515.

176. **Stamatellos I, Apostolides A, Stamatopoulos P, et al.** Pregnancy rates after hysteroscopic polypectomy depending on the size or number of the polyps. *Arch Gynecol Obstet* 2008;277:395–399.

177. **Brill AI.** What is the role of hysteroscopy in the management of abnormal uterine bleeding? *Clin Obstet Gynecol* 1995;38:319–345.

178. **Emanuel MH, Wamsteker K, Hart AA, et al.** Long-term results of hysteroscopic myomectomy for abnormal uterine bleeding. *Obstet Gynecol* 1999;93:743–748.

179. **Hart R, Molnar BG, Magos A.** Long term follow up of hysteroscopic myomectomy assessed by survival analysis. *Br J Obstet Gynaecol* 1999;106:700–705.

180. **Indman PD.** Hysteroscopic treatment of menorrhagia associated with uterine leiomyomas. *Obstet Gynecol* 1993;81:716–720.

181. **O'Connor H, Magos A.** Endometrial resection for the treatment of menorrhagia. *N Engl J Med* 1996;335:151–156.

182. **Vercellini P, Zaina B, Yaylayan L, et al.** Hysteroscopic myomectomy: long-term effects on menstrual pattern and fertility. *Obstet Gynecol* 1999;94:341–347.

183. **Wamsteker K, Emanuel MH, de Kruif JH.** Transcervical hysteroscopic resection of submucous fibroids for abnormal uterine bleeding: results regarding the degree of intramural extension. *Obstet Gynecol* 1993;82:736–740.

184. **Anonymous.** A Scottish audit of hysteroscopic surgery for menorrhagia: complications and follow up. Scottish Hysteroscopy Audit Group. *Br J Obstet Gynaecol* 1995;102:249–254.

185. **Brooks PG.** Hysteroscopic surgery using the resectoscope: myomas, ablation, septae and synechiae. Does pre-operative medication help? *Clin Obstet Gynecol* 1992;35:249–255.

186. **Sowter MC, Singla AA, Lethaby A.** Pre-operative endometrial thinning agents before hysteroscopic surgery for heavy menstrual bleeding. *Cochrane Database Syst Rev* 2000;2:CD001124.

187. **Vercellini P, Oldani S, Yaylayan L, et al.** Randomized comparison of vaporizing electrode and cutting loop for endometrial ablation. *Obstet Gynecol* 1999;94:521–527.

188. **Murakami T, Shimizu T, Katahira A, et al.** Intraoperative injection of prostaglandin F2alpha in a patient undergoing hysteroscopic myomectomy. *Fertil Steril* 2003;79:1439–1441.

189. **Crosignani PG, Vercellini P, Mosconi P, et al.** Levonorgestrel-releasing intrauterine device versus hysteroscopic endometrial resection in the treatment of dysfunctional uterine bleeding. *Obstet Gynecol* 1997;90:257–263.

190. **Istre O, Trolle B.** Treatment of menorrhagia with the levonorgestrel intrauterine system versus endometrial resection. *Fertil Steril* 2001;76:304–309.

191. **Cooper J, Gimpelson R, Laberge P, et al.** A randomized, multicenter trial of safety and efficacy of the NovaSure system in the treatment of menorrhagia. *J Am Assoc Gynecol Laparosc* 2002;9:418–428.

192. **Cooper KG, Bain C, Parkin DE.** Comparison of microwave endometrial ablation and transcervical resection of the endometrium for treatment of heavy menstrual loss: a randomised trial. *Lancet* 1999;354:1859–1863.

193. **Corson SL.** A multicenter evaluation of endometrial ablation by Hydro ThermAblator and rollerball for treatment of menorrhagia. *J Am Assoc Gynecol Laparosc* 2001;8:359–367.

194. **Duleba AJ, Heppard MC, Soderstrom RM, et al.** Randomized study comparing endometrial cryoablation and rollerball electroablation for treatment of dysfunctional uterine bleeding. *J Am Assoc Gynecol Laparosc* 2003;10:17–26.

195. **Meyer WR, Walsh BW, Grainger DA, et al.** Thermal balloon and rollerball ablation to treat menorrhagia: a multicenter comparison. *Obstet Gynecol* 1998;92:98–103.

196. **Magos AL, Baumann R, Lockwood GM, et al.** Experience with the first 250 endometrial resections for menorrhagia. *Lancet* 1991;337:1074–1078.

197. **Wortman M, Daggett A.** Hysteroscopic endomyometrial resection. *JSLS* 2000;4:197–207.

198. **Overton C, Hargreaves J, Maresh M.** A national survey of the complications of endometrial destruction for menstrual disorders: the MISTLETOE study. Minimally invasive surgical techniques—laser, EndoThermal or endoresection. *Br J Obstet Gynaecol* 1997;104:1351–1359.

199. **Munro MG.** Complications of hysteroscopic and uterine resectoscopic surgery. *Obstet Gynecol Clin North Am* 2010;37:399–425.

200. **Lethaby A, Shepperd S, Cooke I, et al.** Endometrial resection and ablation versus hysterectomy for heavy menstrual bleeding. *Cochrane Database Syst Rev* 2000;2:CD000329.

201. **Pinion SB, Parkin DE, Abramovich DR, et al.** Randomised trial of hysterectomy, endometrial laser ablation, and transcervical endometrial resection for dysfunctional uterine bleeding. *BMJ* 1994;309:979–983.

202. **Eskandar MA, Vilos GA, Aletebi FA, et al.** Hysteroscopic endometrial ablation is an effective alternative to hysterectomy in women with menorrhagia and large uteri. *J Am Assoc Gynecol Laparosc* 2000;7:339–345.

203. **Alexander DA, Naji AA, Pinion SB, et al.** Randomised trial comparing hysterectomy with endometrial ablation for dysfunctional uterine bleeding: psychiatric and psychosocial aspects. *BMJ* 1996;312:280–284.

204. **Castano PM, Adekunle L.** Transcervical sterilization. *Semin Reprod Med* 2010;28:103–109.

205. **Sugimoto O.** Diagnostic and therapeutic hysteroscopy for traumatic intrauterine adhesions. *Am J Obstet Gynecol* 1978;131:539–547.

206. **March CM, Israel R.** Gestational outcome following hysteroscopic lysis of adhesions. *Fertil Steril* 1981;36:455–459.

207. **Schlaff WD, Hurst BS.** Preoperative sonographic measurement of endometrial pattern predicts outcome of surgical repair in patients with severe Asherman's syndrome. *Fertil Steril* 1995;63:410–413.

208. **Cooper NA, Smith P, Khan KS, et al.** Vaginoscopic approach to outpatient hysteroscopy: a systematic review of the effect on pain. *BJOG* 2010;117:532–539.

209. **Cooper NA, Khan KS, Clark TJ.** Local anaesthesia for pain control during outpatient hysteroscopy: systematic review and meta-analysis. *BMJ* 2010;340:c1130.

210. **Cicinelli E, Didonna T, Schonauer LM, et al.** Paracervical anesthesia for hysteroscopy and endometrial biopsy in postmenopausal

women. A randomized, double-blind, placebo-controlled study. *J Reprod Med* 1998;43:1014–1018.

211. **Munro MG, Brooks PG.** Use of local anesthesia for office diagnostic and operative hysteroscopy. *J Minim Invasive Gynecol* 2010;17:709–718.

212. **Preutthipan S, Herabutya Y.** Vaginal *misoprostol* for cervical priming before operative hysteroscopy: a randomized controlled trial. *Obstet Gynecol* 2000;96:890–894.

213. **Thomas JA, Leyland N, Durand N, et al.** The use of oral *misoprostol* as a cervical ripening agent in operative hysteroscopy: a double-blind, placebo-controlled trial. *Am J Obstet Gynecol* 2002;186:876–879.

214. **Waddell G, Desindes S, Takser L, et al.** Cervical ripening using vaginal *misoprostol* before hysteroscopy: a double-blind randomized trial. *J Minim Invasive Gynecol* 2008;15:739–744.

215. **Oppegaard KS, Lieng M, Berg A, et al.** A combination of *misoprostol* and *estradiol* for preoperative cervical ripening in postmenopausal women: a randomised controlled trial. *BJOG* 2010;117:53–61.

216. **Phillips DR, Nathanson H, Milim SJ.** The effect of dilute 0.25% *vasopressin* solution on the linear force necessary for cervical dilatation. *J Am Assoc Gynecol Laparosc* 1996;3:S38–S39.

217. **Nezhat CH, Fisher DT, Datta S.** Investigation of often-reported ten percent hysteroscopy fluid overfill: is this accurate? *J Minim Invasive Gynecol* 2007;14:489–493.

218. **Hoekstra PT, Kahnoski R, McCamish MA, et al.** Transurethral prostatic resection syndrome—a new perspective: encephalopathy with associated hyperammonemia. *J Urol* 1983;130:704–707.

219. **Brill AI.** Energy systems for operative hysteroscopy. *Obstet Gynecol Clin North Am* 2000;27:317–326.

220. **Windle ML.** Local anesthetic agents, infiltrative administration. eMedicine, Clinical Procedures 2009. Available online at: http:/emedicine.medscape.com/article/149178-overview

221. **Obenhaus T, Maurer W.** [CO2 embolism during hysteroscopy]. *Anaesthesist.* 1990;39:243–246.

222. **Stoloff DR, Isenberg RA, Brill AI.** Venous air and gas emboli in operative hysteroscopy. *J Am Assoc Gynecol Laparosc* 2001;8:181–192.

223. **Vo Van JM, Nguyen NQ, Le Bervet JY.** [A fatal gas embolism during a hysteroscopy-curettage]. *Cah Anesthesiol* 1992;40:617–618.

224. **Perlitz Y, Oettinger M, Karam K, et al.** Anaphylactic shock during hysteroscopy using *Hyskon* solution: case report and review of adverse reactions and their treatment. *Gynecol Obstet Invest* 1996;41:67–69.

225. **Ellingson TL, Aboulafia DM.** *Dextran* syndrome. Acute hypotension, noncardiogenic pulmonary edema, anemia, and coagulopathy following hysteroscopic surgery using 32% *dextran 70. Chest* 1997;111:513–518.

226. **Choban MJ, Kalhan SB, Anderson RJ, et al.** Pulmonary edema and coagulopathy following intrauterine instillation of 32% *dextran-70 (Hyskon). J Clin Anesth* 1991;3:317–319.

227. **Golan A, Siedner M, Bahar M, et al.** High-output left ventricular failure after dextran use in an operative hysteroscopy. *Fertil Steril* 1990;54:939–941.

228. **Loffer FD, Bradley LD, Brill AI, et al.** Hysteroscopic fluid monitoring guidelines. The ad hoc committee on hysteroscopic training guidelines of the American Association of Gynecologic Laparoscopists. *J Am Assoc Gynecol Laparosc* 2000;7:167–168.

229. **Phillips DR, Nathanson HG, Milim SJ, et al.** The effect of dilute *vasopressin* solution on blood loss during operative hysteroscopy: a randomized controlled trial. *Obstet Gynecol* 1996;88:761–766.

230. **Istre O.** Fluid balance during hysteroscopic surgery. *Curr Opin Obstet Gynecol* 1997;9:219–225.

24 Hysterectomy

Tommaso Falcone
Thomas G. Stovall

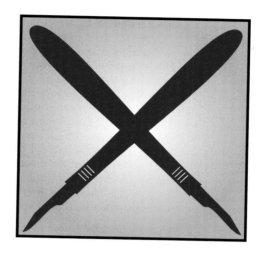

- **Hysterectomy is one of the most commonly performed surgical procedures in the United States.**

- **Vaginal hysterectomy is the procedure of choice in parous women unless this route is contraindicated.**

- **Laparoscopic hysterectomy is associated with faster postoperative recovery and shorter hospital stay compared with abdominal hysterectomy.**

- **There are no randomized clinical trials demonstrating an advantage of robotic or single-port hysterectomy over conventional laparoscopic hysterectomy.**

- **There appears to be no advantage to the routine use of supracervical hysterectomy when compared with total hysterectomy.**

- **Salpingo-oophorectomy at the time of hysterectomy for benign disease in premenopausal women at average risk for ovarian malignancy is associated with an increase in long-term patient mortality from cardiovascular disease, and ovarian conservation should be strongly considered in these patients.**

Hysterectomy is one of the most common surgical procedures performed. After cesarean delivery, it is the second most frequently performed major surgical procedure in the United States (1). According to the National Hospital Discharge survey, the rate of hysterectomy during the 5-year study period was 5.4 per 1,000 women per year in 2000 and declined to 5.1 per 1,000 per year in 2004. These data do not represent hysterectomies performed in ambulatory settings. **The highest rate of hysterectomy is between the ages of 40 and 49 years with an average age of 46.1 years** (1). The highest rates of hysterectomy are for women living in the southern United States and they occur at a younger age. The lowest rates are consistently in the northeastern portion of the United States. Lower socioeconomic status is associated with increased hysterectomy rates (2). Hysterectomy rates are higher for black women (3). Reports on the effect of physician gender conflict with data that shows no overall impact (4). Bilateral salpingo-oophorectomy decreased between 2000 and 2004 from 53.8% to 49.5% (1). The frequency was the highest with abdominal hysterectomy and the lowest with vaginal hysterectomy.

Indications

The indications for hysterectomy are listed in Table 24.1. **Uterine leiomyomas are consistently the leading indication for hysterectomy. As expected, the indications differ with the patient's age** (1). Hospitalization rates for hysterectomy in women between the ages of 15 and 54 years decreased from 1998 to 2005 for all indications except for menstrual disorders (5).

Leiomyomas

The proportion of hysterectomies performed for leiomyomas decreased over time (1) (see Chapter 15). Fertility-preserving surgical management (myomectomy) is possible in most patients with leiomyomas. **The decision to perform a hysterectomy for leiomyomas is usually based on the need to treat symptoms**—abnormal uterine bleeding, pelvic pain, or pelvic pressure. Other indications for intervention have included "rapid" uterine enlargement, ureteral compression, or uterine growth after menopause. There is no clearly reproducible definition of rapid growth. **The concept of rapid growth was challenged because these patients did not demonstrate clearly malignant conditions** (6). Refuted reasons for hysterectomy in patients with leiomyomas are size greater than 12 weeks of gestation without symptoms, inability to palpate the ovaries on bimanual examination, and increased morbidity at hysterectomy with increased uterine size. If the procedures are performed abdominally, there is no difference in surgical morbidity between patients with a 12-week-sized uterus and those with a 20-week-sized uterus (7). **Therefore, hysterectomy for leiomyomas should be considered only in symptomatic patients who do not desire future fertility** (7).

To reduce uterine size before hysterectomy, patients with large leiomyomas may be pretreated with a gonadotropin-releasing hormone (GnRH) agonist (8,9). In many cases, the reduction of uterine size is sufficient to permit vaginal hysterectomy when an abdominal hysterectomy would otherwise be necessary. In one prospective trial, premenopausal patients with leiomyomas the size of 14 to 18 weeks' gestation were randomized to receive either 2 months of preoperative depot GnRH agonist or no GnRH agonist (8). Treatment with a short course (8 weeks) of *leuprolide acetate* before surgery enabled the procedures to be converted safely from an abdominal hysterectomy to a vaginal hysterectomy (9). This preoperative regimen was associated with a rise in hematocrit before surgery and a shorter hospital stay and convalescent period because patients were more likely to have a vaginal rather than an abdominal hysterectomy.

Dysfunctional Uterine Bleeding

Excessive uterine bleeding is the indication for about 20% of hysterectomies. Dysfunctional uterine bleeding assumes abnormal bleeding without an obvious anatomic cause (see Chapter 14). **Anovulatory uterine bleeding is typically associated with polycystic ovary syndrome (PCOS), a condition in which anovulatory cycles are common.** The bleeding can be controlled by medical intervention with *progestin, estrogen,* or a combination of *progestin* and *estrogen* given as oral contraceptives. Ovulatory abnormal uterine bleeding can be controlled by nonsteroidal anti-inflammatory agents, hormonal intervention, *tranexamic acid,* or the *levonorgestrel* intrauterine device. In these patients, endometrial sampling should be performed before hysterectomy (10). **Dilation and curettage is not an effective means of controlling bleeding and is not necessary before hysterectomy. Hysterectomy should be reserved for**

Table 24.1 Indications for Hysterectomy (Percentage): United States 2000–2004	
Uterine leiomyoma	40.7
Endometriosis	17.7
Other (includes cervical dysplasia and menstrual disorders)	15.2
Uterine prolapse	14.5
Cancer	9.2
Endometrial hyperplasia	2.7

From **Whiteman MK, Hillis SD, Jamieson DJ, et al.** Inpatient hysterectomy surveillance in the United States, 2000–2004. *Obstet Gynecol* 2008;34.e1–e7, with permission.

patients who do not respond to or cannot tolerate medical therapy. Alternatives to hysterectomy (e.g., endometrial ablation or resection) should be considered in selected patients because these operations may be cost-effective and have a lower morbidity rate. However, in a clinical trial that randomized endometrial ablation to hysterectomy, 29% of patients assigned to the ablation underwent hysterectomy by 60 months (11).

Intractable Dysmenorrhea

About 10% of adult women are incapacitated for up to 3 days per month as a result of dysmenorrhea (see Chapter 16) (12). **Dysmenorrhea can be treated with nonsteroidal anti-inflammatory agents used alone or in combination with oral contraceptives or other hormone agents to reduce or ablate menstrual flow** (12). The *levonorgestrel* intrauterine device effectively reduces dysmenorrhea symptoms. Hysterectomy is rarely required for the treatment of primary dysmenorrhea. In patients with secondary dysmenorrhea, the underlying condition (e.g., leiomyomas, endometriosis) should be treated primarily. **Hysterectomy should be considered only if medical therapy fails or if the patient does not want to preserve fertility** (12).

Pelvic Pain

In a review of 418 women in whom hysterectomy was performed for a variety of nonmalignant conditions, 18% had chronic pelvic pain. Preoperative laparoscopy was performed in only 66% of these patients. After hysterectomy, there was a significant reduction in symptoms that was associated with an improvement in the patient's quality of life (13). In a review of 104 patients who underwent hysterectomy for chronic pelvic pain that was believed to be of uterine origin, 78% experienced improvement in their pain after follow-up for a mean of 21.6 months (14). However, 22% of patients had no improvement in or exacerbation of their pain. **Hysterectomy should be performed only in those patients whose pain is of gynecologic origin and does not respond to nonsurgical treatments** (12) (see Chapter 16).

Cervical Intraepithelial Neoplasia

In the past, hysterectomy was performed as primary treatment of cervical intraepithelial neoplasia. **More conservative treatments, such as laser or loop electrosurgical excision procedure (LEEP), can be effective in treating the disease, making hysterectomy unnecessary in most women with these conditions** (see Chapter 19). For patients with recurrent high-grade dysplasia who do not desire to preserve fertility, hysterectomy may be an appropriate treatment option. After hysterectomy, these patients are at increased risk for vaginal intraepithelial neoplasia.

Genital Prolapse

Hysterectomy for symptomatic genital prolapse accounts for about 14.5% of hysterectomies performed in the United States (1). **Unless there is an associated condition requiring an abdominal incision, vaginal hysterectomy is the preferred approach for genital prolapse.** Uterine prolapse typically is not an isolated event and most often is associated with a variety of pelvic support defects. Each defect must be corrected to optimize the surgical outcome and decrease the risk of developing future pelvic support defects.

Obstetric Emergency

Most emergency hysterectomies are performed because of postpartum hemorrhage resulting from uterine atony. Other indications include uterine rupture that cannot be repaired or a pelvic abscess that does not respond to medical therapy. Hysterectomy may be required for patients with placenta accreta or placenta increta.

Pelvic Inflammatory Disease

Pelvic inflammatory disease can be treated successfully with antibiotics. The uterus, tubes, and ovaries rarely need to be removed in a patient with pelvic inflammatory disease that is refractory to intravenous antibiotic therapy (see Chapter 18). Whether one proceeds with conservative surgical management, abscess drainage, or organ removal is a subjective decision that must be based on the individual. If accessible, some pelvic abscesses may be drained successfully by percutaneous catheter drainage guided by ultrasonography or computed tomography (CT) scanning. Surgical intervention is necessary if the patient has acute abdominal findings associated with peritonitis and signs of sepsis in the presence of a ruptured tubo-ovarian abscess. **For the patient who desires future fertility, consideration should be given to unilateral salpingectomy or**

salpingo-oophorectomy or bilateral salpingo-oophorectomy without hysterectomy. For the patient in whom bilateral salpingo-oophorectomy is required, the uterus can be left in place for possible ovum donation and *in vitro* fertilization.

Endometriosis

Medical and conservative surgical procedures are successful for treatment of endometriosis (15). **Bilateral salpingo-oophorectomy, with or without hysterectomy, should be performed only in patients who do not respond to conservative surgical (resection or ablation of endometriotic implants) or medical therapy** (see Chapter 17). Most patients with endometriosis who require hysterectomy have unrelenting pelvic pain or dysmenorrhea. Other less common situations include patients who do not desire future fertility and who have endometriosis involving other pelvic organs, such as the ureter or colon. Hysterectomy with or without salpingo-oophorectomy provides significant pain relief to the majority of patients. At the time of hysterectomy for endometriosis, consideration should be given to conserving normal ovaries (16).

Pelvic Mass or Benign Ovarian Tumor

If a pelvic mass is palpated on pelvic examination, a transvaginal ultrasound should be performed (see Chapter 14). If the mass is suspicious, appropriate consultation with a gynecologic oncologist is recommended. Benign ovarian tumors that are persistent or symptomatic require surgical treatment. If the patient desires fertility, the uterus should be conserved. If fertility is not an issue or if the patient is perimenopausal or postmenopausal, a decision must be made regarding whether the uterus should be removed. In one study, 100 patients who underwent bilateral salpingo-oophorectomy plus hysterectomy for benign adnexal disease were compared with a group of risk-matched women who underwent bilateral salpingo-oophorectomy without hysterectomy for the same indication (17). There was a significant increase in operative morbidity, estimated blood loss, and the length of hospital stay for patients in whom hysterectomy was performed.

Preoperative Considerations

The preoperative discussion should include an informed consent that documents the options, risks, benefits, outcome, and personnel involved with the procedure. The medical record should reflect the completion of childbearing and that adequate trial of medical or nonsurgical management was offered, attempted, or refused.

Health Assessment

An assessment of a patient's health status is important in order to obtain an optimal outcome after hysterectomy for benign disease. There are no routinely recommended tests, although individual hospitals may have their own requirements. The patient should be evaluated for risk factors associated with venous thromboembolic events (18). Age, medical history, such as inherited or acquired thrombophilias, obesity, smoking, and hormonal medication, including contraceptives or hormone therapy, may increase the risk.

It is important to assess and correct underlying anemias before surgery. Blood product use can be minimized with preoperative iron supplementation or use of GnRH agonists.

Hysterectomy versus Supracervical Hysterectomy

There is a trend toward retention of the cervix at hysterectomy because of the perception that several outcome parameters, including sexual function and pelvic support, are better after a supracervical hysterectomy. Three prospective randomized clinical trials as summarized in a Cochrane review challenge this perception (19). There was no evidence to support the concept that leaving the cervix improves sexual function or lower rates of incontinence or constipation. All of these studies included hysterectomies that were performed by laparotomy. Surgical time was decreased by approximately 11 minutes.

This decreased surgical time may be more significant for laparoscopic cases, as the most difficult part of the surgery is the detachment of the cervix from the lateral ligaments and from the vagina. This is where most ureteral injuries occur during laparoscopic hysterectomy. This advantage should be balanced with the potential risk of ongoing cyclic bleeding from the cervix that is reportedly between 5% to 20% from the randomized clinical trials and 19% from a prospective observational laparoscopic trial (20). With conservation of the cervix, the patient should be told there is a potential 1% to 2% risk for reoperation to remove the cervix and that trachelectomy is associated with a risk of intraoperative complications. Patients with suspected gynecologic cancers or cervical dysplasia are not candidates for supracervical hysterectomy.

Prophylactic Salpingo-oophorectomy

The decision to remove the ovaries and tubes should be based on assessment of risk and not the route of hysterectomy (21). **Premenopausal women who are at average risk of ovarian cancer (approximate lifetime risk of 1.4%) should be considered for ovarian preservation when they are undergoing hysterectomy for benign conditions where the ovaries and fallopian tubes are healthy** (22). Parous women who have used oral contraceptives may have a substantially lower risk (22). Elective removal of the ovaries and fallopian tubes has declined since 2002 (23).

Salpingo-oophorectomy is performed prophylactically to prevent ovarian cancer and to eliminate the potential for further surgery for either benign or malignant disease. Arguments against prophylactic salpingo-oophorectomy center on the need for earlier and more prolonged hormone therapy and the potential increase risk of cardiovascular disease and bone loss (24,25). There is no overall survival benefit of prophylactic salpingo-oophorectomy in women at average risk for ovarian cancer. **In premenopausal women before age 50 years at average risk for ovarian cancer who underwent bilateral salpingo-oophorectomy, there was a significant increase in mortality from cardiovascular disease compared to women who had ovarian preservation** (25). A Markov decision analysis model was used to estimate the best strategy for maximizing a woman's survival when salpingo-oophorectomy is considered in women at average risk for ovarian cancer who are undergoing hysterectomy for benign disease, and in the **women who had salpingo-oophorectomy before age 55 years, there was an 8.58% excess mortality by age 80** (26). **Both the American College of Obstetricians and Gynecologists and the Society of Gynecologic Oncologists recommend carefully assessing risk, and consideration should be given to conservation of the ovaries in premenopausal women who are at average risk of ovarian cancer** (21,22).

Although *estrogen* therapy is well tolerated and provides good short-term symptomatic relief, recent publications demonstrate that the increased risk of breast cancer in women taking estrogen after hysterectomy makes women reluctant to use it, and long-term compliance with posthysterectomy *estrogen* therapy is low (27).

In women at risk for ovarian or breast cancer, a formal evaluation with genetic counseling should be offered (see Chapter 37). Salpingo-oophorectomy is associated with a reduced risk of ovarian and breast cancer. **Women with a strong family history of ovarian and breast cancer and those who carry germline mutations, BRCA1 or BRCA2 should undergo risk-reducing salpingo-oophorectomy as their lifetime risk is between 10% and 50%** (21,22,28,29).

Based on the finding that many serous carcinomas arise in the fallopian tube rather than in the ovary, it was proposed that bilateral salpingectomy with ovarian conservation should be performed in patients with these high penetrance germline mutations while awaiting more definitive surgical intervention (30,31). One could consider this in women at average risk for these tumors when they undergo hysterectomy for benign disease. It is unknown whether this would substantially decrease the risk of developing these malignancies.

Although salpingo-oophorectomy can be accomplished by laparoscopy or laparotomy in virtually 100% of cases, the success rate for vaginal hysterectomy ranges from 65% to 95% for experienced vaginal surgeons (32,33).

Concurrent Surgical Procedures

Appendectomy

Appendectomy may be performed concurrently with hysterectomy to prevent appendicitis and to remove disease that may be present. The former use is of limited value because the peak incidence of appendicitis is between 20 and 40 years of age, whereas the peak age for hysterectomy is 10 to 20 years later (34). **There is no increase in morbidity associated with appendectomy performed at the time of hysterectomy** (35). Incidental appendectomies in all abdominal hysterectomies could reduce the morbidity of appendicitis at a later time (35).

Appendectomy is performed with vaginal hysterectomy without additional intraoperative or postoperative morbidity (36).

Cholecystectomy

Gallbladder disease is about four times more common in women than men, and its highest incidence occurs between 50 and 70 years of age, when hysterectomy is most often performed. Women may require both procedures. A combined procedure does not appear to result in increased febrile morbidity or length of hospital stay (37).

Abdominoplasty

Abdominoplasty performed at the time of hysterectomy is associated with a shorter hospital stay, a shorter operating time, and a lower intraoperative blood loss than when the two operations are performed separately (38,39). Liposuction can be performed safely at the time of vaginal hysterectomy (40).

Choice of Surgical Access: Vaginal, Abdominal, or Laparoscopic Hysterectomy

From 2000 to 2004, approximately 68% of all hysterectomies were performed abdominally and 32% were performed vaginally. One-third of the vaginal cases were performed with the assistance of the laparoscope (laparoscopically assisted vaginal hysterectomy) (1). There are no specific criteria that can be used to determine the route of hysterectomy. The route chosen should be based on the individual patient, but vaginal access is preferred. An alternative access is preferred if there is a narrow pubic arch (less than 90 degrees), and a narrow vagina (narrower than two fingerbreadths, especially at the apex), or if the there is an undescended immobile uterus. The presence of an adnexal mass, cul-de-sac disease, pelvic adhesions, or the assessment of chronic pain may require the addition of laparoscopy for assessment. A previous cesarean section or nulliparity does not contraindicate a vaginal approach (41).

A Cochrane review validated the perception that vaginal hysterectomy is the surgical route of choice for hysterectomy (42). This review included 3,643 patients from 27 randomized trials. It compared abdominal hysterectomy with vaginal hysterectomy and three types of laparoscopic hysterectomies. The main observations were the shorter length of hospital stay, faster postoperative recovery, and decreased febrile morbidity of vaginal and laparoscopic hysterectomy compared with abdominal hysterectomy. **The report concludes that there are improved outcomes with vaginal hysterectomy, and, when vaginal access is not possible, laparoscopic hysterectomy appears to have advantages over abdominal hysterectomy.** Cost-analysis trials demonstrate that laparoscopic hysterectomy can be cost-effective relative to abdominal procedure but not compared with vaginal hysterectomy (43,44). The main cost determinants are the length of hospital stay and the use of disposable surgical devices.

Risk of complication from each type of procedure provides insight into the proper options for the patient. The eVALuate study comprised two parallel randomized multicenter trials, with one comparing laparoscopic with abdominal hysterectomy and the other comparing laparoscopic with vaginal hysterectomy for nonmalignant disease (45). Patients with a uterine mass less than 12-week pregnancy were included. The primary end points were assessment of complications. A total of 1,380 patients were recruited. The trial included conversion to laparotomy for the laparoscopic and vaginal groups as a major complication. If you include conversion to laparotomy as a major complication, the number needed to treat to harm would be 20 for the laparoscopic group. If you exclude conversion to laparotomy as a complication, then the complication rates are similar between all groups. All six ureter injuries reported in this series occurred in the laparoscopic group. The overall lower urinary tract complication rate is three times higher with the laparoscopic group compared with vaginal or abdominal procedures. A minor complication, mostly postoperative fever or infection, occurred in approximately 25% of each group.

Perioperative Checklist

It is important to systematically go through a checklist of perioperative measures to effectively reduce potential complications (Table 24.2). If excessive blood loss is expected, intraoperative blood salvage techniques should be considered. All patients undergoing hysterectomy for benign disorders are at moderate risk for venous thromboembolism and require prophylaxis (18). Unfractionated *heparin* (5,000 U every 12 hours) or low molecular weight *heparin* (e.g.,

Table 24.2 Perioperative Checklist
1. Is the informed consent signed?
2. Is there a recent Pap test documented in the chart?
3. Has pregnancy been ruled out?
4. Are blood products available if needed?
5. Will prophylactic antibiotics be initiated within 1 hour of incision?
6. Was the appropriate antibiotic selected according to American College of Obstetricians and Gynecologists guidelines?
7. Was the appropriate prophylaxis for venous thromboembolic events chosen?
8. Document that prophylactic antibiotics will be discontinued within 24 hours after surgery.

Enoxaparin, 40 mg) or intermittent pneumatic compression device is recommended. Patients on oral contraceptives up to the time of hysterectomy should be considered for pharmacologic treatment. Mechanical bowel preparation for prevention of infection complications from bowel injury is no longer recommended (46).

Technique

Abdominal Hysterectomy

General Preparation

To reduce the colony count of skin bacteria, the patient is asked to shower. Hair surrounding the incision area may be removed at the time of surgery or before surgery using a depilatory agent. Hair clipping is preferable to shaving because it decreases the incidence of incisional infection, and if shaving is done, it should be performed in the operating room just prior to the surgery (34).

Patient Positioning   For most abdominal cases, the patient is placed in the dorsal supine position for the operation. After the patient is anesthetized adequately, her legs are placed in the stirrups and a pelvic examination is performed to validate the in-office pelvic examination findings. A Foley catheter is placed in the bladder, and the vagina is cleansed with an iodine solution. The patient's legs are straightened.

Skin Preparation   Several methods for skin cleaning can be recommended, including a 5-minute iodine solution scrub followed by application of iodine solution, iodine solution scrub followed by alcohol with application of an iodine-impregnated occlusive drape, or an iodine-alcohol combination with or without application of an iodine-impregnated occlusive drape. *Chlorhexidine*-alcohol solutions are also used for abdominal preparations. Povidone-iodine solution is FDA approved for vaginal use, and *chlorhexidine gluconate* can be used in the vagina of patients who are iodine allergic.

Surgical Technique

Incision   **The choice of incision should be determined by the following considerations:**

1. Simplicity of the incision
2. Need for exposure
3. Potential need for enlarging the incision
4. Strength of the healed wound
5. Cosmesis of the healed incision
6. Location of previous surgical scars

The skin is opened with a scalpel, and the incision is carried down through the subcutaneous tissue and fascia. With traction applied to the lateral edges of the incision, the fascia is divided.

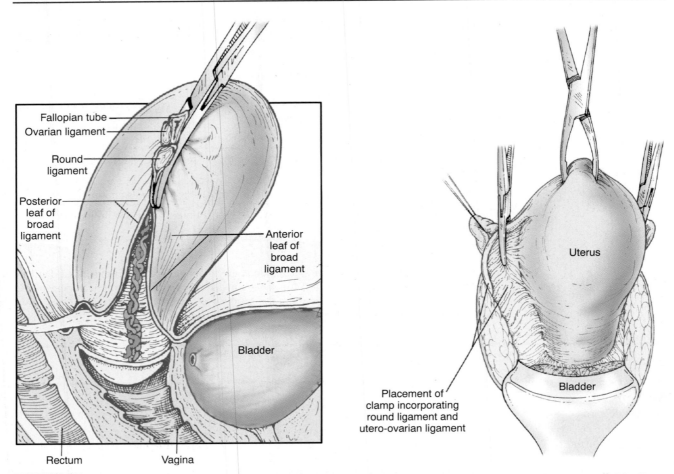

Figure 24.1   **The uterus is elevated by placement of clamps across the broad ligament.** (From **Mann WA, Stovall TG.** *Gynecologic surgery.* New York: Churchill Livingstone, 1996, with permission.)

The peritoneum is opened similarly. This technique minimizes the possibility of inadvertent enterotomy, entering the abdominal cavity.

Abdominal Exploration   Cytologic sampling of the peritoneal cavity, if needed, should be performed before abdominal exploration. The upper abdomen and the pelvis are explored systematically. The liver, gallbladder, stomach, kidneys, para-aortic lymph nodes, and large and small bowel should be examined and palpated.

Retractor Choice and Placement   A variety of retractors were designed for pelvic surgery. The Balfour and the O'Connor-O'Sullivan retractors are used most often. The Bookwalter retractor has a variety of adjustable blades that can be helpful, particularly in obese patients.

Elevation of the Uterus   The uterus is elevated by placing broad ligament clamps at each cornu so that it crosses the round ligament. The clamp tip may be placed close to the internal os. This placement provides uterine traction and prevents back bleeding (Fig. 24.1).

Round Ligament Ligation or Transection   The uterus is deviated to the patient's left side, stretching the right round ligament. With the proximal portion held by the broad ligament clamp, the distal portion of the round ligament is ligated with a suture ligature or simply transected with Bovie cautery (Fig. 24.2). The distal portion can be grasped with forceps, and the round ligament is cut to separate the anterior and posterior leaves of the broad ligament. The anterior leaf of the broad ligament is incised with Metzenbaum scissors or electrocautery along the vesicouterine fold, separating the peritoneal reflection of the bladder from the lower uterine segment (Fig. 24.3).

Ureter Identification   **The retroperitoneum is entered by extending the incision cephalad on the posterior leaf of the broad ligament.** Care must be taken to remain lateral to both the infundibulopelvic ligament and iliac vessels. The external iliac artery courses along the

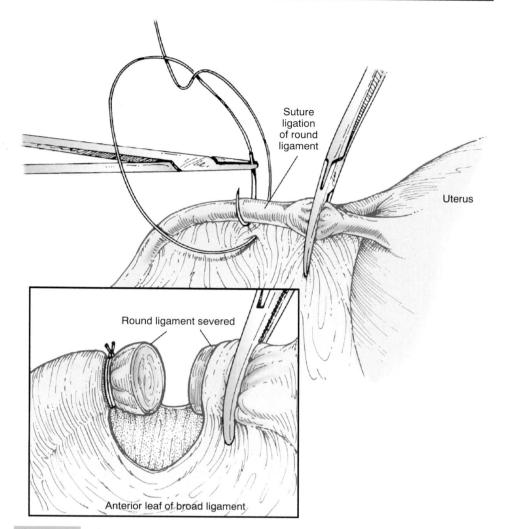

Suture
ligation
of round
ligament

Uterus

Round ligament severed

Anterior leaf of broad ligament

Figure 24.2 **The round ligament is transected and the broad ligament is incised and opened.** (From **Mann WA, Stovall TG.** *Gynecologic surgery.* New York: Churchill Livingstone, 1996, with permission.)

medial aspect of the psoas muscle and is identified by bluntly dissecting the loose alveolar tissue overlying it. **By following the artery cephalad to the bifurcation of the common iliac artery, the ureter is identified crossing the common iliac artery. The ureter should be left attached to the medial leaf of the broad ligament to protect its blood supply** (Fig. 24.4).

Utero-ovarian Vessel and Ovarian Vessel (Infundibulopelvic Ligament) Ligation If the ovaries are to be preserved, the uterus is retracted toward the pubic symphysis and deviated to one side, placing tension on the contralateral ovarian vessels (the so-called infundibulopelvic ligament), the tube, and the ovary. **With the ureter under direct visualization, a window is created in the peritoneum of the posterior leaf of the broad ligament under the utero-ovarian ligament and fallopian tube.** The tube and utero-ovarian ligament are clamped on each side with a curved Heaney or Ballantine clamp, cut, and ligated with both a free-tie and a suture ligature. The medial clamp at the uterine cornu should control back bleeding; if it does not, the clamp should be repositioned to do so (Fig. 24.5).

If the ovaries are to be removed, the peritoneal opening is enlarged and extended cephalad to the ovarian vessels (infundibulopelvic ligament) and caudad to the uterine artery. This opening allows proper exposure of the uterine artery, the ovarian vessels, and the ureter. In this manner, the ureter is released from its proximity to the uterine vessels and uterine vessels.

A curved Heaney or Ballantine clamp is placed lateral to the ovary (Fig. 24.6); care is taken to ensure that the entire ovary is included in the surgical specimen. The uterine vessels on each side

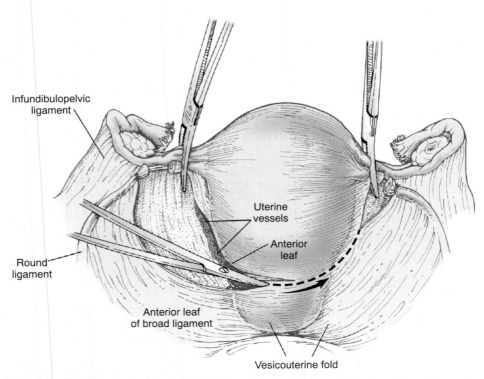

Figure 24.3 The incision in the anterior broad ligament is extended along the vesicouterine fold. (From **Mann WA, Stovall TG.** *Gynecologic surgery.* New York: Churchill Livingstone, 1996, with permission.)

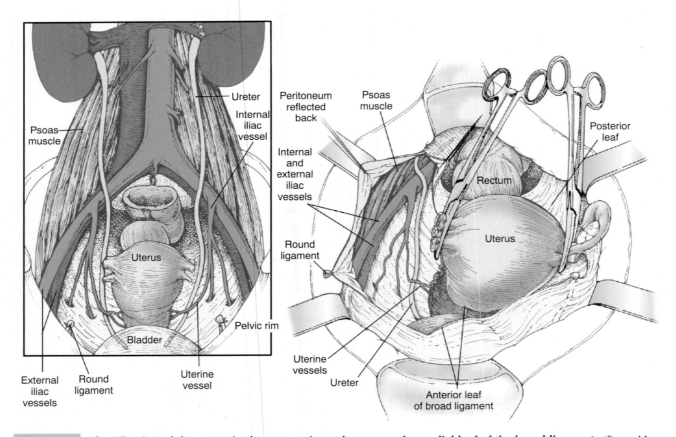

Figure 24.4 Identification of the ureter in the retroperitoneal space on the medial leaf of the broad ligament. (From **Mann WA, Stovall TG.** *Gynecologic surgery.* New York: Churchill Livingstone, 1996, with permission.)

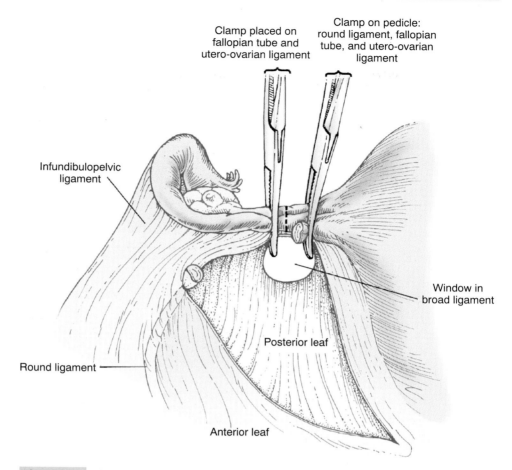

Figure 24.5 Ligation of the utero-ovarian ligament. (From **Mann WA, Stovall TG.** *Gynecologic surgery.* New York: Churchill Livingstone, 1996, with permission.)

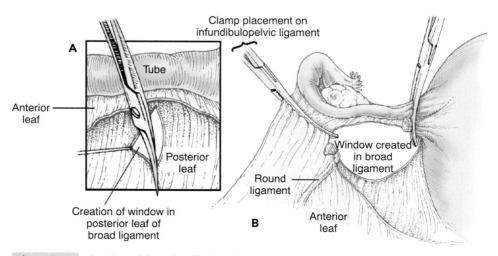

Figure 24.6 Ligation of the infundibulopelvic ligament. (From **Mann WA, Stovall TG.** *Gynecologic surgery.* New York: Churchill Livingstone, 1996, with permission.)

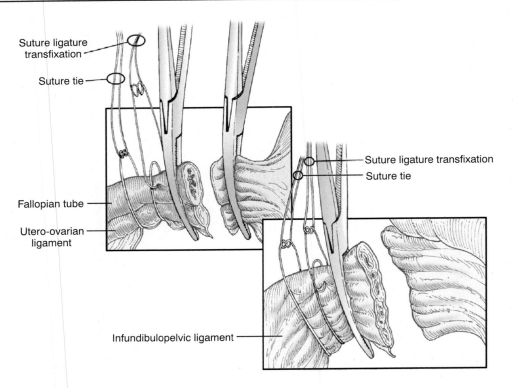

Suture ligature transfixation

Suture tie

Suture ligature transfixation

Suture tie

Fallopian tube

Utero-ovarian ligament

Infundibulopelvic ligament

Figure 24.7   Transection of the infundibulopelvic ligament. (From **Mann WA, Stovall TG.** *Gynecologic surgery.* New York: Churchill Livingstone, 1996, with permission.)

are doubly ligated and cut (Fig. 24.7). Alternatively, free ties can be passed around the uterine vessels, two cephalad and one caudad, before they are cut.

Bladder Mobilization   Using Metzenbaum scissors or Bovie, the bladder is dissected from the lower uterine segment and cervix. An avascular plane, which exists between the lower uterine segment and the bladder, allows for this mobilization. Tonsil clamps may be placed on the bladder edge to provide countertraction and easier dissection (Fig. 24.8).

Uterine Vessel Ligation   The uterus is retracted cephalad and deviated to one side of the pelvis, stretching the lower ligaments. The uterine vasculature is dissected or "skeletonized" from any remaining areolar tissue, and a curved Zeppelin or Heaney clamp is placed perpendicular to the uterine artery at the junction of the cervix and body of the uterus. Care is taken to place the tip of the clamp adjacent to the uterus at this anatomic narrowing. The vessels are cut, and the pedicle is ligated. The same procedure is repeated on the opposite side (Fig. 24.9).

Incision of Posterior Peritoneum   If the rectum is to be mobilized from the posterior cervix, the posterior peritoneum between the uterosacral ligaments just beneath the cervix and rectum may be incised (Fig. 24.10). A relatively avascular tissue plane exists in this area, allowing mobilization of the rectum inferiorly out of the operative field.

Cardinal Ligament Ligation   The cardinal ligament is divided by placing a straight Zeppelin or Heaney clamp medial to the uterine vessel pedicle for a distance of 2 to 3 cm parallel to the uterus. The ligament is cut, and the pedicle is suture ligated. This step is repeated on each side until the junction of the cervix and vagina is reached (Fig. 24.11).

Removal of the Uterus   The uterus is placed on traction cephalad, and the tip of the cervix is palpated. Curved Heaney clamps are placed bilaterally, incorporating the uterosacral ligament and upper vagina just below the cervix. **Care should be taken to avoid foreshortening the vagina.** The uterus is then removed with scalpel or curved scissors (Fig. 24.12).

Vaginal Cuff Closure   A figure-of-eight suture of 0 braided absorbable material is placed at the angle of the vagina for both traction and hemostasis. The pedicles are sutured with a Heaney

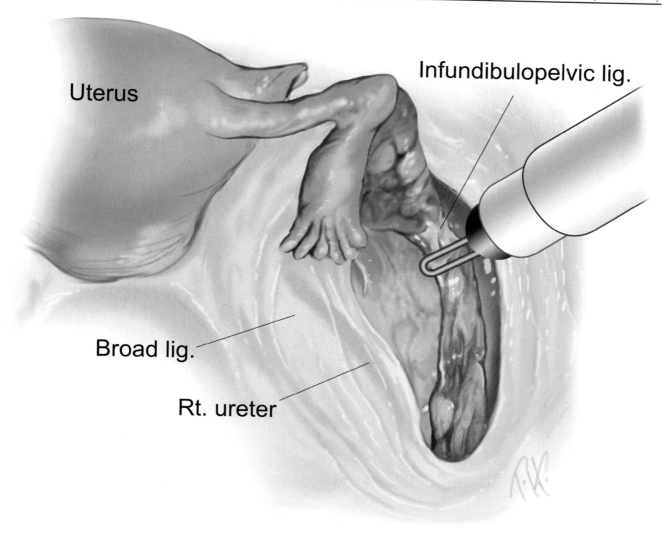

Figure 24.8 **Dissection of the vesicouterine plane to mobilize the bladder.** (From **Mann WA, Stovall TG.** *Gynecologic surgery.* New York: Churchill Livingstone, 1996, with permission.)

stitch, incorporating the uterosacral and cardinal ligament at the angle of the vagina (Fig. 24.13). A running-locked suture can be used for hemostasis along the cuff edge (Fig. 24.14).

Irrigation and Hemostasis   The pelvis is thoroughly irrigated with saline. Meticulous hemostasis in the pelvis, particularly of the vascular pedicles, should be ensured. Ureteral position and integrity are checked to ensure that they are intact and do not appear dilated.

Peritoneal Closure   The pelvic peritoneum is not reapproximated. Research using animal models suggests that reapproximation may increase tissue trauma and promote adhesion formation (47).

Fascia Closure   The parietal peritoneum is not reapproximated as a separate layer. Fascia can be closed with an interrupted or continuous 0 or 1 monofilament absorbable suture. A prospective randomized trial did not show any advantage of interrupted versus continuous fascial closure (48). Bites should be taken about 1 cm from the cut edge of the fascia and about 1 cm apart to prevent wound dehiscence.

Skin Closure   The subcutaneous tissue should be irrigated, with careful hemostasis. Wound disruption seems to be decreased with closure of the subcutaneous fat layer in women with 2 cm or more fat (49). Skin staples or subcuticular sutures are used to reapproximate the skin edges. A dressing is applied and left in place for about 24 hours.

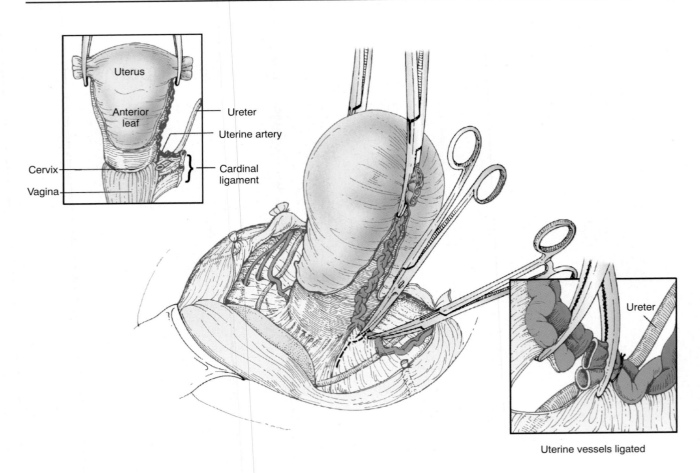

Figure 24.9   Ligation of the uterine blood vessels. (From **Mann WA, Stovall TG.** *Gynecologic surgery.* New York: Churchill Livingstone, 1996, with permission.)

Intraoperative Complications

Every surgeon must be prepared to recognize and repair operative injuries, because despite a high level of attention to detail, injuries and complications, recognized and unrecognized, can still occur.

Ureteral Injuries

Injury to the pelvic ureter is one of the most formidable complications of hysterectomy (50). It is always essential to be aware of the proximity of the ureter to the other pelvic structures. **Most ureteral injuries can be avoided by opening the retroperitoneum and directly identifying the ureter.** The use of ureteral catheters as a substitute for direct visualization is often of little help in patients with extensive fibrosis or scarring resulting from endometriosis, pelvic inflammatory disease, or ovarian cancer. In these instances, a false sense of security may increase an already high risk for ureteral injury. The use of ureteral catheters are associated with hematuria and acute urinary retention, although their complications are usually transitory in nature.

Direct visualization is accomplished by opening the retroperitoneum lateral to the external iliac artery. Blunt dissection of the loose areolar tissue is performed to visualize the artery directly. The artery may be traced cephalad to the bifurcation of the internal and external iliac arteries. The ureter crosses the common iliac artery at its bifurcation and may be followed throughout its course in the pelvis.

Despite these precautions, ureteral injuries may occur. Prompt consultation is necessary if the surgeon is not trained in ureteral repair. If a ureteral obstruction is suspected, confirmation may be obtained by intravenous injection of 1 ampule of *indigo carmine* dye and performance of

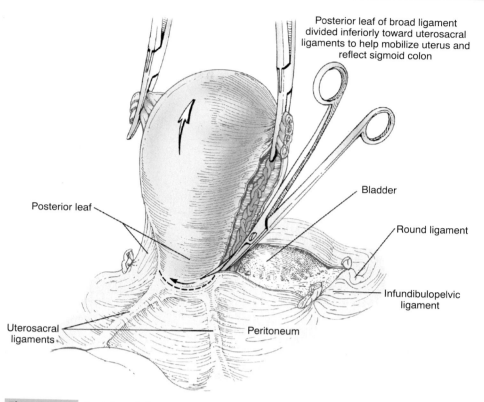

Figure 24.10   **Incision of the rectouterine peritoneum and mobilization of the rectum from the posterior cervix.**   (From **Mann WA, Stovall TG.** *Gynecologic surgery.* New York: Churchill Livingstone, 1996, with permission.)

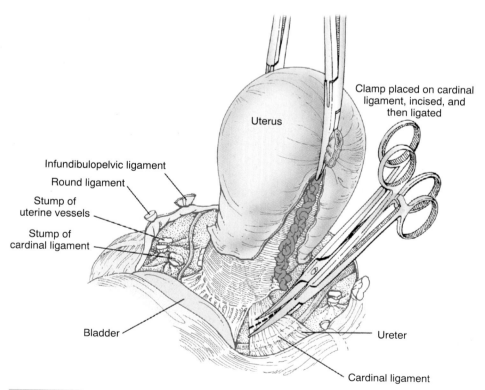

Figure 24.11   **Ligation of the cardinal ligament.**   (From **Mann WA, Stovall TG.** *Gynecologic surgery.* New York: Churchill Livingstone, 1996, with permission.)

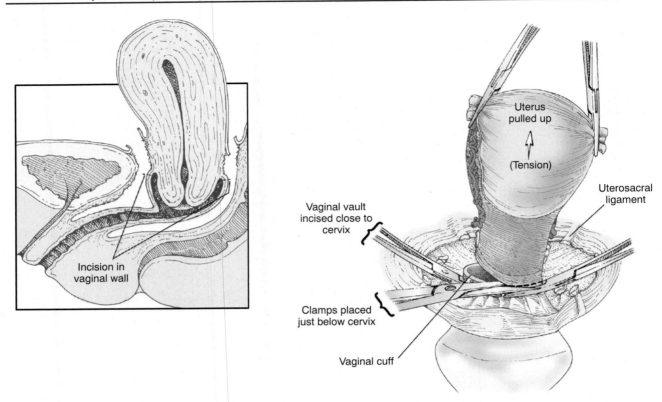

Figure 24.12 **Removal of the uterus by transection of the vagina.** (From **Mann WA, Stovall TG.** *Gynecologic surgery.* New York: Churchill Livingstone, 1996.)

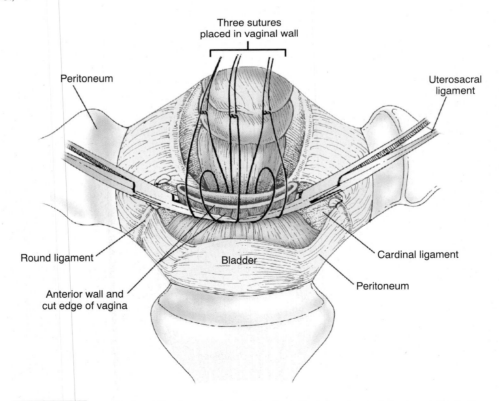

Figure 24.13 **Vaginal cuff closure incorporating the uterosacral and cardinal ligaments.** (From **Mann WA, Stovall TG.** *Gynecologic surgery.* New York: Churchill Livingstone, 1996, with permission.)

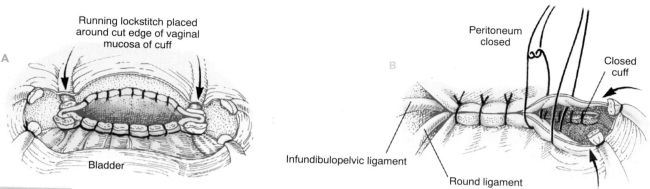

Figure 24.14   A: Vaginal cuff left open with a running suture along the cuff. B: Peritoneum closed. (From **Mann WA, Stovall TG.** *Gynecologic surgery.* New York: Churchill Livingstone, 1996, with permission.)

a cystoscopic evaluation. The integrity of the ureters should be confirmed by the presence or absence of bilateral spill of tinted urine.

Bladder Injury

Because of the close anatomic relationship of the bladder, uterus, and upper vagina, the bladder is the segment of the lower urinary tract that is most vulnerable to injury. **Bladder injury may occur on opening the peritoneum or, more frequently, during the dissection of the bladder off the cervix and upper vagina.** Unless there is involvement of the bladder trigone, a bladder laceration is easily repaired. In the nonirradiated bladder, a one- or two-layer closure with a small-caliber braided absorbable suture such as a 3-0 polyglycolic acid is adequate. The bladder should be drained postoperatively. The length of time that drainage is required is controversial. If the bladder is not compromised, drainage should be continued at least until gross hematuria clears, which may occur as soon as 48 hours postoperatively. A more conservative practice is to continue drainage for 3 to 14 days depending on the type of injury (50). Elective incision into the dome of the bladder is performed in the same manner. If the trigone is involved, a surgeon trained in complicated urologic repair should be consulted, because reimplantation of the ureter may be necessary.

Bowel Injury

Small bowel injuries are the most common intestinal injuries in gynecologic surgery. Small defects of the serosa or muscularis may be repaired using a single layer of continuous or interrupted 3-0 braided absorbable suture. Although single-layer closure of the small bowel has proved adequate, it is safer to close defects involving the lumen in two layers using a 3-0 braided absorbable suture. **The defect should be closed in a direction perpendicular to the intestinal lumen.** If a large area is injured, resection with reanastomosis may be necessary. Because the bacterial flora of the ascending colon is similar to that of the small bowel, injuries can be repaired in a similar manner. The transverse colon rarely is injured in normal gynecologic procedures because it is well outside the operative field. However, the descending colon and the rectosigmoid colon are intimately involved with the pelvic structures and are at significant risk for injury during gynecologic surgery. Injuries not involving the mucosa may be repaired with a single running layer of 2-0 or 3-0 braided absorbable suture. If the laceration involves the mucosa, it may be closed as with small bowel injuries.

Hemorrhage

Significant arterial bleeding usually arises from the uterine arteries or the ovarian vessels near the insertion of the infundibulopelvic ligaments. Blind clamping of these vessels presents a risk for ureteral injury; therefore, the ureters should be identified in the retroperitoneal space and traced to the area of bleeding to avoid inadvertent ligation. **It is best to apply a pressure pack to tamponade the bleeding and slowly remove the pack in an effort to visualize, isolate, and individually clamp the bleeding vessels.** Mass ligatures should be avoided. The use of surgical clips may be helpful. Venous bleeding is less dramatic but often is more difficult to manage, particularly in the presence of extensive adhesions and fibroids. This type of bleeding can be controlled with pressure alone or with suture ligation. Bleeding from peritoneal edges or denuded surfaces may be controlled with pressure, application of topical agents such as thrombin or collagen, or Bovie cautery. A variety of laser techniques are used to control bleeding, such as the use of the Argon beam laser.

Postoperative Management

Bladder Drainage   Overdistention of the bladder resulting from bladder trauma or the patient's reluctance to initiate the voluntary phase of voiding is one of the most common complications after abdominal hysterectomy. An indwelling bladder catheter should be used for the first few postoperative hours until the patient is able to ambulate and urinate.

If retropubic urethropexy was performed, a suprapubic catheter, which allows postvoid residual levels to be checked without repetitive catheterizations, can be considered. This catheter may be removed when satisfactory postvoid residual levels of less than 100 mL are obtained.

Diet   As soon as the patient is alert, diet is resumed, offering solid foods as tolerated with return of appetite. This dietary regimen assumes minimal intraoperative bowel manipulation and dissection. **Early postoperative feeding was shown to be safe and to speed return of bowel function and recovery.** In patients who had pelvic and para-aortic lymphadenectomy, bowel surgery, or other extensive dissections, a slower return to normal bowel function may occur, so the diet is administered as tolerated when the patient's appetite returns.

Activity   **Early ambulation decreases the incidence of thrombophlebitis and pneumonia.** Patients are encouraged to begin ambulation on their first postoperative day if possible and to increase their time out of bed progressively as their strength improves. **On discharge, the patient is instructed to avoid lifting more than 20 pounds for 6 weeks, thereby minimizing stress on fascia to allow full healing. Sexual intercourse is not recommended until at least 6 weeks after surgery, when the vaginal cuff is fully healed.** Patients are instructed to avoid driving until full mobility returns because postoperative pain and tenderness may hinder sudden braking or steering maneuvers in emergency situations. With these exceptions, the patient is encouraged to return to normal activities as soon as she feels comfortable doing so.

Wound Care   The abdominal incision normally requires little attention, except for ordinary hygienic measures. The wound is kept covered with a sterile dressing for the first 24 hours after surgery, by which time the incision has sealed. After the dressing is removed, the incision should be cleaned daily with mild soap and water and kept dry.

Vaginal Hysterectomy

Preoperative Evaluation

Evaluation of Pelvic Support   The most important observation in determining the feasibility of a vaginal hysterectomy is the demonstration of uterine mobility (51). A vaginal approach should be chosen only if the uterus is freely mobile. Pelvic support structures are elevated at the initial pelvic examination. In patients with no apparent prolapse, poor pelvic support can often be demonstrated by observing descent of the uterus with a series of Valsalva maneuvers. Although vaginal hysterectomy is easier to perform when the uterine supporting ligaments are lax, it is not an absolute requirement. T**he practice of applying traction to the cervix with a tenaculum to demonstrate descent of an apparently well-supported uterus is not recommended.** Some gynecologists advocate the application of a tenaculum to the anterior cervical lip, with subsequent traction applied as the patient bears down. This exercise may give some indication of uterine mobility, but it is uncomfortable and not necessarily predictive of the success of vaginal hysterectomy.

Evaluation of the Pelvis   After assessment of pelvic support, the bony pelvis should be evaluated. Ideally, the angle of the pubic arch should be 90 degrees or greater, the vaginal canal should be ample, and the posterior vaginal fornix should be wide and deep. The surgeon may use a closed fist to approximate the bituberous diameter, which should exceed 10 cm. The size and shape of the female pelvis contributes to increased exposure. The importance of a wide pubic arch was underscored by the result of a study of 25 failed vaginal hysterectomies that were compared with 50 successful vaginal hysterectomies. Risk factors, such as age, parity, body weight, surgical indication, uterine size, presence of leiomyomata in the anterior lower uterine segment, previous pelvic surgeries, adhesions, location and length of the cervix, and narrow pubic arch (less than 90 degrees), were examined. In the study, only the presence of a narrow pubic arch increased the risk of vaginal hysterectomy (52).

Surgical Considerations

Patient Positioning   When the patient is in the dorsal lithotomy position, the buttocks should be positioned just over the table's edge. Several stirrup types are available, including those that support the entire leg and those that suspend the legs in straps. **To avoid nerve injury, adequate padding should be used; marked flexion of the thigh and pressure points should be avoided.** Trendelenburg (10- to 15-degree) positioning aids in the intravaginal visualization needed during surgery.

Vaginal Preparation   A povidone-iodine solution or chlorhexideine-alcohol is applied to the vagina, the bladder is drained, and the catheter is removed. Several methods for draping are proposed, including individual or single-piece drapes; the method chosen is at the surgeon's discretion. There is usually no need to shave or clip the pubic hair. Individual drapes with an adhesive barrier should be used to hold them in place and prevent the pubic hair from compromising the field.

Instruments   Instruments specific to and useful in performing a vaginal hysterectomy include right-angled retractors, narrow Deaver retractors, weighted specula, Heaney needle holders, and an assortment of Breisky–Navratil vaginal retractors. Heaney and Heaney–Ballantine hysterectomy clamps are preferable. Several other clamps are commonly used, including the Masterson clamp.

Lighting   Overhead high-intensity lamps should be used and positioned to direct light over the operator's shoulder. The surgeon may use a headlight, which can be worn to provide direct horizontal lighting. A fiberoptic-lighted irrigating suction system can provide additional light and transilluminate tissue planes.

Suture Material   Various suture materials are advocated for gynecologic surgery. The type of suture material chosen is based on the surgeon's preference. A synthetic delayed absorbable polyglactin or polyglycolic acid suture and atraumatic needles are preferable.

Procedure

The patient is examined while anesthetized to confirm prior findings and to assess uterine mobility and descent. The decision whether to proceed vaginally or abdominally is made.

Grasping and Circumscribing the Cervix   The anterior and posterior lips of the cervix are grasped with a single- or double-toothed tenaculum. With downward traction applied on the cervix, a circumferential incision is made in the vaginal epithelium at the junction of the cervix (Fig. 24.15).

Dissection of Vaginal Mucosa   After the initial incision is made with a scalpel or a Bovie, the vaginal epithelium may be dissected sharply from the underlying tissue or pushed bluntly with an open sponge (Fig. 24.16). **If the initial incision is made too close to the external cervical os, a greater amount of dissection is required and causes associated bleeding.** This circumscribing incision should be made just below the bladder reflection. It is important to continue the dissection in the correct cleavage plane to minimize blood loss.

Posterior Cul-de-Sac Entry   **The peritoneal reflection of the posterior cul-de-sac (cul-de-sac of Douglas) can be identified by stretching the vaginal mucosa and underlying connective tissue with forceps** (Fig. 24.17). If difficulty is encountered (e.g., if the cervix is elongated and the peritoneum is not evident), the vaginal mucosa may be incised vertically to the point at which the cul-de-sac becomes more apparent.

If the vaginal mucosa is dissected in the wrong plane, the hysterectomy may begin extraperitoneally by clamping and cutting the uterosacral and cardinal ligaments close to the cervix. The posterior cul-de-sac will be readily identifiable. If the peritoneal reflection of the posterior cul-de-sac cannot be identified, entry into the anterior peritoneum is attempted, and a finger is hooked into the posterior cul-de-sac to place tension on the peritoneum. The peritoneum is opened with Mayo scissors. An interrupted suture is placed to approximate the peritoneum and vaginal cuff and provide hemostasis (Fig. 24.18). The posterior pelvic cavity is examined for pathologic alterations of the uterus or adhesive disease of the cul-de-sac. The weighted speculum is placed into the posterior cul-de-sac.

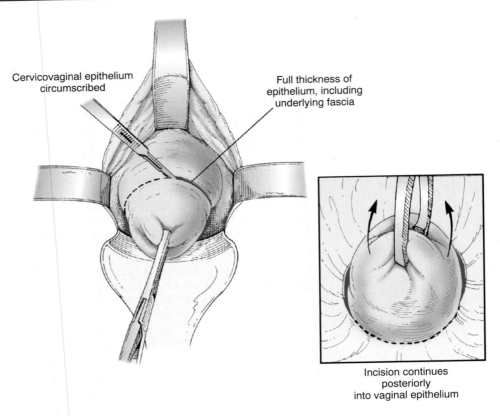

Figure 24.15 **Circumferential incision in the vagina to infiltrate a vaginal hysterectomy.** (From **Mann WA, Stovall TG.** *Gynecologic surgery.* New York: Churchill Livingstone, 1996, with permission.)

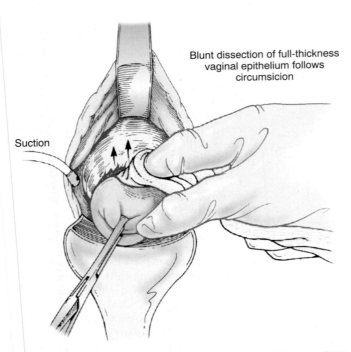

Figure 24.16 **Dissection of the vaginal mucosa.** (From **Mann WA, Stovall TG.** *Gynecologic surgery.* New York: Churchill Livingstone, 1996, with permission.)

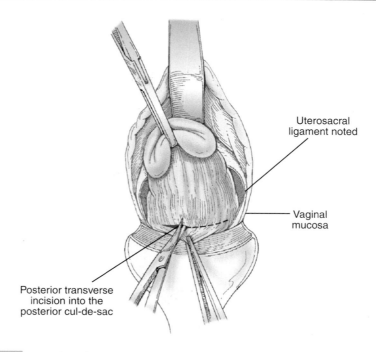

Figure 24.17 **Entry into the posterior cul-de-sac.** (From **Mann WA, Stovall TG.** *Gynecologic surgery.* New York: Churchill Livingstone, 1996, with permission.)

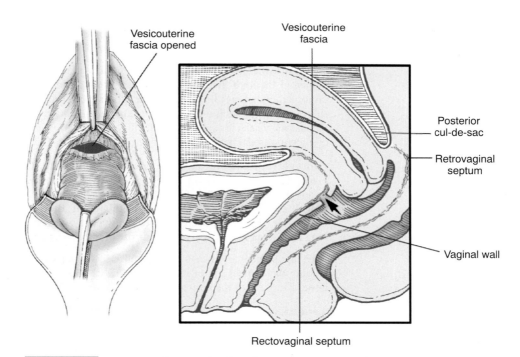

Figure 24.18 **Interrupted suture is placed on posterior vaginal cuff and peritoneum for hemostasis.** (From **Mann WA, Stovall TG.** *Gynecologic surgery.* New York: Churchill Livingstone, 1996, with permission.)

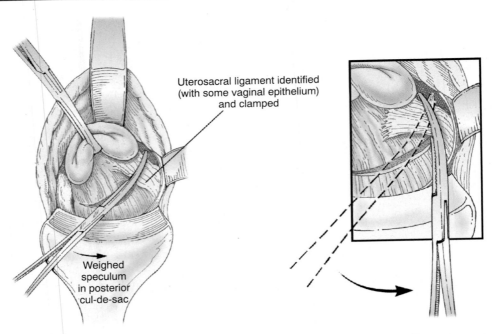

Figure 24.19 **Ligation of the uterosacral ligaments.** (From **Mann WA, Stovall TG.** *Gynecologic surgery.* New York: Churchill Livingstone, 1996, with permission.)

Uterosacral Ligament Ligation   With retraction of the lateral vaginal wall and countertraction on the cervix, the uterosacral ligaments are clamped with the tip of the clamp incorporating the lower portion of the cardinal ligaments (Fig. 24.19). The clamp is placed perpendicular to the uterine axis, and the pedicle is cut and sutured close to the clamp. A small pedicle (0.5 cm) distal to the clamp is optimal because a larger pedicle becomes necrotic and the tissue sloughs, which may become a culture medium for micro-organisms. The pedicle should be incised no more than one-half to three-fourths of the way around the tip of the clamp. Limiting the incision prevents the next pedicle, which may be vascular, from being cut.

When suturing any pedicle, the needle point is placed at the tip of the clamp, and the needle is passed through the tissue by a rolling motion of the operator's wrist. Once ligated, the uterosacral ligaments may be transfixed to the posterolateral vaginal mucosa (Fig. 24.20). This suture may lend additional support to the vagina and provide hemostasis at this point on the vaginal mucosa. This suture is held with a hemostat to facilitate location of any bleeding at the completion of the procedure and to aid in the closure of vaginal mucosa.

Entry versus Nonentry into the Vesicovaginal Space (Cul-de-Sac)   Downward traction is placed on the cervix. Using either Mayo scissors, with the points directed toward the uterus, or an open moistened 4 × 4 gauze sponge, the bladder is advanced. **If the vesicovaginal peritoneal reflection is easily identified at this point, the vesicovaginal space may be entered. Otherwise, it may be preferable to delay entry. There is no danger in delaying entry so long as the operator ascertains that the bladder was advanced.**

After the bladder is advanced, a curved Deaver or Heaney retractor is placed in the midline, holding the bladder out of the operative field. This process precedes each step of the vaginal hysterectomy until the vesicovaginal space is entered.

Cardinal Ligament Ligation   With traction on the cervix continued, the cardinal ligaments are identified, clamped, and cut. The suture is ligated (Fig. 24.21).

Advancement of Bladder   The bladder again is advanced out of the operative field. A blunt dissection technique may be used; sharp dissection may be helpful if the patient had previous surgery, such as cesarean delivery, which may have scarred the bladder reflection.

Uterine Artery Ligation   Contralateral and downward traction are placed on the cervix. **With an effort to incorporate the anterior and posterior leaves of the visceral peritoneum, the**

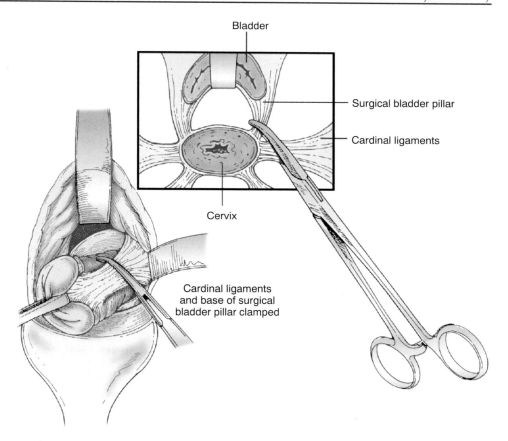

Figure 24.20 **Transfixion of the uterosacral ligament to the posterolateral vaginal mucosa.** (From **Mann WA, Stovall TG.** *Gynecologic surgery.* New York: Churchill Livingstone, 1996, with permission.)

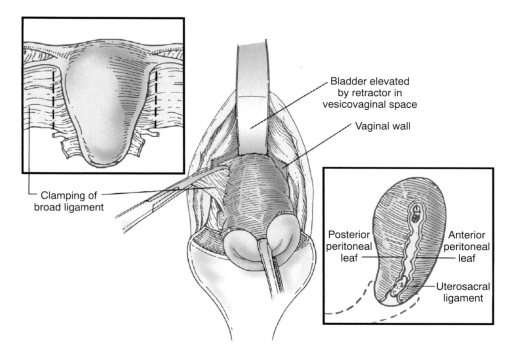

Figure 24.21 **Ligation of the cardinal ligament.** (From **Mann WA, Stovall TG.** *Gynecologic surgery.* New York: Churchill Livingstone, 1996, with permission.)

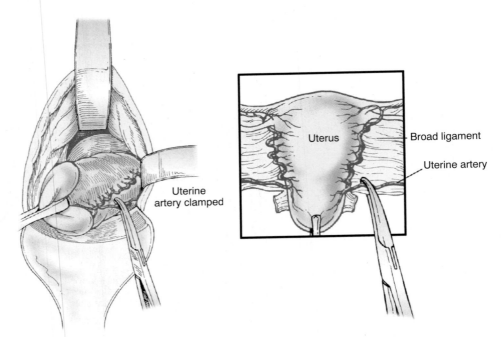

Figure 24.22 **Ligation of the uterine artery.** (From **Mann WA, Stovall TG.** *Gynecologic surgery.* New York: Churchill Livingstone, 1996.)

uterine vessels are identified, clamped, and cut, and the pedicle is suture ligated (Fig. 24.22). **A single suture and single clamp technique is adequate and decreases the potential risk for ureteral injury.** When the uterus is large or when a fibroid distorts the anatomic relationships, a second suture may be required to ligate any remaining branches of the uterine artery.

Entry into the Vesicovaginal Space **The anterior peritoneal fold can be identified just before or after clamping and suture ligation of the uterine arteries. The anterior peritoneal cavity should not be opened blindly because of the increased risk of bladder injury** (Fig. 24.23). The peritoneum is grasped with forceps, tented, and opened using scissors with the tips pointed toward the uterus. A Heaney or Deaver retractor is placed, and the peritoneal contents are identified. This retractor serves to keep the bladder out of the operative field.

Delivery of the Uterus A tenaculum is placed onto the uterine fundus in a successive fashion to deliver the fundus posteriorly (Fig. 24.24). The operator's index finger is used to identify the utero-ovarian ligament and aid in clamp placement.

Utero-ovarian and Round Ligament Ligation With the posterior and anterior peritoneum opened, the remainder of the broad ligament and utero-ovarian ligaments are clamped, cut, and ligated (Fig. 24.25). The utero-ovarian and round ligament complexes are double ligated with a suture tie followed by a ligature medial to the first suture. A hemostat is placed on the second suture to aid in the identification of any bleeding and to assist with peritoneal closure. A hemostat should not be placed on the first suture or any other vascular pedicle to avoid the risk for loosening the tie.

Removal of the Ovaries During the removal of the adnexa, the round ligaments should be removed separately from the adnexal pedicles. Traction is placed on the utero-ovarian pedicle. The ovary is drawn into the operative field by grasping it with a Babcock clamp. A Heaney clamp is placed across the ovarian vessels (infundibulopelvic ligament), and the ovary and tube are excised (Fig. 24.26). A transfixion tie and suture ligature are placed on the ovarian vessels. The surgeon should not be reluctant to remove the fallopian tube separately from the ovary if taking them together risks loss of the tissue pedicle or injury to the ureter or nearby blood vessels.

Hemostasis A retractor or tagged sponge is placed into the peritoneal cavity, and each of the pedicles is visualized and inspected for hemostasis. If additional sutures are required, they should be placed precisely, with care to avoid the ureter or bladder.

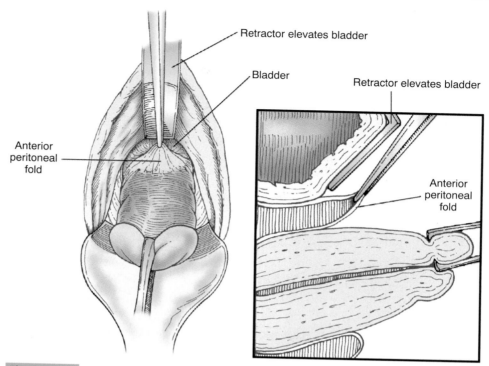

Figure 24.23   Entry into the vesicovaginal space. (From **Mann WA, Stovall TG.** *Gynecologic surgery.* New York: Churchill Livingstone, 1996, with permission.)

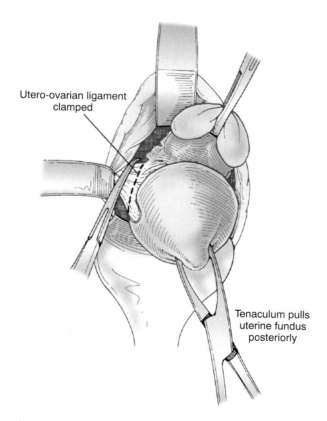

Figure 24.24   Delivery of the uterine fundus posteriorly. (From **Mann WA, Stovall TG.** *Gynecologic surgery.* New York: Churchill Livingstone, 1996, with permission.)

827

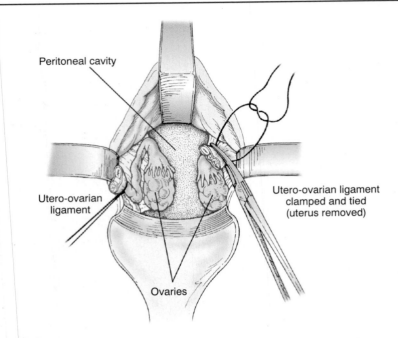

Figure 24.25 **Ligation of the utero-ovarian and round ligaments.** (From **Mann WA, Stovall TG.** *Gynecologic surgery.* New York: Churchill Livingstone, 1996, with permission.)

Peritoneal Closure **Because the pelvic peritoneum does not provide support and re-forms within 24 hours after surgery, the peritoneum need not be reapproximated routinely.** If it is important, the anterior peritoneal edge is identified and grasped with forceps. A continuous absorbable 0 suture is begun at the 12-o'clock position. The suture is continued in a purse-string fashion and incorporates the distal portion of the left upper pedicle and the left uterosacral ligament (Fig. 24.27). At the beginning of the procedure tension is applied to the suture that

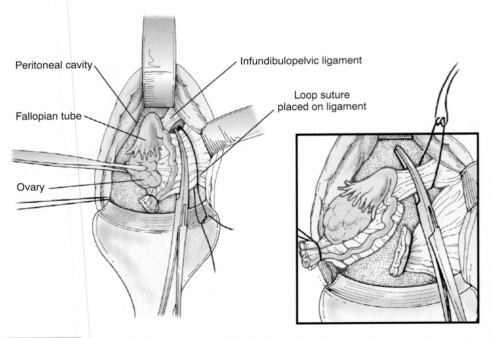

Figure 24.26 **Removal of the ovaries and fallopian tubes by clamping across the ovarian vessels (infundibulopelvic ligament).** (From **Mann WA, Stovall TG.** *Gynecologic surgery.* New York: Churchill Livingstone, 1996, with permission.)

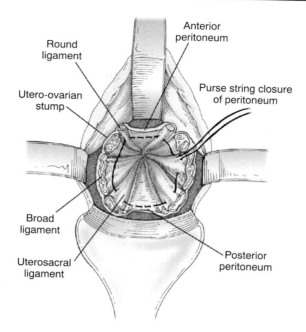

Figure 24.27 **Closure of the peritoneum.** (From **Mann WA, Stovall TG.** *Gynecologic surgery.* New York: Churchill Livingstone, 1996, with permission.)

incorporates the posterior peritoneum and vaginal mucosa. This allows for high posterior reperitonealization, which shortens the cul-de-sac and helps prevent future enterocele formation. The right uterosacral ligament and the distal portion of the right upper pedicle are incorporated, and this continuous suture ends at the point on the anterior peritoneum where it began.

Vaginal Mucosa Closure **The vaginal mucosa can be reapproximated in a vertical or horizontal manner, using either interrupted or continuous sutures** (Fig. 24.28). The vaginal mucosa is, in this case, reapproximated horizontally with interrupted absorbable sutures. The

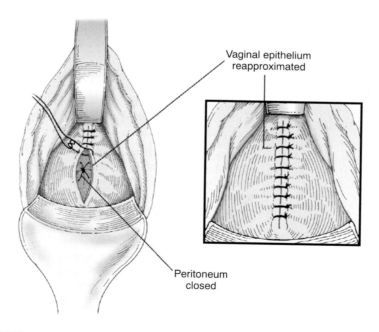

Figure 24.28 **Closure of the vaginal mucosa.** (From **Mann WA, Stovall TG.** *Gynecologic surgery.* New York: Churchill Livingstone, 1996, with permission.)

sutures are placed through the entire thickness of the vaginal epithelium, with care taken to avoid entering the bladder anteriorly. These sutures will obliterate the underlying dead space and produce an anatomic approximation of the vaginal epithelium, thereby decreasing the postoperative formation of granulation tissue.

Bladder Drainage   After completion of the procedure, the bladder is drained. Unless an anterior or posterior colporrhaphy or other reconstructive procedure is performed, neither bladder catheter nor vaginal packing is mandatory.

Surgical Techniques for Selected Patients

Injection of Vaginal Mucosa   **The use of paracervical and submucosal injection of 20 to 30 mL of 0.5% *lidocaine* with 1:200,000 *epinephrine* before incision of the vaginal mucosa may decrease postoperative pain and facilitate identification of surgical planes.** There is no need to inject the cervix. Areas to be injected include the bladder pillars, lower portion of the cardinal ligament, uterosacral ligaments, and paracervical tissue. The incidence of cuff cellulitis and cuff abscess formation is increased when *epinephrine* is injected into the cervicovaginal mucosa.

Morcellation of the Large Uterus   Uterine morcellation is a well-known but underutilized surgical procedure whereby the uterus is removed piecemeal. Several methods of uterine morcellation were described, including hemisection or bivalving, wedge or "V" incisions, and intramyometrial coring (53). Before beginning any morcellation procedure, the uterine vessels must be ligated, and the peritoneal cavity must be entered. When uterine hemisection or bivalving is performed, the cervix is split at the midline, and the uterus is cut into halves, which are removed separately (53). This method seems best suited for fundal, midline leiomyomas.

Wedge morcellation is best suited for anterior or posterior fibroids or for fibroids in the other broad ligaments (i.e., when the fibroids are away from the midline). The cervix is amputated, and the myometrium is grasped with clamps. Wedge-shaped portions of myometrium are removed from the anterior or posterior uterine wall. The apex of the wedge is kept in the midline, thereby reducing the bulk of the myometrium. This process is repeated until the uterus can be removed or until a pseudocapsule of a fibroid can be grasped with a Leahy clamp or towel clip. Traction is applied, and a "myomectomy" is performed.

When the intramyometrial coring technique is used, the myometrium above the site of the ligated vessels is incised parallel to the axis of the uterine cavity and serosa of the uterus. This incision is continued around the full circumference of the myometrium in a symmetrical fashion beneath the uterine serosa. Traction is maintained on the cervix, and the avascular myometrium is cut to allow the undisturbed endometrial cavity, with a thick layer of myometrium, to be delivered with the cervix. As a result, the inside of the uterus with its unopened endometrial cavity is brought closer to the operator. Incision of the lateral portions of the myometrium medial to the remaining attachment of the broad ligament results in considerable additional descent of the uterus and greatly increases the mobility of the uterine fundus. The uterus is converted from a globular to an elongated tissue mass. The cored uterus is removed by clamping the utero-ovarian pedicle and fallopian tubes.

In a retrospective comparison of 383 patients undergoing abdominal hysterectomy or vaginal hysterectomy with uterine morcellation, length of stay and perioperative complications were significantly increased with abdominal hysterectomy. It appears that vaginal hysterectomy with uterine morcellation is safe and allows an increased number of women to undergo vaginal hysterectomy (54).

McCall Culdoplasty

Although McCall culdoplasty is thought to help decrease future enterocele formation, the accuracy of this belief remains open to debate. An absorbable suture is placed through the full thickness of the posterior vaginal wall at the point of the highest portion of the vaginal vault. The patient's left uterosacral ligament pedicle is grasped and sutured. The suture incorporates the posterior peritoneum, between the uterosacral ligaments and the right uterosacral ligament. The suture is completed by passing the needle from the inside to the outside at the same point at which it was begun. The suture is tied, thereby approximating the uterosacral ligaments and the posterior peritoneum.

Schuchardt Incision

When vaginal exposure is difficult, the Schuchardt incision may be used. If the surgeon is right handed, the incision is made on the patient's left side. To decrease blood loss, the area can be infiltrated with *lidocaine*-containing *epinephrine*. The incision follows a curved line from the 4-o'clock position at the hymenal margin to a point halfway between the anus and the ischial tuberosity. The incision may be continued into the vaginal vault as high as necessary to gain exposure. The depth of the incision is the medial portion of the pubococcygeus muscle, which may be divided in extreme cases. The incision must be closed in layers at the completion of the procedure.

Intraoperative Complications

Bladder Injury

Injury to the urinary bladder is one of the most common intraoperative complications associated with hysterectomy. **If the bladder is inadvertently entered, repair should be performed when the injury is discovered and not delayed until completion of surgery.** When bladder injury is recognized, the edges of the wound should be mobilized to assess the full extent of the injury and allow repair without tension. This assessment should include visualization of the trigone to exclude injury to that area. The bladder may be repaired with a single- or double-layered closure with a small-caliber absorbable suture. *Methylene blue, indigo carmine,* or a dye of sterile milk formula can be instilled into the bladder to ensure that the repair is adequate.

Bowel Injury

Because patients with suspected pelvic adhesions or obvious pelvic disease are excluded as candidates for vaginal hysterectomy, bowel injuries do not occur often. Bowel injuries are associated with the performance of a posterior colporrhaphy and are usually confined to the rectum.

If the rectum is entered, the injury is repaired with a single- or double-layer closure using a small-caliber absorbable suture, followed by copious irrigation. Postoperatively, the patient should be given a stool softener and a low-residue diet.

Hemorrhage

Intraoperative hemorrhage invariably is the result of failure to ligate securely a significant blood vessel, bleeding from the vaginal cuff, slippage of a previously placed ligature, or avulsion of tissue before clamping. Most intraoperative bleeding can be avoided with adequate exposure and good surgical technique. Using square knots with attention to proper knot-tying mechanisms will prevent bleeding in most cases. The use of Heaney-type sutures may minimize ligature slippage and subsequent bleeding from bulky pedicles. When bleeding does occur, blind clamping, which may endanger the ureter, should be avoided. The bleeding vessel should be identified and precisely ligated, with visualization of the ureter if necessary. **If the location of the ureter is in question, it should be visualized before suturing a bleeding vessel.**

Perioperative Care

Bladder Drainage Postoperative bladder drainage should be employed after any procedure in which spontaneous, complete voiding is not anticipated. Reasons to consider closed bladder drainage include significant local pain, additional vaginal reparative procedures, surgery for stress incontinence, the use of a vaginal pack, and patient anxiety.

After vaginal hysterectomy without additional repair, most patients can void spontaneously, and catheter drainage is not required. The relative amount of pain after a vaginal hysterectomy is less than with abdominal hysterectomy and, in the absence of additional repairs or a pack, no obstructive effect should be present.

If the patient does not tolerate pain well postoperatively or is extremely anxious, the transurethral insertion of a 16-Fr. catheter after completing surgery is warranted. This catheter may be inserted postoperatively if the patient is unable to void spontaneously on two attempts. Closed-catheter drainage after vaginal hysterectomy usually is not necessary for longer than 24 hours. The catheter is removed without clamping, and there is no need to obtain a urine specimen for culture and sensitivity.

Diet   Although little manipulation of the bowel occurs during vaginal hysterectomy, there is some slowing of gastrointestinal motility. This slowing rarely occurs to a degree that limits some form of oral intake soon after surgery. Most patients experience some degree of nausea after surgery, which, combined with drowsiness from analgesics, usually makes them disinterested in food on the evening after surgery. A clear liquid diet is suitable during the first night after surgery, and on the first full postoperative day, a regular diet can usually be consumed. **The patient is often the best judge of what she can tolerate as her appetite returns.**

Laparoscopic Hysterectomy

Preoperative Preparation

The main limitations to a laparoscopic approach are medical or anesthetic disorders that do not allow adequate pneuomperitoneum or proper ventilation (34). Extensive and dense pelvic abdominal adhesions from previous surgery and very large uterine size are relative contraindications, although this decision can be made after assessing the peritoneal cavity (see Chapter 23). If the uterine size limits access to the uterine vessels, laparoscopic hysterectomy may not be possible. Obesity is not a contraindication to laparoscopic hysterectomy. The increased morbidity from laparotomy in patients with high body mass (BMI) can be minimized with laparoscopy.

Different classifications were proposed for the types of laparoscopic hysterectomy. Laparoscopic hysterectomy is defined as a laparoscopic-assisted vaginal hysterectomy (LAVH) if the uterine vessels are occluded vaginally. The Cochrane review authors recommended that if the vessels are occluded laparoscopically, or if part of the operation is performed vaginally, the procedure be called *laparoscopic hysterectomy,* and, if no component is performed vaginally, the procedure should be called a *total laparoscopic hysterectomy* (41).

Patient Positioning   The patient is placed in dorsal lithotomy position with legs placed in Allen or Yellowfin stirrups (Allen Medical Systems, Acton, MA). Attention to proper leg placement will avoid nerve injury. Hyperflexion of the hips should be avoided because this may cause femoral nerve palsy. The patient should be placed on an egg crate mattress or beanbag cushion to limit patient movement in the Trendelenburg position. The arms are tucked on the patients' side and protected with egg crate–type material. No shaving or clipping is necessary. Shoulder braces should not be used as they are associated with brachial plexus injury.

The steps to follow before introducing the first trocar are:

- Perform an examination under anesthesia.

- Place a Foley catheter to drain the bladder.

- Introduce a uterine manipulator (e.g., Koh colpotomizer [Cooper Surgical Inc., Trumbull, CT] or VCare [Conmed Corp., Utica NY]).

- Place an oral gastric tube.

Instrumentation   **The most important instrument is the one used to occlude blood vessels.** A multitude of energy forms exist, including electrosurgery, lasers, and ultrasonic scalpel (see Chapter 23). Some surgeons use stapling devices, although the cost of these stapling devices is high, and an energy-occluding device is needed to access areas that a stapler cannot. The versatility of the devices with energy makes them the method of choice to occlude vessels. **There are no valid clinical data showing that one instrument is safer than another.** The preferred one involves bipolar energy because gynecologists are experienced with this form of energy.

Surgical Technique of Laparoscopic Hysterectomy

Peritoneal Access

The most important technical consideration for all laparoscopic surgery is port placement (see Chapter 23). The umbilical site typically is used in patients without a previous history of surgery or intra-abdominal infection. In cases of previous surgery where there was a midline incision or a history of a pelvic-abdominal incision, an open laparoscopy is recommended or an alternative site is chosen to introduce the primary cannula. The open laparoscopy is essentially a mini-laparotomy at the umbilicus. The alternative site is the left upper quadrant. The standard closed technique involves the use of pneumoperitoneum needle (Verres needle), insufflation, and primary trocar insertion. An alternative technique is the direct trocar insertion (no insufflation prior to trocar insertion). A meta-analysis showed no advantage of one technique over the other (24). Gynecologists should use the approach with which they have most experience.

If the left upper quadrant is used, the surgeon should be aware of the closest anatomic structures to the left costal margin (see Chapter 23, Fig. 23.3). Typically the cannula is introduced below the left costal margin in the midclavicular line. The closest structures to this area are the stomach and the left lobe of the liver. Therefore, an oral gastric tube should be introduced to empty the stomach before starting the procedure.

The patient is kept in a horizontal (not Trendelenburg) position until proper peritoneal access is confirmed. The angle of insertion of the primary trocar will depend on the size of the patient. Typically for nonobese or overweight patients a 45-degree angle from the horizontal is used and with obese patients a 60- to 80-degree angle or open technique is used.

Proper placement of accessory ports is critical to allow the steps of a laparoscopic hysterectomy. The authors typically use three lateral accessory ports and do not use a suprapubic port. Lateral ports offer the surgeon an ergonomic approach in which both hands can be used comfortably. **The most important step when placing lateral ports is to avoid the inferior epigastric vessels, which are branches of the external iliac artery and vein.** (see Chapter 23, Fig. 23.3). Direct visualization is best. These vessels (typically two veins and an artery) are seen through the peritoneum medial to the insertion of the round ligament in the deep inguinal ring. They cannot be transilluminated. Ports are placed approximately 8 cm from the midline and 8 cm above the pubic symphysis.

Laparoscopic hysterectomy requires traction and countertraction to identify the vascular pedicles and the ureter, which is accomplished with the uterine manipulator. In the case of a large uterus, a laparoscopic tenaculum is required. The procedure starts with coagulating and transecting the round ligament (Fig. 24.29). The incision is carried anteriorly to create a bladder peritoneal flap by sharp dissection of the loose areolar cervicovesical tissue. The retroperitoneal space is opened and the ureter identified on the medial leaf of the broad ligament (Fig. 24.30). The ovarian vessels (infundibulopelvic ligament) or the utero-ovarian ligaments are coagulated and transected, depending on whether the ovaries will be removed (Fig. 24.31). The surgeon can proceed vaginally (LAVH), but there will not be any improved uterine descent because the transected tissue has no major role in uterine support.

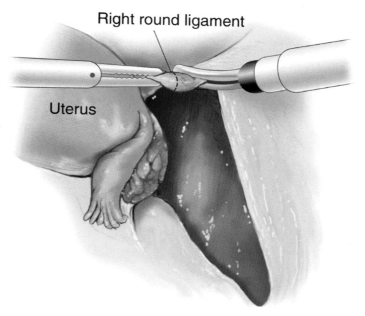

Right round ligament

Uterus

Figure 24.29   The right round ligament is grasped and desiccated with a bipolar device.

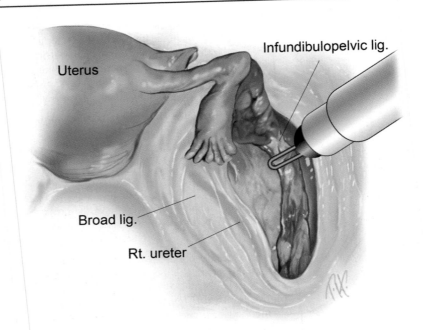

Figure 24.30   The round ligament has been transected, the peritoneum is opened lateral to the right ureter, which is identified in the retroperitoneal space.

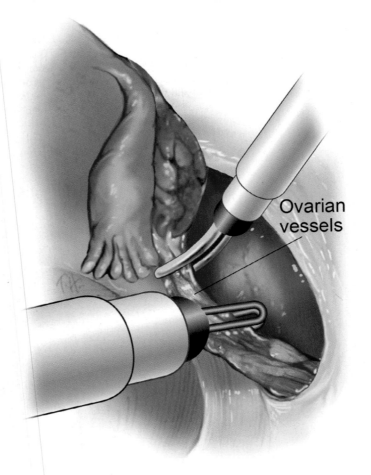

Figure 24.31   The right infundibulopelvic ligament is grasped with a bipolar device, desiccated and cut.

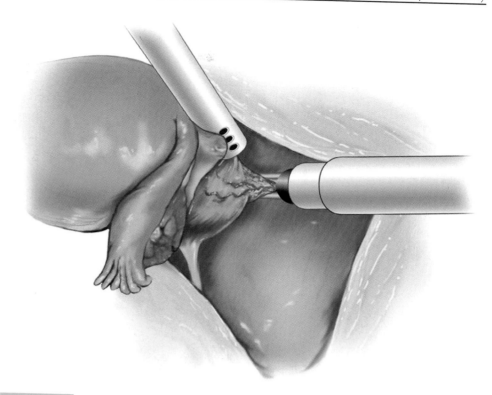

Figure 24.32 After the bladder peritoneum is sharply dissected down to the level of the cervix, the uterine vessels are grasped with the bipolar devise and desiccated.

The uterus is then torqued away from the uterine artery to be occluded. The uterine artery is skeletonized by cutting the posterior peritoneum up to the uterosacral ligament, coagulated, and transected. The procedure is carried out on the other side. This area of occlusion is approximately the level of the internal os. If a supracervical hysterectomy was performed, the uterus can now be amputated. When this is done, the remaining endocervical canal should be cauterized.

The anterior dissection should be completed so that the bladder is completely off the anterior fornix area of the vagina (Fig. 24.32). Using a vaginal device such as the Koh, the surgeon can identify this area. Ensuring that no CO_2 escapes from the vagina, and an incision is made on the vagina circumferentially around the cervix (Fig. 24.33). The uterus can be pulled out though the vagina or can be morcellated first, and then removed either vaginally or laparoscopically, whichever is easier.

The vaginal cuff is closed laparoscopically or vaginally with interrupted or continuous delayed absorbable suture (2-0 on CT-1 needle). To give added pelvic support, the uterosacral ligaments are reattached to the vagina (McCall's culdoplasty) with delayed absorbable suture. Intravenous *indigo carmine* is given and the integrity of the bladder and ureters confirmed with cystoscopy, if desired, by the surgeon.

At the end of the procedure, the secondary ports should be removed under direct visualization to ensure that there is no bleeding. In order to minimize the risk of herniation, the fascia should be closed at port sites that are greater than 8 mm and at those sites where smaller ports have been used but there has been prolonged manipulation.

The patient is kept in the short stay unit and discharged within 24 hours if there are no complications. A regular diet as tolerated is given on the same day as the surgery. Ambulation is encouraged as soon as possible. Median time to return to work is 3 to 4 weeks (42).

Robotic-Assisted Laparoscopic Hysterectomy

A surgical robot consists of a surgeon's console with the instrument manipulators and view screen, a robot tower with telerobotic arms that are attached to the patient, and the computer interface equipment, which is housed in a separate tower (see Chapter 25 for a more complete discussion). Robotic assistance at laparoscopy has some advantages, including a three-dimensional

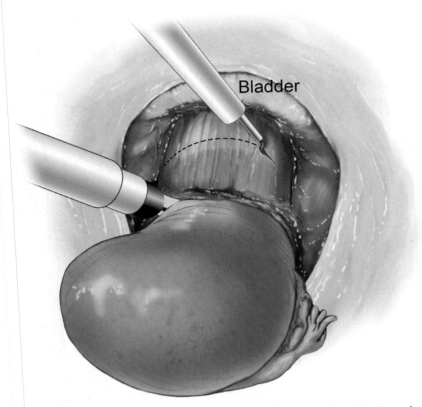

Figure 24.33   **The vagina over the anterior fornix is identified and incision is made.**

view, instruments with articulating tips that offer seven degrees of movement, scaling of movement, and more precise movements. The disadvantages are the bulky device around the patient that limits the assistant's movements, the lack of haptic feedback, and the high cost of the robot. The robot device uses a 12-mm laparoscope and instruments that require 8 mm ports.

The robotic tower can be docked between the legs or on the patient's side (side docked). Side docking allows access to the perineum and vagina so that the assistant can comfortably manipulate the uterus. A robot-assisted hysterectomy goes through the same steps as a laparoscopic hysterectomy. A right-handed surgeon should have the monopolar scissors or harmonic scalpel through a right robotic port and a vessel-sealing device such as a bipolar instrument through a left-sided robotic port. If a fourth robotic arm is used, the additional port is placed on the right side for right-handed surgeons.

Observational studies showed that outcomes for robotic-assisted hysterectomy can be similar to laparoscopic hysterectomy but with less blood loss and possibly fewer conversions to laparotomy (55,56). The learning curve to stabilize operative times for skilled laparoscopic surgeons is about 50 cases (57). Although these case series demonstrated equivalent operative times, an analysis of the Premier hospital database of over 36,000 laparoscopic or robotic hysterectomies demonstrated longer surgical times and higher costs with the robot-assisted procedures compared with conventional laparoscopy with little difference in perioperative and postoperative outcomes (58). Robotic-assisted laparoscopic hysterectomy is associated with delayed vaginal cuff dehiscence around 7 to 8 weeks after hysterectomy, although one case series showed an increased frequency with conventional laparoscopy (59,60). The frequency of other complications is similar to conventional laparoscopy. A more complete discussion of this subject is in Chapter 25.

Laparoendoscopic Single-Site Surgery

Another modification of laparoscopic hysterectomy is the introduction of laparoendoscopic single-site surgery or single-port surgery. Because some surgeons use multiple ports at one site, laparoendoscopic single-site surgery is probably the best term. The role of single-site access to hysterectomy is unclear, and there are only case reports (61). Specifically designed umbilical port systems that admit multiple instrument access have enabled the development of this technique. The availability of flexible instruments and flexible tip laparoscopes allows the surgeon to perform a hysterectomy by reducing instrument crowding and clashing at the umbilicus. The basic hysterectomy steps are the same.

Intraoperative Complications: Laparoscopic Hysterectomy

The intraoperative complications of a laparoscopic hysterectomy are similar to an open hysterectomy. These are injury to the ureter, bladder, and bowel and hemorrhage. Recognition and management are similar. **Because there is an increased frequency of injury to the ureter and bladder, a cystoscopic evaluation after injection of intravenous indigo carmine dye is recommended** (62).

Intraoperative bleeding during a laparoscopic procedure is handled by use of a bipolar instrument. The same principles apply as with an open case. Cautery should not be used without proper localization of the ureters. If it is not apparent where the bleeding is occurring, the procedure should be converted to an open one.

Perioperative Care

Many surgeons remove the bladder catheter at the end of the laparoscopic hysterectomy. Patients can resume a regular diet the same day as the surgery. Transition to oral analgesics can be made the same day.

Postoperative Complications of Hysterectomy

A comprehensive discussion of postoperative complications after gynecologic surgery is presented in Chapter 22.

Wound Infections

Wound infections occur after 4% to 6% of abdominal hysterectomies (33). Measures believed to reduce the incidence of wound infections include a preoperative shower, no removal of hair, or if hair removal is necessary, removal of hair with clippers in the operating room, use of adhesive drapes and prophylactic antibiotics, and delayed primary closure (see Chapter 22).

Incisional Pain

Incisional pain can occur at trocar sites, especially if located in the region of the ilioinguinal or iliohypogastric nerves. Pfannenstiel incisions can be a source of chronic pain at the incision site as a result of nerve entrapment (63).

Hemorrhage

Immediately after hysterectomy, hemorrhage may become apparent in one of two ways. **Bleeding from the vagina may first be noted by the nursing staff or physician within the first few hours after surgery. Second, the patient may be noted to have little bleeding from the vagina but deteriorating vital signs manifested by low blood pressure and rapid pulse, falling hematocrit level, and flank or abdominal pain. The first presentation is in the form of bleeding from the vaginal cuff or one of the pedicles. The second presentation may be a retroperitoneal hemorrhage.** Each situation is approached differently in its evaluation and treatment, but both involve the same general principles of rapid diagnosis, stabilization of vital signs, appropriate fluid and blood replacement, and constant surveillance of the patient's overall condition.

After vital signs are assessed, attention should be directed to the amount of bleeding. A small amount of bleeding is expected after any vaginal hysterectomy. **Steady bleeding 2 to 3 hours after surgery suggests lack of hemostasis.** The patient should be taken promptly to the examining room, where the operative site is viewed using a large speculum and good lighting. If bleeding is not excessive, the vaginal cuff can be inspected, and in many instances, bleeding from the cuff edge will be found. Hemostasis can easily be achieved with one or two sutures placed through the mucosa.

If bleeding is excessive or appears to be coming from above the cuff, or if the patient is too uncomfortable to tolerate adequate examination, she should be taken to the operating room.

General anesthesia should be administered and the vaginal operative site should be thoroughly explored. Any bleeding point may be sutured or ligated. Bleeding that is coming from above the cuff or is extremely heavy usually cannot be controlled through the vaginal route. An exploratory laparotomy is necessary to examine the pelvic floor, identify and isolate the bleeding vessel, and achieve hemostasis. **The ovarian vessels and uterine arteries should be thoroughly inspected because they often are the source of excessive vaginal bleeding.** If it is difficult to localize bleeding to a specific pelvic vessel, or if these maneuvers do not work, ligation of the hypogastric artery may be performed.

In the patient with little vaginal bleeding in whom vital signs have deteriorated, retroperitoneal hemorrhage should be suspected. Input and output should be monitored. Hematocrit assessment, along with cross-matching of packed red blood cells, should be performed immediately. Examination may reveal tenderness and dullness in the flank. In cases of intraperitoneal bleeding, abdominal distention may occur. Diagnostic radiologic studies can be used to confirm the presence of retroperitoneal or intra-abdominal bleeding. Ultrasonography is one option for viewing low pelvic hematomas; CT provides better visualization of retroperitoneal spaces and can delineate a hematoma.

If the patient's condition stabilizes rapidly with intravenous fluids, one of two approaches may be used for continued care. The first is to give the patient a transfusion and follow serial hematocrit assessments and vital signs. In many instances, retroperitoneal bleeding will tamponade and stop, forming a hematoma that may eventually be resorbed. The risk with this approach is that the hematoma will become infected, necessitating surgical drainage. In some instances when the patient's condition is stable, radiologic embolization may be considered.

Another option is to perform abdominal exploratory surgery while the patient's condition is stable. This approach adds the morbidity of a second procedure but avoids the possibility of the patient's condition deteriorating with continued delay or the formation of a pelvic abscess. Once adequate exposure is obtained, the peritoneum over the hematoma should be opened and the blood evacuated. All bleeding vessels should be identified and ligated. If bleeding is difficult to control, consideration should be given to unilateral or bilateral ligation of the anterior division of the internal iliac artery. Once hemostasis is achieved, the pelvis should be drained using a closed system.

Urinary Tract Complications

Urinary Retention

Urinary retention after hysterectomy is an uncommon occurrence. If the urethra is unobstructed and retention occurs, it is usually the result of either pain or bladder atony resulting from anesthesia. Both are temporary effects.

If a catheter was not placed after surgery, retention can be relieved initially with the insertion of a Foley catheter for 12 to 24 hours. Most patients are able to void after the catheter is removed 1 day later. If the patient still has trouble voiding and urethral spasm is suspected, success can be achieved with a skeletal muscle relaxant such as *diazepam* (2 mg twice a day). In most cases, waiting is the best course, and voiding usually occurs spontaneously.

Ureteral Injury

In patients who develop flank pain soon after hysterectomy, ureteral obstruction should be suspected. The incidence of ureteral injury is lower with vaginal hysterectomy than with abdominal hysterectomy and higher with laparoscopic hysterectomy (41,44). One risk factor for its occurrence is total uterine prolapse, in which the ureters are drawn outside the bony pelvis.

In a patient with flank pain in whom ureteral obstruction is suspected, a CT urogram and a urinalysis should be performed. **If obstruction is noted on CT scan, it is usually present near the ureterovesical junction. The immediate step is attempted passage of a catheter through the ureter under cystoscopic guidance.** If a catheter can be passed through the ureter, it should be left in place for at least 4 to 6 weeks, allowing sutures to absorb and the obstruction or kinking to release. **If the catheter cannot be passed through the ureter, the best course is to perform abdominal exploratory surgery and repair the ureter at the site of obstruction.**

Vesicovaginal Fistula

Vesicovaginal fistulas occur most often after total abdominal hysterectomy for benign gynecologic disease (50). Intraoperative steps to avoid the formation of a vesicovaginal fistula include correct identification of the proper plane between the bladder and cervix, sharp rather than blunt dissection of the bladder, and care in clamping and suturing the vaginal cuff. The development of a postoperative vesicovaginal fistula after hysterectomy is rare; the incidence is as low as 0.2%.

Patients who have a postoperative vesicovaginal fistula develop a watery vaginal discharge 10 to 14 days after surgery. Some fistulas resulting from surgery are noted as early as the first 48 to 72 hours after surgery. After vaginal examination with a speculum, the diagnosis can usually be confirmed with the insertion of a cotton tampon into the vagina followed by the instillation of *methylene blue* or *indigo carmine* dye through a transurethral catheter. If the tampon stains blue, a vesicovaginal fistula is present. If no staining occurs, the presence of a ureterovaginal fistula must be ruled out by the intravenous injection of 5 mL of *indigo carmine* dye. Within 20 minutes, the tampon should stain blue if a ureterovaginal fistula is present. A CT urogram should be performed to rule out ureteral obstruction.

If a vesicovaginal fistula is diagnosed, a Foley catheter should be inserted for prolonged drainage. Up to 15% of fistulas close spontaneously with 4 to 6 weeks of continuous bladder drainage. If closure has not occurred by 6 weeks, operative correction is necessary. Waiting 3 to 4 months from the time of diagnosis before operative repair is recommended to allow reduction of inflammation and to improve vascular supply. After vaginal hysterectomy, the fistula site is above the bladder trigone and away from the ureters. Vaginal repair can be anticipated in most patients. The surgical correction is undertaken in a four-layered closure: the bladder mucosa, the seromuscular layer, the endopelvic fascia, and the vaginal epithelium.

Incidental cystotomy at the time of hysterectomy is more common than vesicovaginal fistula. When identified and repaired correctly, cystotomy rarely results in the development of a fistula.

Prolapse of the Fallopian Tube

Posthysterectomy prolapse of the fallopian tube is a rare event and can be confused with granulation tissue at the vaginal apex. Predisposing factors for the development of fallopian tube prolapse include development of a hematoma and an abscess at the vaginal apex. Approximately one-half of patients undergoing vaginal hysterectomy form some granulation tissue at the vaginal vault. **In patients in whom granulation tissue persists after attempts to cauterize it or pain is experienced with attempts to remove it, fallopian tube prolapse should be suspected.** A biopsy of the area is warranted and usually reveals tubal epithelium if a fallopian tube is present.

If fallopian tube prolapse is diagnosed, it should be repaired with surgery. The surrounding vaginal mucosa should be opened and undermined widely. The tube is ligated high and removed, followed by closure of the vaginal mucosa.

Vaginal Cuff Dehiscence

Patients with cuff dehiscence present with pain, vaginal bleeding, vaginal discharge or gush of fluid 2 to 5 months after surgery. The most common initiating event is coitus. Immediate examination for cuff integrity is necessary. Treatment typically requires surgical repair in the operating room.

Discharge Instructions

Before discharging the patient, instructions should be reviewed. Printed postoperative instructions are helpful to the patient and a suggested set of instructions are as follows:

1. Avoid strenuous activity for the first 2 weeks, and increase activity level gradually.
2. Avoid heavy lifting, douching, or sexual intercourse until instructed by the physician.
3. Bathe as needed using shower or tub baths.
4. Follow a regular diet.
5. Avoid straining for a bowel movement or urination. For constipation, use *Milk of Magnesia* or *Metamucil* (1 tsp in juice).

6. Call the physician if excessive vaginal bleeding or fever occurs.

7. Schedule a return appointment at the time specified by the physician.

The physician should provide telephone numbers for emergencies both during and after office hours. Typically, the first postoperative visit is scheduled about 4 weeks after discharge from the hospital. At the time of that visit, the patient should be ambulating well, and vaginal discharge or bleeding should be minimal. Speculum examination of the cuff should be gentle and cursory, but the patient should be assured that the healing process is proceeding normally. Finally, the patient's questions should be answered and advice given on increasing her activity level, including sexual activity, work, and normal household activity.

General Pelvic Symptoms and Quality of Life

Patient satisfaction after hysterectomy is related to the initial indication for surgery and patient expectation. The Maine Women's Health Study evaluated the effect of hysterectomy for non-malignant disorders on quality of life (13). They documented a marked improvement in pelvic pain, urinary symptoms, and psychological and sexual symptoms at 1 year in the majority of patients. In the Maryland Women's Health Study patients were followed for up to 2 years after hysterectomy for nonmalignant conditions (64). Symptoms related to the underlying indication for surgery, and associated symptoms of depression and anxiety and quality of life, improved after hysterectomy. Each study reported that about 8% of patients had new symptoms, such as depression and lack of interest in sex or lack of improvement in quality of life. Although women with pelvic pain and depression did not show the same level of improvement as other groups, there was significant improvement over baseline. Patient satisfaction is very high after hysterectomy (64).

Sexual Function

There is considerable debate in the lay literature about the effect of hysterectomy on sexual function, although **evidence consistently suggests that the majority of women have unchanged or improved sexual function 1 to 2 years after hysterectomy** (13,64). Few women who had a hysterectomy had a measurable worsening in sexual function during this time period. The long-term effects of hysterectomy on sexual function remain largely unknown. Studies have addressed the short-term effects of hysterectomy on dyspareunia, frequency of intercourse, orgasm, libido or sexual interest, vaginal dryness, and overall sexual function. The Maine Women's Health Study demonstrated a significant decrease in the number of women who reported dyspareunia 12 and 24 months after hysterectomy compared to the preoperative period (13). Eighty-one percent of the women who experienced dyspareunia preoperatively had an improvement in this symptom at 24 months after hysterectomy, while only 1.9% of women without preoperative dyspareunia developed it by 24 months after surgery. In this study, 39% of women reported dyspareunia preoperatively, and only 8% had this complaint 12 months after hysterectomy. Women who were managed nonsurgically showed no decline in the mean frequency of dyspareunia (13).

Most studies report that hysterectomy has little impact on the frequency of intercourse, libido, and sexual interest. Orgasmic function before and after hysterectomy is somewhat more controversial, but the largest study by Carlson et al. reported a slight increase in the proportion of women who experienced orgasms after a hysterectomy (13). It is plausible that removal of the uterus and/or cervix (especially if the ovaries are also removed) may adversely affect sexual function in some women, but this may be offset by the improvement in sexual function that could result from cessation of abnormal or heavy vaginal bleeding, dysmenorrhea, or symptoms of prolapse. It is likely that vaginal dryness is not affected by hysterectomy and depends more on age and postoperative hormonal status. Body image and sexual function are improved after vaginal, abdominal, and laparoscopic hysterectomy, but no differences were found between the three routes (13,63).

References

1. **Whiteman MK, Hillis SD, Jamieson DJ, et al.** Inpatient hysterectomy surveillance in the United States, 2000–2004. *Obstet Gynecol* 2008;34.e1–e7.

2. **Cooper R, Lucke J, Lawlor DA, et al.** Socioeconomic position and hysterectomy: a cross-cohort comparison of women in Australia

and Great Britain. *J Epidemiol Community Health* 2008;62:1057–1063.

3. **Jacoby VL, Fujimoto VY, Giudice LC, et al.** Racial and ethnic disparities in benign gynecologic conditions and associated surgeries. *Obstet Gynecol* 2010;202:514–521.

4. **Gretz H, Bradley WH, Zakashansky K, et al.** Effect of physician gender and specialty on utilization of hysterectomy in New York, 2001–2005. *Am J Obstet Gynecol* 2008;199:347.e1–e6.

5. **Whiteman MK, Kuklina E, Jamieson DJ, et al.** Inpatient hospitalization for gynecologic disorders in the United States. *Obstet Gynecol* 2010;541.e1–e6.

6. **Parker WH, Fu YS, Berek JS.** Uterine sarcoma in patients operated for presumed leiomyomata and presumed rapidly growing leiomyoma. *Obstet Gynecol* 1994;83:814–878.

7. **Friedman AJ, Haas ST.** Should uterine size be an indication for surgical intervention in women with myomas? *Am J Obstet Gynecol* 199;168:751–755.

8. **Lethaby A, Vollenhoven B, Sowter M.** Pre-operative GnRH analogue therapy before hysterectomy or myomectomy for uterine fibroids. *Cochrane Database Syst Rev* 2000;2:CD000547.

9. **Stovall TG, Ling FW, Henry LC.** A randomized trial evaluating leuprolide acetate prior to hysterectomy for leiomyomata. *Am J Obstet Gynecol* 1991;164:1420–1425.

10. **ACOG Committee on Practice Bulletins—Gynecology. American College of Obstetricians and Gynecologists.** ACOG Practice Bulletin No. 14. Management of anovulatory bleeding. *Int J Gynaecol Obstet* 2001;72:263–271.

11. **Dichersin K, Munro MG, Clark M, et al.** Hysterectomy compared with endometrial ablation for dysfunctional uterine bleeding: a randomized controlled trial. *Obstet Gynecol* 2007;110:1279–1289.

12. **ACOG Committee on Practice Bulletins—Gynecology.** ACOG Practice Bulletin No. 51. Chronic pelvic pain. *Obstet Gynecol* 2004; 103:589–605.

13. **Carlson KJ, Miller BA, Fowler FJ Jr.** The Maine Women's Health Study: I Outcomes of hysterectomy. *Obstet Gynecol* 1994;83:556–565.

14. **Stovall TG, Ling FW, Crawford DA.** Hysterectomy for chronic pelvic pain of presumed uterine etiology. *Obstet Gynecol* 1990;75: 676–679.

15. **ACOG Committee on Practice Bulletins—Gynecology.** ACOG Practice Bulletin No. 113. Management of endometriosis. *Obstet Gynecol* 2010;116:223–236.

16. **Shakiba K, Bena JF, McGill KM, et al.** Surgical treatment of endometriosis: a 7-year follow-up on the requirement for further surgery. *Obstet Gynecol* 2008;111:1285–1292.

17. **Gambone JC, Reiter RC, Lench JB.** Short-term outcome of incidental hysterectomy at the time of adnexectomy for benign disease. *J Womens Health* 1992;1:197–200.

18. **American College of Obstetricians and Gynecologists.** ACOG Practice Bulletin No. 84. Prevention of deep vein thrombosis and pulmonary embolism. *Obstet Gynecol* 2007;110:429–440.

19. **Lethaby A, Ivanova V, Johnson NP.** Total versus subtotal hysterectomy for benign gynecological conditions. *Cochrane Database Syst Rev* 2006;2:CD004993.

20. **Ghomi A, Hantes J, Lotze EC.** Incidence of cyclical bleeding after laparoscopic supracervical hysterectomy. *J Minim Invasive Gynecol* 2005;12:201–205.

21. **American College of Obstetricians and Gynecologists.** ACOG Practice Bulletin No. 89. Elective and risk reducing salpingo-oophorectomy. *Obstet Gynecol* 2008;111:231–241.

22. **Berek JS, Chalas E, Edelson M, et al.** Prophylactic and risk-reducing bilateral salpingo-oophorectomy: recommendations based on risk of ovarian cancer. *Obstet Gynecol* 2010;116:733–743.

23. **Asante A, Whiteman MK, Kulkarni A, et al.** Elective oophorectomy in the United States. Trends and in-hospital complications, 1998–2006. *Obstet Gynecol* 2010;116:1088–1095.

24. **Parker WH, Broder MS, Chang E, et al.** Ovarian conservation at the time of hysterectomy and long-term health outcomes in the Nurses' Health Study. *Obstet Gynecol* 2009;113:1027–1037.

25. **Ingelsson E, Lundholm C, Johansson ALV, et al.** Hysterectomy and risk of cardiovascular disease: a population based cohort study. *Eur Heart J* 2011;32:745–750.

26. **Parker WH, Broder MS, Liv Z, et al.** Ovarian conservation at the time of hysterectomy for benign disease. *Obstet Gynecol* 2005;106: 219–226.

27. **Ryan PJ, Harrison R, Blake GM, et al.** Compliance with hormone replacement therapy (HRT) after screening for postmenopausal osteoporosis. *Br J Obstet Gynaecol* 1992;99:1325–1328.

28. **Kauff ND, Satagopan JM, Robson ME, et al.** Risk-reducing salpingo-oophorectomy in women with a BRCA1 or BRCA2 mutation. *N Engl J Med* 2002;346:1609–1615.

29. **Rebbeck TR, Lynch HT, Neuhausen SL, et al.** Prevention and Observation of Surgical End Points Study Group. Prophylactic oophorectomy in carriers of BRCA1 or BRCA2 mutations. *N Engl J Med* 2002;346:1616–1622.

30. **Levanon K, Crum C, Drapkin R.** New Insights into the pathogenesis of serous ovarian cancer and its clinical import. *J Clin Oncol* 2008;26:5284–5293.

31. **Greene MH, Mai PL, Schwartz PE.** Does bilateral salpingectomy with ovarian retention warrant consideration as a temporary bridge to risk-reducing bilateral oophorectomy in BRCA1/2 mutation carriers? *Am J Obstet Gynecol* 2011;204:19.e1–e6

32. **Sheth SS.** The place of oophorectomy at vaginal hysterectomy. *Br J Obstet Gynaecol* 1991;98:662–666.

33. **Ballard LA, Walters MD.** Transvaginal mobilization and removal of ovaries and fallopian tubes after vaginal hysterectomy. *Obstet Gynecol* 1996;87:35–39.

34. **Falcone T, Walters MD.** Hysterectomy for benign disease. *Obstet Gynecol* 2008;111:753–767.

35. **Salom EM, Schey D, Penalver M, et al.** The safety of incidental appendectomy at the time of abdominal hysterectomy. *Am J Obstet Gynecol* 2003;189:1563–1568.

36. **Kovac SR, Cruikshank SH.** Incidental appendectomy during vaginal hysterectomy. *Int J Gynaecol Obstet* 1993;43:62–63.

37. **Murray JM, Gilstrap LC, Massey FM.** Cholecystectomy and abdominal hysterectomy. *JAMA* 1980;244:2305–2306.

38. **Hester TR, Baird W, Bostwick J, et al.** Abdominoplasty combined with other major surgical procedures: safe or sorry? *Plast Reconstr Surg* 1989;83:997–1004.

39. **Voss SC, Sharp HC, Scott JR.** Abdominoplasty combined with gynecologic surgical procedures. *Obstet Gynecol* 1986;67:181–186.

40. **Kovac SR.** Vaginal hysterectomy combined with liposuction. *Mo Med* 1989;86:165–168.

41. **Le Tohic A, Dhainaut C, Yazbeck C, et al.** Hysterectomy for benign uterine pathology among women without previous vaginal delivery. *Obstet Gynecol* 2008;111:829–837.

42. **Johnson N, Barlow D, Lethaby A, et al.** Surgical approach to hysterectomy for benign gynecological disease. *Cochrane Database Syst Rev* 2006;2:CD 003677.

43. **Falcone T, Paraiso MF, Mascha E.** Prospective randomized clinical trial of laparoscopically assisted vaginal hysterectomy versus total abdominal hysterectomy. *Am J Obstet Gynecol* 1999;180:955–961.

44. **Sculpher M, Manca A, Abbott J, et al.** Cost effectiveness of laparoscopic hysterectomy compared with standard hysterectomy: results from a randomized trial. *BMJ* 2004;328:134–140.

45. **Garry R, Fountain J, Mason S, et al.** The eVALuate study: two parallel randomized trials, one comparing laparoscopic with abdominal hysterectomy, the other comparing laparoscopic with vaginal hysterectomy. *BMJ* 2004;328:129–136.

46. **Guenaga KF, Matos D, Castro AA, et al.** Mechanical bowel preparation for elective colorectal surgery. *Cochrane Database Syst Rev* 2003;2:CD001544.

47. **Tulandi T, Al-Jaroudi D.** Nonclosure of peritoneum: a reappraisal. *Am J Obstet Gynecol* 2003;89:609–612.

48. **Orr JW Jr, Orr PF, Barrett JM, et al.** Continuous or interrupted fascial closure: a prospective evaluation of no. 1 Maxon suture in 402 gynecologic procedures. *Am J Obstet Gynecol* 1990;163:1485–1489.

49. **Kore S, Vyavaharkar M, Akolekar R, et al.** Comparison of closure of subcutaneous tissue versus non-closure in relation to wound disruption after abdominal hysterectomy in obese patients. *J Postgrad Med* 2000;46:26–28.

50. **Walters MD, Barber MD.** Complications of hysterectomy. In: **Walters MD, Barber MD, eds.** *Hysterectomy for benign disease.* Philadelphia, PA: Saunders, Elsevier, 2010:195–212.

51. **Walters MD.** Vaginal hysterectomy and trachelectomy: basic surgical techniques. In: **Walters MD, Barber MD, eds.** *Hysterectomy for benign disease.* Philadelphia, PA: Saunders, Elsevier, 2010:123–134.

52. **Harmanli OH, Khilnani R, Dandolu V, et al.** Narrow pubic arch and increased risk of failure for vaginal hysterectomy. *Obstet Gynecol* 2004;104:697–700.

53. **Barber MD.** Difficult vaginal hysterectomy. In: **Walters MD, Barber MD, eds.** *Hysterectomy for benign disease.* Philadelphia, PA: Saunders, Elsevier, 2010:135–160.

54. **Taylor SM, Romero AA, Krammerer-Doak N, et al.** Abdominal hysterectomy for the enlarged myomatous uterus compared with vaginal hysterectomy with morcellation. *Am J Obstet Gynecol* 2003;189:1579–1583.

55. **Payne TN, Dauterive R.** A comparison of total laparoscopic hysterectomy to robotically assisted hysterectomy: surgical outcomes in a community practice. *J Minim Invasive Gynecol* 2008;15:286–291.

56. **Gaia G, Holloway RW, Santoro L, et al.** Robotic-Assisted hysterectomy for endometrial cancer compared with traditional laparoscopic and laparotomy approaches. *Obstet Gynecol* 2010;116:1422–1431.

57. **Lenihan JP, Kovanda C, Seshadri-Kreaden U.** What is the learning curve for robotic assisted gynecologic surgery? *J Minim Invasive Gynecol* 2008;15:589–594.

58. **Pasic RP, Rizzo JA, Fang H, et al.** Comparing robot-assisted with conventional laparoscopic hysterectomy: Impact on cost and clinical outcomes. *J Minim Invasive Gynecol* 2010;17:729–738.

59. **Hur HC.** Vaginal cuff dehiscence after hysterectomy. *Up to Date* 2010. Available online at: http://www.uptodate.com/contents/vaginal-cuff-dehiscence-after-hysterectomy

60. **Kho RM, Akl MN, Cornella JL, et al.** Incidence and characteristics of patients with vaginal cuff dehiscence after robotic procedures. *Obstet Gynecol* 2009;114:231–235.

61. **Escobar PF, Starks D, Nickles Fader A, et al.** Single port and natural orifice surgery in gynecology. *Fertil Steril* 2010;94:2497–2502.

62. **Jelovsek JE, Chiung C, Chen G, et al.** Incidence of lower urinary tract injury at the time of total laparoscopic hysterectomy. *JSLS* 2007;11:422–427.

63. **Loos MJ, Scheltinga MR, Mulders LG, et al.** The Pfannenstiel incision as a source of chronic pain. *Obstet Gynecol* 2008;111:839–846.

64. **Hartman KE, Ma C, Lamvu GM, et al.** Quality of life and sexual function after hysterectomy in women with preoperative pain and depression. *Obstet Gynecol* 2004;104:701–709.

25 Robotic Operations

Javier F. Magrina

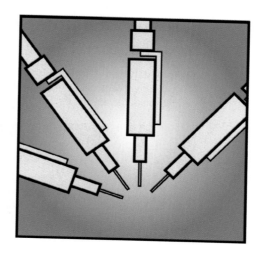

- **Robotic surgery is a form of facilitated laparoscopy that utilizes robotic technology to enhance the performance of the operation by placing a computerized interface between patient and surgeon.**

- **Two of the most important differences between conventional laparoscopic instruments and robotic instruments are articulation and intuitive movements.**

- **The robotic system offers advantages for the surgeon, but it is particularly useful in four circumstances: obese patients, long surgeries, and operations requiring extensive suturing or high precision.**

- **High precision and absence of tremor are useful for retroperitoneal lymphadenectomy, adhesiolysis, parametrial ureteral dissection, and accurate suturing, in such procedures as ureteral anastomosis or reimplantation, and genitourinary fistula repair.**

- **Applications of robotic technology include simple hysterectomy, myomectomy, appendectomy (in conjunction with other procedures), adnexectomy, excision of severe endometriosis, tubal anastomosis, and rectovaginal or vesicovaginal fistulas, especially those in the upper vagina.**

- **Studies show the feasibility of robotics for the treatment of patients with cervical, endometrial, tubal, and ovarian cancer, with apparent similar or better perioperative outcomes compared to laparoscopy and with improved outcomes compared to laparotomy.**

Robotic technology as applied to laparoscopy utilizes robotic technology to facilitate the performance of the operation by placing a computerized interface between patient and surgeon. Although originally designed for cardiovascular surgery and approved for that use by the U.S. Food and Drug Administration (FDA) in 2003, it has found applications in urology and gynecology, and more recently in otolaryngology and colorectal surgery.

There are studies showing that the use of robotic technology for the performance of preset laboratory exercises results in faster performance times, increased accuracy, enhanced dexterity, easier and faster suturing, and a lower number of errors when compared to conventional laparoscopic instrumentation (1–4). The physical stress for medical students learning robotics is significantly less than what they encounter when learning the same tasks by laparoscopy (5). The technological advantages of robotics can facilitate learning surgical techniques when compared to acquiring similar skills in laparoscopy, as demonstrated by a shorter learning curve for robotic surgery. There is a flattening of the operating time after 20 to 50 robotic hysterectomies, while for laparoscopically assisted vaginal hysterectomy (LAVH) a similar facility with the requisite skills does not occur until after 80 procedures (6–9). In gynecologic oncology, a flattening of the operating time was noted after 20 procedures for endometrial cancer when using the robotic technology (10).

Robotic Technology and Differences with Laparoscopy

There is only one robotic system available, brand-named Da Vinci (Intuitive Inc, Sunnyvale, CA), which received FDA approval for the performance of hysterectomy in 2005. A second generation of the device, the Da Vinci S, was released in 2006, and the third generation of the Da

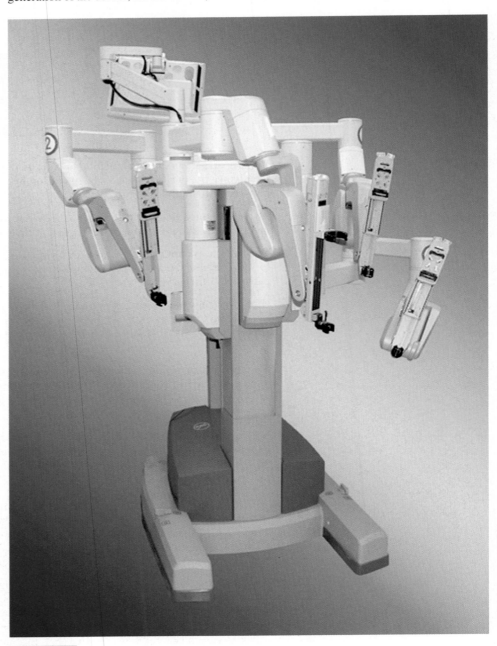

Figure 25.1   Robotic column with robotic arms.

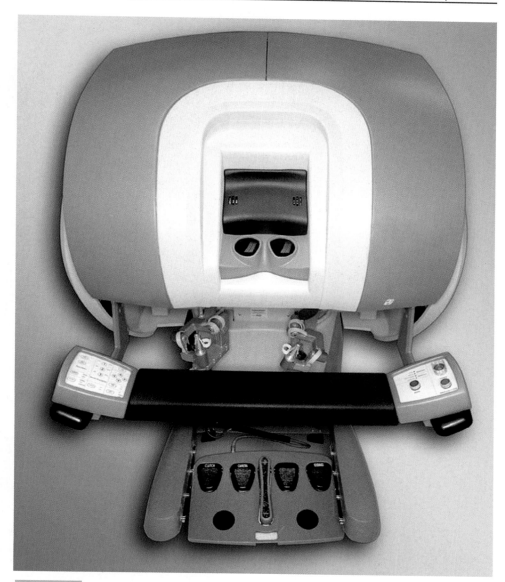

Figure 25.2 Robotic console with hand controls and foot switches.

Vinci robotic system, the SI model, was released in 2009 and incorporates a resident teaching console. A robotic system is composed primarily of a robotic column, which holds the robotic arms (Fig. 25.1) and a surgeon's console (Fig. 25.2). The robotic arms that hold the robotic instruments (Fig. 25.3) are fastened to the robotic trocars (Fig. 25.4). Commonly used robotic instruments for gynecologic surgeries are shown in Figure 25.5A-F.

Robotic Column

The robotic column has three or four robotic arms, depending on the selection at the time of purchase (Fig. 25.1). The fourth arm is extremely useful for assisting with tissue retraction. The robotic arms always function in the direction toward the robotic column and not away from it. For this reason the robotic column must be positioned strategically in response to the location of the surgery that will be performed.

For pelvic surgery the robotic column is commonly situated between the patient's legs (Fig. 25.6), **while for upper abdominal surgery it is positioned at the patient's head. For procedures to the right or left of the abdomen, the robotic column is positioned at the opposite side of the patient.** For instance, for extraperitoneal left aortic lymphadenectomy, the robotic column is at the patient's right side. For procedures where easy access to the entrance of

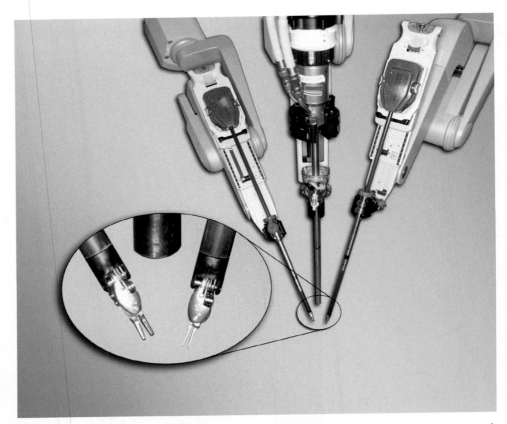

Figure 25.3 **Robotic laparoscope and two robotic arms with robotic instruments inserted.** The tip of the instruments can be appreciated in the insert.

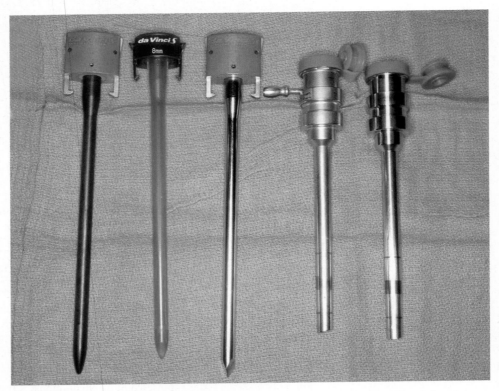

Figure 25.4 **The robotic trocars are metallic and can be seen to the right of the picture.** The escape valve was added because the original trocars did not have it. The three types of available trocar obturators are on the left of the picture: blunt (*left*), tissue-spreading (*middle*) and cutting (*right*).

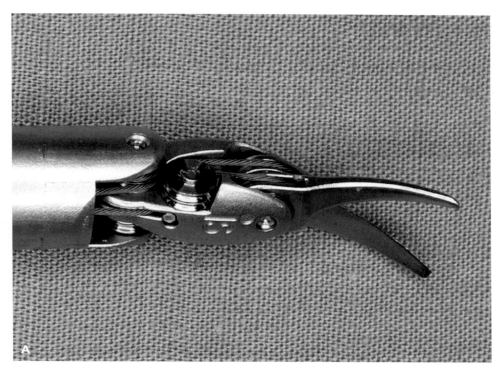

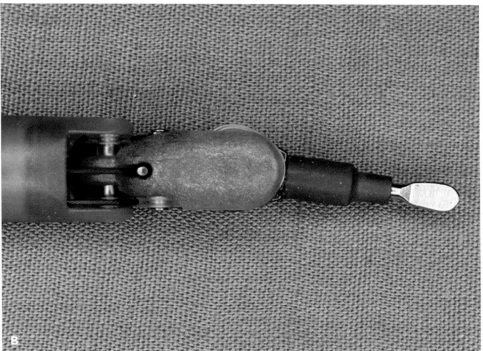

Figure 25.5 **Robotic instruments commonly used in gynecologic surgeries.** A: Monopolar curved scissors. B: Monopolar spatula.

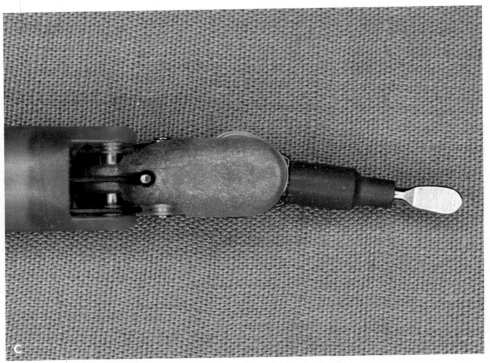

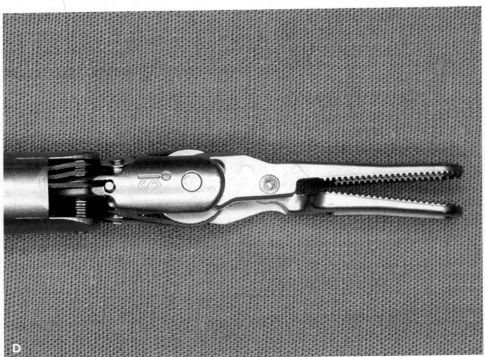

Figure 25.5 *(Continued)* C: PK (plasma kinetic) dissecting forceps, bipolar. D: Prograsp forceps, bipolar.

the vagina and rectum is necessary, the robotic column is positioned lateral to the right or to the left of the patient's legs.

Robotic Console

The surgeon sits at the console (Fig. 25.2) **away from the patient** (Fig. 25.7) **and the assistant sits next to the patient** (Fig. 25.6). **The surgeon has a stereoscopic image, which is different from the laparoscopic image,** and controls the movements of the robotic arms using two hand

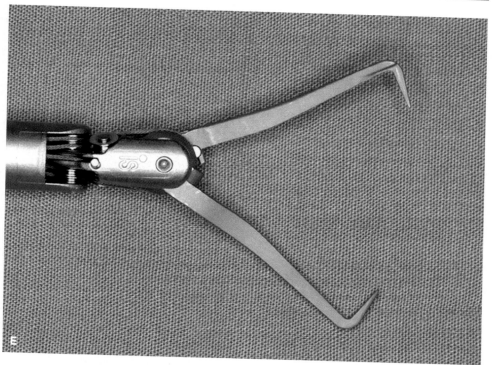

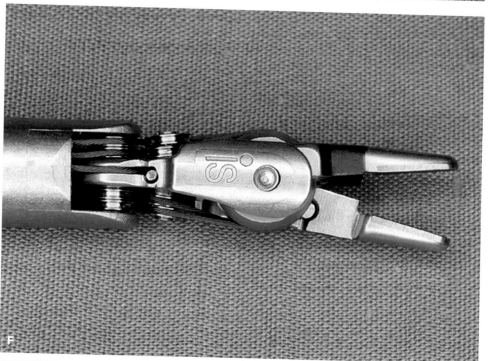

Figure 25.5   *(Continued)* **E:** Tenaculum forceps used for myomectomy. **F:** Needle grasper used for suturing.

controls and five foot switches: clutch, camera, focusing, monopolar (cutting and coagulating), and bipolar. The surgeon's arms and hands can be maintained in a comfortable working position, because pressing the clutch foot switch disengages the robotic arms from the surgeon hands. This allows the surgeon to reposition the arms to an appropriate and comfortable position without moving the portion of the robotic arms connected to the patient.

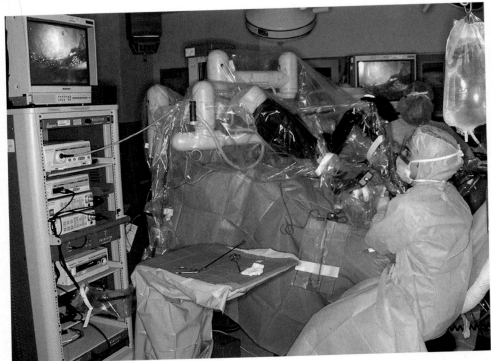

Figure 25.6   **The robotic column is usually positioned between the patient legs for pelvic surgery.** The assistant is seated to the left of the patient and is scrubbed for the procedure.

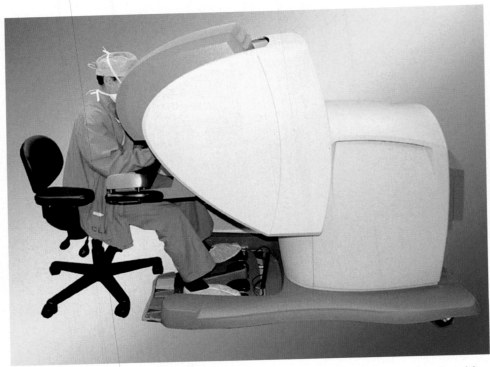

Figure 25.7   **The surgeon is seated at the console and is able to maintain a relaxed position for the arms and legs.**

Because the surgeon is separated from the patient, there is a time delay that permits the performance of telesurgery, as long as the latency time does not exceed 150 milliseconds. The surgeon can control the movements of the robotic arms and instruments in a patient located at a different geographic location (11). Telementoring allows the mentor surgeon to guide another surgeon through a surgical procedure at a remote location by using superimposed electronic signals (telestration), direct voice commands, and control of the laparoscope via joystick and the electrosurgical instruments (12). **Robotic movements are intuitive; the tip of the instrument mimics the movement of the surgeon's hands, in contrast to the experience in laparoscopy when the movements of the tip of the instrument are counterintuitive, opposite to the movements of the surgeon's hands.**

Other technological advantages include downscaling of movements, absence of tremor, and stillness. In laparoscopy the amplitude of movement of the tip of the instrument is the same as the amplitude of the movement of the surgeon's hands, whereas in robotics it can be downsized, resulting in increased precision. **The computerized interface between surgeon hands and robotic instruments eliminates unwanted tremor, increasing precision.** When placed in a specific position, such as for retracting bowel or uterus, the robotic instruments remain in place until repositioned, which can be a difference from human assistance.

The lack of tactile feedback (haptics) is a drawback for the neophyte, but the stereoscopic view rapidly compensates for it. There is a degree of resistance felt at the hand controls of the console, which, coupled with the stereoscopic view, allows the surgeon to determine the consistency of tissues, whether soft or hard, such as "to palpate" the rim of the cervical cup of a uterine manipulator, or "feel" a hard probe introduced in the rectum. The lack of tactile feedback is an advantage when operating in obese patients, because the surgeon cannot feel the resistance of the instruments being inserted through a thick abdominal wall, a difference from laparoscopy.

Another potential advantage of the robotic laparoscopy technique compared to laparoscopy without the assistance of robotics is that it may decrease the number of injuries in surgeons. There are multiple reports of laparoscopic-related surgeon morbidity syndromes, resulting from the unnatural forced position of wrists, fingers, elbows, and shoulders and the awkward standing position of the surgeon (13). A recent study revealed a lower number of surgeon injuries and lower perception of surgeon's pain, numbness, and fatigue using robotics compared to conventional laparoscopy (14).

Instrumentation

Two of the most important differences between conventional laparoscopic instruments and robotic instruments are articulation and intuitive movements. The tip of a laparoscopic instrument is rigid and the instrument only has 4 degrees of freedom. The tip of robotic instruments are articulated with 7 degrees of freedom, reproducing the movements of the human wrist and fingers (Fig. 25.3) (EndoWrist instruments, Intuitive Surgery Inc, Sunnyvale, CA). The articulation allows the performance of complex maneuvers in small spaces; it accommodates the instrument to the correct plane of dissection (instead of forcing the tissue to the direction of the instrument as in laparoscopy), eliminates changing instruments from one port to another as in conventional laparoscopy, and facilitates suturing and intracorporeal knot tying. As indicated above, the movement of the robotic instruments is intuitive, following the movement of the surgeon hands.

Types of Instruments

Robotic instruments useful for gynecological surgery include ProGrasp forceps, PK dissecting forceps, tenaculum forceps, SutureCut needle driver, monopolar curved scissors, and monopolar cautery spatula (Fig. 25.5A-F).

Trocars

The robotic trocars are metallic and have three different types of obturators: blunt, tissue-spreading, and cutting (Fig. 25.4). **The robotic trocars are placed in a different configuration than conventional laparoscopy trocars because of technical limitations imposed by the robotic arms.** They are usually placed at the level of the umbilicus or higher for pelvic surgery and must be 10 cm apart from each other and from the laparoscope to prevent collision of the

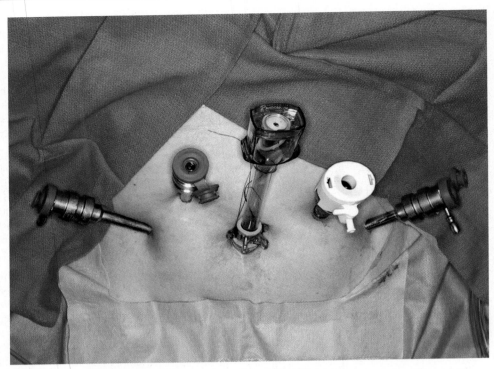

Figure 25.8 **Trocar position for robotic pelvic surgery.** The optical trocar is at the umbilicus. Two robotic trocars are placed 10 cm lateral to the right and left of the umbilicus, respectively. The assistant white trocar is 3 cm cranial and equidistant between the umbilical and left robotic trocar. An additional robotic trocar is 3 cm cranial and equidistant between the umbilical and the right robotic trocar.

robotic arms (Fig. 25.8). At least one assistant trocar is necessary, which must be placed 3 to 5 cm away from any of the other trocars.

Docking

***Docking* is a robotic term defined as the attachment of the robotic arms to the robotic trocars inserted in the patient.** A mean docking time of about 3 minutes was reported in an initial study of 88 patients undergoing robotic hysterectomy (6). Docking times improved progressively after groups of 10 patients each.

Certification and Credentialing in Robotics

There is a mandatory training course of 2 days to obtain certification in robotics provided by the manufacturing company Intuitive, Inc (Sunnyvale, CA) in centers located in the United States, Europe, and Asia. The gynecologist learns the robotic system and logs about 8 hours of dry and animal laboratory tasks. Residents or fellows completing training programs with robotics must demonstrate proficiency with documented basic robotic training and successfully perform a minimum of 10 robotic surgeries, preferably of the same type, and obtain a letter from the program director attesting to their level of robotic proficiency. Credentialing is dependent on each hospital credentialing body and is different for each institution: while some require robotic practice in five animals and having a proctor for the first five robotic surgeries, others mandate having a proctor for only two to five robotic procedures prior to obtaining robotic privileges.

Assistant

An assistant is needed for docking, switching robotic instruments, solving robotic arm collision, retrieving small specimens, retracting tissue, and for the use of instruments not available with robotic technology, such as a vessel-sealing device and suction and irrigation.

The assistant must be trained in robotics and be very knowledgeable about the procedure, because the surgeon is seated in a separate place and not scrubbed.

Teaching Robotics

The robotic teaching console allows the surgeon and the resident or fellow to each have his or her own console while having dual control. The surgeon is able to demonstrate the performance of a specific task to the trainee, or to assist the resident with one robotic arm, or prevent an imminent injury by disengaging the robotic arms from the resident's hands, while both surgeon and resident are seated and viewing the stereoscopic image. The benefits of the teaching console were not compared to standard laparoscopic teaching to evaluate advantages. The half million dollar cost of the teaching console is a large disadvantage.

Previous laparoscopic experience was considered an advantage to learning robotics. Multiple reports show that transitioning from laparotomy to robotics is easier than transitioning from laparoscopy to robotics (15). A large number of gynecologic oncologists and gynecologists incorporated robotics into their daily practice without having incorporated laparoscopy into their practice or performing advanced laparoscopic procedures. In one study the initiation of robotics in a gynecologic oncology program reduced laparotomy from 78% to 35% in the first year of implementation and it increased the number of minimally invasive procedures from 22% performed by laparoscopy to 65% being robotic assisted (15). Thus, robotic technology is relatively easy to use, associated with a short learning curve, and comfortable for the surgeon (15–17). It is less stressful to learn robotics than laparoscopy. Reduced stress and ease of learning with robotics compared to laparoscopy was demonstrated when 16 medical students were exposed to both techniques (5).

Robotic Applications in Benign Gynecology

The robotic system offers advantages for the surgeon, but it is particularly useful in four circumstances: obese patients, long surgeries, and operations requiring extensive suturing or high precision. There is no resistance felt by the surgeon hands to the movement of the robotic instruments, regardless of the thickness of the patient's abdominal wall. Suturing and intracorporeal knot tying are greatly facilitated by the articulation of the robotic instruments. Surgeon's fatigue is decreased when seated for long operations. **High precision and absence of tremor is useful for retroperitoneal lymphadenectomy, adhesiolysis, parametrial ureteral dissection, and accurate suturing, such as for ureteral anastomosis or reimplantation and genitourinary fistula repair. Applications of robotic technology include simple hysterectomy, myomectomy, appendectomy (in conjunction with other procedures), adnexectomy, excision of severe endometriosis, tubal anastomosis, and rectovaginal or vesicovaginal fistulas, especially those in the upper vagina** (1,4). Robotic surgery is associated with a similar or shorter surgical time than conventional laparoscopy for the performance of simple hysterectomy and myomectomy, with a reduced blood loss, complication rates, and hospital stays (2,4).

Hysterectomy

Laparoscopic-assisted vaginal hysterectomy was introduced in 1989. By 2005, only 14% of hysterectomies in United States were laparoscopic (18). By contrast, 3 years after FDA approval of robotic hysterectomy in 2005, 10% of hysterectomies were performed robotically in 2008 (Intuitive, Inc).

A report on 91 patients undergoing a robotic simple hysterectomy demonstrated a mean surgical time of 127.8 minutes, blood loss of 78.6 mL, and hospital stay of 1.4 days. One enterotomy was repaired robotically. There were no conversions to laparoscopy or laparotomy. Postoperative complications included single instances of exacerbation of congestive heart failure, ileus, vaginal cuff abscess, and *Clostridium difficile* colitis (19). **A retrospective comparison of robotic and laparoscopic hysterectomy showed a longer operating time for robotics (27 minutes) but a lower blood loss and shorter hospital stay** (19). Postoperative complications were similar. The conversion rate was higher for laparoscopy compared to robotic operations (9% vs. 4%, respectively).

Myomectomy

Laparoscopic myomectomy provides less morbidity and a shorter recovery time compared to open myomectomy in two prospective randomized studies (20,21). Similarly, robotic myomectomy morbidity and recovery times appear preferable to open myomectomy. In a comparison of both techniques, robotic patients experienced less blood loss, no blood transfusions, lower postoperative complications, and shorter hospital stays. The operating time and cost were increased in the robotic group (22). In an initial series of 35 patients undergoing robotic myomectomy, the mean operating time was 230.8 minutes, mean blood loss was 169 mL, and median hospital stay was 1 day (23). Two patients (8.6%) required conversion to laparotomy, resulting from inadequate robotic instrumentation for myomectomy.

Robotic myomectomy provided comparable perioperative results to laparoscopy in two retrospective studies of patients with symptomatic myomas (24,25). No significant differences were noted between both groups for blood loss, complications, and hospital stay. The robotic operating time was longer than laparoscopy in one of the studies and no different in the other (24,25). In our comparison study, we noted differences favorable to the robotic group relative to operating time (141 vs. 166 minutes), blood loss (100 vs. 250 mL), and hospital stay over 2 days (12% vs. 23%). There were no significant differences between groups when patients were adjusted for uterine size and myoma weight. There were no differences in intra- or postoperative complications. Postmyomectomy pregnancy rates, uterine rupture, and late operative complications using robotics remain undetermined.

Adnexectomy

Numerous studies show the benefits of laparoscopy over laparotomy for patients with an adnexal mass. Robotics provides similar perioperative outcomes when compared to laparoscopy for patients with an adnexal mass. Outcomes were improved with robotics for obese patients (body mass index [BMI] ≥30) with an adnexal mass. In a comparison series of 176 patients with an adnexal mass, 85 operations were by robotics and 91 by laparoscopy (26). The operating time was 12 minutes longer for the entire robotic group (83 vs. 71 minutes), but it was similar to laparoscopy when comparing only patients with a BMI 30 or more (80 vs. 71 minutes). Blood loss was similar for both groups (39.1 vs. 41.2 mL), but lower for the robotic group when comparing only obese patients (BMI ≥30) (39 vs. 60 mL). The length of hospital stay, as measured by the number of patients staying longer than 2 days (0 vs. 3) was similar for both groups.

Tubal Reversal

Robotic tubal reversal may be preferable to laparotomy. In a prospective study comparing both techniques on patients with a previous tubal ligation, the operating time was longer using robotics (201 vs. 155 minutes), but the hospital stay (4 hours vs. 1.3 days), and recovery time to normal activities (11.1 vs. 28.1 days) were improved for robotic patients (27). Both groups had similar pregnancy rates (62.5% vs. 50%). In another retrospective case-control study of outpatient tubal anastomosis performed by robotics or minilaparotomy, perioperative outcomes were similar except for a longer operating time, increased cost, and a shorter time to patient's recovery with robotics (28).

Appendectomy

Reported results on 107 robotic appendectomies performed in conjunction with other pelvic procedures had a mean time for appendectomy of 3.4 minutes. No perioperative complications related to appendectomy were encountered. Increased abnormal pathological findings were observed in patients with pelvic pain compared to those without pain (37% vs. 15%, respectively). Appendiceal metastases were found in 43% of patients with ovarian malignancy (29).

Sacrocolpopexy

The robotic approach to sacrocolpopexy may be better than conventional laparoscopy because of the ease of suturing and of intracorporeal knot tying. A report of feasibility experience with 80 patients demonstrated total operating time of 197.9 minutes, and most patients underwent additional procedures at the same surgical setting (30). There was a 25.4% decrease of the operating time after the first 10 surgeries. Complications were minimal. Other reported operating times are 317 and 328 minutes (31,32).

Robotic sacrocolpopexy may be preferable to laparotomy because of improved perioperative outcomes and similar anatomical results. A comparison of 73 robotic with 105 laparotomy sacrocolpopexies for vaginal and uterine prolapse revealed a longer operating time (328 vs. 225 minutes) but reduced blood loss (103 vs. 255 mL) and shorter hospital stay (1.3 vs. 2.7 days) for the robotic group. Anatomical improvement was similar for both groups as determined by pelvic organ prolapse quantification (POP-Q) C point (−9 vs. −8) (see Chapter 27) (32). Late complications, such as erosion rate and long-term anatomical results of robotic sacrocolpopexy are unknown.

Gynecologic Oncology

Studies show the feasibility of robotics for the treatment of patients with cervical, endometrial, tubal, and ovarian cancer, with apparent similar or better perioperative outcomes, compared to conventional laparoscopy and with improved outcomes compared to laparotomy (33–39). A survey of Society of Gynecologic Oncologists members indicated 24% are regular users of robotics and 66% believed their use would increase (33).

Endometrial Cancer

Laparoscopy provides similar or longer operative times, less blood loss, fewer postoperative complications, shorter hospital stay and recovery times, with similar recurrence and survival rates compared to laparotomy (34–39). Robotic technology may be preferable to conventional laparoscopy in selected patients for surgery for endometrial cancer, especially in morbidly obese patients. In expert hands, the use of minimally invasive techniques—laparoscopy and robotics—may facilitate the operations.

Studies comparing robotics to laparotomy suggest improved perioperative outcomes for robotics. Operative times are similar or longer, blood loss and hospital stay are reduced, the number of lymph nodes is comparable or higher, and postoperative complications are similar or decreased with robotics (15–17,40–44). Studies comparing robotics with conventional laparoscopy for endometrial cancer show similar or superior results for robotics. Some showed reduced blood loss, shorter hospital stay, increased lymph node yield, and lower morbidity with robotics compared to conventional laparoscopy (41). Others reported longer operating time but reduced blood loss, lower transfusion rate, lower conversion rate to laparotomy, and reduced hospital stay, even though the robotic patients had a higher BMI compared to laparoscopy (44). Robotics, as with laparoscopy, resulted in a shorter recovery time for endometrial cancer patients compared to laparotomy (40,45).

In an initial review of 38 patients with robotics operations, the perioperative outcomes were similar to patients treated by laparoscopy (n = 22). Results were similar to patients treated by laparotomy (n = 16) other than a larger blood loss and longer hospital stay for this group of patients. The operating times were similar for the three groups, blood loss was lower for the robotic and laparoscopy groups (283, 222, and 517 mL), and length of hospital stay was shorter for the robotic and laparoscopy groups (2, 2.5, and 6 days). There was no difference relative to the number of lymph nodes removed (18.4, 26.3, and 18.4, for robotics, laparoscopy, and laparotomy, respectively), number of lymph node metastases, positive cytological findings, or tumor recurrence. Postoperative complications were comparable among the three groups.

Boggess et al. compared 103 robotic patients with 81 laparoscopy patients and 138 laparotomy patients (41). The operating times for robotic and laparoscopy procedures were similar, but longer than laparotomy (191.2 minutes, 213.4 minutes, and 146.5 minutes, respectively). The blood loss, hospital stay, and number of nodes were all improved for the robotic group. Bell et al. compared a group of 40 robotic patients with 30 patients operated by laparoscopy and 40 patients operated by laparotomy (40). Robotic and laparoscopy operating times were comparable (184 minutes and 171 minutes, respectively) and longer than laparotomy (108.6 minutes). Blood loss was similar to laparoscopy, and both were lower than the laparotomy group. The number of lymph nodes removed was similar among the three groups. Postoperative complications were lower in the robotic group compared to the other two groups (7.5%, 27.5%, and 20%, respectively).

Another study evaluated the results of robotics and conventional laparoscopy for obese and morbidly obese patients (BMI 30–60) with endometrial cancer (42). Robotics was found to be preferable to the laparoscopic approach because of a shorter operative time, reduced blood loss, increased number of lymph nodes removed, and shorter hospital stay. The benefits of robotics for obese patients was noted with simple robotic hysterectomy, where the operating time remained unchanged in spite of the patient's increased BMI (6). This may result from the absent awareness of the resistance of the robotic instruments being inserted through a thick abdominal wall because of the lack of tactile feedback.

The application of robotics for endometrial cancer can result in improvements of the perioperative outcomes (43). The operating time decreased by 47 minutes, vaginal cuff delayed healing decreased from 16% to 0%, and the number of pelvic and aortic lymphadenectomies and number of nodes retrieved increased per quarter analyzed from the initiation of robotics.

The increased costs of this technology is a criticism of robotics. Because cost is tied to frequency of use, when used on a regular basis the cost becomes similar to laparoscopy and less expensive than laparotomy as a result of shorter hospital stay. A comparison study of costs for robotics, conventional laparoscopy, and laparotomy for endometrial cancer showed a significantly reduced cost for robotics and laparoscopy compared to laparotomy and comparable costs for robotics and laparoscopy (40).

Cervical Cancer

Early Cervical Cancer

Robotic and laparoscopic radical hysterectomy may provide patient benefits over a laparotomy approach relative to blood loss, blood transfusions, and length of hospital stay. Operating times and postoperative complications are lower or similar (46–52). Recurrence and survival rates remain unchanged when comparing the results of both techniques (46–48,51,52). A prospective randomized trial is under way comparing laparoscopic or robotic radical hysterectomy with laparotomy (53).

The surgical technique for robotic radical hysterectomy is described elsewhere (54). A rapid learning curve is noted with robotic radical hysterectomy, with a 44-minute reduction in operating time after the first 34 procedures in association with a low complication rate and high nodal count (55).

In several retrospective studies comparing laparotomy with robotic radical hysterectomy, there was a shorter, similar, or longer operating time; reduced blood loss; shorter hospital stay; lower, similar, or higher number of lymph nodes removed; and similar rate of postoperative complications (49,56–58). In comparison with laparoscopy, robotics is associated with a shorter, similar, or longer operating time; reduced blood loss; shorter hospital stay; similar or lower postoperative complications; and comparable or higher number of nodes (49,50,57).

Tumor recurrence does not appear increased with robotics compared to laparoscopy. At a mean length of follow-up of 31.1 months (range, 10 to 50 months), none of the patients in the robotic group experienced recurrence, and there was no difference with the laparoscopy group (50).

Other Applications of Robotics for Cervical Cancer

Radical parametrectomy is a surgical option for patients with an undiagnosed invasive cervical carcinoma discovered on a simple hysterectomy specimen with negative margins and with no gross visible disease. The feasibility of robotic radical parametrectomy was reported by Ramirez et al. in five patients with acceptable complications (59). There are no comparison studies of robotic radical parametrectomy with laparoscopy or laparotomy.

Radical trachelectomy for cancer of the residual cervical stump is preferable to pelvic irradiation in some patients because of the increased risk of bowel complications from intestinal adhesions to the remaining cervix. The laparoscopic approach is previously reported (60). The use of robotic radical trachelectomy in a patient with a "cut-through" endometrial cancer discovered in the subtotal hysterectomy specimen was reported (61). Radical trachelectomy is an alternative to radical hysterectomy for cervical cancer in young patients desiring fertility and with a tumor size of 2 cm or less, no lymphatic invasion or nodal metastases, and potential for preservation of the upper portion of the cervix. The feasibility of robotic radical trachelectomy was demonstrated in two patients with early stage cervical cancer (62). The operative times were longer (387 and 358 minutes), because of the novelty of the procedure and the required waiting time for the frozen section. No intra- or postoperative complications were observed. There are no comparison studies of robotic radical trachelectomy with laparoscopy or laparotomy. A review of eight reported patients up to May 2009 showed a median operating time of 339 minutes, median blood loss of

62.5 mL, no intraoperative complications, no blood transfusions, no conversions to laparotomy, and a median length of hospital stay of 1.5 days (63). The median number of pelvic lymph nodes removed was 20.

Retroperitoneal Lymphadenectomy for Advanced Cervical Cancer

The laparoscopic approach to pelvic and aortic lymphadenectomy prior to chemoirradiation for patients with advanced cervical cancer is well documented, both transperitoneal and extraperitoneal (64–69). There are many studies discussing robotic pelvic and aortic lymphadenectomy included in the treatment of patients with different types of gynecologic malignancies, including cervical, endometrial, and ovarian malignancies (16,49,50,55–58,70,71).

A novel technique and the results of robotic transperitoneal infrarenal aortic lymphadenectomy in 33 patients with different gynecologic cancers was reported (72). The requirement of this technique was the placement of the robotic column at the patient's head, which mandated the rotation of the operating table 180 degrees after completion of the robotic pelvic operation and the insertion of additional trocars in the lower pelvis (72). The mean console time was 42 minutes, the mean number of nodes 12.9, and the mean number of positive nodes 2.6. There was one conversion to laparotomy caused by bleeding. These results are comparable to those reported with laparoscopic aortic lymphadenectomy. Placing the robotic column at the patient's head and inserting additional trocars in the lower pelvis were requirements to remove the infrarenal aortic nodes with robotics. Previous attempts to remove the left infrarenal aortic lymph nodes in a frozen cadaver were unsuccessful when the robotic column was stationed at the level of the patient's feet.

The feasibility of the extraperitoneal robotic approach to aortic lymphadenectomy was reported (73,74). The development of the robotic extraperitoneal technique in frozen cadavers, successfully applied to a patient with cervical cancer stage IB2 presenting with enlarged left aortic lymph nodes, is reported (73). It was noted that appropriate placement of the robotic trocars and the robotic column is necessary to prevent robotic arm collision and to reach the different aortic lymph nodal areas. The operating, docking, and console times were 103, 3.5, and 49 minutes, respectively. The blood loss was 30 mL. Selective removal of five enlarged aortic lymph nodes revealed no evidence of metastases.

Another study by Vergote et al. reported the development of their technique for inframesenteric aortic lymphadenectomy in five patients (74). All console times were less than 1 hour. The operating times and number of aortic lymph nodes in both studies are within the range of those reported with the laparoscopic approach. Both studies concluded that the robotic approach was technically easier than the conventional laparoscopy procedure (73,74).

Robotic Pelvic Exenteration for Recurrent Cervical Cancer

Robotic anterior pelvic exenteration was described in three patients with recurrent cervical cancer (75). The operating times (range, 480 to 600 minutes) are longer than for laparotomy, but blood loss (range, 200 to 500 mL) is markedly lower. The length of hospital stay was similar or longer than by laparotomy (range, 25 to 53 days). Patients required a pararectal incision (10 cm) for the pouch construction, and one patient with vaginal reconstruction had a perineal phase. Whether the robotic approach to pelvic exenteration will become preferable to laparotomy is unknown.

Ovarian Cancer

Surgery for ovarian cancer requires access to all four abdominal quadrants. The ability to operate in all four quadrants using robotics can only be achieved by rotating the operating table and positioning the robotic column at the patient's head. In this position it is possible to excise the aortic lymph nodes to the level of the renal vessels and to perform resection of upper abdominal metastases, including small bowel, diaphragm, liver, and supracolic omental disease. Initial experience with 21 patients with ovarian cancer who underwent operations by robotics was reported (76). Included were 12 primary, 4 interval, and 5 secondary cytoreductive surgeries for ovarian cancer. In addition to primary tumor excision, major procedures included modified posterior pelvic exenteration, rectosigmoid resection, small bowel resection, diaphragm resection, and resection of liver metastases. The operating times had a wide range (103 to 454 minutes) resulting from the extent of procedures. Blood loss was low (25 to 300 mL). Postoperative complications were low but increased with the number of procedures.

There are reports of robotics for ovarian cancer consisting of an occasional patient included within a series of patients with different types of gynecologic cancers and with no comparison to laparoscopy or laparotomy (77–81). Robotics may be useful for selected patients with ovarian cancer. Because of the need for operating table rotation and the insertion of additional trocars, it may not become widely accepted. The use of the surgical robotic system can be advocated in the case of isolated recurrences of ovarian cancer, such as in the pelvis, or in the upper abdomen, diaphragm, liver, and spleen. Isolated left liver metastases were removed successfully in three patients with recurrent ovarian cancer with no complications (82).

In conclusion, robotics and laparoscopy have advantages compared to laparotomy for selected patients with cervical, endometrial and early ovarian cancer. Although prospective randomized trials are desirable, the retrospective evidence supports the selected use of minimally invasive surgery for endometrial and cervical cancer patients and selected patients with primary or recurrent ovarian cancer.

Complications Unique to Robotics

Because there is no tactile feedback, the robotic arms can injure any organ not under visual control. The potential for injury is higher with the fourth retracting arm when out of the visual field and repositioned without visual control. Constant visual control of the robotic instrument position is mandatory for the prevention of injuries. Collision of the robotic arms is felt as an unwanted resistance, which is realized when the instruments are brought under view.

Constant pressure of the robotic arms on the patient thighs or arms may result in injury. This can be prevented during positioning of the trocars and robotic arms. A rapid move by the surgeon on any robotic instrument may result in hitting the assistant near the operating table with the robotic arm. Moving a robotic arm by anyone other than the surgeon may result in patient internal injury.

Because the robotic trocars are fastened to the robotic arms, and the arms are fixed to the robotic column, any sudden loss of the pneumoperitoneum may result in the instruments being pulled off the anterior abdominal wall as it becomes flattened. Similarly, any sliding of the patient on the operating table as a result of the Trendelenburg position will result in pressure at the trocars site and potential injury or increased postoperative trocar site pain. The robotic column must be positioned at the level of the patient's feet or lateral to the legs in order to prevent access to the vagina, rectum, or urethra.

Disadvantages of Robotics

The present robotic system has limited surgical field reach. It allows for pelvic or abdominal surgery, but not both, unless the robotic column is repositioned from the patient's feet to the patient's head. This repositioning increases surgical time and requires the insertion of additional trocars.

The available robotic instrumentation is appropriate for gynecological surgery, but there is no vessel sealing cutting device or suction-irrigation device. An assistant is necessary, at the surgical site away from the surgeon, and therefore, all orders or corrections are verbal.

Although the grasping pressure of the robotic instruments is high and can damage tissue, tissue traction is not as efficient as with conventional laparoscopic instruments. Because there is no tactile feedback when grasping a tissue, there is only visual control of the traction exerted upon any structure. **The lack of tactile feedback is an advantage in obese patients (see above technology), but can be a disadvantage when the instruments are not in the visual field.**

Cost is a common reason why many institutions have delayed the initiation of robotic programs. The initial purchase of the robotic system is high, about $1.5 million, with an additional annual maintenance fee, and all robotic instruments become functionless after ten uses, so they are disposed.

The robotic column and its arms are bulky, with a total weight of 1,200 lb. An operating room must have adequate space, preferably about 600 square feet. There must be a dedicated team for robotic surgery and preferably a specific team for each surgical specialty. The surgical assistant must be versed in robotic technology and be able to provide the required maneuvers without direct interaction because the surgeon is away at a console and not in a surgical sterile condition.

References

1. **Moorthy K, Munz Y, Dosis A, et al.** Dexterity enhancement with robotic surgery. *Surg Endosc* 2004;18:790–795.

2. **Prasad SM, Prasad SM, Maniar HS, et al.** Surgical robotics: impact of motion scaling on task performance. *J Am Coll Surg* 2004;199:863–868.

3. **Sarle R, Tewari A, Shrivastava A, et al.** Surgical robotics and laparoscopic training drills. *J Endourol* 2004;18:63–67.

4. **Yohannes P, Rotariu P, Pinto P, et al.** Comparison of robotic versus laparoscopic skills: is there a difference in the learning curve? *Urology* 2002;60:39–45.

5. **van der Schatte Olivier RH, Van't Hullenaar CD, Ruurda JP, et al.** Ergonomics, user comfort, and performance in standard and robot-assisted laparoscopic surgery. *Surg Endosc* 2009;23:1365–1371.

6. **Kho RM, Hilger WS, Hentz JG, et al.** Robotic hysterectomy: technique and initial outcomes. *Am J Obstet Gynecol* 2007;197:113.e111–e114.

7. **Kreiker GL, Bertoldi A, Larcher JS, et al.** Prospective evaluation of the learning curve of laparoscopic-assisted vaginal hysterectomy in a university hospital. *J Am Assoc Gynecol Laparosc* 2004;11:229–235.

8. **Lenihan JP, Jr., Kovanda C, Seshadri-Kreaden U.** What is the learning curve for robotic assisted gynecologic surgery? *J Minim Invasive Gynecol* 2008t;15:589–594.

9. **Pitter MC, Anderson P, Blissett A, et al.** Robotic-assisted gynaecological surgery-establishing training criteria; minimizing operative time and blood loss. *Int J Med Robot* 2008;4:114–120.

10. **Seamon LG, Fowler JM, Richardson DL, et al.** A detailed analysis of the learning curve: robotic hysterectomy and pelvic-aortic lymphadenectomy for endometrial cancer. *Gynecol Oncol* 2009;114:162–167.

11. **Anvari M, McKinley C, Stein H.** Establishment of the world's first telerobotic remote surgical service: for provision of advanced laparoscopic surgery in a rural community. *Ann Surg* 2005;241:460–464.

12. **Rodrigues Netto N Jr, Mitre AI, Lima SV, Fugita OE, et al.** Telementoring between Brazil and the United States: initial experience. *J Endourol* 2003;17:217–220.

13. **Reyes DA, Tang B, Cuschieri A.** Minimal access surgery (MAS)-related surgeon morbidity syndromes. *Surg Endosc* 2006;20:1–13.

14. **Gofrit ON, Mikahail AA, Zorn KC, et al.** Surgeons' perceptions and injuries during and after urologic laparoscopic surgery. *Urology* 2008;71:404–407.

15. **Peiretti M, Zanagnolo V, Bocciolone L, et al.** Robotic surgery: changing the surgical approach for endometrial cancer in a referral cancer center. *J Minim Invasive Gynecol* 2009;16:427–431.

16. **DeNardis SA, Holloway RW, Bigsby GEt, et al.** Robotically assisted laparoscopic hysterectomy versus total abdominal hysterectomy and lymphadenectomy for endometrial cancer. *Gynecol Oncol* 2008;111:412–417.

17. **Veljovich DS, Paley PJ, Drescher CW, et al.** Robotic surgery in gynecologic oncology: program initiation and outcomes after the first year with comparison with laparotomy for endometrial cancer staging. *Am J Obstet Gynecol* 2008;198:679.e671–e679.

18. **Jacoby VL, Autry A, Jacobson G, et al.** Nationwide use of laparoscopic hysterectomy compared with abdominal and vaginal approaches. *Obstet Gynecol* 2009;114:1041–1048.

19. **Payne TN, Dauterive FR.** A comparison of total laparoscopic hysterectomy to robotically assisted hysterectomy: surgical outcomes in a community practice. *J Minim Invasive Gynecol* 2008;15:286–291.

20. **Mais V, Ajossa S, Guerriero S, et al.** Laparoscopic versus abdominal myomectomy: a prospective, randomized trial to evaluate benefits in early outcome. *Am J Obstet Gynecol* 1996;174:654–658.

21. **Seracchioli R, Rossi S, Govoni F, et al.** Fertility and obstetric outcome after laparoscopic myomectomy of large myomata: a randomized comparison with abdominal myomectomy. *Hum Reprod* 2000;15:2663–2668.

22. **Advincula AP, Xu X, Goudeau St, et al.** Robot-assisted laparoscopic myomectomy versus abdominal myomectomy: a comparison of short-term surgical outcomes and immediate costs. *J Minim Invasive Gynecol* 2007;14:698–705.

23. **Advincula AP, Song A, Burke W, et al.** Preliminary experience with robot-assisted laparoscopic myomectomy. *J Am Assoc Gynecol Laparosc* 2004;11:511–518.

24. **Bedient CE, Magrina JF, Noble BN, et al.** Comparison of robotic and laparoscopic myomectomy. *Am J Obstet Gynecol* 2009;201:566.e561–e565.

25. **Nezhat C, Lavie O, Hsu S, et al.** Robotic-assisted laparoscopic myomectomy compared with standard laparoscopic myomectomy—a retrospective matched control study. *Fertil Steril* 2009;91:556–569.

26. **Magrina JF, Espada M, Munoz R, et al.** Robotic adnexectomy compared with laparoscopy for adnexal mass. *Obstet Gynecol* 2009;114:581–584.

27. **Dharia Patel SP, Steinkampf MP, Whitten SJ, et al.** Robotic tubal anastomosis: surgical technique and cost effectiveness. *Fertil Steril* 2008;90:1175–1179.

28. **Rodgers AK, Goldberg JM, Hammel JP, et al.** Tubal anastomosis by robotic compared with outpatient minilaparotomy. *Obstet Gynecol* 2007;109:1375–1380.

29. **Akl MN, Magrina JF, Kho RM, et al.** Robotic appendectomy in gynaecological surgery: technique and pathological findings. *Int J Med Robot* 2008;4:210–213.

30. **Akl MN, Long JB, Giles DL, et al.** Robotic-assisted sacrocolpopexy: technique and learning curve. *Surg Endosc* 2009;23:2390–2394.

31. **Daneshgari F, Kefer JC, Moore C, et al.** Robotic abdominal sacro-colpopexy/sacrouteropexy repair of advanced female pelvic organ prolapse (POP): utilizing POP-quantification-based staging and outcomes. *BJU Int* 2007;100:875–879.

32. **Visco AG, Advincula AP.** Robotic gynecologic surgery. *Obstet Gynecol* 2008;112:1369–1384.

33. **Mabrouk M, Frumovitz M, Greer M, et al.** Trends in laparoscopic and robotic surgery among gynecologic oncologists: a survey update. *Gynecol Oncol* 2009;112:501–505.

34. **Magrina JF, Weaver AL.** Laparoscopic treatment of endometrial cancer: five-year recurrence and survival rates. *Eur J Gynaecol Oncol* 2004;25:439–441.

35. **Malur S, Possover M, Michels W, et al.** Laparoscopic-assisted vaginal versus abdominal surgery in patients with endometrial cancer—a prospective randomized trial. *Gynecol Oncol* 2001;80:239–244.

36. **Nezhat F, Yadav J, Rahaman J, et al.** Analysis of survival after laparoscopic management of endometrial cancer. *J Minim Invasive Gynecol* 2008;15:181–187.

37. **Cho YH, Kim DY, Kim JH, et al.** Laparoscopic management of early uterine cancer: 10-year experience in Asian Medical Center. *Gynecol Oncol* 2007;106:585–590.

38. **Magrina JF.** Outcomes of laparoscopic treatment for endometrial cancer. *Curr Opin Obstet Gynecol* 2005;17:343–346.

39. **Magrina JF, Mutone NF, Weaver AL, et al.** Laparoscopic lymphadenectomy and vaginal or laparoscopic hysterectomy with bilateral salpingo-oophorectomy for endometrial cancer: morbidity and survival. *Am J Obstet Gynecol* 1999;181:376–381.

40. **Bell MC, Torgerson J, Seshadri-Kreaden U, et al.** Comparison of outcomes and cost for endometrial cancer staging via traditional laparotomy, standard laparoscopy and robotic techniques. *Gynecol Oncol* 2008;111:407–411.

41. **Boggess JF, Gehrig PA, Cantrell L, et al.** A comparative study of 3 surgical methods for hysterectomy with staging for endometrial cancer: robotic assistance, laparoscopy, laparotomy. *Am J Obstet Gynecol* 2008;199.e361–e369.

42. **Gehrig PA, Cantrell LA, Shafer A, et al.** What is the optimal minimally invasive surgical procedure for endometrial cancer staging in the obese and morbidly obese woman? *Gynecol Oncol* 2008;111:41–45.

43. **Holloway RW, Ahmad S, DeNardis SA, et al.** Robotic-assisted laparoscopic hysterectomy and lymphadenectomy for endometrial cancer: analysis of surgical performance. *Gynecol Oncol* 2009;115:447–452.

44. **Seamon LG, Cohn DE, Henretta MS, et al.** Minimally invasive comprehensive surgical staging for endometrial cancer: robotics or laparoscopy? *Gynecol Oncol* 2009;113:36–41.

45. **Zullo F, Palomba S, Russo T, et al.** A prospective randomized comparison between laparoscopic and laparotomic approaches in women with early stage endometrial cancer: a focus on the quality of life. *Am J Obstet Gynecol* 2005;193:1344–1352.

46. Frumovitz M, dos Reis R, Sun CC, et al. Comparison of total laparoscopic and abdominal radical hysterectomy for patients with early-stage cervical cancer. *Obstet Gynecol* 2007;110:96–102.

47. Holloway RW, Finkler NJ, Pikaart DP, et al. Comparison of total laparoscopic and abdominal radical hysterectomy for patients with early-stage cervical cancer. *Obstet Gynecol* 2007;110:1174–1175.

48. Magrina JF. Robotic surgery in gynecology. *Eur J Gynaecol Oncol* 2007;28:77–82.

49. Magrina JF, Kho RM, Weaver AL, et al. Robotic radical hysterectomy: comparison with laparoscopy and laparotomy. *Gynecol Oncol* 2008;109:86–91.

50. Nezhat FR, Datta MS, Liu C, et al. Robotic radical hysterectomy versus total laparoscopic radical hysterectomy with pelvic lymphadenectomy for treatment of early cervical cancer. *JSLS* 2008;12:227–237.

51. Puntambekar SP, Palep RJ, Puntambekar SS, et al. Laparoscopic total radical hysterectomy by the Pune technique: our experience of 248 cases. *J Minim Invasive Gynecol* 2007;14:682–689.

52. Zakashansky K, Lerner DL. Total laparoscopic radical hysterectomy for the treatment of cervical cancer. *J Minim Invasive Gynecol* 2008;15:387–388.

53. Obermair A, Gebski V, Frumovitz M, et al. A phase III randomized clinical trial comparing laparoscopic or robotic radical hysterectomy with abdominal radical hysterectomy in patients with early stage cervical cancer. *J Minim Invasive Gynecol* 2008;15:584–588.

54. Magrina JF, Kho R, Magtibay PM. Robotic radical hysterectomy: technical aspects. *Gynecol Oncol* 2009;113:28–31.

55. Persson J, Reynisson P, Borgfeldt C, et al. Robot assisted laparoscopic radical hysterectomy and pelvic lymphadenectomy with short and long term morbidity data. *Gynecol Oncol* 2009;113:185–190.

56. Boggess JF, Gehrig PA, Cantrell L, et al. A case-control study of robot-assisted type III radical hysterectomy with pelvic lymph node dissection compared with open radical hysterectomy. *Am J Obstet Gynecol* 2008;199:357.e351–e357.

57. Estape R, Lambrou N, Diaz R, et al. A case matched analysis of robotic radical hysterectomy with lymphadenectomy compared with laparoscopy and laparotomy. *Gynecol Oncol* 2009;113:357–361.

58. Maggioni A, Minig L, Zanagnolo V, et al. Robotic approach for cervical cancer: comparison with laparotomy: a case control study. *Gynecol Oncol* 2009;115:60–64.

59. Ramirez PT, Schmeler KM, Wolf JK, et al. Robotic radical parametrectomy and pelvic lymphadenectomy in patients with invasive cervical cancer. *Gynecol Oncol* 2008;111:18–21.

60. Diaz-Feijoo B, Gil-Moreno A, Puig O, et al. Total laparoscopic radical trachelectomy with intraoperative sentinel node identification for early cervical stump cancer. *J Minim Invasive Gynecol* 2005;12:522–524.

61. Zanagnolo V, Magrina JF. Robotic radical trachelectomy after supracervical hysterectomy for cut-through endometrial adenocarcinoma stage IIB: a case report. *J Minim Invasive Gynecol* 2009;16:655–657.

62. Persson J, Kannisto P, Bossmar T. Robot-assisted abdominal laparoscopic radical trachelectomy. *Gynecol Oncol* 2008;111:564–567.

63. Ramirez PT, Schmeler KM, Malpica A, et al. Safety and feasibility of robotic radical trachelectomy in patients with early-stage cervical cancer. *Gynecol Oncol* 2010;116:512–515.

64. Burnett AF, O'Meara AT, Bahador A, et al. Extraperitoneal laparoscopic lymph node staging: the University of Southern California experience. *Gynecol Oncol* 2004;95:189–192.

65. Gil-Moreno A, Franco-Camps S, Diaz-Feijoo B, et al. Usefulness of extraperitoneal laparoscopic paraaortic lymphadenectomy for lymph node recurrence in gynecologic malignancy. *Acta Obstet Gynecol Scand* 2008;87:723–730.

66. Kehoe SM, Abu-Rustum NR. Transperitoneal laparoscopic pelvic and paraaortic lymphadenectomy in gynecologic cancers. *Curr Treat Options Oncol* 2006;7:93–101.

67. Marnitz S, Kohler C, Roth C, et al. Is there a benefit of pretreatment laparoscopic transperitoneal surgical staging in patients with advanced cervical cancer? *Gynecol Oncol* 2005;99:536–544.

68. Querleu D, Dargent D, Ansquer Y, et al. Extraperitoneal endosurgical aortic and common iliac dissection in the staging of bulky or advanced cervical carcinomas. *Cancer* 2000;88:1883–1891.

69. Tillmanns T, Lowe MP. Safety, feasibility, and costs of outpatient laparoscopic extraperitoneal aortic nodal dissection for locally advanced cervical carcinoma. *Gynecol Oncol* 2007;106:370–374.

70. Fanning J, Fenton B, Purohit M. Robotic radical hysterectomy. *Am J Obstet Gynecol* 2008;198:649.e641–e644.

71. Kim YT, Kim SW, Hyung WJ, et al. Robotic radical hysterectomy with pelvic lymphadenectomy for cervical carcinoma: a pilot study. *Gynecol Oncol* 2008;108:312–316.

72. Magrina JF, Long JB, Kho RM, et al. Robotic transperitoneal infrarenal aortic lymphadenectomy: technique and results. *Int J Gynecol Cancer* 2010;20:184–187.

73. Magrina JF, Kho R, Montero RP, et al. Robotic extraperitoneal aortic lymphadenectomy: development of a technique. *Gynecol Oncol* 2009;113:32–35.

74. Vergote I, Pouseele B, Van Gorp T, et al. Robotic retroperitoneal lower para-aortic lymphadenectomy in cervical carcinoma: first report on the technique used in 5 patients. *Acta Obstet Gynecol Scand* 2008;87:783–787.

75. Lambaudie E, Narducci F, Leblanc E, et al. Robotically-assisted laparoscopic anterior pelvic exenteration for recurrent cervical cancer: report of three first cases. *Gynecol Oncol* 2010;116:582–583.

76. Bandera CA, Magrina JF. Robotic surgery in gynecologic oncology. *Curr Opin Obstet Gynecol* 2009;21:25–30.

77. Diaz-Arrastia C, Jurnalov C, Gomez G, et al. Laparoscopic hysterectomy using a computer-enhanced surgical robot. *Surg Endosc* 2002;16:1271–1273.

78. Field JB, Benoit MF, Dinh TA, et al. Computer-enhanced robotic surgery in gynecologic oncology. *Surg Endosc* 2007;21:244–246.

79. Lambaudie E, Houvenaeghel G, Walz J, et al. Robot-assisted laparoscopy in gynecologic oncology. *Surg Endosc* 2008;22:2743–2747.

80. Reynolds RK, Burke WM, Advincula AP. Preliminary experience with robot-assisted laparoscopic staging of gynecologic malignancies. *JSLS* 2005;9:149–158.

81. van Dam PA, van Dam PJ, Verkinderen L, et al. Robotic-assisted laparoscopic cytoreductive surgery for lobular carcinoma of the breast metastatic to the ovaries. *J Minim Invasive Gynecol* 2007;14:746–749.

82. Choi SB, Park JS, Kim JK, et al. Early experiences of robotic-assisted laparoscopic liver resection. *Yonsei Med J* 2008;49:632–638.

UROGYNECOLOGY AND PELVIC RECONSTRUCTIVE SURGERY

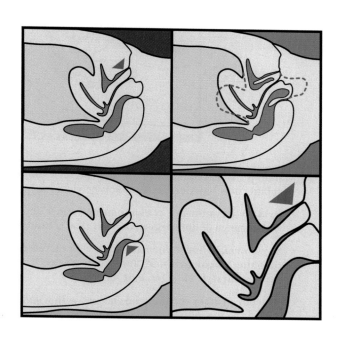

26 Lower Urinary Tract Disorders

Shawn A. Menefee
Ingrid Nygaard

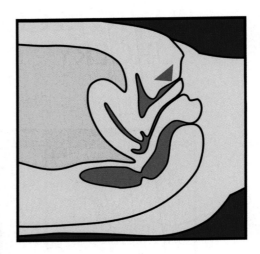

- **Bladder storage and emptying depend on a complex interplay between the brain, spinal cord, bladder, urethra, and pelvic floor.**

- **Urinary incontinence is common in women and generally is treated successfully with a range of nonsurgical and surgical treatments.**

- **Stress urinary incontinence occurs with increases in abdominal pressure (such as coughing, running, lifting) and can be treated with pelvic muscle exercises, vaginal devices, lifestyle changes, and surgery.**

- **Urgency urinary incontinence occurs with a sudden sense of urgency (such as on the way to the bathroom or when washing hands) and can be treated with bladder training, medications, lifestyle changes, and neuromodulation.**

- **Bladder pain remains a challenging and poorly understood entity.**

Physiology of Micturition

The bladder is a complex organ that has a relatively simple function: to store urine effortlessly, painlessly, and without leakage and to discharge urine voluntarily, effortlessly, completely, and painlessly. To meet these demands, the bladder must have normal anatomic support and normal neurophysiologic function.

Normal Urethral Closure

Normal urethral closure is maintained by a combination of intrinsic and extrinsic factors. The *extrinsic* factors include the levator ani muscles, the endopelvic fascia, and their attachments to the pelvic sidewalls and the urethra. This structure forms a hammock beneath the urethra that responds to increases in intra-abdominal pressure by tensing, allowing the urethra to be closed against the posterior supporting shelf (Fig. 26.1). When this supportive mechanism becomes faulty for some reason—the endopelvic fascia has detached from its normal points of fixation, muscular support has weakened, or a combination of these two processes—normal support is lost and anatomic hypermobility of the urethra and bladder neck develops. For many women, this loss of support is severe enough to cause loss of closure during

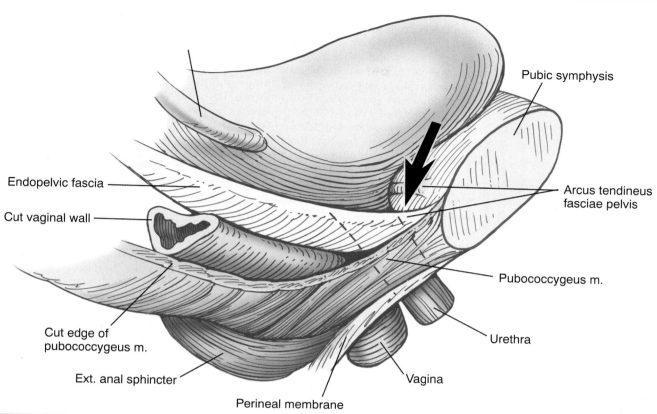

Endopelvic fascia

Cut vaginal wall

Cut edge of
pubococcygeus m.

Ext. anal sphincter

Perineal membrane

Pubic symphysis

Arcus tendineus
fasciae pelvis

Pubococcygeus m.

Urethra

Vagina

Figure 26.1 **Lateral view of the pelvic floor drawn from a three-dimensional reconstruction with the urethra, vagina, and fascial tissues transected at the level of the vesical neck.** Note how the urethra is compressed against the underlying supportive tissues by the downward force (*arrow*) generated by a cough or sneeze. (From **Delancey J.** Structural support of the urethra as it relates to stress urinary incontinence: the hammock hypothesis. *Am J Obstet Gynecol* 1994;170:1718, with permission.)

periods of increased intra-abdominal pressure, resulting in stress incontinence. However, many women remain continent in spite of loss of urethral support (1).

The *intrinsic* **factors contributing to urethral closure include the striated muscle of the urethral wall, vascular congestion of the submucosal venous plexus, the smooth muscle of the urethral wall and associated blood vessels, the epithelial coaptation of the folds of the urethral lining, urethral elasticity, and the tone of the urethra as mediated by α-adrenergic receptors of the sympathetic nervous system.**

Effective urethral closure is maintained by the interaction of extrinsic urethral support and intrinsic urethral integrity, each of which is influenced by several factors (muscle tone and strength, innervation, fascial integrity, urethral elasticity, coaptation of urothelial folds, urethral vascularity). In the clinical setting, damaged urethral support is manifested clinically by urethral hypermobility, which often results in incompetent urethral closure during physical activity and presents as stress urinary incontinence. Intrinsic urethral functioning is more complicated and is not understood nearly as well as incontinence related to loss of urethral support (2).

Clinical appreciation of the importance of extrinsic support and intrinsic urethral function led to the separation of stress incontinence into two broad types:

1. **Incontinence caused by anatomic hypermobility of the urethra**
2. **Incontinence caused by intrinsic sphincteric weakness or deficiency**

Surgical approaches are based on this arbitrary distinction, with a pubovaginal sling recommended for women with intrinsic sphincter deficiency and a colposuspension (also known as retropubic urethropexy) for those with hypermobility. This rationale was based initially on a small study in which women younger than age 50 years with urethral closure pressure less than

20 cm H_2O had a higher failure rate after a Burch colposuspension than did women with a closure pressure greater than 20 cm H_2O (3). No difference in outcome was seen in women older than 50 years. This dichotomy was called into question, based on the observation that all women with stress incontinence have some degree of sphincter weakness, regardless of whether they have hypermobility. **Minimally invasive synthetic midurethral slings have largely replaced pubovaginal slings and retropubic urethropexy as the most commonly performed surgical procedures for stress urinary incontinence.** The use of midurethral slings would seem to lessen the impact of a poorly functioning urethra; however, a similar debate is ongoing about the impact of poor urethral function with both retropubic and transobturator slings. **It appears that women with poor urethral function are more likely to experience treatment failure irrespective of the type of procedure performed** (4).

The Bladder

The bladder is a bag of smooth muscle that stores urine and contracts to expel urine under voluntary control. It is a low-pressure system that expands to accommodate increasing volumes of urine without an appreciable rise in pressure. This function appears to be mediated primarily by the sympathetic nervous system. During bladder filling, there is an accompanying increase in outlet resistance. The bladder muscle (the detrusor) should remain inactive during bladder filling, without involuntary contractions. When the bladder has filled to a certain volume, fullness is registered by tension-stretch receptors, which signal the brain to initiate a micturition reflex. This reflex is controlled by cortical control mechanisms, depending on the social circumstances and the state of the patient's nervous system. Normal voiding is accomplished by voluntary relaxation of the pelvic floor and urethra, accompanied by sustained contraction of the detrusor muscle, leading to complete bladder emptying.

Innervation

The lower urinary tract receives its innervation from three sources: (i) the sympathetic and (ii) parasympathetic divisions of the autonomic nervous system, and (iii) the neurons of the somatic nervous system (external urethral sphincter). The *autonomic nervous system* consists of all efferent pathways with ganglionic synapses that lie outside the central nervous system. The sympathetic system primarily controls bladder storage, and the parasympathetic nervous system controls bladder emptying. The somatic nervous system plays only a peripheral role in neurologic control of the lower urinary tract through its innervation of the pelvic floor and external urethral sphincter.

The sympathetic nervous system originates in the thoracolumbar spinal cord, principally T11 through L2 or L3 (see Chapter 6). The ganglia of the sympathetic nervous system are located close to the spinal cord and use acetylcholine as the preganglionic neurotransmitter. The postganglionic neurotransmitter in the sympathetic nervous system is norepinephrine, and it acts on **two types of receptors: α-receptors, located principally in the urethra and bladder neck, and β-receptors, located principally in the bladder body. Stimulation of α-receptors increases urethral tone and thus promotes closure, whereas α-adrenergic receptor blockers have the opposite effect. Stimulation of β-receptors decreases tone in the bladder body.**

The parasympathetic nervous system controls bladder motor function—bladder contraction and bladder emptying. The parasympathetic nervous system originates in the sacral spinal cord, primarily in S2 to S4, as does the somatic innervation of the pelvic floor, urethra, and external anal sphincter. Sensation in the perineum is also controlled by sensory fibers that connect with the spinal cord at this level. For this reason, examination of perineal sensation, pelvic muscle reflexes, and pelvic muscle or anal sphincter tone is relevant to clinical evaluation of the lower urinary tract. The parasympathetic neurons have long preganglionic neurons and short postganglionic neurons, which are located in the end organ. Both the preganglionic and postganglionic synapses use acetylcholine as their neurotransmitter, acting on muscarinic receptors. **Because acetylcholine is the main neurotransmitter used in bladder muscle contraction, virtually all drugs used to control detrusor muscle overactivity have anticholinergic properties.**

Bladder storage and bladder emptying involve the interplay of the sympathetic and parasympathetic nervous systems. The modulation of these activities appears to be influenced by a variety of nonadrenergic, noncholinergic neurotransmitters and neuropeptides, which fine tune the system at various facilitative and inhibitory levels in the spinal cord and higher areas of the central nervous system (5–7). Neuropathology at almost any level of the neurourologic axis can have an adverse effect on lower urinary tract function.

Micturition

Micturition is triggered by the peripheral nervous system under the control of the central nervous system. It is useful to consider this event as occurring at a micturition threshold, a bladder volume at which reflex detrusor contractions occur. The threshold volume is not fixed; rather, it is variable and can be altered depending on the contributions made by sensory afferents from the perineum, bladder, colon, rectum, and input from the higher centers of the nervous system. The micturition threshold is, therefore, a floating threshold that can be altered or reset by various influences.

The spinal cord and higher centers of the nervous system have complex patterns of inhibition and facilitation. The most important facilitative center above the spinal cord is the pontine-mesencephalic gray matter of the brainstem, often called the *pontine micturition center,* which serves as the final common pathway for all bladder motor neurons. Transection of the tracts below this level leads to disturbed bladder emptying, whereas destruction of tracts above this level leads to detrusor overactivity. The cerebellum serves as a major center for coordinating pelvic floor relaxation and the rate, force, and range of detrusor contractions, and there are multiple interconnections between the cerebellum and the brainstem reflex centers. Above this level, the cerebral cortex and related structures exert inhibitory influences on the micturition reflex. Thus, the upper cortex exerts facilitative influences that release inhibition, permitting the anterior pontine micturition center to send efferent impulses down the complex pathways of the spinal cord, where a reflex contraction in the sacral micturition center generates a detrusor contraction that causes bladder emptying.

A normal lower urinary tract is one in which the bladder and urethra store urine without pain until a socially acceptable time and place arises, at which point voiding occurs in a coordinated and complete fashion. Lower urinary tract disorders include disorders of storage (such as urinary incontinence), emptying (such as urinary hesitancy and retention), and sensation (such as urgency or pain). Current definitions for these disorders are depicted in Table 26.1.

Urinary Incontinence

Definitions

Defining urinary incontinence would seem an easy task: women who leak urine must be "incontinent." **A joint report from the International Urogynecological Association and the International Continence Society made recommendations on the terminology of female pelvic floor dysfunction in an attempt to update the definitions by a female-specific approach and clinically based consensus. This report defined incontinence as "the complaint of any involuntary leakage of urine"** (8). This definition does not take into account the wide variation in this symptom and the disruption it causes. For example, half of young nulliparous women report occasional minor urine leakage; for most this is neither a bother nor a symptom for which they would seek treatment. At the other extreme, 5% to 10% of adult women have severe leakage daily. These women often dramatically alter their lives because of leakage, curtailing activities, social outings, and intimacy. Many suffer marked deterioration in self-esteem. In between these two extremes lies another one-third of adult women who report leakage at least weekly, but without the same degree of life-altering severity as the women previously noted.

Collectively, these women assume a substantial cost burden. The total annual cost to care for patients with incontinence in the United States is estimated at $11.2 billion in the community and $5.2 billion in nursing homes (9). In the United States, much of this cost is borne directly by women in the form of incontinence pads and excess laundry costs. Despite the burden imposed by leakage, many women do not discuss this symptom with a health care professional. For some women, this is because the leakage does not bother them, whereas others are embarrassed and suffer in silence. Still others do not raise this issue because they mistakenly believe the only treatment option is surgical. It is incumbent on the provider to ask women about leakage.

Studies show that there is little relationship between the volume of urine lost and the distress that it causes a patient (10). The degree to which women are bothered by leakage is influenced by various factors, including cultural values and expectations regarding urinary continence and incontinence. **If the leakage is distressing to the patient, evaluation and treatment should be offered. Incontinence can almost always be improved and frequently can be cured, often using relatively simple, nonsurgical interventions.**

Table 26.1 Classification and Definition of Lower Urinary Symptoms in Women

I. Abnormal Storage	Symptoms and Signs
Incontinence (symptom)	Any involuntary leakage of urine
Stress urinary incontinence (symptom)	Involuntary leakage on effort or exertion, or on sneezing or coughing
Stress urinary incontinence (sign)	Observation of involuntary leakage from the urethra, synchronous with exertion/effort, or sneezing or coughing
Urgency urinary incontinence (symptom)	Involuntary loss of urine associated with urgency
Mixed incontinence	Involuntary loss of urine associated with urgency and also with effort or physical exertion or on sneezing or coughing
Continuous urinary incontinence	Continuous involuntary loss of urine
Frequency	Number of voids per day, from waking in the morning until falling asleep at night
Increased daytime urinary frequency	Micturition occurs more frequently during waking hours than previously deemed normal by women (traditionally defined as more than seven episodes)
Nocturia	Interruption of sleep one or more times because of the need to micturate (each void is preceded and followed by sleep)
Nocturnal enuresis	Involuntary loss of urine that occurs during sleep
Urgency	Sudden, compelling desire to pass urine, which is difficult to defer
Postural urinary incontinence	Involuntary loss of urine associated with change of body position, for example, rising from a seated or lying position
Insensible urinary incontinence	Urinary incontinence where the women has been unaware of how it occurred
Coital incontinence	Involuntary loss of urine with coitus. This symptoms might be further divided into that occurring with penetration or intromission and that occurring at organism.
Overactive bladder syndrome (OAB)	Urinary urgency, usually accompanied by frequency and nocturia, with or without urgency urinary incontinence, in the absence of urinary tract infection or other obvious pathology
II. Abnormal Sensory Symptoms	
Increased bladder sensation	Desire to void during bladder filling occurs earlier or is more persistent from that previous experienced (differs from urgency by the fact that micturition can be postpone despite the desire to void)
Reduced bladder sensation	Definite desire to void occurs later than that previously experienced, despite an awareness that the bladder is filling
Absent bladder sensation	Absence of the sensation of bladder filling and a definite desire to void
III. Abnormal Emptying	
Hesitancy	Delay in initiating micturition
Straining to void	Need to make an intensive effort (by abdominal straining, Valsalva or suprapubic pressure) to initiate, maintain, or improve urinary stream
Slow stream	Urinary stream perceived as slower compared to previous performance or in comparison with others
Intermittency	Urine flow that stops and starts on one or more occasions during voiding
Feeling of incomplete bladder emptying	Bladder does not feel empty after micturition
Postmicturition leakage	Involuntary passage of urine following the completion of micturition
Spraying of urinary stream	Urine passage is a spray or split rather than a single discrete stream
Position-dependent micturition	Requiring specific positions to be able to micturate spontaneously or to improve bladder emptying, for example, leaning forward or backward on the toilet seat or voiding in a semistanding position
Urinary retention	Inability to pass urine despite persistent effort

From **Haylen BT, de Ridder D, Freeman RM, et al.** An International Urogynecological Association (IUGA)/International Continence Society (ICS) Joint Report on the terminology for female pelvic floor dysfunction. *Neurourol Urodyn* 2010;29:4–20, with permission.

Types of Disorders

Stress Urinary Incontinence

Stress urinary incontinence occurs during periods of increased intra-abdominal pressure (e.g., sneezing, coughing, or exercise) when the intravesical pressure rises higher than the pressure that the urethral closure mechanism can withstand. Some advocate the term "activity-related incontinence" in some languages to avoid the confusion with psychological stress (8). Stress urinary incontinence is the most common form of urinary incontinence in women and is particularly common in younger women. Active women are more likely to notice symptoms of stress urinary incontinence. In a survey of 144 collegiate female varsity athletes, 27% reported stress incontinence while participating in their sport (11). The activities most likely to produce urinary loss were jumping, high-impact landings, and running.

Stress incontinence is an interesting "disease" as the same symptoms have varying effects on different women. This condition is best considered in a biobehavioral model that examines the interaction of three variables: (i) the biologic strength of the urethral sphincteric mechanism, (ii) the level of physical stress placed on the closure mechanism, and (iii) the woman's expectations about urinary control. This model explains the enormous variation that exists among the symptoms, the degree of demonstrable leakage, and a patient's response to her stress incontinence. Modification of any one of these factors may influence the patient's clinical status; for example, many patients give up certain physical activities (e.g., running, dancing, aerobics) when they experience stress incontinence. Limiting their activities may eliminate the incontinence problem, but it does so at a certain cost to their quality of life. Other women learn to cope with stress incontinence by adopting new body postures during physical activities that prevent them from leaking or by strengthening their pelvic muscles to compensate for increased exertion. Other women may be profoundly relieved to find out that the small amount of leakage they experience from time to time is not abnormal. In any case, the interaction of these three biopsychosocial factors opens up a variety of strategies for the management of stress incontinence. **Surgical intervention is only one strategy, and it addresses only the biologic competence of the sphincteric mechanism rather than either of the other factors that interact to produce the clinical problem.**

Urgency Urinary Incontinence and Overactive Bladder

Although stress incontinence is the most common type of urinary continence in all women, urgency incontinence is the most common form of incontinence in older women (12). **Urgency urinary incontinence is the involuntary leakage of urine accompanied by or immediately preceded by urgency. The new joint report from the International Urogynecological Association and International Continence Society recommended this symptom be called *urgency urinary incontinence* to differentiate between the normal urge experienced when the bladder is full from the abnormal response that may require treatment.** This is a symptom-based diagnosis; the cause may or may not be detrusor overactivity, based on urodynamic observation characterized by involuntary detrusor contractions during the filling phase.

Women may have other related problems such as urgency, nocturia, and increased daytime frequency. The definition of nocturia is quantifiable: The woman wakes one or more times a night to void (8). Increased daytime frequency occurs when the patient considers that she voids too often. The term *pollakisuria* is used to describe this condition in many countries.

Urgency is the sudden compelling desire to pass urine that is difficult to defer. Most women have experienced these symptoms during times of voluntary delays in voiding or increased fluid intake. However, urinary urgency implies more than just the feeling that all normal women have if they voluntarily delay voiding beyond a reasonable time (8). When a woman presents for treatment, she generally reports an intrusive, bothersome, persistent need to urinate that takes her attention away from other activities. Increased daytime frequency is often brought up as an issue when a woman experiences a change in her own voiding pattern.

There is very little information about what is "normal" in terms of voiding frequency. Overactive bladder (OAB) is frequently defined in studies of pharmacologic agents as more than eight voids per 24 hours, a definition that was based on the 95th percentile of voids in a small sample of Scandinavian women (13). **Data from a broader sample of women in the United States** suggest that the median number of voids per day is eight, and 95% of so-called normal women void 12 or fewer times per day (14).

Overactive detrusor function is defined as a urodynamic diagnosis characterized by involuntary detrusor contractions during the filling phase, which may be spontaneous or provoked. It is divided into *neurogenic detrusor overactivity, resulting from a relevant neurologic condition* and *idiopathic detrusor overactivity, when there is no clear cause* (15).

The term *overactive bladder syndrome* is defined as urinary urgency, usually accompanied by frequency and nocturia, with or without urgency urinary incontinence, in the absence of urinary tract infection or other obvious pathology (8). It is often referred to as *OAB-dry* when women with these symptoms do not leak urine, and *OAB-wet* when it is accompanied by incontinence. It is important to note that a woman with severe urgency and a sense of impending leakage who remains dry may have the exact same bladder pathology as one with severe urgency and concomitant leakage. A woman with a strong urethral sphincteric mechanism may be able to avoid leakage during uninhibited bladder contractions, and although one with a strong sphincter may remain dry, she still may be disturbed by the urgency and impending sense of leakage.

Mixed Incontinence

As implied by the name, women with mixed incontinence have symptoms of both stress and urge urinary incontinence. Younger women are more likely to have stress incontinence alone, whereas in older women mixed and urge incontinence predominate. In a review of 15 population-based studies of women of all ages with urinary incontinence, a median of 49% (range 24% to 75%) had stress urinary incontinence, 21% (range 7% to 49%) had urge urinary incontinence, and 29% (range 11% to 61%) had mixed urinary incontinence (16).

Functional and Transient Incontinence

Functional incontinence is more common in elderly women and refers to incontinence that occurs because of factors unrelated to the physiologic voiding mechanism. A woman who cannot get to the bathroom quickly enough may often become incontinent. Functional incontinence can be related to such factors as decreased mobility, musculoskeletal pain, or poor vision. Factors leading to transient urinary incontinence are, as the name implies, medically reversible conditions. A useful mnemonic to help remember these factors is DIAPPERS (17,18) (Table 26.2). These factors argue strongly for the inclusion of a thorough medical evaluation as part of the workup of any patient with urinary incontinence.

Extraurethral Incontinence

Although most urinary incontinence represents unwanted urine loss through the urethra (transurethral incontinence), urine loss can also occur through abnormal openings. These openings can be created by congenital defects or some form of trauma. The congenital causes of urinary incontinence are not common and usually are easy to diagnose. The most extreme cases are caused by *bladder exstrophy,* in which there is a congenital absence of the lower anterior abdominal wall and anterior portion of the bladder, resulting in the entire bladder opening directly

Table 26.2 Reversible Causes of Incontinence
D Delirium
I Infection
A Atrophic urethritis and vaginitis
P Pharmacologic causes
P Psychological causes
E Excessive urine production
R Restricted mobility
S Stool impaction

From **Resnick NM, Yalla SV.** Management of urinary incontinence in the elderly. *N Engl J Med* 1985;313: 800–805, with permission.

to the outside (19). Such cases are diagnosed at birth. Before the advent of modern reconstructive surgery, these infants usually died very early in life from sepsis.

Ectopic ureter, a subtle congenital anomaly causing extraurethral urine loss, generally is detected early in life, but occasionally may escape detection until adolescence or early adulthood (20). In infancy, an ectopic ureter should be suspected when a mother seeks care for her baby, whom she says is never dry. Normally, infants have periods of dryness interspersed with periods of wetness. Most commonly, the ectopic ureter drains into the vagina, but occasionally, it may drain into the urethra distal to the point of continence. This condition can be diagnosed by excretory urography.

A traumatic opening between the urinary tract and the outside is called a *fistula*. Vesico-vaginal fistulas, located between the bladder and urethra, are most common, but fistulas may occur between the vagina, uterus, or bowel, and the urethra, ureter, or bladder.

Worldwide, the most common cause of vesicovaginal fistulas is obstructed labor. This was true in the Western world 150 years ago, but advances in the provision of basic obstetric services and advanced obstetric intervention have virtually eliminated this problem in developed countries.

Obstructed labor can occur in rural areas where girls are married young (sometimes as early as 9 to 10 years of age) and where transportation is poor and access to medical services is limited. In such circumstances, pregnancy often occurs shortly after menstruation begins and before maternal skeletal growth is complete. When labor begins, cephalopelvic disproportion is common and little can be done to correct fetal malpresentations. Women may be in labor as long as 5 to 6 days without intervention, and if they survive, they usually give birth to a stillborn infant. In such cases, the soft tissues of the pelvis are crushed by constant pressure from the fetal head, leading to an ischemic vascular injury and subsequent tissue necrosis. When this tissue sloughs, a genitourinary or rectovaginal fistula develops. Many of these patients have complex or multiple fistulas, involving total destruction of the urethra and sloughing of the entire bladder base (Fig. 26.2). Obstetric fistulas are frequently as large as 5 to 6 cm in diameter.

After such fistulas develop, the lives of these young women (most of whom are younger than 20 years of age) are ruined unless they can gain access to curative surgical services. The constant, uncontrolled dribble of urine makes them offensive to their husbands and family members and they are often ostracized from their families. Most of them eventually become destitute social outcasts—and yet these are otherwise healthy young women. **The social and economic costs of this problem are enormous, yet the world medical community largely ignores it. The morbidity associated with obstetric fistulas remains, along with the related maternal mortality, one of the single most neglected issues in international women's health care.**

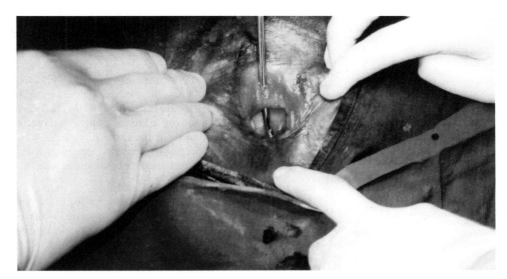

Figure 26.2 **Moderate-sized obstetric vesicovaginal fistula.** A metal probe has been placed through the urethra and is clearly visible through the bladder base. (Copyright Worldwide Fistula Fund, used by permission.)

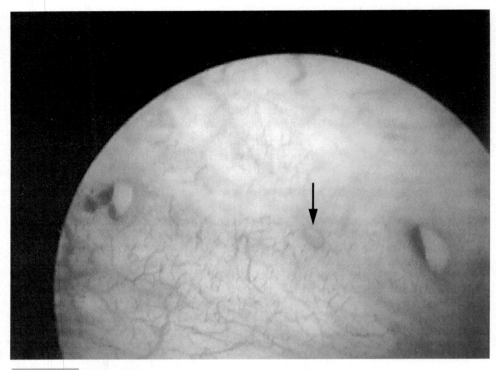

Figure 26.3 **Posthysterectomy fistulas.** Note three small fistulas in a row.

In the industrialized world, **the most common causes of genitourinary fistulas are surgery, malignancy, and radiation therapy, alone or in combination. Most often a vesicovaginal fistula develops after an otherwise uncomplicated vaginal or abdominal hysterectomy in which a small portion of the bladder was inadvertently trapped in a surgical clamp or was transfixed by a suture.** These fistulas most often occur at the vaginal apex and are no larger than 1 to 2 mm. The amount of urine that can leak through a fistula of any size, however, is enormous. Figure 26.3 shows a cystoscopic view of three small vesicovaginal fistulae, lined up where the cuff suture line would have been. With traditional vaginal and abdominal hysterectomy, many surgeons recommend universal cystoscopy at the completion of the surgical case to assess for urinary tract injury and potentially decrease the incidence of urinary tract fistula. A review of 839 patients undergoing hysterectomy for benign disease followed by universal cystoscopy at completion of the procedure revealed lower urinary tract injury in 4.3%, including bladder injury in 2.9% and ureteral injury in 1.8% (21).

With the increase in minimally invasive techniques for pelvic surgery, including hysterectomy, the use of electrocautery devices is commonplace. This more frequent use of electrocautery for ligation of vessels and the resulting thermal spread increases concern about the possibility of ureteral damage that may lead to ureterovaginal fistula. **When significant urine leakage occurs, often 10 to 14 days following a laparoscopic hysterectomy, ureterovaginal fistula should be strongly considered in the differential diagnosis.** As with abdominal and vaginal surgery, careful attention to the location of the ureter, especially in proximity to the uterine arteries, must be a standard precaution. The incidence of ureterovaginal fistula after laparoscopic hysterectomy appears to be 1% to 4% (22).

Although rare, vesicouterine fistulas are increasing in incidence as the rate of cesarean deliveries increases. Such fistulas are almost always associated with repeat cesarean deliveries. **The classic triad of vaginal urinary leakage, cyclic hematuria, and amenorrhea is known as Youssef's syndrome** (23).

Nocturia

Nocturia is the number of voids recorded during a night's sleep; each void is preceded and followed by sleep. To sort out whether nocturia results from heightened urine production at night, the nocturnal urinary volume can be assessed from a bladder chart. Nocturnal urinary volume is defined as the total volume of urine passed between the time the woman goes to bed with the intention of sleeping and the time of waking with the intention of rising. Thus, it excludes the last void before going to bed but includes the first void after rising in the morning. Nocturia can be the result of nocturnal polyuria potentially related to delayed mobilization of fluid especially in the elderly, sleep problems (e.g., sleep apnea), or low volume voids. Nocturnal polyuria is present when an increased proportion of the 24-hour output occurs at night.

Risk Factors for Urinary Incontinence

Most of the data about risk factors for urinary incontinence come from clinical trials or cross-sectional studies using survey design. Some risk factors were more rigorously studied than others. Thus, the information available is limited in its general applicability and one cannot infer causality from it. Despite these limitations, **there is some evidence that age, pregnancy, childbirth, obesity, functional impairment, and cognitive impairment are associated with increased rates of incontinence or incontinence severity** (16). Some factors pertain more to certain age groups than others. For example, in studies of older women, childbirth no longer increases the risk of incontinence, possibly because of the presence of comorbidities and other factors that promote incontinence. Medical diagnoses that were associated with urinary incontinence include diabetes, strokes, and spinal cord injuries. Other factors about which less is known or findings are contradictory include hysterectomy, constipation, occupational stressors, smoking, and genetics.

Pregnancy and delivery predispose women to stress urinary incontinence, at least during their younger years. Of women who have not borne children, those who are pregnant leak more often than their nonpregnant counterparts; about half of women report symptoms of stress urinary incontinence during pregnancy, but in most, the symptom resolves after delivery. In a prospective study, 32% of 305 primiparas developed stress urinary incontinence during pregnancy and 7% after delivery. By 1 year, only 3% reported stress urinary incontinence (24). However, 5 years later, 19% of women with no symptoms after the first delivery had stress urinary incontinence. Of women reporting stress urinary incontinence 3 months postpartum (in most of whom it had resolved by 1 year), 92% had such leakage 5 years later. Transient postpartum leakage may be a marker for future incontinence.

Various changes happen after delivery that may predispose women to stress urinary incontinence. Levator ani muscle strength decreases (25). **About 20% of women develop a visible defect in the levator ani muscles after vaginal delivery** (26). **The bladder neck descends, and the pelvic muscles undergo partial denervation with pudendal neuropathy** (27). **In most studies, parity is strongly associated with urinary incontinence in younger women** (28). **In studies of women 60 years and older, parity is no longer an independent risk factor for incontinence** (29). The reason for this is not well elucidated, but it may be because the changes in muscle, nerve, connective tissue, and hormonal function that occur with aging make other women "catch up" to those who developed incontinence at a younger age because of delivery trauma. Alternately, it may be that medical problems more common in older women account for a larger proportion of incontinence risk as women age.

Obesity deserves special mention for its role in causing or exacerbating stress incontinence. Many researchers report an association (that remains after adjusting for age and parity) between increased weight and body mass index (BMI) and urinary incontinence. For example, a dose–response relationship between BMI and severe urinary incontinence was described (30). Compared with women with a BMI less than 25 kg/m^2, odds ratios (OR) for the following BMI groups were: 25 to 29, OR 2.0 (range 1.7–2.3); 30 to 34, OR 3.1 (2.6–3.7); 35 to 39, OR 4.2 (3.3–5.3); 40+ 5.0 (3.4–7.3). A prospective randomized study evaluating overweight and obese women with at least 10 urinary incontinence episodes per week undergoing an intensive 6-month weight-loss program versus structured education program found that women in the weight-loss program had a mean weight loss of 8.0% and decreased their leakage episodes by 47% compared to mean weight loss of 1.6% and 28% reduction in leakage episodes in the education program group (31).

Initial Evaluation

The initial evaluation of patients with incontinence requires a systematic approach to consider possible causes. The basic evaluation should include the following items: history (including assessment of quality of life and degree of bother from symptoms), physical examination, and simple primary care level tests. Most women can begin nonsurgical treatment after this basic evaluation.

History

A thorough medical history should be obtained from every incontinent patient. The history should include a review of symptoms, general medical history, review of past surgery, and current medications. The woman's most troubling symptoms must be ascertained—how often she leaks urine, how much urine she leaks, what provokes urine loss, what improves or worsens the problem, and what treatment (if any) she had in the past. It is essential to keep the patient's chief symptom at the forefront to avoid inappropriate management. Consider, for example, a woman whose chief concern is that once a month, while leading a business seminar, she has a sudden, overwhelming urge to void followed by complete bladder emptying. She finds this leakage devastating and is considering quitting her job because of her acute embarrassment. On occasion, she leaks a few drops of urine during exercise, but this minor leakage does not bother her. During the evaluation, urodynamics reveal minimal stress urinary incontinence at capacity during strong coughing. No detrusor overactivity is seen. The patient is offered, and undergoes, a surgical procedure for her documented urodynamic stress incontinence. Not surprisingly, her chief symptom is not improved and she is devastated.

The general medical history may reveal systemic illnesses that have a direct bearing on urinary incontinence, such as diabetes mellitus (which produces osmotic diuresis if glucose control is poor), vascular insufficiency (which can lead to incontinence at night when peripheral edema is mobilized into the vascular system, resulting in increased diuresis), chronic pulmonary disease (which can lead to stress incontinence from chronic coughing), or a wide variety of neurologic conditions that can affect the neurourologic axis at any point from the cerebral cortex to the peripheral nervous system. Medications that may affect the lower urinary tract are summarized in Table 26.3 (32–35).

Quality-of-Life Measures

Physicians caring for incontinent women should ask them about the way the incontinence specifically affects their lives and to what degree the incontinence bothers them. There often is discord between the objective symptom severity and subjective bother. Only by understanding each woman's situation can treatment be appropriately planned and response evaluated. Some women may be completely satisfied if they are able to sit through a movie without running to the bathroom, even if they leak urine at other times. Others may be satisfied only if they are 100% dry. Given that the latter is likely an unrealistic goal, knowing that the patient feels this way gives the provider the opportunity to educate her about the likely outcome of treatment.

Physicians may use one of several well-designed, validated quality-of-life measures. An expert summary of the literature in this area conducted for the International Consultation on Incontinence recommended the instruments summarized in Table 26.4. These instruments were found to be valid, reliable, and responsive to change following standard psychometric testing.

Table 26.3 Medications that May Affect the Urinary Tract

1. Sedatives such as the benzodiazepines may cause confusion and secondary incontinence, particularly for elderly patients.

2. Alcohol may have similar effects to benzodiazepines and also impairs mobility and causes diuresis.

3. Anticholinergic drugs may impair detrusor contractility and may lead to voiding difficulty and overflow incontinence. Drugs with anticholinergic properties are widespread and include antihistamines, antidepressants, antipsychotics, opiates, antispasmodics, and drugs used to treat Parkinson's disease.

4. α-Agonists, which are often found in over-the-counter cold remedies, increase outlet resistance and may lead to voiding difficulty.

5. α-Blockers, sometimes used to treat hypertension (e.g., *prazosin, terazosin*), may decrease urethral closure pressure and lead to stress incontinence.

6. Calcium-channel blockers may reduce bladder smooth muscle contractility and lead to voiding problems or incontinence; they may also cause peripheral edema, which may lead to nocturia or nighttime urine loss.

7. Angiotensin-converting enzyme inhibitors may result in a chronic and bothersome cough that can result in increasing stress urinary incontinence in an otherwise asymptomatic patient.

Table 26.4 Questionnaires to Assess Urinary Incontinence

The following questionnaires have been recommended by the International Consultation on Incontinence to assess symptoms of incontinence and impact of incontinence on quality of life in women.[a]

Symptoms

Urogenital Distress Inventory.
Shumaker SA, Wyman JF, Uebersax JS, et al. Health-related quality of life measures for women with urinary incontinence: the Incontinence Impact Questionnaire and the Urogenital Distress Inventory. *Qual Life Res* 1994;3:291–306.

Urogenital Distress Inventory (UDI)-6 (short form).
Uebersax JS, Wyman JF, Shumaker SA, et al. Short forms to assess life quality and symptom distress for urinary incontinence in women: the incontinence impact questionnaire and the urogenital distress inventory. *Neurourol Urodyn* 1995;14:131–139.

Urge-UDI.
Lubeck DP, Prebil LA, Peebles P, et al. A health related quality of life measure for use in patient with urge urinary incontinence: a validation study. *Qual Life Res* 1999;1999: 337–344.

King's Health Questionnaire.
Kelleher CJ, Cardozo LD, Khullar V, et al. A new questionnaire to assess the quality of life of urinary incontinent women. *Br J Obstet Gynaecol* 1997;104:1374–1379.

Incontinence Severity Index.
Sandvik H, Hunskaar S, Seim A, et al. Validation of a severity index in female urinary incontinence and its implementation in an epidemiological survey. *J Epidemiol Community Health* 1993;47:497–499.

Quality of Life

Quality of life in persons with urinary incontinence (I-QOL).
Wagner TH, Patrick DL, Bavendam TG, et al. Quality of life of persons with urinary incontinence: development of a new measure. *Urology* 1996;47:67–72.

Incontinence Impact Questionnaire.
Wyman JF, Harkins SW, Taylor JR, et al. Psychosocial impact of urinary incontinence in women. *Obstet Gynecol* 1987;70:378–381.

Incontinence Impact Questionnaire (IIQ)-7 (short form).
Uebersax JS, Wyman JF, Shumaker SA, et al. Short forms to assess life quality and symptom distress for urinary incontinence in women. The incontinence impact questionnaire and the urogenital distress inventory. *Neurourol Urodyn* 1995;14:131–139.

Urge-IIQ.
Lubeck DP, Prebil LA, Peebles P, et al. A health related quality of life measure for use in patient with urge urinary incontinence: a validation study. *Qual Life Res* 1999;1999: 337–344.

[a]**Donovan JL, Badia X, Corcos J, et al.** Symptom and quality of life assessment. In: **Abrams P, Cardozo L, Khoury J, et al., eds.** *Incontinence.* Plymouth, UK: Plymbridge Distributors, 2002.

Physical Examination

The physical examination of the patient with incontinence should focus on general medical conditions that may affect the lower urinary tract and problems related to urinary incontinence. Such conditions include cardiovascular insufficiency, pulmonary disease, occult neurologic processes (e.g., multiple sclerosis, stroke, Parkinson's disease, and anomalies of the spine and lower back), abdominal masses, and mobility. Key factors to assess during the physical examination are summarized in Table 26.5. **A cotton swab test has poor predictive value for determining either stress urinary incontinence diagnosis or predicting treatment success** (36). It is used by some clinicians to determine movement of the anterior vaginal wall with Valsalva. A woman with a fixed nonmobile urethra is a poor candidate for a surgery (such as a Burch colposuspension) designed to elevate the urethra. It is not possible to increase support for an already well-supported urethra.

Table 26.5 Physical Examination of a Woman with Lower Urinary Tract Dysfunction
Neurologic
Mental status
Perineal sensation
Perineal reflexes
Patellar reflexes
Abdominal examination
Masses
Cardiovascular
Congestive heart failure
Lower extremity edema
Mobility
Gait assessment
Pelvic examination
Prolapse
Atrophy
Levator muscle palpation (symmetry, ability to squeeze)
Anal sphincter function
Test of urethral mobility (e.g., cotton swab test)

Simple (Primary Care Level) Tests

It is important to realize that formal urodynamics tests are neither the only nor the most important tests of bladder function. Other simple tests that can be performed in the primary care setting provide useful information to guide patient care.

Voiding Diary

A frequency/volume bladder chart (often termed a "bladder diary") is an invaluable aid in the evaluation of patients with urinary incontinence. A frequency/volume chart is a voiding record kept by the patient for several days. Patients are instructed to write down the time of every void on the chart and measure the amount of urine voided. The time of any incontinent episodes, and the specific activities associated with urine loss, should be recorded. If desired, the patient can be instructed to keep a record of fluid intake. Although the type of intake may guide management suggestions, in most cases volume of intake can be estimated with some accuracy from the amount of urine produced.

A frequency/volume bladder chart provides vital information about bladder function that is not provided by formal urodynamics studies: 24-hour urinary output, the total number of daily voids, number of nighttime voids, the average voided volume, and the functional bladder capacity (largest volume voided in normal daily life). This information allows the clinician to confirm reports of urinary frequency with objective data and to determine whether part of the patient's problem is an abnormally high (or low) urinary output. The chart can be used to calculate the volume of urine generated in nighttime hours versus daytime hours. Nighttime volume is calculated by adding output from voids that occur after the woman has fallen asleep for the night and the first morning void on awakening for the day. Older women sometimes have a marked shift in urine production, with more than half of their urine output generated during sleeping hours (Fig. 26.4). Demonstrating this on the voiding diary may lead to further treatment options.

Urinalysis

Examination of the urine by dipstick testing and microscopy is done to exclude infection, hematuria, and metabolic abnormalities. **Hematuria cannot be diagnosed on the results of a dipstick test alone; confirmation by microscopic evaluation is mandatory.**

	Urinate in toilet (time and amount)		Accident (time)	Activity during accident	Fluid intake (time, type, amount)
To Bed →	2200	240 cc			1 glass water
	0300	660 cc	0300	Leak on way to bathroom	
	0500	540 cc	0500	Preparing to urinate	
Up For Day →	0700	150 cc			16 oz coffee 1 cup water
	0845	35 cc			
	1145	160 cc			
	1200				16 oz lemonade
	1540	60 cc			
	1800	100 cc			2 glasses wine 2 cups water
	1940	60 cc			16 oz diet coke 1 glass water

Number of pads changed today ___1___
Type of pad used ___Maxi pad___

Figure 26.4   Voiding diary (also called bladder chart). Daytime frequency is seven. The patient has nocturia (gets up to void two times during sleeping hours) and also has nocturnal polyuria (an increased proportion of the 24-hour output occurs at night; note that nighttime urine output excludes the last void before sleep but includes the first void of the morning). She has urge incontinence, likely caused by the relatively larger bladder volumes voided at night, which in turn may be related to her greater fluid, caffeine, and alcohol consumption in the evening.

If a urinary tract infection is documented by microscopy or culture, it is reasonable to see whether urinary tract symptoms improved with eradication of bacteriuria. Occasionally, a simple urinary tract infection causes the onset or exacerbation of urinary incontinence. **Some women, particularly older ones, have asymptomatic bacteriuria that truly is asymptomatic; thus, if attempted treatment of a woman with bacteriuria but without classic urinary tract infection symptoms (such as dysuria, urgency, or frequency) does not improve incontinence, further antibacterial treatment is generally unnecessary.**

If hematuria and bacteriuria are found, the urine should be rechecked after eradication of the bacteriuria. **Hematuria found in the absence of bacteriuria may need further evaluation to rule out kidney or bladder tumors;** the necessity for and extent of the evaluation depends on concomitant risk factors and the clinical presentation. If malignancy is suspected, bladder biopsy should be performed by the surgeon who would treat the patient in the event a malignancy is discovered.

Routine urinary cytology is not helpful, but testing may be of value in women older than 50 years with irritative urinary tract symptoms, particularly if those symptoms are of sudden onset.

Postvoid Residual Volume   **Incomplete bladder emptying may cause incontinence. Patients with a large postvoid residual (PVR) urine volume have a diminished functional bladder capacity because of the dead space occupied in the bladder by retained urine.** This stagnant pool of urine is a source of urinary tract infections because the major defense of the bladder against infection is frequent, nearly complete emptying.

A large PVR volume can contribute to urinary incontinence in two ways. If the bladder is overdistended, increases in intra-abdominal pressure can force urine past the urethral sphincter, causing stress incontinence (sometimes termed "overflow incontinence" in the context of a large

PVR volume). In some cases, bladder overdistention may provoke an uninhibited contraction of the detrusor muscle, leading to incontinence. These conditions may coexist, further complicating the problem.

The PVR volume can be assessed by either direct catheterization or ultrasonography. Although sufficiently accurate for clinical purposes, ultrasonography measurements of PVR volume have a standard error of 15% to 20%. It is reasonable to confirm an elevated PVR volume detected on ultrasound with a catheterized volume (37). It is important to perform this test within 10 minutes of a void to avoid an artificially elevated result because of diuresis. It is agreed that a PVR level less than 50 mL is normal and greater than 200 mL is abnormal, but there is much debate about values in the midrange. Because many women are unable to void well during an anxiety-ridden first visit, it is helpful to recheck the PVR volume at a future visit before embarking on further diagnostic tests. The value of assessing bladder emptying in neurologically normal women who do not have pelvic organ prolapse or symptoms of voiding dysfunction has not been demonstrated.

Cough Stress Test

Patients should be examined with a full bladder, particularly if stress incontinence is a consideration. Urine egress from the urethra at the time of a cough documents stress incontinence. If leakage is not observed when the woman is supine, she should stand with her feet separated and cough several times.

Pad Tests

Weighing menstrual or bladder pads before and after activity provides another objective way to measure urinary leakage. Such pad tests are widely used in patient-oriented research to assess treatment effectiveness, but rarely are they used in clinical practice. Pad tests can be divided into short-term tests, usually performed under standardized office conditions, and long-term tests, usually performed at home for 24 to 48 hours. Pad tests are generally performed with a symptomatically full bladder or with a certain volume of saline instilled into the bladder before beginning the series of exercises. A pad weight gain of 1 g or more is considered positive for a 1-hour test, and a pad weight gain greater than 4 g is positive for a 24-hour test.

Advanced Testing

Urodynamics

At its most basic level, a urodynamic study is anything that provides objective evidence about lower urinary tract function (38). In this sense, measurement of a patient's voided urine volume and catheterization to determine her PVR volume are urodynamic studies. A frequency/volume chart is also a valuable urodynamic study. **Obtaining clinically valuable information does not always require the use of expensive, complex technology. After basic testing, further testing is recommended in the following circumstances: the diagnosis is uncertain (for example, because of major discrepancies between the history, the voiding diary, and symptom scales); surgery is being considered; an elevated PVR volume, a neurologic condition that may complicate treatment (such as multiple sclerosis), marked pelvic organ prolapse, or numerous prior surgical attempts at correction. Bladder and kidney imaging should be considered if the patient has hematuria in the absence of an infection.** Current urodynamic definitions are summarized in Table 26.6.

Uroflowmetry

To assess voiding function, urodynamic testing usually begins with uroflowmetry, a study in which the volume of urine voided is plotted over time. Flow time, peak flow rate, and time to peak flow usually increase as the voided volume increases.

Filling Cystometry

Cystometry is done to assess bladder and urethral function during bladder filling. Simple (or single-channel) cystometry is performed when bladder pressure only is measured during filling. Because the bladder is an intra-abdominal organ, the pressure recorded in the bladder is a combination of several other pressures, most notably the pressure created by the activity of the detrusor muscle itself and the pressure exerted on the bladder by the weight of the surrounding intra-abdominal contents (e.g., uterus, intestines, straining, or exertion). For this reason, the **technique of complex (also called multichannel or subtracted) cystometry is used to try to approximate the actual pressure exerted in the bladder by the activity of the detrusor muscle alone. The detrusor pressure (P_{det}) is obtained by measuring**

Table 26.6 Urodynamic Definitions

I. Bladder sensation

A. *First sensation*	First becomes aware of bladder filling
B. *First desire to void*	Feeling that would lead the person to void at next convenient moment, but voiding can be delayed if necessary
C. *Strong desire to void*	Persistent desire to void without the fear of leakage
D. *Sensation*	Classified as:
	1. Increased
	2. Reduced
	3. Absent
	4. Nonspecific bladder sensations (other symptoms make person aware of bladder filling, like abdominal fullness)
	5. Bladder pain (is abnormal)
	6. Urgency (sudden compelling desire to void)

II. Detrusor function

A. *Normal*	Allows bladder filling with little or no change in pressure; no involuntary phasic contractions
B. *Detrusor overactivity*	Involuntary detrusor contractions during filling
1. *Phasic*	Characteristic wave form; may or may not lead to incontinence
2. *Terminal*	Single involuntary detrusor contractions occurring at cystometric capacity, which cannot be suppressed, and results in incontinence usually resulting in bladder emptying
3. *Detrusor overactivity incontinence*	Incontinence that is due to an involuntary leakage episode
4. *Neurogenic detrusor overactivity*	There is a relevant neurologic condition (replaces term *detrusor hyperreflexia*)
5. *Idiopathic detrusor overactivity*	No definite cause (replaces term *detrusor instability*)
C. *Bladder compliance*	Fill volume/change in detrusor pressure (P_{det})
	1. Calculate at start of bladder filling (usually 0)
	2. At cystometric capacity (excluding any detrusor contraction)
D. *Bladder capacity*	
1. *Cystometric capacity*	Volume at end of cystometrogram; capacity is volume voided together with any residual urine
2. *Maximum cystometric capacity*	Volume at which person feels she can no longer delay voiding

III. Urethral function

A. *Normal urethral closure mechanism*	Maintains a positive urethral closure pressure during bladder filling
B. *Incompetent urethral closure mechanism*	Allows leakage of urine in the absence of a detrusor contraction
C. *Urethral relaxation incontinence*	Leakage that is due to urethral relaxation in the absence of raised abdominal pressure or detrusor overactivity
D. *Urodynamic stress incontinence*	Involuntary leakage of urine during increased abdominal pressure, in the absence of detrusor contraction (replaces term *genuine stress incontinence*)
E. *Urethral pressure (P_{ura})*	Fluid pressure needed to open closed urethra
1. *Pressure profile*	Pressure along length of urethra
2. *Urethral closure pressure*	$P_{ura} - P_{ves}$
3. *Maximum urethral closure pressure (MUCP)*	Maximum difference between P_{ura} and P_{ves}
4. *Pressure transmission ratio*	Increment in urethral pressure on stress as percentage of simultaneously recorded increment in intravesical pressure

(Continued)

Table 26.6 (*Continued*)	
F. *Abdominal leak point pressure*	Intravesical pressure at which urine leakage occurs because of increased abdominal pressure
IV. Pressure flow studies	
A. *Urine flow*	Defined as:
1. Continuous	
2. Intermittent	
a. *Flow rate*	Volume voided/unit time
b. *Voided volume*	Total volume voided
c. *Maximum flow rate*	
d. *Voiding time*	Includes interruptions
e. *Flow time*	Time over which measurable flow actually occurs
f. *Average flow rate*	Voided volume/flow time
g. *Closing pressure*	Pressure measured at end of measured flow
h. *Detrusor function during voiding*	Classified as:
1. Normal	
2. *Detrusor underactivity*	Contraction of reduced strength resulting in prolonged bladder emptying and/or a failure to achieve complete bladder emptying
3. *Acontractile*	Cannot be demonstrated to contract
i. *Urethral function during voiding*	Classified as:
1. *Normal*	Continuously relaxed
2. *Dysfunctional voiding*	Intermittent and/or fluctuating flow rate that is due to involuntary intermittent contractions of the periurethral striated muscle during voiding in neurologically normal people
3. *Detrusor sphincter dyssynergia*	Detrusor contraction concurrent with an involuntary contraction of the urethral and/or periurethral striated muscle
4. *Nonrelaxing urethral sphincter obstruction*	Usually occurs in people with a neurologic lesion

From **Abrams P, Cardozo L, Fall M, et al.** The standardization of terminology of lower urinary tract function: report from the Standardization Sub-committee of the International Continence Society. *Neurourol Urodyn* 2002;21:167–178, with permission.

total intravesical pressure (P_{ves}) **with a bladder pressure catheter, approximating** *intra-abdominal pressure* (P_{abd}) **with a rectal or vaginal catheter, and then electronically subtracting the latter from the former:**

$$P_{det} = P_{ves} - P_{abd}.$$

Measurements can be obtained using electronic microtip transducer pressure catheters, fluid-filled pressure lines, fiberoptic catheters, or air-charged catheters. All are acceptable for clinical use, but it is important to realize that when different types of catheters are used, the correlation between numbers is imperfect. Other technical factors that influence cystometry results include the choice of distending medium, filling rate, and patient position. The steps involved in a multichannel urodynamic study are outlined in Table 26.7. Normal cystometric values for women are shown in Table 26.8.

An example of detrusor overactivity seen during complex cystometry is shown in Figure 26.5. Surface or needle electromyography may be performed during filling and voiding to assess muscle activity of the urethral sphincter or pelvic floor. Electromyography as generally performed did not prove useful in neurologically intact women with symptoms of only stress urinary incontinence, and is not required in this patient population.

Both false-positive and false-negative results can occur with urodynamic studies. False-positive results occur in patients with asymptomatic detrusor overactivity, detrusor overactivity

Table 26.7 Steps in Conducting a Multichannel Urodynamic Study
1. ***Insert pressure and filling catheter into bladder*** (may be two catheters or dual catheter) to measure intravesical pressure and to fill bladder. Insert pressure catheter into upper vagina or rectum to approximate abdominal pressure.
2. ***Infuse fluid (usually sterile water or saline, sometimes radiographic contrast dye) at a rate of 50 to 100 mL/min.*** Record the volume infused and the pressure measurements continuously. The patient's bladder may be filled with her lying supine, in a modified lithotomy position, sitting, or standing. When possible, do cystometry in the standing position as most patients with incontinence report this problem more when they are erect.
3. ***Note the point at which any leakage occurs.***
4. ***During filling, record the first desire to void (that is, the feeling that would lead her to void at the next convenient moment, but voiding can be delayed if necessary) and the strong desire to void (that is, the persistent desire to void without the fear of leakage).*** The maximum cystometric capacity, in women with normal sensation, is the volume at which the woman can no longer delay micturition; filling should not be continued to the point of pain or severe discomfort.
5. ***If no detrusor overactivity is noted during filling, have the patient do provocative maneuvers at maximum capacity, such as coughing, heel-bouncing, and listening to the sound of running water to provoke uninhibited detrusor contractions,*** which may be the cause of the patient's symptoms.

that is irrelevant to the symptom, or detrusor overactivity that is situational (e.g., caused by test anxiety). False-negative results can occur because a 20- to 40-minute cystometrogram is not always an accurate measure of 24-hour bladder activity. Looking for detrusor overactivity with such a test is like looking for an episodic cardiac arrhythmia using 12-lead electrocardiography, as opposed to looking for the arrhythmia using a 24-hour Holter monitor. The sensitivity of the latter test is far greater than that of the former. Ambulatory urodynamics can be performed and are more likely to detect detrusor overactivity than office-based studies.

Tests of Urethral Function

Several tests of urethral function, including urethral pressure profilometry, Valsalva leak-point pressures, and the fluoroscopic and cystoscopic assessment of the bladder neck, are used in attempts to guide therapy in women with stress urinary incontinence. **Women with poor urethral function, evidenced by low Valsalva leak-point pressures, low maximal urethral closure pressures, or a visualized open bladder neck, are thought to be at higher risk of treatment**

Table 26.8 Approximate Normal Values of Female Bladder Function
• Residual urine <50 mL
• First desire to void occurs between 150 and 250 mL infused
• Strong desire to void does not occur until after 250 mL
• Cystometric capacity between 400 and 600 mL
• Bladder compliance between 20 and 100 mL/cm H_2O measured 60 sec after reaching cystometric capacity
• No uninhibited detrusor contractions during filling, despite provocation
• No stress or urge incontinence demonstrated, despite provocation
• Voiding occurs as a result of a voluntarily initiated and sustained detrusor contraction
• Flow rate during voiding is >15 mL/sec with a detrusor pressure of <50 cm H_2O

From **Wall LL, Norton P, Delancey J.** *Practical urogynecology.* Baltimore, MD: Williams & Wilkins, 1993, with permission.

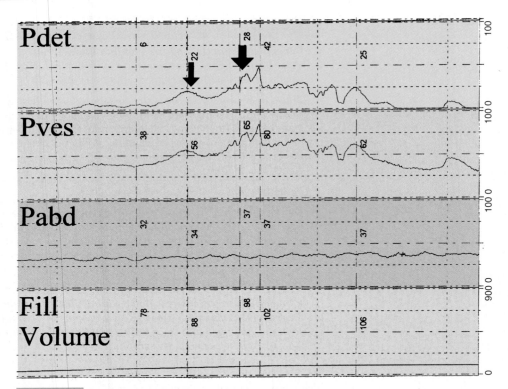

Figure 26.5   Detrusor overactivity on filling cystometrography. The patient begins to sense urgency, accompanied by an unstable bladder contraction, when 88 mL of water are instilled into the bladder. The detrusor pressure rises, and when 96 mL of water are instilled, she leaks. P_{abd}, abdominal pressure; P_{ves}, vesical pressure; P_{det}, detrusor pressure.

failure using standard retropubic urethropexy (Fig. 26.6). Cutoff values for these tests are poorly defined and remain controversial. Although women with stress urinary incontinence have, on average, significantly lower maximal urethral closure pressures than those without incontinence, there is wide overlap in the values between such women, and no lower limit of urethral closure pressure or leak point pressure is established that diagnoses stress urinary incontinence.

The urethral pressure profile is a test designed to measure urethral closure. Because continence requires the pressure in the urethra to be higher than the pressure in the bladder, it was believed that measuring the pressure differential between the two would provide useful clinical information. The urethral pressure profile is determined by slowly pulling a pressure-sensitive catheter through the urethra from the bladder.

The urethral closure pressure (P_{close}) is the difference between the urethral pressure (P_{ure}) and the bladder pressure:

$$(P_{ves}): P_{close} = P_{ure} - P_{ves}.$$

It was suggested that women with stress incontinence with low urethral closure pressure (<20 cm H_2O) have a poorer prognosis for surgical outcome than women who do not have this condition; however, this area is the subject of considerable debate (3,39,40). Because stress incontinence, by definition, occurs during increases in intra-abdominal pressure that are generated by some kind of physical activity, it is not obvious why measurement of resting urethral pressure should be relevant to stress-related leakage, which is a dynamic event. One review concluded that urethral pressure profilometry is not a useful diagnostic test for stress incontinence in women and that its use in clinical management is unsupported by current evidence (41).

Leak-point pressure (LPP) is a urodynamic measure of the minimum intra-abdominal or intravesical pressure required to cause incontinence during abdominal strain or cough.

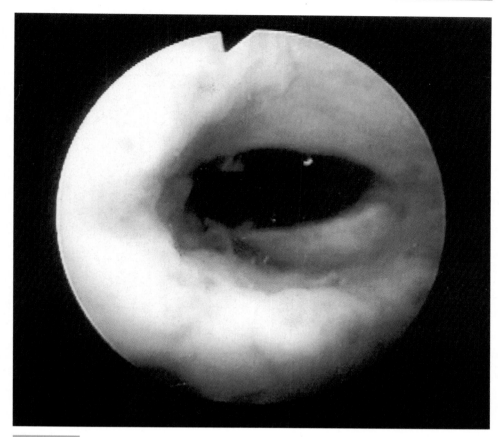

Figure 26.6   Open and scarred bladder neck in an elderly woman who has undergone three anterior colporrhaphies for stress urinary incontinence in the past.

There is no consensus about whether it should be measured from the resting supine baseline (generally near 0) or from the standing resting baseline (which increases depending on body mass). Other factors that may affect the results include the catheter's type, caliber, and placement (vaginal, rectal, or intravesical), the bladder volume at which the measurement is obtained, the mechanism by which intra-abdominal pressure is increased (coughing versus straining), and patient position (42).

Leak point pressure measurements often are performed at a bladder volume of 200 or 300 mL. Patients are asked to cough with gradually increasing force (cough leak-point pressure) and finally to strain slowly (Valsalva) to increase intravesical pressure gradually. The lowest pressure at which leakage occurs is recorded as the cough or the Valsalva leak-point pressure (Fig. 26.7). If leakage is not demonstrated, the highest pressure that was obtained can be recorded with the notation "no leakage" to the specified pressure as measured in centimeters of water pressure. Many clinicians use a cutoff point of 60 cm water pressure to separate women who have intrinsic sphincter deficiency from those who do not. This is problematic for two reasons: (i) the marked variability of results that depend on all the aforementioned factors and (ii) the lack of prospective studies that demonstrate the predictive value of leak point pressure values on surgical outcomes. Results from this and other urodynamics tests must be evaluated as one piece of the patient's puzzle, along with the history, physical examination, voiding diary, and other tests. Medicare guidelines require that when bulking agents, such as collagen, are considered to treat stress incontinence, the intra-abdominal leak point pressure when the bladder has been filled with at least 150 mL of fluid must be less than 100 cm H_2O.

Fluoroscopy and cystourethroscopy were used to visualize the bladder neck because many clinicians and investigators believe that a closed bladder neck is important in maintaining continence. However, studies of continent women reveal that many individuals with normal urethral function

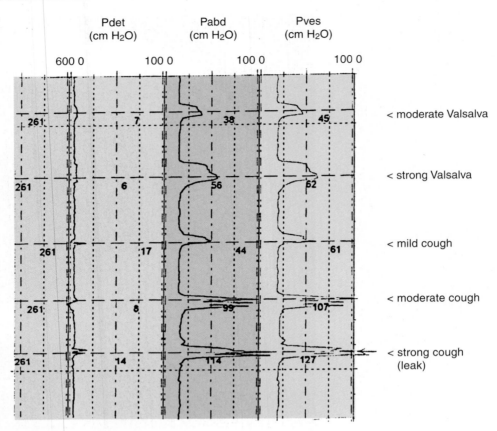

Figure 26.7   Leak point pressure. The abdominal leak point pressure (LPP) is 114 cm H_2O (the abdominal pressure at which the patient leaked urine).

show evidence of bladder neck opening with physical stress (43). Neither test is recommended in the routine evaluation of women with straightforward incontinence.

Voiding Cystometrogram

Urodynamic testing usually concludes with an instrumented voiding study (also known as a pressure-flow study or voiding cystometrogram), in which the vesical, abdominal, and urethral pressures are measured simultaneously during bladder emptying (Fig. 26.8). Various studies identified Valsalva voiding, low preoperative flow rate, and high preoperative detrusor pressures during voiding as risk factors for postoperative voiding dysfunction; however, findings often are contradictory.

Imaging Tests

The role of imaging techniques in studying female urinary incontinence is not yet established. Researchers are evaluating the potential roles of ultrasonography, fluoroscopy, functional neuroimaging, and magnetic resonance imaging (MRI). These tests should not be done routinely but are useful in certain conditions. If the patient's symptoms (easily remembered by the three Ds: dysuria, dribbling, and dyspareunia) or examination suggests a urethral diverticulum, MRI is the test of choice (44).

Neurophysiologic Tests

The neuromuscular function of the pelvic floor is dependent on the integrity of the nervous system. Injury can theoretically occur anywhere along these nerves, from the cell body located in Onuf's nucleus in the ventral part of the spinal cord, along its axon, to the neuromuscular junction. Pelvic floor neurophysiology utilizes techniques applied to nerves and skeletal muscles elsewhere in the body to document neuromuscular integrity or evidence of injury. **These tests are not routinely used in the clinical evaluation of most incontinent women.**

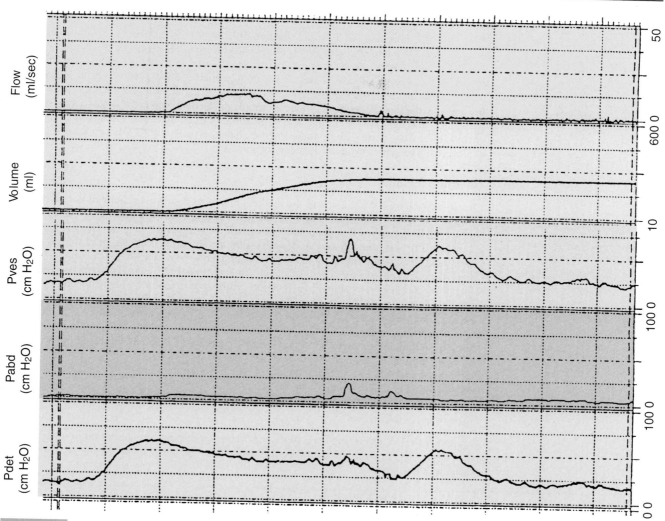

Figure 26.8 **Voiding cystometrogram.** This patient voids in an uninterrupted flow pattern by means of a prolonged bladder contraction. She does not strain to void, with the exception of minimal straining toward the end of the flow.

Pudendal Nerve Terminal Motor Latency

The pudendal nerve terminal motor latency (PNTML) indirectly assesses the integrity and patency of the terminal portion of the pudendal nerve, its neuromuscular junction, and the muscle it serves. Using a specialized electrode affixed over the index finger, the pudendal nerve is electrically stimulated near the ischial spine (either transrectally or transvaginally), and the resulting muscular response is measured. The response, termed a *compound muscle action potential* (CMAP), is detected at the anal sphincter. The interval between the stimulation and the onset of the CMAP is measured. A prolonged latency is noted with injury to large and heavily myelinated axons. The latency time may be within the normal range when only smaller nerve fibers are affected; thus, neurologic dysfunction may exist in the presence of a normal latency time.

Sacral Reflexes

Only the distal efferent arm of the pudendal nerve is analyzed in the PNTML. Similar to the clinically obtained anal wink or bulbocavernosus reflex, electrically induced sacral reflexes can gather information about both the afferent and efferent arc in the pelvic nerves. A short train of dual impulses delivered next to the clitoris and measured at the anal sphincter is termed the clitoroanal reflex and provides information about the integrity of the afferent and efferent arm of the somatic pudendal nerve. A stimulating electrode placed in the bladder sends these signals along the visceral, autonomic fibers to the spinal cord, and a reflex signal will return along the pudendal nerve to the anal sphincter.

Somatosensory Evoked Potentials

Normal pelvic floor and pelvic organ function ultimately is controlled by higher centers in the central nervous system, including the cerebral cortex. Recording electrodes located on the scalp near the motor cortex allow the signal transmission speed between a skeletal muscle and the brain to be measured. Repeated electrical stimuli, called somatosensory evoked potentials, at a muscle of interest are used to assess the integrity of the central afferent limb. In a reverse fashion, electrical or magnetically induced stimuli can be delivered at the motor cortex (or along the spine), and the induced muscle action potentials can be detected. Prolonged latencies not attributable to the peripherally studied nerves (such as with a PNTML or sacral reflex) are evidence of a central nervous system conduction flaw.

Electromyography

Electromyography (EMG) assesses the inherent electrical potentials generated during neuronal activation of skeletal muscle. It can be performed using surface electrodes or needle electrodes. Surface EMG measures the summation of muscle activity in the general area of the applied electrode. It is best used for simply describing the pattern and coordination of muscle activity but is less useful in providing more specific assessments. Needle EMG of the pelvic floor can "map" the anatomic location of muscles but is mostly replaced by ultrasonography. The major value of needle EMG is its ability to assess nerve injury and determine whether the injury is acute and ongoing or chronic. Single-fiber EMG can quantify the ratio of muscle fibers to nerve fibers (the so-called fiber density). An increase in fiber density is evidence of previous nerve injury with successful reinnervation. Concentric needle EMG is more widely available and allows for further neurophysiologic evaluation. Abnormal electrical activity associated with acute injury may be seen, and motor unit action potentials (MUAPs) can be assessed and quantified. Following nerve injury and reinnervation, MUAP parameters—such as duration, amplitude, number of phases, and turns—are typically larger.

Emerging Technologies

Positron emission tomography and functional magnetic resonance imaging studies are yielding preliminary insights into the neural control of continence; these technologies are used in the research setting only.

Nonsurgical Treatment	**Treatment of urinary incontinence can be either nonsurgical or surgical. The approach to treatment is based on the clinical findings and the degree of discomfort experienced by the patient, who should be fully informed of the risks and expected outcome.**
Lifestyle Changes	**Lifestyle interventions can decrease stress urinary incontinence in many women** (45). There is good level 1 evidence that weight loss in both morbidly and moderately obese women decreases both stress and urge urinary incontinence (31). Postural changes (such as crossing the legs during periods of increased intra-abdominal pressure) often prevent stress urinary incontinence. There is some evidence that decreasing caffeine intake improves continence; however, fluid intake in general seems to play a minor role in the pathogenesis of incontinence. Although smokers are at greater risk for incontinence, no data were reported on whether smoking cessation resolves incontinence.
Physical Therapy	Medical evidence from well-designed randomized clinical trials shows that supervised pelvic floor muscle training (Kegel exercises) is an effective treatment for stress urinary incontinence. **The Cochrane Incontinence Group concluded that pelvic floor muscle training is consistently better than no treatment or placebo treatment for stress incontinence and should be offered as first-line conservative management to women.** Intensive training sessions that include personal contact with a health care professional to teach and supervise pelvic floor muscle training may be more beneficial than standard care. Biofeedback provides no added benefit over pelvic floor muscle training alone in women with stress urinary incontinence (46). **Several factors improve the likelihood that pelvic muscle training will relieve stress urinary incontinence. The woman must do the exercises correctly, regularly, and for an adequate duration. Based on exercise training of skeletal muscles elsewhere in the body, many**

physical therapists recommend training sessions three to four times per week, with three repetitions of eight to ten sustained contractions each time.

Electrical stimulation therapy was used to treat incontinence by delivering low levels of current via a probe placed in the vagina or rectum. When compared with sham devices and pelvic floor exercises, electrostimulation produced mixed results in the treatment of stress urinary incontinence but may be more helpful in women with overactive bladders (47–50). Further research is needed to determine what niche this treatment may fill for women with urinary incontinence.

Behavioral Therapy and Bladder Training	Bladder training focuses on modifying bladder function by changing voiding habits. Behavioral therapy focuses on improving voluntary control rather than bladder function (51). The key component to bladder training is a scheduled toileting program. After reviewing the patient's voiding diary, an initial voiding interval is chosen that represents the longest interval between voiding that is comfortable. She is instructed to empty her bladder when she awakes, and then every time during the day that the interval is reached (for example, every 30 to 60 minutes). When the patient feels the urge to void during that interval, she is instructed to use urge-suppression strategies, such as distraction or relaxation techniques, until she gets to the stated interval. Effective distraction strategies include mental exercises (such as mathematical problems), deep breathing, or "singing" the words to a song silently. The main goal is to avoid running to the bathroom at the moment of severe urgency. Another strategy is to quickly contract the pelvic muscle several times in a row ("freeze and squeeze"), which often lessens urgency. Gradually, the interval is increased (usually weekly) until the patient voids every 2 to 3 hours. Bladder training is most effective when women record every void and check in (by telephone or in person) with a health care provider weekly. This program lasts for about 6 weeks. Bladder training is effective; in a trial in which bladder training was compared with treatment with *oxybutynin,* 73% of women in the bladder training group were clinically cured (52).

The primary technique of behavioral training is pelvic floor muscle training, as described previously, but with a focus on urge inhibition. Mastering voluntary pelvic floor muscle contractions helps to strengthen the outlet (decreasing leakage) and inhibit detrusor contractions. Other components of therapy may include voiding schedules, urge-inhibitions strategies, and fluid management.

Patients with neurogenic detrusor overactivity, rather than idiopathic detrusor overactivity, do not respond as well to behavioral therapy because the problem is actually one of neural pathway destruction rather than the need to reestablish cortical control mechanisms. Frequently, these patients have a trigger volume of urine that sets off a contraction that they cannot control voluntarily. They may benefit from a timed schedule in which they void at regular intervals (such as every 2 hours) to keep their bladder volume below the trigger point. Attempting to lengthen the interval between voids often does not work well.

Less-intensive treatments also decrease incontinence episodes. In a randomized trial, the guidance of a simple self-help booklet was only somewhat less effective in reducing leakage (mean reduction in leakage episodes 43%) than behavioral training (mean reduction 69%) or behavioral training plus electrical stimulation (mean reduction 72%) (53).

Vaginal and Urethral Devices	Vaginal devices (pessaries) and urethral inserts are available for treating stress urinary incontinence. In a tertiary care population, approximately two-thirds of women with stress urinary incontinence offered a trial of vaginal devices chose to undergo pessary fitting (54). Most (89%) achieved a successful fit. Of those who took a pessary home to manage their stress urinary incontinence, approximately one-half used it for more than 6 months. Women who stopped using the pessary generally did so within the first month. In an intent-to-treat analysis of a recent large multisite randomized trial, 3 months after beginning either pessary or behavioral therapy, 40% of those randomized to pessary and 49% of those doing behavioral therapy were "very much" or "much" better. By 12 months there were no group differences in outcomes and patient satisfaction was greater than 50% for each group (55). Some women are pleased to be able to avoid surgery or to use a "crutch" while waiting for the effect of pelvic muscle training; others prefer a treatment option (like surgery) that does not require daily intervention. Examples of some vaginal devices are shown in Figure 26.9.

Urethral inserts are sterile inserts placed into the urethra by the patient and removed before a void, after which a new sterile insert is placed. Such inserts are appropriate for women with

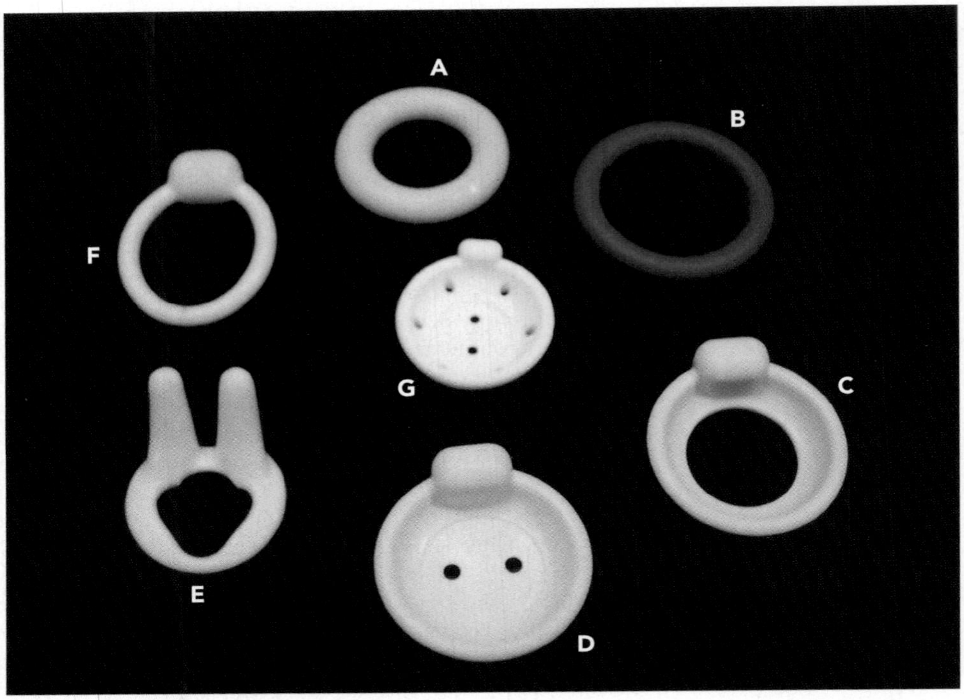

Figure 26.9   **Vaginal incontinence pessaries:** (clockwise from top): **A:** Suarez ring (Cook Urological, Spencer, IN), **B:** PelvX ring (DesChutes Medical Products, Bend, OR), **C:** Incontinence dish (Milex Inc., Chicago, IL), **D:** Incontinence dish with support (Mentor Corp., Santa Barbara, CA), **E:** Introl prosthesis (was Johnson and Johnson; currently not available), **F:** Incontinence ring with support (Milex Inc., Chicago, IL), (middle): **G:** Incontinence dish with support (Milex Inc., Chicago, IL).

relatively pure stress incontinence, no history of recurrent urinary tract infections, and no serious contraindications to bacteriuria (e.g., artificial heart valves). The *FemSoft* device was U.S. Food and Drug Administration (FDA) approved in 1997 and is the only urethral insert that is available in the United States. Several other urethral inserts and urethral occlusion devices were marketed with good effectiveness but were withdrawn from the market. In a 5-year, multicenter trial involving 150 women with a mean follow-up of 15 months, a statistically significant reduction in incontinence episodes and pad weight were observed with 93% of the women having a negative pad test at 12 months. However, urinary tract infections were common and found in 31.3% of the subjects (56). Urethral inserts have not developed a widespread acceptance but may offer a viable treatment option for some select patients.

Medications

Stress Incontinence

The tone of the urethra and bladder neck is maintained in large part by α-adrenergic activity from the sympathetic nervous system. For this reason, many pharmacologic agents are used with varying degrees of success to treat stress incontinence. These drugs include *imipramine* (which has a concomitant relaxing effect on the detrusor), *ephedrine, pseudoephedrine, phenylpropanolamine,* and *norepinephrine.* Many of these compounds increase vascular tone and may, therefore, lead to problems with hypertension, a condition that afflicts many postmenopausal women with stress incontinence. There is an increased risk for hemorrhagic cerebral vascular accident in women taking *phenylpropanolamine,* and while the risk is very low, it is not possible to predict who is at risk for this complication (57). The use of these agents in the treatment of stress urinary incontinence appears to be more limited than originally thought (58). No drugs are cleared by the FDA to treat stress incontinence.

Based on a biologic rationale, it was thought that *estrogen* could effectively treat urinary incontinence, given the presence of estrogen receptors in the bladder, urethra, and levator muscles.

In early uncontrolled case series, women using various *estrogen* preparations experienced less incontinence. However, in several large randomized trials, women assigned to receive *estrogen* and *progesterone* did not have less leakage, and were more likely to experience the onset of incontinence or worsening of baseline symptoms (59). In over 23,000 women enrolled in the Women's Health Initiative double-blind, placebo-controlled, randomized clinical trial, use of menopausal hormone therapy (*conjugated estrogen* alone in women with a prior hysterectomy, *conjugated estrogen* and *medroxyprogesterone acetate* in women with a uterus) increased the incidence of all types of urinary incontinence at 1 year among women who were continent at baseline (60). Among women who reported urinary incontinence at baseline, both frequency and severity of incontinence worsened at 1 year in women taking either hormone preparation compared with those in the placebo group. Thus, **conjugated estrogen with or without *progestin* should not be prescribed for the prevention or relief of urinary incontinence.**

Urge Incontinence and Overactive Bladder

The drugs used for treating detrusor overactivity can be grouped into different categories according to their pharmacologic characteristics; **these drugs are anticholinergic agents that exert their effects on the bladder by blocking the activity of acetylcholine at muscarinic receptor sites.** All of these drugs have side effects, the most common of which are dry mouth resulting from decreased saliva production, increased heart rate because of vagal blockade, feelings of constipation resulting from decreased gastrointestinal motility, and occasionally, blurred vision caused by blockade of the sphincter of the iris and the ciliary muscle of the lens of the eye.

Medications commonly used to treat these conditions are listed in Table 26.9. The introduction of several new drugs for overactive bladder resulted in significant attention being given to urinary incontinence in the media.

The newer drugs have some advantages over *oxybutynin,* which was available for decades. These advantages include once- (or sometimes twice-) daily dosing, rather than three to four times per day and, to some degree, a less severe side-effect profile. The latter results from changes in the delivery system and to more selectivity of muscarinic receptors (so that, for example, the bladder may be targeted more than the salivary glands). In addition, quaternary amines (such as *trospium chloride*) are not distributed into the central nervous system because of their large molecular size and hydrophilicity. The primary disadvantage of the newer agents is cost.

In 2009, the Agency for Healthcare Research and Quality carried out an evidence-based review of the large body of literature on pharmacologic therapies for urinary urgency incontinence and overactive bladder (61). Estimates from their meta-analysis models suggest that immediate-release forms of medications (*oxybutynin,* short-acting *tolterodine*) decreased incontinence episodes and voids by 1.46 and 2.16 per day, respectively. Extended-release forms of medications (*tolterodine, trospium chloride, solifenacin, oxybutynin*) decreased incontinence episodes and voids by 1.78 and 2.24 per day, respectively. However, placebo also impacted continence, decreasing incontinence episodes and voids by 1.08 and 1.48 per day, respectively. **Whether or not the improvements observed with medication are clinically significant depends on patients' perceptions and initial level of severity.** In the randomized trials reviewed, baseline episodes of incontinence ranged from 1.6 to 5.3; decreasing this by one or two may or may not constitute a successful outcome for a given patient.

When initiating therapy with generic *oxybutynin,* it is best to start with a lower dose (particularly for elderly patients) and increase it as needed to a higher, more frequent dosage. Patients should be encouraged to titrate their medication to their symptoms and to vary the dosage (within acceptable limits) according to their needs. If this is not effective, the next step is to move to one of the other anticholinergic agents. Some women may respond better to one agent than another. A 2-week trial is sufficient to determine effectiveness. It is helpful to ask patients to record daily episodes of incontinence or urgency before and during therapy so effectiveness can be more accurately determined.

Patients should be warned of the side effects of anticholinergic agents. Patients should be particularly advised about the symptom of a dry mouth and told that this is not caused by thirst. Some patients increase their fluid intake to combat this problem, with a subsequent worsening of their incontinence. If dry mouth is a problem, patients should relieve it by chewing gum, sucking on a piece of hard candy, or eating a piece of moist fruit.

Table 26.9 Commonly Used Medications for Urge Incontinence

Drug	Oral Dose Range
Generic and Brand Names	
Oxybutynin	
Ditropan[a]	2.5–5 mg tid–qid
Ditropan syrup[a]	1 tsp (5 mg)
Ditropan XL[a]	5, 10, or 15 mg qd
Oxytrol patch[b]	1 patch 2 times per week
Oxybutynin gel (Gelnique)[b]	1 sachet qd
Tolterodine[c]	
Detrol	1–2 mg bid (immediate release)
Detrol LA	4 mg qd (extended release)
Fesoterodine (Toviaz)	4 or 8 mg qd
Trospium chloride[d]	
Sanctura	20 mg bid
Sanctura XR	60 mg qd
Solifenacin succinate[e]	
Vesicare	5–20 mg qd (one daily dose; usual dosing is 5–10 mg qd)
Darifenacin[f]	
Enablex	7.5 or 15 mg by mouth qd

tid, three times a day; qid, four times a day; qd, every day; bid, twice a day.
[a]Available as generic.
[b]Watson Pharmaceuticals.
[c]Pfizer.
[d]Allergan.
[e]Astellas Pharmaceuticals.
[f]7.5 or 15 mg by mouth

Nocturia and Nocturnal Enuresis

Medications that treat nocturia and nocturnal enuresis have one of three aims: (i) to reduce urine output, (ii) to increase bladder capacity and reduce unstable bladder contractions, and (iii) to act centrally on sleep and micturition centers.

An analogue of arginine vasopressin, *DDAVP*, is used extensively to treat children with nocturnal enuresis. Some studies suggest that it may be useful in adults (62,63). It is available as a nasal spray and as an oral preparation. When taken orally, the dose required is approximately 10 times greater because of the increased availability of the nasal preparation. Complications associated with the *DDAVP* include hyponatremia, particularly in patients with excessive fluid intake; therefore, it is essential in higher-risk patients to measure serum sodium levels periodically.

There are few clinical trials that specifically investigate the use of anticholinergic medications to treat nocturia or nocturnal enuresis. Anecdotal evidence supports a trial of a long-acting or extended-release form of an anticholinergic, taken approximately 1 hour before bedtime.

The most extensively studied medications for the treatment of nocturnal enuresis are tricyclic antidepressants, particularly *imipramine*. These agents may work by altering the sleep mechanism, by providing anticholinergic or antidepressant effects, or by affecting antidiuretic hormone excretion. The typical starting dose of *imipramine* is 25 mg at bedtime, which may be increased to as high as 75 mg. In the elderly, *imipramine* should be used cautiously because it increases the risk of hip fracture, presumably related to the potential side effect of orthostatic hypertension (64).

In a randomized, placebo-controlled study comparing nighttime doses of placebo and 1 mg of *bumetanide* (a loop diuretic), *bumetanide* decreased nocturia episodes by 25% compared with placebo (65). Patients who produce half of their total urine at night often benefit from the use of a diuretic (e.g., 20 mg *furosemide*) in the late afternoon to move fluid through the system and decrease their nighttime urine production.

Surgical Treatment for Stress Incontinence

Historically, the body of literature concerning surgical therapy for stress urinary incontinence, while large, is hampered by poor methods, short follow-up, biased outcome observations, and little attention paid to the patients' perceptions of symptoms and quality of life (66). Over the past decade, scientific research in this area evolved; while much of the literature continues to reflect small short-term case series, randomized trials with rigorous follow-up are becoming more common.

Several shifts occurred in recommendations regarding surgical therapy in the past generation. In 1997, the American Urological Association convened a clinical guidelines panel to analyze published outcomes data on surgical procedures to treat female stress urinary incontinence and to produce practice recommendations to guide surgical decision making (67). **The panel concluded that colposuspension (e.g., Burch, Marshall-Marchetti-Krantz [MMK]) and slings were more effective than transvaginal needle suspensions or anterior repairs for long-term success (48-month cure/dry rates).** The median probability estimates for cure/dry rates at 48 months and longer were 84% (95% confidence interval [CI], 79%–88%) for colposuspension and 83% (95% CI, 75%–88%) for sling procedures, compared with 67% (95% CI, 53%–79%) for transvaginal needle suspensions and 61% (95% CI, 47%–72%) for anterior repairs. **Thus, the latter two procedures are no longer recommended as adequate treatments for stress urinary incontinence.**

Historical Perspective

Anterior vaginal repair (also termed *anterior colporrhaphy*) was described by Howard Kelly in 1914, and this operation remained the standard first approach to stress incontinence until the middle of the 20th century (68). Many different operations are lumped together under the term *anterior colporrhaphy*, including simple plication of the bladder neck, elevation of the bladder neck by plicating the fascia under the urethra, and elevation and fixation of the bladder neck by passing sutures lateral to the urethra and driving the needles anteriorly into the back of the pubic symphysis for fixation. As noted previously, the problem with most techniques of anterior colporrhaphy is that they do not hold up well over time (69–71). In essence, this operation attempts to take weak support from below and push it back up from below, with hope that these structures will maintain their strength and position over time. Although there were excellent long-term results shown with anterior colporrhaphy, most of these cases involve specific techniques requiring skillful dissection of the endopelvic fascia, deep bold bites of suture, and fixation of permanent sutures to the pubic bone from below: in essence, a transvaginal retropubic bladder neck suspension (72,73). Most surgical series that evaluated techniques of anterior colporrhaphy for stress incontinence show long-term success rates of only 35% to 65%, a figure that most would regard as unacceptably low. **Anterior colporrhaphy should be reserved primarily for patients requiring cystocele repair who do not have significant stress incontinence.**

Needle suspension procedures are so named because they suspend the urethra and bladder neck through a technique that involves passage of sutures between the vagina and anterior abdominal wall using a specially designed long needle carrier. Although initial cure rates are between 70% to 90%, rates decrease significantly over time in many series, with 5-year success rates of 50% or less (67,74–77). Therefore, these operations are no longer recommended.

Retropubic Urethropexy (Colposuspension)

The modern era of retropubic surgery for stress incontinence began in 1949, when Marshall et al. described their technique for urethral suspension in a man with postprostatectomy incontinence (78). A variety of modifications of this operation were described, all of which share at least two characteristics: They are performed through an open low abdominal incision or with laparoscopically assisted exposure of the space of Retzius, and they all involve attachment of the periurethral or perivesical endopelvic fascia to some other supporting structure in the anterior pelvis (Fig. 26.10). In the MMK operation, the periurethral fascia is attached to the back of the pubic symphysis. Another approach, the Burch colposuspension, involves the attachment of the fascia at the level of the bladder neck to the iliopectineal ligament (Cooper's ligament) (79,80). With the paravaginal repair, the lateral endopelvic fascia along the urethra and bladder is reattached to the arcus tendineus fascia pelvis (81,82). In the Turner-Warwick vagino-obturator shelf procedure, the endopelvic fascia, vagina, or both are attached to the fascia of the obturator internus muscle (83,84).

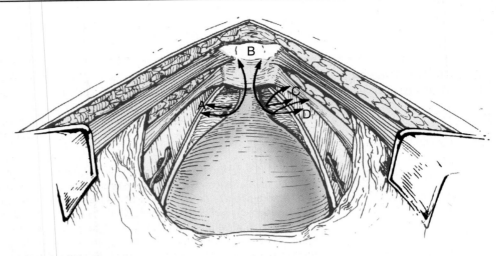

Figure 26.10 Points of reattachment of the endopelvic fascia during retropubic bladder neck suspensions. A: Arcus tendineus fascia pelvis (for paravaginal repair). **B:** Periosteum of pubic symphysis (for Marshall-Marchetti-Krantz procedure). **C:** Ileopectineal, or Cooper's, ligament (for Burch colposuspension). **D:** Obturator internus fascia (also used for paravaginal, or obturator shelf, repair).

A 2009 Cochrane review found that 69% to 88% of women treated with Burch colposuspension were largely continent, and 5 years after surgery the continence rate remained high at 70%. Twelve trials were available that compared colposuspension with various forms of suburethral slings; there were no significant differences in failure rates between slings and colposuspension at any time interval studied (85).

The long-term success of laparoscopic colposuspension is unclear, but there is limited evidence to suggest the results are less favorable than with open colposuspension, although this may reflect a learning effect and be unreliable in isolation (86).

Traditional Pubovaginal Sling

Sling operations traditionally were performed using a combined vaginal and abdominal approach (Fig. 26.11). The anterior vagina is opened, the space of Retzius is dissected on each side of the bladder neck, and a sling is passed around the bladder neck and urethra and then attached to the anterior rectus fascia or some other structure to cradle the urethra in a supporting hammock. This supports the urethra and allows it to be compressed during periods of increased intra-abdominal pressure (87–97). The sling can be made of organic or inorganic materials. Organic materials can be autologous tissues harvested from the patient (e.g., fascia lata, rectus fascia, tendon, round ligament, rectus muscle, vagina), processed allografts from human donors (e.g., fascia lata, dermis), or heterologous tissues harvested from another species and processed for surgical use (e.g., ox dura mater, porcine dermis). Synthetic materials (e.g., *Silastic, Gore-Tex, Marlex*) are popular because of their consistent strength and availability, but historically these substances were plagued by problems with erosion and infection when used around the urethra (67,98,99).

The multicenter Urinary Incontinence Treatment Network conducted a randomized clinical trial comparing Burch colposuspension and fascial pubovaginal sling in 655 women with stress urinary incontinence (100). The primary outcome, success, was rigorously defined as a negative pad test, no urinary incontinence (as recorded in a 3-day diary), a negative cough and Valsalva stress test, no self-reported symptoms, and no retreatment for the condition. At 24 months, success rates were higher for women who underwent the sling procedure than for those who underwent the Burch procedure for the overall category of success (47% vs. 38%; $p = .01$). However, more women who underwent the sling procedure later had urinary tract infections, difficulty voiding, and postoperative urge incontinence. This study highlights the wide range in success depending on how it is defined: for example, based on a cough stress test, success rates were 71% in the Burch group and 87% in the sling group, while based on a pad test, rates were 84% and 85%, respectively.

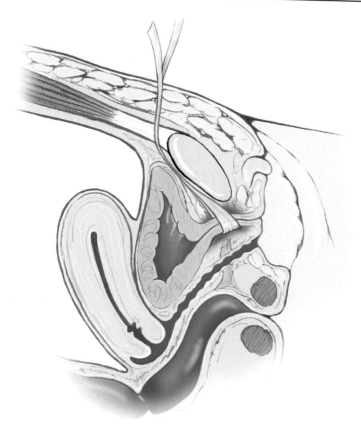

Figure 26.11 **A completed traditional suburethral sling procedure with the fascia located at the bladder neck with the ends of the sling tied to or above the rectus fascia.** The classic procedure uses autologous fascia; however, some surgeons use allograft or xenograft tissue performed in a similar fashion. (Redrawn from original by Jasmine Tan.)

Minimally Invasive Sling

In the 1990s, various orthopedic bone anchors were marketed to implant into the pubic bone to suspend the urethra with sutures or slings. Despite a lack of medical evidence to support either the bone anchor or the allograft use, bone anchor systems became the quick and minimally invasive method to suspend allograft slings (101). Although bone anchors were not superior to standard fixation techniques, their use led to increased complications in several series.

In 1996, Falconer et al. described the tension-free vaginal tape (TVT) for correcting stress urinary incontinence (102). In this technique, polypropylene mesh is placed under the midurethra with minimal tension (Fig. 26.12 A, B). To perform this operation, a small midurethral incision is made in the vaginal epithelium mucosa. A 40- by 1-cm mesh tape covered by a plastic sheath and attached to two 5-mm curved trocars is passed lateral to the urethra and through the endopelvic fascia into the retropubic space. The trocar is passed along the back of the pubic bone, through the rectus fascia, and into two small suprapubic skin incisions. The tension on the tape is adjusted, the sheath is removed, and the remaining tape is cut off at the level of the skin. This technique has the advantage of being performed quickly using limited anesthesia (fewer than 30 minutes in experienced hands). The procedure requires the use of a catheter guide to deviate the urethra and cystoscopy to ensure that bladder or urethral perforations are recognized immediately because the trocar is passed blindly.

Numerous modifications of the TVT were proposed and marketed. Such devices generally circumvent the stringent regulatory control provided by the FDA by gaining approval through a Premarket Notification 510(k). This mechanism is a submission to the FDA demonstrating that a new device is substantially equivalent either to a legally marketed or "predicate" device introduced before 1976 in the United States or to one approved by the FDA through the 510(k)

891

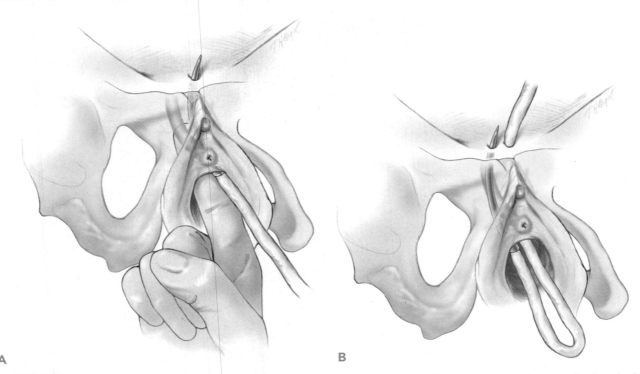

A   B

Figure 26.12 **Midurethral synthetic slings involve the use of large pore, monofilament polypropylene mesh placed after minimal dissection at the midurethra followed by placement of a trocar through the retropubic route.** Some surgeons prefer placing the trocar by a suprapubic route beginning with a small abdominal incision. **A:** The trocar is guided into the previously performed midurethral incision with care to place the trocar against the pubic bone to avoid entry into the peritoneal cavity. The trocar handle has been removed in this view after perforation through the abdominal incision. **B:** The synthetic sling should rest in the midurethra location and is brought through two stab incisions above the pubic symphysis. (Redrawn from original by Jasmine Tan.)

process itself. Substantial equivalence means the new device has the same intended use as the predicate device *and* has the same technological characteristics *or* different technological characteristics, but it is as safe and effective as the predicate device. **Surgeons should be aware that most new devices for urinary incontinence are not tested in clinical trials before they are marketed.**

Since its introduction, there were scores of articles published suggesting that TVT is effective and safe and similar in effectiveness to colposuspension. Larger, multicenter trials provide the most realistic look at outcomes of a surgical procedure performed by many surgeons with varying experience on a wide array of patients. A report of the 2-year follow-up of 344 women with urodynamic stress incontinence enrolled from 14 centers in a multicenter randomized clinical trial compared TVT and open Burch colposuspension. The objective cure rates (defined as a negative 1-hour pad test) ranged from 63% to 85% for the TVT procedure and 51% to 87% for open colposuspension, depending on how missing data were handled, leading the authors to conclude that "TVT may be better, worse, or the same as open colposuspension in the cure of stress incontinence" (103). Subjectively, only 43% of women in the TVT group and 37% of women in the open colposuspension group reported cure of their stress leakage. Women undergoing the TVT were more likely to have a cystocele after surgery, whereas those undergoing the Burch colposuspension were more likely to have apical prolapse. Two years after the index procedure, seven women (4.8%) in the Burch colposuspension group underwent surgery for pelvic organ prolapse, compared with no women in the TVT group. There was no difference in the number of women that underwent repeat surgery for stress incontinence (1.8% in the TVT group and 3.4% in the Burch group). Women who underwent TVT were less likely to have voiding disorders requiring intermittent self-catheterization than those who underwent colposuspension (0% vs. 2.7%).

Another form of minimally invasive sling is the transobturator tape procedure (also known as a TOT) or transobturator suburethral tape. This modification was designed to reduce complications associated with retropubic needle passage. Inserting the trocar through the obturator space theoretically lessens the risk of bladder, bowel, or vascular injury because the procedure involves passing the polypropylene midurethral sling through the obturator membrane along its ischiorectal fossa path, bypassing the pelvic cavity altogether (104,105). In a multicenter trial, 183 women from seven sites underwent a transobturator tape procedure for stress and mixed urinary incontinence. At 1-year follow-up 80.5% patients were cured (defined as absence of subjective report of stress urine leakage and negative cough stress test). Perioperative complications included one bladder perforation, two urethral perforations, and one lateral vaginal perforation. Tape erosion necessitating removal occurred in five cases (three vaginal and two urethral) (106).

A 2009 Cochrane review identified 62 trials with over 7,000 women in which minimally invasive sling was studied in at least one arm (107). Most were of poor to moderate quality with short follow-up. Minimally invasive synthetic suburethral sling operations appeared to be as effective as traditional suburethral slings but with shorter operating time and less postoperative voiding dysfunction and *de novo* urgency symptoms. Similarly, minimally invasive synthetic suburethral slings were as effective as open retropubic colposuspension with fewer perioperative complications, less postoperative voiding dysfunction, shorter operative time and hospital stay, but significantly more bladder perforations (6% vs. 1%). A retropubic bottom-to-top route was more effective than top-to-bottom route and was associated with significantly less voiding dysfunction, fewer bladder perforations, and tape erosions. At the time of this review, 17 trials comprising 2,434 women compared the transobturator route with the retropubic route of sling placement. The transobturator route had a slightly lower objective cure rate (84% vs. 88%) but had less voiding dysfunction, blood loss, bladder perforation, and shorter operating time.

After the publication of this Cochrane review, the largest (597 women) randomized equivalence trial to date comparing retropubic and transobturator sling approaches was published by the Urinary Incontinence Treatment Network (108). Women were randomized in the operating room and were followed for 1 year. The primary outcome was treatment success at 12 months according to both objective criteria (a negative stress test, a negative pad test, and no retreatment) and subjective criteria (self-reported absence of symptoms, no leakage episodes recorded, and no retreatment). Objective success rates were 80.8% and 77.7% and subjective success rates were 62.2% and 55.8%, in the retropubic and transobturator groups, respectively. Women in the retropubic group had more voiding dysfunction (2.7% vs. 0%), while those in the transobturator group had a higher rate of neurologic symptoms (9.4% vs. 4.0%). **There were no significant differences between groups in postoperative urge incontinence, satisfaction with the results of the procedure, or quality of life.**

A third generation of minimally invasive slings was developed, the so-called minislings. Insertion of the minisling requires only a single vaginal incision, less dissection, and the potential to be placed in a clinic setting. Data are mixed, with some finding equivalent success rates and others up to eightfold higher failure rates in the minisling group than in the full-length synthetic sling (109,110).

Bulking Agents

Injectable (so-called bulking) agents are less invasive than surgery, and although they are less likely than surgery to result in cure, they relieve symptoms in many women. In the United States, glutaraldehyde cross-linked bovine collagen (*Contigen*), carbon beads (*Durasphere*), cross-linked polydimethylsiloxane (*Macroplastique*), and calcium hydroxylapatite (*Coaptite*) are approved for use to treat stress urinary incontinence and can be injected either peri- or transurethrally. The newer agents were studied primarily by transurethral injection. Injecting a material around the periurethral tissues facilitates coaptation of the urethra under conditions of increased intra-abdominal pressure (111–116). In a 15-article review, the short-term cure or improvement rate was 75% (117). *Contigen* can be passed easily through small-bore needles under local anesthesia but requires preoperative skin testing to check for possible allergic reactions (3%). *Durasphere* is nonantigenic (thus no skin testing is required) and does not migrate. As compared with collagen, *Durasphere* appears to have similar reduction in leakage episodes and is more likely to require only a single injection (112). This bulking agent does require a larger-gauge needle for injection and is somewhat more difficult to inject than collagen. *Macroplastique* is approved for use in the United States. This material appears to offer better outcomes as defined by improvement and cure rates than *Contigen* at 12 months (113). A follow-up 24-month study revealed that 84% of patients maintained improvement from the 12-month assessment (114). A recent prospective randomized trial of *Coaptite* versus *Contigen* revealed similar improvement and safety profile at 12 months when compared *Contigen*. *Coaptite* required less material per injection (4 mL vs. 6.6 mL) and was more likely to require only a single injection (115). These techniques may require several injections to achieve continence, and the long-term success of these operations remains poorly studied.

Complications

In choosing surgical management, surgeons must weigh the chance of cure against the chance of severe complications. In the aforementioned randomized trial comparing TVT and Burch, women undergoing TVT were more likely to experience a bladder perforation than those undergoing the Burch procedure (9% vs. 2%, respectively) but less likely to have a fever (1% vs. 5%) or prolonged catheterization more than 29 days (3% vs. 13%) (118). Less common complications require a large sample size to detect differences. Severe complications reported on the FDA manufacturer and user facility device experience (MAUDE) database include vascular injuries, bowel injuries, and patient deaths after retropubic midurethral slings and groin and leg pain, visceral injuries, and severe infections from transobturator approaches (119). Even though these serious life-threatening complications are rare, surgeons must be cognizant of the risks and use intraoperative safety measures to prevent their occurrence.

Actual complication rates are often difficult to discern because denominators often are not available. In a nationwide analysis of 367 complications associated with 1,455 TVT procedures performed in Finland, there was a 1.9% rate (95% CI, 1.2–2.7) of blood loss over 200 mL, a 1.9% rate (95% CI, 1.2–2.7) of retropubic hematoma, a 0.5% rate (95% CI, 0.2–1.0) of hematoma outside the retropubic area, a 0.1% rate (95% CI, 0.0–0.4) of injury to the epigastric vessel, a 0.1% rate (95% CI, 0.0–0.4) of injury to the obturator nerve, and a 3.8% rate (95% CI, 2.9–5.0) of bladder perforation (120).

A prospective, randomized trial of retropubic versus transobturator slings (the TOMUS trial) involving 597 patients revealed more bladder perforations in the retropubic group (15 vs. 0), more patients with elevated PVR volume (>100 mL at time of discharge), and higher rate of sling release or catheterization for voiding dysfunction after 6 weeks (8 vs. 0). The transobturator group had more vaginal perforations (13 vs. 6) and neurologic symptoms including lower extremity weakness and numbness found immediately following surgery to 6 weeks (31 vs. 15). Otherwise, serious adverse events were similar in both groups (108).

Erosion is unique to surgeries in which a graft is placed, and the rate depends largely on the type of graft used. **Tension-free vaginal tape is associated with a low rate of graft erosion, compared with a much higher rate of erosion with certain synthetics previously used for pubovaginal slings.** Most midurethral synthetic slings used at this time are made of polypropylene; the main differences in the character of the mesh involve elasticity and rigidity and not the material itself. **In the randomized trial comparing TVT to TOT described above, of the 597 women who underwent a sling procedure, 1.8% of the patients were noted to have a mesh erosion or exposure** (108).

The most common adverse events (5% to 10% rate for each) after all surgeries for stress urinary incontinence include urinary tract infection, failure to cure, new onset detrusor overactivity, voiding dysfunction, genital prolapse, and bladder perforation. When new onset detrusor overactivity occurs after surgery for incontinence, cystoscopy should be considered to rule out a foreign body in the bladder (Fig. 26.13). Less common events (2% to 5% for each) include excessive blood loss, wound infection, pain, or nerve injury. Events such as sinus tracts and fistulae are rare. Erosion rates depend on the material implanted and, as noted previously, are rare for the midurethral slings. In addition, medical events, such as thromboembolic, cardiac, or pulmonary events, are rare.

As midurethral slings largely replace pubovaginal slings and retropubic urethropexies as the primary procedure for stress urinary incontinence, the comparison of complications of these procedures becomes more important. Given the debate on the effectiveness of the different approaches for midurethral slings, the severity and incidence of complications for midurethral slings will become more important when determining the best primary procedure for stress urinary incontinence. Likewise, the uncommon occurrence of intraoperative and long-term complications of these procedures and underreporting of complications demonstrates the need for reliable large registries for midurethral slings and other promising procedures to assess the safety of these procedures.

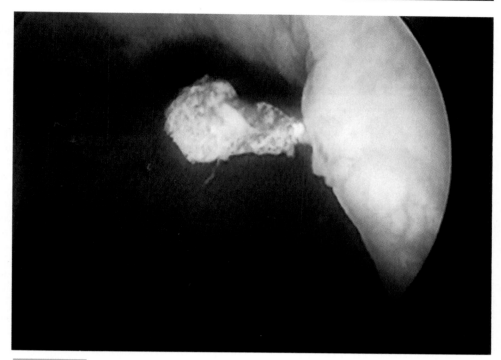

Figure 26.13   Cystoscopic view of encrusted suture penetrating bladder wall following sling urethropexy.

Procedures for Urgency Urinary Incontinence

Neuromodulation

Even with the development of newer anticholinergic medications with fewer side effects, there continues to be a select group of patients with overactive bladders who remain refractory to standard medical and behavioral treatment. Surgical treatment of this condition traditionally involved substantial morbidity and major urinary denervation, reconstruction, or both to achieve therapeutic benefits. The development of implantable sacral nerve root stimulators led to FDA approval of sacral root neuromodulation in patients with refractory urinary urgency and frequency, urge incontinence, and voiding dysfunction. This therapy offers patients with severe symptoms an alternative to urinary augmentation or diversion. **Sacral nerve stimulation therapy** is performed in two phases. In the first phase, a **percutaneous nerve evaluation test** is performed to determine which patients respond to this type of therapy. **Those who respond are implanted with a permanent electrode lead adjacent to the third sacral nerve root connected to a pulse generator.**

A multicenter prospective study demonstrated that 63% of test patients responded to the initial procedure. After implantation, 47% of patients became completely dry, and 77% were successful in eliminating "heavy" leakage episodes. Despite substantial success in nearly 80% of patients who received implants, 30% of patients required further surgical revision because of pain or other complications at the generator or implant site. No permanent injuries or nerve damage was reported in the initial trials (121,122).

In a group of 96 patients with implants (who responded favorably during the test stimulation period), reductions in urge incontinence episodes and severity were still seen at an average of 31 months after implantation. The device was removed in 11 of the 96 patients because of lack of efficacy, pain, or bowel dysfunction. There were no permanent injuries (123). The technique for this procedure evolved to include the location of a generation implant site on the back and the performance of the procedure in two stages with initial percutaneous implantation of a quadpolar instead of a unipolar stimulator. These modifications may improve success rates and decrease the morbidity associated with these procedures. A recent systematic review evaluating eight randomized trials concluded that continuous sacral neural stimulation offers benefits for carefully selected patients with overactive bladder and urinary retention in the absence of obstruction, but many implants did not work or required revisions. The review recommended trials to assess effectiveness directly compared to other treatment options (124).

Percutaneous Tibial Nerve Stimulation

Percutaneous tibial nerve stimulation (PTNS) was first described in 1987 to treat lower urinary tract symptoms and FDA approved in 2000 for overactive bladder. This therapy uses peripheral neurostimulation technique with small (34-gauge) needle electrode inserted at a 60-degree angle approximately 5 cm cephalad to the medial malleolus and slightly posterior to the tibia. The treatment course typically consists of a weekly 30-minute session for 12 weeks. A multicenter, double-blind, randomized control trial involved 220 women with overactive bladder symptoms randomized 1:1 to 12 weeks of treatment with weekly PTNS or sham therapy. The PTNS treatment group achieved statistically significant improvement in bladder symptoms, with 55% reporting moderate to marked improvement compared to 21% in the sham arm compared to baseline (125). The OrBIT (Overactive Bladder Innovative Therapy) trial compared PTNS to extended-release *tolterodine* in the treatment of OAB and found similar improvements in both groups (126). A large portion of responders in this trial (96%) had sustained improvement in OAB symptoms at 12-month follow-up when receiving periodic treatments (127,128). PTNS may represent a viable treatment option for patients who cannot tolerate side effects from anticholinergic medications, who do not responded to behavioral therapy, or who decline implantable neurostimulators.

Botox Injections

Botulinum toxin A (BtxA), a neurotoxin produced by the anaerobic bacteria *Clostridium botulinum*, acts on peripheral cholinergic nerve endings to inhibit calcium-mediated release of acetylcholine vesicles at the presynaptic neuromuscular junctions. In a report from a multicenter study, a 73% continence rate occurred in 180 patients with neurogenic detrusor overactivity incontinence who underwent cystoscopic *Botox* injections (129). A recent prospective placebo-controlled trial in patients with refractory idiopathic urge incontinence demonstrated a 60% clinical response using the Patient Global Impression of Improvement score of 4 or greater with a median duration of response of 373 days. The *Botox* group did experience an increase in postvoid residual in 75% of the subjects (130). The off-label use of Botulinum A cystoscopic detrusor injections to treat refractory urge incontinence in women with and without neurologic impairment is gaining popularity. The procedure is done via cystoscopy and involves injecting 15 to 30 different detrusor muscle sites under direct visualization, sparing the bladder trigone and ureteral orifices.

Augmentation Cystoplasty and Urinary Diversion

Surgery to replace the function of a diseased bladder has been done for more than a century and over the past several decades has gained some popularity in treating people with intractable detrusor overactivity not responsive to any other form of management. **These surgical options include (i) conduit diversion (creation of various intestinal conduits to the skin) or continent diversion (which includes a rectal reservoir or continent cutaneous diversion), (ii) bladder reconstruction, or (iii) replacement of the bladder with various intestinal segments.** For a discussion of these techniques, both historical and current, the interested reader is referred to a review by Greenwell et al. (131). A Cochrane review found only two randomized trials that were of sufficient quality to include and concluded that there were no major differences in outcomes between the techniques and that higher quality research was needed (132). With the advent of sacral neuromodulation and cystoscopic injection with Botulinum A, these procedures are done much less often to treat women with detrusor overactivity.

Surgical Treatment of Fistulae

A wide variety of techniques are available for fistula repair (133,134). Traditionally, fistula repair was performed after a waiting period to allow the resolution of inflammation and formation of scar tissue. This is particularly important in the case of obstetric fistulas, in which the extent of the vascular injury to the soft tissues of the pelvis may not be apparent for many weeks. However, there is a recent trend toward early closure of small gynecologic fistulas (135). **The** keys to closure of a vesicovaginal fistula include wide mobilization of tissue planes so that the fistula edges can be approximated without any tension, close approximation of tissue edges, closure of the fistula in several layers, and meticulous attention to postoperative bladder drainage for 10 to 14 days. The closure of large fistulas will be enhanced by the use of tissue grafts (e.g., Martius labial fat-pad grafts, gracilis muscle flaps) that provide an additional blood supply to nourish an area that has sustained vascular injury. The Latzko procedure used to close a vesicovaginal fistula is shown in Figure 26.14.

Cystoscopy

Scientific evidence does not support routine cystoscopy in women with stress urinary incontinence in the absence of other pathologies (136). Cystoscopy cannot be used to predict intrinsic sphincteric deficiency, stress incontinence, or detrusor overactivity. Cystoscopy can be considered in the following circumstances: (i) in women with urge incontinence to rule out other disorders, especially in women with microscopic hematuria, (ii) in the evaluation of vesicovaginal fistulae, and (iii) intraoperatively to evaluate possible ureteral or vesical injury.

Urologists often use flexible cystoscopy in men; however, women tolerate a rigid cystoscope well, given their short urethras and absence of prostate glands. The view afforded by a rigid cystoscope is clearer than that obtained with a flexible scope, and less technical skill is required to view the entire bladder using a rigid scope. However, with advancement in technology, the efficacy divide between rigid and flexible cystoscopes continues to narrow. **Cystoscopes are available with several viewing angles: 0 degree (straight), 30 degrees (forward-oblique), 70 degrees (lateral), and 120 degrees (retroview). The last scope is rarely used in women.** Zero-degree lenses are essential for viewing the urethra, whereas a 30-degree lens provides the best view of the bladder base and posterior wall, and the 70-degree lens generally provides the best view of the anterior and lateral walls. For diagnostic cystoscopy, sterile water is an ideal medium because it is readily available and inexpensive.

To evaluate the urethra, the cystoscope, typically with a 0-degree or 30-degree lens, should be advanced with distension medium flowing, keeping the center of the urethral lumen in the center of the visual field. The mucosa is normally pink and smooth and the urethral folds close.

After insertion of the cystoscope into the bladder with a 70-degree lens, an air bubble will be present at the bladder dome, which may assist in proper orientation. Then the remainder of the bladder is examined systematically by making a series of sweeps, slowly rotating the cystoscope between the dome and urethrovesical junction. To view the trigone, the light cord should be oriented toward the ceiling (keeping the camera in an upright position). The scope is pulled back until it is almost in the urethra and the base of the bladder is viewed. Because the trigone is a zone of metaplasia, it looks different from the rest of the urothelium (Fig. 26.15).

Vaginal and abdominal hysterectomies are associated with a 0.02% to 0.85% incidence of ureteral injury (137). The injury rate increases in reconstructive pelvic surgeries, reaching as high as 11% after uterosacral ligament suspension (138). In a study of 46 women who underwent proximal uterosacral ligament vaginal vault suspension, three of the five women with cystoscopic evidence of obstruction were treated successfully by removing and replacing the sutures. This finding emphasizes the importance of confirming ureteral integrity at surgery. **The value of cystoscopy to evaluate ureteral injury after minimally invasive hysterectomy is unknown because this injury is often thought to occur in association with thermal injury, and it is unclear whether obstruction or decreased flow will be apparent intraoperatively.**

Administering indigo carmine dye intravenously 5 minutes before cystoscopy aides in the assessment of ureteral patency. Quick efflux of stained urine should be seen bilaterally. Sluggish efflux should prompt further investigation. However, preexisting ureteral obstruction may be responsible for lack of flow. In 157 women who underwent complex urogynecologic procedures, 5 cases (3.2%) of unsuspected ureteral obstruction were identified with intraoperative cystoscopy (139). One was caused by ureteral ligation, and the remaining four represented chronic ureteral obstruction resulting from pelvic organ prolapse (two cases), ureteropelvic junction obstruction (one case), and ureterovesical junction stenosis after prior transurethral resection of bladder cancer (one case).

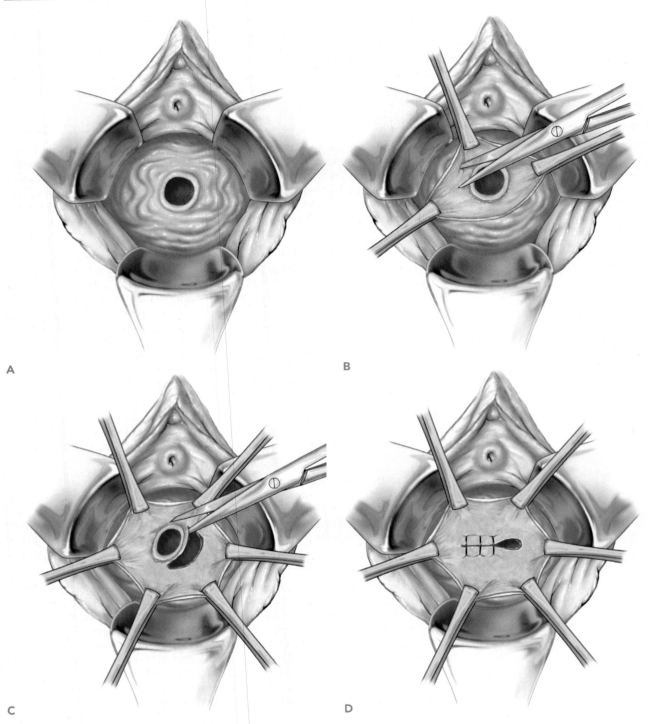

Figure 26.14   Repair of apical vesicovaginal fistula.   A: The fistula at the vaginal apex is exposed with adequate retraction. A pediatric foley can be placed into the fistula tract to aid in traction and dissection. **B:** The vaginal epithelium is dissected from the fistula to mobilize the tissue to allow for tension-free closure. In the classic Latzko procedure, the vaginal epithelium 2 cm around the opening of the fistula is removed. **C:** The fistula tract may either be completely excised, or in the Latzko procedure, the fistula edge may freshened up slightly but is not excised. **D:** Interrupted absorbable sutures are placed in an extramucosal location in an interrupted fashion. An additional layer of interrupted sutures is often placed to invert the initial suture line. The vaginal epithelium is then closed over the repair. In the classic Latzko procedure, the initial layer involves closure of the vagina over the fistula tract, then two additional layers with the vaginal epithelium result in an apical colpocleisis. (Redrawn from original by Jasmine Tan.)

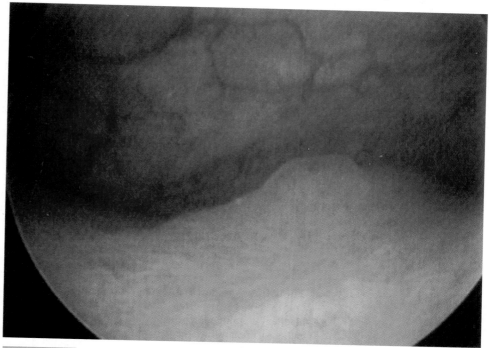

Figure 26.15 Cystoscopic view of normal-appearing trigone with left ureteral orifice visible.

Voiding Dysfunction and Bladder Pain Syndromes

Voiding Dysfunction

Women are afflicted less commonly than men with voiding difficulties, but these disorders do occur in women and can be defined as emptying dysfunction resulting from relaxation of the pelvic floor musculature or failure of the detrusor muscle to contract appropriately. True outflow obstruction (defined as a detrusor pressure of more than 50 cm H_2O in association with a urine flow rate of less than 15 mL/sec) is rare in women and, when seen, is usually found in those who underwent obstructive bladder neck surgery for stress incontinence (140,141). **For normal voiding to occur, the pelvic floor and urethral sphincter must relax, which should happen in conjunction with a coordinated contraction of the detrusor muscle that leads to complete bladder emptying.** The bladder may be emptied by other mechanisms, such as by abdominal straining in the absence of a detrusor contraction or simply by relaxation of the pelvic floor. Complete bladder emptying is not the same as normal voiding. Some women may empty their bladders completely but only by expending great effort over several minutes. In such cases, voiding is clearly abnormal, even though the bladder is empty when voiding ceases. In the worst cases, voiding is both difficult and incomplete.

Causes

Neurologic diseases, such as multiple sclerosis, may cause voiding difficulty as a result of *detrusor-sphincter dyssynergia,* in which the urethral sphincter contracts at the same time as the detrusor (143). Great effort is required to overcome urethral resistance; the patient voids with an interrupted stop-and-start stream and usually has a significant amount of residual urine.

Other causes of voiding difficulty include medications (such as antihistamines and anticholinergic agents), infections (in particular, herpes simplex virus, and urinary tract infections), obstruction (following bladder neck surgery, or in women with advanced pelvic organ prolapse), overdistension, severe constipation (particularly in the elderly), and, rarely, psychogenic factors. Fowler's syndrome refers to unexplained urinary retention occurring as an isolated phenomenon (144). Such women usually are between 20 and 35 years of age. Commonly the first retention episode will be triggered by an event such as surgery or childbirth. Retention rarely resolves but is not associated with the development of other disorders.

Evaluation

Evaluation of a woman with voiding difficulty begins with a careful physical examination. **Advanced pelvic organ prolapse may contribute to urinary retention, but it is unlikely that prolapse above the level of the vaginal introitus will be the sole cause of retention.** When in doubt, the woman can wear a pessary for a week to see whether elevating the prolapse reduces the voiding difficulty. Occasionally pelvic masses—in particular, low anterior myomas—may cause urinary retention. Abnormal findings detected during neurologic examination of the perineum and lower extremities may suggest the need to focus on the spine. Urodynamic evaluation will help determine whether the woman has an obstruction (manifested by high detrusor pressures during voiding or by no urethral relaxation during voiding) or whether the detrusor muscle is not contracting. The latter is not necessarily indicative of a neurogenic disorder in women, because a large minority of normal healthy women void by urethral and pelvic floor muscle relaxation alone, with no detrusor contraction. Cystourethroscopy may reveal an obstructing lesion, such as a polyp, tumor, ureterocele, or ball-valve stone. Usually, the evaluation reveals no obvious source, and treatment can commence.

Treatment

The mainstay in the treatment of voiding difficulty is clean, intermittent self-catheterization (145). The most important protection against urinary tract infection is frequent and complete bladder emptying rather than avoiding the introduction of a foreign body into the bladder. Self-catheterization allows the patient to accomplish this task using a small (14-Fr) plastic catheter that she inserts through the urethra into the bladder, draining its contents. The catheter is then removed, washed with soap and water, dried, and stored in a clean, dry place. Elaborate sterile procedures are not necessary. Bacteria are introduced into the bladder in this process, and the urine of women after self-catheterization regimens will always be colonized with bacteria; however, this condition should not be treated unless symptomatic infection occurs.

In addition to decreasing urinary urgency and incontinence caused by detrusor overactivity, neuromodulation of the sacral nerve roots may help women with nonobstructive urinary retention (122). In a trial of 177 patients with idiopathic urinary retention, those who had greater than 50% improvement in baseline voiding symptoms during a test stimulation period qualified for surgical implantation of *InterStim*. Of these, 37 were randomly assigned to early implantation, whereas 31 in the control group delayed implantation for 6 months. Improved voiding occurred in 83% of the implant group compared with 9% of the control group at 6 months (146). It appears that the long-term success rates of *InterStim* for urinary retention remain high. In a trial following patients for 5-years after implantation, 71% of the patients with urinary retention had successful outcomes (147). Although this technology requires a surgical procedure, many women favor this therapy over lifelong self-catheterization.

Mild sedatives are sometimes helpful in this process, as are α-blockers (e.g., *prazosin, phenoxy-benzamine, tamsulosin*), which reduce urethral tone. Although cholinergic medications such as *bethanechol chloride* are successful in making strips of bladder muscle contract in a laboratory, there is little evidence that such drugs are helpful clinically (148).

Bladder Pain Syndromes

Most patients with disorders of bladder sensation experience pain rather than lack of bladder sensation. As with the treatment of most chronic pain disorders, the cause of most painful bladder conditions is unknown, and the therapies used are only partially successful. As a result, disorders of bladder sensation are among the most frustrating urogynecologic conditions to manage.

Terminology and Prevalence

Bladder pain syndrome, often termed *interstitial cystitis,* is a poorly defined heterogeneous syndrome, and diagnostic criteria are changing continuously. **The International Continence Society standardization report recommends adapting the term *bladder pain syndrome,* rather than *interstitial cystitis,* and defines painful bladder syndrome as "an unpleasant sensation (pain, pressure, discomfort) perceived to be related to the urinary bladder associated with lower urinary tract symptom(s) of more than 6 weeks duration, in the absence of infection or other identifiable causes"** (15). **Urgency and pain are the defining characteristics of bladder pain syndrome** (149). Several factors have inhibited advances in the understanding of interstitial cystitis, including the lack of specific diagnostic criteria, the lack of specific histopathologic changes, the unpredictable fluctuation in symptoms, and the marked variability among patients in terms of symptoms, objective findings, and treatment responses (150).

The National Institute of Diabetes, Digestive, and Kidney Diseases (NIDDK) developed a research definition for interstitial cystitis that requires objective findings of glomerulations or a classic Hunner's ulcer during hydrodistention of the bladder and subjective symptoms of bladder pain or urinary urgency in the absence of other urogenital pathology (151). Strict application of NIDDK criteria in one study would have misdiagnosed more than 60% of patients thought to definitely or possibly have interstitial cystitis (152). Many clinicians have challenged the clinical utility of the NIDDK research criteria, and most conceptualize interstitial cystitis as the end point on the spectrum of painful bladder disorders (153).

The prevalence of bladder pain syndrome varies widely depending on the diagnostic criteria utilized. When mild and moderately severe cases are considered, the syndrome is not rare (154). Estimates of prevalence in the United States range from 52 per 100,000 women in the population-based Nurses Health Study to as high as 1 in 4.5 women "with accurate diagnostic records" (155,156). The prevalence appears to be 6 to 15 times more common among women than men (155,157). The identification of risk factors for bladder pain syndrome is particularly challenging because of the typically long delay in diagnosis (154). The Interstitial Cystitis Database study confirms many of the previous epidemiologic observations: affected individuals are predominately female (92%), white (91%), and report an average age of symptom onset of 32.2 years (150,155).

Diagnosis

A careful history should be obtained, along with a sterile urine specimen for analysis and culture. Many women treated repetitively for chronic cystitis take multiple courses of antibiotics on the basis of symptoms without ever having the presence of an infection confirmed by cultures. Detrusor overactivity may be the cause of frequency, urgency, and urge incontinence, but that is not usually a factor in dysuria or painful urination. **Women older than 50 years (particularly those who smoke or are exposed to chemicals at work) are at risk for bladder cancer, and this possibility must be considered, especially if hematuria is present.** Urinary cytologic assessment is sometimes helpful in detecting early tumors of the urinary tract, and cystoscopy and intravenous urography are mandatory in the evaluation of patients with hematuria.

Other possible causes for painful voiding must be considered in the differential diagnosis, including urethral diverticula; vulvar disease; endometriosis; chemical irritation from soaps, bubble bath, or feminine hygiene products; urinary stones; urogenital atrophy from estrogen deprivation; and sexually transmitted disease.

The diagnosis of bladder pain syndrome or interstitial cystitis is largely one of exclusion. The ideal diagnostic test for interstitial cystitis is not determined, and there are myriad proposed tests.

Treatment

Typically, the evaluation of bladder pain syndrome results in no definitive diagnosis, and management focuses on the treatment of symptoms.

Frequency–urgency syndromes should be managed with a careful voiding regimen (similar to that used in the treatment of urgency urinary incontinence) and local care.

The use of urinary tract analgesics such as *Prosed DS* may be helpful in reducing urethral irritation. *Prosed DS* is a polypharmaceutical agent containing a mixture of *methenamine, methylene blue, phenyl salicylate, benzoic acid,* and *hyoscyamine* that has a soothing effect on many irritative urinary tract symptoms.

There is no scientific evidence linking diet to painful bladder syndrome, but many doctors and patients find that alcohol, tomatoes, spices, chocolate, caffeinated and citrus beverages, and high-acid foods may contribute to bladder irritation and inflammation. Some patients note that their symptoms worsen after eating or drinking products containing artificial sweeteners. Patients may try eliminating various items from their diet and reintroducing them one at a time to determine which, if any, affect their symptoms. Instruction in the basics of vulvar and perineal hygiene is important (thorough drying; avoidance of most body powders, perfumes, or colored irritating soaps; avoidance of tight-fitting undergarments) to avoid other factors that may contribute to painful voiding.

Hydrodistention of the bladder (usually under anesthesia) is recommended as a treatment option and can result in clinical improvement in some patients. Likewise, bladder installations are commonly used for acute treatment of bladder pain syndrome. The medications used range from local anesthetics to bladder specific medications including *resiniferatoxin, dimethyl sulfoxide, BCG, pentosan polysulfate,* and *oxybutynin.* Some patients benefit from the instillation into the bladder of 50 mL of a 50% solution of *dimethylsulfoxide (DMSO)* for 20 to 30 minutes every other week for four or five sessions. A recent Cochran review found that evidence is limited and randomized controlled trials are needed to adequately assess outcomes. Intravesical installations of *BCG* and *oxybutynin* are reasonably well tolerated, and evidence is the most promising for these agents (157).

Tricyclic antidepressants are commonly used in patients with pain. A trial by the Interstitial Cystitis Collaborative Research Network found that *amitriptyline* plus education and behavioral modification did not significantly improve symptoms in the treatment of naive patients with bladder pain syndrome, but the network did suggest that it may be beneficial in those patients who could tolerate a daily dose of 50 mg or greater (158).

Pentosan polysulfate (Elmiron) is an FDA-approved oral agent with heparin-like activity that attempts to replace the glycosaminoglycan sulfate layer that is believed deficient in these patients. The FDA-recommended oral dosage of *pentosan polysulfate* is 100 mg, three times a day. Patients may not feel relief from pain for the first 2 to 4 months, and it may take up to 6 months for a decrease in urinary frequency to occur.

It is theorized that bladder pain may result from increased histamine release, and some patients benefit from medications that block these inflammatory mediators, such as *diphenhydramine hydrochloride,* 25 to 50 mg orally three times per day, in combination with 300 mg of *cimetidine* three times per day. Tricyclic antidepressants help some women by modulating sensory nerve pain.

Transcutaneous electrical nerve stimulation (TENS), through wires placed on the lower back or just above the symphysis, may help some women, though the mechanism of action is unclear. Ongoing preliminary research suggests that some women with severe bladder pain syndrome may find relief following sacral neuromodulation (*InterStim*), acupuncture, or intravesical *Botox* injection associated with hydrodistension.

References

1. **DeLancey JO.** Structural support of the urethra as it relates to stress urinary incontinence: the hammock hypothesis. *Am J Obstet Gynecol* 1994;170:1713–1723.
2. **Wall LL, Helms M, Peattie AB, et al.** Bladder neck mobility and the outcome of surgery for genuine stress urinary incontinence: a logistic regression analysis of lateral bead-chain cystourethrograms. *J Reprod Med* 1994;39:429–435.
3. **Sand PK, Bowen LD, Panganiban R, et al.** The low pressure urethra as a factor in failed retropubic urethropexy. *Obstet Gynecol* 1987; 69:399–402.
4. **Stay K, Dwyer PL, Rosamilia L, et al.** Risk factors of treatment failure of midurethral sling procedures for women with urinary stress incontinence. *Urogynecol J Pelvic Floor Dysfunct* 2010;21:149–155.
5. **Burnstock G.** Nervous control of smooth muscle by transmitters, cotransmitters and modulators. *Experientia* 1985;41:869–874.
6. **Burnstock G.** The changing face of autonomic neurotransmission. *Acta Physiol Scand* 1986;126:67–91.
7. **Daniel EE, Cowan W, Daniel VP.** Structural bases of neural and myogenic control of human detrusor muscle. *Can J Physiol Pharmacol* 1983;61:67–91.
8. **Haylen BT, de Ridder D, Freeman RM, et al.** An International Urogynecological Association (IUGA)/International Continence Society (ICS) joint report on the terminology for female pelvic floor dysfunction. *Neurourol Urodyn* 2010;29:4–20.
9. **U.S. Department of Health and Human Services.** Urinary incontinence in adults: acute and chronic management. In: **U.S. Public Health Service.** Agency for Health Care Policy and Research. No. 96–0682. AHCPR Publications, 1996.
10. **Frazer MI, Haylen BT, Sutherst JR.** The severity of urinary incontinence in women: comparison of subjective and objective tests. *Br J Urol* 1989;63:14–15.
11. **Nygaard I, DeLancey JO, Arnsdorf L, et al.** Exercise and incontinence. *Obstet Gynecol* 1990;75:848–851.
12. **Wall LL.** Diagnosis and management of urinary incontinence due to detrusor instability. *Obstet Gynecol Surv* 1990;45:1S–47S.
13. **Larrson G, Victor A.** Micturition patterns in a healthy female population, studies with a frequency/volume chart. *Scand J Urol Nephrol Suppl* 1998;114:53–57.
14. **Fitzgerald MP, Stablein U, Brubaker L.** Urinary habits among asymptomatic women. *Am J Obstet Gynecol* 2002;187:1384–1388.
15. **Abrams P, Andersson KE, Birder L, et al.** Fourth international consultation on incontinence recommendations of the International Scientific Committee: evaluation and treatment of urinary incontinence, pelvic organ prolapse, and fecal incontinence. *Neurourol Urodyn* 2010;29:213–240.
16. **Hunskaar S, Burgio K, Diokno A, et al.** Epidemiology and natural history of urinary incontinence. In: **Abrams P, Cardozo L, Khoury S, et al., eds.** *Incontinence.* Plymouth, UK: Plymbridge Distributors Ltd, 2002:165–201.
17. **Resnick NM, Yalla SV.** Management of urinary incontinence in the elderly. *N Engl J Med* 1985;313:800–805.
18. **Resnick NM, Yalla SV, Laurine E.** An algorithmic approach to urinary incontinence in the elderly. *Clin Res* 1986;34:832–837.
19. **Stanton SL.** Gynecologic complications of epispadias and bladder exstrophy. *Am J Obstet Gynecol* 1974;119:749–754.

20. **Mitchell RJ.** An ectopic vaginal ureter. *J Obstet Gynaecol Br Commw* 1961;68:299–302.

21. **Ibeanu OA, Chesson RR, Echols KT, et al.** Urinary tract injury during hysterectomy based on universal cystoscopy. *Obstet Gynecol* 2009;113:6–10.

22. **Tamussino KF, Lang PF, Breini E.** Ureteral complication with operative gynecologic laparoscopy. *Am J Obstet Gynecol* 1998;178:967–970.

23. **Porcaro AB, Zicari M, Zecchini Antoniolli S, et al.** Vesicouterine fistulas following cesarean section: report on a case, review and update of the literature. *Int Urol Nephrol* 2002;34:335–344.

24. **Viktrup L, Lose G, Rolff M, et al.** The symptom of stress incontinence caused by pregnancy or delivery in primiparas. *Obstet Gynecol* 1992;79:945–949.

25. **Peschers UM, Schaer GN, DeLancey JO, et al.** Levator ani function before and after childbirth. *BJOG* 1997;104:1004–1008.

26. **DeLancey JO, Kearney R, Chou Q, et al.** The appearance of levator ani muscle abnormalities in magnetic resonance images after vaginal delivery. *Obstet Gynecol* 2003;101:46–53.

27. **Snooks SJ, Swash M, Mathers SE, et al.** Effect of vaginal delivery on the pelvic floor: a 5-year follow-up. *Br J Surg* 1990;77:1358–1360.

28. **Chiarelli P, Brown W, McElduff P.** Leaking urine: prevalence and associated factors in Australian women. *Neurourol Urodyn* 1999;18:567–571.

29. **Brown JS, Grady D, Ouslander JG, et al.** Prevalence of urinary incontinence and associated risk factors in postmenopausal women. Heart and Estrogen/Progestin Replacement Study (HERS) Research Group. *Obstet Gynecol* 1999;94:66–70.

30. **Hannestad YS, Rortveit G, Dalveit AK, et al.** Are smoking and other lifestyle factors associated with female urinary incontinence? The Norwegian EPINCONT study. *Br J Obstet Gynaecol* 2003;110:247–254.

31. **Subak LL, Wing R, Smith West D.** Weight loss to treat urinary incontinence in overweight and obese women. *N Engl J Med* 2009;360:481–490.

32. **Bissada NK, Finkbeiner AE.** Urologic manifestations of drug therapy. *Urol Clin North Am* 1988;15:725–736.

33. **Ostergard DR.** The effects of drugs on the lower urinary tract. *Obstet Gynecol Surv* 1979;34:424–432.

34. **Wall LL, Addison WA.** Prazosin-induced stress incontinence. *Obstet Gynecol* 1990;75:558–560.

35. **Menefee SA, Chesson R, Wall LL.** Stress urinary incontinence due to prescription medications: alpha-blockers and angiotensin converting enzyme inhibitors. *Obstet Gynecol* 1998;91:853–854.

36. **Walters MD, Diaz K.** Q-tip test: a study of continent and incontinent women. *Obstet Gynecol* 1987;70:208–211.

37. **Artibani W, Andersen JT, Gajewski JB, et al.** *Imaging and other investigations.* Plymouth, UK: Plymbridge Distributors Ltd, 2002.

38. **Wall LL, Norton PA, DeLancey JOL.** *Practical urodynamics.* Baltimore, MD: Williams & Wilkins, 1993.

39. **Richardson DA, Ramahi A, Chalas E.** Surgical management of stress incontinence in patients with low urethral pressure. *Obstet Gynecol Invest* 1991;150:106–109.

40. **Hilton P, Stanton SL.** Urethral pressure measurement by microtransducer: the results in symptom-free women and in those with genuine stress incontinence. *Br J Obstet Gynaecol* 1983;90:919–933.

41. **Weber AM.** Is urethral pressure profilometry a useful diagnostic test for stress urinary incontinence? *Obstet Gynecol Surv* 2001;56:720–735.

42. **Culligan PJ, Goldberg RP, Blackhurst DW, et al.** Comparison of microtransducer and fiberoptic catheters for urodynamic studies. *Obstet Gynecol* 2001;98:253–257.

43. **Versi E, Cardozo LD, Studd JW, et al.** Internal urinary sphincter in maintenance of female continence. *BMJ* 1986;292:166–167.

44. **Neitlich JD, Foster HE Jr, Glickman MG, et al.** Detection of urethral diverticula in women: comparison of a high resolution fast spin echo technique with double balloon urethrography. *J Urol* 1998;159:408–410.

45. **Hay Smith J, Berghman B, Burgio K, et al.** Adult conservative management. In: **Abrams P CL, Khoury S, Wein A, eds.** *Incontinence.* 4th ed. Paris, France: Health Publications, 2009:1025–1120

46. **Dumoulin C, Hay-Smith J.** Pelvic floor muscle training versus no treatment, or inactive control treatment, for urinary incontinence in women for urinary incontinence in women. *Cochrane Database Syst Rev* 2010;1:CD005654.

47. **Luber KM, Wolde-Tsadik G.** Efficacy of functional electrical stimulation in treating genuine stress urinary incontinence: a randomized clinical trial. *Neurourol Urodyn* 1997;16:543–551.

48. **Sand PK, Richardson DA, Staskin DR, et al.** Pelvic floor electrical stimulation in the treatment of genuine stress urinary incontinence: a multicenter, placebo-controlled trial. *Am J Obstet Gynecol* 1995;173:72–79.

49. **Brubaker L, Benson JT, Bent AE, et al.** Transvaginal electrical stimulation for female urinary incontinence. *Am J Obstet Gynecol* 1997;177:536–540.

50. **Yamanishi T, Yasuda K, Sakakibara R, et al.** Randomized, double-blind study of electrical stimulation for urinary incontinence due to detrusor overactivity. *Urology* 2000;55:353–357.

51. **Burgio K.** Current perspectives on management of urgency using bladder and behavioral training. *J Am Acad Nurse Pract* 2004;16:4–9.

52. **Burgio KL, Locher JL, Goode PS, et al.** Behavioral vs drug treatment for urge urinary incontinence in older women: a randomized controlled trial. *JAMA* 1998;280:1995–2000.

53. **Goode PS, Burgio KL, Locher JL, et al.** Effect of behavioral training with or without pelvic floor electrical stimulation on stress incontinence in women: a randomized controlled trial. *JAMA* 2003;290:345–352.

54. **Donnelly MJ, Powell-Morgan S, Olsen AL, et al.** Vaginal pessaries for the management of stress and mixed urinary incontinence. *Int Urogynecol J Pelvic Floor Dysfunct* 2004;15:302–307.

55. **Richter HE, Burgio KL, Brubaker L, et al.** Continence pessary compared with behavioral therapy or combined therapy for stress incontinence: a randomized controlled trial. *Obstet Gynecol* 2010;115:609–617.

56. **Sirls LT, Foote JE, Kaufman JM, et al.** Long-term results of the FemSoft urethral insert for the management of female stress urinary incontinence. *Intern Urogynecol J Pelv Floor Dys* 2002;13:88–95.

57. **Kernan WN, Viscoli CM, Brass LM, et al.** Phenylpropanolamine and risk of hemorrhagic stroke. *N Engl J Med* 2000;343:1826–1832.

58. **Nygaard I, Kreder KJ.** Pharmacologic therapy of lower urinary tract dysfunction. *Clin Obstet Gynecol* 2004;47:83–92.

59. **Grady D, Brown JS, Vittinghoff E, et al.** The HERS Research Group. Postmenopausal hormones and incontinence: the Heart and Estrogen/Progestin Replacement Study. *Obstet Gynecol* 2001;97:116–120.

60. **Hendrix SL, Cochrane BB, Nygaard IE, et al.** Effects of estrogen with and without progestin on urinary incontinence. *JAMA* 2005;293:935–948.

61. **Hartmann KE, McPheeters ML, Biller DH, et al.** Treatment of overactive bladder in women. *Evid Rep Technol Assess (Full Rep)* 2009:1–120

62. **Janknegt RA, Zweers HM, Delaere KP, et al.** Oral desmopressin as a new treatment modality for primary nocturnal enuresis in adolescents and adults: a double-blind, randomized, multicenter study. Dutch Enuresis Study Group. *J Urol* 1997;157:513–517.

63. **Valiquette G, Abrams GM, Herbert J.** DDAVP in the management of nocturia in multiple sclerosis. *Ann Neurol* 1992;31:577.

64. **Ray WA, Griffin MR, Schaffner W, et al.** Psychotropic drug use and the risk of hip fracture. *N Engl J Med* 1987;316:363–369.

65. **Pedersen PA, Johansen PB.** Prophylactic treatment of adult nocturia with bumetanide. *Br J Urol* 1988;62:145–147.

66. **Black NA, Downs SH.** The effectiveness of surgery for stress incontinence in women: a systematic review. *Br J Urol* 1996;78:497–510.

67. **Leach GE, Dmochowski RR, Appell RA, et al.** Female Stress Urinary Incontinence Clinical Guidelines Panel summary report on surgical management of female stress urinary incontinence. The American Urological Association. *J Urol* 1997;158:875–880.

68. **Kelly HA, Dumm WM.** Urinary incontinence in women without manifest injury to the bladder. *Surg Gynecol Obstet* 1914;18:444–450.

69. **Stanton SL, Cardozo LD.** A comparison of vaginal and suprapubic surgery in the correction of incontinence due to urethral sphincter incompetence. *Br J Urol* 1979;51:497–499.

70. **Bailey KV.** A clinical investigation into uterine prolapse with stress incontinence treatment by modified Manchester colporrhaphy. I. *J Obstet Gynaecol Br Emp* 1954;61:291–301.

71. **Colombo M, Vitobello D, Proietti F, et al.** Randomised comparison of Burch colposuspension versus anterior colporrhaphy in women with stress urinary incontinence and anterior vaginal wall prolapse. *Br J Obstet Gynaecol* 2000;107:544–551.

72. **Beck RP, McCormick S.** Treatment of urinary stress incontinence with anterior colporrhaphy. *Obstet Gynecol* 1982;59:269–274.

73. **Beck RP, McCormick S.** A 25-year experience with 519 anterior colporrhaphy procedures. *Obstet Gynecol* 1991;78:1011–1018.

74. **Bergman A, Elia G.** Three surgical procedures for genuine stress incontinence: five-year follow-up of a prospective randomized study. *Am J Obstet Gynecol* 1995;173:66–71.

75. **O'Sullivan DC, Chilton CP, Munson KW.** Should Stamey colposuspension be our primary surgery for stress incontinence? *Br J Urol* 1995;75:457–460.

76. **Trockman BA, Leach GE, Hamilton J, et al.** Modified Pereyra bladder neck suspension: 10-year mean follow-up using outcomes analysis in 125 patients. *J Urol* 1995;154:1841–1847.

77. **Tebyani N, Patel H, Yamaguchi R, et al.** Percutaneous needle bladder neck suspension for the treatment of stress urinary incontinence in women: long-term results. *J Urol* 2000;163:1510–1512.

78. **Marshall VF, Marchetti AA, Krantz KE.** The correction of stress incontinence by simple vesicourethral suspension. *Surg Gynecol Obstet* 1949;88:509–518.

79. **Burch J.** Urethrovaginal fixation to Cooper's ligament for correction of stress incontinence, cystocele and prolapse. *Am J Obstet Gynecol* 1961;81:281–290.

80. **Burch J.** Cooper's ligament urethrovesical suspension for stress incontinence: a nine-year experience—results, complications, technique. *Am J Obstet Gynecol* 1968;100:764–774.

81. **Richardson AC, Lyon JB, Williams NL.** Treatment of stress urinary incontinence due to paravaginal fascial defect. *Obstet Gynecol* 1981;57:357–362.

82. **Shull BL, Baden WF.** A six-year experience with paravaginal defect repair for stress urinary incontinence. *Am J Obstet Gynecol* 1989;160:1432–1440.

83. **Turner-Warwick R.** *Turner-Warwick vagino-obturator shelf urethral repositioning procedure.* New York: Springer-Verlag, 1988.

84. **German KA, Kynaston H, Weight S, et al.** A prospective randomized trial comparing a modified needle suspension procedure with the vagina/obturator shelf procedure for genuine stress incontinence. *Br J Urol* 1994;74:188–190.

85. **Lapitan MC, Cody JD, Grant A.** Open retropubic colposuspension for urinary incontinence in women. *Cochrane Database Syst Rev* 2009;2:CD002912.

86. **Moehrer B, Ellis G, Carey M, et al.** Laparoscopic colposuspension for urinary incontinence in women. *Cochrane Database Syst Rev* 2002;1:CD002239.

87. **Parker RT, Addison WA, Wilson CJ.** Fascia lata urethrovesical suspension for recurrent stress urinary incontinence. *Am J Obstet Gynecol* 1979;135:843–852.

88. **Beck RP, McCormick S, Nordstrom L.** The fascia lata sling procedure for treating recurrent genuine stress incontinence of urine. *Obstet Gynecol* 1988;72:699–703.

89. **Beck RP, Lai AR.** Results in treating 88 cases of recurrent urinary stress incontinence with the Oxford fascia lata sling procedure. *Am J Obstet Gynecol* 1982;142:649–651.

90. **Chaikin DC, Rosenthal J, Blaivas JG.** Pubovaginal fascial sling for all types of stress urinary incontinence: long-term analysis. *J Urol* 1998;160:1312–1316.

91. **Cross CA, Cespedes RD, McGuire EJ.** Our experience with pubovaginal slings in patients with stress urinary incontinence. *J Urol* 1998;159:1195–1198.

92. **Breen JM, Geer BE, May GE.** The fascia lata suburethral sling for treating recurrent urinary stress incontinence. *Am J Obstet Gynecol* 1997;92:747–750.

93. **Stanton SL, Brindley GS, Holmes DM.** Silastic sling for urethral sphincter incompetence. *Br J Obstet Gynaecol* 1985;92:747–750.

94. **Horbach NS, Blanco JS, Ostergard DR, et al.** A suburethral sling procedure with polytetrafluoroethylene for the treatment of genuine stress incontinence in patients with low urethral closure pressure. *Obstet Gynecol* 1988;71:648–652.

95. **Rottenberg RD, Weil A, Brioschi PA, et al.** Urodynamic and clinical assessment of the Lyodura sling operation for urinary stress incontinence. *Br J Obstet Gynaecol* 1985;92:829–834.

96. **Wright EJ, Iselin CE, Carr LK, et al.** Pubovaginal sling using cadaveric allograft for the treatment of intrinsic sphincter deficiency. *J Urol* 1998;160:759–762.

97. **Amundsen CL, Visco AG, Ruiz H, et al.** Outcome in 104 pubovaginal slings using freeze-dried allograft fascia lata from a single tissue bank. *Urology* 2000;56:2–8.

98. **Kobashi KC, Dmochowski R, Mee S.** Erosion of polyester pubovaginal sling. *J Urol* 1999;162:2070–2072.

99. **Clemons JQ, DeLancey JO, Faerber GJ, et al.** Urinary tract erosions after synthetic pubovaginal slings: diagnosis and management strategy. *Urology* 2000;56:589–595.

100. **Albo ME, Richter HE, Brubaker L, et al.** Burch colposuspension versus fascial sling to reduce urinary stress incontinence. *N Engl J Med* 2007;356:2143–2155.

101. **Heit M.** What is the scientific evidence for bone anchor use during bladder neck suspension? *Int Urogynecol J Pelvic Floor Dysfunct* 2002;13:143–144.

102. **Falconer C, Ekman-Ordeberg G, Malmstrom A, et al.** Clinical outcome and changes in connective tissue metabolism after intravaginal slingplasty in stress incontinent women. *Int Urogynecol J Pelvic Floor Dysfunct* 1996;7:133–137.

103. **Ward KL, Hilton P.** A prospective multicenter randomized trial of tension-free vaginal tape and colposuspension for primary urodynamic stress incontinence: two-year follow-up. *Am J Obstet Gynecol* 2004;190:324–331.

104. **Dargent D, Bretones S, George P, et al.** [Insertion of a sub-urethral sling through the obturating membrane for treatment of female urinary incontinence.] *Gynecol Obstet Fertil* 2002;30:576–582.

105. **Delorme E, Droupy S, de Tayrac R, et al.** Transobturator tape (Uratape): a new minimally-invasive procedure to treat female urinary incontinence. *Eur Urol* 2004;45:203–207.

106. **Costa P, Gris P, Droupy S, et al.** Surgical treatment of female stress urinary incontinence with a trans-obturator-tape (TOT): short term results of a prospective multicentric study. *Eur Urol* 2004;46:102–106.

107. **Ogah J, Cody JD, Rogerson L.** Minimally invasive synthetic suburethral sling operations for stress urinary incontinence in women. *Cochrane Database Syst Rev* 2009;4:CD006375.

108. **Richter HE, Albo ME, Zyczynski HM, et al.** Retropubic versus transobturator midurethral slings for stress incontinence. *N Engl J Med* 2010;362:2066–2076.

109. **De Ridder D, Berkers J, Deprest J, et al.** Single incision mini-sling versus a transobturator sling: a comparative study on MiniArc and Monarc slings. *Int Urogynecol J Pelvic Floor Dysfunct* 2010;21:773–778.

110. **Basu M, Duckett J.** A randomised trial of a retropubic tension-free vaginal tape versus a mini-sling for stress incontinence. *BJOG* 2010;117:730–735.

111. **Murless BC.** The injection treatment of stress incontinence. *J Obstet Gynaecol Br Emp* 1938;45:67–73.

112. **Lightner D, Calvosa C, Andersen R, et al.** A new injectable bulking agent for treatment of stress urinary incontinence: results of a multicenter, randomized, controlled, double-blind study of Durasphere. *Urology* 2001;58:12–15.

113. **Ghoniem G, Corcos J, Comiter C, et al.** Cross-linked polydimethylsiloxane injection for female stress urinary incontinence: results of a multicenter, randomized, controlled, single-blind study. *J Urol* 2009;204–210.

114. **Ghoniem G, Corcos J, Comiter, et al.** Durability of urethral bulking agent injection for female stress urinary incontinence: 2-year multicenter study results. *J Urol* 2010;183:1444–1449.

115. **Mayer RD, Domochowski RR, Appell RA, et al.** Multicenter prospective randomized 52-week trial of calcium hydroxlapatite versus bovine dermal collagen for treatment of stress urinary incontinence. *Urology* 2007;69:876–880.

116. **Lightner D, Diokno A, Synder J.** Study of Durasphere in the treatment of stress urinary incontinence: a multicenter, double blind randomized, comparative study. *J Urol* 2000;163:166.

117. **Smith ARB, Daneshgari F, Dmochowski R.** Surgical treatment of incontinence in women. In: **Abrams P, Cardozo L, Khoury J, et al., eds.** *Incontinence.* Plymouth, UK: Plymbridge Distributors, 2002.

118. **Ward K, Hilton P.** Prospective multicentre randomised trial of tension-free vaginal tape and colposuspension as primary treatment for stress incontinence. *BMJ* 2002;325:67.

119. **Deng DY, Rutman M, RAz S, et al.** Presentations ad management of major complications of midurethral slings: are complication underreported. *Neurourol Urodyn* 2007;26:46–52.

120. **Kuuva N, Nilsson CG.** A nationwide analysis of complications associated with the tension-free vaginal tape (TVT) procedure. *Acta Obstet Gynecol Scand* 2002;81:72–77.

121. **Schmidt RA, Jonas U, Oleson KA, et al.** Sacral nerve stimulation for treatment of refractory urinary urge incontinence. Sacral Nerve Stimulation Study Group. *J Urol* 1999;162:352–357.

122. **Siegel SW, Catanzaro F, Dijkema HE, et al.** Long-term results of a multicenter study on sacral nerve stimulation for treatment of urinary urge incontinence, urgency-frequency, and retention. *Urology* 2000;56:87–91.

123. **Janknegt RA, Hassouna MM, Siegel SW, et al.** Long-term effectiveness of sacral nerve stimulation for refractory urge incontinence. *Eur Urol* 2001;39:101–106.

124. **Herbison GP, Arnold EP.** Sacral neuromodulation with implanted devices for urinary storage and voiding dysfunction. *Cochrane Database Syst Rev* 2009;2:CD004202.

125. **Peters KM, Carrico DJ, Perez-Marrero RA, et al.** Randomized trial of percutaneous tibial nerve stimulation versus sham efficacy in the treatment of overactive bladder syndrome: results of the SUmiT trial. *J Urol* 2010;183:1438–1443.

127. **Peters KM, MacDiarmid SA, Wooldridge, et al.** Randomized trial of percutaneous tibial nerve stimulation versus extended-release tolterodine: results from the Overactive Bladder Innovative Therapy trial. *J Urol* 2009;182:1055–1061.

128. **MacDiarmid SA, Peters K, Shobeiri SA, et al.** Long-term durability of percutaneous tibial nerve stimulation for the treatment of overactive bladder. *J Urol* 2010;183:234–240.

129. **Reitz A, Stohrer M, Kramer G, et al.** European experience of 200 cases treated with botulinum-A toxin injections into the detrusor muscle for urinary incontinence due to neurogenic detrusor overactivity. *Eur Urol* 2004;45:510–515.

130. **Brubaker L, Richter HE, Visco A, et al.** Refractory idiopathic urge incontinence and botulinum A injection. *J Urol* 2008;180:217–222.

131. **Greenwell TJ, Venn SN, Mundy AR.** Augmentation cystoplasty. *BJU Int* 2001;88:511–525.

132. **Yong SM, Dublin N, Pickard R, et al.** Urinary diversion and bladder reconstruction/replacement using intestinal segments for intractable incontinence or following cystectomy. *Cochrane Database Syst Rev* 2003;1:CD003306.

133. **Fitzpatrick C, Elkins TE.** Plastic surgical techniques in the repair of vesicovaginal fistulas: a review. *Int Urogynecol J Pelvic Floor Dysfunct* 1993;4:403–406.

134. **Arrowsmith SD.** Genitourinary reconstruction in obstetric fistula. *J Urol* 1994;152:287–295.

135. **Menefee SA, Elkins T.** Urinary fistula. *Curr Opin Obstet Gynecol* 1996;8:380–383.

136. **Andersen JT, Gajewski JB, Ostergard DR.** *Imaging and other investigations.* Plymouth, UK: Plymbridge Distributors, 2002.

137. **Gilmour DT, Dwyer PL, Carey MP.** Lower urinary tract injury during gynecologic surgery and its detection by intraoperative cystoscopy. *Obstet Gynecol* 1999;94:883–889.

138. **Barber MD, Visco AG, Weidner AC, et al.** Bilateral uterosacral ligament vaginal vault suspension with site-specific endopelvic fascia defect repair for treatment of pelvic organ prolapse. *Am J Obstet Gynecol* 2000;183:1402–1411.

139. **Handa VL, Maddox MD.** Diagnosis of ureteral obstruction during complex urogynecologic surgery. *Int Urogynecol J Pelvic Floor Dysfunct* 2001;12:345–348.

140. **Lose G, Jorgensen L, Mortensen SO, et al.** Voiding difficulties after colposuspension. *Obstet Gynecol* 1987;69:33–38.

141. **Carlson KV, Rome S, Nitti VW.** Dysfunctional voiding in women. *J Urol* 2001;165:143–148.

142. **Leng WW, Davies BJ, Tarin T, et al.** Delayed treatment of bladder outlet obstruction after sling surgery: association with irreversible bladder dysfunction. *J Urol* 2004;172:1379–1381.

143. **Rackley RR, Appell RA.** Evaluation and management of lower urinary tract disorders in women with multiple sclerosis. *Int Urogynecol J Pelvic Floor Dysfunct* 1999;10:139–143.

144. **Swinn MJ, Fowler CJ.** Isolated urinary retention in young women, or Fowler's syndrome. *Clin Auton Res* 2001;11:309–311.

145. **Lapides J, Diokno AC, Silber SJ, et al.** Clean, intermittent self-catheterization in the treatment of urinary tract disease. *J Urol* 1972;107:458–461.

146. **Jonas U, Fowler CJ, Chancellor MB, et al.** Efficacy of sacral nerve stimulation for urinary retention: results 18 months after implantation. *J Urol* 2001;165:15–19.

147. **van Kerrebroeck PE, van Voskuilen AC, Heesakkers JP, et al.** Results of sacral neuromodulation for urinary voiding dysfunction: outcomes of a prospective, worldwide clinical study. *J Urol* 2007;178:2029–2034.

148. **Finkbeiner AE.** Is bethanechol chloride clinically effective in promoting bladder emptying? A literature review. *J Urol* 1985;134:443–449.

149. **O'Leary MP, Sant GR, Fowler FJ Jr, et al.** The interstitial cystitis symptom index and problem index. *Urology* 1997;49:58–63.

150. **Simon LJ, Landis JR, Erickson DR, et al.** The Interstitial Cystitis Data Base Study: concepts and preliminary baseline descriptive statistics. *Urology* 1997;49:64–75.

151. **Gillenwater JY, Wein AJ.** Summary of the National Institute of Arthritis, Diabetes, Digestive and Kidney Diseases Workshop on Interstitial Cystitis, National Institutes of Health, Bethesda, Maryland, August 28–29, 1987. *J Urol* 1988;140:203–206.

152. **Hanno PM, Landis JR, Matthews-Cook Y, et al.** The diagnosis of interstitial cystitis revisited: lessons learned from the National Institutes of Health Interstitial Cystitis Database study. *J Urol* 1999;161:553–557.

153. **Clemons JL, Arya LA, Myers DL.** Diagnosing interstitial cystitis in women with chronic pelvic pain. *Obstet Gynecol* 2002;100:337–341.

154. **Oravisto KJ.** Epidemiology of interstitial cystitis. *Ann Chir Gynaecol Fenn* 1975;64:75–77.

155. **Curhan GC, Speizer FE, Hunter DJ, et al.** Epidemiology of interstitial cystitis: a population based study. *J Urol* 1999;161:549–552.

156. **Parsons CL, Dell J, Stanford EJ, et al.** Increased prevalence of interstitial cystitis: previously unrecognized urologic and gynecologic cases identified using a new symptom questionnaire and intravesical potassium sensitivity. *Urology* 2002;60:573–578.

157. **Dawson TE, Jamison J.** Intravesical treatment for painful bladder syndrome/interstitial cystitis. *Cochrane Database Syst Rev* 2007;4:CD006113.

158. **Foster HE, Hanno PM, Nickel JC, et al.** Effects of amitriptyline on symptoms in treatment naive patients with interstitial cystitis/painful bladder syndrome. *J Urol* 2010;183:1853–1858.

27 Pelvic Organ Prolapse

Jonathan L. Gleason
Holly E. Richter
R. Edward Varner

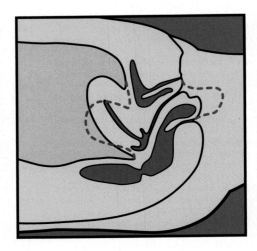

- Pelvic organ prolapse is an increasingly common condition seen in women with the aging of the population.

- Causes of pelvic organ prolapse are multifactorial and contribute to the weakening of the pelvic support connective tissue and muscles as well as nerve damage.

- Patients may be asymptomatic or have significant symptoms such as those related to the lower urinary tract, pelvic pain, defecatory problems, fecal incontinence, back pain, and dyspareunia.

- Physical examination includes thoughtful attention to all parts of the vagina, including the anterior, apical, and posterior compartments, levator muscle, and anal sphincter complex.

- Nonsurgical treatment options include pelvic floor muscle training and the use of intravaginal devices.

- Surgical treatment involves an individualized, multicompartmental approach consistent with the patient's previous treatment attempts, activity level, and health status.

- Studies are needed to determine the characteristics of those patients who would derive long-term benefit from vaginal versus abdominal approaches to the surgical repair of pelvic organ prolapse.

Pelvic organ prolapse (POP) is a bulge or protrusion of pelvic organs and their associated vaginal segments into or through the vagina (1). It is a common and costly affliction of older women (2,3). **It has been estimated that over the next 30 years, the demand for treatment of POP will increase 45%, commensurate with an increase in the population of women older than 50 years of age** (4,5). As this problem grows in significance, it becomes increasingly important to comprehend the pathophysiology and risk factors associated with pelvic organ prolapse and try to prevent its occurrence. Furthermore, continued efforts are needed to understand factors that result in long-lasting, robust repair of pelvic organ prolapse for those patients undergoing surgical management. Despite extensive anecdotal experience, the optimal surgical approach to apical and other compartment prolapse remains elusive (6).

In the United States, 11% of women up to the age of 80 years have surgery for pelvic organ prolapse or urinary incontinence, and nearly one-third of procedures are repeat surgery (3). Data from the Women's Health Initiative revealed anterior pelvic organ prolapse in 34.3%, posterior wall prolapse in 18.6%, and uterine prolapse in 14.3% of women in the study (7). In this study, a significant risk factor associated with prolapse was vaginal delivery. After adjusting for age, ethnicity, and body mass index, women with at least one vaginal delivery were twice as likely as nulliparous women to have pelvic organ prolapse. Causes of pelvic support disorders are most likely multifactorial, however; factors other than vaginal delivery also are associated with the development of these disorders. One study found that the incidence of prolapse doubled with each decade of life between the ages of 20 and 59 years (8). In another study, each year of increasing age was associated with a 12% increase in the risk of developing prolapse (9). Other associated risk factors for the development of POP include history of hysterectomy (8), obesity (7,10,11), history of previous prolapse operations, and race (11).

Pathophysiology

Pelvic organ prolapse results from attenuation of the supportive structures, whether by actual tears or "breaks" or by neuromuscular dysfunction or both. Support of the vaginal canal is provided by the enveloping endopelvic connective tissue and its condensations at the vaginal apex, which form the cardinal uterosacral ligament complex. The endopelvic connective tissue is the first line of support, buttressed intimately with the pelvic diaphragm, composed of the levator ani and coccygeus muscles. These muscles provide a supportive diaphragm through which the urethra, vagina, and rectum egress (Fig. 27.1). The muscular support provides basal tonicity and support of the pelvic structures; when contracted, as in the setting of increased abdominal pressure, the rectum, vagina, and urethra are pulled anteriorly toward the pubis.

The support system for the uterus and vagina has been described as consisting of three levels (12).

Level I refers to the uterosacral/cardinal ligament complex, which serve to maintain the vaginal length and axis.

Level II support consists of the paravaginal attachments of the lateral vagina and endopelvic fascia to the arcus tendineus that maintain the midline position of the vagina.

Level III support pertains to the distal vagina and is made up of the muscles and connective tissue surrounding the distal vagina and perineum.

Definitions

The more common pelvic support disorders include rectoceles and cystoceles (Fig. 27.2), **enteroceles** (Fig. 27.3), **and uterine prolapse** (Fig. 27.4); reflecting displacement of the rectum, small bowel, bladder, and uterus, respectively; resulting from failure of the endopelvic connective tissue, levator ani muscular support, or both (12).

A **rectocele** is a protrusion of the rectum into the vaginal lumen resulting from weakness in the muscular wall of the rectum and the paravaginal musculoconnective tissue, which holds the rectum in place posteriorly.

An **enterocele** is a herniation of the peritoneum and small bowel and is the only true hernia among the pelvic support disorders. Most enteroceles occur downward between the uterosacral ligaments and the rectovaginal space, but they may also occur primarily apically, especially in the setting of a previous hysterectomy.

A **cystocele** is descent of the urinary bladder with the anterior vaginal wall. Cystoceles usually occur when the pubocervical musculoconnective tissue weakens midline or detaches from its lateral or superior connecting points.

Uterine prolapse is generally the result of poor cardinal or uterosacral ligament apical support, which allows downward protrusion of the cervix and uterus toward the introitus.

Procidentia, **which involves prolapse of the uterus and vagina, and** *total vaginal vault prolapse,* **which can occur after hysterectomy, represent eversion of the entire vagina** (Fig. 27.5).

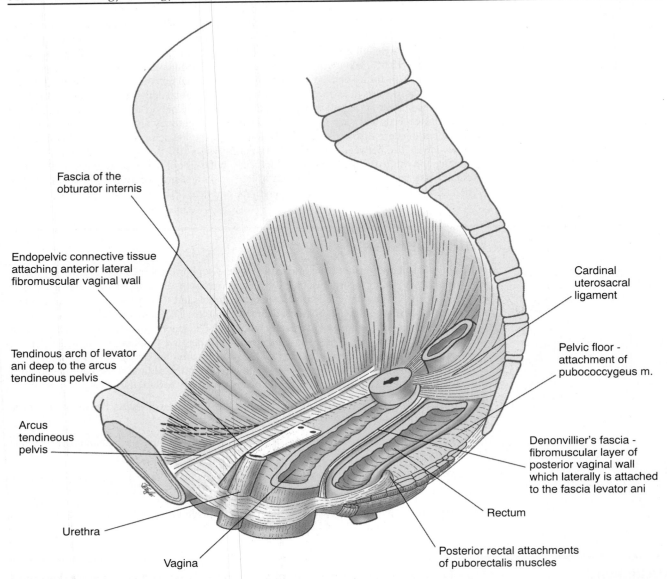

Fascia of the
obturator internis

Endopelvic connective tissue
attaching anterior lateral
fibromuscular vaginal wall

Tendinous arch of levator
ani deep to the arcus
tendineous pelvis

Arcus
tendineous
pelvis

Urethra

Vagina

Cardinal
uterosacral
ligament

Pelvic floor -
attachment of
pubococcygeus m.

Denonvillier's fascia -
fibromuscular layer of
posterior vaginal wall
which laterally is attached
to the fascia levator ani

Rectum

Posterior rectal attachments
of puborectalis muscles

Figure 27.1 **A sagittal view of the female pelvis with bladder and uterus removed (ureters, trigone, and cervix intact) illustrating anterior and posterior vaginal fibromuscular planes, their endopelvic fascial attachments, and a functional pelvic floor.**
(Redrawn by J. Taylor from **Skandalakis JE, ed.** *Hernia: surgical anatomy and technique.* New York: McGraw-Hill: 244–250.)

These descriptive terms are somewhat inaccurate and misleading, focusing on the bladder, rectum, small bowel, or uterus rather than the specific defects responsible for the alterations in
vaginal support. Specific defect support issues will be discussed in the setting of the surgical
management section.

Surgical Anatomy

Pelvic support structures include:

1. The muscles and connective tissue of the pelvic floor

2. The fibromuscular tissue of the vaginal wall

3. The endopelvic connective tissue

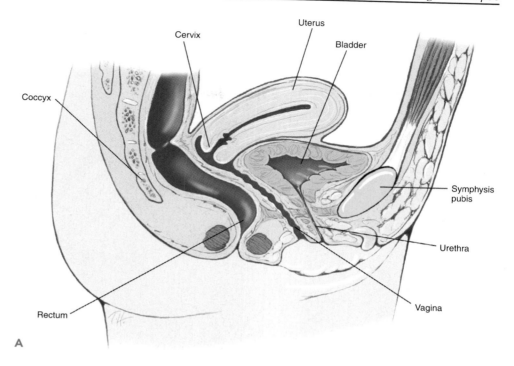

A

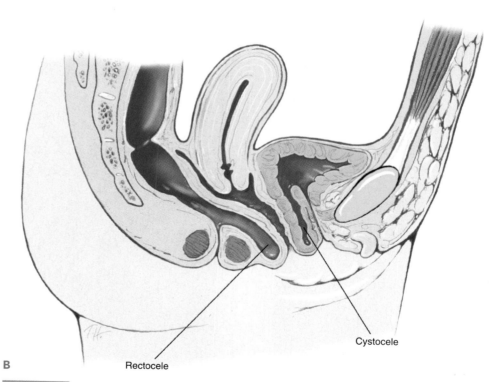

B

Figure 27.2 A: Sagittal section of the pelvis showing normal anatomy. B: Cystocele and rectocele.

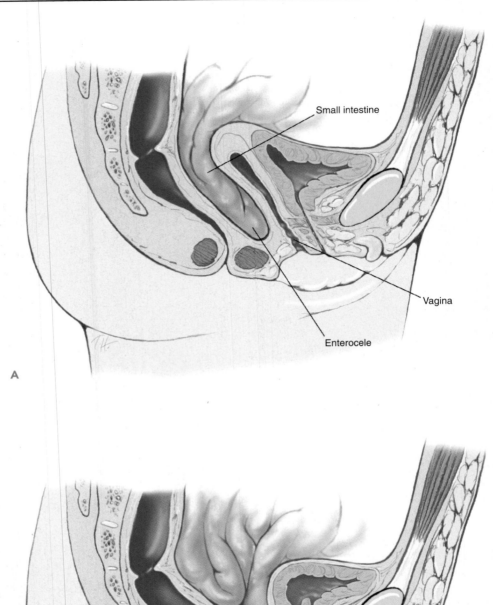

Small intestine

Vagina

Enterocele

A

Small intestine

Enterocele

B

Figure 27.3   A: **Posterior enterocele without eversion.** B: **Enterocele with eversion.**

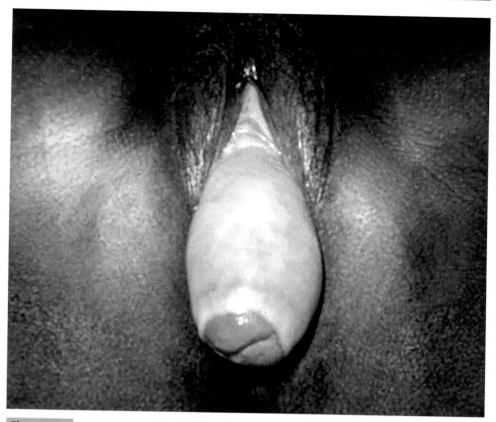

Figure 27.4   Uterine prolapse with apical detachment from the uterosacral ligament complex and lateral wall detachment from the endopelvic connective tissue.

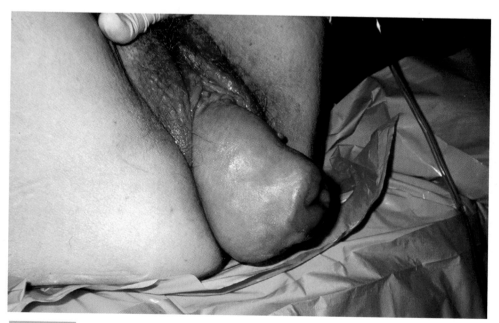

Figure 27.5   Procidentia of the uterus and vagina.

Endopelvic connective tissue includes:

1. The cardinal/uterosacral complex, which attaches the upper vagina and cervix posteriorly

2. Lateral connective tissue attachments of the anterior vaginal wall to the arcus tendineus pelvis and of the posterior vaginal wall to the fascia of the levator ani and to the posterior arcus tendineus near the ischial spine

3. Less dense areolar connective tissue surrounding retroperineal portion of the pelvic organs

The orientation of these structures is noted in Figure 27.1. In general, an intact pelvic floor, including a functional puborectalis muscle and an intact cardinal/uterosacral complex, should prevent pelvic organ prolapse by allowing posterior deflection of the rectum and vagina and compression of these structures against the pelvic floor in the upright position (Fig. 27.6). The fibromuscular layer of the vaginal wall and the other endopelvic connective tissue attachments augment the support structure and are particularly important when pelvic floor function is compromised.

Apical Compartment

Normal apical support includes the integrity of the cardinal/uterosacral ligaments, the upper paravaginal fibromuscular connective tissue, and, when the uterus is present, the paracervical fascia. The fibromuscular tissue of the upper vagina blends in with the paracervical fascia. Both of these are attached laterally and posterior laterally to the cardinal ligaments and uterosacral ligaments (Fig. 27.1). The vaginal fibromuscular tissue is also

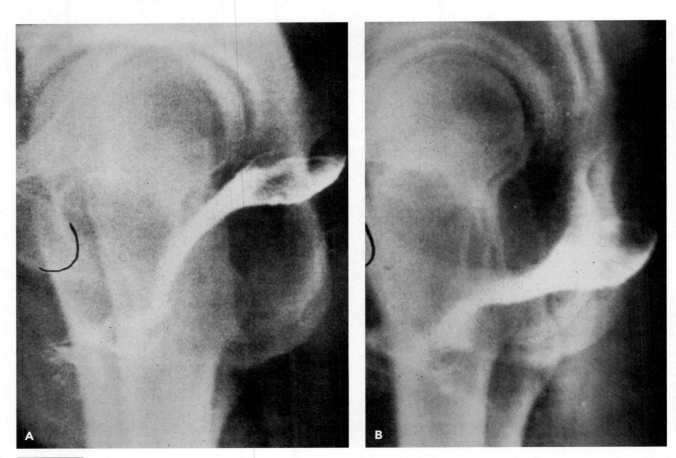

Figure 27.6 **Vaginograms from the same patient at rest (A) and during Valsalva maneuver (B).** Illustrates posterior vaginal deflection maintained by apical cardinal/uterosacral posterior suspension and the anterior sling effect of the puborectalis muscle and more distal perineal structures. (From **Nichols DH, Randall CL.** *Vaginal surgery.* 4th ed. Baltimore, MD: Williams & Wilkins, 1996:4–5, with permission.)

attached to the upper anterior rectum at its sigmoid junction and forms the inferior border of the cul-de-sac of Douglas. The cardinal and uterosacral ligaments are condensations of areolar connective tissue and they contribute level I support for the vagina. Their origin is at the lateral borders of sacral vertebra 2 to 4, and they travel retroperitoneally to their insertion at the upper vagina and cervix (Fig. 27.1). They serve as the anterior and lateral borders of the cul-de-sac and cross at or just anterior to the ischial spines. The ureter is closest to the uterosacral ligament at or just posterior to its insertion on the posterior lateral cervix. If anterior cephalad traction is placed on the ureter or cervix, frequently the cardinal uterosacral ligaments will stand out as ridges lateral to the cul-de-sac; however, peritoneal folds may have similar appearance. Therefore, placement of sutures in such structures based on visual appearance may not be reliable.

Defects in apical support include:

1. The loss of cardinal/uterosacral support with resultant cervical/uterine or vaginal cuff descent

2. The detachment of the fibromuscular vagina from the anterior rectum with resultant enterocele or, at times, sigmoidocele into the rectovaginal space

3. Tears or attenuation of the upper fibromuscular tissue, usually after hysterectomy, leading to a central apical descent that frequently presents as a ballooning defect

Often, these defects occur concurrently. Defects in cardinal/uterosacral attachment are at sites close to their insertion into the cervix and upper vagina where breaks or tears occur; in those with apical descent, condensations of cardinal/uterosacral tissue can be found adjacent to the peritoneum just cephalad to the ischial spines (13).

Anterior Compartment

The anterior vaginal compartment includes the anterior vaginal wall, its attachments, the urethra, and the bladder. The support structure for the bladder is the rhomboid-shaped anterior vaginal wall (specifically its fibromuscular layer), which is attached laterally to the arcus tendineus fascia (Fig. 27.7). Inferiorly, the fibromuscular layer blends in with the connective tissue, which spans the two bands of puborectalis and pubococcygeus muscles

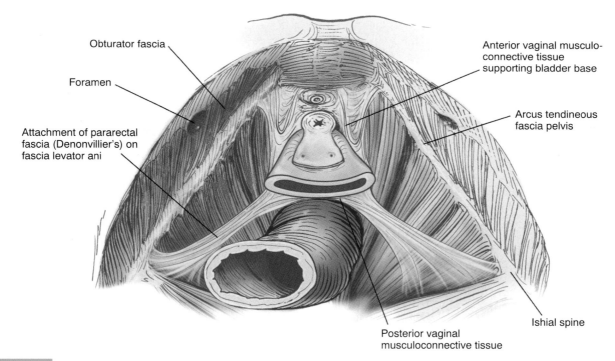

Figure 27.7 **View of the pelvic cavity with bladder, upper vagina, and sigmoid colon removed.** The fibromuscular wall of the anterior vagina is attached to the arcus tendineus fascia pelvis by endopelvic connective tissue and supports the bladder. The pararectal fascia (Denonvillier's fascia) includes the fibromuscular tissue of the posterior vagina and its lateral attachment to the fascia levator ani.

and the pubic rami. The urethra appears to be preferentially supported by these connective tissues as well as by the pubourethral ligaments. In the apical area, the vaginal fibromuscular layer blends in with the precervical fascia and the connective tissue of the cardinal ligament complex. In the upright position, the rhomboid-shaped anterior vaginal wall is oriented approximately 30 degrees from the horizon (from pubis to ischial spines). There is some downward bulge of the central area of the rhomboid plate, which should be minimized by the back-stop effect of the posterior vagina and rectum if the pelvic floor anatomy and function are normal.

Defects of this support structure may include tears or attenuation of the vaginal fibromuscular wall, or detachment from the pelvic sidewalls, the cervix or cardinal ligament complex, or from the pubis. Specific sites of fibromuscular tears are frequently difficult to recognize.

Physical examination may reveal the following findings:

1. The presence of a central ballooning-type defect
2. Descent of the area of the vaginal wall below the bladder neck
3. Descent of the cervix or apical vaginal area
4. The presence or absence of sulci extending lateroanteriorly, which would indicate that lateral detachment to the arcus is maintained or lost.

Posterior Compartment

The support of the rectum and posterior vagina includes the pelvic floor musculature and connective tissue posteriorly and Denonvillier's (pararectal) fascia, which is the fibromuscular layer of the posterior vaginal wall and its lateral attachments to the lateral pelvic floor (levator) musculature and its fascia (Fig. 27.8). This lateral attachment site, the fascia levator ani, fuses with the arcus tendineus fascia pelvis at the middle to upper level of the vagina

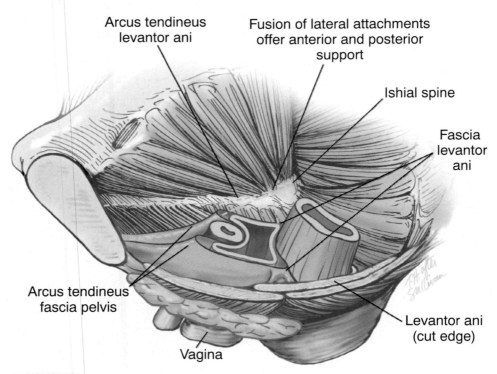

Figure 27.8 **Sagittal oblique view of the distal midvagina illustrating lateral connection of the posterior musculoconnective tissue wall to the fascia levator ani and anterior wall to the arcus tendineus pelvis.** The attachment sites fuse together at a point closer to the ischial spine where the vagina assumes a more oval shape. (Modified by J. Taylor from illustration by Lianne Krueger Sullivan. From **Cundiff GW, Fenner D.** Evaluation and treatment of women with rectocele: focus on associated defecatory and sexual dysfunction. *Obstet Gynecol* 2004;104:1403–1421, erratum in *Obstet Gynecol* 2005;105:222, with permission.)

and continues to the level of the ischial spine. Less dense, areolar, connective tissue surrounds the rectum and vagina and may supply some support to these structures as well.

The fibromuscular layer at the upper vagina fuses with the paracervical fascia and the fan-shaped cardinal ligament structure. The integrity of the attachment of this posterior vaginal layer to the anterior rectal wall just below the rectal sigmoid junction prevents enterocele formation. In the distal vagina, the fibromuscular layer fuses laterally with the fascia of the puborectalis and then the bulbocavernous muscle and centrally with the perineal connective tissue. Thus, normal posterior support includes a plate of connective tissue that is attached laterally as noted, posteriorly toward sacral segments 2 to 4, and inferiorly to the perineum. This fibromuscular plane not only holds the rectum in place posteriorly, but also aids in preventing perineal descent by suspending the perineum to the sacrum. The constant resting tone of the pelvic floor muscles, particularly the puborectalis, serve to close the genital hiatus, pulling the distal vagina and anorectal junction toward the pubic symphysis and creating an anorectal angle and a posterior deflection of the rectum, vagina, and bladder base.

It has been hypothesized, based on careful cadaveric dissections, that most rectoceles were due to discrete tears in the Denonvillier's fascia at its lateral, apical, and perineal attachments and centrally within the fascia itself (14). Perineal detachment, along with a defect in the perineal membrane, has been described as a perineal rectocele, which is most commonly associated with reports of difficulty with defecation. Apical attachment defects are generally associated with enteroceles and occasionally sigmoidoceles.

Evaluation

Although as many as 50% of women older than age 50 have some degree of pelvic organ prolapse (15), fewer than 20% seek treatment (16). This may result from a number of causes, including lack of symptoms, embarrassment, or misperceptions about available treatment options. Although pelvic organ prolapse is not life threatening, it can impose a significant burden of social and physical restrictions of activities, impact on psychological well-being, and overall quality of life.

Symptoms

Pelvic organ prolapse often is accompanied by symptoms of voiding dysfunction, including urinary incontinence, obstructive voiding symptoms, urinary urgency and frequency, and, at the extreme, urinary retention and upper renal compromise with resultant pain or anuria. Other symptoms often associated with POP include pelvic pain, defecatory problems (e.g., constipation, diarrhea, tenesmus, fecal incontinence), back and flank pain, overall pelvic discomfort, and dyspareunia. Patients seeking care for prolapse may have one or several of these symptoms involving the lower pelvic floor. **Choice of treatment usually depends on severity of the symptoms and the degree of prolapse consistent with the patient's general health and level of activity** (16).

Data relating pelvic floor symptoms to the extent and location of prolapse are weak (17–19). Any symptoms associated with physical findings of lower stage prolapse require careful evaluation, especially if surgery is being considered. A recent retrospective study of 330 patients reported that women with more advanced prolapse were less likely to have symptoms of stress incontinence and more likely to use manual reduction of the prolapse to void. Therefore, careful consideration of lower urinary tract symptoms is important. Prolapse severity was not associated with bowel or sexual problems in this study (20).

Physical Examination

In evaluating patients with pelvic organ prolapse, it is particularly useful to divide the pelvis into compartments, each of which may exhibit specific defects. The use of a Graves speculum or Baden retractor can help to evaluate the apical compartment of the vagina. The anterior and posterior compartments are best examined with the use of a univalve or Sims speculum. The speculum is placed posteriorly to retract the posterior wall downward when examining the anterior compartment and placed anteriorly to retract the anterior wall upward when examining the posterior compartment. A rectovaginal examination may be useful in evaluating the posterior compartment to distinguish a posterior vaginal wall defect from a dissecting apical enterocele or a combination of both.

If an anterior lateral detachment defect is suspected, an open ring forceps (or a Baden retractor) may be placed in the vagina at a 45-degree angle posteriorly cephalad to hold the lateral fornices adjacent to the pelvic sidewall.

During the evaluation of each compartment, the patient is encouraged to perform Valsalva so the full extent of the prolapse can be ascertained. If the findings determined with Valsalva are inconsistent with the patient's description of her symptoms, it may be helpful to perform a standing straining examination with the bladder empty (20,21).

Pelvic Organ Prolapse Quantitation System

Many systems for staging prolapse have been described. Typically it is graded on a scale of 0 to 3 or 0 to 4, with the grade increasing with the severity of prolapse (22). **Currently the system approved by the International Continence Society is the Pelvic Organ Prolapse Quantification system, or POP-Q** (23). This standardized quantification system facilitates communication between physicians in practice and research and enables progression of these conditions to be followed accurately. In this system, anatomic descriptions of specific sites in the vagina are used in place of traditional terms. The system identifies nine locations in the vagina and vulva in centimeters relative to the hymen, which are used to assign a stage (from 0 to IV) of prolapse at its most advanced site (Fig. 27.9). Although probably more detailed than necessary for general practice, clinicians should be familiar with the POP-Q system because most published studies use it to describe research results. Its two most important advantages over previous grading systems are (i) it allows the use of a standardized technique with quantitative measurements at straining relative to a constant reference point (i.e., the hymen), and (ii) its ability to assess prolapse at multiple vaginal sites.

The classification uses six points along the vagina (two points on the anterior, middle, and posterior compartments) measured in relation to the hymen. The anatomic position of the six defined points should be measured in centimeters proximal to the hymen (negative number) or distal to the hymen (positive number), with the plane of the hymen representing zero. Three other measurements in the POP-Q examination include the genital hiatus, perineal body, and the total vaginal length (23).

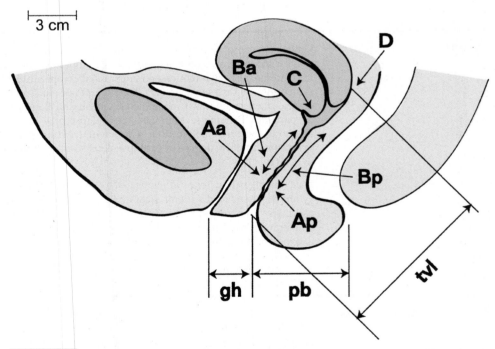

Figure 27.9   Standardization of terminology for female pelvic organ prolapse (POP-Q) classification. This diagram demonstrates the anatomic position of the POP-Q sites, including six sites involving the anterior (Aa, Ba), middle (C, D), and posterior (Ap, Bp) compartments with the genital hiatus (gh), perineal body (pb), and total vaginal length (tvl). (From **Bump RC, Mattiason A, Bo K, et al.** The standardization of terminology of female pelvic organ prolapse and pelvic floor dysfunction. *Am J Obstet Gynecol* 1996;175:12, with permission.)

The genital hiatus is measured from the middle of the external urethral meatus to the posterior midline hymen. The perineal body is measured from the posterior margin of the genital hiatus to the midanal opening. The total vaginal length is the greatest depth of the vagina in centimeters when the vaginal apex is reduced to its full normal position. All measurements except the total vaginal length are measured during maximal straining.

The anterior vaginal wall measurements are termed Aa and Ba, with the Ba point moving depending on the amount of anterior compartment prolapse. Point Aa represents a point on the anterior vagina 3 cm proximal to the external urethral meatus, which corresponds to the bladder neck. By definition, the range of position of this point is −3 to +3. Point Ba represents the most distal or dependent point of any portion of the anterior vaginal wall from point Aa to just anterior to the vaginal cuff or anterior lip of the cervix. This point can vary depending on the nature of the patient's support defect. For example, point Ba is −3 in the absence of any prolapse (it is never less than −3) to a positive value equal to the total vaginal length in a patient with total eversion of the vagina.

The middle compartment consists of points C and D. Point C represents the most dependant edge of the cervix or vaginal cuff after hysterectomy. Point D is the location of the posterior fornix; it is omitted if the cervix is absent. This point represents the level of the attachment of the uterosacral ligament to the posterior cervix. It is intended to differentiate suspensory failure from cervical elongation.

The posterior compartment is measured similarly to the anterior compartment: the corresponding terms are Ap and Bp. The nine measurements can be recorded as a simple line of numbers (i.e., −3, −3, −8, −10, −3, −3, 11, 4, 3 for points Aa, Ba, C, D, Ap, Bp, total vagina length, genital hiatus, and perineal body, respectively). The six vaginal sites have possible ranges that depend on the total vaginal length (Table 27.1). After collection of the site-specific measurements, stages are assigned according to the most dependent portion of the prolapse (Table 27.2).

The POP-Q examination often appears confusing on initial review; however, a measuring device (i.e., a marked ring forceps or marked cotton-tip applicator) can assist in instructing those unfamiliar with this staging system. **The POP-Q examination provides a standardized measurement system to allow for more accurate assessments of postoperative outcome and to ensure uniform, reliable, and site-specific descriptions of pelvic organ prolapse.** There is interest in using the POP-Q examination to measure prolapse as a continuous variable rather than in stages because it would provide greater statistical power in clinical research (24). The American Urogynecology Society provides a video (25) that describes the POP-Q exam and demonstrates its use.

In a clinical setting, at least three measurements should be obtained: the most advanced extent of the prolapse in centimeters relative to the hymen that affects the anterior vagina, the posterior vagina, and the cervix or vaginal apex.

As noted previously, whether the older staging systems or the POP-Q system is used, it is important to document the most pertinent findings on examination. This will help in documenting the baseline extent of prolapse and the results of treatment.

Table 27.1 Possible Ranges of the Six Site-Specific Pelvic Organ Prolapse Quantitative Examination Measurements

Points	Description	Range
Aa	Anterior wall 3 cm from hymen	−3 cm to +3 cm
Ba	Most dependent portion of rest of anterior wall	−3 cm to +TVL
C	Cervix or vaginal cuff	± TVL
D	Posterior fornix (if no prior hysterectomy)	± TVL or omitted
Ap	Posterior wall 3 cm from hymen	−3 cm to +3 cm
Bp	Most dependent portion of rest of posterior wall	−3 cm to +TVL

TVL, total vaginal length.
Adapted from **Bump RC, Mattiasson A, Bo K, et al.** The standardization of terminology of female pelvic organ prolapse and pelvic floor dysfunction. *Am J Obstet Gynecol* 1996;175:11–12, with permission.

Table 27.2 Stages of Pelvic Organ Prolapse	
Stage 0	No prolapse is demonstrated. Points Aa, Ap, Ba, Bp are all at −3 cm, and point C is between total vaginal length (TVL) and −(TVL −2 cm).
Stage I	The most distal portion of the prolapse is greater than 1 cm above the level of the hymen.
Stage II	The most distal portion of the prolapse is less than 1 cm proximal or distal to the plane of the hymen.
Stage III	The most distal portion of the prolapse is less than 1 cm below the plane of the hymen but no further than 2 cm less than the total vaginal length.
Stage IV	Complete to nearly complete eversion of the vagina. The most distal portion of the prolapse protrudes to greater than (TVL −2) cm.

From **Bump RC, Mattiassion A, Bo K, et al.** The standardization of terminology of female pelvic organ prolapse and pelvic floor dysfunction. *Am J Obstet Gynecol* 1996;175:13, with permission.

Pelvic Muscle Function Assessment

Pelvic muscle function should be assessed during the pelvic examination. Following bimanual examination with the patient in the lithotomy position, the examiner can palpate the puborectalis and pubococcygeus muscles inside the hymen along the pelvic sidewalls at approximately the 4 and 8 o'clock positions. One can appreciate basal muscle tone and whether there is increased tone with contraction as well as strength, duration, and symmetry of contraction (26). **A rectovaginal examination should also be performed to assess basal and contraction muscle tone of the anal sphincter complex.**

As a part of the pelvic organ prolapse examination, urethral mobility often is measured. **Many women with prolapse will have urethral hypermobility (defined as a resting urethral angle greater than 30 degrees or a maximal strain angle greater than 30 degrees).** The presence of urethral mobility in combination with symptoms of stress incontinence may help determine whether an incontinence procedure should be performed. However, studies have shown that nearly all women with stage II to IV prolapse have urethral hypermobility, and asymptomatic parous women have an average maximum straining angle of 54 degrees (27,28). During pelvic examination, the urethra is typically swabbed with *Betadin*e, and *lidocaine* jelly is placed in the urethra or on a cotton tip swab. The swab is placed in the urethra at the urethrovesical junction and, with the use of a goniometer (Fig. 27.10), the baseline urethral angle from the horizontal and maximal strain angles is measured.

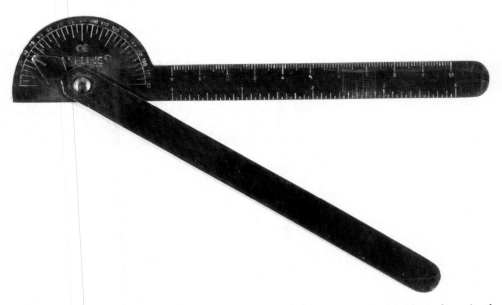

Figure 27.10 Goniometer, which is used to measure baseline urethral angle and maximal strain angle of the urethra with a cotton tip swab in place.

Bladder Function Evaluation

Patients with prolapse exhibit the full range of lower urinary tract symptoms. Despite the fact that some patients may not have significant symptoms, it is important to obtain objective information about bladder and urethral function. With severe POP, the urethral kinking effect of the prolapse may mask a potential urine leakage problem; therefore, basic office bladder testing with prolapse reduction should be performed to mimic bladder and urethral function if the prolapse were treated. At a minimum, the following assessments should be performed: a clean catch or catheterized urine sample to test for infection, a postvoid residual (PVR) volume, and assessment of bladder sensation, which can be performed as a part of office cystometrics. Although there is no consensus as to what constitutes an abnormal PVR volume, provided the patient has voided 150 mL or more, a PVR less than or equal to 100 mL is acceptable (27). Reduction stress testing at the time of simple office cystometrics can be performed with the use of a pessary, large cotton swab, ring forceps, or the posterior blade of a speculum. Care should be taken that the urethra not be overly straightened (with a resultant false-positive test result) or obstructed (with a resultant false-negative test result), or that tension is not placed on the puborectalis muscles by excessive posterior retraction. These risks can be minimized by orienting the vaginal apex toward the sacrum.

Bowel Function Evaluation

Once a decision is made to perform surgical repair of the posterior compartment based on symptoms, type, and location of defects, an appropriate approach should be determined and the patient should be made aware of the expected outcomes and potential adverse effects such as pain and sexual dysfunction. **If the patient has defecatory dysfunction with a rectocele and symptoms of constipation, pain with defecation, fecal or flatal incontinence, or any signs of levator spasm or anal sphincter spasm, appropriate evaluation and conservative management of concurrent conditions could be initiated before repair of the rectocele and continued postoperatively** (28).

Imaging

Diagnostic imaging of the pelvis in women with pelvic organ prolapse is not routinely performed. However, if clinically indicated, tests that may be performed include fluoroscopic evaluation of bladder function, ultrasound of the pelvis, and defecography for patients in whom intussusception or rectal mucosal prolapse are suspected. Magnetic resonance imaging is increasingly being used for the evaluation of pelvic pathology such as mullerian anomalies and pelvic pain; however, generalized use in women with prolapse is not currently clinically indicated and is used primarily for research purposes.

Treatment

Nonsurgical Therapy

Nonsurgical therapy of pelvic organ prolapse includes conservative behavioral management and the use of mechanical devices. **A nonsurgical treatment approach usually is considered in women with mild to moderate prolapse, those who desire preservation of future childbearing, those in whom surgery may not be an option, or those who do not desire surgical intervention.**

Conservative Management

Conservative management approaches include alteration of lifestyle or physical intervention such as **pelvic floor muscle training** (PFMT). These approaches are used mainly in cases of mild to moderate prolapse; however, their true role in managing prolapse and associated symptoms is unclear (29,30). **The goals of a conservative therapy approach to the treatment of prolapse are as follows** (31):

- Prevent worsening prolapse

- Decrease the severity of symptoms

- Increase the strength, endurance, and support of the pelvic floor musculature

- Avoid or delay surgical intervention

Lifestyle intervention includes such activities as weight loss and reduction of those activities that increase intra-abdominal pressure. This interaction is typically anecdotal in practice. No case series, prospective studies, or randomized control trials exist that have examined the effectiveness of this approach to the treatment of prolapse.

Pelvic floor muscle exercises may limit the progression of mild prolapse and related symptoms (32,33); however, a lower response rate has been noted when prolapse extends beyond the vaginal introitus (34).

The efficacy of biofeedback therapy in the treatment of impaired defecation associated with a rectocele has been determined (35). Thirty-two female patients, median age 52 years (range, 34–77 years), experiencing impaired rectal evacuation with a rectocele greater than 2 cm at proctography underwent a structured behavioral retraining. Immediate and medium-term follow-up results were reported (median 10 months; range 2–30 months). Fifty-six percent of patients (n = 14) felt a little and 16% (n = 4) felt major improvement in symptoms, including 3 (12%) with complete symptom relief. Immediately after biofeedback there was a modest reduction in need to strain (67; 50%), feeling of incomplete evacuation (73; 59%), and need to assist defecation digitally (79; 63%) that was maintained at follow-up. Bowel movement frequency was significantly normalized at follow-up (p = .02). These investigators concluded that **behavioral retraining, including biofeedback therapy, may be an effective primary therapy for some patients with a rectocele associated with impaired defecation.**

Mechanical Devices

The use of mechanical devices such as pessaries is usually considered for women who cannot undergo surgery for medical reasons, desire to avoid surgery, or have a significant degree of prolapse that makes other nonsurgical approaches unfeasible. Some practitioners extend indications to include pregnancy-related prolapse as well as prolapse and incontinence in elderly women. Reports have shown that age older than 65 years, the presence of severe medical comorbidity, and sexual activity were associated with successful pessary user (36,37). Unsuccessful use or a preference for surgery has been associated with a shortened vaginal length (≤6 cm), a wide vaginal introitus, sexual activity, stress incontinence, stage III or IV posterior compartment prolapse, and desire for surgery at a first office visit (38). Few literature-based reviews and reports recommend pessaries as first-line treatment for women with POP, and there is little consensus regarding choice of pessary and management of pessary usage (39). Most of the information on pessary use is derived primarily from descriptive and retrospective studies, relatively small prospective series, manufacturer's recommendations, and anecdotal experience.

Pessaries provide pelvic organ support within the vaginal vault. **Two categories of pessaries— support and space filling—exist for prolapse (39). The ring pessary (with diaphragm) is a commonly used support pessary, and the Gelhorn pessary is a commonly used space-filling pessary. The ring and other support pessaries are recommended for stage I and II prolapse, whereas the space-filling pessaries are used for stage III and IV prolapse** (40). It is unclear whether pessaries can prevent the progression of POP with regular use. A prospective cohort study addressed this issue in a series of 56 women who were fitted with a pessary, of which 33.9% (n = 19) continued use for at least 1 year (41). Baseline and follow-up pelvic examinations were performed using the POP-Q system (23). The women removed the pessary 48 hours before one visit, but there was no information to ascertain adherence to pessary use. No woman had worsening of the prolapse, and four women (21.1%; 95% confidence interval [CI], 0.2%–43.7%) had an improvement. Improvement overall was noted in women with anterior compartment prolapse.

In women with stages I and II prolapse with stress urinary incontinence, a continence pessary may be considered and has been shown to produce patient satisfaction above 50% at 12 months (42). There are no randomized controlled trials of pessary use in women with POP (43). Likewise, there are no consensus guidelines on the care of pessaries (i.e., intervals between changes), the role of local estrogens, or the type of pessary indicated for specific types of POP (43). Manufacturers recommendations and different pessary types can be seen in Figure 27.11. Effective and satisfactory outcomes have been reported for stage II or greater prolapse using the Gelhorn and ring diaphragm pessary (36). After 2 to 6 months, 77% to 92% of women with a successful pessary fitting were satisfied and, using intention-to-treat analysis, 44% to 67% of all women who were treated initially with a pessary for prolapse were satisfied. There are few other series describing pessary use for prolapse with greater than 4 weeks follow-up (36,38,44,45).

Possible complications associated with pessary use include vaginal discharge and odor. Failure to retain the pessary may occur or, conversely, the pessary may be too large, which could lead to excoriation or irritation. With reduction of vaginal prolapse, *de novo* or

UTERINE PROLAPSE

I. 1st & 2nd DEGREE
- **O** Ring with Support
- **U** Ring without Support
- **R** Shaatz
- **I** Regula

II. 3rd DEGREE
- **X** Donut
- **L,M,N** Gellhorns
- **W** Inflatoball
- **G** Cube
- **F** Tandem-Cube

CYSTOCELE and/or RECTOCELE
- **J** Gehrung
- **I** Regula

CYSTOCELE + SUI
- **K** Gehrung with Knob

SUI

I. SIMPLE
- **T** Ring Incontinence
- **A,D,E,H** Hodge

II. + MILD PROLAPSE
- **P,Q** Ring with or without Support + Knob
- **V** Incontinence Dish

III. + PROLAPSE & CYSTOCELE
- **S** Dish with Support
- **Q** Ring with Support + Knob

INCOMPETENT CERVIX
- **E** Hodge ⎫ Used with or without ⎱
- **C** Smith ⎩ cerclage ⎰

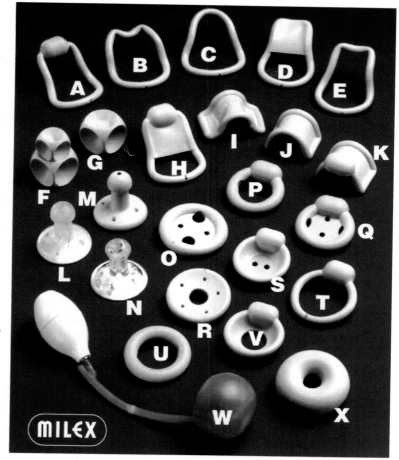

A Hodge with Knob (Silicone) **B** Risser (Silicone) **C** Smith (Silicone) **D** Hodge with Support (Silicone) **E** Hodge (Silicone) **F** Tandem-Cube (Silicone) **G** Cube (Silicone) **H** Hodge with Support+Knob (Silicone) **I** Regula (Silicone) **J** Gehrung (Silicone) **K** Gehrung with Knob (Silicone) **L** Gellhorn 95% Rigid (Silicone) **M** Gellhorn Flexible (Silicone) **N** Gellhorn Rigid (Acrylic) **O** Ring with Support (Silicone) **P** Ring with Knob (Silicone) **Q** Ring with Support+Knob (Silicone) **R** Shaatz (Silicone) **S** Incontinence Dish with Support (Silicone) **T** Ring Incontinence (Silicone) **U** Ring (Silicone) **V** Incontinence Dish (Silicone) **W** Inflatoball (Latex) **X** Donut (Silicone)

Figure 27.11 **Pessaries used to treat the various degrees of prolapse.** (Milex Company, a Division of Cooper Surgical.)

increased stress incontinence may occur, and in rare instances, more severe complications, including vesicovaginal or rectovaginal fistula, small bowel entrapment, hydronephrosis, and urosepsis, have been described (46–48).

Placement and Management

Pessary placement involves consideration of a number of issues, primarily the patient's desire and motivation to use this type of device. Typically, if she has had previous surgery or strongly desires to avoid surgery, she may be motivated enough for a primary attempt at pessary placement. Other issues include current sexual function status, type and duration of exercise in which the patient engages, and the status of the vaginal walls and cervix. In hypoestrogenic women, treatment of the vagina with estrogen and maintenance of intravaginal estrogen treatment is recommended.

Fitting a Pessary

The patient should be examined in the lithotomy position after emptying her bladder. The clinician should use a dry glove to better grasp the pessary and water-soluble lubricants as needed. The size of the pessary is estimated after a digital examination and use of ring forceps to reduce the prolapse or bladder neck. Once the approximate size is determined, the appropriate type is selected based on the patient's needs and activity level. **When fitted, the patient is asked to stand, perform Valsalva, and cough to ensure the pessary is retained.** The pessary should be assessed to ensure it is providing the desired support and leakage control. The patient should be able to void with the pessary in place before leaving the office. Proper size is ensured by the ability to sweep the index finger between the pessary and the vaginal wall. The patient should feel comfortable with the pessary in place.

Insertion of the pessary is eased by using a water-soluble lubricant for insertion, folding or collapsing the pessary to reduce its size, and when it is inside the vagina, pushing it high to an area behind the symphysis pubis and inserting the device more posteriorly to avoid the urethra. Instructing the patient how to insert and remove the pessary may be done with the patient in a standing or supine position, depending on her dexterity (49).

Ring pessaries, with or without support, are the most commonly used type. They are the easiest to fold, insert, and remove. **Gellhorn** and **cube** pessaries are typically more difficult to insert and remove by the patient. They are held in place by significant space occupation and suction and offer strong support. The suction of the cube pessary needs to be broken, facilitating removal. Cube pessaries should be removed daily; Gelhorns can stay in longer (up to 6–8 weeks). **Donut pessaries,** which are very popular, are considered a space-fitting pessary for large vaginal vault prolapse, complete procidentia with decreased perineal support, and good introital integrity. **The patient should be questioned about a latex allergy and instructed to remove and clean the device every 2 to 3 days.** Continence pessaries, rings, and dishes with support typically also are easy to fold, insert, and remove (50).

Follow-Up Recommendations

After the initial fitting, the patient should return in 1 to 2 weeks and then at 4 to 6 weeks, depending on her independence with the pessary, her proficiency in placement and removal, and her cognitive and motor abilities (44). After this initial follow-up, follow-up should continue at 6- to 12-month intervals at the discretion of the provider and depending on the patient's ability to insert and remove the pessary effectively. If the patient needs to return to the provider for removal and cleaning of the pessary, 4- to 12-week intervals are more appropriate.

On follow-up visits, proper placement of the pessary and support of the prolapse as well as continence efficacy should be ensured. Because pessaries are fitted through a process of trial and error, it is not uncommon to change the size or type at least once after the initial fitting. The pessary's integrity should be checked, and the tissues should be evaluated for irritation, pressure sores, ulceration, and lubrication (44).

Surgical Management

The primary aims of surgery are to relieve symptoms, which may be caused by prolapse, and, in most cases, to restore vaginal anatomy so that sexual function may be maintained or improved without significant adverse effects or complications. Occasionally, when sexual function is not desired, obliterative or constrictive surgery is more appropriate and also may relieve symptoms. There is no steadfast rule as to when surgery is indicated. Many patients with more advanced prolapse have few or no symptoms, whereas some with lesser degrees of prolapse have what they describe as severe symptoms. This is confounded by the observation that many of the "symptoms" may not be specifically related to the anatomic defect or may be worsened by anxiety. In general, surgery should be offered to patients who have tried conservative therapy and were not satisfied with the results or who do not desire conservative therapy. The prolapse should be symptomatic or should be greater than or equal to stage II with apparent progression. All patients should be given the alternative of trying conservative treatments when applicable (51).

Approaches to surgery include vaginal, abdominal, and laparoscopic routes, or a combination of approaches. Depending on the extent and location of prolapse, surgery may involve a combination of repairs directed to the anterior vagina, vaginal apex, posterior vagina, and perineum. Concomitant surgery may be planned for urinary or fecal incontinence. The surgical route is chosen based on the type and severity of prolapse, the surgeon's training and experience, the patient's preference, and the expected or desired surgical outcome.

Procedures for prolapse can be broadly categorized into three groups: (i) restorative, which use the patient's endogenous support structures; (ii) compensatory, which attempt

to replace deficient support with permanent graft material; and (iii) obliterative, which close or partially close the vagina (51).

These groupings are somewhat arbitrary and not entirely exclusive. For example, grafts may be used to reinforce repairs, such as colporrhaphy, or to replace support that is deficient or lacking. Graft use in sacrocolpopexy substitutes for the connective tissues attachments (cardinal and uterosacral ligaments) that would normally support the vaginal apex. In addition to the primary goal of relieving symptoms related to prolapse, urinary, defecatory, and sexual function must be considered in choosing the appropriate procedures.

Whether to repair all defects is controversial. Restorative repairs may be less successful than compensatory repairs in patients with generally "poor tissue," and at times one defect repair may exert more tension on the repair of another defect. Management should be based on the patient's presentation, expectations, the specific anatomical defects noted (preoperatively and, at times, intraoperatively), and on the presence or absence of lower urinary and bowel dysfunction (51).

Vaginal Procedures

The Apical Compartment

Examination for apical defects is at times difficult. Such defects may be missed when large anterior or posterior defects are present. In cases when apical defects are suspected but not confirmed, surgeons should evaluate the apical support intraoperatively and plan for management of these defects when they are found. Traction on the cervix with a tenaculum or on the vaginal cuff both centrally and laterally with Allis clamps may reveal otherwise unrecognized defects.

Transvaginal repairs include extraperitoneal procedures such as sacrospinous suspensions, iliococcygeal suspensions, and high paravaginal suspensions of the apical vaginal fornices to the arcus tendineus at the level of the ischial spine or to the endopelvic fascia, and intraperitoneal suspensions such as uterosacral suspensions and McCall culdoplasties (51). Accepted practice is that the vaginal apex should be resuspended in a posterior cephalad direction to a site or sites posterior and caudad to the sacral promontory. Anterior apical suspensions change the direction of the vaginal axis and may be fraught with a greater incidence of posterior compartment defects, including rectoceles, enteroceles, and sigmoidoceles.

The general principles of the repair should include management of the specific apical defects:

1. If present, the attenuated part of the upper vaginal wall (fibromuscular defect) should be repaired or covered by graft material.
2. The vaginal cuff or, in some instances, the cervix should be suspended without excessive tension.
3. Any defect in the attachment of the upper vagina to the rectum at or below its sigmoid junction should be corrected.

Enterocele repairs may include:

1. Removal of the peritoneal sac with closure of the peritoneal defect, followed by closure of the fascial or fibromuscular defect or both below it
2. Dissection and reduction of the peritoneal sac and closure of the defect
3. Obliteration of the peritoneal sac from within with transabdominal Halban or Moschcowitz type procedures or transvaginal McCall or Halban procedures (52).

Historically, the treatment for symptomatic uterine prolapse has been hysterectomy, which is performed vaginally or abdominally in combination with an apical suspension procedure, and repair of coexisting defects. Apical support procedures that have been described for use when the uterus or cervix is to be kept in place include Manchester and Gilliam procedures and fixation of the cervix to the sacrospinous ligament . The other procedures described in this section may also be used in women who desire uterine conservation. Adequate outcome data on such uterine-sparing procedures are not yet available. When the cervix is absent, in addition to repair of fibromuscular defects, both fibromuscular planes anterior and posterior to the vaginal cuff should be attached to whatever suspension is employed.

Sacrospinous Ligament Fixation

The fixation of the vaginal apex to the sacrospinous ligament, the tendineus component of the coccygeus muscle, was first described in 1958 and was subsequently modified in Europe and the United States (53–56). **Access is traditionally extraperitoneal via the rectovaginal space with penetration of the pararectal (Denonvillier's fascia) at the level of the ischial spine to expose the muscle and ligament. Variations in this approach to the ligament include entrances through an anterior lateral access, an apical passage posterior to the uterosacral ligament, and a laparoscopic approach** (57–59). Bilateral sacrospinous ligament suspensions have also been advocated; however, these techniques may impose a greater degree of tension on the sutures and, at times, create a band of apical vagina across the rectum at the level of the suspension (60,61). Whether this can cause defecatory dysfunction remains unknown. The advantages of the sacrospinous fixation procedure include (i) its transvaginal extraperitoneal approach, (ii) resultant posterior vaginal deflection, and (iii) the fact that it is a durable repair if performed correctly. Reported success for apical support has been good (89%–97%) with follow-up times ranging from 1 month to 11 years (51,62). However, there have been subsequent reports of high rates of anterior vaginal prolapse (63,64). It is not clear whether this observation is related to the procedure and its exaggerated posterior vaginal deflection or to the fact that many patients with apical descent also have defects in the upper vaginal fibromuscular tissue. Failure to address an anterior defect concurrently with suspension of the posterior apical vagina may predispose the patient to such a defect postoperatively. Other disadvantages of the procedure include (i) relative difficulty in adequately exposing the ligament, (ii) an unnatural lateral vaginal deflection toward the fixation site, (iii) an inability to perform without excessive tension when the vaginal length is compromised, as may be the case in repeat procedures, (iv) potential risk for injury to the sciatic nerve or pudendal nerve or vessel, and (v) occasional need to shorten or narrow the upper vagina when a fibromuscular defect involves much of the apical area.

Iliococcygeal Vaginal Suspension

Iliococcygeal vaginal suspension involves the attachment, usually bilaterally, of the vaginal apex to the iliococcygeus muscle and fascia (61,65,66). Extraperitoneal access is achieved via the posterior vagina. Compared with other vaginal suspension procedures, the iliococcygeal suspension has the fewest case series in the literature (65–67); however, cure rates appear comparable to the sacrospinous suspension technique (51). The dissection of the area to the ischial spine is approached from a midline posterior vaginal wall incision using the ischial spine as a landmark for identifying the sacrospinous ligament and the iliococcygeal fascia anteriorly and caudad to it. A no. 1 polydioxanone suture is placed through the fascia and attached to the vaginal apex as a pulley stitch. This procedure is more easily performed bilaterally than the sacrospinous suspension and should be considered preferentially in the presence of a shortened vagina. Risk of major vessel, nerve, or ureteral injury should be relatively low compared with other transvaginal suspensions.

Uterosacral Ligament Suspension

Surgical variations of the uterosacral ligament suspension originally described in 1938 have been used prophylactically during hysterectomy or therapeutically for vaginal apical suspension (68). **A therapeutic procedure in which the vaginal apex is suspended to the uterosacral ligaments above the level of the ischial spines had excellent success rates in an observational study of 302 participants** (69). When access to the posterior cul-de-sac is attained, the uterosacral ligament remnant can usually be found adjacent to the pelvic sidewall peritoneum just cephalad to the palpable ischial spine. Up to three sutures are placed in each ligament and incorporated into the anterior and posterior fibromuscular layer of the vagina. Some surgeons approximate the ligaments in the midline to close the cul-de-sac with the intention to treat or prevent enterocele formation (70). Other surgeons suspend the right and left vaginal apex to the ipsilateral uterosacral ligament, leaving the cul-de-sac open to avoid impinging on the rectum and adversely affecting bowel function.

Outcome studies have shown that recurrent apical prolapse occurs in 2% to 5% of cases within the first few years following the procedure, which is a rate comparable or superior to other transvaginal apical repairs, and the incidence of recurrent anterior defects may be less than that reported with sacrospinous suspensions (69,71). The most common serious complication was ureteral obstruction secondary to ureteral kinking or incorporation of an ureter in a suspension stitch. This occurred in as many as 11% of cases (71). Intraoperative cystoscopy—

with documentation of ureteral patency after administration of indigo carmine dye, whereby such a problem can be corrected—is recommended.

Multiple sutures may increase the incidence of tissue devascularization and necrosis, thus resulting in failure of the suspension. One case series of bilateral single suture uterosacral suspensions demonstrated a 15% stage I and no stage II recurrence among 71 women with a mean follow-up of 21.3 months (72). Exposure can be accomplished through the vaginal cuff after hysterectomy, a transverse incision at the vaginal cuff in cases of vaginal vault prolapse or descent, and, rarely, through a posterior colpotomy when uterine or cervical conservation is desired. When the apical vaginal wall is attenuated, it is excised. The pelvic sidewall, lateral to the sigmoid colon, is exposed using Breisky-Navratil retractors and a pack to hold the small bowel cephalad and to place the sigmoid colon and sidewall peritoneum on stretch (Fig. 27.12A). After palpation of the ischial spine, single permanent sutures of 0 or 1 polypropylene are placed through the peritoneum and adjacent ligament approximately 1 cm cephalad to and at the same posterior level as the ischial spines. Traction on the sutures and palpation of the site should reveal that the sutures are firmly attached to the ligamentous structures. The sutures are tagged for use after repair of defects of the anterior compartment. The peritoneum is

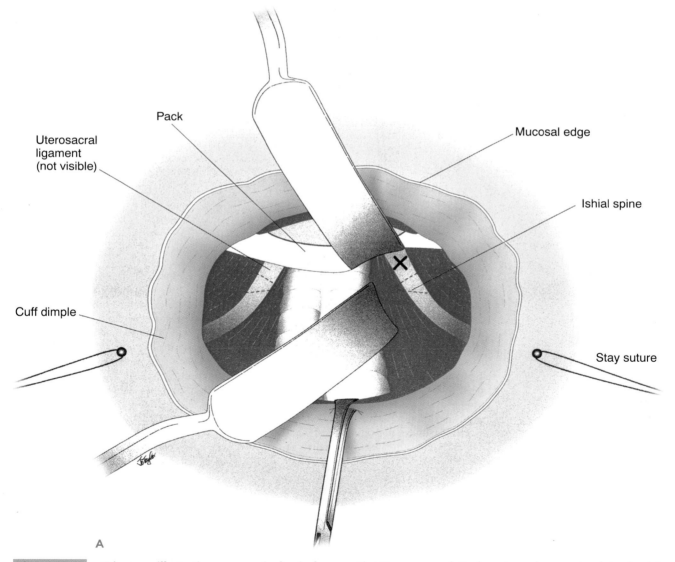

Figure 27.12 **Diagrams illustrating open vaginal apical area** with (**A**) exposure of site for suture placement or lateral pelvic side wall and (**B**) suture placement through ligament then through the posterior and anterior paravaginal tissue where they are locked to enable pulley action to the ligaments when tied. (Redrawn from an image by J. Taylor.)

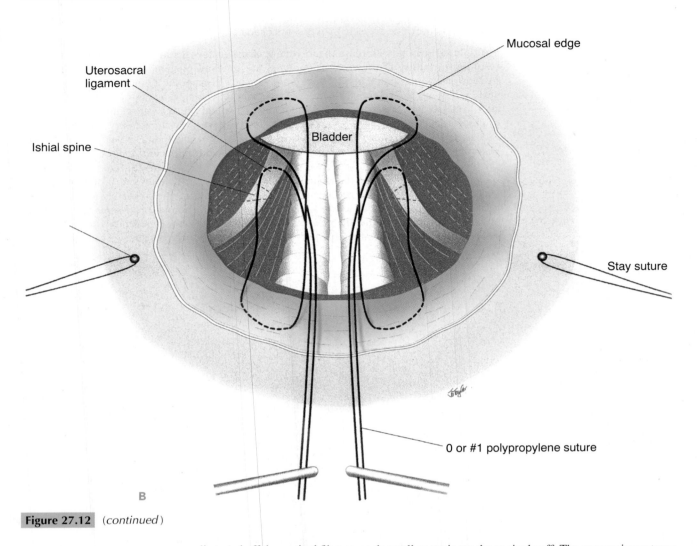

Uterosacral
ligament

Ishial spine

Mucosal edge

Bladder

Stay suture

0 or #1 polypropylene suture

B

Figure 27.12   (*continued*)

dissected off the vaginal fibromuscular wall posterior to the vaginal cuff. The suspension sutures
are then secured with large bites into the posterior vaginal fibromuscular tissue and anterior
fibromuscular tissue, then locked in place to approximate anterior to posterior connective tissue and to fix the suture to the vaginal apex so that it may be moved up to the ligament (Fig.
27.12B). If a rectovaginal enterocele is present, it is dissected, reduced, and closed, approximating the prerectal fascia or anterior rectal wall to the posterior fibromuscular vaginal tissue
just caudad to the suspension sutures. Absorbable cuff closure sutures are placed at each cuff
angle and one to two bites are taken to approximate anterior to posterior vaginal cuff over the
suspension suture sites. When indicated, plication of the central cuff anterior to the posterior
fibromuscular tissue with a box stitch is also performed. These sutures are secured after the
suspension (pulley) sutures are tied, then cuff closure is completed from each side with the
absorbable sutures in a running fashion. Cystoscopy is performed to document ureteral patency.
Ureteral compromise has been noted in only 2 of 150 cases performed. The procedure provides adequate support of POP-Q point C and D in all 58 subjects evaluated more than 1 year
postoperatively (72).

The Anterior Compartment

Anterior Vaginal Colporrhaphy

**Anatomic correction of an anterior defect or cystocele will generally relieve symptoms
of protrusion and pressure and usually will improve micturition function when abnormal micturition is associated temporally with the defect and if there is no associated**

neuropathy. If a single, well-defined midline defect is recognized, excision of the weak vaginal wall and an imbricating closure of the defect may be performed. Most central anterior defects require a more extensive dissection of the vesicovaginal space. Following this dissection, many surgeons then separate the vaginal mucosa and submucosal layers from the fibromuscular layer out to a point lateral to the defect, followed by midline plication of this tissue, then excision of excess epithelium, and closure (72–78). It appears important to maintain the continuum of repaired fibromuscular tissue to a well-supported vaginal apex. If the repair is being performed simultaneously with a vaginal apical suspension, the anterior colporrhaphy is typically performed after the apical support sutures have been placed and prior to tying them down. The dissection is carried out starting from the everted vaginal cuff edge and dissecting toward the bladder neck. A high central defect may also be corrected via a transabdominal approach by dissecting between the base of the bladder and the upper one-third of the anterior vaginal wall. The defective tissue may then be wedged out and the defect closed with running or interrupted sutures. This approach may be of use when performing transabdominal procedures for apical suspension.

If the patient has significant stress incontinence (based on report or the presence of occult or potential incontinence), an appropriate bladder neck suspension may be performed simultaneously with the anterior repair. When performing midurethral sling procedures, it may be preferable not to extend the repair procedure below the urethra, but instead to make a separate incision for the sling. Maintaining some degree of the urethrovesical angle may improve the results of any incontinence procedure. If the patient has voiding dysfunction (reports of incomplete emptying and a high residual urine) and stress incontinence, appropriate urodynamic evaluation should be performed before a procedure is selected, and the patient should be made aware of the potential for continued problems after surgery (78).

Recurrence rates of traditional "fibromuscular plication" anterior repairs vary from 3% to 92%; however, studies define recurrence in numerous ways, from minimal prolapse to stage III descent (63,73–81). The clinical significance of recurrent mild cystoceles (stage I) that are asymptomatic is debatable because many of these defects do not progress to larger ones. When traditional anterior repairs are performed in patients with POP-Q stage II or greater cystoceles (frequently concurrently with other procedures), a 20% recurrence rate of stage II or greater prolapse is not uncommon, although overall recurrence rates as low as 3% have been reported (76). Many studies do not define how the participants were evaluated postoperatively and vary with respect to patient populations, type and severity of defects, presence of concurrent defects, surgical technique, and follow-up time and length. Some studies have suggested higher recurrence rates when these repairs are performed concurrently with sacrospinous suspensions and hypothesize that this type of apical suspension may predispose the repaired anterior wall to greater pressure transmission (63,64). These studies may show higher failure rates because patients having such concurrent repairs may be more likely to have more complicated forms of prolapse or more extensive pelvic floor defects than other patients.

Paravaginal Repair

The paravaginal or "lateral defect" repair involves reattachment of the anterior lateral vaginal sulcus to the obturator internus fascia and, in some cases, muscle at the level of the arcus tendineus pelvis ("white line") (82,83). It is usually performed as a bilateral procedure via transvaginal or retropubic (abdominal or laparoscopic) access. The procedure essentially restores normal anatomy; however, because it is not practical to rebuild the defective endopelvic–fascial bridge to the pelvic sidewall, it attaches the vaginal wall itself. Observational studies have reported good success with this procedure (80%–95%); however, long-term data on durability and function are lacking (12,84–88). Most women with anteriolateral detachments usually have separation of the upper vaginal fornices from the arcus tendineus immediately adjacent to the ischial spine (Fig. 27.13) (89). Thus, it is important to resuspend those specific areas.

It is difficult to achieve optimal results when the paravaginal repair is used in combination with traditional central repairs because of the creation of tension on opposing suture lines. A repair that removes a weakened central vaginal wall may decrease the side-to-side dimensions of the anterior vaginal wall, making it difficult to suspend its lateral points more laterally. When large central defects coexist with lateral defects, one option is an extensive central repair accompanied by an apical support procedure. This changes the shape of the vagina to a more cylindrical structure. Another choice is placement of a graft to span the entire anterior rhomboid-shaped plate, thus augmenting anterior paravaginal tissue strength. The graft with tension adjusted may

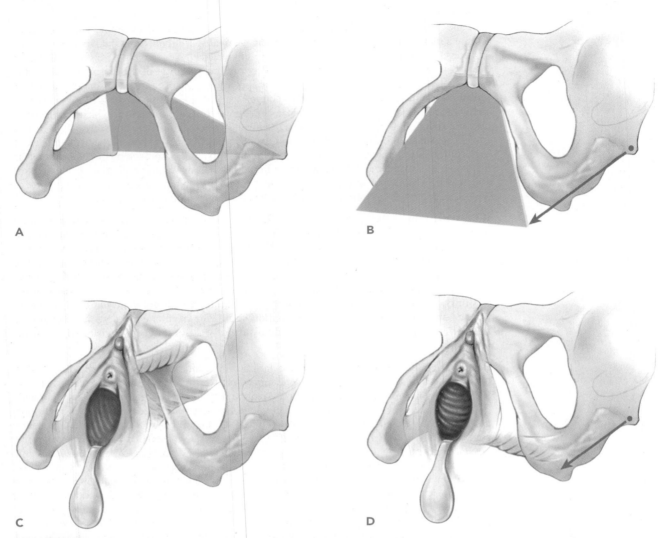

Figure 27.13   **Schematics illustrating normal attachments of the anterior fibromuscular vaginal plane (A and C) and bilateral detachments of that plane from the arcus tendineus up to the level of the ischial spines (B and D).** Note: For B and D to occur, there will either be concurrent apical descent or a detachment of the upper fibromuscular plane from the apical structures. (From **Delancey JO.** Fascial and muscular abnormalities in women with urethral hypermobility and anterior vaginal wall prolapse. *Am J Obstet Gynecol* 2002;187:93–98, with permission.)

be anchored to the arcus tendineus along with the adjacent vaginal wall from the level of the pubic rami to the ischial spine (88).

Although most reports indicate that repair of anterior defects with all of these procedures relieves symptoms directly related to prolapse, there are very few data on patient satisfaction and quality-of-life improvement over time (88).

The Posterior Compartment

Traditional Posterior Colporrhaphy

The first description of the **posterior colporrhaphy** involved plication of the pubococcygeus muscles across the anterior rectum as well as perineal body reconstruction (90). The technique has subsequently been modified in attempts to preserve sexual function. Typically a midline incision is extended from the perineal body to the vaginal apex or to the cephalad border of a small or distal rectocele. **The Denonvillier's fascia is mobilized from the vaginal epithelium, leaving** as much of this tissue as possible attached laterally to the levator fascia. After obvious defects in the rectal muscularis are repaired, the fascia is then plicated in the midline with interrupted or continuous sutures. The authors prefer delayed absorbable sutures for this plication. Permanent nonbraided suture material also can be used. Braided permanent suture material is associated with a greater incidence of stitch infection and formation of granulation tissue (91). The vaginal epithelium is trimmed and closed with absorbable sutures.

When a defective perineal body or perineal membrane is present, reconstruction is performed after accompanying posterior colporrhaphy. The superficial muscles of the perineum and bulbocavernous fascia are plicated in the midline and the skin closed as in an episiotomy repair. Detachments of the inferior portion of the Denonvillier's fascia from the perineal body are also corrected. The puborectalis muscles are plicated concurrently with these procedures by some surgeons, but this approach is associated with a high incidence of sexual dysfunction and thus is not recommended routinely (91). It may be worth consideration in patients who have severe prolapse accompanied by a large genital hiatus with palpable levator weakness or who are unable to contract their pelvic floor muscles. Sutures should be placed carefully through the puborectalis muscles at least 3 cm or greater posterior to their insertion on the pubic rami, thereby decreasing the tension of the plication. For those women with an enlarged hiatus and weakened puborectalis muscles who desire sexual function, an attempt can be made to plicate the muscles far enough posteriorly to allow two fingers to easily pass through the vaginal introitus and to reconstruct the distal posterior vagina and perineum, whereby there will not be a ledge at the site of the puborectalis plication (91). Outcome data on such procedures are inadequate to make conclusions regarding its efficacy; however, it is reasonable to postulate that pelvic floor defects producing an enlarged genital hiatus are common reasons for failure of support procedures, and puborectalis plication may decrease the incidence of such failures.

A complete review of rectocele, anorectal functional disorders, and various repairs can be found elsewhere (92). Reported anatomic cure rates for traditional posterior colporrhaphy have ranged from 76% to 90% with variable follow-up intervals (93–97). Most studies show a benefit in ease of defecation if patients are using splinting preoperatively; however, overall defecatory dysfunction (defined as constipation) was not relieved in most patients and increased (approximately 30%) after the procedure in one study (95). These repairs appear to have little to no benefit in the treatment of fecal incontinence. It is not surprising that the repairs are not particularly effective for defecatory dysfunction related to disorders of constipation or for fecal incontinence because these problems have multifactorial causes. *De novo* dyspareunia is reported to occur in 8% to 26% of sexually active patients who have traditional posterior colporrhaphy and is not always associated with levator plication procedures (93–96,98,99). Potential causes for dyspareunia, other than vaginal strictures or introital tightness, include scarring with immobility of the vaginal wall, levator spasm, and neuralgia associated with sutures or dissection. Dyspareunia also may occur when a Burch procedure or other procedures that anteriorly displace the vaginal canal are combined with a posterior repair (96). Careful surgical technique and appropriate choice of procedure should decrease the incidence of postoperative dyspareunia.

Defect Specific Posterior Repair

Defect or site-specific posterior repairs are restorative procedures by which posterior defects are corrected. These repairs begin with midline posterior vaginal incision through the epithelium and continue with separation of the epithelium from the fibromuscular wall. After irrigation to provide better exposure, a finger is inserted into the rectum to help define defects of the rectal wall and the fibromuscular layer that has been dissected from the vaginal wall submucosa. The specific defects are closed with either interrupted or running sutures (preferably the delayed absorbable type). Defect closure is accomplished in such a way as to minimize tension on the surrounding tissue and may involve vertical, horizontal, or oblique approximation. When fibromuscular tissue has separated from the perineum, the upper anterior rectum, or a well-supported cervix or vaginal cuff, it is important to reapproximate these connections. Repairs of coexistent perineal and apical support defects are important. The object of the surgery is to reestablish an intact plane of connective tissue that positions the rectum against the pelvic floor and obliterates any potential space between a well-supported cervix or vaginal cuff and the cephalad edge of the tissue plane and upper rectum. The technique should minimize tension and potential strictures, which may be more likely to occur with traditional posterior colporrhaphy (97).

Initial case series reveal anatomical cure rates with mean follow-up times less than 18 months from 82% to 100% and *de novo* dyspareunia rates of 2% to 7%, which are much lower than those seen with traditional repairs (99–103). Symptom relief appears to be as good or better than that seen with traditional repairs. The greatest concern with these and other procedures has been durability. A recent report indicates that the recurrence rate of rectocele beyond the midvaginal plane was higher with defect-specific posterior repairs than with side-to-side plication procedures using laterally attached fascia pulled to the midline (33% vs. 14%) and beyond the hymenal ring (11% vs. 4%) (97). The study was not randomized; however, the procedures were performed during the same period with consistent follow-up evaluations 1 year after surgery. Symptoms (dyspareunia, constipation, and fecal incontinence) after surgery did not differ between the two groups. Long-term follow-up of previously reported case series that had good short-term success or prospective randomized trials looking at modifications of traditional repairs versus defect-specific repairs should clearly delineate durability of these procedures.

Transanal Posterior Repair

The aim of transanal rectocele repair, usually performed by colorectal surgeons rather than gynecologists, is to remove or plicate redundant rectal mucosa, to decrease the size of the rectal vault, and to plicate the rectal muscularis. The rectovaginal adventitia and septum are plicated as well, probably along with the posterior vaginal muscularis. The vaginal epithelium is not incised or excised with this procedure, which probably accounts for the reported lack of adverse affects on sexual function in contrast to the vaginal approach to posterior repair. Two randomized trials and several case series from transanal repairs with mean follow-up intervals of 12 to 52 months report anatomic cure rates of 70% to 98%, improved constipation and fecal incontinence, with less need for vaginal digitation to expel stool (104–108). Complications included infections and rectovaginal fistulas, which are surprisingly rare in the reported series. From the gynecologic perspective, transanal posterior repair is an option only when the procedure is performed for defecatory dysfunction and not for prolapse of the posterior vaginal wall. The question remains whether the transanal approach with defect excision and repair improves defecatory dysfunction better than a defect-specific transperineal or transvaginal approach with imbrication of tissues to correct palpable weakness in the rectal wall and its adjacent connective tissues.

Transvaginal Mesh Procedures

Graft materials have been employed in repairing defects or hernias throughout the body. The purpose of grafts is to either completely replace "weak" tissue by spanning across that tissue or to provide a scaffold for fibroblast infiltration. The patient's own connective tissue may grow into the graft, and, if the graft is degradable, replace the graft as a supportive structure. An ideal graft material should (i) be nonantigenic, (ii) exhibit a low infection rate, (iii) decrease or negate recurrence of anatomic defects, (iv) cause no harm with respect to bowel or renal function, and (v) be relatively inexpensive. Graft materials include autologous tissues, cadaveric allografts and fascia, dermis and other connective tissues, xenografts from animal sources, and various synthetic materials. Allografts and xenografts are treated with processes to remove living cells, thus negating their antigenic potential and allowing them to serve as a temporary connective tissue scaffold. It is assumed that fresh, autologous grafts work similarly; however, there may be some fibroblast survival in fresh harvested tissue. Autologous grafts have limitations in size and shape compared with tissue taken from cadaveric or animal sources. Synthetic grafts are permanent and, as long as the tissues to which they are secured retain their position and strength, they should be durable. Autografts, allografts, and xenografts depend on adequate tissue growth from the subject and potentially may have higher failure rates than synthetic ones. **Synthetic grafts are more subject to erosion. Graft erosion may produce bothersome discharge, pain, and sexual dysfunction with vaginal scarring.** This may be more likely to occur in women with attenuated, scarred, or less vascular tissue at the time of the repair. More loosely woven polypropylene meshes appear to exhibit fewer problems with erosion and infection than the synthetic graft material that was previously used (109–113).

Midurethral sling procedures that use such mesh have reported erosion rates of 1% or less as compared with rates as high as 6% with more tightly woven polypropylene and polyethylene grafts (109–113). A greater incidence of graft infection has been reported when other synthetic grafts are used. One would expect higher rates of erosion and infection when large pieces of graft material are used adjunctively to the vaginal wall; however, there have been favorable reports in which loosely woven polypropylene mesh was used in this manner. Small areas of eroded polypropylene graft may be removed with the surrounding tissue to the point where there is good tissue growth into the graft, and the defect can then be closed. Graft erosion into the bladder, urethra, or rectum is less common than into the vagina. When erosion occurs, however, management is more difficult and long-term adverse effects more common. Numerous surgeons have been reticent to use synthetic graft materials to augment paravaginal musculoconnective tissue support because of complications from erosion. There remains a need for long-term follow-up on patients who have repairs with graft material, not only to assess anatomical results and complications, but also to assess subsequent sexual function, presence and absence of pain, and patient satisfaction.

Synthetic transvaginal mesh kits have become commonplace in the treatment of pelvic organ prolapse. These devices were quickly adopted by many surgeons in an effort to improve outcomes, particularly in patients who had failed native tissue repairs. Studies have provided mixed results as to the effectiveness of these devices. There may be a lower recurrence rate in the anterior compartment when compared with native tissue repairs; however, mesh erosions occur in 2% to 19% of those treated (109–113). The severity of mesh erosions ranges from subclinical to severe dyspareunia requiring surgical resection. Small mesh erosions are sometimes successfully managed with vaginal *estrogen* alone. As with anterior compartment procedures, graft materials have been used to improve the success of posterior compartment repairs. One recent systematic review concluded that there is insufficient evidence to evaluate the use of synthetic mesh in the repair of pelvic organ prolapse (114). It is also notable that the U.S. Food and Drug Administration (FDA) has recently released a warning about complications that may arise from the use of transvaginal mesh procedures for pelvic organ prolapse.

The FDA recommendations are that physicians should:

1. Obtain specialized training for each mesh placement technique, and be aware of its risks.

2. Be vigilant for potential adverse events from the mesh, especially erosion and infection.

3. Watch for complications associated with the tools used in transvaginal placement, especially bowel, bladder, and blood vessel perforations.

4. Inform patients that implantation of surgical mesh is permanent, and that some complications associated with the implanted mesh may require additional surgery that may or may not correct the complication.

5. Inform patients about the potential for serious complications and their effect on quality of life, including pain during sexual intercourse, scarring, and narrowing of the vaginal wall (in POP repair).

In summary, transvaginal mesh procedures that are currently in use utilize predominantly synthetic materials. These devices may reduce recurrence of pelvic organ prolapse and are associated with some risk of vaginal mesh extrusion and chronic pain or dyspareunia. Patients should be counseled extensively about the risks and benefits of the use of these devices. Surgeons who use these devices should carefully follow their cases to identify complications.

Abdominal Procedures

Abdominal Uterosacral Suspension

Abdominal uterosacral colposuspension has been used prophylactically after hysterectomy and therapeutically for apical prolapse with cardinal/uterosacral defects (115). It can be performed through laparotomy incisions or by laparoscopic techniques. For the therapeutic procedure, a no. 1 polypropylene or delayed absorbable suture is placed cephalad and at the same level posterior as the ischial spines, which may be palpated transabdominally or with a vaginal finger to push a vaginal fornix to the spine under observation with a laparoscope. One technique is to place one or two permanent sutures through one ligament, then, after reefing across the cul-de-sac peritoneum at the sigmoid border, through the contralateral ligament, and then through the fibromuscular tissue just anterior to the vaginal cuff. Tying the suture suspends the vaginal cuff and obliterates any enterocele defect. Another technique employs separate sutures placed at the same level into each uterosacral ligament and anchored anteriorly and posteriorly to the ipsilateral side of the vaginal cuff, similar to procedures performed transvaginally. Cystoscopy is performed after the procedure to document ureteral patency. One study found subjective and objective recurrence rates to be low (12% and 5%, respectively) (115).

Abdominal Approach to Posterior Repair

When abdominal sacrocolpopexy is planned for apical vaginal prolapse and concomitant rectocele is present, some have advocated extending the posterior graft down the posterior vaginal wall to correct the defect (116). The technique of sacral colpoperineopexy is used to replace the normal vaginal suspensory ligaments and to augment or replace the posterior fibromuscular plane with graft material that runs from the sacrum to the perineal body (116). Its purpose is to correct the posterior compartment defects and to suspend the perineal body, thus preventing descent and opening of the genital hiatus. It has been performed transabdominally or as a combined abdominal and vaginal procedure with both Mersilene mesh and dermal allografts (116,117). Mesh erosion occurred frequently when the vagina was open: 16% for vaginal placed sutures and 40% for transvaginally placed mesh (117). The use of dermal allografts results in an anatomical cure rate of 82% with short-term follow-up and a mean of 12 months following surgery (116,117). Significant improvements also were seen in bowel symptoms. One author reported results on 205 of 236 subjects who underwent an abdominal sacral colpoperineopexy with polypropylene mesh (Marlex) without opening the vagina (118). This procedure included two straps of mesh attached from the lateral anterior vagina to Cooper's ligament. Ten-year satisfaction rates were 68%, and erosion rates were 5%.

Laparoscopic Approach to Posterior Repair

Laparoscopic rectocele repair involves the dissection of the rectovaginal space to the perineal body with either plication of levator fascia or suturing absorbable or permanent mesh in place (119,120). A few small case series have been reported with variable results.

Abdominal Sacrocolpopexy

The standard approach to transabdominal apical vaginal suspension procedures is the abdominal sacrocolpopexy. A complete review of published data on these procedures developed by the Pelvic Floor Disorders Network, which is sponsored by the National Institute of Child Health and Human Development (NICHD), has been published (121). These procedures use graft material attached to the prolapsed region of the anterior and posterior vaginal walls at or encompassing the vaginal apex and suspended to the anterior longitudinal ligament of the sacrum. Cervical sacral suspensions may also be performed when uterine or cervical conservation is desired. Surgical variations abound and include configuration of the graft on the vagina, the extent to which the anterior and posterior vagina are attached to the graft, variable graft and suture materials, presence or absence of peritoneal closure over the graft, and obliteration of the cul-de-sac for treatment or prevention of the enterocele or sigmoidocele. **A thorough preoperative evaluation is important to exclude more distal defects or stress incontinence, which should be repaired concurrently, and other lower urinary tract or anorectal problems.** In published reports, cure rates for apical prolapse range from 78% to 100% (most greater than 90%); when cure is defined as no postoperative prolapse, the range widens from 56% to 100%, although subsequent anterior or posterior vaginal prolapse has not been as consistently reported as has apical prolapse (122–131). Potential advantages of this procedure over transvaginal procedures are less paravaginal scarring and denervation than may be present with transvaginal approaches, and fixation of the entire vaginal apical area by a permanent piece of material to a stable structure (the anterior sacral ligament), which may be more durable than the transvaginal techniques that use the patient's own connective tissue.

Complications of these procedures include (i) erosions of graft material or suture material, which may be caused by graft or suture infection usually secondary to vaginal wall penetration, or performing the procedure adjacent to a vaginal incision, or securing the graft to an attenuated avascular wall with inadequate fibromuscular tissue (3.4%); (ii) significant intraoperative hemorrhage (especially in the presacral space) (4.8%); (iii) postoperative ileus, which may be secondary to the need for excessive packing of the bowel or to extensive Halban or Moschcowitz culdoplasty procedures (3.6%); (iv) small bowel obstruction, requiring reoperation (1.1%); (v) development of intra-abdominal adhesions with resultant pain and bowel dysfunction (unknown incidence); and (vi) wound complications, such as seromas and infections (4.6%) (120).

Several management techniques have been advocated to minimize these problems. Empiric ways to prevent graft erosions include (i) preoperative tissue optimization with vaginal administration of estrogen and treatment of vaginitis and infection of eroded areas; (ii) the use of small-gauge monofilament sutures placed in the fibromuscular tissue, thus avoiding full thickness passage; and (iii) excision of a portion of the vaginal apex when the vaginal wall is thin and depleted of its fibromuscular layer and vascularity. Graft attachment to "healthy" fibromuscular tissue rather than to thin avascular tissue should help prevent erosion. **If such excision is necessary, or if the suspension is to be performed concurrently with a hysterectomy, good approximation of the fibromuscular layers above the mucosa, thorough irrigation, prophylactic use of antibiotics, and avoidance of graft placement across the suture line may decrease the likelihood of graft erosion. Choice of graft material may also be important.** One would expect synthetic grafts to have greater durability than tissue grafts; however, erosion rates are more serious with the synthetic grafts. Anecdotally, some surgeons are convinced that less porous graft material, such as GORE-TEX, has a greater likelihood of becoming infected and eroding than do macroporous, filamentous polypropylene meshes. Numerous case series report serious episodes of hemorrhage from the presacral venous plexus (mean incidence 4.8%; range 0.18%–16.9% of sacrocolpopexies requiring, at a minimum, transfusion) (121). This problem is less likely if dissection and graft fixation is limited to the level of S1 and S2 just caudad to the promontory and with the use of good light and meticulous dissection techniques to expose the anterior sacral ligament.

Careful tissue handling and packing technique may minimize postoperative ileus and adhesions. Incorporation of the sigmoid into a closure of the cul-de-sac posterior to the graft may also slow bowel function postoperatively. Small bowel obstruction has resulted from direct adhesive processes involving grafts to small bowel (120). Complete extra peritonealization of the graft using flaps of peritoneum dissected from the prolapsed area and the peritoneum anterior to the sacral promontory and lateral to the right side of the sigmoid colon should prevent this complication. However, loops of bowel have been seen to prolapse through small defects in peritoneal closure with the same effect. Careful technique with adherence to basic surgical principles may help prevent this and other complications related to laparotomy.

Laparoscopic and Robotic Techniques

As with most pelvic operations, sacrocolpopexy has been successfully accomplished by the laparoscopic and robotic route and has the potential to offer patients the benefits of less postoperative discomfort and faster recovery as well as potential lower risks for adhesions and ileus. Outcomes depend on the expertise and experience of the surgeon; "cutting corners" to shorten the procedure could affect anatomical success. The applicability of the laparoscopic technique is limited by the need for a relatively high level of technical skill. In the authors' experience, ipsilateral suturing (through same sided ports) is preferred to contralateral suturing. The authors have also found that straight self-righting needle drivers and non-self-righting curved needle drivers are useful in attaching the mesh to the vagina. The Carter-Thompson suturing device is sometimes helpful to aid in elevating the sigmoid colon away from the pelvic cul-de-sac by tagging the peritoneal edge. The robot has provided an easier platform for a minimally invasive approach to the sacrocolpopexy. Data about its use are limited to several case series that demonstrate comparable short-term results with open and laparoscopic techniques (121).

For sacrocolpopexy, whether through laparotomy or laparoscopy, the pelvis should be completely exposed with the lower sigmoid colon stretched cephalad (Fig. 27.14).

1. With a vaginal obturator (an EEA sizer) placed vaginally to visualize the area that is not covered by the bladder or rectum, the peritoneum is dissected from the underlying vaginal fibromuscular layer anteriorly to bladder reflection and posteriorly at least to the level of the sigmoid rectal junction, creating bilateral peritoneal flaps. Laterally, vascular bundles are visible.

2. Two separate loosely woven polypropylene mesh grafts are shaped similar to boat paddles. The "paddle" portions are shaped to cover the areas anterior to the apex and posterior to the apex, respectively, and the "handles," which are approximately 8 to 10 cm in length and 1 cm wide, are anchored to the anterior sacral ligament. The paddle portions are secured circumferentially to the fibromuscular layers anteriorly and posteriorly with six to eight monofilament 3-0 nylon sutures and one or two sutures placed centrally (Fig. 27.14A).

3. When the fibromuscular tissue in the area is attenuated, a portion of the vaginal wall is excised and closed, as noted previously.

4. The peritoneum overlying sacral vertebrae 1 and 2 is incised while retracting the sigmoid colon to the left, and careful dissection is employed down to the anterior ligament. Care is taken to stay well medial to the right ureter and hypogastric vessels.

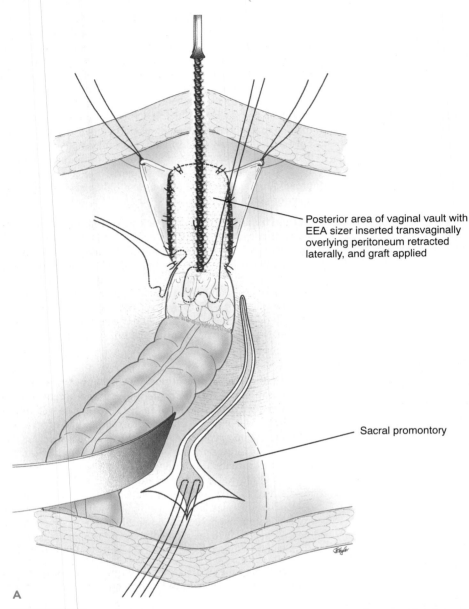

Posterior area of vaginal vault with EEA sizer inserted transvaginally overlying peritoneum retracted laterally, and graft applied

Sacral promontory

A

Figure 27.14   Sacrocolpopexy. A: Illustrates (i) graft attachment to the posterior area of pro-lapsed vagina to or below the rectal-sigmoid junction after the overlying peritoneum has been dissected and flapped laterally and (ii) exposure of the presacral space with suture placement through the anterior sacral ligament. An appropriately shaped second graft is placed anteriorly. **B:** Illustrates attachment of both grafts without tension to the sacrum. Prevention of subsequent enterocele and/or sigmoidocele is accomplished by box closure of the cul-de-sac peritoneum lateral to the left side of the sigmoid, attachment of the presigmoid fat to the graft centrally, and reperitorealization of the graft through the right side of the cul-de-sac. EEA, end-to-end anastomosis sizer. (Redrawn by J. Taylor.)

5. Hemoclips are placed caudad and cephalad on the middle sacral vessels if it is felt that this will allow more optimal suture placement. The peritoneal incision is extended into the right cul-de-sac area adjacent to the sigmoid.

6. Closure of the cul-de-sac lateral to the sigmoid on the left and approximation of the distal presigmoid fat to the distal edge of the posterior graft is accomplished with box stitches of 0-delayed absorbable sutures. It is thought that these procedures and the retroperitonealization of the graft through the right side of the cul-de-sac will prevent posterior enterocele and sigmoidocele as well as a Halban or Moschcowitz procedure.

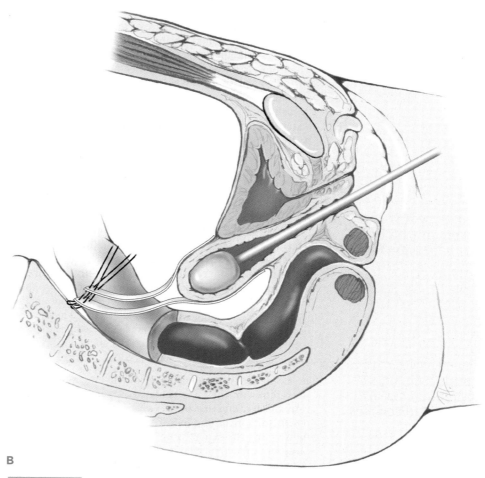

B

Figure 27.14   *(continued)*

7. The two "handle" ends of the graft are then brought to the point of sacral attachment, where their length is adjusted to remove any tension on the vaginal sutures and secured to the anterior sacral ligament with no. 1 permanent braided nylon sutures (Fig. 27.14B).

8. Reperitonealization of the graft is then performed using the right cul-de-sac peritoneum and peritoneal flaps dissected from the vaginal apical area; occasionally presigmoid fat is used.

Following this procedure, adjunctive procedures, such as paravaginal repair, Burch procedure, midurethral sling, and any transvaginal procedure that is indicated, are performed. When rectocele and pelvic floor defects are present, one option is the sacral colpoperineopexy, as discussed in the posterior compartment section (116). A vaginal pack is inserted for approximately 24 hours to ensure that the graft is well applied to the fibromuscular layer at points other than where sutures are placed.

Vaginal Obliterative Procedures

Colpocleisis or vaginal narrowing procedures may be appropriate choices for debilitated patients who do not desire vaginal function, because complete vaginal reconstructive procedures may last several hours and are associated with potentially higher blood loss and increased morbidity (132,133). Many variations exist, from partial colpocleisis (where some portion of the vaginal epithelium is left to provide drainage tracts for cervical or upper genital discharge) to total colpectomy (where all of the vaginal epithelium is removed from the hymen posteriorly to within 0.5–2 cm of the external urethral meatus anteriorly). If hysterectomy is performed, blood loss is greater and operative time is longer than procedures without hysterectomy (134). These techniques should include a high perineorrhaphy and often a plication of the puborectalis muscles to reinforce posterior support and to reduce the genital hiatus, with the goal of decreasing the chance of recurrent prolapse. Case series have reported success rates as high as 100%, although the population of patients, by nature of their relatively short life expectancy and limited activity, are probably at lower risk for recurrence. In some instances in which most of the defects are anterior and posterior, a modified anterior and posterior colporrhaphy may be performed, whereby relatively large portions of the anterior and posterior vaginal wall are removed and closed, creating a narrow (1–2 cm diameter) cylindrical vagina. As with the colpocleisis, the success of the procedure is augmented by an extensive perineorrhaphy and puborectalis plication. Such a procedure may be performed quickly and with relatively low morbidity. The prevention or treatment of stress incontinence, voiding dysfunction, and colorectal dysfunction in the context of these procedures can be problematic. Careful preoperative history and evaluation, if indicated, is important so that additional conservative therapies or operative techniques such as pubourethral plications or less invasive tension-free slings may be employed.

Management of Urinary Symptoms with Pelvic Organ Prolapse Repair

All women who are undergoing surgery for repair of pelvic organ prolapse should be evaluated for urinary incontinence. Women who report stress urinary incontinence and who demonstrate it on preoperative examination and have no contraindications to a continence procedure should have concomitant procedures for the treatment of these symptoms. Women who do not report stress urinary incontinence may also benefit from a prophylactic procedure if they demonstrate incontinence with reduction of their prolapse. There is also evidence that the addition of a continence procedure in the absence of any evidence of urinary incontinence may improve outcomes without significantly increasing the number of complications (135). The addition of continence procedures to prolapse procedures in patients who have both significant stress incontinence and voiding dysfunction remains controversial.

Comparison of Abdominal versus Vaginal Approaches

In recent years there has been controversy as to whether transvaginal or transabdominal procedures are best for prolapse. One cannot discern which is optimal from reports of retrospective and prospective case series because of the considerable differences in numerous factors, including follow-up, characteristics of the subjects, definitions of success and failure, and the expertise or experience of the surgeons performing the procedures. Three prospective randomized trials have compared sacrocolpopexy and sacrospinous suspension procedures (136–138). All three trials showed some increased durability in the sacrocolpopexy group; however, in one of these studies the differences were not statistically significant (138). In the study in which sexual function was examined, there was a greater incidence of dyspareunia in the transvaginal group (137). Most case series reveal that the incidence of serious complications, such as small bowel obstructions, significant hemorrhage, presacral graft infections, pulmonary embolus, and short-term problems (i.e., ileus, hernias, wound seromas or infections, and longer hospitalizations), are more likely to occur in the group undergoing sacrocolpopexy. Vaginal scarring, strictures, and vaginal wall erosions or granulation tissue appear more likely in the group undergoing transvaginal surgery. To date, there is no randomized comparison of vaginal procedures using high uterosacral suspensions and innovative repairs of the fibromuscular tissues, which are less likely to produce strictures than was the case 10 or more years ago.

Most pelvic surgeons would agree that **(i) older, less healthy individuals who are more likely to have surgical and medical complications and cannot or will not tolerate a pessary would derive greater benefit from transvaginal approaches and occasionally obliterative approaches, and (ii) relatively healthy, sexually active women with relatively short vaginas and apical prolapse or with isolated apical defects would derive greater benefit from sacrocolpopexy.** For the remainder of the patients with apical prolapse, with or without more distal defects, it would be ideal if surgeons were equally skilled, knowledgeable, and experienced in both abdominal and vaginal approaches to provide care that is truly individualized, rather than emphasizing one approach to the exclusion of another.

References

1. **American College of Obstetricians and Gynecologists.** Pelvic organ prolapse. ACOG Technical Bulletin. *Int J Gynaecol Obstet* 1996;52:197–205.
2. **Subak LL, Waetjen LE, van den Eeden S, et al.** Cost of pelvic organ prolapse surgery in the United States. *Obstet Gynecol* 2001;98:646–651.
3. **Olsen AL, Smith VJ, Bergstrom JO, et al.** Epidemiology of surgically managed pelvic organ prolapse and urinary incontinence. *Obstet Gynecol* 1997;89:501–506.
4. **Boyles SH, Weber AM, Meyn L.** Procedures for pelvic organ prolapse in the United States 1979–1997. *Am J Obstet Gynecol* 2003;189:70–75.

5. **Luber KM, Boero S, Choe JY.** The demographics of pelvic floor disorders: current observations and future projections. *Am J Obstet Gynecol* 2001;184:1496–1501.

6. **Brubaker L.** Controversies and uncertainties: abdominal versus vaginal surgery for pelvic organ prolapse. *Am J Obstet Gynecol* 2005;192:690–693.

7. **Hendrix SL, Clark A, Nygaard I, et al.** Pelvic organ prolapse in the Women's Health Initiative: gravity and gravidity. *Am J Obstet Gynecol* 2002;186:1160–1166.

8. **Gurel H, Gurel SA.** Pelvic relaxation and associated risk factors: the results of logistic regression analysis. *Acta Obstet Gynecol Scand* 1999;78:290–293.

9. **Swift SE, Pound T, Dias JK.** Case-control study of etiologic factors in the development of severe pelvic organ prolapse. *Int Urogynecol J Pelvic Floor Dysfunct* 2001;12:187–192.

10. **Fornell EU, Wingren G, Kjolhede P.** Factors associated with pelvic floor dysfunction with emphasis on urinary and fecal incontinence and genital prolapse: an epidemiologic study. *Acta Obstet Gynecol Scand* 2004;83:383–389.

11. **Moalli PA, Ivy SJ, Meyn LA, et al.** Risk factors associated with pelvic floor disorders in women undergoing surgical repair. *Obstet Gynecol* 2003;101:869–874.

12. **Young SB, Daman JJ, Bony LG.** Vaginal paravaginal repair: one-year outcomes. *Am J Obstet Gynecol* 2001;185:1360–1366.

13. **Richardson AC, Lyon JB, Williams NL.** A new look at pelvic relaxation. *Am J Obstet Gynecol* 1976;126:568–573.

14. **Richardson AC.** The rectovaginal septum revisited: its relationship to rectocele and its importance in rectocele repair. *Clin Obstet Gynecol* 1993;36:976–983.

15. **Samuelsson EC, Arne Victor FT, Tibblin G, et al.** Signs of genital prolapse in a Swedish population of women 20 to 59 years of age and possible related factors. *Am J Obstet Gynecol* 1999;180:299–305.

16. **Beck RP.** Pelvic relaxational prolapse. In: **Kase NG, Weingold AB, eds.** *Principles and practice of clinical gynecology.* New York: John Wiley & Sons, 1983:677–685.

17. **Brubaker L, Bump R, Jacquetien B, et al.** Pelvic organ prolapse. In: Abrams P, Cardozo L, Khoury S, et al., eds. *Incontinence,* 21st ed. Paris: Health Publications, 2005:243–265.

18. **Mouritsen L, Larsen JP.** Symptoms, bother and POPQ in women referred with pelvic organ prolapse. *Int Urogynecol J Pelvic Floor Dysfunct* 2003;14:122–127.

19. **Ellerkman RM, Cundiff GW, Melick CF, et al.** Correlation of symptoms with location and severity of pelvic organ prolapse. *Am J Obstet Gynecol* 2001;185:1332–1338.

20. **Burrows LJ, Meyn LA, Walters MD, et al.** Pelvic symptoms in women with pelvic organ prolapse. *Obstet Gynecol* 2004;104:982–988.

21. **Silva WA, Kleeman S, Segal J, et al.** Effects of a full bladder and patient positioning on pelvic organ prolapse assessment. *Obstet Gynecol* 2004;104:37–41.

22. **Baden WF, Walker T.** Genesis of the vaginal profile. *Clin Obstet Gynecol* 1972;15:1048–1054.

23. **Bump RC, Mattiasson A, Bo K, et al.** The standardization of terminology of female pelvic organ prolapse and pelvic floor dysfunction. *Am J Obstet Gynecol* 1996;175:10–17.

24. **Lemos NL, Auge AP, Lunardelli JL, et al.** Validation of the pelvic organ prolapse quantification index (POPQ-I): a novel interpretation of the POP-Q system for optimization of POP research. *Int Urogynecol J Pelvic Floor Dysfunct* 2008;19:995–997.

25. **The American Urogynecology Society.** Available at www.augs.org.

26. **Brinks CA, Wells TJ, Samprelle CM, et al.** A digital test for pelvic muscle strength in women with urinary incontinence. *Nurs Res* 1994;43:352–356.

27. **Noblett K, Lane FL, Driskill CS.** Does pelvic organ prolapse quantification exam predict urethral mobility in stages 0 and 1 prolapse? *Int Urogynecol J* 2005;16:268.

28. **Walters MD, Diaz K.** Q-tip test: a study of continent and incontinent women. *Obstet Gynecol* 1987;70:208.

29. **Poma PA.** Nonsurgical management of genital prolapse: a review and recommendations for clinical practice. *J Reprod Med* 2000;45:789–797.

30. **Bump RC, Norton PA.** Epidemiology and natural history of pelvic floor dysfunction. *Obstet Gynecol Clin North Am* 1998;25:723–747.

31. **Hagen S, Stark D, Maher C, et al.** Conservative management of pelvic organ prolapse in women. *Cochrane Database Syst Rev* 2004;2:CD003882.

32. **Davilla GW, Bernier F.** Multimodality pelvic physiotherapy treatment of urinary incontinence in adult women. *Int Urogynecol J* 1995;6:187–194.

33. **Thakar R, Stanton S.** Management of genital prolapse. *BMJ* 2004;324:1258–1262.

34. **Davilla GW.** Vaginal prolapse management with nonsurgical techniques. *Postgrad Med* 1996;99:171–185.

35. **Mimura T, Roy AJ, Storrie JB, et al.** Treatment of impaired defecation associated with rectocele by behavioral retraining (biofeedback). *Dis Colon Rectum* 2000;43:1267–1272.

36. **Clemons J, Aguilar VC, Tillinghast TA, et al.** Patient satisfaction and changes in prolapse and urinary symptoms in women who were fitted successfully with a pessary for pelvic organ prolapse. *Am J Obstet Gynecol* 2004;190:1025–1029.

37. **Brincat C, Kenton K, Fitzgerald MP, et al.** Sexual activity predicts continued pessary use. *Am J Obstet Gynecol* 2004;191:198–200.

38. **Clemons JL, Aguilar VC, Tillinghast TA, et al.** Risk factors associated with an unsuccessful pessary fitting trial in women with pelvic organ prolapse. *Am J Obstet Gynecol* 2004;190:345–350.

39. **Cundiff GW, Weidner AC, Visco AG, et al.** A survey of pessary use by members of the American Gynecologic Society. *Obstet Gynecol* 2000;95:931–935.

40. **Sulak PJ, Kuehl TJ, Shull BJ.** Vaginal pessaries and their use in pelvic relaxation. *J Reprod Med* 1993;38:919–923.

41. **Handa VL, Jones M.** Do pessaries prevent the progression of pelvic organ prolapse? *Int Urogynecol J* 2002;13:349–352.

42. **Richter HE, Burgio KL, Brubaker L, et al.** Continence pessary compared with behavioral therapy or combined therapy for stress incontinence: a randomized controlled trial. *Obstet Gynecol* 2010;115:609–617.

43. **Adams E, Thomson A, Maher C, et al.** Mechanical devices for pelvic organ prolapse in women. *Cochrane Database Syst Rev* 2004;2:CD004010.

44. **Wu V, Farrell SA, Basket TF, et al.** A simplified protocol for pessary management. *Obstet Gynecol* 1997;90:990–994.

45. **Farrell SA, Singh B, Aldakhil L.** Continence pessaries in the management of urinary incontinence in women. *J Obstet Gynaecol Can* 2004;26:113.

46. **Harris TA, Bent AE.** Genital prolapse with and without urinary incontinence. *J Reprod Med* 1990;35:792–798.

47. **Meinhardt W, Schuitemaker NEW, Smeets MJGH, et al.** Bilateral hydronephrosis with urosepsis due to neglected pessary. *Scand J Urol Nephrol* 1993;27:419–420.

48. **Ott R, Richter H, Behr J, et al.** Small bowel prolapse and incarceration caused by a vaginal ring pessary. *Br J Surg* 1993;80:1157–1159.

49. **Palumbo MV.** Pessary placement and management. *Ostomy Wound Manage* 2000;46:40.

50. **Bush K.** Review of vagina pessaries. *Obstet Gynecol Surv* 2000;55:465.

51. **Sze EHM, Karram MM.** Transvaginal repair of vault prolapse: a review. *Obstet Gynecol* 1997;89:466–475.

52. **Shull BL, Bachofen CG.** Enterocele and rectocele. In: Walters M, Karram MM, eds. Urogynecology and reconstructive pelvic surgery. 2nd ed. St. Louis, MO: Mosby, 1999:221–234.

53. **Sederl J.** Zur operation des prolapses der blind endigenden sheiden. *Geburtshilfe Frauenheilkd* 1958;18:824–828.

54. **Richter K, Albright W.** Long term results following fixation of the vagina on the sacrospinous ligament by the vaginal route. *Am J Obstet Gynecol* 1981;141:811–816.

55. **Randall C, Nichols D.** Surgical treatment of vaginal inversion. *Obstet Gynecol* 1971;38:327–332.

56. **Nichols D.** Sacrospinous fixation for massive eversion of the vagina. *Am J Obstet Gynecol* 1982;142:901–904.

57. **Miyazaki FS.** Miya tool ligature carrier for sacrospinous ligament suspension. *Obstet Gynecol* 1987;70:286–288.

58. **Morley GW, DeLancey JO.** Sacrospinous ligament fixation for eversion of the vagina. *Am J Obstet Gyencol* 1988;158:872–881.

59. **Sharp TR.** Sacrospinous suspension made easy. *Obstet Gynecol* 1993;82:873–875.

60. **Imparato E, Aspesi G, Rovetta E, et al.** Surgical management and prevention of vaginal vault prolapse. *Surg Gynecol Obstet* 1992;175:233–237.

61. **Nichols D.** Massive eversion of the vagina. In: **Nichols DH, ed.** Gynecologic and obstetric surgery. St, Louis, MO: Mosby, 1993:431–464.

62. **Morgan DM, Rogers MA, Huebner M, et al.** Heterogeneity in anatomic outcome of sacrospinous ligament fixation for prolapse: a systematic review. *Obstet Gynecol* 2007;109:1424–1433.

63. **Holley RL, Varner RE, Gleason BP, et al.** Recurrent pelvic support defects after sacrospinous ligament fixation for vaginal vault prolapse. *J Am Coll Surg* 1995;180:444–448.

64. **Shull BL, Capen CV, Riggs MW, et al.** Preoperative and postoperative analysis of site-specific pelvic support defects in 81 women treated with sacrospinous ligament suspension and pelvic reconstruction. *Am J Obstet Gynecol* 1992;166:1764–1771.

65. **Inmon WB.** Pelvic relaxation and repair including prolapse of vagina following hysterectomy. *South Med J* 1963;56:577–582.

66. **Shull BT, Capen CV, Riggs MW, et al.** Bilateral attachment of the vaginal cuff to iliococcygeus fascia: an effective method of cuff suspension. *Am J Obstet Gynecol* 1993;168:1669–1677.

67. **Meeks GR, Washburne JF, McGeher RP, et al.** Repair of vaginal vault prolapse by suspension of the vagina to iliococcygeus (prespinous) fascia. *Am J Obstet Gynecol* 1994;171:1444–1454.

68. **McCall ML.** Posterior culdoplasty: surgical correction of enterocele during vaginal hysterectomy: a preliminary report. *Am J Obstet Gynecol* 1938;36:94–99.

69. **Shull BL, Bachofen C, Coates KW, et al.** A transvaginal approach to repair of apical and other associated sites of pelvic organ prolapse with uterosacral ligaments. *Am J Obstet Gynecol* 2000;183:1365–1373.

70. **Karram M, Goldwasser S, Kleeman S, et al.** High uterosacral vaginal vault suspension with fascial reconstruction for vaginal repair of enterocele and vaginal vault prolapse. *Obstet Gynecol* 2001;185:1339–1342.

71. **Barber MD, Visco AG, Weidner AC, et al.** Bilateral uterosacral ligament vaginal vault suspension with site specific endopelvic fascia defect repair for treatment of pelvic organ prolapse. *Am J Obstet Gynecol* 2000;183:1402–1411.

72. **Wheeler TL 2nd, Gerten KA, Richter HE, Duke AG, Varner RE.** Outcomes of vaginal vault prolapse repair with a high uterosacral suspension procedure utilizing bilateral single sutures. *Int Urogynecol J Pelvic Floor Dysfunct* 2007;18:1207–1213.

73. **Goff BF.** An evaluation of the Bissell operation for uterine prolapse: a follow-up study. *Surg Gynecol Obstet* 1933;57:763–771.

74. **Macer GA.** Transabdominal repair of cystocele, a 20 year experience, compared with the traditional vaginal approach. *Am J Obstet Gynecol* 1978;131:203–207.

75. **Stanton SL, Hilton P, Norton C, et al.** Clinical and urodynamic effects of anterior colporrhaphy and vaginal hysterectomy for prolapse with and without incontinence. *Br J Obstet Gynaecol* 1982;89:459–463.

76. **Porges RF, Smilen SW.** Long-term analysis of the surgical management of pelvic support defects. *Am J Obstet Gynecol* 1994;171:1518–1528.

77. **Kohli N, Sze EHM, Roat TW, et al.** Incidence of recurrent cystocele after anterior colporrhaphy with and without concomitant transvaginal needle suspension. *Am J Obstet Gynecol* 1996;175:1476–1482.

78. **Weber AM, Walters MD.** Anterior vaginal prolapse: review of anatomy and technique of surgical repair. *Obstet Gynecol* 1997;89:311–318.

79. **Smilen SW, Saini J, Wallach SJ, et al.** The risk of cystocele after sacrospinous ligament fixation. *Am J Obstet Gynecol* 1998;179:1465–1472.

80. **Weber AM, Walters MD, Piedmonte MR, et al.** Anterior colporrhaphy: a randomized trial of three surgical techniques. *Am J Obstet Gynecol* 2001;185:1299–1306.

81. **Sand PK, Koduri A, Lobel RW, et al.** Prospective randomized trial of polyglactin 910 mesh to prevent recurrence of cystoceles and rectoceles. *Am J Obstet Gynecol* 2001;184:1357–1364.

82. **White GR.** Cystocele: a radical cure by suturing lateral sulci of vagina to white line of pelvic fascia. *JAMA* 1909;21:1707–1710.

83. **Richardson AC, Edmonds PB, Williams NL.** Treatment of stress urinary incontinence due to paravaginal fascial defect. *Obstet Gynecol* 1981;57:357–362.

84. **Goetsch C.** Suprapubic vesicourethral suspension as a primary means of correcting stress incontinence and cystocele. *West J Surg* 1954;62:201–204.

85. **Shull BL, Baden WF.** A six-year experience with paravaginal defect repair for stress urinary incontinence. *Am J Obstet Gynecol* 1989;160:1432–1435.

86. **Shull BL, Benn SJ, Kuehl TJ.** Surgical management of prolapse of the anterior vaginal segment: an analysis of support defects, operative morbidity, and anatomic outcome. *Am J Obstet Gynecol* 1994;171:1429–1436.

87. **Bruce RG, El-Galley RES,** Galloway NTM. Paravaginal defect repair in the treatment of female stress urinary incontinence and cystocele. *Urology* 1999;54:647–651.

88. **Mallipeddi PK, Steele AC, Kohli N, et al.** Anatomic and functional outcome of vaginal paravaginal repair in the correction of anterior vaginal wall prolapse. *Int Urogynecol J* 2001;12:83–88.

89. **DeLancey JOL.** Fascial and muscular abnormalities in women with urethral hypermobility and anterior vaginal wall prolapse. *Am J Obstet Gynecol* 2002;18:93–98.

90. **Jeffcoate TN.** Posterior colpoperineorrhaphy. *Am J Obstet Gynecol* 1959;77:490–502.

91. **Varner RE, Holley RL, Richter HE, et al.** Infections related to placement of permanent braided and mono-filament suture material through vaginal mucosa. *J Pelvic Surg* 1998;4:71–74.

92. **Cundiff GW, Fenner D.** Evaluation and treatment of women with rectocele: focus on associated defecatory and sexual dysfunction. *Obstet Gynecol* 2004;104:1403–1421.

93. **Arnold MW, Stewart WR, Aguilar PS.** Rectocele repair: four years' experience. *Dis Colon Rectum* 1990;33:684–687.

94. **Mellgren A, Anzen B, Nilsson BY, et al.** Results of rectocele repair: a prospective study. *Dis Colon Rectum* 1995;38:7–13.

95. **Kahn MA, Stanton SL.** Posterior colporrhaphy: its effects on bowel and sexual function. *Br J Gynaecol Obstet* 1997;104:82–86.

96. **Weber AM, Walters MD, Piedmonte MR.** Sexual function and vaginal anatomy in women before and after surgery for pelvic organ prolapse and urinary incontinence. *Am J Obstet Gynecol* 2000;182:1610–1615.

97. **Abramov Y, Gandhi S, Goldberg RP, et al.** Site-specific rectocele repair compared with standard posterior colporrhaphy. *Obstet Gynecol* 2005;105:314–318.

98. **Francis WJA, Jeffcoate TNA.** Dyspareunia following vaginal operations. *J Opt Soc Am* 1961;68:1–10.

99. **Cundiff GW, Weidner AC, Visco AG, et al.** An anatomic and functional assessment of the discrete defect rectocele repair. *Am J Obstet Gynecol* 1998;179:1451–1457.

100. **Porter WE, Steele A, Walsh P, et al.** The anatomic and functional outcomes of defect-specific rectocele repairs. *Am J Obstet Gynecol* 1999;181:1353–1359.

101. **Kenton K, Shott S, Brubaker L.** Outcome after rectovaginal fascia reattachment for rectocele repair. *Am J Obstet Gynecol* 1999;181:1360–1364.

102. **Glavind K, Madsen H.** A prospective study of the discrete fascial defect rectocele repair. *Acta Obstet Gynecol Scand* 2000;79:145–147.

103. **Singh K, Cortes E, Reid WMN.** Evaluation of the fascial technique for surgical repair of isolated posterior vaginal wall prolapse. *Obstet Gynecol* 2003;101:320–324.

104. **Kahn MA, Kumar D, Stanton SL.** Posterior colporrhaphy vs. transanal repair of the rectocele: an initial follow up of a prospective randomized trial. *Br J Obstet Gynaecol* 1998;105:57.

105. **Nieminen K, Hiltunen KM, Laitinen J, et al.** Transanal or vaginal approach to rectocele repair: a prospective randomized pilot study. *Dis Colon Rectum* 2004;47:1636–1642.

106. **Janssen LWM, van Dijke CF.** Selection criteria for anterior rectal wall repair in symptomatic rectocele and anterior rectal wall prolapse. *Dis Colon Rectum* 1994;37:1100–1107.

107. **Van Dam JH, Huisman WM, Hop WCJ, et al.** Fecal continence after rectocele repair: a prospective study. *Int J Colorectal Dis* 2000;15:54–57.

108. **Ayabaca SM, Zbar AP, Pescatori M.** Anal continence after rectocele repair. *Dis Colon Rectum* 2002;45:63–69.

109. **Nieminen K, Hiltunen R, Takala T, et al.** Outcomes after anterior vaginal wall repair with mesh: a randomized, controlled trial with a 3 year follow-up. *Am J Obstet Gynecol* 2010;203:235.e1–e8.

110. **Takahashi S, Obinata D, Sakuma T, et al.** Tension-free vaginal mesh procedure for pelvic organ prolapse: a single-center experience of 310 cases with 1-year follow up. *Int J Urol* 2010;17:353–358.

111. **Hiltunen R, Nieminen K, Takala T, et al.** Low-weight polypropylene mesh for anterior vaginal wall prolapse: a randomized controlled trial. *Obstet Gynecol* 2007;110:455–462.

112. **Nguyen JN, Burchette RJ.** Outcome after anterior vaginal prolapse repair: a randomized controlled trial. *Obstet Gynecol* 2008;111:891–898.

113. **Carey M, Higgs P, Goh J, et al.** Vaginal repair with mesh versus colporrhaphy for prolapse: a randomized controlled trial. *BJOG* 2009;116:1380–1386.

114. **Sung VW, Rogers RG, Schaffer JI, et al.** Graft use in transvaginal pelvic organ prolapse repair: a systematic review. *Obstet Gynecol* 2008;112:1131–1142.

115. **Lowenstein L, Fitz A, Kenton K, et al.** Transabdominal uterosacral suspension: outcomes and complications. *Am J Obstet Gynecol* 2009;200:656.e1–e5.

116. **Cundiff GW, Harris RL, Coates K, et al.** Abdominal sacral colpoperineopexy: a new approach for correction of posterior compartment defects and perineal descent associates with vaginal vault prolapse. *Am J Obstet Gynecol* 1997;177:1345–1355.

117. **Visco AG, Weidner AC, Barber MD, et al.** Vaginal mesh erosion after abdominal sacral colpopexy. *Am J Obstet Gyencol* 2001;184:297–302.

118. **Sullivan ES, Longaker CJ, Lee PY.** Total pelvic mesh repair; a ten-year experience. *Dis Colon Rectum* 2001;44:857–863.

119. **Lyons TL, Winer WK.** Laparoscopic rectocele repair using polyglactin mesh. *J Am Assoc Gynecol Laparosc* 1997;4:381–384.

120. **Seracchioli R, Hourcubie JA, Vianello F, et al.** Laparoscopic treatment of pelvic floor defects in women of reproductive age. *J Am Assoc Gynecol Laparosc* 2004;11:332–335.

121. **Nygaard IE, McCreery R, Brubaker L, et al.** Abdominal sacrocolpopexy: a comprehensive review. *Obstet Gynecol* 2004;104:805–823.

122. **Arthure HG.** Vault suspension. *Proc R Soc Med* 1949;42:388–390.

123. **Lane FE.** Repair of posthysterectomy vaginal-vault prolapse. *Obstet Gynecol* 1962;20:72–77.

124. **Birnbaum SJ.** Rational therapy for the prolapse vagina. *Am J Obstet Gynecol* 1973;115:411–419.

125. **Addison WA, Livengood CH III, Sutton GP, et al.** Abdominal sacral colpopexy with Mersilene mesh in the retroperitoneal position in the management of posthysterectomy vaginal vault prolapse and enterocele. *Am J Obstet Gynecol* 1985;153:140–146.

126. **Snyder TE, Krantz KE.** Abdominal retroperitoneal sacral colpopexy for the correction of vaginal prolapse. *Obstet Gynecol* 1991;77:944–949.

127. **Addison WA, Timmons MC.** Abdominal approach to vaginal eversion. *Clin Obstet Gynecol* 1993;36:995–1004.

128. **Pilsgaard K, Mouritsen L.** Follow-up after repair of vaginal vault prolapse with abdominal colposacropexy. *Acta Obstet Gynecol Scand* 1999;78:66–70.

129. **Culligan PJ, Murphy M, Blackwell L, et al.** Long-term success of abdominal sacral colpopexy using synthetic mesh. *Am J Obstet Gynecol* 2002;187:1473–1480.

130. **Brizzolara S, Pillai-Allen A.** Risk of mesh erosion with sacral colpopexy and concurrent hysterectomy. *Obstet Gynecol* 2003;102:306–310.

131. **Timmons MC, Addison WA, Addison SB, et al.** Abdominal sacral colpopexy in 163 women with posthysterectomy vaginal vault prolapse and enterocele: evolution of operative techniques. *J Reprod Med* 1992;37:323–327.

132. **Harmanli OH, Dandolu V, Chatwani AJ, et al.** Total colpocleisis for severe pelvic organ prolapse. *J Reprod Med* 2003;48:703–706.

133. **Von Pechmann WS, Mutone MD, Fyffe J, et al.** Total colpocleisis with high levator plication for the treatment of advanced pelvic organ prolapse. *Am J Obstet Gynecol* 2003;189:121–126.

134. **Hoffman MS, et al.** Vaginectomy with pelvic herniorrhaphy for prolapse. *Am J Obstet Gynecol* 2003;189:364–371.

135. **Brubaker L, Nygaard I, Richter HE, et al.** Two-year outcomes after sacrocolpopexy with and without burch to prevent stress urinary incontinence. *Obstet Gynecol* 2008;112:49–55.

136. **Benson JT, Lucente V, McClellan E.** Vaginal versus abdominal reconstructive surgery for the treatment of pelvic support defects: a prospective randomized study with long-term outcome evaluation. *Am J Obstet Gynecol* 1996;175:1418–1422.

137. **Lo T-S, Wang AC.** Abdominal colposacropexy and sacrospinous ligament suspension for severe uterovaginal prolapse: a comparison. *J Gynecol Surg* 1998;14:59–64.

138. **Maher CF, Qatawneh AM, Dwyer PL, et al.** Abdominal sacrocolpopexy or vaginal sacrospinous colpopexy for vaginal vault prolapse: a prospective randomized study. *Am J Obstet Gynecol* 2004;190:20–26.

28 Anorectal Dysfunction

Robert E. Gutman
Geoffrey W. Cundiff

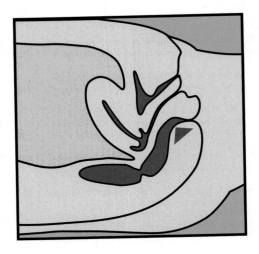

- Defecatory dysfunction and fecal incontinence are common conditions for women that have tremendous psychosocial and economic implications.

- The differential diagnosis for anorectal dysfunction is broad and can be classified into systemic factors, anatomic and structural abnormalities, and functional disorders.

- A thorough history and physical examination are critical for the evaluation of fecal incontinence and defecatory dysfunction, as well as appropriate ancillary testing.

- Treatment of anorectal dysfunction should focus on treatment of the underlying condition, with nonsurgical management attempted before surgery.

- Overlapping sphincteroplasty is the procedure of choice for fecal incontinence caused by a disrupted anal sphincter.

Anorectal dysfunction encompasses a variety of conditions that disrupt normal anorectal function. Such conditions can be subdivided as those that cause defecatory dysfunction and fecal incontinence. Although anorectal dysfunction transcends any individual medical specialty, the pathophysiology, evaluation, and management of conditions relevant to obstetricians/gynecologists are presented in this chapter.

Normal Colorectal Function

Anal continence and defecation are complex physiologic processes that require intact and coordinated neurologic and anatomic function, including colonic absorption and motility, rectal compliance, anorectal sensation, and the multifaceted continence mechanism. An understanding of normal physiology and pathophysiology is essential to the treatment of women with anorectal dysfunction.

Stool Formation and Colonic Transit

The colon plays an important role in absorption and regulation of water and electrolytes. **As much as 5 L of water and associated electrolytes can be absorbed in one day.** Parasympathetic-mediated peristaltic contraction of colonic smooth muscle transfers fecal material to the rectum. A delay in stool transit at the rectosigmoid region of the colon allows for maximal absorption of water and sodium.

Storage

As stool accumulates in the rectosigmoid, rectal distention triggers a transient decrease in the internal anal sphincter (IAS) tone and an increase in the external anal sphincter (EAS) tone, known as the *rectoanal inhibitory reflex.* **Exposure of the anal canal to fecal matter facilitates** *sampling,* **whereby the anal canal and its abundant sensory nerves determine stool consistency (i.e., solid, liquid, or gas).** *Accommodation* **occurs as the normally compliant rectal vault relaxes in response to increased volume. This cycle, combined with increased rectal distention, stimulates an urge to defecate.** This urge can be voluntarily suppressed through cortical control, resulting in further accommodation and activation of the continence mechanism.

Continence Mechanism

Muscles

The key muscles of the continence mechanism are the puborectalis, IAS, and EAS. The puborectalis muscle originates from the pubic rami at the level of the arcus tendineus levator ani and passes laterally to the vagina and rectum in a U-shaped configuration, creating a sling around the genital hiatus. Contraction of the puborectalis muscle narrows the genital hiatus, developing the near 90-degree anorectal angle. The resting tone of the puborectalis muscle serves as the primary continence mechanism for solid stool. The IAS and EAS are essential for continence of flatus and liquid stool. The internal sphincter maintains most of the resting tone for the sphincter complex through autonomic reflex arcs and is essential for passive continence. Although the external sphincter also maintains constant resting tone, it is ultimately responsible for preventing fecal urgency and stress incontinence associated with sudden increases in intra-abdominal pressure. This function is under both voluntary and involuntary control. The anal cushions act as the final anatomic barrier. They fill with blood, causing occlusion of the anal canal.

Nerves

Many pathologic states disrupt normal function through denervation. **The IAS receives its sympathetic supply from L5, which passes through the pelvic plexus via the hypogastric plexus.** The parasympathetic supply from S2-4 synapses at the pelvic plexus, where it joins the sympathetic nerves. In addition to the parasympathetic and sympathetic components, the autonomic nervous system of the gut has an enteric nervous system (ENS). The ENS provides local circuitry that can contract or relax the gut muscles, as well as impact absorption and secretion. The autonomic ganglia of the ENS, located in the gut, are interconnected to provide local integration and processing of information. The IAS acts through reflex arcs at the spinal cord without voluntary control. The puborectalis (levator ani) is innervated by branches of the S2-4 sacral roots and does not receive direct innervation from the pudendal nerve (1). The EAS is innervated bilaterally by the pudendal nerve (S2-4) via Alcock's canal. The pudendal nerve fibers cross over at the level of the spinal cord, allowing preservation of EAS function in the event of unilateral damage. The rich sensory supply from the anal canal travels along the inferior rectal branch of the pudendal nerve.

Evacuation

Initiation of defecation is normally under cortical control. As previously discussed, delivery of stool to the rectum stimulates the rectoanal inhibitory reflex, permitting sampling followed by accommodation. Further rectal distention results in an urge to defecate. Evacuation occurs with voluntary relaxation of the pelvic floor muscles (puborectalis muscle and EAS) in conjunction with increased intra-abdominal and intrarectal pressure from Valsalva. This results in widening of the anorectal angle and shortening of the anal canal, which facilitates emptying. Coordinated peristaltic activity of the rectosigmoid assists evacuation. After this process is complete, the closing reflex is initiated, resulting in contraction of the pelvic floor muscles and activation of the continence mechanism.

Epidemiology

The epidemiology of anorectal dysfunction has been best defined in terms of the incidence and prevalence of fecal incontinence. Few studies have been done to assess the incidence and prevalence of defecatory dysfunction.

Defecatory Dysfunction

The term *defecatory dysfunction* often is used synonymously with the symptom of constipation. **Constipation is an imprecise term used by patients to report a variety of symptoms, including infrequent stools, dyschezia, straining, variation in stool consistency and caliber, incomplete emptying, bloating, and abdominal pain. The most common symptoms associated with constipation are straining and hard stools** (2,3). **Defecatory dysfunction is defined by many physicians as infrequent stools, typically fewer than three bowel movements per week.** This definition is based on stool frequency studies in which 95% of women have more than three bowel movements per week. Using this definition, the prevalence of constipation should be 5% (4). However, the prevalence of constipation has been estimated to range from 2% to 28%, depending on the definition applied (5–7).

There is an increased prevalence of constipation among women and elderly individuals, nonwhite individuals, and those with low income and low education levels (5–7). Based on an estimated 2.5 million visits to US physicians per year for constipation, with an average cost of $2,752 per patient, the annual cost for evaluation of constipation would be approximately $6.9 billion (8,9). An estimated 85% of physician visits results in a prescription; including drug costs would increase this amount substantially (8). More recently, evaluation of 76,854 California Medicaid patients without supplemental insurance found somewhat lower annual total direct costs to care for constipation at almost $19 million ($246 per patient) for this subset of the US population (10). Constipation has a detrimental effect on health-related quality of life (3,10). Constipation contributed to decreased mental and physical scores for quality of life on the SF-36 Health Survey in a Canadian-based population (11).

Fecal Incontinence

The reported prevalence of fecal incontinence varies between 2% and 3% for community-dwelling individuals, 3% to 17% for those of increased age, and 46% to 54% for nursing home residents (12). A prevalence of 28% has been reported among patients seeking benign gynecologic care and 36% of primary care patients surveyed (13,14). The prevalence of fecal incontinence in the United States is expected to increase 59% from 10.6 million in 2010 to 16.8 million in 2050 as the population ages (15). Epidemiologic studies of fecal incontinence are compromised by social stigmata and the lack of a uniform definition. Definitions of fecal incontinence vary with respect to the type of material passed (solid, liquid, or gas), the frequency and duration of events (once in a lifetime to twice a week), and the impact on quality of life. Most authors agree that the true prevalence of this condition is underestimated in the current scientific literature. A large health survey in the United States found age, female gender, physical limitations, and poor general health to be independent risk factors associated with fecal incontinence (16).

Fecal incontinence has tremendous psychosocial and economic implications for individuals and society as a whole. The loss of such a basic function can be emotionally devastating, leading to poor self-esteem, depression, social isolation, and decreased quality of life (13,14,17). **Fecal incontinence is the second leading reason for nursing home placement in the United States, even though less than one-third of individuals with this condition seek medical attention** (13,17). The overall annual cost to treat fecal incontinence is difficult to pinpoint, but accounts for more than $400 million per year in the cost of adult incontinence products alone (17).

Symptom-Based Approach to Colorectal Disorders

Several medical conditions cause defecatory dysfunction, fecal incontinence, or combined symptoms. Following is the differential diagnosis—a proposed classification system based on systemic factors, anatomic and structural abnormalities, and functional disorders.

Differential Diagnosis

Disordered Defecation

Causes of defecatory dysfunction have traditionally been divided into systemic disorders and idiopathic constipation (all nonsystemic causes). Idiopathic constipation can be subdivided into anatomic and structural abnormalities and functional disorders (Table 28.1).

Diabetes, hypothyroidism, and pregnancy are the most common endocrinologic systemic factors that cause constipation, and all have a component of decreased gastrointestinal motility and intestinal transit. In one study, gastrointestinal symptoms were present in 76% of patients with diabetes, including constipation, which occurred in 60% (18). In patients with diabetes, constipation is believed to be secondary to intestinal autonomic neuropathy, resulting in delayed or absent gastrocolic reflex and decreased bowel motility. This enteric neuropathy may also cause gastroparesis and diarrhea. Although diabetes has been classified with the endocrinologic causes, it should also be grouped with the enteric neuropathies. Pregnancy is not considered a disease state; however, there is an 11% to 38% prevalence of constipation that is believed to result from the effect of progesterone on smooth muscle (19,20). Iron supplements and prior constipation treatment are also associated with constipation during pregnancy (20).

The neurologic systemic factors can be divided into central and peripheral processes. Spinal cord lesions, multiple sclerosis, and Parkinson disease affect the autonomic nervous system. Trauma to the sacral nerves often leads to severe constipation from decreased left-sided colonic motility, decreased rectal tone and sensation, and increased distention. These findings are also seen in patients with meningomyelocele, damage to the lumbosacral spine, and pelvic floor trauma (21,22). Higher spinal cord lesions result in delayed sigmoid transit and decreased rectal compliance. In these upper motor neuron lesions, colonic reflexes are intact, and defecation can be initiated by digital stimulation of the anal canal (23,24). Individuals with multiple sclerosis can have no gastrocolic reflex, decreased colonic motility, decreased rectal compliance, and even rectosphincteric dyssynergia (25,26). Constipation worsens with the duration of illness and may be compounded by the side effects of medical therapy. Similar findings of rectosphincteric dyssynergia and medication side effects are present with Parkinson disease.

Among the peripheral neurogenic disorders, dysfunction occurs at the level of the ENS. The ultimate example of this is congenital aganglionosis (Hirschsprung disease). The absence of intramural ganglion cells in the submucosal and myenteric plexuses of the rectum causes loss of the rectosphincteric inhibitory reflex. Patients with this illness usually present with functional obstruction and proximal colonic dilation. In most patients, the condition is diagnosed within 6 months of age, although milder cases can be seen later in life.

Other systemic factors to consider are collagen vascular and muscle disorders. Importantly, some of the most commonly used prescription and over-the-counter medications, including aluminum antacids, beta-blockers, calcium channel blockers, anticholinergics, antidepressants, and opiates, cause defecatory dysfunction (Table 28.2). Lifestyle issues, such as inadequate fiber intake and insufficient fluid intake, can exert similar effects independently or in conjunction with other disorders.

Structural abnormalities refer to the obstructive disorders, such as pelvic organ prolapse, perineal descent, intussusception, rectal prolapse, and tumors. Functional disorders are those that do not have an identifiable anatomic or systemic etiology. Most functional disorders are motility disorders, such as slow-transit constipation or colonic inertia, irritable bowel syndrome (constipation predominant), and functional constipation. The Rome III criteria created strict definitions for these idiopathic conditions that are believed to result from the complex interaction of psychosocial factors and altered gut physiology via the gut-brain-gut axis (27). Patients also may have functional limitations, such as decreased mobility and

Table 28.1 Causes of Defecatory Dysfunction and Fecal Incontinence

Fecal Incontinence		Defecatory Dysfunction
	Systemic Factors	
	Metabolic/Endocrine	
•	Diabetes mellitus	•
•	Thyroid disease	•
	Hypercalcemia	•
	Hypokalemia	•
	Neurological	
•	Central Nervous System	•
	Multiple sclerosis, Parkinson disease, stroke, tumor, dementia	
•	Peripheral Nervous System	•
	Hirschsprung disease, spina bifida, autonomic neuropathy, pudendal neuropathy	
	Infectious	
•	Bacterial, viral, parasitic diarrhea	
	Collagen Vascular/Muscle Disorder	
	Systemic sclerosis, amyloidosis, myotonic dystrophy, dermatomyositis	•
	Idiopathic/Autoimmune	
•	Inflammatory bowel disease	
•	Food allergy	
	Medications	
•	Prescription, over the counter	•
	Anatomical/Structural Abnormalities	
	Pelvic Outlet Obstruction	
•	Pelvic organ prolapse	•
•	Descending perineum syndrome	•
•	Anismus/rectosphincteric dyssynergia	•
•	Intussusception, rectal prolapse	•
•	Volvulus	•
•	Neoplasia	•
•	Benign strictures	•
•	Hemorrhoids	•
	Anal Sphincter Disruption/Fistula	
•	Obstetrical trauma	
•	Surgical trauma	
•	Anal intercourse	
•	Injury (trauma, radiation proctitis)	
	Functional	
	Motility Disorders	
	Global motility disorder	•
	Colonic inertia/slow-transit constipation	•
•	Irritable bowel syndrome	•
	Functional constipation	•
•	Functional diarrhea	
	Functional Limitations	
•	Decreased mobility	•
•	Decreased cognition	•

Table 28.2 Drugs Associated with Constipation	
Over-the-Counter Medications	
Antidiarrheals (*loperamide, Kaopectate*)	
Antacids (with aluminum or calcium)	
Iron supplements	
Prescription Medications	
Anticholinergics	*Others*
Antidepressants	Iron
Antipsychotics	Barium sulfate
Antispasmodics	Metallic intoxication (arsenic, lead, mercury)
Antiparkinsonian drugs	Opiates
Antihypertensives	Nonsteroidal anti-inflammatory agents
Calcium channel blockers	Anticonvulsants
Beta-blockers	Vinca alkaloids
Diuretics	5HT3 antagonists (*ondansetron, granisetron*)
Ganglionic blockers	

cognition. It is important to understand that this classification system is somewhat arbitrary, and several of these conditions are interrelated.

Fecal Incontinence

Anal continence depends on a complex interaction of cognitive, anatomic, neurologic, and physiologic mechanisms. The continence mechanism can often compensate for a deficiency in one of these processes, but it can be overwhelmed with increased severity or decreased function over time. Systemic etiologies of fecal incontinence often are due to disease states that cause diarrhea. The rapid transport of large volumes of liquid stool to the rectum can produce urgency and incontinence even in healthy individuals (28). Fecal incontinence frequently results from infectious diarrhea caused by bacteria (e.g., *Clostridium, Escherichia coli, Salmonella, Shigella, Yersinia, Campylobacter*), viruses (e.g., Rotavirus, Norwalk, HIV), and parasites (e.g., *Entamoeba, Giardia, Cryptosporidium, Ascaris*). Numerous medications and dietary items cause diarrhea and fecal incontinence (Table 28.3). Endocrine factors that can lead to fecal incontinence include diabetes mellitus and hyperthyroidism. With diabetes, diarrhea can develop from autonomic dysfunction, bacterial overgrowth, osmotic diarrhea with sugar substitutes, and pancreatic insufficiency. Inflammatory bowel disease is considered an idiopathic or autoimmune systemic factor. Ulcerative colitis and Crohn disease cause fecal incontinence during exacerbations with bouts of bloody diarrhea. Inflammatory bowel disease can also result in structural abnormalities, such as anal fissures, fistulas, abscesses, and operative complications that lead to fecal incontinence.

As with defecatory dysfunction, neurologic causes of fecal incontinence can be divided into central and peripheral disorders. Among the central nervous system disorders, upper motor neuron lesions above the level of the defecation center (located in the sacral cord) cause spastic bowel dysfunction. Cortical communication is disrupted, resulting in impaired cognitive control and sensory deficit. The anal sphincter is under spastic contraction, but digital stimulation can be performed to initiate reflex evacuation. **Head trauma, neoplasms, and cerebral vascular accidents that damage portions of the frontal lobe result in loss of control of both micturition and defecation.** Greater loss of inhibition is present when the lesion is located more anteriorly in the frontal lobe. Spinal cord trauma and lower motor neuron lesions above the defecation center tend to cause permanent loss of cortical control. For 2 to 4 weeks following spinal cord injury, "spinal shock" occurs, resulting in a temporary loss of reflexes below the level of the lesion, flaccid bowel function, constipation, and fecal impaction. After the

Table 28.3 Drugs and Dietary Items Associated with Diarrhea	
Over-the-Counter Medications	
Laxatives	
Antacids (with magnesium)	
Prescription Medications	
Laxatives	Chemotherapy
Diuretics	*Colchicine*
Thyroid preparations	*Cholestyramine*
Cholinergics	*Neomycin*
Prostaglandins	*Para-aminosalicylic acid*
Dietary Items	
Dietetic foods, candy or chewing gum, and elixirs with *sorbitol, mannitol,* or *xylitol*	
Olestra	
Caffeine	
Ethanol	
Monosodium glutamate	

initial shock, spastic paralysis ensues with hyperactive bowel function. The gastrocolic reflex, along with digital stimulation, initiates reflex evacuation in the absence of cortical inhibition. Fortunately, IAS tone is maintained despite the loss of EAS control for stress and urge situations. Both constipation and fecal incontinence can occur in these patients.

The demyelination that is seen in multiple sclerosis is randomly distributed and can occur at any level in the central nervous system. In addition to the somatic disruption that is similar to spinal cord injury, autonomic dysfunction frequently is present. **People with dementia and other degenerative disorders that cause cognitive impairment frequently have fecal incontinence caused by overflow incontinence.** Although sensory nerves are functioning properly, these individuals lack the cognitive awareness necessary to inhibit defecation until a socially acceptable time, and they develop overflow incontinence.

Lower motor neuron lesions occurring at or below the level of the defecation center in the sacral cord cause flaccid bowel dysfunction. Cortical communication is disrupted, resulting in impaired cognitive control and sensory deficit. The bowel reflexes, including the bulbocavernosus and anal reflexes, are interrupted. The anal sphincter is flaccid, and fecal retention with overflow incontinence usually occurs. Digital disimpaction and Valsalva often are required for evacuation. Digital stimulation has no effect, and medications tend to work poorly. Examples of motor neuron lesions include tumor or trauma to the cauda equina, tabes dorsalis, spina bifida, and peripheral neuropathy.

The classic example of peripheral neuropathy is congenital aganglionosis (Hirschsprung disease), which was discussed earlier. The most common peripheral neuropathy occurs with diabetes. **Approximately 20% of individuals with diabetes have fecal incontinence** (29). The cause tends to be multifactorial with the exact mechanism uncertain. Fecal incontinence can occur with diabetic diarrhea or years later from progressive disease. Individuals with diabetes frequently experience intestinal autonomic neuropathy, an abnormal gastrocolic reflex, and chronic constipation. The subsequent pelvic floor denervation causes fecal incontinence by sensory neuropathy, failure of the rectoanal inhibitory reflex, and sphincter dysfunction (30). Consequently, fecal incontinence from peripheral neuropathy can be the result of defective sampling, a disrupted rectoanal inhibitory reflex, or pudendal neuropathy with sphincter dysfunction. Patients may experience stress or urge incontinence as well as overflow incontinence.

Anatomic and structural causes of fecal incontinence are usually due to obstetric or surgical trauma. Damage or dysfunction of the IAS, EAS, and puborectalis can result in varying degrees of fecal incontinence. Those with impaired resting tone from a defective IAS will have passive incontinence (incontinence at rest), which is worse during sleep because of decreased EAS activity (31). An inability to respond to sudden distention and to suppress defecation is often seen with external sphincter dysfunction. External and internal sphincter dysfunction often causes incontinence of liquid stool. Incontinence of solid stool is usually seen with widening of the anorectal angle from damage to the puborectalis muscles. Damage to the anal cushions usually causes minor soiling. Other anatomic and structural abnormalities associated with fecal incontinence include obstructive disorders such as pelvic organ prolapse, descending perineum syndrome, anismus, and intussusception; fistulas from diverticulitis, inflammatory bowel disease, cancer, or surgical trauma; and decreased rectal compliance from inflammatory bowel disease, cancer, and radiation. Decreased compliance results in higher intraluminal pressures with smaller volumes of stool, poor storage capacity, urgency, and incontinence (32).

Functional disorders associated with fecal incontinence include irritable bowel syndrome (diarrhea variant), functional diarrhea, decreased mobility, and decreased cognition.

Combined Disorders of Defecation and Fecal Incontinence	Several conditions have the potential to cause both defecatory dysfunction and fecal incontinence (Table 28.1). Most of these disorders cause combined symptoms through the development of fecal impaction followed by overflow incontinence. This situation can be seen with many of the neurologic conditions, pelvic outlet obstructive disorders, functional disorders of irritable bowel syndrome, decreased mobility, and decreased cognition. The cause of these symptoms is often multifactorial.

Structural versus Functional Disorders

Disordered Defecation	Disordered defecation can result from outlet obstruction or functional motility disorders.

Outlet Obstruction

Anismus/Rectosphincteric Dyssynergia   Anismus is otherwise known as rectosphincteric dyssynergia, pelvic floor dyssynergia, spastic floor syndrome, and paradoxical puborectalis syndrome. The anorectal angle narrows as a result of paradoxical contraction of the puborectalis and external anal sphincter during defecation. Frequent symptoms include dyschezia, straining, hard stools, incomplete emptying, and tenesmus. A recent prospective study of 120 patients with dyssynergic defecation found a higher prevalence in women (77%) (33,34). The need for digital assistance (digital disimpaction or splinting) to evacuate the rectum occurs in up to 58% of patients. **Psychosocial factors, such as a history of sexual abuse, depression, eating disorder, obsessive-compulsive disorder, and stress, may play an important role in this disease.** In this study, 22% reported a history of sexual abuse, and 31% reported a history of physical abuse. One-third believed the problem began during childhood, and 24% reported a precipitating illness or surgery was related to a particular event. Five percent of women claimed that pregnancy or childbirth was a precipitating factor. This condition also is seen in young children with constipation and dyschezia. The response to biofeedback and pelvic floor physical therapy, as well as the aforementioned patient characteristics, indicate a learned response mechanism is involved (33,34). Although this is often categorized as an outlet obstruction, the Rome III criteria for functional gastrointestinal disorders places this in the category of functional defecation disorders. The specific Rome III diagnostic criteria for dyssynergic defecation includes "inappropriate contraction of the pelvic floor or less than 20% relaxation of basal resting sphincter pressure with adequate propulsive forces during attempted defecation" (35).

Pelvic Organ Prolapse   **Pelvic organ prolapse bears special mention because it is often seen by gynecologists but inconsistently associated with defecatory dysfunction. Prolapse is very common, although many women with this condition are asymptomatic.** Those with symptoms may report incomplete evacuation and the need to apply digital pressure to the posterior vaginal wall or perineum to aid in evacuation of stool (digitation or splinting). It is important to rule out other causes of constipation, because these symptoms are nonspecific, and rectocele can result from chronic straining and increased intra-abdominal pressure due to other etiologies of defecatory dysfunction. **Defecatory dysfunction related to pelvic organ prolapse can result from rectocele, enterocele, or perineal descent, either individually or in combination.**

Rectocele **is a herniation of the rectal mucosa through a defect in the rectovaginal septum.** These site-specific defects can be transverse or longitudinal through the inferior, middle, or superior regions of the rectovaginal septum (36). *Enterocele* **is a herniation of a peritoneal sac and bowel through the pelvic floor, typically between the uterus or vaginal cuff and rectum. It is more common following hysterectomy and retropubic urethropexy.** There are two theories surrounding the formation of an enterocele. The first theory implicates a defect in the fibromuscular endopelvic fascia of the vagina, allowing peritoneum and bowel to herniate. The second theory attributes its formation to a support defect with full thickness protrusion, including endopelvic fascia (37). Ultimately, the mechanism might be attributed to a combination of the two theories because some support defects are secondary to superior breaks in the rectovaginal and pubocervical fascia. **Patients with rectocele and enterocele may have similar symptoms, including pelvic pressure, vaginal protrusion, obstipation, fecal incontinence, and sexual dysfunction.** Although associations have been made between defecatory dysfunction and advanced stages of pelvic organ prolapse, a causal relationship remains to be established. Controversy remains as to whether anatomic herniation is the cause of these symptoms or the effect of underlying colonic dysfunction, chronic constipation, and straining.

Descending perineum syndrome **is defined as descent of the perineum (at the level of the anal verge) beyond the ischial tuberosities during Valsalva.** Excessive perineal descent was first described in the colorectal literature by Parks et al. in 1966 (38,39). It occurs as a result of inferior detachment of the rectovaginal septum from the perineal body. As the condition progresses, the patient can develop pudendal neuropathy from stretch injury. Perineal descent has been associated with a variety of defecatory disorders, including constipation, fecal incontinence, rectal pain, solitary rectal ulcer syndrome, rectocele, and enterocele (40).

Rectal Intussusception   **Rectal intussusception or intrarectal prolapse is the circumferential prolapse of the upper rectal wall into the rectal ampulla but not through the anal verge.** It occurs most often in women in their fourth and fifth decades. The most common symptoms are obstructive, including incomplete emptying, manual disimpaction, splinting, pain with defecation, and bleeding. Other symptoms include fecal incontinence, decreased urge to defecate, inability to distinguish between gas and feces, and mucus discharge with pruritus ani. Bleeding often originates from a solitary rectal ulcer or localized proctitis of the involved bowel segment (41). **Intussusception is seen in as many as one-third of women with defecatory dysfunction and other symptoms, such as constipation, rectal pain, and fecal incontinence** (42). It has also been seen in 29% of asymptomatic patients (43). The intussusception rarely develops into total rectal prolapse (44).

Functional Motility Disorders

Functional Bowel Disorders   **Functional bowel disorders, as defined by the Rome III criteria, consist of irritable bowel syndrome, functional bloating, functional constipation, functional diarrhea, and unspecified functional bowel disorders.** In this section we will focus primarily on irritable bowel syndrome (45).

Irritable bowel syndrome (IBS) has been estimated to have a prevalence of 10% to 20% and is more common in women and younger individuals. It accounts for 25% to 50% of all referrals to gastrointestinal clinics. Irritable bowel syndrome has distinct diagnostic criteria, including the exclusion of structural or metabolic abnormalities. **These patients often have other gastrointestinal, genitourinary, and psychological illness, including gastroesophageal reflux disease, fibromyalgia, headache, backache, chronic pelvic pain, sexual dysfunction, lower urinary tract dysfunction, depression, and anxiety.** Stressful life events seem to correlate with the onset and exacerbation of symptoms. A detailed history frequently reveals past physical or sexual abuse (46). Currently, specific criteria allow for classification of IBS into diarrhea-, constipation-, and pain-predominant categories (Table 28.4). The constipation variant is most commonly associated with defecatory dysfunction, whereas the diarrhea variant causes fecal incontinence. The pain or spastic variant causes predominantly abdominal discomfort but can also be associated with both defecatory dysfunction and fecal incontinence. After excluding

Table 28.4 Irritable Bowel Syndrome

Diagnostic Criterion[a]

Recurrent abdominal pain or discomfort[b] at least 3 days per month in the last 3 months associated with two or more of the following:

1. Improved with defecation

2. Onset associated with a change in frequency of stool

3. Onset associated with a change in form (appearance) of stool

[a]Criterion fulfilled for the last 3 months with symptom onset at least 6 months prior to diagnosis.
[b]"Discomfort" means an uncomfortable sensation not described as pain.
In pathophysiology research and clinical trials, a pain/discomfort frequency of at least 2 days a week during the screening evaluation is recommended for subject eligibility.
From **Drossman DA, Corazziari E, Talley NJ, et al., eds.** *Rome III: the functional gastrointestinal disorders.* 3nd ed. McLean, VA: Degnon Associates, 2006:885–897, Appendix A, with permission.

organic disease, the criteria listed in Table 28.4 have a sensitivity of 65%, specificity of 100%, positive predictive value of 100%, and negative predictive value of 76% (47).

***Functional constipation* is a term created by the Rome II criteria as a unifying definition of constipation** (Table 28.5). The rationale for the criteria listed in Table 28.5 stems from the variability in patient definitions of constipation (46).

Functional Defecation Disorders **Functional defecation disorders are divided into *dyssynergic defecation* and *inadequate defecatory propulsion* (colonic inertia). (For the purposes of this chapter, dyssynergic defecation has been included in the structural category of outlet obstruction; however, it is important to recognize that Rome III considers it a functional disorder.) Both of the functional defecation disorders require the presence of functional constipation.** Table 28.6 lists the criteria for diagnosing these conditions.

Colonic Inertia/Slow-Transit Constipation **Severe constipation, defined as fewer than three stools per week and refractory to therapy, is relatively rare; however, these patients frequently suffer from motility disorders such as *global motility disorder* and *colonic inertia*. Women are more likely to be affected than men.** Colonic inertia or slow-transit constipation

Table 28.5 Functional Constipation

Diagnostic Criteria[a]*

1. Must include two or more of the following:

    a. Straining during at least 25% of defecations

    b. Lumpy or hard stools in at least 25% of defecations

    c. Sensation of incomplete evacuation for at least 25% of defecations

    d. Sensation of anorectal obstruction/blockage for at least 25% of defecations

    e. Manual maneuvers to facilitate at least 25% of defecations (e.g., digital evacuation, support of the pelvic floor)

    f. Fewer than three defecations per week

2. Loose stools are rarely present without the use of laxatives, and there are insufficient criteria for IBS.

3. Insufficient criteria for irritable bowel syndrome

[a]Criteria fulfilled for the last 3 months with symptom onset at least 6 months prior to diagnosis.
From **Drossman DA, Corazziari E, Talley NJ, et al., eds.** *Rome III: the functional gastrointestinal disorders.* 3nd ed. McLean, VA: Degnon Associates, 2006:885–897, Appendix A, with permission.

Table 28.6 Functional Defecation Disorders

Diagnostic Criteria [a]

1. The patient must satisfy diagnostic criteria for functional constipation (Table 28.5)

2. During repeated attempts to defecate must have at least two of the following:

   a. Evidence of impaired evacuation, based on balloon expulsion test or imaging

   b. Inappropriate contraction of the pelvic floor muscles (i.e., anal sphincter or puborectalis) or less than 20% relaxation of basal resting sphincter pressure by manometry, imaging, or EMG

   c. Inadequate propulsive forces assessed by manometry or imaging

[a]Criteria fulfilled for the last 3 months with symptom onset at least 6 months prior to diagnosis.
From **Drossman DA, Corazziari E, Talley NJ, et al., eds.** *Rome III: the functional gastrointestinal disorders.* 3nd ed. McLean, VA: Degnon Associates, 2006:885–897, Appendix A, with permission.

is defined as the delayed passage of radiopaque markers through the proximal colon without retropulsion of markers from the left colon and in the absence of systemic or obstructive disorders. The cause remains unclear. Patients with this disorder have impaired phasic colonic motor activity and diminished gastrocolic reflexes (48,49). Studies on the role of laxatives, absorption, hormones, psychological abnormalities, and endogenous opioids have been inconclusive. Current literature suggests a possible neurologic or smooth muscle disorder (49,50).

Fecal Incontinence

Sphincter Disruption

In young women, obstetric injury is the most common cause of fecal incontinence. The mechanism of injury can be from anatomic disruption of the anal sphincter complex, pelvic floor denervation, or a combination of the two conditions. The risk factors for anal sphincter laceration are primiparity, high birth weight, forceps delivery, and episiotomy (51–53). Recent work suggests that women with anal sphincter injuries have slower labor, without the normal deceleration phase, and with late descent of the fetal head (54). Although there are limited long-term prospective studies demonstrating the natural history of anal sphincter injury, pelvic floor neuropathy, and the progression of these conditions to fecal incontinence, current literature supports the relationship of early-onset symptoms to sphincter damage and delayed-onset symptoms to neuropathy (55). This relationship would account for the large discrepancy in the prevalence of fecal incontinence between younger men and women that decreases as the population ages (56).

Obstetric Trauma   **Third- and fourth-degree lacerations at delivery are associated with an increased risk of fecal incontinence (odds ratio [OR] 3.09)** (55). Whereas the incidence of clinically documented third- and fourth-degree anal sphincter tears is between 0.5% and 5.9% (51,53,57), occult third- and fourth-degree defects are present in 28% to 35% of primiparous women and 44% of multiparous women, and approximately one-third of these patients have symptoms of anal incontinence. **Patients with occult anal sphincter tears are 8.8 times more likely to have fecal incontinence** (53,58). Forceps-assisted vaginal delivery significantly increases this risk, but the data on vacuum-assisted delivery are less conclusive (52,59,60). Elective cesarean delivery, in contrast with emergency cesarean delivery, was believed to prevent anal incontinence, but recent studies argue against any protective effect with cesarean delivery, irrespective of timing (46,51,53,59,61,62). A recent Cochrane review concludes that there is insufficient evidence to support primary elective cesarean delivery for the purpose of preserving fecal continence (63). **Midline episiotomy is strongly linked to sphincter damage and fecal incontinence** (52,64). One study of a large population found conflicting results, with an overall protective effect seen with episiotomy (OR 0.89). The likelihood of fourth-degree laceration was increased (OR 1.12) and of third-degree laceration was decreased (OR 0.81) (51). A Cochrane review supports the restrictive use of both midline and mediolateral episiotomy due to less posterior perineal trauma, less suturing, and fewer healing complications. There were no differences in severe trauma, pain, dyspareunia, or urinary incontinence, but there was an increase in anterior perineal trauma with restrictive use (65). An important finding in another study was that one-half of patients who underwent immediate repair of a third-degree laceration had symptoms of anal incontinence, and 85% had persistent sphincter defects on endoanal ultrasonography (66).

Surgical Trauma   **Iatrogenic injury follows obstetric trauma as the second most common cause of direct sphincter damage.** Surgical procedures that have been associated with fecal incontinence include anal fistula repair, anal sphincterotomy, hemorrhoidectomy, and anal dilation. Fistulotomy is the most common procedure that results in fecal incontinence. Rectovaginal or anovaginal fistulas can develop after obstetric injury, operative complications during pelvic surgery, and inflammatory bowel disease exacerbations. Fistulas cause fecal incontinence, and the degree of postoperative dysfunction depends on the location of the fistula and the amount of sphincter that is disrupted during the surgical repair. It also depends on the preoperative level of sphincter function and pudendal nerve function. Anal sphincterotomy to treat painful anal fissures can lead to incontinence by disruption of rectal sensory innervation and anal cushions and transection of the anal sphincter (67,68). Hemorrhoidectomy often results in minor soiling as a result of resection of the anal cushions, which act as the final mucosal barrier. Similar to sphincterotomy, rectal sensory innervation can be disrupted, and injury to the internal sphincter can occur during sharp dissection (68,69).

Sphincter Denervation

Idiopathic (primary neurogenic) fecal incontinence results from denervation of both the anal sphincter and pelvic floor muscles. Denervation injury related to obstetric trauma accounts for approximately three of four cases of idiopathic fecal incontinence and is the most common overall cause of fecal incontinence (70,71).

Obstetric Trauma   The two proposed mechanisms of pudendal neuropathy are stretch injury during the second stage of labor and compression of the nerve as it exits Alcock's canal (70). **Established risk factors for pelvic floor neuropathy include multiparity, high birth weight, forceps delivery, prolonged active second stage, and third-degree laceration** (72,73). Several studies have shown increased pudendal nerve terminal motor latencies following vaginal delivery, especially after sphincter laceration (53,71,74). Most women will recover function within a few months postpartum. Others will have evidence of injury several years later, which may represent the cumulative effects of subsequent deliveries (71,75). However, fecal incontinence will develop in only a fraction of patients with neuropathy (73).

Descending Perineum Syndrome   **As noted previously, prolonged straining for any reason could cause descending perineum syndrome. This syndrome is defined as descent of the perineum beyond the ischial tuberosities during Valsalva** (38,39). Pudendal neuropathy results from stretching and entrapment of the pudendal nerve. This diagnosis is supported by findings of elongation of the pudendal nerve, prolonged pudendal nerve motor terminal latency, and decreased anal sensation in women with perineal descent (76–78). As pudendal neuropathy progresses, it ultimately leads to fecal incontinence (40,79).

Functional Bowel Disorders

Functional Fecal Incontinence   **The Rome III criteria established well-defined guidelines for functional causes of fecal incontinence** (Table 28.7). The criteria essentially exclude systemic and anatomic abnormalities; however, minor abnormalities of sphincter innervation or structure are permitted.

Irritable Bowel Syndrome   **The diarrhea variant of irritable bowel syndrome is often associated with fecal incontinence as well as disordered defecation.** The criteria for diagnosis are presented in Table 28.4.

Functional Diarrhea   **The Rome III criteria create a unifying definition of diarrhea called functional diarrhea** (Table 28.8). The rationale for the criteria listed in Table 28.8 stems from the variability in patients' descriptions of diarrhea (46).

Table 28.7 Functional Fecal Incontinence

Diagnostic Criteria[a]

1. Recurrent uncontrolled passage of fecal material in an individual with a developmental age of at least 4 years and one or more of the following:

   a. Abnormal functioning of normally innervated and structurally intact muscles

   b. Minor abnormalities of sphincter structure and/or innervation

   c. Normal or disordered bowel habits, (i.e., fecal retention or diarrhea)

   d. Psychological causes

AND

2. Exclusion of all of the following

   a. Abnormal innervation caused by lesion(s) within the brain (e.g., dementia), spinal cord, or sacral nerve roots, or mixed lesions (e.g., multiple sclerosis), or as part of a generalized peripheral or autonomic neuropathy (e.g., due to diabetes)

   b. Anal sphincter abnormalities associated with a multisystem disease (e.g., scleroderma)

   c. Structural or neurogenic abnormalities believed to be the major or primary cause of fecal incontinence.

[a]Criteria fulfilled for the last 3 months
From **Drossman DA, Corazziari E, Talley NJ, et al., eds.** *Rome III: the functional gastrointestinal disorders.* 3nd ed. McLean, VA: Degnon Associates, 2006:885–897, Appendix A, with permission.

Pitfalls for the Pelvic Floor Surgeon

It sometimes is easy to overlook or misinterpret signs and symptoms of constipation and defecatory dysfunction. Any acute change in bowel habits must be evaluated thoroughly, and malignancy must be considered in the differential diagnosis. Even in the presence of chronic disease, malignancy must still be excluded. Persistent symptoms after an empiric trial of medical therapy should prompt further evaluation, including colonoscopy or flexible sigmoidoscopy. It is also possible to mistakenly attribute symptoms of defecatory dysfunction and constipation to pelvic organ prolapse when prolapse is actually the result of an underlying bowel disorder. In this case, surgical treatment of prolapse will have little lasting benefit if the underlying bowel disorder remains untreated.

History and Physical Examination

History

A thorough history and physical examination are critical to the evaluation of fecal incontinence and defecatory dysfunction. The history of present illness should focus on the bowel habits, including frequency and consistency of bowel movements (hard vs. soft, formed vs. unformed, diarrhea vs. constipation). Determining the duration and severity of symptoms, as well as exacerbating factors, is important for understanding the impact on quality of life. Patients should be questioned about straining with bowel movements, symptoms of incomplete emptying, and splinting of the perianal region, perineal body, or posterior vaginal wall to assist

Table 28.8 Functional Diarrhea

Diagnostic Criterion[a]

Loose (mushy) or watery stools without pain occurring in at least 75% of stools

[a]Criteria fulfilled for the last 3 months with symptom onset at least 6 months prior to diagnosis
From **Drossman DA, Corazziari E, Talley NJ, et al., eds.** *Rome III: the functional gastrointestinal disorders.* 3nd ed. McLean, VA: Degnon Associates, 2006:885–897, Appendix A, with permission.

with evacuation. Patients should also be asked about the need to perform digital disimpaction because they are unlikely to volunteer this information. With respect to fecal incontinence, information should be obtained about leakage with solids, liquid, and flatus and the ability to discriminate between these different types of stool (sampling). Similar to urinary incontinence, fecal incontinence can be stress related, urge related, or unconscious. Questions about alternating diarrhea and constipation, mucus or blood in the stools, constitutional symptoms, and changes in stool caliber can help the investigator uncover systemic and functional etiologies. Finally, it is important to ask about adaptive behaviors, incontinence product usage, and past and present treatments, including surgery, physical therapy, and medications.

A large amount of information can be obtained efficiently through questionnaires. Validated questionnaires quantify symptoms, which are subjective in nature, to objectively measure response to treatment. **A valuable survey to assess defecatory dysfunction is the Colorectal-Anal Distress Inventory (CRADI), which has been incorporated into the Pelvic Floor Distress Inventory (PFDI)** (80). The latter is a useful tool for evaluating symptoms of prolapse, urinary incontinence, fecal incontinence, voiding dysfunction, and defecatory dysfunction. Other useful symptom scales and bother scores for fecal incontinence include the Wexner Score, Fecal Incontinence Severity Index, and Fecal Incontinence Quality of Life Scale (81–83).

The medical history, surgical history, family history, and review of systems should focus on uncovering potential systemic and obstructive disorders shown in Table 28.1. **A complete obstetric history should include the number of vaginal deliveries, operative vaginal deliveries, or presence of a third- or fourth-degree laceration, which is critical for patients with fecal incontinence.** Length of the second stage of labor, birth weight, and the use of episiotomy should be ascertained because they may pose risk factors for sphincter damage and denervation. The sexual history should include questions about rape, anal intercourse, and dyspareunia. Use of over-the-counter, prescription, and illegal drugs should be recorded as well as food allergies.

Physical Examination

The evaluation of anorectal dysfunction requires a basic general examination as well as a focused abdominal and pelvic examination. The general physical survey should include a global assessment of mobility and cognitive function. Routine examination of the abdomen involves inspection, palpation, and auscultation to rule out the presence of masses, organomegaly, and areas of peritoneal irritation. This examination should be followed by a detailed evaluation of the vagina, perineum, and anorectum. The goals of the pelvic examination are to define objectively the degree of prolapse and determine the integrity of the connective tissue, neurologic function, and muscular support of the pelvic organs.

Neurologic Examination

Important elements of the neurologic examination are assessment of cranial nerve function, sensation and strength of the lower extremities, and reflexes for the lower extremities, bulbocavernosus, and anal wink. These examinations evaluate the function of the lower lumbar and sacral nerve roots, recognizing the importance of the second through fourth sacral nerve roots in pelvic floor dysfunction. The perineal reflexes can be elicited by stroking the labia majora and perianal skin or tapping the clitoris with a cotton-tipped swab. The anal wink, bulbocavernosus, and cough reflexes all test the integrity of motor innervation to the external anal sphincter (S2–4). Sensation over the inner thigh, vulva, and perirectal areas should be tested for symmetry to light touch and pinprick.

Muscle Strength

The integrity of the pelvic floor muscles should be assessed at rest and with voluntary contraction to determine strength, duration, and anterior lift. The ability to relax these muscles and tenderness on palpation should also be evaluated. Several standardized systems have been described to objectively measure muscle strength, but none has been accepted as a standard. The puborectalis muscle should be readily palpable posteriorly as it creates a 90-degree angle between the anal and rectal canals. Voluntary contraction of this muscle "lifts" the examining finger anteriorly toward the pubic rami. An intact external anal sphincter muscle that has decreased tone and contractility often indicates pudendal neuropathy. Similarly, neuropathy affecting the puborectalis can be recognized by an obtuse anorectal angle and weak voluntary contraction. Similar to the urethral axis, the anorectal angle can also be tested using a cotton-tipped swab, although this test is rarely performed. Deflection is measured in the supine position at rest, with strain, and with squeeze.

Vaginal Support

The salient points of pelvic organ prolapse (see Chapter 27 **for patients with defecatory dysfunction are the support of the vaginal apex, posterior wall, and perineal body, although some experts believe anterior wall defects can also affect defecatory dysfunction.** The posterior wall is assessed while supporting the vaginal apex and anterior wall with a Sims speculum. This permits the examiner to focus on identifying specific locations of rectovaginal fascial defects. A rectovaginal examination aids in identification of defects in the rectovaginal fascia or perineal body. Loss of vaginal rugation has also been reported overlying the site of a rectovaginal fascial tear (84). This technique is especially useful for enteroceles, which have a smooth, thin epithelium over the enterocele sac or peritoneum.

Normally, the perineum should be located at the level of the ischial tuberosities, or within 2 cm of this landmark. A perineum below this level, either at rest or with straining, represents perineal descent. Subjective findings of perineal descent include widening of the genital hiatus and perineal body, as well as a flattening of or a convex appearance of the intergluteal sulcus. Women with perineal descent also tend to have less severe stages of pelvic organ prolapse based on the **Pelvic Organ Prolapse Quantification (POP-Q) staging system** because it measures descent from the hymenal ring (85). An increase in the length of the perineal body and genital hiatus consistent with straining suggests perineal descent. The degree of perineal descent can also be measured objectively with a St. Mark's perineometer, although a thin ruler placed in the posterior introitus at the level of the ischial tuberosities also can be used. Descent is measured as the distance the perineal body moves when the patient strains. Although pelvic floor fluoroscopy is the standard technique for measuring perineal descent, this technique is most useful in patients with symptoms of severe defecatory dysfunction and evidence of perineal descent on pelvic examination.

Anorectal Examination

Visual and digital inspection of the vagina and anus will help to identify structural abnormalities such as prolapse, fistulas, fissures, hemorrhoids, or prior trauma. As previously mentioned, a rectovaginal examination provides useful information regarding the integrity of the rectovaginal septum and can demonstrate laxity in the support of the perineal body. The rectovaginal examination is helpful in the diagnosis of enteroceles, which can be felt as protrusion of bowel between the vaginal and rectal fingers with straining. Digital rectal examination should be performed at rest, with squeeze, and while straining. The presence of fecal material in the anal canal may suggest fecal impaction or neuromuscular weakness of the anal continence mechanism. Circumferential protrusion of the upper rectum around the examining finger during straining suggests intussusception, which often occurs in combination with laxity of the posterior rectal support along the sacrum.

The integrity of the external anal sphincter and puborectalis muscle can be evaluated by observation and palpation of these structures during voluntary contraction. Evidence of dovetailing of the perianal skin folds and the presence of a perineal scar with an asymmetric contraction often indicates a sphincter defect. When a patient is asked to contract her pelvic floor muscles, two motions should be present: The external anal sphincter should contract concentrically, and the anal verge should be pulled inward. These actions should also be apparent on digital rectal examination. As mentioned previously, the 90-degree angle created by the puborectalis should be readily palpable posteriorly and, with voluntary contraction, the examining finger should be lifted anteriorly toward the pubic rami. Both the puborectalis and external anal sphincter should relax during Valsalva effort. Patients with anismus may experience a paradoxical contraction of these muscles during straining. Finally, defects in the anterior aspects of the external anal sphincter may be detected by digital examination.

Testing

Sophisticated diagnostic testing is currently being used in clinical research and in anorectal physiology laboratories to quantify the function of the colon and anorectum. Following is a description of these techniques as they relate to the management of fecal incontinence and disordered defecation.

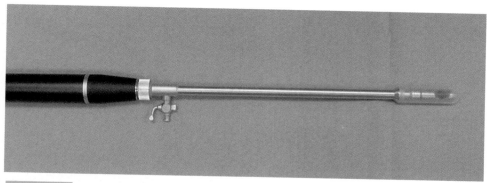

Figure 28.1   **Bruel-Kjaer (Copenhagen, Denmark) ultrasound probe** (type 1850) with a 7.0 MHz transducer (focal length, 2 to 5 cm) housed with a plastic cone.

Fecal Incontinence

Endoanal Ultrasonography

Endoanal ultrasonography permits accurate imaging of both the internal and external anal sphincters. It can assess the continuity and thickness of the muscle and currently is considered the single best method for detecting anal sphincter defects. Endoanal ultrasonography is performed using a Bruel-Kjaer (Copenhagen, Denmark) ultrasound scanner with a 360-degree rectal endoprobe (type 1850) with a 7.0 MHz transducer (focal length, 2–5 cm) housed within a plastic cone (Fig. 28.1). The normal IAS is a continuous hypoechoic band of smooth muscle surrounded by the thick echogenic layer of the striated EAS. A sphincter defect occurs when there is disruption in these muscle bands. Location and severity of the defect can be described by circumferential distance in degrees, percentage of thickness, and distance from the anal verge (Fig. 28.2). Measurements are usually taken in the proximal, middle, and distal anal canal. It is important to recognize the physiologic split in the proximal EAS as it merges with the puborectalis muscle of the levator ani. Misinterpretation of this finding as a sphincter defect can result in an increased prevalence of reported defects. The puborectalis muscle appears as a U-shaped or V-shaped thick echogenic layer outside the IAS in the proximal anal canal. Magnetic resonance imaging (MRI) may be equally as effective or better at diagnosing sphincter defects, especially with the use of a vaginal or rectal coil. For this purpose, MRI is more expensive, and currently its use is largely investigational. It may be beneficial in cases in which endoanal ultrasonography results are inconclusive or the quality of the study is poor.

Electromyography

Electromyography (EMG) is used to evaluate neuromuscular integrity of the EAS following a traumatic injury such as childbirth, as well as to document the presence of pelvic floor neuropathy (86). This technique measures the electrical activity arising in muscle fibers during contraction and at rest. Different types of electrodes may be employed, including surface electrodes, concentric needle electrodes, and single-fiber electrodes. Surface electrodes are less invasive because they are applied near or within the anal canal, but they are capable only of recording basic anal sphincter activity. This technique often is used in conjunction with biofeedback therapy. Concentric needle electrodes are most commonly used in anorectal physiology laboratories to selectively survey an individual muscle's activity. Insertion of the thin needle-like cannulas containing steel wire electrodes can be painful. Even smaller single-fiber EMG electrodes are used to record the activity of single muscle fibers, which can be quantified to calculate fiber density. Following denervation injury, increased muscle fiber density occurs during reinnervation. Thus, single-fiber EMG can provide indirect evidence of neurologic injury by mapping the EAS and identifying injured areas. This technique is used rarely in clinical practice. Endoanal ultrasonography offers increased patient comfort and more reliable results than EMG and has replaced this technique for the detection of EAS disruption because of increased patient comfort and more reliable results.

Motor nerve conduction studies provide another means of measuring pelvic floor neuropathy. The axon of a nerve is stimulated, and the time it takes the action potential to reach the muscle supplied by the nerve is recorded. The delay between stimulation and the muscle

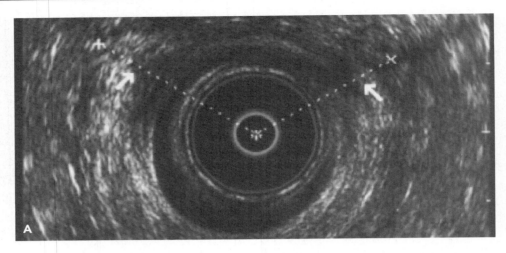

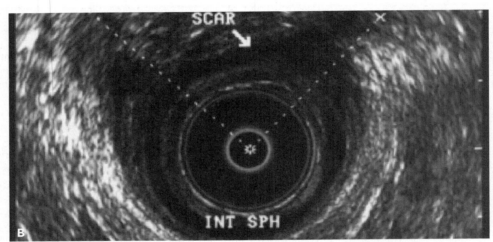

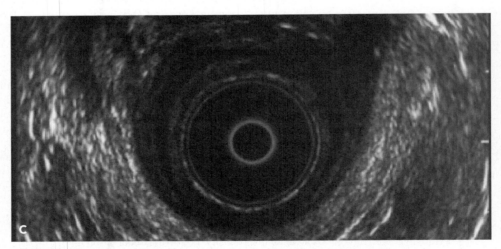

Figure 28.2   **A: Endoanal ultrasound image from the distal anal canal** demonstrating defects in the internal sphincter from 10 to 3 o'clock and the external sphincter from 10 to 2 o'clock. **B: Endoanal ultrasound image from the middle anal canal** demonstrating defects in the internal sphincter from 12 to 2 o'clock and the external sphincter from 10 to 1 o'clock. **C: Endoanal ultrasound image from the proximal anal canal** demonstrating an intact IAS and a normal physiologic split in the external sphincter.

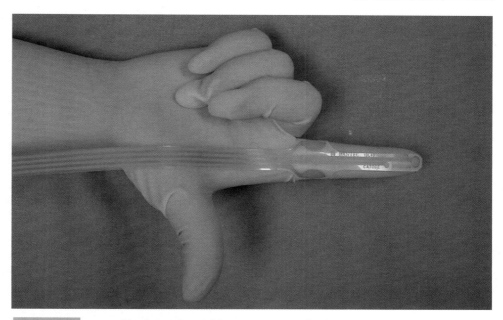

Figure 28.3 St. Mark's electrode used for measuring pudendal nerve motor terminal latency. The stimulating electrode is on the fingertip, and the receiving electrode is on the proximal finger near the knuckle.

response is called the nerve latency. Pudendal nerve terminal motor latency (PNTML) can be determined by transrectal stimulation of the pudendal nerve using a St. Mark's electrode (87). A nerve stimulator is mounted on an examination glove at the fingertip (Fig. 28.3) and positioned transrectally over each ischial spine. A stimulus of up to 50 mV for 0.1 milliseconds is applied, and the latency of the EAS muscle contraction is measured. A value of 2.2 milliseconds or less is considered normal. A recent study evaluating normative values for pudendal and perineal nerve latencies observed increased latencies with increased age (88). Prolongation of the PNTML is indicative of damage to that nerve or the presence of a demyelinating condition. Pudendal nerve function has prognostic value in the surgical repair of traumatic sphincter injuries and is useful in preoperative counseling (89).

Anal Manometry

Anal manometry is used to quantify function of the anal sphincter mechanism. Water-perfused manometry catheters or water-filled balloons are most often used to measure anal canal pressures. Resting anal canal pressures reflect IAS function, and pressures in the lower anal canal during maximal voluntary contraction reflect EAS function. Vector analysis can be used to detect asymmetry within the anal sphincter. Anal manometry provides indirect evidence of sphincter injury; low resting tone indicates IAS injury, and decreased maximum squeeze pressure indicates EAS injury. Anal pressures are influenced by a variety of factors, including tissue compliance and muscular tone. Consequently, anal manometry results are difficult to interpret and correlate poorly with the specific anatomic defect. Interpretation is further complicated by the wide variation of normal pressure values that change with age and parity. Significant overlaps occur between manometric values for incontinent patients and those without incontinence. Thus, anal manometry may be of limited value in the evaluation and treatment of anal sphincter defects and fecal incontinence.

Proctoscopy and Flat Tire Test

Proctoscopy has an important role in the evaluation of fecal incontinence. It can be performed independently or during colonoscopy, flexible sigmoidoscopy, and the flat tire test. **Proctoscopy can detect anorectal pathology, such as prolapsing hemorrhoids, intussusception, ulcerative or radiation proctitis, or a solitary rectal ulcer.** The flat tire test is added when a rectovaginal or colovaginal fistula is suspected but cannot be visualized on routine office evaluation. This test usually is performed under anesthesia but can also be done in the office setting. Saline or water is placed in the vagina with the patient in Trendelenburg position. Using a proctoscope or rigid sigmoidoscope, air is instilled into the rectum. Vaginal retractors provide visualization of the posterior vaginal epithelium and vaginal apex. Observation of bubbling into the vaginal fluid confirms the diagnosis and location of a rectovaginal or colovaginal fistula. The rectal site of the fistula usually is identifiable, depending on the size and location of the fistula as well as the quality of the bowel preparation.

Disordered Defecation

Sitzmark Study

Colonic transit studies are performed using ingested radiopaque markers followed by serial abdominal radiography. Patients are asked to follow a high-fiber diet over the test period and avoid the use of laxatives, suppositories, or enemas. A capsule containing 20 to 24 markers is ingested initially, and abdominal radiography is performed either daily or on the fourth day, the seventh day, and every 3 days thereafter until all the markers are gone. Segmental transit times are then calculated using a mathematical formula. Colonic transit study results are used to classify patients with constipation into delayed transit, normal transit, and outlet obstruction. After day 6, there should be fewer than five markers remaining in the colon. With slow transit, more than five markers are scattered throughout the colon. With outlet obstruction, more than five markers are in the rectosigmoid region, and transit is normal throughout the rest of the colon.

Pelvic Floor Fluoroscopy and Magnetic Resonance Imaging

Pelvic fluoroscopy permits radiological evaluation of pelvic floor and anorectal anatomy and physiology. It is particularly useful in obstructive defecation disorders, such as intussusception, rectocele, enterocele, anismus, and perineal descent. The patient is placed on a radiolucent commode, and contrast material is instilled into the rectum. The addition of vaginal, bladder, and oral contrast material is helpful diagnostically when multicompartmental prolapse is suspected. A series of lateral still images or continuous imaging using videography are made with fluoroscopy while the patient is at rest, during defecation, and with contraction of the anal sphincter. Similar films can be obtained for evacuation of the bladder. Pelvic fluoroscopy has many names, including defecography, defecating proctography, defecating cystoproctography, and colpocystoproctography, depending on the technique used. The measurements obtained include size of the rectal ampulla, length of the anal canal, anorectal angle, puborectalis motion, and pelvic floor descent. Severity of prolapse and pelvic floor descent is quantified in relation to the pubococcygeal line. Pelvic fluoroscopy is superior to physical examination for diagnosing enterocele, and this technique has the advantage of being able to distinguish enteroceles from sigmoidoceles (90). Rectosphincteric dyssynergia may be present when the patient experiences incomplete relaxation of the puborectalis muscle during rectal evacuation, the anorectal angle is preserved, and there is incomplete emptying. Pelvic fluoroscopy is considered the definitive test for diagnosing intussusception, and it is the preferred technique for quantifying perineal descent (91).

Dynamic MRI with luminal contrast is an imaging modality similar to pelvic fluoroscopy. Its ability to detect prolapse is similar to that of fluoroscopy, but MRI can visualize pelvic floor musculature and soft tissue, thus giving it the advantage of detecting ballooning of the levator muscles and levator ani hernias. The supine position of the testing is a drawback; however, there are isolated reports of upright dynamic MRI using open scanners that show results comparable to fluoroscopy for detection of anorectal pathology (92). Fluoroscopy and dynamic MRI can be used in situations involving severe multicompartmental prolapse or in which the severity of the symptoms is disproportionate to examination findings.

Anal Manometry

Anal manometry is used to determine maximum resting pressure, maximum squeeze pressure, rectal sensation and compliance, as well as the presence of an intact rectoanal inhibitory reflex. With disordered defecation, it can be used to diagnose Hirschsprung disease and anismus. The addition of surface EMG to document relaxation helps exclude anismus as a cause of obstructed defecation. Failure of the anal sphincter to relax with defecation and increased electrical activity of the EAS and puborectalis are seen in patients with anismus. In contrast, there should be no increase in the electrical activity measured by surface electrodes for patients with Hirschsprung disease. A rectal balloon expulsion test can also be of assistance in the evaluation of rectal emptying and may be valuable during physiotherapy for diagnosing dyssynergic defecation.

| Colonoscopy and Proctoscopy | Standard gastrointestinal evaluation for patients with symptoms of disordered defecation should include a barium enema or colonoscopy to eliminate the possibility of colorectal malignancy. Proctoscopy should be included as part of the routine examination because it may reveal anorectal pathology. |

Therapeutic Approach to Fecal Incontinence

Treatment of fecal incontinence should first focus on nonsurgical options, including dietary modification, medical therapy, and biofeedback. Any underlying systemic conditions or gastrointestinal disorders should be treated before initiating an extensive evaluation for other causes of fecal incontinence. If symptoms persist, further investigation should be undertaken. If the evaluation discloses an underlying EAS defect and conservative therapy has been unsuccessful, it is reasonable to proceed with surgical treatment.

Following is an overview of treatment options and the efficacy of each approach. The lack of consistent outcome measures makes it difficult to compare efficacy among treatments. Some studies base success on strict conformity with criteria for continence, but the results vary for continence of flatus, liquid, or solid stool. Other studies base success on more subjective criteria, such as improvement following treatment. Daily diaries can be maintained, but the results may be unreliable. Even if a validated symptom survey and quality-of-life scale are employed, few studies use the same outcome measure.

| Nonsurgical Treatment | **Nonsurgical management focuses on maximizing the continence mechanism through alteration of stool characteristics or behavioral modification.** Stool consistency and volume can be manipulated by dietary and pharmacologic means to achieve passage of one to two well-formed stools per day. The rationale for this approach is that formed stool is easier to control than liquid stool. Additionally, behavior modification can be employed using bowel regimens that focus on the predictable elimination of feces. Physical therapy and biofeedback can also be useful for strengthening the continence mechanism. |

| Pharmacologic Approaches | ### Dietary Modification and Fiber |

Dietary modification for treatment of fecal incontinence frequently involves avoidance of foods that precipitate loose stools and diarrhea. Common dietary irritants include spicy foods, coffee and other caffeinated beverages, beer and alcohol, and citrus fruits. Avoidance of dairy products or the addition of lactase dietary supplements is essential for those with lactose intolerance. The addition of fiber may improve fecal incontinence by functioning as a stool bulking agent to increase volume and density. The average individual in the United States consumes less than half the recommended daily fiber intake (25–35 g). Various fiber sources are listed in Table 28.9, with the highest content found in high-fiber cereals. It is difficult to consume the recommended daily amount from diet alone, and fiber supplements often are required. Although the increased stool volume and density helps many individuals maintain continence, excessive fiber with inadequate fluid intake may predispose elderly patients to fecal impaction.

Constipating Agents

Constipating agents have the most value in patients with chronic loose stools or diarrhea. They can also help improve symptoms in patients with fecal frequency and urgency. *Loperamide (Imodium)* and *diphenoxylate hydrochloride with atropine (Lomotil)* are the most commonly used agents. *Loperamide* has been shown to prolong transit time and stimulate anal sphincter function. With either of these agents, careful titration is recommended to prevent the primary side effect of constipation. It is generally preferable to begin using 2 to 4 mg of *loperamide* daily and then titrate up to 4 mg three to four times per day. A 4-mg dose before meals has been shown to increase anal tone and improve continence (93). *Lomotil* is started at a dose of one to two tablets every day or every other day and titrated up to one to two tablets three to four times a day as needed. Caution should be exercised for patients taking other anticholinergic medications. Anticholinergic side effects include dry mouth, drowsiness, lightheadedness, and tachycardia. *Codeine* can also be used as a constipating agent. It should be used judiciously in those with chronic disorders and in

Table 28.9 Fiber Sources			
Cereals		*Fiber Supplements*	
All-Bran Extra Fiber (1/2 c)	15 g	Konsyl (1 tsp)	6.0 g
Fiber One (1/2 c)	14 g	Perdiem (1 tsp)	4.0 g
Raisin Bran (1/2 c)	7 g	Metamucil (1 tsp)	3.4 g
All Bran (1/2 c)	6 g	Maalox w/fiber (1 tbs)	3.4 g
Fruit & Fiber (2/3 c)	5 g	Mylanta w/fiber (1 tsp)	3.4 g
Frosted Mini Wheats (1/2 c)	3 g	Citrucel (1 tbs)	2.0 g
Breads		*Vegetables*	
Whole wheat (1 slice)	2.0 g	Lettuce (1 c)	1.4 g
White (1 slice)	0.5 g	Celery (1)	0.5 g
Bagel (1)	1.0 g	Tomato, raw (1)	1.0 g

Modified from **Ellerkmann MR, Kaufman H.** Defecatory dysfunction. In: **Bent AE, Ostergard DR, Cundiff GW, et al, eds.** *Ostergard's urogynecology.* 5th ed. Philadelphia, PA: Lippincott Williams & Wilkins, 2002:362, with permission.

elderly patients because of side effects common to narcotics, including addiction with prolonged usage and central nervous system and respiratory depression. A study of 82 geriatric patients documented the efficacy of pharmacologic treatment for fecal incontinence (94). Patients were treated based on the underlying cause. Those with fecal impaction received *lactulose* and enemas, whereas those with neurogenic fecal incontinence received *codeine* phosphate as a constipating agent and enemas. The rate of cure for fecal incontinence was 60% in the treatment group versus 32% for controls ($P < .001$).

Medications for Irritable Bowel Syndrome

Dietary treatment of IBS consists of avoiding foods that are associated with symptoms, including alcohol, caffeine, sorbitol, and foods that increase gas production. Although increased dietary fiber or fiber supplementation has been shown to improve the constipation-predominant form of this illness, fiber supplementation has little effect on the diarrhea variant associated with fecal incontinence. Pharmacologic therapy is directed toward the predominant symptom. *Loperamide* and *Lomotil* tend to be useful first-line agents for treating diarrhea. Tricyclic antidepressants improve abdominal discomfort and are also valuable in diarrhea-predominant patients because of their constipating effect. The serotonin type 3 (5HT3) antagonist *alosetron* (*Lotronex*) has been approved by the U.S. Food and Drug Administration (FDA) for the treatment of severe diarrhea-predominant IBS refractory to treatment. It has shown improvement in global assessment measures, but its use is limited because of multiple isolated case reports of ischemic colitis. The recommended dose is 1 mg once or twice daily. It does not appear to be effective for the spastic-pain variant of IBS. Anticholinergics (*dicyclomine, hyoscyamine*) and antispasmodics (*mebeverine, pinaverine*) are targeted at the pain and bloating symptoms but may also be useful for the diarrhea variant because of their constipating side effects. Studies comparing anticholinergic medications to placebo show inconclusive results with only modest benefits. Antispasmodic agents may also be of value and are available in many countries but are not approved for use in the United States. Currently, additional 5HT3 antagonists and 5HT4 antagonists are under development and are approved for use in Europe but not in the United States. Most studies are poorly designed and difficult to interpret because of a high placebo response rate that often exceeds 30% (95,96).

Behavioral Approaches

Biofeedback

Biofeedback can be an effective therapeutic modality provided patients are motivated and comprehend instructions. The two proposed mechanisms through which biofeedback improves fecal continence are afferent and efferent training. *Afferent training* focuses on improving sensation in the anorectal canal through recruitment of adjacent neurons to decrease the sensory threshold of volume stimulation. The goal of this training is to enhance and restore anal sensation and the rectoanal inhibitory reflex. *Efferent training* enhances and restores voluntary contraction of the EAS, which permits additional recruitment of motor units and stimulates muscle hypertrophy. These two methods of training can be performed independently but are often combined for additional therapeutic benefit. The most common training method uses an intrarectal balloon. The balloon acts to stimulate rectal distention and provide pressure feedback from coordinated or synchronized contraction of the pelvic floor muscles. Other techniques focus on strength training of the EAS alone using anal pressure feedback or EMG or afferent training alone using an intrarectal balloon without pelvic floor muscle contraction in response to the stimulus.

More than 35 studies have been done to evaluate the efficacy of biofeedback for treatment of fecal incontinence, and several excellent review articles and meta-analyses have determined the effects of individual treatments and predictors of patient response to treatment (97–99). The results of all of these studies uniformly agree that biofeedback and pelvic floor exercises improve fecal incontinence and have a role in clinical practice. They also agree that the existing literature is fraught with methodologic problems and lacks validated outcomes and controls. Thus it is difficult to compare directly the study results.

Biofeedback is an ideal first-line therapy because it offers an effective, minimally invasive treatment without any reported adverse events. Biofeedback also appears to provide a higher probability of successful outcome than standard medical care for treating functional fecal incontinence (67% vs. 36%, respectively, $P < .001$) (97).

A Cochrane review of biofeedback and exercises for treatment of fecal incontinence found only five randomized or quasi-randomized control trials that qualified for inclusion (100). The authors concluded that **there is insufficient evidence to evaluate the efficacy of exercises and biofeedback for treatment of fecal incontinence.** Specifically, they were not able to determine which patients were suitable for treatment nor which method of treatment was optimal. A meta-analysis of biofeedback techniques included a review of 13 studies using strength training alone, 4 studies with sensory training alone, and 18 with coordinated sensory and strength training (99). The authors found no advantages between coordinated training (67% improved) and strength training (70% improved). However, strength training using EMG appeared to be better than strength training with anal canal pressure biofeedback (74% vs. 64% improved, respectively, $P < .04$). The limitations of this study and the literature were acknowledged.

A large randomized control trial of biofeedback for fecal incontinence in 171 patients, divided into four treatment groups, showed no significant benefit when comparing standard care to similar care with the addition of biofeedback (54% vs. 53% improvement, respectively) (101). In all groups, there was a high median rating of change of symptoms and median satisfaction with benefits relatively maintained at 1-year follow-up. All groups displayed improvement in the validated symptom surveys and quality-of-life measures as well as in anal sphincter function. The authors concluded that interactions with the therapist, patient education, and development of better coping strategies seem to be the most important factors for improvement rather than pelvic muscle exercises or biofeedback. Additional benefit may be derived with augmented biofeedback using electrical stimulation (102).

There are no clear indicators to predict which patients will benefit from biofeedback. Potential factors include age, duration and severity of incontinence, prior treatments or surgery, and severity of neurologic or physical damage. Controversy exists as to whether response to biofeedback is dependent on the presence of a structurally intact anal sphincter or normal pudendal nerve function (103–106). Similarly, there is insufficient evidence that electrical stimulation improves fecal incontinence (107). There is an obvious need for well-designed control trials using validated symptom surveys and quality-of-life instruments. More objective measures are desirable, and studies should carefully document duration of treatment and length of follow-up.

Bowel Regimens

The goal of bowel regimens is to achieve predictable elimination of feces. This can be accomplished by using the gastrocolic reflex as well as by dietary and pharmacologic means. Defecation immediately following meals involves the physiologic response of the gastrocolic reflex to facilitate predictable emptying. The strength of the gastrocolic reflex varies among individuals and may be hypoactive or hyperactive with certain systemic disorders, such as diabetes and multiple sclerosis. This technique can be especially useful in the morning to give the individual freedom from fecal incontinence throughout the day. The use of suppositories or enemas in the morning or at night in conjunction with the gastrocolic reflex may provide further relief of daytime symptoms. The goal is to leave the rectum empty between evacuations. Enema use, typically once or twice daily, should be titrated to the patient's baseline colonic activity. **Regular toileting in elderly patients in nursing homes can improve fecal incontinence caused by overflow incontinence from fecal impaction.** The use of cone-tip colostomy-irrigation catheters is reserved for patients in whom other therapeutic modalities have failed. These catheters avoid the risk of rectal perforation and provide a dam to prevent efflux of the irrigating solutions (108).

Surgical Treatment

In general, surgical treatment should be employed after conservative measures have failed. Although there may be exceptions to this principle, most surgeons follow this recommendation because of the poor long-term outcomes and high complication rates with surgery for fecal incontinence.

Overlapping Sphincteroplasty

Overlapping sphincteroplasty is the procedure of choice for fecal incontinence caused by a disrupted anal sphincter. Most authorities believe that an overlapping technique is superior to an end-to-end repair, although there are few direct comparisons in the literature. The rationale for the overlapping technique is that a more secure repair can be accomplished by placing sutures through the scarred connective tissue rather than the sphincter muscle. Sutures should be less likely to tear through or pull out of connective tissue than muscle. Therefore, the key component of the overlapping technique is preservation of the scarred ends of the ruptured EAS for suture placement.

Technique

The initial step involves wide mobilization of the ruptured EAS without excision of the scarred ends of the sphincter. This is accomplished through an inverted semilunar perineal incision or a transverse incision near the posterior vaginal fourchette with inferiolateral extension. The latter incision facilitates repair in patients with damage to the rectovaginal septum attachment to the perineal body. Patients with EAS defects have either a band of intervening fibrous scar tissue between the viable muscular ends of sphincter or a complete separation with scar tissue present only on the ruptured ends of the sphincter. In the presence of complete separation of scar tissue, perineal body reconstruction usually is indicated at the time of repair to restore normal anatomy. A Peña muscle stimulator aids in identification of the distal ends of the EAS and differentiates viable muscle tissue from scar tissue. The stimulator can be used to outline the sphincter before incision as well as during the dissection. It is important to apprise the anesthesiologist of the stimulator usage so that paralytic agents are avoided.

Excessive lateral dissection of the EAS past the 3 and 9 o'clock positions should be avoided as this is where the inferior rectal branches of the pudendal nerve innervate the EAS. Moderate bleeding often is encountered during this dissection, and the use of needlepoint electrocautery can maximize hemostasis. Controversy exists regarding the need to separate the EAS and IAS before repair. Identification of the intersphincteric groove facilitates dissection of the EAS. Dissection in this plane is relatively simple and avoids damage to either sphincter. Defects in the IAS can be more difficult to visualize because this muscle is intimately associated with the rectal mucosa. Examination with a finger in the anal canal is often helpful.

The reconstruction begins with repair of an existing IAS defect using a 3-0 delayed absorbable monofilament suture. Next, the EAS defect is repaired with the primary goal of overlapping at least 2 to 3 cm to ensure adequate bulk of sphincter muscle encircling the anal canal. The EAS is overlapped using three to four mattress sutures of 2-0 delayed absorbable monofilament suture through the distal scar tissue. Once the sutures are tied, there should be resistance palpable with placement of a finger in the anal canal. Copious irrigation is performed throughout the procedure. Following sphincter repair, a perineal body reconstruction and rectocele repair should be undertaken, if indicated, to maximize the normal continence mechanism. Finally, the perineal skin is closed with interrupted absorbable monofilament sutures. Closure frequently requires modification of the initial incision because of changes in the perineal architecture that result from the repair. The most common approach is an inverted Y-shaped closure of the incision (Fig. 28.4).

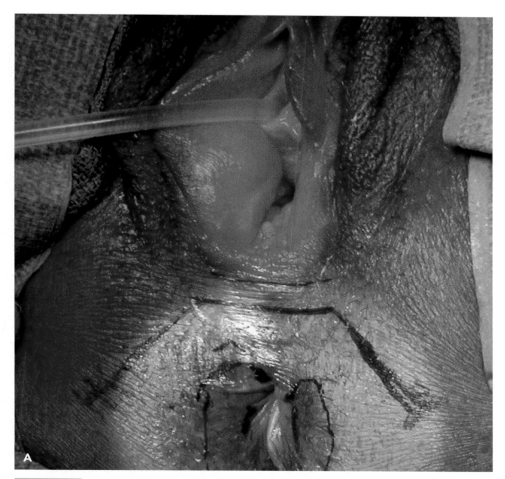

Figure 28.4 **Overlapping sphincteroplasty procedure.** **A:** Inverted semilunar perineal incision with the distal ends of the external sphincter outlined using the Peña muscle stimulator. **B:** The external sphincter has been dissected, the scar divided in the midline, and the internal sphincter repaired. **C:** The external sphincter is overlapped using three mattress sutures of 2–0 delayed absorbable monofilament suture through the distal scar tissue. **D:** The sutures are tied. **E:** The skin is closed.

Some surgeons recommend the overlapping repair regardless of whether it is performed immediately postpartum, delayed postpartum, or several years after obstetric injury. Performance of the overlapping technique is difficult immediately postpartum and requires adequate anesthesia, exposure, and equipment. Many surgeons believe that this can only be accomplished in the operating room. This repair lacks the theoretical advantage of using scar tissue to improve suture holding; however, it maximizes surface area for scarification of the sphincter ends. For a delayed postpartum repair, it is recommended to wait 3 to 6 months to permit complete resolution of inflammation and reinnervation.

Four randomized control trials compared end-to-end approximation to overlapping sphincteroplasty after acute obstetrical injury (109–112). Fitzpatrick et al. randomized 112 primiparous women undergoing immediate repair of a third- or fourth-degree sphincter tear (109). The authors did not detect any significant differences in objective or subjective outcomes between either of the two repairs at 3 months follow-up. Approximately one-half of the women had minor alteration in fecal continence, whereas 7 (6%) had daily soiling. Despite good symptomatic results, 74 (66%) had full-thickness EAS defects on endoanal ultrasonography. Williams et al. randomized 112 women to overlapping or end-to-end repair with either polyglactin (Vicryl) or polydioxanone (PDS) (110). They, too, found no difference in outcomes between the different methods of repair or type of suture used. Fernando et al. randomized 64 women and discovered a lower rate of fecal incontinence symptoms and fecal urgency after overlapping repair compared to end-to-end

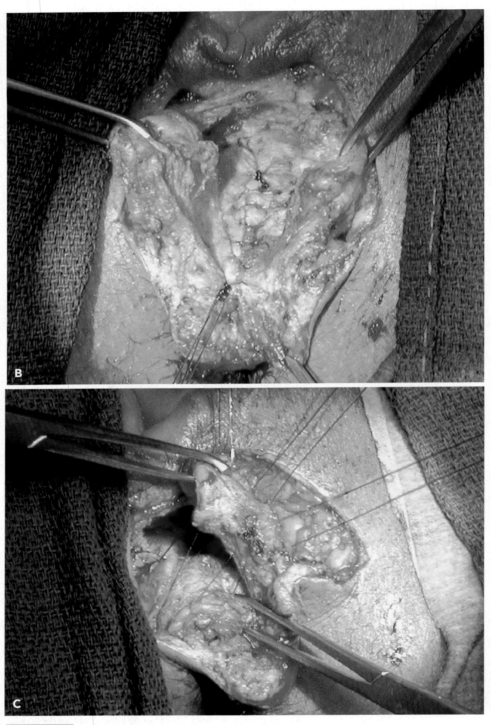

Figure 28.4   *(continued)*

repair (111). Farrell et al. randomized 149 women to one of the two techniques and was the only study to discover higher rates of fecal incontinence of flatus in the overlapping group compared to the end-to-end group (61% vs. 39%; OR 2.44) (112). There was a trend toward overall higher rates of fecal incontinence; however, these were not statistically different (15% vs. 8%) (112). A Cochrane review that included the first three randomized controlled trials concluded that the overlapping repair technique resulted in less fecal incontinence and fecal urgency, but the data were insufficient to recommend one repair over the other (113). Another randomized controlled

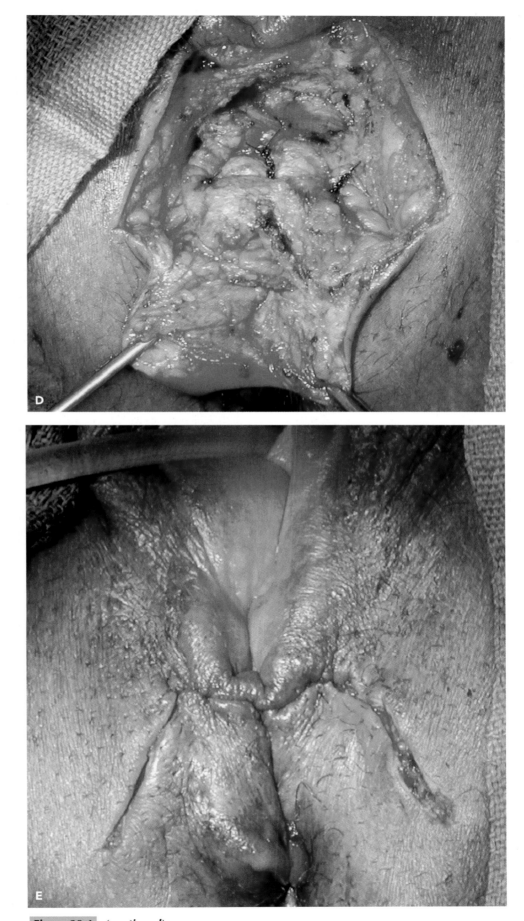

Figure 28.4 *(continued)*

trial involved a delayed repair in 23 patients more than 1 year following delivery (114). The scar was preserved for each repair, and a puborectalis plication was performed. At a median follow-up of 18 months, there were no detectable differences in continence scores; however, the study was clearly underpowered. Consequently, the authors believe there is no definitive evidence to support an overlapping technique at the time of acute obstetrical injury and repair but prefer an overlapping technique as a delayed repair.

Efficacy

Despite the many large series reporting the outcomes of overlapping sphincteroplasty, almost all are retrospective in nature and lack validated measures of symptom severity and quality-of-life considerations. Several overlapping sphincteroplasty series with a total of 891 patients were evaluated from 1984 to 2001. Although the length of follow-up was variable, the results showed excellent and good outcomes in approximately two-thirds of patients (median 67%, range 52%–83%) (115). None of these studies had long-term outcomes.

More recent studies suggest poor long-term outcomes for the overlapping sphincteroplasty. In a series of 55 women who underwent overlapping sphincteroplasty for fecal incontinence secondary to obstetric trauma, researchers contacted 47 (86%) patients by postal questionnaire and telephone interview with a median time since surgery of 77 months (range 60–96 months) (116). The investigators observed less symptomatic improvement when compared with the results at 15 months postoperative evaluation. After excluding one patient because of Crohn disease, eight (17%) failed because they required additional surgery, such as colostomy, postanal repair, and artificial bowel sphincter. Among the remaining 38 patients, 27 (71%) reported improved bowel control, 5 (13%) were unimproved, and 6 (16%) were worse. No patient was fully continent to solid and liquid stool and flatus. Only 23 (50%) patients had "good" outcomes defined as not requiring further continence surgery and fecal incontinence less than once per month.

In another study, investigators contacted 49 (69%) of 71 patients by telephone interview (117). All underwent overlapping sphincteroplasty with a median follow-up of 62.5 months (range 47–141 months). Only 6 (12%) patients were totally continent, and another 18 (37%) were continent to liquid and solid stool. More than half of the patients had incontinence to liquid or solid stool. The largest series with long-term follow-up involved contact of 130 (71%) of 191 patients using a postal or telephone questionnaire (118). The median time from surgery for respondents was 10 years (range 7–16 years). Of those who responded, 6% had no incontinence, 16% were incontinent of flatus only, 19% had soiling only, and 57% were incontinent of solid stool. These outcomes were significantly worse than the previously reported 3-year assessment (119). Despite the fact that 61% had a poor outcome defined as having fecal incontinence or requiring additional surgery for incontinence, 62% still considered their bowel control to be better than before surgery, and 74% were satisfied with the results of their surgery. Although control may be improved when compared with preoperative status, continence outcomes do not seem to be maintained at long-term follow-up.

The cause of this deterioration in long-term outcomes is unknown. Possible explanations include weakening of the muscles with normal aging, repair breakdown, and underlying nerve damage from either obstetric injury or the repair itself. A problem with most studies is the lack of a follow-up ultrasonography to determine whether the repair was still intact. The effect of pudendal nerve function on overlapping sphincteroplasty is somewhat controversial. Significantly lower success rates have been shown in a comparison of those with normal pudendal nerve terminal motor latencies to those with abnormal latencies (63% vs. 17%; $P < .01$) (120). Other studies have confirmed this finding (79,89,106,107,121,122), but the more recent studies fail to show a difference based on preoperative neurophysiologic testing (116,118). Other controversial factors that may affect outcome include age, duration of fecal incontinence, size of the defect, and anal manometry results.

Although there are many controversial aspects to overlapping sphincteroplasty, the literature is in agreement that **diverting colostomy is not necessary;** bowel confinement does not improve outcomes; clinical improvement correlates with postoperative endoanal ultrasonography results; and prior sphincteroplasty does not affect outcomes (114,116,120,123–128).

Subsequent Deliveries

Multiple studies confirm the impact of anal sphincter laceration during the first delivery on the risk of a sphincter laceration in a second delivery (129–132). These studies have calculated odds ratios ranging between 2.5 and 5.3 for a second sphincter disruption. Two recent population-based studies revealed adjusted odds ratios of 4.2 (95% confidence interval [CI], 3.9–4.6) and 4.3 (95% CI, 3.8–4.8) (130,131). These odds ratios probably represent underestimates because they do not take into account higher cesarean delivery rates in subsequent births for women with a history of sphincter laceration. Both of these studies observed significantly increased risk of recurrent sphincter laceration associated with increased birth weight. The studies estimated that approximately 25 cesarean deliveries have to be performed to prevent one recurrent sphincter laceration. In fact, only 10% of women with anal sphincter lacerations at second delivery had a history of prior sphincter laceration. **Although a history of prior sphincter laceration increases the risk of recurrent sphincter laceration, the risk remains relatively small.** It is important to accurately counsel expectant mothers about their risk of sphincter laceration. Using this information, they can decide whether the risk of recurrent laceration outweighs the risk of elective cesarean birth. The risk of subsequent vaginal delivery on symptoms of fecal incontinence is unknown for women with a repaired anal sphincter. The presence or absence of preexisting fecal incontinence, as well as the estimated fetal weight, should be considered in counseling for a subsequent pregnancy.

Gracioplasty

Surgical reconstruction with a muscle flap should be considered in cases in which there is insufficient muscle to repair the EAS and all conservative measures have failed. Insufficient muscle can be caused by trauma or severe atrophy that results from denervation injury and congenital disease. Most patients considering this procedure have already undergone an overlapping sphincteroplasty that failed. Graciloplasty, first described by Pickrell et al. in 1952, is a skeletal muscle transposition procedure that uses the gracilis to create a new anal sphincter (133). There are three suitable muscles for this type of procedure: the gracilis, sartorius, and gluteus maximus. The muscle should be easily mobilized and transposed but not essential for locomotion or posture. The sartorius and gluteus maximus are suboptimal because the sartorius receives segmental vascularization, which restricts rotation, and the gluteus maximus is important in daily activities such as running, climbing stairs, and rising from a sitting position. **The gracilis is a better choice because it can easily be mobilized without damage.** As the most superficial adductor, it receives neurovascular supply proximally and has no important independent function.

Technique

Either one long incision or three small incisions are made in the medial thigh. The gracilis muscle is identified and mobilized toward its insertion onto the medial aspect of the tibia where the tendon is divided. Anterior and posterior perianal incisions are made approximately 1.5 cm from the anal verge. Tunnels are developed in the extrasphincteric space and from the proximal thigh to the anterior perianal incision. The gracilis muscle is then gently delivered to the anterior perianal incision, guided around the anus to the posterior perianal incision, and returned to the anterior incision encircling the anal canal. The distal tendon of the gracilis is passed behind the muscle and anchored to the contralateral periosteum of the ischium. In cases when there is inadequate length, it can be sutured to the ipsilateral ischium. This procedure can also be performed bilaterally. In patients with a large rectovaginal fistula or cloaca, a myocutaneous flap can be mobilized and used to help close the defect. Improvement of fecal incontinence is caused by passive increase of the resistance of the anal canal by the bulk of the encircling muscle (Fig. 28.5).

Experimental efforts to improve the efficacy of this procedure have focused on developing resting tone in the transposed muscle through the use of an implanted neurostimulator. The intent of the stimulated graciloplasty is to convert the fast-twitch muscle fibers into slow-twitch muscle fibers, which are more fatigue resistant. Initially, implantation of the pacemaker was performed at 6 weeks after the graciloplasty, but now most are performed concomitantly. Stimulation can be applied directly to the obturator nerve or intramuscularly to the nerve branches inside the muscle. The muscle is stimulated at a cyclic frequency, with gradual increases every 2 weeks. After 2 months, continuous stimulation is performed. Stimulation is adjusted to maintain tonic contraction around the anus, and it is interrupted or turned off to defecate.

Efficacy

An exhaustive review of the published literature identified 37 articles on patients undergoing dynamic graciloplasty (134). Most of these articles were case series, and there were no randomized trials or cohort studies evaluating safety and efficacy. Mortality rate was 1% (range

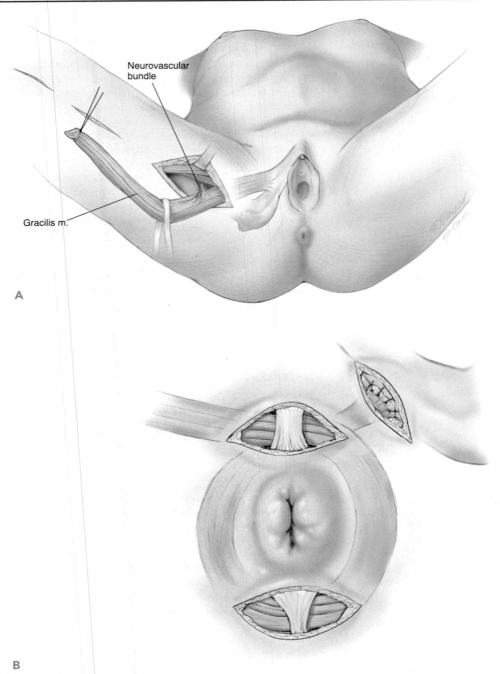

Figure 28.5 **Graciloplasty.** **A:** The gracilis muscle is identified and mobilized toward its insertion onto the medial aspect of the tibia where the tendon is divided. **B:** Anterior and posterior perianal incision are made approximately 1.5 cm from the anal verge. The muscle is then tunneled around the extrasphincteric space circumferentially. The distal tendon is passed behind the muscle and anchored to the contralateral periosteum of the ischium.

0%–13%; 95% CI, 1%–3%) after excluding cancer deaths. There was a high rate of morbidity (1.12 events per patient). Most patients will have at least one adverse event, and several will have multiple complications. There is also a very high reoperation rate. The most common complications were infections (28%), stimulator and lead faults (15%), and leg pain (13%). Satisfactory continence was achieved 42% to 85% of the time, although satisfaction was not defined consistently across studies. The authors concluded that dynamic graciloplasty appeared to have equal or better efficacy than colostomy but carried a higher morbidity rate. Another review of

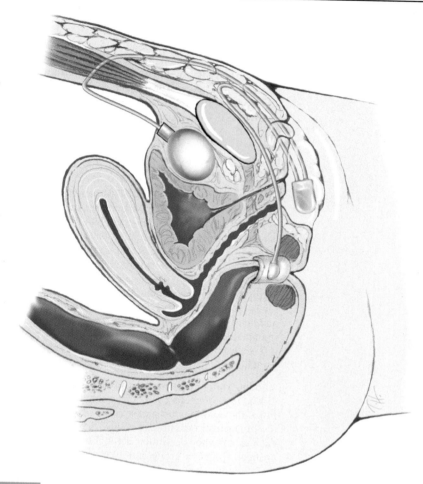

Figure 28.6 **Acticon® Neosphincter.** This device includes an inflatable cuff placed around the anal canal, a balloon reservoir stored behind the pubic bone, and a pump located in the labia. (Courtesy of American Medical Systems, Inc. Minnetonka, Minnesota, www.AmericanMedicalSystems.com.)

the three largest case series found success rates ranging from 55% to 78% (135–137). Major infections were found in 13% to 29%, pain in 27% to 28%, and device or lead problems in 12% to 18%. More recent series containing large numbers of patients found similar results for efficacy, morbidity, and reoperation rate (138,139). High rates of disturbed evacuation also were reported.

Artificial Sphincter

The artificial anal sphincter is an alternative to a graciloplasty. This is a modification of the device originally designed to treat urinary incontinence. The current device is the Acticon® Neosphincter (American Medical Systems, Minnetonka, Minnesota) (Fig. 28.6). The indications for its use are similar to those for the graciloplasty.

Technique

Implantation of the artificial anal sphincter is performed, similar to the graciloplasty, through perianal tunnels. A silastic inflatable cuff is placed around the native sphincter to occlude the anal canal. A pressure-regulating balloon containing radio-opaque solution is situated in the retropubic space, and a control pump is positioned in the labia majora. Activation of the control pump deflates the cuff, permitting defecation (Fig. 28.6).

Efficacy

An extensive review of the literature summarized 13 case series and one case report from 1996 to 2003. There were no randomized trials or cohort studies (140). The largest series consisted of 112 patients (141). There was one series with 53 patients, and all others had fewer than 28 patients each (142). Explantation was required in 17% to 41% of patients. Reasons for explantation included infection, erosion, device malfunction, pain, incontinence, and dissatisfaction, with infection being the most common. Surgical revision was necessary in 13% to 50% of the reports. Almost everyone had at least one adverse event, and more than one-third of these events required surgical intervention. Reasons for surgical revision were similar to those for explantation. Rates of fecal impaction ranged from 6% to 83%. All studies recorded statistically and clinically significant improvement in continence scores for patients with a functional artificial sphincter; however, most did not report the continence status for those in whom the device was explanted. The proportion of patients with a functional device ranged from 49% to 85%. The authors concluded that there is insufficient evidence on the safety and effectiveness of the artificial sphincter for fecal incontinence.

One randomized control trial of 14 patients compared an artificial sphincter with a program of supportive care (143). Supportive care included all aspects of conservative management, such as physiotherapy, dietary advice, pharmacotherapy, and advice regarding skin care, odor management, anxiety reduction, and use of incontinence aids or appliances. Significant improvements in continence scores and quality-of-life measures were seen in the artificial sphincter group but not in the control group at 6 months follow-up. Explantation rate was 14% (one of seven patients). Two other patients had complications, including severe fecal impaction and perineal wound erosion requiring reoperation. The authors conclude that the **artificial sphincter is safe and effective compared with supportive care alone.** They anticipate perioperative and late complications, which may require explantation in up to one-third of patients. It is also remarkable that only one patient (14%) whose condition was managed conservatively had significant improvement based on continence scores, whereas the status of all others was relatively unchanged.

Another study compared the effectiveness of artificial sphincter with dynamic graciloplasty (144). Two surgeons each performed four consecutive operations with each technique to minimize the learning curve of a new operation. Each started with a different procedure to avoid discrepancies in the time of follow-up. This prospective cohort study involved eight patients in each group who had similar demographic variables. Length of follow-up was 44 months in the artificial sphincter group and 39 months in the dynamic graciloplasty group. Early postoperative complications were similar in each group at 50%, as were late complications, with both groups reporting a high reoperation rate of 63%. There were six (75%) late complications in the artificial sphincter group, of which three (38%) were nonreversible and required explantation. Postoperative continence scores were significantly lower with the artificial sphincter than with graciloplasty. The authors conclude that **artificial sphincter has better efficacy and similar morbidity compared with dynamic graciloplasty.** The rate of late complications for the artificial sphincter exceeded that reported in the literature, which may indicate poor long-term durability. Postoperative continence scores reflect those reported for artificial sphincter but are far worse than those for dynamic graciloplasty. The authors feel that the learning curve with the artificial sphincter is less important than that with graciloplasty.

Sacral Nerve Root Stimulator

Sacral neuromodulation (InterStim®, Medtronic, Minneapolis, Minnesota) **was approved by the FDA for treatment of urinary urge incontinence in 1997 and for nonobstructive urinary retention and urgency in 1999. It has been employed experimentally for the treatment of fecal incontinence and is currently undergoing FDA approval for this intervention. In Europe, it was approved for treatment of both urinary and fecal incontinence in 1994.** The exact mechanism of action has not been fully elucidated. The goal of sacral nerve stimulation is to recruit residual function of the continence mechanism through electrical stimulation of its peripheral nerve supply. Initially, indications were confined to patients with deficient EAS and levator ani function without gross morphologic defects and intact neuromuscular connections. More recently, the acceptable indications have expanded to include deficiency of the IAS, limited structural defects, and functional deficits of the internal and external anal sphincter.

Technique

The device is instilled exactly the same way as for treatment of urinary incontinence. Current application is performed as a two-stage outpatient surgical procedure. The first stage involves instillation of the electrodes. The electrode is placed through the S2-4 foramen using minimally invasive surgical technique. During the test phase, multiple electrodes can be employed either bilaterally or at different levels to determine the site with the best response. Proper location is confirmed intraoperatively using fluoroscopy as well as visualization of an appropriate pelvic floor muscle response (bellows) with minimal plantar flexion of the first and second toes, which usually corresponds to S3 stimulation. An interval testing phase utilizes an external pulse generator that typically lasts 1 to 2 weeks. Those with a good response (decrease in fecal incontinence episodes of at least 50% documented by bowel-habit diary) will proceed to the second stage, implantation of the permanent pulse generator (IPG). Typically only one electrode is left in place at the end of the second stage. Once the permanent pulse generator is implanted, all adjustments are made using telemetry. The patient has a basic remote control that enables her to turn the device on or off and adjust the amplitude of the stimulation.

Efficacy

By the end of 2003, sacral nerve stimulation had been used to treat more than 1,300 patients with fecal incontinence (145). Despite this large number, the analysis of the results was limited to several small case series. In all studies, significant improvements in continence scores lasting up to 99 months occurred. Most patients experienced at least a 75% improvement in continence scores, and improvement also occurred in the frequency of incontinence episodes, the ability to postpone defecation, and bowel emptying. Intent-to-treat analysis revealed 80% to 100% therapeutic success. There also were significant improvements in quality-of-life measures using validated measurement scales. Complications occurred in 0% to 50% of patients, with the most common complications consisting of pain at the electrode or IPG site, electrode migration, infection, or worsening of bowel symptoms. No permanent sequelae occurred, however. Effects of anorectal physiology varied among the published studies, highlighting the fact that the precise mechanism of action remains unclear.

A Cochrane review of three crossover trials concluded that the limited data suggest improvement in both fecal incontinence and constipation with sacral nerve stimulation (146). Large multi-center trials have been conducted to evaluate the efficacy of sacral nerve stimulation for fecal incontinence. Wexner et al. prospectively followed 120 patients (110 female, 10 male) for a mean of 28 (2-70) months (147,148). Participants completed validated quality-of-life measures and bowel diaries. Success, defined as a 50% or greater improvement and reduction in fecal incontinence episodes per week, was achieved in 83% at 1 year and 85% at 2 years. Forty-one percent achieved total continence at 1 year, and mean incontinent episodes decreased from 9.4 to 1.9 per week. The same group reported an overall 10.8% infection rate (13/120), with nine occurring within the first month and four occurring after 1 year. Among the early infections, five responded to antibiotics, one resolved spontaneously, and three were treated surgically. For the late infections, all four had to be removed. Another large multicenter study of 200 patients revealed decreased severity scores and improved quality of life with sacral nerve stimulation (149). Loose stool consistency and low stimulation intensity were predictive of successful outcomes on multivariate analysis. Ultrasound findings, manometry, age and gender did not impact outcomes. Tjandra et al. performed a randomized controlled trial of 120 participants with 1-year follow-up comparing sacral nerve stimulation to best supportive therapy consisting of pelvic floor exercises, bulking agent, and dietary manipulation (150). Fecal incontinence outcomes improved dramatically in the stimulation group, with 47% achieving complete continence. In contrast, there were no significant improvements observed in the supportive therapy group. **Thus, sacral nerve stimulation appears to be a promising new treatment for fecal incontinence with relatively limited complications. FDA approval for fecal incontinence seems likely in the near future, and the minimally invasive nature of this procedure makes it a desirable first-line surgical option.**

Therapeutic Approach to Constipation

As with fecal incontinence, it is imperative to attempt conservative management of constipation and defecatory dysfunction before performing surgery. Initial evaluation should focus on identifying any underlying systemic conditions (Table 28.1) associated with disordered defecation and optimizing treatment for these conditions. In the absence of systemic etiologies, it is reasonable to proceed with empiric, nonsurgical management, such as diet, fiber supplementation, and toileting behavior changes. Biofeedback and laxatives can be used in more severe cases. Initially, disimpaction with regular enemas or laxatives is essential if the patient

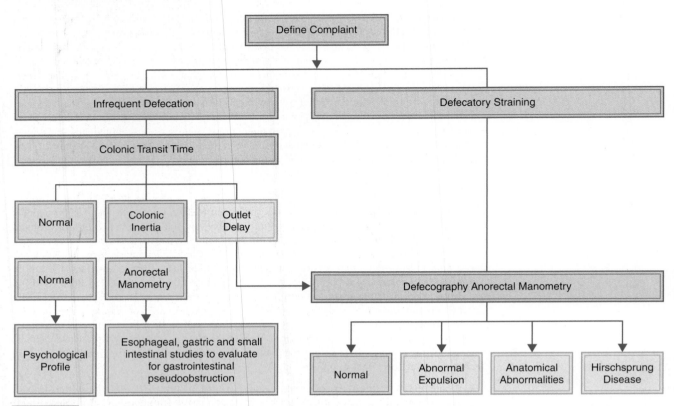

Figure 28.7   **Diagnostic Algorithm for Idiopathic Constipation.** (From **Ellerkmann MR, Kaufman H.** Defecatory dysfunction. In: **Bent AE, Ostergard DR, Cundiff GW, et al., eds.** *Ostergard's urogynecology and pelvic floor dysfunction.* 5th ed. Philadelphia, PA: Lippincott Williams & Wilkins, 2002:358, with permission.)

has fecal impaction. **Symptoms that persist despite a trial of conservative management indicate the need for further evaluation of colonic and anorectal function.** A diagnostic algorithm for idiopathic (nonsystemic) constipation is given in Figure 28.7. Treatment should then be tailored to the underlying cause. Some conditions associated with disordered defecation are best treated using nonsurgical techniques, whereas others may benefit from surgery once conservative management has failed. As with fecal incontinence, the lack of consistent outcome measures in the published literature makes it difficult to compare efficacy among treatments.

Nonsurgical Treatment

Nonsurgical management focuses on maximizing anorectal function through alteration of stool characteristics or behavioral modification. Stool consistency and volume can be manipulated by dietary and pharmacologic means to achieve passage of one stool every day or every other day. Additionally, behavior modification can be employed using regular toileting to prevent fecal impaction. Physical therapy and biofeedback can also be useful for coordinating pelvic floor and anal sphincter relaxation with defecation.

Pharmacologic Approaches

Dietary Modification and Fiber

The role of increased fluid and fiber intake for the treatment of constipation is controversial. It has been a commonly accepted belief that constipation is caused by low fluid intake and can be improved by increasing consumption. Several studies showed no association between fluid intake and constipation (151–153). However, one large study of 21,012 nursing home residents found a weak association between decreased fluid intake and constipation with an odds ratio of 1.49 (154). In one interventional study, increased fluid intake failed to improve stool frequency, consistency, or defecatory dysfunction in children (155). Another interventional study using fiber and mineral water displayed an increase in stool frequency and a decrease in laxative use in adults with constipation (156). This study lacked baseline data collection resulting in recall bias, and the use of mineral water containing magnesium may confound the results because of its mild laxative effect. Overall, the existing data do not support increased fluid intake to treat constipation unless there is evidence of dehydration (151).

The addition of fiber may decrease constipation through several mechanisms. Fiber acts as a stool bulking agent and improves stool consistency through water absorption. It can also act as a substrate for bacterial proliferation and gas production. These mechanisms of action are believed to result in increased colonic motility, decreased transit time, and increased stool frequency.

Fiber therapy appears to have a beneficial effect in the treatment of diverticular disease, constipation of pregnancy, and possibly IBS (19,157,158). Its efficacy for idiopathic (nonsystemic) constipation remains uncertain. Dietary fiber intake for patients with constipation was similar to that of controls in several studies (152,153). A meta-analysis of 36 randomized trials using laxatives or fiber therapy for the treatment of constipation showed that the use of fiber or laxatives resulted in increased stool frequency and improved symptoms without the presence of severe side effects (159). Conversely, another meta-analysis showed an inability to restore transit time and stool weight in constipated patients using dietary fiber (158). Approximately half of the patients in another study responded to fiber treatment, but a much better response occurred in patients without an identifiable structural or motility disorder (160). Consequently, a low-fiber diet may be a contributing factor in chronic constipation, and an empiric trial of fiber therapy can be expected to help some patients. Side effects of increased gas production may limit compliance with treatment, so doses should be slowly titrated. Fiber therapy should be avoided in patients with impaction, megacolon or megarectum, or obstructive gastrointestinal lesions. Fiber therapy should also be used with caution in patients with cognitive dysfunction (dementia), difficulty with ambulation, and underlying neurogenic disease for fear of worsening the condition. There is no evidence to substantiate the recommendation for extra water intake with fiber supplements (161).

Laxatives

Laxatives are commonly used to treat constipation and disordered defecation. Many classes of laxatives are available over the counter.

Bulk-Forming Laxatives   These come in natural forms (*psyllium*) as well as synthetic form (*Metamucil, Konsyl, Citrucel*) and are felt to be the safest laxatives. They have mechanisms of action and side effects similar to that of fiber (162).

Hyperosmolar Laxatives   These consist of poorly absorbed substances that increase intraluminal osmolarity and water absorption. This action results in greater stool volume with decreased consistency. Examples include nonabsorbable sugars (*lactulose* and *sorbitol*), *glycerin*, and *polyethylene glycol* (*GoLytely, MiraLAX*). *Polyethylene glycol* is a common preoperative bowel preparation. Side effects are diarrhea, increased flatus, and abdominal cramping (162).

Emollient Laxatives   These agents are divided into two subsets: *docusate salts* and mineral oil. The *docusate salts* have hydrophilic and hydrophobic properties similar to detergents. They soften stool and decrease surface tension by increasing stool water and lipid content. Examples include *docusate calcium* (*Surfak*), *docusate potassium* (*Dialose, Kasof*), and *docusate sodium* (*Colace, Comfolax*). They also improve the absorption of other laxatives and are combined in preparations with stimulant laxatives such as *Correctol, Peri-Colace,* and *Feen-a-Mint.* The limited absorption of mineral oil allows it to penetrate and soften the stool. It can be used orally or rectally. Prolonged daily use can lead to decreased absorption of the fat-soluble vitamins A, D, E, and K. Use of mineral oil should be avoided in elderly and debilitated patients, as well as in those with esophageal motility disorders because of the potential for aspiration pneumonia. Side effects include diarrhea, anal leakage, and pruritus ani (162–164).

Saline Laxatives   These usually contain magnesium cations and phosphate anions that are relatively nonabsorbable and produce an osmotic gradient with increased water absorption. They also stimulate intestinal motility by increasing cholecystokinin release. Fast-acting effects can be seen with both oral (2–6 hours) and rectal (15 minutes) preparations. Examples include *magnesium citrate, magnesium hydroxide* (*Milk of Magnesia*), *magnesium sulfate, sodium phosphate,* and *biphosphate* (*Phospho-soda, Fleet enema*). Although generally well tolerated, electrolyte abnormalities can occur. These side effects should be avoided in patients with renal insufficiency because of the potential for magnesium toxicity (162–164).

Stimulant Laxatives   These are found in three basic types: *castor oil,* anthraquinones, and diphenylmethanes. A metabolite of *castor oil, ricinoleic acid,* increases intestinal motility and secretion. Anthraquinones (*cascara sagrada, senna* [*Senokot*], *casanthranol* [*aloe*], and *danthron*) are absorbed by the small intestine and stimulate motility by increasing intraluminal fluid and electrolyte content. Diphenylmethanes (*phenolphthaleins* [*Feen-a-Mint, Correctol*] and *bisacodyl* [*Dulcolax*]) have a mechanism of action similar to anthraquinones. These agents are potent and are intended for short-term use in cases refractory to bulk or osmotic laxatives. It has been a long-standing belief that prolonged use can lead to a dilated atonic colon known as cathartic colon syndrome, melanosis coli, or neuronal degeneration. A recent article refutes the theory that stimulant laxatives damage the autonomic nervous system when used at recommended doses (151). Other side effects include cramping, nausea, and abdominal pain (162–164).

Prokinetic Agents

Medications that stimulate gastrointestinal motility primarily through neuromodulation of acetycholine levels include *metoclopramide, cisapride,* cholinergic agonists (*bethanechol*), cholinesterase inhibitors (*neostigmine*), and serotonin agonists. Their efficacy in the treatment of chronic idiopathic constipation is uncertain. *Metoclopramide* is better for upper gastrointestinal motility disorders, whereas *cisapride* appears to exert its effect at the level of the colon (162–164).

Behavioral Approaches

Behavioral techniques such as **biofeedback** and **bowel regimens** may have a role in certain conditions associated with constipation and defecatory dysfunction. Overall, these approaches have far less application to disordered defecation than to fecal incontinence. **Biofeedback is important in the treatment of dyssynergic defecation. Relaxation techniques and behavioral modification may be helpful for IBS. Bowel regimens in conjunction with laxatives, suppositories, and enemas can facilitate emptying by optimizing the gastrocolic reflex and increased peristaltic activity.**

Efficacy of Nonsurgical Treatment

Irritable Bowel Syndrome

The most commonly used first-line treatment for the constipation variant of IBS is fiber supplementation and osmotic laxatives. The efficacy of bulking agents for this condition is controversial, and many studies, including meta-analyses, exhibit an effect similar to placebo. There may be benefit to the use of fiber because of the high placebo effect with IBS treatment and lack of serious adverse events associated with its use. However, patients may experience exacerbation of bloating and abdominal discomfort with fiber therapy. Randomized trials and meta-analysis revealed a beneficial effect of *polyethylene glycol* (*MiraLAX*) over placebo for the treatment of chronic constipation. In addition, *polyethylene glycol* was better than *tegaserod* and *lactulose* for chronic constipation (165–167). They can be useful as adjunctive treatment options, but can also exacerbate abdominal pain and discomfort. A newer class of drugs, serotonin 5HT4 agonist *tegaserod* (*Zelnorm*), stimulates peristalsis, increases colonic motility, decreases intestinal transit times, and reduces visceral hypersensitivity. The recommended dose is 6 mg twice daily. Randomized trials have consistently shown an approximately 10% greater improvement in global IBS symptoms when compared with placebo. Improvement in the bloating and pain symptoms also occurred. No episodes of ischemic colitis or cardiac toxicity have been reported with the use of this medication, and the most common side effects are diarrhea and headache. *Cisapride,* a 5HT4 agonist with partial 5HT3 antagonist actions, has been withdrawn from use secondary to rare cardiac toxicity. Additional 5HT4 agonists, 5HT3 agonists, and cholecystokinin antagonists are in development (95,96).

Colonic Inertia and Slow-Transit Constipation

Patients with slow-transit constipation tend to respond poorly to fiber supplementation, although most have already tried an empiric trial of fiber before testing to confirm the diagnosis (160). Some patients may benefit from regular toileting, either in the morning or after meals when there is increased colonic motor activity. Biofeedback may have modest short-term benefits, but the long-term effect is questionable (168). Enemas and suppositories can be used in conjunction with bowel regimens. It is also reasonable to attempt a trial of any of the laxatives listed in Table 28.10. Stimulant laxatives are commonly used, but questions remain about the development

Table 28.10 Laxatives for the Treatment of Disordered Defecation			
Type of Laxative	*Adult Dose*	*Onset of Action*	*Side Effects*
Bulk-Forming Laxatives			
Natural (*psyllium*)	7 g PO	12–72 h	Impaction above strictures
Synthetic (*methylcellulose*)	4–6 g PO	12–72 h	Fluid overload
Emollient Laxatives			
Docusate salts	50–500 mg PO	24–72 h	Skin rashes
Mineral oil	15–45 mL PO	6–8 h	Decreased vitamin absorption
			Lipid pneumonia
Hyperosmolar Laxatives			
Polyethylene glycol	3–22 L PO	1 h	Abdominal bloating
Lactulose	15–60 mL PO	24–48 h	Abdominal bloating
Sorbitol	120 mL 25% solution PO	24–48 h	Abdominal bloating
Glycerine	3 g suppository	15–60 min	Rectal irritation
	5–15 mL enema	15–30 min	Rectal irritation
Saline Laxatives			
Magnesium sulfate	15 g PO	0.5–3 h	Magnesium toxicity
Magnesium phosphate	10 g PO	0.5–3 h	
Magnesium citrate	200 mL PO	0.5–3 h	
Stimulant Laxatives			
Castor oil	15–60 mL PO	2–6 h	Nutrient malabsorption
Diphenylmethanes			
Phenolphthalein	60–100 mg PO	6–8 h	Skin rashes
Bisacodyl	30 mg PO	6–10 h	Gastric irritation
	10 mg PR	0.25–1 h	Rectal stimulation
Anthraquinones			
Cascara sagrada	1 mL PO	6–12 h	Melanosis coli
Senna	2 mL PO	6–12 h	Degeneration of Meissner and Auerbach plexuses
Aloe (Casanthrol)	250 mg PO	6–12 h	
Danthron	75–150 mg PO	6–12 h	Hepatotoxicity (w/*docusate*)

PO, by mouth; PR, per rectum.
From **Wald A.** Approach to the patient with constipation. In: **Yamada T, ed.** *Textbook of gastroenterology.* 3rd ed. Philadelphia, PA: Lippincott Williams & Wilkins, 1999:921, with permission.

of neuronal degeneration with prolonged usage. It is imperative that patients adhere to and not exceed the recommended dosages. Data regarding laxative use for this condition have failed to show a significantly better response than placebo. Prokinetic agents are intuitively the ideal choice to stimulate colonic motility. Currently there is only one available prokinetic agent, *tegaserod*, approved for the treatment of constipation that improves colonic transit. Its data are almost entirely based on treatment of IBS, and there is a lack of information for its use in slow-transit constipation. Other prokinetic agents in various stages of testing include *bethanechol, neostigmine, cholecystokinin antagonists, misoprostol, colchicine, neurotrophin-3,* and other 5HT4 agonists such as *prucalopride* and *mosapride* (49).

Dyssynergic Defecation

As with slow-transit constipation, initial management using bowel regimens, laxatives, enemas, suppositories, and fiber supplementation is appropriate for patients with dyssynergic defecation, yet many will have already tried conservative management before undergoing testing to confirm the diagnosis. These treatments are relatively well tolerated with few serious side effects. They have not been shown to have greater efficacy when compared with placebo, and their role in the treatment of dyssynergic defecation remains uncertain. Specific treatment for this condition tends to focus on biofeedback because of studies indicating that this is an acquired behavioral disorder of defecation. Modalities such as diaphragmatic muscle training, simulated defecation, and manometric or electromyography-guided anal sphincter and pelvic muscle relaxation have been employed independently or combined with other techniques. These techniques have yielded symptomatic improvement in approximately 60% to 80% of patients. Many patients with dyssynergic defecation also have abnormal rectal sensation, so rectal sensory conditioning may provide additional benefit (33,49,169,170). Others have tried *botulinum toxin* injections to paralyze the puborectalis and anal sphincter muscle. Small case series have shown modest early improvement, but the results do not appear to be long lasting (171,172). A recent randomized trial of 48 participants comparing *botulinum toxin* to biofeedback retraining found better initial improvement with the *botulinum toxin* (70% vs. 50%) but no difference at 1 year (33% vs. 25%) (173).

Pessary for Treatment of Pelvic Organ Prolapse

Pessaries of various shapes and sizes have been used for centuries to treat pelvic organ prolapse (174). **They are a safe alternative to surgery, with the most common complications being increased vaginal discharge and erosion or ulceration of the vaginal wall.** Although pessaries represent a common therapeutic modality, there are limited data regarding fitting and management (175). Even less is known about which type of pessary is better for enteroceles and rectoceles, although the site of prolapse does not appear to affect the ability to retain a pessary (176). Pessaries can be divided into subtypes of supportive and space occupying (177). Some of the space-occupying pessaries, such as the Gellhorn and cube, use a suction mechanism to maintain vaginal retention, whereas others, like the donut, do not. In theory, space-occupying pessaries and those that exert forces against the posterior wall and vaginal apex (donut, inverted Gehrung) should aid in treatment of rectoceles and enteroceles. However, there are few data regarding the efficacy of pessaries for relieving symptoms of disordered defecation. One prospective study found that stage III or IV posterior vaginal wall prolapse was an independent predictor for discontinuation of pessary use in favor of surgical repair (178). The only randomized crossover trial comparing different types of pessaries (ring and Gelhorn) found improvement in quality-of-life measures with each pessary that did not differ. Protrusion and voiding dysfunction symptoms were most improved (179). More research is needed to determine the role of pessaries for treatment of rectoceles and enteroceles as well as symptoms that are likely to be improved using a pessary.

Surgical Treatment

Following is a review of the efficacy of various surgical treatments for specific conditions associated with constipation and disordered defecation.

Slow Transit/Colonic Inertia

Subtotal colectomy with ileosigmoid or ileorectal anastomosis is considered by many to be the surgical treatment of choice for slow-transit constipation refractory to medical management. Most surgeons restrict the use of this surgical procedure to the most extreme cases and typically operate on fewer than 10% of patients. Strict criteria for surgery include the following: chronic, severe, disabling symptoms unresponsive to medical therapy; slow transit in the proximal colon; no evidence of pseudo-obstruction; and normal anorectal function (162). Success rates are variable and depend on several factors. An extensive review of colectomy for slow-transit constipation analyzed 32 studies from 1981 to 1988 and found satisfaction rates ranged from 39% to 100% (180). Higher success rates occurred in studies in the United States (n = 11, median 94%, range 75%–100%) and prospective studies (n = 16, median 90%, range 50%–100%). Superior outcomes occurred in those who had a complete physiologic evaluation and proven slow-transit constipation. Patients with anismus had higher rates of recurrent symptoms and lower satisfaction levels (181). Poorer outcomes occurred with ileosigmoid and cecorectal anastomosis than with ileorectal anastomosis. Those with segmental resection (hemi-colectomy) had the worst outcome. None of the studies had a comparison group, and outcomes were variable and lacking validated measures. Morbidity associated with the operation included small bowel obstruction (median 18%, range 2%–71%), need for reoperation (median 14%, range 0%–50%), diarrhea (median 14%, range 0%–46%), fecal incontinence (median 14%, range 0%–52%), recurrent constipation (median 9%, range 0%–33%), persistent abdominal pain (median 41%, range 0%–90%), and permanent ileostomy (median 5%, range 0%–28%). Mortality ranged from 0%–6% (182). A quality-of-life study revealed that the score correlated poorly with frequency of bowel movements. However, a lower score was seen in those patients who had persistent abdominal pain, diarrhea, fecal incontinence, and permanent ileostomies. Overall satisfaction with the procedure was very high and correlated with the quality-of-life score (183).

Surgical alternatives to subtotal colectomy include ileostomy, cecostomy with antegrade continence enemas, and sacral nerve stimulation. Subtotal colectomy has never been directly compared with ileostomy, but those who had a permanent diversion after subtotal colectomy had lower quality-of-life scores. Patients undergoing cecostomy with antegrade continence enemas can expect to have satisfactory function approximately half of the time, with most requiring additional revision procedures secondary to stomal complications (184). Although sacral nerve stimulation has primarily been used for fecal incontinence, the results of a few small studies evoke optimism for its use in chronic constipation and slow-transit constipation (146,185–187).

Pelvic Organ Prolapse

The variety of surgical treatment techniques for the repair of rectocele include posterior colporrhaphy, defect-directed repair, posterior fascial replacement, transanal repair, and abdominal repair with sacral colpopexy. When an enterocele is present, a culdoplasty is usually performed. In cases of perineal descent, abdominal sacral colpoperineopexy is the procedure of choice. Suture rectopexy can be performed in conjunction with sacral colpoperineopexy if rectal prolapse is present. Despite the routine use of these procedures, data are limited regarding symptomatic improvement of disordered defecation. Greater detail regarding the specific techniques for many of these procedures is provided in Chapter 27 This section will focus on surgical outcomes, including anatomic cure of prolapse, improvement of defecatory dysfunction symptoms, and morbidity associated with the procedure.

Posterior Colporrhaphy

Posterior colporrhaphy has been the surgical procedure for rectocele repair preferred by gynecologic surgeons for more than 100 years. Traditional posterior colporrhaphy narrows the vaginal caliber through plication of the rectovaginal septum and usually includes a perineorrhaphy, which narrows the introitus. Despite it broad use, there are few data regarding long-term anatomic success, symptomatic improvement, and sexual function following the procedure. The outcomes of several studies are summarized in Table 28.11 (189–207). Anatomic cure and relief of vaginal bulge occurred in 76% to 96% of patients. In these studies, the procedure was ineffective at treating constipation, vaginal digitations (splinting), and fecal incontinence. Dyspareunia developed in 8% to 26% of patients with and without levator plication (188–192,207). As early as 1961, high rates of dyspareunia have been reported with this procedure in as many as 50% of patients (208).

Many feel that the successful anatomic support obtained with this procedure is offset by the modest relief of functional symptoms and high rate of *de novo* dyspareunia. However, a recent prospective case series of 38 women undergoing posterior colporrhaphy along with concomitant procedures for rectocele and obstructed defecation revealed markedly different results (209). Fascial plication was performed without levator plication, and perineal body reconstruction rather than routine perineorrhaphy was employed when indicated. Anatomic cure rate was 87% at 12 months and 79% at 24 months. Subjective cure rate was 97% at 12 months and 89% at 24 months. There was significant improvement in preoperative and postoperative symptoms for constipation (76% vs. 24%), digitations (100% vs. 16%), awareness of prolapse (100% vs. 5%), obstructed defecation (100% vs. 13%), and dyspareunia (37% vs. 5%). There was no difference in fecal incontinence and only one case of *de novo* dyspareunia. The authors attribute their improved anatomic and functional outcomes and combined improvement in dyspareunia to exclusion of levator plication, perineorrhaphy, and excision of vaginal epithelium. An additional benefit may be derived during mobilization of the vaginal epithelium, when scar tissue from prior episiotomy or surgery is divided. They also found that preoperative defecating proctography was

Table 28.11 Rectocele Repairs

Posterior Colporrhaphy

	Arnold (189)		Mellgren (190)[a]		Kahn (191)		Weber (192)[a]		Sand (193)[a]	
	Preop	Postop	Preop	Postop	Preop	Postop	Preop	Postop	Preop	Postop
N	29		25	25	231	171	53	53	70	67
Follow-up (mean) months				12		42		12		12
Levator plication		Yes		Yes		Yes		No		No
Anatomical cure (%)		80		96		76				90
Constipation (%)	75	54	100	88	22	33				
Protrusion (%)			21	4	64	31				
Splinting/digitations (%)	20		50	0		33				
Fecal incontinence (%)		36	8	8	4	11				
De novo dyspareunia[b] (%)		23		8		16		26		

Defect-Directed Repair

	Cundiff (194)		Porter (195)		Kenton (196)		Glavind (197)		Singh (198)[a]	
	Preop	Postop	Preop	Postop	Preop	Postop	Preop	Postop	Preop	Postop
N	69	61	125	72	66	46	67	67	42	33
Follow-up (mean) months		12		6		12		3		18
Anatomic cure		82		82		90		100		92
Constipation (%)	46	13	60	50	41	57				
Difficult defecation	32	15	61	44	53	46	40	4	57	27
Protrusion (%)	100	18	38	14	86	9			78	7
Splinting/digitations (%)	39	25	24	14	30	15				
Fecal incontinence (%)	13	8	24	21	30				9	5
Dyspareunia (%)	29	19	67	46	28	8	12	3	31	15
De novo dyspareunia[b] (%)		2		4		7		3		0

Repairs with Grafts

	Oster (199)		Sand (193)[a]		Goh (200)[a]		Kohli (201)		Mercer-Jones (202)[a]	
	Preop	Postop	Preop	Postop	Preop	Postop	Preop	Postop	Preop	Postop
Graft route	Autologous Transvaginal		Polygalactin mesh Transvaginal		Polypropylene Transvaginal		Porcine dermis Transvaginal		Polypropylene Transperineal	
N	15	15	73	65	43	43	43	30	22	22
Follow-up (mean) months		30		12		12		12		12
Anatomic cure		100		92		100		93		95
Constipation (%)		33							50	14
Difficult defecation	47	0							95	32
Protrusion (%)	80	0			100	0			86	23
Splinting/digitations (%)	100	12							64	23
Fecal incontinence (%)										5
Dyspareunia (%)		20								

(continued)

Table 28.11 (*Continued*)

Transanal Repair

	Sullivan (203)		Sehapavak (204)		Jenssen (205)[a]		Van Dam (206)[a,c]		Ayabaca (207)[a]	
	Preop	*Postop*	*Preop*	*Postop*	*Preop*	*Postop*	*Preop*	*Postop*	*Preopv*	*Postop*
N	137	117	355	204	64	64	89	89	49	34
Follow-up (mean) months		18				12		52		48
Anatomic cure		96		98		70		72		90
Constipation (%)			82	15			63	33	83	32
Difficult defecation	58	2			72	16	92	27		
Protrusion (%)	27				38	3	40	28		
Splinting/digitations (%)			26		26	4	23	0	38	
Fecal incontinence (%)	39	3			40	9	10	16	71	27
Dyspareunia (%)		0		20			28	44		

[a]Prospective.
[b]In sexually active patients.
[c]Combined transanal and transvaginal repair.

of limited value and have stopped its routine use as part of the preoperative evaluation for women with symptomatic rectoceles and obstructive defecation.

Defect-Directed Repair

The goal of a defect-directed repair or site-specific repair is to restore normal anatomy (36). This procedure can be combined with a perineal body reconstruction, if necessary, but usually does not routinely involve perineorrhaphy. Table 28.11 lists the anatomic and functional outcomes for this type of repair. **Anatomic cure rates range from 82% to 100%, which are similar to those for posterior colporrhaphy. This procedure also resulted in modest improvement for symptoms of difficult evacuation, vaginal bulge, and vaginal digitations, which appear to be slightly better than for posterior colporrhaphy** (193–197,207). Constipation symptoms significantly decreased in only one study (193). All studies reported low rates of *de novo* dyspareunia with good functional and anatomic outcomes, but the long-term durability of the procedure is unknown. All but one of these studies included concomitant prolapse and urinary incontinence procedures.

A randomized clinical trial of 106 women with stage II or greater posterior vaginal wall prolapse compared posterior colporrhaphy, defect-directed rectocele repair, and defect-directed repair augmented with a porcine small intestinal submucosal (210). Participants completed validated pelvic floor instruments at baseline and 6 months, 1 year, and 2 years after surgery. Anatomic failure was defined as POP-Q system point Bp greater than or equal to -2 at 1 year. There was a significant improvement in prolapse and colorectal scales in all groups with no differences between groups. The proportion of subjects with functional failures was 15% overall and not significantly different between groups. Posterior colporrhaphy and defect-directed repairs resulted in similar anatomic and functional outcomes, although the addition of a porcine-derived graft did not improve anatomic outcomes. On average, all bowel symptoms evaluated were significantly improved 1 year after surgery, with no differences between treatment groups. The development of new "bothersome" bowel symptoms after surgery was uncommon (11%). After controlling for age, treatment group, comorbidities, and preoperative bowel symptoms, corrected postoperative vaginal support (stage 0 or I) was associated with a reduced risk of postoperative straining (adjusted OR 0.17; 95% CI, 0.03–0.9) and feeling of incomplete emptying (adjusted OR 0.1; 95% CI, 0.01–0.52). This led the authors to conclude that resolution or improvement in bowel symptoms can be expected in the majority of women after rectocele repair (211).

Transanal Repair

Transanal repair involves repair of the rectocele through a transanal incision with excision of redundant rectal mucosa and plication of the rectovaginal septum and rectal wall. The

procedure was developed and is primarily used by colorectal surgeons to treat constipation or obstructed defecation associated with "low" or distal rectoceles. The advantages of this approach include excision of redundant rectal mucosa and the ability to treat other anorectal pathology, such as hemorrhoids or anterior rectal wall prolapse (212). Disadvantages include the inability to repair higher rectoceles, enteroceles, cystoceles, uterine prolapse, and defects in the perineal body or anal sphincter (213). Major complications of infection (6%) and rectovaginal fistula (3%) are relatively rare (203). Most studies did not require vaginal bulging or protrusion symptoms as a prerequisite for surgery. The results of several studies are summarized in Table 28.11. The anatomic cure rate was 70% to 98%, and symptoms of constipation, difficult evacuation, and vaginal digitations appear to improve (202–207).

Recent reviews have compared transanal with transvaginal rectocele repair using the results of two small, randomized control trials (214–217). Women with compromised sphincter function and other symptomatic prolapse were excluded. **The results for transvaginal repair were superior to those for transanal repair with respect to subjective failure rate** (relative risk [RR] 0.36; 95% CI, 0.13–1.0) and objective failure rate (RR 0.24; 95% CI, 0.09–0.64) (214). In one study, a significant decrease occurred in the depth of rectocele on postoperative defecography for the transvaginal group compared with the transanal group (2.73 vs. 4.13 cm, respectively) (217). The transvaginal group had fewer problems with bowel evacuation, but this finding was not statistically significant. In one study, researchers discovered that 38% of patients developed fecal incontinence following transanal repair (188). In the two randomized trials, no significant differences were seen in the rate of fecal incontinence or dyspareunia, but the studies were underpowered to detect a difference (216,217). **Although a vaginal approach has been considered superior to a transanal approach for rectocele repair, studies are retrospective and impossible to compare because the indications for transanal repairs are generally different from those for transvaginal repairs.** A prospective, randomized trial with adequate power to evaluate symptomatic outcomes of bowel and sexual function along with anatomic cure is warranted.

Posterior Fascial Reinforcement

Rectocele repair with graft augmentation is becoming more common, despite a paucity of supporting evidence indicating its benefits over standard procedures. The reason for its emergence is the theory that vaginal hernia repairs behave similar to abdominal hernia repairs, which have a documented decrease in recurrence when augmented with grafts. A variety of graft materials have been employed with posterior colporrhaphy and defect-directed repairs including autograft, allograft, xenograft, and synthetic mesh. There are no comparison data to aid in selecting the optimal graft. The purpose of the graft is debatable. It can either be intended to replace existing fascia as a permanent barrier or to provide an absorbable scaffold for collagen deposition, scar formation, and remodeling. The ideal material should have a low erosion rate, be relatively inexpensive, and decrease recurrence rates without causing bowel or sexual dysfunction. The outcomes for rectocele repair using graft materials placed either vaginally or abdominally appear in Table 28.11. High anatomic cure rates of 89% to 100% occurred, and symptoms of constipation, difficult evacuation, and vaginal bulge also appeared to improve.

One randomized trial used absorbable vaginal mesh for rectocele repair (192). Patients were randomly assigned to fascial replacement with polyglactin 910 mesh at the time of anterior and posterior colporrhaphy. There were no differences in recurrence rates when comparing 70 women with a traditional colpoperineorrhaphy with 73 women having a traditional repair plus mesh: 10% versus 8%, respectively. This study did not describe changes in bowel or sexual function, and there were no mesh-related adverse events. As previously noted, the randomized controlled trial comparing posterior colporrhaphy, defect-directed repair, and defect-directed repair with porcine small intestine submucosal graft augmentation revealed higher anatomical failure rates in the graft-augmented group compared to the site-specific alone or the posterior colporrhaphy group (46% vs. 22% and 14%, respectively; $P = .02$), with no difference in symptom outcomes (210). Importantly, the risks of vaginal mesh erosion and severe complications may be relatively low but carry significant morbidity, including rectovaginal fistula, persistent vaginal bleeding and discharge, dyspareunia, and the need for additional surgery (199,207). **Nonsynthetic grafts appear to be safer, with fewer erosions compared with synthetic grafts; however, there is no evidence to suggest that the addition of a graft to the posterior compartment improves outcomes** (210,218,219).

Abdominal Rectocele Repair

The abdominal approach to rectocele repair may be of value when a superior defect in the rectovaginal fascia occurs in a patient with accompanying enterocele, uterine prolapse, or vault prolapse. If a patient is undergoing an abdominal or laparoscopic procedure such as a sacral colpopexy, the graft can be extended along the posterior vaginal wall to correct proximal defects in the rectovaginal septum (220). There are limited data regarding the efficacy of abdominal rectocele repair. The indication for this procedure, as well as the need for additional vaginal repair of distal defects, is often determined intraoperatively. An ancillary study from the Pelvic Floor Disorders Network evaluating bowel symptoms 1 year after sacrocolpopexy found that the majority of bothersome bowel symptoms resolve after this procedure. There was no difference in postoperative bowel symptoms among those who underwent a concomitant rectocele repair and those who did not. It is important to note that the study was not developed to evaluate the impact of concomitant rectocele repair on bowel symptom resolution, and those who underwent a rectocele repair had more severe baseline bowel symptoms including worse obstructive symptom (221). ·

Sacral Colpoperineopexy for Perineal Descent

Sacral colpoperineopexy is a modification of sacral colpopexy aimed at correction of apical prolapse combined with rectocele and perineal descent (39). A continuous graft is placed from the anterior longitudinal ligament of the sacrum down to the perineal body. This procedure can be accomplished either through a total abdominal approach or a combined abdominal and vaginal procedure. **If performing a total abdominal approach, the rectovaginal space is opened, and the rectum is dissected off the posterior vaginal wall and rectovaginal septum toward the perineal body. The graft is then sutured to the perineal body or as close to it as possible.** A rectovaginal examination with the surgeon's nondominant hand facilitates this attachment by supporting the perineal body. The graft is secured to additional points along the posterior vaginal wall and apex, and sacral colpopexy is completed in the usual fashion.

If performing a combined abdominal and vaginal approach, the graft is secured to the perineal body vaginally. The posterior vaginal wall is opened, and a defect-directed rectocele repair is performed. Sacral colpopexy is accomplished in the usual fashion except that the vaginal dissection is opened superiorly, creating a window to the abdominal dissection. The graft can then be passed down from the abdominal field to the vaginal field and anchored inferiorly to the perineal body and laterally to the arcus tendineus fascia rectovaginalis (Fig. 28.8).

Short-term outcomes for 19 patients who underwent sacral colpoperineopexy indicated good anatomic results for apical and posterior support as well as for perineal descent (39). Complete cessation of defecatory dysfunction symptoms was accomplished in 66% of patients. In a report of outcomes for a slightly different variation of the sacral colpoperineopexy, the authors' technique involved attachment of Marlex mesh to the perineal body using a needle carrier (222). The failure rate was 25% and mesh erosion rate was 5% for 205 patients with up to 10-year follow-up. A study of Mersilene mesh erosion rates related to sacral colpopexy and sacral colpoperineopexy noted similar erosion rates between sacral colpopexy and colpoperineopexy when the vagina was not opened (3.2% vs. 4.5%, respectively) (223). However, the erosion rate was 16% with vaginal suture placement and 40% when the mesh was placed vaginally. The use of nonsynthetic grafts such as dermal allograft and xenograft may help prevent high erosion rates. In a case series of 11 patients, researchers performed sigmoid resection (if indicated) and suture rectopexy in conjunction with sacral colpoperineopexy using AlloDerm for women with coexistent rectal prolapse, perineal descent, and defecatory dysfunction. Early follow-up (12.5 ± 7.7 months) revealed excellent improvement of defecatory dysfunction symptoms and quality-of-life considerations, with an 82% cure of perineal descent (224). A recently published retrospective cohort of 38 women revealed high satisfaction following abdominal sacral colpoperineopexy, despite the persistence of obstructed defecation symptoms 5 years after surgery (225). **Sacral colpoperineopexy may have value for a select group of patients,** but larger prospective series with long-term anatomic and symptomatic outcomes are necessary to evaluate the durability of this procedure.

Rectal Prolapse

Numerous surgical procedures have been described for the treatment of rectal prolapse and are broadly categorized into perineal or abdominal approaches. Most surgeons prefer an abdominal procedure because of lower recurrence rates, reserving perineal procedures for more debilitated patients.

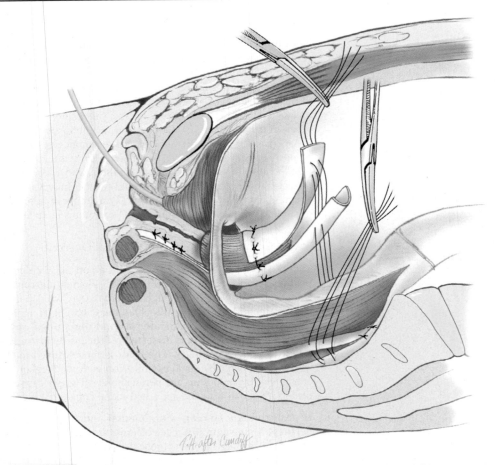

Figure 28.8 **Abdominal sacral colpoperineopexy with sigmoid resection and suture rectopexy.** This sagittal view shows the posterior graft sutured to the rectovaginal fascia and perineal body after defect-directed rectocele repair. The anterior graft is sutured to the pubocervical fascia. Both sheets will be secured to the sacral periosteum to the right of the rectum. Rectopexy sutures (*left*) have not yet been tied and secured. (Courtesy of Geoffrey W. Cundiff, M.D.)

Abdominal Procedures

Abdominal procedures vary with respect to the extent of rectal mobilization, method of rectal fixation, and inclusion or exclusion of bowel resection. During abdominal rectopexy, the mesorectal plane is developed and the rectum mobilized down to the pelvic floor posteriorly, with care taken to identify and preserve the hypogastric nerves. Division of the lateral ligaments may or may not be performed. The concern is that division of the lateral ligaments will lead to rectal denervation and increased postoperative constipation. If performing a suture rectopexy, the fascia propria of the rectum is secured to the sacral periosteum from S-1 to S-3 (226). If performing a sigmoid resection with the rectopexy (Frykman-Goldberg resection rectopexy), the bowel resection is performed after mobilization and before suturing (227). The theoretical advantages of a rectosigmoid resection are creation of a dense area of fibrosis between the anastomotic suture line and the sacrum; removal of abundant rectosigmoid, avoiding torsion or volvulus; additional fixation through straightening of the left colon and decreased mobility from the phrenocolic ligament; and relief of constipation in select patients. It is typically reserved for patients with a long redundant sigmoid colon, although specific criteria have not been proposed. Mesh rectopexies are usually avoided because of concern for increased complications and infections associated with placement of a foreign body at the time of bowel resection. There are two basic types of mesh rectopexy: **posterior mesh rectopexy** and **anterior sling rectopexy (Ripstein procedure)** (228,229). A variety of materials have been used for this procedure, including absorbable and permanent mesh. The assumption is that placement of this material will provide increased support through increased fibrous tissue formation. During the Ripstein procedure, an anterior sling of fascia lata or synthetic mesh is placed in front of the rectum and sutured to the sacrum. Most surgeons avoid this procedure because of fear of obstructed defecation. Modifications using a posterolateral wrap have been developed to resolve this problem.

In a series of more than 10 patients, there were five open series and five laparoscopic reports for suture rectopexy (230). The recurrence rates ranged between 0% and 9%. Most reports showed an improvement in fecal incontinence symptoms, but the results for constipation were variable. There were no mortalities noted and no difference between laparoscopic and open results. For posterior mesh rectopexy, there were 14 open series and five laparoscopic reports. The recurrence rates ranged between 0% and 6%. As with suture rectopexy, there was general improvement in fecal incontinence, mixed results for constipation, and no differences between laparoscopic and open outcomes. The mortality rate was between 0% and 3%, with increased rates of infection if resection rectopexy was performed. For anterior sling rectopexy (Ripstein procedure), there were eight studies with a recurrence rate between 0% and 12%. Again, there was a trend toward improvement of fecal incontinence and mixed response for constipation. Mortality ranged from 0% to 3%. For resection rectopexy (Frykman-Goldberg procedure), there were nine open series and three laparoscopic reports. Recurrence ranged between 0% and 5%. There was general improvement in continence as well as an overall reduction in constipation observed in most studies. Mortality rate was 0% for all studies but one, in which it was 6.7% (231). This study was a small, randomized trial comparing 15 patients undergoing resection rectopexy to 15 patients undergoing absorbable mesh rectopexy. The patient who died was in the resection group and had a myocardial infarction. The authors concluded that sigmoid resection did not seem to increase operative morbidity but tended to diminish postoperative constipation, possibly by causing less outlet obstruction. The study was underpowered to detect a difference in morbidity or mortality.

The laparoscopic series demonstrated similar safety and efficacy to the open techniques, and the effect on continence and constipation tended to mirror the type of rectopexy performed. **In a small, randomized trial, there were significant short-term benefits with laparoscopic rectopexy compared with open rectopexy, including earlier ambulation, more rapid return to normal diet, shorter hospital stay, and lower morbidity** (232). Most surgeons believe that there are no differences in recurrence rates between suture and mesh rectopexy. Consequently, the role of mesh in these procedures is suspect. The role of division of the lateral ligaments is somewhat controversial. A Cochrane review performed in 2008 concluded that division of the lateral ligaments was associated with less recurrent prolapse but more postoperative constipation (233). The authors acknowledged the limitations of their review, which consisted of very few trials with small sample sizes and methodological weakness. A review of seven open and four laparoscopic series involving division of the lateral ligaments revealed a general improvement in fecal incontinence and either no change or worsening of constipation (230). Conversely, there were 15 open and 4 laparoscopic series with preservation of the ligaments that displayed improved continence and a trend toward reduced constipation. This study suggests that preservation of the lateral ligaments is associated with an improvement in fecal incontinence and constipation symptoms.

Perineal Procedures

Perineal procedures are more easily tolerated because they avoid laparotomy. Thus, they are ideal for patients at high risk for perioperative and postoperative morbidity and mortality. There are basically two perineal procedures: the *Delorme procedure* and *perineal rectosigmoidectomy* (Altemeier operation). Perianal encirclement procedures such as the Thiersch procedure are not recommended because of poor success rates, high recurrence rates, and fecal impaction.

The **Delorme procedure** was first described in 1900 and involves separation of the rectal mucosa from the sphincter and muscularis propria, followed by resection of the rectal mucosa and plication of the distal rectal wall (muscularis propria) (234) (Fig. 28.9). A review of 10 series found a recurrence rate ranging between 4% and 38% and mortality rates of 0% to 4% (230). The low mortality rates are impressive considering the higher-risk population; however, the recurrence rates make it a less desirable procedure among healthy patients. There was a general improvement in fecal incontinence and constipation. Fecal incontinence (presumably indicating anal sphincter disruption or denervation), chronic diarrhea, and severe perineal descent are associated with failure of this procedure (235). The Delorme operation may be preferred in cases when

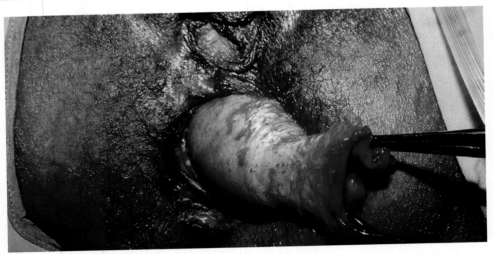

Figure 28.9   Delorme's procedure. After mucosal stripping to the full extent of the prolapse, the circular smooth muscle or the rectum is plicated. A mucosa-to-mucosa anastomosis is then performed.

the prolapsing segment is shorter than 3 to 4 cm or there is no circumferential full-thickness prolapse, making perineal rectosigmoidectomy difficult to perform (230,236).

Perineal rectosigmoidectomy (Altemeier operation) has become the perineal procedure of choice (237). Among 12 studies, performance of full thickness excision of the rectosigmoid was associated with recurrence rates from 0% to 16% and mortality rates of 0% to 5%. Patients generally have minimal pain and a relatively uneventful postoperative course. Recurrent prolapse probably reflects inadequate resection. Incontinence results are modest at best but seem to improve substantially with the addition of levatorplasty. The addition of levatorplasty also appears to decrease the short-term recurrence rate, but there is no significant change in constipation with this procedure (238). Most agree that perineal rectosigmoidectomy with levatorplasty is the best procedure for very elderly patients and those with profound comorbidity. This is the preferred approach for patients with incarcerated, strangulated, or even gangrenous prolapsed rectal segment who are not candidates for abdominal rectopexy. Although there is a general consensus that abdominal rectopexy is better than perineal rectosigmoidectomy, there is only one small, prospective, randomized controlled trial comparing these procedures. This study did not have the power to detect a difference in recurrence rates but found that patients undergoing abdominal resection rectopexy had less fecal incontinence and better physiological results than patients who had perineal rectosigmoidectomy (233,239).

References

1. **Barber MD, Bremer RE, Thor KB, et al.** Innervation of the female levator ani muscles. *Am J Obstet Gynecol* 2002;187:64–71.
2. **Harari D, Gurwitz JH, Avorn J, et al.** How do older persons define constipation? Implications for therapeutic management. *J Gen Intern Med* 1997;12:63–66.
3. **Glia A, Lindberg G.** Quality of life in patients with different types of functional constipation. *Scand J Gastroenterol* 1997;32:1083–1089.
4. **Cundiff GW, Nygaard I, Bland DR, et al.** Proceedings of the American Urogynecologic Society Multidisciplinary Symposium on Defecatory Disorders. *Am J Obstet Gynecol* 2000;182:S1–S10.
5. **Higgins PD, Johanson JF.** Epidemiology of constipation in North America: a systematic review. *Am J Gastroenterol* 2004;99:750–759.
6. **Sonnenberg A, Koch TR.** Epidemiology of constipation in the U.S. *Dis Colon Rectum* 1989;32:1–8.
7. **Drossman DA, Li Z, Andruzzi E, et al.** U.S. household survey of functional gastrointestinal disorders: prevalence, sociodemography and health impact. *Dig Dis Sci* 1993;38:1569–1580.
8. **Sonnenberg A, Koch TR.** Physician visits in the United States for constipation: 1958 to 1986. *Dig Dis Sci* 1989;34:606–611.
9. **Rantis PC Jr, Vernava AM III, Daniel GL, et al.** Chronic constipation—is the work-up worth the cost? *Dis Colon Rectum* 1997;40:280–286.
10. **Singh G, Lingala V, Wang H, et al.** Use of health care resources and cost of care for adults with constipation. *Clin Gastroenterol Hepatol* 2007;5:1053–1058.
11. **Irvine EJ, Ferrazzi S, Pare P, et al.** Health-related quality of life in functional GI disorders: focus on constipation and resource utilization. *Am J Gastroenterol* 2002;97:1986–1993.
12. **Nelson RL.** Epidemiology of fecal incontinence. *Gastroenterology* 2004;126:S3–S7.
13. **Boreham MK, Richter HE, Kenton KS, et al.** Anal incontinence in women presenting for gynecologic care: prevalence, risk factors, and impact upon quality of life. *Am J Obstet Gynecol* 2005;192:1637–1642.
14. **Dunivan GC, Heymen S, Palsson OS, et al.** Fecal incontinence in primary care: prevalence, diagnosis, and health care utilization. *Am J Obstet Gynecol* 2010;202:493.e1–e6.
15. **Wu J, Hundley AF, Fulton RG, et al.** Forecasting the prevalence of

pelvic floor disorders in U.S. Women: 2010 to 2050. *Obstet Gynecol* 2009;114:1278–1283

16. **Nelson R, Norton N, Cautley E, et al.** Community-based prevalence of anal incontinence. *JAMA* 1995;274:559–561.

17. **Johanson JF, Lafferty J.** Epidemiology of fecal incontinence: the silent affliction. *Am J Gastroenterol* 1996;91:33–36.

18. **Feldman M, Schiller LR.** Disorders of gastrointestinal motility associated with diabetes mellitus. *Ann Intern Med* 1983;98:378–384.

19. **Jewell DJ, Younge G.** Interventions for treating constipation in pregnancy. *Cochrane Database Syst Rev* 2001;2:CD001142.

20. **Bradley CS, Kennedy CM, Turcea AM, et al.** Constipation in pregnancy: prevalence, symptoms and risk factors. *Obstet Gynecol* 2007;110:1351–1357.

21. **Devroede G, Lamarche J.** Functional importance of extrinsic parasympathetic innervation to the distal colon and rectum in man. *Gastroenterology* 1974;66:273–280.

22. **Devroede G, Arhan P, Duguay C, et al.** Traumatic constipation. *Gastroenterology* 1979;77:1258–1267.

23. **Read NW, Timms JM.** Defecation and the pathophysiology of constipation. *Clin Gastroenterol* 1986;15:937–965.

24. **Glick ME, Meshkinpour H, Haldeman S, et al.** Colonic dysfunction in patients with thoracic spinal cord injury. *Gastroenterology* 1984;86:287–294.

25. **Weber J, Grise P, Roquebert M, et al.** Radiopaque markers transit and anorectal manometry in 16 patients with multiple sclerosis and urinary bladder dysfunction. *Dis Colon Rectum* 1987;30:95–100.

26. **Glick ME, Meshkinpour H, Haldeman S, et al.** Colonic dysfunction in multiple sclerosis. *Gastroenterology* 1982;83:1002–1007.

27. **Longstreth GF, Thompson WG, Chey WD, et al.** Functional bowel disorders. *Gastroenterology* 2006;130:1480–1491.

28. **Barnett JL.** Anorectal diseases. In: **Yamada T, ed.** Textbook of gastroenterology. 3rd ed. Philadelphia, PA: Lippincott Williams & Wilkins, 1999.

29. **Wald A, Tunuguntla AK.** Anorectal sensorimotor dysfunction in fecal incontinence and diabetes mellitus: modification with biofeedback therapy. *N Engl J Med* 1984;310:1282–1287.

30. **Schiller LR, Santa Ana CA, Schumulen AC, et al.** Pathogenesis of fecal incontinence in diabetes mellitus: evidence for internal-anal-sphincter dysfunction. *N Engl J Med* 1982;307:1666–1671.

31. **Harris RL, Cundiff GW.** Anal incontinence. *Postgrad Obstet Gynecol* 1997;17:1–6.

32. **Ihre T.** Studies on anal function in continent and incontinent patients. *Scand J Gastroenterol* 1974;9:1–80.

33. **Rao SS.** Dyssynergic defecation. *Gastroenterol Clin North Am* 2001;30:97–114.

34. **Rao SS, Tuteja AK, Vellema T, et al.** Dyssynergic defecation: demographics, symptoms, stool patterns, and quality of life. *J Clin Gastroenterol* 2004;38:680–685.

35. **Drossman DA.** The functional gastrointestinal disorders and the Rome III process. *Gastroenterology* 2006;130:1377–1390.

36. **Richardson AC.** The rectovaginal septum revisited: its relationship to rectocele and its importance in rectocele repair. *Clin Obstet Gynecol* 1993;36:976–982.

37. **Tulikangas PK, Walters MD, Brainard JA, et al.** Enterocele: is there a histologic defect? *Obstet Gynecol* 2001;98:634–637.

38. **Parks AG, Porter NH, Hardcastle J.** The syndrome of the descending perineum. *Proc R Soc Med* 1966;59:477–482.

39. **Henry MM, Parks AG, Swash M.** The pelvic floor musculature in the descending perineum syndrome. *Br J Surg* 1982;69:470–472.

40. **Cundiff GW, Harris RL, Coates K, et al.** Abdominal sacral colpoperineopexy: a new approach for correction of posterior compartment defects and perineal descent associated with vaginal vault prolapse. *Am J Obstet Gynecol* 1997;177:1345–1355.

41. **Ihre T.** Intussusception of the rectum and the solitary ulcer syndrome. *Ann Med* 1990;22:419–423.

42. **Thompson JR, Chen AH, Pettit PD, et al.** Incidence of occult rectal prolapse in patients with clinical rectoceles and defecatory dysfunction. *Am J Obstet Gynecol* 2002;187:1494–1500.

43. **Freimanis MG, Wald A, Caruana B, et al.** Evacuation proctography in normal volunteers. *Invest Radiol* 1991;26:581–585.

44. **Mellgren A, Schultz I, Johansson C, et al.** Internal rectal intussusception seldom develops into total rectal prolapse. *Dis Colon Rectum* 1997;40:817–820.

45. **Bharucha AE, Wald, A, Enck P, et al.** Functional anorectal disorders. *Gastroenterology* 2006;130:1510–1518.

46. **Thompson WG, Longstreth GF, Drossman DA, et al.** Functional bowel disorders and functional abdominal pain. In: **Drossman DA, Corazziari E, Talley NJ, et al., eds.** *Rome II: the functional gastrointestinal disorders.* 2nd ed. McLean, VA: Degnon Associates, 2000:351–432.

47. **Vanner SJ, Depew WT, Paterson WG, et al.** Predictive value of the Rome criteria for diagnosing the irritable bowel syndrome. *Am J Gastroenterol* 1999;94:2912–2917.

48. **Bassotti G, Imbimbo B, Betti C, et al.** Impaired colonic motor response to eating in patients with slow-transit constipation. *Am J Gastroenterol* 1992;87:504–508.

49. **Rao SS.** Constipation: evaluation and treatment. *Gastroenterol Clin North Am* 2003;32:659–683.

50. **Knowles CH, Martin JE.** Slow transit constipation: a model of human gut dysmotility. Review of possible aetologies. *Neurogastroenterol Motil* 2000;12:181–196.

51. **Handa VL, Danielsen BH, Gilbert WM.** Obstetric anal sphincter lacerations. *Obstet Gynecol* 2001;98:225–230.

52. **Fenner DE, Genberg B, Brahma P, et al.** Fecal and urinary incontinence after vaginal delivery with anal sphincter disruption in an obstetrics unit in the United States. *Am J Obstet Gynecol* 2003;189:1543–1550.

53. **Sultan AH, Kamm MA, Hudson CN, et al.** Anal-sphincter disruption during vaginal delivery. *N Engl J Med* 1993;329:1905–1911.

54. **Nguyen T, Handa VL, Hueppchen N, et al.** Labour curve findings associated with fourth degree sphincter disruption: the impact of labour progression on perineal trauma. *J Obstet Gynaecol Can* 2010;32:21–27.

55. **De Leeuw JW, Vierhout ME, Struijk PC, et al.** Anal sphincter damage after vaginal delivery: functional outcome and risk factors for fecal incontinence. *Acta Obstet Gynecol Scand* 2001;80:830–834.

56. **Nygaard IE, Rao SS, Dawson JD.** Anal incontinence after anal sphincter disruption: a 30-year retrospective cohort study. *Obstet Gynecol* 1997;89:896–901.

57. **Kamm MA.** Faecal incontinence. *BMJ* 1998;316:528–532.

58. **Faltin DL, Boulvain M, Irion O, et al.** Diagnosis of anal sphincter tears by postpartum endosonography to predict fecal incontinence. *Obstet Gynecol* 2000;95:643–647.

59. **MacArthur C, Glazener CM, Wilson PD, et al.** Obstetric practice and faecal incontinence three months after delivery. *Br J Obstet Gynaecol* 2001;108:678–683.

60. **Sultan AH, Johanson RB, Carter JE.** Occult anal sphincter trauma following randomized forceps and vacuum delivery. *Int J Gynaecol Obstet* 1998;61:113–119.

61. **Lal M, Mann CH, Callender R, et al.** Does cesarean delivery prevent anal incontinence? *Obstet Gynecol* 2003;101:305–312.

62. **Borello-France D, Burgio KL, Richter HE, et al.** Pelvic Floor Disorders Network. Fecal and urinary incontinence in primiparous women. *Obstet Gynecol* 2006;108:863–872.

63. **Nelson RL, Furner SE, Westercamp M, et al.** Cesarean delivery for the prevention of anal incontinence. *Cochrane Database Syst Rev* 2010;2:CD006756.

64. **Signorello LB, Harlow BL, Chekos AK, et al.** Midline episiotomy and incontinence. *BMJ* 2000;320:86–90.

65. **Carroli G, Mignini L.** Episiotomy for vaginal birth. *Cochrane Database Syst Rev* 2009;1:CD000081.

66. **Sultan AH, Kamm MA, Hudson CN, et al.** Third degree obstetric anal sphincter tears: risk factors and outcome of primary repair. *BMJ* 1994;308:887–891.

67. **Walker WA, Rothenberger DA, Goldberg SM.** Morbidity of internal sphincterotomy for anal fissure and stenosis. *Dis Colon Rectum* 1985;28:832–835.

68. **Zbar AP, Beer-Gabel M, Chiappa AC, et al.** Fecal incontinence after minor anorectal surgery. *Dis Colon Rectum* 2001;44:1610–1623.

69. **Read MG, Read NW, Haynes WG, et al.** A prospective study of the effect of haemorrhoidectomy on sphincter function and faecal incontinence. *Br J Surg* 1982;69:396–398.

70. **Snooks SJ, Henry MM, Swash M.** Faecal incontinence due to external anal sphincter division in childbirth is associated with damage to the innervation of the pelvic floor musculature: a double pathology. *Br J Obstet Gynaecol* 1985;92:824–828.

71. Snooks SJ, Setchell M, Swash M, et al. Injury to the innervation of the pelvic floor sphincter musculature in childbirth. *Lancet* 1984;1:546–550.

72. Ryhammer AM, Bek KM, Laurberg S. Multiple vaginal deliveries increase the risk of permanent incontinence of flatus and urine in normal premenopausal women. *Dis Colon Rectum* 1995;38:1206–1209.

73. Handa VL, Harris TA, Ostergard DR. Protecting the pelvic floor: obstetric management to prevent incontinence and pelvic organ prolapse. *Obstet Gynecol* 1996;88:470–478.

74. Allen RE, Hosker GL, Smith AT, et al. Pelvic floor damage and childbirth: a neurophysiological study. *Br J Obstet Gynaecol* 1990;97:770–779.

75. Smith ARB, Hosker GL, Warrell DW. The role of partial denervation of the pelvic floor in the aetiology of genitourinary prolapse and stress incontinence of urine: a neurophysiologic study. *Br J Obstet Gynaecol* 1989;96:24–28.

76. Henry MM, Parks AG, Swash M. The anal reflex in idiopathic fecal incontinence: an electrophysiological study. *Br J Surg* 1980;67:781–783.

77. Ho YH, Goh HS. The neurophysiological significance of perineal descent. *Int J Colorectal Dis* 1995;10:107–111.

78. Gee AS, Mills A, Durdey P. What is the relationship between perineal descent and anal mucosal electrosensitivity? *Dis Colon Rectum* 1995;38:419–423.

79. Berkelmans I, Heresbach D, Leroi AM, et al. Perineal descent at defecography in women with straining at stool: a lack of specificity or predictive value for future anal incontinence. *Eur J Gastroenterol Hepatol* 1995;7:75–79.

80. Barber MD, Kuchibhatla MN, Pieper CF, et al. Psychometric evaluation of 2 comprehensive condition-specific quality of life instruments for women with pelvic floor disorders. *Am J Obstet Gynecol* 2001;185:1388–1395.

81. Jorge JM, Wexner SD. Etiology and management of fecal incontinence. *Dis Colon Rectum* 1993;36:77–97.

82. Rockwood TH, Church JM, Fleshman JW, et al. Patient and surgeon ranking of the severity of symptoms associated with fecal incontinence: the fecal incontinence severity index. *Dis Colon Rectum* 1999;42:1525–1532.

83. Rockwood TH, Church JM, Fleshman JW, et al. Fecal incontinence quality of life scale: quality of life instrument for patients with fecal incontinence. *Dis Colon Rectum* 2000;43:9–17.

84. Richardson AC. Female pelvic floor support defects [editorial]. *Int Urogynecol J Pelvic Floor Dysfunct* 1996;7:241.

85. Bump RC, Mattiasson A, Bo K, et al. The standardization of terminology of female pelvic organ prolapse and pelvic floor dysfunction. *Am J Obstet Gynecol* 1996;175:10–17.

86. Swash M. Electromyography in pelvic floor disorders. In: Henry MM, ed. *Coloproctology and the pelvic floor.* 2nd ed. London: Butterworth-Heinemann, 1992:184–195.

87. Swash M, Snooks SJ. Motor nerve conduction studies of the pelvic floor innervation. In: Henry MM, ed. *Coloproctology and the pelvic floor.* 2nd ed. London: Butterworth-Heinemann, 1992:196–206.

88. Olsen AL, Ross M, Stansfield RB, et al. Pelvic floor nerve conduction studies: establishing clinically relevant normative data. *Am J Obstet Gynecol* 2003;189:1114–1119.

89. Laurberg S, Swash M, Henry MM. Delayed external sphincter repair for obstetric tear. *Br J Surg* 1988;75:786–788.

90. Hock D, Lombard R, Jehaes C, et al. Colpocystodefecography. *Dis Colon Rectum* 1993;36:1015–1021.

91. Kelvin FM, Maglinte DD, Hornback JA, et al. Pelvic prolapse: assessment with evacuation proctography (defecography) *Radiology* 1992;184:547–551.

92. Lamb GM, de Jode MG, Gould SW, et al. Upright dynamic MR defaecating proctography in an open configuration MR system. *Br J Radiol* 2000;73:152–155.

93. Read M. Effects of loperamide on anal sphincter function in patients complaining of chronic diarrhea with fecal incontinence and urgency. *Dig Dis Sci* 1982;27:807–814.

94. Tobin GW, Brocklehurst JC. Fecal incontinence in residential homes for the elderly: prevalence, aetiology and management. *Age Ageing* 1986;15:41–46.

95. Talley NJ. Pharmacologic therapy for the irritable bowel syndrome. *Am J Gastroenterol* 2003;98:750–758.

96. Schoenfeld P. Efficacy of current drug therapies in irritable bowel syndrome: what works and does not work. *Gastroenterol Clin North Am* 2005;34:319–335.

97. Palsson OS, Heymen S, Whitehead WE. Biofeedback treatment for functional anorectal disorders: a comprehensive efficacy review. *Appl Psychophysiol Biofeedback* 2004;29:153–174.

98. Norton C. Behavioral management of fecal incontinence in adults. *Gastroenterology* 2004;126:S64–S70.

99. Heymen S, Jones KR, Ringel Y, et al. Biofeedback treatment of fecal incontinence: a critical review. *Dis Colon Rectum* 2001;44:728–736.

100. Norton C, Hosker G, Brazzelli M. Biofeedback and/or sphincter exercises for the treatment of faecal incontinence in adults. *Cochrane Database Syst Rev* 2000;2:CD002111.

101. Norton C, Chelvanayagam S, Wilson-Barnett J, et al. Randomized controlled trial of biofeedback for fecal incontinence. *Gastroenterology* 2003;125:1320–1329.

102. Fynes MM, Marshall K, Cassidy M, et al. A prospective, randomized study comparing the effect of augmented biofeedback with sensory biofeedback alone on fecal incontinence after obstetric trauma. *Dis Colon Rectum* 1999;42:753–758.

103. Norton C, Kamm MA. Outcome of biofeedback for fecal incontinence. *Br J Surg* 1999;86:1159–1163.

104. Leroi AM, Dorival MP, Lecouturier MF, et al. Pudendal neuropathy and severity of incontinence but not presence of an anal sphincter defect may determine the response to biofeedback therapy in fecal incontinence. *Dis Colon Rectum* 1999;42:762–769.

105. Rieger NA, Wattchow DA, Sarre RG, et al. Prospective trial of pelvic floor retraining in patients with fecal incontinence. *Dis Colon Rectum* 1997;40:821–826.

106. van Tets WF, Juijpers JH, Bleijenberg G. Biofeedback treatment is ineffective in neurogenic fecal incontinence. *Dis Colon Rectum* 1996;39:992–994.

107. Hosker G, Cody JD, Norton CC. Electrical stimulation for faecal incontinence in adults. *Cochrane Database Syst Rev* 2007;3:CD001310

108. Madoff RD, Williams JG, Caushaj PF. Fecal incontinence. *N Engl J Med* 1992;326:1002–1007.

109. Fitzpatrick M, Behan M, O'Connell PR, et al. A randomized clinical trial comparing primary overlap with approximation repair of third-degree obstetric tears. *Am J Obstet Gynecol* 2000;183:1220–1224.

110. Williams A, Adams EJ, Tincello DG, et al. How to repair an anal sphincter injury after vaginal delivery: results of a randomized controlled trial. *BJOG* 2006;113:201–207.

111. Fernando RJ, Sultan AH, Kettle C, et al. Repair techniques for obstetrical anal sphincter injuries: a randomized controlled trial. *Obstet Gynecol* 2006;107:1261–1268.

112. Farrell SA, Gilmour D, Turnbull GK, et al. Overlapping compared with end-to-end repair of third- and fourth-degree obstetric anal sphincter tears: a randomized controlled trial. *Obstet Gynecol* 2010;116:16–24.

113. Fernando R, Sultan AH, Kettle C, et al. Methods of repair of obstetric anal sphincter injury. *Cochrane Database Syst Rev* 2006;3:CD002866

114. Tjandra JJ, Han WR, Goh J, et al. Direct repair vs. overlapping sphincter repair: a randomized, controlled trial. *Dis Colon Rectum* 2003;46:937–942.

115. Madoff RD. Surgical treatment options for fecal incontinence. *Gastroenterology* 2004;126:S48–S54.

116. Malouf AJ, Norton CS, Engel AF, et al. Long-term results of overlapping anterior anal-sphincter repair for obstetric trauma. *Lancet* 2000;355:260–265.

117. Halverson AL, Hull TL. Long-term outcome of overlapping anal sphincter repair. *Dis Colon Rectum* 2002;45:345–348.

118. Bravo Gutierrez A, Madoff RD, Lowry AC, et al. Long-term results of anterior sphincteroplasty. *Dis Colon Rectum* 2004;47:727–731.

119. Buie WD, Lowry AC, Rothenberger DA, et al. Clinical rather than laboratory assessment predicts continence after anterior sphincteroplasty. *Dis Colon Rectum* 2001;44:1255–1260.

120. Gilliland R, Altomare DF, Moreira H Jr, et al. Pudendal neuropathy is predictive of failure following anterior overlapping sphincteroplasty. *Dis Colon Rectum* 1998;41:1516–1522.

121. Londono-Schimmer EE, Garcia-Duperly R, Nicholls RJ, et al. Overlapping anal sphincter repair for faecal incontinence due to sphincter trauma: five year follow-up results. *Int J Colorectal Dis* 1994;9:110–113.

122. Sangwan YP, Coller JA, Barrett RC, et al. Unilateral pudendal neuropathy: impact on outcome of anal sphincter repair. *Dis Colon Rectum* 1996;39:686–689.

123. Rosenberg J, Kehlet H. Early discharge after external anal sphincter repair. *Dis Colon Rectum* 1999;42:457–459.

124. Hasegawa H, Yoshioka K, Keighley MR. Randomized trial of fecal diversion for sphincter repair. *Dis Colon Rectum* 2000;43:961–964.

125. Nessim A, Wexner SD, Agachan F, et al. Is bowel confinement necessary after anorectal reconstructive surgery? A prospective, randomized, surgeon-blinded trial. *Dis Colon Rectum* 1999;42:16–23.

126. Pinedo G, Vaizey CJ, Nicholls RJ, et al. Results of repeat anal sphincter repair. *Br J Surg* 1999;86:66–69.

127. Savoye-Collett C, Savoye G, Koning E, et al. Anal endosonography after sphincter repair: specific patterns related to clinical outcome. *Abdom Imaging* 1999;24:569–573.

128. Giordano P, Renzi A, Efron J, et al. Previous sphincter repair does not affect the outcome of repeat repair. *Dis Colon Rectum* 2002;45:635–640.

129. Peleg D, Kennedy CM, Merrill D, et al. Risk of repetition of a severe perineal laceration. *Obstet Gynecol* 1999;93:1021–1024.

130. Elfaghi I, Johansson-Erneste B, Rydhstroem H. Rupture of the sphincter ani: the recurrence rate in second delivery. *Br J Obstet Gynaecol* 2004;111:1361–1364.

131. Spydslaug A, Trogstad LI, Skrondal A, et al. Recurrent risk of anal sphincter laceration among women with vaginal deliveries. *Obstet Gynecol* 2005;105:307–313.

132. Lowder JL, Burrows LJ, Krohn MA, et al. Risk factors for primary and subsequent anal sphincter lacerations: a comparison of cohorts by parity and prior mode of delivery. *Am J Obstet Gynecol* 2007;196:344.e1–e5.

133. Pickrell KL, Broadbent TR, Masters FW, et al. Construction of a rectal sphincter and restoration of anal continence by transplanting the gracilis muscle; a report of four cases in children. *Ann Surg* 1952;135:853–862.

134. Chapman AE, Geerdes B, Hewett P, et al. Systematic review of dynamic graciloplasty in the treatment of faecal incontinence. *Br J Surg* 2002;89:138–153.

135. Madoff RD, Rosen HR, Baeten CG, et al. Safety and efficacy of dynamic muscle plasty for anal incontinence: lessons from a prospective multicenter trial. *Gastroenterology* 1999;116:549–556.

136. Baeten CG, Bailey HR, Bakka A, et al. Safety and efficacy of dynamic graciloplasty for fecal incontinence: report of a prospective multicenter trial. Dynamic Graciloplasty Therapy Study Group. *Dis Colon Rectum* 2000;43:743–751.

137. Geerdes BP, Heineman E, Konsten J, et al. Dynamic graciloplasty: complications and management. *Dis Colon Rectum* 1996;39:912–917.

138. Rongen MJ, Uluday O, El Naggar K, et al. Long-term follow-up of dynamic graciloplasty for fecal incontinence. *Dis Colon Rectum* 2003;46:716–721.

139. Penninckx F, Belgian Section of Colorectal Surgery. Belgian experience with dynamic graciloplasty for faecal incontinence. *Br J Surg* 2004;91:872–878.

140. Mundy L, Merlin TL, Maddem GJ, et al. Systemic review of safety and effectiveness of an artificial bowel sphincter for faecal incontinence. *Br J Surg* 2004;91:665–672.

141. Wong WD, Congliosi SM, Spencer MP, et al. The safety and efficacy of the artificial bowel sphincter for fecal incontinence: results from a multicenter cohort study. *Dis Colon Rectum* 2002;45:1139–1153.

142. Devesa JM, Rey A, Hervas PL, et al. Artificial anal sphincter: complications and functional results of a large personal series. *Dis Colon Rectum* 2002;45:1154–1163.

143. O'Brien PE, Dixon JB, Skinner S, et al. A prospective, randomized, controlled clinical trial of placement of the artificial bowel sphincter (Acticon Neosphincter) for the control of fecal incontinence. *Dis Colon Rectum* 2004;47:1852–1860.

144. Ortiz H, Armendariz P, DeMiguel M, et al. Prospective study of artificial anal sphincter and dynamic graciloplasty for severe anal incontinence. *Int J Colorectal Dis* 2003;18:349–354.

145. Matzel KE, Stadelmaier U, Hohenberger W. Innovations in fecal incontinence: sacral nerve stimulation. *Dis Colon Rectum* 2004;47:1720–1728.

146. Mowatt G, Glazener C, Jarrett M. Sacral nerve stimulation for faecal incontinence and constipation in adults. *Cochrane Database Syst Rev* 2007;3:CD004464.

147. Wexner SD, Coller JA, Devroede G, et al. Sacral nerve stimulation for fecal incontinence: results of a 120-patient prospective multicenter study. *Ann Surg* 2010;251:441–449.

148. Wexner SD, Hull T, Edden Y, et al. Infection rates in a large investigational trial of sacral nerve stimulation for fecal incontinence. *J Gastrointest Surg* 2010;14:1081–1089.

149. Gallas S, Michot F, Faucheron JL, et al. Predictive factors for successful sacral nerve stimulation in the treatment of fecal incontinence: Results of trial stimulation in 200 patients. *Colorectal Dis* 2011;13:689–696..

150. Tjandra JJ, Chan MK, Yeh CH, et al. Sacral nerve stimulation is more effective than optimal medical therapy for severe fecal incontinence: a randomized, controlled study. *Dis Colon Rectum* 2008;51:494–502.

151. Muller-Lissner SA, Kamm MA, Scarpignato C, et al. Myths and misconceptions about chronic constipation. *Am J Gastroenterol* 2005;100:232–242.

152. Preston DM, Lennard-Jones JE. Severe chronic constipation of young women: "idiopathic slow transit constipation." *Gut* 1986;27:41–48.

153. Towers AL, Burgio KL, Locher JL, et al. Constipation in the elderly: influence of dietary, psychological, and physiological factors. *J Am Geriatr Soc* 1994;42:701–706.

154. Robson KM, Kiely DK, Lembo T. Development of constipation in nursing home residents. *Dis Colon Rectum* 2000;43:940–943.

155. Young RJ, Beerman LE, Vanderhoof JA. Increasing oral fluids in chronic constipation in children. *Gastroenterol Nurs* 1998;21:156–161.

156. Anti M, Pignataro G, Armuzzi A, et al. Water supplementation enhances the effect of high-fiber diet on stool frequency and laxative consumption in adult patients with functional constipation. *Hepatogastroenterology* 1998;45:727–732.

157. Brodribb AJ. Treatment of symptomatic diverticular disease with a high-fiber diet. *Lancet* 1977;1:664–666.

158. Muller-Lissner SA. Effect of wheat bran on weight of stool and gastrointestinal transit time: a meta analysis. *BMJ* 1988;296:615–617.

159. Tramonte SM, Brand MB, Mulrow CD, et al. The treatment of chronic constipation in adults: a systematic review. *J Gen Intern Med* 1997;12:15–24.

160. Voderholzer WA, Schatke W, Muhldorfer BE, et al. Clinical response to dietary fiber treatment of chronic constipation. *Am J Gastroenterol* 1997;92:95–98.

161. Ziegenhagen DJ, Tewinkel G, Kruis W, et al. Adding more fluid to wheat bran has no significant effects on intestinal functions of healthy subjects. *J Clin Gastroenterol* 1991;13:525–530.

162. Wald A. Constipation. *Med Clin North Am* 2000;84:1231–1246.

163. Ellerkmann MR, Kaufman H. Defecatory dysfunction. In: Bent AE, ed. Ostergard's Urogynecology. 5th ed. Philadelphia, PA: Lippincott Williams & Wilkins, 2002:355–389.

164. Wald A. Approach to the patient with constipation. In: Yamada T, ed. Textbook of gastroenterology. 3rd ed. Philadelphia, PA: Lippincott Williams & Wilkins, 1999.

165. Belsey JD, Geraint M, Dixon TA. Systematic review and meta analysis: polyethylene glycol in adults with non-organic constipation. *Int J Clin Pract* 2010;64:944–955.

166. Dipalma JA, Cleveland MV, McGowan J, et al. A randomized, multicenter, placebo-controlled trial of polyethylene glycol laxative for chronic treatment of chronic constipation. *Am J Gastroenterol* 2007;102:1436–1441.

167. Dipalma JA, Cleveland MV, McGowan J, et al. A randomized, multicenter comparison of polyethylene glycol laxative and tegaserod in treatment of patients with chronic constipation. *Am J Gastroenterol* 2007;102:1964–1971.

168. **Battaglia E, Serra AM, Buonafede G, et al.** Long-term study on the effects of visual biofeedback and muscle training as a therapeutic modality in pelvic floor dyssynergia and slow-transit constipation. *Dis Colon Rectum* 2004;47:90–95.

169. **Ho YH, Tan M, Goh HS.** Clinical and physiologic effects of biofeedback in outlet obstruction constipation. *Dis Colon Rectum* 1996;39:520–524.

170. **Enck P.** Biofeedback training in disordered defecation: a critical review. *Dig Dis Sci* 1993;38:1953–1960.

171. **Ron Y, Avni Y, Lukovetski A, et al.** Botulinum toxin type-A in therapy of patients with anismus. *Dis Colon Rectum* 2001;44:1821–1826.

172. **Friedenberg F, Gollamudi S, Parkman HP.** The use of botulinum toxin for the treatment of gastrointestinal motility disorders. *Dig Dis Sci* 2004;49:165–175.

173. **Farid M, El Monem HA, Omar W, et al.** Comparative study between biofeedback retraining and botulinum neurotoxin in the treatment of anismus patients. *Int J Colorectal Dis* 2009;24:115–120.

174. **Shah SM, Sultan AH, Thakar R.** The history and evolution of pessaries for pelvic organ prolapse. *Int Urogynecol J Pelvic Floor Dysfunct* 2006;17:170–175.

175. **Adams E, Thomson A, Maher C, et al.** Mechanical devices for pelvic organ prolapse in women. *Cochrane Database Syst Rev* 2004;2:CD004010.

176. **Clemons JL, Aguilar VC, Tillinghast TA, et al.** Risk factors associated with an unsuccessful pessary fitting trial in women with pelvic organ prolapse. *Am J Obstet Gynecol* 2004;190:235–250.

177. **Cundiff GW, Weidner AC, Visco AG, et al.** A survey of pessary use by members of the American Urogynecological Society. *Obstet Gynecol* 2000;95:931–935.

178. **Clemons JL, Aguilar VC, Sokol ER, et al.** Patient characteristics that are associated with continued pessary use versus surgery after 1 year. *Am J Obstet Gynecol* 2004;191:159–164.

179. **Cundiff GW, Amundsen CL, Bent AE, et al.** The PESSRI study: symptom relief outcomes of a randomized crossover trial of the ring and Gellhorn pessaries. *Am J Obstet Gynecol* 2007;196:405.e1–e8.

180. **Knowles CH, Scott M, Lunniss PJ.** Outcomes of colectomy for slow transit constipation. *Ann Surg* 1999;230:627–638.

181. **Bernini A, Madoff RD, Lowry AC, et al.** Should patients with combined colonic inertia and nonrelaxing pelvic floor undergo subtotal colectomy? *Dis Colon Rectum* 1998;41:1363–1366.

182. **Walsh PV, Peebles-Brown DA, Watkinson G.** Colectomy for slow transit constipation. *Ann R Coll Surg Engl* 1987;69:71–75.

183. **FitzHarris GP, Garcia-Aguilar J, Parker SC, et al.** Quality of life after subtotal colectomy for slow-transit constipation: both quality and quantity count. *Dis Colon Rectum* 2003;46:433–440.

184. **Lees NP, Hodson P, Hill J, et al.** Long-term results of the antegrade continent enema procedure for constipation in adults. *Colorectal Dis* 2004;6:362–368.

185. **Malouf AJ, Wiesel PH, Nicholls T, et al.** Short-term effects of sacral nerve stimulation for idiopathic slow transit constipation. *World J Surg* 2002;26:166–170.

186. **Kenefick NJ, Vaizey CJ, Cohen CR, et al.** Double-blind placebo-controlled crossover study of sacral nerve stimulation for idiopathic constipation. *Br J Surg* 2002;89:1570–1571.

187. **Holzer B, Rosen HR, Novi G, et al.** Sacral nerve stimulation in patients with severe constipation. *Dis Colon Rectum* 2008;51:524–529.

188. **Arnold MW, Stewart WR, Aguilar PS.** Rectocele repair: four years' experience. *Dis Colon Rectum* 1990;33:684–687.

189. **Mellgren A, Anzen B, Nillson BY, et al.** Results of rectocele repair: a prospective study. *Dis Colon Rectum* 1995;38:7–13.

190. **Kahn MA, Stanton SL.** Posterior colporrhaphy: its effects on bowel and sexual function. *Br J Obstet Gynaecol* 1997;104:82–86.

191. **Weber AM, Walters MD, Piedmonte MR.** Sexual function and vaginal anatomy in women before and after surgery for pelvic organ prolapse and urinary incontinence. *Am J Obstet Gynecol* 2000;182:1610–1615.

192. **Sand PK, Koduri A, Lobel RW, et al.** Prospective randomized trial of polyglactin 910 mesh to prevent recurrence of cystoceles and rectoceles. *Am J Obstet Gynecol* 2001;184:1357–1364.

193. **Cundiff GW, Weidner AC, Visco AG, et al.** Anatomic and functional assessment of the discrete defect rectocele repair. *Am J Obstet Gynecol* 1998;179:1451–1457.

194. **Porter WE, Steele A, Walsh P, et al.** The anatomic and functional outcomes of defect-specific rectocele repairs. *Am J Obstet Gynecol* 1999;181:1353–1359.

195. **Kenton K, Shott S, Brubaker L.** Outcome after rectovaginal fascia reattachment for rectocele repair. *Am J Obstet Gynecol* 2000;79:1360–1364.

196. **Glavind K, Madsen H.** A prospective study of the discrete fascial defect rectocele repair. *Acta Obstet Gynecol Scand* 2000;79:145–147.

197. **Singh K, Cortes E, Reid WM.** Evaluation of the fascial technique for surgical repair of isolated posterior vaginal wall prolapse. *Obstet Gynecol* 2003;101:320–324.

198. **Oster S, Astrup A.** A new vaginal operation for recurrent and large rectocele using dermis transplant. *Acta Obstet Gynecol Scand* 1981;60:493–495.

199. **Goh JT, Dwyer PL.** Effectiveness and safety of polypropylene mesh in vaginal prolapse surgery. *Int Urogynecol J* 2001;12:S90.

200. **Kohli N, Miklos JR.** Dermal graft-augmented rectocele repair. *Int Urogynecol J Pelvic Floor Dysfunct* 2003;14:146–149.

201. **Mercer-Jones MA, Sprowson A, Varma JS.** Outcome after transperineal mesh repair of rectocele: a case series. *Dis Colon Rectum* 2004;47:864–868.

202. **Sullivan ES, Leaverton GH, Hardwick CE.** Transrectal perineal repair: an adjunct to improved function after anorectal surgery. *Dis Colon Rectum* 1968;11:106–114.

203. **Sehapayak S.** Transrectal repair of rectocele: an extended armamentarium of colorectal surgeons. A report of 355 cases. *Dis Colon Rectum* 1985;28:422–433.

204. **Janssen LW, van Dijke CF.** Selection criteria for anterior rectal wall repair in symptomatic rectocele and anterior rectal wall prolapse. *Dis Colon Rectum* 1994;37:1100–1107.

205. **van Dam JH, Huisman WM, Hop WC, et al.** Fecal continence after rectocele repair: a prospective study. *Int J Colorectal Dis* 2000;15:54–57.

206. **Ayabaca SM, Zbar AP, Pescatori M.** Anal continence after rectocele repair. *Dis Colon Rectum* 2002;45:63–69.

207. **Cundiff GW, Fenner D.** Evaluation and treatment of women with rectocele: focus on associated defecatory and sexual dysfunction. *Obstet Gynecol* 2004;104:1403–1421.

208. **Francis WJ, Jeffcoate TN.** Dyspareunia following vaginal operations. *J Opt Soc Am* 1961;68:1–10.

209. **Maher CF, Qatawneh AM, Baessler K, et al.** Midline rectovaginal fascial plication for repair of rectocele and obstructed defecation. *Obstet Gynecol* 2004;104:685–689.

210. **Paraiso MF, Barber MD, Muir TW, Walters MD.** Rectocele repair: a randomized trial of three surgicval techniques including graft augmentation. *Am J Obstet Gynecol* 2006;195:1762–1771.

211. **Gustilo-Ashby AM, Paraiso MF, Jelovsek JE, et al.** Bowel symptoms 1 year after surgery for prolapse: further analysis of a randomized trial of rectocele repair. *Am J Obstet Gynecol* 2007;197:76.e1–e5.

212. **Zbar AP, Leinemann A, Fritsch H, et al.** Rectocele: pathogenesis and surgical management. *Int J Colorectal Dis* 2003;18:369–384.

213. **Goh JT, Tjandra JJ, Carey MP.** How could management of rectoceles be optimized? *ANZ J Surg* 2002;72:896–901.

214. **Maher C, Baessler K, Glazener CM, et al.** Surgical management of pelvic organ prolapse in women. *Cochrane Database Syst Rev* 2010;4:CD004014.

215. **Maher C, Baessler K.** Surgical management of posterior vaginal wall prolapse: an evidence-based literature review. *Int Urogynecol J Pelvic Floor Dysfunct* 2006;17:84–88.

216. **Kahn MA, Stanton SL, Kumar D, et al.** Posterior colporrhaphy is superior to the transanal repair for treatment of posterior vaginal wall prolapse. *Neurourol Urodyn* 1999;18:70–71.

217. **Nieminen K, Hiltunen K, Laitinen J, et al.** Transanal or vaginal approach to rectocele repair: a prospective randomized pilot study. *Dis Colon Rectum* 2004;47:1636–1642.

218. **Watson SJ, Loder PB, Halligan S, et al.** Transperineal repair of symptomatic rectocele with Marlex mesh: a clinical, physiological and radiologic assessment of treatment. *J Am Coll Surg* 1996;183:257–261.

219. **Murphy M, Society of Gynecologic Surgeons Systematic Review Group.** Clinical practice guidelines on vaginal graft use from the society of gynecologic surgeons. *Obstet Gynecol* 2008;112:1123–1130.

220. **Addison WA, Cundiff GW, Bump RC, et al.** Sacral colpopexy is the preferred treatment for vaginal vault prolapse. *J Gynecol Tech* 1996;2:69–74.

221. **Gutman RE, Bradley CS, Ye W, et al.** Pelvic Floor Disorders Network. Effects of colpocleisis on bowel symptoms among women with severe pelvic organ prolapse. *Int Urogynecol J Pelvic Floor Dysfunct* 2010;21:461–466.

222. **Sullivan ES, Longaker CJ, Lee PY.** Total pelvic mesh repair: a ten-year experience. *Dis Colon Rectum* 2001;44:857–863.

223. **Visco AG, Weidner AC, Barber MD, et al.** Vaginal mesh erosion after abdominal sacral colpopexy. *Am J Obstet Gynecol* 2001;184:297–302.

224. **Kaufman HS, Cundiff G, Thompson J, et al.** Suture rectopexy and sacral colpoperineopexy with Alloderm® for perineal descent. *Dis Colon Rectum* 2000;43:A16.

225. **Grimes CL, Quiroz LH, Gutman RE, et al.** Long-term impact of abdominal sacral colpoperineopexy on symptoms of obstructed defecation. *Female Pelvic Med Reconstr Surg* 2010;16:234–237.

226. **Cutait D.** Sacro-promontory fixation of the rectum for complete rectal prolapse. *Proc R Soc Med* 1959;52[Suppl]:105.

227. **Frykman HM, Goldberg SM.** The surgical treatment of rectal procidentia. *Surg Gynecol Obstet* 1969;129:1225–1230.

228. **Ripstein CB.** Treatment of massive rectal prolapse. *Am J Surg* 1952;83:68–71.

229. **Ripstein CB.** Surgical care of muscle rectal prolapse. *Dis Colon Rectum* 1965;8:34–38.

230. **Madiba TE, Baig MK, Wexner SD.** Surgical management of rectal prolapse. *Arch Surg* 2005;140:63–73.

231. **Luukkonen P, Mikkonen U, Jarvinen H.** Abdominal rectopexy with sigmoidectomy vs rectopexy alone for rectal prolapse: a prospective, randomized study. *Int J Colorectal Dis* 1992;7:219–222.

232. **Solomon MJ, Young CJ, Eyers AA, et al.** Randomized clinical trial of laparoscopic versus open abdominal rectopexy for rectal prolapse. *Br J Surg* 2002;89:35–39.

233. **Tou S, Brown SR, Malik AI, et al.** Surgery for complete rectal prolapse in adults. *Cochrane Database Syst Rev* 2008;4:CD001758.

234. **Delorme R.** Sur le traitement des prolapses du rectum totaux pour l'excision de la muscueuse rectale ou rectocolique. *Bull Mem Soc Chir Paris* 1900;26:499–518.

235. **Sielezneff I, Malouf A, Cesari J, et al.** Selection criteria for internal rectal prolapse repair by Delorme's transrectal excision. *Dis Colon Rectum* 1999;42:367–373.

236. **Takesue Y, Yokoyama T, Murakami Y, et al.** The effectiveness of perineal rectosigmoidectomy for the treatment of rectal prolapse. *Surg Today* 1999;29:290–293.

237. **Altemeier WA, Culbertson WR, Schwengerdt C, et al.** Nineteen years' experience with the one-stage perineal repair of rectal prolapse. *Ann Surg* 1971;173:993–1007.

238. **Agachan F, Reissman P, Pfeifer J, et al.** Comparison of three perineal procedures for the treatment of rectal prolapse. *South Med J* 1997;90:925–932.

239. **Deen KI, Grant E, Billingham C, et al.** Abdominal resection rectopexy with pelvic floor repair versus perineal rectosigmoidectomy and pelvic floor repair for full-thickness rectal prolapse. *Br J Surg* 1994;81:302–304.

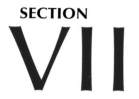
REPRODUCTIVE ENDOCRINOLOGY

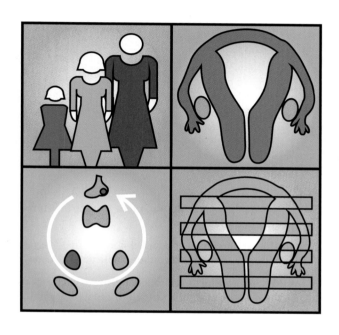

29

Puberty

Robert W. Rebar
Arasen A. V. Paupoo

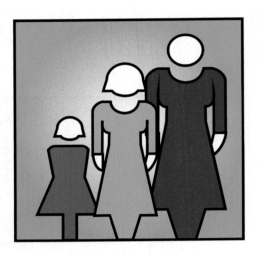

- Normal pubertal development occurs in a predictable orderly sequence over a definite time frame.

- The major causes of delayed puberty include anatomic genital tract abnormalities and hypo- and hypergonadotropic amenorrhea.

- When pubertal development occurs asynchronously with development of breasts in the absence of significant pubic and axillary hair, the diagnosis is usually androgen insensitivity.

- The most common cause of precocious puberty is constitutional (idiopathic), but more serious causes must be ruled out and therapy geared toward optimizing adult height.

- The most common cause of heterosexual development at the expected age of puberty is polycystic ovary syndrome.

Puberty is the period during which secondary sexual characteristics develop and the capability of sexual reproduction is attained. The physical changes accompanying pubertal development result directly or indirectly from maturation of the hypothalamus, stimulation of the sex organs, and secretion of sex steroids. Hormonally, puberty in humans is characterized by the resetting of the classic negative gonadal steroid feedback loop, alterations in circadian and ultradian (frequent) gonadotropin rhythms, and the acquisition in the woman of a positive estrogen feedback loop, which controls the monthly rhythm as an interdependent expression of gonadotropins and ovarian steroids.

The ability to evaluate and treat aberrations of pubertal development requires an understanding of the normal hormonal and physical changes that occur at puberty. An understanding of these changes is important in evaluating young women with amenorrhea.

Normal Pubertal Development

Factors Affecting Time of Onset

The major determinant of the timing of the onset of puberty is no doubt genetic, but a number of other factors appear to influence both the age at onset and the progression of pubertal development. Among these influences are nutritional state, general health, geographic location, exposure to light, and psychological state (1). **The concordance of the age of menarche in mother–daughter pairs and between sisters and in ethnic populations illustrates the importance of genetic factors** (1). Typically, the age of menarche is earlier than average in children with moderate obesity (up to 30% above normal weight for age), whereas delayed menarche is common in those with severe malnutrition. Children who live in urban settings, closer to the equator, and at lower altitudes typically begin puberty earlier than those who live in rural areas, farther from the equator, and at higher elevations. The risk of earlier onset of puberty is 10 to 20 times greater after international adoption for unclear reasons (2). Other risk factors implicated for precocious puberty include exposure to estrogenic endocrine-disrupting chemicals and the absence of a father in the home (3,4). Blind girls apparently undergo menarche earlier than sighted girls, suggesting some influence of light (5).

In Western Europe, the age of menarche declined 4 months each decade between 1850 and 1960 (1). Data suggest that the trend toward earlier pubertal development may be continuing among girls (but not boys) who live in the United States (6). It is presumed that these changes represent improved nutritional status and healthier living conditions.

One of the more controversial hypotheses centers on the role of total body weight and body composition on the age of menarche. It is argued that a girl must reach a critical body weight (47.8 kg) before menarche can occur (7). Body fat must increase to 23.5% from the typical 16% of the prepubertal state, which presumably is influenced by nutritional status (8). This hypothesis is supported by observations that menarche occurs earliest in obese girls, followed by normal-weight girls, then underweight girls, and lastly anorectic girls (Fig. 29.1). The importance of other factors is indicated by observations that menarche is often delayed in morbidly obese girls, those with diabetes, and those who exercise intensely but are of normal body weight and body fat percentage. Girls with precocious puberty may undergo menarche even if they have a low body fat percentage, and other girls show no pubertal development with a body fat percentage of 27% (9). **The hypothesis linking menarche to body weight and composition does not always seem valid because menarche is a late event in pubertal development.**

Physical Changes during Puberty

The changes associated with puberty occur in an orderly sequence over a definite time frame. Any deviation from this sequence or time frame should be regarded as abnormal. The pubertal changes, their relationship to one another, and the ages at which they occur are distinctly different in girls than in boys. Although this chapter focuses on girls, changes in boys are considered briefly.

Tanner Stage

In girls, pubertal development typically takes place over 4.5 years (Fig. 29.2). The first sign of puberty is accelerated growth, and breast budding is usually the first recognized pubertal change, followed by the appearance of pubic hair, peak growth velocity, and menarche. The stages initially described by Marshall and Tanner are often used to describe breast and pubic hair development (10).

With regard to breast development (Fig. 29.3), *Tanner stage 1* refers to the prepubertal state and includes no palpable breast tissue, with the areolae generally less than 2 cm in diameter. The nipples may be inverted, flat, or raised. In *Tanner stage 2*, breast budding occurs, with a visible and palpable mound of breast tissue. The areolae begin to enlarge, the skin of the areolae thins, and the nipple develops to varying degrees. *Tanner stage 3* is reflected by further growth and elevation of the entire breast. When the individual is seated and viewed from the side, the nipple is generally at or above the midplane of breast tissue. In most girls, *Tanner stage 4* is defined by projection of the areola and papilla above the general breast contour in a secondary mound. Breast development is incomplete until *Tanner stage 5*, in which the breast is mature in contour and proportion. In most women, the nipple is more pigmented at this stage than earlier in

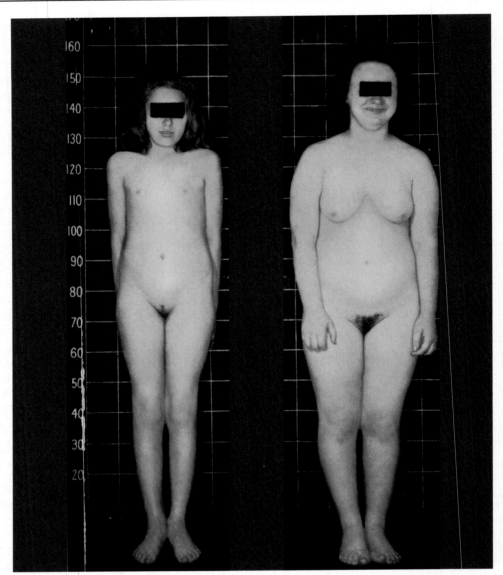

Figure 29.1   Normal twins at 12 years of age. The heavier twin (weighing 143 lb) is clearly more advanced in puberty than the lighter twin (weighing 87 lb). Anecdotal photographs and data such as these served to provide the basis for the theory that body fat, body mass, and menarche are linked. (From **Wilkins L.** *The diagnosis and treatment of endocrine disorders in childhood and adolescence.* 3rd ed. Springfield, IL: Charles C Thomas, 1965, with permission.)

development, and Montgomery's glands are visible around the circumference of the areola. The nipple is generally below the midplane of breast tissue when the woman is seated and viewed from the side. Full breast development usually occurs over 3 to 3.5 years, but it may occur in as little as 2 years or not progress beyond stage 4 until the first pregnancy. Breast size is no indication of breast maturity.

Pubic hair staging is related both to quantity and distribution (Fig. 29.4). In **Tanner stage 1**, there is no sexually stimulated pubic hair present, but some nonsexual hair may be present in the genital area. **Tanner stage 2** is characterized by the first appearance of coarse, long, crinkly pubic hair along the labia majora. In **Tanner stage 3**, coarse, curly hair extends onto the mons pubis. **Tanner stage 4** is characterized by adult hair in thickness and texture, but the hair is not distributed as widely as in adults and typically does not extend onto the inner aspects of the thighs. Except in certain ethnic groups, including Asians and American Indians, pubic hair extends onto the thighs in **Tanner stage 5**.

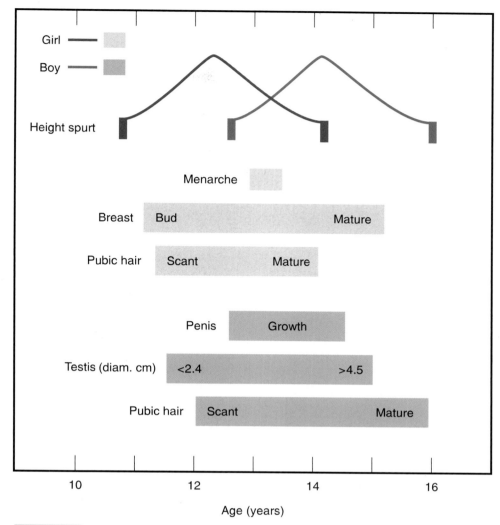

Figure 29.2   **Schematic sequence of events at puberty.** An idealized average girl and an idealized average boy are represented. (From **Rebar RW.** Practical evaluation of hormonal status. In: **Yen SSC, Jaffe RB, eds.** *Reproductive endocrinology: physiology, pathophysiology and clinical management.* 3rd ed. Philadelphia, PA: WB Saunders, 1991:830, with permission; based on data from **Marshall WA, Tanner JM.** Variations in patterns of pubertal changes in girls. *Arch Dis Child* 1969;44:291–303, and **Marshall WA, Tanner JM.** Variation in the pattern of pubertal changes in boys. *Arch Dis Child* 1970;45:13–23, with permission.)

The staging of male pubertal sexual maturation is based on genital size and pubic hair development. *Tanner stage 1* is prepubertal. *Tanner stage 2* of genital growth begins when testicular enlargement is first evident. Testis length along the longitudinal axis ranges from 2.5 to 3.2 cm. The size of the penis increases. Pigmented, curly pubic hair is first visible around the base of the penis. In *Tanner stage 3*, there is further growth of the penis in both length and diameter, the scrotum develops further, and testis length increases to 3.3 to 4 cm. Thicker, curly hair extends above the penis. *Tanner stage 4* involves further growth of the genitalia, with testis length ranging from 4 to 4.5 cm. Extension of pubic hair over the genital area continues, but the volume is less than in the adult. At this stage, the prostate gland is palpable by rectal examination. In *Tanner stage 5*, the genitalia are within the adult range in size. Average flaccid penile length in adult men ranges between 8.6 and 10.5 cm from tip to base. Pubic hair spreads laterally onto the medial thighs. Hair may or may not extend from the pubic area toward the umbilicus and anus.

Pigmented pubic hair is often the first recognized sign of male puberty even though it typically occurs 6 months after genital growth begins. Tanner stage 3 puberty often is accompanied by

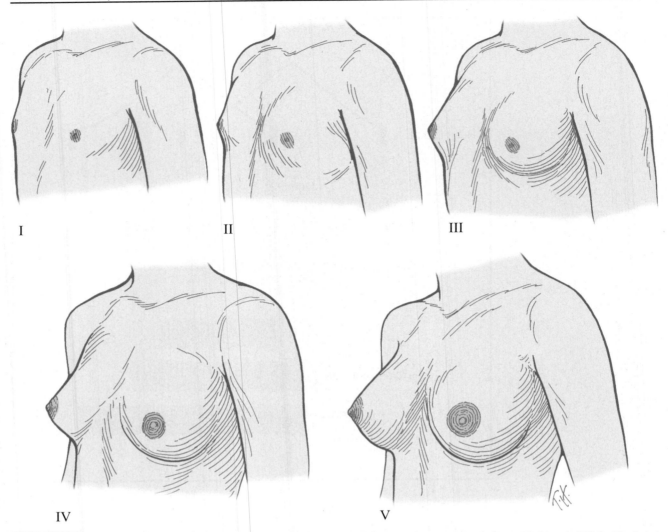

I II III

IV V

Figure 29.3 **Diagrammatic depiction of Tanner breast stages in adolescent women.** (From **Ross GT, Van de Wiele RL, Frantz AG.** *The ovaries and the breasts.* In: **Williams RH, ed.** *Textbook of endocrinology.* 6th edition. Philadelphia, PA: WB Saunders, 1981:355, with permission; adapted from **Marshall WA, Tanner JM.** Variations in patterns of pubertal changes in girls. *Arch Dis Child* 1969;44:291–303).

symmetric or asymmetric gynecomastia, and mature sperm first can be identified with microscopic urinalysis.

Height and Growth Rate

Plotting height increments (i.e., growth velocity) against the phases of puberty allows one to see relationships during puberty (Fig. 29.2). Girls reach peak height velocity early in puberty before menarche. As a consequence, they have limited growth potential after menarche. In contrast, boys reach peak height velocity about 2 years later than girls. Boys grow an average of 28 cm during the growth spurt, in comparison to a mean of 25 cm for girls. Adult men eventually are an average of 13 cm taller than adult women because they are taller at the onset of the growth spurt. Hormonal control of the pubertal growth spurt is complex. Growth hormone (GH), insulinlike growth factor 1 (IGF-1), and gonadal steroids play major roles. Adrenal androgens appear to be less important. Mutations limiting conversion of androgens to estrogens in males confirmed that estrogen is the major stimulus to the pubertal growth spurt in both boys and girls (11).

During the growth spurt associated with puberty, the long bones in the body lengthen and the epiphyses ultimately close. The bone or skeletal age of any individual can be estimated closely by comparing x-rays documenting the development of bones in the nondominant hand (most commonly), knee, or elbow to standards of maturation for the normal population. The Greulich and Pyle atlas is used most often for this purpose (12). Skeletal age is more closely

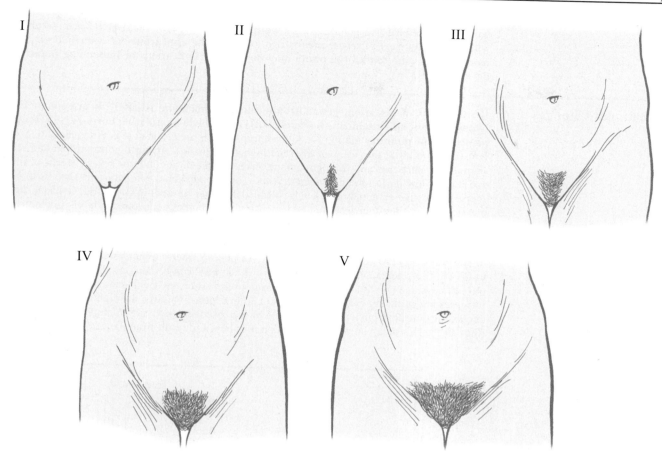

Figure 29.4 Diagrammatic depiction of Tanner pubic hair staging in adolescent women. (From **Ross GT, VandeWiele RL, Frantz AG.** The ovaries and the breasts. In: **Williams RH, ed.** *Textbook of endocrinology.* 6th ed. Philadelphia, PA: WB Saunders, 1981:355, with permission; adapted from **Marshall WA, Tanner JM.** Variations in patterns of pubertal changes in girls. *Arch Dis Child* 1969;44:291–303.)

correlated with pubertal stage than with chronologic age during puberty. **With height and chronologic age, an individual's bone age can be used to predict final adult height using the Bayley-Pinneau tables** (13). Bone age determinations can be used to assess the degree of delay, monitor subsequent development, and estimate final adult height.

Another practical clinical approach to predicting adult height uses midparental height. **The adjusted midparental height is calculated by adding 13 cm to the mother's height (for boys) or subtracting 13 cm from the father's height (for girls) and then determining the mean of the heights of the parents, including the adjusted height of the opposite-sex parent. Adding and subtracting 8.5 cm to the calculated predicted height approximates the target range of the 3rd to the 97th percentile for the anticipated adult height of the child.** This quick calculation can be of assistance in evaluating individuals with delayed or precocious pubertal development and those with short stature.

Several changes in body composition occur during pubertal development. **Although lean body mass, skeletal mass, and body fat are equal in prepubertal boys and girls, by maturity, men have 1.5 times the lean body mass and almost 1.5 times the skeletal mass of women, whereas women have twice as much body fat as men** (1). **The changes in body contour in girls, with accumulation of fat at the thighs, hips, and buttocks, occur during the pubertal growth spurt. In this regard, testosterone is a potent anabolic steroid and is responsible for the major changes in boys, whereas estrogen increases total body fat in a characteristic distribution at the thighs, buttocks, and abdomen in girls.**

Other physical changes show sexual dimorphism at puberty. In boys both the membranous and cartilaginous portions of the vocal cords lengthen much more than they do in girls, accounting for deepening of the voice. Comedones, acne, and seborrhea of the scalp begin because of increased secretion of adrenal and gonadal steroids at puberty. In general, early-onset acne correlates with the development of severe acne later in puberty. **The appearance of comedones in the nasal creases and behind the pinna may be the first indications of impending pubertal development.**

Hormonal Changes

By 10 weeks of gestation, gonadotropin-releasing hormone (GnRH) is present in the hypothalamus, and luteinizing hormone (LH) and follicle-stimulating hormone (FSH) are present in the pituitary gland (14). Gonadotropin levels are elevated in both female and male fetuses before birth; the levels of FSH are higher in females. At birth, gonadotropin and sex steroid concentrations are still high, but the levels decline during the first several weeks of life and remain low during the prepubertal years. The hypothalamic–pituitary unit appears to be suppressed by the extremely low levels of gonadal steroids present in childhood. Gonadal suppression of gonadotropin secretion is demonstrated by higher gonadotropin levels in children with gonadal dysgenesis and those who undergo gonadectomy before puberty (15).

Several of the hormonal changes associated with pubertal development begin before any of the physical changes are obvious. Early in puberty, there is increased sensitivity of LH to GnRH. Sleep-entrained increases in both LH and FSH can be documented early in puberty (16). In boys, the nocturnal increases in gonadotropin levels are accompanied by simultaneous increases in circulating testosterone levels (17). In contrast, in girls, the nighttime increases in circulating gonadotropin levels are followed by increased secretion of estradiol the next day (18) (Fig. 29.5). This delay in estradiol secretion is believed to result from the additional synthetic

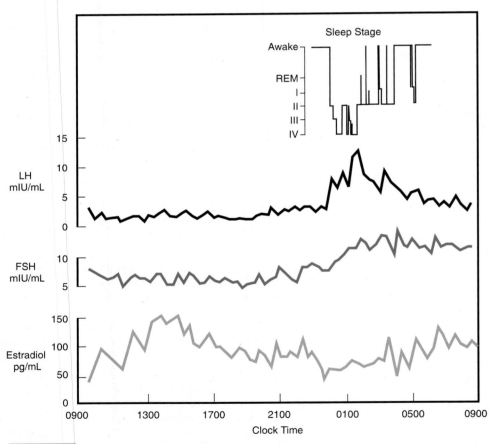

Figure 29.5 Patterns of circulating luteinizing hormone (LH), follicle-stimulating hormone (FSH), and estradiol in a stage 3 pubertal girl over a 24-hour period with the encephalographic stage of sleep indicated. (From **Boyar RM, Wu RHK, Roffwarg H, et al.** Human puberty: 24-hour estradiol patterns in pubertal girls. *J Clin Endocrinol Metab* 1976;43:1418-421, with permission.)

steps required in the aromatization of estrogens from androgens. Basal levels of both FSH and LH increase through puberty. The patterns differ in boys and girls, with LH levels (measured in mIU/mL) eventually becoming greater than FSH levels (19) (Fig. 29.6). Although it now appears that gonadotropins are always secreted in an episodic or pulsatile fashion, even before puberty, the pulsatile secretion of gonadotropins is more easily documented as puberty progresses and basal levels increase (20).

Increased adrenal androgen secretion is important in stimulating adrenarche, the appearance of pubic and axillary hair, in both boys and girls. Pubarche specifically refers to the appearance of pubic hair. Progressive increases in circulating levels of the major adrenal androgens, dehydroepiandrosterone (DHEA) and its sulfate (DHEAS), begin as early as 2 years of age, accelerate at 7 to 8 years of age, and continue until 13 to 15 years of age (21–23). The accelerated increases in adrenal androgens begin about 2 years before the increases in gonadotropin and gonadal sex steroid secretion when the hypothalamic–pituitary–gonadal unit is still functioning at a low prepubertal level.

In girls, mean levels of estradiol, secreted predominantly by the ovaries, increases steadily during puberty (19). Although, as noted, increases in estradiol first appear during the daytime hours, basal levels eventually increase during both the day and night. Estrone, which is secreted in part by the ovaries and arises in part from extraglandular conversion of estradiol and androstenedione, increases early in puberty but plateaus by midpuberty. Thus, **the ratio of estrone to estradiol decreases throughout puberty, indicating that ovarian production of estradiol becomes increasingly important and peripheral conversion of androgens to estrone becomes less important during maturation.**

In boys, most of the testosterone in the circulation arises from direct secretion by the Leydig cells of the testis. Testosterone induces development of a male body habitus and voice change, whereas dihydrotestosterone (DHT), produced following 5α reduction within target cells, induces enlargement of the penis and prostate gland, beard growth, and temporal hair recession during puberty. Mean plasma testosterone levels rise progressively during puberty, with the greatest increase occurring during Tanner stage 2 (24).

Growth hormone secretion increases along with increased gonadotropin secretion at the onset of puberty. It is believed that the increase in GH is mediated by estrogen, which in boys is dependent on aromatization of testosterone to estradiol and reflects increasing sex steroid production at puberty. Nonetheless, there are profound sex differences in GH secretion during puberty. Girls have higher basal levels of GH throughout puberty, reaching maximal levels around the time of menarche and decreasing thereafter. In contrast, basal concentrations of GH remain constant throughout puberty in boys. Growth hormone secretion is highly pulsatile, with most pulses occurring during sleep and with sex steroids increasing pulse amplitude rather than altering pulse frequency.

Growth hormone stimulates production of IGF-1 in all tissues, with concentrations found in the circulation spilling over from the liver. During puberty the negative feedback effect of IGF-1 on GH secretion must be reduced because both IGF-1 and GH levels are high. GH and IGF-1 play significant roles in the changes in body composition that occur at puberty because both hormones are potent anabolic agents.

In the final stages of puberty in both boys and girls, GH secretion begins to diminish, returning to prepubertal levels in adult life, despite continued exposure to high levels of gonadal steroids.

Mechanisms Underlying Puberty

The mechanisms responsible for the numerous hormonal changes that occur during puberty are poorly understood, although it is recognized that a "central nervous system program" must be responsible for initiating puberty. It appears that the hypothalamic–pituitary–gonadal axis in girls develops in two distinct stages during puberty. First, sensitivity to the negative or inhibitory effects of the low levels of circulating sex steroids present in childhood decreases early in puberty. Second, late in puberty, there is maturation of the positive or stimulatory feedback response to estrogen, which is responsible for the ovulatory midcycle surge of LH.

Current evidence suggests that the central nervous system inhibits the onset of puberty until the appropriate time (25). Based on this theory, the neuroendocrine control of puberty is mediated by GnRH-secreting neurons in the medial basal hypothalamus, which together

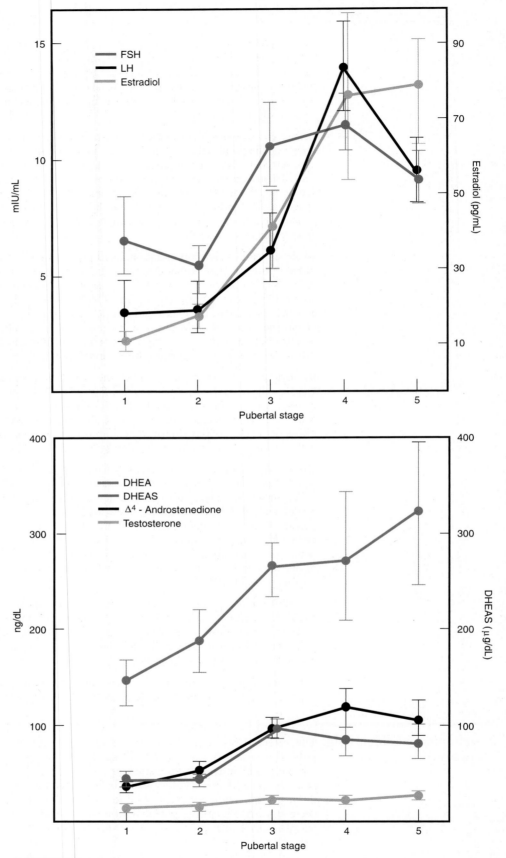

Figure 29.6 **Increases (± standard error) in circulating levels of gonadotropins and adrenal and gonadal steroids through puberty in girls.** DHEA, dehydroepiandrosterone; DHEAS, dehydroepiandrosterone sulfate. (From **Emans SJH, Goldstein DP.** The physiology of puberty. In: **Emans SJH, Goldstein DP, eds.** *Pediatric and adolescent gynecology.* 3rd ed. Boston, MA: Little, Brown, 1990:95, with permission.)

act as an endogenous pulse generator. At puberty, the GnRH pulse generator is reactivated (i.e., disinhibited), leading to increased amplitude and frequency of GnRH pulses. In turn, the increased GnRH secretion results in increased gonadotropin and then gonadal steroid secretion. What causes this "disinhibition" of GnRH release is unknown.

The relationship between body mass and the onset of puberty focused attention on leptin, produced by adipocytes, as a candidate for the factor initiating puberty. In the infertile leptin-deficient mouse, leptin therapy can induce sexual maturation and maintain fertility. Observations of two patients with leptin receptor mutations who failed to enter puberty suggest that leptin may have a similar role in humans (25).

Longitudinal studies of leptin secretion noted that there is increased leptin secretion around the time of pubertal onset. Leptin levels are increased throughout puberty in girls but not in boys. There is speculation that leptin is a trigger for pubertal onset, but a more widely held view is that leptin plays a more permissive role in regulating pubertal onset (25).

Aberrations of Pubertal Development

Classification

Several aberrations of pubertal development, as detailed in Table 29.1, can occur in girls. Pubertal aberrations can be classified in four broad categories:

1. **Delayed or interrupted puberty exists in girls who fail to develop any secondary sex characteristics by age 13, have not had menarche by age 15 (95th percentile is 14.5 yr), or have not attained menarche 5 or more years since the onset of pubertal development.**

Table 29.1 Aberrations of Pubertal Development

I. Delayed or interrupted puberty

   A. Anatomic abnormalities of the genital outflow tract

      1. Müllerian dysgenesis (Rokitansky-Küster-Hauser syndrome)

      2. Distal genital tract obstruction

         a. Imperforate hymen

         b. Transverse vaginal septum

   B. Hypergonadotropic (follicle-stimulating hormone >30 mIU/mL) hypogonadism (gonadal "failure")

      1. Gonadal dysgenesis with stigmata of Turner syndrome

      2. Pure gonadal dysgenesis

         a. 46,XX

         b. 46,XY

      3. Early gonadal "failure" with apparent normal ovarian development

   C. Hypogonadotropic (luteinizing hormone and follicle-stimulating hormone <10 mIU/mL) hypogonadism

      1. Constitutional delay

      2. Isolated gonadotropin deficiency

         a. Associated with midline defects (Kallmann syndrome)

         b. Independent of associated disorders

         c. Prader-Labhart-Willi syndrome

         d. Laurence-Moon-Bardet-Biedl syndrome

         e. Many other rare syndromes

(Continued)

Table 29.1 *Continued*

3. Associated with multiple hormone deficiencies

4. Neoplasms of the hypothalamic–pituitary area

   a. Craniopharyngiomas

   b. Pituitary adenomas

   c. Other

5. Infiltrative processes (Langerhans cell–type histiocytosis)

6. After irradiation of the central nervous system

7. Severe chronic illnesses with malnutrition

8. Anorexia nervosa and related disorders

9. Severe hypothalamic amenorrhea (rare)

10. Antidopaminergic and gonadotropin-releasing hormone–inhibiting drugs (especially psychotropic agents, opiates)

11. Primary hypothyroidism

12. Cushing syndrome

13. Use of chemotherapeutic (especially alkylating) agents

II. Asynchronous pubertal development

   A. Complete androgen insensitivity syndrome (testicular feminization)

   B. Incomplete androgen insensitivity syndrome

III. Precocious puberty

   A. Central (true) precocious puberty

     1. Constitutional (idiopathic) precocious puberty

     2. Hypothalamic neoplasms (most commonly hamartomas)

     3. Congenital malformations

     4. Infiltrative processes (Langerhans cell–type histiocytosis)

     5. After irradiation

     6. Trauma

     7. Infection

   B. Precocious puberty of peripheral origin (precocious pseudopuberty)

     1. Autonomous gonadal hypersecretion

       a. Cysts

       b. McCune-Albright syndrome

     2. Congenital adrenal hyperplasia

       a. 21-Hydroxylase (P450c21) deficiency

       b. 11β-Hydroxylase (P450c11) deficiency

       c. 3β-Hydroxysteroid dehydrogenase deficiency

     3. Iatrogenic ingestion/absorption of estrogens or androgens

     4. Hypothyroidism

     5. Gonadotropin-secreting neoplasms

       a. Human chorionic gonadotropin secreting

         i. Ectopic germinomas (pinealomas)

(Continued)

Table 29.1 *Continued*

ii. Choriocarcinomas
iii. Teratomas
iv. Hepatoblastomas
b. Luteinizing hormone–secreting (pituitary adenomas)
6. Gonadal neoplasms
a. Estrogen-secreting
i. Granulosa–theca cell tumors
ii. Sex-cord tumors
b. Androgen-secreting
i. Sertoli-Leydig cell tumors (arrhenoblastomas)
ii. Teratomas
7. Adrenal neoplasms
a. Adenomas
b. Carcinomas
IV. Heterosexual puberty
A. *Polycystic ovarian syndrome*
B. *Nonclassic forms of congenital adrenal hyperplasia*
C. *Idiopathic hirsutism*
D. *Mixed gonadal dysgenesis*
E. *Rare forms of male pseudohermaphroditism (Reifenstein syndrome, 5a-reductase deficiency)*
F. *Cushing syndrome (rare)*
G. *Androgen-secreting neoplasms (rare)*

2. *Asynchronous pubertal development* **is characterized by pubertal development that deviates from the normal pattern of puberty.**

3. *Precocious puberty* **is defined as pubertal development beginning before the age of 7 years in white girls and before the age of 6 years in African American girls** (6). This new definition is controversial and is challenged because some feel that evaluation for breast or pubic hair development before 9 or 8 years of age in white or African American girls, respectively, may be warranted (26). It is clear that, in most cases, development nearer to the mean age of puberty is less likely to have a pathologic basis. Precocious pubertal development is characterized in several ways. In *isosexual* precocious puberty, the early changes are common to the phenotypic sex of the individual. In *heterosexual* precocious puberty, the development is characteristic of the opposite sex. Precocious puberty is sometimes termed "true" when it is of central origin with activation of the hypothalamic–pituitary unit. In precocious pseudopuberty, also known as *precocious puberty of peripheral origin,* secretion of hormones in the periphery (commonly by neoplasms) stimulates pubertal development.

4. *Heterosexual puberty* **is characterized by a pattern of development that is typical of the opposite sex occurring at the expected age of normal puberty.**

Disorders of sexual development and amenorrhea may be considered in relation to this classification of the aberrations of puberty. It is very helpful to document the growth of the individual and to plot the individual's height and weight on one of several commonly available growth charts (Fig. 29.7).

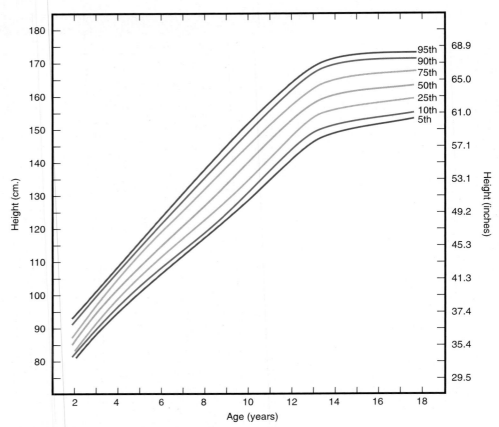

Figure 29.7 **Growth chart showing stature by age percentiles for girls aged 2 to 18 years.** Weight can be plotted in a similar fashion. Several excellent growth charts are available to clinicians, including those from Ross Laboratories (Columbus, OH), Serono Laboratories (Randolph, MA), and Genentech, Inc. (South San Francisco, CA). (From **Hamill PVV, Drizd TA, Johnson CL, et al.** Physical growth: National Center for Health Statistics percentiles. *Am J Clin Nutr* 1979;32:607–629, with permission; based on data from the National Center for Health Statistics.)

Delayed or Interrupted Puberty

The history and physical examination, with particular attention to growth, are most important in the evaluation of individuals with delayed puberty. **Pubertal delay is much more common in boys than in girls. It is important to remember that puberty may be delayed in any child suffering from any severe chronic disease,** including celiac disease, Crohn disease, sickle cell anemia, and cystic fibrosis. Chronic illness should be reviewed during the history and physical examination. One possible approach to evaluation is depicted in Figure 29.8.

Anatomic Abnormalities of the Genital Outflow Tract

Those girls who have mature secondary sex characteristics and any of a number of disorders of the outflow tract and uterus, often termed müllerian agenesis and dysgenesis, are most often identified on examination (Fig. 29.9). One of the most logical classification schemes that was proposed is shown in Table 29.2 (27). The incidence of these anomalies was estimated to be 0.02% of the female population several, but the incidence may have increased as a result of the maternal ingestion of diethylstilbestrol (DES) and the resultant increase in anomalies of the lumen of the uterus (class VI) (28,29). Of the disorders unrelated to drug use, the septate uterus (class V) is most common.

Disorders of the outflow tract and uterus often occur as a part of a syndrome of malformations that include abnormalities of the skeletal and renal systems (***Mayer-Rokitansky-Küster-Hauser syndrome***). Familial aggregates of the most common disorders of müllerian differentiation in girls—müllerian aplasia and incomplete müllerian fusion—are best explained on the basis of polygenic and multifactorial inheritance (30). It is clear that the *HOX* genes, a family of regulatory

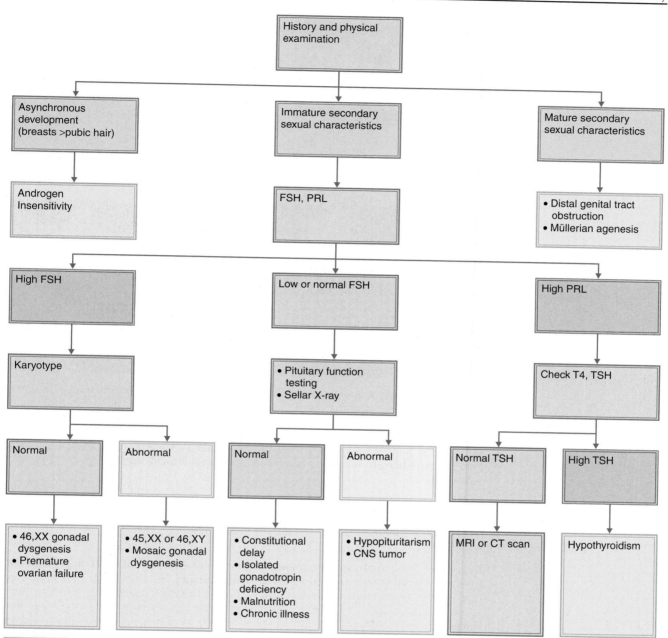

Figure 29.8 **Flow diagram for the evaluation of delayed or interrupted pubertal development, including primary amenorrhea, in phenotypic girls.** Girls with asynchronous development often present because of failure to menstruate. FSH, follicle-stimulating hormone; PRL, prolactin; T4, thyroxine; TSH, thyroid-stimulating hormone; CNS, central nervous system; MRI, magnetic resonance imaging; CT, computed tomography. (From **Rebar RW.** Normal and abnormal sexual differentiation and pubertal development. In: **Moore TR, Reiter RC, Rebar RW, et al., eds.** *Gynecology and obstetrics: a longitudinal approach.* New York: Churchill Livingstone, 1993:97–133, with permission.)

genes that encode for transcription factors, are essential for proper development of the müllerian tract in the embryonic period, and *HOXA 13* is altered in hand–foot–genital syndrome (31). *WNT4* may be involved in uterine development, as a *WNT4* mutation was described in cases involving a Mayer-Rokitansky-Küster-Hauser-like syndrome with hyperandrogenism (32).

The most common single anatomic disorder of puberty is the imperforate hymen, which prevents the passage of endometrial tissue and blood. These products can accumulate in the vagina (*hydrocolpos*) or uterus (*hydrometrocolpos*) and result in a bulging hymen that is often bluish in color. The affected individual often has a history of vague abdominal pain with

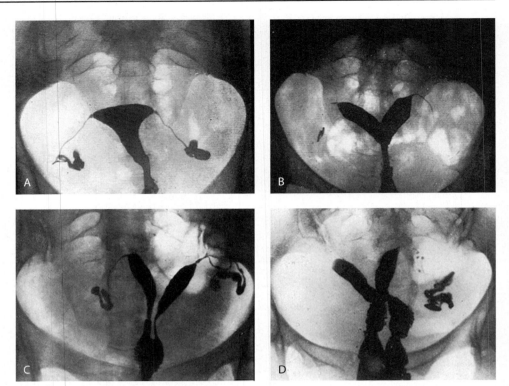

Figure 29.9   **Hysterosalpingograms of normal and abnormal female genital tracts.** The radiographic photographs have been reversed to accentuate the uterine cavities. **A:** Normal study with bilateral spill. **B:** Bicornuate uterus. **C:** Uterus didelphis. **D:** Uterus didelphis with double vagina. (Courtesy of **Dr. A. Gerbie;** from **Spitzer IB, Rebar RW.** Counselling for women with medical problems: ovary and reproductive organs. In: **Hollingsworth D, Resnik R, eds.** *Medical counselling before pregnancy.* New York: Churchill Livingstone, 1988:213–248, with permission.)

approximately monthly exacerbations. It is sometimes difficult to distinguish an imperforate hymen from a transverse vaginal septum, and in most situations, examination under anesthesia is required.

Regardless of the cause, uterine anomalies not involving segmental müllerian agenesis or hypoplasia (class I) are compatible with normal pregnancy. However, increased fetal wastage is reported in the presence of these anomalies (33). Uterine malformations are associated with spontaneous abortion, preterm labor, abnormal presentations, and complications of labor (i.e., retained placenta). Many of these uterine anomalies can be identified with hysterosalpingography (Fig. 29.9). Hysterosalpingography, laparoscopy, and hysteroscopy are used to differentiate a septate uterus (class V) from a bicornuate uterus (class IV). Magnetic resonance imaging (MRI) and endovaginal ultrasonography (sometimes with sonohysterography) are as accurate as these invasive techniques in identifying the abnormality (34).

Obstruction or malformation of the distal genital tract must be distinguished from androgen insensitivity. Individuals with androgen insensitivity have breast development in the absence of significant pubic and axillary hair development; the vagina may be absent or foreshortened in these women.

Hypergonadotropic and Hypogonadotropic Hypogonadism

Basal levels of FSH and prolactin should be determined in individuals in whom secondary sex characteristics have not developed to maturity (Fig. 29.8). Bone age should be estimated from x-rays of the nondominant hand. If prolactin levels are elevated, thyroid function should be assessed to determine whether the individual has primary hypothyroidism. Paradoxically, primary hypothyroidism can result in precocious puberty. If thyroid function is normal, a hypothalamic or pituitary neoplasm is possible, and careful evaluation of the hypothalamic and pituitary area by MRI or computed tomography (CT) is indicated.

Table 29.2 Classification of Müllerian Anomalies

Class I. Segmented müllerian agenesis or hypoplasia

A. Vaginal

B. Cervical

C. Fundal

D. Tubal

E. Combined

Class II. Unicornuate uterus

A. With a rudimentary horn

  1. With a communicating endometrial cavity

  2. With a noncommunicating cavity

  3. With no cavity

B. Without any rudimentary horn

Class III. Uterus didelphys

Class IV. Bicornuate uterus

A. Complete to the internal os

B. Partial

C. Arcuate

Class V. Septate uterus

A. With a complete septum

B. With an incomplete septum

Class VI. Uterus with internal luminal changes

Adapted from **Buttram VC Jr, Gibbons WE.** Müllerian anomalies: a proposed classification (an analysis of 144 cases). *Fertil Steril* 1979;32:40, with permission.

The karyotype should be determined in any individual with delayed puberty and increased basal FSH concentrations. Regardless of the karyotype, the individual with hypergonadotropic hypogonadism has some form of ovarian "failure" (i.e., primary hypogonadism).

Forms of Gonadal Failure

Turner Syndrome   The diagnosis of Turner syndrome requires the presence of characteristic features in phenotypic females coupled with complete or partial absence of the second sex chromosome, with or without cell line mosaicism. **Most affected individuals have a 45,X karyotype, while others have mosaic karyotypes (i.e., 45,X/46,XX; 45,X/46,XY).** Intrauterine growth restriction is common in infants with a 45,X karyotype. After birth, these patients generally grow slowly, beginning in the second or third year of life. They typically have many of the associated stigmata, including lymphedema and sometimes large cystic hygromas of the neck at birth; a webbed neck; multiple pigmented nevi; disorders of the heart, kidneys (most commonly horseshoe), and great vessels (most commonly coarctation of the aorta); and small hyperconvex fingernails (35) (Fig. 29.10). Diabetes mellitus, thyroid disorders, essential hypertension, and other autoimmune disorders are often present in individuals with 45,X karyotypes.

Most 45,X patients have normal intelligence, but many affected individuals have an unusual cognitive defect characterized by an inability to appreciate the shapes and relations of objects with respect to one another (i.e., space-form blindness). Patients with a small ring X chromosome have an increased risk of mental retardation (36). As they grow older, affected children typically are shorter than normal. Although they do not develop breasts at puberty, some pubic or axillary hair may develop because appropriate adrenarche can occur with failure of thelarche (i.e., breast development).

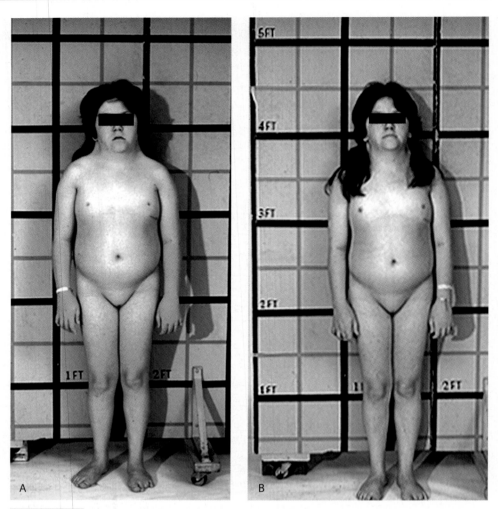

Figure 29.10   **Typical appearance of two individuals with 45,X gonadal dysgenesis. A:** This 16-year-old individual has obvious short stature, a webbed neck, shortened fourth metatarsals, and a thoracotomy scar from the repair of the coarctation of the aorta that was performed at 13 years of age. **B:** This 11-year-old individual also has obvious short stature and stigmata of Turner syndrome. Note that these two individuals look more like each other than they might look like any genetic siblings.

Although less severe short stature and some adolescent development may occur with chromosomal mosaicism, it is reasonable to assume that any short, slowly growing, sexually infantile girl has Turner syndrome until proved otherwise because this disorder is so prevalent (about 1 in 2,500 newborn phenotypic females). In fact, the 45,X karyotype is the single most frequent chromosomal disorder in humans, but most affected fetuses are aborted spontaneously early in pregnancy. However, trisomy is the most common chromosomal type or category of abnormality in first-trimester losses.

The short stature commonly associated with the Turner phenotype appears to result from the loss of a homeobox-containing gene (which encodes for an osteogenic gene) located on the pseudoautosomal region (PAR 1) of the short arms of the X (Xp22) and Y (Yp11.3) chromosomes (37). This gene, which is called either *SHOX* (short stature homeobox-containing gene) or *PHOG* (pseudoautosomal homeobox osteogenic gene), escapes X inactivation because of its pseudoautosomal location. The gene appears to account for about two-thirds of the height deficit commonly associated with Turner syndrome.

Even in the presence of typical Turner stigmata, a karyotype is indicated to eliminate the possibility of the presence of any portion of a Y chromosome. Analysis of pooled data suggests that the presence of Y chromosome material is associated with a 12% risk of a gonadoblastoma (38). If a Y chromosome is identified, laparoscopic prophylactic gonadectomy is recommended at the time of diagnosis to eliminate the risk of malignancy. Although gonadoblastomas are benign tumors with no metastatic potential that can arise spontaneously in gonads containing a portion of a Y chromosome, they can be precursors to germ cell malignancies, such as dysgerminomas (most commonly), teratomas, embryonal carcinomas, or endodermal sinus tumors (39). In individuals in whom there is no evidence of neoplastic dissemination, the uterus may be left *in situ* for donor *in vitro* fertilization and embryo transfer.

Individuals with Turner syndrome are at increased risk of sudden death from aortic rupture or dissection resulting from cystic medial necrosis during pregnancy, and the risk may be as great as 2% or more (40). In addition, this may occur even if the aortic root diameter is normal. Because of their small stature, ascending aortic diameters of less than 5 cm may represent significant dilatation. Thus, the use of the aortic size index (ascending aortic diameters measured by MRI at the level of the right pulmonary artery normalized to body surface area) is preferred (41). Patients with an aortic size index greater than 2.0 cm/m^2 require close cardiovascular surveillance and those with an aortic size index of 2.5 cm/m^2 or more are at highest risk for aortic dissection. In fact, the risk of acute aortic dissection is increased by more than 100-fold in young and middle-aged women with Turner syndrome. **If pregnancy is being considered, preconception assessment must include cardiologic evaluation with MRI of the aorta.**

The evaluation of other commonly involved organ systems should include a careful physical examination, with special attention to the cardiovascular system, and thyroid function tests (including antibody assessment), fasting blood glucose, renal function tests, and intravenous pyelography or a renal ultrasonography.

Treatment of Turner Syndrome   To increase final adult height, commonly accepted treatment strategies include use of *exogenous GH* (42–44). With recombinant human GH use, the average height gain varied from 4 to 16 cm. It appears that early initiation of therapy (between 2–8 years of age), gradually increasing the dose, and continuing treatment for a mean of 7 years can lead to achievement of a final height greater than 150 cm in most patients (43). Weekly doses of *GH* of 0.375 mg/kg divided into seven daily doses are typical. Therapy may be continued until a satisfactory height is attained or until little growth potential remains (bone age ≥14 years and growth velocity <2 cm per year). It is not clear if a nonaromatizable anabolic steroid such as *oxandrolone* will provide additional growth. In girls older than 8 years of age or those with extreme short stature, consideration can be given to using higher doses of GH and adding *oxandrolone* (45). The dose of *oxandrolone* should be 0.05 mg/kg per day or less, as higher doses will result in virilization and more rapid skeletal maturation. In addition, liver enzymes should be monitored.

The gonadal steroid treatment of patients with Turner syndrome is as follows:

1. **To promote sexual maturation, therapy with** *exogenous estrogen* **should be initiated when the patient is psychologically ready, at about 12 to 13 years of age, and after** *GH* **therapy was administered for several years. Low-dose** *estrogen* **can be introduced at this time without compromising final adult height** (46).

2. **Because the intent is to mimic normal pubertal development, therapy with low-dose** *estrogen* **alone** (such as 0.025 mg per day *transdermal estradiol* or 0.3–0.625 mg *conjugated estrogens* orally each day) **should be initiated.**

3. **Progestins** (5–10 mg *medroxyprogesterone acetate* or 200 mg *micronized progesterone* orally for 12 to 14 days every 1 to 2 months) **can be added to prevent endometrial hyperplasia after the patient first experiences vaginal bleeding or after 6 to 12 months of unopposed** *estrogen* **use if the patient has not yet had any bleeding.**

4. **The dose of** *estrogen* **is increased slowly over 1 to 2 years until the patient is taking about twice as much** *estrogen* **as the amount administered to postmenopausal women.**

5. **Girls with gonadal dysgenesis must be monitored carefully for the development of hypertension with estrogen therapy.**

6. **The patients and their parents should be counseled regarding the emotional and physical changes that will occur with therapy.**

7. **It is important to educate the patient that hormone replacement therapy is usually required until the time of normal menopause to maintain feminization and prevent osteoporosis** (47).

Mosaic Forms of Gonadal Dysgenesis   **Individuals with rare mosaic forms of gonadal dysgenesis may develop normally at puberty.** The decision to initiate therapy with exogenous estrogen should be based mainly on circulating FSH levels. Levels in the normal range for the patient's age imply the presence of functional gonads.

These individuals can become pregnant, with success rates of more than 50% using donor oocytes (48). The increased risk of sudden death during pregnancy resulting from aortic rupture should be assumed to be similar to that of other women with the Turner phenotype (40).

Pure Gonadal Dysgenesis   **The term *pure gonadal dysgenesis* refers to 46,XX or 46,XY phenotypic females who have streak gonads. This condition may occur sporadically or may be inherited as an autosomal recessive trait or as an X-linked trait in XY gonadal dysgenesis** (Fig. 29.11). Affected girls typically are of average height and have none of the stigmata of Turner syndrome, but they have elevated levels of FSH because the streak gonads produce neither steroid hormones nor inhibin. **When gonadal dysgenesis occurs in 46,XY individuals, it is sometimes termed *Swyer syndrome*. Surgical extirpation is warranted in individuals with a 46,XY karyotype to prevent development of germ cell neoplasms.** Both 46,XX and 46,XY forms of gonadal dysgenesis benefit from exogenous estrogen and are potential candidates for donor oocytes.

In early gonadal failure, the ovaries apparently develop normally but contain no oocytes by the expected age of puberty. These disorders are considered further in the discussion delineating the evaluation of amenorrhea (see Chapter 30).

Hypogonadotropic Hypogonadism

Hypothalamic–pituitary disturbances are usually associated with low levels of circulating gonadotropins (with both LH and FSH levels less than or equal to 10 mIU/mL) (49). There are both sporadic and familial causes of hypogonadotropic hypogonadism, and the differential diagnosis is extensive. **Mutations in several genes cause hypogonadotropic hypogonadism in humans** (50). This condition can arise from abnormalities in hypothalamic GnRH secretion, impaired release of gonadotropins from the pituitary gland, or both.

At least 17 different single-gene mutations are identified as being associated with delayed or absent puberty in humans (51). They are estimated to account for about 30% of individuals with disorders of puberty. These genes include *KAL1* (X-linked Kallmann syndrome), *FGFR1* (autosomal Kallmann syndrome), *DAX1* (the gene for X-linked congenital adrenal hypoplasia), *GNRHR* (the gene for the GnRH receptor), *PC1* (the gene for prohormone convertase 1), and *GPR54* (encoding a G-protein coupled receptor). Delayed puberty may result from mutations in genes affecting gonadotrophs specifically (*GnRHR, LHβ, FSHβ*) or in genes involved more generally in the development and functioning of the pituitary gland (*LHX3, PROP1, HESX1*).

Constitutional Delay   It is important to remember that low levels of LH and FSH are normally present in the prepubertal years; thus, girls with constitutionally delayed puberty may mistakenly be presumed to have hypogonadotropic hypogonadism. **Constitutional delay is the most common cause of delayed puberty.** In a normal population, 2% to 3% of normal children will be classified as having pubertal delay, and this finding may be considered a normal variant. **Constitutional delayed growth and adolescence can be diagnosed only after careful evaluation excludes other causes of delayed puberty and normal sexual development is documented by longitudinal follow-up.** The farther below the third percentile for height that the young girl is, the less likely it is that the cause is constitutional. Because some children are severely handicapped socially by constitutional pubertal delay, some physicians occasionally provide *exogenous estrogen* in low doses for 3 to 4 months to stimulate some pubertal development. However, the benefits of treatment are not well documented, and there is little evidence to support the idea that treatment improves psychosocial function.

Kallmann Syndrome   As originally described in 1944, *Kallmann syndrome* **consisted of the triad of anosmia, hypogonadism, and color blindness in men** (52). **Women may be affected, and other associated defects may include cleft lip and palate, cerebellar ataxia, nerve deafness, and abnormalities of thirst and vasopressin release.** The frequency approximates

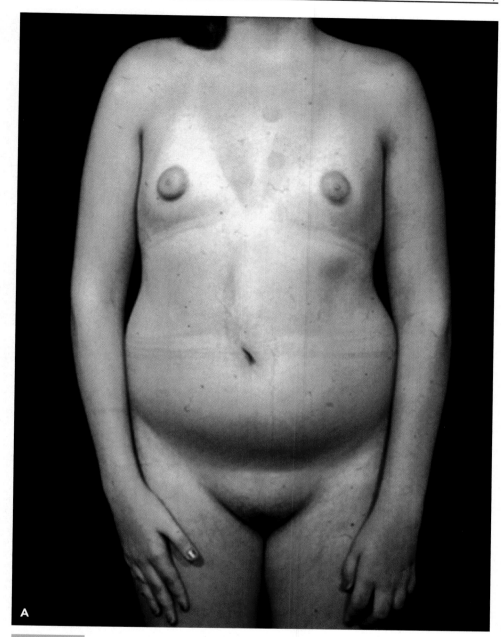

Figure 29.11   A: A 16-year-old individual with 46,XX gonadal dysgenesis and primary amenorrhea. Circulating follicle-stimulating hormone (FSH) levels were markedly elevated. The small amount of breast development (Tanner stage 2) is unusual, but some pubertal development may occur in such patients.

1 in 10,000 men and 1 in 50,000 women. Sporadic cases are more common than inherited forms. Inheritance is described as being X-linked recessive, autosomal dominant, and autosomal recessive. Because autopsy studies show partial or complete agenesis of the olfactory bulb, the term *olfactogenital dysplasia* is used to describe the disorder. These anatomic findings coincide with embryologic studies documenting that GnRH neurons originally develop in the epithelium of the olfactory placode and normally migrate into the hypothalamus (53). In some affected individuals, gene defects were found in one protein, anosmin-1, that facilitates this neuronal migration, thus leading to an absence of GnRH neurons in the hypothalamus and olfactory bulbs and consequent hypogonadotropic hypogonadism and anosmia (Kallmann syndrome) (54). The gene defect resulting in loss of this adhesion protein is localized to the Xp22.3

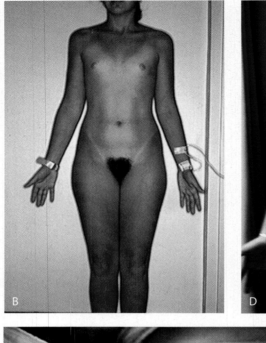

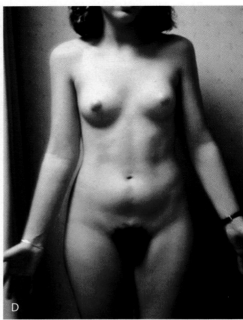

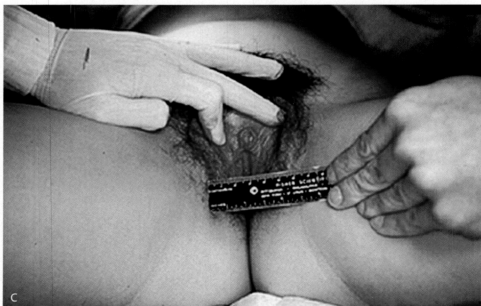

Figure 29.11   (*Continued*) **B:** A 16-year-old individual with 46,XY gonadal dysgenesis who presented with primary amenorrhea and markedly elevated FSH levels. Most affected individuals do not present with as much pubic and axillary hair development. The right gonad contained a dysgerminoma, but there was no evidence of metastases. (From **Rebar RW.** Normal and abnormal sexual differentiation and pubertal development. In: **Moore TR, Reiter RC, Rebar RW, et al., eds.** *Gynecology and obstetrics: a longitudinal approach.* New York: Churchill Livingstone, 1993:97–133, with permission.) **C:** Clitoromegaly noted in the girl with 46,XY gonadal dysgenesis depicted in Figure 29.11B. **D:** The same individual as depicted in Figure 29.11B and D with 46,XY gonadal dysgenesis 1 year after gonadectomy and replacement with exogenous estrogen.

locus in an X-linked form of the syndrome, and this locus is designated *KAL1*. Other features of X-linked Kallmann syndrome include unilateral renal agenesis, bimanual synkinesia, and sensorineural hearing loss. In some cases of autosomal dominant Kallmann syndrome, inactivating mutations of the gene encoding the fibroblast growth factor receptor-1 (*FGFR1* or *KAL2*) were reported. The disorder is so heterogeneous that it appears likely that it forms a structural continuum with other midline defects. Septo-optic dysplasia represents the most severe form of the disorder.

Clinically, affected individuals typically present with sexual infantilism and an eunuchoid habitus, but some degree of breast development may occur (Fig. 29.12). Primary amenorrhea is the rule. The ovaries are usually small, with follicles seldom developing beyond the primordial stage. Circulating gonadotropin levels are usually very low but almost invariably measurable. Affected individuals respond readily to pulsatile administration of exogenous GnRH, and this is the most physiologic approach to ovulation induction (48). For women not seeking pregnancy, therapy with exogenous estrogen and progestin is indicated.

Isolated gonadotropin deficiency can occur in association with the *Prader-Labhart-Willi syndrome,* which is characterized by obesity, short stature, hypogonadism, small hands and feet (acromicria), mental retardation, and infantile hypotonia. When the syndrome occurs in association with the Laurence-Moon-Bardet-Biedl syndrome, retinitis pigmentosa, postaxial polydactyly, obesity, and hypogonadism may be present. Prader-Labhart-Willi syndrome apparently results from rearrangements of chromosome 15q11 to q13, an imprinted region of the human genome (55). Laurence-Moon-Bardet-Biedl syndrome, inherited in an autosomal recessive manner, is apparently heterogeneous, with at least four involved gene loci having been mapped to date (56).

Multiple pituitary hormone deficiencies, which are usually hypothalamic in origin, may be congenital and either part of an inherited constellation of findings or sporadic. If GH or thyroid-stimulating hormone (TSH) concentrations are subnormal, growth and pubertal development will be affected. Thus, the condition should be diagnosed before the age of puberty. Because individuals with hypopituitarism have a high mortality rate, predominantly caused by vascular and respiratory disease, it is important to identify affected individuals. Later age at diagnosis, female sex, and above all craniopharyngioma are identified as significant independent risk factors (57). Untreated gonadotropin deficiency is an important risk factor for early mortality.

Tumors of the Hypothalamus and Pituitary   **Several different tumors of the hypothalamic and pituitary regions may lead to hypogonadotropic hypogonadism** (58) (Fig. 29.13A). **Except for craniopharyngiomas, these tumors are relatively uncommon in children. A craniopharyngioma is a tumor of the Rathke's pouch. It is the most common neoplasm associated with delayed puberty, and it accounts for 10% of all childhood central nervous system tumors. Craniopharyngiomas are usually suprasellar in location and may be asymptomatic well into the second decade of life.** Such tumors may present as headache, visual disturbances, short stature or growth failure, delayed puberty, or diabetes insipidus. Visual field defects (including bilateral temporal hemianopsia), optic atrophy, or papilledema may be seen on physical examination. Laboratory evaluation should document hypogonadotropism and may reveal hyperprolactinemia as a result of interruption of hypothalamic dopamine inhibition of prolactin release. Radiographically, the tumor may be either cystic or solid and may show areas of calcification. Appropriate therapy for hypothalamic–pituitary tumors may involve surgical excision or radiotherapy (with adequate pituitary hormone replacement therapy) and are best managed by a team of physicians that includes an endocrinologist, a neurosurgeon, and a radiotherapist.

Other Central Nervous System Disorders   Other central nervous system disorders that may lead to delayed puberty include infiltrative diseases, such as Langerhans cell-type histiocytosis, particularly the form known previously as *Hand-Schüller-Christian disease* (Fig. 29.13B and 29.13C). Diabetes insipidus is the most common endocrinopathy (because of infiltration of the supraoptic nucleus in the hypothalamus), but short stature resulting from GH deficiency and delayed puberty caused by gonadotropin deficiency are not uncommon in this disorder (59).

Irradiation of the central nervous system for treatment of any neoplasm or leukemia may result in hypothalamic dysfunction. Although GH deficiency is the most frequent finding, partial or complete gonadotropin deficiency may develop in some patients.

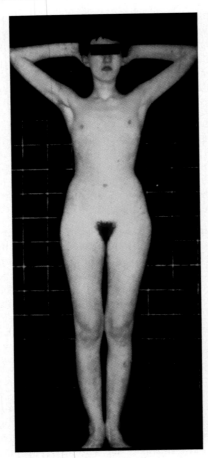

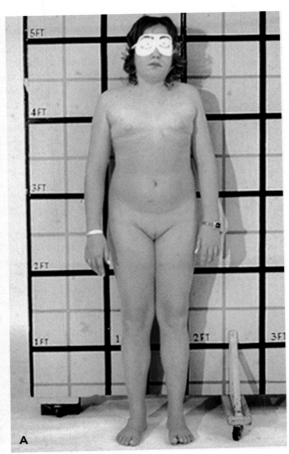

Figure 29.12   Left **A 21.-year-old woman with Kallmann syndrome.** Note that the patient has some pubic and axillary hair. Bone age was 16 years. It is rare to see affected individuals today who were not given oral contraceptive agents to induce menses (with some consequent breast development). (From **Wilkins L.** *The diagnosis and treatment of endocrine disorders in childhood and adolescence.* 3rd ed. Springfield, IL: Charles C Thomas, 1965, with permission.)

Figure 29.13   Right **A: A 16-year-old girl with delayed puberty.** Breast budding began at 11 years of age, but there was no further development. During the year before presentation, her scholastic performance in school deteriorated, she gained 25 lb, she became increasingly lethargic, and nocturia and polydypsia were noted. Initial evaluation documented low follicle-stimulating hormone, elevated prolactin, and a bone age of 10.5 years. Computed tomography scanning documented a large hypothalamic neoplasm that proved to be an ectopic germinoma. The patient was also documented to be hypothyroid and hypoadrenal and to have diabetes insipidus. Despite the elevated prolactin, she had no galactorrhea because of the minimal breast development. (From **Rebar RW.** Normal and abnormal sexual differentiation and pubertal development. In: **Moore TR, Reiter RC, Rebar RW, et al., eds.** *Gynecology and obstetrics: a longitudinal approach.* New York: Churchill Livingstone, 1993:97–133, with permission.)

Severe chronic illnesses, often accompanied by malnutrition, may lead to slowed growth in childhood and delayed adolescence. Regardless of the cause, weight loss to less than 80% to 85% of ideal body weight often results in hypothalamic GnRH deficiency. If adequate body weight and nutrition are maintained in chronic illnesses such as Crohn disease or chronic pulmonary or renal disease, sufficient gonadotropin secretion usually is present to initiate and maintain pubertal development.

Anorexia Nervosa and Bulimia   **Significant weight loss and psychological dysfunction occur simultaneously with anorexia nervosa (60,61).** Although many anorectic girls experience amenorrhea after pubertal development begins, if the disorder begins sufficiently early,

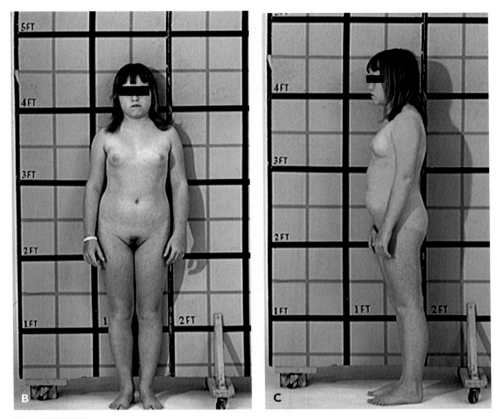

Figure 29.13 B: **A 16-year-old girl (frontal view) with primary amenorrhea who progressed in puberty until about 12 years of age.** Breast budding occurred at about 10 years of age. The patient's short stature is obvious. She proved to have hypopituitarism. Classic radiographic findings established the diagnosis of Langerhans cell–type histiocytosis (Hand-Schüller-Christian disease). C: **Side view of girl shown in Figure 29.13B.**

pubertal development may be delayed or interrupted (Fig. 29.14). **The following constellation of associated findings confirms anorexia nervosa in most individuals:**

1. **Relentless pursuit of thinness**
2. **Amenorrhea, sometimes preceding the weight loss**
3. **Extreme inanition**
4. **Obsessive-compulsive personality often characterized by overachievement**
5. **Distorted and bizarre attitude toward eating, food, or weight**
6. **Distorted body image**

Because normal body weight is commonly maintained in bulimia, it is unusual for bulimic patients to experience either delayed development or amenorrhea. Girls with anorexia nervosa may have, in addition to hypogonadotropic hypogonadism, partial diabetes insipidus, abnormal temperature regulation, hypotension, chemical hypothyroidism with low serum triiodothyronine (T_3) and high reverse T_3 levels, and elevated circulating cortisol levels in the absence of evidence of hypercortisolism (62). Other common features include hypokalemia, anemia, hypoalbuminemia, high β-carotene levels, and high cholesterol levels. All features of anorexia nervosa are reversible with weight gain, except for amenorrhea (which persists in 30% to 47%) and osteopenia (i.e., it now seems that any bone lost cannot be fully recovered). **Management of patients with anorexia nervosa is notoriously difficult. A team approach involving the primary clinician, psychiatrist, and nutritionist is most effective. In fact, anorexia nervosa has the highest mortality of any psychiatric disorder. Deaths are often sudden and unexpected. Cause of death (often unknown) can include hypoglycemia and electrolyte imbalance.**

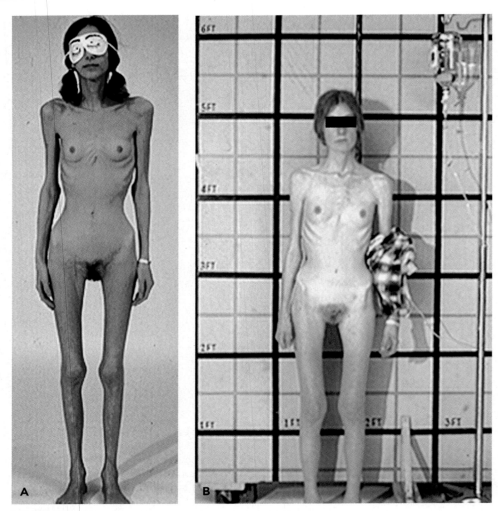

Figure 29.14   A: A 20-year-old college woman with anorexia nervosa. B: A 16-year-old student with anorexia nervosa. In both cases, as is true of most such patients, pubertal development had been completed and menses initiated before anorexia led to marked weight loss.

Fear of obesity, a syndrome of self-induced malnutrition common among teenage gymnasts and ballet dancers, may slow growth and delay pubertal development (63). These children voluntarily reduce their caloric intake as much as 40%, leading to nutritional growth retardation. An additive role for endurance training in the delayed development is possible, but the mechanisms are unclear at this point. These conditions are essentially severe forms of hypothalamic amenorrhea. Inevitably delayed puberty will occur unless adequate caloric intake is provided.

Hyperprolactinemia   **Low levels of LH and FSH may be associated with hyperprolactinemia.** As noted, galactorrhea cannot occur in the absence of complete breast development. Pituitary prolactinomas are rare during adolescence but must be considered when certain signs and symptoms are present. **Many individuals with prolactinomas have a history of delayed menarche.** The association between the ingestion of certain drugs (most often psychotropic agents and opiates in this age group) is well established. Primary hypothyroidism is associated with hyperprolactinemia because increased levels of thyrotropin-releasing hormone (TRH) stimulate secretion of prolactin. The *empty sella syndrome*, in which the sella turcica is enlarged but is replaced by cerebrospinal fluid, may be associated with hyperprolactinemia.

Use of Chemotherapeutic Agents   **As survival rates following treatment for childhood malignancy improve, the effects of cancer therapy become more important. Both radiation** therapy to the abdomen and systemic chemotherapeutic agents, particularly alkylating agents, have toxic effects on germ cells. Although prepubertal gonads appear less vulnerable than those of adults, ovarian failure is common. An argument can be made for endocrine assessment as early as 1 year following completion of therapy to identify children who will suffer from hypogonadism. Spontaneous ovarian activity can resume even years after therapy.

Asynchronous Puberty

Asynchronous pubertal development is characteristic of androgen insensitivity (i.e., testicular feminization). Affected individuals typically present with breast development (usually only to Tanner stage 3) out of proportion with the amount of pubic and axillary hair present (Fig. 29.15). In this disorder, 46,XY individuals have bilateral testes, female external genitalia, a blindly ending vagina (often foreshortened and sometimes absent), and no müllerian derivatives (i.e., uterus and fallopian tubes) (64). Infrequently, patients may have clitoral enlargement and labioscrotal fusion at puberty, which is referred to as *incomplete androgen insensitivity.*

Asynchronous puberty is heterogeneous but is always related to some abnormality of the androgen receptor or of androgen action (65). In perhaps 60% to 70% of cases, androgen receptors cannot be detected (i.e., the patient is receptor negative). In the remaining cases, androgen receptors are present (i.e., receptor positive), but mutations in the androgen receptor are detected or there is a defect at a more distal step in androgen action (i.e., a postreceptor defect). Receptor-positive individuals are indistinguishable clinically from receptor-negative individuals. Several different mutations in the androgen receptor gene, most of which occur within the androgen-binding domain of the receptor, are identified in affected individuals who are receptor positive. Severe X-linked androgen receptor gene mutations cause complete androgen insensitivity, whereas mild mutations impair virilization with or without infertility, and moderate mutations result in a wide phenotypic spectrum of expression among siblings (66).

Because the Sertoli cells of the testes make antimüllerian hormone (AMH), müllerian derivatives are absent in this disorder; thus, müllerian regression occurs normally. The testes are often normal in size and may be located anywhere along the path of embryonic testicular descent—in the abdomen, inguinal canal, or labia. Half of all individuals with androgen insensitivity develop inguinal hernias. Recognizing that most such girls will be 46,XX, it is important to determine the karyotype in prepubertal girls with inguinal hernias, especially if a uterus cannot be detected with certainty by ultrasound.

The risk of germ cell malignancy is 2% in complete androgen insensitivity syndrome (67). Most clinicians believe the risk for gonadal neoplasia is low before 25 years of age; thus, the **testes should be left in place until after pubertal feminization, especially because the risk of neoplasia appears to increase with age.** Exogenous estrogen should be provided after gonadectomy.

The diagnosis is often suspected by the typical physical findings and strongly suggested by normal (or even somewhat elevated) male levels of testosterone, normal or somewhat elevated levels of LH, and normal levels of FSH. The diagnosis is confirmed by a 46,XY karyotype.

Interacting with the patient and family requires sensitivity and care. It may be inadvisable to begin by informing the patient of the karyotype; the psychological implications may be devastating because the patient was reared as a girl. Family members should be informed initially that müllerian aplasia occurred and that the risk for neoplasia mandates gonadectomy after puberty. Because the disorder can be inherited in an X-linked recessive fashion, families should undergo appropriate genetic counseling and screening to identify the possible existence of other affected family members.

Precocious Puberty

Although precocious pubertal development may be classified in several ways, it is perhaps simplest to think of the development as gonadotropin dependent (in which case it is almost invariably of central origin) or gonadotropin independent (of peripheral origin). Precocious puberty is 20 times more common in girls than in boys. In fully 90% of girls, the precocious development is idiopathic, whereas this appears to be true for only 10% of boys. Family history, the rapidity with which secondary sexual characteristics are developing, the rate of growth, and the presence or absence of central nervous system disease should all be considered

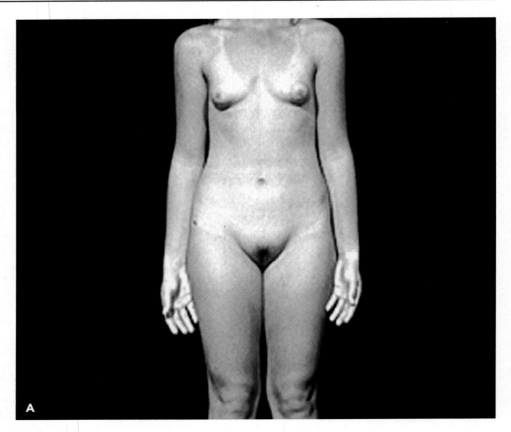

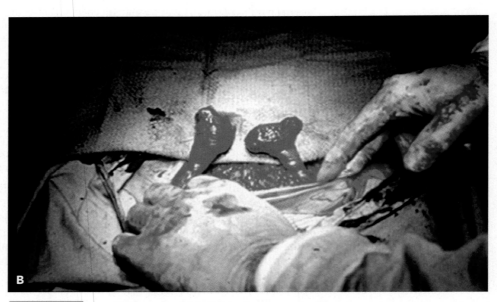

Figure 29.15   A: **This 17-year-old individual presented with primary amenorrhea and was found to have a blind-ending vagina and bilateral inguinal masses.** Circulating levels of testosterone were at the upper limits of the normal range for men and the karyotype was 46,XY, confirming androgen insensitivity. B: **Two inguinal testes were found at surgery.** (From **Simpson JL, Rebar RW.** Normal and abnormal sexual differentiation and development. In: **Becker KL, ed.** *Principles and practice of endocrinology and metabolism.* 2nd ed. Philadelphia, PA: JB Lippincott, 1995:788–822, with permission.)

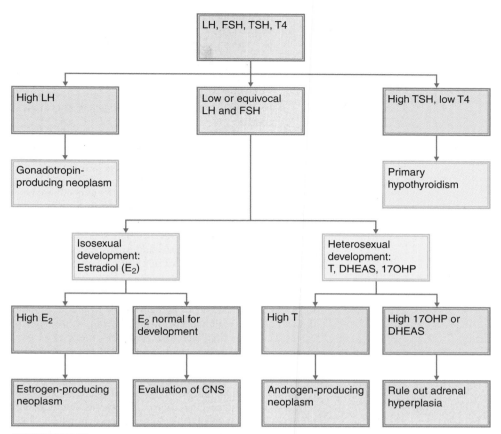

Figure 29.16   Flow diagram for the evaluation of precocious puberty in phenotypic females. LH, luteinizing hormone; FSH, follicle-stimulating hormone; TSH, thyroid-stimulating hormone; T4, thyroxine; T, testosterone; DHEAS, dehydroepiandrosterone sulfate; 17OHP, 17-hydroxyprogesterone; CNS, central nervous system. (From **Rebar RW.** Normal and abnormal sexual differentiation and pubertal development. In: **Moore TR, Reiter RC, Rebar RW, et al., eds.** *Gynecology and obstetrics: a longitudinal approach.* New York: Churchill Livingstone, 1993:97–133, with permission.)

in deciding whether to pursue evaluation of a girl for precocious puberty. The evaluation of precocious puberty is as follows:

1. **Measurement of basal gonadotropin levels is the first step in the evaluation of a child with sexual precocity** (Fig. 29.16).

2. **Thyroid function should be evaluated** to rule out primary hypothyroidism as the cause of precocious development.

3. **High levels of LH (which really may be human chorionic gonadotropin detected because of cross-reactivity with LH in immunoassays) suggest a gonadotropin-producing neoplasm,** most often a pinealoma (ectopic germinoma) or choriocarcinoma or, less often, a hepatoblastoma. (Gonadotropin-producing neoplasms are the only causes of precocious puberty in which the gonadotropin dependence does not equate with central precocious puberty.)

4. **Low or pubertal levels of gonadotropins indicate the need to determine circulating estradiol concentrations in girls with isosexual development** and to assess androgen levels, specifically testosterone, DHEAS, and 17α-hydroxyprogesterone in girls with heterosexual development.

5. **Increased estradiol levels suggest an estrogen-secreting neoplasm, probably of ovarian origin.**

6. **Increased testosterone levels suggest an androgen-producing neoplasm of the ovary or the adrenal gland.** Such neoplasms may be palpable on abdominal or rectal exam-

ination. Increased 17α-hydroxyprogesterone levels are diagnostic of 21-hydroxylase deficiency (i.e., congenital adrenal hyperplasia [CAH]). Levels of DHEAS are elevated in various forms of CAH.

7. **If the estradiol levels are compatible with the degree of pubertal development observed, evaluation of the central nervous system by MRI or CT scanning is warranted.**

8. **Bone age should always be assessed in evaluating an individual with sexual precocity.**

9. **A GnRH stimulation test can be used to confirm central precocious puberty. After 100 μg GnRH, an LH peak of greater than 15 mIU/mL is suggestive of gonadotropin-dependent precocious puberty** (68).

Perhaps the most difficult decision for the gynecologist is determining how much evaluation is warranted for the young girl brought in by her mother for precocious breast budding only (*precocious thelarche*) or the appearance of pubic or axillary hair alone (*precocious pubarche* or *adrenarche*) (Fig. 29.17). In such cases, it is acceptable to many clinicians to follow the patient at frequent intervals and to proceed with evaluation if there is evidence of pubertal progression. The feasibility of this approach may depend on the concerns of the parents.

Premature Thelarche

Premature thelarche is unilateral or bilateral breast enlargement without other signs of sexual maturation. There is no significant nipple or areola development. It usually occurs by 2 years of age and rarely after age 4. It may be caused by increased sensitivity of the breasts to low levels of estrogen or to increased estradiol secretion by follicular cysts. It is a benign self-limited disorder and thus only reassurance and follow-up are required. In most cases, onset of puberty, adult height, and adult reproductive function are normal (69). Rarely, premature thelarche can be a harbinger of progressive gonadarche. It is suggested that measurement of uterine volume (anteroposterior diameter × longitudinal diameter × transverse diameter × 0.523) may be the most sensitive and specific discriminator between premature thelarche and early true precocious puberty (70). If needed, breast ultrasound can help distinguish unilateral premature thelarche from fibroadenomas, cysts, neurofibromas, or other lesions.

Premature Adrenarche

Premature adrenarche or pubarche may be caused by increased sensitivity to low levels of androgens and must be distinguished from late-onset (nonclassic) CAH. If there is no evidence of breast development or of progression, these conditions are virtually always benign.

Girls with premature adrenarche are at increased risk of developing polycystic ovary syndrome (PCOS), hyperinsulinemia, acanthosis nigricans, and dyslipidemia in adolescence and adult life, especially if fetal growth was reduced and birth weight was low (71). Although mean androgen levels are within the normal range, a significant minority have an exaggerated response to corticotropin stimulation. The magnitude of this response is inversely related to insulin sensitivity. Thus, premature adrenarche may be the first sign of insulin resistance or PCOS in some individuals. Treatment of coexisting obesity and long-term follow-up are indicated to address potential complications of PCOS and insulin resistance.

Isolated Premature Menarche

Isolated premature menarche is vaginal bleeding at age 1 to 9 years in the absence of other signs of puberty. The bleeding is usually limited to a few days. It can recur for 1 to 6 years and then cease. The etiology is uncertain. Most cases are associated with subsequent normal pubertal development and fertility. The differential diagnosis includes vaginal foreign bodies, trauma, sexual abuse, vaginal infection, or neoplasms such as rhabdomyosarcoma, McCune-Albright syndrome (in which menarche may occur before other manifestations of sexual precocity), and primary hypothyroidism.

Central (True) Precocious Puberty

In central precocious puberty, GnRH prematurely stimulates increased gonadotropin secretion. Central precocious puberty may occur in children in whom there is no structural abnormality, in which case it is termed *constitutional* or *idiopathic*. **Constitutional (idiopathic) sexual precocity is the most common cause of precocious puberty.** It is often familial and represents the so-called tail of the Gaussian curve (i.e., the early 2.5% for the age distribution for the onset of puberty). In many of these girls, puberty is slowly progressive, but in a few, development progresses rapidly. The major complication of sexual precocity is limitation of height. Thus, therapy may be warranted to prevent this consequence.

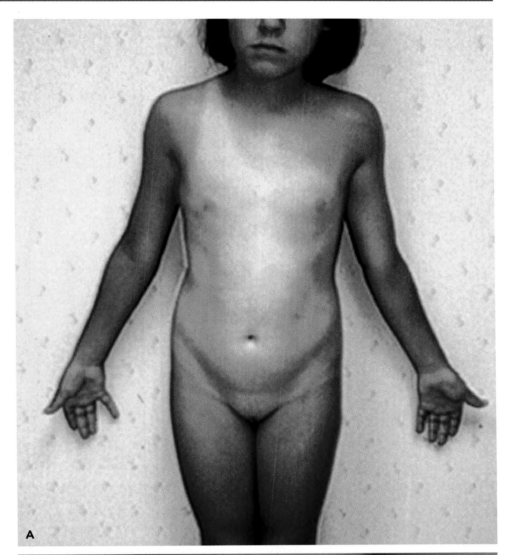

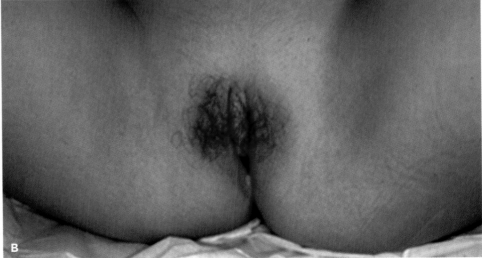

Figure 29.17 **Five-year-old girl with development of pubic hair (A) as shown more closely in (B) (precocious adrenarche).** Gonadotropin levels were prepubertal, and bone age was appropriate for age. No further development occurred until breast budding at approximately age 9.

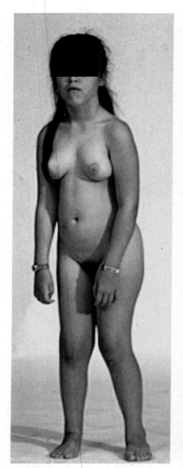 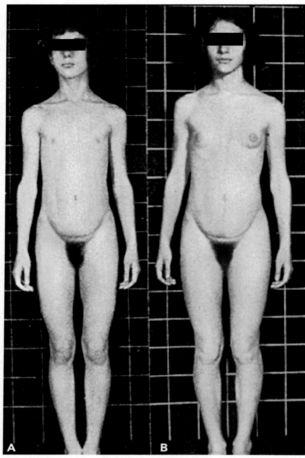

Figure 29.18   Left: **A 7$^1/_2$-year-old girl with Tanner stage 4 pubertal development who began menstruating 1 month earlier.** She was 57 inches tall (above the 95th percentile). Luteinizing hormone and follicle-stimulating hormone levels were consistent with her development. A large neoplasm that proved to be a hypothalamic hamartoma was present on computed tomography scan. Pubertal development began at about 5 years of age.

Figure 29.19   Right: **A: A 10$^1/_2$-year-old girl with 21-hydroxylase deficiency before treatment.** 17-Ketosteroid (KS) excretion was 34 mg per day. **B: The same patient after 9 months of therapy with cortisone** (17-KS excretion: 4.6 mg per day). (From **Wilkins L.** *The diagnosis and treatment of endocrine disorders in childhood and adolescence.* 3rd ed. Springfield, IL: Charles C Thomas, 1965:439, with permission.)

Alternatively, central precocious puberty may result from a tumor, infection, congenital abnormality, or traumatic injury affecting the hypothalamus. A number of congenital malformations, including hydrocephalus, craniostenosis, arachnoid cysts, and septo-optic dysplasia, can be associated with precocious puberty (and with sexual infantilism).

A common etiology (2% to 28%) of central precocious puberty is a hypothalamic hamartoma. It is a congenital malformation composed of a heterotopic mass of nerve tissue containing GnRH neurosecretory neurons, fiber bundles, and glial cells. It is not a true neoplasm and it generally does not change over time based on long-term follow-up studies with periodic CT or MRI scans. Hamartomas appear as isodense, abnormal fullnesses that do not enhance with contrast material. Extreme precocity (usually before 3 years of age) and the absence of tumor markers, such as β-human chorionic gonadotropin and α-fetoprotein, suggest a hamartoma (72). Hamartomas can be associated with laughing (gelastic) seizures, behavioral disturbances, mental retardation, and dysmorphic syndromes. It appears that hamartomas produce GnRH in a pulsatile manner and thus stimulate gonadotropin secretion (Fig. 29.18) (73). Precocious pubertal development can be controlled with GnRH-agonist therapy (74). Because deaths were reported after neurosurgical extirpation, the latter should be reserved for management of hamartomas associated with intractable seizures or hydrocephalus (75).

The efficacy of gonadotropin-releasing hormone analogues (GnRHa) in increasing adult height is undisputed only in early-onset (girls less than 6 years old) central precocious puberty (76). Concerns of weight gain and long-term decrease in bone mineral density with the use of GnRHa do not seem to be warranted. The most important clinical criterion for initiating GnRHa treatment is documented progression of pubertal development over a 3- to 6-month period. This observational period may not be necessary if the child is at or past Tanner stage 3, particularly with advanced skeletal maturation. It appears that discontinuation of GnRHa at a chronological age of about 11 years and a bone age of about 12 years is associated with maximum adult height (77–79). There are a variety of GnRHa formulations, and the choice of a particular agent depends on patient and physician preference.

Precocious Puberty of Peripheral Origin

In gonadotropin-independent precocious puberty, production of estrogens or androgens from the ovaries, adrenals, or rare steroid-secreting neoplasms leads to early pubertal development. Small functional ovarian cysts, typically asymptomatic, are common in children and may cause transient sexual precocity (80). **Simple cysts (with a benign ultrasonographic appearance) can be observed and usually resolve over time.** Of the various ovarian neoplasms that can secrete estrogens, granulosa-theca cell tumors occur most frequently but are still rare (81). Although such tumors may grow rapidly, more than two-thirds are benign.

Exposure to exogenous estrogens can mimic gonadotropin-independent precocious puberty. Ingestion of oral contraceptives, other estrogen-containing pharmaceutical agents, and estrogen-contaminated foods, and the topical use of estrogens, are implicated in cases of precocious development in infants and children. Ingestion of exogenous steroids over a considerable length of time is required to induce changes typical of complete precocious development.

McCune-Albright Syndrome

The *McCune-Albright syndrome* is characterized by the classic triad of polyostotic fibrous dysplasia of bone, irregular café-au-lait spots on the skin, and GnRH-independent sexual precocity. The café-au-lait spots are usually large, do not cross the midline, and have irregular "coast of Maine" margins. They are often located on the same side as the bony lesions. Sexual precocity often begins in the first 2 years and usually presents with menstrual bleeding. Girls develop sexual precocity as a result of functioning ovarian cysts. Serum estradiol is elevated. Other endocrinopathies may include hyperthyroidism, hypercortisolism, hyperprolactinemia, acromegaly, and hyperparathyroidism. Osteomalacia, hepatic abnormalities, and cardiac arrhythmia may occur. Mutations of the $G_{s\alpha}$ subunit of the G protein, which couples extracellular hormonal signals to the activation of adenylate cyclase, are responsible for the autonomous hyperfunction of the endocrine glands and, presumably, for the other defects present in this disorder (82). Treatment with a GnRH agonist is not effective because the precocious pubertal development is GnRH independent. Treatment with aromatase inhibitors, such as *testolactone* and *fadrozole,* has mixed results. A multicenter trial showed that *tamoxifen* decreases vaginal bleeding, growth rate, and the rate of bone age advancement (83).

Primary Hypothyroidism

Longstanding primary hypothyroidism is associated with sexual precocity. It can present with premature breast development or isolated vaginal bleeding. If serum prolactin is elevated, galactorrhea may be present. On pelvic ultrasound, solitary or multiple ovarian cysts may be found. Primary hypothyroidism is the only cause of precocious puberty that is associated with a delayed bone age. These features return to normal within a few months of initiation of *levothyroxine* therapy.

Congenital Adrenal Hyperplasia

Heterosexual precocious puberty **is always of peripheral origin and is most often caused by CAH.** In most untreated or poorly treated adolescent girls and in some adolescent boys, spontaneous true isosexual pubertal development does not occur until proper treatment is instituted. In most patients treated satisfactorily from early life, the onset of puberty occurs at the expected chronological age. Three adrenal enzyme defects—21-hydroxylase deficiency, 11β-hydroxylase deficiency, and 3β-hydroxysteroid dehydrogenase deficiency—can lead to heterosexual precocity and to virilization of the external genitalia because of increased androgen production beginning *in utero* (84). The clinical presentation of the various forms of CAH depends on the following factors: (i) the affected enzyme, (ii) the extent of residual enzymatic activity, and (iii) the physiologic consequences of deficiencies in the end products and excesses of precursor steroids.

21-Hydroxylase Deficiency   **Most patients with classic CAH have 21-hydroxylase deficiency** (Fig. 29.19). All forms of 21-hydroxylase deficiency are caused by homozygous or compound heterozygous mutations in the human *CYP21A2* gene, which encodes the 21-hydroxylase enzyme; in the carrier, heterozygote state, only one allele is mutated (85). Two *CYP21A2* genes, a 3' *CYP21A2B* gene encoding the functional enzyme and a pseudogene termed *CYP21A2A,* are situated very close to each other within the major histocompatibility locus on the short arm of chromosome 6. At least one-fourth of cases of 21-hydroxylase deficiency result from unequal crossover and genetic recombination between the two genes during meiosis. Severe mutations do not correlate with severe phenotype, and phenotypic variability likely depends on the activity of other interacting genes.

Neonatal screening suggests an incidence of about 1 in 15,000 births. Because of the location of the gene within the major histocompatibility locus, siblings with 21-hydroxylase deficiency usually have identical human leukocyte antigen (HLA) types. There are various forms of 21-hydroxylase deficiency, including simple virilizing (typically identified at birth because of genital ambiguity), salt-wasting (in which there is impairment of mineralocorticoid and glucocorticoid secretion), and late-onset or nonclassic (in which heterosexual development occurs at the expected age of puberty). The so-called classic form includes the simple virilizing and salt-wasting forms. The nonclassic form is discussed in the following section on heterosexual pubertal development.

Deficiency of 21-hydroxylase results in the impairment of the conversion of 17α-hydroxyprogesterone to 11-deoxycortisol and of progesterone to deoxycorticosterone (Fig. 29.20). As a consequence, precursors accumulate, and there is increased conversion to adrenal androgens. Because the development of the external genitalia is controlled by androgens, in the classic form of this disorder, girls are born with ambiguous genitalia, including an enlarged clitoris and fusion of the labioscrotal folds and the urogenital sinus. The internal female organs (including the uterus, fallopian tubes, and ovaries) develop normally because they are not affected by the increased androgen levels. In three-quarters of cases with classic 21-hydroxylase deficiency, salt-wasting occurs, as defined by hyponatremia, hyperkalemia, and hypotension. It is important to recognize that the extent of virilization may be the same in simple virilizing and salt-wasting CAH. Thus, **even a mildly virilized newborn with 21-hydroxylase deficiency should be observed for signs of a potentially life-threatening crisis within the first weeks of life.** During childhood, untreated girls with the classic form grow rapidly but have advanced bone ages, enter puberty early, experience early closure of their epiphyses, and ultimately are short in stature as adults. CAH, with appropriate therapy, is the only inherited disorder of sexual differentiation in which normal pregnancy and childbearing are possible. **The classic forms of 21-hydroxylase deficiency are easily diagnosed based on the presence of genital ambiguity and markedly elevated levels of 17α-hydroxyprogesterone.** Some states in the US initiated neonatal screening programs to detect 21-hydroxylase deficiency at birth.

3β-Hydroxysteroid Dehydrogenase   Deficiency of 3β-hydroxysteroid dehydrogenase (3β-HSD), caused by mutations in the *HSD3B2* gene that encodes the 3β-HSDII enzyme, affects the synthesis of glucocorticoids, mineralocorticoids, and sex steroids. Typically, levels of 17-hydroxypregnenolone and DHEA are elevated (Fig. 29.20). The classic form of the disorder, detectable at birth, is quite rare, and affected girls may be masculinized only slightly. In severe cases, salt wasting may be present.

A nonclassic form of this disorder may be associated with heterosexual precocious pubertal development (as is the classic form if untreated), but postpubertal hyperandrogenism occurs more often. The androgen excess in individuals with nonclassic 3β-HSD deficiency appears to result from androgens derived from the peripheral conversion of increased serum concentrations of DHEA. This disorder is inherited in autosomal recessive fashion, with allelism at the *3β-HSD* gene on chromosome 1 believed to be responsible for the varying degrees of enzyme deficiency.

11-Hydroxylase Deficiency   **The classic form of 11-hydroxylase deficiency is believed to constitute 5% to 8% of all cases of CAH.** Deficiency in 11-hydroxylase, caused by mutations in the *CYP11B1* gene, results in the inability to convert 11-deoxycortisol to cortisol and the consequent accumulation of androgen precursors (Fig. 29.20). Markedly elevated levels of 11-deoxycortisol and deoxycorticosterone are present in the disorder. Because deoxycorticosterone acts as a mineralocorticoid, many individuals with this disorder become hypertensive. A mild

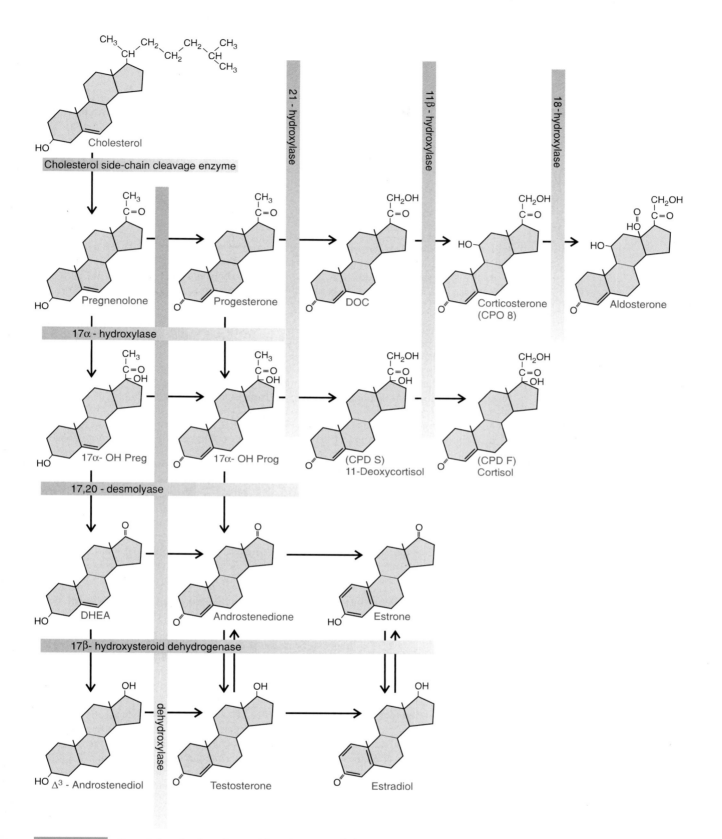

Figure 29.20 **Gonadal and adrenal steroid pathways and the enzymes required for steroid conversion.** DOC, deoxycorticosterone; 17α-OH Preg, 17α-hydroxypregnenolone; 17α-OH Prog, 17α-hydroxyprogesterone; DHEA, dehydroepiandrosterone sulfate. (From **Rebar RW, Kenigsberg D, Hodgen GD.** The normal menstrual cycle and the control of ovulation. In: **Becker KL, ed.** *Principles and practice of endocrinology and metabolism.* 2nd ed. Philadelphia, A: JB Lippincott, 1995:868–880, with permission.)

nonclassic form of 11-hydroxylase deficiency was reported but apparently is very uncommon (84).

Treatment of Congenital Adrenal Hyperplasia   **The treatment of CAH involves providing replacement doses of the deficient steroid hormones.** *Hydrocortisone* (10 to 20 mg/m^2 body surface area) or its equivalent is given daily in divided doses to suppress the elevated levels of pituitary corticotropin present and thus suppress the elevated androgen levels. With such treatment, signs of androgen excess should regress. In children, growth velocity, bone age, and hormone levels should be monitored carefully because both overreplacement and underreplacement can result in premature closure of the epiphyses and short stature. Data now indicate that early diagnosis and compliance with therapy lead to adult height within 1 standard deviation of the anticipated target height in girls with 21-hydroxylase deficiency (86).

Mineralocorticoid replacement is generally required in individuals with 21-hydroxylase deficiency whether or not they are salt losing. The intent of glucocorticoid therapy should be to suppress morning 17α-hydroxyprogesterone levels to between 300 and 900 ng/dL. Sufficient *fludrocortisone* should be given daily to suppress plasma renin activity to less than 5 mg/mL per hour.

It is possible to diagnose 21-hydroxylase deficiency prenatally in patients known to be at risk (84). The diagnosis is established by documenting elevated levels of 17α-hydroxyprogesterone or 21-deoxycortisol in amniotic fluid. Genetic diagnosis using specific probes and cells obtained by chorionic villus sampling or amniocentesis is possible. *Dexamethasone* (20 μg/kg/day in three divided doses) can be administered to the pregnant women beginning before the ninth week of gestation because the urogenital sinus begins to form at nine weeks of gestation. If the fetus is determined to be a male or an unaffected female upon DNA analysis, treatment is discontinued. Otherwise, treatment is continued to term. Human studies found that this treatment regimen is effective in reducing virilization in the genetic female so that genitoplasty was not needed in the majority of cases (87,88). The majority of studies proved that this management scheme is effective for both mother and the child. Maternal complications, including hypertension, massive weight gain, and overt Cushing syndrome, were noted in about 1% of pregnancies in which the mothers are given low doses of *dexamethasone*. All maternal complications disappear after delivery. The long-term effects of this treatment strategy on the physical and neurodevelopmental health of the offspring remains unclear. A recent systematic review concluded that *dexamethasone* seems to reduce virilization without significant adverse maternal or fetal effects, though the available data allow merely weak inferences to be made (89). Despite the risks and the nonuniformity of beneficial outcome to affected female fetuses, many parents may choose prenatal medical treatment because of the psychological impact of ambiguous genitalia.

Girls with ambiguous genitalia may require reconstructive surgery, including clitoral recession and vaginoplasty. Timing of such surgery is debated, but the girl must be of appropriate size to ensure the surgery is as simple as possible.

Heterosexual Pubertal Development

The most common cause of heterosexual development at the expected age of puberty is PCOS (Fig. 29.21). Because the syndrome is heterogeneous and poorly defined, clinical difficulties result in diagnosis and management (90). For the sake of simplicity, **PCOS may be defined as LH-dependent hyperandrogenism** (91). The Rotterdam criteria are commonly used to identify individuals with PCOS and require the presence of at least two of the following: oligo- or anovulation, clinical and/or biochemical signs of hyperandrogenism, and polycystic ovaries, with exclusion of other etiologies (CAH, androgen-secreting tumors, Cushing syndrome) (92). Polycystic ovaries ultrasonically are defined as the presence of 12 or more follicles in each ovary measuring 2 to 9 mm in diameter and/or increased ovarian volume (>10 mL). Most clinical manifestations arise as a consequence of the hyperandrogenism and often include hirsutism beginning at or near puberty and irregular menses from the age of menarche because of oligo-ovulation or anovulation. **Clinical manifestations are as follows:**

1. **Affected girls may be but are not necessarily somewhat overweight.**
2. **In rare instances, menarche may be delayed, and primary amenorrhea may occur.**
3. **Basal levels of LH tend to be elevated in most affected individuals, and androgen production is invariably increased, even though circulating levels of androgens may be near the upper limits of the normal range in many affected women.**

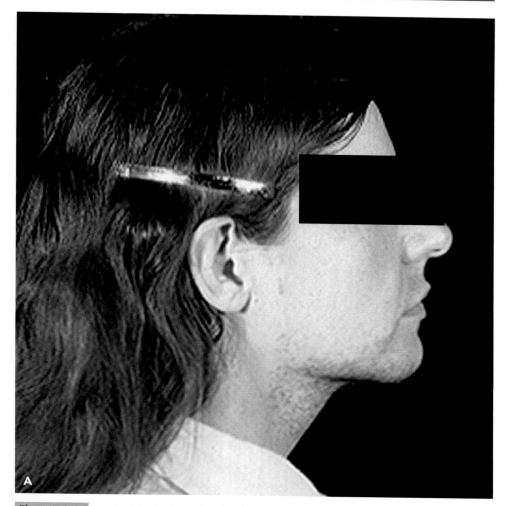

Figure 29.21   Typical facial hirsutism in three women with polycystic ovarian syndrome. A: 25-year-old.

4. In anovulatory women, estrone levels are typically greater than estradiol levels.

5. Because circulating levels of estrogens are not diminished in PCOS and androgen levels are only mildly elevated, affected girls become both feminized and masculinized at puberty. This is an important feature because girls with classic forms of CAH who do not experience precocious puberty (and even those who do) only become masculinized at puberty (i.e., they do not develop breasts).

6. Some degree of insulin resistance may be present, even in the absence of overt glucose intolerance (93).

7. Polycystic ovaries are frequently, but not always present in ultrasound examination.

Differential Diagnosis and Evaluation

Distinguishing PCOS from the nonclassic forms of CAH is problematic and controversial (94,95). The evaluation is as follows:

1. **Some clinicians advocate measurement of 17α-hydroxyprogesterone in all women who develop hirsutism.** Although values of 17α-hydroxyprogesterone are commonly elevated more than 100-fold in individuals with classic 21-hydroxylase deficiency, they may or may not be elevated in nonclassic late-onset forms of the disorder.

2. **Measurement of 17α-hydroxyprogesterone can identify women with various forms of 11-hydroxylase deficiency.**

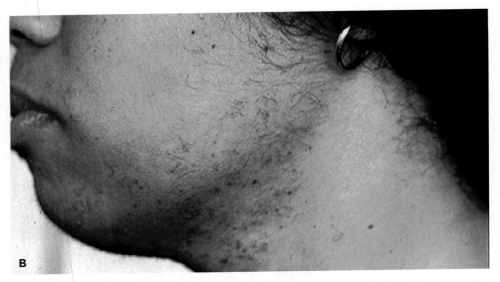

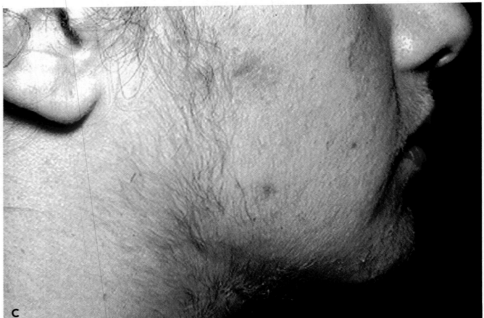

Figure 29.21 (*Continued*) **B:** 21-year-old **C:** 17-year-old.

3. **Basal levels of DHEAS and 17α-hydroxyprogesterone may be moderately elevated in patients with PCOS, making the diagnosis even more difficult.**

4. **To screen for CAH, 17α-hydroxyprogesterone should be measured in early morning.**

5. **In women with regular cyclic menses, it is important to measure 17α-hydroxyprogesterone only in the follicular phase because basal levels increase at midcycle and in the luteal phase.**

Measurements of 17α-hydroxyprogesterone appear to be of value in populations at high risk for nonclassic late-onset 21-hydroxylase deficiency. In the white population, the gene occurs in only about 1 in 1,000 individuals, but it occurs in 1 in 27 Ashkenazi Jews, 1 in 40 Hispanics, 1 in 50 Yugoslavs, and 1 in 300 Italians (84). The incidence is increased among Eskimos and French Canadians. Alternatively, screening might be restricted to hirsute teenagers presenting with the more "typical" features of nonclassic 21-hydroxylase deficiency, including severe hirsutism beginning at puberty, "flattening" of the breasts (i.e., defeminization), shorter

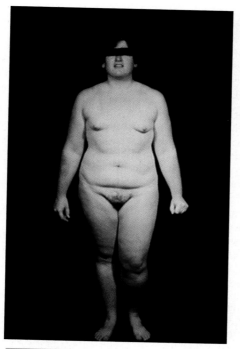

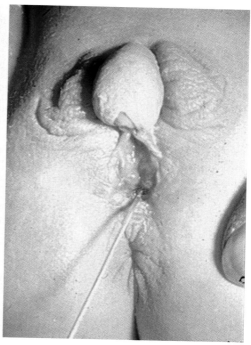

Figure 29.22 Left: **A 19-year-old girl with secondary amenorrhea and severe acne and hirsutism beginning at the normal age of puberty.** Stimulatory testing with corticotropin documented nonclassic 21-hydroxylase deficiency. Flattening of the breasts is apparent. She was shorter than her one sister and her mother.

Figure 29.23 Right: **Newborn girl with 46,XX karyotype and genital ambiguity.** There is obvious clitoral hypertrophy, paired frenula, so-called scrotalization of the labia, and a common urogenital sinus (shown by the probe). She had 21-hydroxylase deficiency. (From **Rebar RW.** Normal and abnormal sexual differentiation and pubertal development. In: **Moore TR, Reiter RC, Rebar RW, et al., eds.** *Gynecology and obstetrics: a longitudinal approach.* New York: Churchill Livingstone, 1993:97–133, with permission.)

stature than other family members, and increased DHEAS levels (between 5,000 and 7,000 ng/mL). Women with a strong family history of hirsutism or hypertension might be screened (49) (Fig. 29.22).

Basal Levels of 17α-Hydroxyprogesterone   **Basal levels of 17α-hydroxyprogesterone higher than 800 ng/dL are virtually diagnostic of CAH. Levels between 300 and 800 ng/dL require stimulatory testing with corticotropin to distinguish between PCOS and CAH. To complicate the situation even further, nonclassic 21-hydroxylase deficiency may occur even when basal levels of 17α-hydroxyprogesterone are below 300 ng/dL, thus requiring stimulatory testing in those cases.**

Cosyntropin Stimulation Test   **The most commonly used stimulatory test involves measurement of 17α-hydroxyprogesterone 30 minutes after administration of a bolus of 0.25 mg of synthetic cosyntropin (*Cortrosyn*) (96).** In normal women, this value seldom exceeds 400 ng/dL. Patients with classic 21-hydroxylase deficiency achieve peak levels of 3,000 ng/dL or higher. Patients with nonclassic 21-hydroxylase deficiency commonly achieve levels of 1,500 ng/dL or more. Heterozygous carriers achieve peak levels up to about 1,000 ng/dL. In hirsute women with hypertension, 11-deoxycortisol levels can be determined during the test. If both 11-deoxycortisol and 17α-hydroxyprogesterone levels are increased, the rare 11-hydroxylase deficiency is present. Only measurements of several steroid precursors after corticotropin stimulation can identify individuals with nonclassic forms of 3β-HSD deficiency.

The elevated levels of 17α-hydroxyprogesterone present in all forms of 21-hydroxylase deficiency are rapidly suppressed by administration of exogenous corticoids. Even a single dose of a glucocorticoid such as *dexamethasone* will suppress 17α-hydroxyprogesterone in CAH but not in virilizing ovarian and adrenal neoplasms.

Hirsutism   It is suggested that androgen-receptor blockade may be preferable to glucocorticoids as primary treatment of nonclassic 21-hydroxylase deficiency (97). Although menses usually (but not always) become regular shortly after beginning therapy with glucocorticoids, the hirsutism in this disorder is remarkably refractory to glucocorticoids.

Distinguishing nonclassic forms of CAH from idiopathic hirsutism may be problematic. Individuals with idiopathic hirsutism have regular ovulatory menses, thus effectively eliminating PCOS from consideration. Confusion can be created by the fact that some women with nonclassic CAH may continue to ovulate. Basal levels of 17α-hydroxyprogesterone are normal in idiopathic hirsutism, as is the response to adrenocorticotropic hormone stimulation. Idiopathic hirsutism represents enhanced androgen action at the hair follicle (98).

Mixed Gonadal Dysgenesis

The term *mixed gonadal dysgenesis* is used to designate those individuals with asymmetric gonadal development, with a germ cell tumor or a testis on one side and an undifferentiated streak, rudimentary gonad, or no gonad on the other side. Most individuals with this rare disorder have a mosaic karyotype of 45,X/46,XY and are raised as girls who experience virilization at puberty. Gonadectomy is indicated to remove the source of androgens and eliminate any risk for neoplasia.

Rare Forms of Male Pseudohermaphroditism

Individuals who have rare forms of male pseudohermaphroditism, especially 5α-reductase deficiency (the so-called *penis at 12 syndrome*) and the *Reifenstein syndrome*, generally have ambiguous female genitalia with variable virilization at puberty. *Cushing syndrome* may occur rarely during the pubertal years, as may adrenal or ovarian androgen-secreting neoplasms.

Genital Ambiguity at Birth

Ambiguous external genitalia in a newborn constitutes a major diagnostic challenge. Prompt evaluation is of critical importance to identify a possible life-threatening disorder and to assign the appropriate gender. The prime diagnosis until ruled out is CAH because it is the only condition that is life-threatening. Extreme sensitivity is required in interacting with the family, and no attempt should be made to guess the sex of the baby. The incidence of genital ambiguity is 1 in 4,500, although some degree of male undervirilization, or female virilization may be present in as many as 2% of live births (99,100).

Physical Signs

During the 3 to 4 days required for evaluation, it is important to be supportive of the parents. Many clinicians believe that it is important not to attach any unusual significance to the genital ambiguity and to treat the abnormality as just another "birth defect." Physicians should emphasize that the child should undergo normal psychosexual development regardless of the sex-of-rearing selected. Either a name compatible with either sex should be chosen or the naming of the infant should be delayed until the studies are completed.

Although the diagnosis is not usually obvious on examination, there are some helpful distinguishing features (Fig. 29.23). **In normal boys, there is only a single midline frenulum on the ventral side of the phallus; in normal girls, there are two frenula lateral to the midline. A girl with clitoral enlargement still has two frenula, and a boy with hypospadias has a single midline frenulum or several irregular fibrous bands (chordee).** It is important to determine whether any müllerian derivatives are present. Studies suggest that MRI may be the most effective way of evaluating the infant for the presence of müllerian tissue (101).

The location or consistency of the gonad may be helpful in deducing its composition. A gonad located in the labial or inguinal regions almost always contains testicular tissue. A testis is generally softer than an ovary or a streak gonad and is more apt to be surrounded by blood vessels imparting a reddish cast. An ovary is more often white, fibrous, and convoluted. A gonad that varies in consistency may be an ovotestis or a testis or a streak gonad that underwent neoplastic transformation. If a well-differentiated fallopian tube is absent on only one side, the side without the tube probably contains a testis or ovotestis.

Diagnosis and Management

The fact that there is uncertainty about the sex of one's baby is devastating and incomprehensible for most parents. Parents require reassurance that either a male or female gender will be assigned ultimately. Optimum clinical management should comprise of the following (67):

1. **Gender assignment must be avoided before expert evaluation of newborns.**
2. **Evaluation and long-term management must be performed at a center with an experienced multidisciplinary team (pediatric endocrinologist, pediatric urologist, geneticist, clinical psychologist, and gynecologist).**
3. **All individuals should receive a gender assignment after appropriate assessment.**
4. **Open communication with patients and families is essential, and participation in decision making should be encouraged.**
5. **Patient and family concerns should be respected and addressed in strict confidence.**

First-line testing in newborns includes:

1. **Karyotyping with X- and Y-specific probe detection (even when prenatal karyotype is available)**
2. **Measurement of serum 17-hydroprogesterone, testosterone, gonadotropins, antimüllerian hormone, and electrolytes**
3. **Abdominopelvic ultrasound (to assess anatomy of the vagina, uterus, or urogenital sinus, exclude renal anomalies, and locate any inguinal gonads)**
4. **Urinalysis (to check for protein as a screen for any associated renal anomaly)**

The results of these investigations are generally available within 48 hours and sufficient to develop a working diagnosis. If needed, additional testing may include (102):

1. **Human chorionic gonadotropin- and adrenocorticotropin-stimulation tests to assess testicular and adrenal steroid biosynthesis**
2. **Urinary steroid analysis by gas chromatography mass spectroscopy**
3. **Imaging studies**
4. **Biopsies of gonadal material**
5. **Genetic testing**

Although genital ambiguity is usually identified at birth, it may not be recognized for several years. Questions about changing the sex-of-rearing may arise. It was believed that sex-of-rearing may be changed before 2 years of age without psychologically damaging the child, but experience with individuals with 5α-reductase deficiency suggests that gender changes may be made after 2 years of age in certain instances (103). In any case, **surgery for genital ambiguity to make the external genitalia (and development) as compatible with the sex-of-rearing of the child is warranted but was not always successful.** Clitoral recession and clitorectomy are the most frequently performed surgical procedures.

Masculinized external genitalia can be classified into five "Prader" stages. Excessive androgen exposure results in virilization to varying degrees, including clitoral enlargement, labial fold fusion, and rostral migration of the urethral/vaginal perineal orifice. Prader stage V defines virilization resulting in complete labioscrotal fusion, a penile phallus with the urethra opening on the glans. Clitoroplasty is required at an early stage after it is established that a Prader stage V "male" has CAH and needs to be reassigned to the female sex (104).

Teratogens

It is important to recognize that ambiguous genitalia can result from the maternal ingestion of various teratogens, most of which are synthetic steroids (Table 29.3). Exposure to the teratogen must occur early in pregnancy, during genital organogenesis. Not all exposed fetuses manifest the same anomalies or even the presence of any anomalies. In principle, most synthetic steroids with androgenic properties, including weakly androgenic progestins, can affect female genital differentiation. The doses required to produce genital ambiguity are generally so great that the concern is only theoretical. **The one agent that can lead to genital ambiguity when ingested in**

Table 29.3 Androgens and Progestogens Potentially Capable of Producing Genital Ambiguity[a]

Proved	No Effect	Insufficient Data
Testosterone enanthate	Progesterone	Ethynodiol diacetate
Testosterone propionate	17α-Hydroxyprogesterone	Dimethisterone
Methylandrostenediol	Medroxyprogesterone	Norgestrel
6α-Methyltestosterone	Norethynodrel	Desogestrel
Ethisterone		Gestodene
Norethindrone		Norgestimate
Danazol		

[a]Those agents proved to cause genital ambiguity do so only when administered in relatively high doses. Insufficient data exist regarding effects of *dimethisterone* and *norgestrel*. In low doses (e.g., as in oral contraceptives), progestins, even including *norethindrone,* seem unlikely to virilize a female fetus.

clinically used quantities is *danazol*. There is no evidence that inadvertent ingestion of oral contraceptives, which contain relatively low doses of either *mestranol* or *ethinyl estradiol* and a 19-nor-steroid, results in virilization (105,106).

References

1. **Tanner JM.** *Growth at adolescence.* 2nd ed. Oxford, UK: Blackwell Scientific Publications, 1962.
2. **Teilmann G, Pedersen CB, Skakkebaek NE, et al.** Increased risk of precocious puberty in internationally adopted children in Denmark. *Pediatrics* 2006;118:e391–e399.
3. **Parent AS, Teilmann G, Juul A, et al.** The timing of normal puberty and the age limits of sexual precocity: variations around the world, secular trends, and changes after migration. *Endocr Rev* 2003;24:668–693.
4. **Matchock RL, Susman EJ.** Family composition and menarcheal age: anti-inbreeding strategies. *Am J Hum Biol* 2006;18:481–491.
5. **Zacharias L, Wurtman RJ.** Blindness: its relation to age of menarche. *Science* 1964;144:1154–1155.
6. **Kaplowitz PB, Oberfield SE,** for the Drug and Therapeutics and Executive Committees of the Lawson Wilkins Pediatric Endocrine Society. Reexamination of the age limit for defining when puberty is precocious in girls in the United States: implications for evaluation and treatment. *Pediatrics* 1999;104:936–941.
7. **Frisch RE.** Body fat, menarche, and reproductive ability. *Semin Reprod Endocrinol* 1985;3:45–49.
8. **Maclure M, Travis LB, Willett W, et al.** A prospective cohort study of nutrient intake and age at menarche. *Am J Clin Nutr* 1991;54:649–656.
9. **deRidder CM, Thijssen JHH, Bruning PF, et al.** Body fat mass, body fat distribution, and pubertal development: a longitudinal study of physical and hormonal sexual maturation of girls. *J Clin Endocrinol Metab* 1992;75:442–446.
10. **Marshall WA, Tanner JM.** Variations in patterns of pubertal changes in girls. *Arch Dis Child* 1969; 44:291–303.
11. **Cutler GB Jr.** The role of estrogen in bone growth and maturation during childhood and adolescence. *J Steroid Biochem Mol Biol* 1997;61:141–144.
12. **Greulich WW, Pyle SI.** *Radiographic atlas of skeletal development of the hand and wrist.* 2nd ed. London, England: Oxford University Press, 1959.
13. **Bayley N, Pinneau SR.** Tables for predicting adult height from skeletal age: revised for use with the Greulich-Pyle hand standards. *J Pediatr* 1952;40:423–441.
14. **Kaplan SL, Grumbach MM, Aubert ML.** The ontogeny of pituitary hormones and hypothalamic factors in the human fetus: maturation of central nervous system regulation of anterior pituitary function. *Recent Prog Horm Res* 1976;32:161–243.
15. **Conte FA, Grumbach MM, Kaplan SL.** A diphasic pattern of gonadotropin secretion in patients with the syndrome of gonadal dysgenesis. *J Clin Endocrinol Metab* 1975;40:670–674.
16. **Boyar RM, Finkelstein JW, Roffwarg HP, et al.** Synchronization of augmented luteinizing hormone secretion with sleep during puberty. *N Engl J Med* 1972;287:582–586.
17. **Boyar RM, Rosenfeld RS, Kapen S, et al.** Simultaneous augmented secretion of luteinizing hormone and testosterone during sleep. *J Clin Invest* 1974;54:609–618.
18. **Boyar RM, Wu RHK, Roffwarg H, et al.** Human puberty: 24-hour estradiol patterns in pubertal girls. *J Clin Endocrinol Metab* 1976;43:1418–1421.
19. **Grumbach MM.** The neuroendocrinology of puberty. In: Krieger DT, Hughes JC, eds. Neuroendocrinology. Sunderland, MA: Sinauer Associates, 1980:249–258.
20. **Penny R, Olambiwonnu NO, Frasier SD.** Episodic fluctuations of serum gonadotropins in pre- and post-pubertal girls and boys. *J Clin Endocrinol Metab* 1977;45:307–311.
21. **Korth-Schutz S, Levine LS, New MI.** Serum androgens in normal prepubertal and pubertal children and in children with precocious adrenarche. *J Clin Endocrinol Metab* 1976;42:117–124.
22. **Ducharme J-R, Forest MG, DePeretti E, et al.** Plasma adrenal and gonadal sex steroids in human pubertal development. *J Clin Endocrinol Metab* 1976;42:468–476.
23. **Lee PA, Xenakis T, Winer J, et al.** Puberty in girls: correlation of serum levels of gonadotropins, prolactin, androgens, estrogens and progestin with physical changes. *J Clin Endocrinol Metab* 1976;43:775–784.
24. **Judd HL, Parker DC, Siler TM, et al.** The nocturnal rise of plasma testosterone in pubertal boys. *J Clin Endocrinol Metab* 1974;38:710–713.
25. **Grumbach MM, Kaplan SL.** The neuroendocrinology of human puberty: an ontogenetic perspective. In: **Grumbach MM, Sizonenko PC, Aubert ML, eds.** *Control of the onset of puberty.* Baltimore, MD: Williams & Wilkins, 1990:1–62.
26. **Rosenfield RL.** Current age of onset of puberty. *Pediatrics* 2000;105:622.
27. **Buttram VC Jr, Gibbons WE.** Müllerian anomalies: a proposed classification (an analysis of 144 cases). *Fertil Steril* 1979;32:40–46.
28. **Smith FR.** The significance of incomplete fusion of the müllerian ducts in pregnancy and parturition with a report on 35 cases. *Am J Obstet Gynecol* 1931;22:714–728.

29. **Herbst AL, Hubby MM, Azizi F, et al.** Reproductive and gynecological surgical experience in diethylstilbestrol-exposed daughters. *Am J Obstet Gynecol* 1981;141:1019–1028.

30. **Simpson JL.** Genetics of the female reproductive ducts. *Am J Med Genet* 1999;89:224–239.

31. **Taylor HS.** The role of HOX genes in the development and function of the female reproductive tract. *Semin Reprod Med* 2000;18:81–89.

32. **Philibert P, Biason-Lauber A, Rouzier R, et al.** Identification and functional analysis of a new WNT4 gene mutation among 28 adolescent girls with primary amenorrhea and mullerian duct abnormalities: a French collaborative study. *J Clin Endocrinol Metab* 2008;93:895–900.

33. **Buttram VC Jr, Reiter RC.** *Surgical treatment of the infertile female.* Baltimore, MD: Williams & Wilkins, 1985:89.

34. **Pellerito JS, McCarthy SM, Doyle MB, et al.** Diagnosis of uterine anomalies: relative accuracy of MR imaging, endovaginal sonography, and hysterosalpingography. *Radiology* 1992;183:795–800.

35. **Simpson JL.** Localizing ovarian determinants through phenotypic-karyotypic deductions: progress and pitfalls. In: **Rosenfield R, Grumbach M, eds.** Turner syndrome. New York: Marcel Dekker, 1990:65–77.

36. **Van Dyke DL, Wiktor A, Palmer CG, et al.** Ullrich-Turner syndrome with a small ring X chromosome and the presence of mental retardation. *Am J Med Genet* 1992;43:996–1005.

37. **Ellison JW, Wardak Z, Young MF, et al.** PHOG, a candidate gene for involvement in the short stature of Turner syndrome. *Hum Mol Genet* 1997;6:1341–1347.

38. **Cools M, Drop SL, Wolffenbuttel KP, et al.** Germ cell tumors in the intersex gonad: old paths, new directions, moving frontiers. *Endocr Rev* 2006;27:468–484.

39. **Bremer GL, Land JA, Tiebosch A, et al.** Five different histological subtypes of germ cell malignancies in an XY female. *Gynecol Oncol* 1993;50:247–248.

40. **Karnis MF, Zimon AE, Lalwani SI, et al.** Risk of death in pregnancy achieved through oocyte donation in patients with Turner syndrome: a national survey. *Fertil Steril* 2003;80:498–501.

41. **Matura LA, Ho VB, Rosing DR, et al.** Aortic dilatation and dissection in Turner syndrome. *Circulation* 2007; 116:1663–1670.

42. **Rosenfeld RG, Frane J, Attie KM, et al.** Six-year results of a randomized prospective trial of human growth hormone and oxandrolone in Turner syndrome. *J Pediatr* 1992;121:49–55.

43. **Sas TC, de Muinck Keizer-Schrama S, Stijnen T, et al.** Normalization of height in girls with Turner syndrome after long-term growth hormone treatment: results of a randomized dose-response trial. *J Clin Endocrinol Metab* 1999;84:4607–4612.

44. **Sas TC, Gerver WJ, De Bruin R, et al.** Body proportions during long-term growth hormone treatment in girls with Turner syndrome participating in a randomized dose-response trial. *J Clin Endocrinol Metab* 1999;84:4622–4628.

45. **Rosenfeld RG, Attie KM, Frane J, et al.** Growth hormone therapy of Turner's syndrome: beneficial effect on adult height. *J Pediatr* 1998;132:319–324.

46. **Chernausek SD, Attie KM, Cara JF, et al.** Growth hormone therapy of Turner syndrome: the impact of age of estrogen replacement on final height. Genentech, Inc., Collaborative Study Group. *J Clin Endocrinol Metab* 2000;85:2439–2445.

47. **Hogler W, Briody J, Moore B, et al.** Importance of estrogen on bone health in Turner syndrome: a cross-sectional and longitudinal study using dual-energy x-ray absorptiometry. *J Clin Endocrinol Metab* 2004;89:193–199.

48. **Rebar RW, Cedars MI.** Hypergonadotropic amenorrhea. In: **Filicori M, Flamigni C, eds.** *Ovulation induction: basic science and clinical advances.* Amsterdam, Netherlands: Elsevier Science B.V., 1994:115–121.

49. **Kustin J, Rebar RW.** Hirsutism in young adolescent girls. *Pediatr Ann* 1986;15:522.

50. **Achermann JC, Jameson JL.** Advances in the molecular genetics of hypogonadotropic hypogonadism. *J Pediatr Endocrinol Metab* 2001;14:3–15.

51. **Herbison AE.** Genetics of puberty. *Horm Res* 2007;68:75–79.

52. **Kallmann FJ, Schoenfeld WA, Barrera SE.** The genetic aspects of primary eunuchoidism. *Am J Ment Defic* 1944;48:203–236.

53. **Schwanzel-Fukuda M, Jorgenson KL, Bergen HT, et al.** Biology of normal luteinizing hormone-releasing hormone neurons during and after their migration from olfactory placode. *Endocr Rev* 1992;13:623–634.

54. **Crowley WF Jr, Jameson JL.** Clinical counterpoint: gonadotropin-releasing hormone deficiency: perspectives from clinical investigation. *Endocr Rev* 1992;13:635–640.

55. **Henek M, Wevrick R.** The role of genomic imprinting in human developmental disorders: lessons from Prader-Willi syndrome. *Clin Genet* 2001;59:156–164.

56. **Beales PL, Warner AM, Hitman GA, et al.** Bardet-Biedl syndrome: a molecular and phenotypic study of 18 families. *J Med Genet* 1997;34:92–98.

57. **Tomlinson JN, Holden N, Hills RK, et al.** Association between premature mortality and hypopituitarism. West Midlands Prospective Hypopituitary Study Group. *Lancet* 2001;357:425–431.

58. **Vance ML.** Hypopituitarism. *N Engl J Med* 1994;330:1651–1662.

59. **Braunstein GD, Whitaker JN, Kohler PO.** Cerebellar dysfunction in Hand-Schüller-Christian disease. *Arch Intern Med* 1973;132:387–390.

60. **Spitzer R.** *Diagnostic and statistical manual of mental disorders.* 4th ed. Washington, DC: American Psychiatric Association, 1994:53.

61. **Vigersky RA, Loriaux DL, Andersen AE, et al.** Anorexia nervosa: behavioral and hypothalamic aspects. *J Clin Endocrinol Metab* 1976;5:517–535.

62. **Gold PW, Gwirtsman H, Avgerinos PC, et al.** Abnormal hypothalamic-pituitary-adrenal function in anorexia nervosa: pathophysiologic mechanisms in underweight and weight-corrected patients. *N Engl J Med* 1986;314:1335–1342.

63. **Vigersky RA, Andersen AE, Thompson RH, et al.** Hypothalamic dysfunction in secondary amenorrhea associated with simple weight loss. *N Engl J Med* 1977;297:1141–1145.

64. **Morris JM.** The syndrome of testicular feminization in male pseudohermaphrodites. *Am J Obstet Gynecol* 1953;65:1192.

65. **Griffin JE.** Androgen resistance—the clinical and molecular spectrum. *N Engl J Med* 1992;326: 611–618.

66. **Gottlieb B, Pinsky L, Beitel LK, et al.** Androgen insensitivity. *Am J Med Genet* 1999;89:210–217.

67. **Lee PA, Houk CP, Ahmed SF, Hughes IA.** Consensus statement on management of intersex disorders. *Pediatrics* 2006;118:e488–e500.

68. **Oerter KE, Uriarte MM, Rose SR, et al.** Gonadotropin secretory dynamics during puberty in normal girls and boys. *J Clin Endocrinol Metab* 1990;71:1251.

69. **Van Winter JT, Noller KL, Zimmerman D, et al.** Natural history of premature thelarche in Olmsted County, Minnesota, 1940 to 1984. *J Pediatr* 1990;116:278.

70. **Haber HP, Wollmann HA, Ranke MB.** Pelvic ultrasonography: early differentiation between isolated premature thelarche and central precocious puberty. *Eur J Pediatr* 1995;154:182–186.

71. **Ibanez L, DiMartino-Nardi J, Potau N, et al.** Premature adrenarche—normal variant of forerunner of adult disease? *Endocr Rev* 2000;21:671–696.

72. **Partsch CJ, Heger S, Sippell WG.** Management and outcome of central precocious puberty. *Clin Endocrinol* 2002;56:129–148.

73. **Mahachoklertwattana P, Kaplan SL, Grumbach MM.** The luteinizing hormone-releasing hormone-secreting hypothalamic hamartoma is a congenital malformation: natural history. *J Clin Endocrinol Metab* 1993;77:118–124.

74. **Feuillan PP, Jones JV, Barnes K, et al.** Reproductive axis after discontinuation of gonadotropin-releasing hormone analog treatment of girls with precocious puberty: a long term follow-up comparing girls with hypothalamic hamartoma and idiopathic precocious puberty. *J Clin Endocrinol Metab* 1999;84:44–49.

75. **Hochman HI, Judge DM, Reichlin S.** Precocious puberty and hypothalamic hamartoma. *Pediatrics* 1981;67:236–244.

76. **Carel JC, Eugster EA, Rogol A, et al.** Consensus statement on the use of gonadotropin-releasing hormone analogs in children. *Pediatrics* 2009;123:e752–e762.

77. **Carel JC, Roger M, Ispas S, et al.** Final height after long-term treatment with triptorelin slow-release for central precocious puberty: importance of statural growth after interruption of treatment. *J Clin Endocrinol Metab* 1999;84:1973–1978.

78. **Arrigo T, Cisternino M, Galluzzi F, et al.** Analysis of the factors affecting auxological response to GnRH agonist treatment and final height outcome in girls with idiopathic central precocious puberty. *Eur J Endocrinol* 1999;141:140–144.

79. **Oostdijk W, Rikken B, Schreuder S, et al.** Final height in central precocious puberty after long term treatment with a slow release GnRH agonist. *Arch Dis Child* 1996;75:292–297.

80. **Lyon AJ, DeBruyn R, Grant DB.** Transient sexual precocity and ovarian cysts. *Arch Dis Child* 1985;60:819–822.

81. **Ein SH, Darte JM, Stephens CA.** Cystic and solid ovarian tumors in children: a 44-year review. *J Pediatr Surg* 1970;5:148–156.

82. **Weinstein LS, Shenker A, Gejman PV, et al.** Activating mutations of the stimulatory G protein in the McCune-Albright syndrome. *N Engl J Med* 1991;325:1688–1695.

83. **Eugster EA, Rubin SD, Reiter EO,et al.** *Tamoxifen* treatment for precocious puberty in McCune-Albright syndrome: a multicenter trial. *J Pediatr* 2003;143:60–66.

84. **Speiser PW.** Congenital adrenal hyperplasia. In: **Becker KL, ed.** *Principles and practice of endocrinology and metabolism.* 2nd ed. Philadelphia, PA: JB Lippincott, 1995:686–695.

85. **White PC, Speiser PW.** Congenital adrenal hyperplasia due to 21-hydroxylase deficiency. *Endocr Rev* 2000;21:245–291.

86. **Engster EA, Dimeglio LA, Wright JC, et al.** Height outcome in congenital adrenal hyperplasia caused by 21-hydroxylase deficiency: a meta-analysis. *J Pediatr* 2001;138:3–5.

87. **Lajic S, Wedell A, Bui T, et al.** Long-term somatic follow-up of pre-natally treated children with congenital adrenal hyperplasia. *J Clin Endocrinol Metab* 1998;83:3872–3880.

88. **New MI, Carlson A, Obeid J, et al.** Extensive personal experience: prenatal diagnosis for congenital adrenal hyperplasia in 532 pregnancies. *J Clin Endocrinol Metab* 2001;86:5651–5657.

89. **Fernández-Balsells MM, Muthusamy K, Smushkin G, et al.** Prenatal dexamethasone use for the prevention of virilization in pregnancies at risk for classical congenital adrenal hyperplasia due to 21 hydroxylase (CYP21A2) deficiency: a systematic review and meta-analyses. *Clin Endocrinol (Oxf)* 2010;73:436–444.

90. **Futterweit W.** Pathophysiology of polycystic ovarian syndrome. In: **Redmond GP, ed.** Androgenic disorders. New York: Raven Press, 1995:77–166.

91. **Rebar RW.** Disorders of menstruation, ovulation, and sexual response. In: **Becker KL, ed.** *Principles and practice of endocrinology and metabolism.* 2nd ed. Philadelphia, PA: Lippincott, 1995:880–899.

92. **The Rotterdam ESHRE/ASRM-Sponsored PCOS Consensus Workshop Group.** Revised 2003 consensus on diagnostic criteria and long-term health risks related to polycystic ovary syndrome. *Fertil Steril* 2004;81:19–25.

93. **Lewy VD, Danadian K, Witchel SF, et al.** Early metabolic abnormalities in adolescent girls with polycystic ovarian syndrome. *J Pediatr* 2001;138:38–44.

94. **Lobo RA, Goebelsmann U.** Adult manifestation of congenital hyperplasia due to incomplete 21-hydroxylase deficiency mimicking polycystic ovarian disease. *Am J Obstet Gynecol* 1980;138:720–726.

95. **Chrousos GP, Loriaux DL, Mann DL, et al.** Late-onset 21-hydroxylase deficiency mimicking idiopathic hirsutism or polycystic ovarian disease. *Ann Intern Med* 1982;96:143–148.

96. **New MI, Lorenzen F, Lerner AJ, et al.** Genotyping steroid 21-hydroxylase deficiency: hormonal reference data. *J Clin Endocrinol Metab* 1983;57:320–326.

97. **Spritzer P, Billaud L, Thalabard J-C, et al.** Cyproterone acetate versus hydrocortisone treatment in late-onset adrenal hyperplasia. *J Clin Endocrinol Metab* 1990;70:642–646.

98. **Horton R, Hawks D, Lobo R.** 3a, 17b-Androstanediol glucuronide in plasma: a marker of androgen action in idiopathic hirsutism. *J Clin Invest* 1982;69:1203–1206.

99. **Hamerton JL, Canning N, Ray M, et al.** A cytogenetic survey of 14,069 newborn infants. Incidence of chromosome abnormalities. *Clin Genet* 1975;4:223–243.

100. **Blackless M, Charuvastra A, Derryck A, et al.** How sexually dimorphic are we? *Am J Hum Biol* 2000;12:151–166.

101. **Hricak H, Chang YCF, Thurner S.** Vagina: evaluation with MR imaging. I. Normal anatomy and congenital anomalies. *Radiology* 1991;179:593.

102. **Ogilvy-Stuart AL, Brain CE.** Early assessment of ambiguous genitalia. *Arch Dis Child* 2004;89:401–407.

103. **Imperato-McGinley J, Guerrero L, Gautier T, et al.** Steroid 5a-reductase deficiency: an inherited form of male pseudo-hermaphroditism. *Science* 1974;186:1213–1215.

104. **Hughes IA.** Congenital adrenal hyperplasia: a lifelong disorder. *Horm Res* 2007;68:84–89.

105. **Schardein JL.** Congenital abnormalities and hormones during pregnancy: a clinical review. *Teratology* 1980;22:251–270.

106. **Bracken MB.** Oral contraception and congenital malformations in offspring: a review and meta-analysis of the prospective studies. *Obstet Gynecol* 1990;76:552–557.

30 Amenorrhea

Valerie L. Baker
Wendy J. Schillings
Howard D. McClamrock

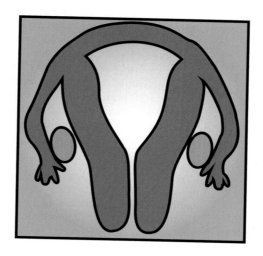

- Girls experienced menarche at increasingly younger ages during the past century. Primary amenorrhea is defined as absence of menses at age 13 years when there is no visible development of secondary sexual characteristics or age 15 years in the presence of normal secondary sexual characteristics.

- Absent or irregular menses may be an indication that a woman has a medical condition that can affect her overall health. The health implications can vary depending on the etiology of the amenorrhea. Therefore, a cause for amenorrhea should be established whenever possible.

- When gonadal failure occurs in conjunction with primary amenorrhea, it is associated with a high incidence of abnormal karyotype.

- The anatomic causes of amenorrhea are relatively few, and the majority may be diagnosed by history and physical examination.

- The most important elements in the diagnosis of amenorrhea include physical examination for secondary sexual characteristics and anatomic abnormalities, measurement of human chorionic gonadotropin (hCG) to rule out pregnancy, serum prolactin and thyroid stimulating hormone (TSH) levels, and assessment of follicle-stimulating hormone (FSH) levels to differentiate between hypergonadotropic and hypogonadotropic forms of hypogonadism.

- Therapeutic measures may include specific therapies (medical or surgical) aimed at correcting the primary cause of amenorrhea, hormone therapy to initiate and maintain secondary sexual characteristics and provide symptomatic relief, treatments to maximize and maintain peak bone mass including hormone therapy, calcium, and vitamin D for cases where circulating estrogen levels are low, and ovulation induction for patients desiring pregnancy.

A complex hormonal interaction must take place in order for normal menstruation to occur. The hypothalamus must secrete gonadotropin-releasing hormone (GnRH) in a pulsatile fashion, which is modulated by neurotransmitters and hormones. The GnRH stimulates secretion of follicle-stimulating hormone (FSH) and luteinizing hormone (LH) from the pituitary, which promotes ovarian follicular development and ovulation. A normally functioning ovarian follicle secretes estrogen; after ovulation, the follicle is converted to corpus luteum, and progesterone is secreted in addition to estrogen. These hormones stimulate endometrial development. If pregnancy does not occur, estrogen and progesterone secretion decrease and withdrawal bleeding begins. If any of the components (hypothalamus, pituitary, ovary, uterus, and outflow tract) are nonfunctional, bleeding cannot occur.

The mean age of menarche became younger during this century. Therefore, the definition of primary amenorrhea changed: Primary amenorrhea is defined as the absence of menses by 13 years of age when there is no visible development of secondary sexual characteristics or by 15 years of age in the presence of normal secondary sexual characteristics. The ages defining primary amenorrhea were decreased by 1 year to continue to represent two standard deviations above the mean age of developing secondary sexual characteristics and menses (1). Failure to begin breast development by age 13 warrants investigation. A woman who previously menstruated can develop secondary amenorrhea, which is defined as absence of menstruation for three normal menstrual cycles (2). A woman with regular cycles and a delay of menses of even a week may warrant assessment with a pregnancy test. It is reasonable to evaluate a woman who has fewer than nine cycles per year. With a few exceptions, the causes of primary amenorrhea are similar to the causes of secondary amenorrhea.

Patients may develop slight alterations in the hypothalamic–pituitary–ovarian axis that are not severe enough to cause amenorrhea but instead cause irregular menses (oligomenorrhea) associated with absent or infrequent ovulation. These patients may bleed excessively during menstruation because estrogen is unopposed. The etiologies of oligomenorrhea overlap with the etiologies of amenorrhea, with the exception that certain anatomic (e.g., absent uterine development) and karyotypic abnormalities (e.g., Turner syndrome), are largely associated with primary amenorrhea.

The World Health Organization (WHO) described three classes of amenorrhea. WHO Group I includes women with no evidence of endogenous estrogen production, normal or low FSH levels, normal prolactin levels, and no lesion in the hypothalamic-pituitary region. WHO Group II is associated with evidence of estrogen production and normal levels of prolactin and FSH. WHO Group III includes individuals with elevated serum FSH indicating gonadal insufficiency or failure.

To detect the cause of amenorrhea, it is useful to determine whether secondary sexual characteristics are present (Fig. 30.1). The absence of secondary sexual characteristics indicates that a woman was never exposed to estrogen.

Amenorrhea without Secondary Sexual Characteristics

Although the diagnosis and treatment of disorders associated with hypogonadism were discussed in another chapter (see Chapter 29), they will be mentioned here because these conditions may present as primary amenorrhea. **Because breast development is the first sign of estrogen exposure in puberty, patients without secondary sexual characteristics typically have primary, not secondary, amenorrhea (Fig 30.1).** It is helpful to categorize the causes of amenorrhea in the absence of breast development on the basis of gonadotropin status.

Causes of Primary Amenorrhea

Hypergonadotropic Hypogonadism Associated with Absence of Secondary Sexual Characteristics

Gonadal dysgenesis is a term typically used to describe abnormal development of the gonads, typically resulting in streak gonads. Gonadal dysgenesis is associated with high levels of LH and FSH because the gonad fails to produce the steroids and inhibin that would normally feed back to the pituitary gland to suppress pituitary production of LH and FSH. Karyotypic abnormalities are common in women with primary amenorrhea associated with gonadal failure (Table 30.1). **In one series, approximately 30% of patients with primary amenorrhea had an associated karyotypic abnormality (3). Turner syndrome (45,X) and its variants represent the most common form of hypergonadotropic hypogonadism in women with primary amenorrhea.**

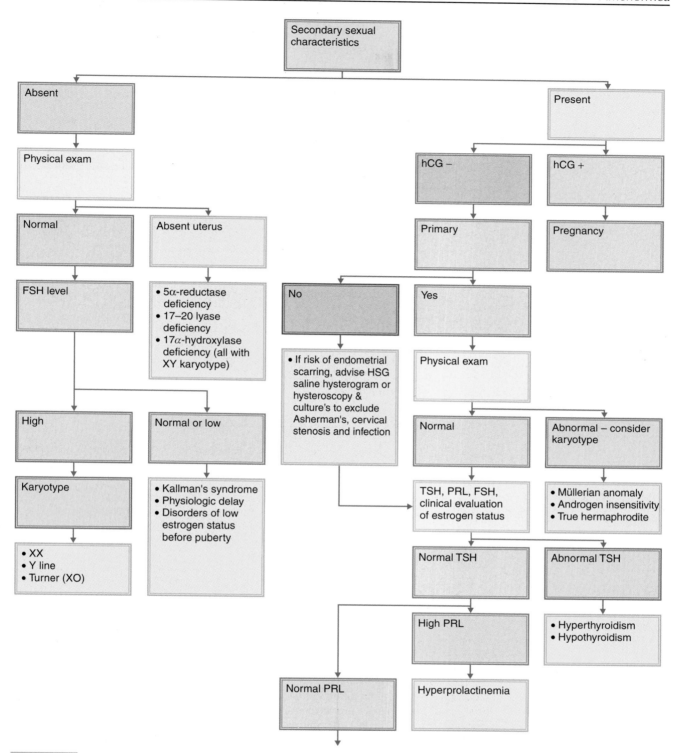

Figure 30.1 Decision tree for evaluation of amenorrhea. FSH, follicle-stimulating hormone; HCG, human chorionic gonadotropin; HSG, hysterosalpingogram; TSH, thyroid-stimulating hormone; PRL, prolactin; CT, computed tomography; MRI, magnetic resonance imaging; EEG, electroencephalogram; SHG, saline hysterogram.

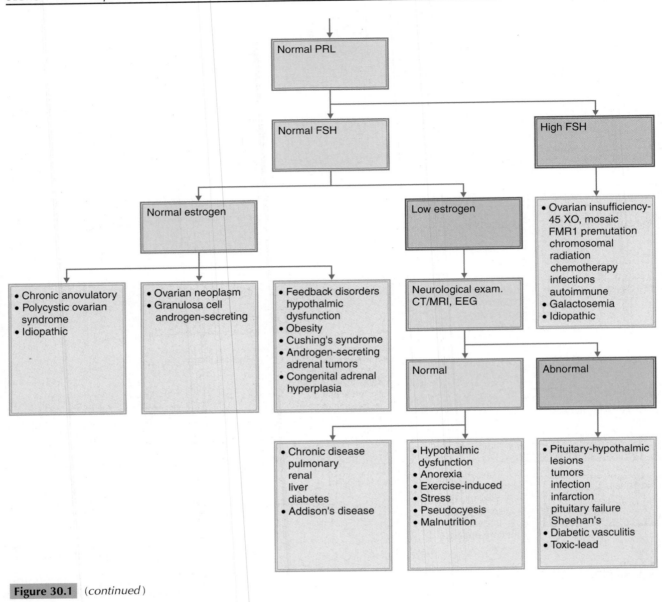

Figure 30.1   *(continued)*

Other disorders associated with primary amenorrhea include structurally abnormal X chromosomes, mosaicism (e.g., 45,X in some cells and another karyotype such as 46,XX or 46,XXX in other cells), pure gonadal dysgenesis (46,XX and 46,XY individuals with gonadal streaks resulting from lack of gonad development), enzyme deficiencies that prevent normal estrogen production, and gonadotropin-receptor inactivating mutations. Individuals with these conditions have gonadal failure and cannot synthesize ovarian steroids. Therefore, gonadotropin levels are elevated because of the lack of negative estrogen feedback on the hypothalamic–pituitary axis. **Most patients with these conditions have primary amenorrhea and lack secondary sexual characteristics.** Occasionally patients with a partial deletion of the X chromosome, mosaicism, or pure gonadal dysgenesis (46,XX) may synthesize enough estrogen in early puberty to induce breast development and a few episodes of uterine bleeding and thus have secondary amenorrhea. Ovulation and, occasionally, pregnancy are possible.

Genetic Disorders

Turner Syndrome   **Turner syndrome (45,X) is the most common karyotypic abnormality causing gonadal failure and primary amenorrhea** (3,4). It appears that patients with Turner

Table 30.1 Amenorrhea Associated with a Lack of Secondary Sexual Characteristics

Abnormal pelvic examination

5α-reductase deficiency, 17, 20-lyase deficiency, or 17α-hydroxylase deficiency in XY individual

Congenital lipoid adrenal hyperplasia

Luteinizing hormone receptor defect

Hypergonadotropic hypogonadism

Gonadal dysgenesis

Follicle-stimulating hormone receptor defect

Partial deletion of X chromosome

Sex chromosome mosaicism

Environmental and therapeutic ovarian toxins

17α-hydroxylase deficiency in XX individual

Galactosemia

Congenital lipoid adrenal hyperplasia in XX individual

Hypogonadotropic hypogonadism

Physiologic delay

Kallmann syndrome

Central nervous system tumors

Hypothalamic/pituitary dysfunction

syndrome initially have normal ovarian development *in utero*. Amenorrhea is the result of accelerated atresia of the follicles. The fibrotic ovaries are called streak ovaries.

In addition to gonadal failure, there are associated stigmata with Turner syndrome that include short stature, webbed neck, shield chest, cubitus valgus (increased carrying angle of the arms), low hair line, high arched palate, multiple pigmented nevi, and short fourth metacarpals (4). X inactivation is a process that inactivates most of the genes on one X chromosome. Of the genes on the X chromosome, 20% escape X inactivation, and it is believed that loss of the second copy of these genes in a 45,X patient causes the stigmata associated with Turner syndrome (5).

After the diagnosis of Turner syndrome is confirmed by karyotype, studies should be performed to ensure that cardiac (30% have coarctation of the aorta), renal (especially horseshoe kidney), and autoimmune (thyroiditis) abnormalities are diagnosed and treated. Cardiac magnetic resonance imaging (MRI) should be used in addition to echocardiography (6). Evaluation should be performed in childhood to identify potential attention-deficit or nonverbal learning disorders. **Women with Turner syndrome should be screened for diabetes mellitus, aortic enlargement, hypertension, and hearing loss throughout their lives** (6).

Abnormal X Chromosome   **Those 46,XX individuals with partial deletions of the X chromosome have variable phenotypes depending on the amount and location of the missing genetic material.** Patients with a deletion of the long arm of the X chromosome (Xq−) from Xq13 to Xq26 have sexual infantilism, normal stature, no somatic abnormalities, and streak gonads (7). Some patients may be eunuchoid in appearance and have delayed epiphyseal closure. Patients with a deletion of the short arm of the X chromosome (Xp) usually are phenotypically similar to individuals with Turner syndrome (8). Many genes on the Xp chromosome escape X inactivation and act similarly to genes on autosomes. The effective monosomy created by the deletion results in the phenotypic features of Turner syndrome (5). Most patients with a ring X have ovarian failure and phenotypes similar to Turner syndrome, although some are able to reproduce successfully. These patients differ from those with Turner syndrome in that they are more likely to have intellectual disability and have syndactyly. Patients with isochrome of the long arm of the X chromosome (i[Xq]) are similar to XO patients, with the exception that autoimmune disorders are more common. Half of the women with balanced translocations of the X chromosome to an autosome have gonadal failure. Typically, the normal X is inactivated to preserve the balance of autosomal genes. The gonadal failure can be caused by the chromosomal break occurring in a gene that is required for ovarian function, abnormal meiosis, or X inactivation of the translocated X and adjacent autosomal genes (5,9).

Mosaicism   **Primary amenorrhea is associated with various mosaic states, the most common of which is 45,X/46,XX** (10). The clinical findings in 45,X/47,XXX and 45,X/46,XX/47,XXX are similar to those in 45,X/46,XX and vary in estrogen and gonadotropin production, depending on the number of follicles in the gonads. When compared with the pure 45,X cell line, individuals with 45,X/46,XX are taller and have fewer abnormalities, although 80% of those with 45,X/46,XX mosaics are shorter than their peers, and 66% have some somatic abnormalities. Spontaneous menstruation occurs in approximately 20% of these patients (10).

Pure Gonadal Dysgenesis   **Individuals who are phenotypically female with sexual infantilism, primary amenorrhea, normal stature, and no karyotypic abnormalities (46,XX or 46,XY) have pure gonadal dysgenesis.** The gonads are usually streaks, but there may be some development of secondary sexual characteristics, and a few episodes of uterine bleeding. Pure gonadal dysgenesis in a 46,XY individual (previously known as Swyer syndrome) can occur when mutations in the SRY (sex-determining region gene on the Y chromosome) located at Yp11 result in XY females without proper gonad development (11,12).

Mutations in many other genes such as SOX9, DAX1, WT-1, and SF1, which affect testicular differentiation and inhibit antimüllerian hormone production, result in XY pure gonadal dysgenesis (13). The SOX9 gene located at 17q24 has a role in testis differentiation and promotes antimüllerian hormone secretion. Some but not all mutations in the *SOX9* gene cause XY sex reversal, along with camptomelic dysplasia (severe skeletal abnormalities) (14,15). Duplications of the DAX1 gene at Xp21 cause dose-sensitive XY sex reversal (16). DAX1 is hypothesized to antagonize the *SRY* gene, preventing testis development. Transgenic XY mice with overexpression of the *DAX1* gene develop as phenotypic females, supporting this hypothesis (17). Mutation in the WT1 gene (Wilms' tumor suppressor gene 1) located at 11p13 causes several different syndromes, depending on where the mutation in the gene occurs. In Frasier syndrome, there is alternative splicing, which causes the protein product to lack a highly conserved KTS triplet repeat. The normal +KTS isoform of the protein is believed to synergize with SF1 (steroidogenic factor 1) to promote the expression of antimüllerian hormone (AMH). Lack of the +KTS isoform in an XY patient results in normal female internal and external genitalia, streak gonads, and progressive glomerulopathy. These women frequently develop gonadoblastomas but rarely develop Wilms' tumor, which is associated with mutations in other locations in the *WT1* gene. XX patients with the mutation that prevents the +KTS isoform have similar kidney abnormalities but develop normal ovaries and genitalia (17–19). One XY patient with a heterozygous mutation of the *SF1* gene had adrenal failure and sex reversal (20). SF1 is an orphan nuclear receptor that regulates AMH expression and regulates all the cytochrome P450 steroid hydroxylase enzymes (19). Duplication of 1p, which encodes the *WNT4* gene, causes XY sex reversal. WNT4 may upregulate DAX1 transcripts. A TRX mutation causes XY sex reversal. Other genes that cause XY gonadal dysgenesis are likely to be identified. Mutations at 9p24 and 10q cause XY sex reversal, but the exact genes causing the defects are not elucidated (17,19,21).

XX pure gonadal dysgenesis can be caused by the presence of small Y chromosome fragments in the genome. It is estimated that 5% to 40% of patients with Ullrich-Turner syndrome have Y sequences by polymerase chain reaction (PCR), depending on the DNA sequences targeted for testing (22,23). If Y sequences are present, gonadectomy is advised because of the risk of gonadoblastoma (22).

In other patients with XX gonadal dysgenesis, the condition is likely to be caused by gene mutations that lead to ovarian insufficiency before pubertal development or after the development of secondary sexual characteristics, as discussed later in this chapter.

Mixed Gonadal Dysgenesis   **Most patients with mixed gonadal dysgenesis are XY and have ambiguous genitalia with a streak gonad on one side and a malformed testis on the opposite. A small proportion of these patients have mutations in the *SRY* gene** (17).

Rare Enzyme Deficiencies

Congenital Lipoid Adrenal Hyperplasia   **Patients with this autosomal recessive disorder are unable to convert cholesterol to pregnenolone, which is the first step in steroid hormone biosynthesis.** A defect was not found in the *P450scc* gene, which is the conversion enzyme responsible for this step in the pathway. Instead, 15 different mutations were identified in the steroidogenic acute regulatory protein (StAR), which facilitates the transport of cholesterol from the outer to the inner mitochondrial membrane. This protein appears to be the rate-limiting step for steroid hormone biosynthesis stimulated by tropic hormones. These patients present in infancy with hyponatremia, hyperkalemia, and acidosis. Both XX and XY individuals are phenotypically female. Genetic clusters of the disorder are found in the Japanese, Korean, and Palestinian Arab populations. With appropriate mineralocorticoid and glucocorticoid replacement, these patients can survive into adulthood. Most patients are XY and do not have a uterus. Without hormone replacement, they remain sexually infantile. XX patients may acquire secondary sexual characteristics at puberty but develop large ovarian cysts and early ovarian failure (24,25).

17á-Hydroxylase and 17,20-lyase Deficiency   **Mutations in the *CYP17* gene cause abnormalities in both the 17α-hydroxylase and 17,20-lyase functions of the protein that is active in the adrenal and gonadal steroidogenic pathways.** More than 20 mutations that alter the reading frame of the gene are identified, even though very few people have the disorder (26). Patients have either 46,XX or 46,XY karyotypes. The uterus is absent in individuals with 46,XY karyotype, a feature distinguishing them from individuals with the 46,XX karyotype. Individuals with CYP17 mutations have primary amenorrhea, no secondary sexual characteristics, female phenotype, hypertension, and hypokalemia (27). The diminished levels of 17α-hydroxylase that characterize this disorder lead to a reduction in cortisol production, which in turn causes an increase in adrenocorticotropic hormone (ACTH). 17-hydroxylase is not required for production of mineralocorticoids; thus, excessive amounts of mineralocorticoid are produced, resulting in sodium retention, loss of potassium, and hypertension. **Patients with 17α-hydroxylase deficiency have primordial follicles, but gonadotropin levels are elevated because the enzyme deficiency prevents synthesis of sex steroids.**

Aromatase Deficiency   This very rare autosomal recessive abnormality prevents the affected individual from aromatizing androgens to estrogen (28). **This syndrome may be suspected even before birth because most mothers of affected children become virilized during pregnancy.** This occurs because the placenta cannot convert the fetal androgens to estrogen and they diffuse into the maternal circulation. At birth, a female child has clitoromegaly and posterior labioscrotal fusion (ambiguous genitalia). At puberty, there is no breast development, primary amenorrhea, worsening virilization, absent growth spurt, delayed bone age, and multicystic ovaries. The diagnostic hormonal pattern consists of an elevation of FSH, LH, testosterone, and dehydroepiandrosterone sulfate (DHEAS) levels, and undetectable levels of estradiol. Estrogen therapy improves the ovarian and skeletal abnormalities but must be titrated to mimic normal estrogen levels. Estrogen administration should be minimal during childhood and increased at puberty (29,30).

Galactosemia   **In girls, galactosemia often is associated with ovarian failure, but this condition usually is detected by newborn screening programs.** A galactose-1 phosphate uridyl transferase level can be measured to assess the patient for galactosemia or carrier status.

Rare Gonadotropin Receptor Mutations

Luteinizing Hormone Receptor Mutation   **Inactivation of LH receptors is identified in XY pseudohermaphrodites with primary amenorrhea in the absence of secondary sexual characteristics** caused by homozygous premature stop codon, deletions, and missense mutations in the LHR gene located on chromosome 2. The Leydig cells in these individuals are unable to respond to LH, causing Leydig cell hypoplasia. This leads to early testicular failure and prevents masculinization. XX siblings with the same mutations develop normal secondary sexual characteristics but are amenorrheic with elevated LH levels, normal FSH levels, and cystic ovaries (31,32).

Follicle-Stimulating Hormone Receptor Mutation   An autosomal recessive single amino acid substitution in the extracellular domain of the FSH receptor, which prevents FSH binding, was identified in six families in Finland. This condition leads to primary or early secondary amenorrhea, variable development of secondary sexual characteristics, and high levels of FSH and LH (33).

Other Causes of Primary Ovarian Failure without Secondary Sexual Characteristics

Severe damage to the ovaries before the onset of puberty can lead to ovarian insufficiency and failure to develop secondary sexual characteristics. Ovarian dysfunction can occur in association with irradiation of the ovaries, chemotherapy with alkylating agents (e.g., *cyclophosphamide*), or combinations of radiation and other chemotherapeutic agents (34,35). Other causes of premature ovarian failure (also known as primary ovarian insufficiency) are more commonly associated with amenorrhea after the development of secondary sexual characteristics, as described below.

Hypogonadotropic Hypogonadism Associated with the Absence of Secondary Sex Characteristics

Primary amenorrhea resulting from hypogonadotropic hypogonadism occurs when the hypothalamus fails to secrete adequate amounts of GnRH or when a pituitary disorder associated with inadequate production or release of pituitary gonadotropins is present.

Physiologic Delay   **Physiologic or constitutional delay of puberty is the most common manifestation of hypogonadotropic hypogonadism. Amenorrhea may result from the lack of physical development caused by delayed reactivation of the GnRH pulse generator.** Levels of GnRH are functionally deficient in relation to chronologic age but normal in terms of physiologic development.

Kallmann Syndrome   **The second most common hypothalamic cause of primary amenorrhea associated with hypogonadotropic hypogonadism is insufficient pulsatile secretion of GnRH (Kallmann syndrome), which has varied modes of genetic transmission.** Insufficient pulsatile secretion of GnRH leads to deficiencies in FSH and LH (36). Kallmann syndrome is often associated with anosmia (inability to perceive odors), although a woman may not be aware of her impaired sense of smell. The hypogonadism and anosmia arise because of failure of proper neuronal migration during fetal development.

Other Causes of Gonadotropin-Releasing Hormone Deficiency   Deficiencies in GnRH may be caused by developmental or genetic defects, inflammatory processes, tumors, vascular lesions, or trauma. **Central nervous system tumors that lead to primary amenorrhea, the most common of which is craniopharyngioma, are usually extracellular masses that interfere with the synthesis and secretion of GnRH or stimulation of pituitary gonadotropins.** Virtually all of these patients have disorders in the production of other pituitary hormones and LH and FSH (37,38). Prolactin-secreting pituitary adenomas are rare in childhood and more commonly occur after development of secondary sexual characteristics.

Genetic Disorders

5α-Reductase Deficiency   5α-Reductase deficiency should be considered a cause of amenorrhea (39). Patients with this disorder are genotypically XY, frequently experience virilization at puberty, have testes (because of functioning Y chromosomes), and have no müllerian structures as a result of functioning AMH. 5α-Reductase converts testosterone to its more potent form, dihydrotestosterone. **Patients with 5-reductase deficiency differ from patients with androgen insensitivity because they do not develop breasts at puberty** (Fig. 30.2). **These patients have low gonadotropin levels as a result of testosterone levels that are sufficient to suppress breast development and allow normal feedback mechanisms to remain intact.** Normal male differentiation of the urogenital sinus and external genitalia do not occur because dihydrotestosterone is required for this development. Normal internal male genitalia derived from the wolffian ducts are present because this development requires only testosterone. Male pattern hair growth, muscle mass, and voice deepening are testosterone dependent.

Gonadotropin-Releasing Hormone Receptor Mutations   Several mutations are identified in the GnRH receptor gene that causes abnormal GnRH function. Most affected patients are compound heterozygotes, but homozygous autosomal recessive mutations are identified. The GnRH receptor is a G-protein–coupled receptor. Functional studies show that the mutations cause marked decrease in binding of GnRH to its receptor or prevent second-messenger signal transduction. Without a functional signal transduction, FSH and LH are not stimulated and are unable to promote follicular growth (40). All patients are normosomic. Receptor mutations in GnRH cause 17% of sporadic cases of idiopathic hypogonadotropic hypogonadism with normal olfaction (41).

Follicle-Stimulating Hormone Deficiency   **Patients with FSH deficiency usually seek treatment for delayed puberty and primary amenorrhea associated with hypoestrogenism.**

They are distinguished from other hypoestrogenic patients by having decreased FSH levels and increased LH levels. These patients have low serum androgen levels despite the abnormal LH-to-FSH ratio, indicating that FSH-stimulated follicular development is a prerequisite for thecal cell androgen production. In some of these patients, autosomal recessive mutations in the FSHβ subunit, which impair dimerization of α and β subunits and prevent binding to the FSH receptor, are identified (42). Pregnancy was achieved in one patient after induction of ovulation with injectable gonadotropins (43).

Other Hypothalamic/ Pituitary Dysfunctions	**Functional gonadotropin deficiency results from malnutrition, malabsorption, weight loss or anorexia nervosa, excessive exercise, chronic disease, neoplasias, and marijuana use, although these conditions are more commonly associated with amenorrhea accompanied by secondary sexual characteristics that developed before the onset of the problem, which is discussed in detail below (44–48). Hypothyroidism, polycystic ovarian syndrome (PCOS), Cushing syndrome, hyperprolactinemia, and infiltrative disorders of the central nervous system are more commonly associated with amenorrhea in the presence of development of secondary sexual characteristics, but can lead to amenorrhea accompanied by delayed puberty (49,50). Constitutional delay without underlying causes is less common in girls than in boys, and the reason for lack of development should be vigorously pursued (51).**

Evaluation of Women with Amenorrhea Associated with the Absence of Secondary Sexual Characteristics	**A careful history and physical examination are necessary to appropriately diagnose and treat primary amenorrhea associated with hypogonadism. The physical examination may be particularly helpful in patients with Turner syndrome.** A history of short stature but consistent growth rate, a family history of delayed puberty, and normal physical findings (including assessment of smell, optic discs, and visual fields) may suggest physiologic delay. Headaches, visual disturbances, short stature, symptoms of diabetes insipidus, and weakness of one or more limbs suggest central nervous system lesions (38). Galactorrhea may be seen with prolactinomas, a condition more commonly associated with secondary amenorrhea in the presence of normal secondary sexual characteristics.

The diagnostic workup is summarized as follows:

1. **The initial laboratory test should be assessment of serum FSH and LH levels unless the history and physical examination suggest otherwise in order to differentiate hypergonadotropic and hypogonadotropic forms of hypogonadism.** If the FSH level is elevated, a karyotype should be obtained. An elevated FSH level in combination with a 45,X karyotype confirms the diagnosis of Turner syndrome. Partial deletion of the X chromosome, mosaicism, pure gonadal dysgenesis, and mixed gonadal dysgenesis are diagnosed by obtaining a karyotype.

2. **Because of the association with coarctation of the aorta (up to 30%) and thyroid dysfunction, patients with Turner syndrome should undergo echocardiography every 3 to 5 years and thyroid function studies yearly. Cardiac MRI is considered an important component of the cardiac evaluation** (6). Patients with Turner syndrome should be evaluated for hearing loss, renal malformations, diabetes, and hypertension.

3. **If the karyotype is abnormal and contains the Y chromosome, as in gonadal dysgenesis, the gonads should be removed to prevent tumors** (13).

4. **If the karyotype is normal and the FSH level is elevated, it is important to consider the diagnosis of 17-hydroxylase deficiency because it may be a life-threatening disease if untreated.** This diagnosis should be considered when testing indicates elevated serum progesterone (>3.0 ng/mL) level, a low 17α-hydroxyprogesterone (0.2 ng/mL) level, and an elevated serum deoxycorticosterone level (52). The diagnosis is confirmed with an ACTH stimulation test. After ACTH bolus administration, affected individuals have markedly increased levels of serum progesterone compared with baseline levels and no change in serum 17α-hydroxyprogesterone levels.

5. **If the screening FSH level is low, the diagnosis of hypogonadotropic hypogonadism is established. Central nervous system lesions should be ruled out by imaging using computed tomography (CT) or MRI, especially if galactorrhea, headaches, or visual field defects are identified.** Suprasellar or intrasellar calcification in an abnormal sella is found in approximately 70% of patients with craniopharyngioma (38).

6. **Physiologic delay is a diagnosis of exclusion that is difficult to distinguish from insufficient GnRH secretion.** The diagnosis can be supported by a history suggesting

physiologic delay, an x-ray showing delayed bone age, and the absence of a central nervous system lesion on CT or MRI scanning.

Treatment of Amenorrhea Associated with the Absence of Secondary Sexual Characteristics

Individuals with primary amenorrhea associated with all forms of gonadal failure and hypergonadotropic hypogonadism need cyclic estrogen and progestogen therapy to initiate, mature, and maintain secondary sexual characteristics. Prevention of osteoporosis is an additional benefit of estrogen therapy:

1. **Therapy is usually initiated with 0.3 to 0.625 mg per day of *conjugated estrogens* or 0.5 to 1 mg per day of *estradiol*.**

2. **If the patient is short in stature, higher doses should not be used because premature closure of the epiphyses should be avoided.** Most of these patients are of normal height, and higher *estrogen* doses may be used initially and reduced to the maintenance doses after several months.

3. **Estrogen can be given daily in combination with progestogen (*medroxyprogesterone acetate* or *progesterone*) to prevent hyperplasia that could result from unopposed estrogen stimulation of the endometrium in patients with a uterus.** *Medroxyprogesterone* acetate may be administered at a dose of 2.5 mg daily every day of the month or 5 to 10 mg for 12 to 14 days per month. Oral micronized *progesterone* may be administered at a daily dose 100 mg every day of the month or 200 mg daily for 12 to 14 days per month. Cyclic hormone therapy (with 12 to 14 days of *progestogen* per month) more closely mimics the natural menstrual cycle. Progesterone suppositories may be administered at a dose of 50 mg daily or 100 mg for 12 to 14 days monthly.

4. **Occasionally, individuals with mosaicism and gonadal streaks may ovulate and be able to conceive either spontaneously or after the institution of *estrogen* therapy.**

5. **If 17α-hydroxylase deficiency is confirmed, treatment is instituted with corticosteroid replacement and** estrogen. *Progestogen* should be added to protect the endometrium from hyperplasia.

If possible, therapeutic measures are aimed at correcting the primary cause of amenorrhea:

1. **Craniopharyngiomas may be resected with a transsphenoidal approach or during craniotomy,** depending on the size of the tumor. Some studies show improved prognosis with radiation therapy used in combination with limited tumor removal (38,53).

2. **Germinomas are highly radiosensitive, and surgery is rarely indicated** (54).

3. **Prolactinomas and hyperprolactinemia often may respond to dopamine agonists (*bromocriptine* or *cabergoline*)** (55).

4. **Specific therapies are directed toward malnutrition, malabsorption, weight loss, anorexia nervosa, exercise amenorrhea, neoplasia, and chronic diseases.** Logically, it would appear that patients with hypogonadotropic hypogonadism of hypothalamic origin should be treated with long-term administration of pulsatile *GnRH*. This form of therapy is impractical because it requires the use of an indwelling catheter and a portable pump for prolonged periods and the lack of availability of this equipment in the United States. The primary focus of treatment should be to correct the underlying problem that is causing the menstrual dysfunction (e.g., malnutrition). If a patient is unable to correct the underlying condition, she may be treated with cyclic *estrogen* and *progestogen* therapy at least until sexual maturity is achieved. Once sexual maturation is achieved, hormone therapy can be continued to treat hypoestrogenic symptoms until the underlying disorder leading to amenorrhea can be adequately treated.

5. **Patients with Kallmann syndrome, and patients with other etiologies for hypothalamic amenorrhea, can be treated with hormone replacement,** as described above. For individuals with anorexia, intensive treatment to achieve weight gain and emotional well-being is preferable to long-term treatment with hormone therapy (56).

6. **If the patient has physiologic delay of puberty, the only management required is reassurance** that the anticipated development will occur eventually.

Individuals whose karyotypes contain a Y cell line (45,X/46,XY mosaicism, or pure gonadal dysgenesis 46,XY) are predisposed to gonadal ridge tumors, such as gonadoblastomas, dys-

germinomas, and yolk sac tumors. The gonads of these individuals should be removed when the condition is diagnosed to prevent malignant transformation. There is some evidence that hirsute individuals without Y chromosomes should undergo gonad removal. One patient with hirsutism and the karyotype 45,X was noted to have a streak gonad; the contralateral gonad was dysgenic and contained developing follicles, well-differentiated seminiferous tubules, and Leydig cells. This patient was found to be HY antigen–positive (57).

Clomiphene citrate is most often ineffective for inducing ovulation in patients with hypogonadism who desire pregnancy because such patients are hypoestrogenic. In patients with hypogonadism, ovulation induction with injectable gonadotropins is generally successful. In patients without ovarian function, oocyte donation may be appropriate. **There are reports of deaths in pregnant patients with Turner syndrome resulting from aortic dissection and rupture** (58). Careful counseling and investigation should be undertaken in patients with Turner syndrome before treating them with donated oocytes.

Amenorrhea with Secondary Sexual Characteristics and Abnormalities of Pelvic Anatomy

Causes

Outflow and Müllerian Anomalies

Amenorrhea occurs if there is blockage of the outflow tract, if the outflow tract is missing, or if there is no functioning uterus (Table 30.2) In order for menses to occur, the endometrium must be functional and there must be patency of the cervix and vagina. Most women with müllerian abnormalities will have normal ovarian function and thus will have normal secondary sexual characteristic development.

Table 30.2 Anatomic Causes of Amenorrhea

Secondary sexual characteristics present

Müllerian anomalies
Imperforate hymen
Transverse vaginal septum
Mayer-Rokitansky-Küster-Hauser syndrome
Androgen insensitivity
True hermaphrodism
Absent endometrium
Asherman syndrome
Secondary to prior uterine or cervical surgery
Curettage, especially postpartum
Cone biopsy
Loop electroexcision procedure
Secondary to infections
Pelvic inflammatory disease
Intrauterine devise–related
Tuberculosis
Schistosomiasis

Transverse Blockages

Any transverse blockage of the müllerian system will cause amenorrhea (59). **Such outflow obstructions include imperforate hymen, transverse vaginal septum, and absence of the cervix or vagina.** Transverse blockage of the outflow tract with an intact endometrium frequently causes cyclic pain without menstrual bleeding in adolescents. The blockage of blood flow can cause hematocolpos, hematometra, or hemoperitoneum, and endometriosis.

Müllerian Anomalies

Mayer-Rokitansky-Küster-Hauser syndrome includes vaginal agenesis with variable müllerian duct abnormalities accompanied in some cases by renal, skeletal, and auditory abnormalities (60). Müllerian agenesis accounts for approximately 10% of cases of primary amenorrhea (2). Of the patients with this syndrome, 15% have an absent, pelvic, or horseshoe kidney, 40% have a double urinary collecting system, and 5% to 12% have skeletal abnormalities (61–63). Mayer-Rokitansky-Küster-Hauser syndrome is associated with abnormal galactose metabolism (64).

Absence of Functioning Endometrium

Amenorrhea may occur if there is no functioning endometrium. When the findings of the physical examination are normal, anatomic abnormalities of the uterine cavity should be considered. A congenitally absent endometrium is a rare finding in patients with primary amenorrhea. **Asherman syndrome, which is more common with secondary amenorrhea or hypomenorrhea, may occur in patients with risk factors for endometrial or cervical scarring** (Fig. 30.3). Such risk factors include a history of uterine or cervical surgery, infections related to use of an intrauterine device, and severe pelvic inflammatory disease. Asherman syndrome is found in 39% of patients undergoing hysterosalpingography who previously underwent postpartum curettage (65). Infections such as tuberculosis and schistosomiasis may cause Asherman syndrome but are not common for women who have lived their whole lives in the United States. Cervical stenosis resulting from surgical removal of dysplasia (cone biopsy, loop electroexcision procedure) may lead to amenorrhea.

Androgen Insensitivity

Phenotypic females with complete congenital androgen insensitivity (previously called testicular feminization) develop secondary sexual characteristics but do not have menses (Fig. 30.2). **Genotypically, they are male (XY) but have a defect that prevents normal androgen receptor function, leading to the development of the female phenotype. Serum testosterone is in the normal male range. The vagina may be absent or short.**

Defects in the androgen receptor gene located on the X chromosome include absence of the gene that encodes for the androgen receptor and abnormalities in the binding domains of the receptor. Androgen receptor deficits are diverse and may result from diminished receptor function or concentration. The diversity of androgen receptor mutations may be related to diversity in phenotype. More than 250 extremely diverse mutations are described, with amino acid substitution being by far the most common (66,67). Postreceptor defects can exist (68). Total serum testosterone concentration is in the range of normal males. Because antimüllerian hormone is present and functions normally in these patients, internal female (müllerian) structures such as a uterus, vagina, and fallopian tubes are absent. **Testes rather than ovaries are present in the abdomen or in inguinal hernias because of the presence of normally functioning genes on the Y chromosome. Patients have a blind vaginal pouch and scant or absent axillary and pubic hair.** These patients experience abundant breast development at puberty; however, the nipples are immature and the areolae are pale. Testosterone is not present during development to suppress the formation of breast tissues; at puberty, the conversion of testosterone to estrogen stimulates breast growth. Patients are unusually tall with eunuchoidal tendency (long arms with big hands and feet).

True Hermaphroditism

True hermaphroditism is a rare condition that should be considered as a possible cause of amenorrhea. Both male and female gonadal tissues are present in these patients, in whom XX, XY, and mosaic genotypes are found. Two-thirds of the patients menstruate, but menstruation was never reported in XY genotypes. The external genitalia usually are ambiguous, and breast development frequently occurs in these individuals. **Fifteen percent of XX true hermaphrodites have *SRY* translocations, and another 10% have Y chromosomal mosaicism within the gonad** (17).

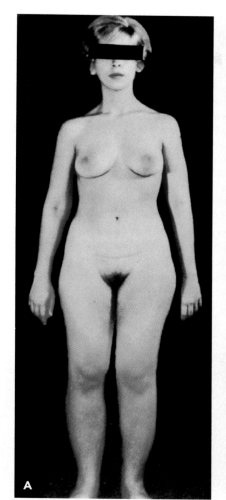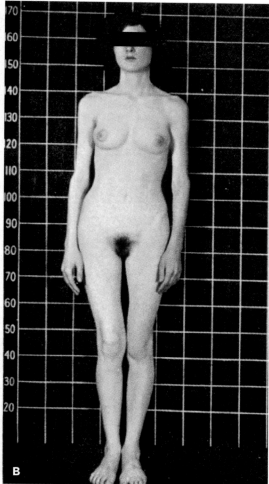

Figure 30.2   A: **A well-developed patient with complete androgen insensitivity.** Note the characteristic paucity of pubic hair and well-developed breasts. (From **Yen SSC, Jaffe RB.** *Reproductive endocrinology.* 3rd ed. Philadelphia, PA: WB Saunders, 1991:497, with permission.) B: **Another patient with androgen insensitivity syndrome with a contrasting thin body hiatus.** This is a 17-year-old twin 46,XY. (From **Jones HW Jr, Scott WW.** *Hermaphrodism, genital anomalies, and related endocrine disorders.* 2nd ed. Baltimore, MD: Williams & Wilkins, 1971, with permission.)

Evaluation of Women with Amenorrhea, Normal Secondary Sexual Characteristics, and Suspected Anatomic Abnormalities

Most congenital abnormalities can be diagnosed by physical examination:

1. **An imperforate hymen is diagnosed by the presence of a bulging membrane that distends during Valsalva maneuver.** Ultrasonography or MRI is useful to identify the müllerian anomaly when the abnormality cannot be found by physical examination. The patient should be examined for skeletal malformations and assessed with intravenous pyelography or renal ultrasound to detect concomitant renal abnormalities. These abnormalities occur less frequently than in müllerian agenesis (63).

2. **It is difficult to differentiate a transverse septum or complete absence of the cervix and uterus in a female from a blind vaginal pouch in a male pseudohermaphrodite by examination alone. Androgen insensitivity is likely when pubic and axillary hair is absent.** To confirm the diagnosis, a karyotype determination should be performed to see whether a Y chromosome is present. In some patients, the defect in the androgen receptor is not complete and virilization occurs.

3. **An absent endometrium is an outflow tract abnormality that cannot be diagnosed by physical examination in a patient with primary amenorrhea.** This abnormality is so rare that in a patient with normal physical findings (normal vagina, cervix, and uterus), it may be advisable to proceed with evaluation of endocrine abnormalities. Although in most cases performance of the progestogen challenge test is not recommended, this test may be of value to confirm the rare diagnosis of congenitally absent endometrium. In this case, progestogen can be administered to a woman who appears to have normal estrogen production (or if estrogen status is questioned, 2.5 mg *conjugated estrogen* or 2 mg *micronized estradiol* can be given for 25 days with 5 to 10 mg of *medroxyprogesterone acetate* added for the last 10 days). Congenital absence of the endometrium is confirmed if no bleeding occurs with this regimen in a patient with primary amenorrhea and no physical abnormalities. This is a very rare diagnosis and routine performance of progestogen challenge is not recommended. Transvaginal ultrasound to assess endometrial thickness may be helpful, with a thickened endometrial lining indicating endometrial response to estrogen.

4. *Asherman syndrome* **cannot be diagnosed by physical examination. It is diagnosed by performing hysterosalpingography, saline infusion sonography (also known as saline hysterogram), or hysteroscopy.** These tests will show either complete obliteration or multiple filling defects caused by synechiae. If tuberculosis or schistosomiasis is suspected, endometrial cultures should be performed.

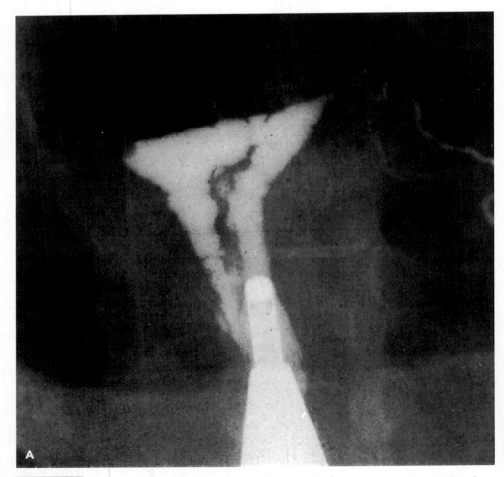

Figure 30.3 A: Intrauterine adhesion seen on hysterosalpingogram in a patient with Asherman syndrome. (From **Donnez J, Nisolle M.** *The encyclopedia of visual medicine series—an atlas of laser operative laparoscopy and hysteroscopy.* New York: Parthenon, 1994:306, with permission.)

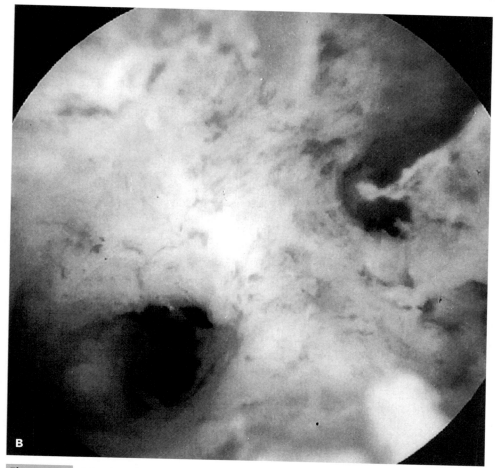

Figure 30.3 (*Continued*) B: **Hysteroscopic view of intrauterine adhesion in a patient with Asherman syndrome.**

Treatment of Women with Amenorrhea, Normal Secondary Sexual Characteristics, and Abnormalities of Pelvic Anatomy

The treatment of congenital anomalies can be summarized as follows:

1. **Treatment of an imperforate hymen involves making a cruciate incision to open the vaginal orifice.** Most imperforate hymens are not diagnosed until a hematocolpos forms. It is unwise to place a needle into a hematocolpos without completely removing the obstruction because a pyocolpos may occur.

2. **If a transverse septum is present, surgical removal is required.** Forty-six percent of transverse septa occur in the upper third of the vagina, and 40% occur in the middle third of the vagina (69). Frank dilators should be used to distend the vagina until it is healed to prevent vaginal adhesions (70). Patients have a fully functional reproductive system after surgery; however, patients with repaired high transverse septa may have lower pregnancy rates (71).

3. **Hypoplasia or absence of the cervix in the presence of a functioning uterus is more difficult to treat than other outflow obstructions.** Surgery to repair the cervix is rarely successful, and hysterectomy is typically required (72). Endometriosis is a common finding, and it is questionable whether this condition should be treated initially with surgery or if it will resolve spontaneously after surgical repair of the obstruction. The ovaries should be retained to provide the benefits of estrogen and to allow for the possibility of future childbearing by removing mature oocytes for *in vitro* fertilization and transfer of embryos to a gestational carrier.

4. **If the vagina is absent or short, progressive dilation is usually successful in making it functional** (70,73). If dilation fails or the patient is unable to perform dilation, the McIndoe split thickness graft technique may be performed (62,74,75). Controversy

exists as to the best technique (60). The initial use of vaginal dilators is required to maintain a functional vagina.

5. **In patients with complete androgen insensitivity, the testes should be removed after pubertal development is complete to prevent malignant degeneration** (76). In patients with testes, 52% develop a neoplasia, most often a gonadoblastoma. Almost one-half of the testicular neoplasms are malignant (dysgerminomas), but transformation usually does not occur until after puberty (77). In patients who develop virilization and have an XY karyotype, the testes should be removed immediately to preserve the female phenotype and to promote female gender identity. Bilateral laparoscopic gonadectomy is the preferred procedure for removal of intra-abdominal testes.

6. **Adhesions in the cervix and uterus (Asherman syndrome) can be removed using hysteroscopic resection with scissors or electrocautery.** It is reasonable to place a pediatric Foley catheter in the uterine cavity for 7 to 10 days postoperatively (along with systemic administration of broad-spectrum antibiotic therapy). A 2-month course of high-dose estrogen therapy with monthly progestogen withdrawal is used to prevent reformation of adhesions. Eighty percent of patients thus treated achieve pregnancy, but complications including miscarriage, preterm labor, placenta previa, and placenta accreta can occur (78). Cervical stenosis can be treated by cervical dilation.

Amenorrhea with Secondary Sexual Characteristics and Normal Pelvic Anatomy

Although the complete list of potential causes is long, as noted below, the most common causes of amenorrhea in women with normal secondary sexual characteristics and normal pelvic are pregnancy, polycystic ovarian syndrome, hyperprolactinemia, primary ovarian insufficiency (also known as premature ovarian failure), and hypothalamic dysfunction. Pregnancy must be considered in all women of reproductive age with amenorrhea.

Causes

Polycystic Ovarian Syndrome

PCOS is a medical condition associated with hyperandrogenism, ovulatory dysfunction, and polycystic ovaries (79). All definitions of PCOS exclude patients with significantly elevated prolactin, significant thyroid dysfunction, adult-onset congenital adrenal hyperplasia, and androgen-secreting neoplasms from being classified as PCOS. **The National Institutes of Health (NIH) 1990 criteria included hyperandrogenism and oligomenorrhea or amenorrhea as required for PCOS diagnosis. The Rotterdam 2003 criteria required two of three of the following for PCOS diagnosis: hyperandrogenism, oligomenorrhea or amenorrhea, polycystic ovaries by ultrasound** (80). Although insulin resistance is noted among women with PCOS, it is not included in any of the diagnostic criteria. Obesity is common, but approximately 20% of women with PCOS are not obese. Women with PCOS are often subfertile caused by infrequent or absent ovulation. PCOS can have other general health implications, including increased risk for endometrial hyperplasia and cancer, diabetes, and possibly cardiovascular disease.

Even though **PCOS usually causes irregular bleeding rather than amenorrhea, it remains one of the most common causes of amenorrhea** (2). The etiology of PCOS remains largely unknown.

In patients who are hirsute and amenorrheic and appear to have PCOS, androgen-secreting adrenal tumors and congenital adrenal hyperplasia should be considered. Elevations in androgens (e.g., Sertoli-Leydig, hilus, and lipoid cell tumors) and estrogens (e.g., granulosa cell tumors) by ovarian tumors may lead to abnormal menstrual patterns, including amenorrhea. A history of rapid onset of hirsutism is suggestive of a tumor.

Hyperprolactinemia

Hyperprolactinemia is a common cause of anovulation in women. Elevation of prolactin produces abnormal GnRH secretion, which can lead to menstrual disturbances (81). Prolactin levels rise in pregnancy, but typically return to normal within 6 months after delivery in nursing mothers and within weeks in nonnursing mothers. Dopamine release suppresses prolactin secretion. Levels of prolactin can be increased by pituitary adenomas that produce prolactin, by other central nervous system (CNS) lesions that disrupt the normal transport of dopamine down the pituitary stalk, and by medications that interfere with normal dopamine secretion (such as antidepressants, antipsychotics including *risperidone, metoclopramide,* some antihypertensives, opiates, and H_2-receptor blockers).

If elevated TSH and elevated prolactin levels are found together, the hypothyroidism should be treated before hyperprolactinemia is treated. Often, the prolactin level will normalize with treatment of hypothyroidism because thyroid-releasing hormone, which is elevated in hypothyroidism, stimulates prolactin secretion.

Primary Ovarian Insufficiency (Premature Ovarian Failure)

Primary ovarian insufficiency is suggested as the preferred term for the condition that otherwise was referred to as premature ovarian failure or premature menopause (82,83). Overt primary ovarian insufficiency (POI) is defined as the presence of amenorrhea for 4 months or more accompanied by two serum FSH levels in the menopausal range for a woman who is less than 40 years of age. Ovarian "insufficiency" is suggested to be more appropriate than "failure" in part because ovarian function can wax and wane, and function can resume even after it appears that a woman transitioned into menopause. Ovarian insufficiency may be caused by decreased follicular endowment or accelerated follicular atresia (82). Over 75% of women with POI will have at least intermittent symptoms including hot flushes, night sweats, and emotional lability (84). Symptoms are uncommon among women with primary amenorrhea who never received estrogen.

If the ovary does not develop or stops its hormone production before puberty, the patient will not develop secondary sexual characteristics without exogenous hormone therapy. If ovarian insufficiency begins later in life, the woman will have normal secondary sexual characteristics.

POI clearly compromises the chance of a woman conceiving with autologous oocytes. However, 5% to 10% of women with a diagnosis of premature ovarian failure achieve pregnancy, with approximately 80% of these pregnancies resulting in the delivery of a healthy child (85). It can be difficult to determine which women will be able to conceive. Published studies of testing for ovarian reserve have not specifically focused on the POI populations, and pregnancies may occur despite very unfavorable results for tests of ovarian reserve such as serum FSH, estradiol, and AMH.

POI is a heterogenous disorder with many potential causes. POI may be caused by sex chromosome disorders, mutations of single genes, and by *FMR1* premutations. Radiation or chemotherapy may lead to POI. The cause of POI may be autoimmune. **The cause remains unknown in a majority of cases** (Table 30.3).

Sex Chromosome and Single Gene Disorders Associated with Primary Ovarian Insufficiency   **Deletion of the X chromosome (Turner syndrome) is associated with primary ovarian insufficiency, despite normal development of the ovaries, because of accelerated atresia of the follicles** (86). Although Turner syndrome may often be associated with primary

Table 30.3 Causes of Ovarian Insufficiency or Failure after Development of Secondary Sexual Characteristics
Chromosomal etiology (e.g., Turner mosaic)
FMR1 premutation
Iatrogenic causes: radiation, chemotherapy, surgical damage to ovarian blood supply or ovary
Infections
Autoimmune-lymphocytic autoimmune oophoritis
Infections
Galactosemia
Perrault syndrome
Idiopathic (80%–90% of cases)

amenorrhea with absence of secondary sexual characteristics, breast development may occur if ovarian function is initially present. Mosaicism of an XO or XY cell line may cause ovarian insufficiency. **Individuals with a 47,XXX karyotype may develop ovarian failure** (87). The most common physical features of 47,XXX are tall stature, epicanthal folds, hypotonia, and clinodactyly.

A deletion of a portion of the X chromosome may be present in patients with POI. The Xq21-28 region is critical (7,88). Several genes in this region are identified as the cause of early ovarian insufficiency in humans. Examples include the *POF1B* gene located at Xq21, the *DIAPH2* gene located at distal Xq21, and the *XPNPEP2* gene located at Xq25 (89,90). The specific functions of these genes require further investigation. In addition, a mutation of the *BMP15* gene located at Xp11.2 is identified in patients with premature ovarian failure (91).

An autosomal recessive form of premature ovarian failure is associated with hearing loss in Perrault syndrome (92). Mutations in *FOXL2* causes ovarian failure and ptosis (93). Familial ovarian failure is inherited by dominant Mendelian inheritance in rare cases (94). Numerous genetic mutations leading to ovarian insufficiency are identified and many more are likely to be discovered (95,96). Other than the *FMR1* premutation described next, no one mutation is particularly common.

Fragile X Carriers   **Fragile X syndrome, the most common cause of inherited (X-linked) intellectual disability, is caused by inactivation of the *FMR1* (fragile X mental retardation 1) gene located on Xq27.3. This inactivation occurs as a result of expansion of a cytosine-guanine-guanine (CGG) triplet repeat of more than 200 copies** (97). *FMR1* **premutation carriers (typically defined as greater than 55 but under 200 CGG repeats) may have primary ovarian insufficiency and impaired fertility.** The prevalence of POI in women who carry the *FMR1* premutation is estimated to be between 13% and 26%. The risk of having POI appears to increase with increasing premutation repeat size between 59 and 99. It is possible that there is an increased risk of POI among women who carry intermediate-size allele (approximately 41 to 58 repeats), but this is not conclusively proven. The risk plateaus or decreases for women with repeat sizes of 100. Interestingly, women with full mutations (200 or more CGG repeats) are not at higher risk for POI. It is hypothesized that expression of abnormal *FMR1* mRNA produced by patients with the premutation causes dysfunction in the ovary, which does not occur when the *FMR1* gene is inactivated and not transcribed. The incidence of having a premutation is 0.8% to 7.5% of women with sporadic POI and up to 13% of women with familial POI.

FMR1 **premutations carried by women are unstable and can expand in the next generation to transmit fragile X syndrome to male offspring,** especially if women have more than 100 repeats. The smallest repeat to expand to the full mutation in one generation is approximately 59. In contrast to potential expansion in women, the repeat sequence is transmitted from fathers to daughters in a relatively stable manner.

Iatrogenic Causes of Primary Ovarian Insufficiency   **Radiation, chemotherapy (especially alkylating agents such as *cyclophosphamide*)** (98), **surgical interference with ovarian blood supply, and infections can cause ovarian failure from early loss of follicles. A radiation dose of 800 cGy causes sterility in most individuals. Ovarian failure can be caused by as little as 150 cGy in some patients, especially if they are older than 40 years of age with limited ovarian reserve.** In an evaluation of ovarian function in 100 childhood cancer survivors, 17 had premature ovarian failure. Those with spontaneous menses had smaller ovarian volume, fewer antral follicles, and lower inhibin B levels when compared with controls (99). Ovarian suppression with GnRH agonists and oral contraceptives to reduce the risk of ovarian failure was attempted with limited success (100,101). Cigarette smoking decreases the age at which menopause will occur. But smoking would not be expected to be the primary cause of amenorrhea occurring before the age of 40.

Infections   **In rare cases, mumps was associated with premature ovarian failure** (102). Women with human immunodeficiency virus (HIV) infection may prematurely lose ovarian function compared to women without HIV infection (103). Cytomegalovirus was shown postmortem to cause oophoritis, but premature ovarian failure had not yet developed clinically in the patient, so the relationship of cytomegalovirus to ovarian failure remains unclear (104).

Autoimmune Disorders   **In one series, 4% of women with POI were noted to have steroidogenic cell immunity with lymphocytic oophoritis as the mechanism for follicle dysfunction** (105). **Autoimmune lymphocytic oophoritis is associated with a theca cell infiltrate** that spares granulosa cells (106). Ultrasound examination reveals the presence of numerous ovarian follicles, despite elevated serum FSH levels and hypoestrogenism (82). Ovarian antibody testing is not clinically reliable for diagnosing the disorder, as women with biopsy-proven autoimmune oophoritis may have a negative test for ovarian antibody. However, women with autoimmune lymphocytic oophoritis appear to reliably test positive for adrenal antibodies. The most readily available antibody is the 21-hydroxylase antibody (by immunoprecipitation). Ideally, antibody to the adrenal gland itself, as assessed by indirect immunofluorescence, is reasonable to test if available. Testing for 21-hydroxylase antibody is strongly recommended for women who are determined to have POI because women who test positive for this antibody are at risk for potentially fatal hypoadrenalism. Signs that suggest a risk for potentially fatal adrenal insufficiency include hyperpigmentation, weakness, nausea, vomiting, diarrhea, and weight loss.

POI may be part of a polyglandular autoimmune syndrome. Antibodies are present in a variable number of patients with POI, depending on the autoimmune studies performed. One study showed that 92% of patients with premature ovarian failure had autoantibodies (107). Only 20% of these patients exhibited signs of immunologic dysfunction, most frequently in the form of a thyroid disorder that is common in the general population of women who do not have POI. **Presence of antithyroid antibodies does not confirm that there is an autoimmune cause for POI.** Rarely, POI is associated with myasthenia gravis, idiopathic thrombocytopenia purpura, rheumatoid arthritis, vitiligo, autoimmune hemolytic anemia, diabetes mellitus, and other autoimmune disorders (108–110).

Galactosemia   Galactosemia is caused by a lack of functional galactose-1-phosphate uridyl transferase. Galactosemia is a rare cause of POI and is typically diagnosed in childhood prior to presentation with amenorrhea. Galactose metabolites appear to have toxic effects on ovarian follicles, causing their premature destruction (111). Cataracts and mental retardation are associated with galactosemia. There is evidence that heterozygote carriers of this disorder may have suboptimal ovarian function (112). Early dietary modification may delay but not prevent the ovarian failure (26).

Pituitary and Hypothalamic Lesions

Hypothalamic Tumors   **For normal menstruation to occur, the hypothalamus must be able to secrete GnRH, and the pituitary must be able to respond with production and release of FSH and LH. Tumors of the hypothalamus or pituitary, such as craniopharyngiomas, germinomas, tubercular or sarcoid granulomas, or dermoid cysts, may prevent appropriate hormonal secretion.** Patients with these disorders may have neurologic abnormalities, and secretion of other hypothalamic and pituitary hormones may be abnormal. Craniopharyngiomas are the most common tumors. They are located in the suprasellar region and frequently cause headaches and visual changes. The surgical and radiologic treatment of tumors may in itself cause further abnormalities in hormone secretion (Table 30.4).

Pituitary Lesions   **Hypopituitarism is rare because a large portion of the gland must be destroyed before decreased hormonal secretion affects the patient clinically.** The pituitary gland may be destroyed by tumors (nonfunctioning or hormone secreting), infarction, or infiltrating lesions such as lymphocytic hypophysitis, granulomatous lesions, and surgical or radiologic ablations. **Sheehan syndrome is associated with postpartum necrosis of the pituitary resulting from a hypotensive episode that, in its severe form (pituitary apoplexy), presents with the patient in shock.** The patient may develop a localized, severe, retro-orbital headache or abnormalities in visual fields and visual acuity. Patients with a mild form of postpartum pituitary necrosis cannot lactate, lose pubic and axillary hair, and do not menstruate after delivery.

Diabetic vasculitis and sickle cell anemia rarely manifest as pituitary failure. Hypopituitarism is associated with hyposecretion of ACTH and thyroid-stimulating hormone (TSH) and gonadotropins; therefore, thyroid and adrenal function must be evaluated. **If hypopituitarism occurs before puberty, menses and secondary sexual characteristics will not develop.**

Growth hormone (GH), TSH, ACTH, and prolactin are secreted by the pituitary, and the excess production of each by pituitary tumors causes menstrual abnormalities. The menstrual abnormalities are caused by adverse effects of these hormones on the GnRH pulse generator and not by direct effects on the ovary. Prolactinomas are the most common hormone-secreting tumors in the pituitary, as described above.

Table 30.4 Pituitary and Hypothalamic Lesions
Pituitary and hypothalamic
Craniopharyngioma
Germinoma
Tubercular granuloma
Sarcoid granuloma
Dermoid cyst
Pituitary
Nonfunctioning adenomas
Hormone-secreting adenomas
Prolactinoma
Cushing's disease
Acromegaly
Infarction
Lymphocytic hypophysitis
Surgical or radiologic ablations
Sheehan's syndrome
Diabetic vasculitis

Altered Hypothalamic Gonadotropin-Releasing Hormone Secretion

Abnormal secretion of GnRH accounts for one-third of patients with amenorrhea (113). Chronic disease, malnutrition, stress, psychiatric disorders, eating disorders, and exercise inhibit GnRH pulses, thus altering the menstrual cycle (Table 30.5). Other hormonal systems that produce excess or insufficient hormones can cause abnormal feedback and adversely affect GnRH secretion. In hyperprolactinemia, Cushing disease (excess ACTH), and acromegaly (excess GH), excess pituitary hormones are secreted that inhibit GnRH secretion. It is uncommon to have functional hypothalamic amenorrhea without a secondary cause. Prognosis for recovery is better if the precipitating cause of the amenorrhea can be reversed (114).

When the decrease in GnRH pulsatility is severe, amenorrhea results. With less severe alterations in GnRH pulsatility, anovulation and oligomenorrhea can occur. The pulsatile secretion of GnRH is modulated by interactions with neurotransmitters and peripheral gonadal steroids. Endogenous opioids, corticotropin-releasing hormones (CRH), melatonin, and α-aminobutyric acid (GABA) inhibit the release of GnRH, whereas catecholamines, acetylcholine, and vasoactive intestinal peptide stimulate GnRH pulses. Dopamine and serotonin have variable effects (115).

Decreased leptin levels are associated with hypothalamic amenorrhea, regardless of whether it is caused by exercise, eating disorders, or idiopathic factors (116,117). Leptin is a hormone secreted by adipocytes that is involved in energy hemostasis. Receptors are found in the hypothalamus and bone, making it an excellent candidate for a modulator of menstrual function and bone mass. Levels correlate with nutritional changes and body mass index. Administration of leptin to women with hypothalamic amenorrhea increased levels of LH, estradiol, insulinlike growth factor-1 (IGF-1), and thyroid hormone. Ovulation and increased bone mass occurred in these patients (117). Weight loss occurring with leptin administration limits the utility of using leptin as a therapeutic agent.

Eating Disorders

Anorexia nervosa is an eating disorder that affects 5% to 10% of adolescent women in the United States. The criteria for diagnosis of anorexia nervosa are refusal to maintain body weight above 15% below normal, an intense fear of becoming fat, altered perception of one's body image (i.e., patients see themselves as fat despite being underweight), and

Table 30.5 Abnormalities Affecting Release of Gonadotropin-Releasing Hormone

Variable estrogenstatus [a]

Anorexia nervosa

Exercise-induced

Stress-induced

Pseudocyesis

Malnutrition

Chronic diseases

> Diabetes mellitus

> Renal disorders

> Pulmonary disorders

> Liver disease

> Chronic infections

> Addison's disease

Hyperprolactinemia

Thyroid dysfunction

Euestrogenic states

Obesity

Hyperandrogenism

> Polycystic ovary syndrome

> Cushing syndrome

> Congenital adrenal hyperplasia

> Androgen-secreting adrenal tumors

> Androgen-secreting ovarian tumors

Granulosa cell tumor

Idiopathic

[a]Severity of the condition determines estrogen status—the more severe, the more likely to manifest as hypoestrogenism.

amenorrhea. Patients attempt to maintain their low body weight by food restriction, laxative abuse, and intense exercise. **This is a life-threatening disorder with a mortality rate as high as 9%.** Amenorrhea may precede, coincide, or follow the weight loss. Multiple hormonal patterns are altered. The 24-hour patterns of FSH and LH may show constantly low levels as seen in childhood or increased LH pulsatility during sleep consistent with the pattern seen in early puberty. Hypercortisolism is present despite normal ACTH levels, and the ACTH response to CRH administration is blunted. Circulating triiodothyronine (T_3) is low, yet circulating inactive reverse T_3 concentrations are high (118). Patients may develop cold and heat intolerance, lanugo hair, hypotension, bradycardia, and diabetes insipidus. They may have yellowish discoloration of the skin resulting from elevated levels of serum carotene caused by altered vitamin A metabolism.

Binge eating is associated with bulimia consisting of vomiting, laxative abuse, and diuretics to control weight. Signs of bulimia include tooth decay, parotid gland hypertrophy (chipmunk jowls), hypokalemia, and metabolic alkalosis (119).

Weight Loss and Dieting

Weight loss can cause amenorrhea even if weight does not decrease below normal. Loss of 10% body mass in 1 year is associated with amenorrhea. Some but not all of these women have an underlying eating disorder. Prognosis is good for the return of menses if the patients recover from the weight loss. Dieting without weight loss and changes in diet can lead to amenorrhea (114).

Exercise

In patients with exercise-induced amenorrhea, there is a decrease in the frequency of GnRH pulses, which is assessed by measuring a decreased frequency of LH pulses. These patients are usually hypoestrogenic, but less severe alterations may cause minimal menstrual dysfunction (anovulation or luteal phase defect). The decrease in GnRH pulsatility can be caused by hormonal alterations, such as low levels of leptin or high levels of ghrelin, neuropeptide Y and corticotrophin-releasing hormone (120). Runners and ballet dancers are at higher risk for amenorrhea than swimmers (121). It was previously suggested that a minimum of 17% body fat is required for the initiation of menses and 22% body fat for the maintenance of menses (122). Studies suggest that inappropriately low caloric intake during strenuous exercise is more important than body fat (123). **Higher-intensity training, poor nutrition, stress of competition, and associated eating disorders increase an athlete's risk for menstrual dysfunction (124). Osteoporosis may result in stress fractures during training and lifelong increased fracture risk.** Stress fractures most commonly occur in the weight-bearing cortical bone such as the tibia, metatarsal, fibula, and femur. These athletes may fail to reach peak bone mass and have abnormal bone mineralization.

Stress

Stress-related amenorrhea can be caused by abnormalities in neuromodulation in hypothalamic GnRH secretion, similar to those that occur with exercise and anorexia nervosa. Excess endogenous opioids and elevations in CRH secretion inhibit the secretion of GnRH (115). These mechanisms are not fully understood but appear to be the common link between amenorrhea and chronic diseases, pseudocyesis, and malnutrition.

Obesity

Most obese patients have normal menstrual cycles, but the percentage of women with menstrual disorders increases for women with obesity compared with women of normal weight. The menstrual disorder is more often irregular uterine bleeding with anovulation rather than amenorrhea. **Obese women have an excess number of fat cells in which extraglandular aromatization of androgen to estrogen occurs. They have lower circulating levels of sex hormone–binding globulin, which allows a larger proportion of free androgens to be converted to estrone. Excess estrogen creates a higher risk for endometrial cancer for these women.** The decrease in sex hormone–binding globulin allows an increase in free androgen levels, which initially are eliminated by an increased rate of metabolic clearance. This compensatory mechanism diminishes over time, and hirsutism can develop. Frequently, these patients are classified as having PCOS. Alterations in the secretion of endorphins, cortisol, insulin, growth hormone, and IGF-1 may interact with the abnormal estrogen and androgen feedback to the GnRH pulse generator to cause menstrual abnormalities.

Other Hormonal Factors

The secretion of hypothalamic neuromodulators can be altered by feedback from abnormal levels of peripheral hormones. Excesses or deficiencies of thyroid hormone, glucocorticoids, androgens, and estrogens can cause menstrual dysfunction. Excess secretion of GH, TSH, ACTH, and prolactin from the pituitary gland can cause abnormal feedback inhibition of GnRH secretion, leading to amenorrhea. **Growth hormone excess causes acromegaly, which may be associated with anovulation, hirsutism, and polycystic-appearing ovaries as a result of stimulation of the ovary by IGF-1. More commonly, GH excess is accompanied by amenorrhea, low gonadotropin levels, and elevated prolactin levels. Acromegaly is recognized by enlargement of facial features, hands, and feet; hyperhidrosis; visceral organ enlargement; and multiple skin tags. Cushing disease is caused by an ACTH-secreting pituitary tumor, which is manifested by truncal obesity, moon facies, hirsutism, proximal weakness, depression, and menstrual dysfunction.**

Evaluation for Women with Amenorrhea in the Presence of Normal Pelvic Anatomy and Normal Secondary Sexual Characteristics

A pregnancy test (urine or serum human chorionic gonadotropin [hCG]) should be performed in a reproductive-age woman who has amenorrhea with normal secondary sexual characteristics and a normal pelvic examination. If the results of the pregnancy test are negative, the evaluation of amenorrhea is as follows:

1. **Clinical assessment of estrogen status**
2. **Serum TSH**
3. **Serum prolactin**

4. **Serum FSH level**
5. **Vaginal ultrasound for assessment of antral follicle count in the ovaries can be considered (may help establish the diagnosis of PCOS or suggest POI)**
6. **Imaging of the pituitary and hypothalamic assessment if prolactin is elevated or if hypothalamic amenorrhea is suspected (particularly if CNS symptoms are present or there is no clear explanation for hypothalamic amenorrhea).**

Assessment of Estrogen Status

The presence of vaginal dryness or hot flashes increases the likelihood of a diagnosis of hypoestrogenism. A sample of vaginal secretions can be obtained during the physical examination, and mucosal estrogen response can be demonstrated by the presence of superficial cells. A serum estradiol level higher than 40 pg/mL is considered indicative of significant estrogen production, but interassay discrepancies often exist and serum estrogen levels can vary greatly on a day-to-day basis for a given woman. Vaginal ultrasound demonstrating a thin endometrium suggests that a patient is hypoestrogenic, unless there is reason to suspect that the patient lacks functional endometrium. A DEXA (dual-energy x-ray absorptiometry) scan to determine bone mineral density should be considered for a patient in whom long-term hypoestrogenism is suspected.

There is little utility in routine performance of a progestogen challenge test to determine the patient's estrogen status. False positives and false negatives are common.

Thyroid and Prolactin Disorders	**Consideration should be given to thyroid disorders and hyperprolactinemia in women with amenorrhea because of the relatively common incidence of these conditions.**

1. **Sensitive TSH assays can be used to evaluate hypothyroidism and hyperthyroidism.** Further evaluation of a thyroid disorder is required if abnormalities in TSH levels are found. Mild degrees of thyroid dysfunction are unlikely to cause amenorrhea. Given the general health implications of thyroid dysfunction and readily available treatments, routine assessment of TSH is reasonable for women with amenorrhea.
2. **Prolactin is most accurately obtained in a patient who is fasting and who has not had any recent breast stimulation to avoid concluding that a patient is hyperprolactinemic on the basis of a transient prolactin elevation.** If a patient still has some menstrual cycles, it is advisable to obtain the prolactin level in the follicular phase.

Follicle-Stimulating Hormone Levels	Assessment of serum FSH levels is required to determine whether the patient has hypergonadotropic, hypogonadotropic, or eugonadotropic amenorrhea. **A circulating FSH level of greater than 25 to 40 mIU/mL indicated on at least two blood samples is indicative of hypergonadotropic amenorrhea.** Hypergonadotropism implies that the cause of amenorrhea is ovarian insufficiency. The history should establish whether the cause of ovarian insufficiency is chemotherapy or radiation therapy.

One test that is likely to be performed increasingly frequently is serum AMH. AMH is a product of the granulosa cells. **AMH levels are low in women with POI and high in women with PCOS.** AMH may be used more commonly in the evaluation of amenorrhea, but its assessment is not yet part of routine evaluation.

If the diagnosis of POI is confirmed, the patient should be tested for:

1. *FMR1* **premutation**
2. **Karyotype**
3. **21-hydroxylase antibody.**

FMR1 premutation testing will reveal women at risk for bearing a child with fragile X syndrome, which may be important information for other family members. The goal of the peripheral blood karyotype is to identify an absent or abnormal X chromosome and to identify whether or not any portion of a Y chromosome is present. *In situ* hybridization studies may prove the existence of Y chromosomal material with a Y-specific probe when the karyotype is normal and should be assessed if there are clinical signs to suggest that a Y-bearing cell line is present despite normal routine peripheral blood karyotype (125). It is important to identify Y chromosomal material so it may be removed to prevent malignant degeneration. Although commonly suggested that karyotype only be performed if the patient is under age 30, it should be noted that rare patients with Turner syndrome developed amenorrhea after age 35. In addition, some patients who present over the age of 30 may have actually had the onset of POI at a younger age but were unaware because of the use of oral contraceptives. Therefore, consideration should be given to performance of karyotype, regardless of the patient's age. Testing for 21-hydroxylase antibody will identify women at risk for adrenal crisis.

If a diagnosis of PCOS is suspected, the patient should have:

1. Documentation of hyperandrogenism (either by serum total testosterone and sex hormone binding globulin or free testosterone and/or by presence of physical findings such as acne, hirsutism, and androgenic alopecia),

2. Serum 17-hydroxyprogesterone to exclude congenital adrenal hyperplasia resulting from 21-hydroxylase deficiency, particularly if the patient is at increased risk (highest prevalence is among Ashkenazi Jews, Hispanics, Yugoslavs, Native American Inuits in Alaska, and Italians) (79),

3. If the diagnosis of PCOS is made, the patient should undergo a 2-hour oral glucose tolerance test and a fasting lipid profile.

Assessment of the Pituitary and Hypothalamus

If the patient is hypoestrogenic and the FSH level is not high, pituitary and hypothalamic lesions should be excluded.

1. **A complete neurologic examination** may help localize a lesion.

2. **Either CT or MRI scanning should be performed** to confirm the presence or absence of a tumor. MRI will identify smaller lesions than CT; if a lesion is too small for identification by CT, it may be clinically insignificant. MRI offers the advantage of avoiding exposure to x-ray.

3. **The patient's history** of weight changes, exercise, eating habits, and body image is an important factor in determining whether anorexia nervosa, malnutrition, obesity, exercise, or stress may be responsible for amenorrhea.

Patients with certain specific clinical findings should undergo screening for other hormonal alterations:

1. **Androgen levels should be assessed** in any hirsute patient to ensure that adrenal and ovarian tumors are not present and to aid in the diagnosis of PCOS.

2. **Acromegaly** is suggested by coarse facial features, large doughy hands, and hyperhidrosis and **may be confirmed by measuring IGF-1 levels.**

3. In patients with truncal obesity, hirsutism, hypertension, and erythematous striae, **Cushing syndrome should be ruled out** by assessing 24-hour urinary cortisol levels or performing a 1-mg overnight *dexamethasone* suppression test or late night salivary cortisol (126). It is important to confirm that the patient is not taking exogenous glucocorticoid.

Treatment for Women with Amenorrhea in the Presence of Normal Pelvic Anatomy and Normal Secondary Sexual Characteristics

The treatment of nonanatomic causes of amenorrhea associated with normal secondary sexual characteristics varies widely according to the cause. The underlying disorder should be treated whenever possible. Patients who are pregnant may be counseled regarding the options for continued care. When thyroid abnormalities are detected, thyroid hormone, radioactive iodine, or antithyroid drugs may be administered as appropriate. When hyperprolactinemia is present, treatment may include discontinuation of contributing medications, treatment with dopamine agonists such as *bromocriptine* or *cabergoline,* and, rarely, surgery for particularly large pituitary tumors. When POI causes amenorrhea, hormone replacement may be considered to diminish symptoms and to prevent osteoporosis. Counseling regarding the risks and benefits of hormone replacement therapy is indicated. Gonadectomy is required when a Y cell line is present.

Surgical removal, radiation therapy, or a combination of both is advocated for treatment of CNS tumors other than prolactinomas. It may be necessary to treat individuals who have panhypopituitarism with various replacement regimens after all the deficits are elucidated. These regimens include estrogen and progestogen replacement for lack of gonadotropins, corticosteroid replacement for lack of ACTH, thyroid hormone for lack of TSH, and *desmopressin acetate* (*1-deamino-8-D-AVP* [*DDAVP*]) to replace vasopressin.

The treatment of amenorrhea associated with hypothalamic dysfunction depends on the underlying cause:

1. Hormonally active ovarian tumors are surgically removed (rare).

2. Obesity, malnutrition or chronic disease, Cushing syndrome, and acromegaly should be specifically treated.

3. Stress-induced amenorrhea may respond to psychotherapy.

4. Exercise-induced amenorrhea may improve with moderation of activity and weight gain, when appropriate. If hypoestrogenism persists, higher doses of estrogen may be needed in these women than in older menopausal women to maintain bone density. In addition, 1,200 to 1,500 mg of calcium and 400 to 800 IU of vitamin D daily are advised. Bisphosphonates do not improve bone density in amenorrheic athletes because it is lack of bone formation rather than increased resorption that causes the osteopenia. In addition, the use of bisphosphonates is not advised because they can be deposited into the bone, and long-term effects, especially during pregnancy, are unknown.

5. Treatment of eating disorders such as anorexia nervosa generally demands a multidisciplinary approach, with severe cases requiring hospitalization (127).

Chronic anovulation associated with PCOS may be treated after identifying the desires of the patient. Patients may be concerned about their lack of menstruation, not hirsutism, or infertility. The endometrium of these individuals should be protected from the environment of unopposed estrogen that accompanies the anovulatory state. Oral contraceptives are a good alternative for those patients who require contraception. For those patients who are not candidates for oral contraceptive use, cyclic administration of progestogen is advised. Progestogen withdrawal will occur if there is an adequate estrogenic environment to induce proliferation of the endometrium, and it is not sufficient to cause withdrawal bleeding in patients who are hypoestrogenic (e.g., those who have amenorrhea associated with anorexia nervosa). Women with PCOS may require treatment for insulin resistance, dyslipidemia, and obesity. Regular periodic screening with an oral glucose load test and lipid panel is recommended for women with PCOS. Reduction in weight in obese women with PCOS leads to improved pregnancy rates, decreases hirsutism, and improves glucose and lipid levels (79). Insulin-sensitizing medications such as *metformin* and cholesterol-lowering medications such as statins can be considered. Ovulation induction is performed if pregnancy is desired, as described below.

A common progestogen used to induce withdrawal bleeding and thus protect the endometrium from hyperplastic transformation is *medroxyprogesterone acetate* (10 mg for 12 to 14 days per month). Occasionally, ovulation may occur; therefore, patients should be made aware that pregnancy is possible, and appropriate contraceptive measures should be used. Because there is theoretical concern that *medroxyprogesterone acetate* used in early pregnancy may increase the incidence of pseudohermaphroditism, a pregnancy test should be obtained if a woman fails to have a withdrawal bleed (128). Alternatively, *progesterone* suppositories (50 to 100 mg) or oral *micronized progesterone* (200 mg) can be given for 12 to 14 days per month to protect the endometrium from hyperplasia and induce withdrawal bleeding. No increased incidence of birth defects is associated with the use of natural progesterone (129).

In hypoestrogenic individuals such as those with POI, estrogen replacement must be added to the progestogen for successful menstrual regulation and prevention of osteoporosis. The doses of estrogen needed for relief of symptoms in young women with POI are often higher than those that are used for older menopausal women (130). Women with POI (who would normally still be making hormone if the ovaries were functioning normally) are different from those reaching menopause at a median age of 51. Therefore, data regarding hormone therapy that were collected from women reaching menopause at the median age should not be extrapolated to younger women. Although there are no comparative data and no long-term prospectively collected data regarding hormone therapy for women with POI, the risks of hormone therapy are likely to be lower and the benefits potentially greater for younger women than for older women reaching menopause after the age of 50 (131).

When chronic anovulation is caused by congenital adrenal hyperplasia, glucocorticoid administration (i.e., *dexamethasone* 0.5 mg at bedtime) is sometimes successful in restoring the normal feedback mechanisms, thereby permitting regular menstruation and ovulation.

Hirsutism

Patients who have oligomenorrhea or amenorrhea resulting from chronic anovulation may have hirsutism. The most common cause of hirsutism and oligo-ovulation is PCOS. After ruling out androgen-secreting tumors and congenital adrenal hyperplasia, treatment may be aimed at decreasing coarse hair growth.

Oral Contraceptives   Oral contraceptives may be effective for hirsutism by decreasing ovarian androgen production and increasing circulating levels of sex hormone–binding globulin, leading to decreased free androgen in the circulation.

Antiandrogens   *Spironolactone* decreases androgen production and competes with androgens at the androgen receptor. Side effects include diuresis and dysfunctional uterine bleeding. The use of spironolactone is typically combined with oral contraceptives to avoid irregular bleeding and to prevent pregnancy from occurring while on *spironolactone*. *Flutamide* is approved by the U.S. Food and Drug Administration (FDA) for adjuvant therapy in prostatic cancer and for treatment of hirsutism. Its effects are similar to those of *spironolactone* (132). Liver function should be monitored because of the rare complication of hepatotoxicity. *Cyproterone acetate,* a strong progestin and antiandrogen, is used abroad but is not available in the United States. It is usually administered in combination with *ethinyl estradiol* in an oral contraceptive. By decreasing circulating androgen and LH levels, and by inducing antagonism of androgen effects at the peripheral level, *cyproterone acetate* is effective in treating hirsutism (133). *Finasteride,* a 5α-reductase inhibitor, is approved by the FDA for the treatment of benign prostatic hypertrophy (*Proscar*) and male pattern baldness (*Propecia*). It is effective in treating hirsutism, although perhaps is no more effective than other available agents (134,135). Its major advantage is that it is exceptionally well tolerated and may be used when side effects preclude the use of other therapeutic options for hirsutism.

All antiandrogens are teratogenic as they may lead to feminization of the external genitalia of a male fetus (ambiguous genitalia) if the patient should conceive while taking the medication. Therefore, antiandrogens are typically used in combination with oral contraceptives.

GnRH Agonist   Administration of GnRH agonist agents virtually eliminates ovarian steroid production, and estrogen-progestogen add-back therapy allows long-term administration and protection against osteoporosis.

Eflornithine Hydrochloride   *Eflornithine hydrochloride* is a topical cream that is approved by the FDA for use on the face and chin. Improvements in facial hirsutism may be seen in 4 to 8 weeks of twice-daily applications.

Ovulation Induction

A large subset of patients with amenorrhea or oligomenorrhea and chronic anovulation seek care because they are unable to conceive (see Chapter 32). Ovulation induction therapy is generally the treatment of choice for such patients, but pretreatment counseling should be provided in sufficient detail to ensure realistic expectations. The patient should be provided with information regarding the chances of a successful pregnancy (considering age of the patient and treatment modality), potential complications (hyperstimulation and multiple gestation), expense, time, and psychological impact involved in completing the course of therapy. Treatment should be individualized (136).

Earlier studies raised the possibility of a relationship between ovulation induction and the risk of ovarian cancer (137,138). Ongoing studies are attempting to address this issue conclusively, but **data support an increase of approximately 2.5-fold in ovarian cancer in patients with infertility, which appears unrelated to the use of ovulation-inducing drugs (139140). There is no conclusive evidence to link fertility drug use and ovarian cancer;** thus, no change in current ovulation induction practices seems warranted at present (141). **Pregnancy and use of oral contraceptives before or after childbearing may protect against ovarian cancer.**

Clomiphene citrate **is the usual first choice for ovulation induction in most patients because of its relative safety, efficacy, route of administration (oral), and relatively low cost** (142). *Clomiphene citrate* is indicated primarily in patients with adequate levels of estrogen and normal levels of FSH and prolactin. It is generally ineffective in hypogonadotropic patients who already have a poor estrogen supply (143). Patients with inappropriate gonadotropin release (an increased LH-to-FSH ratio), such as that which occurs in PCOS, are candidates for therapy with *clomiphene citrate.* **As many as 80% of certain patients can be expected to ovulate after** clomiphene citrate **therapy.** Contraindications to the use of *clomiphene citrate* include pregnancy, liver disease, and preexisting ovarian cysts. Side effects include hot flashes and poorly understood visual symptoms, which generally were viewed as an indication to discontinue subsequent *clomiphene citrate* use. The risk of multiple pregnancy is increased with *clomiphene citrate* compared with an overall of risk of approximately 8% (142). The majority of multiple gestations are twins; triplets and higher order multiple gestations are rare.

The most commonly recommended treatment regimen for *clomiphene citrate* is 50 mg daily for 5 days, beginning on the third to fifth day of menstrual or withdrawal bleeding. Cycles may be monitored by measuring midluteal progesterone levels to assess ovulation. Ovulation may be confirmed by an appropriate rise of basal body temperature and menses occurring at the expected time after the temperature rise. Ultrasonographic monitoring to assess folliculogenesis may be helpful, especially when *hCG* is used to induce ovulation. Endometrial thinning caused by the antiestrogenic effects of *clomiphene citrate* may be detected with midcycle ultrasound. With these data, it is possible to immediately adjust the dose in the subsequent cycle if a given regimen is ineffective. Dosage increases of 50 mg per day are usually used, and more than 70% of conceptions occur at doses no higher than 100 mg per day for 5 days (144). Dosages higher than 150 mg per day for 5 days are usually ineffective, and patients who remain anovulatory with this dosage should undergo further evaluation accompanied by changes in the therapeutic plan. Longer courses of *clomiphene citrate* therapy, and adjunctive therapy with glucocorticoids, are suggested if a patient does not ovulate with standard therapy (145).

Although a large randomized trial demonstrated that *clomiphene* alone is superior to *metformin* alone in achieving live birth in women with PCOS, a meta-analysis suggests that for some patients with PCOS, *metformin* and *clomiphene* combined may increase the likelihood of ovulation compared with *clomiphene* alone (146,147). Thinning of the endometrium at midcycle in the face of adequate midcycle estradiol and lack of success with repeated cycles of *clomiphene* are generally indications to consider injectable gonadotropins. Aromatase inhibitors, such as *letrozole*, were suggested as an option for ovulation induction (148).

Women with PCOS who do not ovulate or become pregnant with *clomiphene citrate,* and women with hypogonadotropic hypoestrogenic anovulation, may be candidates for therapy with injectable gonadotropins. Available preparations include recombinant FSH and LH and products purified from the urine of menopausal women (FSH or FSH-LH combinations). Administration protocols and dosages vary widely and should be adjusted to individual needs. Safe administration requires careful monitoring of ovarian response with ultrasonography and, in some cases, serial estradiol measurements. In general, gonadotropins are administered at a dose of 50 to 150 IU per day by subcutaneous injection for 3 to 5 days, after which time estradiol and follicular monitoring commence. In most cycles, gonadotropin is administered for 7 to 12 days. Ovulation is triggered by subcutaneous or intramuscular injection of 5,000 to 10,000 IU *hCG* or subcutaneous injection of 250 μg of *recombinant hCG* once the lead follicle reaches 16 to 20 mm in diameter based on ultrasonographic assessments. Ovulation generally occurs approximately 38 to 40 hours after *hCG* administration. Luteal phase support is sometimes provided with the administration of *progesterone* supplementation or with additional injections of *hCG*.

The two major complications associated with induction of ovulation with gonadotropins are multiple pregnancy (10% to 30%) and ovarian hyperstimulation syndrome. The incidence of both of these complications can be reduced but not eliminated by careful monitoring. Cycles complicated by the recruitment of numerous follicles or by high estradiol levels may be canceled by withholding the ovulatory dose of *hCG*. Selected patients may be converted safely to *in vitro* fertilization. Because severe ovarian hyperstimulation syndrome is life-threatening and may lead to prolonged hospitalization, ovulation induction with gonadotropins generally is performed by experienced practitioners who devote a significant portion of their practice to the treatment of infertility.

Ovulation induction with pulsatile *GnRH* may be effective in patients who have chronic anovulation associated with low levels of estrogen and gonadotropins. For therapy to be successful, a functional ovary and pituitary gland must be present. Patients with ovarian or pituitary failure do not respond to *GnRH* therapy. To be effective, *GnRH* must be administered in a pulsatile fashion, either intravenously or subcutaneously by a programmable pump. Ovulation induction with *GnRH*, as compared with gonadotropins, is associated with a relatively low incidence of ovarian hyperstimulation and multiple births. In addition, the need for appropriate timing of the ovulatory dose of *hCG* is avoided because patients treated with pulsatile *GnRH* have an appropriately timed endogenous LH surge. Disadvantages are mainly related to maintaining the programmable pump and injection site and lack of availability of an appropriate pump in the United States. After ovulation, luteal phase support is necessary and may be provided with *hCG, progesterone,* or continuation of the *GnRH* therapy.

For women with overt POI (also known as premature ovarian failure, as noted above), there is no good evidence to suggest that any treatment can increase the chance of conception with autologous oocytes (85). Treatments that were tried include ovulation induction with *clomiphene* or *gonadotropin,* pretreatment with high-dose estrogen or gonadotropin-releasing hormone agonist followed by expectant management or gonadotropin stimulation, standard-dose hormone therapy followed by gonadotropin, and corticosteroid pretreatment followed by gonadotropin. Administration of *dehydroepiandrosterone (DHEA)* is suggested for women with POI (149). It is uncertain whether the benefit seen in preliminary reports will stand the test of time.

If POI is diagnosed while a patient still has a significant supply of oocytes, fertility preservation could be considered if the patient is not able to consider conception at the time of diagnosis. In most cases, patients with prolonged amenorrhea are not diagnosed at a time when significant numbers of reproductively competent oocytes are present. Fertility preservation is an option for patients about to undergo gonadotoxic chemotherapy or if a patient is known (e.g., based on family history) to be at risk for POI. Either embryos or oocytes can be cryopreserved. There is more worldwide experience with cryopreservation of embryos. Improvements are occurring in techniques of oocyte and ovarian tissue cryopreservation (150,151).

Patients with POI who desire pregnancy will in most cases have a high chance of having a child with the help of oocyte donation. Oocytes from donors may be harvested after ovulation induction, fertilized with sperm from the intended father, and transferred into the recipient's uterus after the endometrium is appropriately prepared with estrogen and progesterone. Special concern is warranted for women with Turner syndrome who appear to have a maternal mortality of at least 2% (58). Rupture of the aorta may occur even if an echocardiogram shows no dilatation (152). It is suggested that all women with Turner syndrome undergo a full cardiac evaluation, including a cardiac MRI at a center with expertise in cardiovascular imaging, and that pregnancy be contraindicated if the patient has known congenital cardiovascular disease (e.g., bicuspid aortic valve or aortic coarctation) or with aortic size greater than 2 cm/m^2 (153).

References

1. **Hoffman B, Bradshaw K.** Delayed puberty and amenorrhea. *Semin Reprod Med* 2003;4:353–362.
2. **The Practice Committee of the American Society for Reproductive Medicine.** Current evaluation of amenorrhea. *Fertil Steril* 2008;90:S219–S225.
3. **Rosen GF, Kaplan B, Lobo RA.** Menstrual function and hirsutism in patients with gonadal dysgenesis. *Obstet Gynecol* 1988;17:677–680.
4. **Turner HH.** A syndrome of infantilism, congenital webbed neck, and cubitus-valgus. *Endocrinology* 1938;23:566–574.
5. **Leppig KA, Disteche CM.** Ring X and other structural X chromosome abnormalities: X inactivation and phenotype. *Semin Reprod Med* 2001;19:147–157.
6. **Bondy CA, Turner Syndrome Study Group.** Care of girls and women with Turner syndrome: a guideline of the Turner Syndrome Study Group. *J Clin Endocrinol Metab* 2007;92:10–25.
7. **Therman E, Susman B.** The similarity of phenotypic effects caused by Xp and Xq deletion in the human female: a hypothesis. *Hum Genet* 1990;85:175–183.
8. **Zinn AR, Tonk VS, Chen Z, et al.** Evidence for a Turner syndrome locus or loci at Xp11.2-p22.1. *Am J Hum Genet* 1998;63:1757–1766.
9. **Schmidt M, Du Sart D.** Functional disomies of the X chromosome influence the cell selection and hence the X inactivation pattern in females with balanced X–autosome translocations: a review of 122 cases. *Am J Med Genet* 1992;42:161–169.
10. **Ferguson-Smith MA.** Karyotype-phenotype correlations in gonadal dysgenesis and their bearing on the pathogenesis of malformations. *J Med Genet* 1965;2:142–155.
11. **Hawkins JR.** Mutational analysis of SRY in XY females. *Hum Mutat* 1993;2:347–350.
12. **Timmreck L, Reindollar R.** Contemporary issues in primary amenorrhea. *Obstet Gynecol Clin North Am* 2003;30:287–302.
13. **Jorgensen PB, Kjartansdóttir KR, Fedder J.** Care of women with XY karyotype: a clinical practice guideline. *Fertil Steril* 2010;94:105–115.
14. **Foster JW, Dominguez-Steglich MA, Guioli S, et al.** Campomelic dysplasia and autosomal sex reversal caused by mutations in an SRY-related gene. *Nature* 1994;372:525–530.
15. **Wagner T, Wirth J, Meyer J, et al.** Autosomal sex reversal and campomelic dysplasia are caused by mutations in and around the SRY-related gene SOX9. *Cell* 1994;79:1111–1120.
16. **Zanaria E, Bardoni B, Dabovic B, et al.** Xp duplications and sex reversal. *Philos Trans R Soc Lond B Biol Sci* 1995;350:291–296.
17. **Cotinot C, Pailhoux E, Jaubert F, et al.** Molecular genetics of sex determination. *Semin Reprod Med* 2002;20:157–167.
18. **Barbaux S, Niaudet P, Gubler MC, et al.** Donor splice-site mutations in WTI are responsible for Frasier syndrome. *Nat Genet* 1997;17:467–470.
19. **MacLaughlin DT, Donahoe PK.** Mechanisms of disease: sex determination and differentiation. *N Engl J Med* 2004;350:367–378.
20. **Achermann JC, Ito M, Hindmarsh PC, et al.** A mutation in the gene encoding steroidogenic factor-1 causes XY sex reversal and adrenal failure in humans. *Nat Genet* 1999;22:125–126.
21. **Warne GL, Kanumakala S.** Molecular endocrinology of sex differentiation. *Semin Reprod Med* 2002;20:169–179.

22. **Damiani D, Guedes DR, Fellous M, et al.** Ullrich-Turner syndrome: relevance of searching for Y chromosome fragments. *J Pediatr Endocrinol* 1999;12:827–831.

23. **Osipova GR, Karmanov ME, Kozlova SI, et al.** PCR detection of Y-specific sequences in patients with Ullrich-Turner syndrome: clinical implications and limitations. *Am J Med Genet* 1998;76:283–287.

24. **Bose HS, Sugawara T, Strauss J, et al.** The pathophysiology and genetics of congenital lipoid adrenal hyperplasia. *N Engl J Med* 1996;335:1870–1878.

25. **Touraine P, Beau I, Gougeon A, et al.** New natural inactivation mutations of the follicle-stimulating hormone receptor: correlations between receptor function and phenotype. *Mol Endocrinol* 1999;13:1844–1854.

26. **Adashi EY, Hennebold JD.** Mechanisms of disease: single gene mutations resulting in reproductive dysfunction in women. *N Engl J Med* 1999;340:709–718.

27. **Goldsmith O, Soloman DH, Horton R.** Hypogonadism and mineralocorticoid excess: the 17-hydroxylase deficiency syndrome. *N Engl J Med* 1967;277:673–677.

28. **Zirilli L, Rochira V, Diazzi C, et al.** Human models of aromatase deficiency. *J Steroid Biochem Molecular Biol* 2008;109:212–218.

29. **Bulun SE.** Clinical review 78: aromatase deficiency in women and men: would you have predicted the phenotypes? *J Clin Endocrinol Metab* 1996;81:867–871.

30. **Mullis PE, Yoshimura N, Kuhlmann B, et al.** Aromatase deficiency in a female who is compound heterozygote for two new point mutations in the P450arom gene: impact of estrogens on hypergonadotropic hypogonadism, multicystic ovaries and bone densitometry in childhood. *J Clin Endocrinol Metab* 1997;82:1739–1745.

31. **Latronico AC, Anasti M, Arnhold I, et al.** Testicular and ovarian resistance to luteinizing hormone caused by inactivating mutations of the luteinizing hormone-receptor gene. *N Engl J Med* 1996;334:507–512.

32. **Latronico AC.** Naturally occurring mutations of the luteinizing hormone receptor gene affecting reproduction. *Semin Reprod Med* 2000;18:17–20.

33. **Tapanainen JS, Vaskivup T, Aittomaki K, et al.** Inactivating FSH receptor mutations and gonadal dysfunction. *Mol Cell Endocrinol* 1998;145:129–135.

34. **Barrett A, Nicholls J, Gibson B.** Late effects of total body irradiation. *Radiother Oncol* 1987;9:131–135.

35. **Ahmed SR, Shalet SM, Campbell RH, et al.** Primary gonadal damage following treatment of brain tumors in childhood. *J Pediatr* 1983;103:562–565.

36. **Fechner A, Fong S, McGovern P.** A review of Kallmann syndrome: genetics pathophysiology, and clinical management. *Obstet Gynecol Sur* 2008;63:189–194.

37. **Banna M.** Craniopharyngioma: based on 160 cases. *Br J Radiol* 1976;49:206–223.

38. **Thomsett JJ, Conte FA, Kaplan SL, et al.** Endocrine and neurologic outcome in childhood craniopharyngioma: review of effective treatment in 42 patients. *J Pediatr* 1980;97:728–735.

39. **Peterson RE, Imperato-McGinley J, Gautier T, et al.** Male pseudohermaphroditism due to steroid 5α reductase deficiency. *Am J Med* 1977;62:170–191.

40. **Cohen DP.** Molecular evaluation of the gonadotropin-releasing hormone receptor. *Semin Reprod Med* 2000;18:11–16.

41. **Beranova M, Oliveira LM, Bedecarrats GY, et al.** Prevalence, phenotypic spectrum and modes of inheritance of gonadotropin-releasing hormone receptor mutations in idiopathic hypogonadotropic hypogonadism. *J Clin Endocrinol Metab* 2001;86:1580–1588.

42. **Layman LC, Lee EJ, Peak DB, et al.** Brief report: delayed puberty and hypogonadism caused by mutations in the follicle-stimulating hormone (beta)-subunit gene. *N Engl J Med* 1997;337:607–611.

43. **Matthews CH, Borgato S, Beck-Peccoz P.** Primary amenorrhea and infertility due to a mutation in the beta-subunit of follicle-stimulating hormone. *Nat Genet* 1993;5:83–86.

44. **Kulin HE, Bwibo N, Mutie D, et al.** Gonadotropin excretion during puberty in malnourished children. *J Pediatr* 1984;105:325–328.

45. **Cumming DC, Rebar RW.** Exercise in reproductive function in women. *Am J Intern Med* 1983;4:113–125.

46. **Ferraris J, Saenger P, Levine L, et al.** Delayed puberty in males with chronic renal failure. *Kidney Int* 1980;18:344–350.

47. **Siris ES, Leventhal BG, Vaitukaitis JL.** Effects of childhood leukemia and chemotherapy on puberty and reproductive function in girls. *N Engl J Med* 1976;294:1143–1146.

48. **Copeland KC, Underwood LE, Van Wyk JJ.** Marijuana smoking and pubertal arrest. *Pediatrics* 1980;96:1079–1080.

49. **Patton ML, Woolf PD.** Hyperprolactinemia and delayed puberty: a report of three cases and their response to therapy. *Pediatrics* 1983;71:572–575.

50. **Asherson RA, Jackson WPU, Lewis B.** Abnormalities of development associated with hypothalamic calcification after tuberculous meningitis. *BMJ* 1965;2:839–843.

51. **Alper MM, Garner PR, Seibel MM.** Premature ovarian failure. *J Reprod Med* 1986;8:699–708.

52. **Davajan V, Kletzky OA.** Primary amenorrhea: phenotypic female external genitalia. In: **Mishell DR, Davajan V, Lobo RA,** eds. Infertility contraception and reproductive endocrinology. 3rd ed. Cambridge, MA: Blackwell Scientific Publications, 1991:356–371.

53. **Lichter AS, Wara WM, Sheline GE, et al.** The treatment of craniopharyngiomas. *Int J Radiat Oncol* 1977;2:675–683.

54. **Wara WM, Fellows FC, Sheline GE, et al.** Radiation therapy for pineal tumors and suprasellar germinomas. *Radiology* 1977;124:221–223.

55. **Koenig MP, Suppinger K, Leichti B.** Hyperprolactinemia as a cause of delayed puberty: successful treatment with bromocriptine. *J Clin Endocrinol Metab* 1977;45:825–828.

56. **Golden NH.** Eating disorders in adolescence: what is the role of hormone replacement therapy? *Curr Opinion Obstet Gynecol* 2007;19:434–439.

57. **Rosen GF, Vermesh M, d'Ablain GG, et al.** The endocrinologic evaluation of a 45X true hermaphrodite. *Am J Obstet Gynecol* 1987;157:1272–1273.

58. **Karnis MF, Zimon AE, Lalwani SI, et al.** The risk of death in pregnancy achieved through oocyte donation in patients with Turner syndrome: a national survey. *Fertil Steril* 2003;80:498–501.

59. **Buttram VC Jr, Gibbons WE.** Müllerian anomalies: a proposed classification. *Fertil Steril* 1979;32:40–46.

60. **Laufer MR.** Congenital absence of the vagina: in search of the perfect solution. When, and by what technique, should a vagina be created? *Curr Opin Obstet Gynecol* 2002;14:441–444.

61. **Fore SR, Hammond CB, Parker RT, et al.** Urology and genital anomalies in patients with congenital absence of the vagina. *Obstet Gynecol* 1975;46:410–416.

62. **Gell JS.** Müllerian anomalies. *Semin Reprod Med* 2003;21:375–388.

63. **Griffin JE, Edwards C, Madden JD, et al.** Congenital absence of the vagina. *Ann Intern Med* 1976;85:224–236.

64. **Cramer DW, Goldstein DP, Fraer C, et al.** Vaginal agenesis (Mayer-Rokitansky-Kuster-Hauser syndrome) associated with the N314D mutation of galactose-1-phosphate uridyl transferase (GALT). *Mol Hum Reprod* 1996;2:145–148.

65. **Klein SM, Garcia CR.** Asherman's syndrome: a critique and current review. *Fertil Steril* 1973;24:722–735.

66. **Suttan C, Lumbroso S, Paris F, et al.** Disorders of androgen action. *Semin Reprod Med* 2002;20:217–224.

67. **McPhaul MJ.** Androgen receptor mutations and androgen insensitivity. *Mol Cell Endocrinol* 2002;198:61–67.

68. **Amrhein JA, Meyer WJ III, Jones HW Jr, et al.** Androgen insensitivity in man: evidence of genetic heterogeneity. *Proc Natl Acad Sci U S A* 1976;73:891–894.

69. **Rock JA.** Anomalous development of the vagina. *Semin Reprod Endocrinol* 1986;4:1–28.

70. **Frank RT.** The formation of an artificial vagina. *Am J Obstet Gynecol* 1938;35:1053–1055.

71. **Rock JA, Zacur HA, Diugi AM, et al.** Pregnancy success following surgical correction of imperforate hymen and complete transverse vaginal septum. *Obstet Gynecol* 1982;59:448–451.

72. **Williams EA.** Uterovaginal agenesis. *Ann R Coll Surg Engl* 1976;58:266–277.

73. **Ingram JN.** The bicycle seat stool in the treatment of vaginal agenesis and stenosis: a preliminary report. *Am J Obstet Gynecol* 1982;140:867–873.

74. **McIndoe A.** The treatment of congenital absence and obliterative condition of the vagina. *Br J Plast Surg* 1950;2:254–267.

75. **Rock JA, Breech LL.** Surgery for anomalies of the Müllerian ducts. In: Rock JA, Jones HW, eds. TeLinde's operative gynecology. 10th ed. Philadelphia, PA: JB Lippincott, Williams & Wilkins, 2008.

76. **Conte FA, Grumbach MM.** Pathogenesis, classification, diagnosis, and treatment of anomalies of sex. In: **De Groot LJ,** ed. **Endocrinology.** Philadelphia, PA: WB Saunders, 1989:1810–1847.

77. **Manuel M, Katayama KP, Jones HW Jr.** The age of occurrence of gonadal tumors in intersex patients with a Y chromosome. *Am J Obstet Gynecol* 1976;124:293–300.

78. **Doody KM, Carr BR.** Amenorrhea. *Obstet Gynecol Clin North Am* 1990;17:361–387.

79. **ACOG Committee on Practice Bulletins—Gynecology.** ACOG Practice Bulletin No. 108: polycystic ovary syndrome. *Obstet Gynecol* 2009;114:936–949.

80. **The Rotterdam ESHRE/ASRM-Sponsored PCOS Consensus Workshop Group.** Revised 2003 consensus on diagnostic criteria and long-term health risks related to polycystic ovary syndrome. *Fertil Steril* 2004;81:19–23.

81. **Klibanski A.** Clinical practice. Prolactinomas. *N Engl J Med* 2010;362:1219–1226.

82. **Nelson LM.** Clinical practice. Primary ovarian insufficiency. *N Engl J Med* 2009;360:606–614.

83. **Welt CK.** Primary ovarian insufficiency: a more accurate term for premature ovarian failure. *Clin Endocrinol* 2008;68:499–509.

84. **Rebar RW, Connolly HV.** Clinical features of young women with hypergonadotropic amenorrhea. *Fertil Steril* 1990;53:804–810.

85. **van Kasteren YM, Schoemaker J.** Premature ovarian failure: a systematic review on therapeutic interventions to restore ovarian function and achieve pregnancy. *Hum Reprod Update* 1999;5:483–492.

86. **Singh RP, Carr DH.** The anatomy and histology of XO human embryos and fetuses. *Anat Rec* 1966;155:369–383.

87. **Tartaglia N, Howell S, Sutherland A, et al.** A review of trisomy X (47,XXX). *Orphanet J Rare Dis* 2010;5:8.

88. **Krauss CM, Tarskoy RN, Atkins L, et al.** Familial premature ovarian failure due to interstitial deletion of the long arm of the X chromosome. *N Engl J Med* 1987;317:125–131.

89. **Bione S, Sala C, Manzini C, et al.** A human homologue of the *Drosophila melanogaster* diaphanous gene is disrupted in a patient with premature ovarian failure: evidence for conserved function in oogenesis and implications for human sterility. *Am J Hum Genet* 1998;62:533–541.

90. **Pruiett RL, Ross JL, Zinn AR.** Physical mapping of nine Xq translocation breakpoints and identification of XPNPEP2 as a premature ovarian failure candidate gene. *Cytogenet Cell Genet* 2000;89:44–50.

91. **DiPasquale E, Beck-Peccoz P, Persani L.** Hypergonadotropic ovarian failure associated with an inherited mutation of hormone loss morphogenetic protein-15(BMP15) gene. *Am J Hum Genet* 2004;75:106–111.

92. **Nishi Y, Hamamoto K, Kafiyama M, et al.** The Perrault syndrome: clinical report and review. *Am J Med Genet* 1988;31:623–629.

93. **Crisponi L, Deiana M, Loi A, et al.** The putative forkhead transcription factor FOXL2 is mutated in blepharophimosis/ptosis/epicanthus inversus syndrome. *Nat Genet* 2001;27:159–166.

94. **Mattison DR, Evan MI, Schwimmer WB.** Familial premature ovarian failure. *Am J Hum Genet* 1984;36:1341–1348.

95. **Simpson JL.** Genetic and phenotypic heterogeneity in ovarian failure: overview of selected candidate genes. *Ann N Y Acad Sci* 2008;1135:146–154.

96. **Skillern A, Rajkovic A.** Recent developments in identifying genetic determinants of premature ovarian failure. *Sex Dev* 2008;2:228–243.

97. **Wittenberger MD, Hagerman RJ, Sherman SL, et al.** The FMR1 premutation and reproduction. *Fertil Steril* 2007;87:456–465.

98. **Stillman RJ, Schinfeld JS, Schiff I, et al.** Ovarian failure in long term survivors of childhood malignancy. *Am J Obstet Gynecol* 1981;139:62–66.

99. **Larsen EC, Muller J, Schmiegelow K, et al.** Reduced ovarian function in long-term survivors of radiation- and chemotherapy-treated childhood cancer. *J Clin Endocrinol Metab* 2003;88:5307–5314.

100. **Whitehead E, Shalet SM, Blackledge G, et al.** The effect of combination chemotherapy on ovarian function in women treated for Hodgkin's disease. *Cancer* 1983;52:988–993.

101. **Waxman JH, Ahmed R, Smith D, et al.** Failure to preserve fertility in patients with Hodgkin's disease. *Cancer Chemother Pharmacol* 1987;19:159–162.

102. **Morrison JC, Givens JR, Wiser WL, et al.** Mumps oophoritis: a cause of premature ovarian failure. *Fertil Steril* 1975;26:655–659.

103. **Santoro N, Fan M, Maslow B, Schoenbaum E.** Women and HIV infection: the makings of a midlife crisis. *Maturitas* 2009;64:160–164.

104. **Williams DJ, Connor P, Ironside JW.** Premenopausal cytomegalovirus oophoritis. *Histopathology* 1990;16:405–407.

105. **Bakalov VK, Anasti JN, Calis KA, et al.** Autoimmune oophoritis as a mechanism of follicular dysfunction in women with 46,XX spontaneous premature ovarian failure. *Fertil Steril* 2005;84:958–965.

106. **Welt CK.** Autoimmune oophoritis in the adolescent. *Ann N Y Acad Sci* 2008;1135:118–122.

107. **Mignot MH, Shoemaker J, Kleingel M, et al.** Premature ovarian failure. I: the association with autoimmunity. *Eur J Obstet Gynecol Reprod Biol* 1989;30:59–66.

108. **Jones GS, de Moraes-Ruehsen M.** A new syndrome of amenorrhea in association with hypergonadotropism and apparently normal ovarian follicular apparatus. *Am J Obstet Gynecol* 1969;104:597–600.

109. **Kim MH.** "Gonadotropin-resistant ovaries" syndrome in association with secondary amenorrhea. *Am J Obstet Gynecol* 1974;120:257–263.

110. **de Moraes-Ruehsen M, Blizzard RM, Garcia-Bunuel R, et al.** Autoimmunity and ovarian failure. *Am J Obstet Gynecol* 1972;112:693–703.

111. **Kaufman FR, Kogut MD, Donnell GN, et al.** Hypergonadotropic hypogonadism in female patients with galactosemia. *N Engl J Med* 1981;304:994–998.

112. **Cramer DW, Harlow BL, Barbieri RL, et al.** Galactose-1-phosphate uridyl transferase activity associated with age at menopause and reproductive history. *Fertil Steril* 1989;51:609–615.

113. **Reindollar RH, Novak M, Tho SP.** Adult onset amenorrhea: a study of 262 patients. *Am J Obstet Gynecol* 1986;155:531–543.

114. **Perkins RB, Hall JE, Martin KA.** Aetiology, previous menstrual function and patterns of neuro-endocrine disturbance as prognostic indicators in hypothalamic amenorrhea. *Hum Reprod* 2001;16:2198–2205.

115. **Genazzani AR, Petragtia F, DeRamundo BM, et al.** Neuroendocrine correlates of stress-related amenorrhea. *Ann N Y Acad Sci* 1991;626:125–129.

116. **Warren MP, Voussoughian F, Geer EB, et al.** Functional hypothalamic amenorrhea: hypoleptinemia and disordered eating. *J Clin Endocrinol Metab* 1999;84:873–877.

117. **Welt CK, Chan JL, Bullen J, et al.** Recombinant human leptin in women with hypothalamic amenorrhea. *N Engl J Med* 2004;351:987–997.

118. **Herzog DB, Copeland PM.** Eating disorders. *N Engl J Med* 1985;313:295–303.

119. **Mehler PS.** Clinical practice: bulimia nervosa. *N Engl J Med* 2003;349:875–881.

120. **Gordon CM.** Functional hypothalmic amenorrhea. *N Engl J Med* 2010;363:365–371.

121. **Desouza MJ, Metzger DA.** Reproductive dysfunction in amenorrheic athletic and anorexic patients: a review. *Med Sci Sports Exerc* 1991;23:995–1007.

122. **Frisch RE, McArthur JW.** Menstrual cycles: fatness as a determinant of minimum weight for height necessary for their maintenance or onset. *Science* 1974;185:949–995.

123. **Laughlin GA, Yen SS.** Nutritional and endocrine-metabolic aberrations in amenorrheic athletes. *J Clin Endocrinol Metab* 1997;81:4301–4309.

124. **Highet R.** Athletic amenorrhea: an update on a etiology, complications and management. *Sports Med* 1989;7:82–108.

125. **Medlej R, Laboaccaro JM, Berta P, et al.** Screening for Y-derived sex determining gene SRY in 40 patients with Turner syndrome. *J Clin Endocrinol Metab* 1992;75:1289–1292.

126. **Newell-Price J.** Diagnosis/differential diagnosis of Cushing's syndrome: a review of best practice. *Best Pract Res Clin Endocrinol Metab* 2009;23:S5–S14.

127. **Andersen AE, Ryan GL.** Eating disorders in the obstetric and gynecologic patient population. *Obstet Gynecol* 2009;114:1353–1367.

128. **Schardein JL.** Congenital abnormalities and hormones during pregnancy: a clinical review. *Teratology* 1980;22:251–270.

129. **Resseguie LJ, Hick JF, Bruen JA, et al.** Congenital malformations among offspring exposed *in utero* to progestins, Olmsted County, Minnesota, 1936–1974. *Fertil Steril* 1985;43:514–519.

130. **Rebar RW.** Premature ovarian failure. *Obstet Gynecol* 2009; 113:1355–1363.

131. **North American Menopause Society.** Estrogen and progestogen use in postmenopausal women: 2010 position statement of the North American Menopause Society. *Menopause* 2010;17:242–255.

132. **Cusan L, Dupont A, Gomez JL, et al.** Comparison of *flutamide* and *spironolactone* in the treatment of hirsutism: a randomized controlled trial. *Fertil Steril* 1994;61:281–287.

133. **Belisle S, Love EJ.** Clinical efficacy and safety of *cyproterone acetate* in severe hirsutism: results of a multicentered Canadian study. *Fertil Steril* 1986;46:1015–1020.

134. **Rittmaster RS.** *Finasteride. N Engl J Med* 1994;330:120–125.

135. **Price TM.** *Finasteride* for hirsutism: there's new approach to treating hirsutism—but is it any better or even as effective as conventional therapy? *Contemp Obstet Gynecol* 1999;44:73–84.

136. **van Santbrink EJP, Eijkemans MJ, Laven JSE, et al.** Patient-tailored conventional ovulation induction algorithms in anovulatory infertility. *Trend Endocrinol Metabol* 2005;16:381–389.

137. **Whittemore AS, Harris R, Itnyre J, et al.** Characteristics relating to ovarian cancer risk: collaborative analysis of 12 US case-control studies. *Am J Epidemiol* 1992;136:1184–1203.

138. **Rossing MA, Daling JR, Weiss NL, et al.** Ovarian tumors in a cohort of infertile women. *N Engl J Med* 1994;331:771–776.

139. **Venn A, Watson L, Lumley J, et al.** Breast and ovarian cancer incidence after infertility and *in vitro* fertilization. *Lancet* 1995;346:995–1000.

140. **Mosgaard BJ, Lidegaard O, Kjaer SK, et al.** Infertility, fertility drugs, and invasive ovarian cancer: a case control study. *Fertil Steril* 1997;67:1005–1012.

141. **Brinton LA, Moghissi K, Scoccia B.** Ovulation induction and cancer risk. *Fertil Steril* 2005;83:261–274.

142. **Practice Committee of the American Society for Reproductive Medicine.** Use of *clomiphene citrate* in women. *Fertil Steril* 2006;86:S187–S193.

143. **McClamrock HD, Adashi EY.** Ovulation induction. I. Appropriate use of clomiphene citrate. *Female Patient* 1988;13:92–106.

144. **Rust LA, Israel R, Mishell DR Jr.** An individualized graduated therapeutic regimen for *clomiphene citrate. Am J Obstet Gynecol* 1974;120:785–790.

145. **Lobo RA, Granger LR, Davajan V, et al.** An extended regimen of *clomiphene citrate* in women unresponsive to standard therapy. *Fertil Steril* 1982;37:762–766.

146. **Legro RS, Barnhart HX, Schlaff WD, et al.** *Clomiphene, metformin,* or both for infertility in the polycystic ovary syndrome. *N Engl J Med* 2007;356:551–566.

147. **Creanga AA, Bradley HM, McCormick C, et al.** Use of *metformin* in polycystic ovary syndrome: a meta-analysis. *Obstet Gynecol* 2008;111:959–968.

148. **Polyzos NP, Tzioras S, Badawy AM, et al.** Aromatase inhibitors for female infertility: a systematic review of the literature. *Reprod Biomed Online* 2009;19:456–471.

149. **Mamas L, Mamas E.** Premature ovarian failure and dehydroepiandrosterone. *Curr Opin Obstet Gynecol* 2009;21:306–308.

150. **Noyes N, Porcu E, Borini A.** Over 900 oocyte cryopreservation babies born with no apparent increase in congenital anomalies. *Reprod Biomed Online* 2009;18:769–776.

151. **Oktay K, Oktem O.** Ovarian cryopreservation and transplantation for fertility preservation for medical indications: report of an ongoing experience. *Fertil Steril* 2010;93:762–768.

152. **Boissonnas CC, Davy C, Bornes M, et al.** Careful cardiovascular screening and follow-up of women with Turner syndrome before and during pregnancy is necessary to prevent maternal mortality. *Fertil Steril* 2009;91:929.e5–e7.

153. **Bondy C, Rosing D, Reindollar R.** Cardiovascular risks of pregnancy in women with Turner syndrome. *Fertil Steril* 2009;91: e31–e32.

31

Endocrine Disorders

Oumar Kuzbari
Jessie Dorais
C. Matthew Peterson

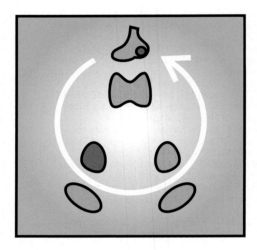

- Hyperandrogenism most often presents as hirsutism, which usually arises as a result of androgen excess related to abnormalities of function in the ovary or adrenal glands. By contrast, virilization is rare and indicates marked elevation in androgen levels.

- The most common cause of hyperandrogenism and hirsutism is polycystic ovarian syndrome (PCOS). There are only two major criteria for the diagnosis of PCOS: anovulation and the presence of hyperandrogenism as established by clinical or laboratory means. Patients with PCOS frequently exhibit insulin resistance and hyperinsulinemia.

- Combination oral contraceptives (OCs) decrease adrenal and ovarian androgen production and reduce hair growth in nearly two-thirds of hirsute patients.

- Because hyperinsulinemia appears to play a role in PCOS-associated anovulation, treatment with insulin sensitizers may shift the endocrine balance toward ovulation and pregnancy, either alone or in combination with other treatment modalities.

- Excluding cases that are of iatrogenic or factitious etiology, adrenocorticotropic hormone–independent forms of *Cushing syndrome* are adrenal in origin. Adrenal tumors are usually very large by the time Cushing syndrome is manifest.

- *Congenital adrenal hyperplasia* is transmitted as an autosomal recessive disorder. Deficiency of 21-hydroxylase is responsible for more than 90% of cases of adrenal hyperplasia resulting from an adrenal enzyme deficiency.

- Patients with severe hirsutism, virilization, or recent and rapidly progressing signs of androgen excess require careful investigation for the presence of an androgen-secreting neoplasm. Ovarian neoplasms are the most frequent androgen-producing tumors.

- Elevations in prolactin may cause amenorrhea or galactorrhea. Amenorrhea without galactorrhea is associated with hyperprolactinemia in approximately 15% of women. In patients with both galactorrhea and amenorrhea, approximately two-thirds will have hyperprolactinemia; of those, approximately one-third will have a pituitary adenoma. **In more than one-third of women with hyperprolactinemia, a radiologic abnormality consistent with a microadenoma (>1 cm) is found.**

- **Because levels of thyroid-stimulating hormone (TSH) are sensitive to excessive or deficient levels of circulating thyroid hormone, and because most disorders of hyperthyroidism and hypothyroidism are related to dysfunction of the thyroid gland, TSH levels are used to screen for these disorders. The most common thyroid abnormalities in women, autoimmune thyroid disorders, represent the combined effects of the multiple antibodies produced. Severe primary hypothyroidism is associated with amenorrhea or anovulation. The classic triad of exophthalmos, goiter, and hyperthyroidism in Graves disease is associated with symptoms of hyperthyroidism.**

The endocrine disorders encountered most frequently in gynecologic patients are those related to disturbances in the regular occurrence of ovulation and accompanying menstruation. The most prevalent are those characterized by androgen excess, often with insulin resistance, including what is arguably the most common endocrinopathy in women—polycystic ovary syndrome (PCOS). Other conditions leading to ovulatory dysfunction, hirsutism, or virilization, and common disorders of the pituitary and thyroid glands associated with reproductive abnormalities, are reviewed in this chapter.

Hyperandrogenism

Hyperandrogenism most often presents as hirsutism, which arises as a result of androgen excess related to abnormalities of function in the ovary or adrenal glands, constitutive increase in expression of androgen effects at the level of the pilosebaceous unit, or a combination of the two. **By contrast, virilization is rare and indicates marked elevations in androgen levels.** An ovarian or adrenal neoplasm that may be benign or malignant commonly causes virilization.

Hirsutism

Hirsutism, the most frequent manifestation of androgen excess in women, is defined as excessive growth of terminal hair in a male distribution. This refers particularly to midline hair, side burns, moustache, beard, chest or intermammary hair, and inner thigh and midline lower back hair entering the intergluteal area. The response of the pilosebaceous unit to androgens in these androgen responsive areas transforms vellus hair (fine, nonpigmented, short) that is normally present into terminal hair (coarse, stiff, pigmented, and long).

Androgen effects on hair vary in relation to specific regions of the body surface. Hair that shows no androgen dependence includes lanugo, eyebrows, and eyelashes. The hair of the limbs and portions of the trunk exhibits minimal sensitivity to androgens. Pilosebaceous units of the axilla and pubic region are sensitive to low levels of androgens, such that the modest androgenic effects of adult levels of androgens of adrenal origin are sufficient for substantial expression of terminal hair in these areas. Follicles in the distribution associated with male patterns of facial and body hair (midline, facial, inframammary) require higher levels of androgens, as seen with normal testicular function or abnormal ovarian or adrenal androgen production. Scalp hair is inhibited by gonadal androgens, in varying degrees, as determined by age and genetic determination of follicular responsiveness, resulting in the common frontal-parietal balding seen in some males and in virilized females. **Hirsutism results from both increased androgen production and skin sensitivity to androgens. Skin sensitivity depends on the genetically determined local activity of 5α-reductase, the enzyme that converts testosterone to dihydrotestosterone (DHT), the bioactive androgen in hair follicles.**

Hair demonstrates cyclic activity between growth (anagen), involution (catagen), and resting (telogen) phases. The durations of both the growth and resting phases vary according to region of the body, genetic factors, age, and hormonal effects. The cycles of growth, rest, and shedding are normally asynchronous, but when synchronous entry into telogen phase is triggered by major metabolic or endocrine events, such as pregnancy and delivery, or severe illness, dramatic (although transient) hair loss may occur in the following months (telogen effluvium).

Hirsutism is a relative, rather than absolute, designation. What is normal in one setting may be considered abnormal in others; social and clinical reactions to hirsutism can vary significantly, reflecting ethnic variation in skin sensitivity to androgens and cultural ideals. Androgen-dependent hair (excluding pubic and axillary hair) occurs in only 5% of premenopausal white women and is considered abnormal by white women of North America, whereas considerable facial and male pattern hair in other areas may be more common and more often considered acceptable and normal among such groups as the Inuit and women of Mediterranean background.

Hypertrichosis and Virilization

Two conditions should be distinguished from hirsutism. *Hypertrichosis* **is the term reserved for androgen-independent terminal hair in nonsexual areas, such as the trunk and extremities.** This may be the result of an autosomal-dominant congenital disorder, a metabolic disorder (such as anorexia nervosa, hyperthyroidism, porphyria cutanea tarda), or medications (e.g., *acetazolamide,* anabolic steroids, androgenic progestins, androgens, *cyclosporine, diazoxide,* dehydroepiandrosterone (DHEA), heavy metals, *interferon, methyldopa, minoxidil, penicillamine, phenothiazines, phenytoin, streptomycin, reserpine, valproic acid*). **Virilization is a marked and global masculine transformation that includes coarsening of the voice, increase in muscle mass, clitoromegaly (normal clitoral dimensions $\pm$ standard deviation [SD] are 3.4 + 1 mm width by 5.1 + 1.4 mm length) and features of defeminization (loss of breast volume and body fat contributing to feminine body contour)** (1). Although hirsutism accompanies virilization, **the presence of virilization indicates a high likelihood of more serious conditions than are common with hirsutism alone and should prompt evaluation to exclude ovarian or adrenal neoplasm.** Although rare, these diagnoses become likely when onset of androgen effects is rapid or sufficiently pronounced to produce the picture of virilization.

The history should focus on the age of onset and rate of progression of hirsutism or virilization. **A rapid rate of progression or virilization is associated with a more severe degree of hyperandrogenism and should raise suspicion of ovarian and adrenal neoplasms or Cushing syndrome.** This is true whether rapid progression or virilization occurs before, during, or after puberty. Anovulation, manifesting as amenorrhea or oligomenorrhea, increases the probability that there is underlying hyperandrogenism. Hirsutism occurring with regular cycles is more commonly associated with normal androgen levels and thus is attributed to increased genetic sensitivity of the pilosebaceous unit and is termed *idiopathic hirsutism.* When virilization is present, anovulation virtually always occurs.

In determining the extent of hirsutism, a sensitive and tactful approach by the physician is mandatory and should include questions regarding the use and frequency of shaving and/or chemical or mechanical depilatories. Typically, clinical evaluation of the degree of hirsutism is subjective. Most physicians arbitrarily classify the degree of hirsutism as mild, moderate, or severe. Objective assessment is helpful, especially in establishing a baseline from which therapy can be evaluated. The Ferriman–Gallwey Scoring System for Hirsutism quantitates the extent of hair growth in the most androgen sensitive sites. It is a scoring scale of androgen-sensitive hair in nine body areas rated on a scale of 0 to 4 (2). A total score higher than 8 is defined as hirsutism (Fig. 31.1) (3). Although widely used, this scoring system has limitations, one of which is the fact that the scale does not include the sideburn, buttocks, and perineal areas. Substantial hirsutism may be confined to one or two areas without exceeding the cutoff value in total hirsutism score. The score does not reflect the extent to which hirsutism affects a woman's well being (3,4).

A family history should be obtained to disclose evidence of idiopathic hirsutism, PCOS, congenital or adult onset adrenal hyperplasia (CAH or AOAH), diabetes mellitus, and cardiovascular disease. A history of drug use should be obtained. In addition to drugs that commonly cause hypertrichosis, anabolic steroids and testosterone derivatives may cause hirsutism and even virilization. During the physical examination, attention should be directed to obesity, hypertension, galactorrhea, male-pattern baldness, acne (face and back), and hyperpigmentation. With virilization, the presence of an androgen-producing ovarian neoplasm or Cushing syndrome must be considered. In many cases of Cushing syndrome, the patient's presenting symptom is hirsutism. This devastating disorder may masquerade as other disorders such as AOAH and PCOS. Before making these diagnoses, the physician should search for the physical signs of the syndrome such as "moon face," plethora, purple striae, dorsocervical and supraclavicular fat pads, and proximal muscle weakness. A moon-shaped face, upper body obesity, muscle weakness, and the development of a pad of fat between the shoulder blades are particularly notable to both patients and diagnosticians considering the diagnosis of Cushing syndrome.

Role of Androgens

Androgens and their precursors are produced by both the adrenal glands and the ovaries in response to their respective trophic hormones, adrenocorticotropic hormone (ACTH)

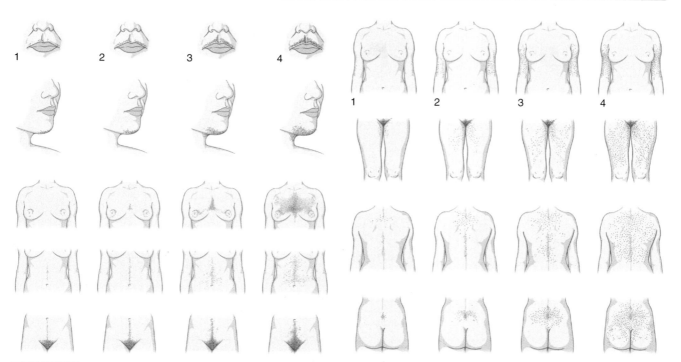

Figure 31.1 **Ferriman-Gallwey hirsutism scoring system.** Each of the nine body areas most sensitive to androgen is assigned a score from 0 (no hair) to 4 (frankly virile), and these separate scores are summed to provide a hormonal hirsutism score. (Reproduced from **Hatch R, Rosefield RL, Kim MH, et al.** Hirsutism: implications, etiology, and management. *Am J Obstet Gynecol* 1981;140:815–830. ©Elsevier.)

and luteinizing hormone (LH), respectively (Fig. 31.2). Biosynthesis begins with the rate-limiting conversion of cholesterol to pregnenolone by side-chain cleavage enzyme. Thereafter, pregnenolone undergoes a two-step conversion to the 17-ketosteroid DHEA along the Δ-5 steroid pathway. This conversion is accomplished by CYP17, an enzyme with both 17α-hydroxylase and 17,20-lyase activities. In a parallel fashion, progesterone undergoes transformation to androstenedione in the Δ-4 steroid pathway. The metabolism of Δ-5 to Δ-4 intermediates is accomplished via a Δ-5-isomerase, 3β-hydroxysteroid dehydrogenase (3β-HSD).

Adrenal 17-Ketosteroids

Secretion of adrenal 17-ketosteroids increases prepubertally and independently of pubertal maturation of the hypothalamic–pituitary–ovarian axis. This alteration in adrenal steroid secretion is termed *adrenarche* and is characterized by a dramatic change in the response of the adrenal cortex to ACTH and with preferential secretion of Δ-5 steroids, including 17-hydroxypronenolone, DHEA, and dehydroepiandrosterone sulfate (DHEAS). The basis for this action is related to the increase in the zona reticularis and in the increased activity of the 17-hydroxylase and the 17,20-lyase enzymes. Independent of the increase in ovarian androgen secretion accompanying puberty, the increase in adrenal androgens owing to adrenarche can account for significant increases in pubic and axillary hair and sweat production by the axillary pilosebaceous units.

Testosterone

Approximately half of a woman's serum testosterone is derived from peripheral conversion of secreted androstenedione and the other half is derived from direct glandular (ovarian and adrenal) secretion. The ovaries and adrenal glands contribute almost equally to testosterone production in women. The contribution of the adrenals is achieved primarily through secretion of androstenedione.

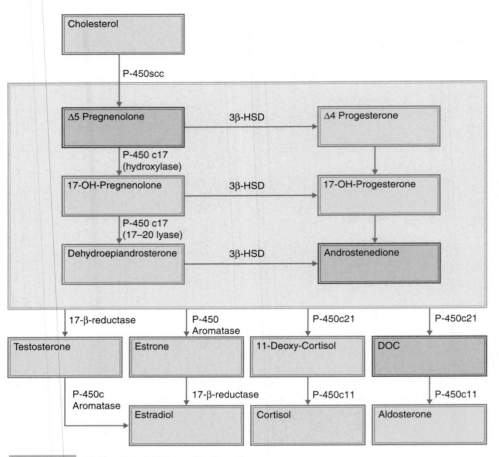

Figure 31.2   **Major steroid biosynthesis pathway.**

Approximately 66% to 78% of circulatory testosterone is bound to sex hormone–binding globulin (SHBG) and is considered biologically inactive. Most of the proportion of serum testosterone that is not bound to SHBG is weakly associated with albumin (20% to 32%). A small percentage (1% to 2%) of testosterone is entirely unbound or free. **The fraction of circulating testosterone that is unbound by SHBG has an inverse relationship with the SHBG concentration.** Increased SHBG levels are noted in conditions associated with high estrogen levels. Pregnancy, the luteal phase, use of estrogen (including oral contraceptives), and conditions causing elevated thyroid hormone levels and cirrhosis of the liver are associated with reduced fractions of free testosterone caused by elevated SHBG levels. Conversely, levels of SHBG decrease and result in elevated free testosterone fractions in response to androgens, androgenic disorders (PCOS, adrenal hyperplasia or neoplasm, Cushing syndrome), androgenic medications (i.e., progestational agents with androgenic biologic activities, such as *danazol,* glucocorticoids, and growth hormones), hyperinsulinemia, obesity, and prolactin.

Laboratory Assessment of Hyperandrogenemia

In hyperandrogenic states, increases in testosterone production are not proportionately reflected in increased total testosterone levels because of the depression of SHBG levels that occurs concomitant with increasing androgen effects on the liver. Therefore, when moderate hyperandrogenism, characteristic of many functional hyperandrogenic states, occurs, elevations in total testosterone levels may remain within the normal range, and only free testosterone levels will reveal the hyperandrogenism. **Severe hyperandrogenism, as occurs in virilization and that results from neoplastic production of testosterone, is reliably detected by measures of total testosterone.** Therefore, in practical clinical evaluation of the hyperandrogenic patient, determination of the total testosterone level in concert with clinical assessment is frequently sufficient for diagnosis and management. When more precise delineation of the degree of hyperandrogenism is desired, measurement or estimation of free testosterone levels can be undertaken and will more reliably reflect increases in testosterone production. These measurements are not necessary in evaluating the majority of patients, but they are common in clinical research studies and may be useful in some clinical settings. Because many practitioners measure some form of testosterone level, they should understand the methods used and their accuracy. Although equilibrium dialysis is the gold standard for measuring free testosterone, it is expensive, complex, and usually limited to research settings. In a clinical setting, free testosterone levels can be estimated by assessment of testosterone binding to albumin and SHBG.

Testosterone, that is nonspecifically bound to albumin (AT), is linearly related to free testosterone (FT) by the equation:

$$AT = K_a\,[A] \times FT,$$

where AT is the albumin-bound testosterone, K_a is the association constant of albumin for testosterone, and [A] is the albumin concentration.

In many cases of hirsutism, albumin levels are within a narrow physiologic range and thus do not significantly affect the free testosterone concentration. When physiologic albumin levels are present, the free testosterone level can be estimated by measuring the total testosterone and SHBG. In individuals with normal albumin levels, this method has reliable results compared with those of equilibrium dialysis. It provides a rapid, simple, and accurate determination of the total and calculated free testosterone level and the concentration of SHBG.

The bioavailable testosterone level is based on the relationship of albumin and free testosterone and incorporates the actual albumin level with the total testosterone and SHBG. This combination of total testosterone, SHBG, and albumin level measurements can be applied to derive a more accurate estimate of available bioactive testosterone and thus the androgen effect derived from testosterone. Bioactive testosterone determined in this manner provides a superior estimate of the effective androgen effect derived from testosterone (5).

Pregnancy can alter the accuracy of measurements of bioavailable testosterone. During pregnancy, estradiol, which shares with testosterone a high affinity for SHBG, occupies a large proportion of SHBG binding sites, so that measurement of SHBG levels can overestimate the binding capacity of SHBG for testosterone. Derived estimates of free testosterone, as opposed to direct measure by equilibrium dialysis, are therefore inaccurate during pregnancy. Testosterone measurements in pregnancy are primarily of interest when autonomous secretion by tumor or luteoma is in question, and for these, total testosterone determinations provide sufficient information for diagnosis.

For testosterone to exert its biologic effects on target tissues, it must be converted into its active metabolite, DHT, by 5α-reductase (a cytosolic enzyme that reduces testosterone and androstenedione). Two isozymes of 5α-reductase exist: type 1, which predominates in the skin, and type 2, or acidic 5α-reductase, which is found in the liver, prostate, seminal vesicles, and genital skin. The type 2 isozyme has a 20-fold higher affinity for testosterone than type 1. Both type 1 and 2 deficiencies in males result in ambiguous genitalia, and both isozymes may play a role in androgen effects on hair growth. Dihydrotestosterone is more potent than testosterone, primarily because of its higher affinity and slower dissociation from the androgen receptor. Although DHT is the key intracellular mediator of most androgen effects, measurements of circulating levels are not clinically useful.

The relative androgenicity of androgens is as follows:

> **DHT = 300**
> **Testosterone = 100**
> **Androstenedione = 10**
> **DHEAS = 5.**

Until adrenarche, androgen levels remain low. Around 8 years of age, adrenarche is heralded by a marked increase in DHEA and DHEAS. The half-life of free DHEA is extremely short (about 30 minutes) but extends to several hours if DHEA is sulfated. Although no clear role is identified for DHEAS, it is associated with stress and levels decline steadily throughout adult life. **After menopause, ovarian estrogen secretion ceases, and DHEAS levels continue to decline,**

whereas testosterone levels are maintained or may even increase. Although postmenopausal ovarian steroidogenesis contributes to testosterone production, testosterone levels retain diurnal variation, reflecting an ongoing and important adrenal contribution. Peripheral aromatization of androgens to estrogens increases with age, but because small fractions (2% to 10%) of androgens are metabolized in this fashion, such conversion is rarely of clinical significance.

Laboratory Evaluation

The 2008 Endocrine Society Clinical Practice Guidelines suggest testing for elevated androgen levels in women with moderate (Ferriman–Gallwey hirsutism score 9 or greater) or severe hirsutism or hirsutism of any degree when it is sudden in onset, rapidly progressive, or associated with other abnormalities such as menstrual dysfunction, infertility, significant acne, obesity, or clitoromegaly. These guidelines suggest against testing for elevated androgen levels in women with isolated mild hirsutism because the likelihood of identifying a medical disorder that would change management or outcome is extremely low (Fig. 31.3) (4). Medications that cause hirsutism are listed and should be considered (Table 31.1).

When laboratory testing for the assessment of hirsutism is indicated, either a bioavailable testosterone level (includes a total testosterone, SHBG, and albumin level) or a calculated free testosterone level (if albumin levels are assumed to be normal) provides the most accurate assessment of the androgen effect derived from testosterone. In clinical situations requiring a testosterone evaluation, the addition of 17-hydroxyprogesterone will screen for adult onset adrenal hyperplasia, when indicated (Table 31.2). When hirsutism is accompanied by absent or abnormal menstrual periods, assessment of prolactin and thyroid-stimulating hormone (TSH) values are required to diagnose an ovulatory disorder. Hypothyroidism and hyperprolactinemia may result in reduced levels of SHBG and may increase the fraction of unbound testosterone levels, occasionally resulting in hirsutism. In cases of suspected Cushing syndrome, patients should undergo screening with a 24-hour urinary cortisol (most sensitive and specific) assessment or an overnight *dexamethasone* suppression test. For this test, the patient takes 1 mg of *dexamethasone* at 11 p.m., and a blood cortisol assessment is performed at 8 a.m. the next day. **Cortisol levels of 2 μg/dL or higher after overnight *dexamethasone* suppression require a further workup for evaluation of Cushing syndrome.** Elevated 17-hydroxyprogesterone (17-OHP) levels identify patients who may have AOAH, found in 1% to 5% of hirsute women. The 17-OHP levels can vary significantly within the menstrual cycle, increasing in the periovulatory period and luteal phase, and may be modestly elevated in PCOS. Standardized testing requires early morning testing during the follicular phase.

According to the Endocrine Society clinical guidelines, patients with morning follicular phase 17-OHP levels of less than 300 ng/dL (10 nmol/L) are likely unaffected. When levels are greater than 300 ng/dL but less than 10,000 ng/dL (300 nmol/L), ACTH testing should be performed to distinguish between PCOS and AOAH. Levels greater than 10,000 ng/dL (300 nmol/L) are virtually diagnostic of congenital adrenal hyperplasia.

Precocious pubarche precedes the diagnosis of adult onset congenital adrenal hyperplasia in 5% to 20% of cases. Measurement of 17-OHP should be performed in patients presenting with precocious pubarche, and a subsequent ACTH stimulation test is recommended if basal 17-OHP is greater than 200 ng/dL. A study using a 200 ng/dL threshold for basal 17-OHP plasma levels to prompt ACTH stimulation testing offered 100% (95% confidence interval [CI], 69–100) sensitivity and 99% (95% CI, 96–100) specificity for the diagnosis of adult onset congenital adrenal hyperplasia within the cohort with precocious puberty (6).

Because increased testosterone production is not reliably reflected by total testosterone levels, the clinician may choose to rely on typical male pattern hirsutism as confirmation of its presence, or may elect measures that reflect levels of free or unbound testosterone (bioavailable or calculated free testosterone levels). Total testosterone does serve as a reliable marker for testosterone-producing neoplasms. **Total testosterone levels greater than 200 ng/dL should prompt a workup for ovarian or adrenal tumors.**

Although the ovary is the principal source of androgen excess in most of PCOS patients, 20% to 30% of patients with PCOS will demonstrate supranormal levels of DHEAS. Measuring circulating levels of DHEAS has limited diagnostic value, and overinterpretation of DHEAS levels should be avoided (7).

In the past, testing for androgen conjugates (e.g., 3α-androstenediol G [3α-diol G] and androsterone G [AOG] as markers for 5α-reductase activity in the skin) was advocated. Routine

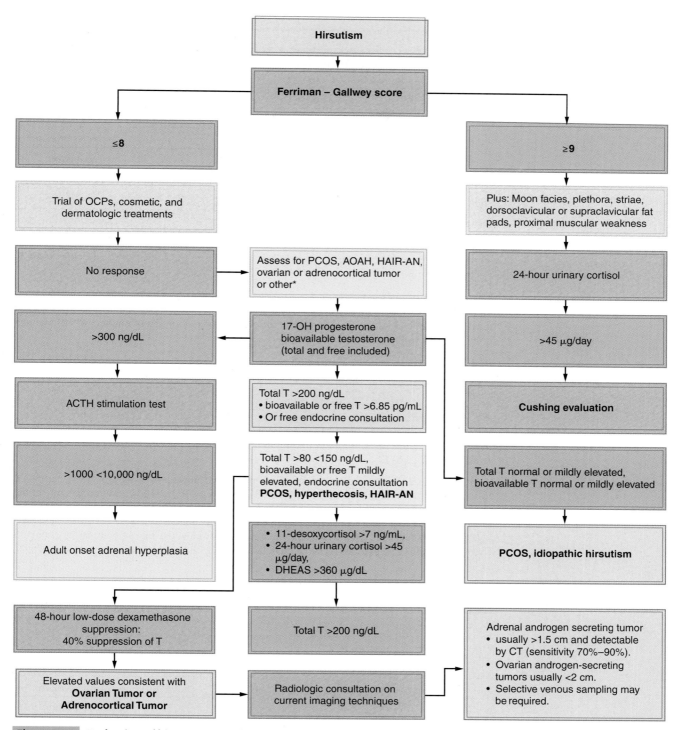

Figure 31.3 Evaluation of hirsute women for hyperandrogenism. Evaluation includes more than the assessment of the degree of hirsutism. When hirsutism is moderate (>9) or severe or if mild hirsutism is accompanied by features that suggest an underlying disorder, elevated androgen levels should be ruled out. Disorders to be considered include endocrinopathies, of which PCOS is the most common, and neoplasms. Plasma testosterone is best assessed in the early morning on day 4 to 10 in regularly cycling women. A 17-hydroxyprogesterone is also indicated when symptoms warrant a bioavailable testosterone measurement.
*3β-hydroxysteroid dehydrogenase deficiency in severe forms presents with mineralocorticoid and cortisol deficiency. Mild forms are diagnosed with a mean post-ACTH(1-24) stimulation: 17-hydroxypregnenolone/17-hydroxyprogesterone ratio of 11 compared to 3.4 in normals. 11β-hydroxylase deficiency presents with hypertension in the first years of life in two thirds of patients. The mild form presents with vitalization or precocious puberty without hypertension. Undiagnosed adults demonstrate hirsutism, acne, and amenorrhea. Diagnosis is confirmed with an 11-desoxycortisol level >25 ng/mL 60 minutes after ACTH(1-24) stimulation. ACTH, adrenocorticotropic hormone; AOAH, adult-onset adrenal hyperplasia; DHEAS, dehydroepiandrosterone sulfate; HAIR-AN, hyperandrogenemia, insulin resistance- acanthosis nigricans. (See references 2–11,15.)

Table 31.1 Medications Associated with Hirsutism	
Acetazolamide	methyldopa
anabolic steroids	minoxidil
androgenic progestins	penicillamine
androgens	phenothiazines
Cyclosporine	phenytoin
Diazoxide	streptomycin
DHEA	reserpine
heavy metals	valproic acid
Interferon	

determination of androgen conjugates to assess hirsute patients is not recommended, because hirsutism itself is an excellent bioassay of free testosterone action on the hair follicle and because these androgen conjugates arise from adrenal precursors and are likely markers of adrenal and not ovarian steroid production (8).

In the zona reticularis layer of the adrenal cortex, DHEAS is generated by *SULT2A1* (9). This layer of the adrenal cortex is thought to be the primary source of serum DHEAS. DHEAS levels decline as a person ages and the reticularis layer diminishes in size. In most laboratories, the upper limit of a DHEAS level is 350 μg/dL (9.5 nmol/L). A random sample is sufficient because the level of variation is minimized as a result of the long half-life characteristic of sulfated steroids. DHEAS is used as a screen for androgen-secreting adrenocortical tumors; however, moderate elevations are a common finding in the presence of PCOS, obesity, and stress, which reduces specificity (10).

A study of women with androgen-secreting adrenocortical tumors (ACT-AS) (N = 44), compared to women with nontumor androgen excess (NTAE) (N = 102), sheds additional light on the choice of hormones used to screen for an adrenocortical tumor. In the study, the demographics and the prevalence of hirsutism, acne, oligomenorrhea and amenorrhea were not different in each group. Free testosterone (free T) was the most commonly elevated androgen in ACT-AS (94%), followed by androstenedione (A) (90%), DHEAS (82%), and total testosterone (total T) (76%),

Table 31.2 Normal Values for Serum Androgens[a]	
Testosterone (total)	20–80 ng/dL
Free testosterone (calculated)	0.6–6.8 pg/mL
Percentage free testosterone	0.4–2.4%
Bioavailable testosterone	1.6–19.1 ng/dL
SHBG	18–114 nmol/L
Albumin	3,300–4,800 mg/dL
Androstenedione	20–250 ng/dL
Dehydroepiandrosterone sulfate	100–350 μg/dL
17-hydroxyprogesterone (follicular phase)	30–200 ng/dL

SHBG, sex hormone–binding globulin.

[a]Normal values may vary among different laboratories. Free testosterone is calculated using measurements for total testosterone and sex hormone–binding globulin, whereas bioavailable testosterone is calculated using measured total testosterone, sex hormone–binding globulin, and albumin. Calculated values for free and bioavailable testosterone compare well with equilibrium dialysis methods of measuring unbound testosterone when albumin levels are normal. Bioavailable testosterone includes free plus very weakly bound (non-SHBG, nonalbumin) testosterone. Bioavailable testosterone is the most accurate assessment of bioactive testosterone in the serum without performing equilibrium dialysis.

Table 31.3 Sensitivity and Specificity of Basal Hormone Levels in the Evaluation of Female Patients with Androgen-secreting Adrenocortical Tumors (ACT-AS) and Nontumor Causes of Androgen Excess (NTAE)

	ACT-AS (n)	NTAE (n)	Sensitivity% (CIª)	Specificity% (CIª)
Total testosterone >1.25 ng/mL	42	102	60 (45–74)	94 (90–99)
Free testosterone >6.85 pg/mL	17	77	82 (57–96)	97 (91–100)
Androstenedione >4.65 ng/mL	38	99	66 (49–80)	80 (71–87)
DHEAS >3.6 µg/mL	39	97	79 (64–91)	79 (70–87)
17OHP >1.95 ng/mL	36	79	67 (49–81)	86 (76–93)
11-desoxycortisol >7 ng/mL	27	35	89 (71–98)	100 (90–100)

Thresholds were selected using Youden's index, as described in the methods.
ªCI: 95% confidence intervals.
(Reprinted with permission from **d'Alva CB, Abiven-Lepage G, Viallon V, et al.** Sex steroids in androgen-secreting adrenocortical tumors: clinical and hormonal features in comparison with non-tumoral causes of androgen excess. *Eur J Endocrinol* 2008;159:641–647.

and all three androgens were simultaneously elevated in 56% of the cases. Serum androgen levels became subnormal in all ACT-AS patients after the tumor was removed. In nontumor androgen excess alone, the most commonly elevated androgen was androstenedione (93%), while all three androgens (T, A, and DHEAS) were elevated in only 22% of the cases. Free testosterone values above 6.85 pg/mL (23.6 pmol/L) had the best diagnostic value for ACT-AS (sensitivity 82%; CI, 57%–96%; specificity 97%, CI, 91%–100%) (Table 31.3). The large overlap of androstenedione, testosterone, and DHEAS levels between ACT-AS and androgen excess groups suggests that thoughtful consideration should be employed when choosing hormone studies for this evaluation (11).

The heterogeneity of hormone secretion patterns in the adrenocortical tumor group reveals the complexities of hormone level screening for adrenocortical tumors: 7 of 44 patients (15.9%) had tumors secreting androgens alone, 2 of 44 (4.5%) had tumors secreting androgens and estrogens, 28 of 44 (63.6%) had tumors secreting both androgens and cortisol, and 7 of 44 (15.9%) had tumors secreting androgens, cortisol, and estrogens. Compound S or 11-desoxycortisol was increased ($\geq$10 ng/mL or 28.9 nmol/L) in 23 of 27 ACT-AS patients (85%); 20 of 21 patients with malignant tumors, and 3 of 6 patients with apparently benign tumors, although 11-desoxycortisol was normal and inferior to 6 ng/mL (17.3 nmol/L) in 35 of 35 nontumor androgen excess patients (100%). Youden's index displayed that a 11-desoxycortisol level above 7 ng/mL (20.2 nmol/L) has a sensitivity of 89% (95% CI, 71%–98%) and a specificity of 100% (95% CI, 90%–100%) for the detection of ACT-AS (11,12).

When clinical signs of androgen excess reach the point of virilization or the free testosterone level is above 6.85 pg/mL (23.6 pmol/L), follow-up testing with a 11-desoxycortisol (>7 ng/mL), DHEAS (>3.6 µg/mL), and 24-hour urinary cortisol (>45 µg per day) are the most sensitive and specific for the detection of an androgen-secreting adrenocortical tumor. Careful consideration of the sensitivity and specificity, diurnal variation, and age-related variation of potentially measureable androgens will aid in choosing the most useful measurements (Table 31.3).

Polycystic Ovary Syndrome

PCOS is arguably one of the most common endocrine disorders in women of reproductive age, affecting 5% to 10% of women worldwide. This familial disorder appears to be inherited as a complex genetic trait (13). It is characterized by a combination of hyperandrogenism (either clinical or biochemical), chronic anovulation, and polycystic ovaries. It is frequently associated with insulin resistance and obesity (14). PCOS receives considerable attention because of its high prevalence and possible reproductive, metabolic, and cardiovascular consequences. **It is the most common cause of hyperandrogenism, hirsutism, and anovulatory infertility in developed countries** (15,16). The association of amenorrhea with bilateral polycystic ovaries and obesity was first described in 1935 by Stein and Leventhal (17). Its genetic origins are likely polygenic and/or multifactorial (18).

Diagnostic Criteria

In an international conference on PCOS organized by the National Institutes of Health (NIH) in 1990, diagnostic criteria for PCOS were based on consensus rather than clinical trial evidence. Their diagnostic criteria recommended clinical and/or biochemical evidence of hyperandrogenism, chronic anovulation, and exclusion of other known disorders. These criteria were an important initial step in standardizing diagnosis and led to a number of landmark randomized clinical trials in PCOS (19).

Since the 1990 NIH-sponsored PCOS conference, evolving perception is that the syndrome may constitute a broader spectrum of signs and symptoms of ovarian dysfunction than those set forth in the original NIH diagnostic criteria. The 2003 Rotterdam Consensus Workshop concluded that PCOS is a syndrome of ovarian dysfunction along with the cardinal features hyperandrogenism and polycystic ovary (PCO) morphology (Table 31.4).

It is recognized that women with regular cycles, hyperandrogenism, and PCO morphology may be part of the syndrome. Some women with the syndrome will have PCO morphology without clinical evidence of androgen excess, but will display evidence of ovarian dysfunction with irregular cycles. In this new schema, PCOS remains a diagnosis of exclusion with the need to rule out other disorders that mimic the PCOS phenotype (19).

Using the Rotterdam PCOS Diagnostic Criteria, the presence of two of the three criteria is sufficient to diagnosis PCOS: menstrual cycle anomalies (amenorrhoea, oligomenorrhea), clinical and/or biochemical hyperandrogenism, and/or the ultrasound appearance of polycystic ovaries after all other diagnoses are ruled out. Other pathologies that can result in a POCS phenotype include AOAH, adrenal or ovarian neoplasm, Cushing syndrome, hypo- or hypergonadotropic disorders, hyperprolactinemia, and thyroid disease (Fig. 31.4).

All other frequently encountered manifestations offer less consistent findings and therefore qualify only as minor diagnostic criteria for PCOS. They include elevated LH-to-FSH (follicle-stimulating hormone) ratio, insulin resistance, perimenarchal onset of hirsutism, and obesity.

Clinical hyperandrogenism includes hirsutism, male pattern alopecia, and acne (19). Hirsutism occurs in approximately 70% of patients with PCOS in the United States and in only 10% to 20% of patients with PCOS in Japan (20,21). A likely explanation for this discrepancy is the genetically determined differences in skin 5α-reductase activity (22,23).

Nonclassic adrenal hyperplasia and PCOS may present with similar clinical features. It is important to measure the basal follicular phase 17-hydroxyprogesterone level in all women presenting

Table 31.4 Revised Diagnostic Criteria of Polycystic Ovary Syndrome
1990 Criteria (both 1 and 2)
1. Chronic anovulation and
2. Clinical and/or biochemical signs of hyperandrogenism and exclusion of other etiologies.
Revised 2003 criteria (2 out of 3)
1. Oligoovulation or anovulation
2. Clinical and/or biochemical signs of hyperandrogenism
3. Polycystic ovaries and exclusion of other etiologies (congenital adrenal hyperplasia, androgen-secreting tumors, Cushing's syndrome)

From **Rotterdam ESHRE/ASRM-Sponsored PCOS Consensus Workshop Group.** Revised 2003 consensus on diagnostic criteria and long-term health risks related to polycystic ovary syndrome. *Fertil Steril* 2004;81:19–25, with permission.

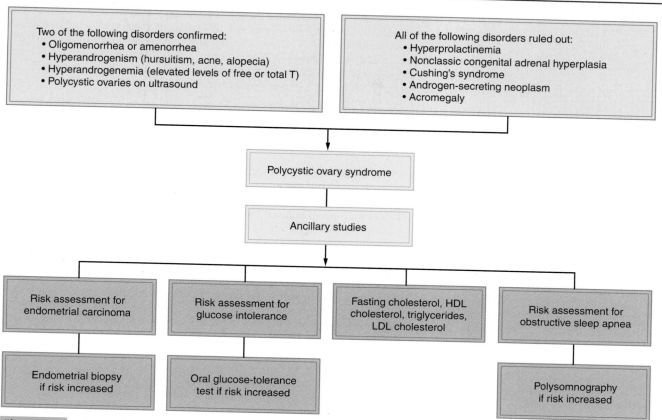

Figure 31.4 **Diagnostic algorithm for polycystic ovary syndrome.** (From **Rosenfield RL.** Clinical practice. Hirsutism. *N Engl J Med* 2005;353:2578–2588, with permission.)

with hirsutism to exclude the presence of nonclassic congenital adrenal hyperplasia, regardless of the presence of polycystic ovaries or metabolic dysfunction (24).

The menstrual dysfunction in PCOS arises from anovulation or oligo-ovulation and ranges from amenorrhea to oligomenorrhea. Regular menses in the presence of anovulation in PCOS is uncommon, although one report found that among hyperandrogenic women with regular menstrual cycles, the rate of anovulation is 21% (25). **Classically, the disorder is lifelong, characterized by abnormal menses from puberty with acne and hirsutism arising in the teens. It may arise in adulthood, concomitant with the emergence of obesity, presumably because this is accompanied by increasing hyperinsulinemia** (26).

The sonographic criteria for PCO requires the presence of 12 or more follicles in either ovary measuring 2 to 9 mm in diameter and/or increased ovarian volume (>10 mL). A single ovary meeting these criteria is sufficient to affix the PCO diagnosis (19). The appearance of PCO on ultrasound scanning is common. Only a fraction of those with PCO appearance have the clinical and/or endocrine features of PCOS. A PCO appearance is found in about 23% of women of reproductive age, while estimates of the incidence of PCOS vary between 5% and 10% (27). Polycystic appearing ovaries in women with PCOS was not associated with increased cardiovascular disease risk, independent of body mass index (BMI), age, and insulin levels (28). An English study demonstrated that without symptoms of polycystic ovary syndrome, a PCO appearance alone is not associated with impaired fecundity or fertility (29).

Obesity occurs in more than 50% of patients with PCOS. The body fat is usually deposited centrally (android obesity), and a higher waist-to-hip ratio is associated with insulin resistance indicating an increased risk of diabetes mellitus and cardiovascular disease (30). Among women with PCOS, there is widespread variability in the degree of adiposity by geographic location and ethnicity. In studies in Spain, China, Italy, and the United States, the percentage of obese women with PCOS were 20%, 43%, 38%, and 69%, respectively (31).

Insulin resistance resulting in hyperinsulinemia is commonly exhibited in PCOS. Insulin resistance may eventually lead to the development of hyperglycemia and type 2 diabetes mellitus (32). About one-third of obese PCOS patients have impaired glucose tolerance (IGT), and 7.5% to 10% have type 2 diabetes mellitus (33). These rates are mildly increased in nonobese women who have PCOS (10% IGT; 1.5% diabetes, respectively), compared with the general population of the United States (7.8% IGT; 1% diabetes, respectively) (34,35).

Abnormal lipoproteins are common in PCOS and include elevated total cholesterol, triglycerides, and low-density lipoproteins (LDL); and,low levels of high-density lipoproteins (HDL), and apoprotein A-I (30,36). According to one report, the most characteristic lipid alteration is decreased levels of $HDL_{2\alpha}$ (37).

Other observations in women with PCOS include impaired fibrinolysis, as shown by elevated circulating levels of plasminogen activator inhibitor, an increased incidence of hypertension over the years (which reaches 40% by perimenopause), a greater prevalence of atherosclerosis and cardiovascular disease, and an estimated sevenfold increased risk for myocardial infarction (36,38–41).

Pathology

Macroscopically, ovaries in women with PCOS are two to five times the normal size. A cross-section of the surface of the ovary discloses a white, thickened cortex with multiple cysts that are typically less than a centimeter in diameter. Microscopically, the superficial cortex is fibrotic and hypocellular and may contain prominent blood vessels. In addition to smaller atretic follicles, there is an increase in the number of follicles with luteinized theca interna. The stroma may contain luteinized stromal cells (42).

Pathophysiology and Laboratory Findings

The hyperandrogenism and anovulation that accompany PCOS may be caused by abnormalities in four endocrinologically active compartments: (i) the ovaries, (ii) the adrenal glands, (iii) the periphery (fat), and (iv) the hypothalamus–pituitary compartment (Fig. 31.5).

In patients with PCOS, the ovarian compartment is the most consistent contributor of androgens. Dysregulation of CYP17, the androgen-forming enzyme in both the adrenals and the ovaries, may be one of the central pathogenetic mechanisms underlying hyperandrogenism in PCOS (43). The ovarian stroma, theca, and granulosa contribute to ovarian hyperandrogenism and are stimulated by LH (44). This hormone relates to ovarian androgenic activity in PCOS in a number of ways.

1. Total and free testosterone levels correlate directly with LH levels (45).
2. The ovaries are more sensitive to gonadotropic stimulation, possibly as a result of CYP17 dysregulation (43).
3. Treatment with a gonadotropin-releasing hormone (GnRH) agonist effectively suppresses serum testosterone and androstenedione levels (46).
4. Larger doses of a GnRH agonist are required for androgen suppression than for endogenous gonadotropin-induced estrogen suppression (47).

The increased testosterone levels in patients with PCOS are considered ovarian in origin. The serum total testosterone levels are usually no more than twice the upper normal range (20 to 80 ng/dL). However, in ovarian hyperthecosis, values may reach 200 ng/dL or more (48). The adrenal compartment plays a role in the development of PCOS. Although the hyperfunctioning CYP17 androgen-forming enzyme coexists in both the ovaries and the adrenal glands, DHEAS is increased in only about 50% of patients with PCOS (49,50). The hyperresponsiveness of DHEAS to stimulation with ACTH, the onset of symptoms around puberty, and the observation of 17,20-lyase activation (one of the two CYP17 enzymes) are key events in adrenarche that led to the hypothesis that PCOS arises as an exaggeration of adrenarche (48).

The *peripheral compartment,* defined as the skin and the adipose tissue, manifests its contribution to the development of PCOS in several ways.

1. The presence and **activity of 5α-reductase** in the skin largely **determines the presence or absence of hirsutism** (22,23).
2. Aromatase and 17β-hydroxysteroid dehydrogenase activities are increased in fat cells and **peripheral aromatization is increased with increased body weight** (51,52).

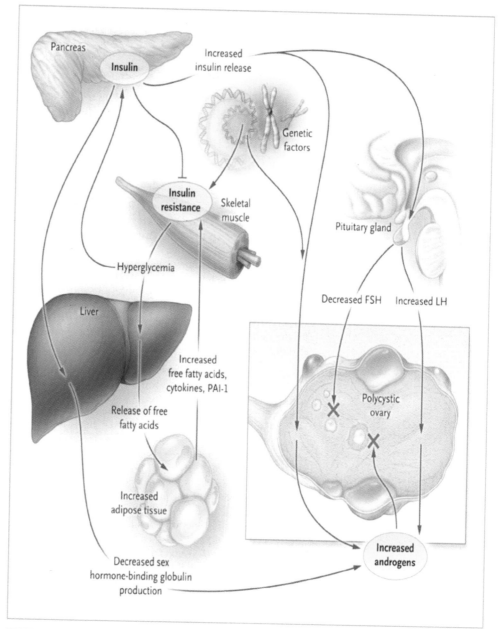

Figure 31.5 **Pathophysiological characteristics of the polycystic ovary syndrome (PCOS).** Insulin resistance results in a compensatory hyperinsulinemia, which stimulates ovarian androgen production in an ovary genetically predisposed to PCOS. Arrest of follicular development (red "X") and anovulation could be caused by the abnormal secretion of gonadotropins such as follicle-stimulating hormone (FSH) or luteinizing hormone (LH) (perhaps induced by hyperinsulinemia), intraovarian androgen excess, direct effects of insulin, or a combination of these factors. Insulin resistance, in concert with genetic factors, may also lead to hyperglycemia and an adverse profile of cardiovascular risk factors. (From **Rosenfield RL.** Clinical practice. Hirsutism. *N Engl J Med* 2005;353:2578–2588, with permission.)

3. With obesity the **metabolism of estrogens,** by way of reduced 2-hydroxylation and 17α-oxidation, **is decreased** and metabolism via estrogen active 16-hydroxyestrogens (estriol) is increased (53).

4. Whereas estradiol (E2) is at a follicular phase level in patients with PCOS, **estrone (E1) levels are increased as a result of peripheral aromatization of androstenedione** (54).

5. A **chronic hyperestrogenic state,** with reversal of the E1-to-E2 ratio, results and is unopposed by progesterone.

The **hypothalamic–pituitary compartment** participates in aspects critical to the development of PCOS.

1. An **increase in LH pulse frequency** relative to those in the normal follicular phase is the result of increased GnRH pulse frequency (55).

2. This increase in LH pulse frequency explains the frequent observation of an **elevated LH and LH-to-FSH ratio.**

3. **FSH is not increased** with LH, likely because of the combination of increased gonadotropin pulse frequency and the synergistic negative feedback of chronically elevated estrogen levels and normal follicular inhibin.

4. About 25% of patients with PCOS exhibit **mildly elevated prolactin levels,** which may result from abnormal estrogen feedback to the pituitary gland. In some patients with PCOS, *bromocriptine* has reduced LH levels and restored ovulatory function (56).

Polycystic ovary syndrome is a complex multigenetic disorder that results from the interaction between multiple genetic and environmental factors. **Genetic studies of PCOS reported allele sharing in large PCOS patient populations and linkage studies focused on candidate genes most likely to be involved in the pathogenesis of PCOS. These genes can be grouped in four categories: (i) insulin resistance–related genes, (ii) genes that interfere with the biosynthesis and the action of androgens, (iii) genes that encode inflammatory cytokines, and (iv) other candidate genes** (57).

Linkage studies identified the follistatin, *CYP11A, Calpain 10,* IRS-1 and IRS-2 regions and loci near the insulin receptor (19p13.3), SHBG, *TCF7L2,* and the insulin genes, as likely PCOS candidate genes (58–64). A polymorphic variant, *D19S884,* in *FBN3* was found to be associated with risk of PCOS (65). Using theca cells derived from women with PCOS elevated mRNA levels was noted for *CYP11A, 3BHSD2,* and *CYP17* genes with corresponding overproduction of testosterone, 17-α-hydroxyprogesterone, and progesterone. Despite the characteristically heightened steroidogenesis in POCS, the *STARB* gene was not overexpressed (58). Microarray data using theca cells from PCOS women did not identify any genes near the 19p13.3 locus that were differentially expressed; however, the mRNAs of several genes that map to 19p13.3, including the insulin receptor, p114-Rho-GEF, and several expressed sequence tags, were detected in both PCOS and normal theca cells. Those studies identified new factors that might impact theca cell steroidogenesis and function, including *cAMP-GEFII,* genes involved in all-transretinoic acid (atRA) synthesis signaling, genes that participate in the Wnt signal transduction pathway, and transcription factor GATA6. These findings suggest that a 19p13.3 locus or some other candidate gene may be a signal transduction gene that results in overexpression of a suite of genes downstream that may affect steroidogenic activity (66). Polymorphisms in major folliculogenesis genes, *GDF9, BMP15, AMH,* and *AMHR2,* are not associated with PCOS susceptibility (67).

Insulin Resistance

Patients with PCOS frequently exhibit insulin resistance and hyperinsulinemia. Insulin resistance and hyperinsulinemia participate in the ovarian steroidogenic dysfunction of PCOS. Insulin alters ovarian steroidogenesis independent of gonadotropin secretion in PCOS. Insulin and insulin-like growth factor I (IGF-I) receptors are present in the ovarian stromal cells. A specific defect in the early steps of insulin receptor–mediated signaling (diminished autophosphorylation) was identified in 50% of women with PCOS (68).

Insulin has direct and indirect roles in the pathogenesis of hyperandrogenism in PCOS. Insulin in collaboration with LH enhances the androgen production of theca cells. Insulin inhibits the hepatic synthesis of sex hormone–binding globulin, the main circulating protein that binds to testosterone, thus increasing the proportion of unbound or bioavailable testosterone (13).

The most common cause of insulin resistance and compensatory hyperinsulinemia is obesity, but despite its frequent occurrence in PCOS, obesity alone does not explain this important association (56). The insulin resistance associated with PCOS is not solely the result of hyperandrogenism based on the following:

1. Hyperinsulinemia is not a characteristic of hyperandrogenism in general but is uniquely associated with PCOS (69).

2. In obese women with PCOS, 30% to 45% have glucose intolerance or frank diabetes mellitus, whereas ovulatory hyperandrogenic women have normal insulin levels and glucose tolerance (69). It seems that the associations between PCOS and obesity on the action of insulin are synergistic.

3. Suppression of ovarian steroidogenesis in women with PCOS with long-acting GnRH analogues does not change insulin levels or insulin resistance (70).

4. Oophorectomy in patients with hyperthecosis accompanied by hyperinsulinemia and hyperandrogenemia does not change insulin resistance, despite a decrease in androgen levels (70,71).

Acanthosis nigricans **is a reliable marker of insulin resistance in hirsute women. This thickened, pigmented, velvety skin lesion is most often found in the vulva and may be present on the axilla, over the nape of the neck, below the breast, and on the inner thigh (72). The HAIR-AN syndrome consists of hyperandrogenism (HA), insulin resistance (IR), and acanthosis nigricans (AN) (68,73).** These patients often have high testosterone levels (>150 ng/dL), fasting insulin levels of greater than 25 μIU/mL (normal <20 to 24 μIU/mL), and maximal serum insulin responses to glucose load (75 gm) exceeding 300 μIU/mL (normal is <160 μIU/m: at 2 hours postglucose load).

Screening Strategies for Diabetes and Insulin Resistance

The 2003 Rotterdam Consensus Group recommends that obese women with PCOS and nonobese PCOS patients with risk factors for insulin resistance, such as a family history of diabetes, should be screened for metabolic syndrome, including glucose intolerance with an oral glucose tolerance test (19). The standard 2-hour oral glucose tolerance test (OGTT) provides an assessment of both the degrees of hyperinsulinemia and glucose tolerance and yields the highest amount of information for a reasonable cost and risk (7).

Multiple other testing or screening schema were proposed to assess the presence of hyperinsulinemia and insulin resistance. In one, the fasting glucose-to-insulin ratio is determined, and values less than 4.5 indicate insulin resistance. Using the 2-hour GTT with insulin levels, 10% of nonobese and 40% to 50% of obese PCOS women have impaired glucose tolerance (IGT = 2-hour glucose level $\geq$140 but $\leq$199 mg/dL) or overt type 2 diabetes mellitus (any glucose level >200 mg/dL). Some research studies utilized a peak insulin level of over 150 μIU/mL or a mean level of over 84 μIU/mL over the three blood draws of a 2-hour GTT as a criteria to diagnoses hyperinsulinemia.

The documentation of hyperinsulinemia using either the glucose to insulin ratio or the 2-hour GTT with insulin is problematic. When compared to the gold standard measure for insulin resistance, the hyperinsulemic-euglycemic clamp, it shows that the glucose-to-insulin ratio does not always accurately portray insulin resistance. When hyperglycemia is present, a relative insulin secretion deficit is present. This deficient insulin secretion exacerbates the effects of insulin resistance and renders inaccurate the use of hyperinsulinemia as an index of insulin resistance. Thus, routine measurements of insulin levels may not be particularly useful.

Although detection of insulin resistance, *per se,* is not of practical importance to the diagnosis or management of PCOS, **testing women with PCOS for glucose intolerance is of value because their risk of cardiovascular disease correlates with this finding.** An appropriate frequency for such screening depends on age, BMI and waist circumference, all of which increase risk.

Interventions

Two-Hour Glucose Tolerance Test Normal Glucose Ranges (World Health Organization criteria, after 75-gm glucose load)

- **Fasting**   **64 to 128 mg/dL**

- **One hour**   **120 to 170 mg/dL**

- **Two hour**   **70 to 140 mg/dL**

Two-Hour Glucose Values for Impaired Glucose Tolerance and Type 2 Diabetes (World Health Organization criteria, after 75-gm glucose load)

- **Normal (2-hour)** $<$**140 mg/dL**
- **Impaired (2-hour)** $=$ **140 to 199 mg/dL**
- **Type 2 diabetes mellitus (2-hour)** $\geq$**200 mg/dL**

Abnormal glucose metabolism may be significantly improved with weight reduction, which may reduce hyperandrogenism and restore ovulatory function (74). In obese, insulin-resistant women, caloric restriction that results in weight reduction will reduce the severity of insulin resistance (a 40% decrease in insulin level with a 10-kg weight loss) (75). This decrease in insulin levels should result in a marked decrease in androgen production (a 35% decrease in testosterone levels with a 10-kg weight loss) (76). Exercise reduces insulin resistance, independent from any associated weight loss, but data on the impact of exercise on the principal manifestations of PCOS are lacking.

In addition to addressing the increased risk for diabetes, the clinician should recognize insulin resistance or hyperinsulinemia as a cluster syndrome called *metabolic syndrome* or *dysmetabolic syndrome X*. Recognition of the importance of insulin resistance or hyperinsulinemia as a risk factor for cardiovascular disease led to diagnostic criteria for the dysmetabolic syndrome. The more dysmetabolic syndrome X criteria are present, the higher the level of insulin resistance and its downstream consequences. The presence of three of the following five criteria confirm the diagnosis, and an insulin-lowering agent and/or other interventions may be warranted (19).

Metabolic Syndrome Diagnostic Criteria

- **Female waist** $>$**35 inches**
- **Triglycerides** $>$**150 mg/dL**
- **HDL** $<$**50 mg/dL**
- **Blood pressure** $>$**130/85 mmHg**
- **Fasting glucose:**   **110–126 mg/dL**
- **Two-hour glucose (75 gm OGTT):**   **140–199 mg/dL**

Risk factors for the dysmetabolic syndrome include nonwhite race, sedentary lifestyle, BMI greater than 25, age over 40 years, cardiovascular disease, hypertension, PCOS, hyperandrogenemia, insulin resistance, HAIR-AN syndrome, nonalcoholic steatohepatitis (NASH), and a family history of type 2 diabetes mellitus, gestational diabetes, or impaired glucose tolerance.

Long-Term Risks and Interventions

Comprehensive treatment of PCOS addresses reproductive, metabolic and psychological features.

Metabolic Syndrome

A report by the Androgen Excess and PCOS Society concluded that lifestyle management, either alone or combined with antiobesity pharmacologic and/or surgical treatments, should be used as the primary therapy in overweight and obese women with PCOS (31). Lifestyle management of obesity in PCOS is multifactorial. Dietary management of obesity should focus on reducing body weight, maintaining a lower long-term body weight, and preventing weight gain. An initial weight loss of greater than or equal to 5% to 10% is recommended. In obese and overweight women with PCOS, dietary interventions with a resultant weight reduction of more than 5% to less than 15% over the starting body weight is associated with a reduction in either total or free testosterone, adrenal androgens, and improvement in SHBG levels. Metabolic improvements in fasting insulin, glucose, glucose tolerance, total cholesterol, triglycerides, plasminogen activator inhibitor-1, and free fatty acids are reported. Clinically, hirsutism, menstrual function, and ovulation are all improved (31).

Structured exercise improves insulin resistance and offers significant benefits in PCOS. The incorporation of structured exercise, behavior modification, and stress management strategies

Table 31.5 Lifestyle Modification Principles Suggested for Obesity Management in Polycystic Ovary Syndrome (PCOS)

Guidelines for dietary and lifestyle intervention in PCOS

1. Lifestyle modification is the first form of therapy, combining behavioral (reduction of psychosocial stressors), dietary, and exercise management.

2. Reduced-energy diets (500–1,000 kcal/day reduction) are effective options for weight loss and can reduce body weight by 7% to 10% over a period of 6 to 12 months.

3. Dietary plans should be nutritionally complete and appropriate for life stage and should aim for <30% of calories from fat, <10% of calories from saturated fat, with increased consumption of fiber, whole-grain breads and cereals, and fruit and vegetables.

4. Alternative dietary options (increasing dietary protein, reducing glycemic index, reducing carbohydrate) may be successful for achieving and sustaining a reduced weight but more research is needed in PCOS specifically.

5. The structure and support within a weight-management program is crucial and may be more important than the dietary composition. Individualization of the program, intensive follow-up and monitoring by a physician, and support from the physician, family, spouse, and peers will improve retention.

6. Structured exercise is an important component of a weight-loss regime; aim for >30 min/day.

Reprinted with permission from **Moran LJ, Pasquali R, Teede HJ, et al.** Treatment of obesity in polycystic ovary syndrome: a position statement of the Androgen Excess and Polycystic Ovary Syndrome Society. *Fertil Steril* 2009;92:1966–1982.

as fundamental components of lifestyle management increases the success of the weight loss strategy (Table 31.5).

Even though lifestyle management strategies should be used as the primary therapy in obese and overweight women with PCOS, they are difficult to maintain long term. Alternative approaches to the treatment of obesity include the use of pharmacologic agents, such as *orlistat, sibutramine,* and *rimonabant,* or bariatric surgery (31). The NIH clinical recommendations advise bariatric surgery when BMI is greater than 40 kg/m^2 or greater than 35 kg/m^2 in patients with a high-risk, obesity-related condition after failure of other treatments for weight control (31,77).

Dyslipidemia is one of the most common metabolic disorders seen in PCOS patients (up to 70% prevalence in a US PCOS population) (78). It is associated with insulin resistance and hyperandrogenism in combination with environmental (diet, physical exercise) and genetic factors. Various abnormal patterns include decreased levels of HDL, elevated levels of triglycerides, decreased total and LDL levels, and altered LDL quality (79,80).

To assess cardiovascular risks and prevent disease in patients with PCOS, the Androgen Excess and Polycystic Ovary Syndrome (AE-PCOS) Society recommend the following monitoring activities (80):

1. Waist circumference and BMI measurement at every visit, using the National Health and Nutrition Examination Survey method.

2. A complete lipid profile based using the American Heart Association guidelines (Fig. 31.6). If the fasting serum lipid profile is normal, it should be reassessed every 2 years or sooner if weight gain occurs.

3. A 2-hour post-75-g oral glucose challenge measurement in PCOS women with a BMI greater than 30 kg/m^2, or alternatively in lean PCOS women with advanced age (40 years), personal history of gestational diabetes, or family history of type 2 diabetes.

4. Blood pressure measurement at each visit. The ideal blood pressure is 120/80 or lower. Prehypertension should be treated because blood pressure control has the largest benefit in reducing cardiovascular diseases.

5. Regular assessment for depression, anxiety, and quality of life.

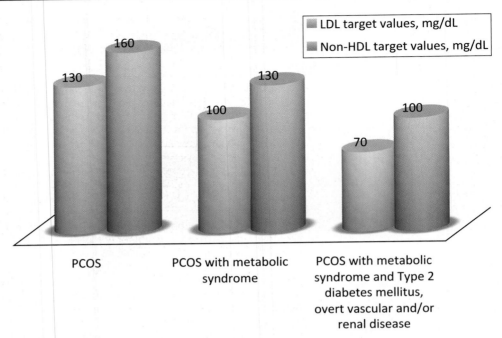

Figure 31.6 **Lipid guidelines in PCOS to prevent cardiovascular disease risk (values in mg/dL).** (Non-HDL = Total Cholesterol − HDL, if TG <400 mg/dL). (Data for figure derived from **Wild RA, Carmina E, Diamanti-Kandarakis E, et al.** Assessment of cardiovascular risk and prevention of cardiovascular disease in women with the polycystic ovary syndrome: a consensus statement by the Androgen Excess and Polycystic Ovary Syndrome (AE-PCOS) Society. *J Clin Endocrinol Metab* 2010;95(5):2038–2049.)

A significant proportion of the population and particularly the obese population have inadequate vitamin D levels. Because vitamin D plays a role in many metabolic activities, assessment and supplementation when indicated are recommended.

25-hydroxy Vitamin D Levels

- Deficient: 8 ng/mL or less (≤20 nmol/L)
- Insufficient: 8–20 ng/mL (20–50 nmol/L)
- Optimal: 20–60 ng/mL (50–150 nmol/L; 40–50 ng/mL is treatment goal)
- High: 60–90 ng/mL (150–225 nmol/L)
- Toxic: >90 ng/mL or greater (≥225 nmol/L)

Supplementation Facts

1. The body uses 3,000 to 5,000 IU D_3 per day.
2. In the absence of the sun, 600 IU of D_3 are required to maintain vitamin D levels.
3. D_2 is more rapidly metabolized and is less potent than D_3.
4. Patients receiving 50,000 IU of vitamin D_2 once a week for 8 weeks will usually correct a vitamin D deficiency, and this can be followed by giving 50,000 U of vitamin D_2 once every other week to maintain vitamin D sufficiency.
5. D_3 is more potent and appropriate dosing to correct levels is still under investigation.

Cancer

In chronic anovulatory patients with PCOS, persistently elevated estrogen levels, which are uninterrupted by progesterone, increase the risk of endometrial carcinoma (81,82). **These endometrial cancers are usually well differentiated, stage I lesions with a cure rate of more than 90%** (see Chapter 35). Endometrial biopsy should be considered in PCOS patients, because they may occasionally harbor these cancers as early as the third decade of life. Abnormal bleeding, increasing weight, and age are factors that should lower the threshold for endometrial sampling. **Prevention of endometrial cancer is a core management goal for patients with**

PCOS. If other dimensions of management do not induce regular ovulation (e.g. *clomiphene*) or impose continuous progestation influence (e.g., oral contraceptives), regular secrectory transformation and menstruation should be induced with periodic administration of a progestational agent. Even though the hyperestrogenic state is associated with an increased risk of breast cancer, studies examining the relationship between PCOS and breast cancer have not always identified a significantly increased risk (82–86). **The risk of ovarian cancer is increased two- to threefold in women with PCOS** (82,87).

Depression and Mood Disorders

The clinical features of PCOS, such as infertility, acne, hirsutism, and obesity, promote psychological morbidity. Women with PCOS face challenges to their feminine identity that can lead to loss of self-esteem, anxiety, poor body image, and depression (88).

A study examining the prevalence of depression and other mood disorders in women with PCOS reported a significantly increased prevalence of depression (35% to 40%) when compared with controls (10.7%), after adjusting for BMI, and a family history of depression and/or infertility. Other mood disorders such as anxiety and eating disorders were common in women with PCOS (89). **The high prevalence of depression and other mental health disorders in women with PCOS suggests that assessment and treatment of mental health disorders should be included in the evaluation and management plan** (89). Lifestyle management improves quality of life and depression in obese and overweight and women with PCOS (88).

Treatment of Hyperandrogenism and PCOS

Treatment depends on a patient's goals. Some patients require hormonal contraception, whereas others desire ovulation induction. In all cases where there is significant ovulatory dysfunction, progestational interruption of the unopposed estrogen effects on the endometrium is necessary. This may be accomplished by periodic luteal function resulting from ovulation induction, progestational suppression via contraceptive formulations, or intermittent administration of progestational agents for endometrial or menstrual regulation. **Interruption of the steady state of hyperandrogenism and control of hirsutism usually can be accomplished simultaneously. Patients desiring pregnancy are an exception, and for them effective control of hirsutism may not be possible.** Treatment regimens for hirsutism are listed in Table 31.6. The induction of ovulation and treatment of infertility are discussed in Chapter 32.

Table 31.6 Medical Treatment of Hirsutism	
Treatment Category	*Specific Regimens*
Weight loss	
Hormonal suppression	Oral contraceptives
	Medroxyprogesterone
	Gonadotropin-releasing hormone analogues
	Glucocorticoids
Steroidogenic enzyme inhibitors	Ketoconazole
5α-reductase inhibitors	Finasteride
Antiandrogens	Spironolactone
	Cyproterone acetate
	Flutamide
Insulin sensitizer	Metformin
Mechanical	Temporary
	Permanent
	Electrolysis
	Laser hair removal

Weight Reduction

Weight reduction is the initial recommendation for patients with accompanying obesity because it promotes health, reduces insulin, SHBG, and androgen levels, and may restore ovulation either alone or combined with ovulation-induction agents (75). Weight loss of as little as 5% to 7% over a 6-month period can reduce the bioavailable or calculated free testosterone level significantly and restore ovulation and fertility in more than 75% of women (90). Exercise involving large muscle groups reduces insulin resistance and can be an important component of nonpharmacologic, lifestyle-modifying management.

Oral Contraceptives

Combination oral contraceptives (OCs) decrease adrenal and ovarian androgen production and reduce hair growth in nearly two-thirds of hirsute patients (91–94). Treatment with OCs offers the following benefits:

1. The **progestin component suppresses LH,** resulting in diminished ovarian androgen production.
2. The **estrogen component increases hepatic production of SHBG,** resulting in decreased free testosterone concentration (95,96).
3. **Circulating androgen levels are reduced,** including those of DHEAS, which to some extent is independent of the effects of both LH and SHBG (30,97).
4. **Estrogens decrease conversion of testosterone to DHT** in the skin by inhibition of 5α-reductase.

When an OC is used to treat hirsutism, a balance must be maintained between the decrease in free testosterone levels and the intrinsic androgenicity of the progestin. Three progestin compounds that are present in OCs (*norgestrel, norethindrone,* and *norethindrone acetate*) are believed to be androgen dominant. The androgenic bioactivity of these steroids may be a factor of their shared structural similarity with 19-nortestosterone steroids (98). Oral contraceptives containing the so-called new progestins (*desogestrel, gestodene, norgestimate,* and *drospirenone*) have minimized androgenic activity. However, there is limited evidence of clinically measurable differences in outcome resulting from the disparity of *in vitro* estimates of androgenic potency.

The use of OCs alone may be relatively ineffective (<10% success rate) in the treatment of hirsutism in women with PCOS, and the OCs may exacerbate insulin resistance in these patients (99,100). Effective protocols for pharmacologic management of significant hirsutism with OCs usually include coadministration of agents that impede androgen action.

Medroxyprogesterone Acetate

Oral or intramuscular administration of *medroxyprogesterone acetate* (*MPA*) successfully treats hirsutism (101). It directly affects the hypothalamic–pituitary axis by decreasing GnRH production and the release of gonadotropins, thereby reducing testosterone and estrogen production by the ovary. Despite a decrease in SHBG, total and free androgen levels are decreased significantly (102). **The recommended oral dose for GnRH suppression is 20 to 40 mg daily in divided dosages or 150 mg given intramuscularly every 6 weeks to 3 months in the depot form.** Hair growth is reduced in up to 95% of patients (103). Side effects of the treatment include amenorrhea, bone mineral density loss, depression, fluid retention, headaches, hepatic dysfunction, and weight gain. MPA is not commonly used for hirsutism.

Gonadotropin-Releasing Hormone Agonists

Administration of GnRH agonists may allow the differentiation of androgen produced by adrenal sources from that of ovarian sources (47). It was shown to suppress ovarian steroids to castrate levels in patients with PCOS (104). Treatment with *leuprolide acetate* given intramuscularly every 28 days decreases hirsutism and hair diameter in both idiopathic hirsutism and hirsutism secondary to PCOS (105). Ovarian androgen levels are significantly and selectively suppressed. The addition of OC or estrogen replacement therapy to GnRH agonist treatment (add-back therapy) prevents bone loss and other side effects of menopause, such as hot flushes and genital atrophy. The hirsutism-reducing effect is retained (102,106). Suppression of hirsutism is not potentiated by the addition of estrogen replacement therapy to GnRH agonist treatment (107).

Glucocorticoids

Dexamethasone may be used to treat patients with PCOS who have either adrenal or mixed adrenal and ovarian hyperandrogenism. Doses of *dexamethasone* as low as 0.25 mg nightly or every other night are used initially to suppress DHEAS concentrations to less than 400 μg/dL. **Because *dexamethasone* has 40 times the glucocorticoid effect of cortisol, daily doses greater** than 0.5 mg every evening should be avoided to prevent the risk of adrenal suppression and severe side effects that resemble Cushing syndrome. To avoid oversuppression of the pituitary–adrenal axis, morning serum cortisol levels should be monitored intermittently (maintain at >2 μg/dL). Reduction in hair growth rate was reported, and significant improvement in acne associated with adrenal hyperandrogenism (108).

Ketoconazole

Ketoconazole inhibits the key steroidogenic cytochromes. Administered at a low dose (200 mg per day), it can significantly reduce the levels of androstenedione, testosterone, and calculated free testosterone (109). It is rarely used for the chronic inhibition of androgen production in women with hyperandrogenism because of the serious risk of adrenocortical suppression and development of adrenal crisis (15).

Spironolactone

Spironolactone is a specific antagonist of aldosterone, which competitively binds to the aldosterone receptors in the distal tubular region of the kidney. It is an effective potassium-sparing diuretic that originally was used to treat hypertension. The effectiveness of *spironolactone* in the treatment of hirsutism is based on the following mechanisms:

1. Competitive inhibition of DHT at the intracellular receptor level (22).
2. Suppression of testosterone biosynthesis by a decrease in the CYP enzymes (110).
3. Increase in androgen catabolism (with increased peripheral conversion of testosterone to estrone).
4. Inhibition of skin 5α-reductase activity (22).

Although total and free testosterone levels are reduced significantly in patients with both PCOS and idiopathic hirsutism (hyperandrogenism with regular menses) after treatment with *spironolactone,* total and free testosterone levels in patients with PCOS remain higher than those with idiopathic hirsutism (hyperandrogenism with regular menses) (111). In both groups, SHBG levels are unaltered. The reduction in circulating androgen levels observed within a few days of *spironolactone* treatment partially accounts for the progressive regression of hirsutism.

At least a modest improvement in hirsutism can be anticipated in 70% to 80% of women using at least 100 mg of *spironolactone* per day for 6 months (112). *Spironolactone* reduces the daily linear growth rate of sexual hair, hair shaft diameters, and daily hair volume production (113). Combination therapy with spironolactone and oral contraceptives seems effective via their differing but synergistic activities (15,114).

The most common dose is 50 to 100 mg twice daily. Women treated with 200 mg per day show a greater reduction in hair shaft diameter than women receiving 100 mg per day (115). Maximal inhibition of hirsutism is noted between 3 and 6 months but continues for 12 months. Electrolysis can be recommended 9 to 12 months after the initiation of *spironolactone* for permanent hair removal.

The most common side effect of *spironolactone* is menstrual irregularity (usually metrorrhagia), which may occur in over 50% of patients with a dosage of 200 mg per day (115). Normal menses may resume with reduction of the dosage. Infrequently, other side effects such as mastodynia, urticaria, or scalp hair loss may occur. Nausea and fatigue can occur with high doses (112). Because spironolactone can increase serum potassium levels, its use is not recommended in patients with renal insufficiency or hyperkalemia. Periodic monitoring of potassium and creatinine levels is suggested.

Return of normal menses in amenorrheic patients is reported in up to 60% of cases (111). Patients must be counseled to use contraception while taking *spironolactone* because it theoretically can feminize a male fetus.

Cyproterone Acetate

Cyproterone acetate is a synthetic progestin derived from 17-OHP, which has potent antiandrogenic properties. The primary mechanism of *cyproterone acetate* is competitive inhibition of testosterone and DHT at the level of the androgen receptor (116). This agent induces hepatic enzymes and may increase the metabolic clearance rate of plasma androgens (117).

A European formulation of *ethinyl estradiol* with *cyproterone acetate* significantly reduces plasma testosterone and androstenedione levels, suppresses gonadotropins, and increases SHBG levels (118). *Cyproterone acetate* shows mild glucocorticoid activity (and may reduce DHEAS levels) (116,119). Administered in a reverse sequential regimen (*cyproterone acetate* 100 mg per day on days 5 to 15, and *ethinyl estradiol* 30 to 50 mg per day on cycle days 5 to 26), this cyclic schedule allows regular menstrual bleeding, provides excellent contraception, and is effective in the treatment of even severe hirsutism and acne (120).

Side effects of *cyproterone acetate* include fatigue, weight gain, decreased libido, irregular bleeding, nausea, and headaches. These symptoms occur less often when *ethinyl estradiol* is added. *Cyproterone acetate* administration is associated with liver tumors in beagles and is not approved by the U.S. Food and Drug Administration (FDA) for use in the United States.

Flutamide

Flutamide, a pure nonsteroidal antiandrogen, is approved for treatment of advanced prostate cancer. Its mechanism of action is inhibition of nuclear binding of androgens in target tissues. Although it has a weaker affinity to the androgen receptor than *spironolactone* or *cyproterone acetate*, larger doses (250 mg given two or three times daily) may compensate for the reduced potency. *Flutamide* is a weak inhibitor of testosterone biosynthesis.

In a single, 3-month study of *flutamide* alone, most patients demonstrated significant improvement in hirsutism with no change in androgen levels (121). Significant improvement in hirsutism with a significant drop in androstenedione, DHT, LH, and FSH levels was observed in an 8-month follow-up of *flutamide* and low-dose OCs in women who did not respond to OCs alone (122). The side effects of *flutamide* treatment combined with a low-dose OC included dry skin, hot flashes, increased appetite, headaches, fatigue, nausea, dizziness, decreased libido, liver toxicity, and breast tenderness (123).

In hyperinsulinemic hyperandrogenemic nonobese PCOS adolescents on a combination of *metformin* (850 mg per day) and *flutamide* (62.5 mg per day), the low-dose OC containing *drospirenone* resulted in a more effective and more efficient reduction in total and abdominal fat excess than was demonstrated by those utilizing an OC with *gestodene* as the progestin (124). The combination of *ethinyl-drospirenone, metformin,* and *flutamide* is effective in reducing excess total and abdominal fat and attenuating dysadipocytokinemia in young women with hyperinsulinemic PCOS. The use of the antiandrogen *flutamide* appeared to emphasize effects (125). Many patients taking *flutamide* (50% to 75%) report dry skin, blue-green discoloration of urine, and liver enzyme elevation. Liver toxicity or failure and death are rare but severe side effects of *flutamide* appear to be dose related (126). The 2008 Endocrine Society clinical practice guidelines do not recommend using *flutamide* as first-line therapy for treating hirsutism. If it is used, the lowest effective dose should be given, and the patient's liver function should be monitored closely (4). *Flutamide* should not be used in women desiring pregnancy.

Finasteride

Finasteride is a specific inhibitor of type 2 5α-reductase enzyme activity, approved in the United States at a 5-mg dose for the treatment of benign prostatic hyperplasia, and at a 1-mg dose to treat male-pattern baldness. In a study in which *finasteride* (5 mg daily) was compared with *spironolactone* (100 mg daily), both drugs resulted in similar significant improvement in hirsutism, despite differing effects on androgen levels (127). Most of the improvement in hirsutism with *finasteride* occurred after 6 months of therapy with 7.5 mg of *finasteride* daily (128). The improvement in hirsutism in the presence of rising testosterone levels is convincing evidence that it is the binding of DHT, and not testosterone, to the androgen receptor that is responsible for hair growth. *Finasteride* does not prevent ovulation or cause menstrual irregularity. The increase in SHBG caused by OCs further decreases free testosterone levels; OCs in combination with *finasteride* are more effective in reducing hirsutism than *finasteride* alone. As with *spironolactone* and *flutamide, finasteride* could theoretically feminize a male fetus; therefore, both of these agents are used only with additional contraception.

Ovarian Wedge Resection

Bilateral ovarian wedge resection is associated with only a transient reduction in androstenedione levels and a prolonged minimal decrease in plasma testosterone (129,130). In patients with hirsutism and PCOS who had wedge resection, hair growth was reduced by approximately 16% (17,131). Although Stein and Leventhal's original report cited a pregnancy rate of 85% following wedge resection and maintenance of ovulatory cycles, subsequent reports show lower pregnancy rates and a concerning incidence of periovarian adhesions (17,132). Instances of premature ovarian failure and infertility were reported (133).

Laparoscopic Electrocautery

Laparoscopic ovarian electrocautery is used as an alternative to wedge resection in patients with severe PCOS whose condition is resistant to *clomiphene citrate*. In a recent series, ovarian drilling was achieved laparoscopically with an insulated electrocautery needle, using 100-W cutting current to assist entry and 40-W coagulating current to treat each microcyst over 2 seconds (8-mm needle in ovary) (134). In each ovary, 10 to 15 punctures were created. This led to spontaneous ovulation in 73% of patients, with 72% conceiving within 2 years. Of those who underwent a follow-up laparoscopy, 11 of 15 were adhesion free. To reduce adhesion formation, a technique that cauterized the ovary in only four points led to a similar pregnancy rate, with a miscarriage rate of 14% (135). Other laparoscopic techniques using laser instead of electrocautery for laparoscopic ovarian drilling were described (136). Most series report a decrease in both androgen and LH concentrations and an increase in FSH concentrations (137,138). The beneficial endocrinological effects of laparoscopic ovarian drilling and the improvement in hirsutism were sustained for up to 9 years in patients with PCOS (139). Unilateral diathermy results in bilateral ovarian activity (140). Further studies are anticipated to define candidates who may benefit most from such a procedure. **The risk of adhesion formation should be discussed with the patient.**

Physical Methods of Hair Removal

Depilatory creams remove hair only temporarily. They break down and dissolve hair by hydrolyzing disulfide bonds. Although depilatories can have a dramatic effect, many women cannot tolerate these irritative chemicals. The topical use of corticosteroid cream may prevent contact dermatitis. *Eflornithine hydrochloride* cream, also known as *difluoromethylornithine* (*DMFO*), irreversibly blocks ornithine decarboxylase (ODC), the enzyme in hair follicles that is important in regulating hair growth. It is effective in the treatment of unwanted facial hair (141). Noticeable results take about 6 to 8 weeks of therapy. Treatment must be continued while inhibition of hair growth is desired, and when the cream is discontinued, hair returns to pretreatment levels after about 8 weeks (4).

Shaving is effective and, contrary to common belief, it does not change the quality, quantity, or texture of hair. Plucking, if done unevenly and repeatedly, may cause inflammation and damage to hair follicles and render them less amenable to electrolysis. Waxing is a grouped method of plucking in which hairs are plucked out from under the skin surface. The results of waxing last longer (up to 6 weeks) than shaving or depilatory creams (142).

Bleaching removes the hair pigment through the use of *hydrogen peroxide* (usually 6% strength), which is sometimes combined with *ammonia*. Although hair lightens and softens during oxidation, this method is frequently associated with hair discoloration or skin irritation and is not always effective (141).

Electrolysis and laser hair removal are the only permanent means recommended for hair removal. Under magnification, a trained technician destroys each hair follicle individually. When a needle is inserted into a hair follicle, galvanic current, electrocautery, or both used in combination (blend) destroy the hair follicle. After the needle is removed, a forceps is used to remove the hair. Hair regrowth ranges from 15% to 50%. Problems with electrolysis include pain, scarring, and pigmentation. Cost can be an obstacle (143). Laser hair removal destroys the hair follicle through photoablation. These methods are most effective after medical therapy arrests further growth.

Insulin Sensitizers

Because hyperinsulinemia appears to play a role in PCOS-associated anovulation, treatment with insulin sensitizers may shift the endocrine balance toward ovulation and pregnancy, either alone or in combination with other treatment modalities.

Metformin (*Glucophage*) is an oral biguanide antihyperglycemic drug used extensively for non–insulin-dependent diabetes. *Metformin* is pregnancy category B drug with no known human teratogenic effect. It lowers blood glucose mainly by inhibiting hepatic glucose production and by enhancing peripheral glucose uptake. *Metformin* enhances insulin sensitivity at the postreceptor level and stimulates insulin-mediated glucose disposal (144).

Metformin has been used extensively to treat oligo-ovulatory infertility, insulin resistance, and hyperandrogenism in PCOS patients. *Metformin* is used to treat PCOS oligo-ovulatory infertility either alone or in combination with dietary restriction, *clomiphene,* or gonadotropins. In randomized control studies, *metformin* improves the odds of ovulation in women with PCOS when compared with placebo (145,146). **A large multicenter, randomized control trial in women with PCOS concluded that *clomiphene* is superior to *metformin* in achieving live births in infertile women with PCOS.** When ovulation was used as the outcome, the combination of *metformin* and *clomiphene* was superior to either *clomiphene* alone or *metformin* alone (147). Multiple births are a complication of *clomiphene* therapy.

The most common side effects are gastrointestinal, including nausea, vomiting, diarrhea, bloating, and flatulence. Because the drug caused fatal lactic acidosis in men with diabetes who have renal insufficiency, **baseline renal function testing is suggested** (148). **The drug should not be given to women with elevated serum creatinine levels** (144).

Concepts regarding the role of obesity and insulin resistance or hyperinsulinemia in PCOS suggest that the primary intervention should be recommending and assisting with weight loss (5% to 10% of body weight). In those with an elevated BMI, *orlistat* proved helpful in initiating and maintaining weight loss. A percentage of PCOS patients will respond to weight loss alone with spontaneous ovulation. In those who do not respond to weight loss alone or who are unable to lose weight, the sequential addition of *clomiphene citrate* followed by an insulin sensitizer, followed by the combination of these agents may promote ovulation without resorting to injectable gonadotropins.

A prevailing concern over the increased incidence of spontaneous abortions in women with PCOS and the potential reduction afforded by insulin sensitizers suggests that insulin sensitizers may be beneficial in combination with gonadotropin therapy for ovulation induction or *in vitro* fertilization (149). Women with early pregnancy loss have a low level of insulin-like growth factor (IGF) binding protein-1 (IGFBP-1), and of circulating glycodelin, which has immunomodulatory effects protecting the developing fetus. Use of *metformin* increased levels of both factors, which might explain early findings suggesting that *metformin* use may reduce the high spontaneous abortion rates seen among women with PCOS (150).

A number of observational studies suggested that *metformin* reduces the risk of pregnancy loss (151,152). However, there are no adequately designed and sufficiently powered randomized control trials to address this issue. In the prospective randomized pregnancy and PCOS (PPCOS) trial, there was a concerning nonsignificant trend toward a greater rate of miscarriages in the *metformin* only group (151). This trend was not noted in other trials.

There are no conclusive data to support a beneficial effect of *metformin* on pregnancy loss, and the trend toward a higher miscarriage rate in the PPCOS trial, which used extended release *metformin,* is of some concern (145,147).

The incidence of ovarian hyperstimulation syndrome is reduced with adjuvant *metformin* in PCOS patients at risk for severe ovarian hyperstimulation syndrome (153).

Cushing Syndrome

The adrenal cortex produces three classes of steroid hormones: glucocorticoids, mineralocorticoids, and sex steroids (androgen and estrogen precursors). Hyperfunction of the adrenal gland can produce clinical signs of increased activity of any or all of these hormones. Increased glucocorticoid action results in nitrogen wasting and a catabolic state. This causes muscle weakness, osteoporosis, atrophy of the skin with striae, nonhealing ulcerations and ecchymoses, reduced immune resistance that increases the risk of bacterial and fungal infections, and glucose intolerance resulting from enhanced gluconeogenesis and antagonism to insulin action.

Although most patients with Cushing syndrome gain weight, some lose it. **Obesity is typically central, with characteristic redistribution of fat over the clavicles around the neck and on the trunk, abdomen, and cheeks.** Cortisol excess may lead to insomnia, mood disturbances, depression, and even overt psychosis. With overproduction of sex steroid precursors, women may exhibit hyperandrogenism (hirsutism, acne, oligomenorrhea or amenorrhea, thinning of scalp hair). Masculinization is rare, and its presence suggests an autonomous adrenal origin, most often an adrenal malignancy. With overproduction of mineralocorticoids, patients may manifest arterial hypertension and hypokalemic alkalosis. The associated fluid retention may cause pedal edema (Table 31.7) (154).

Characteristic clinical laboratory findings associated with hypercortisolism are confined mainly to a complete blood count showing evidence of granulocytosis and reduced levels of lymphocytes and eosinophils. Increased urinary calcium secretion may be present.

Table 31.7 Overlapping Conditions and Clinical Features of Cushing Syndrome

Symptoms	Signs	Overlapping Conditions
Features that best discriminate Cushing syndrome; most do not have a high sensitivity		
	Easy bruising	
	Facial plethora	
	Proximal myopathy (or proximal muscle weakness)	
	Striae (especially if reddish purple and >1 cm wide)	
	In children, weight gain with decreasing growth velocity	
Cushing syndrome features in the general population that are common and/or less discriminatory		
Depression	Dorsocervical fat pad ("buffalo hump")	Hypertension*
Fatigue	Facial fullness	Incidental adrenal mass
Weight gain	Obesity	Vertebral osteoporosis*
Back pain	Supraclavicular fullness	Polycystic ovary syndrome
Changes in appetite	Thin skin*	Type 2 diabetes*
Decreased concentration	Peripheral edema	Hypokalemia
Decreased libido	Acne	Kidney stones
Impaired memory (especially short term)	Hirsutism or female balding	Unusual infections
Insomnia	Poor skin healing	
Irritability		
Menstrual abnormalities		
In children, slow growth	In children, abnormal genital virilization	
	In children, short stature	
	In children, pseudoprecocious puberty or delayed puberty	

Features are listed in random order.
*Cushing's syndrome is more likely if onset of the feature is at a younger age.

Causes

The six recognized noniatrogenic causes of Cushing syndrome can be divided between those that are ACTH dependent and those that are ACTH independent (Table 31.8). **The ACTH-dependent causes can result from ACTH secreted by pituitary adenomas or from an ectopic source. The hallmark of ACTH-dependent forms of Cushing syndrome is the presence of normal or high plasma ACTH concentrations with increased cortisol levels. The adrenal glands are hyperplastic bilaterally. Pituitary ACTH-secreting adenoma, or Cushing disease, is the most common cause of endogenous Cushing syndrome** (154). These pituitary adenomas are usually microadenomas (<10 mm in diameter) that may be as small as 1 mm. They behave as though they are resistant, to a variable degree, to the feedback effect of cortisol. Like the normal gland, these tumors secrete ACTH in a pulsatile fashion; unlike the

Table 31.8 Causes of Cushing Syndrome

Category	Cause	Relative Incidence
ACTH-dependent	Cushing syndrome	60%
	Ectopic ACTH-secreting tumors	15%
	Ectopic CRH-secreting tumors	Rare
ACTH-independent	Adrenal cancer	15%
	Adrenal adenoma	10%
	Micronodular adrenal hyperplasia	Rare
	Iatrogenic/factitious	Common

ACTH, adrenocorticotropic hormone; CRH, corticotropin-releasing hormone.
ACTH-dependent Cushing syndrome may be caused by pituitary adenoma, basophil hyperplasia, nodular adrenal hyperplasia, or cyclic Cushing syndrome.

normal gland, the diurnal pattern of cortisol secretion is lost. **Ectopic ACTH syndrome most often is caused by malignant tumors** (155). About one-half of these tumors are small-cell carcinomas of the lung (156). Other tumors include bronchial and thymic carcinomas, carcinoid tumors of the pancreas, and medullary carcinoma of the thyroid.

Ectopic corticotropin-releasing hormone (CRH) tumors are rare and include such tumors as bronchial carcinoids, medullary thyroid carcinoma, and metastatic prostatic carcinoma (156). The presence of an ectopic CRH-secreting tumor should be suspected in patients whose dynamic testing suggests pituitary ACTH-dependent disease but who have rapid disease progression and very high plasma ACTH levels.

The most common cause of ACTH-independent Cushing syndrome is exogenous or iatrogenic (i.e., superphysiologic therapy with corticosteroids) or factitious (self-induced). Corticosteroids are used in pharmacologic quantities to treat a variety of diseases with an inflammatory component. Over time, such therapy will result in Cushing syndrome. When corticosteroids are taken by the patient but not prescribed by a physician, the diagnosis may be especially challenging. The diagnostic workup for Cushing syndrome focuses on the ability to suppress autonomous cortisol secretion and whether ACTH is elevated or suppressed. According to the 2008 Endocrine Society's clinical practice guidelines for the diagnosis of Cushing syndrome, the initial use of one test with high diagnostic accuracy (24-hour urine free cortisol, late night salivary cortisol, 1 mg overnight or 2 mg 48-hour *dexamethasone* suppression test) is recommended. The 24-hour urine-free cortisol (UFC) should be used to diagnose Cushing syndrome in pregnant women and in patients with epilepsy, whereas the 1-mg overnight *dexamethasone* suppression test, rather than UFC, should be used for initial testing for Cushing syndrome in patients with severe renal failure and adrenal incidentaloma. The 2-mg 48-hour *dexamethasone* suppression test is the optimal test in conditions that are associated with overactivation of the hypothalamic–pituitary–adrenal (HPA) axis: depression, morbid obesity, alcoholism, and diabetes mellitus.

Patients with an abnormal result should see an endocrinologist and undergo a second test, either one of the above or, in some cases, a serum midnight cortisol or *dexamethasone* CRH test. These guidelines are summarized in (Fig. 31.7) (154).

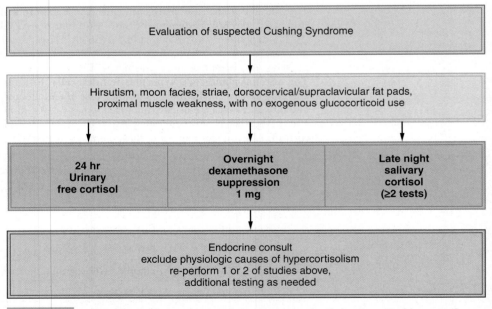

Figure 31.7 **Algorithm for testing patients suspected of having Cushing syndrome (CS).** Diagnostic criteria that suggest Cushing syndrome are a urinary-free cortisol (UFC) greater than the normal range for the assay, serum cortisol greater than 1.8 μg/dL (50 nmol/L) after 1 mg dexamethasone (1 mg DST), and a late night salivary cortisol greater than 145 ng/dL (4 nmol/L). (Based on recommendations from **Nieman LK, Biller BM, Findling JW, et al.** The diagnosis of Cushing's syndrome: an Endocrine Society Clinical Practice Guideline. *J Clin Endocrinol Metab* 2008;93:1526–1540.)

Treatment of ACTH-independent Forms of Cushing Syndrome

Excluding cases that are of iatrogenic or factitious etiology, ACTH-independent forms of Cushing syndrome are adrenal in origin. Adrenal cancers are usually very large by the time Cushing syndrome is manifest. This is because the tumors are relatively inefficient synthesizers of steroid hormones. Tumors are larger than 6 cm in diameter and are easily detectable by computed tomography (CT) scanning or magnetic resonance imaging (MRI). Adrenal cancers often produce steroids other than cortisol. Thus, when Cushing syndrome is accompanied by hirsutism or virilization in women or feminization in men, adrenal cancer should be suspected.

An adrenal tumor that appears large and irregular on radiologic imaging is suggestive of carcinoma. In these cases, a unilateral adrenalectomy through an abdominal exploratory approach is preferable. In most malignant tumors, complete resection is virtually impossible. However, a partial response to postoperative chemotherapy or radiation may be achieved. Most patients with malignancy die within 1 year. When administered immediately after surgery, *mitotane* (O,P-DDD, an adrenocorticolytic drug) may be of benefit in preventing or delaying recurrent disease (157). Manifestations of Cushing syndrome in these patients are controlled by adrenal enzyme inhibitors.

Adrenal adenomas are smaller than carcinomas and average 3 cm in diameter. These tumors are usually unilateral and infrequently associated with other steroid-mediated syndromes. Micronodular adrenal disease is a disorder of children, adolescents, and young adults. The adrenal glands contain numerous small (>3 mm) nodules, which often are pigmented and secrete sufficient cortisol to suppress pituitary ACTH. This condition can be sporadic or familial.

Surgical removal of a neoplasm is the treatment of choice (158,159). If a unilateral, well-circumscribed adenoma is identified by MRI or CT scanning, the flank approach may be the most convenient. The cure rate following surgical removal of adrenal adenomas approaches 100%. Because normal function of the HPA axis is suppressed by autonomous cortisol production, cortisol replacement follows surgery and is titrated downward over several months, during which recovery of normal adrenal function is monitored.

Treatment of Cushing Disease

The main goals of treatment in ACTH-dependent Cushing syndrome are reversal of clinical features, normalization of biochemical changes with minimal morbidity, and long-term control without recurrence (155).

The treatment of choice for Cushing disease is transsphenoidal resection. The remission rate is approximately 70% to 90% and the recurrence rate is 5% to 10% at 5 years and 10% to 20% at 10 years in patients with microadenomas who undergo surgery by an experienced surgeon (160–164). Patients with macroadenoma have lower remission rates (<60%) and higher recurrence rates (12% to 45%) (165–167). Following surgery, transient diabetes insipidus and enduring compromise of anterior pituitary secretion of growth hormone, gonadotropins, and TSH are common (167,168).

Radiation Therapy

Fractionated external beam radiotherapy or stereotactic radiosurgery is used to treat patients with Cushing disease in whom transsphenoidal microsurgery was not successful or in patients who are poor surgical candidates. This therapy can achieve control of hypercortisolemia in approximately 50% to 60% of patients within 3 to 5 years (155,169,170). Hypopituitarism is the most common side effect of pituitary irradiation, and long-term follow-up is essential to detect relapse, which can occur after an initial response to radiotherapy.

High-voltage external pituitary radiation (4,200 to 4,500 cGy) is given at a rate not exceeding 200 cGy per day. Only 15% to 25% of adults show total improvement, but approximately 80% of children respond (168,171).

Medical Therapy

Mitotane can be used to induce medical adrenalectomy during or after pituitary radiation (157). The role of medical therapy is to prepare the severely ill patient for surgery and to maintain normal cortisol levels while a patient awaits the full effect of radiation. Occasionally, medical therapy is used for patients who respond to therapy with only partial remission. Adrenal enzyme inhibitors include *aminoglutethimide, metyrapone, trilostane,* and *etomidate.*

A combination of *aminoglutethimide* and *metyrapone* may cause a total adrenal enzyme block, requiring corticosteroid-replacement therapy. *Ketoconazole*, an FDA-approved antifungal agent, inhibits adrenal steroid biosynthesis at the side arm cleavage and 11β-hydroxylation steps. The dose of *ketoconazole* for adrenal suppression is 600 to 800 mg per day for 3 months to 1 year (172). *Ketoconazole* is effective for long-term control of hypercortisolism of either pituitary or adrenal origin.

Nelson syndrome results from adenomatous progression of ACTH-secreting cells in patients with Cushing syndrome treated by bilateral adrenalectomy. The macroadenoma that causes this syndrome produces sellar pressure symptoms of headaches, visual field disturbances, and ophthalmoplegia. Extremely high ACTH levels in Nelson syndrome are associated with severe hyperpigmentation (melanocyte-stimulating hormone activity). The treatment is surgical removal or radiation. The offending adenomatous tissue is often resistant to complete surgical removal (173). This syndrome reportedly complicates 10% to 50% of bilateral adrenalectomy cases. Measuring pituitary MRI and ACTH plasma levels at regular intervals after bilateral adrenalectomy will allow detection of the early progression of corticotroph tumors and the possibility of cure by surgery, particularly with microadenomas (155). Nelson syndrome is less common today because bilateral adrenalectomy is less frequently used as initial treatment.

Congenital Adrenal Hyperplasia

CAH is transmitted as an autosomal recessive disorder. Several adrenocortical enzymes necessary for cortisol biosynthesis may be affected. Failure to synthesize the fully functional enzyme has the following effects:

1. A relative decrease in cortisol production.
2. A compensatory increase in ACTH levels.
3. Hyperplasia of the zona reticularis of the adrenal cortex.
4. An accumulation of the precursors of the affected enzyme in the bloodstream.

21-Hydroxylase Deficiency

Deficiency of 21-hydroxylase is responsible for over 90% of all cases of adrenal hyperplasia due to adrenal synthetic enzyme deficiency. The disorder produces a spectrum of conditions; CAH, with or without salt wasting, and milder forms that are expressed as hyperandrogenism of pubertal onset (adult onset adrenal hyperplasia, AOAH). Salt-wasting CAH, the most severe form, affects 75% of patients with congenital manifestations during the first 2 weeks of life and results in a life-threatening hypovolemic salt-wasting crisis, accompanied by hyponatremia, hyperkalemia, and acidosis. The salt-wasting form results from a severity of enzyme deficiency sufficient to result in ineffective aldosterone synthesis. With or without salt-wasting and newborn adrenal crisis, the condition is usually diagnosed earlier in affected female newborns than in males as genital virilization (e.g., clitoromegaly, labioscrotal fusion, and abnormal urethral course) is apparent at birth.

In simple virilizing CAH, affected patients are diagnosed as virilized newborn females or as rapidly growing masculinized boys at 3 to 7 years of age. Diagnosis is based on basal levels of the substrate for 21-hydroxylase, 17-OHP; in cases of congenital adrenal hyperplasia caused by 21-hydroxylase deficiency and in milder forms of the disorder with manifestations later in life (acquired, late onset, or adult-onset adrenal hyperplasia), diagnosis depends on basal and ACTH-stimulated levels of 17-OHP.

Patients with morning follicular phase 17-OHP levels of less than 300 ng/dL (10 nmol/L) are likely unaffected. When levels are greater than 300 ng/dL, but less than 10,000 ng/dL (300 nmol/L), ACTH testing should be performed to distinguish between 21-hydroxylase deficiency and other enzyme defects or to make the diagnosis in borderline cases. Levels greater than 10,000 ng/dL (300 nmol/L) are virtually diagnostic of congenital adrenal hyperplasia.

Nonclassic Adult Onset Congenital Adrenal Hyperplasia

The nonclassic type of 21-hydroxylase deficiency represents partial deficiency in 21-hydroxylation, which produces a late-onset, milder hyperandrogenemia. Its occurrence depends on some degree of functional deficit resulting from mutations affecting both alleles for the 21-hydroxylase enzyme. Heterozygote carriers for mutations in the 21-hydroxylase enzyme will demonstrate normal basal and modestly elevated stimulated levels of 17-OHP, but no abnormalities in circulating androgens. Some women with mild gene defects in both alleles demonstrate modest elevations in circulating 17-OHP concentrations, but no clinical symptoms or signs.

The hyperandrogenic symptoms of AOAH are mild and typically present at or after puberty. The three phenotypic varieties are (174):

1. Those with ovulatory abnormalities and features consistent with PCOS (39%)
2. Those with hirsutism alone without oligomenorrhea (39%)
3. Those with elevated circulating androgens but without symptoms (cryptic) (22%).

Precocious puberty reveals late-onset congenital adrenal hyperplasia in 5% to 20% of cases that mainly are caused by nonclassic 21-hydroxylase deficiency.

Measurement of 17-OHP should be performed in patients presenting with precocious puberty, and a subsequent ACTH stimulation test is recommended if basal 17-OHP is greater than 200 ng/dL.

The need for screening patients with hirsutism for adult-onset adrenal hyperplasia depends on the patient population. The frequency of some form of the disorder varies by ethnicity and is estimated at 0.1% of the general population, 1% to 2% of Hispanics and Yugoslavs, and 3% to 4% of Ashkenazi Jews (175).

Genetics of 21-Hydroxylase Deficiency

1. The 21-hydroxylase gene is located on the short arm of chromosome 6, in the midst of the HLA region.
2. The 21-hydroxylase gene is now termed *CYP21*. Its homologue is the pseudogene *CYP21P* (176).
3. Because *CYP21P* is a pseudogene, the lack of transcription renders it nonfunctional. The *CYP21* is the active gene.
4. The *CYP21* gene and the *CYP21P* pseudogene alternate with two genes called *C4B* and *C4A*, both of which encode for the fourth component (C4) of serum complement (176).
5. The close linkage between the 21-hydroxylase genes and HLA alleles allowed the study of 21-hydroxylase inheritance patterns in families through blood HLA typing (e.g., linkage of HLA-B14 was found in Ashkenazi Jews, Hispanics, and Italians) (177).

Prenatal Diagnosis and Treatment

Women with congenital and adult-onset forms of the disorder are at a significant risk for having affected infants, owing to the high frequency of 21-hydroxylase mutations in the general population. This presents an important rationale for screening hyperandrogenic women for this disorder when they anticipate childbearing. **In families at risk for CAH and in instances where one partner expresses the congenital or adult onset form of the disease, first-trimester prenatal screening using chorionic villus sampling is advocated** (176). The fetal DNA is used for specific amplification of the *CYP21* gene using polymerase chain reaction (PCR) amplification (178). When the fetus is at risk for CAH, maternal *dexamethasone* treatment can suppress the fetal HPA axis and prevent genital virilization in affected females (179). The dose is 20 μg/kg in three divided doses administered as soon as pregnancy is recognized and no later than 9 weeks of gestation. This is done prior to performing chorionic villus sampling or amniocentesis in the second trimester. *Dexamethasone* crosses the placenta and suppresses ACTH in the fetus. If the fetus is determined to be an unaffected female or a male, treatment is discontinued. If the fetus is an affected female, *dexamethasone* therapy is continued.

The practice of prenatal *dexamethasone* treatment for women whose fetuses are at risk for CAH is controversial; seven of eight pregnancies will be treated with *dexamethasone* unnecessarily, albeit briefly, to prevent one case of ambiguous genitalia. The efficacy and safety of prenatal *dexamethasone* treatment is not established, and long-term follow-up data on the offspring of treated pregnancies are lacking (180).

Numerous studies in experimental animal models showed that prenatal *dexamethasone* exposure could impair somatic growth, brain development, and blood pressure regulation. A human study of 40 fetuses at risk for CAH who were treated prenatally with *dexamethasone* to prevent virilization of affected females reported long-term effects on neuropsychological functions and scholastic performance (179,181).

The 2010 Endocrine Society guidelines conclude that prenatal *dexamethasone* therapy should be pursued only through institutional review boards' approved protocols at centers capable of collecting sufficient outcome data (182).

11β-Hydroxylase Deficiency

In a small percentage of patients with CAH, hypertension, rather than mineralocorticoid deficiency, develops. The hypertension responds to corticosteroid replacement (183–186). Many of these patients have a deficiency in 11β-hydroxylase (184,185). In most populations, 11β-hydroxylase deficiency accounts for 5% to 8% of the cases of CAH, or 1 in 100,000 births (187). A much higher incidence, 1 in 5,000 to 7,000, was described in Moroccan Jewish immigrants (186).

Two 11β-hydroxylase isoenzymes are responsible for cortisol and aldosterone synthesis, respectively, CYP11-B1 and CYP11-B2. They are encoded by two genes on the middle of the long arm of chromosome 8 (187–189).

Inability to synthesize a fully functional 11β-hydroxylase enzyme causes a decrease in cortisol production, a compensatory increase in ACTH secretion, and increased production of androstenedione, 11-deoxycortisol, 11-deoxycorticosterone, and DHEA. The diagnosis of 11β-hydroxylase-deficient late-onset adrenal hyperplasia is determined when 11-deoxycortisol levels are higher than 25 ng/mL 60 minutes after ACTH(1–24) stimulation (190).

Patients with 11β-hydroxylase deficiency may present with either a classic pattern of the disorder or symptoms of a mild deficiency. The severe classic form is found in about two-thirds of the patients with mild-to-moderate hypertension during the first years of life. In about one-third of the patients it is associated with left ventricular hypertrophy, with or without retinopathy, and occasionally death is reported from cerebrovascular accident (183). Signs of androgen excess are common in the severe form and are similar to those seen in the 21-hydroxylase deficiency.

In the mild, nonclassic form, children have virilization or precocious puberty but not hypertension. Adult women will seek treatment for postpubertal onset of hirsutism, acne, and amenorrhea.

3β-Hydroxysteroid Dehydrogenase Deficiency

Deficiency of 3β-hydroxysteroid dehydrogenase occurs with varying frequency in hirsute patients (191,192). The enzyme is found in both the adrenal glands and ovaries (unlike 21- and 11-hydroxylase) and is responsible for transforming Δ-5 steroids into the corresponding Δ-4 compounds, a step integral to the synthesis of glucocorticoids, mineralocorticoids, and testosterone and estradiol. In severe forms, cortisol and mineralocorticoids are deficient. The clinical spectrum of 3β-hydroxysteroid dehydrogenase deficiency ranges from the classic salt wasting, hypogonadism, and ambiguous genitalia in males and females, to nonclassic hyperandrogenic symptoms in children and young women (193). In mild forms, elevated ACTH levels overcome these critical deficiencies, and the diagnosis of this disorder relies on the relationship of Δ-5 and Δ-4 steroids. A marked elevation of DHEA and DHEAS in the presence of normal, or mildly elevated, testosterone or androstenedione can suggest the initiation of a screening protocol for 3β-hydroxysteroid dehydrogenase deficiency using exogenous ACTH stimulation (191). Following intravenous administration of a 0.25-mg ACTH(1-24) bolus, within 60 minutes 17-hydroxypregnenolone levels rise significantly in women with 3β-hydroxysteroid dehydrogenase deficiency, compared with normal women (2,276 ng/dL compared with normal of 1,050 ng/dL). The mean poststimulation ratio between 17-hydroxypregnenolone and 17-OHP is markedly elevated (mean ratio of 11 compared with 3.4 in normal controls and 0.4 in 21-hydroxylase deficiency). The rarity of this disorder indicates that routine screening of hyperandrogenic patients is not justified (191,192).

Treatment of Adult-Onset Congenital Adrenal Hyperplasia

Many patients with congenital AOAH do not need treatment. Glucocorticoid treatment should be avoided in asymptomatic patients with AOAH because the potential adverse effects of glucocorticoids probably outweigh any benefits (180,182).

Glucocorticoid therapy is recommended only to reduce hyperandrogenism for those with significant symptoms. *Dexamethasone* and antiandrogen drugs (both cross the placenta) should be used with caution and in conjunction with oral contraceptives in adolescent girls and young women with signs of virilization or irregular menses. When fertility is desired, ovulation induction might be necessary, and a glucocorticoid that does not cross the placenta (e.g., *prednisolone* or *prednisone*) should be used (179).

Many patients who are undiagnosed but who actually have AOAH are treated with therapies for ovarian hyperandrogenism and/or PCOS, with progestins for endometrial regulation, *clomiphene* or gonadotropins for ovulation induction, or progestins and antiandrogens for control of hirsutism. These therapies may be appropriate, as an alternative to glucocorticoid therapy, even when AOAH is recognized as the cause for the patient's symptoms.

Androgen-Secreting Ovarian and Adrenal Tumors

Patients with severe hirsutism, virilization, or recent and rapidly progressing signs of androgen excess require careful investigation for the presence of an androgen-secreting neoplasm. The two most common sources of androgen-secreting tumors are the adrenal glands and the ovaries. To assess the symptoms, serum and urine tests for androgens and their metabolites should be obtained along with modern abdominal imaging techniques such as CT, MRI, and ultrasound scans (194). In prepubertal girls, virilizing tumors may cause signs of heterosexual precocious puberty in addition to hirsutism, acne, and virilization. In patients suspected of harboring an adrenal or ovarian tumor because of rapidly progressing or severe hyperandrogenism, the bioavailable testosterone level (free testosterone level above 6.85 pg/mL; 23.6 pmol/L), followed by an 11-desoxycortisol (above 7 ng/mL; 20.2 nmol/L), DHEAS (>3.6 μg/mL) and a 24-hour urinary cortisol (>45 μg per day) are the most sensitive and specific for the detection of an androgen-secreting adrenocortical tumor (Table 31.3). A markedly elevated free testosterone level (2.5 times the upper normal range) is considered typical of an adrenal androgen-secreting tumor, while moderately elevated free testosterone levels are often ovarian in origin. A DHEAS level greater than 800 μg/dL is typical of an adrenal tumor. An adrenal tumor is unlikely when serum DHEAS and urinary 17-ketosteroid excretion measurements are in the normal basal range and the serum cortisol concentration is less than 3.3 μg/dL after *dexamethasone* administration (195). The results of other dynamic tests, especially testosterone suppression and stimulation, are unreliable (196).

A vaginal and abdominal ultrasonographic examination is the first step in the evaluation of findings suggesting ovarian neoplasm. Duplex Doppler scanning may increase the accuracy of tumor diagnosis and localization (197).

CT scanning can reveal tumors larger than 10 mm (1 cm) in the adrenal gland but may not help to distinguish among different types of solid tumors or benign incidental nodules (198). In the ovaries, CT scanning cannot help differentiate hormonally active from functional tumors (197,198).

MRI is comparable, if not superior, to CT scanning in detecting ovarian neoplasms, but is neither more sensitive than high-quality ultrasound nor more useful in clinical decision making when ultrasound identifies a likely neoplasm. Nuclear medicine imaging of the abdomen and pelvis after injection with NP-59 ((131-iodine) 6-beta-iodomethyl-19-norcholesterol), preceded by adrenal and thyroid suppression, may facilitate tumor localization. In the rare circumstances when imaging fails to provide clear evidence for a neoplastic source of excess androgens, selective venous catheterization with measurement of site-specific androgen levels to identify an occult source of for androgen excess may be utilized (199). If all four vessels are catheterized transfemorally, selective venous catheterization allows direct localization of the tumor. Samples are obtained for hormonal analysis, with positive localization defined as a 5:1 testosterone gradient compared with lower vena cava values (200). Under such circumstances specificity approaches 80%, but this rate should be weighed against the 5% rate of significant complications, such as adrenal hemorrhage and infarction, venous thrombosis, hematoma, and radiation exposure (201).

Androgen-Producing Ovarian Neoplasms

Ovarian neoplasms are the most frequent androgen-producing tumors. Granulosa cell tumors constitute 1% to 2% of all ovarian tumors and occur mostly in adult women (in postmenopausal more frequently than in premenopausal women) (see Chapter 37). Usually associated with estrogen production, they are the most common functioning tumors in children and can lead to isosexual precocious puberty (202). Patients can present with vaginal bleeding caused by endometrial hyperplasia or endometrial cancer resulting from prolonged exposure to tumor-derived estrogen (203). Total abdominal hysterectomy and bilateral salpingo-oophorectomy are the treatments of choice. If fertility is desired, a more conservative approach involving unilateral salpingo-oophorectomy with careful staging can be performed in women with stage IA (the cancer does not extend outside the involved ovary and a concomitant uterine cancer is excluded) (203). The malignant potential of these lesions is variable. The 10-year survival rates vary from 60% to 90%, depending on the stage, tumor size, and histologic atypia (202).

Thecomas are rare and occur in older patients. In one study only 11% were androgenic, even in the presence of steroid-type cells (luteinized thecomas) (202). They are unilateral in more than 90% of the cases and rarely malignant. A unilateral oophorectomy is adequate treatment (204).

Sclerosing stromal tumors are benign neoplasms that usually occur in patients younger than 30 years (202). A few cases with estrogenic or androgenic manifestations were reported.

Sertoli-Leydig cell tumors, previously classified as androblastoma or arrhenoblastoma, account for 11% of solid ovarian tumors. They contain various proportions of Sertoli cells, Leydig cells, and fibroblasts (202). Sertoli-Leydig cell tumors are the most common virilizing tumors in women of reproductive age; however, masculinization occurs in only one-third of patients. The tumor is bilateral in 1.5%. In 80% of cases, it is diagnosed at stage IA (202). Sertoli-Leydig cell tumors are frequently low-grade malignancies, and their prognosis is related to their degree of differentiation and stage of disease (205). Treatment with unilateral salpingo-oophorectomy is justified in patients with stage IA disease who desire fertility. Total abdominal hysterectomy, bilateral salpingo-oophorectomy, and adjuvant therapy are recommended for postmenopausal women who have advanced-stage disease.

Pure Sertoli cell tumors are usually unilateral. For a premenopausal woman with stage I disease, a unilateral salpingo-oophorectomy is the treatment of choice. Malignant tumors are rapidly fatal (206).

Gynandroblastomas are benign tumors with well-differentiated ovarian and testicular elements. A unilateral oophorectomy or salpingo-oophorectomy is sufficient treatment.

Sex cord tumors with annular tubules (SCTAT) are frequently associated with Peutz-Jeghers syndrome (gastrointestinal polyposis and mucocutaneous melanin pigmentation) (207). Their morphologic features range between those of the granulosa cell and Sertoli cell tumors.

Whereas SCTAT with Peutz-Jeghers syndrome tend to be bilateral and benign, SCTAT without Peutz-Jeghers syndrome is almost always unilateral and malignant in one-fifth of cases (202).

Steroid Cell Tumors

According to Young and Scully, **steroid cell tumors are composed entirely of steroid-secreting cells subclassified into stromal luteoma, Leydig cell tumors (hilar and nonhilar), and steroid cell tumors that are not otherwise specific** (202). Virilization or hirsutism is encountered with three-fourths of Leydig cell tumors, with one-half of steroid cell tumors not otherwise specific, and with 12% of stromal luteomas.

Nonfunctioning Ovarian Tumors

Ovarian neoplasms that do not directly secrete androgens are occasionally associated with androgen excess, resulting from excess secretion by adjacent ovarian stroma, and include serous and mucinous cystadenomas, Brenner tumors, Krukenberg tumors, benign cystic teratomas, and dysgerminomas (208). Gonadoblastomas arising in the dysgenetic gonads of patients with a Y chromosome are rarely associated with androgen and estrogen secretion (209,210).

Stromal Hyperplasia and Stromal Hyperthecosis

Stromal hyperplasia is a nonneoplastic proliferation of ovarian stromal cells. Stromal hyperthecosis is defined as the presence of luteinized stromal cells at a distance from the follicles (211). Stromal hyperplasia, which is typically seen in patients between 60 and 80 years of age, may be associated with hyperandrogenism, endometrial carcinoma, obesity, hypertension, and glucose intolerance (211,212). Hyperthecosis is seen in a mild form in older patients. In patients of reproductive age, hyperthecosis may demonstrate severe clinical manifestations of virilization, obesity, and hypertension (213). Hyperinsulinemia and glucose intolerance may occur in up to 90% of patients with hyperthecosis and may play a role in the etiology of stromal luteinization and hyperandrogenism (72). **Hyperthecosis is found in many patients with HAIR-AN syndrome (hyperandrogenemia, insulin resistance, and acanthosis nigricans).**

In patients with hyperthecosis, levels of ovarian androgens, including testosterone, DHT, and androstenedione, are increased, usually in the male range. The predominant estrogen, as in PCOS, is estrone, which is derived from peripheral aromatization. The E1-to-E2 ratio is increased. Unlike in PCOS, gonadotropin levels are normal (214). Ovaries with stromal hyperthecosis have variable sonographic appearances (215).

Wedge resection for the treatment of mild hyperthecosis was successful and resulted in resumption of ovulation and in a pregnancy (216). In cases of more severe hyperthecosis and high total testosterone levels, the ovulatory response to wedge resection is transient (214). In a study in which bilateral oophorectomy was used to control severe virilization, hypertension and glucose intolerance sometimes disappeared (217). When a GnRH agonist was used to treat patients with severe hyperthecosis, ovarian androgen production was dramatically suppressed (218).

Virilization During Pregnancy

Luteomas of pregnancy are frequently associated with maternal and fetal masculinization. This is not a true neoplasm but rather a reversible hyperplasia, which usually regresses postpartum. A review of the literature reveals a 30% incidence of maternal virilization and a 65% incidence of virilized female newborns in the presence of a pregnancy luteoma and maternal masculinization (219–221).

Other tumors causing virilization in pregnancy include (in descending order of frequency) Krukenberg tumors, mucinous cystic tumors, Brenner tumors, serous cystadenomas, endodermal sinus tumors, and dermoid cysts (202).

Virilizing Adrenal Neoplasms

The most common virilizing adrenal neoplasms are adrenal carcinomas. Adrenocortical carcinomas are rare aggressive tumors that have a bimodal age incidence, with most cases presenting at ages 40 to 50 years (222). Virilization was reported in 20% to 30% of adults with functional adrenocortical carcinoma (223).

When these malignancies virilize, frequently they are associated with elevations in 11-deoxycortisol, cortisol, and DHEAS. These tumors are commonly large and often detectable on abdominal examination. Adrenal tumors that secrete androgens exclusively, whether benign or malignant, are extraordinarily rare (194,224). Modern imaging techniques, such as CT, ultrasonography, MRI, or venous sampling, are extremely useful for distinguishing between an ovarian and an adrenal tumor as a cause of virilization (222).

Prolactin Disorders

Prolactin was first identified as a product of the anterior pituitary in 1933 (225). It is found in nearly every vertebrate species. Its presence in humans was long inferred by the association of the syndrome of amenorrhea and galactorrhea in the presence of pituitary macroadenomas, though it was not definitively identified as a human hormone until 1971. The specific activities of human prolactin (hPRL) were defined by the separation of its activity from growth hormone and subsequently by the development of radioimmunoassays (226–228). **Although the initiation and maintenance of lactation is the primary function of prolactin, many studies document roles for prolactin activity both within and beyond the reproductive system.**

Prolactin Secretion

There are 199 amino acids within human prolactin, with a molecular weight (MW) of 23,000 D (Fig. 31.8). Although human growth hormone and placental lactogen have significant lactogenic activity, they have only a 16% and 13% amino acid sequence homology with prolactin, respectively. In the human genome, a single gene on chromosome 6 encodes prolactin. The prolactin gene (10 kb) has five exons and four introns, and its transcription is regulated in the pituitary by a proximal promotor region and in extrapituitary locations by a more upstream promotor (229).

In the basal state three forms are released: a monomer, a dimer, and a multimeric species, called little, big, and big-big prolactin, respectively (230–232). The two larger species can be degraded to the monomeric form by reducing disulfide bonds (233). The proportions of each of these prolactin species vary with physiologic, pathologic, and hormonal stimulation (233–236). The heterogeneity of secreted forms remains an active area of research. Studies indicate that little

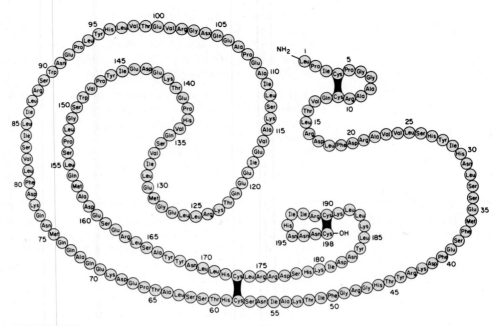

Figure 31.8   Amino acid sequence of prolactin. Three cysteine disulfide bands are located within the molecule. (From **Bondy PK.** *Rosenberg leukocyte esterase: metabolic control and disease,* 8th ed. Philadelphia: WB Saunders, 1980, with permission.)

prolactin (MW 23,000 D) constitutes more than 50% of all combined prolactin production and is most responsive to extrapituitary stimulation or suppression (233,235,236). **Clinical assays for prolactin measure the little prolactin, and in all but extremely rare circumstances, these measures are sufficient to assess diseases of abnormal pituitary production of the hormone.** Prolactin, and its relatives growth hormone and placental lactogen, do not require glycosylation for most of their primary activities, as is the case for the gonadotropins and TSH. Glycosylated forms are secreted, and glycosylation does affect the bioactivity and immunoreactivity of little prolactin (237–240). It appears that the glycosylated form is the predominant species secreted, but the most potent biologic form appears to be the 23,000-D nonglycosylated form of prolactin (239). Prolactin has over 300 known biological activities. Prolactin's most recognized activities include those associated with reproduction (lactation, luteal function, reproductive behavior) and homeostasis (immune responsivity, osomoregulation, and angiogenesis) (241). Despite these many activities, **the only recognized disorder associated with deficiency of prolactin secretion is inability to lactate.**

To some degree, the physical heterogeneity of prolactin may explain the biologic heterogeneity of this hormone, and although this complicates the physiologic evaluation of prolactin's myriad effects, it is of little import to the diagnosis and management of hyperprolactinemic states.

In contrast to other anterior pituitary hormones, which are controlled by hypothalamic-releasing factors, prolactin secretion is primarily under inhibitory control mediated by dopamine. **Multiple lines of evidence suggest that dopamine, which is secreted by the tuberoinfundibular dopaminergic neurons into the portal hypophyseal vessels, is the primary prolactin-inhibiting factor.** Dopamine receptors were found on pituitary lactotrophs, and treatment with dopamine or dopamine agonists suppresses prolactin secretion (242–248). The dopamine antagonist *metoclopramide* abolishes the pulsatility of prolactin release and increases serum prolactin levels (244,245,249). **Interference with dopamine transit from the hypothalamus to the pituitary by mass lesions, or blockade of the dopamine receptor as occurs with antipsychotic and other medications, increases serum prolactin levels.** Thyrotropin-releasing hormone (TRH) causes prolactin release when present at supraphysiologic levels (as in primary hypothyroidism), but does not appear to play an important modulatory role in the normal physiologic regulation of prolactin secretion. γ-Aminobutyric acid (GABA) and other neurohormones and neurotransmitters may function as prolactin-inhibiting factors (250–253). Several hypothalamic polypeptides that modulate prolactin-releasing activity are listed in Table 31.9. It appears that dopamine and

Table 31.9 Chemical Factors Modulating Prolactin Release and Conditions that Result in Hyperprolactinemia

Inhibitory factors

Dopamine

γ-Aminobutyric acid

Histidyl-proline diketopiperazine

Pyroglutamic acid

Somatostatin

Stimulatory factors

β-Endorphin

17β-Estradiol

Enkephalins

Gonadotropin-releasing hormone

Histamine

Serotonin

Substance P

Thyrotropin-releasing hormone

Vasoactive intestinal peptide

Physiologic conditions

Anesthesia

Empty sella syndrome

Idiopathic

Intercourse

Major surgery and disorders of chest wall (burns, herpes, chest percussion)

Newborns

Nipple stimulation

Pregnancy

Postpartum (nonnursing: days 1–7; nursing: with suckling)

Sleep

Stress

Postpartum

Hypothalamic conditions

Arachnoid cyst

Craniopharyngioma

Cystic glioma

Cysticercosis

Dermoid cyst

Epidermoid cyst

Histiocytosis

Neurotuberculosis

(*Continued*)

Table 31.9 *Continued*
Pineal tumors
Pseudotumor cerebri
Sarcoidosis
Suprasellar cysts
Tuberculosis
Pituitary conditions
Acromegaly
Addison disease
Craniopharyngioma
Cushing syndrome
Hypothyroidism
Histiocytosis
Lymphoid hypophysitis
Metastatic tumors (especially of the lungs and breasts)
Multiple endocrine neoplasia
Nelson syndrome
Pituitary adenoma (microadenoma or macroadenoma)
Post—oral contraception
Sarcoidosis
Thyrotropin-releasing hormone administration
Trauma to stalk
Tuberculosis
Metabolic dysfunction
Ectopic production (hypernephroma, bronchogenic sarcoma)
Hepatic cirrhosis
Renal failure
Starvation refeeding
Drug conditions
α *Methyldopa*
Antidepressants (*amoxapine, imipramine, amitriptyline*)
Cimetidine
Dopamine antagonists (phenothiazines, thioxanthenes, *butyrophenone, diphenylbutylpiperidine, dibenzoxazepine, dihydroindolone, procainamide, metoclopramide*)
Estrogen therapy
Opiates
Reserpine
Sulpiride
Verapamil

TRH act as primary neurohormones, while others (i.e., neuropeptide Y, galanin, and enkephalin) act as modulators. It is likely that under differing physiologic conditions (i.e., pregnancy, lactation, stress, aging) a modulator may become a principal regulator of hormone secretion.

The prolactin receptor is a member of the class 1 cytokine receptor superfamily and is encoded by a gene on chromosome 5 (254). Transcriptional regulation of the prolactin receptor is accomplished through three tissue-specific promoter regions; promoter I for the gonads, promoter II for the liver, and promoter III, a generic promoter that includes the mammary gland (255).

Hyperprolactinemia

Physiologic disturbances, pharmacologic agents, or markedly compromised renal function may cause elevations in prolactin levels, and transient elevations occur with acute stress or painful stimuli. The most common cause of elevated prolactin levels is likely pharmacologic; most patients using antipsychotic medications and many other patients using agents with antidopaminergic properties will exhibit moderately elevated prolactin levels. Drug-related and physiologic conditions resulting in hyperprolactinemia do not always require direct intervention to normalize prolactin levels.

Evaluation

Plasma levels of immunoreactive prolactin are 5 to 27 ng/mL throughout the normal menstrual cycle. Samples should not be drawn soon after the patient awakes or after procedures. Prolactin is secreted in a pulsatile fashion with a pulse frequency ranging from about 14 pulses per 24 hours in the late follicular phase to about 9 pulses per 24 hours in the late luteal phase. There also is a diurnal variation, with the lowest levels occurring in midmorning. Levels rise 1 hour after the onset of sleep and continue to rise until peak values are reached between 5 and 7 a.m. (256,257). The pulse amplitude of prolactin appears to increase from early to late follicular and luteal phases (258–260). Because of the variability of secretion and inherent limitations of radioimmunoassay, an elevated level should always be rechecked. This sample preferably is drawn midmorning and not after stress, previous venipuncture, breast stimulation, or physical examination, all of which transiently increase prolactin levels.

When prolactin levels are found to be elevated, hypothyroidism and medications should first be ruled out as a cause. Prolactin and TSH determinations are basic evaluations in infertile women. Infertile men with hypogonadism should be tested. Likewise, prolactin levels should be measured in the evaluation of amenorrhea, galactorrhea, hirsutism with amenorrhea, anovulatory bleeding, and delayed puberty (Fig. 31.9).

Physical Signs

Elevations in prolactin may cause amenorrhea, galactorrhea, both, or neither. Amenorrhea without galactorrhea is associated with hyperprolactinemia in approximately 15% of women (261–263). The cessation of normal ovulatory processes resulting from elevated prolactin levels is primarily caused by the suppressive effects of prolactin, via hypothalamic mediation, on GnRH pulsatile release (243,261,262,264–272). In addition to causing a hypogonadotropic state, prolactin elevations may secondarily impair the mechanisms of ovulation by causing a reduction in granulosa cell number and FSH binding, inhibition of granulosa cell 17β-estradiol production by interfering with FSH action, and by causing inadequate luteinization and reduced luteal secretion of progesterone (273–278). Other etiologies for amenorrhea are detailed in Chapter 30.

Although isolated galactorrhea is considered indicative of hyperprolactinemia, prolactin levels are within the normal range in nearly 50% of such patients (279–281) (Fig. 31.9). In these cases, whether caused by a prior transient episode of hyperprolactinemia or other unknown factors, the sensitivity of the breast to the lactotrophic stimulus engendered by normal prolactin levels is sufficient to result in galactorrhea. This situation is very similar to that observed in nursing mothers in whom milk secretion, once established, continues and even increases despite progressive normalization of prolactin levels. Repeat testing is occasionally helpful in detecting hyperprolactinemia. **Approximately one-third of women with galactorrhea have normal menses. Conversely, hyperprolactinemia commonly occurs in the absence of galactorrhea (66%), which may result from inadequate estrogenic or progestational priming of the breast.**

In patients with both galactorrhea and amenorrhea (including the syndromes described and named by Forbes, Henneman, Griswold, and Albright in 1951, Argonz and del Castilla in 1953, and Chiari and Frommel in 1985), **approximately two-thirds will have hyperprolactinemia;**

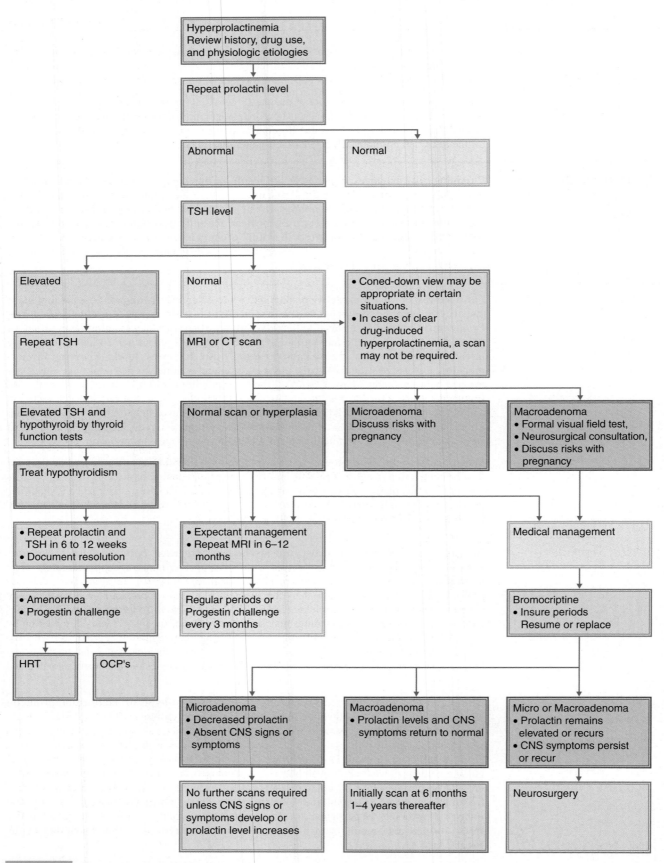

Figure 31.9 **Workup for hyperprolactinemia.** TSH, thyroid-stimulating hormone; MRI, magnetic resonance imaging; CT, computed tomography; HRT, hormone replacement therapy; OCPs, oral contraceptive pills; CNS, central nervous system.

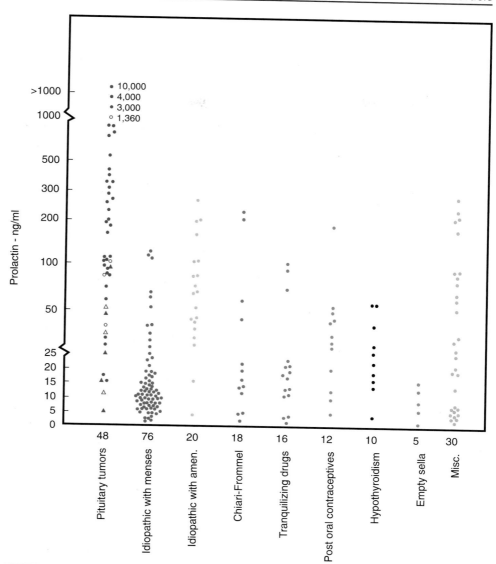

Figure 31.10   Prolactin levels in 235 patients with galactorrhea. Among patients with a tumor, open triangles denote associated acromegaly, and solid circles and solid triangles denote previous radiotherapy or surgical resection, respectively. (From **Kleinberg DL, Noel GL, Frantz AG.** Galactorrhea: a study of 235 cases, including 48 with pituitary tumors. *N Engl J Med* 1977;296:589–600, with permission.)

in that group, approximately one-third will have a pituitary adenoma (282). In anovulatory women, 3% to 10% of women diagnosed with polycystic ovary disease have coexistent and usually modest hyperprolactinemia (283,284) (Fig. 31.10).

Prolactin and TSH levels should be measured in all patients with delayed puberty. Pituitary abnormalities, including craniopharyngiomas and adenomas, should be considered in all cases of delayed puberty accompanied by low levels of gonadotropins, regardless of whether prolactin levels are elevated. When prolactin-secreting pituitary adenomas are present, the condition of multiple endocrine neoplasia type 1 (MEN-1) syndrome (gastrinomas, insulinoma, parathyroid hyperplasia, and pituitary neoplasia) should be considered, although symptoms of pituitary adenoma are rarely the presenting symptom. Patients who have a pituitary adenoma and a family history of multiple adenomas warrant special attention (285). Prolactinomas are noted in approximately 20% of patients with MEN-1. The *MEN-1* gene is localized to chromosome 11q13 and appears to act as a constitutive tumor suppressor gene. An inactivating mutation results in development of the tumor. It is thought that prolactin-secreting pituitary adenomas that occur in patients with MEN-1 may be more aggressive than sporadic cases (286).

When an elevated prolactin level is documented and medications or hypothyroidism as the underlying cause is excluded, knowledge of neuroanatomy and imaging techniques and their interpretation is essential to further evaluation (see Chapter 7). **Pituitary hyperprolactinemia is most often caused by a microadenoma or associated with normal imaging findings. These patients can be reassured that the probable course of their condition is benign. Macroadenomas or juxtasellar lesions are less common and require more complex evaluation and treatment, including surgery, radiation, or both.** Levels of TSH should be measured in all patients with hyperprolactinemia (Fig. 31.9).

Imaging Techniques

In patients with larger microadenomas and macroadenomas, prolactin levels usually are higher than 100 ng/mL. However, levels lower than 100 ng/mL may be associated with smaller microadenomas, macroadenomas that produce a "stalk section" effect, and suprasellar tumors that may be missed on a "coned-down" view of the sella turcica. Modest elevations of prolactin can be associated with microadenomas or macroadenomas, nonlactotroph pituitary tumors, and other central nervous system abnormalities; thus, imaging of the pituitary gland must be considered when otherwise unexplained and persistent prolactin elevation is present. **In patients with a clearly identifiable drug-induced or physiologic hyperprolactinemia, imaging is not necessary unless accompanied by symptoms suggesting a mass lesion (headache, visual field deficits).** MRI with gadolinium enhancement of the sella and pituitary gland appears to provide the best anatomic detail (287). The cumulative radiation dose from multiple CT scans may cause cataracts, and the "coned-down" views or tomograms of the sella are very insensitive and expose the patient to radiation. For patients with hyperprolactinemia who desire future fertility, MRI is indicated to differentiate a pituitary microadenoma from a macroadenoma and to identify other potential sellar-suprasellar masses. Although rare, when pregnancy-related complications of a pituitary adenoma occur, they occur more frequently in the presence of macroadenomas.

In over 90% of untreated women, microadenomas do not enlarge over a 4- to 6-year period. The argument that medical therapy will prevent a microadenoma from growing is false. Although prolactin levels correlate with tumor size, both elevations and reductions in prolactin levels may occur without any change in tumor size. If during follow-up a prolactin level rises significantly or central nervous system symptoms (headache, visual changes) are noted, repeat imaging may be indicated. Treatment is discussed below.

Hypothalamic Disorders

Dopamine was the first of many substances whose production was demonstrated in the arcuate nucleus. Dopamine-releasing neurons innervate the external zone of the median eminence. When released into the hypophyseal portal system, dopamine inhibits prolactin release in the anterior pituitary. Lesions that disrupt dopamine release can result in hyperprolactinemia. Such lesions may arise from the suprasellar area, pituitary gland, and infundibular stalk, and from adjacent bone, brain, cranial nerves, dura, leptomeninges, nasopharynx, and vessels. Numerous pathologic entities and physiologic conditions in the hypothalamic–pituitary region can disrupt dopamine release and cause hyperprolactinemia.

Pituitary Disorders

Microadenoma

In over one-third of women with hyperprolactinemia, a radiologic abnormality consistent with a microadenoma (<1 cm) is found. Release of pituitary stem cell growth inhibition via activation or loss-of-function mutations results in cell cycle dysregulation and is critical to the development of pituitary microadenomas and macroadenomas. Microadenomas are monoclonal in origin. Genetic mutations are thought to release stem cell growth inhibitors and result in autonomous anterior pituitary hormone production, secretion, and cell proliferation. Additional anatomic factors that may contribute to adenoma formation include reduced dopamine concentrations in the hypophyseal portal system and vascular isolation of the tumor or both. Recently, the heparin-binding secretory-transforming (*HST*) gene was noted in a variety of cancers and in prolactinomas (288). Patients with microadenomas can be reassured of a probable benign course, and many of these lesions exhibit gradual spontaneous regression (289,290).

Both microadenomas and macroadenomas are monoclonal in origin. Pituitary prolactinomas and lactotrope adenomas are sparsely or densely granulated histologically. The sparsely granulated lactotrope adenomas have trabecular, papillary, or solid patterns. Calcification of these tumors may take the form of a psammoma body or a pituitary stone. Densely granulated lactotrope adenomas are strongly acidophilic tumors and appear to be more aggressive than sparsely granulated lactotrope adenomas. Unusual acidophil stem cell adenomas can be associated with hyperprolactinemia, with some clinical or biochemical evidence of growth hormone excess.

Microadenomas rarely progress to macroadenomas. Six large series of patients with microadenomas reveal that, with no treatment, the risk of progression for microadenoma to a macroadenoma is only 7% (291). Treatments include expectant, medical, or, rarely, surgical therapy. All affected women should be advised to notify their physicians of chronic headaches, visual disturbances (particularly tunnel vision consistent with bitemporal hemianopsia), and extraocular muscle palsies. Formal visual field testing is rarely helpful, unless imaging suggests compression of the optic nerves.

Autopsy and radiographic series reveal that 14.4% to 22.5% of the US population harbor microadenomas, and approximately 25% to 40% stain positively for prolactin (292). Clinically significant pituitary tumors requiring some type of intervention affect only 14 per 100,000 individuals (292)

Expectant Management   **In women who do not desire fertility, expectant management can be used for both microadenomas and hyperprolactinemia without an adenoma while menstrual function remains intact.** Hyperprolactinemia-induced estrogen deficiency, rather than prolactin itself, is the major factor in the development of osteopenia (293). Therefore, **estrogen replacement with typical hormone replacement regimens or hormonal contraceptives is indicated for patients with amenorrhea or irregular menses. Patients with drug-induced hyperprolactinemia can be managed expectantly with attention to the risks of osteoporosis. In the absence of symptoms of pituitary enlargement, imaging may be repeated in 12 months, and if prolactin levels remain stable, less frequently thereafter, to assess further growth of the microadenoma.**

Medical Treatment   Ergot alkaloids are the mainstay of therapy. In 1985, *bromocriptine* was approved for use in the United States to treat hyperprolactinemia caused by a pituitary adenoma. These agents act as strong dopamine agonists, thus decreasing prolactin levels. Effects on prolactin levels occur within hours, and lesion size may decrease within 1 or 2 weeks. *Bromocriptine* decreases prolactin synthesis, DNA synthesis, cell multiplication, and overall size of prolactinomas. *Bromocriptine* treatment results in normal prolactin blood levels or return of ovulatory menses in 80% to 90% of patients.

Because ergot alkaloids, like *bromocriptine,* are excreted via the biliary tree, caution is required when using it in the presence of liver disease. The major adverse effects include nausea, headaches, hypotension, dizziness, fatigue and drowsiness, vomiting, headaches, nasal congestion, and constipation. **Many patients tolerate *bromocriptine* when the dose is increased gradually, by 1.25 mg (one-half tablet) daily each week until prolactin levels are normal or a dose of 2.5 mg twice daily is reached. A proposed regimen is as follows: one-half tablet every evening (1.25 mg) for 1 week, one-half tablet morning and evening (1.25 mg) during the second week, one-half tablet in the morning (1.25 mg) and a full tablet every evening (2.5 mg) during the third week, and one tablet every morning and every evening during the fourth week and thereafter (2.5 mg twice a day).** The lowest dose that maintains the prolactin level in the normal range is continued (1.25 mg twice daily often is sufficient to normalize prolactin levels in individuals with levels less than 100 ng/mL). Pharmacokinetic studies show peak serum levels occur 3 hours after an oral dose, with a nadir at 7 hours. Because little detectable *bromocriptine* is in the serum by 11 to 14 hours, twice-a-day administration is required. Prolactin levels can be checked soon (6 to 24 hours) after the last dose.

One rare, but notable, adverse effect of *bromocriptine* is a psychotic reaction. Symptoms include auditory hallucinations, delusional ideas, and changes in mood that quickly resolve after discontinuation of the drug (294).

Many investigators report no difference in fibrosis, calcification, prolactin immunoreactivity, or the surgical success in patients pretreated with *bromocriptine* compared to those not receiving *bromocriptine* (291).

An alternative to oral administration is the vaginal administration of *bromocriptine* tablets, which is well tolerated, and actually results in increased pharmacokinetic measures (295). *Cabergoline,* another ergot alkaloid, has a very long half-life and can be given orally twice per week. Its long duration of action is attributable to slow elimination by pituitary tumor tissue, high affinity binding to pituitary dopamine receptors, and extensive enterohepatic recirculation.

Cabergoline, which appears to be as effective as *bromocriptine* in lowering prolactin levels and in reducing tumor size, has substantially fewer adverse effects than *bromocriptine.* Very rarely, patients experience nausea and vomiting or dizziness with *cabergoline;* they may be treated with intravaginal *cabergoline* as with *bromocriptine.* A gradually increasing dosage helps avoid the side effects of nausea, vomiting, and dizziness. *Cabergoline* at 0.25 mg twice per week is usually adequate for hyperprolactinemia with values less than 100 ng/mL. If required to normalize prolactin levels, the dosage can be increase by 0.25 mg per dose on a weekly basis to a maximum of 1 mg twice weekly.

Recent studies reveal an increased risk of cardiac valve regurgitation in patients with Parkinson disease who were treated with high doses of *cabergoline* or *pergolide* but not with *bromocriptine* (296,297). Higher doses and a longer duration of therapy were associated with a higher risk of valvulopathy. It is postulated that 5HT2b-receptor stimulation leads to fibromyoblast proliferation (298). A recent cross-sectional study showed a higher rate of asymptomatic tricuspid regurgitation among *cabergoline*-treated patients compared to untreated patients with newly diagnosed prolactinomas as well as normal controls (299,300).

The demonstrated relative safety of *bromocriptine* in reproductive-aged women and during more than 2,500 pregnancies suggest *bromocriptine* is the first choice for hyperprolactinemia and micro- and macroadenomas (301).

When *bromocriptine* or *cabergoline* cannot be used, other medications such as *pergolide* or *metergoline* may be used. In patients with a microadenoma who are receiving *bromocriptine* therapy, a repeat MRI scan may be performed 6 to 12 months after prolactin levels are normal, if indicated. Further MRI scans should be performed if new symptoms appear.

Discontinuation of *bromocriptine* therapy after 2 to 3 years may be attempted in a select group of patients who have maintained normoprolactinemia while on therapy (302,303). In a retrospective series of 131 patients treated with *bromocriptine* for a median of 47 months, normoprolactinemia was sustained in 21% at a median follow-up of 44 months after treatment discontinuation (303). Discontinuation of *cabergoline* therapy was successful in patients treated for 3 to 4 years who maintained normoprolactinemia (304). In *cabergoline* discontinuers who met stringent inclusion criteria, a recurrence rate of 64% was noted (305). A recent meta-analysis involving 743 patients noted sustained normoprolactinemia in only a minority of patients (21%) after discontinuation. Patients with 2 years or more of therapy before discontinuation and no demonstrable tumor visible on MRI had the highest chance of persistent normoprolactinemia (306). Recurrence rates are higher for macroadenomas (as compared to microadenomas or hyperprolactinemia without adenoma) after cessation of *bromocriptine* or *cabergoline,* warranting close follow-up with serum prolactin and MRI after cessation of therapy. In patients with macroadenomas, withdrawal of therapy should proceed with caution, as rapid tumor reexpansion may occur.

Macroadenomas

Macroadenomas are pituitary tumors that are larger than 1 cm in size. *Bromocriptine* is the best initial and potentially long-term treatment option, but transsphenoidal surgery may be required. High-dose *cabergoline* therapy was used in *bromocriptine* resistant or intolerant macroadenoma patients with success; however, cautions remain regarding the development of cardiac valve abnormalities (307).

Evaluation for pituitary hormone deficiencies may be indicated. Symptoms of macroadenoma enlargement include severe headaches, visual field changes, and, rarely, diabetes insipidus and blindness. After prolactin has reached normal levels following ergot alkaloid treatment, a repeat MRI is indicated within 6 months to document shrinkage or stabilization of the size of the macroadenoma. This examination may be performed earlier if new symptoms develop or if there is no improvement in previously noted symptoms.

Medical Treatment   Treatment with *bromocriptine* decreases prolactin levels and the size of macroadenomas; nearly one-half show a 50% reduction in size, and another one-fourth show a 33% reduction after 6 months of therapy. Because tumor regrowth occurs in more than 60% of cases after discontinuation of bromocriptine therapy, long-term therapy is usually required.

After stabilization of tumor size is documented, the MRI scan is repeated 6 months later and, if stable, yearly for several years. This examination may be performed earlier if new symptoms develop or if there is no improvement in symptoms. Serum prolactin levels are measured every 6 months. **Because tumors may enlarge despite normalized prolactin values, a reevaluation of symptoms at regular intervals (6 months) is prudent. Normalized prolactin levels or resumption of menses should not be taken as absolute proof of tumor response to treatment** (306,308).

Surgical Intervention   **Tumors that are unresponsive to *bromocriptine* or that cause persistent visual field loss require surgical intervention.** Some neurosurgeons have noted that a short (2- to 6-week) preoperative course of *bromocriptine* increases the efficacy of surgery in patients with larger adenomas (291). Unfortunately, despite surgical resection, recurrence of hyperprolactinemia and tumor growth is common. Complications of surgery include cerebral carotid artery injury, diabetes insipidus, meningitis, nasal septal perforation, partial or panhypopituitarism, spinal fluid rhinorrhea, and third nerve palsy. Periodic MRI scanning after surgery is indicated, particularly in patients with recurrent hyperprolactinemia.

Metabolic Dysfunction and Hyperprolactinemia

Occasionally, patients with hypothyroidism exhibit hyperprolactinemia with remarkable pituitary enlargement caused by thyrotroph hyperplasia. These patients respond to thyroid replacement therapy with reduction in pituitary enlargement and normalization of prolactin levels (309).

Hyperprolactinemia occurs in 20% to 75% of women with chronic renal failure. Prolactin levels are not normalized through hemodialysis but are normalized after transplantation (310–312). Occasionally, women with hyperandrogenemia also have hyperprolactinemia. Elevated prolactin levels may alter adrenal function by enhancing the release of adrenal androgens such as DHEAS (313).

Drug-Induced Hyperprolactinemia

Numerous drugs interfere with dopamine secretion and can be responsible for hyperprolactinemia and its attendant symptoms (Table 31.9). **If medication can be discontinued, resolution of hyperprolactinemia is uniformly prompt. If not, endocrine management should be directed at estrogen replacement and normalization of menses for those with disturbed or absent ovulation. Treatment with dopamine agonists may be utilized if ovulation is desired and the drug-inducing hyperprolactinemia cannot be discontinued.**

Use of Estrogen in Hyperprolactinemia

In rodents, pituitary prolactin-secreting adenomas occur with high-dose estrogen administration (314). Elevated levels of estrogen, as found in pregnancy, are responsible for hypertrophy and hyperplasia of lactotrophic cells and account for the progressive increase in prolactin levels in normal pregnancy. The increase in prolactin during pregnancy is physiologic and reversible; adenomas are not fostered by the hyperestrogemia of pregnancy. Pregnancy may have a favorable influence on preexisting prolactinomas (315,316). Estrogen administration is not associated with clinical, biochemical, or radiologic evidence of growth of pituitary microadenomas or the progression of idiopathic hyperprolactinemia to an adenoma status (317–320). **For these reasons, estrogen replacement or OC use is appropriate for hypoestrogenic patients with hyperprolactinemia secondary to microadenoma or hyperplasia.**

Monitoring Pituitary Adenomas During Pregnancy

Prolactin-secreting microadenomas rarely create complications during pregnancy. Monitoring of patients with serial gross visual field examinations and funduscopic examination is recommended. If persistent headaches, visual field deficits, or visual or funduscopic changes occur, MRI scanning is advisable. **Because serum prolactin levels progressively rise throughout pregnancy, prolactin measurements are rarely of value.**

For those women who become pregnant while taking *bromocriptine* to treat a return of spontaneous ovulations, discontinuation of *bromocriptine* is recommended. This does not preclude subsequent use of *bromocriptine* during the pregnancy to treat symptoms (visual field defects, headaches) that arise from further enlargement of the microadenoma (301,321–323).

Bromocriptine did not exhibit teratogenicity in animals, and observational data do not suggest harm to pregnancy or fetus in humans.

Pregnant women with previous transsphenoidal surgery for microadenomas or macroadenomas may be monitored with monthly Goldman perimetry visual field testing. Periodic MRI scanning may be necessary in women with symptoms or visual changes. **Breastfeeding is not contraindicated in the presence of microadenomas or macroadenomas** (301,321–323). The use of *bromocriptine* and presumably other dopaminergic agents that may cause blood pressure elevation during the postpartum period is contraindicated (324–328).

Thyroid Disorders

Thyroid disorders are 10 times more common in women than men. Approximately 1% of the female population of the United States will develop overt hypothyroidism (329). Even prior to the discovery of the long-acting thyroid stimulator (LATS) in women with Graves disease in 1956, numerous investigations demonstrated a link between these autoimmune thyroid disorders and reproductive physiology and pathology (330).

Thyroid Hormones

Iodide is a critical component of the class of hormones known as thyronines, among which the most important are triiodothyronine (T_3) and thyroxine (T_4). Iodide obtained from dietary sources is actively transported into the thyroid follicular cell for the synthesis of these hormones. The sodium–iodide symporter (NIS) is a key molecule in thyroid function. It allows the accumulation of iodide from the circulation into the thyrocyte against an electrochemical gradient. The NIS requires energy that is supplied by Na-K ATPase, and iodine uptake is stimulated by TSH or thyrotropin. The enzyme thyroid peroxidase (TPO) then oxidizes iodide near the cell-colloid surface and incorporates it into tyrosyl residues within the thyroglobulin molecule, which results in the formation of monoiodotyrosine (MIT) and diiodotyrosine (DIT). T_3 and T_4, formed by secondary coupling of MIT and DIT, are catalyzed by TPO. The membrane-bound, heme-containing oligomer, TPO, is localized in the rough endoplasmic reticulum, Golgi vesicles, lateral and apical vesicles, and on the follicular cell surface. Thyroglobulin, the major protein formed in the thyroid gland, has an iodine content of 0.1% to 1.1% by weight. About 33% of the iodine is present in thyroglobulin in the form of T_3 and T_4, and the remainder is present in MIT and DIT or found as unbound iodine. Thyroglobulin provides a storage capacity capable of maintaining a euthyroid state for nearly 2 months without the formation of new thyroid hormones. The thyroid antimicrosomal antibodies found in patients with autoimmune thyroid disease are directed against the TPO enzyme (331,332).

TSH regulates thyroidal iodine metabolism by activation of adenylate cyclase. This facilitates endocytosis as a component of iodide uptake, digestion of thyroglobulin-containing colloid, and the release of thyroid hormones T_4, T_3, and reverse T_3. T_4 is released from the thyroid at 40 to 100 times the concentration of T_3. The concentration of reverse T_3, which has no intrinsic thyroid activity, is 30% to 50% of T_3, and 1% of T_4 concentration. Of thyroid hormones released, 70% are bound by circulating thyroid-binding globulin (TBG). T_4 is present in higher concentrations in the circulating storage pool and has a slower turnover rate than T_3. Approximately 30% of T_4 is converted to T_3 in the periphery. Reverse T_3 participates in regulation of the conversion of T_4 to T_3. T_3 is the primary physiologically functional thyroid hormone at the cellular level. T_3 binds the nuclear receptor with 10 times the affinity of T_4. Thyroid hormone effects on cells include increased oxygen consumption, heat production, and metabolism of fats, proteins, and carbohydrates. Systemically, thyroid hormone activity is responsible for the basal metabolic rate. It balances fuel efficiency with performance. Hyperthyroid states result in excessive fuel consumption with marginal performance.

Iodide Metabolism

Normal function of the thyroid gland is dependent on iodine. The World Health Organization recommends 150 μg of iodine per day in women of reproductive age and 250 μg per day is recommended during pregnancy and nursing. Adequate iodination of household salt is defined as salt containing 15 to 40 mg of iodine per kilogram of salt (333).

Optimal iodine intake to prevent disease lies within a relatively narrow range around the recommended daily consumption. Extreme iodine deficiency states are associated with cretinism, goiter, and hypothyroidism, while iodine sufficiency is associated with autoimmune thyroid disease and reduced remission rates in Graves disease (334).

Risk Factors for Autoimmune Thyroid Disorders

Environmental factors associated with the occurrence of autoimmune thyroid diseases include pollutants (plasticizers, polychlorinated biphenyls) and exposure to infections such as yersinia enterocolitica, coxsackie B, *Helicobacter pylori,* and hepatitis C (335,336). For reasons not entirely known, women experience a 5- to 10-fold increased incidence of autoimmune thyroid disease (337). This difference is postulated to be the result of differences in sex steroid hormone levels, differences in environmental exposures, innate differences in female and male immune systems, and inherent chromosomal differences in the sexes (338,339). The immunoglobulins produced against the thyroid are polyclonal, and the multiple combinations of various antibodies consolidate to create the clinical spectrum of autoimmune thyroid diseases that may affect health and reproductive function.

Evaluation

Thyroid Function

Measurements of free serum T_4 and T_3 are complicated by the low levels of free hormone in systemic circulation, with only 0.02% to 0.03% of T_4 and 0.2% to 0.3% of T_3 circulating in the unbound state (340). Of the T_4 and T_3 in circulation, approximately 70% to 75% is bound to TBG, 10% to 15% attached to prealbumin, 10% to 15% bound to albumin, and a minor fraction (<5%) is bound to lipoprotein (340,341). Total thyroid measurements are dependent on levels of TBG, which are variable and affected by many conditions such as pregnancy, oral contraceptive pill use, estrogen therapy, hepatitis, and genetic abnormalities of TBG. Thus, assays for the measurement of free T_4 and T_3 are more clinically relevant than measuring total thyroid hormone levels.

There are many different laboratory techniques to measure estimated free serum T_4 and T_3. These methods invariably measure a portion of free hormone that is dissociated from the *in vivo* protein bound moiety. This is of little clinical significance assuming the same proportions are measured for all assays and considered in the calibration of the assay (342). The T_3 resin uptake test is an example of one laboratory method used to estimate free T_4 in the serum. **The T_3 resin uptake (T_3 RU) determines the fractional binding of radiolabeled T_3, which is added to a serum sample in the presence of a resin that competes with TBG for T_3 binding.** The binding capacity of TBG in the sample is inversely proportional to the amount of labeled T_3 bound to the artificial resin. Therefore, a low T_3 resin uptake indicates high TBG T_3 receptor site availability and implies high circulating TBG levels.

The free T_4 index (FTI) is obtained by multiplying the serum T_4 concentration by the T_3 resin uptake percentage, yielding an indirect estimate of the levels of free T_4:

$$T_3 \text{ RU\%} \times T_4 \text{ total} = \text{free } T_4 \text{ index}.$$

A high T_3 RU percentage indicates reduced TBG receptor site availability and high free T_4 index and thus hyperthyroidism, whereas a low T_3 resin uptake percentage is a result of increased TBG receptor site binding and thus hypothyroidism. Equilibrium dialysis and ultrafiltration techniques may be used to determine the free T_4 directly. Free T_4 and T_3 may also be determined by radioimmunoassay. Most available laboratory methods used for determining estimations of free T_4 are able to correct for moderate variations in serum TBG but are prone to error in the setting of large variations of serum TBG, when endogenous T_4 antibodies are present, and in the setting of inherent albumin abnormalities (340).

Because most disorders of hyperthyroidism and hypothyroidism are related to dysfunction of the thyroid gland and TSH levels are sensitive to excessive or deficient levels of circulating thyroid hormone, TSH levels are used to screen for these disorders. Current thyrotropin or TSH sandwich immunoassays are extremely sensitive and capable of differentiating low-normal from pathologic or iatrogenically subnormal values and elevations. TSH measurements provide the best way to screen for thyroid dysfunction and accurately predict thyroid hormone dysfunction in about 80% of cases (343). Reference values for TSH are traditionally based on the central 95% of values for healthy individuals, and some controversy exists regarding the upper limit of normal. Values in the upper limit of normal may predict future thyroid disease (342,344). In a longitudinal study, women with positive thyroid antibodies (TPOAbs or TgAbs), the prevalence of hypothyroidism at follow-up was 12.0% (3.0% to 21.0%; 95% CI) when baseline TSH was 2.5 mU/L or less, 55.2% (37.1%–73.3%) for TSH between 2.5 and 4.0 mU/L, and 85.7% (74.1%–97.3%) for TSH above 4.0 mU/L (345). Physicians ordering thyrotropin

Table 31.10 Thyroid Autoantigens

Antigen	Location	Function
Thyroglobulin (Tg)	Thyroid	Thyroid hormone storage
Thyroid peroxidase (TPO) (microsomal antigen)	Thyroid	Transduction of signal from TSH
TSH receptor (TSHR)	Thyroid, lymphocytes, fibroblasts, adipocytes (including retro-orbital), and cancers	Transduction of signal from TSH
Na^+/I^- symporter (NIS)	Thyroid, breast, salivary or lacrimal gland, gastric or colonic mucosa, thymus, pancreas	ATP-driven uptake of I^- along with Na^1

TSH, thyroid-stimulating hormone; ATP, adenosine triphosphate

values should be aware of their limitations in the setting of acute illness, central hypothyroidism, the presence of heterophile antibodies, and TSH autoantibodies. In the setting of heterophile antibodies or TSH autoantibodies, TSH values will be falsely elevated (342). In cases of central hypothyroidism, decreased sialylation of TSH results in a longer half-life and a reduction in bioactivity (346,347). TSH levels may be elevated or normal when the patient remains clinically hypothyroid in states of central hypothyroidism, and successful treatment is often associated with low or undetectable TSH levels.

Immunologic Abnormalities

Many antigen–antibody reactions affecting the thyroid gland can be detected. Antibodies to TgAb, the TSH receptor (TSHRAb), TPOAb, the sodium iodine symporter (NISAb), and to thyroid hormone were identified and implicated in autoimmune thyroid disease states (348). A number of recognized thyroid autoantigens are listed in Table 31.10. Antibody production to thyroglobulin depends on a breach in normal immune surveillance (349,350). The incidence of thyroid autoantibodies in various autoimmune thyroid disorders is shown in Table 31.11.

Antithyroglobulin antibodies are predominantly in the noncomplement fixing, polycolonal, immunoglobulin-G (IgG) class. Antithyroglobulin antibodies are found in 35% to 60% of patients with hypothyroid autoimmune thyroiditis, 12% to 30% of patients with Graves disease, and 3% of the general population (351–353). Antithyroglobulin antibodies are associated with acute thyroiditis, nontoxic goiter, and thyroid cancer (348).

Previously referred to as antimicrosomal antibodies, TPO antibodies are directed against thyroid peroxidase and are found in Hashimoto thyroiditis, Graves disease, and postpartum thyroiditis. The antibodies produced are characteristically cytotoxic, complement-fixing IgG antibodies. In patients with thyroid autoantibodies, 99% will have positive anti-TPO antibodies, whereas only 36% will have positive antithyroglobulin antibodies, making anti-TPO a more sensitive test for autoimmune thyroid disease (353). Anti-TPO antibodies are present in 80% to 99% of patients with hypothyroid autoimmune thyroiditis, 45% to 80% of patients with Graves disease, and 10% to 15% of the general population (352–354). These antibodies can cause artifact in the measurement of thyroid hormone levels. Antithyroid peroxidase antibodies are used clinically in

Table 31.11 Prevalence of Thyroid Autoantibodies and Their Role in Immunopathology

Antibody	General Population	Hypothyroid Autoimmune Thyroiditis	Graves Disease
Antithyroglobulin (TgAb)	3%	35%–60%	12%–30%
Antimicrosomal thyroid peroxidase (TPOAb)	10%–15%	80%–99%	45%–80%
Anti-TSH receptor (TSHRAb)	1%–2%	6%–60%	70%–100%
Anti-Na/I symporter (NISAb)	0%	25%	20%

TSH, thyroid-stimulating hormone.

Table 31.12 Nomenclature of Anti-TSH Receptor Antibodies

Abbreviation	Term	Assay Used	Refers To
LATS	Long-acting thyroid stimulator	In vivo assay of stimulation of mouse thyroid	Original description of serum molecule able to stimulate mouse thyroid; no longer used
TSHRAb, TRAb	TSHR antibodies	Competitive and functional assays described below	All antibodies recognizing the TSH receptor (includes TBII (competitive), and TSI, TBI and TNI (functional) based on assay method
TBII	TSHR-binding inhibitory immunoglobulin	Competitive binding assays with TSH	Antibodies able to compete with TSH for TSH receptor binding irrespective of biologic activity
TSI (also TSAb)	TSHR-stimulating immunoglobulins	Competitive and functional bioassays of TSH receptor activation	Antibodies able to block TSH receptor binding, induce cAMP production and nonclassical signaling cascades
TBI (also TSBAb, TSHBAb	TSHR stimulation-blocking antibodies	Functional bioassays of TSH receptor activation	Antibodies able to block TSH receptor binding, induce cAMP production with +/− effects on nonclassical cascades
TNI	TSHR nonbinding immunoglobulin	Binding and functional assays	No TSH binding, no effect on cAMP levels and variable effects on nonclassical cascades

TSH, thyroid-stimulating hormone.

the diagnosis of Graves disease, the diagnosis of chronic autoimmune thyroiditis, in conjunction with TSH testing as a means to predict future hypothyroidism in subclinical hypothyroidism, and to assist in the diagnosis of autoimmune thyroiditis in euthyroid patients with goiter or nodules (348).

Another group of antibodies important in autoimmune thyroid disease bind the TSH receptor (TSHR). The TSHR belongs to the family of G-protein coupled receptors. TSHRAb are pathogenic and capable of activating (TSI) or blocking (TBI) TSH receptor functions. TBIs are detectable in two varieties: those that block TSH binding and those that block both pre- and postreceptor processes. Several investigators detected such blocking antibodies in patients with primary hypothyroidism and atrophic thyroid glands (355,356). The nomenclature and detection assay of TSH receptor antibodies are listed in Table 31.12. Anti-TSH receptor antibodies were reported in 6% to 60% of patients with hypothyroid autoimmune thyroiditis, 70% to 100% of patients with Graves disease, and 1% to 2% of the general population (357–361). Untreated Graves disease patients tested with third-generation immunometric assays are uniformly positive (362). TSHRAb are classified as binding inhibitory immunoglobulins by competitive binding assays (TBII); and in functional assays: stimulating (TSI)—according to their capacity to increase cyclic adenosine monophosphate (cAMP) production; blocking (TBI)—which possesses the capacity to reduce TSH effects; and, neutral (TNI)—with no effect on TSH binding or alteration of cAMP levels. A number of competitive and functional assays are available to determine the levels of each antibody type, which, *in toto*, correlate with severity of disease, extraglandular signs, risk of fetal effects, and chances for remission and recurrence. TSHRAb are used clinically to distinguish postpartum thyroiditis from Graves disease, to predict the risk of fetal and neonatal thyrotoxicosis in women with prior ablative treatment or current thionamide therapy in the setting of Graves disease, and in the diagnosis of euthyroid Graves ophthalmopathy (348). These assays will increasingly optimize individual patient testing and treatment (363).

Antibodies to the NIS are prevalent in a number of thyroid conditions. Anti-NISAbs were detected in 24% of patients with Hashimoto disease and 22% of patients with Graves disease (364). Anti-NISAbs are used experimentally (348).

Autoimmune Thyroid Disease

The most common thyroid abnormalities in women, autoimmune thyroid disorders, represent the combined effects of the multiple thyroid autoantibodies (365). The various antigen–antibody reactions result in the wide clinical spectrum of these disorders. Transplacental transmission of some of these immunoglobulins may affect thyroid function in the fetus. **The presence of autoimmune thyroid disorders, particularly Graves disease, is associated with other autoimmune conditions: Hashimoto thyroiditis, Addison disease, ovarian failure, rheumatoid arthritis, Sjögren syndrome, diabetes mellitus (type 1), vitiligo, pernicious anemia, myasthenia gravis, and idiopathic thrombocytopenic purpura.** Other factors that are associated with the development of autoimmune thyroid disorders include low birth weight, iodine excess and deficiency, selenium deficiency, parity, oral contraceptive pill use, reproductive age span, fetal microchimerism, stress, seasonal variation, allergy, smoking, radiation damage to the thyroid, and viral and bacterial infections (366).

Recommendations for Testing and Treatment

Overt and subclinical hypothyroidism are defined as an elevated TSH with a low T_4 and an elevated TSH and normal T_4, respectively, using appropriate patient ranges (nonpregnant and pregnant). A number of professional organizations published various recommendations for thyroid function assessment via a TSH in women. Because of the long interval from development of disease to diagnosis, the nonspecific nature of symptoms, and the potential adverse neonatal and maternal outcomes associated with untreated hypothyroidism in pregnancy, the American Association of Clinical Endocrinologists (AACE) recommended screening women prior to conceiving or at the first prenatal appointment (367,368). The AACE also recommended screening for the presence of hypothyroidism in patients with type 1 diabetes mellitus (threefold increased risk of postpartum thyroid dysfunction and 33% prevalence overall), patients taking lithium therapy (35% prevalence), and consideration of testing in patients presenting with infertility (>12% prevalence) or depression (10% to 12% prevalence), as these populations are at an increased risk of hypothyroidism (368). A screening TSH was recommended in women starting at the age of 50 because of the increased prevalence of hypothyroidism in this population (369). Thyroid function testing at 6-month intervals was recommended for patients taking *amiodarone*, as hyperthyroidism or hypothyroidism occurs in 14% to 18% of these patients (368). Any woman with a history of postpartum thyroiditis should be offered annual surveillance of thyroid function, as 50% of these patients will develop hypothyroidism within 7 years of diagnosis (370). Because there is a high prevalence of hypothyroidism in women with Turner and Down syndromes, an annual check of thyroid function is recommended for these patients (371,372).

Alternatively, the Endocrine Society's clinical practice guidelines regarding the management of thyroid dysfunction during pregnancy and postpartum recommends **targeted screening for the following individuals: history of thyroid disorder, family history of thyroid disease, goiter, thyroid autoantibodies, clinical signs or symptoms of thyroid disease, autoimmune disorders, infertility, head and/or neck radiation, and preterm delivery** (373). **The American Congress of Obstetricians and Gynecologists accepted these recommendations for TSH testing** (374). **Because of the (i) potentially significant neurologic affects on the fetus and other adverse pregnancy events; (ii) physiologic rise in TBG and the TSH-like activity of hCG in pregnancy, and (iii) potential for the targeted screening groups to have overt or subclinical hypothyroidism defined by the reference ranges for pregnancy (TSH <2.5, 3.1, and 3.5 μIU/mL for the first, second, and third trimesters, respectively), targeted maternal testing for hypothyroidism is encouraged.** The targeted screening protocol allows that 30% of subclinical hypothyroidism cases may be missed. According to these recommendations, preconceptionally diagnosed hypothyroid women (overt or subclinical) should have their T_4 dosage adjusted such that the TSH value is less than 2.5 μIU/mL before pregnancy. The T_4 dosage in women already on replacement will routinely require a dose escalation (30% to 50%) at 4 to 6 weeks gestation in order to maintain a TSH value less than 2.5 μIU/mL. Pregnant women with overt hypothyroidism should be normalized as rapidly as possible to maintain TSH at less than 2.5 and 3 μIU/mL in the first, second, and third trimesters, respectively. Euthyroid women with thyroid autoantibodies are at risk of hypothyroidism and should have TSH screening in each trimester. After delivery, hypothyroid women need a reduction in T_4 dosage used during pregnancy. Because subclinical hypothyroidism is associated with adverse outcomes for mother and the fetus, T_4 replacement is recommended.

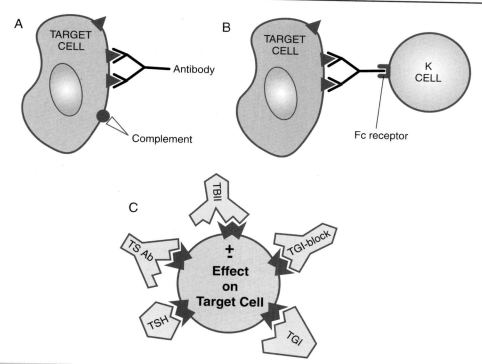

Figure 31.11   **Types of autoimmune injury found in Hashimoto thyroiditis.** **A:** Complement-mediated cytotoxicity, which can be abolished by inactivating the complement system. **B:** Antibody-dependent cell-mediated cytotoxicity (ADCC) function through killer T cells, monocytes, and natural killer cells that have immunoglobulin G fragment receptors. **C:** Stimulation of blockade of hormone receptors leading to hyperfunction or hypofunction or growth, depending on the types of immunoglobulins acting on the target cell. TBII, TSH-binding inhibitor immunoglobulin; TGI, thyroid growth–promoting immunoglobulin; TSAb, thyroid-stimulating antibodies; TSH, thyroid-stimulating hormone. (From **Coulam CB, Faulk WP, McIntyre JA.** *Immunologic obstetrics.* New York: Norton Medical Books, 1992:658, with permission.)

Hashimoto Thyroiditis

Hashimoto thyroiditis, or chronic lymphocytic thyroiditis, was first described in 1912 by Dr. Hakaru Hashimoto. Hashimoto thyroiditis can manifest as hyperthyroidism, hypothyroidism, euthyroid goiter, or diffuse goiter. High levels of antimicrosomal and antithyroglobulin antibody are usually present, and TSHRAb may be present (353,375,376). Typically, glandular hypertrophy is found, but atrophic forms are also present. Three classic types of autoimmune injury are found in Hashimoto thyroiditis: (i) complement-mediated cytotoxicity, (ii) antibody-dependent cell-mediated cytotoxicity, and (iii) stimulation or blockade of hormone receptors, which results in hypo- or hyperfunction or growth (Fig. 31.11).

The histologic picture of Hashimoto thyroiditis includes cellular hyperplasia, disruption of follicular cells, and infiltration of the gland by lymphocytes, monocytes, and plasma cells. Occasionally, adjacent lymphadenopathy may be noted. Some epithelial cells are enlarged and demonstrate oxyphilic changes in the cytoplasm (Askanazy cells or Hürthle cells, which are not specific to this disorder). The interstitial cells show fibrosis and lymphocytic infiltration. Graves disease and Hashimoto thyroiditis may cause very similar histologic findings manifested by a similar mechanism of injury.

Clinical Characteristics and Diagnosis of Hashimoto Thyroiditis

Patients with Hashimoto thyroiditis may present with typical symptoms of hypothyroidism or may be relatively asymptomatic. Patients often present with a goiter, which can involve the parietal lobe. At later stages of the disease, hypothyroidism can be found without a goiter. Notable clinical manifestations associated with Hashimoto thyroiditis include fatigue, weight gain, hyperlipidemia, dry hair, dry skin, cold intolerance, depression, menstrual irregularities, bradycardia, and or memory impairment. Hashitoxicosis, the hyperthyroid manifestation of

Table 31.13 Potential Causes of Hypothyroidism
Primary
Congenital absence of thyroid gland
External thyroid gland radiation
Familial disorders and thyroxine synthesis
Hashimoto thyroiditis
Iodine-131 ablation for Graves disease
Ingestion of antithyroid drugs
Iodine deficiency
Idiopathic myxedema (autoimmune)
Surgical removal of thyroid gland
Secondary
Hypothalamic thyrotropin-releasing hormone deficiency
Pituitary or hypothalamic tumors or disease

Hashimoto thyroiditis, may occur after a hypothyroid state and development into a euthyroid or hyperthyroid state and is thought to be the result of development of TSH-stimulating antibodies (TSI) associated with Graves disease (368). This variant is estimated to occur in 4% to 8% of patients with Hashimoto thyroiditis. In the setting of Hashitoxicosis, the patient requires frequent follow-up and the potential for adjustments in thyroid supplementation. These patients often become hypothyroid during the course of treatment.

In many cases, an elevated serum TSH is detected during routine screening. Elevated serum anti-TPO antibodies confirm the diagnosis, and free T_4 and T_3 document overt or subclinical hypothyroidsim. The sedimentation rate may be elevated, depending on the course of the disease at the time of recognition. Other causes of hypothyroidism should be considered, as listed in Table 31.13. Progression from subclinical to clinically overt hypothyroidism is reported to vary from 3% to 20%, with a higher risk noted in patients with goiter or thyroid antibodies (329,377). Treatment of subclinical hypothyroidism is somewhat controversial, but clinical studies suggested treatment of subclinical hypothyroidism is associated with a reduction in neurobehavioral abnormalities, a reduction in cardiovascular risk factors, and an improvement in lipid profile (378,379).

Treatment

Thyroxine replacement is initiated in patients with clinically overt hypothyroidism or subclinical hypothyroidism with a goiter. Regression of gland size usually does not occur, but treatment often prevents further growth of the thyroid gland. Treatment is recommended for patients with subclinical hypothyroidism in the setting of a TSH greater than 10 mIU/L on repeat measurements, pregnant patients, a strong habit of tobacco use, signs or symptoms associated with thyroid failure, or patients with severe hyperlipidemia (380). All pregnant patients with an elevated TSH level should be treated with *levothyroxine*. Treatment does not slow progression of the disease. The initial dosage of *levothyroxine* may be as little as 12.5 μg per day up to a full replacement dose. The mean replacement dosage of *levothyroxine* is 1.6 μg/kg of body weight per day, although the dosage varies greatly between patients (368). Aluminum hydroxide (antacids), cholestyramine, iron, calcium, and sucralfate may interfere with absorption. *Rifampin* and *sertraline hydrochloride* may accelerate the metabolism of *levothyroxine*. The half-life of *levothyroxine* is nearly 7 days; therefore, nearly 6 weeks of treatment are necessary before the effects of a dosage change can be evaluated.

Hypothyroidism appears to be associated with decreased fertility resulting from disruption in ovulation, and thyroid autoimmune disease is associated with an increased risk of pregnancy loss with or without overt thyroid dysfunction (381). A meta-analysis of case-control and longitudinal studies performed since 1990 reveals a possible association between miscarriage and thyroid antibodies with an odds ratio of 2.73 (95% CI, 2.20–3.40). This association may be explained by a heightened autoimmune state affecting the fetal allograft or a slightly higher age of women with antibodies compared with those without antibodies (0.7 $\pm$ 1 year, p <.001) (382). Studies suggest that early subclinical hypothyroidism may be associated with menorrhagia (383).

Severe primary hypothyroidism is associated with menstrual irregularities in 23% of women, with oligomenorrhea being the most common (382). Reproductive dysfunction in hypothyroidism may be caused by a decrease in the binding activity of sex hormone–binding globulin, resulting in increased estradiol and free testosterone and from hyperprolactinemia (382). The increase in prolactin levels is the result of enhanced sensitivity of the prolactin-secreting cells to TRH (with elevated TRH seen in primary hypothyroidism) and defective dopamine turnover resulting in hyperprolactinemia (384–387). Hyperprolactinemia-induced luteal phase defects are associated with less severe forms of hypothyroidism (388,389). Replacement therapy appears to reverse the hyperprolactinemia and correct ovulatory defects (390,391).

Combined thyroxine and triiodothyronine therapy is no more effective than thyroxine therapy alone, and patients with hypothyroidism should be treated with thyroxine alone (392). Treatment should target normalizing TSH values, and a daily dose of 0.012 mg up to a full replacement dose of *levothyroxine* (1.6 μg/kg of body weight per day) may be required with dosage dependent on the patient's weight, age, cardiac status, and duration and severity of hypothyroidism (368).

Graves Disease

Graves disease, characterized by exophthalmos, goiter, and hyperthyroidism, was first identified as an association of findings in 1835. A heritable specific defect in immunosurveillance by suppressor T lymphocytes is believed to result in the development of a helper T-cell population that reacts to multiple epitopes of the thyrotropin receptor. This activity induces a B-cell–mediated response, resulting in the clinical features of Graves disease (389). The TSHRAb bind to conformational epitopes in the extracellular domain of the thyrotropin receptor and are uniformly detected in patients with untreated Graves disease (390).

Graves disease is a complex autoimmune disorder in which several genetic susceptibility loci and environmental factors are likely to play a role in the development of the disease. Human leukocyte antigen and polymorphisms in the cytotoxic T-lymphocyte antigen 4 (*CTLA-4*) gene were established as susceptibility loci; however, the magnitude of their contributions seems to vary among patient populations and study groups. Additional loci are likely to be identified by a combination of genome-wide linkage analyses and allelic association analyses of candidate genes. The rate of concordance for Graves disease is only 20% in monozygotic twins and even lower in dizygotic twins, consistent with a multifactorial inheritance pattern highly influenced by environmental factors. Linkage analysis identified loci on chromosomes 14q31, 20q11.2, and Xq21 that are associated with susceptibility to Graves disease (393).

Clinical Characteristics and Diagnosis

The classic triad in Graves disease consists of exophthalmos, goiter, and hyperthyroidism. The symptoms associated with Graves disease include frequent bowel movements, heat intolerance, irritability, nervousness, heart palpitations, impaired fertility, vision changes, sleep disturbances, tremor, weight loss, and lower extremity swelling. Physical findings may include lid lag, nontender thyroid enlargement (two to four times normal), onycholysis, dependent lower extremity edema, palmar erythema, proptosis, staring gaze, and thick skin. A cervical venous bruit and tachycardia may be noted. The tachycardia does not respond to increased vagal tone produced with a Valsalva maneuver. Severe cases may demonstrate acropachy, chemosis, clubbing, dermopathy, exophthalmos with ophthalmoplegia, follicular conjunctivitis, pretibial myxedema, and vision loss.

Approximately 40% of patients with new onset of Graves disease and many of those previously treated have elevated T_3 and normal T_4 levels. Abnormal T_4 or T_3 results are often caused by protein binding changes rather than altered thyroid function; therefore, assessment of free T_4 and free T_3 is indicated in conjunction with TSH. In Graves disease, the TSH levels are suppressed, and levels may remain undetectable for some time even after the initiation of treatment. Thyroid autoantibodies, including TSI, may be useful during pregnancy to more accurately predict fetal risk of thyrotoxicosis (368). Autonomously functioning, benign thyroid neoplasms that exhibit

Table 31.14 Potential Causes of Hyperthyroidism
Factitious hyperthyroidism
Graves disease
Metastatic follicular cancer
Pituitary hyperthyroidism
Postpartum thyroiditis
Silent hyperthyroidism (low radioiodine uptake)
Struma ovarii
Subacute thyroiditis
Toxic multinodular goiter
Toxic nodule
Tumors secreting human chorionic gonadotropin (molar pregnancy, choriocarcinoma)

a similar clinical picture include toxic adenomas and toxic multinodular goiter. A radioactive iodine uptake thyroid scan may help differentiate these two conditions from Graves disease. Rare conditions resulting in thyrotoxicosis include metastatic thyroid carcinoma causing thyrotoxicosis, amiodarone induced thyrotoxicosis, iodine induced thyrotoxicosis, postpartum thyroiditis, a TSH-secreting pituitary adenoma, an hCG-secreting choriocarcinoma, struma ovarii, and "de Quervan's" or subacute thyroiditis (394). Factitious ingestion of thyroxine or desiccated thyroid should be considered in patients with eating disorders. Patients with thyrotoxicosis factitia demonstrate elevated T_3 and T_4, suppressed TSH, and a low serum thyroglobulin level, whereas other causes of thyroiditis and thyrotoxicosis demonstrate high levels of thyroglobulin. Potential causes of hyperthyroidism are listed in Table 31.14.

Treatment

Iodine-131 Ablation   Treatment of women with hyperthyroidism of an autoimmune origin presents unique challenges to the physician who must consider the patient's needs and her reproductive plans. Because the drugs used to treat this disorder have potentially harmful effects on the fetus, special attention must be given to the use of contraception and the potential for pregnancy.

A single dose of radioactive iodine-131 is an effective cure in about 80% of cases and is the definitive treatment in nonpregnant women. Any woman of childbearing age should be tested for pregnancy before undergoing diagnostic or therapeutic administration of iodine. Ablation of a second-trimester fetal thyroid gland and congenital hypothyroidism (cretinism) from treatment during the first trimester were reported (395). Nuclear medicine professionals provide expertise in the administration of the radioactive isotope, and because the effect of the radioactive iodine is not immediate, the endocrinologist continues to provide suppressive medical treatment for 6 to 12 weeks after administration of iodine while the patient remains hyperthyroid. As early as 2 to 3 months after treatment, patients may become hypothyroid and should be supplemented with thyroxine as indicated by serum levels of free thyroid hormone levels (368). TSH testing is not sensitive for predicting thyroid function during this time as changes in TSH lag 2 weeks to several months behind thyroid function changes (368). Failure to respond to iodine 6 months after treatment may require a repeat treatment with radioactive iodine (394). Postablative hypothyroidism develops in 50% of patients within the first year after iodine therapy and in more than 2% of patients per year thereafter.

A higher rate of miscarriage was noted in women treated with iodine therapy in the year preceding therapy, but there is no reported increase in the rate of stillbirths, preterm birth, low birth weight, congenital malformation, or death after therapy (396). Many thyroidologists and nuclear medicine specialists are willing to allow pregnancy earlier than 1 year after therapy if patients receive replacement therapy with *levothyroxine*.

Thyroid-Stimulating Receptor Antibody in Graves Disease   The level of TSHRAb of the TBII class grossly parallels the degree of hyperthyroidism as assessed by the serum levels of thyroid hormones and total thyroid volume. Studies suggest that the combination of a small goiter volume (<40 mL) and a low TBII level (<30 U/L) results in a 45% chance of remission during the 5 years after completion of a 12- to 24-month course of antithyroid drug therapy (397). In contrast, the overall rate of relapse exceeded 70% in patients with a large goiter volume (>70 mL) and a higher TBII level (>30 U/L). The subgroup of patients with larger goiters and higher TBII levels had less than a 10% chance to remain in remission in the 5 years after treatment. Although it is not necessary for the diagnosis of Graves disease, except in some cases of multinodular goiter, a TSHRAb measurement may be a useful marker of disease severity. Used in combination with other clinical factors, it may contribute to initial decisions regarding treatment. See Table 31.12 for a review of the nomenclature and assay methods for TSHRAb.

Measurements of TSHRAb (TBII category) during treatment with antithyroid drugs are predictive of subsequent outcome. In one series, 73% of TBII-negative patients had remission compared with only 28% of TBII-positive patients who achieved remission after 12 months of antithyroid drug therapy (398). The duration of a course of antithyroid drug therapy may potentially be modified according to the TSHRAb status. In patients whose TSHRAb status became negative and antithyroid drug therapy was discontinued, the relapse rate was 41% compared with a rate of 92% for those patients who remained TSHRAb positive (399). Regardless of the rapidity of the disappearance of TSHRAb, it does seem that antithyroid drug therapy should be maintained for 9 to 12 months to minimize the risk of relapse. TSHRAb status appears to determine, in an inverse relationship, the reduction in thyroid volume after radioactive iodine therapy.

Third-generation TSHRAb assays have been developed, and their utility in evaluation and treatment monitoring is being evaluated. Many patients with Graves disease have or will develop antineutrophil cytoplasmic antibodies (ANCA) after treatment, but the significance of this finding is still under study. Smoking appears to be an independent risk factor for relapse after medical therapy and should be considered when planning treatment.

Antithyroid Drugs   Antithyroid drugs of the thioamide class include *propylthiouracil* (PTU) and *methimazole*. Low doses of either agent block the secondary coupling reactions that form T_3 and T_4 from MIT and DIT. At higher doses, they also block iodination of tyrosyl residues in thyroglobulin. *Propylthiouracil* additionally blocks the peripheral conversion of T_4 to T_3. Approximately one-third of patients treated by this approach alone go into remission and become euthyroid (397).

In 2009, the FDA published a warning on the use of *propylthiouracil* because of 32 reported cases of serious liver injury associated with its use (400,401). The average daily dose associated with liver failure was 300 mg, and liver failure was reported to occur anywhere from 6 days to 450 days after initiation of therapy (402). Traditionally *PTU* was the drug of choice to treat hyperthyroidism for the duration of pregnancy because it less readily crosses the placenta, and *methimazole* was associated with an increased risk of choanal atresia and aplasia cutis (403–406). Because of the case reports of *PTU*-related liver failure and the increased risk of birth defects associated with *methimazole* use during embryogenesis, the FDA and the Endocrine Society recommend PTU never be used as first-line medical treatment of hyperthyroidism for nonpregnant patients. It is recommended that its use be limited to pregnant women during the first trimester; situations where surgery or radioactive iodine treatment are contraindicated, and individuals who have developed a toxic reaction to *methimazole* (400,402). The FDA recommends monitoring patients closely for signs and symptoms of liver injury while taking *PTU*. If liver injury is suspected, *PTU* should be promptly discontinued (400). The American Thyroid Association recommends an initial dose of 100 to 600 mg per day in three divided doses with a goal to maintain T_4 in the upper limit of normal using the lowest possible dose. Minor reactions such as pruritus affect 3% to 5% of patients treated with thionamide therapy, and antihistamines may eliminate symptoms and allow continued use. Agranulocytosis is a rare and potentially fatal complication of *PTU* and *methimazole* therapy, and developing in 0.2% of women treated, and it mandates immediate discontinuation of the drug (403). Agranulocytosis most commonly presents with fever and a sore throat followed by sepsis; the occurrence of fever, sore throat, or a viral-like syndrome should prompt an urgent evaluation.

Methimazole is the first-line drug for the treatment of hyperthyroidism, except in the first trimester of pregnancy, as it has been shown to be more effective than *PTU* at controlling severe hyperthyroidism and is associated with higher adherence rates and less toxicity (407). The American Thyroid Associated recommends initial daily doses of 10 to 40 mg per day in a single dose. Like treatment with *PTU*, the goal is to maintain a free T_4 level in the upper limits of normal using the lowest possible dose. Free T_4 levels show improvement 4 weeks after therapy, and TSH levels take 6 to 8 weeks to normalize (403). *Methimazole* use in pregnancy is associated with an 18-fold risk of fetal choanal atresia compared with the general population (95% CI, 3–121) (408). Congenital aplasia cutis was associated with maternal use of *methimazole* during pregnancy; however, it is not known at this time whether the risk (0.03%) is greater than that seen in the general population (409).

Studies suggest a potential role for an intrathyroid *dexamethasone* injection to prevent relapse (410). Other medical therapies include iodide and *lithium*, both of which reduce thyroid hormone release and inhibit the organification of iodine. Iodide leads to the secondary coupling of T_3 and T_4. Iodide inhibition of thyroid metabolism is only transient, and complete escape from inhibition occurs within 1 to 2 weeks of iodide therapy, making this useful only for acute management of severe thyrotoxicosis (394). *Lithium* may be used when thionamide therapy is contraindicated or in combination with *PTU* or *methimazole* (394). To avoid toxicity during treatment, serum *lithium* levels should be monitored. *Lithium* has been associated with fetal Ebstein anomaly, and iodide has been associated with congenital goiter; these medications should not be used in pregnant women and should be used with caution in women of reproductive age. Because of the complications related to medical therapy of hyperthyroidism, women desiring pregnancy should be counseled to strongly consider surgical treatment or radioactive iodine treatment prior to pregnancy (402).

Surgery   **Thyroidectomy was used for the treatment of Graves disease but is now rarely used unless there is a suspicion for coexisting thyroid malignancy** (368). Potential candidates for surgical intervention include pregnant women refusing or not tolerating antithyroid medical therapy, pediatric patients presenting with Graves disease, or patients who refuse radioactive iodine therapy. Surgery is the most rapid and consistent method of achieving a euthyroid state in Graves disease and avoids the possible long-term risks of radioactive iodine. Surgical intervention may be considered in severe Graves ophthalmopathy. Patients should be rendered euthyroid before a thyroidectomy. The risks of surgery include postoperative hypoparathyroidism, recurrent laryngeal nerve paralysis, routine anesthetic and surgical risks, hypothyroidism, and failure to relieve thyrotoxicosis.

β-Blockers   *Propranolol* occasionally is used with or without concurrent antithyroid medications before radioactive iodine or surgery to provide relief of symptoms. Larger and more frequent doses may be required because of a relative resistance to β-adrenergic antagonists in the setting of hyperthyroidism.

Thyroid Storm

Thyroid storm is an acute, life-threatening exacerbation of hyperthyroidism and should be treated as a medical emergency in an intensive care unit setting. Symptoms include tachycardia, tremor, diarrhea, vomiting, fever, dehydration, and altered mental status that may proceed to coma. Patients with poorly controlled hyperthyroidism are most susceptible. Beta-blocker agents, glucocorticoids, *PTU* (the action of which includes inhibition of T_4-T_3 conversion), and iodides are all key elements of therapy.

Hyperthyroidism in Gestational Trophoblastic Disease and Hyperemesis Gravidarum

Because of the weak TSH-like activity of hCG, conditions with high levels of hCG, such as molar pregnancy, may be associated with biochemical and clinical hyperthyroidism. Symptoms regress with removal of the abnormal trophoblastic tissue and resolution of elevated levels of hCG. In a similar fashion, when hyperemesis gravidarum is associated with high levels of hCG, mild biochemical and clinical features of hyperthyroidism may be seen (411,412). Gestational trophoblastic disease is reviewed in Chapter 39.

Thyroid Function in Pregnancy

Physicians should be aware of the changes in thyroid physiology during pregnancy. Pregnancy is associated with reversible changes in thyroid physiology that should be noted before diagnosing thyroid abnormalities (see Fig. 31.12 for pregnancy associated changes in TBG, total T_4, hCG, TSH, and free T_4) (403). **Women with a history of hypothyroidism often require increased thyroxine replacement during pregnancy, and patients should have thyroid function tests performed at the first prenatal visit and during each trimester thereafter.** Evidence suggests that optimal fetal and infant neurodevelopmental outcomes may require careful titration of replacement thyroxine that meets the frequently increased requirements of pregnancy (413,414).

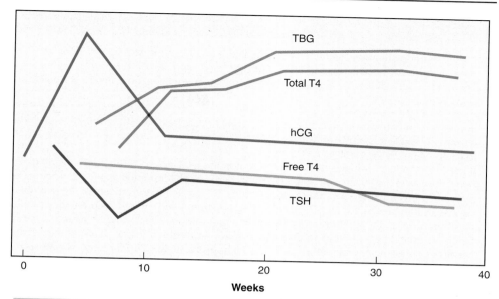

Figure 31.12 **Pregnancy-associated changes in TSH relative to hCG and free T$_4$ in relation to TBG.** Relative serum concentration changes throughout pregnancy highlighting a fall in TSH associated with an increase in hCG early in pregnancy and a fall in free T$_4$ as TBG levels rise during pregnancy. hCG, human chorionic gonadotropin; TSH, thyroid-stimulating hormone; TBG, thyroid-binding globulin, total T$_4$, total thyroxine; free T$_4$, free thyroxine. (Based on data from **Brent GA.** Maternal thyroid function: interpretation of thyroid function tests in pregnancy. *Clin Obstet Gynecol* 1997;40:3–15.)

Postpartum, women should return to their prepregnancy dosage of *levothyroxine* and have a follow-up TSH checked 6 to 8 weeks postpartum.

Reproductive Effects of Hyperthyroidism

High levels of TSAb (TSI) in women with Graves disease are associated with fetal-neonatal hyperthyroidism (415,416). Despite both the inhibition and elevation of gonadotropins seen in thyrotoxicosis, most women remain ovulatory and fertile (387,417). Severe thyrotoxicosis can result in weight loss, menstrual cycle irregularities, and amenorrhea. An increased risk of spontaneous abortion is noted in women with thyrotoxicosis. An increased incidence of congenital anomalies, particularly choanal atresia and possibly aplasia cutis, can occur in the offspring of women treated with methimazole (404,405,408).

Autoimmune hyperthyroid Graves disease may improve spontaneously, in which case antithyroid drug therapy may be reduced or stopped. TSHRAb production may persist for several years after radical radioactive iodine therapy or surgical treatment for hyperthyroid Graves disease. In this circumstance, there is a risk of exposing a fetus to TSHRAb. Fetal–neonatal hyperthyroidism is observed in 2% to 10% of pregnancies occurring in mothers with a current or previous diagnosis of Graves disease, secondary to the transplacental passage of maternal TSHRAb. This is a serious condition with a 16% neonatal mortality rate and a risk of intrauterine fetal death, stillbirth, and skeletal developmental abnormalities, such as craniosynostosis. Caution against overtreatment with antithyroid medication is warranted, as these medications may cross the placenta in sufficient quantities to induce fetal goiter. Guidelines for TSHRAb testing during pregnancy in women with previously treated Graves disease are found in Table 31.15. Fetal goiters and the associated fetal hypo- or hyperthyroid status were diagnosed accurately in mothers with Graves disease using a combination of fetal ultrasonography of the thyroid with Doppler, fetal heart rate monitoring, bone maturation, and maternal TSHRAb and antithyroid drug status (418).

Postpartum Thyroid Dysfunction

Postpartum thyroid dysfunction is much more common than recognized; it is often difficult to diagnose because its symptoms appear 1 to 8 months postpartum and are often confused with postpartum depression and difficulties adjusting to the demands of the neonate and infant. Postpartum thyroiditis appears to be caused by the combination of a rebounding immune system in the postpartum state and the presence of thyroid autoantibodies. Histologically,

Table 31.15 Guidelines for TSHRAb Testing During Pregnancy with Previously Treated Graves Disease

1. In the woman with antecedent Graves disease in remission after ATD treatment, the risk for fetal–neonatal hyperthyroidism is negligible, and systematic measurement of TSHRAb is not necessary.
Thyroid function should be evaluated during pregnancy to detect an unlikely but possible recurrence. In that case, TSHRAb assay is mandatory.

2. In the woman with antecedent Graves disease previously treated with radioiodine or thyroidectomy and regardless of the current thyroid status (euthyroidism with or without thyroxine substitution), TSHRAb should be measured early in pregnancy to evaluate the risk for fetal hyperthyroidism.
If the TSHRAb level is high, careful monitoring of the fetus is mandatory for the early detection of signs of thyroid overstimulation (tachycardia, impaired growth rate, oligohydramnios, goiter). Cardiac echography and measurement of circulatory velocity may be confirmatory. Ultrasonographic measurements of the fetal thyroid have been defined from 20 weeks gestational age but require a well-trained operator, and thyroid visibility may be hindered because of fetal head position. Color Doppler ultrasonography is helpful in evaluating thyroid hypervascularization. Because of the potential risks of fetal-neonatal hyperthyroid cardiac insufficiency and the inability to measure the degree of hyperthyroidism in the mother because of previous thyroid ablation, it may be appropriate to consider direct diagnosis in the fetus. Fetal blood sampling through cordocentesis is feasible as early as 25 to 27 weeks gestation with less than 1% adverse effects (fetal bleeding, bradycardia, infection, spontaneous abortion, in utero death) when performed by experienced clinicians. ATD administration to the mother may be considered to treat the fetal hyperthyroidism.

3. In the woman with concurrent hyperthyroid Graves disease, regardless of whether it has preceded the onset of pregnancy, ATD treatment should be monitored and adjusted to keep free T_4 in the high-normal range to prevent fetal hypothyroidism and minimize toxicity associated with higher doses of these medications.
TSHR-Ab should be measured at the beginning of the last trimester, especially if the required ATD dosage is high. If the TSHRAb assay is negative or the level low, fetal–neonatal hyperthyroidism is rare. If antibody levels are high (TBII ≥ 40 U/L or TSAb $\geq 300\%$), evaluation of the fetus for hyperthyroidism is required. In this condition, there is usually a fair correlation between maternal and fetal thyroid function such that monitoring the ATD dosage according to the mother's thyroid status is appropriate for the fetus. In some cases in which a high dose of ATD >20 mg/d of methimazole or >300 mg/d of propylthiouracil [PTU]) is necessary, there is a risk of goitrous hypothyroidism in the fetus, which might be indistinguishable from goitrous Graves disease. The correct diagnosis relies on the assay of fetal thyroid hormones and TSH, which allows for optimal treatment.

4. In any woman who has previously given birth to a newborn with hyperthyroidism, a TSHR-Ab assay should be performed early in the course of pregnancy.

TSHRAb, thyroid-stimulating hormone receptor antibodies; ATD, autoimmune thyroid disease; T_4, thyroxine; TBII, TSH-binding inhibitory immunoglobulin; TSAb, thyroid-stimulating antibody.

lymphocytic infiltration and inflammation are found and anti-TPO antibodies are often present (419,420). The following are criteria for the diagnosis of postpartum thyroiditis: (i) no history of thyroid hormonal abnormalities either before or during pregnancy, (ii) documented abnormal TSH level (either depressed or elevated) during the first year postpartum, and (iii) absence of a positive TSH-receptor antibody titer (Graves disease) or a toxic nodule. A number of studies describe clinical and biochemical evidence of postpartum thyroid dysfunction in 5% to 10% of new mothers (421,422).

Clinical Characteristics and Diagnosis

Postpartum thyroiditis usually begins with a transient hyperthyroid phase between 6 weeks and 6 months postpartum followed by a hypothyroid phase. Only one-fourth of the cases follow this classic clinical picture, and more than one-third have either hyperthyroidism or hypothyroidism alone. Individuals with type 1 diabetes have a threefold increased risk of developing postpartum thyroiditis. Women with a history of postpartum thyroiditis in a previous pregnancy have nearly a 70% chance of recurrence in a subsequent pregnancy. Although psychotic episodes are rare, postpartum thyroid dysfunction should be considered in all women with postpartum psychosis. The thyrotoxic phase may be subclinical and overlooked, particularly in areas where iodine intake is low (423). Unlike patients with Graves disease, those with the hyperthyroidism caused by postpartum thyroiditis have a low level of radioactive isotope uptake. Women with a history of postpartum thyroiditis should be followed closely as they have a 20% risk of permanent hypothyroidism immediately following the onset of thyroiditis, up to a 60% risk of permanent hypothyroidism over the next 5 to 10 years, and up to a 70% risk of postpartum thyroiditis in future pregnancies (424,425).

The absence of thyroid tenderness, pain, fever, elevated sedimentation rate, and leukocytosis helps to rule out subacute thyroiditis (de Quervain thyroiditis). Evaluation of TSH, T_4, T_3, T_3 resin uptake, and antimicrosomal antibody titer confirms the diagnosis.

Treatment

Most patients are diagnosed during the hypothyroid phase and require 6 to 12 months of thyroxine replacement if they are symptomatic (370). Because approximately 60% of women develop permanent hypothyroidism, TSH should be evaluated following discontinuation of replacement therapy.

Rarely, patients are diagnosed during the hyperthyroid phase (426). Antithyroid medications are not routinely used for these women. *Propranolol* may be used for relief of symptoms but should be used with appropriate counseling in nursing mothers.

Antithyroid Antibodies and Disorders of Reproduction

Women who have antithyroid autoantibodies before and after conception appear to be at an increased risk for spontaneous abortion (427,428). Nonorgan-specific antibody production and pregnancy loss are documented in cases of antiphospholipid abnormalities (429). The concurrent presence of organ-specific thyroid antibodies and nonorgan-specific autoantibody production is not uncommon (429–431). In cases of recurrent pregnancy loss, thyroid autoantibodies may serve as peripheral markers of abnormal T-cell function and further implicate an immune component as the cause of reproductive failure. The clinical implications of these findings in the management of patients with recurrent pregnancy loss are not known. Recurrent pregnancy loss is covered in Chapter 33.

Thyroid Nodules

Thyroid nodules are a common finding on physical examination and are demonstrated by high frequency ultrasonography in over two-thirds of patients (432). Occasionally such nodules are functional, and clinical and laboratory evaluation should be applied to distinguish these nodules from nonfunctional nodules, which are occasionally malignant. For nonfunctional "cold" nodules, fine-needle biopsy and aspiration are required to rule out malignancy. In the case of indeterminate aspirates, 2% to 20% are malignant; therefore, surgical biopsy often is indicated (433). Molecular diagnosis screening of the *BRAF* mutation improves the diagnosis of cancer on fine-needle aspiration (434).

Turner Syndrome and Down Syndrome

Patients with Turner syndrome (and other forms of hypergonadotropic hypogonadism associated with abnormalities of the second sex chromosome) exhibit a high prevalence of autoimmune thyroid disorders. Approximately 50% of adult patients with Turner syndrome have antithyroid peroxidase (anti-TPO) and antithyroglobulin (anti-TG) autoantibodies. Of these patients, approximately 30% will develop subclinical or clinical hypothyroidism. The disorder is indistinguishable from Hashimoto thyroiditis. A susceptibility locus for Graves disease is noted on chromosome X (435). Because of the increased risk of autoimmune thyroid disease, it is recommended that women with Turner syndrome be screened with yearly TSH testing starting at the age of 4 (436).

Down syndrome, caused by an extra chromosome 21, is characterized by an atypical body habitus, mental retardation, cardiac malformations, an increased risk of leukemia, and a reduced life expectancy. The extra chromosome is almost always of maternal origin. Autoimmune thyroid disorders are more common in patients with Down syndrome than in the general population. The gene for autoimmune polyglandular syndrome I (*APECED*) was mapped to chromosome 21 and is thought to be a transcription factor involved in immune regulation (AIRE). This gene may play a role in the development of autoimmune thyroid disease in these patients (437). Hashimoto thyroiditis is the most common type of thyroid disease in individuals with Down syndrome. Hypothyroidism develops in as many as 50% of patients older than age 40 with Down syndrome. These clinical syndromes and other evidence suggest part of the genetic susceptibility to Hashimoto thyroiditis may reside on chromosomes X and 21. Because of the increased frequency of hypothyroidism associated with Down syndrome, it is recommended to screen individuals at 6 months, 12 months, and then annually thereafter (372).

References

1. **Verkauf BS, Von Thron J, O'Brien WF.** Clitoral size in normal women. *Obstet Gynecol* 1992;80:41–44.

2. **Ferrimann D, Gallway JD.** Clinical assessment of body hair growth in women. *J Clin Endocrinol Metab* 1961;21:1440.

3. **Rosenfield RL.** Clinical practice. Hirsutism. *N Engl J Med* 2005; 353:2578–2588.

4. **Martin KA, Chang RJ, Ehrmann DA, et al.** Evaluation and treatment of hirsutism in premenopausal women: an endocrine society clinical practice guideline. *J Clin Endocrinol Metab* 2008;93:1105–1120.

5. **Vermeulen A, Verdonck L, Kaufman JM.** A critical evaluation of simple methods for the estimation of free testosterone in serum. *J Clin Endocrinol Metab* 1999;84:3666–3672.

6. **Armengaud JB, Charkaluk ML, Trivin C, et al.** Precocious pubarche: distinguishing late-onset congenital adrenal hyperplasia from premature adrenarche. *J Clin Endocrin Metab* 2009;94:2835–2840.

7. **Azziz R, Carmina E, Dewailly D, et al.** The Androgen Excess and PCOS Society criteria for the polycystic ovary syndrome: the complete task force report. *Fertil Steril* 2009;91:456–488.

8. **Rittmaster RS.** Clinical relevance of testosterone and dihydrotestosterone metabolism in women. *Am J Med* 1995;98:17S–21S.

9. **Rainey WE, Nakamura Y.** Regulation of the adrenal androgen biosynthesis. *J Steroid Biochem Mol Biol* 2008;108:281–286.

10. **Siegel SF, Finegold DN, Lanes R, et al.** ACTH stimulation tests and plasma dehydroepiandrosterone sulfate levels in women with hirsutism. *N Engl J Med* 1990;323:849–854.

11. **d'Alva CB, Abiven-Lepage G, Viallon V, et al.** Sex steroids in androgen-secreting adrenocortical tumors: clinical and hormonal features in comparison with non-tumoral causes of androgen excess. *Eur J Endocrinol* 2008;159:641–647.

12. **Youden WJ.** Index for rating diagnostic tests. *Cancer* 1950;3:32–35.

13. **Ehrmann DA.** Polycystic ovary syndrome. *N Engl J Med* 2005;352:1223–1236.

14. **Toulis KA, Goulis DG, Kolibianakis EM, et al.** Risk of gestational diabetes mellitus in women with polycystic ovary syndrome: a systematic review and a meta-analysis. *Fertil Steril* 2009;92:667–677.

15. **Practice Committee of the American Society of Reproductive Medicine.** The evaluation and treatment of androgen excess. *Fertil Steril* 2006;86:S173–S180.

16. **Nestler JE.** Metformin for the treatment of the polycystic ovary syndrome. *N Engl J Med* 2008;358:47–54.

17. **Stein IF, Leventhal ML.** Amenorrhea associated with bilateral polycystic ovaries. *Am J Obstet Gynecol* 1935;29:181–191.

18. **Zawadzki JK, Danif A.** Diagnostic criteria for polycystic ovary syndrome towards a rational approach. In: **Dunaif A, Givens JR, Hasetine FP, et al., eds.** *Polycystic ovary syndrome.* Cambridge: Blackwell Science, 1992:377–384.

19. **Rotterdam ESHRE/ASRM-Sponsored PCOS Consensus Workshop Group.** Revised 2003 consensus on diagnostic criteria and long-term health risks related to polycystic ovary syndrome. *Fertil Steril* 2004;81:19–25.

20. **Goldzieher JW, Axelrod LR.** Clinical and biochemical features of polycystic ovarian disease. *Fertil Steril* 1963;14:631–653.

21. **Aono T, Miyazaki M, Miyake A, et al.** Responses of serum gonadotrophins to LH-releasing hormone and oestrogens in Japanese women with polycystic ovaries. *Acta Endocrinol (Copenh)* 1977;85:840–849.

22. **Serafini P, Ablan F, Lobo RA.** 5-Alpha-reductase activity in the genital skin of hirsute women. *J Clin Endocrinol Metab* 1985;60:349–355.

23. **Lobo RA, Goebelsmann U, Horton R.** Evidence for the importance of peripheral tissue events in the development of hirsutism in polycystic ovary syndrome. *J Clin Endocrinol Metab* 1983;57:393–397.

24. **Pall M, Azziz R, Beires J, et al.** The phenotype of hirsute women: a comparison of polycystic ovary syndrome and 21-hydroxylase-deficient nonclassic adrenal hyperplasia. *Fertil Steril* 2010;94:684–689.

25. **Carmina E, Lobo RA.** Do hyperandrogenic women with normal menses have polycystic ovary syndrome? *Fertil Steril* 1999;71:319–322.

26. **Peserico A, Angeloni G, Bertoli P, et al.** Prevalence of polycystic ovaries in women with acne. *Arch Dermatol Res* 1989;281:502–503.

27. **Polson DW, Adams J, Wadsworth J, et al.** Polycystic ovaries—a common finding in normal women. *Lancet* 1988;1:870–872.

28. **Loucks TL, Talbott EO, McHugh KP, et al.** Do polycystic-appearing ovaries affect the risk of cardiovascular disease among women with polycystic ovary syndrome? *Fertil Steril* 2000;74:547–552.

29. **Hassan MA, Killick SR.** Ultrasound diagnosis of polycystic ovaries in women who have no symptoms of polycystic ovary syndrome is not associated with subfecundity or subfertility. *Fertil Steril* 2003;80:966–975.

30. **Wild RA.** Obesity, lipids, cardiovascular risk, and androgen excess. *Am J Med* 1995;98:27S–32S.

31. **Moran LJ, Pasquali R, Teede HJ, et al.** Treatment of obesity in polycystic ovary syndrome: a position statement of the Androgen Excess and Polycystic Ovary Syndrome Society. *Fertil Steril* 2009;92:1966–1982.

32. **Kenny SJ, Aubert RE, Geiss LS.** Prevalence and incidence of non-insulin-dependent diabetes. In: **Harris MI ed.** *Diabetes in America.* Washington, DC: US National Institutes of Health, NIH Publication. No.95-1468, Bethesda MD, 1995:179–220.

33. **Ehrmann DA, Barnes RB, Rosenfield RL, et al.** Prevalence of impaired glucose tolerance and diabetes in women with polycystic ovary syndrome. *Diabetes Care* 1999;22:141–146.

34. **Legro RS, Kunselman AR, Dodson WC, et al.** Prevalence and predictors of risk for type 2 diabetes mellitus and impaired glucose tolerance in polycystic ovary syndrome: a prospective, controlled study in 254 affected women. *J Clin Endocrinol Metab* 1999;84:165–169.

35. **Harris MI, Hadden WC, Knowler WC, et al.** Prevalence of diabetes and impaired glucose tolerance and plasma glucose levels in U.S. population aged 20–74 yr. *Diabetes* 1987;36:523–534.

36. **Dahlgren E, Johansson S, Lindstedt G, et al.** Women with polycystic ovary syndrome wedge resected in 1956 to 1965: a long-term follow-up focusing on natural history and circulating hormones. *Fertil Steril* 1992;57:505–513.

37. **Conway GS, Agrawal R, Betteridge DJ, et al.** Risk factors for coronary artery disease in lean and obese women with the polycystic ovary syndrome. *Clin Endocrinol (Oxf)* 1992;37:119–125.

38. **Andersen P, Seljeflot I, Abdelnoor M, et al.** Increased insulin sensitivity and fibrinolytic capacity after dietary intervention in obese women with polycystic ovary syndrome. *Metabolism* 1995;44:611–616.

39. **Guzick DS, Talbott EO, Sutton-Tyrrell K, et al.** Carotid atherosclerosis in women with polycystic ovary syndrome: initial results from a case-control study. *Am J Obstet Gynecol* 1996;174:1224–1229; discussion 9–32.

40. **Birdsall MA, Farquhar CM, White HD.** Association between polycystic ovaries and extent of coronary artery disease in women having cardiac catheterization. *Ann Intern Med* 1997;126:32–35.

41. **Danigren E, Janson PO, Johansson S, et al.** Polycystic ovary syndrome and risk for myocardial infarction. *Acta Obstet Cynecol Scand* 1992;71:559–604.

42. **Clement PB.** Nonneoplastic lesions of the ovary. In: **Kurman RJ, ed.,** *Blaustein's pathology of the female genital tract,* 4th ed. New York: Springer-Verlag, 1994:559–604.

43. **Rosenfield RL, Barnes RB, Cara JF, et al.** Dysregulation of cytochrome P450-17 α as the cause of polycystic ovarian syndrome. *Fertil Steril* 1990;53:785–791.

44. **McNatty KP, Makris A, DeGrazia C, et al.** The production of progesterone, androgens, and estrogens by granulosa cells, thecal tissue, and stromal tissue from human ovaries *in vitro. J Clin Endocrinol Metab* 1979;49:687–699.

45. **Lobo RA, Kletzky OA, Campeau JD, et al.** Elevated bioactive luteinizing hormone in women with the polycystic ovary syndrome. *Fertil Steril* 1983;39:674–678.

46. **Chang RJ, Laufer LR, Meldrum DR, et al.** Steroid secretion in polycystic ovarian disease after ovarian suppression by a long-acting gonadotropin-releasing hormone agonist. *J Clin Endocrinol Metab* 1983;56:897–903.

47. **Biffignandi P, Massucchetti C, Molinatti GM.** Female hirsutism: pathophysiological considerations and therapeutic implications. *Endocr Rev* 1984;5:498–513.

48. **Rittmaster RS.** Differential suppression of testosterone and estradiol in hirsute women with the superactive gonadotropin-releasing hormone agonist leuprolide. *J Clin Endocrinol Metab* 1988;67:651–655.

49. **Lobo RA.** Hirsutism in polycystic ovary syndrome: current concepts. *Clin Obstet Gynecol* 1991;34:817–826.

50. **Hoffman DI, Klove K, Lobo RA.** The prevalence and significance of elevated dehydroepiandrosterone sulfate levels in anovulatory women. *Fertil Steril* 1984;42:76–81.

51. **Lobo RA.** The role of the adrenal in polycystic ovary syndrome. *Semin Reprod Endocrinol* 1984:251–264.

52. **Deslypere JP, Verdonck L, Vermeulen A.** Fat tissue: a steroid reservoir and site of steroid metabolism. *J Clin Endocrinol Metab* 1985;61:564–570.

53. **Edman CD, MacDonald PC.** Effect of obesity on conversion of plasma androstenedione to estrone in ovulatory and anovulatory young women. *Am J Obstet Gynecol* 1978;130:456–461.

54. **Schneider J, Bradlow HL, Strain G, et al.** Effects of obesity on estradiol metabolism: decreased formation of nonuterotropic metabolites. *J Clin Endocrinol Metab* 1983;56:973–978.

55. **Judd HL.** Endocrinology of polycystic ovarian disease. *Clin Obstet Gynecol* 1978;21:99–114.

56. **Bracero N, Zacur HA.** Polycystic ovary syndrome and hyperprolactinemia. *Obstet Gynecol Clin North Am* 2001;28:77–84.

57. **Deligeoroglou E, Kouskouti C, Christopoulos P.** The role of genes in the polycystic ovary syndrome: predisposition and mechanisms. *Gynecol Endocrinol* 2009;25:603–609.

58. **Urbanek M, Legro RS, Driscoll DA, et al.** Thirty-seven candidate genes for polycystic ovary syndrome: strongest evidence for linkage is with follistatin. *Proc Natl Acad Sci U S A* 1999;96:8573–8578.

59. **Gharani N, Waterworth DM, Batty S, et al.** Association of the steroid synthesis gene CYP11a with polycystic ovary syndrome and hyperandrogenism. *Hum Mol Genet* 1997;6:397–402.

60. **Ehrmann DA, Schwarz PE, Hara M, et al.** Relationship of calpain-10 genotype to phenotypic features of polycystic ovary syndrome. *J Clin Endocrinol Metab* 2002;87:1669–1673.

61. **Tucci S, Futterweit W, Concepcion ES, et al.** Evidence for association of polycystic ovary syndrome in Caucasian women with a marker at the insulin receptor gene locus. *J Clin Endocrinol Metab* 2001;86:446–449.

62. **Hogeveen KN, Cousin P, Pugeat M, et al.** Human sex hormone-binding globulin variants associated with hyperandrogenism and ovarian dysfunction. *J Clin Invest* 2002;109:973–981.

63. **Biyasheva A, Legro RS, Dunaif A, et al.** Evidence for association between polycystic ovary syndrome (PCOS) and TCF7L2 and glucose intolerance in women with PCOS and TCF7L2. *J Clin Endocrinol Metab* 2009;94:2617–2625.

64. **Waterworth DM, Bennett ST, Gharani N, et al.** Linkage and association of insulin gene VNTR regulatory polymorphism with polycystic ovary syndrome. *Lancet* 1997;349:986–990.

65. **Ewens KG, Stewart DR, Ankener W, et al.** Family-based analysis of candidate genes for polycystic ovary syndrome. *J Clin Endocrinol Metab* 2010;95:2306–2315.

66. **Wood JR, Nelson VL, Ho C, et al.** The molecular phenotype of polycystic ovary syndrome (PCOS) theca cells and new candidate PCOS genes defined by microarray analysis. *J Biol Chem* 2003;278:26380–26390.

67. **Sproul K, Jones MR, Mathur R, et al.** Association study of four key folliculogenesis genes in polycystic ovary syndrome. *BJOG* 2010;117:756–760.

68. **Barbieri RL, Ryan KJ.** Hyperandrogenism, insulin resistance, and acanthosis nigricans syndrome: a common endocrinopathy with distinct pathophysiologic features. *Am J Obstet Gynecol* 1983;147:90–101.

69. **Seibel MM.** Toward understanding the pathophysiology and treatment of polycystic ovary disease. *Semin Reprod Endocrinol* 1984;2:297.

70. **Dunaif A, Graf M, Mandeli J, et al.** Characterization of groups of hyperandrogenic women with acanthosis nigricans, impaired glucose tolerance, and/or hyperinsulinemia. *J Clin Endocrinol Metab* 1987;65:499–507.

71. **Dunaif A, Green G, Futterweit W, et al.** Suppression of hyperandrogenism does not improve peripheral or hepatic insulin resistance in the polycystic ovary syndrome. *J Clin Endocrinol Metab* 1990;70:699–704.

72. **Nagamani M, Van Dinh T, Kelver ME.** Hyperinsulinemia in hyperthecosis of the ovaries. *Am J Obstet Gynecol* 1986;154:384–389.

73. **Grasinger CC, Wild RA, Parker IJ.** Vulvar acanthosis nigricans: a marker for insulin resistance in hirsute women. *Fertil Steril* 1993;59:583–586.

74. **Dunaif A.** Hyperandrogenic anovulation (PCOS): a unique disorder of insulin action associated with an increased risk of non-insulin-dependent diabetes mellitus. *Am J Med* 1995;98:33S–39S.

75. **Kiddy DS, Hamilton-Fairley D, Bush A, et al.** Improvement in endocrine and ovarian function during dietary treatment of obese women with polycystic ovary syndrome. *Clin Endocrinol (Oxf)* 1992;36:105–111.

76. **Pasquali R, Antenucci D, Casimirri F, et al.** Clinical and hormonal characteristics of obese amenorrheic hyperandrogenic women before and after weight loss. *J Clin Endocrinol Metab* 1989;68:173–179.

77. **Escobar-Morreale HF, Botella-Carretero JI, Alvarez-Blasco F, et al.** The polycystic ovary syndrome associated with morbid obesity may resolve after weight loss induced by bariatric surgery. *J Clin Endocrinol Metab* 2005;90:6364–6369.

78. **Legro RS, Kunselman AR, Dunaif A.** Prevalence and predictors of dyslipidemia in women with polycystic ovary syndrome. *Am J Med* 2001;111:607–613.

79. **Valkenburg O, Steegers-Theunissen RP, Smedts HP, et al.** A more atherogenic serum lipoprotein profile is present in women with polycystic ovary syndrome: a case-control study. *J Clin Endocrinol Metab* 2008;93:470–476.

80. **Wild RA, Carmina E, Diamanti-Kandarakis E, et al.** Assessment of cardiovascular risk and prevention of cardiovascular disease in women with the polycystic ovary syndrome: a consensus statement by the Androgen Excess and Polycystic Ovary Syndrome (AE-PCOS) Society. *J Clin Endocrinol Metab* 2010;95:2038–2049.

81. **Jafari K, Javaheri G, Ruiz G.** Endometrial adenocarcinoma and the Stein-Leventhal syndrome. *Obstet Gynecol* 1978;51:97–100.

82. **Chittenden BG, Fullerton G, Maheshwari A, et al.** Polycystic ovary syndrome and the risk of gynaecological cancer: a systematic review. *Reprod BioMed Online* 2009;19:398–405.

83. **Balen A.** Polycystic ovary syndrome and cancer. *Hum Reprod Update* 2001;7:522–525.

84. **Wild S, Pierpoint T, Jacobs H, et al.** Long-term consequences of polycystic ovary syndrome: results of a 31 year follow-up study. *Hum Fertil* 2000;3:101–105.

85. **Cowan LD, Gordis L, Tonascia JA, et al.** Breast cancer incidence in women with a history of progesterone deficiency. *Am J Epidemiol* 1981;114:209–217.

86. **Brinton LA, Moghissi KS, Westhoff CL, et al.** Cancer risk among infertile women with androgen excess or menstrual disorders (including polycystic ovary syndrome). *Fertil Steril* 2010;94:1787–1792.

87. **Schildkraut JM, Schwingl PJ, Bastos E, et al.** Epithelial ovarian cancer risk among women with polycystic ovary syndrome. *Obstet Gynecol* 1996;88(Pt 1):554–559.

88. **Thomson RL, Buckley JD, Lim SS, et al.** Lifestyle management improves quality of life and depression in overweight and obese women with polycystic ovary syndrome. *Fertil Steril* 2009;94:1812–1916.

89. **Kerchner A, Lester W, Stuart SP, et al.** Risk of depression and other mental health disorders in women with polycystic ovary syndrome: a longitudinal study. *Fertil Steril* 2009;91:207–212.

90. **Futterweit W.** An endocrine approach obesity. In: **Simopoulos AP, Vanltallie TB, Gullo SP, et al., eds.** *Obesity: new directions in assessment and management.* New York: Charles Press, 1994: 96–121.

91. **Givens JR, Andersen RN, Wiser WL, et al.** The effectiveness of two oral contraceptives in suppressing plasma androstenedione, testosterone, LH, and FSH, and in stimulating plasma testosterone-binding capacity in hirsute women. *Am J Obstet Gynecol* 1976;124:333–339.

92. **Raj SG, Raj MH, Talbert LM, et al.** Normalization of testosterone levels using a low estrogen-containing oral contraceptive in women with polycystic ovary syndrome. *Obstet Gynecol* 1982;60:15–19.

93. **Wiebe RH, Morris CV.** Effect of an oral contraceptive on adrenal and ovarian androgenic steroids. *Obstet Gynecol* 1984;63:12–14.

94. **Wild RA, Umstot ES, Andersen RN, et al.** Adrenal function in hirsutism. II. Effect of an oral contraceptive. *J Clin Endocrinol Metab* 1982;54:676–681.

95. **Marynick SP, Chakmakjian ZH, McCaffree DL, et al.** Androgen excess in cystic acne. *N Engl J Med* 1983;308:981–986.

96. **Schiavone FE, Rietschel RL, Sgoutas D, et al.** Elevated free testosterone levels in women with acne. *Arch Dermatol* 1983;119:799–802.

97. **Amin ES, El-Sayed MM, El-Gamel BA, et al.** Comparative study of the effect of oral contraceptives containing 50 microgram of estrogen and those containing 20 microgram of estrogen on adrenal cortical function. *Am J Obstet Gynecol* 1980;137:831–833.

98. **Goldzieher JW.** Polycystic ovarian disease. *Fertil Steril* 1981; 35:371–394.

99. **Rittmaster RS.** Clinical review 73: medical treatment of androgen-dependent hirsutism. *J Clin Endocrinol Metab* 1995;80:2559–2563.

100. **Godsland IF, Walton C, Felton C, et al.** Insulin resistance, secretion, and metabolism in users of oral contraceptives. *J Clin Endocrinol Metab* 1992;74:64–70.

101. **Ettinger B, Golditch IM.** Medroxyprogesterone acetate for the evaluation of hypertestosteronism in hirsute women. *Fertil Steril* 1977;28:1285–1288.

102. **Jeppsson S, Gershagen S, Johansson ED, et al.** Plasma levels of medroxyprogesterone acetate (MPA), sex-hormone binding globulin, gonadal steroids, gonadotrophins and prolactin in women during long-term use of depo-MPA (Depo-Provera) as a contraceptive agent. *Acta Endocrinol (Copenh)* 1982;99:339–343.

103. **Gordon GG, Southern AL, Calanog A, et al.** The effect of medroxyprogesterone acetate on androgen metabolism in the polycystic ovary syndrome. *J Clin Endocrinol Metab* 1972,35:444–447.

104. **Meldrum DR, Chang RJ, Lu J, et al.** "Medical oophorectomy" using a long-acting GNRH agonist—a possible new approach to the treatment of endometriosis. *J Clin Endocrinol Metab* 1982;54:1081–1083.

105. **Falsetti L, Pasinetti E.** Treatment of moderate and severe hirsutism by gonadotropin-releasing hormone agonists in women with polycystic ovary syndrome and idiopathic hirsutism. *Fertil Steril* 1994;61:817–822.

106. **Morcos RN, Abdul-Malak ME, Shikora E.** Treatment of hirsutism with a gonadotropin-releasing hormone agonist and estrogen replacement therapy. *Fertil Steril* 1994;61:427–431.

107. **Tiitinen A, Simberg N, Stenman UH, et al.** Estrogen replacement does not potentiate gonadotropin-releasing hormone agonist-induced androgen suppression in treatment of hirsutism. *J Clin Endocrinol Metab* 1994;79:447–451.

108. **Cunningham SK, Loughlin T, Culliton M, et al.** Plasma sex hormone-binding globulin and androgen levels in the management of hirsute patients. *Acta Endocrinol (Copenh)* 1973;104:365–371.

109. **Gal M, Orly J, Barr I, et al.** Low dose ketoconazole attenuates serum androgen levels in patients with polycystic ovary syndrome and inhibits ovarian steroidogenesis *in vitro. Fertil Steril* 1994;61:823–832.

110. **Menard RH, Guenthner TM, Kon H, et al.** Studies on the destruction of adrenal and testicular cytochrome P-450 by spironolactone. Requirement for the 7alpha-thio group and evidence for the loss of the heme and apoproteins of cytochrome P-450. *J Biol Chem* 1979;254:1726–1733.

111. **Cumming DC, Yang JC, Rebar RW, et al.** Treatment of hirsutism with spironolactone. *JAMA* 1982;247:1295–1298.

112. **Rittmaster R.** Evaluation and treatment of hirsutism. *Infert Reprod Med Clin North Am* 1991,2:511–545.

113. **Barth JH, Cherry CA, Wojnarowska F, et al.** Spironolactone is an effective and well tolerated systemic andiandrogen therapy for hirsute women. *J Clin Endocrinol Metab* 1989;68:966–970.

114. **Pittaway DE, Maxson WS, Wentz AC.** Spironolactone in combination drug therapy for unresponsive hirsutism. *Fertil Steril* 1985;43:878–882.

115. **Lobo RA, Shoupe D, Serafini P, et al.** The effects of two doses of spironolactone on serum androgens and anagen hair in hirsute women. *Fertil Steril* 1985;43:200–205.

116. **Calaf-Alsina J, Rodriguez-Espinosa J, Cabero-Roura A, et al.** Effects of a cyproterone-containing oral contraceptive on hormonal levels in polycystic ovarian disease. *Obstet Gynecol* 1987;69:255–258.

117. **Helfer EL, Miller JL, Rose LI.** Side-effects of spironolactone therapy in the hirsute woman. *J Clin Endocrinol Metab* 1988;66:208–211.

118. **Miller JA, Jacobs HS.** Treatment of hirsutism and acne with cyproterone acetate. *Clin Endocrinol Metab* 1986;15:373–389.

119. **Mowszowicz I, Wright F, Vincens M, et al.** Androgen metabolism in hirsute patients treated with cyproterone acetate. *J Steroid Biochem* 1984;20:757–761.

120. **Girard J, Baumann JB, Buhler U, et al.** Cyproteroneacetate and ACTH adrenal function. *J Clin Endocrinol Metab* 1978;47:581–586.

121. **Marcondes JA, Minnani SL, Luthold WW, et al.** Treatment of hirsutism in women with flutamide. *Fertil Steril* 1992;57:543–547.

122. **Ciotta L, Cianci A, Marletta E, et al.** Treatment of hirsutism with flutamide and a low-dosage oral contraceptive in polycystic ovarian disease patients. *Fertil Steril* 1994;62:1129–1135.

123. **Cusan L, Dupont A, Belanger A, et al.** Treatment of hirsutism with the pure antiandrogen flutamide. *J Am Acad Dermatol* 1990;23(Pt 1):462–469.

124. **Ibanez L, De Zegher F.** Flutamide-metformin plus an oral contraceptive (OC) for young women with polycystic ovary syndrome: switch from third- to fourth-generation OC reduces body adiposity. *Hum Reprod* 2004;19:1725–1727.

125. **Ibanez L, Valls C, Cabre S, et al.** Flutamide-metformin plus ethinylestradiol-drospirenone for lipolysis and antiatherogenesis in young women with ovarian hyperandrogenism: the key role of early, low-dose flutamide. *J Clin Endocrinol Metab* 2004;89:4716–4720.

126. **Osculati A, Castiglioni C.** Fatal liver complications with flutamide. *Lancet* 2006;367:1140–1141.

127. **Wong IL, Morris RS, Chang L, et al.** A prospective randomized trial comparing finasteride to spironolactone in the treatment of hirsute women. *J Clin Endocrinol Metab* 1995;80:233–238.

128. **Ciotta L, Cianci A, Calogero AE, et al.** Clinical and endocrine effects of finasteride, a 5 alpha-reductase inhibitor, in women with idiopathic hirsutism. *Fertil Steril* 1995;64:299–306.

129. **Judd HL, Rigg LA, Anderson DC, et al.** The effects of ovarian wedge resection on circulating gonadotropin and ovarian steroid levels in patients with polycystic ovary syndrome. *J Clin Endocrinol Metab* 1976;43:347–355.

130. **Katz M, Carr PJ, Cohen BM, et al.** Hormonal effects of wedge resection of polycystic ovaries. *Obstet Gynecol* 1978;51:437–444.

131. **Goldzieher JW, Green JA.** The polycystic ovary. I. Clinical and histologic features. *J Clin Endocrinol Metab* 1962;22:325–338.

132. **Adashi EY, Rock JA, Guzick D, et al.** Fertility following bilateral ovarian wedge resection: a critical analysis of 90 consecutive cases of the polycystic ovary syndrome. *Fertil Steril* 1981;36:320–325.

133. **Toaff R, Toaff ME, Peyser MR.** Infertility following wedge resection of the ovaries. *Am J Obstet Gynecol* 1976;124:92–96.

134. **Felemban A, Tan SL, Tulandi T.** Laparoscopic treatment of polycystic ovaries with insulated needle cautery: a reappraisal. *Fertil Steril* 2000;73:266–269.

135. **Armar NA, Lachelin GC.** Laparoscopic ovarian diathermy: an effective treatment for anti-oestrogen resistant anovulatory infertility in women with the polycystic ovary syndrome. *Br J Obstet Gynaecol* 1993;100:161–164.

136. **Pirwany I, Tulandi T.** Laparoscopic treatment of polycystic ovaries: is it time to relinquish the procedure? *Fertil Steril* 2003;80:241–251.

137. **Armar NA, McGarrigle HH, Honour J, et al.** Laparoscopic ovarian diathermy in the management of anovulatory infertility in women with polycystic ovaries: endocrine changes and clinical outcome. *Fertil Steril* 1990;53:45–49.

138. **Rossmanith WG, Keckstein J, Spatzier K, et al.** The impact of ovarian laser surgery on the gonadotrophin secretion in women with polycystic ovarian disease. *Clin Endocrinol (Oxf)* 1991;34:223–230.

139. **Amer SA, Banu Z, Li TC, et al.** Long-term follow-up of patients with polycystic ovary syndrome after laparoscopic ovarian drilling: endocrine and ultrasonographic outcomes. *Hum Reprod* 2002;17:2851–2857.

140. **Balen AH, Jacobs HS.** A prospective study comparing unilateral and bilateral laparoscopic ovarian diathermy in women with the polycystic ovary syndrome. *Fertil Steril* 1994;62:921–925.

141. **Schrode K, Huber F, Staszak J, et al.** Randomized, double blind, vehicle controlled safety and efficacy evaluation of eflornithine 15% cream in the treatment of women with excessive facial hair. Presented at American Academy of Dermatology annual meeting, 2000.

142. **Lynfield YL, Macwilliams P.** Shaving and hair growth. *J Invest Dermatol* 1970;55:170–172.

143. **Wagner RF Jr.** Physical methods for the management of hirsutism. *Cutis* 1990;45:319–321.

144. **Kim LH, Taylor AE, Barbieri RL.** Insulin sensitizers and polycystic ovary syndrome: can a diabetes medication treat infertility? *Fertil Steril* 2000;73:1097–1098.

145. **Mathur R, Alexander CJ, Yano J, et al.** Use of metformin in polycystic ovary syndrome. *Am J Obstet Gynecol* 2008;199:596–609.

146. **Creanga AA, Bradley HM, McCormick C, et al.** Use of metformin in polycystic ovary syndrome: a meta-analysis. *Obstet Gynecol* 2008;111:959–968.

147. **Legro RS, Barnhart HX, Schlaff WD, et al.** Clomiphene, metformin, or both for infertility in the polycystic ovary syndrome. *N Engl J Med* 2007;356:551–566.

148. **Hasegawa I, Murakawa H, Suzuki M, et al.** Effect of troglitazone on endocrine and ovulatory performance in women with insulin resistance-related polycystic ovary syndrome. *Fertil Steril* 1999;71:323–327.

149. **Stadtmauer LA, Toma SK, Riehl RM, et al.** Metformin treatment of patients with polycystic ovary syndrome undergoing *in vitro* fertilization improves outcomes and is associated with modulation of the insulin-like growth factors. *Fertil Steril* 2001;75:505–509.

150. **Jakubowicz DJ, Seppala M, Jakubowicz S, et al.** Insulin reduction with metformin increases luteal phase serum glycodelin and insulin-like growth factor-binding protein 1 concentrations and enhances uterine vascularity and blood flow in the polycystic ovary syndrome. *J Clin Endocrinol Metab* 2001;86:1126–1133.

151. **Glueck CJ, Wang P, Goldenberg N, et al.** Pregnancy outcomes among women with polycystic ovary syndrome treated with metformin. *Hum Reprod* 2002;17:2858–2864.

152. **Glueck CJ, Phillips H, Cameron D, et al.** Continuing metformin throughout pregnancy in women with polycystic ovary syndrome appears to safely reduce first-trimester spontaneous abortion: a pilot study. *Fertil Steril* 2001;75:46–52.

153. **Tang T.** The use of metformin for women with PCOS undergoing IVF treatment. *Hum Reprod* 2006;21:1416–1425.

154. **Nieman LK, Biller BM, Findling JW, et al.** The diagnosis of Cushing's syndrome: an Endocrine Society Clinical Practice Guideline. *J Clin Endocrinol Metab* 2008;93:1526–1540.

155. **Biller BM, Grossman AB, Stewart PM, et al.** Treatment of adrenocorticotropin-dependent Cushing's syndrome: a consensus statement. *J Clin Endocrinol Metab* 2008;93:2454–2462.

156. **Orth DN.** Ectopic hormone production. In: **Felig P, Baster JD, Broadus AE, et al., eds.** *Endocrinology and metabolism.* New York: McGraw-Hill, 1987:1692–1735.

157. **Schteingart DE, Tsao HS, Taylor CI, et al.** Sustained remission of Cushing's disease with mitotane and pituitary irradiation. *Ann Intern Med* 1980;92:613–619.

158. **Orth DN, Liddle GW.** Results of treatment in 108 patients with Cushing's syndrome. *N Engl J Med* 1971;285:243–247.

159. **Valimaki M, Pelkonen R, Porkka L, et al.** Long-term results of adrenal surgery in patients with Cushing's syndrome due to adrenocortical adenoma. *Clin Endocrinol (Oxf)* 1984;20:229–236.

160. **Hammer GD, Tyrrell JB, Lamborn KR, et al.** Transsphenoidal microsurgery for Cushing's disease: initial outcome and long-term results. *J Clin Endocrinol Metab* 2004;89:6348–6357.

161. **Boggan JE, Tyrrell JB, Wilson CB.** Transsphenoidal microsurgical management of Cushing's disease. Report of 100 cases. *J Neurosurg* 1983;59:195–200.

162. **Swearingen B, Biller BM, Barker FG 2nd, et al.** Long-term mortality after transsphenoidal surgery for Cushing disease. *Ann Intern Med* 1999;130:821–824.

163. **Hofmann BM, Fahlbusch R.** Treatment of Cushing's disease: a retrospective clinical study of the latest 100 cases. *Front Horm Res* 2006;34:158–184.

164. **Sonino N, Zielezny M, Fava GA, et al.** Risk factors and long-term outcome in pituitary-dependent Cushing's disease. *J Clin Endocrinol Metab* 1996;81:2647–2652.

165. **Bigos ST, Somma M, Rasio E, et al.** Cushing's disease: management by transsphenoidal pituitary microsurgery. *J Clin Endocrinol Metab* 1980;50:348–354.

166. **De Tommasi C, Vance ML, Okonkwo DO, et al.** Surgical management of adrenocorticotropic hormone-secreting macroadenomas:

outcome and challenges in patients with Cushing's disease or Nelson's syndrome. *J Neurosurg* 2005;103:825–830.

167. **Blevins LS Jr, Christy JH, Khajavi M, et al.** Outcomes of therapy for Cushing's disease due to adrenocorticotropin-secreting pituitary macroadenomas. *J Clin Endocrinol Metab* 1998;83:63–67.

168. **Aron DC, Findling JW, Tyrrell JB.** Cushing's disease. *Endocrinol Metab Clin North Am* 1987;16:705–730.

169. **Devin JK, Allen GS, Cmelak AJ, et al.** The efficacy of linear accelerator radiosurgery in the management of patients with Cushing's disease. *Stereo Funct Neurosurg* 2004;82:254–262.

170. **Estrada J, Boronat M, Mielgo M, et al.** The long-term outcome of pituitary irradiation after unsuccessful transsphenoidal surgery in Cushing's disease. *N Engl J Med* 1997;336:172–177.

171. **Jennings AS, Liddle GW, Orth DN.** Results of treating childhood Cushing's disease with pituitary irradiation. *N Engl J Med* 1977;297:957–962.

172. **Loli P, Berselli ME, Tagliaferri M.** Use of ketoconazole in the treatment of Cushing's syndrome. *J Clin Endocrinol Metab* 1986;63:1365–1371.

173. **Nelson DH, Meakin JW, Dealy JB, et al.** ACTH-producing tumor of the pituitary gland. *N Engl J Med* 1958;85:731–734.

174. **Azziz R, Zacur HA.** 21-Hydroxylase deficiency in female hyperandrogenism: screening and diagnosis. *J Clin Endocrinol Metab* 1989;69:577–584.

175. **New MI, Lorenzen F, Lerner AJ, et al.** Genotyping steroid 21-hydroxylase deficiency: hormonal reference data. *J Clin Endocrinol Metab* 1983;57:320–326.

176. **Speiser PW, Dupont B, Rubinstein P, et al.** High frequency of nonclassical steroid 21-hydroxylase deficiency. *Am J Hum Genet* 1985;37:650–667.

177. **New MI.** Steroid 21-hydroxylase deficiency (congenital adrenal hyperplasia). *Am J Med* 1995;98:2S–8S.

178. **Speiser PW, New MI, White PC.** Molecular genetic analysis of nonclassic steroid 21-hydroxylase deficiency associated with HLA-B14,DR1. *N Engl J Med* 1988;319:19–23.

179. **Merke DP, Bornstein SR.** Congenital adrenal hyperplasia. *Lancet* 2005;365:2125–2136.

180. **Speiser PW, White PC.** Congenital adrenal hyperplasia. *N Engl J Med* 2003;349:776–788.

181. **Hirvikoski T, Nordenstrom A, Lindholm T, et al.** Cognitive functions in children at risk for congenital adrenal hyperplasia treated prenatally with dexamethasone. *J Clin Endocrinol Metab* 2007;92:542–548.

182. **Speiser PW, Azziz R, Baskin LS, et al.** A summary of the Endocrine Society clinical practice guidelines on congenital adrenal hyperplasia due to steroid 21-hydroxylase deficiency. *Int J Pediat Endocrinol* 2010;2010:1–6.

183. **White PC.** Steroid 11 beta-hydroxylase deficiency and related disorders. *Endocrinol Metab Clin North Am* 2001;30:61–79.

184. **Nimkarn S, New MI.** Steroid 11[beta]- hydroxylase deficiency congenital adrenal hyperplasia. *Trends Endocrinol Metab* 2008;19:96–99.

185. **White PC, Curnow KM, Pascoe L.** Disorders of steroid 11 beta-hydroxylase isozymes. *Endocr Rev* 1994;15:421–438.

186. **Rosler A, Leiberman E, Cohen T.** High frequency of congenital adrenal hyperplasia (classic 11 beta-hydroxylase deficiency) among Jews from Morocco. *Am J Med Genet* 1992;42:827–834.

187. **Mornet E, Dupont J, Vitek A, et al.** Characterization of two genes encoding human steroid 11 beta-hydroxylase (P-450(11) beta). *J Biol Chem* 1989;264:20961–20967.

188. **Taymans SE, Pack S, Pak E, et al.** Human CYP11B2 (aldosterone synthase) maps to chromosome 8q24.3. *J Clin Endocrinol Metab* 1998;83:1033–1036.

189. **Parajes S, Loidi L, Reisch N, et al.** Functional consequences of seven novel mutations in the CYP11B1 gene: four mutations associated with nonclassic and three mutations causing classic 11[beta]-hydroxylase deficiency. *J Clin Endocrinol Metab* 2010;95:779–788.

190. **Azziz R, Boots LR, Parker CR Jr, et al.** 11 beta-hydroxylase deficiency in hyperandrogenism. *Fertil Steril* 1991;55:733–741.

191. **Pang SY, Lerner AJ, Stoner E, et al.** Late-onset adrenal steroid 3 beta-hydroxysteroid dehydrogenase deficiency. I. A cause of hirsutism in pubertal and postpubertal women. *J Clin Endocrinol Metab* 1985;60:428–439.

192. **Azziz R, Bradley EL Jr, Potter HD, et al.** 3 beta-hydroxysteroid dehydrogenase deficiency in hyperandrogenism. *Am J Obstet Gynecol* 1993;168(Pt 1):889–895.

193. **Carbunaru G, Prasad P, Scoccia B, et al.** The hormonal phenotype of nonclassic 3[beta]-hydroxysteroid dehydrogenase (HSD3B) deficiency in hyperandrogenic females is associated with insulin-resistant polycystic ovary syndrome and is not a variant of inherited HSD3B2 deficiency. *J Clin Endocrinol Metab* 2004;89:783–794.

194. **Cordera F, Grant C, van Heerden J, et al.** Androgen-secreting adrenal tumors. *Surgery* 2003;134:874–880.

195. **Derksen J, Nagesser SK, Meinders AE, et al.** Identification of virilizing adrenal tumors in hirsute women. *N Engl J Med* 1994;331:968–973.

196. **Ettinger B, Von Werder K, Thenaers GC, et al.** Plasma testosterone stimulation-suppression dynamics in hirsute women. *Am J Med* 1971;51:170–175.

197. **Surrey ES, de Ziegler D, Gambone JC, et al.** Preoperative localization of androgen-secreting tumors: clinical, endocrinologic, and radiologic evaluation of ten patients. *Am J Obstet Gynecol* 1988;158(Pt 1):1313–1322.

198. **Korobkin M.** Overview of adrenal imaging/adrenal CT. *Urol Radiol* 1989;11:221–226.

199. **Taylor L, Ayers JW, Gross MD, et al.** Diagnostic considerations in virilization: iodomethyl-norcholesterol scanning in the localization of androgen secreting tumors. *Fertil Steril* 1986;46:1005–1010.

200. **Moltz L, Pickartz H, Sorensen R, et al.** Ovarian and adrenal vein steroids in seven patients with androgen-secreting ovarian neoplasms: selective catheterization findings. *Fertil Steril* 1984;42:585–593.

201. **Wentz AC, White RI Jr, Migeon CJ, et al.** Differential ovarian and adrenal vein catheterization. *Am J Obstet Gynecol* 1976;125:1000–1007.

202. **Young RH, Scully RE.** Sex-cord stromal steroid cell and other ovarian tumors with endocrine, paraendocrine, and paraneoplastic manifestations. In: **Kurman RJ, ed.** *Blaustein's pathology of the female genital tract*, 4th ed. New York: Springer-Verlag, 1994:783–847.

203. **Schumer ST, Cannistra SA.** granulosa cell tumor of the ovary. *J Clin Oncol* 2003;21:1180–1189.

204. **Nocito AL, Sarancone S, Bacchi C, et al.** Ovarian thecoma: clinico-pathological analysis of 50 cases. *Ann Diag Pathol* 2008;12:12–16.

205. **Colombo N, Parma G, Zanagnolo V, et al.** Management of ovarian stromal cell tumors. *J Clin Oncol* 2007;25:2944–2951.

206. **Young RH, Scully RE.** Ovarian Sertoli cell tumors: a report of 10 cases. *Int J Gynecol Pathol* 1984;2:349–363.

207. **Young RH, Welch WR, Dickersin GR, et al.** Ovarian sex cord tumor with annular tubules: review of 74 cases including 27 with Peutz-Jeghers syndrome and four with adenoma malignum of the cervix. *Cancer* 1982;50:1384–1402.

208. **Aiman J.** Virilizing ovarian tumors. *Clin Obstet Gynecol* 1991;34:835–847.

209. **Scully RE.** Gonadoblastoma. A review of 74 cases. *Cancer* 1970;25:1340–1356.

210. **Ireland K, Woodruff JD.** Masculinizing ovarian tumors. *Obstet Gynecol Surv* 1976;31:83–111.

211. **Boss JH, Scully RE, Wegner KH, et al.** Structural variations in the adult ovary. Clinical significance. *Obstet Gynecol* 1965;25:747–764.

212. **Jongen VH, Hollema H, van der Zee AG, et al.** Ovarian stromal hyperplasia and ovarian vein steroid levels in relation to endometrioid endometrial cancer. *BJOG* 2003;110:690–695.

213. **Krug E, Berga SL.** Postmenopausal hyperthecosis: functional dysregulation of androgenesis in climacteric ovary. *Obstet Gynecol* 2002;99(Pt 2):893–897.

214. **Judd HL, Scully RE, Herbst AL, et al.** Familial hyperthecosis: comparison of endocrinologic and histologic findings with polycystic ovarian disease. *Am J Obstet Gynecol* 1973;117:976–982.

215. **Brown DL, Henrichsen TL, Clayton AC, et al.** Ovarian stromal hyperthecosis: sonographic features and histologic associations. *J Ultrasound Med* 2009;28:587–593.

216. **Karam K, Hajj S.** Hyperthecosis syndrome. Clinical, endocrinologic and histologic findings. *Acta Obstet Gynecol Scand* 1979; 58:73–79.

217. **Braithwaite SS, Erkman-Balis B, Avila TD.** Postmenopausal virilization due to ovarian stromal hyperthecosis. *J Clin Endocrinol Metab* 1978;46:295–300.

218. **Steingold KA, Judd HL, Nieberg RK, et al.** Treatment of severe androgen excess due to ovarian hyperthecosis with a long-acting gonadotropin-releasing hormone agonist. *Am J Obstet Gynecol* 1986;154:1241–1248.

219. **Garcia-Bunuel R, Berek JS, Woodruff JD.** Luteomas of pregnancy. *Obstet Gynecol* 1975;45:407–414.

220. **Cronje HS.** Luteoma of pregnancy. *S Afr Med J* 1984;66:59–60.

221. **Mazza V, Di Monte I, Ceccarelli PL, et al.** Prenatal diagnosis of female pseudohermaphroditism associated with bilateral luteoma of pregnancy: case report. *Hum Reprod* 2002;17:821–824.

222. **Ng L, Libertino JM.** Adrenocortical carcinoma: diagnosis, evaluation and treatment. *J Urol* 2003;169:5–11.

223. **Latronico AC, Chrousos GP.** Adrenocortical tumors. *J Clin Endocrinol Metab* 1997;82:1317–1324.

224. **Gaudio AD, Gaudio GAD.** Virilizing adrenocortical tumors in adult women. Report of 10 patients, 2 of whom each had a tumor secreting only testosterone. *Cancer* 1993;72:1997–2003.

225. **Riddle O, Bates RW, Dykshorn S.** The preparation, identification and assay of prolactin. A hormone of the anterior pituitary. *Am J Physiol* 1933;105:191–196.

226. **Frantz AG, Kleinberg DL.** Prolactin: evidence that it is separate from growth hormone in human blood. *Science* 1970;170:745–747.

227. **Lewis UJ, Singh RN, Sinha YN, et al.** Electrophoretic evidence for human prolactin. *J Clin Endocrinol Metab* 1971;33:153–156.

228. **Hwang P, Guyda H, Friesen H.** Purification of human prolactin. *J Biol Chem* 1972;247:1955–1958.

229. **Freeman ME, Kanyicska B, Lerant A, et al.** Prolactin: structure, function, and regulation of secretion. *Physiol Rev* 2000;80:1523–1631.

230. **Suh HK, Frantz AG.** Size heterogeneity of human prolactin in plasma and pituitary extracts. *J Clin Endocrinol Metab* 1974;39:928–935.

231. **Guyda JH.** Heterogeneity of human growth hormone and prolactin secreted *in vitro*: immunoassay and radioreceptor assay correlations. *J Clin Endocrinol Metab* 1975;41:953–967.

232. **Farkouh NH, Packer MG, Frantz AG.** Large molecular size prolactin with reduced receptor activity in human serum: high proportion in basal state and reduction after thyrotropin-releasing hormone. *J Clin Endocrinol Metab* 1979;48:1026–1032.

233. **Benveniste R, Helman JD, Orth DN, et al.** Circulating big human prolactin: conversion to small human prolactin by reduction of disulfide bonds. *J Clin Endocrinol Metab* 1979;48:883–886.

234. **Jackson RD, Wortsman J, Malarkey WB.** Characterization of a large molecular weight prolactin in women with idiopathic hyperprolactinemia and normal menses. *J Clin Endocrinol Metab* 1985;61:258–264.

235. **Fraser IS, Lun ZG, Zhou JP, et al.** Detailed assessment of big big prolactin in women with hyperprolactinemia and normal ovarian function. *J Clin Endocrinol Metab* 1989;69:585–592.

236. **Larrea F, Escorza A, Valero A, et al.** Heterogeneity of serum prolactin throughout the menstrual cycle and pregnancy in hyperprolactinemic women with normal ovarian function. *J Clin Endocrinol Metab* 1989;68:982–987.

237. **Lewis UJ, Singh RN, Sinha YN, et al.** Glycosylated human prolactin. *Endocrinology* 1985;116:359–363.

238. **Markoff E, Lee DW.** Glycosylated prolactin is a major circulating variant in human serum. *J Clin Endocrinol Metab* 1985:1102–1106.

239. **Markoff E, Lee DW, Hollingsworth DR.** Glycosated and nonglycosated prolactin in serum during pregnancy. *J Clin Endocrinol Metab* 1988;67:519–523.

240. **Pellegrini I, Gunz G, Ronin C, et al.** Polymorphism of prolactin secreted by human prolactinoma cells: immunological, receptor binding, and biological properties of the glycosylated and nonglycosylated forms. *Endocrinology* 1988;122:2667–2674.

241. **Bole-Feysot C, Goffin V, Edery M, et al.** Prolactin (PRL) and its receptor: actions, signal transduction pathways and phenotypes observed in PRL receptor knockout mice. *Endocr Rev* 1998;19:225–268.

242. **Goldsmith PC, Cronin MJ, Weiner RI.** Dopamine receptor sites in the anterior pituitary. *J Histochem Cytochem* 1979;27:1205–1207.

243. **Quigley ME, Judd SJ, Gilliland GB, et al.** Effects of a dopamine antagonist on the release of gonadotropin and prolactin in normal women and women with hyperprolactinemic anovulation. *J Clin Endocrinol Metab* 1979;48:718–720.

244. **Quigley ME, Judd SJ, Gilliland GB, et al.** Functional studies of dopamine control of prolactin secretion in normal women and women with hyperprolactinemic pituitary microadenoma. *J Clin Endocrinol Metab* 1980;50:994–998.

245. **De Leo V, Petraglia F, Bruno MG, et al.** Different dopaminergic control of plasma luteinizing hormone, follicle-stimulating hormone and prolactin in ovulatory and postmenopausal women: effect of ovariectomy. *Gynecol Obstet Invest* 1989;27:94–98.

246. **Lachelin GC, Leblanc H, Yen SS.** The inhibitory effect of dopamine agonists on LH release in women. *J Clin Endocrinol Metab* 1977;44:728–732.

247. **Hill MK, Macleod RM, Orcutt P.** Dibutyryl cyclic AMP, adenosine and guanosine blockade of the dopamine, ergocryptine and apomorphine inhibition of prolactin release *in vitro. Endocrinology* 1976 Dec;99(6):1612-7.

248. **Lemberger L, Crabtree RE.** Pharmacologic effects in man of a potent, long-acting dopamine receptor agonist. *Science* 1979; 205:1151–1153.

249. **Braund W, Roeger DC, Judd SJ.** Synchronous secretion of luteinizing hormone and prolactin in the human luteal phase: neuroendocrine mechanisms. *J Clin Endocrinol Metab* 1984;58:293–297.

250. **Grossman A, Delitala G, Yeo T, et al.** GABA and muscimol inhibit the release of prolactin from dispersed rat anterior pituitary cells. *Neuroendocrinology* 1981;32:145–149.

251. **Gudelsky GA, Apud JA, Masotto C, et al.** Ethanolamine-O-sulfate enhances gamma-aminobutyric acid secretion into hypophysial portal blood and lowers serum prolactin concentrations. *Neuroendocrinology* 1983;37:397–399.

252. **Melis GB, Paoletti AM, Mais V, et al.** The effects of the gabaergic drug, sodium valproate, on prolactin secretion in normal and hyperprolactinemic subjects. *J Clin Endocrinol Metab* 1982;54:485–489.

253. **Melis GB, Fruzzetti F, Paoletti AM, et al.** Pharmacological activation of gamma-aminobutyric acid-system blunts prolactin response to mechanical breast stimulation in puerperal women. *J Clin Endocrinol Metab* 1984;58:201–205.

254. **Bazan JF.** Structural design and molecular evolution of a cytokine receptor superfamily. *Proc Natl Acad Sci U S A* 1990;87:6934–6938.

255. **Hu ZZ, Zhuang L, Meng J, et al.** Transcriptional regulation of the generic promoter III of the rat prolactin receptor gene by C/EBPbeta and Sp1. *J Biol Chem* 1998;273:26225–26235.

256. **Sassin JF, Frantz AG, Weitzman ED, et al.** Human prolactin: 24-hour pattern with increased release during sleep. *Science* 1972;177:1205–1207.

257. **Sassin JF, Frantz AG, Kapen S, et al.** The nocturnal rise of human prolactin is dependent on sleep. *J Clin Endocrinol Metab* 1973;37:436–440.

258. **Carandente F, Angeli A, Candiani GB, et al.** Rhythms in the ovulatory cycle. 1st: Prolactin. Chronobiological Research Group on Synthetic Peptides in Medicine. *Chronobiologia* 1989;16:35–44.

259. **Pansini F, Bianchi A, Zito V, et al.** Blood prolactin levels: influence of age, menstrual cycle and oral contraceptives. *Contraception* 1983;28:201–207.

260. **Pansini F, Bergamini CM, Cavallini AR, et al.** Prolactinemia during the menstrual cycle. A possible role for prolactin in the regulation of ovarian function. *Gynecol Obstet Invest* 1987;23:172–176.

261. **Bohnet HG, Dahlen HG, Wuttke W, et al.** Hyperprolactinemic anovulatory syndrome. *J Clin Endocrinol Metab* 1976;42:132–143.

262. **Franks S, Murray MA, Jequier AM, et al.** Incidence and significance of hyperprolactinaemia in women with amenorrhea. *Clin Endocrinol (Oxf)* 1975;4:597–607.

263. **Jacobs HS, Hull MG, Murray MA, et al.** Therapy-orientated diagnosis of secondary amenorrhoea. *Horm Res* 1975;6:268–287.

264. **Boyar RM, Kapen S, Finkelstein JW, et al.** Hypothalamic-pituitary function in diverse hyperprolactinemic states. *J Clin Invest* 1974;53:1588–1598.

265. **Moult PJ, Rees LH, Besser GM.** Pulsatile gonadotrophin secretion in hyperprolactinaemic amenorrhoea an the response to bromocriptine therapy. *Clin Endocrinol (Oxf)* 1982;16:153–162.

266. **Buckman MT, Peake GT, Srivastava L.** Patterns of spontaneous LH release in normo- and hyperprolactinaemic women. *Acta Endocrinol (Copenh)* 1981;97:305–310.

267. **Aono T, Miyake A, Yasuda TS, et al.** Restoration of oestrogen positive feedback effect on LH release by bromocriptine in hyperprolacti-

naemic patients with galactorrhoea-amenorrhoea. *Acta Endocrinol (Copenh)* 1979;91:591–600.

268. **Travaglini P, Ambrosi B, Beck-Peccoz P, et al.** Hypothalamic-pituitary-ovarian function in hyperprolactinemic women. *J Endocrinol Invest* 1978;1:39–45.

269. **Glass MR, Shaw RW, Butt WR, et al.** An abnormality of oestrogen feedback in amenorrhoea-galactorrhoea. *BMJ* 1975;3:274–275.

270. **Koike J, Aono T, Tsutsumi H, et al.** Restoration of oestrogen-positive feedback effect on LH release in women with prolactinoma by transsphenoidal surgery. *Acta Endocrinol (Copenh)* 1982;100:492–498.

271. **Rakoff J, VandenBerg G, Siler TM, et al.** An integrated direct functional test of the adenohypophysis. *Am J Obstet Gynecol* 1974;119: 358–368.

272. **Zarate A, Jacobs LS, Canales ES, et al.** Functional evaluation of pituitary reserve in patients with the amenorrhea-galactorrhea syndrome utilizing luteinizing hormone-releasing hormone (LH-RH), L-dopa and chlorpromazine. *J Clin Endocrinol Metab* 1973;37:855–859.

273. **McNatty KP.** Relationship between plasma prolactin and the endocrine microenvironment of the developing human antral follicle. *Fertil Steril* 1979;32:433–438.

274. **Dorrington J, Gore-Langton RE.** Prolactin inhibits oestrogen synthesis in the ovary. *Nature* 1981;290:600–602.

275. **Cutie E, Andino NA.** Prolactin inhibits the steroidogenesis in mid-follicular phase human granulosa cells cultured in a chemically defined medium. *Fertil Steril* 1988;49:632–637.

276. **Adashi EY, Resnick CE.** Prolactin as an inhibitor of granulosa cell luteinization: implications for hyperprolactinemia-associated luteal phase dysfunction. *Fertil Steril* 1987;48:131–139.

277. **Soto EA, Tureck RW, Strauss JF 3rd.** Effects of prolactin on progestin secretion by human granulosa cells in culture. *Biol Reprod* 1985;32:541–545.

278. **Demura R, Ono M, Demura H, et al.** Prolactin directly inhibits basal as well as gonadotropin-stimulated secretion of progesterone and 17β-estradiol in the human ovary. *J Clin Endocrinol Metab* 1985;54:1246–1250.

279. **Kleinberg DL, Noel GL, Frantz AG.** Galactorrhea: a study of 235 cases, including 48 with pituitary tumors. *N Engl J Med* 1977; 296:589–600.

280. **Tolis G, Somma M, Van Campenhout J, et al.** Prolactin secretion in sixty-five patients with galactorrhea. *Am J Obstet Gynecol* 1974;118:91–101.

281. **Boyd AE 3rd, Reichlin S, Turksoy RN.** Galactorrhea-amenorrhea syndrome: diagnosis and therapy. *Ann Intern Med* 1977;87:165–175.

282. **Schlechte J, Sherman B, Halmi N, et al.** Prolactin-secreting pituitary tumors in amenorrheic women: a comprehensive study. *Endocr Rev* 1980;1:295–308.

283. **Minakami H, Abe N, Oka N, et al.** Prolactin release in polycystic ovarian syndrome. *Endocrinol Jpn* 1988;35:303–310.

284. **Murdoch AP, Dunlop W, Kendall-Taylor P.** Studies of prolactin secretion in polycystic ovary syndrome. *Clin Endocrinol (Oxf)* 1986;24:165–175.

285. **Lythgoe K, Dotson R, Peterson CM.** Multiple endocrine neoplasia presenting as primary amenorrhea: a case report. *Obstet Gynecol* 1995;86(Pt 2):683–686.

286. **Burgess JR, Shepherd JJ, Parameswaran B, et al.** Spectrum of pituitary disease in multiple endocrine neoplasia type 1 (MEN-1): Clinical, biochemical, and radiologic features of pituitary disease in a large MEN-1 kindred. *J Clin Endocrinol Metab* 1996;81:2642–2646.

287. **Bohler HC Jr, Jones EE, Brines ML.** Marginally elevated prolactin levels require magnetic resonance imaging and evaluation for acromegaly. *Fertil Steril* 1994;61:1168–1170.

288. **Gonsky R, Herman V, Melmed S, et al.** Transforming DNA sequences present in human prolactin-secreting pituitary tumors. *Mol Endocrinol* 1991;5:1687–1695.

289. **Sisam DA, Sheehan JP, Sheeler LR.** The natural history of untreated microprolactinomas. *Fertil Steril* 1987;48:67–71.

290. **Schlechte J, Dolan K, Sherman B, et al.** The natural history of untreated hyperprolactinemia: a prospective analysis. *J Clin Endocrinol Metab* 1989;68:412–418.

291. **Weiss MH, Wycoff RR, Yadley R, et al.** Bromocriptine treatment of prolactin-secreting tumors: surgical implications. *Neurosurgery* 1983;12:640–642.

292. **Ezzat S, Asa SL, Couldwell WT, et al.** The prevalence of pituitary adenomas. *Cancer* 2004;101:613–619.

293. **Klibanski A, Biller BM, Rosenthal DI, et al.** Effects of prolactin and estrogen deficiency in amenorrheic bone loss. *J Clin Endocrinol Metab* 1988;67:124–130.

294. **Turner TH, Cookson JC, Wass JA, et al.** Psychotic reactions during treatment of pituitary tumours with dopamine agonists. *Br Med J (Clin Res Ed)* 1984;289:1101–1103.

295. **Katz E, Weiss BE, Hassell A, et al.** Increased circulating levels of bromocriptine after vaginal compared with oral administration. *Fertil Steril* 1991;55:882–884.

296. **Schade R, Andersohn F, Suissa S, et al.** Dopamine agonists and the risk of cardiac-valve regurgitation. *N Engl J Med* 2007;356:29–38.

297. **Zanettini R, Antonini A, Gatto G, et al.** Valvular heart disease and the use of dopamine agonists for Parkinson's disease. *N Engl J Med* 2007;356:39–46.

298. **Roth BL.** Drugs and valvular heart disease. *N Engl J Med* 2007;356:6–9.

299. **Colao A, Galderisi M, Di Sarno A, et al.** Increased prevalence of tricuspid regurgitation in patients with prolactinomas chronically treated with cabergoline. *J Clin Endocrinol Metab* 2008;93:3777–3784.

300. **Bogazzi F, Manetti L, Raffaelli V, et al.** Cabergoline therapy and the risk of cardiac valve regurgitation in patients with hyperprolactinemia: a meta-analysis from clinical studies. *J Endocrinol Invest* 2008;31:1119–1123.

301. **Krupp P, Monka C.** Bromocriptine in pregnancy: safety aspects. *Klin Wochenschr* 1987;65:823–827.

302. **Jeffcoate WJ, Pound N, Sturrock ND, et al.** Long-term follow-up of patients with hyperprolactinaemia. *Clin Endocrinol (Oxf)* 1996;45:299–303.

303. **Passos VQ, Souza JJ, Musolino NR, et al.** Long-term follow-up of prolactinomas: normoprolactinemia after bromocriptine withdrawal. *J Clin Endocrinol Metab* 2002;87:3578–3582.

304. **Colao A, Di Sarno A, Cappabianca P, et al.** Withdrawal of long-term cabergoline therapy for tumoral and nontumoral hyperprolactinemia. *N Engl J Med* 2003;349:2023–2033.

305. **Biswas M, Smith J, Jadon D, et al.** Long-term remission following withdrawal of dopamine agonist therapy in subjects with microprolactinomas. *Clin Endocrinol* 2005;63:26–31.

306. **Dekkers OM, Lagro J, Burman P, et al.** Recurrence of hyperprolactinemia after withdrawal of dopamine agonists: systematic review and meta-analysis. *J Clin Endocrinol Metab* 2010;95:43–51.

307. **Ono M, Miki N, Amano K, et al.** Individualized high-dose cabergoline therapy for hyperprolactinemic infertility in women with micro- and macroprolactinomas. *J Clin Endocrinol Metab* 2010;95:2672–2679.

308. **Mori H, Mori S, Saitoh Y, et al.** Effects of bromocriptine on prolactin-secreting pituitary adenomas. Mechanism of reduction in tumor size evaluated by light and electron microscopic, immunohistochemical, and morphometric analysis. *Cancer* 1985;56:230–238.

309. **Abram M, Brue T, Morange I, et al.** [Pituitary tumor syndrome and hyperprolactinemia in peripheral hypothyroidism]. *Ann Endocrinol (Paris)* 1992;53:215–223.

310. **Chirito E, Bonda A, Friesen HG.** Prolactin in renal failure. *Clin Res* 1972;20:423.

311. **Nagel TC, Freinkel N, Bell RH, et al.** Gynecomastia, prolactin, and other peptide hormones in patients undergoing chronic hemodialysis. *J Clin Endocrinol Metab* 1973;36:428–432.

312. **Olgaard K, Hagen C, McNeilly AS.** Pituitary hormones in women with chronic renal failure: the effect of chronic intermittent haemo- and peritoneal dialysis. *Acta Endocrinol (Copenh)* 1975;80:237–246.

313. **Thorner MO, Edwards CRW, Hanker JP.** Prolactin and gonadotropin interaction in the male. In: **Troen P, Nankin H, eds.** *The testis in normal and infertile men.* New York: Raven Press, 1977:351–366.

314. **Lloyd RV.** Estrogen-induced hyperplasia and neoplasia in the rat anterior pituitary gland. An immunohistochemical study. *Am J Pathol* 1983;113:198–206.

315. **Scheithauer BW, Sano T, Kovacs KT, et al.** The pituitary gland in pregnancy: a clinicopathologic and immunohistochemical study of 69 cases. *Mayo Clin Proc* 1990;65:461–474.

316. **Weil C.** The safety of bromocriptine in hyperprolactinaemic female infertility: a literature review. *Curr Med Res Opin* 1986;10:172–195.

317. **Shy KK, McTiernan AM, Daling JR, et al.** Oral contraceptive use and the occurrence of pituitary prolactinoma. *JAMA* 1983;249:2204–2207.

318. **Corenblum B, Taylor PJ.** Idiopathic hyperprolactinemia may include a distinct entity with a natural history different from that of prolactin adenomas. *Fertil Steril* 1988;49:544–546.

319. **Corenblum B, Donovan L.** The safety of physiological estrogen plus progestin replacement therapy and with oral contraceptive therapy in women with pathological hyperprolactinemia. *Fertil Steril* 1993;59:671–673.

320. **Scheithauer BW, Kovacs KT, Randall RV, et al.** Effects of estrogen on the human pituitary: a clinicopathologic study. *Mayo Clin Proc* 1989;64:1077–1084.

321. **Raymond JP, Goldstein E, Konopka P, et al.** Follow-up of children born of bromocriptine-treated mothers. *Horm Res* 1985;22:239–246.

322. **Ruiz-Velasco V, Tolis G.** Pregnancy in hyperprolactinemic women. *Fertil Steril* 1984;41:793–805.

323. **Turkalj I, Braun P, Krupp P.** Surveillance of bromocriptine in pregnancy. *JAMA* 1982;247:1589–1591.

324. **Katz M, Kroll D, Pak I, et al.** Puerperal hypertension, stroke, and seizures after suppression of lactation with bromocriptine. *Obstet Gynecol* 1985;66:822–824.

325. **Gittelman DK.** Bromocriptine associated with postpartum hypertension, seizures, and pituitary hemorrhage. *Gen Hosp Psychiatry* 1991;13:278–280.

326. **Iffy L, Lindenthal J, McArdle JJ, et al.** Severe cerebral accidents postpartum in patients taking bromocriptine for milk suppression. *Isr J Med Sci* 1996;32:309–312.

327. **Iffy L, McArdle JJ, Ganesh V.** Intracerebral hemorrhage in normotensive mothers using bromocriptine postpartum. *Zentralbl Gynakol* 1996;118:392–395.

328. **Kirsch C, Iffy L, Zito GE, et al.** The role of hypertension in bromocriptine-related puerperal intracranial hemorrhage. *Neuroradiology* 2001;43:302–304.

329. **Tunbridge WM, Evered DC, Hall R, et al.** The spectrum of thyroid disease in a community: the Whickham survey. *Clin Endocrinol (Oxf)* 1977;7:481–493.

330. **Whartona T.** *Adenographoa: sive glandularum totius corporis descripto.* 1659.

331. **Portmann L, Hamada N, Heinrich G, et al.** Anti-thyroid peroxidase antibody in patients with autoimmune thyroid disease: possible identity with anti-microsomal antibody. *J Clin Endocrinol Metab* 1985;61:1001–1003.

332. **Czarnocka B, Ruf J, Ferrand M, et al.** Purification of the human thyroid peroxidase and its identification as the microsomal antigen involved in autoimmune thyroid diseases. *FEBS Lett* 1985;190:147–152.

333. **World Heath Organization.** *Assessment of iodine deficiency disorders and monitoring their elimination. A guide for program managers.* Geneva: WHO, 2007:1–108.

334. **Laurberg P, Cerqueira C, Ovesen L, et al.** Iodine intake as a determinant of thyroid disorders in populations. *Best Pract Res Clin Endocrinol Metab* 2010;24:13–27.

335. **Bahn AK, Mills JL, Snyder PJ, et al.** Hypothyroidism in workers exposed to polybrominated biphenyls. *N Engl J Med* 1980;302:31–33.

336. **Tomer Y, Huber A.** The etiology of autoimmune thyroid disease: a story of genes and environment. *J Autoimmun* 2009;32:231–239.

337. **Wang C, Crapo LM.** The epidemiology of thyroid disease and implications for screening. *Endocrinol Metab Clin North Am* 1997;26:189–218.

338. **McCombe PA, Greer JM, Mackay IR.** Sexual dimorphism in autoimmune disease. *Curr Mol Med* 2009;9:1058–1079.

339. **Brix TH, Knudsen GP, Kristiansen M, et al.** High frequency of skewed X-chromosome inactivation in females with autoimmune thyroid disease: a possible explanation for the female predisposition to thyroid autoimmunity. *J Clin Endocrinol Metab* 2005;90:5949–5953.

340. **Stockigt JR.** Free thyroid hormone measurement. A critical appraisal. *Endocrinol Metab Clin North Am* 2001;30:265–289.

341. **Benvenga S, Cahnmann HJ, Robbins J.** Characterization of thyroid hormone binding to apolipoprotein-E: localization of the binding site in the exon 3-coded domain. *Endocrinology* 1993;133:1300–1305.

342. **Dufour DR.** Laboratory tests of thyroid function: uses and limitations. *Endocrinol Metab Clin North Am* 2007;36:579–594.

343. **Caldwell G, Kellett HA, Gow SM, et al.** A new strategy for thyroid function testing. *Lancet* 1985;1:1117–1119.

344. **Surks MI, Ortiz E, Daniels GH, et al.** Subclinical thyroid disease: scientific review and guidelines for diagnosis and management. *JAMA* 2004;291:228–238.

345. **Walsh JP, Bremner AP, Feddema P, et al.** Thyrotropin and thyroid antibodies as predictors of hypothyroidism: a 13-year, longitudinal study of a community-based cohort using current immunoassay techniques. *J Clin Endocrinol Metab* 2010;95:1095–1104.

346. **Persani L, Borgato S, Romoli R, et al.** Changes in the degree of sialylation of carbohydrate chains modify the biological properties of circulating thyrotropin isoforms in various physiological and pathological states. *J Clin Endocrinol Metab* 1998;83:2486–2492.

347. **Persani L, Ferretti E, Borgato S, et al.** Circulating thyrotropin bioactivity in sporadic central hypothyroidism. *J Clin Endocrinol Metab* 2000;85:3631–3635.

348. **Saravanan P, Dayan CM.** Thyroid autoantibodies. *Endocrinol Metab Clin North Am* 2001;30:315–337.

349. **Boukis MA, Koutras DA, Souvatzoglou A, et al.** Thyroid hormone and immunological studies in endemic goiter. *J Clin Endocrinol Metab* 1983;57:859–862.

350. **Asamer H, Riccabona G, Holthaus N, et al.** [Immunohistologic findings in thyroid disease in an endemic goiter area]. *Arch Klin Med* 1968;215:270–284.

351. **Amino N, Hagen SR, Yamada N, et al.** Measurement of circulating thyroid microsomal antibodies by the tanned red cell haemagglutination technique: its usefulness in the diagnosis of autoimmune thyroid diseases. *Clin Endocrinol (Oxf)* 1976;5:115–125.

352. **Wright-Pascoe R, Smikle MF, Barton EN, et al.** Limited usefulness of antithyroperoxidase and antithyroglobulin assays in Jamaicans with Graves' disease. *Hum Antibodies* 1999;9:161–164.

353. **Nordyke RA, Gilbert FI Jr, Miyamoto LA, et al.** The superiority of antimicrosomal over antithyroglobulin antibodies for detecting Hashimoto's thyroiditis. *Arch Intern Med* 1993;153:862–865.

354. **Mariotti S, Sansoni P, Barbesino G, et al.** Thyroid and other organ-specific autoantibodies in healthy centenarians. *Lancet* 1992;339:1506–1508.

355. **Weetman AP, McGregor AM, Campbell H, et al.** Iodide enhances IgG synthesis by human peripheral blood lymphocytes *in vitro*. *Acta Endocrinol (Copenh)* 1983;103:210–215.

356. **Allen EM, Appel MC, Braverman LE.** The effect of iodide ingestion on the development of spontaneous lymphocytic thyroiditis in the diabetes-prone BB/W rat. *Endocrinology* 1986;118:1977–1981.

357. **Costagliola S, Morgenthaler NG, Hoermann R, et al.** Second generation assay for thyrotropin receptor antibodies has superior diagnostic sensitivity for Graves' disease. *J Clin Endocrinol Metab* 1999;84:90–97.

358. **Takasu N, Oshiro C, Akamine H, et al.** Thyroid-stimulating antibody and TSH-binding inhibitor immunoglobulin in 277 Graves' patients and in 686 normal subjects. *J Endocrinol Invest* 1997;20:452–461.

359. **Zouvanis M, Panz VR, Kalk WJ, et al.** Thyrotropin receptor antibodies in black South African patients with Graves' disease and their response to medical therapy. *J Endocrinol Invest* 1998;21:771–774.

360. **Cho BY, Kim WB, Chung JH, et al.** High prevalence and little change in TSH receptor blocking antibody titres with thyroxine and antithyroid drug therapy in patients with non-goitrous autoimmune thyroiditis. *Clin Endocrinol (Oxf)* 1995;43:465–471.

361. **Tamaki H, Amino N, Kimura M, et al.** Low prevalence of thyrotropin receptor antibody in primary hypothyroidism in Japan. *J Clin Endocrinol Metab* 1990;71:1382–1386.

362. **Davies TF, Ando T, Lin RY, et al.** Thyrotropin receptor-associated diseases: from adenomata to Graves disease. *J Clin Invest* 2005;115:1972–1983.

363. **Lytton SD, Kahaly GJ.** Bioassays for TSH-receptor autoantibodies: an update. *Autoimmun Rev* 2010;10:116–122.

364. **Spitzweg C, Morris JC.** The immune response to the iodide transporter. *Endocrinol Metab Clin North Am* 2000;29:389–398.

365. **Vanderpump M.** *The thyroid: a fundamental and clinical text.* Philadelphia: Lippincott-Raven Publishers, 1996.

366. **Prummel MF, Strieder T, Wiersinga WM.** The environment and autoimmune thyroid diseases. *Eur J Endocrinol* 2004;150:605–618.

367. **Haddow JE, Palomaki GE, Allan WC, et al.** Maternal thyroid deficiency during pregnancy and subsequent neuropsychological development of the child. *N Engl J Med* 1999;341:549–555.

368. **Baskin HJ, Cobin RH, Duick DS, et al.** American Association of Clinical Endocrinologists medical guidelines for clinical practice for the evaluation and treatment of hyperthyroidism and hypothyroidism. *Endocr Pract* 2002;8:457–469.

369. **Pearce EN.** Thyroid dysfunction in perimenopausal and postmenopausal women. *Menopause Int* 2007;13:8–13.

370. **Lazarus JH.** Thyroid disorders associated with pregnancy: etiology, diagnosis, and management. *Treat Endocrinol* 2005;4:31–41.

371. **Livadas S, Xekouki P, Fouka F, et al.** Prevalence of thyroid dysfunction in Turner's syndrome: a long-term follow-up study and brief literature review. *Thyroid* 2005;15:1061–1066.

372. **Hardy O, Worley G, Lee MM, et al.** Hypothyroidism in Down syndrome: screening guidelines and testing methodology. *Am J Med Genet A* 2004;124A:436–437.

373. **Abalovich M, Amino N, Barbour LA, et al.** Management of thyroid dysfunction during pregnancy and postpartum: an Endocrine Society Clinical Practice Guideline. *J Clin Endocrinol Metab* 2007;92(8 Suppl):S1–S47.

374. **American College of Obstetrics and Gynecology.** ACOG practice bulletin. Thyroid disease in pregnancy. Number 37. *Int J Gynaecol Obstet* 2002;79:171–180.

375. **Mariotti S, Caturegli P, Piccolo P, et al.** Antithyroid peroxidase autoantibodies in thyroid diseases. *J Clin Endocrinol Metab* 1990;71:661–669.

376. **Endo T, Kaneshige M, Nakazato M, et al.** Autoantibody against thyroid iodide transporter in the sera from patients with Hashimoto's thyroiditis possesses iodide transport inhibitory activity. *Biochem Biophys Res Commun* 1996;228:199–202.

377. **Cooper DS.** Clinical practice. Subclinical hypothyroidism. *N Engl J Med* 2001;345:260–265.

378. **McDermott MT, Ridgway EC.** Subclinical hypothyroidism is mild thyroid failure and should be treated. *J Clin Endocrinol Metab* 2001;86:4585–4590.

379. **Danese MD, Ladenson PW, Meinert CL, et al.** Clinical review 115: effect of thyroxine therapy on serum lipoproteins in patients with mild thyroid failure: a quantitative review of the literature. *J Clin Endocrinol Metab* 2000;85:2993–3001.

380. **Devdhar M, Ousman YH, Burman KD.** Hypothyroidism. *Endocrinol Metab Clin North Am* 2007;36:595–615.

381. **Poppe K, Glinoer D.** Thyroid autoimmunity and hypothyroidism before and during pregnancy. *Hum Reprod Update* 2003;9:149–161.

382. **Prummel MF, Wiersinga WM.** Thyroid autoimmunity and miscarriage. *Eur J Endocrinol* 2004;150:751–755.

383. **Wilansky DL, Greisman B.** Early hypothyroidism in patients with menorrhagia. *Am J Obstet Gynecol* 1989;160:673–677.

384. **Feek CM, Sawers JS, Brown NS, et al.** Influence of thyroid status on dopaminergic inhibition of thyrotropin and prolactin secretion: evidence for an additional feedback mechanism in the control of thyroid hormone secretion. *J Clin Endocrinol Metab* 1980;51:585–589.

385. **Kramer MS, Kauschansky A, Genel M.** Adolescent secondary amenorrhea: association with hypothalamic hypothyroidism. *J Pediatr* 1979;94:300–303.

386. **Scanlon MF, Chan V, Heath M, et al.** Dopaminergic control of thyrotropin, alpha-subunit, thyrotropin beta-subunit, and prolactin in euthyroidism and hypothyroidism: dissociated responses to dopamine receptor blockade with metoclopramide in hypothyroid subjects. *J Clin Endocrinol Metab* 1981;53:360–365.

387. **Thomas R, Reid RL.** Thyroid disease and reproductive dysfunction: a review. *Obstet Gynecol* 1987;70:789–798.

388. **del Pozo E, Wyss H, Tolis G, et al.** Prolactin and deficient luteal function. *Obstet Gynecol* 1979;53:282–286.

389. **Keye WR, Yuen BH, Knopf RF, et al.** Amenorrhea, hyperprolactinemia and pituitary enlargement secondary to primary hypothyroidism. Successful treatment with thyroid replacement. *Obstet Gynecol* 1976;48:697–702.

390. **Bohnet HG, Fiedler K, Leidenberger FA.** Subclinical hypothyroidism and infertility. *Lancet* 1981;2:1278.

391. **Wurfel W.** [Thyroid regulation pathways and its effect on human luteal function]. *Gynakol Geburtshilfliche Rundsch* 1992;32:145–150.

392. **Walsh JP, Shiels L, Lim EM, et al.** Combined thyroxine/liothyronine treatment does not improve well-being, quality of life, or cognitive function compared to thyroxine alone: a randomized controlled trial in patients with primary hypothyroidism. *J Clin Endocrinol Metab* 2003;88:4543–4550.

393. **Weetman AP.** Graves' disease by any other name? *Thyroid* 2000;10:1071–1072.

394. **Nayak B, Hodak SP.** Hyperthyroidism. *Endocrinol Metab Clin North Am* 2007;36:617–656.

395. **Stoffer SS, Hamburger JI.** Inadvertent 131I therapy for hyperthyroidism in the first trimester of pregnancy. *J Nucl Med* 1976;17:146–149.

396. **Schlumberger M, De Vathaire F, Ceccarelli C, et al.** Exposure to radioactive iodine-131 for scintigraphy or therapy does not preclude pregnancy in thyroid cancer patients. *J Nucl Med* 1996;37:606–612.

397. **Vitti P, Rago T, Chiovato L, et al.** Clinical features of patients with Graves' disease undergoing remission after antithyroid drug treatment. *Thyroid* 1997;7:369–375.

398. **Michelangeli V, Poon C, Taft J, et al.** The prognostic value of thyrotropin receptor antibody measurement in the early stages of treatment of Graves' disease with antithyroid drugs. *Thyroid* 1998;8:119–124.

399. **Edan G, Massart C, Hody B, et al.** Optimum duration of antithyroid drug treatment determined by assay of thyroid stimulating antibody in patients with Graves' disease. *BMJ* 1989;298:359–361.

400. **Anonymous.** Propylthiouracil-related liver toxicity: public workshop. Washington DC: Food and Drug Administration and the American Thyroid Association, 2009.

401. **Rivkees SA.** 63 years and 715 days to the "boxed warning": unmasking of the propylthiouracil problem. *Int J Pediatr Endocrinol* 2010 (in press).

402. **Cooper DS, Rivkees SA.** Putting propylthiouracil in perspective. *J Clin Endocrinol Metab* 2009;94:1881–1882.

403. **Casey BM, Leveno KJ.** Thyroid disease in pregnancy. *Obstet Gynecol* 2006;108:1283–1292.

404. **Milham S Jr.** Scalp defects in infants of mothers treated for hyperthyroidism with methimazole or carbimazole during pregnancy. *Teratology* 1985;32:321.

405. **Mandel SJ, Cooper DS.** The use of antithyroid drugs in pregnancy and lactation. *J Clin Endocrinol Metab* 2001;86:2354–2359.

406. **Karlsson FA, Axelsson O, Melhus H.** Severe embryopathy and exposure to methimazole in early pregnancy. *J Clin Endocrinol Metab* 2002;87:947–949.

407. **Cooper DS.** Antithyroid drugs. *N Engl J Med* 2005;352:905–917.

408. **Barbero P, Valdez R, Rodriguez H, et al.** Choanal atresia associated with maternal hyperthyroidism treated with methimazole: a case-control study. *Am J Med Genet A* 2008;146A:2390–2395.

409. **Van Dijke CP, Heydendael RJ, De Kleine MJ.** Methimazole, carbimazole, and congenital skin defects. *Ann Intern Med* 1987;106:60–61.

410. **Mao X-M, Li H-Q, Li Q, et al.** Prevention of relapse of Graves' disease by treatment with an intrathyroid injection of dexamethasone. *J Clin Endocrinol Metab* 2009;94:4984–4991.

411. **Yoshimura M, Hershman JM.** Thyrotropic action of human chorionic gonadotropin. *Thyroid* 1995;5:425–434.

412. **Padmanabhan LD, Mhaskar R, Mhaskar A, et al.** Trophoblastic hyperthyroidism. *J Assoc Physicians India* 2003;51:1011–1013.

413. **Alexander EK, Marqusee E, Lawrence J, et al.** Timing and magnitude of increases in levothyroxine requirements during pregnancy in women with hypothyroidism. *N Engl J Med* 2004;351:241–249.

414. **Klein RZ, Sargent JD, Larsen PR, et al.** Relation of severity of maternal hypothyroidism to cognitive development of offspring. *J Med Screen* 2001;8:18–20.

415. **Zakarija M, Garcia A, McKenzie JM.** Studies on multiple thyroid cell membrane-directed antibodies in Graves' disease. *J Clin Invest* 1985;76:1885–1891.

416. **Zakarija M, McKenzie JM.** Thyroid-stimulating antibody (TSAb) of Graves' disease. *Life Sci* 1983;32:31–44.

417. **Tanaka T, Tamai H, Kuma K, et al.** Gonadotropin response to luteinizing hormone releasing hormone in hyperthyroid patients with menstrual disturbances. *Metabolism* 1981;30:323–326.

418. **Polak M, Le Gac I, Vuillard E, et al.** Fetal and neonatal thyroid function in relation to maternal Graves' disease. *Best Pract Res Clin Endocrinol Metab* 2004;18:289–302.

419. **Iwatani Y, Amino N, Tamaki H, et al.** Increase in peripheral large granular lymphocytes in postpartum autoimmune thyroiditis. *Endocrinol Jpn* 1988;35:447–453.

420. **Vargas MT, Briones-Urbina R, Gladman D, et al.** Antithyroid microsomal autoantibodies and HLA-DR5 are associated with postpartum thyroid dysfunction: evidence supporting an autoimmune pathogenesis. *J Clin Endocrinol Metab* 1988;67:327–333.

421. **Amino N, Mori H, Iwatani Y, et al.** High prevalence of transient post-partum thyrotoxicosis and hypothyroidism. *N Engl J Med* 1982;306:849–852.

422. **Hayslip CC, Fein HG, O'Donnell VM, et al.** The value of serum antimicrosomal antibody testing in screening for symptomatic postpartum thyroid dysfunction. *Am J Obstet Gynecol* 1988;159:203–209.

423. **Jansson R.** Postpartum thyroid disease. *Mol Biol Med* 1986;3:201–211.

424. **Lucas A, Pizarro E, Granada ML, et al.** Postpartum thyroiditis: long-term follow-up. *Thyroid* 2005;15:1177–1181.

425. **Lazarus JH, Ammari F, Oretti R, et al.** Clinical aspects of recurrent postpartum thyroiditis. *Br J Gen Pract* 1997;47:305–308.

426. **Walfish PG, Chan JY.** Post-partum hyperthyroidism. *Clin Endocrinol Metab* 1985;14:417–447.

427. **Stagnaro-Green A, Roman SH, Cobin RH, et al.** Detection of at-risk pregnancy by means of highly sensitive assays for thyroid autoantibodies. *JAMA* 1990;264:1422–1425.

428. **Glinoer D, Soto MF, Bourdoux P, et al.** Pregnancy in patients with mild thyroid abnormalities: maternal and neonatal repercussions. *J Clin Endocrinol Metab* 1991;73:421–427.

429. **Maier DB, Parke A.** Subclinical autoimmunity in recurrent aborters. *Fertil Steril* 1989;51:280–285.

430. **Magaro M, Zoli A, Altomonte L, et al.** The association of silent thyroiditis with active systemic lupus erythematosus. *Clin Exp Rheumatol* 1992;10:67–70.

431. **LaBarbera AR, Miller MM, Ober C, et al.** Autoimmune etiology in premature ovarian failure. *Am J Reprod Immunol Microbiol* 1988;16:115–122.

432. **Guth S, Theune U, Aberle J, et al.** Very high prevalence of thyroid nodules detected by high frequency (13 MHz) ultrasound examination. *Eur J Clin Invest* 2009;39:699–706.

433. **McHenry CR, Walfish PG, Rosen IB.** Non-diagnostic fine needle aspiration biopsy: a dilemma in management of nodular thyroid disease. *Am Surg* 1993;59:415–419.

434. **Nikiforova MN, Nikiforov YE.** Molecular diagnostics and predictors in thyroid cancer. *Thyroid* 2009;19:1351–1361.

435. **Barbesino G, Tomer Y, Concepcion ES, et al.** Linkage analysis of candidate genes in autoimmune thyroid disease. II. Selected gender-related genes and the X-chromosome. International Consortium for the Genetics of Autoimmune Thyroid Disease. *J Clin Endocrinol Metab* 1998;83:3290–3295.

436. **Davenport ML.** Approach to the patient with Turner syndrome. *J Clin Endocrinol Metab* 2010;95:1487–1495.

437. **Aaltonen J, Bjorses P, Sandkuijl L, et al.** An autosomal locus causing autoimmune disease: autoimmune polyglandular disease type I assigned to chromosome 21. *Nat Genet* 1994;8:83–87.

32 Infertility and Assisted Reproductive Technology

Mira Aubuchon
Richard O. Burney
Danny J. Schust
Mylene W.M. Yao

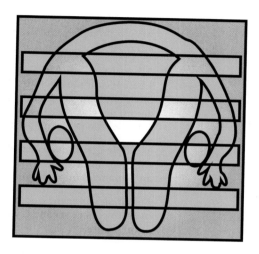

- The physician's initial encounter with the infertile couple is extremely important because it sets the tone for subsequent evaluation and treatment. Factors from either or both partners may contribute to difficulties in conceiving; therefore, it is important to consider all possible diagnoses before pursuing invasive treatment.

- The main causes of infertility include male factor, decreased ovarian reserve, ovulatory disorders (ovulatory factor), tubal injury, blockage, or paratubal adhesions (including endometriosis with evidence of tubal or peritoneal adhesions), uterine factors, systemic conditions (including infections or chronic diseases such as autoimmune conditions or chronic renal failure), cervical and immunologic factors, and unexplained factors (including endometriosis with no evidence of tubal or peritoneal adhesions).

- Basic investigations that should be performed before starting any infertility treatment are semen analysis, confirmation of ovulation, and the documentation of tubal patency.

- Male factor is the sole cause of infertility in 20% of infertile couples and may be a contributing factor in as many as 40% of cases. Treatment of reversible endocrine or infectious causes of subfertility, such as sexually transmitted diseases and thyroid disorders, tends to be efficacious. Intrauterine insemination (IUI) is the best studied and most widely practiced of all the insemination techniques. Intracytoplasmic sperm injection (ICSI) has allowed couples with male factor infertility to achieve assisted reproductive technology (ART) pregnancy outcomes that are comparable with those of couples with non–male factor infertility using conventional *in vitro* fertilization (IVF) treatment.

- An association between the age of the woman and reduced fertility is well documented. The decline in fecundability begins in the early 30s and accelerates during the late 30s and early 40s.

- Disorders of ovulation account for about 20% to 40% of all cases of female infertility. These disorders are generally among the most easily diagnosed and treatable causes of infertility.

- The most common cause of oligo-ovulation and anovulation—both in the general population and among women presenting with infertility—is polycystic ovarian syndrome (PCOS).

- Tubal and peritoneal factors account for 30% to 40% of cases of female infertility. Cervical factor is estimated to be a cause of infertility in no more than 5% of infertile couples. Uterine pathologies constitute the etiologic factor in infertility in as many as 15% of couples seeking treatment and are diagnosed in as many as 50% of infertile patients. Leiomyomas have not been shown to be a direct cause of infertility.

- All methods of ART, by definition, involve interventions to retrieve oocytes. These techniques include IVF, ICSI, gamete intrafallopian transfer (GIFT), zygote intrafallopian transfer (ZIFT), cryopreserved embryo transfers, and the use of donor oocytes. Because of improved success rates associated with IVF-embryo transfer, the performance of GIFT and ZIFT has declined.

- Multiple gestation, especially higher-order multiple gestation, is a serious complication of infertility treatment and has tremendous medical, psychological, social, and financial implications and complications.

- Fortunately, recent studies have not shown an increased risk for breast, uterine, or ovarian cancer secondary to medications used for superovulation in the treatment of infertility.

- Information on the Society for Assisted Reproductive Technology (SART) and registered ART clinics are accessible on the Internet.

Infertility is defined as 1 year of unprotected intercourse without pregnancy (1). This condition may be further classified as *primary infertility*, in which no previous pregnancies have occurred, and *secondary infertility*, in which a prior pregnancy, although not necessarily a live birth, has occurred. About 90% of couples should conceive within 12 months of unprotected intercourse (2). *Subfertility* refers to couples who conceive after 12 months of attempted impregnation (2). *Fecundability* refers to the probability of pregnancy per cycle, which is considered to be at 20% in fertile couples (1). *Fecundity* refers to the probability of achieving a live birth in a single cycle and, by definition, has a value lower than fecundability. The diagnosis of impaired fecundity has been proposed to include couples with 36 months or more without conception or physical inability or difficulty in having a child; however, there is currently no clear consensus on any of these terms (3–5).

Epidemiology

Twenty-one percent of couples in the United States are expected to experience infertility in their lifetimes, with a current prevalence of 7.4% (6). In 2002, over 7 million US women age 22 to 44 reported using infertility services in their lifetimes (7). Once diagnosed, 13% of couples will not pursue treatment (8). The diagnosis of impaired fecundity has been rising, **reaching 15% in 2002 and largely resulting from the trend toward delayed childbearing in developed countries** (3). Worldwide, male factor accounts for 51.2% and tubal blockage for 25% to 35% of infertility and subfertility (conception after attempting for 1 year) (9,10). In Europe, ovulatory dysfunction accounts for 21% to 32%, male factor 19% to 57%, tubal factor 14% to 26%, unexplained 8% to 30%, endometriosis 4% to 6%, and combined male and female factors 34.4% of infertility (11–13). The odds of infertility increase with female age and in general among patients who have not graduated from college (14). The high cost of infertility treatment is a barrier for many in the United States where insurance typically does not cover these services (15). Language and other cultural barriers affect access for many minority groups (15,16). The women most likely to obtain specialized treatment are 30 years of age or older, white, married, and of relatively high socioeconomic status (7).

Initial Assessment

The physician's initial encounter with the infertile couple is of primary importance because it sets the tone for subsequent evaluation and treatment. Ideally, both partners should be present at this first visit. **It cannot be overemphasized that infertility is a problem of the couple.** The presence of both partners, beginning with the initial evaluation, jointly involves them in the therapeutic process. This essential shared involvement demonstrates that the physician is receptive to the partner's needs as well as those of the patient and offers the partner an opportunity to ask questions and voice concerns.

The physician should obtain a complete medical, surgical, and gynecologic history from the woman. Specifically, information regarding menstrual cycle regularity, pelvic pain, and previous pregnancy outcomes is important. Risk factors for infertility, such as a history of pelvic inflammatory disease (PID) or pelvic surgery, should be reviewed. A history of intrauterine exposure to *diethylstilbestrol* (*DES*) is significant. In addition, a review of systems relevant to pituitary, adrenal, and thyroid function is useful. Questions regarding galactorrhea, hirsutism, and changes in weight are particularly relevant. A directed history, including developmental defects such as undescended testes, past genital surgery, infections (including mumps orchitis), previous genital trauma, and medications should be obtained from the male partner. A history of occupational exposures that might affect the reproductive function of either partner is important, as is information about coital frequency, dyspareunia, and sexual dysfunction. Finally, information should be obtained on any family history of infertility, premature ovarian failure, congenital or developmental defects, mental retardation, and hereditary conditions relevant to preconceptional planning, such as cystic fibrosis, thalassemias, and Tay Sachs disease.

The initial interview provides the physician with the opportunity to assess the emotional impact of infertility on the couple. It presents a time for the physician to emphasize the emotional support available to the couple as they proceed with the diagnostic evaluation and suggested treatments. In some cases, referral to a trained social worker or psychologist may be beneficial.

The physical examination of the woman should be thorough, with particular attention given to height, weight, body habitus, hair distribution, thyroid gland, and pelvic examination. Referral of the male partner to a urologist for examination often is beneficial if historic information or subsequent evaluation suggests an abnormality. This initial encounter is an excellent time to outline the general causes of infertility and to discuss subsequent diagnostic and treatment plans (Figs. 32.1–32.3).

The basic investigations that ideally should be performed before starting any infertility treatment are semen analysis, confirmation of ovulation, and the documentation of tubal patency. Other noninfertility assessments should include rubella immunity testing (17). If a patient with severe systemic illness, such as renal failure, liver failure, or cancer, wishes to conceive, careful preconceptional assessment and counseling is advisable because the risks of fertility treatment and pregnancy can be substantial.

Causes of Infertility

The main causes of infertility include:

1. **Male factor**
2. **Decreased ovarian reserve**
3. **Ovulatory factor**
4. **Tubal factor**
5. **Uterine factor**
6. **Pelvic factor**
7. **Unexplained**

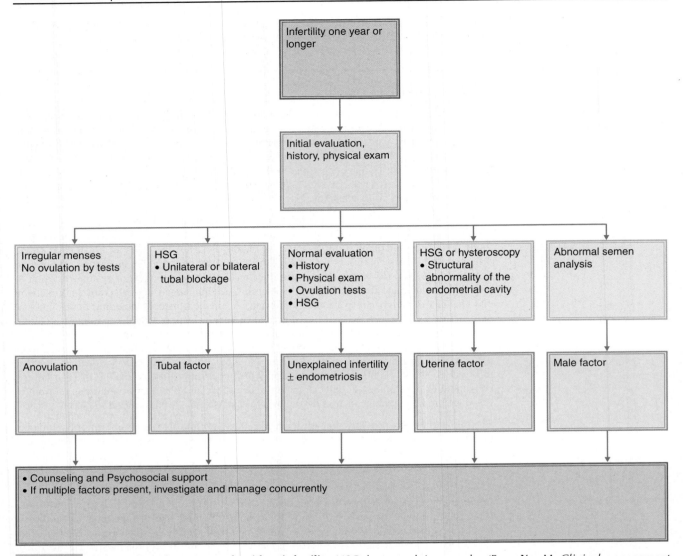

Figure 32.1   **Diagnostic and treatment algorithm: infertility.** HSG, hysterosalpingography. (From **Yao M.** *Clinical management of infertility.* Washington, DC: The Advisory Board: 2000, with permission.)

Factors from either or both partners may contribute to difficulties in conceiving; therefore, it is important to consider all possible diagnoses before pursuing invasive treatments. The relative prevalence of the different causes of infertility varies widely among patient populations (Table 32.1). In many cases, no specific cause is detected despite a thorough evaluation, and the couple's infertility is categorized as unexplained.

Very few couples have absolute infertility, which can result from congenital or acquired irreversible loss of functional gametes in either partner or the absence of reproductive structures in either partner. In these specific instances, couples should be counseled regarding their options for adoption, use of donor gametes, or surrogacy.

Impact of Lifestyle on Fertility

Overweight and obese women have higher rates of ovulatory dysfunction and infertility, along with 30% lower pregnancy rates with *in vitro* fertilization (IVF) compared to normal-weight women (18,19). Obese men have higher rates of hypogonadotropic hypogonadism and sperm DNA damage compared to normal-weight men (20,21). Substance abuse in men is discussed

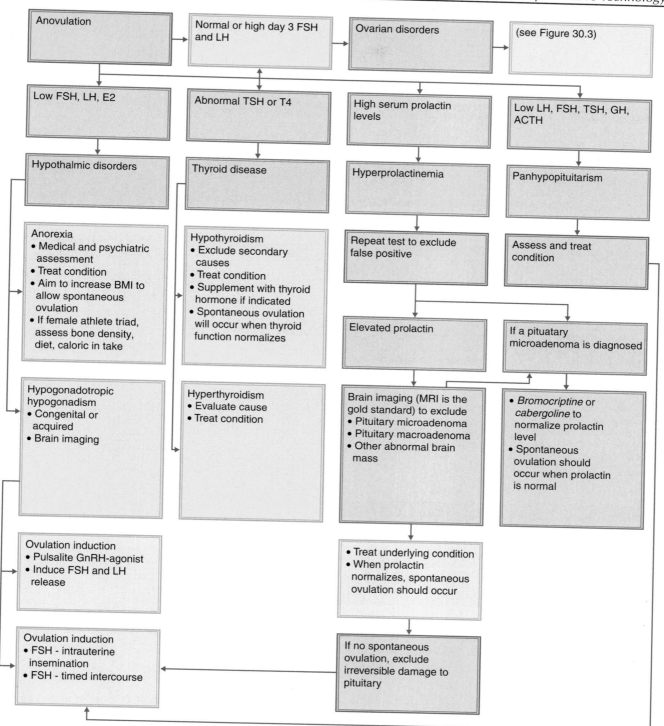

Figure 32.2   Diagnostic and treatment algorithm: anovulation. FSH, follicle-stimulating hormone; LH, luteinizing hormone; E2, estradiol; TSH, thyroid-stimulating hormone; T4, thyroxine; GH, growth hormone; ACTH, adrenocorticotropic hormone; BMI, body mass index; MRI, magnetic resonance imaging; GnRH, gonadotropin-releasing hormone. (From **Yao M.** *Clinical management of infertility.* Washington, DC: The Advisory Board: 2000, with permission.)

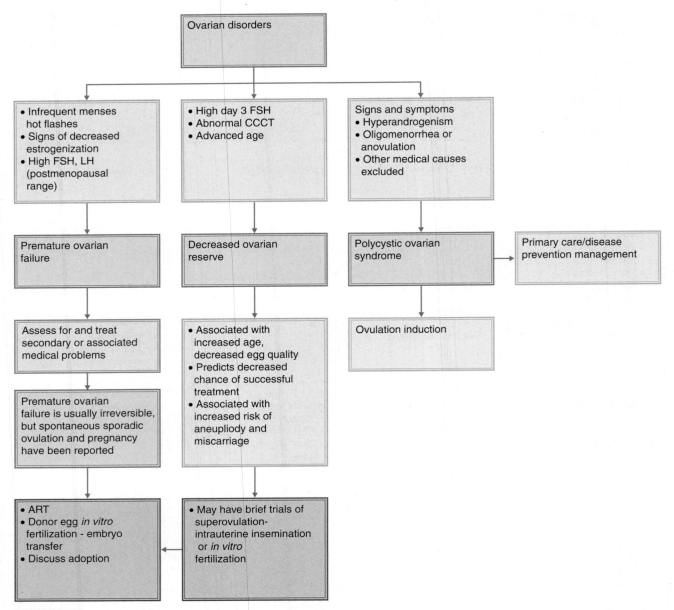

Figure 32.3   Diagnostic and treatment algorithm: ovarian disorders. FSH, follicle-stimulating hormone; LH, luteinizing hormone; CCCT, clomiphene citrate challenge test ART, assisted reproductive technology. (From **Yao M.** *Clinical management of infertility.* Washington, DC: The Advisory Board: 2000, with permission.)

in the next section. Women who smoke need twice the number of IVF cycles to conceive as nonsmokers, but the effect of alcohol on fertility is less clear (18).

Male Factor

Male factor is the only cause of infertility in about 20% of infertile couples, but it may be a contributing factor in as many as 50% of cases (9,11–13). The concept of a global decline in sperm counts is controversial (22,23). A decline in sperm density has been observed in the United States, Europe and Australia, while decreased motility and semen volume have been reported in India (22). Given that decreases in sperm parameters have been noted in fertile men, the clinical relevance for fecundability is unknown (24). However, one simulation model has suggested that if sperm concentrations decline by 21% to 47%, fecundability would decrease by 7% to 15% (25).

Table 32.1 Causes of Infertility	
Relative prevalence of the etiologies of infertility (%)	
Male factor	20–30
Both male and female factors	10–40
Female factor	40–55
Unexplained infertility	10–20
Approximate prevalence of the causes of infertility in the female (%)	
Ovulatory dysfunction	20–40
Tubal or peritoneal factor	20–40
Miscellaneous causes	10–15

Physiology

Spermatogenesis The male reproductive tract consists of the testis, epididymis, vas deferens, prostate, seminal vesicles, ejaculatory duct, bulbourethral glands, and urethra. **Gonadotropin-responsive cells in the testes include Leydig cells (the site of androgen synthesis) and Sertoli cells, which line the seminiferous tubules (the site of spermatogenesis). The pituitary gland secretes luteinizing hormone (LH), which stimulates the synthesis and secretion of testosterone by the Leydig cells, and follicle-stimulating hormone (FSH), which acts with testosterone on the Sertoli cells to stimulate spermatogenesis** (26). In humans, a new cohort of spermatogonia enter the maturation process every 16 days, and the development from spermatogonia stem cells to the mature sperm cells takes about 75 days (27). Spermatogonia undergo mitotic division to give rise to spermatocytes. These diploid spermatocytes subsequently undergo meiosis to produce haploid spermatids, which contain 23 (rather than 46) chromosomes (26). Maturation of spermatids is called *spermiogenesis* and involves condensation of the nucleus, formation of the flagellum, and the formation of the acrosome (a structure derived from the Golgi complex covering the tip or head of the sperm nucleus) (28). The resultant spermatozoa are released into the seminiferous tubule lumen and then enter the epididymis, where they continue to mature and become progressively more motile during the 2 to 6 days that are required to traverse this tortuous structure and reach the vas deferens (29).

Sperm Transport **During ejaculation, mature spermatozoa are released from the vas deferens along with fluid from the prostate, seminal vesicles, and bulbourethral glands.** The released semen is a gelatinous mixture of spermatozoa and seminal plasma; however, this thins out 20 to 30 minutes after ejaculation. This process, called *liquefaction,* is the direct result of proteolytic enzymes within the prostatic fluid (30). **Following ejaculation, the released spermatozoa must undergo capacitation to become competent to fertilize the oocyte.** Capacitation occurs within the cervical mucus and involves removal of inhibitory mediators such as cholesterol from the sperm surface, tyrosine phosphorylation, and calcium ion influx, all of which allow the sperm to recognize additional fertilization cues during travel through the female reproductive tract. When the sperm reach the tubal isthmus they are slowly released into the ampulla, further reducing the number of sperm that reach the oocyte (31). Sperm transport from the posterior vaginal fornix to the fallopian tubes occurs within 2 minutes during the follicular phase of the menstrual cycle (32).

Fertilization **As the capacitated sperm near and pass through cumulus cells surrounding the oocyte, hydrolytic enzymes are released from the acrosome via exocytosis in a process called the *acrosome reaction.*** Both capacitation and the acrosome reaction can be induced *in vitro* (28,31). Following the acrosome reaction, the sperm binds to and penetrates the zona pellucida (the extracellular coat surrounding the oocyte). This allows the sperm to fuse with the plasma membrane of the oocyte, an event that promotes changes in the oocyte and prevent entry by additional sperm (31). **As the first sperm penetrates the zona pellucida, cortical granules are released (the cortical reaction) from the oocyte into the perivitelline space. This stops the oocyte's zona pellucida from binding new sperm and inhibits penetration by previously bound sperm, further reducing the possibility of polyspermy** (33).

Table 32.2 Drugs that Can Impair Male Fertility	
Impaired spermatogenesis	Sulfasalazine, methotrexate, nitrofurantoin, colchicine, chemotherapy
Pituitary suppression	Testosterone injections, gonadotrophin-releasing hormone analogues
Antiandrogenic effects	Cimetidine, spironolactone
Ejaculation failure	α-blockers, antidepressants, phenothiazines
Erectile dysfunction	β-blockers, thiazide diuretics, metoclopramide
Drugs of misuse	Anabolic steroids, cannabis, heroin, cocaine

From **Hirsh A.** Male infertility. *BMJ* 2003;327:669–672, with permission.

Sperm Sensitivity to Toxins   Decreased sperm concentration and motility have been noted in areas of the United States with heavy agriculture and pesticide use, but occupational exposures have not been linked to infertility (24,34). Higher intake of food containing soy is associated with lower sperm concentrations (35). **Alcoholism negatively affects all semen analysis parameters, and either smoked or chewed tobacco is associated with decreased density and motility** (36–39). Marijuana inhibits motility and the acrosome reaction *in vitro,* and cocaine inhibits sperm motility and is associated with male infertility (40–42). Certain drugs may reduce sperm numbers or function or may cause ejaculatory dysfunction (Table 32.2). **Vaginal lubricants such as *Astroglide, KY Jelly,* saliva, and olive oil inhibit sperm motility *in vitro,* while no adverse effects are seen with *hydroxyethylcellulose (Pre-Seed),* mineral oil, or canola oil** (32).

Semen Analysis

The basic semen analysis measures semen volume, sperm concentration, sperm motility, and sperm morphology (30). Recently revised, the normal values suggested by the World Health Organization (WHO) in 2010 are listed along with the previously published guidelines in Table 32.3 (30,43). Both criteria were developed using fertile men whose semen parameters were in the lowest fifth percentile of the group studied, but values above the reference ranges do not guarantee male fertility. Furthermore, since infertile men were not used to develop the criteria, values below the cutoffs may not necessarily indicate infertility (30). However, significant deviations from the reference limits are generally classified as male factor infertility (44). Given regional differences in semen quality and between laboratories, laboratories are encouraged to develop their own reference ranges. Typically, semen is assessed manually, but computer-aided sperm analysis (CASA) may be used. Limitations of CASA include a lack of standardization among instruments, an inability to differentiate intact from nonintact sperm, possible bias from artifacts during preparation, and a paucity of studies on fertility outcomes in large populations (30).

Abstinence   **Abstinence of a minimum of 2 to a maximum of 7 days usually is recommended prior to the semen analysis, but the optimal duration is unknown** (30). The epididymis stores the equivalent of three ejaculations (29). With prolonged abstinence, sperm overflow into the urethra and are flushed out into the urine (30). A study of men attending an infertility clinic found that the total motile sperm count and normal morphology decreased after 10 days' abstinence in normozoospermic men but after 5 days' abstinence in oligozoospermic men (45). There are conflicting reports regarding the impact of shorter abstinence of 1 or 2 days on semen parameters (45,46), but one study suggested intrauterine insemination success rates might be improved by shortening abstinence times prior to specimen collection (46).

Specimen Collection   The specimen should be obtained by masturbation and collected in a clean container kept at ambient temperature (30). The patient should report any loss of the specimen, particularly the first portion of the ejaculate, which contains the highest sperm concentration. Collection may be performed either at home or in a private room near the laboratory. The sample should be taken to the laboratory within 30 minutes to 1 hour of collection to prevent dehydration and degradation. **If masturbation into a container is not possible, condoms specially designed for semen analysis should be used rather than latex condoms, which are toxic to sperm. Intercourse to collect the sample is discouraged because of the risk of contamination.** Even when the specimen is obtained under optimal circumstances, interpretation of the results of the semen analysis is complicated by variability within the same individual and

Table 32.3 Semen Analysis Terminology and Normal Values

Terminology

Normozoospermia	All semen parameters normal
Oligozoospermia	Reduced sperm numbers Mild to moderate: 5–20 million/mL Severe: <5 million/mL
Asthenozoospermia	Reduced sperm motility
Teratozoospermia	Increased abnormal forms of sperm
Oligoasthenoteratozoospermia	Sperm variables all subnormal
Azoospermia	No sperm in semen
Aspermia (anejaculation)	No ejaculate (ejaculation failure)
Leucocytospermia	Increased white cells in semen
Necrozoospermia	All sperm are nonviable or nonmotile

Normal Semen Analysis: World Health Organization

	1992 Guidelines	2010 Guidelines
Volume	2 mL	≥1.5 mL
Sperm concentration	20 million/mL	≥15 million/mL
Sperm motility	50% progressive or >25% rapidly progressive	≥32% progressive
Morphology (strict criteria)	>15% normal forms	≥4% normal forms
White blood cells	<1 million/mL	<1 million/mL
Immunobead or mixed antiglobulin reaction test	<10% coated with antibodies	<50%

Terminology from **Hirsh A.** Male infertility. *BMJ* 2003;327:669–672, with permission.

wide differences in normal semen parameters. Semen parameters may vary widely from one man to another and among men with proven fertility. **In many circumstances, several specimens are necessary to verify an abnormality** (30).

Sperm Volume and pH   **The lower limit of normal semen volume is 1.5 mL or more and the pH should be 7.2 or higher.** These parameters are affected mainly by the balance between the acidic secretions of the prostate gland and the alkaline fluid from the seminal vesicles. Low volume along with pH less than 7 suggests obstruction of the ejaculatory ducts or absence of the vas deferens. Difficulties with collection, retrograde ejaculation, or androgen deficiency can contribute to low volume. High volumes greater than 5 mL suggest inflammation of the accessory glands (30).

Sperm Concentration   Sperm concentration or density is defined as the number of sperm per milliliter in the total ejaculate. **The normal lower limit is 15 million/mL or more, recently revised from 20 million/mL or more** (30,43). Only intact sperm are counted in determining sperm concentration. Fifteen percent to 20% of infertile men are azoospermic (no sperm) and 10% have a density of less than 1 million/mL (30,47).

Sperm Motility and Viability   Sperm motility is the percentage of progressively motile sperm in the ejaculate. **The normal lower limit is 32% or more, recently revised from 50% or more** (30,43). **Viability should be at least 58%.** Progressive motility refers to movement either linearly or in a large circle regardless of speed. Nonprogressive motility describes sperm that display only small movements or twitching or no movement at all (immotile). Assessments of speed of progression, either rapid or slow, have been removed from the revised guidelines because of difficulty in unbiased measurement of this parameter. A reduction in sperm motility is referred to as *asthenozoospermia.* Leukocytes can impair sperm motility through oxidative stress. When a large number of immotile sperm are present or when progressive motility is less than 40%, viability studies should be performed. Viable immotile sperm may have flagellar defects, while the presence of nonviable immotile sperm (necrozoospermia) suggests epididymal pathology. Viable sperm have intact plasma membranes, which will not stain (dye exclusion) but will swell in hypoosmotic solutions (hypoosmotic swelling test) (30).

Sperm Morphology   Morphology refers to anatomic malformations of the sperm. **The lower limit for normal morphology is 4% or more using strict criteria, a change from previous guidelines using a more lenient assessment and a cutoff of 30% or more** (30,43). Assessment of sperm morphology involves fixing and staining of a portion of the specimen. The strict Tygerberg criteria were introduced by Kruger et al. in 1986 to assess sperm morphology (30,48,49). Using this system, the entire spermatozoon—including the head, midpiece, and tail—is assessed, and even mild abnormalities in head forms are classified as abnormal. Most sperm from normal men exhibit minor abnormalities when subjected to Tygerberg standards. An abnormality of sperm morphology is known as *teratozoospermia,* and these sperm have poor fertilizing potential and may have abnormal DNA. A disadvantage to any morphology assessment is that reproducibility may be hampered by the subjective nature of the assessment (30).

Nonsperm Cells   These include epithelial cells, round cells, and isolated sperm heads or tails. **Round cells include immature germ cells and leukocytes.** Immature germ cell elevation suggests testicular damage, while leukocytes (predominantly neutrophils) are associated with inflammation. Leukocytes can be distinguished by peroxidase positive staining, and normal leukocyte concentrations should be less than 1 million/mL. However, the prognostic significance of leukocytes in the semen is controversial (30,50). When bacterial colonization is found, the most common pathogens are *Chlamydia trachomatis* (41.4%), *Ureaplasma urealyticum* (15.5%), and *Mycoplasma hominis* (10.3%) (51).

Antisperm Antibodies   Antisperm antibodies, particularly those found on the surface of sperm, are associated with decreased pregnancy rates. Testing may be indicated with a history of ductal obstruction, prior genital infection, testicular trauma, and prior vasectomy reversal. It may be useful with oligozoospermia in the setting of normal hormonal levels, asthenospermia with normal sperm concentration, sperm agglutination, or unexplained infertility. **Antisperm antibody testing is not needed if the sperm are to be used for intracytoplasmic sperm injection (ICSI)** (44,47). Using the immunobead test, washed spermatozoa are exposed and assessed for binding to labeled beads. In the mixed agglutination reaction, human red blood cells sensitized with human immunoglobulin G (IgG) are mixed with the partner's semen. Spermatozoa that are coated with antibodies form mixed agglutinates with the red blood cells (30).

Other Sperm Tests   Although the standard semen analysis and associated tests provide a fairly reasonable picture of semen quality, they yield little information about sperm function. These specialized tests may be pursued to assess DNA integrity, fertilization potential (zona-free hamster oocyte test), and the effect of cervical mucus on sperm viability and function (postcoital test) (44,52). In general, these tests are not currently considered part of the standard assessment because their prognostic value and impact on management are limited by poor specificity, poor reproducibility, or controversies concerning the interpretation of the results (44,47,52).

Differential Diagnosis of Male Factor

If abnormalities in the semen are detected, further evaluation of the male partner by a urologist is indicated to diagnose the defect. Table 32.4 lists the differential diagnoses for male factor infertility (53). Several groups have attempted to assess the distribution of male infertility diagnoses; two such distributions are shown in Table 32.5 (54,55). The first is the result of a WHO study of 7,057 men with complete diagnoses based on the WHO standard investigation of the infertile couple (54). The figures include data from cases in which the male partner was normal and the presumed cause of the couple's infertility was a female factor. The second distribution is the result of a study of 425 subfertile male patients (54). Although the two studies represent different populations (one is from a study of couples, the other from a urologic practice) and differ in their distribution of male infertility diagnoses, idiopathic male factor and varicocele predominate. Other anatomic and endocrine causes occur less frequently. Same sex female couples or single women without a male partner who desire pregnancy may be considered as part of this category.

Male Age

Men reportedly have fathered children into their 90s, but pregnancy rates are decreased with paternal older than age 40 to 45 and particularly over age 50. Increasing paternal age is associated with a higher frequency of disomic sex chromosomes and structural chromosomal abnormalities in the sperm. With respect to the offspring, paternal age confers higher rates

Table 32.4 Etiologic Factors in Male Infertility	
Pretesticular	*Testicular*
Endocrine	*Genetic*
Hypogonadotropic hypogonadism	Klinefelter's syndrome
Coital disorders	Y chromosome deletions
Erectile dysfunction	Immotile cilia syndrome
Psychosexual	*Congenital*
Endocrine, neural, or vascular	Cryptorchidism
Ejaculatory failure	*Infective (orchitis)*
Psychosexual	*Antispermatogenic agents*
After genitourinary surgery	Heat
Neural	Chemotherapy
Drug related	Drugs
Posttesticular	Irradiation
Obstructive	*Vascular*
Epididymal	Torsion
Congenital	Varicocele
Infective	*Immunologic*
Vasal	*Idiopathic*
Genetic: cystic fibrosis	
Acquired: vasectomy	
Epididymal hostility	
Epididymal asthenozoospermia	
Accessory gland infection	
Immunologic	
Idiopathic	
Postvasectomy	

From **De Kretser DM.** Male infertility. *Lancet* 1997;349:787–790, with permission.

of autosomal dominant diseases such as achondroplasia and craniosynostotic conditions and somewhat higher rates of trisomy 21 (56). In mice, offspring of older fathers have decreased survival (57). Increased paternal age is associated with recurrent pregnancy loss (58).

Treatment of Male Factor Not From Azoospermia

Medical treatment of reversible infectious or endocrine causes of male subfertility, such as sexually transmitted diseases and thyroid disorders, tends to be efficacious. Although injections of exogenous FSH have been reported to improve pregnancy rates, the benefit is less clear for *clomiphene citrate,* an estrogen antagonist at the hypothalamus and pituitary that promotes gonadotropin release. **Exogenous testosterone is not recommended in the treatment of male subfertility because of negative feedback inhibition at the pituitary that results in decreased spermatogenesis, but the combination of testosterone and an antiestrogen may be of benefit.** Antioxidant food supplements have been evaluated (59). Glutathione, carnitine, and vitamin E do not appear to affect semen parameters, but administration of zinc and folic acid were associated with improved sperm concentration and morphology (60). The diagnosis and treatment of azoospermia (no sperm on semen analysis) will be discussed separately from other forms of male factor infertility.

Table 32.5 Frequency of Some Etiologies in Male Factor Infertility			
Cause	*Percentage*	*Cause*	*Percentage*
No demonstrable cause	48.5	Varicocele	37.4
Idiopathic abnormal semen	26.4	Idiopathic	25.4
Varicocele	12.3	Testicular failure	9.4
Infectious factors	6.6	Obstruction	6.1
Immunologic factors	3.1	Cryptorchidism	6.1
Other acquired factors	2.6	Low semen volume	4.7
Congenital factors	2.1	Semen agglutination	3.1
Sexual factors	1.7	Semen viscosity	1.9
Endocrine disturbances	0.6	Other	5.9
TOTAL	103.9[a]		100

[a]More than 100% because of multiple factors.
From **The ESHRE CAPRI Workshop Group.** Male sterility and subfertility: guidelines for management. Hum *Reprod* 1994;9:1260–1264, and **Burkman LJ, Cobbington CC, Franken DR, et al.** The hemizona assay (HZA): development of a diagnostic test for the binding of human spermatozoa to the human hemizona pellucida to predict fertilization potential. *Fertil Steril* 1988;49:688–697, with permission.

Varicocele Repair   **A varicocele is an abnormal dilation of the veins within the spermatic cord.** Varicoceles are present in 15% of normal men and 40% of men seeking infertility treatment, but semen parameters are lower among infertile men with varicoceles (61,62). The pathophysiologic effects of a varicocele appear to be mediated by an associated rise in testicular temperature, reflux of toxic metabolites from the left adrenal or renal veins, or higher reactive oxygen species (61,63). **Although treatment is associated with improved semen parameters in some studies, it is not clear whether varicocele repair definitely improves fertility** (61,64,65). Treatment is typically considered if the varicocele is palpable and the semen analysis is abnormal, but is not indicated if IVF would be required to treat the female partner and the existing semen analysis would be acceptable for ICSI. Treatment methods include surgical repair and percutaneous embolization. Complications of treatment include infection, varicocele persistence, recurrence, and hydrocele formation (61).

Artificial Insemination   Artificial insemination has been used mainly to treat unexplained infertility (usually combined with superovulation) and male factor infertility (including same sex female couples). **All artificial insemination procedures involve the placement of whole semen or processed sperm into the female reproductive tract, which permits sperm–ovum interaction in the absence of intercourse.** The placement of whole semen into the vagina as a mode of fertility treatment is now rarely performed except in cases of severe coital dysfunction. Currently, all of the common forms of artificial insemination involve processed sperm obtained from the male partner or a donor. Many techniques for artificial insemination have been described, but only intracervical and intrauterine inseminations (IUI) have been routinely employed. The success rates with intracervical insemination are lower than those with IUI, particularly when using frozen sperm (66–68).

Insemination Processing   During and after intercourse, seminal fluid usually is prevented from reaching the intrauterine cavity and intra-abdominal space by the cervical barrier. **The introduction of seminal fluid past this barrier may be associated with pelvic infection and severe uterine cramping or anaphylactoid reactions, possibly mediated by seminal factors such as prostaglandins.** Thus, protocols for processing whole semen include the washing of specimens to remove seminal factors and to isolate pure sperm. Additional processing may include centrifugation through density gradients, sperm migration protocols, and differential adherence procedures (66). Finally, phosphodiesterase inhibitors, such as *pentoxiphylline,* have been used during semen processing in an attempt to enhance sperm motility, fertilization capacity, and acrosome reactivity for IVF procedures (60,69).

Intrauterine Insemination **IUI is the best studied and most widely practiced of all the insemination techniques. It involves placement of about 0.3 to 0.5 mL of washed, processed, and concentrated sperm into the intrauterine cavity by transcervical catheterization** (66). Patients should remain immobile for approximately 15 minutes following the procedure (70). Studies of the efficacy of IUI in the treatment of male factor infertility have been difficult to assess because of variations in inclusion criteria and the limitations of sperm function tests. Although it makes intuitive sense that IUI would result in higher pregnancy rates rather than timed intercourse in the case of male factor subfertility, there are conflicting reports of the benefits of IUI (66,71–74). **Ideally, the total motile sperm count in the IUI specimen should be 5 million or 10 million or more** (75–78). Pregnancy rates with semen meeting those thresholds have been reported to be 10.5% per cycle and 38% after 4 to 6 cycles (77,78). No benefit has been found with respect to double IUI versus single IUI during a single cycle (79).

Intracytoplasmic Sperm Injection In general, ICSI has allowed couples with male factor infertility to achieve assisted reproductive technology (ART) pregnancy outcomes that are comparable with those of couples with non–male factor infertility using conventional IVF treatment (80). **ICSI has been used since 1992 to increase the fertilization rate of oocytes retrieved during ART by direct injection of a live sperm into the oocyte, thereby theoretically bypassing limitations imposed by sperm motility and defects in capacitation, the acrosome reaction, and/or sperm binding the zona pellucida** (81). This microsurgical procedure involves stripping the aspirated cumulus complex of all surrounding granulosa cells, followed by insertion of a single viable sperm into the cytoplasm (ooplasm) of the mature metaphase II egg (9,82). **ICSI should be offered if the semen analysis shows less than 2 million motile sperm, less than 5% motility, or if surgically recovered sperm are used.** Its use for abnormal morphology is more controversial (47,83). Immature or round spermatid nucleus injection (ROSNI) for ICSI is considered experimental at this time (84). **Higher pregnancy rates have been noted with fresh compared to frozen specimens and with ejaculated compared to surgically retrieved sperm.** Success rates are affected by the age of the female partner and oocyte quality (47). Non–male factor indications for ICSI include a history of fertilization failure with conventional IVF and the fertilization of oocytes before preimplantation genetic diagnosis (85). Other uses are described under "Unexplained Infertility."

Risks of Intracytoplasmic Sperm Injection In skilled hands, oocyte damage with ICSI is reportedly 10% (81). However, oocyte degeneration can follow even an uncomplicated ICSI procedure, with rates as high as 30% to 50%. This is most likely a function of oocyte quality and/or patient factors rather than the ICSI process itself (82). **Based on data from 5-year-old children, ICSI is associated with a higher congenital anomaly risk (4.2%) when compared with conventional IVF (typically 2% to 3%)** (80). There may be an increased risk of imprinting disorders and hypospadias with ICSI (47). Reports indicate a slightly higher risk of sex chromosome abnormalities (0.8% to 1% ICSI vs. 0.2% IVF) and translocations (0.36% ICSI vs. 0.07% general population). It is unclear whether these relate to the ICSI procedure or inherent gamete defects; men with abnormal semen parameters have higher rates of sperm aneuploidy. Recent studies have not found an association with impaired intellectual or motor development among ICSI children. **In the setting of specific genetic abnormalities such as Y chromosome microdeletions, abnormal karyotypes, cystic fibrosis mutations, or congenital absence of the vas deferens, genetic counseling should be offered to address the possible risk of infertility or other abnormality in the offspring** (80).

Azoospermia: Classification and Treatment

Azoospermia describes the absence of spermatozoa in the ejaculate and is found in 1% of all men and up to 15% to 20% of infertile men. Causes are categorized into pretesticular (nonobstructive), testicular (nonobstructive), and posttesticular (includes obstructive and nonobstructive) etiologies, but in some cases the condition is idiopathic (47,86).

Pretesticular Azoospermia

Pretesticular azoospermia is relatively rare and results from gonadotropin deficiency, which leads to loss of spermatogenesis. The physician should perform a full endocrine history that includes information on puberty and growth and check for low serum levels of LH, FSH, and testosterone (44,47,86). Prolactin levels and pituitary imaging are indicated in cases of hypogonadotropic hypogonadism (47). **Hormonal treatment includes pulsatile gonadotropin-releasing hormone (GnRH), human chorionic gonadotropin, and exogenous gonadotropins**

(44,47,86). The best predictors of good response are postpubertal onset of gonadotropin deficiency and testicular volume greater than 8 mL (47).

Testicular Azoospermia

Gonadal failure is the hallmark of testicular azoospermia. Causes of this condition may be genetic, acquired (e.g., radiation therapy, chemotherapy, testicular torsion, varicocele, or mumps orchitis), or developmental (e.g., testicular maldescent). Testicular atrophy is often present. Because of the low chance of obtaining sperm, testicular biopsy is generally not recommended with hypergonadotropic hypogonadism (elevated levels of LH and FSH with low serum levels of testosterone) and consideration should be given to using donor sperm. Diagnostic testicular biopsies may be indicated in the setting of normal hormonal testing. If sperm are present on diagnostic testing, consideration can be given to using surgically retrieved spermatozoa for ICSI (44,47,86). If no sperm are present, consideration can be given to correcting acquired conditions such as varicocele, which may restore sperm to the ejaculate to permit ICSI or spontaneous pregnancy (87,88). **Chromosomal abnormalities by peripheral karyotype testing are present in about 7% of infertile, 5% of oligospermic, and 10% to 15% in azoospermic men.** Sex chromosome aneuploidies such as Klinefelter syndrome (47,XXY) encompass two-thirds of these infertility-associated chromosome abnormalities. Microdeletions in the Y chromosome have been identified in 10% to 20% of men with idiopathic azoospermia or severe oligospermia with concentration less than 5 million/mL (44,47,86) (Table 32.6). These microdeletions can be transmitted to the male offspring, who may then suffer from infertility. Therefore, screening for genetic causes is indicated in nonacquired cases of testicular azoospermia so that genetic counseling can be provided before treatment (80). The two most commonly implicated candidate gene families are the RNA-binding motif (*RBM*) and the "deleted in azoospermia" (*DAZ*) families, but microdeletions at various loci on the Y chromosome have been described (44,47,86,89–91). For example, microdeletions in Yq11.23 can occur in one or more of three regions: *AZFa* (proximal), *AZFb* (central), and *AZFc* (distal) (44,47,86).

Posttesticular Azoospermia

Posttesticular or obstructive etiologies are associated with normal gonadotropin and testosterone levels and are present in up to 40% of azoospermic men (47,86). Ejaculatory dysfunction is associated with oligospermia or aspermia but rarely azoospermia (86). **Obstructive causes include congenital absence or obstruction of the vas deferens or ejaculatory ducts, acquired obstruction of these ducts, or ductal dysfunction, including retrograde ejaculation** (47,86). In the absence of congenital bilateral absence of the vas deferens (CBAVD) or hypogonadism, men with low volume ejaculate should have a postejaculatory urinalysis to check for retrograde ejaculation, which is associated with diabetes and surgery to the bladder or prostate (44,47). Sperm may be isolated from the neutralized urine of men with retrograde ejaculation and processed for insemination or for ART (30). Transrectal ultrasound may be of use to diagnose

Table 32.6 Genetics and Male Infertility			
Clinical diagnosis	*Genetic tests*	*Most common defects*	*Incidence (%)*
Congenital bilateral absence of vas deferens (CBAVD)	Cystic fibrosis (CFTR gene)	ΔF508, R117H	66
Nonobstructive azoospermia	Karyotype	47, XXY AZFa, AZFb[a], AZFc	15–30 10–15
Severe (<5 M/mL) oligozoospermia	Karyotype Translocation Y chromosome microdeltions	47, XXY Partial AZFb, AZFc	1–2 0.2–0.4 7–10

CFTR, cystic fibrosis transmembrane conductance regulator; AZF, azoospermia factor.
[a] AZFb the most severe (DAZ gene—deleted in azoospermia) causes the most severe defects of spermatogenesis; AZFc causes the mildest defects of spermatogenesis.
From **Hirsh A.** Male infertility. *BMJ* 2003;327:669–672, with permission.

ejaculatory duct obstruction or unilateral vasal agenesis (to demonstrate contralateral atresia) but is generally not needed for CBAVD (86). **Renal imaging is necessary when either unilateral or bilateral vasal absence is diagnosed as a result of the 10% to 25% incidence of renal agenesis.** Most men with CBAVD will have seminal vesicle agenesis, so almost all will have low semen volume, low pH, and low fructose levels (86). Spermatogenesis can be expected to be normal in CBAVD, so generally diagnostic biopsy is not indicated (92). In some cases, testicular biopsy may be indicated to differentiate between testicular and posttesticular causes. At least two-thirds of men with CBAVD have mutations of the cystic fibrosis transmembrane conductance regulator gene (*CFTR*). **However, because many *CFTR* mutations are undetectable, CBAVD patients should be assumed to have a mutation and thus testing of the female partner's carrier status should be performed** (86).

Vasectomy Reversal and Treatment of Obstructive Azoospermia Vasectomy can be reversed effectively using microsurgical vasovasostomy or vasoepididymostomy. These techniques can be used for epidymal obstructions (93). Patency and subsequent pregnancy rates approach 100% and 80%, respectively. Pregnancy typically occurs within 24 months of reversal (94). **Rates of patency and pregnancy vary inversely with the length of time from vasectomy, particularly for reversal procedure performed after 15 years or more** (93,94). Although 60% of reversal patients develop antisperm antibodies, these do not appear to affect fecundability. Following surgery, periodic semen analyses can identify reobstruction, which can range from 3% to 21% depending on which segments were anastamosed. For those patients with azoospermia 6 months after reversal, the procedure is considered a failure and testicular sperm aspiration with ICSI could be considered. However, repeat vasovasostomy is associated with patency rates of 75% and pregnancy rates of 43% (94).

Surgical Sperm Recovery for Intracytoplasmic Sperm Injection Among the many surgical methods for sperm recovery, the most widely described are microsurgical epididymal sperm aspiration (MESA), percutaneous epididymal sperm aspiration (PESA), testicular sperm extraction (TESE), and percutaneous testicular sperm fine-needle aspiration (TESA, also called fine-needle aspiration, or FNA). Both MESA and TESE are open surgical procedures performed with an operating microscope and general or regional anesthesia, whereas the percutaneous procedures need only local anesthesia. The optimal choice for surgical sperm recovery method has not been determined and certainly varies based on patient history. Hematoma risk appears to be low regardless of method. Testicular atrophy is a rare complication of TESE and TESA even when biopsies are obtained from multiple testicular sites (92).

With obstructive azoospermia, pregnancy rates using sperm retrieval and ICSI are 24% and 64%, respectively, and outcomes using either frozen-thawed or fresh sperm are comparable. Because MESA allows for diagnosis and possible reconstruction of ductal pathology and because it usually yields very large numbers of sperm, sperm cryopreservation and avoidance of repeat surgery may be possible (92). If repeat sperm retrievals are needed, the minimum interval between procedures is 3 to 6 months to allow for adequate healing (93).

For nonobstructive (testicular) azoospermia, epididymal aspiration is not an option. Although pregnancies have been reported following testicular sperm retrieval with nonobstructive azoospermia, the likelihood of retrieving sperm is low as are subsequent pregnancy rates (92,95). Patients with obstructive azoospermia must be counseled regarding the risk of transmitting genetic disorders to their offspring (47,86).

Donor Insemination For men with azoospermia, couples with significant male factor infertility who do not desire ART, or women without a male partner who are seeking pregnancy, therapeutic donor insemination offers an effective option (96). **In several prospective randomized or crossover trials, IUI was shown to be superior to intracervical insemination for donor insemination** (68). In patients younger than 30 years of age who have no other infertility factors, delivery rates approach 90% after 12 cycles of IUI treatment with frozen sperm, so patients who do not conceive within 6 to 12 months should be assessed for female factors and encouraged to terminate treatment or proceed with alternative forms of therapy. The concomitant use of *clomiphene citrate* or *gonadotropin* (hMG) for controlled ovarian hyperstimulation (COH) did not result in higher fecundity rates in these patients (97). **Psychological counseling should be offered because of the potential repercussions of using donor gametes** (96).

Donor Sperm Screening Although the use of fresh donor semen is associated with higher pregnancy rates than the use of frozen specimens, both the Centers for Disease Control and

Prevention and the American Society for Reproductive Medicine recommend the use of frozen samples (96,98,99). **This recommendation stems from the increasing incidence of human immunodeficiency virus (HIV) infection in the general population and the lag time between HIV infection and seroconversion.** Currently, semen donors are screened for HIV infection, hepatitis B, hepatitis C, syphilis, gonorrhea, chlamydia, and cytomegalovirus infections, all of which may be transmitted through semen. All cryopreserved samples are quarantined for 6 months, and the donor is retested for HIV before clinical use of the specimen. Donors are likewise questioned about any family history of genetically transmitted disorders, including both Mendelian (e.g., hemophilia, Tay-Sachs disease, thalassemia, cystic fibrosis, congenital adrenal hyperplasia, Huntington disease) and polygenic or multifactorial conditions (e.g., mental retardation, diabetes, heart malformation, spina bifida). Those with a positive family history of these conditions are eliminated as donor candidates (96).

Female Age and Decreased Ovarian Reserve

Decreased Fecundability

Most women will experience a decline in fecundability as they age that is physiologic rather than pathologic. **This decline begins in the early 30s and accelerates during the late 30s and early 40s, reflecting declines in oocyte quantity and quality.** Among populations that do not practice contraception, fertility peaks at age 20, declines somewhat at age 32, steeply declines after the age of 37, and is rare after age 45 (100). Wives of azoospermic husbands who received donor IUI had cumulative pregnancy rates over 12 cycles of 74% (age <31 years), 62% (age 31 to 35), and 54% (age >35) (101). Chronologic aging of the endometrium does not seem to play an appreciable role in reduced fertility, given the excellent pregnancy and live birth rates using donor oocytes (Fig. 32.4) (102,103). IVF success rates similarly decrease with age and will be further discussed later in the chapter (100). Reproductive aging is related to the stock of primordial follicles that are established early in fetal life and decline to near zero at menopause (104).

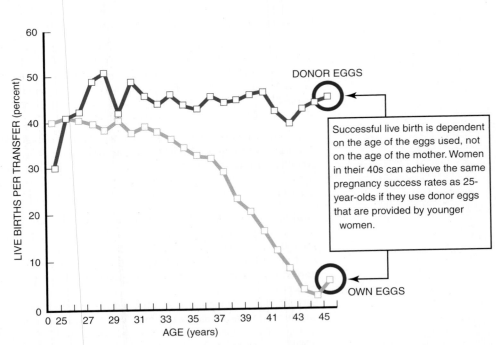

Figure 32.4 **Live births per embryo transfer comparing use of a patient's own versus donor oocytes.** (Adapted from CDC Reproductive Health. 2009 Assisted Reproductive Technology Success Rates. National Summary and Fertility Clinic Reports. http://www.cdc.gov/nccdphp/drh/art.htm.)

Spontaneous Pregnancy Loss

Reproductive aging is associated with abnormalities in the oocyte meiotic spindles that lead to chromosome alignment errors and increase rates of conceptus aneuploidies, particularly trisomies. This serves to increase the risk for spontaneous pregnancy loss and thereby decrease live birth rates in older women (100,105). A large study based on the Danish national registry estimated the rates of clinically recognized spontaneous pregnancy loss for various age groups to be 13.3% (12 to 19 years), 11.1% (20 to 24 years), 11.9% (25 to 29 years), 15.0% (30 to 34 years), 24.6% (35 to 39 years), 51.0% (40 to 44 years), and 93.4% (older than 45 years) (106). In addition, using sensitive hCG assays in women during their reproductive years, 22% of all pregnancies were found to be lost before they could be clinically diagnosed (107).

Ovarian Reserve

Ovarian reserve refers to the size of the nongrowing, or resting, primordial follicle population in the ovaries. This, in turn, presumably determines the number of growing follicles and the "quality" or reproductive potential of their oocytes (105). Tests of ovarian reserve are often used, but the predictive values of these tests for fertility potential are limited, particularly when normal testing is found in older women and abnormal testing is documented in younger women. The tests appear to be better suited for determining how the ovaries will respond to pharmacologic doses of exogenous gonadotropins in terms of follicle count, the number of oocytes produced, serum estradiol levels during stimulation, the duration of stimulation, and the quantity of exogenous gonadotropins required in a given cycle (108). However, unlike age, the results of ovarian reserve testing are poorly predictive of pregnancy outcomes (109–111). **These tests appear to be more indicative of oocyte quantity rather than quality** (110).

Serum Day 3 Follicule Stimulating Hormone   As women age, FSH physiologically rises in the early follicular phase (cycle day 3), with levels of 5.74 IU/L at age 35 to 39 and 14.34 IU/L at age 45 to 59. Higher levels are seen after unilateral oophorectomy. In women in their 40s, levels greater than 20 IU/L are predictive of menopause. **Because the incidence of abnormal values is lower in younger women, testing is typically performed for women aged 35 or older** (108). In subfertile women with an FSH 8 IU/L or more, spontaneous pregnancy rates decrease by 7% per unit of FSH increase, with a 40% reduction at 15 IU/L and 58% at 20 IU/L (112). FSH levels vary widely by assay, laboratory, and population (109). Because of the poor sensitivity of high basal FSH values in determining fecundability, they should not be used as the sole basis for excluding women from consideration for ART (113). Likewise, the poor specificity of low basal FSH values in determining fecundability makes them unreliable when used to reassure patients, particularly those of increased reproductive age (109).

Basal Estradiol Level   Basal day 3 FSH is often combined with estradiol (E2) testing. Estradiol levels on day 3 of the menstrual cycle reflect follicular growth rather than the number of antral follicles (114). Elevations in FSH and decreases in inhibin B (see below) that accompany aging results in advanced follicular growth at the end of the preceding luteal phase. In response, early follicular E2 levels are typically higher in older women and in women with advanced reproductive aging (104).

Clomiphene Citrate Challenge Test   Clomiphene citrate is thought to have antiestrogenic effects on the hypothalamic–pituitary axis, resulting in a decrease in E2-mediated suppression of FSH production by the pituitary. **The *clomiphene citrate* challenge test (CCCT) involves the measurement of serum FSH and estradiol on day 3 of the menstrual cycle, and again on day 10 after administration of *clomiphene citrate* (100 mg orally each day) from days 5 to 9.** The CCCT has been reported to be more sensitive than basal FSH alone in identifying poor response to exogenous gonadotropins, but others report that the predictive values of the tests do not differ substantially (109,110).

Serum Inhibin B   Serum inhibin B is secreted by ovarian granulosa cells starting at the preantral follicle stage and therefore reflects the size of the growing follicular cohort (111). Reduced inhibin B levels are seen with aging even in normal fertile women (114). Inhibin B alone has poor predictive value for ovarian response but improves the predictive value when added to the CCCT (109,110). Unlike basal testing, levels of inhibin B measured on the 5th day of ovarian stimulation were predictive of live birth following IVF/ICSI (115).

Serum Antimüllerian Hormone   Antimüllerian hormone (AMH) is produced by the granulosa cells of preantral and small antral follicles (111,114). The serum level of AMH in women with normal cycles declines with age and becomes undetectable after menopause (114,116).

AMH appears to be a good predictor of both excessive (>3.5 ng/mL) and poor (<1 ng/mL) IVF stimulation response and is strongly correlated to the antral follicle count (111,116,117). **Unlike other serum markers, AMH can be measured at any time in the menstrual cycle** (116).

Antral Follicle Count   Using transvaginal ultrasound in the early follicular phase, all ovarian follicles 2 to 10 mm are counted and the total for both ovaries is called the basal antral follicle count (AFC). The AFC correlates well with chronologic age in normal fertile women and appears to reflect what remains of the primordial follicular pool (104). Decreases in AFC with age are gradual rather than sudden (118). **A total AFC less than 4 is predictive of poor response and higher cancellation rates with IVF** (119,120).

Treatment of Diminished Ovarian Reserve   **Treatments of diminished ovarian reserve include autologous IVF, use of donor oocytes or embryos, and adoption.** Pretreatment of women with diminished ovarian reserve for 4 to 5 months with *dehydroepiandrosterone* (*DHEA;* 25 mg three times daily) has been described to improve oocyte yield and pregnancy rates with IVF (121–123).

Ovulatory Factor

Ovulatory factor accounts for 30% to 40% of all cases of female infertility. Initial diagnoses among women with ovulatory factor infertility may include anovulation (complete absence of ovulation) or oligo-ovulation (infrequent ovulation). Menstrual history may be suggestive if oligomenorrhea, amenorrhea, polymenorrhea, or dysfunctional uterine bleeding is present (124). Menstrual dysfunction is present in 18% to 20% of the general population (125). Figure 32.5 shows the fluctuations of E2, progesterone, FSH, and LH in a normal, 28-day ovulatory cycle. **The normal length of the menstrual cycle in reproductive-age women varies from 21 to 35 days, with a mean of 27 to 29 days** (126). Most of the variability in cycle length occurs during the follicular phase (127), but the luteal phase, often considered to be fixed at 14 days, can range from 7 to 19 days (128). Even women with regular monthly menses may have anovulation, although the presence of moliminal symptoms such as premenstrual breast swelling, bloating, and mood changes are much more suggestive of ovulatory cycles (125).

Methods to Document Ovulation

The "Fertile Window"   **The fertile window is the 6 day interval ending on the day of ovulation, but not after ovulation.** Sperm can survive for up to 6 days in well-estrogenized cervical mucus, but the egg may be fertilizable for less than a day. Daily intercourse during this window may increase the probability of conception (32,127). The average woman is fertile between days 10 and 17 of the menstrual cycle, but many women can conceive outside of this range (128). Therefore, if timed intercourse is too cumbersome, intercourse two to three times weekly throughout the menstrual cycle will likely result in at least some of those occasions

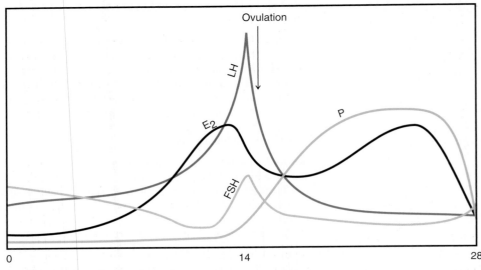

Figure 32.5   **Relative hormonal fluctuations in a normal, ovulatory, 28-day menstrual cycle.**

falling within the fertile window (129). Duration of abstinence prior to the fertile window has not been established, although one author suggests 5 days (127).

Basal Body Temperature   This inexpensive method involves daily recording of oral or rectal temperature using a basal body temperature (BBT) thermometer before the patient arises, eats, or drinks. The secretion of progesterone following ovulation causes a temperature increase of about 0.5 to 1°F over the baseline temperature of 97°F to 98.8°F that is typically recorded during the follicular phase of the menstrual cycle. Ovulation is assumed after 3 consecutive days of raised temperatures. Charting of daily BBTs produces a characteristic biphasic pattern in women with ovulatory cycles (130). **Limitations to BBT include its inability to prospectively predict ovulation and its frequent false-negative results** (131). Smoking and irregular sleep patterns can interfere with accurate BBT testing (130).

Cervical Mucus   **During the fertile window, cervical secretions at the vaginal introitus are slippery and clear, while secretions at other times of the menstrual cycle are dry and sticky** (32,130). The volume of cervical mucus peaks 2 to 3 days prior to ovulation, thus identifying higher day-specific probabilities of conception (32).

Luteinizing Hormone Monitoring   At a mean time of 2 hours following the peak of the serum LH surge, urinary LH can be detected. Commercially available kits for documenting the LH surge are generally accurate, quick, convenient, and relatively inexpensive enzyme-linked immunosorbent assays (ELISA) that use 35 to 50 mIU/mL as their threshold for detection (132,133). **Once the LH surge is detected, ovulation may occur within the next 48 hours** (32,132,133). The positive-predictive and negative-predictive values for these kits have been described to be 92% and 95%, respectively (132,134). Because the duration of the surge may be less than 12 hours, twice daily testing may increase detection rates (133). However, the 2 days of highest probability of conception are the day of and the day prior to the LH surge, so this may actually lead to abstaining from intercourse during a potentially fertile time (127). False-positive rates occur in 7% of cycles, which may reflect urinary clearance of unsustained premature LH surges (32,131,135). The tests cannot be used in patients with irregular cycles (127).

Midluteal Serum Progesterone   When used to document ovulation, serum progesterone measurement should coincide with peak progesterone secretion in the midluteal phase (typically on days 21 to 23 of an ideal 28-day cycle or 7 days following the LH surge). **The lower limit of progesterone levels in the luteal phase varies among laboratories, but a level above 3 ng/mL (10 nmol/L) typically confirms ovulation. However, interpretation of isolated luteal-phase measurements of serum progesterone is complicated by the frequent pulses that characterize the secretion of this hormone.** Although ovulatory levels are often considerably higher than 3 ng/mL, low midluteal serum levels of progesterone are not necessarily diagnostic of anovulation (124).

Ultrasound Monitoring   Ovulation is characterized both by a decrease in the size of a monitored ovarian follicle and by the appearance of fluid in the cul-de-sac using transvaginal ultrasound (124). **Follicles reach a preovulatory diameter of 17 to 19 mm in spontaneous cycles or 19 to 25 mm for clomiphene-induced cycles** (136,137). A combination of LH testing and ultrasound can be used, with LH kit testing starting when the ultrasound-measured follicle size reaches 14 mm (131). Ten percent of the cycles of normally fertile women may have a luteinized unruptured follicle, whereby progesterone is released and the luteal phase progresses normally without visible signs of follicle rupture when daily ultrasounds are performed from cycle days 10 to 20. This incidence is increased to 25% in women with unexplained infertility (138). **Because of the inconvenience and expense of serial measurements, ultrasound monitoring should be reserved for patients who fail less expensive methods for detecting ovulation or for certain types of ovulation induction** (124).

Follow-Up Tests   In women with absent or infrequent ovulation, serum FSH, prolactin, and thyroid-stimulating hormone (TSH) testing should be performed (124).

Polycystic Ovarian Syndrome

The most common cause of oligo-ovulation and anovulation—both in the general population and among women presenting with infertility—is polycystic ovarian syndrome (PCOS) (139). The diagnosis of PCOS is determined by exclusion of other medical conditions such as pregnancy, hypothalamic–pituitary disorders, or other causes of hyperandrogenism (e.g., androgen-secreting tumors or nonclassical congenital adrenal hyperplasia) *and* the presence of two of the following conditions (140):

- **Oligo-ovulation or anovulation (manifested as oligomenorrhea or amenorrhea)**

- **Hyperandrogenemia (elevated levels of circulating androgens) or hyperandrogenism (clinical manifestations of androgen excess)**

- **Polycystic ovaries detected by ultrasonography**

Documentation of elevated serum LH:FSH ratios and hyperinsulinemia are not required for either diagnosis or treatment of PCOS (139,140). Patients with PCOS should be counseled and screened regarding potential metabolic disease and obstetric complications prior to fertility treatment (141).

Ovulation Induction in Women with Polycystic Ovarian Syndrome

Despite the use of similar medications, the indications and goals of ovulation induction should be distinguished from those of superovulation. **The goal of ovulation induction refers to the therapeutic restoration of the release of one egg per cycle in a woman who either has not been ovulating regularly or has not been ovulating at all.** In contrast, the explicit goal of superovulation is to cause more than one egg to be ovulated, thereby increasing the probability of conception in women with unexplained infertility (136).

Weight Loss   Obesity in PCOS patients is associated with poor infertility treatment outcomes (139,142–144), although the impact on pregnancy loss rates is less clear (141,142,145). **Given that even a 5% weight loss may improve pregnancy rates, weight loss should be encouraged in all overweight and obese infertility patients** (139). Generally, lifestyle modification is the first-line therapy, followed by pharmacologic treatment and weight-loss surgery (139). Lifestyle recommendations include a decrease in daily caloric consumption by 500 kcal and regular physical exercise, although the optimal regimen for the latter is unknown (139,146). Weight loss interventions should be undertaken prior to attempting conception in patients with excess body weight (139).

Clomiphene Citrate (Clomid, Serophene) Pharmacology   *Clomiphene citrate* is a weak synthetic estrogen that mimics the activity of an estrogen antagonist when given at typical pharmacologic doses for the induction of ovulation. It is cleared through the liver and excreted into the stool, with 85% clearance in 6 days. **A functional hypothalamic–pituitary–ovarian axis is usually required for appropriate *clomiphene citrate* action.** More specifically, *clomiphene citrate* is thought to bind and block estrogen receptors in the hypothalamus for prolonged periods, thereby decreasing the normal ovarian–hypothalamic estrogen feedback loop. This blockade increases GnRH pulsatility, leading to increased pituitary secretion of gonadotropins, which promote ovarian follicular development (136).

Clomiphene Citrate Outcomes   **Clomiphene is considered a first-line treatment for anovulatory infertility** (147). Over the course of 6 months, *clomiphene* is associated with 49% ovulation, 23.9% pregnancy, and 22.5% live birth rates in women with anovulatory infertility (142). **Clomiphene effectiveness is decreased by obesity, increased age, and hyperandrogenic states** (142,148,149). Side effects of *clomiphene citrate* include vasomotor flushes, mood swings, breast tenderness, pelvic discomfort, and nausea. In a minority of individuals, the antiestrogenic effects of *clomiphene citrate* at the level of the endometrium or the cervix may have adverse effects on fertility. In the presence of visual abnormalities, *clomiphene citrate* should be discontinued promptly. **Multiple gestation rates with *clomiphene citrate* are approximately 8%, most of which are twins** (136). Treatment should be limited to 6 ovulatory cycles or 12 total cycles (141,150,151).

Clomiphene Citrate Dosing   The drug is supplied in 50 mg tablets; the usual starting dose is 50 mg per day, but patients who are very sensitive may respond to 12.5 to 25 mg per day. Therapy is typically begun within the first 5 days after the onset of a spontaneous or progesterone-induced menses and is continued for 5 days (i.e., treatment on days 2 to 6, 3 to 7, or 5 to 9 of the menstrual cycle) (136). It has been reported to be effective when started the day following progesterone withdrawal therapy, without waiting for menses (152). If ovulation does not occur at the initial dosage of *clomiphene citrate,* the dosage is increased in each subsequent cycle by 50 mg per day. **Seventy-four percent of women will ovulate with 100 mg per day, the maximum dose** approved by the U.S. Food and Drug Administration (153). However, some patients need higher doses, which have been safely given up to 250 mg per day (136). A novel stair-step method has been proposed, which increases the dose within a single cycle without intervening menses if there was no follicular response documented by ultrasound 4 to 5 days after the last pill (154). However, this particular protocol raises concern for unknown endometrial and embryonic effects (155).

Ovulation Monitoring during Clomiphene Citrate Therapy   If preovulation monitoring is not performed, patients should be instructed to have intercourse every 2 to 3 days following the last day of therapy and check a serum progesterone weekly for 5 weeks before inducing a withdrawal bleed or increasing the *clomiphene citrate* dose (142). **Although no clear advantage has been demonstrated for any ovulation monitoring technique, regular contact should be maintained with patients to review response to therapy.** The urinary LH surge may be detected 5 to 12 days after treatment is completed. When *clomiphene* is given cycle days 5 to 9, the surge typically occurs on cycle day 16 or 17 and can be confirmed by midluteal serum progesterone testing 7 days later. With ultrasound monitoring, treatment should be withheld if large cysts are seen on baseline testing. Following *clomiphene*, follicles typically reach a preovulatory diameter of 19 to 25 mm by ultrasound, but may be as large as 30 mm (136,137). A combination of LH testing and ultrasound can be used, with LH kits starting when the largest ultrasound-measured follicle reaches 14 mm in diameter (131).

Human Chorionic Gonadotropin   If a dominant follicle develops, but there is no spontaneous LH surge, human chorionic gonadotropin (hCG) can be used to induce final follicular maturation, with ovulation occurring approximately 40 hours following administration (136,156). **Although administration of hCG at midcycle does not appear to improve conception chances in most infertility patients using *clomiphene citrate*, it may be useful for patients with known ovulatory dysfunction** (157–159). The medication may be derived from urine (5,000 to 10,000 IU intramuscularly) or manufactured with recombinant technology (250 μg subcutaneously, equivalent to 5,000 to 6,000 IU urinary) (156).

Timing of Intrauterine Insemination   When IUI is added to the therapeutic protocol, insemination typically is performed 24 hours following the LH surge (157). However, given data that ovulation can occur much later than this, it is not surprising that no differences in pregnancy rates were found when IUI was performed between 24 and 60 hours following the LH surge (160). Although timing of IUI is typically performed 36 hours following hCG administration to coincide with follicle rupture when hCG is added to trigger ovulation, no significant differences in pregnancy or live birth rates are seen whether IUI is performed at 24 or 36 hours following the hCG trigger (161).

Insulin Sensitizers   Insulin resistance is thought to play a central role in the pathogenesis of PCOS (Table 32.7). *Metformin* is an oral biguanide that is approved for the treatment of non–insulin-dependent diabetes and has been used in PCOS to increase the frequency of spontaneous ovulation. *Metformin* acts by several mechanisms, including inhibition of gluconeogenesis in the liver and increasing the uptake of glucose in the periphery (162). **Although the literature is conflicting, larger studies have suggested that the live birth rate with *metformin* alone (7.2%) is lower than that achieved with *clomiphene*, and the combination does not confer additional benefit over *clomiphene* alone** (142,163). Obese patients are less likely to respond to *metformin* (164). It remains unclear whether *metformin* decreases miscarriage rates in PCOS,

Table 32.7 Clinical Findings that Suggest Insulin Resistance and Hyperinsulinemia
Physical findings associated with insulin resistance
Body mass index $>$27 kg/m^2
Waist-to-hip ratio $>$0.85
Waist $>$100 cm
Acanthosis nigricans
Numerous achrochordons (skin tags)

From **Barbieri RL.** Induction of ovulation in infertile women with hyperandrogenism and insulin resistance. *Am J Obstet Gynecol* 2000;183:1412–1418, with permission.

although it appears to be safe when used during pregnancy (142,162). Risks of *metformin* include gastrointestinal upset and rare lactic acidosis, so it should be avoided in settings of hepatic and renal dysfunction and prior to surgery or use of contrast radiologic dye. Reported effective doses include 500 mg three times daily, 850 mg twice daily, or 1,000 mg twice daily (142,162). The medication is best tolerated when started at the lowest dose and increased gradually. Extended release formulations are associated with less gastrointestinal upset (142). **Because regular ovulation may be delayed for 3 to 6 months or may not occur with *metformin* alone, patients may need medications to induce withdrawal bleeding to mitigate the risk of continued anovulation and endometrial hyperplasia** (141). Thiazolidinediones, which include *rosiglitazone* and *pioglitazone,* have been used for ovulation induction in PCOS patients (165–168). They have less associated gastrointestinal upset than *metformin.* All carry the risk of liver toxicity and, in the case of *rosiglitazone,* cardiovascular harm, and they are typically avoided during pregnancy (141).

Dexamethasone   Adjunctive oral *dexamethasone* may improve ovulation rates in patients resistant to *clomiphene* alone (147). These improvements have been reported even in the absence of adrenal hyperandrogenemia, so the mechanism of action remains unclear (169,170). Dose regimens have included 0.5 mg for 5 days starting on the first day of *clomiphene,* 0.5 mg for 6 weeks prior to starting *clomiphene,* and 2 mg for 10 days starting on the first day of *clomiphene* (169–172).

Oral Contraceptive Pretreatment   Administration of oral contraceptives for 2 months prior to beginning a cycle of *clomiphene* may improve ovulation and pregnancy rates in *clomiphene*-resistant patients, perhaps by improving a preexisting hyperandrogenic environment (147,173).

Tamoxifen   *Tamoxifen* is an oral antiestrogen similar in structure to *clomiphene* that is commonly used as an adjuvant therapy for breast cancer but has been used off-label to induce ovulation (174). Ovulation and pregnancy rates are similar with *tamoxifen* and *clomiphene* (147,174). Doses start at 20 mg per day for 5 days (similar in timing to *clomiphene*), and can be increased to 40 or 60 mg per day in subsequent cycles. The mechanism of action for *tamoxifen* in inducing ovulation appears to be similar to that of *clomiphene,* although *tamoxifen* exerts less negative endometrial effects (175).

Aromatase Inhibitors   These drugs include *letrozole* and *anastrazole.* Through their inhibition of aromatase-mediated conversion of androgens to estrogens and subsequent decreases in circulating estradiol, aromatase inhibitors have been approved for treatment of breast cancer. The off-label use of *letrozole* for ovulation induction in *clomiphene*-resistant patients was first reported in 2001 (176). Typical doses are 2.5 to 5 mg of *letrozole* or 1 mg of *anastrazole* daily for 5 days. Timing of administration is similar to that of *clomiphene,* although longer durations of 10 days have been reported (177,178). **Letrozole appears to have less negative effects on endometrial development when compared to *clomiphene*** (176). Although concerns have been raised regarding possible associations between fetal congenital anomalies and the use of aromatase inhibitors, no such increase was observed when *letrozole* was compared to *clomiphene* (179). Patients should be counseled regarding the absence of prospective, sufficiently powered studies to assess safety of off-label use of aromatase inhibitors for ovulation induction (141).

Gonadotropin Therapy   Anovulatory PCOS patients who fail to ovulate or conceive with oral agents should be considered for ovulation induction with exogenous gonadotropin injections. Evening medication administration allows for morning monitoring and midday decision making. Monitoring involves serum estradiol levels and transvaginal ultrasound measurements of follicle development. Typical protocols monitor at baseline, 4 to 5 days after treatment initiation, then every 1 to 3 days until follicular maturation (expected follicle growth is 1 to 2 mm daily after achieving 10 mm diameter) (180). **Given the goal of promoting growth of a single mature follicle, low initial gonadotropin doses of 37.5 to 75 IU per day are generally recommended, with increases in doses by 50% of the previous dose after 7 days if no follicle greater than 10 mm is observed** (141,180). Typical treatment duration is 7 to 12 days, but some patients require longer medications regimens for adequate stimulation. The maximum required gonadotropin dose seldom exceeds 225 units per day. Ovulation triggering with hCG is recommended for gonadotropin cycles and is used when one or two follicles are 16 to 18 mm in diameter and the E2 level per dominant follicle is 150 to 300 pg/mL. Ovulation can be expected 24 to 48 hours after the hCG trigger. GnRH agonists such as *leuprolide* (500 μg subcutaneously) can be used to trigger ovulation, but they require progesterone supplementation following administration. Intercourse should be recommended within 24 to 48 hours of ovulation triggering or IUI

24 to 36 hours after triggering (180). Testing for pregnancy should be performed 15 to 16 days after ovulation triggering and the cycle reviewed if pregnancy testing is negative. Gonadotropin dosage in future cycles should be altered if the prior response was inadequate or excessive.

Gonadotropin Preparations Several gonadotropin preparations are available. *Human menopausal gonadotropin* (HMG) is derived from human urine and includes approximately equivalent FSH and LH (derived from hCG) activity of 75 IU each. Current formulations of HMG and FSH can be administered either subcutaneously or intramuscularly. FSH-only preparations may be derived either from urine or via recombinant methods and are packaged either as lyophilized powder or premixed-liquid cartridges/pens. With the exception of highly purified urinary FSH, which has an FSH activity of 82.5 IU per ampule, all other products contain 75 IU of gonadotropin when supplied in ampules. **All preparations of FSH are highly purified, with minimal to no batch-to-batch variation and a high level of safety regardless of the derived source.** Despite being differentially marketed as *follitropin-α* and *-β*, these recombinant FSH preparations still contain combinations of 1-*α* and 1-*β* glycoprotein chain. Rather, they differ in their posttranslational modifications and processes for purification. *Recombinant LH* is available in syringes delivering 75 IU (156). For PCOS patients, FSH alone (either recombinant or urinary) appears to be sufficient in the gonadotropin preparation, although LH is not harmful (180) (Table 32.8). Contraindications to gonadotropin therapy are listed in Table 32.9.

Gonadotropin Outcomes Cumulative live birth rates are similar when gonadotropins are compared to *clomiphene* for ovulation induction when the goal is monofollicular ovulation and a maximum of six ovulatory cycles is similarly recommended (141). **When compared to other anovulatory patients, PCOS patients using *gonadotropins* are at higher risk for multiple gestations (36%), ovarian hyperstimulation syndrome (4.6%), and cycle cancellation (10%) because of their high numbers of baseline antral follicles** (141, 180, 181). Cancellation should be strongly considered in patients who reach E2 levels 1,000 to 2,500 pg/mL, have three or more follicles 16 mm or larger, or two or more follicles 16 mm or larger plus two or more follicles 14 mm or larger (141). Sequential use of *gonadotropins* and either *clomiphene* or aromatase inhibitors has been associated with lower gonadotropin requirements and lower cancellation rates and treatment duration without compromising pregnancy rates. The addition of aromatase inhibitors is associated with a lower number of dominant follicles and lower maximum E2 levels (182–184).

Table 32.8 Different Types of Available Gonadotropin Preparations

Trade Name	Name of Compound	Source	FSH per Ampule	LH per Ampule	Route of Administration
Repronex (Ferring Pharmaceuticals, Inc.)	Menotropin hMG	Extracted urinary	75 IU	75 IU	IM or SC
Menopur (Ferring Pharmaceuticals, Inc.)	Menotropin urinary hMG	Highly purified	75 IU	75 IU	SC
Bravelle (Ferring Pharmaceuticals, Inc.)	Urofollitropin urinary FSH	Highly purified	75 IU 450u multidose vial 300, 450, and 900 U RFF pen	Negligible	IM or SC
Follistim (Organon Inc.)	Follitropin-beta	Recombinant FSH beta	75 IU 75 and 150 U AQ vial 350, 650, and 975 U AQ cartridge + pen	None	SC
Gonal-F (Serono Laboratories, Inc.)	Follitropin-alpha	Recombinant FSH alpha	75 IU	None	SC
Luveris (Serono Laboratories, Inc.)	Luteinizing hormone	Recombinant LH	None	75 IU	SC

FSH, follicle-stimulating hormone; LH, luteinizing hormone; hMG, human menopausal gonatropin; IM, intramuscularly; SC, subcutaneously; N/A, not applicable.

Table 32.9 Contraindications to Gonadotropins for the Treatment of Infertility in Women

1. Primary ovarian failure with elevated follicle-stimulating hormone levels

2. Uncontrolled thyroid and adrenal dysfunction

3. An organic intracranial lesion such as a pituitary tumor

4. Undiagnosed abnormal uterine bleeding

5. Ovarian cysts or enlargement not caused by polycystic ovary syndrome

6. Prior hypersensitivity to the particular gonadotropin

7. Sex hormone–dependent tumors of the reproductive tract and accessory organs

8. Pregnancy

From ***Physicians desk reference.*** Micromedex (R) Healthcare Series Vol. 107. Thompson PRD and Micromedex Inc., 1974–2004, with permission.

Surgical Treatment   For *clomiphene*-resistant patients, surgical ovarian drilling has been performed as an alternative to the outdated ovarian wedge resection in an effort to decrease ovarian androgen-producing tissue and to promote ovulation without the risk of multiple pregnancy seen with gonadotropin administration (141,185). Drilling 3 to 15 puncture sites per ovary is typically performed via laparoscopy using electrocautery and diathermy or laser, although transvaginal ultrasound-guided and vaginal hydro-laparoscopy procedures have been reported (186–195). Successful drilling has been performed with the harmonic scalpel (190). Within 12 months after ovarian drilling, cumulative ovulation, clinical pregnancy, and live birth rates are 52%, 26% to 48%, and 13% to 32%, respectively. **These outcomes are similar to those using *gonadotropins*, but ovarian drilling carries a lower multiple gestation rate.** Outcomes are not significantly different when diathermy or laser are used for drilling, but they are compromised with patient age greater than 35 years or basal FSH greater than 10 mIU/mL (185,187). The risks of ovarian drilling include surgical complications, adhesions, recurrence of anovulation, and a theoretical risk of ovarian failure (185,196).

Ovulation Induction for Other Anovulatory Disorders

Hyperprolactinemia   Hyperprolactinemia can be associated with oligomenorrhea or amenorrhea and should be evaluated with pituitary magnetic resonance imaging (MRI) to exclude macroadenoma or other intracranial pathology (197). **Dopamine agonists are first-line agents in otherwise asymptomatic oligoovulatiory or anovulatory patients to restore ovulation** (197). *Bromocriptine* normalizes prolactin levels and induces ovulation in 80% to 90% of patients. It is taken two to three times daily, and most patients will respond to a total dose less than 7.5 mg daily. Side effects can be bothersome and include nausea, vomiting, postural hypotension, and headache. *Cabergoline* has similarly high efficacy and the advantage of a 0.25 mg twice-weekly dosing schedule and fewer side effects (198).

Hypogonadotropic Hypogonadism   **Anovulation in the presence of low serum LH, FSH, and estradiol levels defines hypogonadotropic hypogonadism and reflects dysfunction within the hypothalamic–pituitary axis.** Causes of hypogonadotropic hypogonadism, including craniopharyngiomas, pituitary adenomas, arteriovenous malformations, or other central space-occupying lesions, should be excluded using MRI. Stress, extreme weight loss, anorexia, excessive exercise, and low body mass index are all associated with functional hypothalamic suppression, so good nutrition and optimal body weight should be encouraged to restore ovulation (197,199). Leptin is a hormone produced by peripheral adipocytes that reflects energy stores and is deficient in women with diet or exericise-induced amenorrhea (200). Exogenous leptin has been reported to restore ovulation in these women (200,201). **Other conditions of hypothalamic dysfunction, such as congenital hypothalamic failure (Kallmann syndrome), can be treated using pulsatile GnRH therapy or *gonadotropins*. In these patients, both FSH and LH should be administered** (197,202). Pulsatile GnRH agonist therapy (25 ng/kg every 60 to 90 minutes) simulates normal physiology and offers some advantages over gonadotropin injections, including fewer multiple gestations and less ovarian hyperstimulation syndrome (OHSS) while maintaining excellent pregnancy rates (202).

Hypothyroidism The prevalence of hypothyroidism among mid-reproductive aged women is 2% to 4% and is mostly a result of autoimmune factors. Menstrual abnormalities, including those from anovulation, are present in 23% to 68% of overtly hypothyroid women and can be corrected with levothyroxine replacement. **Subclinical hypothyroidism and the presence of antithyroid antibodies (even if euthyroid) are associated with increased rates of infertility and spontaneous pregnancy loss, although there exists a lack of consensus as to appropriate upper normal limits of TSH and selection bias limits interpretation.** In any case, because even very mild or subclinical hypothyroidism can have adverse effects on fetal brain development and subsequent intelligence quotient, it is prudent to screen and treat women with thyroid hormone abnormalities before commencing infertility treatment (203).

Tubal Factor

Tubal factor accounts for 25% to 35% of infertility. Noninfectious causes for tubal factor include tubal endometriosis, salpingitis isthmica nodosa, tubal polyps, tubal spasm, and intratubal mucous debris (10). **The incidence of tubal infertility has been reported to be 8%, 19.5%, and 40% after one, two, and three episodes of PID, respectively** (204). Live birth rates are negatively affected by the severity of a single episode of PID (205). *C. trachomatis* and *Neisseria gonorrhoeae* are common pathogens associated with PID and infertility. *M. hominis* and *U. urealyticum* have been implicated in PID, but their contribution to infertility is less clear (17). Many patients with documented tubal damage have no history of PID and are presumed to have had subclinical chlamydial infections (206,207).

Hysterosalpingography Hysterosalpingography (HSG) is performed after menses but prior to ovulation between cycle days 7 and 12 to avoid potential pregnancy and take advantage of the thinner proliferative phase endometrium. The patient is typically premedicated 30 to 60 minutes prior to the procedure with *ibuprofen* or related medication (208). *Lidocaine* injected intracervically may provide further pain relief (209). With the patient in the dorsal lithotomy position, **either a metal cannula or a balloon catheter is inserted through the cervix and past the internal cervical os. Contrast dye is then injected under fluoroscopy to visualize the uterine cavity, fallopian tube architecture, and tubal patency** (208,210). Certain disease processes, such as salpingitis isthmica nodosa, have a characteristic appearance on HSG, with typical cornual or isthmic honeycombing resulting from contrast-filled diverticular projections (211). Compared to laparoscopy, HSG has a sensitivity and specificity of 86.5% and 79.8% for bilateral tubal patency and 90% and 97% for bilateral tubal occlusion, respectively. The specificity of HSG remains high but the sensitivity drops for unilateral tubal patency (212).

Hysterosalpingography Risks Although use of oil-based contrast has been associated with higher pregnancy rates following HSG when compared to water-based contrast (213,214), water-based contrast is generally preferred to avoid oil embolism or granuloma formation. Furthermore, patients should be screened for and pretreated with glucocorticoids if iodine allergy is found (210). The risk of PID after HSG is 0.3% to 3.1% overall but is greater than 10% in the setting of hydrosalpinges (215,216). **Therefore, HSG should be avoided in the setting of known hydrosalpinges and/or current or suspected PID** (208,216). The role of routine antibiotic prophylaxis for HSG is controversial, but in high-risk patients *doxycycline* could be considered (217). Recommended dosing is 100 mg twice daily, beginning the day before HSG and continuing for 3 to 5 days. If prophylaxis is not used and hydrosalpinges are noted on examination, postprocedure *doxycycline* treatment is recommended. Other rare complications of HSG include vascular intravasation, cervical laceration, uterine perforation, hemorrhage, vasovagal reactions, severe pain, and allergic response to the contrast dye (208).

Chlamydia Serology Chlamydia antibody testing appears to have comparable sensitivity and specificity to HSG but does not localize pathology and the utility of testing is controversial (211). It has been proposed that positive serologies in the setting of normal HSG should still prompt laparoscopy to rule out peritubal adhesions (207).

Laparoscopy **Laparoscopy is considered the gold standard for diagnosing tubal and peritoneal disease.** It allows visualization of all pelvic organs and permits detection and potential concurrent treatment of intramural and subserosal uterine fibroids, peritubal and periovarian adhesions, and endometriosis. Abnormal findings on HSG can be validated by direct visualization on laparoscopy using chromopertubation, which involves the transcervical installation of a dye such as indigo carmine to directly visualize tubal patency and fimbrial architecture (212). **However, even laparoscopy has been reported to have a false-positive rate of 11%**

for proximal tubal occlusion when resected tubal segments are examined pathologically (218).

Other Diagnostic Modalities   Falloposcopy is used in conjunction with hysteroscopy and allows direct fiberoptic visualization of tubal ostia and intratubal architecture for identification of tubal ostial spasm, abnormal tubal mucosal patterns, and even intraluminal debris causing tubal obstruction (218,219). At present, instrumentation availability and technical complications, including tubal perforation, limit its routine use (219). Alternatively, sonohysterography offers a much less invasive method of diagnosing fallopian tubal obstruction. The use of contrast media during sonohysterography is preferred to improve accuracy in documenting fallopian tubal patency, but these contrast agents are not available in the United States. As a substitute, the use of agitated saline (air-saline) during sonohysteroscopy provides good negative predictive value when compared to HSG or laparoscopy (220).

Treatment of Tubal Factor Infertility

As success rates for ART continue to improve, the indications for surgical approaches in the treatment of tubal infertility have become increasingly limited (221). Still, surgery can be effective in several situations and may be the optimal approach in some patients.

Proximal Tubal Occlusion   Proximal tubal catheterization and cannulation performed either via HSG or hysteroscopy can restore tubal patency in up to 85% of obstructions, although the reocclusion rate approaches 30%. **The best candidates for proximal tubal catheterization or cannulation have muscle spasm, stromal edema, amorphous debris, mucosal agglutination, or viscous secretions, while nonresponders include those with luminal fibrosis, failed tubal reanastamosis, fibroids, congenital atresia, or tuberculosis.** Occlusion from salpingitis isthmica nodosa, endometriosis, synechiae, salpingitis, and cornual polyps only occasionally will respond to catheterization or cannulation (10). Catheterization involves passage of a soft catheter into the tubal ostia, while cannulation passes a guidewire thru the ostia and injects contrast media or colored dye. Tubal perforation, typically minor, occurs in 1.9% to 11% of cases (10,211,218). **Catheterization under fluoroscopy during HSG is referred to as selective salpingography** (222). **Visualization of patency with the hysteroscopic approach can be accomplished using laparoscopy or ultrasound** (10,218). Ongoing pregnancy rates following proximal tubal catheterization or cannulation are 12% to 44% regardless of hysteroscopic or HSG approach. If occlusion persists or recurs, IVF is usually recommended. Microsurgical tubocornual anastomosis is an option with small studies reporting pregnancy rates of up to 68% (10). This procedure typically is performed via laparotomy and involves excision of the tubal isthmus, followed by reimplantation of the residual tube into a new opening made through the uterine cornua (211).

Distal Tubal Occlusion (Excluding Sterilization or Hydrosalpinx)   **Distal tubal disease and occlusion are causal in 85% of all tubal infertility and can be secondary to a variety of inflammatory conditions including infection, endometriosis, or prior abdominal or pelvic surgery** (211,223). Patients younger than 35 years of age with mild distal tubal disease, normal tubal mucosa, and absent or minimal pelvic adhesions are the best candidates for corrective microsurgery (223). *In vitro* fertilization should be considered for older patients or those with diminished ovarian reserve, combined proximal and distal tubal disease, severe pelvic adhesions, tubal damage that is not amenable to reconstruction, or additional infertility factors (223,224). Fimbrioplasty involves lysis of fimbrial adhesions or dilation of fimbrial phimosis, whereas salpingostomy (also known as salpingoneostomy) involves the creation of a new tubal opening in an occluded fallopian tube (223). In well-selected patients, pregnancy rates are reported to be 32% to 42.2%, 54.6% to 60%, 30% to 34.6%, and 55.9% for adhesiolysis, fimbrioplasty, salpingostomy, and nonsterilization-related anastamosis, respectively (211,223). **As a group, these procedures are associated with a 7.9% rate of subsequent ectopic pregnancy** (223).

Sterilization Reversal   **Twenty percent of women express regret following sterilization, and 1% to 5% of those will request reversal, often after a change in marital status.** The technique for sterilization reversal involves microsurgical dissection of the occluded ends of the fallopian tube followed by a layered reapposition of the proximal and distal tubal segments. Surgical approaches include minilaparotomy, laparoscopy, and robotic-assisted laparoscopy (224,225). Pregnancy rates following microsurgical tubal reanastamosis for sterilization reversal are 55% to 81%, with most pregnancies occurring within 18 months of surgery (224). Ectopic pregnancy rates following the procedure are generally less than 10% but may approach 18% (223,226). **The main predictors of success are age younger than 35 years, isthmic-isthmic or ampulo-ampullar anastamosis, final anastamosed tubal length greater than 4 cm, and less-destructive sterilization methods such as use of rings or clips** (224,226). Unlike vasectomy reversal, the length of time between fallopian tubal sterilization and reversal does not seem to affect outcome. IVF should be considered in lieu of sterilization reversal for older patients or those with diminished ovarian reserve, severe pelvic adhesions, additional infertility factors, or prior unsuccessful reanastamosis (223,224).

Hydrosalpinx   Distal occlusion may lead to fluid buildup in the fallopian tube, causing a hydrosalpinx. Hydrosalpinx fluid impedes embryo development and implantation (211). A meta-analysis of 14 studies and 1,004 patients with hydrosalpinges concluded that IVF pregnancy rates were significantly lower in the presence of hydrosalpinges (227). **Salpingectomy for hydrosalpinx prior to IVF significantly improves both pregnancy and live birth rates when compared to IVF performed with the fallopian tubes *in situ*, although laparoscopic tubal occlusion appears to be a reasonable alternative** (228–230). There are significantly less outcome data on the use of transvaginal needle drainage and salpingostomy for treatment of hydrosalpinges prior to IVF (211).

Uterine Factors

Pathologies within the uterine cavity are the cause of infertility in as many as 15% of couples seeking treatment and are diagnosed in greater than 50% of infertile patients (231). Therefore, the evaluation of the couple with infertility should consistently include an assessment of the endometrial cavity. Uterine cavity abnormalities include endometrial polyps, endometrial hyperplasia, submucous myomas, intrauterine synechiae, and congenital uterine anomalies (232).

Diagnostic Imaging for Uterine Pathology

Hysteroscopy   **Hysteroscopy is considered the gold standard for uterine cavity evaluation because it allows for direct visualization.** The procedure involves insertion of an endoscope through the cervical canal into the uterine cavity and instillation of distension media to allow for visualization (231–233). **Diagnostic hysteroscopy may be performed in the office using a small-diameter hysteroscope and saline distension, often without need for anesthesia** (232). To optimize visualization of the endometrial cavity and avoid performing the procedure during early pregnancy, hysteroscopy is typically scheduled during the early- to midfollicular phase of the cycle. Disadvantages to the procedure include poor visualization when uterine bleeding is present and the inability to evaluate structures outside the uterine cavity, including those in the myometrium and adnexa. Office hysteroscopy is reported to have a 72% sensitivity for cavity abnormalities when compared to operative hysteroscopy using general anesthesia (231).

Hysterosalpingogram   Insofar as it allows assessment of both tubal and intrauterine pathology, HSG is a reasonable initial imaging technique to use in the basic infertility evaluation. Hysterosalpingogram shows the general configuration of the uterine cavity and indicates endometrial lesions as filling defects or irregularities of the intrauterine wall. **Excessive contrast may lead to false-negative findings, which may account for the 50% sensitivity of HSG compared to hysteroscopy for endometrial polyps.** Inability to discriminate air bubbles, mucous, and debris from true intracavitary pathology may account for HSG's high false-positive rate when compared with hysteroscopy (232,233). Other drawbacks include patient discomfort, use of iodinated contrast, and radiation exposure (232).

Transvaginal Ultrasound   Compared to hysteroscopy, transvaginal ultrasound has a 75% positive predictive value and 96.5% negative predictive value for intracavitary polyps but a 0% positive predictive value for intrauterine adhesions. Similar to HSG, it has a sensitivity of 44% for uterine malformations (233). However, this may be improved significantly with the use of three-dimensional technology.

Sonohysterography   Saline infusion sonography (SIS), synonymous with sonohysterography, involves the transcervical instillation of saline, often via a balloon catheter, during transvaginal ultrasound to distend the uterine cavity and delineate the endometrium. As with office hysteroscopy and HSG, SIS is performed during the follicular phase of the cycle and anesthesia typically is not required. Endometrial polyps appear as hyperechogenic pedunculated lesions, submucous fibroids have mixed echogenicity, and adhesions contain densely echogenic and cystic areas (234). **Compared to hysteroscopy, SIS has 100% sensitivity, specificity, and**

positive and negative predictive values for uterine polyps (233). Because of a smaller volume of distension media used, SIS is generally better tolerated than HSG or hysteroscopy (231,234). Another advantage of SIS is the ability to evaluate the myometrium and the adnexa for fibroids or adenomyosis. When combined with three-dimensional technology, SIS is particularly good at assessing the overall uterine contour and delineating congenital anomalies such as septate uteri (234). Standard SIS has somewhat lower sensitivity of 77.8% in detecting uterine congenital anomalies when compared to hysteroscopy, but this is higher than both two-dimensional transvaginal ultrasound and HSG. Hysterosalpingogram and SIS perform similarly for intrauterine adhesions, each having approximately 50% positive predictive value and greater than 90% negative predictive value (233).

Magnetic Resonance Imaging   Although transvaginal ultrasound, HSG, SIS, and hysteroscopy may suggest congenital uterine anomalies, pelvic MRI is considered the gold standard for imaging and is particularly useful for diagnosing rudimentary uterine horns (235). Pelvic MRI has the best sensitivity and specificity for intramural and submucous myomas compared to pathologic examination and is especially useful for detecting large or multiple fibroids (236,237). MRI has been suggested as a tool to differentiate fibroids from adenomyosis, but routine substitution for ultrasound is not recommended (237,238).

Congenital Anomalies of the Uterus

Congenital uterine anomalies occur in 3% to 4% of women. This increases to 5% to 10% in women with early pregnancy loss and up to 25% in those with second and third trimester pregnancy losses (235). During female embryonic development, the paired paramesonephric or müllerian ducts elongate toward each other and fuse in the midline. This is followed by resorption of the intervening septum to form the upper vagina, cervix, uterus, and fallopian tubes by week 20 of gestation. Failure of any of these steps leads to absent uterine development or development of unicornuate, bicornuate, arcuate, didelphic, or septate uteri. **Because of the proximity of the paramesonephric ducts to the urinary system, renal anomalies often coexist with müllerian anomalies. Appropriate urologic imaging should be performed whenever a müllerian anomaly is diagnosed (235,239). Uterine anomalies are more closely associated with pregnancy wastage and poor obstetric outcomes than with infertility, as the prevalence of congenital uterine defects is generally similar among fertile and infertile women.** The exception to this is müllerian agenesis. Patients with müllerian agenisis can have genetically related children only through the use of IVF and a gestational carrier. The arcuate uterus is the mildest congenital uterine anomaly and typically live birth rates are comparable to those in women with normal uteri (235). **Surgical uterine repair to improve obstetric outcomes is controversial for most anomalies. However, rudimentary uterine horns require removal on diagnosis, and hysteroscopic metroplasty of the septate uteri significantly reduces the rates of pregnancy loss, but not infertility** (235,240). The number of reproductive-age patients presenting with *in utero* exposure to *DES* is declining rapidly and will continue to decline in the future, because the substance was banned in 1971. Women whose mothers were exposed to *DES* have higher rates of uterine malformations (e.g., T-shaped uterus) and associated obstetric complications (235).

Acquired Abnormalities of the Uterus

Leiomyomas   Leiomyomas, also called myomas or fibroids, are benign monoclonal uterine myometrial tumors that affect 25% to 45% of reproductive-age women, particularly African Americans (241). The mechanisms by which fibroids cause infertility are unknown, but may involve altered uterine contractility, impaired gamete transport, or endometrial dysfunction (242). Among women with infertility and uterine leiomyomas, pregnancy rates are primarily affected by leiomyoma location (236,242). **Subserosal fibroids do not appear to affect fertility or obstetric outcomes, while intramural (regardless of cavity distortion) and submucosal myomas are associated with lower implantation and live birth rates** (236,242,243). It remains unclear whether the size of intramural fibroids determines pregnancy rates and obstetric outcomes, because lower or unchanged pregnancy rates have been reported among patients with fibroids of varying sizes including >2cm, >4cm, or 4–8 cm when compared to patients without fibroids (242).

Myomectomy   In women desiring fertility who require treatment for fibroids, myomectomy is the preferred approach, and uterine artery embolization is relatively contraindicated (242). **Removal of cavity-distorting intramural and submucous myomas is generally recommended prior to proceeding with infertility treatment. The utility of surgical removal of non-cavity-distorting intramural fibroids is presently unknown** (236,242, 243).

Myomectomy can be performed hysteroscopically, via laparotomy, laparoscopically (alone or with robotic assistance), or vaginally (237,241,244–246). Hysteroscopic removal is generally preferred for small submucous fibroids without intramural involvement, while use of the other methods generally depends on patient preference, operator skill, or the presence of other pelvic pathology (237,241,244,245). The utility of pretreatment with GnRH agonists prior to surgery is debatable. GnRH agonists may shrink larger fibroids (5 to 6 cm) enough to allow hysteroscopic resection and may decrease the risk of intraoperative blood loss and postoperative anemia. **Fluid overload and uterine perforation are the most common complications of hysteroscopic myomectomy, while bleeding and adjacent organ injury are more often associated with alternative approaches** (237,241). Fibroids that are located low on the uterus and posteriorly are less amenable to laparoscopic resection. Transmyometrial approaches raise concern for uterine rupture during pregnancy, although this risk appears to be very low (241).

Endometrial Polyps   The incidence of asymptomatic endometrial polyps among women with infertility has been reported to range from 6% to 8%, but may be as high as 32% (247–249). Risk factors for polyp development include obesity, unopposed estrogen exposure, and polycystic ovary syndrome. The mechanisms by which endometrial polyps may impair fertility are incompletely described but may relate to disordered endometrial receptivity (250). One report localized 32% of endometrial polyps in infertile women to the posterior uterine wall, indicated that 40.3% of patients had multiple polyps, and stated a 6.9% hyperplasia rate (251). Polypectomy is generally performed via curettage, blind avulsion, or hysteroscopic removal (249). **Although the efficacy of polypectomy prior to infertility treatment has not been clearly established, a prospective randomized trial showed a 2.1-fold higher rate of pregnancy among women who underwent the procedure prior to IUI** (249,252). Higher pregnancy rates have been noted for polyps removed from the uterotubal junction when compared to those removed from other locations (251). Smaller nonrandomized studies provide conflicting data on the negative fertility effects of polyps less than 1.5 to 2 cm (251,253,254).

Intrauterine Synechiae or Asherman's Syndrome   Severe trauma to the basalis layer of the endometrium with subsequent tissue bridge formation leads to intrauterine synechiae or Asherman's syndrome. Symptoms of severe disease include amenorrhea, menstrual irregularities, spontaneous abortion, and recurrent pregnancy loss. **The causes of intrauterine adhesions are often iatrogenic, with patients typically reporting intraoperative or postoperative complications of uterine evacuations for incomplete pregnancy loss, pregnancy termination, or postpartum hemorrhage.** Myomectomy, hysterotomy, diagnostic curettage, cesarean section, tuberculosis, caustic abortifacients, and uterine packing are less-common causes in Western countries (255). In developing countries, Asherman's syndrome resulting from genital tuberculosis is quite common (256). **Hysteroscopic resection of synechiae is the preferred treatment to restore fertility in women with Asherman's syndrome, and success rates are generally very high. Patients with genital tuberculosis have a very poor prognosis.** Postoperative prevention of adhesion reformation disease may involve *estrogen* therapy alone for 1 month or in combination with intraoperative placement of an intrauterine device (such as a small Malecot catheter or pediatric Foley catheter) for 1 to 2 weeks. There is no standard regimen for *estrogen* therapy, but oral *conjugated estrogens* 2.5 mg daily overlapping with *progestin* or *estradiol valerate* 2 mg injections daily have been suggested (255,257).

Luteal-Phase Defect and Progesterone Supplementation

Mechanisms   The luteal phase is normally characterized by progesterone secretion by the corpus luteum and appropriate endometrial secretory transformation that allow for embryonic implantation in the endometrium and support of early pregnancy for the first 7 to 8 weeks of gestation (258,259). **Luteal phase defect (LPD) is a failure to develop a fully mature secretory endometrium during the implantation window and is thought to account for 4% of infertility** (260,261). Proposed mechanisms for LPD include inadequate production of progesterone following ovulation, improper GnRH pulsatility causing insufficient gonadotropin production during the LH surge, and inadequate endometrial responsivity to progesterone (260–262). **ART or gonadotropin ovulation induction medications may induce iatrogenic LPD via disruption of granulosa cells from follicular aspiration and suppression of endogenous LH secretion through a combination of supraphysiologic estradiol levels and GnRH agonist or antagonist therapy** (259,262).

Diagnosis   Diagnostic criteria for LPD have been varyingly defined, but have included a low mid-luteal phase serum progesterone levels of less than 5 to 10 ng/mL, a delay of 2 days or more in endometrial histology when compared to chronologic cycle day in two or more cycles, a BBT rise lasting less than 11 days, and a shortened luteal phase of less than 14 days (259–261). Unfortunately, the characteristic pulsatile secretion of progesterone during the luteal phase of the menstrual cycle combines with wide temporal variations (even within a 60- to 90-minute time span) to make interpretation of midlueal progesterone levels difficult (258). **Similar rates of shortened luteal phase are found in fertile and infertile women, and there is significant variability of luteal phase length from cycle to cycle in an individual woman** (261). **Finally, there is significant interobserver variability in pathologic interpretation of endometrial biopsies from infertile women, and out-of-phase biopsy results poorly discriminate between fertile and infertile women** (263,264).

Treatment   **Progesterone therapy is considered standard practice during ART cycles, but is more controversial during non-ART fertility treatments** (258,259,262). When used, *progesterone* supplementation can be administered via oral, vaginal, or intramuscular routes. Intramuscular *progesterone* is dosed at 25 to 50 mg daily. Most products are delivered in oil, and caution should be used to ascertain the presence of sesame or peanut allergies. Oral micronized *progesterone* is associated with erratic absorption and decreased bioavailability, so it is typically administered via an off-label delivery route—vaginally 200 to 600 mg daily, and often in divided doses. The side effects of this delivery route, however, can include vaginal discharge and irritation. Other vaginal preparations include a once-daily gel and a 100 mg insert that is given two to three times daily. **There remains no consensus regarding the superiority of vaginal versus intramuscular administration.** *Progesterone* therapy typically begins 3 to 4 days following the hCG trigger or LH surge and, if pregnancy occurs, continues for at least 8 to 9 weeks of gestation (258,259,262). Although some *progestins* can stimulate the androgen receptor, there is no evidence of teratogenicity with the *progesterone* supplementation described herein (258).

Pelvic Factor

Endometriosis   Endometriosis affects 6% to 10% of all women during their reproductive years but is present in 25% to 50% of infertile women (212,265). **It is characterized by the presence of endometrial tissue growing outside the uterine cavity and is found primarily on the peritoneum, ovaries, and rectovaginal septum** (265). Fecundability rates in affected patients are estimated at 2% to 10% per month (266). Possible mechanisms for infertility among women with endometriosis include anatomic distortion from adhesions or fibrosis and the known presence of inflammatory mediators that exert toxic effects on gametes, embryos, tubal fimbria, and eutopic endometrium (265,266). **Laparoscopy for direct visualization remains the mainstay in the diagnosis of endometriosis. The disease is staged laparoscopically according to the Revised American Society for Reproductive Medicine's classification, with stages III and IV (moderate to severe) including ovarian endometriomas, dense tubal or ovarian adhesions, and/or cul-de-sac obliteration** (265). However, laparoscopy can miss deep disease that may better be detected by ultrasound (i.e., endometriomas) and rectovaginal examination (267). It is unclear whether the presence of endometriosis negatively affects IVF outcomes, although some reports indicate a worse prognosis for more severe disease (stages III and IV) (221,268).

Endometriosis Infertility Managment   Hormonal suppression of endometriosis typically has a minimal benefit for endometriosis-related infertility (265). In minimal to mild disease, laparoscopic ablation appears to significantly improve pregnancy rates when compared to diagnostic laparoscopy alone, although there remains some dissent (267,269). One major randomized trial reported 31% versus 17% pregnancy rates over 3 years with a subsequent meta-analysis supporting these findings (265,266,270,271). **Although authors have estimated that eight laparoscopies involving treatment of mild or minimal endometriosis would need to be performed for each pregnancy gained, that number is likely to be much higher given that not everyone who undergoes laparoscopy will have endometriosis** (267,270). The benefit of surgical management of endometriosis is even less clear for moderate to severe disease, although removal of endometriomas may be indicated prior to IVF when they would interfere with oocyte retrieval (265–267). Endometrioma resection during IVF or ICSI treatment is associated with decreased ovarian function in up to 13% of cases (272,273). Furthermore, 40% of endometriomas recur postoperatively, and conflicting reports exist that show increases and decreases in pregnancy and live birth rates after surgery (267,272,273). Therefore, IVF is considered a reasonable first-line therapy for endometriosis-associated infertility because of the short time to pregnancy and avoidance of surgery (221).

Adhesions   Adhesions may result from sharp, mechanical, or thermal injury, infection, radiation, ischemia, dessication, abrasion, or foreign body reaction. Adhesiolysis improves pregnancy rates by 12% at 1 year and by 29% at 2 years in infertile women with adnexal adhesions. Use of adhesion barriers reduces adhesion formation following laparoscopy and laparotomy, but there is no evidence to date for improvement in pregnancy rates (274,275).

Unexplained Infertility

Thirty percent of couples are diagnosed with unexplained infertility, in which the basic infertility evaluation reveals normal semen parameters, evidence of ovulation, patent fallopian tubes, and no other obvious cause of infertility. Patients with unexplained infertility may be reassured that even after 12 months of failed attempts, 20% will conceive in the following 12 months and over 50% in the following 36 months. This suggests that in couples with the good prognostic factors of female age less than 30, less than 24 months of infertility, and a previous pregnancy in the same partnership, unexplained infertility may merely reflect the lower extreme of normal fertility. It is likely that current technology is limited in terms of diagnosing all causes for infertility, and the utility of evaluations other than basic testing in an infertile couple has yet to be proven (2,150,276).

Proposed Mechanisms for Unexplained Infertility

Luteinized Unruptured Follicle Syndrome   This condition involves luteinization of a follicle that has failed to rupture and release its oocyte, leading to a normal menstrual cycle but infertility. It is thought to occur in up to 25% of patients with unexplained infertility, more than twice the incidence in fertile women (138). The diagnosis may justify the use of IVF whereby follicles are aspirated and oocyte are retrieved and fertilized *in vitro*.

Immunologic Factors   Although serum antiphospholipid antibodies and antithyroid antibodies are more prevalent among patients with unexplained infertility than among fertile women, the presence of antiphospholipid antibodies has not been found to adversely affect IVF outcomes, so screening is discouraged (277,278). The association between the presence of antithyroid antibodies and infertility is inconsistent, so screening is not recommended (279–282). Unexplained infertility has been associated with antisperm antibodies, but the extent to which these antibodies affect fertility treatment outcomes and whether IUI, ICSI, or glucocorticoids should be used remains unclear (280,282,283). A similar lack of consensus exists concerning the assessment of peripheral natural killer cell number and/or activity in infertility patients (276,282).

Decreased Endometrial Perfusion   Using ultrasound-based endometrial Doppler studies, women with unexplained infertility have been shown to exhibit abnormal endometrial perfusion when compared to fertile women, but, at present, there is no direct link to fertility treatment outcomes and no recommendations to act on these findings (284).

Infection   *C. trachomatis* and related clinical and subclinical infections have been discussed in the "Tubal Factor" section. To date, no consistent associations have been reported between chlamydial species, *M. hominis,* and unexplained infertility in men or women (207,285,286). *U. urealyticum* and *M. genitalium,* however, may be more of a concern (287). Prophylactic *doxycycline* (100 mg twice daily for 4 weeks) given to infertile couples improved pregnancy rates only for those couples in which the male partner was able to clear a ureaplasma infection (288). Antimicrobial prophylaxis is often given for ART, but it is not clear the extent to which clearance of these organisms improves pregnancy rates (287,289).

Undiagnosed Pelvic Pathology   Following a negative infertility workup, laparoscopy has been proposed to evaluate for peritubal adhesions and endometriosis. However, there is a lack of consensus as to the frequency of these abnormalities in women with unexplained infertility, and many practitioners will forgo laparoscopy in lieu of a few cycles of less invasive interventions in such patients (290–292).

Occult Male or Oocyte Factors   Occult male factor despite normal semen analysis and oocyte factors, such as premature zona hardening, mitochondrial dysfunction, and/or aberrant spindle formation, has been suggested as a mechanism for unexplained infertility (293).

Treatment of Unexplained Infertility

It is reasonable to discuss no intervention or expectant management with younger patients presenting with unexplained infertility. Some patients will want to proceed with diagnostic (and potentially therapeutic) laparoscopy. Typical interventions proceed stepwise with superovulation (first with *clomiphene* or *letrozole* for three to four cycles, then *gonadotropins* for three to four cycles) combined with intrauterine insemination, followed by ART (294). ART options for unexplained infertility include conventional IVF, split IVF/ICSI, and full ICSI, even though no male factor has been identified. Risks with *clomiphene, letrozole,* and non-ART *gonadotropins,* as well as gonadotropin preparations, have been discussed above.

Baseline Ovarian Cysts   Prior to beginning therapy, a baseline ultrasound may be performed on cycle day 2 or 3 during menses (or following GnRH agonist suppression) to confirm an optimally thin (<4 mm) endometrium and quiescent ovaries. With *clomiphene citrate* cycles, the presence of ovarian cysts on a baseline scan was associated with decreased rates of ovulation but not of pregnancy, although cyst size was not predictive of response (295). Ovarian cysts on baseline evaluation have been associated with decreased pregnancy rates in ovulation induction cycles employing *gonadotropins* (296). In IVF patients, **functional (estrogen-producing) cysts are seen in 9.3% of women following GnRH agonist suppression** (297). Although nonfunctional ovarian cysts up to 5.3 cm did not affect IVF outcomes, functional ovarian cysts (mean diameter 2 cm and baseline estradiol 180 pg/mL) have been associated with increased gonadotropin requirements (dosing and duration), higher cancellation rates, fewer retrieved oocytes, poorer embryo quality, and lower pregnancy rates per cycle (9.6% vs. 29.7% in cyst-free cycles) (297,298). Ovarian cysts greater than 10 mm that are seen on the baseline scan tend to resolve spontaneously within 1 to 2 months, and oral contraceptive administration does not appear to hasten their resolution (299). However, oral contraceptive pretreatment prior to GnRH agonist cycles is associated with decreased risk of cyst formation (300). Functional cyst aspiration prior to gonadotropin stimulation, which is commonly performed to expedite initiation of treatment, did not improve IVF outcomes in one large study (297).

Superovulation (Controlled Ovarian Hyperstimulation)   **Unlike ovulation induction, in which the goal is to stimulate the release of a single oocyte in a women who was not previously ovulating, the explicit goal of superovulation (for non-ART or ART purposes) is to cause more than one egg to be ovulated, thereby increasing the probability of conception in women with unexplained infertility** (136). In most superovulation protocols, a baseline scan is performed on day 2 of the menstrual cycle to assess antral follicle count and the presence or absence of ovarian cysts. Baseline estrogen and progesterone levels are typically obtained on this day (301). Starting daily doses in superovulation cycles are higher for both *clomiphene* (100 mg for 5 days) and *gonadotropins* (150 to 300 IU daily) than those used for ovulation induction (111,301,302). Superovulation with *clomiphene* is otherwise conducted as described above for ovulation induction. When *gonadotropins* are used for normal responders with unexplained infertility, FSH doses of 225 IU and 300 IU lead to similar outcomes with IVF (111). **The maximal *gonadotropin* dosage is typically 450 IU per day because higher dosages do not increase ovarian response** (301). In most superovulation protocols, *gonadotropins* are started on day 2 or 3 of menses (301–303). The starting dose of *gonadotropins* is maintained each day until cycle day 6 or 7 (stimulation day 4 or 5), when the serum estradiol level and transvaginal ultrasound are first measured to document ovarian response (111,302,303). *Gonadotropin* dosage is increased by 50 to 100 IU per day every 2 to 4 days until a response is evident (304). Estradiol levels typically double every 48 hours, with follicle growth of 1 to 2 mm daily after a 10 mm diameter is reached (305). Triggering of ovulation typically occurs when at least two follicles have reached an average diameter 17 to 18 mm and the endometrial thickness is 8 mm or more (111,302,303,306–308). For non-ART cycles, cancellation should be strongly considered for E2 levels 1,000 to 2,500 pg/mL, for three or more follicles 16 mm or more, or for two or more follicles 16 mm or more plus two or more follicles 14 mm or more (141). Ultrasound monitoring of IVF cycles without estradiol levels can be considered (309).

Treatment Outcomes   It should be noted that pregnancy rates in unexplained infertility patients vary widely among studies, even when the same treatments are used, perhaps as a result of heterogeneity in treatment protocols and patient age. Interpretation of data on the use of *clomiphene* in patients with unexplained infertility is particularly difficult because the studies are heterogeneous and their results conflicting (150,151). **One meta-analysis of 1,159 participants with unexplained infertility involving seven randomized controlled trials of *clomiphene citrate* with and without IUI indicated no improvement in pregnancy or live birth rates when compared to no treatment or placebo** (151). Still, oral therapies continue to be used, and *clomiphene* and *letrozole* have recently been shown to have comparable efficacy when combined with IUI for treating unexplained infertility, with pregnancy rates approximately 18% per cycle (310). Combined therapy with *gonadotropins* and IUI is more likely to result in pregnancy

(9% per cycle) than either superovulation (4%) or IUI (5%) alone (302). Laparoscopy to treat minimal or mild endometriosis is associated with live birth rates similar to those in patients with unexplained infertility who receive COH/IUI (70% over four cycles) (311). **In women over the age of 40, non-ART therapies are much less effective and IVF should be offered as an initial or early treatment option** (312). Pregnancy rates per cycle for unexplained infertility in women who are less than 40 years old have been grouped by treatment modality and reported as follows: (i) *clomiphene*/IUI 7.8%, (ii) *gonadotropin*/IUI 9.8%, and (iii) IVF 30.7% (313). The use of ICSI or splitting sibling oocytes between IVF and ICSI has been proposed as an approach to unexplained infertility patients to diagnose and treat underlying occult male or oocyte factors (293,314). **Although ICSI does improve fertilization rates and reduce fertilization failure, no differences have been noted in pregnancy or live birth rates when comparing IVF to ICSI for unexplained infertility** (314,315).

Cost-Effectiveness   **According to computerized decision-tree modeling, laparoscopy followed by expected management for unexplained infertility may be cost-effective when compared to no intervention, non-ART treatment, or IVF** (294). Given that 15 *gonadotropin*/IUI cycles are needed to produce one additional pregnancy when compared to intracervical insemination alone, IVF seems a reasonable option (150). In Massachusetts, where insurance companies are required to cover infertility treatment, the cost-effectiveness of IVF in the treatment of unexplained infertility was determined. Couples were randomized to accelerated treatment with three cycles of *clomiphene citrate*/IUI followed by up to six cycles of IVF if no pregnancy occurred (n = 256) versus conventional treatment with *clomiphene*/IUI for three cycles, then injectable *gonadotropins*/IUI for three cycles, then IVF for six cycles (n = 247). Median time to pregnancy was 8 months in the accelerated versus 11 months in the conventional treatment groups. The authors used an average cost per cycle with *clomiphene*/IUI of $500, with *gonadotropin*/IUI of $2,500, and assuming IVF costs were less than $17,749 per cycle. They reported that the accelerated treatment protocol resulted in a savings of $2,624 per couple and lowered the per delivery charges by $9,856 compared to conventional treatment regimens. **The study concluded that couples with unexplained infertility who have not achieved pregnancy after three cycles of *clomiphene*/IUI should proceed directly to IVF** (313).

Assisted Reproductive Technologies

Process of Assisted Reproductive Technologies   ART include IVF, ICSI, gamete intrafallopian transfer (GIFT), zygote intrafallopian transfer (ZIFT), cryopreserved embryo transfers, and the use of donor oocytes. Because of improved success rates associated with IVF-embryo transfer, the performance of GIFT and ZIFT has declined in the United States, so this review will focus primarily on IVF and ICSI (316). **Both processes involve:**

- **Prevention of a premature LH surge**
- **Follicle growth**
- **Pretreatment**
- **Adjunctive medications**
- **Oocyte maturation/ovulation triggering**
- **Oocyte retrieval**
- **Luteal support**
- **Fertilization by IVF or ICSI**
- ***In vitro* embryo culture**
- **Transfer of fresh embryos**
- **Cryopreservation of surplus embryos**
- **First trimester pregnancy monitoring**

Prevention of Premature Luteinizing Hormone Surge

Luteinizing Hormone surge and Premature Luteinization   Without GnRH agonist or antagonist suppression, LH surges occur in IVF cycles resulting from high estradiol levels in the early follicular phase. This, in turn, results in a lower oocyte yield and reduced pregnancy rates (317). **Spontaneous ovulation prior to oocyte retrieval is reported to occur in 16% of nonsuppressed IVF cycles** (318). The premature LH rise typically occurs after 5 to 7 days of stimulation (317). **In contrast, premature luteinization is a somewhat misleading term that refers to a rise in serum progesterone (cutoffs vary from 0.8 to 2 ng/mL) observed on the day of hCG administration and occurs in the setting of low LH levels secondary to gonadotropin-suppressive medications** (319). The incidence of premature luteinization has been estimated at 6% to 7% when the progesterone cutoff level is set at greater than 1.5 ng/mL, but it may be as high as 35%. Mechanisms underlying premature luteinization may include incomplete pituitary desensitization, increased granulosa cell receptor sensitivity to LH secondary to aggressive COH or innately poor responders, and/or the presence of multiple follicles each producing a normal amount of progesterone consistent with the late follicular phase (319,320). Although the literature on this subject remains inconsistent, the negative effects of premature luteinization have been attributed to endometrial advancement rather than oocyte or embryonic dysfunction (319–321). Methods proposed to address premature luteinization have included earlier triggering with hCG, less aggressive stimulation protocols, cryopreservation of embryos (freeze-all), and administration of the antiprogestin *mifepristone* at the time of hCG (320,322).

GnRH Agonists   Native GnRH is rapidly degraded in the circulation. Commercial preparations of GnRH agonists consist of decapeptides similar to GnRH but for modification at two amino acid residues, which increase both the half-life and the receptor binding affinities (323). **Over the course of 10 to 14 days, agonists initially bind to and upregulate pituitary GnRH receptor activity, leading to a flare response of increased gonadotropin secretion. This is followed by receptor desensitization (depleted gonadotropin pools along with rapid uncoupling of the GnRH receptor from its regulatory protein and loss of signal transduction) that suppresses circulating levels of pituitary gonadotropins and, with high doses and prolonged use, eventually decreases GnRH receptor numbers** (301,317,323–325). Therefore, prolonged use of GnRH agonists induces a menopause-like state characterized by low estradiol levels and accompanied by common side effects such as hot flashes and moodiness. The flare effect may cause ovarian cyst formation as described in the "Unexplained Infertility" section of this chapter (301). GnRH agonists are commercially available for either depot or daily use and can be administered intranasally (*buserelin* and *nafarelin*) or by intramuscular or subcutaneous injection (*leuprolide, triptorelin,* or *buserelin*). Intranasal preparations have lower absorption rates when compared to injectable agonists and are associated with milder suppression (326). Typical starting daily doses of *leuprolide* are 1 mg, 0.5 mg, or 25 μg (microdose) (324).

Gonadotropin-Releasing Hormone Agonist Protocols   Some of the more commonly used ART medications and protocols are summarized in Fig. 32.6 and Table 32.8. **In the long protocol, a GnRH agonist is started in the luteal phase (day 21) of the previous cycle.** This diminishes the GnRH agonists flare effect and suppresses endogenous FSH and dominant follicle selection to promote synchronous follicular growth (317). After 10 to 14 days of GnRH agonist administration, a pelvic ultrasound and estradiol level are used to confirm suppression and gonadotropin stimulation begins. The GnRH agonist is continued (the dose may be halved or unchanged) throughout the cycle until the hCG trigger (317,324). Mean serum progesterone levels on the day of hCG administration using the long protocol are reportedly 0.84 ng/mL (320). **The long protocol provides for better oocyte yields and pregnancy rates in normal responders when compared with shorter protocols that use later administration or early cessation of agonists** (317). Shorter protocols using lower GnRH agonist doses have been advocated for poor responders in whom excessive suppression may be undesirable, perhaps from direct negative effects of the agonist on the ovary (324). However, long protocols, particularly those using single-dose depot rather than daily GnRH agonist formulations, are associated with higher gonadotropin dose and duration, which themselves have been associated with lower pregnancy rates (327–329). **Alternatively, GnRH microdose flare protocols have been developed that may improve oocyte yield in poor responders. Microdose flare regimens involve pretreatment with 14 to 21 days of combination oral contraceptives. Four days following the**

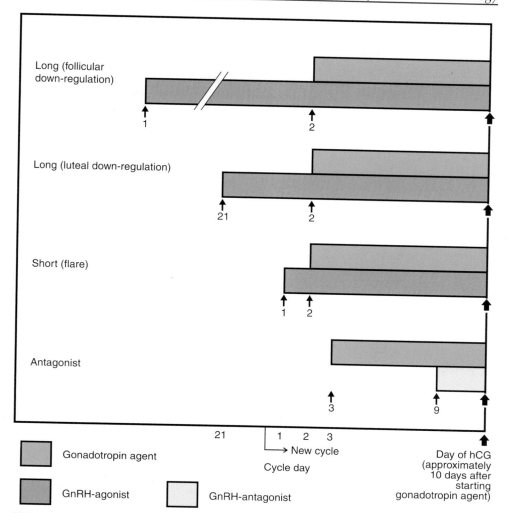

Figure 32.6   *In vitro* **fertilization protocols using gonadotropin-releasing hormone (GnRH) agonist or antagonist with gonadotropins in controlled ovarian hyperstimulation.** hCG, human chorionic gonadotropin.

cessation of the oral contraceptive pills, a microdose (*leuprolide* 25 μg) of agonist is added in the early follicular phase to take advantage of the agonist flare effect. Gonadotropin stimulation is initiated 1 to 2 days later while continuing the agonist (324).

Gonadotropin-Releasing Hormone Antagonists   GnRH antagonists (*cetrorelix* and *ganerelix*) were developed by modifying the GnRH decapeptide at six positions. They compete with endogenous GnRH for binding to pituitary GnRH receptors. **Because they have no agonistic activity, GnRH antagonists lead to almost immediate suppression of FSH and LH and do not require the additional time for pituitary down-regulation that characterizes the GnRH agonists.** With prolonged use, GnRH antagonists down-regulate GnRH receptors (323). At this time, the only delivery method available for GnRH antagonist is subcutaneous injection, although orally active agents are in development. GnRH antagonists can be given as 0.25 mg daily doses or as a single 3 mg dose with no difference in outcome (325). The time between daily injections should not exceed 30 hours (301). With single dose regimens, avoidance of multiple injections is attractive, but additional small doses starting 4 days after initial dose are required in 10% of cycles (325). **Use of GnRH antagonists in ART protocols is typically begun on day 4 to 7 of stimulation. This timing balances the risk for premature LH surges with the need for initiation of endogenous FSH-mediated follicular recruitment and endogenous estradiol production prior to administration** (301,317,325).

Gonadotropin-Releasing Hormone Antagonists Fixed versus Flexible Protocols

Several GnRH antagonist protocols have been developed for use in ART cycles. **Fixed protocols involve starting the antagonist on day 4, 5, 6, or 7 of stimulation regardless of follicular response** (301,308,317,325). Flexible protocols were developed to reduce gonadotropin stimulation dose and duration (317). **In flexible protocols, varying thresholds have been described for antagonist initiation. These include addition of the antagonist when the leading follicle has reached 12 to 16 mm in average diameter or when the estradiol level has risen above 600 pg/mL** (303,307,317,324,325). When flexible protocols are used, pregnancy rates are similar when antagonist is initiated on day 4 or 5 of stimulation but drop significantly when antagonist is initiated after day 6. This suggests that rapid follicular growth may be more important in preventing LH surges and improving pregnancy rates than the day the antagonist is initiated (303). Fixed initiation of a GnRH antagonist on day 6 of stimulation has been associated with higher pregnancy rates when compared to flexible protocols in one meta-analysis involving four randomized trials; however, **the true superiority of one approach over the other remains to be determined** (303,324,325). **Diminished estradiol levels can be expected following GnRH antagonist administration, but this does not appear to affect follicular growth** (308). **The addition of exogenous FSH or LH does not appear to be necessary** (301,324,325).

Gonadotropin-Releasing Hormone Agonists Compared with Antagonists   Because there is no pituitary desensitization period required when GnRH antagonists are used in ART, cycles can begin more quickly than those that employ GnRH agonists (301). **Antagonists are associated with lower duration of stimulation, lower stimulation dose, and reduced rates of ovarian hyperstimulation syndrome** (330). Antagonists are often used in the absence of pretreatment with oral contraceptives. Initiation of antagonist cycles therefore relies on the start of spontaneous menses, often making scheduling easier for GnRH agonist cycles (331). Study and protocol heterogeneity make it difficult to detect consistent differences in IVF pregnancy outcomes after GnRH agonist and antagonist cycles (330,332). **A Cochrane review of 27 randomized controlled trials indicated that while the number of good quality embryos produced for transfer are similar, clinical pregnancy rates are higher by 4.7% in agonist compared to antagonist cycles. They concluded that for every 21 couples, one additional pregnancy would be gained by using a GnRH agonist protocol. The number of oocytes retrieved and the live birth rates favored agonist usage** (330).

Follicular Growth

Follicular Recruitment   Although the inciting stimulus is unclear, cohorts of small antral follicles (<2 mm) become responsive to FSH stimulation only after 45 days of initial growth. They are then considered recruitable and begin to slowly enlarge in the late luteal phase of the cycle preceding ovulation. Once the antral follicle grows beyond 10 mm, FSH induces the appearance of LH receptors on the granulosa cells. At that point, somewhat contrary to the 2-cell-2-gonadotropin model, LH can exert FSH-like actions on the granulosa cell, including stimulation of aromatase. **With complete absence of endogenous LH, such as that seen with hypothalamic hypogonadism, exogenous FSH produces fewer preovulatory follicles, inadequate estradiol, lower ovulation rates, and thinner endometrium when compared to ovaries stimulated with exogenous HMG (FSH and LH).** Therefore, in the setting of normal hypothalamic function, it seems likely that even with suppressive therapy, enough endogenous LH is present to synergize with exogenous FSH to provide adequate stimulation for recruitment (326).

Follicular Waves   Seventy-five percent of unstimulated human menstrual cycles have two waves of follicular development: one major wave in which a dominant follicle is selected to the detriment of other follicles and one minor wave during which all follicles undergo atresia. When progesterone is available to block LH, the first wave is typically minor and occurs one day after ovulation in the previous cycle. The subsequent major wave occurs around the time of menses, with the dominant follicle being selected by its ability to reach a diameter of 10 mm by cycle day 6 or 7, which coincides with an estradiol rise that inhibits FSH. One-quarter of cycles will exhibit an additional wave that occurs 2 days prior to menses and may be minor or major. If the dominant follicle regresses or is removed, a new follicular wave begins 2 days later. In light of this, future efforts toward greater synchrony during stimulation might include ablation of the early dominant follicle using aspiration or administration of exogenous estrogen and progesterone during the follicular phase (333).

Controlled Ovarian Hyperstimulation   The goal of gonadotropin stimulation for ART is the synchronous growth of dominant follicles in quantities greater than that associated with non-ART therapy. FSH is the key hormone in this regard (111). Gonadotropin preparations are described in the "Ovulatory Factor" section, while dosing and the relevance of baseline ovarian cysts are described in the "Unexplained Infertility" section. **ART pregnancy outcomes are not affected by the source of FSH, the delivery system, or the route of administration** (156). In one recent report, women who were predicted to be normal responders using 225 to 300 IU of FSH required 11 days of stimulation, had 11 to 13 follicles 15 mm or larger on the day of hCG trigger, had a peak E2 level of approximately 2,100 pg/mL, and had 10 to 11 oocytes retrieved, of which 82% to 83% were mature (111). Most investigators suggest that the optimal number of retrieved oocytes in a given cycle is between 5 and 15, and the optimal level of estradiol at the time of hCG administration is between 70 and 140 pg/mL per oocyte or follicle (306,329). It should be noted that the utility of estradiol monitoring during ART is controversial, and that ultrasound monitoring alone may be adequate to maximize pregnancy and live birth rates (309). **Cycle cancellation in normal responders occurs in up to 6% of the cycles because of inadequate response and 1.5% of cycles for excessive response** (111). Cycle cancellation increases with older age and decreased ovarian reserve, but is reportedly decreased by 2% for every additional 100 IU *gonadotropins* used (328). There appears to be no benefit of exceeding a total daily gonadotropin dose of 450 IU in any patient (301).

Follicle-Stimulating Hormone versus Human Menopausal Gonadotropin Higher androgen and lower progesterone levels on the day of hCG trigger are observed when HMG is used for stimulation rather than FSH alone, indicating a more favorable endocrine profile with HMG (334). **Concern has been raised that exogenous LH might be needed to address the sudden decrease in endogenous LH that is associated with GnRH antagonist use and the possible excess endogenous LH suppression in long GnRH agonist protocols** (326). However, there is no consensus as to whether the addition of LH to exogenous FSH improves pregnancy and live birth outcomes in women with normal hypothalamic function (156,335,336).

Less Aggressive Stimulation Although it reduces cancellation rates, each additional 100 IU of *gonadotropins* is correspondingly associated with a 2% lower rate of clinical pregnancy and live birth (328). **This seems to support the findings of premature luteinization and lower pregnancy rates when more aggressive FSH stimulation protocols are used** (320). When comparing normal responders using a flexible antagonist protocol and a fixed FSH dose of 150 IU (mild) to those using conventional FSH doses, implantation rates were maximized when a median of 5 oocytes were retrieved in the mild stimulation group, while 10 oocytes were necessary in the conventional dose group. Outcomes were compromised when more than eight oocytes were obtained in the mild group, and only the high dose group experienced poorer outcomes with low oocyte yield. Pregnancy rates seem to level off or decrease when stimulation is pushed beyond a certain threshold, but this threshold is unknown (329).

Pretreatment

Combined oral contraceptives (OCs) are commonly taken for 14 to 28 days prior to GnRH analogues to ease cycle scheduling, synchronize follicular development, further prevent LH surges, reduce the incidence of ovarian cysts, and reduce cancellation rates resulting from hyperstimulation (331,337,338). Patients can begin OCs anytime between days 1 and 5 of menses (337). For antagonist cycles, COH begins 2 to 5 days after stopping OCs (irrespective of menses) (331). During long GnRH agonist protocols, the agonist overlaps the final 5 days of OC use, followed by initiation of COH on the second or third day of withdrawal bleeding (300,338). As previously discussed, microdose flare protocols involve pretreatment with 14 to 21 days of OC, followed 4 days later by a microdose of agonist. COH typically starts 1 to 2 days later (324). **The progestins *norethindrone acetate* 10 mg orally daily, *medroxyprogesterone acetate* 10 mg orally daily, or a single intramuscular dose of *progesterone* (not specified) can be used in place of an OC in ART cycles, but recommendations on the duration of treatment and the timing of initiation vary widely: a duration of 5 to 20 days and initiation anytime between days 1 and 19 of menses have been reported.** A dose of 4 mg of daily micronized *17β estradiol* or *estradiol valerate* has been used in lieu of OCs in ART cycles, with initiation between cycle days 15 and 21 and a duration of 10 to 15 days. Although OC pretreatment for antagonist cycles has been shown to increase both the duration of stimulation and the amount of medication used, its effect on pregnancy rates is controversial (331,337). OC pretreatment during GnRH agonist cycles is associated with higher pregnancy rates than those in cycles without pretreatment (300). *Progestin* and *estradiol* pretreatment do not affect live birth rates in either agonist or antagonist cycles (337).

Adjunctive Medications

Prenatal vitamins should be given to all infertility patients beginning at least 1 month prior to initiation of infertility treatment. Although *aspirin* is commonly used during IVF regimens, recent studies have failed to demonstrate beneficial changes in pregnancy rates (339,340). Antimicrobial prophylaxis using *doxycycline* or *azithromycin* for both partners is often given during ART cycles, particularly those involving assisted hatching procedures, although these medications have not been clearly associated with improved pregnancy rates (287,289,341). Glucocorticoids given to women during the peri-implantation period may improve pregnancy rates in women with autoimmune disease, those undergoing assisted hatching or frozen/thaw embryo transfers, and in women of advanced maternal age (341). *Metformin* may limit ovarian hyperstimulation (OHSS) in PCOS patients, but shows no benefit for pregnancy or live birth rates (342).

Oocyte Maturation/Ovulation Triggering

Physiology of Oocyte Maturation   Prior to maturation, oocytes are arrested in the prophase stage of meiosis I, also known as the germinal vesicle (343,344). Meiosis I oocytes must reach at least the early antral follicle stage to respond to FSH and be competent to resume meiosis. *In vivo,* LH receptors on the follicle are induced by FSH during later stages of follicular development (345). Therefore, only fully grown oocytes respond to the LH surge *in vivo* to begin the cytoplasmic and nuclear maturation that are required for developmental progression toward the metaphase stage of meiosis II. At this point, the developmentally competent oocyte will extrude the first polar body, the oocyte-cumulus complex will detach from the ovarian wall, ovulation will occur, and fertilization is possible (343–346).

Oocyte Maturation during Assisted Reproductive Technology Cycles   **Because spontaneous LH surges occur inconsistently during non-ART gonadotropin cycles and are suppressed in ART cycles, hCG has been used to trigger ovulation. In combination with its long half-life, homology between hCG and LH (identical α subunits) allows for cross-reactivity with the LH receptor and induction of final ococyte maturation and ovulation** (347). hCG is derived from urine (5,000 to 10,000 IU intramuscularly) or through recombinant technology (250 μg subcutaneously, equivalent to 5,000 to 6,000 IU of intramuscular urinary product) (156). The half-life of hCG is 2.32 days, compared to 1 to 5 hours for LH (347). **Ovulation is typically triggered when at least two follicles are 17 to 18 mm or larger in average diameter (but <24 mm) and the endometrial thickness is 8 mm or more** (111,302,303,306–308,348). Similar clinical outcomes have been noted when 5,000 IU or 10,000 IU of hCG (349) and urinary or recombinant preparations are used for triggering (348,350). If there is concern for ovarian hyperstimulation syndrome (OHSS, see below), GnRH agonists can be substituted for hCG to trigger ovulation in antagonist protocols or recombinant LH can be substituted for hCG in agonist protocols; however, both protocols are associated with decreased pregnancy rates in nondonor ART cycles (347,351).

Oocyte Retrieval

Oocyte retrieval is performed via transvaginal ultrasound-guided needle puncture into each follicle followed by aspiration of follicular fluid. Either general anesthesia or intravenous conscious sedation may be used (352). Prophylactic antibiotics such as *ceftriaxone* are recommended at the time of retrieval (353). The vaginal preparation can be performed either with sterile saline alone or with *povidone iodine* followed by vigorous saline flushing (354,355). **The highest oocyte yield is obtained when oocyte retrieval is performed 36 to 37 hours after the hCG injection.** Earlier retrieval (35 hours) is associated with a much lower oocyte yield, and later retrieval risks ovulation; spontaneous follicular rupture appears to occur at a mean of 38.3 hours following hCG administration (348).

Luteal Support

The rationale and regimens for luteal phase support with progesterone are discussed in the "Uterine Factors" section. The timing for luteal *progesterone* support varies, but lower pregnancy rates have been noted with initiation prior to oocyte retrieval or later than 5 days following retrieval (356,357). Luteal phase *estradiol* supplementation is not necessary (358,359).

Fertilization by *In Vitro* Fertilization or Intracytoplasmic Sperm Injection

Following semen collection and sperm processing (described in the "Male Factor" section), sperm are incubated in media for 3 to 4 hours to promote sperm capacitation and the acrosome reaction. Before fertilization, retrieved oocytes are cultured in media. Conventional IVF involves insemination concentrations of 100,000 to 800,000 motile sperm/mL per oocyte with each oocyte in a small droplet of media under oil (9,360,361). For every three cycles done for severe male factor, the use of ICSI prevents one case of fertilization failure when compared to conventional IVF (9). The indications for and the procedure and risks of ICSI are discussed under "Male Factor."

In Vitro Embryo Culture

Embryo Development   **Initial embryo development is typically assessed 15 to 20 hours after insemination or ICSI, when fertilization is characterized by the presence of two pronuclei and the extrusion of the second polar body** (9,361,362). Embryos are examined again for cleavage after 24 to 30 hours of culture (9). The first embryo cleavage occurs approximately 21 hours after fertilization, and subsequent divisions occur every 12 to 15 hours up to the eight-cell stage on the 3rd day of embryo development (363). Compaction to form the 16-cell morula occurs on the 4th day of embryo development, and differentiation of the inner cell mass and trophectoderm to form a blastocyst (containing a fluid-filled area called a blastocele) is completed by the 5th or 6th day (364,365).

Culture Environment   **Sequential media systems are preferred during embryo culture to adjust for each stage of embryo development.** Prior to compaction, the embryo is under genetic control of the oocyte, it uses a pyruvate-based metabolism, it requires at least a few amino acids, and it prefers a relatively oxygenated environment (though much lower than atmospheric oxygen) similar to that found in the fallopian tube. **Following compaction, amino acid needs increase (stable dipeptide glutamine instead of glutamine will avoid toxic ammonium buildup), the embryonic genome is activated, and metabolism requires both glucose and a very low oxygen environment similar as that found in the uterus** (363,366). Supplementation of culture media with hyaluron and albumin is beneficial in postcompaction media preparations (363).

Extended Culture to Blastocyst   Although precompaction human embryos can survive when placed in the uterus, the uterine cavity is a nonphysiological location for them, and there is greater uterine pulsatility during this period that may cause the embryos to be expelled. **Therefore, the blastocyst stage represents a more physiologic time for embryo transfer.** Since nearly 60% of morphologically normal cleavage embryos but only 30% of blastocysts are chromosomally abnormal, extended culture allows for better selection of embryos with improved quality (364,367).

Blastocyst versus Cleavage Transfer Outcomes   **Comparisons involving equal numbers of transferred embryos demonstrate that blastocyst transfer is associated with lower implantation failure, a higher pregnancy rate, and a 7% higher live birth rate than cleavage stage transfer. This is of particular interest in programs that offer elective single embryo transfer** (364,367,368). Given that blastocyst formation rates range from only 28% to 60%, disadvantages of extended culture include the possibility that no embryos will survive to transfer (8.9% vs. 2.8% for cleavage transfer) and a reduced opportunity for embryo cryopreservation. Monozygotic twinning rates may be higher with blastocyst culture, although this has not been a consistent finding (364,369).

Criteria for Extended Culture   There are no established guidelines or criteria that determine when to utilize extended culture. Varying suggestions include maternal age 42 or younger with five or more two pronuclear stage (2PN) embryos on postretrieval day 1; maternal age of 40 or younger and three or more good-quality day 3 embryos having 4 to 10 cells with less than 15% fragmentation; maternal age of 41 to 42 or younger and four or more good-quality day 3 embryos having 4 to 10 cells with less than 15% fragmentation; and age less than 37 with four or more morphologically good embryos on day 3, or four or more embryos with 6 cells and less than 10% fragmentation (362,364,370).

Embryo Transfer

Embryo Morphology   **Embryo morphology guides the choice of embryo for transfer.** Pronuclear embryos are assessed by their distribution and number of nucleoli, the position of the second polar body relative to the first, and cleavage rates (abnormal rates are too fast, too slow, or arrested) (365). Preferred cleavage stage embryos have a normal developmental pattern characterized by early cleavage on day 1, four cells on day 2, and eight cells on day 3. Embryo fragmentation should be 10% or less, the blastomere size should be regular, and there should be no multinucleation (362). The Gardner and Schoolcraft system for scoring blastocysts uses a scale from 1 (worst) to 6 (best), with grades 1 to 3 indicating growth of the blastocele until it completely fills the embryo. Grade 4 blastocysts are expanded with a larger blastocele volume and a thinning zona pellucida. The trophectoderm in a grade 5 blastocyst is starting to hatch though the zona, and the grade 6 blastocyst has completely escaped or hatched from the zona. The inner cell mass is graded A to C based on tightness and cellularity (A is best), and the trophectoderm is assessed from A to C based on cohesiveness and cellularity (A is best) (361).

Number of Embryos to Transfer   High-order multiple pregnancy (three or more fetuses) increases complications for mothers and fetuses, so guidelines have been developed to minimize this adverse outcome (371). **Single embryo transfer should be considered for patients younger than age 35, particularly those undergoing their first ART cycle who have a large quantity of good quality embryos or patients who have conceived in a prior cycle.** Otherwise, transfer should be limited to two embryos in women under 35 years of age. For older women, the maximum number of transferred cleavage-stage embryos should be three in women aged 35 to 37, four in women aged 38 to 40, and five in women older than 40 years of age. Because of their high implantation potential, no more than three blastocysts should be transferred to any woman regardless of her age. Limits on the number of embryos transferred when the embryos were created from donor oocytes should be based on the age of the donor, rather than the recipient (371).

Transfer Procedure   **The goal of transcervical embryo transfer is to atraumatically deliver the embryos to an optimal intrauterine location for implantation. Implantation is more likely after an easy transfer using a soft catheter and when fundal contact is avoided** (353). Trial transfer, although not required, allows advance preparation such as cervical dilation or placement of a traction stitch, although uterine position and depth can be different at the time of the actual procedure. When performed at the time of embryo transfer, trial transfer should not go past the internal os. Trial transfer can be combined with an afterloading technique in which the outer sheath of the transfer catheter is left in place and the transfer catheter is threaded through the trial transfer sheath and into the uterus, although there is no advantage when compared to routine transfer (353,372). Soft catheters such as those made by the Cook or Wallace companies are preferred to rigid catheters to minimize prostaglandin release after cervical and/or endometrial trauma (353). The utility of cervical mucus removal prior to embryo transfer in improving embryo delivery remains controversial (353,372). Although intrauterine infections decrease pregnancy rates, the efficacy of antibiotic administration at the time of transfer is not clear. During a conventional embryo transfer, embryos are suspended in 20 μL of media at the tip of a syringe with air on either side of the fluid. This creates an air–fluid interface easily seen with ultrasound. **Abdominal ultrasound visualization during embryo transfer is useful to ensure deposit of the embryos 1.5 to 2 cm from the uterine fundus.** Once the embryos are deposited, the inner and outer sheath should be removed as a unit to avoid suction within the device (353). No changes in patient position are necessary (372). Following transfer, the catheter is checked for retained embryos. If present, retained embryos should be transferred because there is no detriment in pregnancy rates (353).

Cryopreservation of Embryos

Embryo cryopreservation at the pronuclear, cleavage, and blastocyst stages has allowed for multiple transfer cycles from a single oocyte retrieval. Because transfer of cryopreserved embryos is less expensive than a second fresh cycle, overall fertility treatment costs can be optimized. Embryo cryopreservation can be considered as a means to prevent ovarian hyperstimulation syndrome. Techniques for embryo cryopreservation include slow freezing and rapid freezing or vitrification. Slow freezing protocols use lower concentrations of cryoprotectants but are more time-consuming when compared to vitrification, which uses high-concentration cryoprotectants for rapid cooling and is less expensive. Embryo thawing is accomplished by brief exposure to air and warm water followed by rehydration (373). Although pregnancy rates for freeze/thaw transfer (FET) cycles using the two cryopreservation methods are similar, vitrification is associated with higher postthaw embryo survival (93% vs. 76% with slow freezing) (374). Infant outcomes are reassuring for slow freezing but are more limited for the newer technique of vitrification (375). Overall, use of **frozen embryos results in lower pregnancy rates when compared to fresh transfer cycles, but this may be a result of embryo selection (the best embryos are typically**

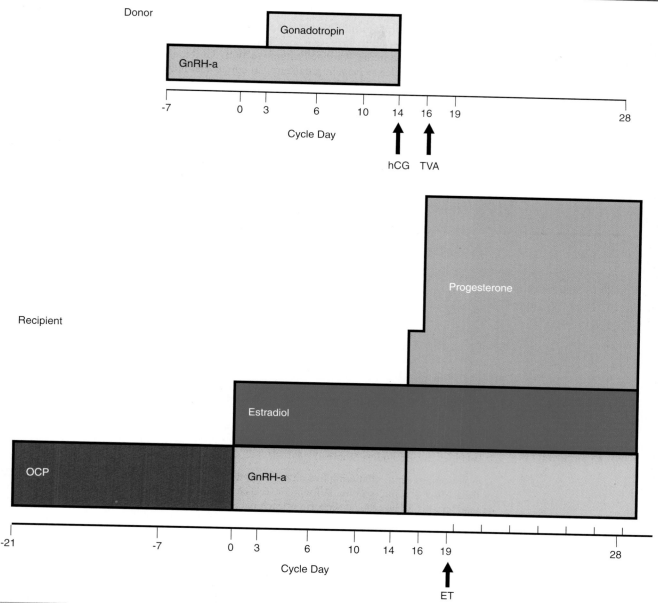

Figure 32.7 **Regimens of ovarian stimulation and hormone replacement used to synchronize the development of ovarian follicles in the oocyte donor and the endometrial cycle in the recipient.** hCG, human chorionic gonadotropin; OCP, oral contraceptive pill; GnRH-a, gonadotropin releasing hormone antagonist; TVA, ultrasound-guided transvaginal aspiration of oocytes. (Adapted from **Chang PL, Sauer MY.** Assisted reproductive techniques. Stenchever MA, ed.; *Atlas of clinical gynecology*, Mishell DR, ed, *Reproductive endocrinology.* Vol. 3. Philadelphia, PA: Current Sciences Group, 1998, with permission.)

used for fresh transfer and lesser quality embryos are frozen) (373,376). Frozen transfer outcomes are heavily dependent on the characteristics of the fresh cycle that generated the frozen embryos; excellent pregnancy rates are noted when the fresh cycle resulted in conception or when all the embryos were frozen from the fresh cycle (376).

Endometrial Preparation for Frozen Embryo Transfer   When FET is combined with a recipient's natural cycle, no exogenous treatment is given, and transfer is timed to spontaneous ovulation. In medicated FET cycles, *estradiol* supplementation begins in the early follicular phase and is continued for 13 to 15 days (373). Multiple *estradiol* preparations have been described for use in FET cycles, but none has been proven superior (377). Transvaginal ultrasound is used to assess endometrial thickness during *estrogen* therapy, and *estrogen* administration continues until an optimal thickness of greater than 8 mm is reached (373). *Progesterone* supplementation begins 48 to 72 hours prior to transfer when cleavage-stage embryos are used and 6 to 7 days prior to transfer when blastocysts will be thawed (373,377). Again, several *progesterone* preparations have been described for use in FET cycles, but none has been proven superior (discussed in the "Uterine Factors" section). GnRH agonists are commonly used during medicated cycles to prevent premature LH surges that might adversely affect endometrial maturation (377) (Fig. 32.7).

First-Trimester Pregnancy Monitoring

The production of hCG by the blastocyst can be detected as early as 7 days posttransfer, and serum quantitative hCG levels may be obtained 11 to 14 days following embryo transfer (373,378). **A serum threshold of 200 mIU/mL of hCG measured 12 days after transfer is 92% and 80% predictive of ongoing pregnancies for day 3 and day 5 embryos, respectively, with levels normally rising approximately 40% per day.** If normally rising hCG levels are detected, transvaginal ultrasound is planned at 6 to 7 weeks of gestation to determine the location of the pregnancy, the number of gestational sacs, and pregnancy viability (378).

Assisted Reproductive Techonology Success Rates

Since 1992, all clinics performing ART in the United States have been required to submit annual success rates to the Centers for Disease Control and Prevention (379). Success rates of IVF vary from program to program. The most comprehensive assessment of the efficacy of ART programs in North America comes from the database of the Society for Assisted Reproductive Technology (SART). Information on SART and registered ART clinics are accessible by the public online. Because ICSI and IVF rates are similar, statistical analyses combine them for the annual SART reports. IVF success rates are largely dependent on maternal age, and data from recent studies, including those from SART, are summarized in Table 32.10 (380). SART statistics should not be used to compare IVF clinics since success rates are largely dependent on patient demographics, including the cause of infertility, which will be different for each individual clinic. Lifestyle factors affecting IVF success are discussed under "Causes of Infertility." Since SART does not publish success rates for non-ART cycles, it can often be helpful for physicians to assist patients in comparing the success rates for *clomiphene, gonadotropins,* and IVF, although rates vary widely between studies (Table 32.11).

A new approach to predicting live birth probabilities focuses on the use of machine learning or the mining of clinic-specific IVF outcomes data to provide a personalized per-cycle prognosis that pertains to the clinical scenario of each patient (381). Briefly, a live birth prediction model was developed by boosted tree analysis of baseline clinical data, uterine response to a patient's first IVF treatment, and embryo developmental parameters, with no preselection of prognostic factors. The model predicted live birth outcomes in a subsequent IVF treatment cycle. Validation by an independent dataset and comparison with a control model that is based on chronological age alone showed that the boosted tree model was more than 1,000 times better in fitting new data and improved discrimination (i.e., the ability to discern among patients with different prognoses) by receiver–operator curve analysis. Approximately 60% of patients were found to have significantly different predicted live birth probabilities when compared to the use of age categories. Further testing across different clinics will be required to determine whether this approach may be generally valid and applicable. Nevertheless, the nonredundant and unique

Table 32.10 *In Vitro* Fertilization Success Rates							
	Donor Egg	**Age Years**					
	All Ages	<35	40	41–42	43	44–45	≥46
CPR/cycle	—	31%–46%	19%–25%	15%–20%	6%–13%	1%–7%	0%–1%
Birth/cycle	50%–60%	40%	10%–17%	5%–13%	2%–8%	1%–3%	0%–1%
Birth/3 cycles	—	59%–67%	25%	19%	10%	2%–6%	0
SAB rate/cycle	—	14%	24%–28%	35%–36%	38%–45%	54%–67%	N/A

CPR, clinical pregnancy rate; Birth, live birth rate; SAB, spontaneous abortion, N/A, not available..
From refs. 379,380,420,421,423.

Table 32.11 Fertility Treatment Success Rates

| | Clinical Pregnancy Rate/Cycle | | | |
	Fertile	Infertile	Age <35	Age ≥40
None	11%–35%	1%–3%	—	2%–4%
CC/TI	—	3%–17%	8%–10%	1%–4%
IUI/TI	—	4–9%	—	—
CC/IUI	—	3%–14%	8%–19%	1%–5%
INJ/IUI	—	13%–19%	9%–20%	5%–9%
IVF	—	35%	31%–46%	13%

CC, clomiphene citrate; TI, timed intercourse; IUI, intrauterine insemination; INJ, injectable gonadotropins; IVF, *in vitro* fertilization.
From refs. 313, 379, 380, 418–422. (looks like these are the correct refs)

contribution of the patient's age to predicting outcomes was found to be limited if data pertaining to the response to *gonadotropins* and embryo development in the first IVF treatment were available. These findings may move prognostic counseling away from an age-centric paradigm and toward a more objective extraction of predictive value from simultaneous analysis of a wide array clinical factors.

Cessation of Therapy

Patients must be accurately informed of estimated success rates and reasonable expectations for all therapeutic interventions. Patients with a very poor prognosis have a 2% to 5% chance of achieving a live birth with fertility therapy, and those with a futile prognosis have a 1% or less chance. Refusing or limiting therapy may be justified if the risk of intervention outweighs the potential benefits (382).

Third Party Reproduction

When gametes and the ability to gestate a pregnancy are compromised through circumstances or disease, other reproductive options can be considered. **These include use of donor sperm** (discussed in "Male Factor"), **donor oocytes, donor embryos, a gestational carrier, or a combination of these approaches.** In contrast to donor gametes (sperm or oocytes), the decision to donate embryos is typically made after the embryos have been generated and there is a known surplus. A gestational carrier receives and gestates birth embryos created from the intended mother's oocytes. Patients who choose to utilize a gestational carrier may have irreparable uterine factor infertility or suffer from medical conditions that contraindicate pregnancy. In true surrogacy, the birth mother is the genetic mother but not the intended mother. Legal and psychosocial counseling are suggested for all parties embarking on any form of third party reproduction.

Donor Oocyte   Patients with ovarian failure, poor oocyte quality, poor ovarian response to stimulation, or failed fertilization or implantation after multiple ART cycles may be candidates to receive donated oocytes. A female same-sex couple may choose to have one partner undergo IVF and place the resulting oocytes fertilized with donor sperm into the other partner (383). **At present, donor oocytes must be used to create embryos during the retrieval cycle, because oocyte freezing is considered experimental** (384). With carefully selected donors, live birth rates per cycle of donor oocyte IVF are 50% to 60% regardless of the recipient's age (Table 32.10). However, recipients must be aware that advanced recipient age is associated with higher risk for preeclampsia, diabetes, and cesarean section (385–387). Oocyte donors must endure all the interventions and risks of the ART process described herein except for embryo transfer and luteal support. Because of the intensity of therapy and the potential infectious disease and genetic risks for donor, recipient, and the resulting offspring, oocyte donors must be screened for infectious and heritable disorders similar to those performed for sperm donors (see "Male Factor") and undergo meticulous informed consent and a comprehensive psychosocial evaluation. Oocyte donors may be anonymous or known to the recipient (96). Oocyte recipients undergo endometrial preparation (as described in the "Process of Assisted Reproductive Technologies" section), but GnRH analogues are not required if there is no endogenous ovarian function. Recipients may initiate *progesterone* one day prior, on the same day, or one day after the donor's oocyte retrieval, but a randomized trial found lower pregnancy rates when progesterone was initiated prior to the retrieval (377). Other topics, such as methods for donor recruitment and financial compensation for the donor, are much more challenging issues (388).

Complications of Assisted Reproductive Technology

Cycle Cancellation

Cycle cancellation in normal responders occurs in up to 6% of cycles because of inadequate stimulation response and in 1.5% of cycles because of excessive response (111). **In 0.2% to 7% of retrievals, no ooctyes will be obtained.** Two proposed explanations include human error during the administration of hCG and early oocyte atresia despite normal follicular response (346).

Oocyte Retrieval

The risks of oocyte retrieval include bleeding requiring transfusion, injury to adjacent structures requiring laparotomy, formation of a pelvic abscess leading to loss of reproductive function despite prophylaxis, and risks related to anesthesia (389).

Multiple Gestation

As the majority of ART cycles involve the transfer of more than one embryo, multiple gestation occurs at higher rates than the 3% rate for spontaneous conception. This has social, medical, emotional, and financial ramifications (379,380). **Although the majority of complications of multiple gestations occur with high-order (three or more) multiples, twins have increased risks for low birth weight, preterm birth, and neurologic deficits when compared to singletons** (380,390). Despite this, 20% of infertile patients view multiple pregnancy as a desired outcome. Because most patients lack insurance coverage for IVF, patients may push their physicians to take greater risks when deciding on the number of embryos to transfer (379). The multiple pregnancy risk is higher in patients under the age of 35 who are undergoing IVF because their embryos are typically of better quality and implantation rates are higher, but multiple pregnancy can occur at any reproductive age (371). From 1998 to 2007, the overall twinning rate in ART cycles remained stable at 29% to 32%, but the rate of high-order multiples decreased from 6% to 2%. **In 2007, the live birth rates for twins and triplets or more for women under the age of 35 who underwent ART in the United States were 33.2% and 3.5%, respectively.** Women aged 43 or 44 had twinning live birth rates of 10.6% and triplet or more live birth rates of 0.8% (380). Most multiple pregnancies arising from ART are dizygotic, but monozygotic twinning occurs in 3.2% of IVF cycles (compared to a background rate of 0.4%) (379). Concerns have been raised that monozygotic twinning might increase after blastocyst culture, but this finding has not been consistent (364,369). With increasing adherence to guidelines suggesting limitations on the number of embryos to transfer in a given ART cycle (discussed in "Process of Assisted Reproductive Technologies") and improved implantation rates that allow single embryo transfer, the multiple pregnancy rates associated with ART should continue to decrease.

Selective Reduction   Ten percent of multifetal pregnancies spontaneously lose at least one gestational sac during the first trimester. This loss rate increases to 21% in women older than 35 years of age. The spontaneous reduction rate to twins or singletons is much higher for triplets (14%) than for quadruplets (3.5%) (391,392). **Selective pregnancy termination or multifetal reduction may be an option for some patients in whom spontaneous reduction does not occur by 11 to 13 weeks.** This involves first karyotyping each fetus through transabdominal chorionic villous sampling to preferentially reduce those that are abnormal, then injecting *potassium chloride* into the heart of the targeted fetus. Although selective reduction carries a 3% to 7% risk of losing the entire pregnancy when performed prior to 19 weeks, this is still lower than the 15% chance of spontaneously losing an entire triplet pregnancy (390,393). Selective fetal reduction is typically considered for triplet or higher pregnancies, but even reduction from twins to singletons may have benefit (390).

Ectopic and Heterotopic Pregnancy

Up to 3.4% of ART pregnancies are ectopic (implantation outside the uterus) and require treatment with either surgery or *methotrexate*. **The absence of an intrauterine pregnancy on transvaginal ultrasound evaluation in conjunction with a maternal serum hCG level above a threshold of 1,500 mIU/mL suggests the diagnosis** (394,395). Heterotopic pregnancy involves concurrent intrauterine and ectopic pregnancy, usually within the fallopian tube, but ovarian implantations have been reported (395,396). The incidence of heterotopic pregnancy, which is normally rare, is particularly high (1%) after IVF treatment. Multiple gestation, smoking, previous tubal surgery, and prior PID are potential risk factors in addition to ART. As with standard ectopic pregnancies, pain and bleeding are the most common presenting findings with heterotopic pregnancies. Heterotopic pregnancies are most often diagnosed in the first 5 to 8 weeks of gestation using laparoscopy or laparotomy. **Only 26% of heterotopic cases can be diagnosed with transvaginal ultrasound, possibly as a result of difficulties in sonographic interpretation in the presence of concomitant ovarian hyperstimulation.** After treatment of a heterotopic gestation with laparoscopy, laparotomy, or ultrasound-guided injection of *potassium chloride* into the extrauterine pregnancy, the overall delivery rate for the intrauterine pregnancy is nearly 70% (395).

Ovarian Hyperstimulation Syndrome

OHSS is a medical complication that is both completely iatrogenic and unique to stimulatory infertility treatment (397). **Its symptoms are the result of ovarian enlargement and fragility, extravascular fluid accumulation, and intravascular volume depletion.** Proposed mechanisms for the characteristic fluid shifts that accompany OHSS include increased protein-rich fluid secretion from the stimulated ovaries, increased renin and prorenin within follicular fluid, and increased capillary permeability mediated by angiotensin. **Vascular endothelial growth factor (VEGF), whose expression in granulosa cells and serum is augmented by hCG, and a variety of other inflammatory cytokines have been implicated in the pathogenesis of this disease** (398). Two distinct patterns of OHSS onset have been described. Early OHSS occurs 3 to 7 days following the hCG trigger and is associated with the administration of exogenous hCG. Late onset disease occurs 12 to 17 days after the hCG trigger; it is the result of endogenous hCG secretion from the pregnancy and tends to be more severe with multiple gestation. Pregnancy outcomes are inconsistently affected by the presence of OHSS, with higher rates of biochemical losses but similar rates of clinical losses when compared to patients without OHSS (399).

Severity Classification   Mild OHSS (grades 1 and 2) is associated with high serum estradiol levels and ovarian enlargement to less than 5 cm and has minimal clinical significance. Grade 3 moderate OHSS is accompanied by mild abdominal distention and has minimal clinical significance (397). Grade 3 OHSS occurs in one-third of all COH cycles (398). Grade 4 moderate OHSS is accompanied by gastrointestinal upset and ovarian enlargement to 5 to 12 cm (397). **The presence of fluid shifts from intra- to extravascular spaces are the hallmark of severe disease, and grade 5 OHSS includes tense ascites or hydrothorax. Grade 6 OHSS is accompanied by hemoconcentration, coagulation abnormalities, respiratory failure, and renal dysfunction** (397). Other markers of severe OHSS include hyponatremia, hyperkalemia, elevated liver function tests, and an elevated white blood cell count (397,398). Concerning symptoms for severe disease include rapid weight gain ($\geq$2 lb per day), increased measurable abdominal girth, hypotension, tachypnea, tachycardia, oliguria, and severe abdominal pain. The latter symptom is suggestive of ovarian cyst rupture or hemorrhage (398).

Risk Factors   Mild OHSS occurs in 13.5% of *clomiphene* cycles, but more severe disease is rare. With gonadotropin injections, the incidence of moderate disease is 3% to 6% and severe OHSS occurs in 0.1% to 2% of patients. Polycystic ovary syndrome, polycystic ovarian morphology with attendant elevated antimüllerian hormone levels (>3.36 ng/mL), and previous episodes of OHSS are major risk factors for the disease; the impact of young age and lean body mass is controversial (351,398,400). Estradiol levels greater than 800 pg/mL on day 9 of stimulation have been associated with a 55.8% risk for the development of OHSS (severity not specified). Estradiol concentrations of greater than 3,500 pg/mL and greater than 6,000 pg/mL at the time of hCG trigger were associated with severe OHSS in 1.5% and 38% of patients, respectively. During antagonist cycles, the presence of 13 or more follicles at 11 mm or greater average diameter was predictive of the development of OHSS. More than 20 preovulatory follicles were associated with a 15% incidence of severe OHSS. When 20 to 29 oocytes were collected at retrieval, 1.4% of patients developed severe OHSS; this raised to 22.7% with 30 or more oocytes (400).

Management   If outpatient management is appropriate, the patient should be instructed to limit her activity, to weigh herself daily, and to monitor her fluid intake (at least 1 L per day of mostly electrolyte-balanced fluid) and output. Daily follow-up by telephone or visit is important and the patient should be reassessed if she notes worsening of the symptoms or if her weight gain increases to more than 2 lb per day. **Indications for hospitalization include an inability to tolerate oral hydration, hemodynamic instability, respiratory compromise, tense ascites, hemoconcentration, leukocytosis, hyponatremia, hyperkalemia, abnormal renal or liver function, and decreased oxygen saturation.** Fluid intake and urine output need to be carefully measured, and admission to an intensive care setting can be considered if the patient has hyperkalemia, renal failure, respiratory failure, or thromboembolic disease. Although intravenous fluids may worsen ascites, they are essential to correct hypovolemia, hypotension, electrolyte abnormalities, and oliguria. Albumin 25% can be dosed 50 to 100 mg intravenously every 4 to 12 hours if further intravascular volume expansion is needed. Diuretics can be considered to improve weight gain and oliguria only after hypovolemia has been corrected. Thromboembolic prophylaxis should be given. Single or repeated transvaginal or transabdominal ultrasound-guided paracentesis may relieve pain, hydrothorax, or persistent oliguria. Rapid large-volume fluid removal can be considered, as compensatory fluid shifts are unlikely to occur in this typically young healthy population as long as the patient is carefully monitored (398).

Prevention   No method will prevent OHSS completely, but steps can be taken to decrease risk. Careful gonadotropin stimulation for monofollicular development is discussed under "Ovulatory Factor." **For ART, stimulation protocols for high-risk patients include lower initial COH doses of 150 IU and GnRH antagonists for LH surge prevention, which reduce the total dosage and duration of gonadotropin stimulation** (401,402). Reintroduction of GnRH antagonists following retrieval may be of benefit (351).

Decreasing the dose of hCG to reduce the incidence of OHSS is controversial (401,402). Exogenous recombinant LH is available for COH, but the dose required to trigger ovulation has not been established (402). **The very short half-life of endogenous LH may in turn reduce the incidence and/or severity of OHSS** (351). **GnRH agonists can be used instead of hCG during antagonist cycles to induce an endogenous LH surge.** As GnRH agonist triggers are associated with lower pregnancy rates, these may be a better option for oocyte donors or for patients who are not planning a fresh embryo transfer (351,402).

Coasting may be considered when estradiol levels are less than 4,500 pg/mL and/or there are 15 to 30 mature follicles present. **During coasting, gonadotropin stimulation is withheld and estradiol levels are checked daily** (351). An initial rise of estradiol is typically observed within the first 48 hours of the coast, but the levels should subsequently plateau or decrease (402). The patient may then be triggered when serum estradiol levels fall to less than 3,500 pg/mL. If GnRH agonists are used for initial LH surge suppression, switching to an antagonist during the coast has been associated with improved outcomes (351).

The cycle should be cancelled and the trigger withheld if there are greater than 30 mature follicles, the coast duration is more than 4 days, or if estradiol levels rise to more than 6,500 pg/mL during coasting (351,402).

The adjunctive use of *metformin* is associated with decreased OHSS rates in PCOS patients (342). *Cabergoline,* **a dopamine agonist that inhibits VEGF production, decreased OHSS rates when given at 0.5 mg daily for 7 or 8 days following retrieval. Long-term use of** *cabergoline* **may be associated with valvular heart disease** (351,401,402). Albumin given at oocyte retrieval does not appear to decrease subsequent rates of OHSS (401).

Cryopreservation of all embryos without transfer will prevent late onset OHSS (402), but pregnancy outcomes vary for frozen/thaw transfers and early onset OHSS may still occur (401,402). More information on embryo crypreservation can be found in the "Process of Assisted Reproductive Technologies" section.

In vitro oocyte maturation completely obviates the need to stimulate the ovaries with gonadotropins. During *in vitro* oocyte maturation cycles, immature follicles are aspirated following hCG administration, and the retrieved oocytes are grown *in vitro* until mature. Mature oocytes are then fertilized by insemination or ICSI. Randomized trials are still needed to further evaluate this technique (403).

Risk of Cancer after Fertility Therapy

Infertility by itself is a predisposing factor for ovarian cancer and breast cancer (404,405). **Although treatments that promote incessant ovulation and elevated estrogen levels offer biologic plausibility for further increased cancer risk, data regarding the impact of infertility therapy on neoplasias have been inconsistent and conflicting** (406). A retrospective cohort study of women in the United States found no association between prior use of *clomiphene* or *gonadotropins* and subsequent development of ovarian or breast cancer, although the authors suggested that very high doses or long duration of administration may warrant closer attention (404,405). A large British cohort of women with ovulatory disorders who were given ovulation-stimulation drugs did not find evidence to suggest causation for cancer of the breast, ovary, colon, skin, or thyroid. However, there was a dose–response relationship between the development of uterine cancer and prior use of *clomiphene*, particularly with a lifetime exposure of 2,250 mg or more (406).

Stress

Stress, as manifested by anxiety or depression, is thought to be increased among women experiencing infertility (407). **Stress is the most common reason for patients, even those with insurance coverage, to terminate fertility treatment** (408). However, it is not clear whether stress worsens infertility, nor is there clear evidence that psychological treatment improves fertility (407). If psychological disorders are present, treatment should be offered regardless of fertility status.

Preimplantation Genetic Diagnosis

The primary indication for preimplantation genetic diagnosis (PGD) is to improve the chances of having healthy infants in families at high risk for a specific genetic disease (409). Following embryo biopsy, genetic testing can be performed on a blastomere (cell from day 3 embryo), polar body, or on blastocyst trophectoderm prior to transferring the embryo. Aneuploidy in embryos most commonly affects chromosomes X, Y, 13, 14, 15, 16, 18, 21, and 22. Fluorescence *in situ* hybridization (FISH) is a technique that assesses aneuploidy, translocation, other structural chromosomal defects and sex chromosome content (410). FISH is technically limited by the number of distinct chromosomes that can be evaluated, which results in an inherently high false-negative rate. Newer methods are being developed that assess the entire genome using comparative genomic hybridization or DNA microarrays (411). One-quarter of the cases of PGD are performed for single gene disorders, most commonly myotonic dystrophy, Huntington disease, cystic fibrosis, fragile X syndrome, spinal muscular atrophy, tuberous sclerosis, Marfan syndrome, thalassemia, and sickle cell anemia. Because polymerase chain reaction (PCR) is required for single gene disorder diagnosis, ICSI is performed during ART to avoid contamination from sperm bound to the zona pellucida. PGD can be used for HLA antigen tissue matching in an effort to produce a child whose cord blood or stem cells could potentially help an existing affected child. Disadvantages to PGD include decreased postbiopsy embryo survival, requirements for extended culture with an associated possibility that no embryos will be available for transfer or cryopreservation, false-positive and false-negative testing results, and controversies regarding disposition of nontransferred embryos (409,410). **PGD is not synonymous with preimplantation genetic screening (PGS), which is performed in couples without known chromosomal anomaly, mutation, or other genetic abnormality.** Although it seems intuitive that replacing only euploid embryos should improve pregnancy and live birth rates in patients with advanced age, recurrent pregnancy loss, or implantation failure, study outcomes have not been consistent (409,410,412–415).

Preservation of Fertility in Cancer Patients

Improved cancer treatments such as chemotherapy, surgery, and radiotherapy have greatly enhanced survival, such that many cancer survivors contemplate parenthood. Unfortunately, those life-saving treatments can diminish fertility potential in both men and women. Cancer itself does not usually affect oocytes, but certain chemotherapeutic drugs or radiation damage may adversely affect ovarian reserve and uterine function, particularly in older women (416). Ovarian transposition prior to radiation therapy seems to be effective in preserving ovarian function (417). It is unclear whether ovarian suppression with GnRH analogues or oral contraceptives before or during chemotherapy or radiation is beneficial. **If time allows prior to commencement of cancer treatment, women can undergo IVF with embryo cryopreservation (oocyte and ovarian tissue preservation are not routine).** In women with cervical cancer, radical trachelectomy allows for retention of the uterus, those with uterine cancer may respond to *progestin* therapy *in lieu* of hysterectomy, and some ovarian tumors are amenable to unilateral oophorectomy if future fertility is desired. In men, cancer directly affects gametogenesis, and cancer treatments cause more fertility damage when given at younger ages. **Semen and sperm cryopreservation prior to cancer treatment are often recommended for fertility preservation in men** (416) .

References

1. **World Health Organization.** *Manual for the standardised investigation and diagnosis of infertile couple.* Cambridge, UK: Cambridge University Press, 2000.

2. **Gnoth C, Godehardt E, Frank-Herrmann P, et al.** Definition and prevalence of subfertility and infertility. *Hum Reprod* 2005;20:1144–1147.

3. **Guzick DS, Swan S.** The decline of infertility: apparent or real? *Fertil Steril* 2006;86:524–526.

4. **Habbema JD, Collins J, Leridon H, et al.** Towards less confusing terminology in reproductive medicine: a proposal. *Hum Reprod* 2004;19:1497–1501.

5. **Homburg R.** Towards less confusing terminology in reproductive medicine: a counter proposal. *Hum Reprod* 2005;20:316–319.

6. **Boivin J, Bunting L, Collins JA, et al.** International estimates of infertility prevalence and treatment-seeking: potential need and demand for infertility medical care. *Hum Reprod* 2007;22:1506–1512.

7. **Chandra A, Stephen EH.** Infertility service use among U.S. women: 1995 and 2002. *Fertil Steril* 2010;93:725–736.

8. **Eisenberg ML, Smith JF, Millstein SG, et al.** Predictors of not pursuing infertility treatment after an infertility diagnosis: examination of a prospective U.S. cohort. *Fertil Steril* 2010;94:2369–2371.

9. **Tournaye H.** Evidence-based management of male subfertility. *Curr Opin Obstet Gynecol* 2006;18:253–259.

10. **Das S, Nardo LG, Seif MW.** Proximal tubal disease: the place for tubal cannulation. *Reprod Biomed Online* 2007;15:383–388.

11. **Maheshwari A, Hamilton M, Bhattacharya S.** Effect of female age on the diagnostic categories of infertility. *Hum Reprod* 2008;23:538–542.

12. **Wilkes S, Chinn DJ, Murdoch A, et al.** Epidemiology and management of infertility: a population-based study in UK primary care. *Fam Pract* 2009;26:269–274.

13. **Thonneau P, Marchand S, Tallec A, et al.** Incidence and main causes of infertility in a resident population (1,850,000) of three French regions (1988–1989). *Hum Reprod* 1991;6:811–816.

14. **Stephen EH, Chandra A.** Declining estimates of infertility in the United States: 1982–2002. *Fertil Steril* 2006;86:516–523.

15. **Fujimoto VY, Jain T, Alvero R, et al.** Proceedings from the conference on reproductive problems in women of color. *Fertil Steril* 2010;94:7–10.

16. **Jain T.** Socioeconomic and racial disparities among infertility patients seeking care. *Fertil Steril* 2006;85:876–881.

17. **Imudia AN, Detti L, Puscheck EE, et al.** The prevalence of ureaplasma urealyticum, *Mycoplasma hominis, Chlamydia trachomatis* and *Neisseria gonorrhoeae* infections, and the rubella status of patients undergoing an initial infertility evaluation. *J Assist Reprod Genet* 2008;25:43–46.

18. **Dondorp W, de Wert G, Pennings G, et al.** Lifestyle-related factors and access to medically assisted reproduction. *Hum Reprod* 2010;25:578–583.

19. **Dokras A, Baredziak L, Blaine J, et al.** Obstetric outcomes after *in vitro* fertilization in obese and morbidly obese women. *Obstet Gynecol* 2006;108:61–69.

20. **Pauli EM, Legro RS, Demers LM, et al.** Diminished paternity and gonadal function with increasing obesity in men. *Fertil Steril* 2008;90:346–351.

21. **Chavarro JE, Toth TL, Wright DL, et al.** Body mass index in relation to semen quality, sperm DNA integrity, and serum reproductive hormone levels among men attending an infertility clinic. *Fertil Steril* 2010;93:2222–2231.

22. **Mukhopadhyay D, Varghese AC, Pal M, et al.** Semen quality and age-specific changes: a study between two decades on 3,729 male partners of couples with normal sperm count and attending an andrology laboratory for infertility-related problems in an Indian city. *Fertil Steril* 2010;93:2247–2254.

23. **Swan SH, Elkin EP, Fenster L.** The question of declining sperm density revisited: an analysis of 101 studies published 1934–1996. *Environ Health Perspect* 2000;108:961–966.

24. **Swan SH.** Semen quality in fertile US men in relation to geographical area and pesticide exposure. *Int J Androl* 2006;29:62–68; discussion 105–108.

25. **Slama R, Kold-Jensen T, Scheike T, et al.** How would a decline in sperm concentration over time influence the probability of pregnancy? *Epidemiology* 2004;15:458–465.

26. **Ruwanpura SM, McLachlan RI, Meachem SJ.** Hormonal regulation of male germ cell development. *J Endocrinol* 2010;205:117–131.

27. **Amann RP.** The cycle of the seminiferous epithelium in humans: a need to revisit? *J Androl* 2008;29:469–487.

28. **Ramalho-Santos J, Schatten G, Moreno RD.** Control of membrane fusion during spermiogenesis and the acrosome reaction. *Biol Reprod* 2002;67:1043–1051.

29. **Turner TT.** De Graaf's thread: the human epididymis. *J Androl* 2008;29:237–250.

30. **World Health Organization.** 2010 Laboratory manual for the examination and processing of human semen. Available online at: http://whqlibdoc.who.int/publications/2010/9789241547789_eng.pdf

31. **Ikawa M, Inoue N, Benham AM, et al.** Fertilization: a sperm's journey to and interaction with the oocyte. *J Clin Invest* 2010;120:984–994.

32. **Practice Committee of American Society for Reproductive Medicine in collaboration with Society for Reproductive Endocrinology and Infertility.** Optimizing natural fertility. *Fertil Steril* 2008;90:S1–S6.

33. **Sun QY.** Cellular and molecular mechanisms leading to cortical reaction and polyspermy block in mammalian eggs. *Microsc Res Tech* 2003;61:342–348.

34. **Gracia CR, Sammel MD, Coutifaris C, et al.** Occupational exposures and male infertility. *Am J Epidemiol* 2005;162:729–733.

35. **Chavarro JE, Toth TL, Sadio SM, et al.** Soy food and isoflavone intake in relation to semen quality parameters among men from an infertility clinic. *Hum Reprod* 2008;23:2584–2590.

36. **Muthusami KR, Chinnaswamy P.** Effect of chronic alcoholism on male fertility hormones and semen quality. *Fertil Steril* 2005;84:919–924.

37. **Gaur DS, Talekar MS, Pathak VP.** Alcohol intake and cigarette smoking: impact of two major lifestyle factors on male fertility. *Indian J Pathol Microbiol* 2010;53:35–40.

38. **Kunzle R, Mueller MD, Hanggi W, et al.** Semen quality of male smokers and nonsmokers in infertile couples. *Fertil Steril* 2003;79:287–291.

39. **Said TM, Ranga G, Agarwal A.** Relationship between semen quality and tobacco chewing in men undergoing infertility evaluation. *Fertil Steril* 2005;84:649–653.

40. **Whan LB, West MC, McClure N, et al.** Effects of delta-9-tetrahydrocannabinol, the primary psychoactive cannabinoid in marijuana, on human sperm function *in vitro. Fertil Steril* 2006;85:653–660.

41. **Bracken MB, Eskenazi B, Sachse K, et al.** Association of cocaine use with sperm concentration, motility, and morphology. *Fertil Steril* 1990;53:315–322.

42. **Yelian FD, Sacco AG, Ginsburg KA, et al.** The effects of *in vitro* cocaine exposure on human sperm motility, intracellular calcium, and oocyte penetration. *Fertil Steril* 1994;61:915–921.

43. **World Health Organization.** *Laboratory manual for the examination of human semen and sperm–cervical mucus interaction.* Cambridge, UK: Cambridge University Press, 1992.

44. **Male Infertility Best Practice Policy Committee of the American Urological Association; Practice Committee of the American Society for Reproductive Medicine.** Report on optimal evaluation of the infertile male. *Fertil Steril* 2006;86:S202–209.

45. **Levitas E, Lunenfeld E, Weiss N, et al.** Relationship between the duration of sexual abstinence and semen quality: analysis of 9,489 semen samples. *Fertil Steril* 2005;83:1680–1686.

46. **Marshburn PB, Alanis M, Matthews ML, et al.** A short period of ejaculatory abstinence before intrauterine insemination is associated with higher pregnancy rates. *Fertil Steril* 2010;93:286–288.

47. **Bhasin S.** Approach to the infertile man. *J Clin Endocrinol Metab* 2007;92:1995–2004.

48. **Kruger TF, Acosta AA, Simmons KF, et al.** Predictive value of abnormal sperm morphology in *in vitro* fertilization. *Fertil Steril* 1988;49:112–117.

49. **Kruger TF, Menkveld R, Stander FS, et al.** Sperm morphologic features as a prognostic factor in *in vitro* fertilization. *Fertil Steril* 1986;46:1118–1123.

50. **Yanushpolsky EH, Politch JA, Hill JA, et al.** Is leukocytospermia clinically relevant? *Fertil Steril* 1996;66:822–825.

51. **Gdoura R, Kchaou W, Znazen A, et al.** Screening for bacterial pathogens in semen samples from infertile men with and without leukocytospermia. *Andrologia* 2008;40:209–218.

52. **Practice Committee of American Society for Reproductive Medicine.** The clinical utility of sperm DNA integrity testing. *Fertil Steril* 2008;90:S178–S180.

53. **de Kretser DM.** Male infertility. *Lancet* 1997;349:787–790.

54. **The ESHRE Capri Workshop Group.** Male sterility and subfertility: guidelines for management. *Hum Reprod* 1994;9:1260–1264.

55. **Burkman LJ, Coddington CC, Franken DR, et al.** The hemizona assay (HZA): development of a diagnostic test for the binding of human spermatozoa to the human hemizona pellucida to predict fertilization potential. *Fertil Steril* 1988;49:688–697.

56. **Kuhnert B, Nieschlag E.** Reproductive functions of the ageing male. *Hum Reprod Update* 2004;10:327–339.

57. **Garcia-Palomares S, Navarro S, Pertusa JF, et al.** Delayed fatherhood in mice decreases reproductive fitness and longevity of offspring. *Biol Reprod* 2009;80:343–349.

58. **Puscheck EE, Jeyendran RS.** The impact of male factor on recurrent pregnancy loss. *Curr Opin Obstet Gynecol* 2007;19:222–228.

59. **Ghanem H, Shamloul R.** An evidence-based perspective to the medical treatment of male infertility: a short review. *Urol Int* 2009;82:125–129.

60. **Oliva A, Dotta A, Multigner L.** Pentoxifylline and antioxidants improve sperm quality in male patients with varicocele. *Fertil Steril* 2009;91:1536–1539.

61. **Practice Committee of American Society for Reproductive Medicine.** Report on varicocele and infertility. *Fertil Steril* 2008;90:S247–249.

62. **Pasqualotto FF, Lucon AM, de Goes PM, et al.** Semen profile, testicular volume, and hormonal levels in infertile patients with varicoceles compared with fertile men with and without varicoceles. *Fertil Steril* 2005;83:74–77.

63. **Pasqualotto FF, Sundaram A, Sharma RK, et al.** Semen quality and oxidative stress scores in fertile and infertile patients with varicocele. *Fertil Steril* 2008;89:602–607.

64. **Marmar JL, Agarwal A, Prabakaran S, et al.** Reassessing the value of varicocelectomy as a treatment for male subfertility with a new meta-analysis. *Fertil Steril* 2007;88:639–648.

65. **Pasqualotto FF, Pasqualotto EB.** Reassessing the value of varicocelectomy as a treatment for male subfertility with a new meta-analysis. *Fertil Steril* 2007;88:1710.

66. **Group ECW.** Intrauterine insemination. *Hum Reprod Update* 2009;15:265–277.

67. **Carroll N, Palmer JR.** A comparison of intrauterine versus intracervical insemination in fertile single women. *Fertil Steril* 2001;75:656–660.

68. **Besselink DE, Farquhar C, Kremer JA, et al.** Cervical insemination versus intra-uterine insemination of donor sperm for subfertility. *Cochrane Database Syst Rev* 2008;2:CD000317.

69. **Kovacic B, Vlaisavljevic V, Reljic M.** Clinical use of pentoxifylline for activation of immotile testicular sperm before ICSI in patients with azoospermia. *J Androl* 2006;27:45–52.

70. **Custers IM, Flierman PA, Maas P, et al.** Immobilisation versus immediate mobilisation after intrauterine insemination: randomised controlled trial. *BMJ* 2009;339:b4080.

71. **Bensdorp AJ, Cohlen BJ, Heineman MJ, et al.** Intra-uterine insemination for male subfertility. *Cochrane Database Syst Rev* 2007;3:CD000360.

72. **Cohlen BJ, Vandekerckhove P, te Velde ER, et al.** Timed intercourse versus intra-uterine insemination with or without ovarian hyperstimulation for subfertility in men. *Cochrane Database Syst Rev* 2000;2:CD000360.

73. **Francavilla F, Sciarretta F, Sorgentone S, et al.** Intrauterine insemination with or without mild ovarian stimulation in couples with male subfertility due to oligo/astheno- and/or teratozoospermia or antisperm antibodies: a prospective cross-over trial. *Fertil Steril* 2009;92:1009–1011.

74. **Ford WC, Mathur RS, Hull MG.** Intrauterine insemination: is it an effective treatment for male factor infertility? *Bailliers Clin Obstet Gynaecol* 1997;11:691–710.

75. **Merviel P, Heraud MH, Grenier N, et al.** Predictive factors for pregnancy after intrauterine insemination (IUI): an analysis of 1038 cycles and a review of the literature. *Fertil Steril* 2010;93:79–88.

76. **Badawy A, Elnashar A, Eltotongy M.** Effect of sperm morphology and number on success of intrauterine insemination. *Fertil Steril* 2009;91:777–781.

77. **Dickey RP, Taylor SN, Lu PY, et al.** Effect of diagnosis, age, sperm quality, and number of preovulatory follicles on the outcome of multiple cycles of clomiphene citrate-intrauterine insemination. *Fertil Steril* 2002;78:1088–1095.

78. **Van Voorhis BJ, Barnett M, Sparks AE, et al.** Effect of the total motile sperm count on the efficacy and cost-effectiveness of intrauterine insemination and *in vitro* fertilization. *Fertil Steril* 2001;75:661–668.

79. **Bagis T, Haydardedeoglu B, Kilicdag EB, et al.** Single versus double intrauterine insemination in multi-follicular ovarian hyperstimulation cycles: a randomized trial. *Hum Reprod* 2010;25:1684–1690.

80. **Practice Committee of American Society for Reproductive Medicine; Practice Committee of Society for Assisted Reproductive Technology.** Genetic considerations related to intracytoplasmic sperm injection (ICSI). *Fertil Steril* 2008;90:S182–S184.

81. **ESHRE Capri Workshop Group.** Male infertility update. *Hum Reprod* 1998;13:2025–2032.

82. **Rosen MP, Shen S, Dobson AT, et al.** Oocyte degeneration after intracytoplasmic sperm injection: a multivariate analysis to assess its importance as a laboratory or clinical marker. *Fertil Steril* 2006;85:1736–1743.

83. **Keegan BR, Barton S, Sanchez X, et al.** Isolated teratozoospermia does not affect *in vitro* fertilization outcome and is not an indication for intracytoplasmic sperm injection. *Fertil Steril* 2007;88:1583–1588.

84. **Practice Committee of American Society for Reproductive Medicine; Practice Committee of Society for Assisted Reproductive Technology.** Round spermatid nucleus injection (ROSNI). *Fertil Steril* 2008;90:S199–S201.

85. **Practice Committee of American Society for Reproductive Medicine.** Intracytoplasmic sperm injection (ICSI). *Fertil Steril* 2008;90:S187.

86. **Practice Committee of American Society for Reproductive Medicine in collaboration with Society for Male Reproduction and Urology.** Evaluation of the azoospermic male. *Fertil Steril* 2008;90:S74–S77.

87. **Lee R, Li PS, Goldstein M, et al.** A decision analysis of treatments for nonobstructive azoospermia associated with varicocele. *Fertil Steril* 2009;92:188–196.

88. **Weedin JW, Khera M, Lipshultz LI.** Varicocele repair in patients with nonobstructive azoospermia: a meta-analysis. *J Urol* 2010;183:2309–2315.

89. **Pryor JL, Kent-First M, Muallem A, et al.** Microdeletions in the Y chromosome of infertile men. *N Engl J Med* 1997;336:534–539.

90. **Ferlin A, Arredi B, Speltra E, et al.** Molecular and clinical characterization of Y chromosome microdeletions in infertile men: a 10-year experience in Italy. *J Clin Endocrinol Metab* 2007;92:762–770.

91. **Reijo R, Alagappan RK, Patrizio P, et al.** Severe oligozoospermia resulting from deletions of azoospermia factor gene on Y chromosome. *Lancet* 1996;347:1290–1293.

92. **Practice Committee of American Society for Reproductive Medicine.** Sperm retrieval for obstructive azoospermia. *Fertil Steril* 2008;90:S213–S218.

93. **Practice Committee of American Society for Reproductive Medicine in collaboration with Society for Male Reproduction and Urology.** The management of infertility due to obstructive azoospermia. *Fertil Steril* 2008;90:S121–S124.

94. **Practice Committee of American Society for Reproductive Medicine.** Vasectomy reversal. *Fertil Steril* 2008;90:S78–S82.

95. **Carpi A, Sabanegh E, Mechanick J.** Controversies in the management of nonobstructive azoospermia. *Fertil Steril* 2009;91:963–970.

96. **Practice Committee of American Society for Reproductive Medicine; Practice Committee of Society for Assisted Reproductive Technology.** 2008 Guidelines for gamete and embryo donation: a Practice Committee report. *Fertil Steril* 2008;90:S30–S44.

97. **De Brucker M, Haentjens P, Evenepoel J, et al.** Cumulative delivery rates in different age groups after artificial insemination with donor sperm. *Hum Reprod* 2009;24:1891–1899.

98. **Payne MA, Lamb EJ.** Use of frozen semen to avoid human immunodeficiency virus type 1 transmission by donor insemination: a cost-effectiveness analysis. *Fertil Steril* 2004;81:80–92.

99. **Subak LL, Adamson GD, Boltz NL.** Therapeutic donor insemination: a prospective randomized trial of fresh versus frozen sperm. *Am J Obstet Gynecol* 1992;166:1597–1604.

100. **Committee on Gynecologic Practice of American College of Obstetricians and Gynecologists; Practice Committee of American Society for Reproductive Medicine.** Age-related fertility decline: a committee opinion. *Fertil Steril* 2008;90:S154–S155.

101. **Schwartz D, Mayaux MJ.** Female fecundity as a function of age: results of artificial insemination in 2193 nulliparous women with azoospermic husbands. Federation CECOS. *N Engl J Med* 1982;306:404–406.

102. **Sauer MV, Kavic SM.** Oocyte and embryo donation 2006: reviewing two decades of innovation and controversy. *Reprod Biomed Online* 2006;12:153–162.

103. **Sauer MV, Paulson RJ, Lobo RA.** Reversing the natural decline in human fertility. An extended clinical trial of oocyte donation to women of advanced reproductive age. *JAMA* 1992;268:1275–1279.

104. **Scheffer GJ, Broekmans FJ, Looman CW, et al.** The number of antral follicles in normal women with proven fertility is the best reflection of reproductive age. *Hum Reprod* 2003;18:700–706.

105. **Practice Committee of the American Society for Reproductive Medicine.** Aging and infertility in women. *Fertil Steril* 2006;86:S248–S252.

106. **Nybo Andersen AM, Wohlfahrt J, Christens P, et al.** Maternal age and fetal loss: population based register linkage study. *BMJ* 2000;320:1708–1712.

107. **Wilcox AJ, Weinberg CR, O'Connor JF, et al.** Incidence of early loss of pregnancy. *N Engl J Med* 1988;319:189–194.

108. **Steiner AZ.** Clinical implications of ovarian reserve testing. *Obstet Gynecol Surv* 2009;64:120–128.

109. **Broekmans FJ, Kwee J, Hendriks DJ, et al.** A systematic review of tests predicting ovarian reserve and IVF outcome. *Hum Reprod Update* 2006;12:685–718.

110. **Hendriks DJ, Broekmans FJ, Bancsi LF, et al.** Repeated clomiphene citrate challenge testing in the prediction of outcome in IVF: a comparison with basal markers for ovarian reserve. *Hum Reprod* 2005;20:163–169.

111. **Jayaprakasan K, Campbell B, Hopkisson J, et al.** A prospective, comparative analysis of anti-mullerian hormone, inhibin-B, and three-dimensional ultrasound determinants of ovarian reserve in the prediction of poor response to controlled ovarian stimulation. *Fertil Steril* 2010;93:855–864.

112. **van der Steeg JW, Steures P, Eijkemans MJ, et al.** Predictive value and clinical impact of basal follicle-stimulating hormone in subfertile, ovulatory women. *J Clin Endocrinol Metab* 2007;92:2163–2168.

113. **van Rooij IA, de Jong E, Broekmans FJ, et al.** High follicle-stimulating hormone levels should not necessarily lead to the exclusion of subfertile patients from treatment. *Fertil Steril* 2004;81:1478–1485.

114. **van Rooij IA, Broekmans FJ, Scheffer GJ, et al.** Serum antimullerian hormone levels best reflect the reproductive decline with age in normal women with proven fertility: a longitudinal study. *Fertil Steril* 2005;83:979–987.

115. **Penarrubia J, Peralta S, Fabregues F, et al.** Day-5 inhibin B serum concentrations and antral follicle count as predictors of ovarian response and live birth in assisted reproduction cycles stimulated with gonadotropin after pituitary suppression. *Fertil Steril* 2010;94:2590–2595.

116. **Kwee J, Schats R, McDonnell J, et al.** Evaluation of anti-mullerian hormone as a test for the prediction of ovarian reserve. *Fertil Steril* 2008;90:737–743.

117. **Nardo LG, Gelbaya TA, Wilkinson H, et al.** Circulating basal anti-mullerian hormone levels as predictor of ovarian response in women undergoing ovarian stimulation for *in vitro* fertilization. *Fertil Steril* 2009;92:1586–1593.

118. **Rosen MP, Sternfeld B, Schuh-Huerta SM, et al.** Antral follicle count: absence of significant midlife decline. *Fertil Steril* 2010;94:2182–2185.

119. **Bancsi LF, Broekmans FJ, Looman CW, et al.** Impact of repeated antral follicle counts on the prediction of poor ovarian response in women undergoing *in vitro* fertilization. *Fertil Steril* 2004;81:35–41.

120. **Hendriks DJ, Mol BW, Bancsi LF, et al.** Antral follicle count in the prediction of poor ovarian response and pregnancy after *in vitro* fertilization: a meta-analysis and comparison with basal follicle-stimulating hormone level. *Fertil Steril* 2005;83:291–301.

121. **Barad DH, Weghofer A, Gleicher N.** Dehydroepiandrosterone treatment of ovarian failure. *Fertil Steril* 2009;91:e14; author reply e5.

122. **Barad D, Gleicher N.** Effect of dehydroepiandrosterone on oocyte and embryo yields, embryo grade and cell number in IVF. *Hum Reprod* 2006;21:2845–2849.

123. **Barad DH, Gleicher N.** Increased oocyte production after treatment with dehydroepiandrosterone. *Fertil Steril* 2005;84:756.

124. **Practice Committee of the American Society for Reproductive Medicine.** Optimal evaluation of the infertile female. *Fertil Steril* 2006;86:S264–S267.

125. **Azziz R, Carmina E, Dewailly D, et al.** The Androgen Excess and PCOS Society criteria for the polycystic ovary syndrome: the complete task force report. *Fertil Steril* 2009;91:456–488.

126. **Cole LA, Ladner DG, Byrn FW.** The normal variabilities of the menstrual cycle. *Fertil Steril* 2009;91:522–527.

127. **Stanford JB, White GL, Hatasaka H.** Timing intercourse to achieve pregnancy: current evidence. *Obstet Gynecol* 2002;100:1333–1341.

128. **Wilcox AJ, Dunson D, Baird DD.** The timing of the "fertile window" in the menstrual cycle: day specific estimates from a prospective study. *BMJ* 2000;321:1259–1262.

129. **Wilcox AJ, Weinberg CR, Baird DD.** Timing of sexual intercourse in relation to ovulation. Effects on the probability of conception, survival of the pregnancy, and sex of the baby. *N Engl J Med* 1995;333:1517–1521.

130. **Pallone SR, Bergus GR.** Fertility awareness-based methods: another option for family planning. *J Am Board Fam Med* 2009;22:147–157.

131. **Guermandi E, Vegetti W, Bianchi MM, et al.** Reliability of ovulation tests in infertile women. *Obstet Gynecol* 2001;97:92–96.

132. **Miller PB, Soules MR.** The usefulness of a urinary LH kit for ovulation prediction during menstrual cycles of normal women. *Obstet Gynecol* 1996;87:13–17.

133. **Nielsen MS, Barton SD, Hatasaka HH, et al.** Comparison of several one-step home urinary luteinizing hormone detection test kits to OvuQuick. *Fertil Steril* 2001;76:384–387.

134. **Grinsted J, Jacobsen JD, Grinsted L, et al.** Prediction of ovulation. *Fertil Steril* 1989;52:388–393.

135. **McGovern PG, Myers ER, Silva S, et al.** Absence of secretory endometrium after false-positive home urine luteinizing hormone testing. *Fertil Steril* 2004;82:1273–1277.

136. **Practice Committee of the American Society for Reproductive Medicine.** Use of clomiphene citrate in women. *Fertil Steril* 2006;86:S187–S193.

137. **Jirge PR, Patil RS.** Comparison of endocrine and ultrasound profiles during ovulation induction with clomiphene citrate and letrozole in ovulatory volunteer women. *Fertil Steril* 2010;93:174–183.

138. **Qublan H, Amarin Z, Nawasreh M, et al.** Luteinized unruptured follicle syndrome: incidence and recurrence rate in infertile women with unexplained infertility undergoing intrauterine insemination. *Hum Reprod* 2006;21:2110–2113.

139. **Thessaloniki ESHRE/ASRM-Sponsored PCOS Consensus Workshop Group.** Consensus on infertility treatment related to polycystic ovary syndrome. *Fertil Steril* 2008;89:505–522.

140. **Rotterdam ESHRE/ASRM-Sponsored PCOS Consensus Workshop Group.** Revised 2003 consensus on diagnostic criteria and long-term health risks related to polycystic ovary syndrome (PCOS). *Hum Reprod* 2004;19:41–47.

141. **Thessaloniki ESHRE/ASRM-Sponsored PCOS Consensus Workshop Group.** Consensus on infertility treatment related to polycystic ovary syndrome. *Hum Reprod* 2008;23:462–477.

142. **Legro RS, Barnhart HX, Schlaff WD, et al.** Clomiphene, metformin, or both for infertility in the polycystic ovary syndrome. *N Engl J Med* 2007;356:551–566.

143. **Jungheim ES, Lanzendorf SE, Odem RR, et al.** Morbid obesity is associated with lower clinical pregnancy rates after *in vitro* fertilization in women with polycystic ovary syndrome. *Fertil Steril* 2009;92:256–261.

144. **McCormick B, Thomas M, Maxwell R, et al.** Effects of polycystic ovarian syndrome on *in vitro* fertilization-embryo transfer outcomes are influenced by body mass index. *Fertil Steril* 2008;90:2304–2309.

145. **Koivunen R, Pouta A, Franks S, et al.** Fecundability and spontaneous abortions in women with self-reported oligo-amenorrhea and/or hirsutism: Northern Finland Birth Cohort 1966 Study. *Hum Reprod* 2008;23:2134–2139.

146. **Palomba S, Giallauria F, Falbo A, et al.** Structured exercise training programme versus hypocaloric hyperproteic diet in obese polycystic ovary syndrome patients with anovulatory infertility: a 24-week pilot study. *Hum Reprod* 2008;23:642–650.

147. **Brown J, Farquhar C, Beck J, et al.** Clomiphene and anti-oestrogens for ovulation induction in PCOS. *Cochrane Database Syst Rev* 2009;4:CD002249.

148. **Rausch ME, Legro RS, Barnhart HX, et al.** Predictors of pregnancy in women with polycystic ovary syndrome. *J Clin Endocrinol Metab* 2009;94:3458–3466.

149. **Imani B, Eijkemans MJ, te Velde ER, et al.** A nomogram to predict the probability of live birth after clomiphene citrate induction of ovulation in normogonadotropic oligoamenorrheic infertility. *Fertil Steril* 2002;77:91–97.

150. **Practice Committee of the American Society for Reproductive Medicine.** Effectiveness and treatment for unexplained infertility. *Fertil Steril* 2006;86:S111–S114.

151. **Hughes E, Brown J, Collins JJ, et al.** Clomiphene citrate for unexplained subfertility in women. *Cochrane Database Syst Rev* 2010;1:CD000057.

152. **Badawy A, Inany H, Mosbah A, et al.** Luteal phase clomiphene citrate for ovulation induction in women with polycystic ovary syndrome: a novel protocol. *Fertil Steril* 2009;91:838–841.

153. **FDA Center for Drug Evaluation and Research, Office of Pharmaceutical Science.** Informatics and Computational Safety Analysis Staff's Maximum Recommended Therapeutic Dose (MRTD) database 2004. Available online at: http://www.fda.gov/aboutfda/centersoffices/cder/ucm092199.htm

154. **Hurst BS, Hickman JM, Matthews ML, et al.** Novel clomiphene "stair-step" protocol reduces time to ovulation in women with polycystic ovarian syndrome. *Am J Obstet Gynecol* 2009;200:510-e1–e4.

155. **Bates GW, Shomento S, McKnight K, et al.** Discussion: "Novel clomiphene protocol in polycystic ovarian syndrome" by Hurst et al. *Am J Obstet Gynecol* 2009;200:e1–e3.

156. **Practice Committee of American Society for Reproductive Medicine, Birmingham, Alabama.** Gonadotropin preparations: past, present, and future perspectives. *Fertil Steril* 2008;90:S13–S20.

157. **Vlahos NF, Coker L, Lawler C, et al.** Women with ovulatory dysfunction undergoing ovarian stimulation with clomiphene citrate for intrauterine insemination may benefit from administration of human chorionic gonadotropin. *Fertil Steril* 2005;83:1510–1516.

158. **Kosmas IP, Tatsioni A, Fatemi HM, et al.** Human chorionic gonadotropin administration vs. luteinizing monitoring for intrauterine insemination timing, after administration of clomiphene citrate: a meta-analysis. *Fertil Steril* 2007;87:607–612.

159. **Cantineau AE, Janssen MJ, Cohen BJ.** Synchronised approach for intrauterine insemination in subfertile couples. *Cochrane Database Syst Rev* 2010;4:CD006942.

160. **Fuh KW, Wang X, Tai A, et al.** Intrauterine insemination: effect of the temporal relationship between the luteinizing hormone surge, human chorionic gonadotrophin administration and insemination on pregnancy rates. *Hum Reprod* 1997;12:2162–2166.

161. **Robb PA, Robins JC, Thomas MA.** Timing of hCG administration does not affect pregnancy rates in couples undergoing intrauterine insemination using clomiphene citrate. *J Natl Med Assoc* 2004;96:1431–1433.

162. **Practice Committee of American Society for Reproductive Medicine.** Use of insulin-sensitizing agents in the treatment of polycystic ovary syndrome. *Fertil Steril* 2008;90:S69–S73.

163. **Tang T, Lord JM, Norman RJ, et al.** Insulin-sensitising drugs (metformin, rosiglitazone, pioglitazone, D-chiro-inositol) for women with polycystic ovary syndrome, oligo amenorrhoea and subfertility. *Cochrane Database Syst Rev* 2010;1:CD003053.

164. **Palomba S, Falbo A, Orio F Jr, et al.** Efficacy predictors for metformin and clomiphene citrate treatment in anovulatory infertile patients with polycystic ovary syndrome. *Fertil Steril* 2009;91:2557–2567.

165. **Cataldo NA, Abbasi F, McLaughlin TL, et al.** Metabolic and ovarian effects of rosiglitazone treatment for 12 weeks in insulin-resistant women with polycystic ovary syndrome. *Hum Reprod* 2006;21:109–120.

166. **Sepilian V, Nagamani M.** Effects of rosiglitazone in obese women with polycystic ovary syndrome and severe insulin resistance. *J Clin Endocrinol Metab* 2005;90:60–65.

167. **Kim CH, Jeon GH, Kim SR, et al.** Effects of pioglitazone on ovarian stromal blood flow, ovarian stimulation, and *in vitro* fertilization outcome in patients with polycystic ovary syndrome. *Fertil Steril* 2010;94:236–241.

168. **Ota H, Goto T, Yoshioka T, et al.** Successful pregnancies treated with pioglitazone in infertile patients with polycystic ovary syndrome. *Fertil Steril* 2008;90:709–713.

169. **Elnashar A, Abdelmageed E, Fayed M, et al.** Clomiphene citrate and dexamethazone in treatment of clomiphene citrate-resistant polycystic ovary syndrome: a prospective placebo-controlled study. *Hum Reprod* 2006;21:1805–1808.

170. **Parsanezhad ME, Alborzi S, Motazedian S, et al.** Use of dexamethasone and clomiphene citrate in the treatment of clomiphene citrate-resistant patients with polycystic ovary syndrome and normal dehydroepiandrosterone sulfate levels: a prospective, double-blind, placebo-controlled trial. *Fertil Steril* 2002;78:1001–1004.

171. **Daly DC, Walters CA, Soto-Albors CE, et al.** A randomized study of dexamethasone in ovulation induction with clomiphene citrate. *Fertil Steril* 1984;41:844–848.

172. **Lobo RA, Paul W, March CM, et al.** Clomiphene and dexamethasone in women unresponsive to clomiphene alone. *Obstet Gynecol* 1982;60:497–501.

173. **Branigan EF, Estes MA.** A randomized clinical trial of treatment of clomiphene citrate-resistant anovulation with the use of oral contraceptive pill suppression and repeat clomiphene citrate treatment. *Am J Obstet Gynecol* 2003;188:1424–1428; discussion 9–30.

174. **Steiner AZ, Terplan M, Paulson RJ.** Comparison of tamoxifen and clomiphene citrate for ovulation induction: a meta-analysis. *Hum Reprod* 2005;20:1511–1515.

175. **Boostanfar R, Jain JK, Mishell DR Jr, et al.** A prospective randomized trial comparing clomiphene citrate with tamoxifen citrate for ovulation induction. *Fertil Steril* 2001;75:1024–1026.

176. **Mitwally MF, Casper RF.** Use of an aromatase inhibitor for induction of ovulation in patients with an inadequate response to clomiphene citrate. *Fertil Steril* 2001;75:305–309.

177. **Badawy A, Mosbah A, Tharwat A, et al.** Extended letrozole therapy for ovulation induction in clomiphene-resistant women with polycystic ovary syndrome: a novel protocol. *Fertil Steril* 2009;92:236–239.

178. **Badawy A, Mosbah A, Shady M.** Anastrozole or letrozole for ovulation induction in clomiphene-resistant women with polycystic ovarian syndrome: a prospective randomized trial. *Fertil Steril* 2008;89:1209–1212.

179. **Tulandi T, Martin J, Al-Fadhli R, et al.** Congenital malformations among 911 newborns conceived after infertility treatment with letrozole or clomiphene citrate. *Fertil Steril* 2006;85:1761–1765.

180. **Practice Committee of American Society for Reproductive Medicine.** Use of exogenous gonadotropins in anovulatory women: a technical bulletin. *Fertil Steril* 2008;90:S7–S12.

181. **Ganesh A, Goswami SK, Chattopadhyay R, et al.** Comparison of letrozole with continuous gonadotropins and clomiphene-gonadotropin combination for ovulation induction in 1387 PCOS women after clomiphene citrate failure: a randomized prospective clinical trial. *J Assist Reprod Genet* 2009;26:19–24.

182. **Jee BC, Ku SY, Suh CS, et al.** Use of letrozole versus clomiphene citrate combined with gonadotropins in intrauterine insemination cycles: a pilot study. *Fertil Steril* 2006;85:1774–1777.

183. **Sipe CS, Davis WA, Maifeld M, et al.** A prospective randomized trial comparing anastrozole and clomiphene citrate in an ovulation

induction protocol using gonadotropins. *Fertil Steril* 2006;86:1676–1681.

184. **Mitwally MF, Casper RF.** Aromatase inhibition reduces the dose of gonadotropin required for controlled ovarian hyperstimulation. *J Soc Gynecol Investig* 2004;11:406–415.

185. **Farquhar C, Lilford RJ, Marjoribanks J, et al.** Laparoscopic "drilling" by diathermy or laser for ovulation induction in anovulatory polycystic ovary syndrome. *Cochrane Database Syst Rev* 2007;3:CD001122.

186. **Palomba S, Falbo A, Battista L, et al.** Laparoscopic ovarian diathermy vs clomiphene citrate plus metformin as second-line strategy for infertile anovulatory patients with polycystic ovary syndrome: a randomized controlled trial. *Am J Obstet Gynecol* 2010;202:577.e1–e8.

187. **Palomba S, Falbo A, Orio F Jr, et al.** Efficacy of laparoscopic ovarian diathermy in clomiphene citrate-resistant women with polycystic ovary syndrome: relationships with chronological and ovarian age. *Gynecol Endocrinol* 2006;22:329–335.

188. **Ott J, Kurz C, Nouri K, et al.** Pregnancy outcome in women with polycystic ovary syndrome comparing the effects of laparoscopic ovarian drilling and clomiphene citrate stimulation in women pre-treated with metformin: a retrospective study. *Reprod Biol Endocrinol* 2010;8:45.

189. **Malkawi HY, Qublan HS.** Laparoscopic ovarian drilling in the treatment of polycystic ovary syndrome: how many punctures per ovary are needed to improve the reproductive outcome? *J Obstet Gynaecol Res* 2005;31:115–119.

190. **Takeuchi S, Futamura N, Takubo S, et al.** Polycystic ovary syndrome treated with laparoscopic ovarian drilling with a harmonic scalpel. A prospective, randomized study. *J Reprod Med* 2002;47:816–820.

191. **Asada H, Kishi I, Kaseda S, et al.** Laparoscopic treatment of polycystic ovaries with the holmium:YAG laser. *Fertil Steril* 2002;77:852–853.

192. **Gladchuk IZ, Shwez VV.** Hormone changes in clomiphene citrate-resistant women with polycystic ovary disease after ovarian cryosurgery and Nd:YAG laser laparoscopy. *J Am Assoc Gynecol Laparosc* 1996;3:S15–S16.

193. **Zhu W, Fu Z, Chen X, et al.** Transvaginal ultrasound-guided ovarian interstitial laser treatment in anovulatory women with polycystic ovary syndrome: a randomized clinical trial on the effect of laser dose used on the outcome. *Fertil Steril* 2010;94:268–275.

194. **Badawy A, Khiary M, Ragab A, et al.** Ultrasound-guided transvaginal ovarian needle drilling (UTND) for treatment of polycystic ovary syndrome: a randomized controlled trial. *Fertil Steril* 2009;91:1164–1167.

195. **Gordts S, Gordts S, Puttemans P, et al.** Transvaginal hydrolaparoscopy in the treatment of polycystic ovary syndrome. *Fertil Steril* 2009;91:2520–2526.

196. **Mercorio F, Mercorio A, Di Spiezio Sardo A, et al.** Evaluation of ovarian adhesion formation after laparoscopic ovarian drilling by second-look minilaparoscopy. *Fertil Steril* 2008;89:1229–1233.

197. **Practice Committee of American Society for Reproductive Medicine.** Current evaluation of amenorrhea. *Fertil Steril* 2008;90:S219–S225.

198. **Gillam MP, Molitch ME, Lombardi G, et al.** Advances in the treatment of prolactinomas. *Endocr Rev* 2006;27:485–534.

199. **Dei M, Seravalli V, Bruni V, et al.** Predictors of recovery of ovarian function after weight gain in subjects with amenorrhea related to restrictive eating disorders. *Gynecol Endocrinol* 2008;24:459–464.

200. **Kelesidis T, Kelesidis I, Chou S, et al.** Narrative review: the role of leptin in human physiology: emerging clinical applications. *Ann Intern Med* 2010;152:93–100.

201. **Welt CK, Chan JL, Bullen J, et al.** Recombinant human leptin in women with hypothalamic amenorrhea. *N Engl J Med* 2004;351:987–997.

202. **Fechner A, Fong S, McGovern P.** A review of Kallmann syndrome: genetics, pathophysiology, and clinical management. *Obstet Gynecol Surv* 2008;63:189–194.

203. **Poppe K, Velkeniers B, Glinoer D.** Thyroid disease and female reproduction. *Clin Endocrinol (Oxf)* 2007;66:309–321.

204. **Westrom L, Joesoef R, Reynolds G, et al.** Pelvic inflammatory disease and fertility. A cohort study of 1,844 women with laparoscopically verified disease and 657 control women with normal laparoscopic results. *Sex Transm Dis* 1992;19:185–192.

205. **Lepine LA, Hillis SD, Marchbanks PA, et al.** Severity of pelvic inflammatory disease as a predictor of the probability of live birth. *Am J Obstet Gynecol* 1998;178:977–981.

206. **Paavonen J, Eggert-Kruse W.** *Chlamydia trachomatis*: impact on human reproduction. *Hum Reprod Update* 1999;5:433–447.

207. **Guven MA, Dilek U, Pata O, et al.** Prevalance of *Chlamydia trachomatis, Ureaplasma urealyticum* and *Mycoplasma hominis* infections in the unexplained infertile women. *Arch Gynecol Obstet* 2007;276:219–223.

208. **Simpson WL Jr, Beitia LG, Mester J.** Hysterosalpingography: a reemerging study. *Radiographics* 2006;26:419–431.

209. **Robinson RD, Casablanca Y, Pagano KE, et al.** Intracervical block and pain perception during the performance of a hysterosalpingogram: a randomized controlled trial. *Obstet Gynecol* 2007;109:89–93.

210. **Baramki TA.** Hysterosalpingography. *Fertil Steril* 2005;83:1595–1606.

211. **Kodaman PH, Arici A, Seli E.** Evidence-based diagnosis and management of tubal factor infertility. *Curr Opin Obstet Gynecol* 2004;16:221–229.

212. **Bulletti C, Panzini I, Borini A, et al.** Pelvic factor infertility: diagnosis and prognosis of various procedures. *Ann N Y Acad Sci* 2008;1127:73–82.

213. **Luttjeboer F, Harada T, Hughes E, et al.** Tubal flushing for subfertility. *Cochrane Database Syst Rev* 2007;3:CD003718.

214. **Vandekerckhove P, Watson A, Lilford R, et al.** Oil-soluble versus water-soluble media for assessing tubal patency with hysterosalpingography or laparoscopy in subfertile women. *Cochrane Database Syst Rev* 2000;2:CD000092.

215. **Stumpf PG, March CM.** Febrile morbidity following hysterosalpingography: identification of risk factors and recommendations for prophylaxis. *Fertil Steril* 1980;33:487–492.

216. **Pittaway DE, Winfield AC, Maxson W, et al.** Prevention of acute pelvic inflammatory disease after hysterosalpingography: efficacy of doxycycline prophylaxis. *Am J Obstet Gynecol* 1983;147:623–626.

217. **Thinkhamrop J, Laopaiboon M, Lumbiganon P.** Prophylactic antibiotics for transcervical intrauterine procedures. *Cochrane Database Syst Rev* 2007;3:CD005637.

218. **Flood JT, Grow DR.** Transcervical tubal cannulation: a review. *Obstet Gynecol Surv* 1993;48:768–776.

219. **Rimbach S, Bastert G, Wallwiener D.** Technical results of falloposcopy for infertility diagnosis in a large multicentre study. *Hum Reprod* 2001;16:925–930.

220. **Lanzani C, Savasi V, Leone FPG, et al.** Two-dimensional HyCoSy with contrast tuned imaging technology and a second-generation contrast media for the assessment of tubal patency in an infertility program. *Fertil Steril* 2009;92:1158–1161.

221. **Feinberg EC, Levens ED, DeCherney AH.** Infertility surgery is dead: only the obituary remains? *Fertil Steril* 2008;89:232–236.

222. **Phillips J, Cochavi S, Silberzweig JE.** Hysterosalpingography with use of mobile C-arm fluoroscopy. *Fertil Steril* 2010;93:2065–2068.

223. **Schippert C, Bassler C, Soergel P, et al.** Reconstructive, organ-preserving microsurgery in tubal infertility: still an alternative to *in vitro* fertilization. *Fertil Steril* 2010;93:1359–1361.

224. **Gomel V.** Reversal of tubal sterilization versus IVF in the era of assisted reproductive technology: a clinical dilemma. *Reprod Biomed Online* 2007;15:403–407.

225. **Dharia Patel SP, Steinkampf MP, Whitten SJ, et al.** Robotic tubal anastomosis: surgical technique and cost effectiveness. *Fertil Steril* 2008;90:1175–1179.

226. **Gordts S, Campo R, Puttemans P, et al.** Clinical factors determining pregnancy outcome after microsurgical tubal reanastomosis. *Fertil Steril* 2009;92:1198–1202.

227. **Camus E, Poncelet C, Goffinet F, et al.** Pregnancy rates after *in-vitro* fertilization in cases of tubal infertility with and without hydrosalpinx: a meta-analysis of published comparative studies. *Hum Reprod* 1999;14:1243–1249.

228. **Strandell A, Lindhard A, Waldenstrom U, et al.** Hydrosalpinx and IVF outcome: cumulative results after salpingectomy in a randomized controlled trial. *Hum Reprod* 2001;16:2403–2410.

229. **Strandell A, Lindhard A, Waldenstrom U, et al.** Hydrosalpinx and IVF outcome: a prospective, randomized multicentre trial in

Scandinavia on salpingectomy prior to IVF. *Hum Reprod* 1999;14:2762–2769.

230. **Johnson N, van Voorst S, Sowter MC, et al.** Surgical treatment for tubal disease in women due to undergo *in vitro* fertilisation. *Cochrane Database Syst Rev* 2010;1:CD002125.

231. **Brown SE, Coddington CC, Schnorr J, et al.** Evaluation of outpatient hysteroscopy, saline infusion hysterosonography, and hysterosalpingography in infertile women: a prospective, randomized study. *Fertil Steril* 2000;74:1029–1034.

232. **Roma Dalfo A, Ubeda B, Ubeda A, et al.** Diagnostic value of hysterosalpingography in the detection of intrauterine abnormalities: a comparison with hysteroscopy. *AJR Am J Roentgenol* 2004;183:1405–1409.

233. **Soares SR, Barbosa dos Reis MM, Camargos AF.** Diagnostic accuracy of sonohysterography, transvaginal sonography, and hysterosalpingography in patients with uterine cavity diseases. *Fertil Steril* 2000;73:406–411.

234. **Tur-Kaspa I, Gal M, Hartman M, et al.** A prospective evaluation of uterine abnormalities by saline infusion sonohysterography in 1,009 women with infertility or abnormal uterine bleeding. *Fertil Steril* 2006;86:1731–1735.

235. **Rackow BW, Arici A.** Reproductive performance of women with mullerian anomalies. *Curr Opin Obstet Gynecol* 2007;19:229–237.

236. **Pritts EA, Parker WH, Olive DL.** Fibroids and infertility: an updated systematic review of the evidence. *Fertil Steril* 2009;91:1215–1223.

237. **Di Spiezio Sardo A, Mazzon I, Bramante S, et al.** Hysteroscopic myomectomy: a comprehensive review of surgical techniques. *Hum Reprod Update* 2008;14:101–119.

238. **Moghadam R, Lathi RB, Shahmohamady B, et al.** Predictive value of magnetic resonance imaging in differentiating between leiomyoma and adenomyosis. *JSLS* 2006;10:216–219.

239. **Breech LL, Laufer MR.** Mullerian anomalies. *Obstet Gynecol Clin North Am* 2009;36:47–68.

240. **Valli E, Vaquero E, Lazzarin N, et al.** Hysteroscopic metroplasty improves gestational outcome in women with recurrent spontaneous abortion. *J Am Assoc Gynecol Laparosc* 2004;11:240–244.

241. **Luciano AA.** Myomectomy. *Clin Obstet Gynecol* 2009;52:362–371.

242. **Klatsky PC, Tran ND, Caughey AB, et al.** Fibroids and reproductive outcomes: a systematic literature review from conception to delivery. *Am J Obstet Gynecol* 2008;198:357–366.

243. **Sunkara SK, Khairy M, El-Toukhy T, et al.** The effect of intramural fibroids without uterine cavity involvement on the outcome of IVF treatment: a systematic review and meta-analysis. *Hum Reprod* 2010;25:418–429.

244. **Advincula AP, Xu X, Goudeau St, et al.** Robot-assisted laparoscopic myomectomy versus abdominal myomectomy: a comparison of short-term surgical outcomes and immediate costs. *J Minim Invasive Gynecol* 2007;14:698–705.

245. **Nezhat C, Lavie O, Hsu S, et al.** Robotic-assisted laparoscopic myomectomy compared with standard laparoscopic myomectomy—a retrospective matched control study. *Fertil Steril* 2009;91:556–559.

246. **Plotti G, Plotti F, Di Giovanni A, et al.** Feasibility and safety of vaginal myomectomy: a prospective pilot study. *J Minim Invasive Gynecol* 2008;15:166–171.

247. **Fatemi HM, Kasius JC, Timmermans A, et al.** Prevalence of unsuspected uterine cavity abnormalities diagnosed by office hysteroscopy prior to *in vitro* fertilization. *Hum Reprod* 2010;25:1959–1965.

248. **Karayalcin R, Ozcan S, Moraloglu O, et al.** Results of 2500 office-based diagnostic hysteroscopies before IVF. *Reprod Biomed Online* 2010;20:689–693.

249. **Lieng M, Istre O, Qvigstad E.** Treatment of endometrial polyps: a systematic review. *Acta Obstet Gynecol Scand* 2010;89:992–1002.

250. **Onalan R, Onalan G, Tonguc E, et al.** Body mass index is an independent risk factor for the development of endometrial polyps in patients undergoing *in vitro* fertilization. *Fertil Steril* 2009;91:1056–1060.

251. **Yanaihara A, Yorimitsu T, Motoyama H, et al.** Location of endometrial polyp and pregnancy rate in infertility patients. *Fertil Steril* 2008;90:180–182.

252. **Perez-Medina T, Bajo-Arenas J, Salazar F, et al.** Endometrial polyps and their implication in the pregnancy rates of patients undergoing intrauterine insemination: a prospective, randomized study. *Hum Reprod* 2005;20:1632–1635.

253. **Isikoglu M, Berkkanoglu M, Senturk Z, et al.** Endometrial polyps smaller than 1.5 cm do not affect ICSI outcome. *Reprod Biomed Online* 2006;12:199–204.

254. **Lass A, Williams G, Abusheikha N, et al.** The effect of endometrial polyps on outcomes of *in vitro* fertilization (IVF) cycles. *J Assist Reprod Genet* 1999;16:410–415.

255. **Robinson JK, Colimon LM, Isaacson KB.** Postoperative adhesiolysis therapy for intrauterine adhesions (Asherman's syndrome). *Fertil Steril* 2008;90:409–414.

256. **Sharma JB, Roy KK, Pushparaj M, et al.** Genital tuberculosis: an important cause of Asherman's syndrome in India. *Arch Gynecol Obstet* 2008;277:37–41.

257. **Roy KK, Baruah J, Sharma JB, et al.** Reproductive outcome following hysteroscopic adhesiolysis in patients with infertility due to Asherman's syndrome. *Arch Gynecol Obstet* 2010;281:355–361.

258. **Practice Committee of American Society for Reproductive Medicine in collaboration with Society for Reproductive Endocrinology and Infertility.** Progesterone supplementation during the luteal phase and in early pregnancy in the treatment of infertility: an educational bulletin. *Fertil Steril* 2008;90:S150–S153.

259. **Erdem A, Erdem M, Atmaca S, et al.** Impact of luteal phase support on pregnancy rates in intrauterine insemination cycles: a prospective randomized study. *Fertil Steril* 2009;91:2508–2513.

260. **Jones HW Jr.** Luteal-phase defect: the role of Georgeanna Seegar Jones. *Fertil Steril* 2008;90:e5–e7.

261. **Bukulmez O, Arici A.** Luteal phase defect: myth or reality. *Obstet Gynecol Clin North Am* 2004;31:727–744.

262. **Hubayter ZR, Muasher SJ.** Luteal supplementation in *in vitro* fertilization: more questions than answers. *Fertil Steril* 2008;89:749–758.

263. **Myers ER, Silva S, Barnhart K, et al.** Interobserver and intraobserver variability in the histological dating of the endometrium in fertile and infertile women. *Fertil Steril* 2004;82:1278–1282.

264. **Coutifaris C, Myers ER, Guzick DS, et al.** Histological dating of timed endometrial biopsy tissue is not related to fertility status. *Fertil Steril* 2004;82:1264–1272.

265. **Giudice LC.** Clinical practice. Endometriosis. *N Engl J Med* 2010;362:2389–2398.

266. **Bulletti C, Coccia ME, Battistoni S, et al.** Endometriosis and infertility. *J Assist Reprod Genet* 2010;27:441–447.

267. **Vercellini P, Somigliana E, Vigano P, et al.** Surgery for endometriosis-associated infertility: a pragmatic approach. *Hum Reprod* 2009;24:254–269.

268. **Kuivasaari P, Hippelainen M, Anttila M, et al.** Effect of endometriosis on IVF/ICSI outcome: stage III/IV endometriosis worsens cumulative pregnancy and live-born rates. *Hum Reprod* 2005;20:3130–3135.

269. **Parazzini F.** Ablation of lesions or no treatment in minimal-mild endometriosis in infertile women: a randomized trial. Gruppo Italiano per lo Studio dell'Endometriosi. *Hum Reprod* 1999;14:1332–1334.

270. **Marcoux S, Maheux R, Berube S.** Laparoscopic surgery in infertile women with minimal or mild endometriosis. Canadian Collaborative Group on Endometriosis. *N Engl J Med* 1997;337:217–222.

271. **Jacobson TZ, Duffy JM, Barlow D, et al.** Laparoscopic surgery for subfertility associated with endometriosis. *Cochrane Database Syst Rev* 2010;1:CD001398.

272. **Somigliana E, Arnoldi M, Benaglia L, et al.** IVF-ICSI outcome in women operated on for bilateral endometriomas. *Hum Reprod* 2008;23:1526–1530.

273. **Esinler I, Bozdag G, Aybar F, et al.** Outcome of *in vitro* fertilization/intracytoplasmic sperm injection after laparoscopic cystectomy for endometriomas. *Fertil Steril* 2006;85:1730–1735.

274. **Practice Committee of American Society for Reproductive Medicine in collaboration with Society of Reproductive Surgeons.** Pathogenesis, consequences, and control of peritoneal adhesions in gynecologic surgery. *Fertil Steril* 2008;90:S144–149.

275. **Ahmad G, Duffy JM, Farquhar C, et al.** Barrier agents for adhesion prevention after gynaecological surgery. *Cochrane Database Syst Rev* 2008;2:CD000475.

276. **Siristatidis C, Bhattacharya S.** Unexplained infertility: does it really exist? Does it matter? *Hum Reprod* 2007;22:2084–2087.

277. **Sauer R, Roussev R, Jeyendran RS, et al.** Prevalence of antiphospholipid antibodies among women experiencing unexplained

infertility and recurrent implantation failure. *Fertil Steril* 2010; 93:2441–2443.

278. **Practice Committee of American Society for Reproductive Medicine**. Anti-phospholipid antibodies do not affect IVF success. *Fertil Steril* 2008;90:S172–S173.

279. **Bellver J, Soares SR, Alvarez C, et al.** The role of thrombophilia and thyroid autoimmunity in unexplained infertility, implantation failure and recurrent spontaneous abortion. *Hum Reprod* 2008;23:278–284.

280. **Cline AM, Kutteh WH.** Is there a role of autoimmunity in implantation failure after *in-vitro* fertilization? *Curr Opin Obstet Gynecol* 2009;21:291–295.

281. **Kilic S, Tasdemir N, Yilmaz N, et al.** The effect of anti-thyroid antibodies on endometrial volume, embryo grade and IVF outcome. *Gynecol Endocrinol* 2008;24:649–655.

282. **Kallen CB, Arici A.** Immune testing in fertility practice: truth or deception? *Curr Opin Obstet Gynecol* 2003;15:225–231.

283. **Omu AE, al-Qattan F, Ismail AA, et al.** Relationship between unexplained infertility and human leukocyte antigens and expression of circulating autogeneic and allogeneic antisperm antibodies. *Clin Exp Obstet Gynecol* 1999;26:199–202.

284. **Edi-Osagie EC, Seif MW, Aplin JD, et al.** Characterizing the endometrium in unexplained and tubal factor infertility: a multiparametric investigation. *Fertil Steril* 2004;82:1379–1389.

285. **Gorini G, Milano F, Olliaro P, et al.** *Chlamydia trachomatis* infection in primary unexplained infertility. *Eur J Epidemiol* 1990;6:335–338.

286. **Gupta A, Gupta A, Gupta S, et al.** Correlation of mycoplasma with unexplained infertility. *Arch Gynecol Obstet* 2009;280:981–985.

287. **Grzesko J, Elias M, Maczynska B, et al.** Occurrence of *Mycoplasma genitalium* in fertile and infertile women. *Fertil Steril* 2009;91:2376–2380.

288. **Toth A, Lesser ML, Brooks C, et al.** Subsequent pregnancies among 161 couples treated for T-mycoplasma genital-tract infection. *N Engl J Med* 1983;308:505–507.

289. **Moore DE, Soules MR, Klein NA, et al.** Bacteria in the transfer catheter tip influence the live-birth rate after *in vitro* fertilization. *Fertil Steril* 2000;74:1118–1124.

290. **Lavy Y, Lev-Sagie A, Holtzer H, et al.** Should laparoscopy be a mandatory component of the infertility evaluation in infertile women with normal hysterosalpingogram or suspected unilateral distal tubal pathology? *Eur J Obstet Gynecol Reprod Biol* 2004;114:64–68.

291. **Cundiff G, Carr BR, Marshburn PB.** Infertile couples with a normal hysterosalpingogram. Reproductive outcome and its relationship to clinical and laparoscopic findings. *J Reprod Med* 1995;40:19–24.

292. **al-Badawi IA, Fluker MR, Bebbington MW.** Diagnostic laparoscopy in infertile women with normal hysterosalpingograms. *J Reprod Med* 1999;44:953–957.

293. **Shveiky D, Simon A, Gino H, et al.** Sibling oocyte submission to IVF and ICSI in unexplained infertility patients: a potential assay for gamete quality. *Reprod Biomed Online* 2006;12:371–374.

294. **Moayeri SE, Lee HC, Lathi RB, et al.** Laparoscopy in women with unexplained infertility: a cost-effectiveness analysis. *Fertil Steril* 2009;92:471–480.

295. **Csokmay JM, Frattarelli JL.** Basal ovarian cysts and clomiphene citrate ovulation induction cycles. *Obstet Gynecol* 2006;107:1292–1296.

296. **Akin JW, Shepard MK.** The effects of baseline ovarian cysts on cycle fecundity in controlled ovarian hyperstimulation. *Fertil Steril* 1993;59:453–455.

297. **Qublan HS, Amarin Z, Tahat YA, et al.** Ovarian cyst formation following GnRH agonist administration in IVF cycles: incidence and impact. *Hum Reprod* 2006;21:640–644.

298. **Penzias AS, Jones EE, Seifer DB, et al.** Baseline ovarian cysts do not affect clinical response to controlled ovarian hyperstimulation for *in vitro* fertilization. *Fertil Steril* 1992;57:1017–1021.

299. **Altinkaya SO, Talas BB, Gungor T, et al.** Treatment of clomiphene citrate-related ovarian cysts in a prospective randomized study. A single center experience. *J Obstet Gynaecol Res* 2009;35:940–945.

300. **Biljan MM, Mahutte NG, Dean N, et al.** Effects of pretreatment with an oral contraceptive on the time required to achieve pituitary suppression with gonadotropin-releasing hormone analogues

and on subsequent implantation and pregnancy rates. *Fertil Steril* 1998;70:1063–1069.

301. **Devroey P, Aboulghar M, Garcia-Velasco J, et al.** Improving the patient's experience of IVF/ICSI: a proposal for an ovarian stimulation protocol with GnRH antagonist co-treatment. *Hum Reprod* 2009;24:764–774.

302. **Guzick DS, Carson SA, Coutifaris C, et al.** Efficacy of superovulation and intrauterine insemination in the treatment of infertility. National Cooperative Reproductive Medicine Network. *N Engl J Med* 1999;340:177–183.

303. **Lainas T, Zorzovilis J, Petsas G, et al.** In a flexible antagonist protocol, earlier, criteria-based initiation of GnRH antagonist is associated with increased pregnancy rates in IVF. *Hum Reprod* 2005;20:2426–2433.

304. **Kolibianakis EM, Albano C, Camus M, et al.** Initiation of gonadotropin-releasing hormone antagonist on day 1 as compared to day 6 of stimulation: effect on hormonal levels and follicular development in *in vitro* fertilization cycles. *J Clin Endocrinol Metab* 2003;88:5632–5637.

305. **Baerwald AR, Walker RA, Pierson RA.** Growth rates of ovarian follicles during natural menstrual cycles, oral contraception cycles, and ovarian stimulation cycles. *Fertil Steril* 2009;91:440–449.

306. **Lass A.** Monitoring of *in vitro* fertilization-embryo transfer cycles by ultrasound versus by ultrasound and hormonal levels: a prospective, multicenter, randomized study. *Fertil Steril* 2003;80:80–85.

307. **Pinto F, Oliveira C, Cardoso MF, et al.** Impact of GnRH ovarian stimulation protocols on intracytoplasmic sperm injection outcomes. *Reprod Biol Endocrinol* 2009;7:5.

308. **de Jong D, Macklon NS, Eijkemans MJ, et al.** Dynamics of the development of multiple follicles during ovarian stimulation for *in vitro* fertilization using recombinant follicle-stimulating hormone (Puregon) and various doses of the gonadotropin-releasing hormone antagonist ganirelix (Orgalutran/Antagon). *Fertil Steril* 2001;75:688–693.

309. **Kwan I, Bhattacharya S, McNeil A, et al.** Monitoring of stimulated cycles in assisted reproduction (IVF and ICSI). *Cochrane Database Syst Rev* 2008;2:CD005289.

310. **Badawy A, Elnashar A, Totongy M.** Clomiphene citrate or aromatase inhibitors for superovulation in women with unexplained infertility undergoing intrauterine insemination: a prospective randomized trial. *Fertil Steril* 2009;92:1355–1359.

311. **Werbrouck E, Spiessens C, Meuleman C, et al.** No difference in cycle pregnancy rate and in cumulative live-birth rate between women with surgically treated minimal to mild endometriosis and women with unexplained infertility after controlled ovarian hyperstimulation and intrauterine insemination. *Fertil Steril* 2006;86:566–571.

312. **Tsafrir A, Simon A, Margalioth EJ, et al.** What should be the first-line treatment for unexplained infertility in women over 40 years of age—ovulation induction and IUI, or IVF? *Reprod Biomed Online* 2009;19(Suppl 4):4334.

313. **Reindollar RH, Regan MM, Neumann PJ, et al.** A randomized clinical trial to evaluate optimal treatment for unexplained infertility: the fast track and standard treatment (FASTT) trial. *Fertil Steril* 2010;94:888–899.

314. **Foong SC, Fleetham JA, O'Keane JA, et al.** A prospective randomized trial of conventional *in vitro* fertilization versus intracytoplasmic sperm injection in unexplained infertility. *J Assist Reprod Genet* 2006;23:137–140.

315. **Bhattacharya S, Hamilton MP, Shaaban M, et al.** Conventional *in-vitro* fertilisation versus intracytoplasmic sperm injection for the treatment of non-male-factor infertility: a randomised controlled trial. *Lancet* 2001;357:2075–2079.

316. **Toner JP.** Progress we can be proud of: U.S. trends in assisted reproduction over the first 20 years. *Fertil Steril* 2002;78:943–950.

317. **Huirne JA, Homburg R, Lambalk CB.** Are GnRH antagonists comparable to agonists for use in IVF? *Hum Reprod* 2007;22:2805–2813.

318. **Kadoch IJ, Al-Khaduri M, Phillips SJ, et al.** Spontaneous ovulation rate before oocyte retrieval in modified natural cycle IVF with and without indomethacin. *Reprod Biomed Online* 2008;16:245–249.

319. **Elnashar AM.** Progesterone rise on the day of HCG administration (premature luteinization) in IVF: an overdue update. *J Assist Reprod Genet* 2010;27:149–155.

320. **Bosch E, Labarta E, Crespo J, et al.** Circulating progesterone levels and ongoing pregnancy rates in controlled ovarian stimulation cycles for *in vitro* fertilization: analysis of over 4000 cycles. *Hum Reprod* 2010;25:2092–3100.

321. **Sonmezer M, Pelin Cil A, Atabekoglu C, et al.** Does premature luteinization or early surge of LH impair cycle outcome? Report of two successful outcomes. *J Assist Reprod Genet* 2009;26:159–163.

322. **Escudero EL, Boerrigter PJ, Bennink HJ, et al.** Mifepristone is an effective oral alternative for the prevention of premature luteinizing hormone surges and/or premature luteinization in women undergoing controlled ovarian hyperstimulation for *in vitro* fertilization. *J Clin Endocrinol Metab* 2005;90:2081–2088.

323. **Ortmann O, Weiss JM, Diedrich K.** Gonadotrophin-releasing hormone (GnRH) and GnRH agonists: mechanisms of action. *Reprod Biomed Online* 2002;5(Suppl 1):1–7.

324. **Reh A, Krey L, Noyes N.** Are gonadotropin-releasing hormone agonists losing popularity? Current trends at a large fertility center. *Fertil Steril* 2010;93:101–108.

325. **Tarlatzis BC, Fauser BC, Kolibianakis EM, et al.** GnRH antagonists in ovarian stimulation for IVF. *Hum Reprod Update* 2006;12:333–340.

326. **Filicori M, Cognigni GE, Samara A, et al.** The use of LH activity to drive folliculogenesis: exploring uncharted territories in ovulation induction. *Hum Reprod Update* 2002;8:543–557.

327. **Albuquerque LE, Saconato H, Maciel MC.** Depot versus daily administration of gonadotrophin releasing hormone agonist protocols for pituitary desensitization in assisted reproduction cycles. *Cochrane Database Syst Rev* 2005;1:CD002808.

328. **Pal L, Jindal S, Witt BR, et al.** Less is more: increased gonadotropin use for ovarian stimulation adversely influences clinical pregnancy and live birth after *in vitro* fertilization. *Fertil Steril* 2008;89:1694–1701.

329. **Verberg MF, Eijkemans MJ, Macklon NS, et al.** The clinical significance of the retrieval of a low number of oocytes following mild ovarian stimulation for IVF: a meta-analysis. *Hum Reprod Update* 2009;15:5–12.

330. **Al-Inany HG, Abou-Setta AM, Aboulghar M.** Gonadotrophin-releasing hormone antagonists for assisted conception: a Cochrane review. *Reprod Biomed Online* 2007;14:640–649.

331. **Griesinger G, Venetis CA, Marx T, et al.** Oral contraceptive pill pretreatment in ovarian stimulation with GnRH antagonists for IVF: a systematic review and meta-analysis. *Fertil Steril* 2008;90:1055–1063.

332. **Lainas TG, Sfontouris IA, Zorzovilis IZ, et al.** Flexible GnRH antagonist protocol versus GnRH agonist long protocol in patients with polycystic ovary syndrome treated for IVF: a prospective randomised controlled trial (RCT). *Hum Reprod* 2010;25:683–689.

333. **Bianchi P, Serafini P, da Rocha AM, et al.** Follicular waves in the human ovary: a new physiological paradigm for novel ovarian stimulation protocols. *Reprod Sci* 2010;17:1067–1076.

334. **Smitz J, Andersen AN, Devroey P, et al.** Endocrine profile in serum and follicular fluid differs after ovarian stimulation with HP-hMG or recombinant FSH in IVF patients. *Hum Reprod* 2007;22:676–687.

335. **Daya S.** Follicle-stimulating hormone and human menopausal gonadotrophin for ovarian stimulation in assisted reproduction cycles. *Cochrane Database Syst Rev* 2009;1.

336. **Coomarasamy A, Afnan M, Cheema D, et al.** Urinary hMG versus recombinant FSH for controlled ovarian hyperstimulation following an agonist long down-regulation protocol in IVF or ICSI treatment: a systematic review and meta-analysis. *Hum Reprod* 2008;23:310–315.

337. **Smulders B, van Oirschot SM, Farquhar C, et al.** Oral contraceptive pill, progestogen or estrogen pre-treatment for ovarian stimulation protocols for women undergoing assisted reproductive techniques. *Cochrane Database Syst Rev* 2010;1:CD006109.

338. **Damario MA, Barmat L, Liu HC, et al.** Dual suppression with oral contraceptives and gonadotrophin releasing-hormone agonists improves *in-vitro* fertilization outcome in high responder patients. *Hum Reprod* 1997;12:2359–2365.

339. **Dirckx K, Cabri P, Merien A, et al.** Does low-dose aspirin improve pregnancy rate in IVF/ICSI? A randomized double-blind placebo controlled trial. *Hum Reprod* 2009;24:856–860.

340. **Lambers MJ, Hoozemans DA, Schats R, et al.** Low-dose aspirin in non-tubal IVF patients with previous failed conception: a prospec-tive randomized double-blind placebo-controlled trial. *Fertil Steril* 2009;92:923–929.

341. **Boomsma CM, Macklon NS.** Does glucocorticoid therapy in the peri-implantation period have an impact on IVF outcomes? *Curr Opin Obstet Gynecol* 2008;20:249–256.

342. **Tso LO, Costello MF, Albuquerque LE, et al.** Metformin treatment before and during IVF or ICSI in women with polycystic ovary syndrome. *Cochrane Database Syst Rev* 2009;2:CD006105.

343. **Zhang M, Ouyang H, Xia G.** The signal pathway of gonadotrophins-induced mammalian oocyte meiotic resumption. *Mol Hum Reprod* 2009;15:399–409.

344. **Marteil G, Richard-Parpaillon L, Kubiak JZ.** Role of oocyte quality in meiotic maturation and embryonic development. *Reprod Biol* 2009;9:203–224.

345. **Mehlmann LM.** Stops and starts in mammalian oocytes: recent advances in understanding the regulation of meiotic arrest and oocyte maturation. *Reproduction* 2005;130:791–799.

346. **Stevenson TL, Lashen H.** Empty follicle syndrome: the reality of a controversial syndrome, a systematic review. *Fertil Steril* 2008;90:691–698.

347. **European Recombinant LH Study Group.** Human recombinant luteinizing hormone is as effective as, but safer than, urinary human chorionic gonadotropin in inducing final follicular maturation and ovulation in *in vitro* fertilization procedures: results of a multicenter double-blind study. *J Clin Endocrinol Metab* 2001;86:2607–2618.

348. **Ludwig M, Doody KJ, Doody KM.** Use of recombinant human chorionic gonadotropin in ovulation induction. *Fertil Steril* 2003;79:1051–1059.

349. **Tsoumpou I, Muglu J, Gelbaya TA, et al.** Symposium: update on prediction and management of OHSS. Optimal dose of HCG for final oocyte maturation in IVF cycles: absence of evidence? *Reprod Biomed Online* 2009;19:52–58.

350. **Al-Inany HG, Aboulghar M, Mansour R, et al.** Recombinant versus urinary human chorionic gonadotrophin for ovulation induction in assisted conception. *Cochrane Database Syst Rev* 2005;2:CD003719.

351. **Garcia-Velasco JA.** How to avoid ovarian hyperstimulation syndrome: a new indication for dopamine agonists. *Reprod Biomed Online* 2009;18(Suppl 2):71–75.

352. **Vlahos NF, Giannakikou I, Vlachos A, et al.** Analgesia and anesthesia for assisted reproductive technologies. *Int J Gynaecol Obstet* 2009;105:201–205.

353. **Mains L, Van Voorhis BJ.** Optimizing the technique of embryo transfer. *Fertil Steril* 2010;94:785–790.

354. **Tsai YC, Lin MY, Chen SH, et al.** Vaginal disinfection with povidone iodine immediately before oocyte retrieval is effective in preventing pelvic abscess formation without compromising the outcome of IVF-ET. *J Assist Reprod Genet* 2005;22:173–175.

355. **van Os HC, Roozenburg BJ, Janssen-Caspers HA, et al.** Vaginal disinfection with povidon iodine and the outcome of *in-vitro* fertilization. *Hum Reprod* 1992;7:349–350.

356. **Sohn SH, Penzias AS, Emmi AM, et al.** Administration of progesterone before oocyte retrieval negatively affects the implantation rate. *Fertil Steril* 1999;71:11–14.

357. **Williams SC, Oehninger S, Gibbons WE, et al.** Delaying the initiation of progesterone supplementation results in decreased pregnancy rates after *in vitro* fertilization: a randomized, prospective study. *Fertil Steril* 2001;76:1140–1143.

358. **Engmann L, DiLuigi A, Schmidt D, et al.** The effect of luteal phase vaginal estradiol supplementation on the success of *in vitro* fertilization treatment: a prospective randomized study. *Fertil Steril* 2008;89:554–561.

359. **Serna J, Cholquevilque JL, Cela V, et al.** Estradiol supplementation during the luteal phase of IVF-ICSI patients: a randomized, controlled trial. *Fertil Steril* 2008;90:2190–2195.

360. **Tournaye H.** Management of male infertility by assisted reproductive technologies. *Baillieres Best Pract Res Clin Endocrinol Metab* 2000;14:423–435.

361. **Gardner DK, Lane M, Stevens J, et al.** Blastocyst score affects implantation and pregnancy outcome: towards a single blastocyst transfer. *Fertil Steril* 2000;73:1155–1158.

362. **Papanikolaou EG, D'Haeseleer E, Verheyen G, et al.** Live birth rate is significantly higher after blastocyst transfer than after

cleavage-stage embryo transfer when at least four embryos are available on day 3 of embryo culture. A randomized prospective study. *Hum Reprod* 2005;20:3198–3203.

363. **Lane M, Gardner DK.** Embryo culture medium: which is the best? *Best Pract Res Clin Obstet Gynaecol* 2007;21:83–100.

364. **Blake DA, Farquhar CM, Johnson N, et al.** Cleavage stage versus blastocyst stage embryo transfer in assisted conception. *Cochrane Database Syst Rev* 2007;4:CD002118.

365. **Ambartsumyan G, Clark AT.** Aneuploidy and early human embryo development. *Hum Mol Genet* 2008;17:R10–R15.

366. **Bavister B.** Oxygen concentration and preimplantation development. *Reprod Biomed Online* 2004;9:484–486.

367. **Papanikolaou EG, Kolibianakis EM, Tournaye H, et al.** Live birth rates after transfer of equal number of blastocysts or cleavage-stage embryos in IVF. A systematic review and meta-analysis. *Hum Reprod* 2008;23:91–99.

368. **Papanikolaou EG, Camus M, Kolibianakis EM, et al.** *In vitro* fertilization with single blastocyst-stage versus single cleavage-stage embryos. *N Engl J Med* 2006;354:1139–1146.

369. **Papanikolaou EG, Fatemi H, Venetis C, et al.** Monozygotic twinning is not increased after single blastocyst transfer compared with single cleavage-stage embryo transfer. *Fertil Steril* 2010;93:592–597.

370. **Reh A, Fino E, Krey L, et al.** Optimizing embryo selection with day 5 transfer. *Fertil Steril* 2010;93:609–615.

371. **Practice Committee of the American Society for Reproductive Medicine; Practice Committee of the Society for Assisted Reproductive Technology.** Guidelines on number of embryos transferred. *Fertil Steril* 2009;92:1518–1519.

372. **Derks RS, Farquhar C, Mol BW, et al.** Techniques for preparation prior to embryo transfer. *Cochrane Database Syst Rev* 2009;4:CD007682.

373. **El-Toukhy T, Coomarasamy A, Khairy M, et al.** The relationship between endometrial thickness and outcome of medicated frozen embryo replacement cycles. *Fertil Steril* 2008;89:832–839.

374. **Kolibianakis EM, Venetis CA, Tarlatzis BC.** Cryopreservation of human embryos by vitrification or slow freezing: which one is better? *Curr Opin Obstet Gynecol* 2009;21:270–274.

375. **Wennerholm UB, Soderstrom-Anttila V, Bergh C, et al.** Children born after cryopreservation of embryos or oocytes: a systematic review of outcome data. *Hum Reprod* 2009;24:2158–2172.

376. **Urman B, Balaban B, Yakin K.** Impact of fresh-cycle variables on the implantation potential of cryopreserved-thawed human embryos. *Fertil Steril* 2007;87:310–315.

377. **Glujovsky D, Pesce R, Fiszbajn G, et al.** Endometrial preparation for women undergoing embryo transfer with frozen embryos or embryos derived from donor oocytes. *Cochrane Database Syst Rev* 2010;1:CD006359:

378. **Kumbak B, Oral E, Karlikaya G, et al.** Serum oestradiol and beta-HCG measurements after day 3 or 5 embryo transfers in interpreting pregnancy outcome. *Reprod Biomed Online* 2006;13:459–464.

379. **Van Voorhis BJ.** Outcomes from assisted reproductive technology. *Obstet Gynecol* 2006;107:183–200.

380. **Centers for Disease Control and Prevention.** 2007 Assisted reproductive technology success rates. Available online at: http://www.cdc.gov/art/ART2007/PDF/COMPLETE_2007_ART.pdf

381. **Banerjee P, Choi B, Shahine LK, et al.** Deep phenotyping to predict live birth outcomes in *in vitro* fertilization. *Proc Natl Acad Sci U S A* 2010;107:13570–13575.

382. **Ethics Committee of the American Society for Reproductive Medicine.** Fertility treatment when the prognosis is very poor or futile. *Fertil Steril* 2009;92:1194–1197.

383. **Marina S, Marina D, Marina F, et al.** Sharing motherhood: biological lesbian co-mothers, a new IVF indication. *Hum Reprod* 2010;25:938–941.

384. **Practice Committee of American Society for Reproductive Medicine; Practice Committee of Society for Assisted Reproductive Technology.** Ovarian tissue and oocyte cryopreservation. *Fertil Steril* 2008;90:S241–S246.

385. **Krieg SA, Henne MB, Westphal LM.** Obstetric outcomes in donor oocyte pregnancies compared with advanced maternal age in *in vitro* fertilization pregnancies. *Fertil Steril* 2008;90:65–70.

386. **Paulson RJ, Boostanfar R, Saadat P, et al.** Pregnancy in the sixth decade of life: obstetric outcomes in women of advanced reproductive age. *JAMA* 2002;288:2320–2323.

387. **Antinori S, Gholami GH, Versaci C, et al.** Obstetric and prenatal outcome in menopausal women: a 12-year clinical study. *Reprod Biomed Online* 2003;6:257–261.

388. **Ethics Committee of the American Society for Reproductive Medicine.** Financial compensation of oocyte donors. *Fertil Steril* 2007;88:305–309.

389. **Sharpe K, Karovitch AJ, Claman P, et al.** Transvaginal oocyte retrieval for *in vitro* fertilization complicated by ovarian abscess during pregnancy. *Fertil Steril* 2006;86:219.e11–e13.

390. **Evans MI, Kaufman MI, Urban AJ, et al.** Fetal reduction from twins to a singleton: a reasonable consideration? *Obstet Gynecol* 2004;104:102–109.

391. **Ulug U, Jozwiak EA, Mesut A, et al.** Survival rates during the first trimester of multiple gestations achieved by ICSI: a report of 1448 consecutive multiples. *Hum Reprod* 2004;19:360–364.

392. **Leondires MP, Ernst SD, Miller BT, et al.** Triplets: outcomes of expectant management versus multifetal reduction for 127 pregnancies. *Am J Obstet Gynecol* 2000;183:454–459.

393. **Brambati B, Tului L, Camurri L, et al.** First-trimester fetal reduction to a singleton infant or twins: outcome in relation to the final number and karyotyping before reduction by transabdominal chorionic villus sampling. *Am J Obstet Gynecol* 2004;191:2035–2040.

394. **Fernandez H, Gervaise A.** Ectopic pregnancies after infertility treatment: modern diagnosis and therapeutic strategy. *Hum Reprod Update* 2004;10:503–513.

395. **Barrenetxea G, Barinaga-Rementeria L, Lopez de Larruzea A, et al.** Heterotopic pregnancy: two cases and a comparative review. *Fertil Steril* 2007;87:417.e9–e15.

396. **Kamath MS, Aleyamma TK, Muthukumar K, et al.** A rare case report: ovarian heterotopic pregnancy after *in vitro* fertilization. *Fertil Steril* 2010;94:1910.e9–e11.

397. **Golan A, Weissman A.** Symposium: update on prediction and management of OHSS. A modern classification of OHSS. *Reprod Biomed Online* 2009;19:28–32.

398. **Practice Committee of American Society for Reproductive Medicine.** Ovarian hyperstimulation syndrome. *Fertil Steril* 2008;90:S188–S193.

399. **Papanikolaou EG, Tournaye H, Verpoest W, et al.** Early and late ovarian hyperstimulation syndrome: early pregnancy outcome and profile. *Hum Reprod* 2005;20:636–641.

400. **Delvigne A.** Symposium: update on prediction and management of OHSS. Epidemiology of OHSS. *Reprod Biomed Online* 2009;19:8–13.

401. **Humaidan P, Quartarolo J, Papanikolaou EG.** Preventing ovarian hyperstimulation syndrome: guidance for the clinician. *Fertil Steril* 2010;94:389–400.

402. **Aboulghar M.** Symposium: update on prediction and management of OHSS. Prevention of OHSS. *Reprod Biomed Online* 2009;19:33–42.

403. **Siristatidis CS, Maheshwari A, Bhattacharya S.** *In vitro* maturation in subfertile women with polycystic ovarian syndrome undergoing assisted reproduction. *Cochrane Database Syst Rev* 2009;1:CD006606.

404. **Brinton LA, Scoccia B, Moghissi KS, et al.** Breast cancer risk associated with ovulation-stimulating drugs. *Hum Reprod* 2004;19:2005–2013.

405. **Brinton LA, Lamb EJ, Moghissi KS, et al.** Ovarian cancer risk after the use of ovulation-stimulating drugs. *Obstet Gynecol* 2004;103:1194–1203.

406. **Silva Idos S, Wark PA, McCormack VA, et al.** Ovulation-stimulation drugs and cancer risks: a long-term follow-up of a British cohort. *Br J Cancer* 2009;100:1824–1831.

407. **Van den Broeck U, D'Hooghe T, Enzlin P, et al.** Predictors of psychological distress in patients starting IVF treatment: infertility-specific versus general psychological characteristics. *Hum Reprod* 2010;25:1471–1480.

408. **Domar AD, Smith K, Conboy L, et al.** A prospective investigation into the reasons why insured United States patients drop out of *in vitro* fertilization treatment. *Fertil Steril* 2010;94:1457–1459.

409. **Practice Committee of Society for Assisted Reproductive Technology; Practice Committee of American Society for Reproductive Medicine.** Preimplantation genetic testing: a Practice Committee opinion. *Fertil Steril* 2008;90:S136–S143.

410. **Simpson JL.** Preimplantation genetic diagnosis at 20 years. *Prenat Diagn* 2010;30:682–695.

411. **Munne S, Howles CM, Wells D.** The role of preimplantation genetic diagnosis in diagnosing embryo aneuploidy. *Curr Opin Obstet Gynecol* 2009;21:442–449.

412. **Schoolcraft WB, Katz-Jaffe MG, Stevens J, et al.** Preimplantation aneuploidy testing for infertile patients of advanced maternal age: a randomized prospective trial. *Fertil Steril* 2009;92:157–162.

413. **Hardarson T, Hanson C, Lundin K, et al.** Preimplantation genetic screening in women of advanced maternal age caused a decrease in clinical pregnancy rate: a randomized controlled trial. *Hum Reprod* 2008;23:2806–2812.

414. **Mersereau JE, Plunkett BA, Cedars MI.** Preimplantation genetic screening in older women: a cost-effectiveness analysis. *Fertil Steril* 2008;90:592–598.

415. **Garrisi JG, Colls P, Ferry KM, et al.** Effect of infertility, maternal age, and number of previous miscarriages on the outcome of preimplantation genetic diagnosis for idiopathic recurrent pregnancy loss. *Fertil Steril* 2009;92:288–295.

416. **Knopman JM, Papadopoulos EB, Grifo JA, et al.** Surviving childhood and reproductive-age malignancy: effects on fertility and future parenthood. *Lancet Oncol* 2010;11:490–498.

417. **Bisharah M, Tulandi T.** Laparoscopic preservation of ovarian function: an underused procedure. *Am J Obstet Gynecol* 2003;188:367–370.

418. **Dovey S, Sneeringer RM, Penzias AS.** Clomiphene citrate and intrauterine insemination: analysis of more than 4100 cycles. *Fertil Steril* 2008;90:2281–2286.

419. **Bedaiwy MA, Shokry M, Mousa N, et al.** Letrozole co-treatment in infertile women 40 years old and older receiving controlled ovarian stimulation and intrauterine insemination. *Fertil Steril* 2009;91:2501–2507.

420. **Serour G, Mansour R, Serour A, et al.** Analysis of 2386 consecutive cycles of *in vitro* fertilization or intracytoplasmic sperm injection using autologous oocytes in women aged 40 years and above. *Fertil Steril* 2010;94:1707–1712.

421. **Klipstein S, Regan M, Ryley DA, et al.** One last chance for pregnancy: a review of 2,705 *in vitro* fertilization cycles initiated in women age 40 years and above. *Fertil Steril* 2005;84:435–445.

422. **Costello MF.** Systematic review of the treatment of ovulatory infertility with clomiphene citrate and intrauterine insemination. *Aust N Z J Obstet Gynaecol* 2004;44:93–102.

423. **Malizia BA, Hacker MR, Penzias AS.** Cumulative live-birth rates after *in vitro* fertilization. *N Engl J Med* 2009;360:236–243.

33 Recurrent Pregnancy Loss

Ruth B. Lathi
Danny J. Schust

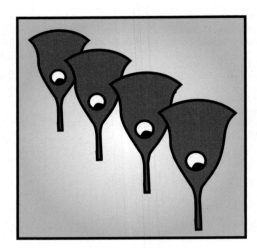

- Isolated spontaneous pregnancy loss is remarkably common. Recurrent pregnancy loss affects between 1 in 300 and 1 in 100 couples.

- After several pregnancy losses, there remains a greater chance of having a viable birth than another loss, even without treatment. Prognosis can improve dramatically with treatment of a known underlying etiology for recurrent pregnancy loss.

- Parental chromosomal abnormalities and the antiphospholipid syndrome (APS) are the only undisputed causes of recurrent pregnancy loss. Other well-described causes include anatomic, endocrine, thrombotic, and possibly other immunologic factors.

- The state of coagulability is a fine balance between pro- and antithrombotic pathways. The hypercoagulability of pregnancy can be attributed to increases in prothrombotic factors and decreases in those that inhibit coagulation.

- The immunologic interactions at the maternal–fetal interface reflect the presence of unique cellular constituents combined with the actions of steroid hormones, protein hormones, and metabolic factors.

- Evaluation of patients with recurrent pregnancy loss should include a detailed patient and family history, an examination focused on endocrine and anatomic abnormalities, and laboratory studies limited to evaluation of treatable etiologies.

- Monitoring early pregnancies in recurrent pregnancy loss patients should include ultrasound, β-human chorionic gonadotropin levels if indicated, frequent visits with psychological support, and the karyotypic analysis of tissues from any pregnancy losses.

- In treating recurrent pregnancy loss, evidence supports repairing anatomic abnormalities, correcting preexisting endocrine disorders, and treating APS and other thrombophilic disorders.

Advances in the ability to document and diagnose early pregnancy reveal that spontaneous pregnancy loss is a common event. **Spontaneous pregnancy loss is, in fact, the most common complication of pregnancy. Approximately 70% of human conceptions fail to achieve viability, and an estimated 50% are lost before the first missed menstrual period** (1). **Most of these pregnancy losses are unrecognized. Studies using sensitive assays for human chorionic gonadotropin (hCG) indicate that the actual rate of pregnancy loss after implantation is 31%** (2). **Loss occurs in 15% of pregnancies that are clinically recognized before 20 weeks of gestation from last menstrual period** (3,4).

Traditionally, recurrent abortion has been defined as the occurrence of three or more clinically recognized pregnancy losses before 20 weeks from the last menstrual period. Using this definition, recurrent pregnancy loss occurs in approximately 1 in 300 pregnancies (2). Clinical investigation of pregnancy loss, however, may be initiated after two consecutive spontaneous abortions, especially when fetal heart activity is identified before any of the pregnancy losses, when the women is older than 35 years of age, or when the couple has had difficulty conceiving (5). A study of over 1,000 patients with recurrent pregnancy loss reported no difference in the prevalence of abnormal results for evidence-based and investigative diagnostic tests when the diagnostic workup was initiated after two versus three or more losses (6). If clinical intervention is undertaken in the form of investigation after two spontaneous abortions, approximately 1% of pregnant women will require evaluation (3). Even with a history of recurrent pregnancy loss, a patient is more likely to carry her next pregnancy successfully to term than to miscarry. **For patients with a history of recurrent pregnancy loss, the risk of subsequent pregnancy loss is estimated to be 24% after two clinically recognized losses, 30% after three losses, and 40% to 50% after four losses** (7). These data make clinical study of recurrent pregnancy loss and its treatment difficult because very large groups of patients must be studied to demonstrate the effects of any proposed therapeutic intervention.

Etiology

Parental chromosomal abnormalities and thrombotic complications of the antiphospholipid antibody syndrome (APS) are the only undisputed causes of recurrent abortion. However, collectively these abnormalities account for less than 10% to 15% of recurrent pregnancy losses. Although the exact proportion of patients diagnosed with a particular abnormality may vary among the populations studied, other associations have been made with anatomic abnormalities (12%–16%), endocrine problems (17%–20%), infections (0.5%–5%), and immunologic factors, including those associated with the APS (20%–50%). Other miscellaneous factors have been implicated and account for approximately 10% of cases. Among women aged 35 or greater who experience recurrent pregnancy loss, spontaneous fetal chromosomal abnormalities are likely to be responsible for the vast majority of losses (8). Even after a thorough evaluation, the potential cause remains unexplained in about one-third to one-half of all cases of recurrent loss (Table 33.1) (3,6,9).

The timing of fetal demise provides etiologic clues and its documentation is important in investigations into causes and treatments for recurrent pregnancy loss. The vast majority of preclinical and early clinical pregnancy losses are the result of *de novo* fetal aneuploidy (10). This is also thought to be the cause of anembryonic pregnancy losses, whereas pregnancy losses occurring after 10 weeks of fetal development are much less likely to derive from fetal aneuploidy. Pregnancy losses resulting from *de novo* fetal aneuploidy, whether early and undocumented or documented through evaluation of chromosomal content in fetal tissues, cloud the results of many published studies. Their presence or absence must be documented in all investigations on recurrent pregnancy loss patients and their potential as a confounding factor discussed. The timing of fetal demise and tissue chromosomal analysis of any collected fetal tissues should be carefully weighed when diagnostic and therapeutic investigations into causes of recurrent pregnancy loss are being considered.

Genetic Factors

The most common inborn parental chromosomal abnormalities contributing to recurrent abortion are balanced translocations (11–14), in which one parent carries an overall normal gene content, but has a piece of one chromosome inappropriately attached to another.

Table 33.1 Proposed Etiologies for Recurrent Spontaneous Abortion	
Etiology	*Proposed Incidence*
Genetic factors	3.5%–5%
1. Chromosomal	
2. Single gene defects	
3. Multifactorial	
Anatomic factors	12%–16%
1. Congenital	
a. incomplete Müllerian fusion or septum resorption	
b. *Diethylstilbestrol* exposure	
c. uterine artery anomalies	
d. cervical incompetence	
2. Acquired	
a. cervical incompetence	
b. synechiae	
c. leiomyomas	
d. adenomyosis	
Endocrine factors	17%–20%
1. Luteal phase insufficiency	
2. Polycystic ovarian syndrome, including insulin resistance and hyperandrogenism	
3. Other androgen disorders	
4. Diabetes mellitus	
5. Thyroid disorders	
6. Prolactin disorders	
Infectious factors	0.5%–5%
1. Bacteria	
2. Viruses	
3. Parasites	
4. Zoonotic	
5. Fungal	
Immunologic factors	20%–50%
1. Cellular mechanisms	
a. Suppressor cell or factor deficiency	
b. Alterations in major histocompatibility antigen expression	
c. Alterations in cellular immune regulation	
1. TH1 immune responses to reproductive antigens (embryo or trophoblast)	
2. TH2 cytokine or growth factor deficiency	

(Continued)

Table 33.1 (*Continued*)	
Etiology	*Proposed Incidence*
3. Hormonal-progesterone, estrogen, prolactin, androgen alterations	
4. *Tryptophan* metabolism	
2. Humoral mechanisms	
a. Antiphospholipid antibodies	
b. Antithyroid antibodies	
c. Antisperm antibodies	
d. Antitrophoblast antibodies	
e. Blocking antibody deficiency	
Thrombotic factors	? incidence
1. Heritable thrombophilias	
a. Single gene defects (*f*VL, MTHFR, factor deficiencies)	
b. Antibody mediated thromboses (APS, anti-β2G1)	Most are included among other categories (e.g., immune, genetic)
Other factors	10%
1. Altered uterine receptivity (integrins, adhesion molecules)	
2. Environmental	
a. Toxins	
b. Illicit drugs	
c. Cigarettes and caffeine	
3. Placental abnormalities (circumvallate, marginate)	
4. Maternal medical illnesses (cardiac, renal hematologic)	
5. Male factors	
6. Exercise	
7. Dyssynchronous fertilization	

TH, T helper; MTHFR, methylene tetrahydrofolate reductase; APS, antiphospholipid antibody syndrome.

Depending on the nature of the translocation (reciprocal or Robertsonian), the gametes produced by the translocation carrier will be normal (reciprocal only), balanced, or unbalanced for the translocated DNA. When fertilized by a chromosomally normal gamete, the resulting embryos may be chromosomally normal (reciprocal only) or may be balanced or unbalanced carriers of the translocation. Most gametes and embryos with abnormal chromosomal status will not survive. Of those that do, live offspring will either be carriers of a balanced translocation or, for Robertsonian translocations, be monosomic or trisomic for the translocated chromosomal DNA.

Among the possible chromosomal monosomies, only that of the X chromosome typically permits viable offspring. On careful examination, however, many of these offspring may, in fact, exhibit mosaicism. Embryonic chromosomal monosomy may be particularly prevalent among patients with histories of recurrent pregnancy loss who are undergoing *in vitro* fertilization (IVF) (15). Compared with monosomies, chromosomal trisomies (e.g., trisomy 13, 18, and 21) appear to be tolerated a bit more readily, although mosaicism also may be implicated with these abnormalities.

Neither family history alone nor a history of prior term births is sufficient to rule out a potential parental chromosomal abnormality. Whereas the frequency of detecting a parental chromosomal abnormality is inversely related to the number of previous spontaneous losses, the chance of detecting a parental chromosomal abnormality is increased among couples who have never experienced a live birth (13). Abnormalities also may be detected upon parental karyotype analysis of some couples with a history of spontaneous abortions interspersed with stillbirths and live births (with or without congenital anomalies). Ultimately the use of parental karyotyping as a screening modality to evaluate the structural chromosomal etiologies of recurrent pregnancy loss may become insufficient. Evidence now suggests that, in some cases, paternal chromosomal abnormalities may be isolated within a particular fertilizing spermatozoon (16,17). Aneuploid spermatozoa may be particularly motile (18). **Other structural chromosome anomalies, such as inversions and insertions, may also contribute to recurrent abortion, as can chromosomal mosaicism and single gene defects.** X-linked disorders uncommonly result in recurrent abortion of male rather than female offspring (19).

Thrombophilias

There is a great deal of interest in the role of inherited thrombophilias in recurrent pregnancy loss (20–22). This heterogeneous group of disorders increases venous or arterial thrombosis. Their associations with pregnancy loss remains controversial and is attributed to hypothetical alterations in placental growth and development, particularly to alterations in placental vascular development (23–28). Abnormal placental vascularization and inappropriate placental thrombosis would link these thrombophilic states to pregnancy loss. Although some thrombophilic states may be acquired, most are heritable. Those heritable thrombophilias most often linked with reference to recurrent pregnancy loss include activated protein C resistance associated with mutations in factor V, deficiencies in proteins C and S, mutations in prothrombin, and mutations in antithrombin III.

Like spontaneous pregnancy loss, inherited and combined inherited or acquired thrombophilias are also surprisingly common. Greater than 15% of whites carry an inherited thrombophilic mutation (21). **The most common of these are the factor V Leiden mutation, a mutation in the promoter region of the prothrombin gene and mutations in the gene encoding methylene tetrahydrofolate reductase (*MTHFR*).** These disorders are present in their heterozygous state in approximately 5%, 2% to 3%, and 11% to 15% of healthy white populations, respectively (22,29–31). These common mutations are associated with mild thrombotic risks. It remains controversial whether homozygous *MTHFR* mutations are associated with vascular disease at all (32). **In contrast, more severe thrombophilic deficiencies, such as those of antithrombin and of protein S, are much less common in the general population.** These epidemiologic data support the hypothesis that a selective genetic advantage may accompany carriage of common heritable thrombophilias. To this point, women with activated protein C resistance because of the factor V Leiden mutation have reduced blood loss at delivery and factor V Leiden carriage is reported to improve pregnancy rates in intracytoplasmic sperm injection or IVF, suggesting a positive role in implantation (33,34). It is important to note that the above epidemiology of factor V Leiden mutations is specific to white populations. Factor V Leiden and prothrombin gene mutations are rare in African and Asian populations, despite similar incidence of venous thromboembolic events (35–38). Protein C, protein S, and antithrombin mutations are the most important risk factors for venous thromboembolic events among many Chinese and other Asian populations (39). These ethnographic differences are important considerations when faced with decisions concerning diagnostic testing in patients with a history of recurrent fetal loss.

The proposed mechanistic basis for the association between adverse fetal outcomes and heritable thrombophilias has focused on impaired placental development and function, secondary to venous and/or arterial thrombosis at the maternal–fetal interface. These findings have been noted in the placentas of women with adverse fetal outcomes and known inherited thrombophilias and have been demonstrated in patients with similar outcomes, but lacking inherited thrombophilic risk (40–44). Discussions of placental thrombosis as causal in early pregnancy losses (<10 weeks gestation) are particularly contentious, citing an elegant series of experiments demonstrating that maternal blood flow into the intervillous spaces of the human placenta does not occur until approximately 10 weeks of gestation (45–48). Prior to establishment of intervillous circulation, nutrient transfer from maternal blood to fetal tissues appears to be dependent on transudation that, in turn, relies on flow through the uterine vasculature. This suggests that maternal or fetal thrombotic episodes in the developing placental vasculature could be equally devastating prior to or after the establishment of intervillous circulation near 10 weeks of gestation. Very early pregnancy losses (biochemical, anembryonic) and known aneuploid fetal losses are unlikely to be altered by the presence of, or treatment for, an underlying thrombophilic state.

The coagulation system relies on a complex cascade of prothrombotic enzymatic activations (often via serine proteases) in delicate balance with antithrombotic pathways. Although pregnancy is most simply described as prothrombotic, the alterations in the coagulation system associated with pregnancy may be described as a state of compensated disseminated intravascular coagulation (DIC) (49). Human hemochorial placentation is unique and inherently unstable. Placental development involves invasion into the maternal decidua and its vasculature and requires precise control of hemostasis and fibrinolysis. Delicate control mechanisms exist locally within the placenta and globally within the pregnant woman (50). Hormonal and related physiologic changes characteristic of pregnancy affect important components of the clotting cascade, the fibrinolytic cascade, and platelet physiology.

Clot formation can be initiated through two pathways, called the extrinsic and intrinsic clotting cascades (Fig. 33.1). **Both respond to blood vessel damage and the release of tissue factor (TF).** Tissue factor is a glycoprotein expressed on the surface of cells surrounding blood vessels. It is not expressed on the endothelium of the blood vessel itself, so exposure of blood to TF is a sensitive indicator of vascular damage. The extrinsic clotting cascade begins with the interaction of newly released TF with factor VII of the clotting cascade. The complex formed by TF and factor VII can either activate factor X directly or activate factor X via the intrinsic pathway. In the intrinsic pathway, the TF/factor VII complex activates factor IX to factor IXa (activated factor IX). Factor IXa then complexes with factor VIIIa. In combination, factors

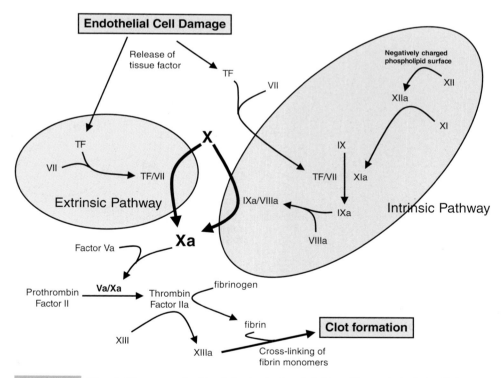

Figure 33.1   The clotting cascade. Physiologic clotting is initiated by endothelial cell damage or abnormal exposure of negatively charged phospholipids to serum and blood components. Procoagulant pathways in black are part of the clotting cascade and are prothrombotic. Both lead to activation of cascades of proteolytic enzymes and cleavage of clotting factors. The extrinsic and intrinsic pathways are initiated by distinct mechanisms. They merge at the activation of factor X to form the common pathway. For all coagulation factors, the subscript letter "a" denotes the activated form of the factor.

IXa and VIIIa activate factor X. Activation of factor XII after binding to negatively charged surfaces can also initiate the intrinsic pathway. Via this route, activated factor XII cleaves factor XI, generating factor XIa. Factor XIa can act as an alternate activator of factor IX. Extrinsic and intrinsic clotting cascades converge in the activation of factor X to factor Xa. Activated factor X (Xa) catalyzes the conversion of prothrombin (factor II) to thrombin (factor IIa). This conversion depends on the presence of activated factor V, which is factor Va. Thrombin, in turn, converts fibrinogen to fibrin, an essential building block for stable clot formation. Thrombin also activates factor XIII, which, in turn, crosslinks fibrin monomers and thereby stabilizes the fibrin clot.

To avoid uncontrolled thrombosis in response to tissue damage or alternate activation of the coagulation cascade, a number of antithrombotic control mechanisms are activated in conjunction with clot formation (Fig. 33.2). Important to this discussion are antithrombin (formerly antithrombin III), protein C, and protein S. Proteins C and S are vitamin K–dependent factors that are activated upon clot formation. Activation is initiated by complexes of thrombomodulin and thrombin at sites of endothelial damage. Complexes of activated protein C and S inactivate factors Va and VIIIa, thereby inhibiting their associated procoagulant activities. Antithrombin is a serine protease inhibitor that binds irreversibly to serine proteases. Proteases that bind antithrombin include factors IXa, Xa, XIa, and XIIa. Antithrombin also accelerates dissociation of factor VIIa/tissue factor complexes, thereby inhibiting intrinsic and extrinsic clotting pathways at their points of initiation. Finally, as its name suggests, antithrombin binds

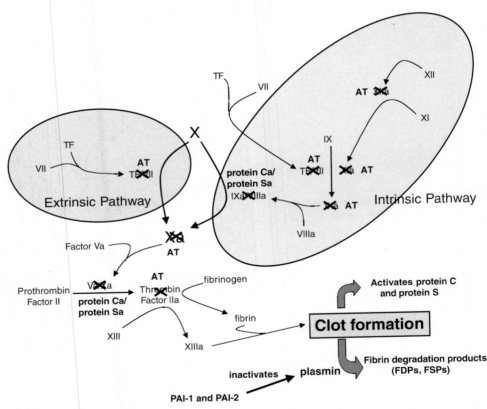

Figure 33.2 Physiologic mechanisms that counteract the clotting cascade. The procoagulant cascade is inhibited by several physiologic mechanisms. The balance between pro- and antithrombotic pathways determines the state of coagulability. Antithrombotic mechanisms include the action of antithrombin (AT) and of proteins C and S. The sites of inhibition by these substances are depicted by an "X." Plasminogen activator inhibitors-1 and -2 (PAI-1 and PAI-2) indirectly inactivate plasmin. Plasmin plays an important role in the dissolution of coagulated blood. For all coagulation factors, the subscript letter "a" denotes the activated form of the factor. FSP, fibrin split products; FDP, fibrin degradation products.

to and inhibits thrombin (factor IIa). Fibrinolysis also acts to delimit uncontrolled coagulation (Fig. 33.3). Mechanisms for fibrinolysis include cleavage of the fibrin clot by plasmin and the formation of fibrin degradation products (FDPs; or fibrin split products [FSPs]). Plasmin activity is, in turn, controlled by plasminogen activator inhibitors (e.g., PAI-1).

Prothrombotic changes associated with pregnancy include increases in the amounts and/or activities of factors in the clotting cascade and decreases in those counteracting clotting. The former includes pregnancy-associated elevations in factors VII, VIII, X, XII, von Willebrand's factor, and fibrinogen levels (49,51,52). All rise throughout gestation. Factor II, factor V, and factor XIII levels also rise early in pregnancy, but return to normal levels after the first trimester (49,53). Normal pregnancy has been associated with the development of activated protein C resistance (acquired APCR, see below) via mechanisms that remain unclear (54). Changes in balancing antithrombotic control mechanisms during pregnancy also favor clot formation. The activities of protein C and antithrombin remain fairly constant during the course of pregnancy. Protein S activity significantly decreases in conjunction with pregnancy-induced increases in the production of C4b-binding protein, a complement factor-binding protein that complexes with protein S, making it unavailable for interaction with activated protein C. This increased binding does not fully explain the level of decrease in protein S activity during pregnancy (55).

Fibrinolysis is impaired during pregnancy, with decreases in fibrinolytic activity beginning at approximately 11 to 15 weeks of gestation (49). A significant factor in this impairment is a marked decrease in plasmin activity, resulting from placental production of the plasmin inhibitor PAI-2 (56,57). In conjunction with these changes, however, FDP levels are seen to rise in pregnancy, beginning at approximately 20 weeks of gestation, and continue their rise

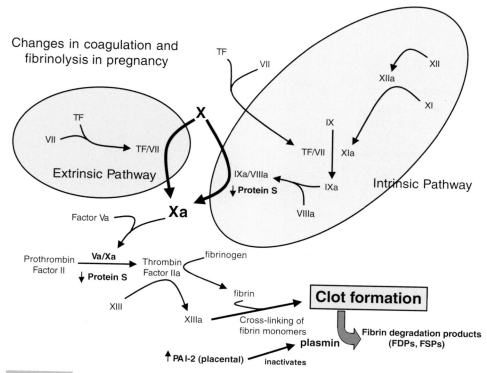

Figure 33.3 **Alterations coagulation and fibrinolysis during normal pregnancy.** Pregnancy is a state of hypercoagulability. Levels of factors VII, VIII, X, and XII are elevated throughout pregnancy, levels of factors II, V, and XIII rise in the first trimester, then return to normal values. The antithrombotic activity mediated by protein S decreases in pregnancy. The placenta produces plasminogen activator inhibitor-2 (PAI-2). For all coagulation factors, the subscript letter "a" denotes the activated form of the factor. FSP, fibrin split products; FDP, fibrin degradation products.

throughout pregnancy (49,56). In normal pregnancy, platelet function and turnover is unchanged. In the third trimester, platelet number typically decreases as the result of increased platelet consumption. This benign gestational thrombocytopenia can reach levels less than $80 \times 10^9/L$ (58). Taken together, pregnancy-associated alterations in the amounts and activities of prothrombotic clotting factors, anticoagulant control mechanisms, and fibrinolysis support the determination of human pregnancy as a state of compensated DIC. Although these changes reverse during the 4 to 6 weeks following delivery, **the vascular damage associated with delivery is an additional significant risk factor for thrombosis, making the immediate postpartum period an important continuation of the prothrombotic state associated with pregnancy** (49,58).

Circulating homocysteine is derived from dietary methionine. Homocysteine, in turn, is metabolized either into cystathionine or back into methionine (Fig. 33.4). The latter process involves the enzyme methionine synthase. Methionine synthase requires donation of a methyl group from 5-methyltetrahydrofolate to produce methionine, and the enzyme *MTHFR* is involved in the production of 5-methyltetrahydrofolate from dietary folate sources (20). The nutritional supplements folic acid, vitamins B_2, B_6, and vitamin B_{12} are all required for proper metabolism of homocysteine; therefore, their deficiency is associated with acquired elevations in circulating homocysteine levels (21,29,59). Although heritable deficiencies in the enzymes required for metabolism of homocysteine have been described for the pathways leading to cystathionine

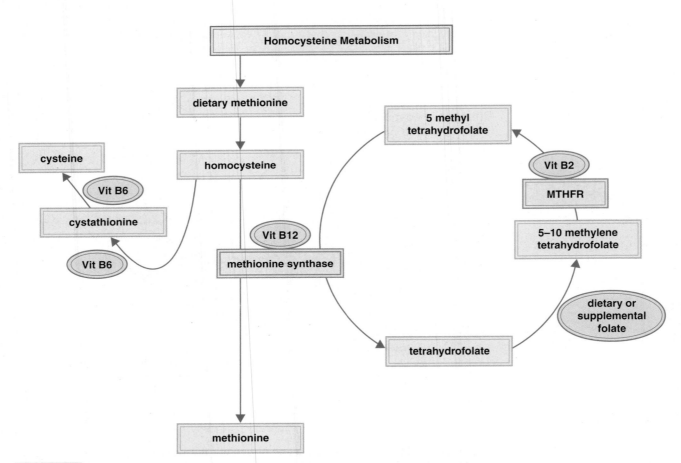

Figure 33.4 **Homocysteine metabolism.** Dietary methionine is metabolized either to cysteine or back into methionine. Homocysteine, a prothrombotic metabolite, is an intermediate in this process. Conversion of homocysteine to methionine requires transfer of a methyl group from 5-methyltetrahydrofolate. The conversion of folate to 5-methyltetrahydrofolate is a multistep process requiring vitamin B_2 as a cofactor for the enzyme, *methylene tetrahydrofolate reductase (MTHFR)*. Vitamin B_{12} is a required cofactor for the enzyme methionine synthase. Vitamin B_6 is also required for metabolism of sulfur containing amino acids such as *methionine*.

formation and those involved in reconversion to methionine, mutations in *MTHFR* have received the most attention (20,59–61). Point mutations in *MTHFR* are surprisingly common, are associated with hyperhomocysteinemia, and are linked to thrombosis (22,29,59–61).

Those heritable thrombophilias most often linked to recurrent pregnancy loss include hyperhomocysteinemia, activated protein C resistance associated with mutations in factor V, deficiencies in proteins C and S, mutations in prothrombin, and mutations in antithrombin. These inherited disorders are mainly autosomal dominant and display a wide variation in prevalence and in the severity of morbidity associated with gene carriage. The latter two characteristics have direct reciprocal correlations in white populations. **In agreement with general thrombotic risk data, carriage of combinations of two or more inherited thrombophilic defects has particularly strong association with adverse pregnancy outcome** (22,24,30,62). Acquired thrombophilias associated with recurrent pregnancy loss include hyperhomocysteinemia and activated protein C resistance. The vast majority of the data linking thrombophilic states to recurrent fetal loss consist of small- to moderate-sized prevalence studies (62–70). Recent attempts to pool these data into meta-analyses have led to more informed recommendations on the testing of patients presenting with recurrent pregnancy loss (71–73). Taken together, these studies suggest that testing for the factor V Leiden mutation, protein S levels, prothrombin promoter mutations, homocysteine levels, and global activated protein C resistance is of use in white patients with a history of repetitive first or second trimester losses. These recommendations do not apply to patients who are nonwhite. Data directly linking hyperhomocysteinemia, folic acid, vitamin B_{12}, and *MTHFR* mutations to recurrent pregnancy loss have been contradictory (41,43,60–62,65,66,68). Studies have evaluated pooled data from previous investigations (one via meta-analysis) and show these disorders to be linked to risk for recurrent pregnancy loss (72).

Anatomic Abnormalities

Anatomic abnormalities of both the uterine cervix and the uterine body have been associated with recurrent pregnancy loss (74,75). These anatomic causes may be either congenital or acquired. During development, the uterus forms via the apposition of a portion of bilateral hollow tubes called the müllerian ducts. The dissolution of the walls of these ducts along their site of apposition allows formation of the intrauterine cavity, the intracervical canal, and the upper vagina. Congenital uterine anomalies may, therefore, include incomplete müllerian duct fusion, incomplete septum resorption, and uterine cervical anomalies. Although the causes underlying many of the congenital anomalies of the female reproductive tract are unclear, it has been well documented that prenatal exposure to maternally ingested *diethylstilbestrol* (*DES*) results in complex congenital uterine, cervical, and vaginal changes.

Historically, all congenital reproductive tract abnormalities have been linked to both isolated spontaneous pregnancy loss and to recurrent pregnancy loss, although the presence of an intrauterine septum and prenatal exposure to DES demonstrate the strongest associations (76–78). Women with an intrauterine septum may have as high as a 60% risk for spontaneous abortion (79). Uterine septum–related losses most frequently occur during the second trimester (80). However, if an embryo implants into the poorly developed endometrium overlying the uterine septum, abnormal placentation and resultant first trimester losses may occur (81). The most common uterine congenital anomaly associated with *in utero DES* exposure is hypoplasia, which may contribute to first- or second-trimester spontaneous abortions, incompetent cervix, and premature labor (82,83). Congenital anomalies of the uterine arteries also may contribute to pregnancy loss via adverse alterations in blood flow to the implanted blastocyst and developing placenta (84).

Acquired anatomic anomalies have likewise been linked to both isolated and recurrent pregnancy losses. These abnormalities include such disparate conditions as intrauterine adhesions, uterine fibroids, and endometrial polyps. Endometrium that develops over an intrauterine synechiae or over a fibroid that impinges in the intrauterine cavity (submucous) may be inadequately vascularized (85). This may promote abnormal placentation for any embryo attempting to implant over such lesions. Although data supporting these concepts are limited, this abnormal placentation may lead to spontaneous pregnancy loss. Less clear is the association between intramural fibroids and recurrent pregnancy loss, but it is suggested that large (>5 cm) intramural fibroids are associated with pregnancy loss and that removal improves outcomes (78,86) (see Chapter 15) .

Endocrine Abnormalities

The endocrinology of normal pregnancy is complex. **Because spontaneous pregnancy is critically dependent on appropriately timed endocrinologic changes of the menstrual cycle, it is not surprising that those endocrine abnormalities that ultimately alter pregnancy maintenance may mediate their effects during the follicular phase of the cycle in which conception occurs, or even earlier.** Modifications in follicular development and ovulation, in turn, may be reflected in abnormalities of blastocyst transport and development, alterations in uterine receptivity to the implanting blastocyst, and improper functioning of the corpus luteum. **Beginning with ovulation and lasting until approximately 7 to 9 weeks of gestation, maintenance of early pregnancy depends on the production of progesterone by the corpus luteum. Normal pregnancies are characterized by a luteal–placental shift at about 7 to 9 weeks gestation, during which the developing placental trophoblast cells take over progesterone production and pregnancy maintenance** (87). Spontaneous pregnancy losses occurring before 10 weeks of gestation may result from a number of alterations in normal progesterone production or utilization. These include failure of the corpus luteum to produce sufficient quantities of progesterone, impaired delivery of progesterone to the uterus, or inappropriate utilization of progesterone by the uterine decidua. Pregnancy failures may also occur near the time of the expected luteal–placental shift if the trophoblast is unable to produce biologically active progesterone following demise of the corpus luteum.

Endocrinologic factors associated with recurrent abortion include luteal phase insufficiency, diabetes mellitus, hypersecretion of luteinizing hormone (LH), thyroid disease, and, potentially, insulin resistance and polycystic ovarian syndrome, hyperprolactinemia and decreased ovarian reserve. Luteal phase insufficiency or luteal phase defects (LPD) are characterized by inadequate luteal milestones and most likely relate to adverse pregnancy outcome via inadequate or improperly timed endometrial development at potential implantation sites. An elegant description of abnormalities at the site of implantation, which may be responsible for some cases of recurrent pregnancy loss, describes impaired decidualization of the endometrium as a mechanism for natural selection of human embryos (88). LPD has many causes, some of which are associated with hypersecretion of luteinizing hormone. Although the mechanism underlying the association of elevated LH levels with recurrent pregnancy loss is incompletely understood, abnormal LH secretion may have direct effects on the developing oocyte (premature aging), on the endometrium (dyssynchronous maturation), or both. Many patients with elevated LH levels also display physical, endocrinologic, and metabolic characteristics of polycystic ovarian syndrome (PCOS). **Some studies report ovarian radiologic evidence of PCOS in as many as 40% to 80% of recurrent pregnancy loss patients** (89,90). In addition to inappropriately elevated LH levels, PCOS patients are frequently obese and often have elevated circulating androgen levels. Although not undisputed, both changes have been linked to recurrent pregnancy loss, and elevated androgen levels have been shown to adversely affect markers of uterine receptivity in women with a history of recurrent pregnancy loss (89–92).

Many women with PCOS have metabolic alterations in glycemic control characterized by insulin resistance. This too may be directly or indirectly related to adverse pregnancy outcome, and it may explain increases in the rate of spontaneous pregnancy loss among women with type 2 diabetes mellitus (93). Women with overt insulin-dependent diabetes mellitus (IDDM) appear to exhibit a threshold of pregestational glycemic control above which spontaneous pregnancy loss is increased (94,95). In fact, hyperglycemia has now been directly linked to embryonic damage (96). In cases of advanced IDDM with accompanying vascular complications, compromised blood flow to the uterus may be mechanistically involved in subsequent pregnancy loss.

Patients with thyroid disease often have concomitant reproductive abnormalities, including ovulatory dysfunction and luteal phase defects. In addition, the metabolic demands of early pregnancy mandate an increased requirement for thyroid hormones. It is therefore not surprising that hypothyroidism has been associated with isolated spontaneous pregnancy loss and with recurrent pregnancy loss (97). The definition of hypothyroidism is itself now under scrutiny with many investigators suggesting that cutoff thyroid-stimulating hormone (TSH) values during pregnancy should be less than 2.5 mIU/mL (98). Others have suggested even lower TSH cutoff values (99). Although it has long been debated whether clinically euthyroid patients with antithyroid antibodies have higher rates of miscarriage and recurrent pregnancy loss, thyroid hormone supplementation was shown to reduce miscarriage in infertility patients with positive antithyroid antibodies undergoing IVF (100–106). The mechanism for an association between antithyroid antibody positivity and recurrent pregnancy loss remains unclear; however, these antibodies could be markers of more generalized autoimmunity or may predict an impaired ability of the thyroid gland to respond to the demands of pregnancy.

Two additional endocrinologic abnormalities have been linked with recurrent pregnancy loss, although support for these associations and their mechanistic pathways remains shrouded in controversy. The relationship of hyperprolactinemia with recurrent pregnancy loss continues to be debated. Animal models suggest that elevated prolactin levels may adversely affect corpus luteal function; however, this concept is not well supported in humans (107,108). Some have suggested that elevated prolactin levels may promote pregnancy wastage via direct effects on the endometrium or indirect immunomodulatory mechanisms (88,109). Most recently, attempts have been made to correlate markers of ovarian reserve (day 3 follicle-stimulating hormone, day 3 estradiol, response to the *clomiphene* challenge test) with recurrent pregnancy loss (89,110,111). At present, no consensus exists concerning this potential association.

Maternal Infection

The association of infection with recurrent abortion is among the most controversial and poorly explored of the potential causes for pregnancy loss. Reproductive tract infection with bacterial, viral, parasitic, zoonotic, and fungal organisms have all been linked theoretically to pregnancy loss; however, mycoplasma, ureaplasma, chlamydia, and β-streptococcus are the most commonly studied pathogens (112,113). More recent data have directly addressed the roles of some of these proposed organisms in recurrent pregnancy loss. One prospective comparison trial involving 70 recurrent pregnancy loss patients reported no elevations in any markers for present or past infection with *Chlamydia trachomatis* when compared with controls (114). In contrast, a very large, prospective trial demonstrated a link between the detection of bacterial vaginosis and a history of second trimester pregnancy loss among 500 recurrent pregnancy loss patients (115). The risk of bacterial vaginosis detection was also positively correlated with cigarette smoking in this study.

The etiologic mechanism linking specific organisms to either isolated or recurrent pregnancy loss remains unclear and must certainly differ among infectious organisms. Certain viral organisms, such as herpes simplex virus (HSV) and human cytomegalovirus (HCMV) can directly infect the placenta and fetus (116,117). The resulting villitis and related tissue destruction may lead to pregnancy disruption. Another theoretic possibility warranting study is that infection-associated early pregnancy loss may result from immunologic activation in response to pathologic organisms. A large body of evidence supports the role of this mechanism in adverse events later in gestation, such as intrauterine growth restriction, premature rupture of membranes, and preterm birth (118,119). Alternatively, mechanisms that protect the fetus from autoimmune rejection also may protect virally infected placental cells from recognition and clearance. This could potentially promote periods of unfettered infectious growth for some of the pathogenic organisms gaining entry to the reproductive tract (120).

Immunologic Phenomena

During the past decade, there has been extensive information published concerning the possible immunologic causes and treatments of recurrent pregnancy loss. **There is a lack of consensus as to the mechanisms and the impact of therapeutic intervention because the detection of a therapeutic effect is difficult in the absence of very large studies.** This situation reflects the fact that many recurrent pregnancy loss patients present after their index pregnancy has expired but prior to its being expelled. In these cases, the physiologic immune reaction to the presence of nonviable tissue may mask any alternative, underlying immune causes for the demise itself. Finally, it is very likely that there are a wide variety of immune alterations that may result in the same end point—isolated or recurrent pregnancy loss. This latter theory is certainly supported by a now classic review article that lists 10 fairly well-supported immune mechanisms that are each potentially important in pregnancy maintenance (121) (Tables 33.1 and 33.2).

Before launching into the most commonly accepted causes of immune-mediated pregnancy loss, a brief review of some of the important concepts in basic immunology is warranted. Although these descriptions are presented in general terms, and are further defined in Chapter 6, they should serve as useful reference for the ensuing information.

Immune responses classically are divided into innate and acquired responses. Innate responses represent the body's first line of defense against pathogenic invasion. They are

Table 33.2 Concepts in Reproductive Immunology

Cellular Immunity

1. Resident endometrial/decidual cells
   a. Few B cells
   b. TCR$\alpha\beta$+ and TCR$\gamma\delta$+ cells are present, TCR$\gamma\delta$+ cells increase in early pregnancy
   c. NK-like, large granular lymphocytes (decidual NK cells) accumulate at sites of implantation
   d. NKT cells and "suppressor" macrophage
   e. Treg cells

2. Immune cell education and homing
   a. Thymic versus extrathymic education
   b. Possible *in situ* education and maintenance
   c. Integrins/vascular ligand pairs and mucosal homing

3. Antigen presentation
   a. MHC class II molecules are not expressed in the placenta
   b. Classical MHC class I molecules HLA-A and HLA-B are not expressed in the placenta
   c. Extravillous cytotrophoblast cells express HLA-C, HLA-E, and HLA-G

4. *In situ* immunoregulation
   a. TH1/TH2 cytokine microenvironments and dysregulation
   b. Hormonal immunomodulation
      1. Progesterone
      2. Estrogen
      3. Human chorionic gonadotropin (hCG)
      4. Prolactin
      5. Androgens
      6. Others
   c. *Tryptophan* metabolism and indolamine 2,3 dioxygenase (IDO)
   d. Leukemia inhibiting factor (LIF)

Humoral Immunity

1. Fetal antigens are recognized by the maternal immune system and humoral responses are mounted

2. Organ nonspecific autoantibodies
   a. Anticardiolipin antibodies
   b. Lupus anticoagulant
   c. Anti-β2 glycoprotein-1 (anti-beta2GP-1) antibodies
   d. Antiphosphatidly serine antibodies

3. Organ specific autoantibodies
   a. Antithyroid antibodies
   b. Antisperm antibodies
   c. Antitrophoblast antibodies
      1. blocking antibodies
      2. HLA sharing
      3. Trophoblast/lymphocyte cross-reactive antibodies (TLX)

Treg, regulatory T cells; TH, T helper; NK, natural killer; NKT, natural killer T; MHC, major histocompatibility complex.

rapid and are not antigen specific. Cell types and mechanisms typically considered vital to innate immunity include complement activation, phagocytosis by macrophage, and lysis by natural killer (NK) and natural killer T (NKT) cells and possibly by TCR $\gamma\delta+$ T cells (see below). **Acquired immune responses, in contrast, are antigen specific and are largely mediated by T cells and B cells. Acquired responses can be further divided into primary (response associated with initial antigen contact) and secondary (rapid and powerful amnestic responses associated with subsequent contact to the same antigen).**

Antigen specificity is generally regulated by two sets of genes in the major histocompatibility complex (MHC), located on chromosome 6 in humans. **MHC class I molecules (HLA-A, -B, and -C) are present on the surface of nearly every cell in the human body and are important in defense against intracellular pathogens, such as viral infection and oncogenic transformation.** MHC class I molecules act as important ligands for both the T-cell receptor on CD8+ cytotoxic/suppressor T cells and for a variety of receptors on NK cells (122). **MHC class II molecules (HLA-DR, HLA-DP, and HLA-DQ), in contrast, are present on the surface of a limited number of antigen-presenting cells, including dendritic cells, macrophage and monocytes, B cells,** and tissue-specific cells such as the Langerhans cells in the skin. These molecules are important in defense against extracellular pathogens, such as bacterial invaders. The major ligand for MHC class II is the T-cell receptor on CD4+ T-helper cells.

One very important concept in immunology that has particular application to pregnancy is that of immune tolerance. The passage of bone marrow–derived T cells through the fetal thymus during early development has been well described. During this developmental interval, the T cells encounter a process termed *thymic education.* During thymic education, T cells that express either the CD4 or the CD8 coreceptor are chosen, and autoreactive cells are effectively eliminated. In short, this education promotes T-cell tolerance, allowing selection and survival only of those T cells that recognize non-self and will not react against self. Recently, a subpopulation of CD4+ T cells has been described that, like all activated lymphocytes, strongly express CD25 on their cell surface (123). These CD4, CD25+ cells are more specifically identified by the intracellular presence of the forkhead box P3 (Fox P3) transcription factor and have been called regulatory T lymphocytes (Treg cells). Treg cells, when activated by autoantigens, can suppress activated inflammatory cells. They secrete regulatory cytokines, including interleukin-10 (IL-10) and transforming growth factor-β (TGF-β) (123–125). They may have particular importance in avoidance of tissue destruction associated with inflammation, possibly with applications to tolerance. In an abortion-prone murine model, adoptive transfer of Treg cells from normal pregnant mice into abortion-prone animals prevented immune-mediated pregnancy wastage (126). In pregnant women, Treg cells suppress autologous peripheral blood mononuclear cell (PBMC) secretion of the inflammatory cytokine, interferon-γ (IFN-γ) when challenged by paternal or unrelated PBMCs (127).

These immunologic characteristics were thoroughly described and investigated for the immune effector cells populating the peripheral immune system. The peripheral immune system consists of the spleen and peripheral blood, and it is generally responsible for protection against blood-borne pathogens. Pathogens that enter the host via the extensive surface areas of the lacrimal ducts, respiratory system, gastrointestinal tract, mammary ducts, and genitourinary tract encounter a very distinct and important immune environment—that of the mucosal immune system. Although the mucosal immune system may be primarily responsible for the initial protection against most exogenous pathogens, an understanding of its immune characteristics lags far behind that of the peripheral immune system. Insight into the specific characteristics of immunity within the reproductive tract is even further limited.

Cellular Immune Mechanisms

Many of the immune theories surrounding the causes of isolated and recurrent spontaneous pregnancy losses have stemmed from attempts to define immunologic rules as they apply specifically to the mucosal reproductive tract. Four main questions summarize much of the theoretical thinking surrounding pregnancy maintenance and reproductive immunology:

1. Which immune cells populate the reproductive tract, particularly at implantation sites?
2. How do these cells arrive at this mucosal immune site and are they educated in the same way as those populating the periphery?
3. How do the characteristics of antigen presentation differ at the maternal–fetal interface?
4. What regulatory mechanisms specifically affect reproductive tract immune cells?

Resident Cells **Immune cells populating the reproductive tract exhibit many characteristics that distinguish them from their peripheral counterparts. In particular, the human endometrium is populated by T cells, macrophage, and NK-like cells, but very few B cells are present.** The relative proportions of these resident cells vary with the menstrual cycle and change dramatically during early pregnancy. In fact, surrounding the time of implantation, one particular cell type comprises between 70% to 80% of the total endometrial lymphocyte populations (128,129). This cell type is called a variety of names, including *decidual granular lymphocytes* (DGLs), *large granular lymphocytes* (LGLs), and *decidual NK cells*. This heterogeneity of names reflects the fact that this particular cell type differs from similar cells isolated from the periphery, although most believe it to be an NK cell variant. While the majority of peripheral NK cells have low cell surface expression of CD56 (CD56^{dim}) and express high levels of CD16, the immunoglobulin receptor responsible for NK-mediated, antibody-dependent cellular cytotoxicity, those in the uterine decidua and at the placental implantation site, are largely CD56^{bright} and CD16^{dim} or CD16− (130). If these unusual endometrial cells are considered NK cells, the implantation site represents the largest accumulation of NK cells in any state of human health or disease. The true function of these cells remains unclear, but their remarkable abundance at the maternal–fetal interface compels further study. These decidual NK cells display fairly poor cytotoxic function but are robust cytokine secretors (131,132). The balance of activating and inhibitory receptors expressed on their cell surfaces determines their ultimate killing versus secretion patterns (133,134). Increases in killer-type activating receptors in comparison to inhibitory receptors were found among patients with a history of recurrent pregnancy loss (135,136). Other immune cells have been described in the periphery as having the characteristics of both NK cells and T cells. These NKT cells demonstrated a role in pregnancy loss in animal models (137). They are present in the decidua in humans and may play an important immunoregulatory role at this site (138).

In the peripheral immune compartment, the vast majority of T cells express a T-cell receptor comprised of an $\alpha\beta$ heterodimer (TCR$\alpha\beta$+). In addition to TCR$\alpha\beta$+ T cells, the human reproductive tract also is populated by a subset of T cells with a distinctive T-cell receptor comprised of the $\gamma\delta$ heterodimer (TCR$\gamma\delta$+), and the numbers of these cells increases in early pregnancy (139–141). TCR$\gamma\delta$+ T cells appear to fulfill functions quite distinct from their $\alpha\beta$+ counterparts; functions that may include direct, non-MHC restricted recognition of antigens within tissues (142). TCR$\gamma\delta$+ T cells may fill a protective niche that is either missed or poorly covered by B cells and TCR$\alpha\beta$+ T cells. The role and importance of TCR$\gamma\delta$+ cells in the reproductive tract and, more particularly, in pregnancy maintenance deserves further attention.

Treg cells are also of the "suppressor" functional phenotype. In pregnant mice and women, these specialized CD4+ cells are systemically expanded in an alloantigen independent fashion and can suppress adverse maternal responses to the fetus (143) and to self (144).

The human decidua contains characteristic immune effector cells. Most investigations into whether alterations in these cells (including T cells, decidual NK cells, and NKT cells) determine pregnancy outcome are hampered by insufficient patient numbers to allow meaningful conclusions. These immune cell populations are reported to be altered in recurrent pregnancy loss patients but not in patients experiencing isolated spontaneous pregnancy losses (141,145–147).

Immune Cell Education and Homing to the Reproductive Tract **The implanting fetus represents the most common model of allograft acceptance. How the maternal immune system avoids rejection of the implanting fetus in an uncomplicated pregnancy invokes the presence of some manifestation of immune tolerance.** This, in turn, begs the questions of how the resident decidual immune effector cells are selected and educated, how they home to reproductive sites, and how they are maintained once they reach this destination. Animal studies have suggested that the rules for selection and maintenance of these cells, in terms of their requirement for MHC and their education within the thymus, may be distinct from those governing either peripheral immune cells or cells within other mucosal sites, including the intestine (148). It appears the human reproductive tract displays similar characteristics—the immunophenotypes of immune cells populating the human reproductive tract are distinct from both the periphery and from other mucosal sites (149,150). The education of TCR$\gamma\delta$+ cells populating epithelial sites may occur outside the thymus and might involve mechanisms that substitute for or modify interaction with MHC (141,151). The development of MHC specificity among NK cells is presently being carefully dissected in animal models with the hope that these investigations will shed light on similar processes in humans and, more specifically, on the selection and maintenance characteristics of decidual NK cells (133,134,152,153).

It is becoming increasingly evident that the cells populating mucosal immune tissues select these sites through interactions between cell surface molecules on the immune cell (integrins) and cell surface molecules on the endothelial cells of blood vessels within the mucosal tissues (e.g., selectins). This cellular recruitment process, called homing, has been most thoroughly described for the intestine (154,155). Both murine and human reproductive tract tissues express these integrin or vascular ligand pairs (155–157). The extension of these findings to pregnancy maintenance will be useful (158,159). Solving the mechanisms of selection, education, and maintenance of reproductive tract immune effector cells is of paramount importance. Until we understand these vital processes in the normal state, we cannot define the effects that alterations will have on human disease nor can we develop therapeutic interventions.

Antigen Presentation at the Maternal–Fetal Interface   Historically, it was proposed that one method by which the implanting trophoblastic allograft potentially could avoid immune detection by the maternal host would be by making itself antigenically invisible. It could downregulate its expression of the MHC-encoded transplantation antigens (some of which would be of paternal origin) and thereby avoid recognition as non-self. Although current knowledge of immunology renders this theory obsolete, the implanting fetus does utilize this strategy to some extent (160). It is certainly true that placental trophoblast cells do not express MHC class II molecules (161,162).

Unlike nearly every other cell in the human body, trophoblast cells do not express the classical MHC class I transplantation antigens HLA-A and -B. Rather, a subpopulation of placental cells, specifically the extravillous cytotrophoblast cells, express the classical MHC class I HLA-C products, and the nonclassical HLA-E and -G products (120,163–167). These extravillous cytotrophoblast cells are of particular interest because they are characterized by remarkable invasive potential (168,169). These cells move from the tips of the anchoring villae of the human placenta, invading deeply into the maternal decidua, and can replace cells within the walls of decidual arterial vessels (168–170). Although the invasive characteristics of extravillous cytotrophoblast may reflect non-MHC–related mechanisms, including well-described integrin switching, the intimate contact of these fetal-derived cells with maternal immune effector cells certainly exposes the fetus to recognition as nonself (171).

It is not known why all placental cells downregulate expression of HLA-A and -B, whereas invasive extravillous cytotrophoblast express HLA-C, -E, and -G. This area of investigation is ripe with hypotheses and study. Because NK cells of the innate immune system recognize and kill cells that express no MHC, the complete downregulation of MHC should cause trophoblast cells to act as targets for those NK cells that are pervasive at sites of implantation (134,160). In addition to possible protection from direct NK cell–mediated killing, the expression of HLA-C, -E, and -G by trophoblast cells may serve a variety of alternate purposes. NK cell receptor-mediated interactions with extravillous cytotrophoblast MHC products modulate cytokine expression profiles at the maternal–fetal interface (131,132). **MHC expression aids in decidual and vascular invasion by the trophoblast, an activity essential for proper placental development** (172). Whereas definitive correlations between placental MHC class I expression patterns and recurrent pregnancy loss have not been reported, trophoblast expression of HLA-G was linked to other disorders of placental invasion, such as preeclampsia (172,173). Genetic mutations at the HLA-G locus have also been linked to recurrent pregnancy loss in some, but not all studies (174–177). Finally, soluble or secreted trophoblast MHC products may aid in the development of maternal immune tolerance toward the placenta (178). Soluble HLA-G was shown to suppress T lymphocyte and NK cell function and to induce the expansion of Treg cells in humans (179).

Aberrant expression of class II MHC determinants, or enhanced expression of MHC class I on syncytiotrophoblast occurring in response to IFN-γ (180) could mediate pregnancy loss by enhancing cytotoxic T-cell attack (181). This theory appears unlikely, because the expression of classical MHC antigens does not seem to be induced on aborted tissues from women experiencing one or more pregnancy losses (181). Finally, MHC class II genotypes appear to affect susceptibility to a variety of diseases, including diabetes and other autoimmune diseases. **A similar link between MHC class II typing and adverse pregnancy outcome was reported for recurrent pregnancy loss** (182,183).

Regulation of Decidual Immune Cells   The characteristics of the interactions between decidual immune effector cells and the implanting fetus may be determined by factors other than those already mentioned. Local regulation of the cells that populate the human decidua will further modify the effects of selection, maintenance, and homing, as well as the distinctive characteristics of antigen presentation at the maternal–fetal interface. As might be predicted, these regulatory effects are often targets for investigative efforts, because they may offer more direct insight into potential therapies for immune-mediated disorders of pregnancy maintenance. **Three such regulatory mechanisms will be discussed here: (i) alterations in T-helper cell phenotypes, (ii) reproductive hormones and immunosuppression, and (iii) tryptophan metabolism.**

As discussed in Chapter 6, antigen-stimulated immune responses involving CD4+ T cells can be divided into two major classes: T helper 1 (TH1) responses and T helper 2 (TH2) responses. This subclassification may be overly simple, but it has been useful in broadly defining types of immune responses based on the characteristics of the CD4+ cells present, as well as their associated cytokines. The production of these responses rests on the environment in which relatively undifferentiated CD4+ TH0 cells become differentiated. Thus, TH0 cells exposed to IFN-γ become TH1-type cells, and those exposed to IL-4 become TH2-type cells (184). TH1 responses are associated with inflammation and primarily involve IFN-γ and IL-12, as well as IL-2, and tumor necrosis factor-β (TNF-β). TH2 cells responses are associated with antibody production and the cytokines IL-10, IL-4, IL-5, and IL-6 (184–186). Although TNF-α can be secreted by both TH1 and TH2 cells, it is most often a characteristic of TH1 response (187,188). **A reciprocal regulating relationship exists between TH1 and TH2 cells and cytokines, with one response supporting its own persistence while averting conversion to the other** (189–191).

One additional T-helper cell subset, TH17 cells, has been recently distinguished, although many of their proinflammatory effects were previously attributed to TH1 cells (192). TH17 cells preferentially produce IL-17 family cytokines (including IL-17A and IL-17F), which upregulate stromal IL-8 and IL-6 and cause local neutrophilic inflammation. These cells are important in sustaining the inflammatory response and are closely associated with several autoimmune diseases (193).

Extending these immune regulatory phenomena to pregnancy, the type of CD4+ cellular response to the implanting fetus is controlled not only by the types of cells (e.g., T-helper cells) in the decidua, but also by the cytokine environment at the maternal–fetal interface. As mentioned previously, the human endometrium and decidua are replete with immune and inflammatory cells capable of cytokine secretion (194–196). Cytokines may affect reproductive events either directly or indirectly, depending on the specific cytokines secreted, their concentrations, and the differentiation stage of potential reproductive target tissues. It is well documented that TH1-type cytokines can be harmful to an implanting embryo (197,198). Further, most agree that some patients with recurrent pregnancy loss exhibit a dysregulation of their T-helper cellular immune response to antigens at the site of implantation, with typical shifts toward TH1 inflammatory responses (199,200). **Depending on the individual series, 60% to 80% of nonpregnant women with a history of otherwise unexplained recurrent spontaneous abortion have been found to have evidence of abnormal *in vitro* TH1 cellular immune responses.** Fewer than 3% of women with normal reproductive histories demonstrate these responses (199,201). Rather, most women with normal pregnancies have a TH2 immune response to trophoblast antigens (199). It has only been recently that the TH17 concept has been applied to pregnancy (202). In humans, a single study demonstrates an increase in the number of TH17 cells in the decidua and peripheral blood of women with otherwise unexplained recurrent pregnancy loss (203). Mechanistically, a dysregulation of TH17 cell control by Treg cells may lead to adverse pregnancy outcomes (204).

Methods for the documentation of cytokine dysregulation among recurrent pregnancy loss patients also varies among investigators; some groups have confirmed this abnormality within the endometrium or among immune cells isolated from the decidua of these patients (205–208). Others use peripheral blood lymphocytes (PBLs) from women with a history of recurrent pregnancy loss and stimulate them *in vitro* with trophoblast antigens (199,209). One study documented aberrant cytokine secretion when PBLs from recurrent pregnancy loss patients were stimulated *in vitro* by HLA-G bearing cells, whereas another study demonstrated that decidual and peripheral immune cells exhibit a shift toward the TH2 phenotype when exposed to HLA-G (210,211). Whether peripheral cytokine levels reflect T-helper cell dysregulation at the maternal–fetal interface and whether this dysregulation affects peripheral as well as local immune response during pregnancy remains controversial (212,213). Finally, as with all immune theories, there seems to be significant redundancy in the necessity for particular cytokines and soluble immunoregulatory factors at the site of implantation. To date, animal models with directed gene deletions have shown few of these factors to be absolutely essential to pregnancy maintenance (e.g., leukemia inhibitory factor [LIF]) (214,215).

Although many mechanisms are aimed at avoiding maternal immune recognition of the implanting fetus, research in both humans and animals indicates that immune responses to fetal antigens can be detected (216–218). **Thus, the regulation of this response at the maternal–fetal interface may be critical.** The concept that successful pregnancy requires some form of generalized suppression of maternal immune response is supported by reports that failure to downregulate maternal responses to recall antigens, such as tetanus toxoid and influenza, is associated with poor pregnancy outcome among recurrent pregnancy loss patients (219). Treg cells appear important in this respect (see above). So too do reproductive hormones. Reproductive hormones have dramatic effects on peripheral cell–mediated immunity, as demonstrated by well-documented and notable gender differences in immune responsiveness (220). The levels of these potentially immunosuppressive hormones are quite elevated in pregnant women. The fact that the levels of these hormones at the maternal–fetal interface may be far above those in the maternal circulation during pregnancy may explain an apparent inconsistency: overall immune responsiveness during pregnancy appears to change little, while local suppression at the maternal–fetal interface may be vital (221).

It has been suggested that the immunosuppressive effects of progesterone within the reproductive tract are at least partially responsible for the maintenance of the semiallogeneic implanting fetus (222). *In vitro* studies have shown that progesterone mediates its suppression of T-cell effector function by altering membrane-resident potassium channels and cell membrane depolarization. This action, in turn, affects intracellular calcium signaling cascades and gene expression and may be mediated by nonclassical steroid receptors or may not involve a receptor at all (223–225). Progesterone-mediated changes in T-cell gene expression have been associated with the development of TH2-type T-helper cell responses and with increased LIF expression (208,226). Because a shift in the intrauterine immune environment from TH2 to TH1 has been linked with early spontaneous pregnancy loss, the elevated intrauterine concentrations of progesterone characteristic of early pregnancy may promote an immune environment favoring pregnancy maintenance (199,208). To this point, *in vitro* evidence indicates that progesterone can inhibit mitogen-induced proliferation of and cytokine secretion by CD8+ T cells and can alter the expression of a transcription factor that drives the development of TH1 cells (227,228).

Levels of estrogen also rise dramatically during pregnancy, and attention has focused on the role of estrogen in immune modulation. A group of animal studies showed that estrogens improve immune responses in males after significant trauma and hemorrhage, suppress cell-mediated immunity after thermal injury, and protect against chronic renal allograft rejection (229–231). *In vitro*, estrogens appear to downregulate delayed-type hypersensitivity (DTH) reactions and promote the development of TH2-type immune responses, particularly at the elevated estrogen concentrations typical of pregnancy (232,233).

One additional regulatory mechanism proposed for the induction of maternal tolerance to the fetal allograft involves the amino acid *tryptophan* and its catabolizing enzyme indolamine 2,3 dioxygenase (IDO). The IDO hypothesis of tolerance in pregnancy rests on data that indicate that T cells need *tryptophan* for activation and proliferation (234), and that local alterations in *tryptophan* metabolism at the maternal–fetal interface could either activate or fail to suppress maternal antifetal immunoreactivity (235). Studies in mice have shown that the inhibition of IDO leads to loss of allogeneic, but not syngeneic, fetuses, and that this effect is mediated by lymphocytes (236). Further support lies in studies demonstrating that hamsters fed diets high in *tryptophan* have increased rates of fetal wastage (237). Extending this theory to humans requires further investigation. However, the demonstration of IDO expression in human uterine decidua, and the documentation of alterations in serum *tryptophan* levels with increasing gestational age during human pregnancy both support further interest in this potential local immunoregulatory mechanism (238,239).

Endometriosis is the growth of both endometrial glands and stroma outside of the intrauterine cavity. Although associations between the development of endometriosis and immunologic abnormalities are now being defined, the link between endometriosis and recurrent pregnancy loss remains contentious (240,241). **The occurrence of recurrent pregnancy loss in the** presence of endometriosis certainly would involve the interaction of complex mechanisms, some of which may involve cellular or humoral immune dysfunction (242,243).

Humoral Immune Mechanisms

Humoral responses to pregnancy-specific antigens exist, and patients with recurrent pregnancy loss can display altered humoral responses to endometrial and trophoblast antigens (Table 33.2) (199,244). Nevertheless, most literature surrounding humoral immune responses and recurrent pregnancy loss focus on organ nonspecific autoantibodies associated with the antiphospholipid antibody syndrome (APS). Historically, these immunoglobulin-G (IgG) and IgM antibodies were considered as directed against negatively charged phospholipids. Those phospholipids most often implicated in recurrent pregnancy loss are cardiolipin and phosphatidylserine. However, antiphospholipid antibodies often are directed against a protein cofactor, $\beta2$ glycoprotein 1, which assists antibody association with the phospholipid (245–249). Antiphospholipid antibodies were originally characterized by prolonged phospholipid-dependent coagulation tests *in vitro* (activated partial thromboplastin time [aPTT], Russell Viper Venom time) and by thrombosis *in vivo*. The association of these antiphospholipid antibodies with thrombotic complications has been termed the antiphospholipid syndrome, and although many of these complications are systemic, some are pregnancy specific—spontaneous abortion, stillbirth, intrauterine growth retardation, and preeclampsia (250,251). A reassessment of the criteria used to diagnose APS resulted in additions to the prior Sapporo criteria for diagnosis of APS and continues to include adverse pregnancy outcomes. These criteria, which have been validated clinically, are as follows (251–253).

For a patient to be diagnosed with antiphospholipid antibody syndrome, one or more clinical and one or more laboratory criteria must be present:

Clinical

1. **One or more confirmed episode of vascular thrombosis of any type:**
   - **Venous**
   - **Arterial**
   - **Small vessel**

2. **Pregnancy complications:**
   - **Three or more consecutive spontaneous pregnancy losses at less than 10 weeks of gestation with exclusion of maternal anatomic and hormonal abnormalities and exclusion of paternal and maternal chromosomal abnormalities**
   - **One or more unexplained deaths of a morphologically normal fetus at or beyond 10 weeks of gestation (normal fetal morphology documented by ultrasound or direct examination of the fetus)**
   - **One or more premature births of a morphologically normal neonate at or before 34 weeks of gestation secondary to severe preeclampsia or placental insufficiency**

Laboratory

Testing must be positive on two or more occasions with evaluations 12 or more weeks apart:

1. **Positive plasma levels of anticardiolipin antibodies of the IgG or IgM isotype at medium to high levels**
2. **Positive plasma levels of lupus anticoagulant**
3. **Anti-$\beta2$ glycoprotein-1 antibodies of the IgG or IgM isotype in titers greater than the 99th percentile**

The presence of antiphospholipid antibodies (anticardiolipin or lupus anticoagulant) and anti-$\beta2$ glycoprotein-1 antibodies during pregnancy is a major risk factor for an adverse pregnancy outcome (245,246,254). In a large series of couples with recurrent abortion, the incidence of the antiphospholipid syndrome was between 3% and 5% (112). The presence of anticardiolipin antibodies among patients with known systemic lupus erythematosus portends less favorable pregnancy outcomes (255).

A number of mechanisms have been proposed by which antiphospholipid antibodies might mediate pregnancy loss (256). Antibodies against phospholipids could increase thromboxane and decrease prostacyclin synthesis within placental vessels. The resultant prothrombotic environment could promote vascular constriction, platelet adhesion, and placental infarction (257–259). Alternatively, *in vitro* evidence from trophoblast cell lines indicates that IgM action against phosphatidylserine inhibits formation of syncytial trophoblast (260). Syncytialization is required for proper placental function. One study demonstrated that both extravillous cytotrophoblast and syncytiotrophoblast cells synthesize β2 glycoprotein-1, the essential cofactor for antiphospholipid antibody binding (261). Although it gives insight into pathophysiology, the prognostic value of serum levels of specific antibodies against β2 glycoprotein-1 with respect to pregnancy outcome among recurrent pregnancy loss patients is contentious and may be poorer than that of standard anticardiolipin antibodies (262–264). Some have proposed that sera from antibody positive recurrent pregnancy loss patients is particularly adept at inhibiting trophoblast adhesion to endothelial cells *in vitro* (265). Others noted rapid development of atherosclerosis in the decidual spiral arteries of patients who test positive for antiphospholipid antibodies (266). Finally, still others have demonstrated that levels of the placental antithrombotic molecule— annexin V—are reduced within the placental villa from those women with recurrent pregnancy loss who are antiphospholipid antibody positive (267). However, placental pathologic evidence supporting causal involvement of the antiphospholipid antibody syndrome in pregnancy loss often is equivocal. The characteristic lesions for this syndrome (placental infarction, abruption, and hemorrhage) are typically missing in women with antiphospholipid antibodies, and these same pathologic lesions can be found in placentae from women with recurrent abortion who do not have biochemical evidence of antiphospholipid antibodies (256,268–270).

One additional group of autoantibodies that have been linked to recurrent pregnancy loss is the antithyroid antibodies (ATA). Although the data remain somewhat controversial, several investigators demonstrated an increased prevalence of these antibodies among women with a history of recurrent pregnancy loss, even in the absence of thyroid endocrinologic abnormalities (98–199,102,103,271–273).

Other antibody-mediated mechanisms for recurrent abortion have been proposed, including antisperm and antitrophoblast antibodies, as well as blocking antibody deficiency. Although each hypothesis has minimal relevance to recurrent pregnancy loss, their discussion is warranted because therapies aimed at these disorders persist. Historically, the blocking antibody deficiency hypothesis has received the most attention (112,181). This hypothesis is based on a supposition that blocking factors (presumably antibodies) were required to prevent a maternal, cell-mediated, antifetal immune response that was believed to occur in all pregnancies. It was therefore proposed that, in the absence of these blocking antibodies, abortion occurred (273). This supposition was not consistently substantiated (274,275). For instance, maternal hyporesponsiveness in mixed lymphocyte culture with paternal stimulator cells was originally proposed to identify women with deficient blocking activity (273). Investigations based on this type of testing were continued by those who proposed that parental HLA sharing resulted in a predisposition to blocking antibody deficiency (276,277). These reports were of limited sample size, were retrospective in nature, and lacked population-based controls. One prospective, population-based control study conclusively demonstrated that HLA heterogeneity was not essential for successful pregnancy (278). However, follow-up studies showed that, in the exceedingly rare case of complete sharing of the entire HLA region, spontaneous pregnancy losses do increase (279). This particular 10-year prospective trial concluded that HLA typing is of no use in outbred populations, because only isolated and significantly inbred populations have such HLA homogeneity. Further evidence refuting the blocking antibody hypothesis for recurrent abortion comes from reports of successful pregnancies among women who do not produce serum factors capable of mixed lymphocyte culture inhibition and also among women who do not produce antipaternal cytotoxic antibodies (273,274). Those mixed lymphocyte culture results that demonstrate hyporesponsiveness in some recurrent pregnancy loss patients are now believed to represent the effect of the pregnancy loss rather than the cause of recurrent abortion (217,273–275).

One final theory that emerged from the blocking antibody investigations involved a novel HLA-linked alloantigen system. The finding that polyclonal rabbit antisera could recognize both lymphocytes and trophoblast cells suggested the existence of trophoblast–lymphocyte cross-reactive alloantigens (called TLX) (280). These TLX were, in turn, linked to maternal blocking antibody deficiency and recurrent pregnancy loss. The TLX hypothesis only has historical relevance. The theory was invalidated when TLX was found to be identical to CD46, a complement receptor that is thought to protect the placenta from complement-mediated attack (281). CD46 was not a novel alloantigen. It can be found on a wide variety of cells, thus explaining the cross-reactive nature of the original rabbit antisera.

It is important to conclude this in-depth discussion of the immune-mediated mechanisms of isolated and recurrent pregnancy loss by suggesting that pregnancy may not require an intact maternal immune system. Supporting this concept are data showing that agammaglobulinemic animals and women can successfully reproduce (282). Further, viable births also occur among women with severe immune deficiencies and in murine models that lack T and B cells (severe combined immunodeficiency [SCID] mice) and those that display a congenital absence of their thymus (nude mice). Still, immune factors may play important roles in a significant proportion of patients with recurrent pregnancy loss, and their presence is the subject of abundant research. Until this role is better defined, an understanding of contemporary immunologic hypotheses fosters the informed consideration of novel findings.

Male Factors

Most publications that review testing and treatment for recurrent pregnancy loss couples, including this chapter, recommend only a single test for the male partner in the couple—a peripheral blood karyotype. The role of the male partner in the etiology of recurrent pregnancy loss is understudied, but there is a growing body of literature suggesting that the development and validation of novel testing and treatment regimens for the male may prove beneficial (283,284). Detailed peripheral chromosomal testing of men whose partners experienced recurrent pregnancy loss revealed an increased incidence of Y chromosome microdeletions when compared to male partners in fertile and infertile couples (285). Small studies demonstrated that male partners in couples experiencing recurrent pregnancy loss have an increased incidence of sperm chromosomal aneuploidy, particularly sex chromosome disomy, when compared to fertile men (16,286). The addition of specialized testing to a standard semen analysis among men in couples with recurrent loss revealed reductions in sperm functional testing (hypo-osmotic swelling, acrosome status, nuclear chromatin decondensation) and increased DNA fragmentation and lipid peroxidation when compared to fertile men or historical controls (287–289). The latter results suggest that these men may have abnormal levels of reactive oxygen species in their semen or that their sperm cells are particularly sensitive to these compounds. To this point, paternal carriage of the *MTHFR* C677T mutation and hyperhomocysteinemia were associated with both DNA damage and recurrent pregnancy loss (290). A single, small, uncontrolled treatment study using antioxidants among male partners in recurrent pregnancy loss couples who had high levels of sperm DNA damage or semen lipid peroxidation suggested favorable treatment outcomes (288).

Other Factors

It is increasingly evident that the implantation of the blastocyst within the uterine decidua involves an exquisitely scripted crosstalk between embryo and mother. Alterations in this dialogue often result in improper implantation and placental development. For instance, recurrent pregnancy loss has been linked to a dysregulation in the expression patterns of vascular endothelial growth factors (VEGFs) on the developing placenta and their requisite receptors within the maternal decidua (291). Cellular and extracellular matrix adhesion properties may also be involved in this dialogue. The concept of uterine receptivity has been emboldened by the description of endometrial integrins and the timing of integrin switching during implantation (292). Others have reported decreased levels of endometrial mucin secretion and reductions in the endometrial release of soluble intercellular adhesion molecule I among women with histories of recurrent pregnancy loss (293,294). Programmed cell death (apoptosis) may also play an essential role in normal placental development. Alterations in two important apoptotic pathways—Fas-Fas ligand and bcl2—have both been linked to recurrent pregnancy loss and poor pregnancy outcome (121,295).

Environmental Factors

A variety of environmental factors have been linked to sporadic and recurrent early spontaneous pregnancy loss. These are difficult studies to perform, because, in humans, they all must be retrospective and all are confounded by alternative or additional environmental exposures. Nevertheless, the following factors have been linked to pregnancy loss: exposure to medications (e.g., antiprogestogens, antineoplastic agents, and inhalation anesthetics), exposure to ionizing radiation, prolonged exposure to organic solvents, and exposure to environmental toxins, especially bisphenol-A and heavy metals (296–299). The latter two exposures have been demonstrated to have both endocrine and immune effects that could lead to poor placentation and subsequent pregnancy loss (300,301). Associations between spontaneous pregnancy loss and exposures to video display terminals, microwave ovens, high-energy electric power lines, and high altitudes (e.g., flight attendants) are not substantiated (302,303). There is no compelling evidence that moderate exercise during pregnancy is associated with spontaneous abortion. In the absence of cervical anatomic abnormalities or incompetent cervix, coitus does not appear to increase the risk for spontaneous pregnancy loss (304,305). **Exposure to three particular substances—alcohol, cigarettes, and caffeine—deserves specific attention.** Although some conflicting data exist, one very large epidemiologic study has shown that **alcohol consumption during the first trimester of pregnancy, at levels as low as three drinks per week, is associated with an increased incidence of spontaneous pregnancy loss** (306–308). **Cigarette smoking has also been linked to early spontaneous pregnancy loss;** however, this is also not without controversy (309–311). **Alcohol and tobacco intake in the male partner correlates with the incidence of domestic violence, which in turn is associated with early pregnancy loss** (312). Finally, recent evidence adds to a growing body of literature that suggests **consumption of coffee and other caffeinated beverages during early pregnancy is linked to adverse pregnancy outcome** (309,313). The most publicized recent report casts doubt on the definition of a lower limit for safe use of caffeine in the first trimester of pregnancy (309). Obesity, stress at work, and use of nonsteroidal anti-inflammatory agents during early pregnancy have all been linked to an increased rate of isolated spontaneous pregnancy loss (314–317).

Preconception Evaluation

Investigative measures that are potentially useful in the evaluation of recurrent spontaneous abortion include obtaining a thorough history from both partners, performing a physical assessment of the woman (with attention to the pelvic examination), and a limited amount of laboratory testing (Table 33.3).

History

A description of all prior pregnancies and their sequence as well as whether histologic assessment and karyotype determinations were performed on previously aborted tissues are important aspects of the history. **Approximately 60% of abortuses lost before 8 weeks of gestation were reported to be chromosomally abnormal; most of these pregnancies are affected by some type of trisomy, particularly trisomy 16** (318,319). **The most common single chromosomal abnormality is monosomy X (45X), especially among anembryonic conceptuses** (320). Aneuploid losses are particularly prevalent among women with recurrent pregnancy loss who are over the age of 35 (8). Although somewhat controversial, the detection of aneuploidy in miscarriage specimens may be less when the couple experiencing recurrent abortions is euploidic. Alternatively, some investigators have suggested that, because aneuploidy is common among miscarriage specimens from patients experiencing both isolated and recurrent spontaneous pregnancy losses, if aneuploidy is documented in fetal tissues from a recurrent pregnancy loss patient, this loss does not affect their prognosis for future pregnancy maintenance (13).

Most women with recurrent pregnancy losses tend to experience spontaneous abortion at approximately the same gestational age in sequential pregnancies (321). Unfortunately, the gestational age when pregnancy loss occurs, as determined by last menstrual period, may not be informative, because there is often a 2- to 3-week delay between fetal demise and signs of pregnancy expulsion (322). The designation of couples experiencing recurrent abortion into either primary or secondary categories is not helpful in either the diagnosis or management of most women with recurrent abortion. Approximately 10% to 15% of couples cannot be classified into either the primary or secondary category because, although their first pregnancy resulted in a loss, it was followed by a term delivery prior to subsequent losses.

It is important to glean any history of subfertility or infertility among couples with recurrent pregnancy loss. This is defined as the inability to conceive after 12 months of unprotected intercourse. By definition, 15% of all couples will meet this criteria; this number increases to 33% among couples with recurrent pregnancy losses. Because many pregnancies are lost before or near the time of missed menses, subfertility among recurrent pregnancy loss patients may in some cases reflect recurrent preclinical losses. Menstrual cycle history may provide information about the possibility of oligo-ovulation or other relevant endocrine abnormalities in recurrent pregnancy loss patients. An assessment of the timing of intercourse relative

Table 33.3 Investigative Measures Useful in the Evaluation of Recurrent Early Pregnancy Loss

History

1. Pattern, trimester, and characteristics of prior pregnancy losses
2. History of subfertility or infertility
3. Menstrual history
4. Prior or current gynecologic or obstetric infections
5. Signs or symptoms of thyroid, prolactin, glucose tolerance and hyperandrogenic disorders (including polycystic ovarian syndrome)
6. Personal or familial thrombotic history
7. Features associated with the antiphospholipid syndrome (thrombosis, false positive test for syphilis)
8. Other autoimmune disorders
9. Medications
10. Environmental exposures, illicit and common drug use (particularly caffeine, alcohol, cigarettes, and *in utero diethylstilbestrol* exposure)
11. Genetic relationship between reproductive partners
12. Family history of recurrent spontaneous abortion, of obstetric complications, or of any syndrome associated with embryonic or fetal losses
13. Previous diagnostic tests and treatments, including, if available, chromosome testing on products of conception.

Physical Examination

1. General physical examination with particular attention to:
   a. Obesity
   b. Hirsutism/acanthosis
   c. Thyroid examination
   d. Breast examination/galactorrhea
   e. Pelvic examination
      1. Anatomy
      2. Infection
      3. Trauma
      4. Estrogenization
      5. Masculinization

Laboratory

1. Parental peripheral blood karyotype
2. Chromosome testing on products of conception
3. Hysterosalpingography, three-dimensional transvaginal sonography, sonohysterography, or office hysteroscopy, followed by hysteroscopy/laparoscopy, if indicated
4. Thyroid stimulating hormone level, serum prolactin level if indicated
5. Anticardiolipin antibody levels (IgG and IgM)
6. Lupus anticoagulant (activated partial thromboplastin time or Russell Viper Venom)
7. Anti-β2-glycoprotein-1 antibodies (IgG and IgM)
8. Complete blood count with platelets
9. Factor V Leiden, G20210A prothrombin gene mutation, protein S activity, homocysteine level, activated protein C resistance (in white patients with suspicious family history)
10. Protein C activity, antithrombin level if personal or family history of venous thromboembolic events

to ovulation should be reviewed with couples in an effort to detect dyssynchronous fertilization that could contribute to pregnancy loss (323). A personal and family history of thrombotic events or renal abnormalities may provide vital information. A family history of pregnancy losses and obstetric complications should be addressed specifically. Detailed information about drug and environmental exposure should also be obtained.

Physical Examination

A general physical examination should be performed to detect signs of metabolic illness, including PCOS, diabetes, hyperandrogenism, and thyroid or prolactin disorders. During the pelvic examination, signs of infection, *DES* exposure, and previous trauma should be ascertained. Estrogenization of mucosal tissues, cervical and vaginal anatomy, and the size and shape of the uterus should also be determined.

Laboratory Assessment

Valuable Tests

Laboratory assessment of couples with recurrent pregnancy losses should include the following:

1. **Chromosome analysis of the products of conception**
2. **Parental peripheral blood karyotyping with banding techniques,**
3. **Assessment of the intrauterine cavity with either office hysteroscopy, sonohysterography, three-dimensional transvaginal sonography, or hysterosalpingography, followed by operative hysteroscopy if a potentially correctable anomaly is found (324),**
4. **Thyroid function testing, including serum thyroid-stimulating hormone levels,**
5. **Anticardiolipin, anti-β2 glycoprotein-1, and lupus anticoagulant testing (aPTT or Russell Viper Venom testing)**
6. **Platelet levels**

Tests with Unproven Utility

A number of laboratory assessment tools are under investigation for use in patients with a history of recurrent pregnancy loss. At present, results are either too preliminary to warrant unfettered recommendation or studies of their use have been too contradictory to allow final determination of their value. **Tests with unproven or unknown utility include:**

1. **Evaluation of ovarian reserve using day 3 serum follicle–stimulating hormone or antimüllerian hormone levels. It appears that decreased ovarian reserve may portend a poor outcome in all patients, including those with recurrent pregnancy loss** (110,111).
2. **Thrombophilia testing:**
   a. **Factor V Leiden, G20210A prothrombin gene mutation, protein S activity**
   b. **Serum homocysteine levels**
   c. **If there is a family or personal history of venous thromboembolic events, obtain protein C activity and antithrombin activity.**
   d. **Consider altering these screening paradigms based on ethnic background. Factor V Leiden and prothrombin promoter mutations are rare in African and Asian populations. Among Asian populations, protein C and protein S are the most common inherited thrombophilias.**
3. **Testing for serologic evidence of PCOS using luteinizing hormone or androgen values may be useful** (89–92).
4. **Testing for peripheral evidence of TH1/TH2 cytokine dysregulation.** Although large studies failed to demonstrate association between peripheral cytokine alterations and pregnancy outcome among patients with recurrent pregnancy loss, smaller studies reported peripheral shifts toward TH1 profiles only in those recurrent pregnancy loss patients who subsequently lose their pregnancy (212,213). One study documented a

shift toward TH1 profiles at the time of fetal demise in these patients; however, it is particularly difficult to determine cause and effect in this situation (325).

5. **Preconceptional testing for the prevalence and activity of peripheral NK cells has been reported in small studies to reflect prognosis and to facilitate patient counseling** (326,327). Still, peripheral NK cells may not adequately reflect those at the site of implantation, and this testing remains unproven.

6. **Testing for antithyroid antibodies among women with recurrent pregnancy loss remains controversial,** but is rapidly gaining support (98–100,103,271–273). Investigators have recently demonstrated an increased prevalence of these antibodies among women with a history of recurrent pregnancy loss, even in the absence of thyroid endocrinologic abnormalities (99,100,102,272).

7. **Testing for the presence of a variety of autoantibodies (other than lupus anticoagulant and anticardiolipin antibody) has been hotly debated, but without consensus** (245,246,249,262,328,329). Testing for some antiphospholipid antibodies, such as antiphosphatidylserine and anti-β2 glycoprotein-1, are particularly attractive because mechanistic connections between their presence and placental pathology were reported (246,260,261,263,264). Measurement of anti-β2 glycoprotein-1 antibodies was formally added to the criteria defining the antiphospholipid syndrome, and data are accumulating for specific relevance to pregnancy loss (245,246,251,330). Among patients with known autoimmune diseases and recurrent pregnancy loss additional antiphospholipid testing may also be warranted (331).

8. **Cervical cultures for mycoplasma, ureaplasma, and chlamydia may be considered.**

9. **Interobserver reproducibility and accuracy are too low to reliably use the Noyes criteria to diagnose a luteal phase defect on timed endometrial biopsy** (332). This tool lacks precision and does not alter clinical management (333). More specific and predictive methodology for diagnosing this disorder is not yet available.

The following investigations have no place in modern clinical care of patients with recurrent spontaneous pregnancy loss:

1. Evaluations that involve extensive testing for serum or site-specific auto- or alloantibodies (including antinuclear antibodies and antipaternal cytotoxic antibodies) are both expensive and unproven. Their use often verifies the statistical tenet that if the number of tests performed reaches a critical limit, the results of at least one will be positive in every patient.

2. Testing for parental HLA profiles is never indicated in outbred populations. Findings that HLA sharing is associated with poor pregnancy outcomes are strictly limited to those specific populations studied, which have very high and sustained levels of marriage within a limited community (279).

3. Use of mixed lymphocyte cultures has not proved useful. Use of other immunologic tests is unnecessary also unless these studies are performed, with informed consent, under a specific study protocol in which the costs of these experimental tests are not borne by the couple or their third-party payers.

4. Further work is necessary before suppressor cell or factor determinations, cytokine, oncogene, and growth factor measurements, or embryotoxic factor assessment can be clinically justified.

Postconception Evaluation

Following conception, close monitoring of patients with histories of recurrent pregnancy loss is advised to provide emotional support and to confirm intrauterine pregnancy and its viability. The incidence of ectopic pregnancy and complete molar gestation is increased in women with a history of recurrent spontaneous pregnancy loss. Although somewhat controversial, some data suggest that the risk of pregnancy complications other than spontaneous abortion are not significantly different between women with and without a history of recurrent losses (102,334–338). Two uncontested exceptions to this observation are those women who have antiphospholipid antibodies and those who have an intrauterine infection.

Determining serum levels of β-hCG may be helpful in monitoring early pregnancy until an ultrasonographic examination can be performed; however, not all investigators have found inadequate β-hCG levels in pregnancies that ultimately abort (339). Other hormonal determinations are rarely of benefit because levels are often normal until fetal death or abortion occurs (340).

The best method for monitoring in early pregnancy is ultrasonography. If used, **serum β-hCG levels should be serially monitored from the time of a missed menstrual period until the level is approximately 1,200 to 1,500 mIU/mL, at which time an ultrasonographic scan is performed and blood sampling is discontinued.** Ultrasonographic assessment may then be performed every 2 weeks until the gestational age at which previous pregnancies were aborted. The prognostic value of serial ultrasonography and a variety of hormonal and biochemical measurements during early pregnancy in women with histories of recurrent losses has been reported (341).

If a pregnancy has been confirmed, but fetal cardiac activity cannot be documented by approximately 6 to 7 weeks of gestation (by sure menstrual or ultrasonographic dating), intervention is recommended to expedite pregnancy termination and to obtain tissue for karyotype analysis. First trimester screening with maternal chemistries and fetal nuchal lucency measurement or chorionic villus sampling are recommended for obstetrical indications. Maternal serum can also be obtained for assessment at 16 to 18 weeks of gestation. Amniocentesis may be recommended to assess the fetal karyotype after the pregnancy has progressed past the time of prior losses.

The importance of obtaining karyotypic analysis from tissues obtained after pregnancy demise in a woman experiencing recurrent losses cannot be overemphasized. Results may suggest karyotypic anomalies in the parents. The documentation of aneuploidy may have important prognostic implications and may direct future interventions. Cost analysis has demonstrated that karyotypic analysis is financially prudent among patients with histories of recurrent pregnancy loss (342). Obtaining karyotypic data from aborted specimens incurs many difficulties in culturing cells from tissues that may have significant inflammation or necrosis and contamination of specimens with maternal cells. Efforts to develop methods that avoid such difficulties include the application of comparative genomic hybridization technology to recurrent pregnancy loss (343). This technology was used successfully on archived and paraffin-embedded pregnancy tissues (344). In the future, fetal karyotype assessment may also be performed using DNA isolated from nucleated fetal erythrocytes in maternal blood (345)

Therapy

Advances in the treatment of patients with recurrent pregnancy loss have been regrettably slow. Despite a rapid expansion in understanding the molecular and subcellular mechanisms involved in implantation and early pregnancy maintenance, extension of these concepts to prevention of recurrent early pregnancy loss has lagged. In addition to these limitations, progress toward treatment of most causes of recurrent pregnancy loss has been hampered by a variety of factors. The condition itself has been inconsistently defined. **The results of clinical trials involving recurrent pregnancy loss patients therefore are nearly impossible to compare and evaluate.** Trial design is frequently substandard, with lack of rationale, lack of appropriate controls, and poor statistical analysis, limiting the ability to draw rational conclusions from reported results. Finally, epidemiologic data indicate that most patients with a history of recurrent pregnancy loss will, in fact, have a successful pregnancy the next time they conceive (7). For these reasons, with few exceptions, most therapies for recurrent pregnancy loss must be considered experimental. Until further study is completed, treatment protocols involving these therapies should be undertaken only with informed consent and in the setting of a well-designed, double-blind, placebo-controlled clinical trial.

Common therapeutic options available for patients with recurrent pregnancy loss include the use of donor oocytes or sperm, the use of preimplantation genetic diagnosis, the use of antithrombotic interventions, the repair of anatomic anomalies, the correction of any endocrine abnormalities, the treatment of infections, and a variety of immunologic

interventions and drug treatments. Psychologic counseling and support should be recommended for all patients.

Genetic Abnormalities

Recent evidence suggests that, in women with a history of three or more spontaneous pregnancy losses, a subsequent pregnancy loss has a 58% chance of chromosomal abnormality (15). Among women with recurrent pregnancy loss who are age 35 or older, the aneuploidy rate is much higher (8). The majority of chromosomal abnormalities identified in miscarriages are autosomal trisomies and considered to result from maternal nondisjunction. Maternal age appears as a consistent and important risk factor for trisomy in the majority of studies. There are several options for patients who suffer from recurrent pregnancy loss who have an identified miscarriage due to trisomy. The first is to conceive again without any specific change in medical management, as these abnormalities are sporadic and unlikely to recur. Studies examining patients with recurrent pregnancy loss show that women who miscarry chromosomally abnormal conceptions are more likely to achieve a live birth with subsequent pregnancy than those who miscarry chromosomally normal conceptions (13,346). A second involves preimplantation genetic diagnosis (PGD) or preimplantation screening, and a third involves the use of donor gametes.

Because chromosomal abnormalities are the most commonly identified cause of miscarriage, some have argued that the use of PGD is indicated for patients with recurrent pregnancy loss. **PGD involves the removal of a single cell from an *in vitro*–matured embryo. Genetic testing can be performed on this cell to examine chromosomal composition for the presence of single gene disorders (e.g., cystic fibrosis) or abnormalities in chromosome number and morphology.** Embryos that are diagnosed with genetic abnormalities would be discarded and only those embryos with normal results would be considered appropriate for transfer into the uterus. Use of PGD in patients with known heritable genetic disorders (e.g., cystic fibrosis, X-linked disorders) is presently in widespread use in internationally recognized assisted reproductive technology centers.

The use of PGD has the potential to reduce the incidence of pregnancy loss arising from a genetic etiology. However, definitive studies in this population have not yet been done. The use of PGD requires the patient to go through an IVF cycle to obtain embryos for biopsy, and the impact of the biopsy technique itself on the embryos' viability is not known at this time. Although there are several retrospective studies showing reduced miscarriage rates with this technique, several prospective trials using the outcome of successful pregnancy per started cycle fail to show any benefit (347–357). IVF is invasive and costly and many patients with recurrent pregnancy loss conceive quickly without intervention and have a high likelihood of live birth with their subsequent pregnancy. Therefore, the optimal control group for a study of IVF PGD in the recurrent pregnancy loss population is debated. Should it be natural conceptions or IVF without PGD? Finally, the prognosis for a patient with recurrent pregnancy loss does seem to be linked to the chromosome analysis of prior miscarriages. Recurrent pregnancy loss patients who miscarry chromosomally abnormal embryos, seem to have better prognosis than those who miscarry chromosomally normal conceptions, again arguing for expectant management for recurrent pregnancy loss patients with a history of aneuploid loss. On the other hand, patients with poorer prognosis are those who miscarry chromosomally normal embryos and therefore would not benefit from PGD. The efficacy of PGD in the treatment of patients with recurrent pregnancy loss continues to be investigated, and the method of embryo biopsy and genetic testing continues to evolve (355,356). As these techniques improve and the understanding of aneuploidy and recurrence improves, there may be a subset of recurrent pregnancy loss patients, such as carriers of parental translocations, who might benefit from this intervention. At this time it cannot be recommended for all patients with a history of recurrent pregnancy loss.

The third approach is to use donor eggs or sperm. This treatment is particularly useful for patients with parental genetic factors and recurrent pregnancy loss, for example, a patient with Robertsonian translocations involving homologous chromosomes. In these patients, their genetic anomaly always results in unbalanced gametes, and the use of donor oocyte or donor sperm is recommended. Use of donor gametes among patients with a history of recurrent pregnancy loss can be useful in other cases where couples are at higher risk for unbalanced offspring because of carrying other forms of chromosomal rearrangements, such as reciprocal translocations or advanced maternal age. In these cases use of donor gametes was demonstrated to be as effective as its use in matched patients without such a history (358). In all cases of balanced translocations or embryonic aneuploidy, genetic counseling is recommended.

Anatomic Anomalies

Hysteroscopic resection represents state-of-the-art therapy for submucous leiomyomas, intrauterine adhesions, and intrauterine septa. This approach appears to limit postoperative sequelae while maintaining efficacy in terms of reproductive outcome (72,76,77,358–362). Use may be safely extended to patients with *DES* exposure, hypoplastic uteri, and complicated septal anomalies (76,77,363). Attempts to improve on standard hysteroscopic metroplasty, which is typically performed in the operating room using general anesthesia, often with laparoscopic guidance, are under investigation. Ultrasonographically guided transcervical metroplasty is reported to be safe and effective (359). Ambulatory, office-based procedures, including septum resection under fluoroscopic guidance, are attractive options (360).

For patients with a history of loss secondary to cervical incompetence, placement of a cervical cerclage is indicated. This is usually performed early in the second trimester after documentation of fetal viability. Cervical cerclage should be considered as a primary intervention for women with *DES*-associated uterine anomalies.

Endocrine Abnormalities

Some investigators have proposed the use of ovulation induction for the treatment of recurrent pregnancy loss (361,362). The theory behind its use in these patients rests on hypotheses that ovulation induction is associated with healthier oocytes. Healthier oocytes, in turn, may decrease the incidence of luteal phase insufficiency, which should result in improved pregnancy maintenance. This approach grossly oversimplifies the mechanisms involved in implantation and early pregnancy maintenance. Until appropriately studied, use of empiric ovulation induction for treatment of unexplained recurrent pregnancy loss should be viewed with caution. Evidence from small studies indicates such use is not effective (361). Still, use of ovulation induction in some subsets of patients with recurrent pregnancy loss could be of benefit. For instance, stimulating folliculogenesis with ovulation induction or luteal phase support with progesterone should be considered for women with luteal phase insufficiency. The efficacy of these therapies, however, is not substantiated (363). Ovulation induction might also be beneficial for women with hyperandrogen and LH hypersecretion disorders, especially following pituitary desensitization with gonadotropin-releasing hormone agonist therapy (112). This treatment remains controversial because the only large, prospective, randomized controlled trial to date reports no therapeutic efficacy; none for prepregnancy pituitary suppression nor for luteal phase progesterone supplementation (364).

Links between PCOS, hyperandrogenism, hyperinsulinemia, and recurrent pregnancy loss make use of insulin-sensitizing agents in the treatment of recurrent pregnancy loss associated with PCOS attractive (89–92). Although further study is needed, there are an increasing number of reports that support its use for this application (365,366). Prepregnancy glycemic control may be particularly important for women with overt diabetes mellitus (93,95). Thyroid hormone replacement with *Synthroid* may be helpful in cases of hypothyroidism. There are data indicating that thyroid hormone therapy may be of some benefit in euthyroid recurrent loss patients with antithyroid antibodies and possibly even in all pregnant women with "euthyroid" TSH levels between 2.5 and 5.0 mIU/L (98–100,272). There does not appear to be a place in the medical management of recurrent pregnancy loss for adding *bromocriptine* in women who do not have a prolactin disorder.

Infections

Empiric antibiotic treatment has been used for couples with recurrent abortion. Its efficacy is unproven. **Elaborate testing for infectious factors among recurrent pregnancy loss patients and use of therapeutic interventions is not justified unless a patient is immunocompromised or a specific infection has been documented (113).** For cases in which an infectious organism has been identified, appropriate antibiotics should be administered to both partners, followed by posttreatment culture to verify eradication of the infectious agent before attempting conception.

Immunologic Factors

Immune-mediated recurrent pregnancy loss has received more attention than any other single etiologic classification of recurrent pregnancy loss. Nevertheless, the diagnosis and subsequent treatment of the majority of cases remains unclear (102,367–370). **Most therapies for proposed immune-related recurrent pregnancy loss must be considered experimental.** As stated earlier, it is known that the developing conceptus contains paternally inherited gene products and tissue-specific differentiation antigens, and that there is maternal recognition of these antigens (216–218). Historically, it has been speculated that either inappropriately weak immune responses to these antigens or unusually strong responses could result in early pregnancy loss. As a consequence, both immunostimulating and immunosuppressive therapies have been proposed, but no conclusions about efficacy can be drawn.

Immunostimulating Therapies: Leukocyte Immunization

Stimulation of the maternal immune system using alloantigens on either paternal or pooled donor leukocytes has been promoted for patients with immunologic recurrent pregnancy loss, and a number of reports support possible mechanisms for potential therapeutic value (371–375). Both individual clinical trials and meta-analyses, however, continue to report conflicting results concerning the efficacy of leukocyte alloimmunization in patients with recurrent pregnancy loss (25,364,365,372,376–379). This most certainly reflects the remarkable heterogeneity in study design, patient selection, and therapeutic protocols, as well as the typically small numbers of enrolled subjects in these investigations. **One of the largest trials evaluating the efficacy of leukocyte immunization in patients with unexplained recurrent pregnancy loss is a part of the Recurrent Miscarriage (REMIS) study (380). This investigation was large (over 90 patients per treatment arm), prospective, placebo controlled, randomized, and double blinded. It demonstrated no efficacy for paternal leukocyte immunization in couples with unexplained recurrent pregnancy loss. The most recent and best of the meta-analyses definitively rejects use of this therapy in patients with recurrent loss** (381). Leukocyte immunization also poses a significant risk to both the mother and her fetus (344,345,382). Several cases of graft-versus-host disease, severe intrauterine growth retardation, and autoimmune and isoimmune complications have been reported (25,378,382–386). In addition, alloimmunization to platelets contained in the paternal leukocyte preparation is associated with cases of potentially fatal fetal thrombocytopenia. **The routine use of this therapy for recurrent abortion cannot be clinically justified at this time. The procedure should be performed only as part of an appropriately controlled trial using informed consent. All costs associated with this treatment should be borne by the investigators until its efficacy has been demonstrated.**

Other immunostimulating therapies have been proposed and abandoned. Intravenous preparations consisting of syncytiotrophoblast microvillus plasma membrane vesicles have been used to mimic the fetal cell contact with maternal blood that normally occurs in pregnancy (387). The efficacy of this therapy has not been established (381,387,388). The use of third-party seminal plasma suppositories has also been attempted, based on the misconception that TLX was part of an idiotype–anti-idiotype control system (389,390). Third-party seminal plasma suppositories for recurrent abortion have no scientifically credible rationale and should not be used.

Immunosuppressive Therapies

Immunosuppressive and other immunoregulating therapies have been advocated for cases in which abortion was believed to result from antiphospholipid antibodies or inappropriate cellular immunity toward the implanting fetus. Again, study design problems, including small numbers of recruited patients, lack of prestratification by maternal age and number of prior losses before randomization, and other methodologic and statistical inaccuracies preclude definitive statements regarding therapeutic efficacy for most of the proposed immunosuppressive approaches.

Intravenous Immunoglobulin   Intravenous immunoglobulins (IVIgs) are composed of pooled samples of immunoglobulins harvested from a large number of blood donors. Studies on the use of IVIg therapy in the treatment of recurrent pregnancy loss are based on the theory that some recurrent pregnancy loss patients have an overzealous immune reactivity to their implanting fetus. IVIgs do have immunosuppressive effects, but the mechanisms underlying this immune modulation are only partially understood. These mechanisms may include decreased autoantibody production and increased autoantibody clearance, T-cell and Fc-receptor regulation, complement inactivation, enhanced T-cell suppressor function, decreased T-cell adhesion to the extracellular matrix, and downregulation of TH1 cytokine synthesis (391–394). **Based on a large number of relatively small studies using a variety of treatment protocols, there remains no conclusive evidence to suggest that use of IVIg in the treatment of patients with unexplained (and presumed immunologic) recurrent pregnancy loss has any benefit** (383,395–399). This includes a recent trial using IVIg in women with secondary recurrent pregnancy loss that was ended early because interim analyses revealed no effect (395). **The Cochrane review of immune therapy for recurrent pregnancy loss also addressed IVIg therapy and reported that its use did**

not alter pregnancy outcomes in patients with otherwise unexplained recurrent pregnancy loss (381,388). Improved posttreatment pregnancy rates may be seen, however, when IVIg is used in those specific patients with autoimmune-mediated pregnancy loss associated with APS (400,401). Therapy with IVIgs for recurrent pregnancy loss is expensive, invasive, and time-consuming, requiring multiple intravenous infusions over the course of pregnancy (402). Side effects of IVIg therapy include nausea, headache, myalgias, and hypotension. More serious adverse effects include anaphylaxis (particularly in patients with IgA deficiency) (403).

Progesterone   As mentioned earlier, progesterone also has known immunosuppressive effects (220–223,227,228). **A number of studies using** *in vitro* **cellular systems relevant to the maternal–fetal interface have now demonstrated that progesterone either inhibits TH1 immunity or causes a shift from TH1- to TH2-type responses** (208,227,228,404). Although the mechanism of action remains unclear, a recent Cochrane review concluded that progesterone supplementation was effective in the treatment of recurrent, but not isolated, spontaneous pregnancy loss (405,406). The review makes no recommendations on dosage, timing of initiation, nor route of progesterone administration. Progesterone has been administered both intramuscularly and intravaginally for the treatment of recurrent pregnancy loss. It is thought that vaginal administration may increase local, intrauterine concentrations of progesterone better than systemic administration. Vaginal formulations may therefore provide a better method of attaining local immunosuppressive levels of progesterone while averting any adverse systemic side effects.

Intralipid Infusion   The relative paucity of inflammatory diseases among the Greenland Inuit population, who consume a diet high in fish oils, led investigators to study the immune modulatory effects of lipid emulsions in total parenteral nutrition preparations for preoperative patients and for burn and trauma victims (406–409). The wide range of demonstrated effects, including lipid preparations that reduced natural killer cell activity, reduced monocytes proinflammatory cytokine production and increased susceptibility to infection, led investigators to hypothesize, as early as 1994, that lipid infusions might promote an immune environment that would favor pregnancy maintenance (410). Since that time, a small number of publications have addressed the effects of lipid infusions (*Intralipid*) in women with a history of pregnancy loss (411,412). These investigations have demonstrated a decrease in peripheral natural killer cell activity in women treated with one to three infusions of *Intralipid*. This effect lasted from 4 to 9 weeks after the last infusion (411). The authors did not address NK cell cytokine secretion patterns nor did they assay decidual NK cell function. **Despite this paucity of data,** *Intralipid* **infusions are being administered to recurrent pregnancy loss patients with increasing frequency. The existing data do not support this practice. At this time,** *Intralipid* **infusions in recurrent pregnancy loss patients should only be administered under an institutional review board–approved protocol and in a study setting. They should not generate clinical income.**

TNF-α Inhibition   Interest in the potent proinflammatory cytokine, TNF-α, as a mediator of pregnancy loss came out of the description of the TH1 and TH2 paradigm (209). Over the past 10 years, there have been several publications that link maternal serum TNF-α levels and activating TNF-α gene promoter polymorphisms to recurrent pregnancy loss (413–415). The development of antagonists of TNF-α in the form of blocking antibodies (*adalimumab, infliximab*) and inhibitory recombinant proteins (*etanercept*) has allowed for successful treatment of several autoimmune disorders, including rheumatoid arthritis, psoriasis, and Crohn's disease. Their use, however, has not been associated with universally positive outcomes and may worsen some disorders, including multiple sclerosis (416). These products are associated with rare but worrisome side effects, including liver failure, aplastic anemia, interstitial lung disease, and anaphylaxis (417). Although there exists only a single, small, retrospective, observational, nonrandomly assigned case series that involved treatment of recurrent pregnancy loss patients with inhibitors of TNF-α, these positive preliminary results have led a growing number of clinics to offer this therapy to patients, often at a significant cost (418). The safety of these compounds in pregnancy has not been appropriately studied, and preliminary reports associating exposure to TNF-α inhibitors during early pregnancy to fetal VACTERL syndrome is concerning (419). **As with** *Intralipid* **therapy, use of TNF-α inhibition for the treatment of recurrent pregnancy loss should only be administered under an institutional review board–approved protocol in a study setting and should not generate clinical income.**

Other immunoregulating therapies theoretically useful in treating recurrent pregnancy loss include the use of *cyclosporine, pentoxifylline,* and *nifedipine,* although maternal and fetal risks with these agents preclude their clinical use. Plasmaphoresis has also been used to treat women with recurrent abortion and antiphospholipid antibodies (420). Generalized immunosuppression with corticosteroids, such as *prednisone,* has been advocated during pregnancy for women with recurrent losses and chronic intervillositis and those with recurrent pregnancy loss and APS (421). Although corticosteroids have shown some treatment promise in these patients, maternal and fetal side effects and the availability of alternative therapies have limited their use (421,422). That said, in response to successful use of *prednisolone* in a woman with 10 prior losses, Quenby et al. have demonstrated that such treatment decreases the number of uterine NK cells in the peri-implantation decidua among women with a history of recurrent loss and have plans for a trial of therapy using live birth as a secondary outcome (423–425). **The efficacy and side effects of *prednisone* plus low-dose *aspirin* was examined in a recent, large, randomized, placebo-controlled trial treating patients with autoantibodies and recurrent pregnancy losses. Pregnancy outcomes for treated and control patients were similar; however, the incidence of maternal diabetes and hypertension and the risk of premature delivery were all increased among those treated with *prednisone* and *aspirin*** (426).

Antithrombotic Therapy

Therapy for patients with recurrent pregnancy losses associated with either APS or other thrombophilic disorders has now shifted toward the use of antithrombotic medications. Unlike immunosuppressive treatments, this approach appears to address the effect (hypercoagulability), but not the underlying cause (e.g., genetic, APS) of recurrent pregnancy loss. However, there are reports that *heparin,* one typical anticoagulant, may exert direct immunomodulatory effects by binding to antiphospholipid antibodies and may decrease movement of inflammatory cells to sites of alloantigen exposure (427,428). **The combined use of low-dose *aspirin* (75 to 80 mg per day) and subcutaneous unfractionated *heparin* (5,000 to 10,000 units twice daily) during pregnancy has been best studied among women with APS and appears to be efficacious** (429–433). A typical regimen for women with antiphospholipid antibody syndrome would include use of *aspirin* (80 mg every day) beginning with any attempts to conceive. After pregnancy has been confirmed, 10,000 IU unfractionated *sodium heparin* is administered subcutaneously twice daily, throughout gestation. An aPTT should be obtained weekly and dosages of *heparin* should be adjusted until anticoagulation is achieved. Patients using this therapy should be treated in conjunction with a perinatologist because of their increased risks for preterm labor, premature rupture of the membranes, intrauterine growth restriction, intrauterine fetal demise, and pre-eclampsia. Other potential risks include gastric bleeding, osteopenia, and abruptio placenta.

Attempts have recently been made to extend the finding that antithrombotic therapy is efficacious when used to treat patients with APS and recurrent pregnancy loss in a number of directions. These directions include the use of *low-molecular weight heparins* (*LMWH*), the use of antithrombotic therapy in non-APS patients with thrombophilia and recurrent pregnancy loss, and even its use among recurrent pregnancy loss patients without thrombophilia (unexplained recurrent losses).

New formulations of heparin, termed *low-molecular weight heparins,* have been demonstrated to be superior to unfractionated heparin in the treatment of many clotting disorders (434–436). *LMWH* has the advantage of an increased antithrombotic ratio when compared with unfractionated heparin. This results in improved treatment of inappropriate clotting but fewer bleeding side effects. In addition, *LMWH* has been associated with a decreased incidence of thrombocytopenia and osteoporosis when compared with its unfractionated counterpart. Finally, *LMWH* has a long half-life and requires less frequent dosing and monitoring, thereby improving patient compliance. ***LMWH* appear to be safe for use in pregnancy, and *LMWH* has shown promise when combined with low-dose aspirin in the treatment of recurrent pregnancy loss associated with APS** (430,435,437). Only a few studies have compared the use of unfractionated heparin and aspirin to LMWH and aspirin in the treatment of women with APS and adverse pregnancy outcomes (433,438). The therapies had similar effects in one study (438). A meta-analysis suggested that unfractionated heparin was superior to LMWH, however, there was significant heterogenicity between studies (433). Efficacy has been suggested for LMWH treatment for patients with recurrent pregnancy loss associated with other thrombophilias, including activated protein C resistance associated with factor V Leiden, mutations in the promoter region of the prothrombin gene, and decreases in protein C and protein S activities (63,439–441). The use of *LMWH* for this indication appears to have an excellent safety profile for mother and fetus (437,442,443) .

The prophylactic use of daily-low dose *aspirin* has become common practice within the lay public based on its perceived cardiovascular effects combined with its low incidence of side effects. Its sole use in the treatment of recurrent pregnancy loss has likewise gained momentum, and many patients with histories of recurrent loss will either be self-prescribing this therapy or will inquire about its usefulness. At present, there are no good data supporting its use either in patients with heritable thrombophilias or in the general recurrent pregnancy loss population. Although studies are small, the use of low-dose *aspirin* alone has not been shown to be effective in the treatment of recurrent pregnancy loss associated with APS (431,444,445). When used in these patients, it should be in combination with unfractionated or *LMWH*. Large randomized prospective trials examining the empiric use of *aspirin* alone or in combination with prophylactic doses of *heparin* have shown no benefit of these therapies in unexplained recurrent pregnancy loss (445). In addition, the use of *aspirin* in early pregnancy has been called into question with reports of an increased incidence of isolated spontaneous pregnancy loss among women who used this medication (316,317). However, these reports are poorly designed and do not adequately address the level of *aspirin* exposure (81 mg vs. 325 mg). **Although reviews have touted the overall safety of *aspirin* in pregnancy, outside of use in combination with *heparin* for patients with recurrent pregnancy loss and APS, this medication should be used only with justification in the well-informed patient during early pregnancy** (446).

More directed antithrombotic therapies have also been described for the treatment of recurrent pregnancy loss among patients with thrombophilias. For instance, the use of protein C concentrates has been reported to be associated with favorable pregnancy outcome in a patient with a history of thrombosis, recurrent fetal losses, and protein C deficiency (447).

As mentioned previously, vitamins B_6, B_{12}, and folate are important in homocysteine metabolism, and hyperhomocysteinemia is linked to recurrent pregnancy loss (21,23,38,66,68,72). Women with recurrent pregnancy loss and isolated fasting hyperhomocysteinemia should be offered supplemental *folic acid* (0.4 to 1.0 mg per day), vitamin B_6 (6 mg per day), and possibly vitamin B_{12} (0.025 mg per day) (448–451). Fasting homocysteine levels should be retested after treatment. If levels are normalized or remain only marginally elevated, no further therapy is necessary. Homocysteine levels will predictably decrease during pregnancy.

Treatment of women with recurrent pregnancy loss and an identified inherited or acquired thrombophilia should be based on accompanying history. Currently, there are no prospective controlled trials examining the benefit of anticoagulation for the prevention of miscarriage in the absence of APS, and, therefore, anticoagulation recommendations for patients with inherited thrombophilias are based on individualized risk of venous thromboembolic events in pregnancy (28).

- **If a venous thromboembolic event occurs during the index pregnancy, posthospitalization management requires therapeutic anticoagulation.**
  UFH: 10,000 to 15,000 U subcutaneous every 8 to 12 hours (monitor to keep aPTT 1.5 to 2.5 times normal) OR
  ***LMWH: enoxaparin* 40 to 80 mg subcutaneous twice a day or *dalteparin* 5,000 to 10,000 U subcutaneous twice a day). Consider monitoring trough factor Xa levels in the third trimester.**

- **If there is a personal history of venous thromboembolic events (particularly in a previous pregnancy or with hormonal contraceptive use) or a strong thrombophilic family history, treat with therapeutic anticoagulation. Thrombotic risk is greatest during the postpartum period.**

- **Anticoagulation should be reinitiated after delivery in doses reflecting predelivery treatment regimens. Postpartum anticoagulation should be continued for 6 to 12 weeks postpartum** (435). Women may continue injectable therapy or transition to oral anticoagulants (e.g., *coumarin*). Use of *heparin* or of *coumarin* derivatives does not prohibit breastfeeding.

Psychological Support

There is no doubt that experiencing both isolated and recurrent losses can be emotionally devastating. The risk of major depression is increased greater than twofold among women with spontaneous pregnancy loss; in most women it arises in the first weeks following delivery (452). A caring and empathetic attitude is prerequisite to all healing. The acknowledgment of the pain and suffering couples have experienced as a result of recurrent abortion can be a cathartic catalyst enabling them to incorporate their experience of loss into their lives rather than their lives into their experience of loss (112). **Referrals to support groups and counselors should be offered.** Self-help measures, such as meditation, yoga, exercise, and biofeedback may also be useful.

Prognosis

The prognosis for successful pregnancy depends both on the potential underlying cause of pregnancy loss and (epidemiologically) on the number of prior losses (Table 33.4). As previously discussed, epidemiologic surveys indicate that the chance of a viable birth even after four prior losses may be as high as 60%. Depending on the study, **the prognosis for successful pregnancy in couples with a cytogenetic etiology for reproductive loss varies from 20% to 80%** (453–455). **Women with corrected anatomical anomalies may expect a successful pregnancy in 60% to 90% of cases** (74,453,456–459). **A success rate higher than 90% has been reported for women with corrected endocrinologic abnormalities** (454). **Between 70% to 90% of pregnancies reported among women receiving therapy for antiphospholipid antibodies have been viable** (460,461).

Many forms of pre- or postconceptional tests have been proposed to help predict pregnancy outcome (201,219,327,462,463); **none have been fully substantiated in large, prospective trials. The documentation of fetal cardiac activity on ultrasound may offer prognostic value; however, it appears that its predictions may be greatly affected by any underlying diagnosis.** In one study, the live birth rate following documentation of fetal cardiac activity between 5 to 6 weeks from the last menstrual period was approximately 77% in women with two or more unexplained spontaneous abortions (464). It may be important to note that the majority of the patients in this study had evidence of inappropriate antitrophoblast cellular immunity. Others have shown that 86% of patients with antiphospholipid antibodies and recurrent pregnancy loss had fetal cardiac activity detected prior to subsequent demise (465). **A prospective, longitudinal, observational study of 325 patients with unexplained recurrent pregnancy losses demonstrated that only 3% of 55 miscarriages occurred following the detection of fetal cardiac activity using transvaginal ultrasonography** (466).

Table 33.4 Prognosis for a Viable Birth	
Following:	
One spontaneous loss	76%
Two spontaneous losses	70%
Three spontaneous losses	65%
Four spontaneous losses	60%
With:	
Genetic factors	20%–80%
Anatomic factors	60%–90%
Endocrine factors	>90%
Infectious factors	70%–90%
Antiphospholipid antibodies	70%–90%
TH1 cellular immunity	70%–87%
Unknown factors	40%–90%
Following detection of fetal cardiac activity:	
Unexplained recurrent pregnancy loss	77%–97%
Antiphospholipid antibody syndrome and recurrent pregnancy loss	Much lower

References

1. **Edmonds DK, Lindsay KS, Miller JF, et al.** Early embryonic mortality in women. *Fertil Steril* 1982;38:447–453.
2. **Wilcox AJ, Weinberg CR, O'Connor JF, et al.** Incidence of early loss of pregnancy. *N Engl J Med* 1988;319:189–194.
3. **Alberman E.** The epidemiology of repeated abortion. In: Beard RW, Sharp F, eds. *Early pregnancy loss: mechanisms and treatment.* New York: Springer-Verlag, 1988:9–17.
4. **Warburton D, Fraser FC.** Spontaneous abortion risks in man: data from reproductive histories collected in a medical genetics unit. *Am J Hum Genet* 1964;16:1–25.
5. **Practice Committee of the American Society for Reproductive Medicine.** Definitions of infertility and recurrent pregnancy loss. *Fertil Steril* 2008;90(Suppl 3):S60.
6. **Jaslow CR, Carney JL, Kutteh WH.** Diagnostic factors identified in 1,020 women with two versus three or more recurrent pregnancy losses. *Fertil Steril* 2010;93:1234–1243.
7. **Regan L, Braude PR, Trembath PL.** Influence of past reproductive performance on risk of spontaneous abortion. *BMJ* 1989;299:541–545.
8. **Marquard K, Westphal LM, Milki AA, et al.** Etiology of recurrent pregnancy loss in women over the age of 35 years. *Fertil Steril* 2010; 94:1473–1477.
9. **Stephenson MD.** Frequency of factors associated with habitual abortion in 197 couples. *Fertil Steril* 1996;66:24–29.
10. **Macklon NS, Geraedts JP, Fauser BC.** Conception to ongoing pregnancy: the "black box" of early pregnancy loss. *Hum Reprod Update* 2002;8:333–343.
11. **Daniel A, Hook EB, Wulf G.** Risks of unbalanced progeny at amniocentesis to carriers of chromosome rearrangements: data from United States and Canadian laboratories. *Am J Med Genet* 1989;33: 14–53.
12. **Fryns JP, Van Buggenhout G.** Structural chromosome rearrangements in couples with recurrent fetal wastage. *Eur J Obstet Gynecol Reprod Biol* 1998;81:171–176.
13. **Ogasawara M, Aoki K, Okada S, et al.** Embryonic karyotype of abortuses in relation to the number of previous miscarriages. *Fertil Steril* 2000;73:300–304.
14. **Warren JE, Silver RM.** Genetics of pregnancy loss. *Clin Obstet Gynecol* 2008;51:84–95.
15. **Simon C, Rubio C, Vidal F, et al.** Increased chromosome abnormalities in human preimplantation embryos after *in-vitro* fertilization in patients with recurrent miscarriage. *Reprod Fertil Dev* 1998;10:87–92.
16. **Carrell DT, Wilcox AL, Lowy L, et al.** Elevated sperm chromosome aneuploidy and apoptosis in patients with unexplained recurrent pregnancy loss. *Obstet Gynecol* 2003;101:1229–1235.
17. **Egozcue S, Blanco J, Vendrell JM, et al.** Human male infertility: chromosome anomalies, meiotic disorders, abnormal spermatozoa and recurrent abortion. *Hum Reprod Update* 2000;6:93–105.
18. **Giorlandino C, Calugi G, Iaconianni L, et al.** Spermatozoa with chromosomal abnormalities may result in a higher rate of recurrent abortion. *Fertil Steril* 1998;70:576–577.
19. **Lanasa MC, Hogge WA.** X chromosome defects as an etiology of recurrent spontaneous abortion. *Semin Reprod Med* 2000;18:97–103.
20. **Girling J, de Swiet M.** Inherited thrombophilia and pregnancy. *Curr Opin Obstet Gynecol* 1998;10:135–144.
21. **Greer IA.** Thrombophilia: implications for pregnancy outcome. *Thromb Res* 2003;109:73–81.
22. **Lockwood CJ.** Inherited thrombophilias in pregnant patients: detection and treatment paradigm. *Obstet Gynecol* 2002;99:333–341.
23. **Nelen WL, Bulten J, Steegers EA, et al.** Hereditary thrombophilia as a cause for fetal loss. *Obstet Gynecol* 2000;95(4 Suppl): S11–S12.
24. **Jivraj S, Rai R, Underwood J, et al.** Genetic thrombophilic mutations among couples with recurrent miscarriage. *Hum Reprod* 2006;21:1161–1165.
25. **Anonymous.** Worldwide collaborative observational study and meta-analysis on allogenic leukocyte immunotherapy for recurrent spontaneous abortion. Recurrent Miscarriage Immunotherapy Trialists Group. *Am J Reprod Immunol* 1994;32:55–72.
26. **Kovac M, Mitic G, Mikovic Z, et al.** Thrombophilia in women with pregnancy-associated complications: fetal loss and pregnancy-related venous thromboembolism. *Gynecol Obstet Invest* 2010;69:233–238.
27. **Anonymous.** Length of hospital stay for gynecologic procedures. ACOG Committee Opinion: Committee on Gynecologic Practice. Number 113—August 1992. *Int J Gynaecol Obstet* 1993;40:262.
28. **American College of Obstetricians and Gynecologists Committee on Practice Bulletins-Obstetrics.** ACOG Practice Bulletin Number 111. Inherited thrombophilias in pregnancy. *Obstet Gynecol* 2010;115:877–887.
29. **Di Stefano G, Provinciali M, Muzzioli M, et al.** Correlation between estradiol serum levels and NK cell activity in endometriosis. *Ann N Y Acad Sci* 1994;741:197–203.
30. **Lockwood CJ.** Inherited thrombophilias in pregnant patients. *Prenat Neonat Med* 2001;6:20–32.
31. **Buchholz T, Thaler CJ.** Inherited thrombophilia: impact on human reproduction. *Am J Reprod Immunol* 2003;50:20–32.
32. **Lane DA, Grant PJ.** Role of hemostatic gene polymorphisms in venous and arterial thrombotic disease. *Blood* 2000;95:1517–1532.
33. **Lindqvist PG, Svensson PJ, Dahlbäck B, et al.** Factor V Q506 mutation (activated protein C resistance) associated with reduced intrapartum blood loss–a possible evolutionary selection mechanism. *Thromb Haemost* 1998;79:69–73.
34. **Gopel W, Ludwig M, Junge AK, et al.** Selection pressure for the factor-V-Leiden mutation and embryo implantation. *Lancet* 2001;358:1238–1239.
35. **Patel RK, Ford E, Thumpston J, et al.** Risk factors for venous thrombosis in the black population. *Thromb Haemost* 2003;90:835–838.
36. **Pepe G, Rickards O, Vanegas OC, et al.** Prevalence of factor V Leiden mutation in non-European populations. *Thromb Haemost* 1997;77:329–331.
37. **Rosendaal FR, Doggen CJ, Zivelin A, et al.** Geographic distribution of the 20210 G to A prothrombin variant. *Thromb Haemost* 1998;79:706–708.
38. **Yamada H, Kato EH, Kobashi G, et al.** Recurrent pregnancy loss: etiology of thrombophilia. *Semin Thromb Hemost* 2001;27:121–129.
39. **Shen MC, Lin JS, Tsay W.** High prevalence of antithrombin III, protein C and protein S deficiency, but no factor V Leiden mutation in venous thrombophilic Chinese patients in Taiwan. *Thromb Res* 1997;87:377–385.
40. **Dizon-Townson DS, Meline L, Nelson LM, et al.** Fetal carriers of the factor V Leiden mutation are prone to miscarriage and placental infarction. *Am J Obstet Gynecol* 1997;177:402–405.
41. **Gris JC, Quéré I, Monpeyroux F, et al.** Case-control study of the frequency of thrombophilic disorders in couples with late foetal loss and no thrombotic antecedent—the Nimes Obstetricians and Haematologists Study5 (NOHA5). *Thromb Haemost* 1999;81:891–899.
42. **Many A, Schreiber L, Rosner S, et al.** Pathologic features of the placenta in women with severe pregnancy complications and thrombophilia. *Obstet Gynecol* 2001;98:1041–1044.
43. **Martinelli I, Taioli E, Cetin I, et al.** Mutations in coagulation factors in women with unexplained late fetal loss. *N Engl J Med* 2000;343:1015–1018.
44. **Mousa HA, Alfirevic Z.** Do placental lesions reflect thrombophilia state in women with adverse pregnancy outcome? *Hum Reprod* 2000;15:1830–1833.
45. **Burton GJ, Hempstock J, Jauniaux E.** Nutrition of the human fetus during the first trimester—a review. *Placenta* 2001;22(Suppl A):S70–S77.
46. **Burton GJ, Jauniaux E, Watson AL.** Maternal arterial connections to the placental intervillous space during the first trimester of human pregnancy: the Boyd collection revisited. *Am J Obstet Gynecol* 1999;181:718–724.
47. **Burton GJ, Watson AL, Hempstock J, et al.** Uterine glands provide histiotrophic nutrition for the human fetus during the first trimester of pregnancy. *J Clin Endocrinol Metab* 2002;87:2954–2959.
48. **Jauniaux E, Burton GJ, Moscoso GJ, et al.** Development of the early human placenta: a morphometric study. *Placenta* 1991;12:269–276.
49. **Stirling Y, Woolf L, North WR, et al.** Haemostasis in normal pregnancy. *Thromb Haemost* 1984;52:176–182.

50. **Lanir N, Aharon A, Brenner B.** Procoagulant and anticoagulant mechanisms in human placenta. *Semin Thromb Hemost* 2003; 29:175–184.

51. **Clark P, Brennand J, Conkie JA, et al.** Activated protein C sensitivity, protein C, protein S and coagulation in normal pregnancy. *Thromb Haemost* 1998;79:1166–1170.

52. **Hellgren M, Blomback M.** Studies on blood coagulation and fibrinolysis in pregnancy, during delivery and in the puerperium. I. Normal condition. *Gynecol Obstet Invest* 1981;12:141–154.

53. **Persson BL, Stenberg P, Holmberg L, et al.** Transamidating enzymes in maternal plasma and placenta in human pregnancies complicated by intrauterine growth retardation. *J Dev Physiol* 1980;2:37–46.

54. **Cumming AM, Tait RC, Fildes S, et al.** Development of resistance to activated protein C during pregnancy. *Br J Haematol* 1995;90:725–727.

55. **Comp PC, Thurnau GR, Welsh J, et al.** Functional and immunologic protein S levels are decreased during pregnancy. *Blood* 1986;68:881–885.

56. **Giavarina D, Mezzena G, Dorizzi RM, et al.** Reference interval of D-dimer in pregnant women. *Clin Biochem* 2001;34:331–333.

57. **Kruithof EK, Tran-Thang C, Gudinchet A, et al.** Fibrinolysis in pregnancy: a study of plasminogen activator inhibitors. *Blood* 1987;69:460–466.

58. **Hellgren M.** Hemostasis during normal pregnancy and puerperium. *Semin Thromb Hemost* 2003;29:125–130.

59. **Ueland PM, Refsum H.** Plasma homocysteine, a risk factor for vascular disease: plasma levels in health, disease, and drug therapy. *J Lab Clin Med* 1989;114:473–501.

60. **Molloy AM, Daly S, Mills JL, et al.** Thermolabile variant of 5, 10-ethylenetetrahydrofolate reductase associated with low red-cell folates: implications for folate intake recommendations. *Lancet* 1997;349:1591–1593.

61. **Murphy RP, Donoghue C, Nallen RJ, et al.** Prospective evaluation of the risk conferred by factor V Leiden and thermolabile methylenetetrahydrofolate reductase polymorphisms in pregnancy. *Arterioscler Thromb Vasc Biol* 2000;20:266–270.

62. **Preston FE, Rosendaal FR, Walker ID, et al.** Increased fetal loss in women with heritable thrombophilia. *Lancet* 1996;348:913–916.

63. **Brenner B, Mandel H, Lanir N, et al.** Activated protein C resistance can be associated with recurrent fetal loss. *Br J Haematol* 1997;97:551–554.

64. **Foka ZJ, Lambropoulos AF, Saravelos H, et al.** Factor V Leiden and prothrombin G20210A mutations, but not methylenetetrahydrofolate reductase C677T, are associated with recurrent miscarriages. *Hum Reprod* 2000;15:458–462.

65. **Holmes ZR, Regan L, Chilcott I, et al.** The C677T MTHFR gene mutation is not predictive of risk for recurrent fetal loss. *Br J Haematol* 1999;105:98–101.

66. **Nelen WL, Blom HJ, Steegers EA, et al.** Homocysteine and folate levels as risk factors for recurrent early pregnancy loss. *Obstet Gynecol* 2000;95:519–524.

67. **Poort SR, Rosendaal FR, Reitsma PH, et al.** A common genetic variation in the 3′-untranslated region of the prothrombin gene is associated with elevated plasma prothrombin levels and an increase in venous thrombosis. *Blood* 1996;88:3698–3703.

68. **Ray JG, Laskin CA.** Folic acid and homocyst(e)ine metabolic defects and the risk of placental abruption, pre-eclampsia and spontaneous pregnancy loss: A systematic review. *Placenta* 1999;20:519–529.

69. **Ridker PM, Miletich JP, Buring JE, et al.** Factor V Leiden mutation as a risk factor for recurrent pregnancy loss. *Ann Intern Med* 1998;128(Pt 1):1000–1003.

70. **Souza SS, Ferriani RA, Pontes AG, et al.** Factor V Leiden and factor II G20210A mutations in patients with recurrent abortion. *Hum Reprod* 1999;14:2448–2450.

71. **Kovalevsky G, Gracia CR, Berlin JA, et al.** Evaluation of the association between hereditary thrombophilias and recurrent pregnancy loss: a meta-analysis. *Arch Intern Med* 2004;164:558–563.

72. **Nelen WL, Blom HJ, Steegers EA, et al.** Hyperhomocysteinemia and recurrent early pregnancy loss: a meta-analysis. *Fertil Steril* 2000;74:1196–1199.

73. **Rey E, Kahn SR, David M, et al.** Thrombophilic disorders and fetal loss: a meta-analysis. *Lancet* 2003;361:901–908.

74. **Rackow BW, Arici A.** Reproductive performance of women with mullerian anomalies. *Curr Opin Obstet Gynecol* 2007;19:229–237.

75. **Reichman DE, Laufer MR.** Congenital uterine anomalies affecting reproduction. *Best Pract Res Clin Obstet Gynaecol* 2010;24:193–208.

76. **Raga F, Bauset C, Remohi J, et al.** Reproductive impact of congenital Mullerian anomalies. *Hum Reprod* 1997;12:2277–2281.

77. **Proctor JA, Haney AF.** Recurrent first trimester pregnancy loss is associated with uterine septum but not with bicornuate uterus. *Fertil Steril* 2003;80:1212–1215.

78. **Propst AM, Hill JA 3rd.** Anatomic factors associated with recurrent pregnancy loss. *Semin Reprod Med* 2000;18:341–350.

79. **Homer HA, Li TC, Cooke ID.** The septate uterus: a review of management and reproductive outcome. *Fertil Steril* 2000;73:1–14.

80. **Saravelos SH, Cocksedge KA, Li TC.** The pattern of pregnancy loss in women with congenital uterine anomalies and recurrent miscarriage. *Reprod Biomed Online* 2010;20:416–422.

81. **Mizuno K, Koske K, Ando K.** Significance of Jones operation on double uterus: vascularity and dating in uterine septum. *Jpn J Fertil Steril* 1978;29:9.

82. **Barnes AB, Colton T, Gundersen J, et al.** Fertility and outcome of pregnancy in women exposed *in utero* to diethylstilbestrol. *N Engl J Med* 1980;302:609–613.

83. **Kaufman RH, Adam E, Hatch EE, et al.** Continued follow-up of pregnancy outcomes in diethylstilbestrol-exposed offspring. *Obstet Gynecol* 2000;96:483–489.

84. **Burchell RC, Creed F, Rasoulpour M, et al.** Vascular anatomy of the human uterus and pregnancy wastage. *Br J Obstet Gynaecol* 1978;85:698–706.

85. **Buttram VC, Jr., Reiter RC.** Uterine leiomyomata: etiology, symptomatology, and management. *Fertil Steril* 1981;36:433–445.

86. **Bajekal N, Li TC.** Fibroids, infertility and pregnancy wastage. *Hum Reprod Update* 2000;6:614–620.

87. **Csapo AI, Pulkkinen MO, Ruttner B, et al.** The significance of the human corpus luteum in pregnancy maintenance. I. Preliminary studies. *Am J Obstet Gynecol* 1972;112:1061–1067.

88. **Salker M, Teklenburg G, Molokhia M, et al.** Natural selection of human embryos: impaired decidualization of endometrium disables embryo-maternal interactions and causes recurrent pregnancy loss. *PLoS One* 2010;5:e10287.

89. **Rai R, Backos M, Rushworth F, et al.** Polycystic ovaries and recurrent miscarriage–a reappraisal. *Hum Reprod* 2000;15:612–615.

90. **Watson H, Kiddy DS, Hamilton-Fairley D, et al.** Hypersecretion of luteinizing hormone and ovarian steroids in women with recurrent early miscarriage. *Hum Reprod* 1993;8:829–833.

91. **Bussen S, Sutterlin M, Steck T.** Endocrine abnormalities during the follicular phase in women with recurrent spontaneous abortion. *Hum Reprod* 1999;14:18–20.

92. **Okon MA, Laird SM, Tuckerman EM, et al.** Serum androgen levels in women who have recurrent miscarriages and their correlation with markers of endometrial function. *Fertil Steril* 1998;69:682–690.

93. **Brydon P, Smith T, Proffitt M, et al.** Pregnancy outcome in women with type 2 diabetes mellitus needs to be addressed. *Int J Clin Pract* 2000;54:418–419.

94. **Greene MF.** Spontaneous abortions and major malformations in women with diabetes mellitus. *Semin Reprod Endocrinol* 1999;17:127–136.

95. **Langer O, Conway DL.** Level of glycemia and perinatal outcome in pregestational diabetes. *J Matern Fetal Med* 2000;9:35–41.

96. **Moley KH, Chi MM, Knudson CM, et al.** Hyperglycemia induces apoptosis in pre-implantation embryos through cell death effector pathways. *Nat Med* 1998;4:1421–1424.

97. **Vaquero E, Lazzarin N, De Carolis C, et al.** Mild thyroid abnormalities and recurrent spontaneous abortion: diagnostic and therapeutical approach. *Am J Reprod Immunol* 2000;43:204–208.

98. **Negro R, Schwartz A, Gismondi R, et al.** Increased pregnancy loss rate in thyroid antibody negative women with TSH levels between 2.5 and 5.0 in the first trimester of pregnancy. *J Clin Endocrinol Metab* 2010;99:E44–48.

99. **Debieve F, Dulière S, Bernard P, et al.** To treat or not to treat euthyroid autoimmune disorder during pregnancy? *Gynecol Obstet Invest* 2009;67:178–182.

100. **De Vivo A, Mancuso A, Giacobbe A, et al.** Thyroid function in women found to have early pregnancy loss. *Thyroid* 2010;20:633–637.

101. **Esplin MS, Branch DW, Silver R, et al.** Thyroid autoantibodies are not associated with recurrent pregnancy loss. *Am J Obstet Gynecol* 1998;179(Pt 1):1583–1586.

102. **Kutteh WH, Yetman DL, Carr AC, et al.** Increased prevalence of antithyroid antibodies identified in women with recurrent pregnancy loss but not in women undergoing assisted reproduction. *Fertil Steril* 1999;71:843–848.

103. **Rushworth FH, Yetman DL, Carr AC, et al.** Prospective pregnancy outcome in untreated recurrent miscarriers with thyroid autoantibodies. *Hum Reprod* 2000;15:1637–1639.

104. **Stagnaro-Green A, Roman SH, Cobin RH, et al.** Detection of at-risk pregnancy by means of highly sensitive assays for thyroid autoantibodies. *JAMA* 1990;264:1422–1425.

105. **Toulis KA, Goulis DG, Venetis CA, et al.** Risk of spontaneous miscarriage in euthyroid women with thyroid autoimmunity undergoing IVF: a meta-analysis. *Eur J Endocrinol* 2010;162:643–652.

106. **Negro R, Mangieri T, Coppola L, et al.** Levothyroxine treatment in thyroid peroxidase antibody-positive women undergoing assisted reproduction technologies: a prospective study. *Hum Reprod* 2005;20:1529–1533.

107. **Li TC, Spuijbroek MD, Tuckerman E, et al.** Endocrinological and endometrial factors in recurrent miscarriage. *BJOG* 2000;107:1471–1479.

108. **Soules MR, Bremner WJ, Steiner RA, et al.** Prolactin secretion and corpus luteum function in women with luteal phase deficiency. *J Clin Endocrinol Metab* 1991;72:986–992.

109. **Hirahara F, Andoh N, Sawai K, et al.** Hyperprolactinemic recurrent miscarriage and results of randomized bromocriptine treatment trials. *Fertil Steril* 1998;70:246–252.

110. **Hofmann GE, Khoury J, Thie J.** Recurrent pregnancy loss and diminished ovarian reserve. *Fertil Steril* 2000;74:1192–1195.

111. **Trout SW, Seifer DB.** Do women with unexplained recurrent pregnancy loss have higher day 3 serum FSH and estradiol values? *Fertil Steril* 2000;74:335–337.

112. **Hill JA.** Sporadic and recurrent spontaneous abortion. *Curr Probl Obstet Gynecol Fertil* 1994;17:114–162.

113. **Summers PR.** Microbiology relevant to recurrent miscarriage. *Clin Obstet Gynecol* 1994;37:722–729.

114. **Paukku M, Tulppala M, Puolakkainen M, et al.** Lack of association between serum antibodies to Chlamydia trachomatis and a history of recurrent pregnancy loss. *Fertil Steril* 1999;72:427–430.

115. **Llahi-Camp JM, Rai R, Ison C, et al.** Association of bacterial vaginosis with a history of second trimester miscarriage. *Hum Reprod* 1996;11:1575–1578.

116. **Robb JA, Benirschke K, Barmeyer R.** Intrauterine latent herpes simplex virus infection: I. Spontaneous abortion. *Hum Pathol* 1986;17:1196–1209.

117. **Altshuler G.** Immunologic competence of the immature human fetus. Morphologic evidence from intrauterine Cytomegalovirus infection. *Obstet Gynecol* 1974;43:811–816.

118. **Heyborne KD, Witkin SS, McGregor JA.** Tumor necrosis factor-alpha in midtrimester amniotic fluid is associated with impaired intrauterine fetal growth. *Am J Obstet Gynecol* 1992;167(Pt 1):920–925.

119. **Romero R, Mazor M, Sepulveda W, et al.** Tumor necrosis factor in preterm and term labor. *Am J Obstet Gynecol* 1992;166:1576–1587.

120. **Furman MH, Ploegh HL, Schust DJ.** Can viruses help us to understand and classify the MHC class I molecules at the maternal-fetal interface? *Hum Immunol* 2000;61:1169–1176.

121. **Thellin O, Coumans B, Zorzi W, et al.** Tolerance to the foeto-placental "graft": ten ways to support a child for nine months. *Curr Opin Immunol* 2000;12:731–737.

122. **Lanier LL.** Activating and inhibitory NK cell receptors. *Adv Exp Med Biol* 1998;452:13–18.

123. **Sakaguchi S, Sakaguchi N.** Regulatory T cells in immunologic self-tolerance and autoimmune disease. *Int Rev Immunol* 2005;24:211–226.

124. **von Herrath MG, Harrison LC.** Antigen-induced regulatory T cells in autoimmunity. *Nat Rev Immunol* 2003;3:223–232.

125. **Banham AH, Powrie FM, Suri-Payer E.** FOXP3+ regulatory T cells: Current controversies and future perspectives. *Eur J Immunol* 2006;36:2832–2836.

126. **Zenclussen AC, Gerlof K, Zenclussen ML, et al.** Regulatory T cells induce a privileged tolerant microenvironment at the fetal-maternal interface. *Eur J Immunol* 2006;36:82–94.

127. **Mjosberg J, Berg G, Ernerudh J, et al.** CD4+ CD25+ regulatory T cells in human pregnancy: development of a Treg-MLC-ELISPOT suppression assay and indications of paternal specific Tregs. *Immunology* 2007;120:456–466.

128. **Johnson PM, Christmas SE, Vince GS.** Immunological aspects of implantation and implantation failure. *Hum Reprod* 1999;14(Suppl 2):26–36.

129. **Vince GS, Johnson PM.** Leucocyte populations and cytokine regulation in human uteroplacental tissues. *Biochem Soc Trans* 2000;28:191–195.

130. **Quenby S, Nik H, Innes B, et al.** Uterine natural killer cells and angiogenesis in recurrent reproductive failure. *Hum Reprod* 2009;24:45–54.

131. **King A, Hiby SE, Gardner L, et al.** Recognition of trophoblast HLA class I molecules by decidual NK cell receptors—a review. *Placenta* 2000;21(Suppl A):S81–S85.

132. **Loke YW, King A.** Decidual natural-killer-cell interaction with trophoblast: cytolysis or cytokine production? *Biochem Soc Trans* 2000;28:196–198.

133. **Bryceson YT, March ME, Ljunggren HG, et al.** Activation, coactivation, and costimulation of resting human natural killer cells. *Immunol Rev* 2006;214:73–91.

134. **Bryceson YT, March ME, Ljunggren HG, et al.** Synergy among receptors on resting NK cells for the activation of natural cytotoxicity and cytokine secretion. *Blood* 2006;107:159–166.

135. **Faridi RM, Das V, Tripthi G, et al.** Influence of activating and inhibitory killer immunoglobulin-like receptors on predisposition to recurrent miscarriages. *Hum Reprod* 2009;24:1758–1764.

136. **Flores AC, Marcos CY, Paladino N, et al.** KIR receptors and HLA-C in the maintenance of pregnancy. *Tissue Antigens* 2007;69(Suppl 1):112–113.

137. **Ito K, Karasawa M, Kawano T, et al.** Involvement of decidual Valpha14 NKT cells in abortion. *Proc Natl Acad Sci U S A* 2000;97:740–744.

138. **Boyson JE, Rybalov B, Koopman LA, et al.** CD1d and invariant NKT cells at the human maternal-fetal interface. *Proc Natl Acad Sci U S A* 2002;99:13741–13746.

139. **Christmas SE, Brew R, Thornton SM, et al.** Extensive TCR junctional diversity of V gamma 9/V delta 2 clones from human female reproductive tissues. *J Immunol* 1995;155:2453–2458.

140. **Mincheva-Nilsson L, Baranov V, Yeung MM, et al.** Immunomorphologic studies of human decidua-associated lymphoid cells in normal early pregnancy. *J Immunol* 1994;152:2020–2032.

141. **Vassiliadou N, Bulmer JN.** Characterization of endometrial T lymphocyte subpopulations in spontaneous early pregnancy loss. *Hum Reprod* 1998;13:44–47.

142. **Hayday AC.** Gamma delta cells: a right time and a right place for a conserved third way of protection. *Annu Rev Immunol* 2000;18:975–1026.

143. **Aluvihare VR, Kallikourdis M, Betz AG.** Tolerance, suppression and the fetal allograft. *J Mol Med* 2005;83:88–96.

144. **Sanchez-Ramon S, Navarro A J, Aristimuño C, et al.** Pregnancy-induced expansion of regulatory T-lymphocytes may mediate protection to multiple sclerosis activity. *Immunol Lett* 2005;96:195–201.

145. **Clifford K, Flanagan AM, Regan L.** Endometrial CD56+ natural killer cells in women with recurrent miscarriage: a histomorphometric study. *Hum Reprod* 1999;14:2727–2730.

146. **Lachapelle MH, Miron P, Hemmings R, et al.** Endometrial T, B, and NK cells in patients with recurrent spontaneous abortion. Altered profile and pregnancy outcome. *J Immunol* 1996;156:4027–4034.

147. **Quenby S, Bates M, Doig T, et al.** Pre-implantation endometrial leukocytes in women with recurrent miscarriage. *Hum Reprod* 1999;14:2386–2391.

148. **Gould DS, Ploegh HL, Schust DJ.** Murine female reproductive tract intraepithelial lymphocytes display selection characteristics distinct from both peripheral and other mucosal T cells. *J Reprod Immunol* 2001;52:85–99.

149. **Pudney J, Quayle AJ, Anderson DJ.** Immunological microenvironments in the human vagina and cervix: mediators of cellular immunity are concentrated in the cervical transformation zone. *Biol Reprod* 2005;73:1253–1263.

150. **Trundley A, Moffett A.** Human uterine leukocytes and pregnancy. *Tissue Antigens* 2004;63:1–12.

151. **McVay LD, Carding SR.** Extrathymic origin of human gamma delta T cells during fetal development. *J Immunol* 1996;157:2873–2882.

152. **Dorfman JR, Raulet DH.** Major histocompatibility complex genes determine natural killer cell tolerance. *Eur J Immunol* 1996;26:151–155.

153. **Salcedo M, Diehl AD, Olsson-Alheim MY, et al.** Altered expression of Ly49 inhibitory receptors on natural killer cells from MHC class I-deficient mice. *J Immunol* 1997;158:3174–3180.

154. **Kruse A, Hallmann R, Butcher EC.** Specialized patterns of vascular differentiation antigens in the pregnant mouse uterus and the placenta. *Biol Reprod* 1999;61:1393–1401.

155. **Schon MP, Arya A, Murphy EA, et al.** Mucosal T lymphocyte numbers are selectively reduced in integrin alpha E (CD103)-deficient mice. *J Immunol* 1999;162:6641–6649.

156. **Perry LL, Feilzer K, Portis JL, et al.** Distinct homing pathways direct T lymphocytes to the genital and intestinal mucosae in chlamydia-infected mice. *J Immunol* 1998;160:2905–2914.

157. **Pudney J, Anderson DJ.** Immunobiology of the human penile urethra. *Am J Pathol* 1995;147:155–165.

158. **Brandtzaeg P.** Function of mucosa-associated lymphoid tissue in antibody formation. *Immunol Invest* 2010;39:303–355.

159. **Kelly KA, Chan AM, Butch A, et al.** Two different homing pathways involving integrin beta7 and E-selectin significantly influence trafficking of CD4 cells to the genital tract following *Chlamydia muridarum* infection. *Am J Reprod Immunol* 2009;61:438–445.

160. **Ljunggren HG, Karre K.** In search of the "missing self": MHC molecules and NK cell recognition. *Immunol Today* 1990;11:237–244.

161. **Mattsson R.** The non-expression of MHC class II in trophoblast cells. *Am J Reprod Immunol* 1998;40:385–394.

162. **Murphy SP, Tomasi TB.** Absence of MHC class II antigen expression in trophoblast cells results from a lack of class II transactivator (CIITA) gene expression. *Mol Reprod Dev* 1998;51:1–12.

163. **King A, Allan DS, Bowen M, et al.** HLA-E is expressed on trophoblast and interacts with CD94/NKG2 receptors on decidual NK cells. *Eur J Immunol* 2000;30:1623–1631.

164. **King, A, Burrows TD, Hiby SE, et al.** Surface expression of HLA-C antigen by human extravillous trophoblast. *Placenta* 2000;21:376–387.

165. **Kovats S, Main EK, Librach C, et al.** A class I antigen, HLA-G, expressed in human trophoblasts. *Science* 1990;248:220–223.

166. **Sernee MF, Ploegh HL, Schust DJ.** Why certain antibodies cross-react with HLA-A and HLA-G: epitope mapping of two common MHC class I reagents. *Mol Immunol* 1998;35:177–188.

167. **Wei XH, Orr HT.** Differential expression of HLA-E, HLA-F, and HLA-G transcripts in human tissue. *Hum Immunol* 1990;29:131–142.

168. **Kam EP, Gardner L, Loke YW, et al.** The role of trophoblast in the physiological change in decidual spiral arteries. *Hum Reprod* 1999;14:2131–2138.

169. **Moffett-King A.** Natural killer cells and pregnancy. *Nat Rev Immunol* 2002;2:656–663.

170. **Damsky CH, Fisher SJ.** Trophoblast pseudo-vasculogenesis: faking it with endothelial adhesion receptors. *Curr Opin Cell Biol* 1998;10:660–666.

171. **Zhou Y, Fisher SJ, Janatpour M, et al.** Human cytotrophoblasts adopt a vascular phenotype as they differentiate. A strategy for successful endovascular invasion? *J Clin Invest* 1997;99:2139–2151.

172. **Lim KH, Zhou Y, Janatpour M, et al.** Human cytotrophoblast differentiation/invasion is abnormal in pre-eclampsia. *Am J Pathol* 1997;151:1809–1818.

173. **Goldman-Wohl DS, Ariel I, Greenfield C, et al.** Lack of human leukocyte antigen-G expression in extravillous trophoblasts is associated with pre-eclampsia. *Mol Hum Reprod* 2000;6:88–95.

174. **Aldrich CL, Stephenson MD, Karrison T, et al.** HLA-G genotypes and pregnancy outcome in couples with unexplained recurrent miscarriage. *Mol Hum Reprod* 2001;7:1167–1172.

175. **Hviid TV, Hylenius S, Hoegh AM, et al.** HLA-G polymorphisms in couples with recurrent spontaneous abortions. *Tissue Antigens* 2002;60:122–132.

176. **Pfeiffer KA, Fimmers R, Engels G, et al.** The HLA-G genotype is potentially associated with idiopathic recurrent spontaneous abortion. *Mol Hum Reprod* 2001;7:373–378.

177. **Yamashita T, Fujii T, Tokunaga K, et al.** Analysis of human leukocyte antigen-G polymorphism including intron 4 in Japanese couples with habitual abortion. *Am J Reprod Immunol* 1999;41:159–163.

178. **Hunt JS, Jadhav L, Chu W, et al.** Soluble HLA-G circulates in maternal blood during pregnancy. *Am J Obstet Gynecol* 2000;183:682–688.

179. **Selmani Z, Naji A, Zidi I, et al.** Human leukocyte antigen-G5 secretion by human mesenchymal stem cells is required to suppress T lymphocyte and natural killer function and to induce CD4+CD25highFOXP3+ regulatory T cells. *Stem Cells* 2008;26:212–222.

180. **Feinman MA, Kliman HJ, Main EK.** HLA antigen expression and induction by gamma-interferon in cultured human trophoblasts. *Am J Obstet Gynecol* 1987;157:1429–1434.

181. **Hill JA.** Immunological mechanisms of pregnancy maintenance and failure: a critique of theories and therapy. *Am J Reprod Immunol* 1990;22:33–41.

182. **Hill JA, Melling GC, Johnson PM.** Immunohistochemical studies of human uteroplacental tissues from first-trimester spontaneous abortion. *Am J Obstet Gynecol* 1995;173:90–96.

183. **Christiansen OB, Andersen HH, Højbjerre M, et al.** Maternal HLA class II allogenotypes are markers for the predisposition to fetal losses in families of women with unexplained recurrent fetal loss. *Eur J Immunogenet* 1995,22:323–334.

184. **O'Garra A, Arai N.** The molecular basis of T helper 1 and T helper 2 cell differentiation. *Trends Cell Biol* 2000;10:542–550.

185. **Kurt-Jones EA, Hamberg S, Ohara J, et al.** Heterogeneity of helper/inducer T lymphocytes. I. Lymphokine production and lymphokine responsiveness. *J Exp Med* 1987;166:1774–1787.

186. **Romagnani S.** Human TH1 and TH2 subsets: doubt no more. *Immunol Today* 1991;12:256–257.

187. **Mosmann TR, Coffman RL.** Heterogeneity of cytokine secretion patterns and functions of helper T cells. *Adv Immunol* 1989;46:111–147.

188. **Romagnani S.** Human TH1 and TH2 subsets: regulation of differentiation and role in protection and immunopathology. *Int Arch Allergy Immunol* 1992;98:279–285.

189. **Maggi E, Parronchi P, Manetti R, et al.** Reciprocal regulatory effects of IFN-gamma and IL-4 on the *in vitro* development of human Th1 and Th2 clones. *J Immunol* 1992;148:2142–2147.

190. **Mosmann TR, Coffman RL.** TH1 and TH2 cells: different patterns of lymphokine secretion lead to different functional properties. *Annu Rev Immunol* 1989;7:145–173.

191. **Mosmann TR, Moore KW.** The role of IL-10 in crossregulation of TH1 and TH2 responses. *Immunol Today* 1991;12:A49–A53.

192. **Nakae S, Iwakura Y, Suto H, et al.** Phenotypic differences between Th1 and Th17 cells and negative regulation of Th1 cell differentiation by IL-17. *J Leukoc Biol* 2007;81:1258–1268.

193. **Harrington LE, Mangan PR, Weaver CT.** Expanding the effector CD4 T-cell repertoire: the Th17 lineage. *Curr Opin Immunol* 2006;18:349–356.

194. **Bulmer JN, Sunderland CA.** Immunohistological characterization of lymphoid cell populations in the early human placental bed. *Immunology* 1984;52:349–357.

195. **Sen DK, Fox H.** The lymphoid tissue of the endometrium. *Gynaecologia* 1967;163:371–378.

196. **Tabibzadeh S.** Human endometrium: an active site of cytokine production and action. *Endocr Rev* 1991;12:272–290.

197. **Berkowitz RS, Hill JA, Kurtz CB, et al.** Effects of products of activated leukocytes (lymphokines and monokines) on the growth of malignant trophoblast cells *in vitro*. *Am J Obstet Gynecol* 1988;158:199–203.

198. **Hill JA, Haimovici F, Anderson DJ.** Products of activated lymphocytes and macrophages inhibit mouse embryo development *in vitro*. *J Immunol* 1987;139:2250–2254.

199. **Hill JA, Polgar K, Anderson DJ.** T-helper 1-type immunity to trophoblast in women with recurrent spontaneous abortion. *JAMA* 1995;273:1933–1936.

200. **Mallmann P, Werner A, Krebs D.** Serum levels of interleukin-2 and tumor necrosis factor-alpha in women with recurrent abortion. *Am J Obstet Gynecol* 1990;163(Pt 1):1367.

201. **Ecker JL, Laufer MR, Hill JA.** Measurement of embryotoxic factors is predictive of pregnancy outcome in women with a history of recurrent abortion. *Obstet Gynecol* 1993;81:84–87.

202. **Saito S, Nakashima A, Shima T, et al.** Th1/Th2/Th17 and regulatory T-cell paradigm in pregnancy. *Am J Reprod Immunol* 2010;63:601–610.

203. **Wang, WJ, Hao CF, Yi-Lin, et al.** Increased prevalence of T helper 17 (Th17) cells in peripheral blood and decidua in unexplained recurrent spontaneous abortion patients. *J Reprod Immunol* 2010;84:164–170.

204. **Wang WJ, Hao CF, Qu QL, et al.** The deregulation of regulatory T cells on interleukin-17-producing T helper cells in patients with unexplained early recurrent miscarriage. *Hum Reprod* 2010;25:2591–2596.

205. **Lea RG, Tulppala M, Critchley HO.** Deficient syncytiotrophoblast tumour necrosis factor-alpha characterizes failing first trimester pregnancies in a subgroup of recurrent miscarriage patients. *Hum Reprod* 1997;12:1313–1320.

206. **Lim KJ, Odukoya OA, Ajjan RA, et al.** The role of T-helper cytokines in human reproduction. *Fertil Steril* 2000;73:136–142.

207. **von Wolff M, Thaler CJ, Strowitzki T, et al.** Regulated expression of cytokines in human endometrium throughout the menstrual cycle: dysregulation in habitual abortion. *Mol Hum Reprod* 2000;6:627–634.

208. **Piccinni MP, Beloni L, Livi C, et al.** Defective production of both leukemia inhibitory factor and type 2 T-helper cytokines by decidual T cells in unexplained recurrent abortions. *Nat Med* 1998;4:1020–1024.

209. **Raghupathy R, Makhseed M, Azizieh F, et al.** Cytokine production by maternal lymphocytes during normal human pregnancy and in unexplained recurrent spontaneous abortion. *Hum Reprod* 2000;15:713–718.

210. **Hamai Y, Fujii T, Yamashita T, et al.** Peripheral blood mononuclear cells from women with recurrent abortion exhibit an aberrant reaction to release cytokines upon the direct contact of human leukocyte antigen-G-expressing cells. *Am J Reprod Immunol* 1998;40:408–413.

211. **Kanai T, Fujii T, Unno N, et al.** Human leukocyte antigen-G-expressing cells differently modulate the release of cytokines from mononuclear cells present in the decidua versus peripheral blood. *Am J Reprod Immunol* 2001;45:94–99.

212. **Jenkins C, Roberts J, Wilson R, et al.** Evidence of a T(H) 1 type response associated with recurrent miscarriage. *Fertil Steril* 2000;73:1206–1208.

213. **Schust DJ, Hill JA.** Correlation of serum cytokine and adhesion molecule determinations with pregnancy outcome. *J Soc Gynecol Investig* 1996;3:259–261.

214. **Chen JR, Cheng JG, Shatzer T, et al.** Leukemia inhibitory factor can substitute for nidatory estrogen and is essential to inducing a receptive uterus for implantation but is not essential for subsequent embryogenesis. *Endocrinology* 2000;141:4365–4372.

215. **Stewart CL, Kaspar P, Brunet LJ, et al.** Blastocyst implantation depends on maternal expression of leukaemia inhibitory factor. *Nature* 1992;359:76–79.

216. **Billington WD, Davies M, Bell SC.** Maternal antibody to foetal histocompatibility and trophoblast-specific antigens. *Ann Immunol (Paris)* 1984;135D:331–335.

217. **Sargent IL, Wilkins T, Redman CW.** Maternal immune responses to the fetus in early pregnancy and recurrent miscarriage. *Lancet* 1988;2:1099–1104.

218. **Tafuri A, Alferink J, Möller P, et al.** T cell awareness of paternal alloantigens during pregnancy. *Science* 1995;270:630–633.

219. **Bermas BL, Hill JA.** Proliferative responses to recall antigens are associated with pregnancy outcome in women with a history of recurrent spontaneous abortion. *J Clin Invest* 1997;100:1330–1334.

220. **Grossman C.** Possible underlying mechanisms of sexual dimorphism in the immune response, fact and hypothesis. *J Steroid Biochem* 1989;34:241–251.

221. **Runnebaum B, Stober I, Zander J.** Progesterone, 20 alpha-dihydroprogesterone and 20 beta-dihydroprogesterone in mother and child at birth. *Acta Endocrinol (Copenh)* 1975;80:569–576.

222. **Siiteri PK, Febres F, Clemens LE, et al.** Progesterone and maintenance of pregnancy: is progesterone nature's immunosuppressant? *Ann N Y Acad Sci* 1977;286:384–397.

223. **Ehring GR, Kerschbaum HH, Eder C, et al.** A nongenomic mechanism for progesterone-mediated immunosuppression: inhibition of K+ channels, Ca2+ signaling, and gene expression in T lymphocytes. *J Exp Med* 1998;188:1593–1602.

224. **Gadkar-Sable S, Shah C, Rosario G, et al.** Progesterone receptors: various forms and functions in reproductive tissues. *Front Biosci* 2005;10:2118–2130.

225. **Schust DJ, Anderson DJ, Hill JA.** Progesterone-induced immunosuppression is not mediated through the progesterone receptor. *Hum Reprod* 1996;11:980–985.

226. **Hunt JS, Miller L, Roby KF, et al.** Female steroid hormones regulate production of pro-inflammatory molecules in uterine leukocytes. *J Reprod Immunol* 1997;35:87–99.

227. **Vassiliadou N, Tucker L, Anderson DJ.** Progesterone-induced inhibition of chemokine receptor expression on peripheral blood mononuclear cells correlates with reduced HIV-1 infectability *in vitro*. *J Immunol* 1999;162:7510–7518.

228. **Kawana K, Kawana Y, Schust DJ.** Female steroid hormones use signal transducers and activators of transcription protein-mediated pathways to modulate the expression of T-bet in epithelial cells: a mechanism for local immune regulation in the human reproductive tract. *Mol Endocrinol* 2005;19:2047–2059.

229. **Knoferl MW, Diodato MD, Angele MK, et al.** Do female sex steroids adversely or beneficially affect the depressed immune responses in males after trauma-hemorrhage? *Arch Surg* 2000;135:425–433.

230. **Gregory MS, Duffner LA, Faunce DE, et al.** Estrogen mediates the sex difference in post-burn immunosuppression. *J Endocrinol* 2000;164:129–138.

231. **Muller V, Szabó A, Viklicky O, et al.** Sex hormones and gender-related differences: their influence on chronic renal allograft rejection. *Kidney Int* 1999;55:2011–2020.

232. **Correale J, Arias M, Gilmore W.** Steroid hormone regulation of cytokine secretion by proteolipid protein-specific CD4+ T cell clones isolated from multiple sclerosis patients and normal control subjects. *J Immunol* 1998;161:3365–3374.

233. **Salem ML, Matsuzaki G, Kishihara K, et al.** beta-estradiol suppresses T cell-mediated delayed-type hypersensitivity through suppression of antigen-presenting cell function and Th1 induction. *Int Arch Allergy Immunol* 2000;121:161–169.

234. **Munn DH, Shafizadeh E, Attwood JT, et al.** Inhibition of T cell proliferation by macrophage tryptophan catabolism. *J Exp Med* 1999;189:1363–1372.

235. **Mellor AL, Munn DH.** Immunology at the maternal-fetal interface: lessons for T cell tolerance and suppression. *Annu Rev Immunol* 2000;18:367–391.

236. **Munn DH, Zhou M, Attwood JT, et al.** Prevention of allogeneic fetal rejection by tryptophan catabolism. *Science* 1998;281:1191–1193.

237. **Meier AH, Wilson JM.** Tryptophan feeding adversely influences pregnancy. *Life Sci* 1983;32:1193–1196.

238. **Kamimura S, Eguchi K, Yonezawa M, et al.** Localization and developmental change of indoleamine 2,3-dioxygenase activity in the human placenta. *Acta Med Okayama* 1991;45:135–139.

239. **Schrocksnadel H, Baier-Bitterlich G, Dapunt O, et al.** Decreased plasma tryptophan in pregnancy. *Obstet Gynecol* 1996;88:47–50.

240. **Lebovic DI, Mueller MD, Taylor RN.** Immunobiology of endometriosis. *Fertil Steril* 2001;75:1–10.

241. **Tomassetti C, Meuleman C, Pexsters A, et al.** Endometriosis, recurrent miscarriage and implantation failure: is there an immunological link? *Reprod Biomed Online* 2006;13:58–64.

242. **Hill JA.** Endometriosis: immune cells and their products. In: **Hunt JS, ed.** Immunobiology of reproduction. Serono Symposium, USA. New York: Springer-Verlag, 1994:23–33.

243. **Somigliana E, Vigano P, Vignali M.** Endometriosis and unexplained recurrent spontaneous abortion: pathological states resulting from aberrant modulation of natural killer cell function? *Hum Reprod Update* 1999;5:40–51.

244. **Eblen AC, Gercel-Taylor C, Shields LB, et al.** Alterations in humoral immune responses associated with recurrent pregnancy loss. *Fertil Steril* 2000;73:305–313.

245. **Alijotas-Reig J, Casellas-Caro M, Ferrer-Oliveras R, et al.** Are anti-beta-glycoprotein-I antibodies markers for recurrent pregnancy loss in lupus anticoagulant/anticardiolipin seronegative women? *Am J Reprod Immunol* 2008;60:229–237.

246. **Alijotas-Reig J, Ferrer-Oliveras R, Rodrigo-Anoro MJ, et al.** Anti-beta(2)-glycoprotein-I and anti-phosphatidylserine antibodies in women with spontaneous pregnancy loss. *Fertil Steril* 2010;93: 2330–2336.

247. **Galli M, Comfurius P, Maassen C, et al.** Anticardiolipin antibodies (ACA) directed not to cardiolipin but to a plasma protein cofactor. *Lancet* 1990;335:1544–1547.

248. **McNeil HP, Simpson RJ, Chesterman CN, et al.** Anti-phospholipid antibodies are directed against a complex antigen that includes a lipid-binding inhibitor of coagulation: beta 2-glycoprotein I (apolipoprotein H). *Proc Natl Acad Sci U S A* 1990;87:4120–4124.

249. **Mezzesimi A, Florio P, Reis FM, et al.** The detection of anti-beta2-glycoprotein I antibodies is associated with increased risk of pregnancy loss in women with threatened abortion in the first trimester. *Eur J Obstet Gynecol Reprod Biol* 2007;133:164–168.

250. **Harris EN.** Syndrome of the black swan. *Br J Rheumatol* 1987;26: 324–326.

251. **Miyakis S, Lockshin MD, Atsumi T, et al.** International consensus statement on an update of the classification criteria for definite antiphospholipid syndrome (APS). *J Thromb Haemost* 2006;4:295–306.

252. **Wilson WA, Gharavi AE, Koike T, et al.** International consensus statement on preliminary classification criteria for definite antiphospholipid syndrome: report of an international workshop. *Arthritis Rheum* 1999;42:1309–1311.

253. **Lockshin MD, Sammaritano LR, Schwartzman S.** Validation of the Sapporo criteria for antiphospholipid syndrome. *Arthritis Rheum* 2000;43:440–443.

254. **Out HJ, Bruinse HW, Christiaens GC, et al.** A prospective, controlled multicenter study on the obstetric risks of pregnant women with antiphospholipid antibodies. *Am J Obstet Gynecol* 1992;167:26–32.

255. **Kutteh WH, Lyda EC, Abraham SM, et al.** Association of anti-cardiolipin antibodies and pregnancy loss in women with systemic lupus erythematosus. *Fertil Steril* 1993;60:449–455.

256. **Meroni PL, Tedesco F, Locati M, et al.** Anti-phospholipid antibody mediated fetal loss: still an open question from a pathogenic point of view. *Lupus* 2010;19:453–456.

257. **Cariou R, Tobelem G, Soria C, et al.** Inhibition of protein C activation by endothelial cells in the presence of lupus anticoagulant. *N Engl J Med* 1986;314:1193–1194.

258. **Freyssinet JM, Wiesel ML, Gauchy J, et al.** An IgM lupus anticoagulant that neutralizes the enhancing effect of phospholipid on purified endothelial thrombomodulin activity—a mechanism for thrombosis. *Thromb Haemost* 1986;55:309–313.

259. **Harris EN, Asherson RA, Gharavi AE, et al.** Thrombocytopenia in SLE and related autoimmune disorders: association with anticardiolipin antibody. *Br J Haematol* 1985;59:227–230.

260. **Lyden TW, Ng AK, Rote NS.** Modulation of phosphatidylserine epitope expression by BeWo cells during forskolin treatment. *Placenta* 1993;14:177–186.

261. **Chamley LW, Allen JL, Johnson PM.** Synthesis of beta2 glycoprotein 1 by the human placenta. *Placenta* 1997;18:403–410.

262. **Bramham K, Hunt BJ, Germain S, et al.** Pregnancy outcome in different clinical phenotypes of antiphospholipid syndrome. *Lupus* 2010;19:58–64.

263. **Lee RM, Emlen W, Scott JR, et al.** Anti-beta2-glycoprotein I antibodies in women with recurrent spontaneous abortion, unexplained fetal death, and antiphospholipid syndrome. *Am J Obstet Gynecol* 1999;181:642–648.

264. **Ogasawara M, Aoki K, Katano K, et al.** Prevalence of autoantibodies in patients with recurrent miscarriages. *Am J Reprod Immunol* 1999;41:86–90.

265. **Bulla R, de Guarrini F, Pausa M, et al.** Inhibition of trophoblast adhesion to endothelial cells by the sera of women with recurrent spontaneous abortions. *Am J Reprod Immunol* 1999;42:116–123.

266. **Rand JH, Wu XX, Andree HA, et al.** Pregnancy loss in the antiphospholipid-antibody syndrome—a possible thrombogenic mechanism. *N Engl J Med* 1997;337:154–160.

267. **Rand JH, Wu XX, Guller S, et al.** Reduction of annexin-V (placental anticoagulant protein-I) on placental villi of women with antiphospholipid antibodies and recurrent spontaneous abortion. *Am J Obstet Gynecol* 1994;171:1566–1572.

268. **Hanly JG, Gladman DD, Rose TH, et al.** Lupus pregnancy. A prospective study of placental changes. *Arthritis Rheum* 1988;31:358–366.

269. **Redline RW.** Placental pathology: a systematic approach with clinical correlations. *Placenta* 2008;29(Suppl A):S86–S91.

270. **Lockshin MD, Druzin ML, Goei S, et al.** Antibody to cardiolipin as a predictor of fetal distress or death in pregnant patients with systemic lupus erythematosus. *N Engl J Med* 1985;313:152–156.

271. **Bussen SS, Steck T.** Thyroid antibodies and their relation to antithrombin antibodies, anticardiolipin antibodies and lupus anticoagulant in women with recurrent spontaneous abortions (antithyroid, anticardiolipin and antithrombin autoantibodies and lupus anticoagulant in habitual aborters). *Eur J Obstet Gynecol Reprod Biol* 1997;74:139–143.

272. **McElduff A, Morris J.** Thyroid function tests and thyroid autoantibodies in an unselected population of women undergoing first trimester screening for aneuploidy. *Aust N Z J Obstet Gynaecol* 2008;48:478–480.

273. **Rocklin RE, Kitzmiller JL, Garvoy MR.** Maternal-fetal relation. II. Further characterization of an immunologic blocking factor that develops during pregnancy. *Clin Immunol Immunopathol* 1982;22:305–315.

274. **Amos DB, Kostyu DD.** HLA—a central immunological agency of man. *Adv Hum Genet* 1980;10:137–208, 385–386.

275. **Coulam CB.** Immunologic tests in the evaluation of reproductive disorders: a critical review. *Am J Obstet Gynecol* 1992;167:1844–1851.

276. **Beer AE, Quebbeman JF, Ayers JW, et al.** Major histocompatibility complex antigens, maternal and paternal immune responses, and chronic habitual abortions in humans. *Am J Obstet Gynecol* 1981; 141:987–999.

277. **McIntyre JA, Faulk WP.** Recurrent spontaneous abortion in human pregnancy: results of immunogenetical, cellular, and humoral studies. *Am J Reprod Immunol* 1983;4:165–170.

278. **Ober CL, Martin AO, Simpson JL, et al.** Shared HLA antigens and reproductive performance among Hutterites. *Am J Hum Genet* 1983;35:994–1004.

279. **Ober C, Hyslop T, Elias S, et al.** Human leukocyte antigen matching and fetal loss: results of a 10 year prospective study. *Hum Reprod* 1998;13:33–38.

280. **McIntyre JA, Faulk WP, Verhulst SJ, et al.** Human trophoblast-lymphocyte cross-reactive (TLX) antigens define a new alloantigen system. *Science* 1983;222:1135–1137.

281. **Purcell DF, McKenzie IF, Lublin DM, et al.** The human cell-surface glycoproteins HuLy-m5, membrane co-factor protein (MCP) of the complement system, and trophoblast leucocyte-common (TLX) antigen, are CD46. *Immunology* 1990;70:155–161.

282. **Rodger JC.** Lack of a requirement for a maternal humoral immune response to establish or maintain successful allogeneic pregnancy. *Transplantation* 1985;40:372–375.

283. **Allison JL, Schust DJ.** Recurrent first trimester pregnancy loss: revised definitions and novel causes. *Curr Opin Endocrinol Diabetes Obest* 2009;16:446–450.

284. **Puscheck EE, Jeyendran RS.** The impact of male factor on recurrent pregnancy loss. *Curr Opin Obstet Gynecol* 2007;19:222–228.

285. **Dewan S, Puscheck EE, Coulam CB, et al.** Y-chromosome microdeletions and recurrent pregnancy loss. *Fertil Steril* 2006;85: 441–445.

286. **Rubio C, Simón C, Blanco J, et al.** Implications of sperm chromosome abnormalities in recurrent miscarriage. *J Assist Reprod Genet* 1999;16:253–258.

287. **Saxena P, Misro MM, Chaki SP, et al.** Is abnormal sperm function an indicator among couples with recurrent pregnancy loss? *Fertil Steril* 2008;90:1854–1858.

288. **Gil-Villa AM, Cardona-Maya W, Agarwal A, et al.** Role of male factor in early recurrent embryo loss: do antioxidants have any effect? *Fertil Steril* 2009;92:565–571.

289. **Gil-Villa AM, Cardona-Maya W, Agarwal A, et al.** Assessment of sperm factors possibly involved in early recurrent pregnancy loss. *Fertil Steril* 2010;94:1465–1472.

290. **Govindaiah V, Naushad SM, Prabhakara K, et al.** Association of parental hyperhomocysteinemia and C677T Methylene tetrahydrofolate reductase (MTHFR) polymorphism with recurrent pregnancy loss. *Clin Biochem* 2009;42:380–386.

291. **Vuorela P, Carpén O, Tulppala M, et al.** VEGF, its receptors and the tie receptors in recurrent miscarriage. *Mol Hum Reprod* 2000;6:276–282.

292. **Lessey BA.** Endometrial integrins and the establishment of uterine receptivity. *Hum Reprod* 1998;13(Suppl 3):247–261.

293. **Aplin JD, Hey NA, Li TC.** MUC1 as a cell surface and secretory component of endometrial epithelium: reduced levels in recurrent miscarriage. *Am J Reprod Immunol* 1996;35:261–266.

294. **Gaffuri B, Airoldi L, Di Blasio AM, et al.** Unexplained habitual abortion is associated with a reduced endometrial release of soluble intercellular adhesion molecule-1 in the luteal phase of the cycle. *Eur J Endocrinol* 2000;142:477–480.

295. **Lea RG, al-Sharekh N, Tulppala M, et al.** The immunolocalization of bcl-2 at the maternal-fetal interface in healthy and failing pregnancies. *Hum Reprod* 1997;12:153–158.

296. **Polifka JE, Friedmann JM.** Environmental toxins and recurrent pregnancy loss. *Infert Reprod Med Clin North Am* 1991;2:195–213.

297. **Sharara FI, Seifer DB, Flaws JA.** Environmental toxicants and female reproduction. *Fertil Steril* 1998;70:613–622.

298. **Valanis B, Vollmer WM, Steele P.** Occupational exposure to antineoplastic agents: self-reported miscarriages and stillbirths among nurses and pharmacists. *J Occup Environ Med* 1999;41:632–638.

299. **Xu X, Cho SI, Sammel M, et al.** Association of petrochemical exposure with spontaneous abortion. *Occup Environ Med* 1998;55:31–36.

300. **Sugiura-Ogasawara M, Ozaki Y, Sonta S, et al.** Exposure to bisphenol A is associated with recurrent miscarriage. *Hum Reprod* 2005;20:2325–2329.

301. **Gerhard I, Waibel S, Daniel V, et al.** Impact of heavy metals on hormonal and immunological factors in women with repeated miscarriages. *Hum Reprod Update* 1998;4:301–309.

302. **Cone JE, Vaughan LM, Huete A, et al.** Reproductive health outcomes among female flight attendants: an exploratory study. *J Occup Environ Med* 1998;40:210–216.

303. **Schnorr TM, Grajewski BA, Hornung RW, et al.** Video display terminals and the risk of spontaneous abortion. *N Engl J Med* 1991;324:727–733.

304. **Kurki T, Ylikorkala O.** Coitus during pregnancy is not related to bacterial vaginosis or preterm birth. *Am J Obstet Gynecol* 1993;169:1130–1134.

305. **Naeye RL.** Coitus and associated amniotic-fluid infections. *N Engl J Med* 1979;301:1198–1200.

306. **Abel EL.** Maternal alcohol consumption and spontaneous abortion. *Alcohol Alcohol* 1997;32:211–219.

307. **Parazzini F, Tozzi L, Chatenoud L, et al.** Alcohol and risk of spontaneous abortion. *Hum Reprod* 1994;9:1950–1953.

308. **Windham GC, Siscovick DS, Raghunathan TE, et al.** Moderate maternal alcohol consumption and risk of spontaneous abortion. *Epidemiology* 1997;8:509–514.

309. **Cnattingius S, Signorello LB, Annerén G, et al.** Caffeine intake and the risk of first-trimester spontaneous abortion. *N Engl J Med* 2000;343:1839–1845.

310. **Ness RB, Grisso JA, Hirschinger N, et al.** Cocaine and tobacco use and the risk of spontaneous abortion. *N Engl J Med* 1999;340:333–339.

311. **Kline J, Levin B, Kinney A, et al.** Cigarette smoking and spontaneous abortion of known karyotype. Precise data but uncertain inferences. *Am J Epidemiol* 1995;141:417–427.

312. **Hedin LW, Janson PO.** Domestic violence during pregnancy. The prevalence of physical injuries, substance use, abortions and miscarriages. *Acta Obstet Gynecol Scand* 2000;79:625–630.

313. **Mills JL, Holmes LB, Aarons JH, et al.** Moderate caffeine use and the risk of spontaneous abortion and intrauterine growth retardation. *JAMA* 1993;269:593–597.

314. **Bellver J, Rossal LP, Bosch E, et al.** Obesity and the risk of spontaneous abortion after oocyte donation. *Fertil Steril* 2003;79:1136–1140.

315. **Brandt LP, Nielsen CV.** Job stress and adverse outcome of pregnancy: a causal link or recall bias? *Am J Epidemiol* 1992;135:302–311.

316. **Li DK, Liu L, Odouli R.** Exposure to non-steroidal anti-inflammatory drugs during pregnancy and risk of miscarriage: population based cohort study. *BMJ* 2003;327:368.

317. **Nielsen GL, Sørensen HT, Larsen H, et al.** Risk of adverse birth outcome and miscarriage in pregnant users of non-steroidal anti-inflammatory drugs: population based observational study and case-control study. *BMJ* 2001;322:266–270.

318. **Boue J, Bou A, Lazar P.** Retrospective and prospective epidemiological studies of 1500 karyotyped spontaneous human abortions. *Teratology* 1975;12:11–26.

319. **Stein Z.** Early fetal loss. *Birth Defects Orig Artic Ser* 1981;17:95–111.

320. **Hook EB, Warburton D.** The distribution of chromosomal genotypes associated with Turner's syndrome: livebirth prevalence rates and evidence for diminished fetal mortality and severity in genotypes associated with structural X abnormalities or mosaicism. *Hum Genet* 1983;64:24–27.

321. **Heuser C, Dalton J, Macpherson C, et al.** Idiopathic recurrent pregnancy loss recurs at similar gestational ages. *Am J Obstet Gynecol* 2010;203:343.e1–e5.

322. **Miller JF, Williamson E, Glue J, et al.** Fetal loss after implantation. A prospective study. *Lancet* 1980;2:554–556.

323. **Boue JG, Boue A.** Increased frequency of chromosomal anomalies in abortions after induced ovulation. *Lancet* 1973;1:679–680.

324. **Olpin, JD, Heilbrun M.** Imaging of Mullerian duct anomalies. *Clin Obstet Gynecol* 2009;52:40–56.

325. **Makhseed M, Raghupathy R, Azizieh F, et al.** Circulating cytokines and CD30 in normal human pregnancy and recurrent spontaneous abortions. *Hum Reprod* 2000;15:2011–2017.

326. **Aoki K, Kajiura S, Matsumoto Y, et al.** Preconceptional natural-killer-cell activity as a predictor of miscarriage. *Lancet* 1995;345:1340–1342.

327. **Emmer PM, Nelen WL, Steegers EA, et al.** Peripheral natural killer cytotoxicity and CD56(pos)CD16(pos) cells increase during early pregnancy in women with a history of recurrent spontaneous abortion. *Hum Reprod* 2000;15:1163–1169.

328. **Branch DW, Silver R, Pierangeli S, et al.** Antiphospholipid antibodies other than lupus anticoagulant and anticardiolipin antibodies in women with recurrent pregnancy loss, fertile controls, and antiphospholipid syndrome. *Obstet Gynecol* 1997;89:549–555.

329. **Yetman DL, Kutteh WH.** Antiphospholipid antibody panels and recurrent pregnancy loss: prevalence of anticardiolipin antibodies compared with other antiphospholipid antibodies. *Fertil Steril* 1996;66:540–546.

330. **Gris JC, Quéré I, Sanmarco M, et al.** Antiphospholipid and antiprotein syndromes in non-thrombotic, non-autoimmune women with unexplained recurrent primary early foetal loss. The Nimes Obstetricians and Haematologists Study—NOHA. *Thromb Haemost* 2000;84:228–236.

331. **Mavragani CP, Ioannidis JP, Tzioufas AG, et al.** Recurrent pregnancy loss and autoantibody profile in autoimmune diseases. *Rheumatology (Oxford)* 1999;38:1228–1233.

332. **Duggan MA, Brashert P, Ostor A, et al.** The accuracy and interobserver reproducibility of endometrial dating. *Pathology* 2001;33:292–297.

333. **Murray MJ, Meyer WR, Zaino RJ, et al.** A critical analysis of the accuracy, reproducibility, and clinical utility of histologic endometrial dating in fertile women. *Fertil Steril* 2004;81:1333–1343.

334. **Coulam CB, Wagenknecht D, McIntyre JA, et al.** Occurrence of other reproductive failures among women with recurrent spontaneous abortion. *Am J Reprod Immunol* 1991;25:96–98.

335. **Fedele L, Acaia B, Parazzini F, et al.** Ectopic pregnancy and recurrent spontaneous abortion: two associated reproductive failures. *Obstet Gynecol* 1989;73:206–208.

336. **Acaia B, Parazzini F, La Vecchia C, et al.** Increased frequency of complete hydatidiform mole in women with repeated abortion. *Gynecol Oncol* 1988;31:310–314.

337. **Hughes N, Hamilton EF, Tulandi T.** Obstetric outcome in women after multiple spontaneous abortions. *J Reprod Med* 1991;36:165–166.

338. **Martius JA, Steck T, Oehler MK, et al.** Risk factors associated with preterm (<37+0 weeks) and early preterm birth (<32+0 weeks): univariate and multivariate analysis of 106,345 singleton births from

the 1994 statewide perinatal survey of Bavaria. *Eur J Obstet Gynecol Reprod Biol* 1998;80:183–189.

339. **Lird T, Whittaker PG.** The endocrinology of early pregnancy loss. In: **Huisjes HJ, Lird T, eds.** Early pregnancy failure. New York: Churchill Livingstone, 1990:39–54.

340. **Westergaard JG, Teisner B, Sinosich MJ, et al.** Does ultrasound examination render biochemical tests obsolete in the prediction of early pregnancy failure? *Br J Obstet Gynaecol* 1985;92:77–83.

341. **Li TC, Spring PG, Bygrave C, et al.** The value of biochemical and ultrasound measurements in predicting pregnancy outcome in women with a history of recurrent miscarriage. *Hum Reprod* 1998;13:3525–3529.

342. **Wolf GC, Horger EO 3rd.** Indications for examination of spontaneous abortion specimens: a reassessment. *Am J Obstet Gynecol* 1995;173:1364–1368.

343. **Tachdjian G, Aboura A, Lapierre JM, et al.** Cytogenetic analysis from DNA by comparative genomic hybridization. *Ann Genet* 2000;43:147–154.

344. **Bell KA, Van Deerlin PG, Feinberg RF, et al.** Diagnosis of aneuploidy in archival, paraffin-embedded pregnancy-loss tissues by comparative genomic hybridization. *Fertil Steril* 2001;75:374–379.

345. **Bianchi DW, Flint AF, Pizzimenti MF, et al.** Isolation of fetal DNA from nucleated erythrocytes in maternal blood. *Proc Natl Acad Sci U S A* 1990;87:3279–3283.

346. **Carp H, Toder V, Aviram A, et al.** Karyotype of the abortus in recurrent miscarriage. *Fertil Steril* 2001;75:678–682.

347. **Garrisi JG, Colls P, Ferry KM, et al.** Effect of infertility, maternal age, and number of previous miscarriages on the outcome of preimplantation genetic diagnosis for idiopathic recurrent pregnancy loss. *Fertil Steril* 2009;92:288–295.

348. **Fischer J, Colls P, Escudero T, et al.** Preimplantation genetic diagnosis (PGD) improves pregnancy outcome for translocation carriers with a history of recurrent losses. *Fertil Steril* 2010;94:283–289.

349. **Munné S, Chen S, Fischer J, et al.** Preimplantation genetic diagnosis reduces pregnancy loss in women aged 35 years and older with a history of recurrent miscarriages. *Fertil Steril* 2005;84:331–335.

350. **Munné S, Fischer J, Warner A, et al.** Preimplantation genetic diagnosis significantly reduces pregnancy loss in infertile couples: a multicenter study. *Fertil Steril* 2006;85:326–332.

351. **Verlinsky Y, Cohen J, Munne S, et al.** Over a decade of experience with preimplantation genetic diagnosis: a multicenter report. *Fertil Steril* 2004;82:292–294.

352. **Mastenbroek S, Twisk M, van Echten-Arends J, et al.** In vitro fertilization with preimplantation genetic screening. *N Engl J Med* 2007;357:9–17.

353. **Twisk M, Mastenbroek S, Hoek A, et al.** No beneficial effect of preimplantation genetic screening in women of advanced maternal age with a high risk for embryonic aneuploidy. *Hum Reprod* 2008;23:2813–2817.

354. **Staessen C, Verpoest W, Donoso P, et al.** Preimplantation genetic screening does not improve delivery rate in women under the age of 36 following single-embryo transfer. *Hum Reprod* 2008;23:2818–2825.

355. **Staessen C, Platteau P, Van Assche E, et al.** Comparison of blastocyst transfer with or without preimplantation genetic diagnosis for aneuploidy screening in couples with advanced maternal age: a prospective randomized controlled trial. *Hum Reprod* 2004;19:2849–2858.

356. **Meyer LR, Klipstein S, Hazlett WD, et al.** A prospective randomized controlled trial of preimplantation genetic screening in the "good prognosis" patient. *Fertil Steril* 2009;91:1731–1738.

357. **Hardarson T, Hanson C, Lundin K, et al.** Preimplantation genetic screening in women of advanced maternal age caused a decrease in clinical pregnancy rate: a randomized controlled trial. *Hum Reprod* 2008;23:2806–2812.

358. **Remohí J, Gallardo E, Levy M, et al.** Oocyte donation in women with recurrent pregnancy loss. *Hum Reprod* 1996;11:2048–3051.

359. **Querleu D, Brasme TL, Parmentier D.** Ultrasound-guided transcervical metroplasty. *Fertil Steril* 1990;54:995–998.

360. **Karande VC, Gleicher N.** Resection of uterine septum using gynaecoradiological techniques. *Hum Reprod* 1999;14:1226–1229.

361. **Raziel A, Herman A, Strassburger D, et al.** The outcome of in vitro fertilization in unexplained habitual aborters concurrent with secondary infertility. *Fertil Steril* 1997;67:88–92.

362. **Fedele L, Bianchi S.** Habitual abortion: endocrinological aspects. *Curr Opin Obstet Gynecol* 1995;7:351–356.

363. **Karamardian LM, Grimes DA.** Luteal phase deficiency: effect of treatment on pregnancy rates. *Am J Obstet Gynecol* 1992;167:1391–1398.

364. **Clifford K, Rai R, Watson H, et al.** Does suppressing luteinising hormone secretion reduce the miscarriage rate? Results of a randomised controlled trial. *BMJ* 1996;312:1508–1511.

365. **Glueck CJ, Wang P, Goldenberg N, et al.** Pregnancy loss, polycystic ovary syndrome, thrombophilia, hypofibrinolysis, enoxaparin, metformin. *Clin Appl Thromb Hemost* 2004;10:323–334.

366. **Jakubowicz DJ, Iuorno MJ, Jakubowicz S, et al.** Effects of metformin on early pregnancy loss in the polycystic ovary syndrome. *J Clin Endocrinol Metab* 2002;87:524–529.

367. **Hill JA.** Immunological mechanisms of pregnancy maintenance and failure: a critique of theories and therapy. *Am J Reprod Immunol* 1990;22:33–41.

368. **Hill JA.** Immunotherapy for recurrent pregnancy loss: "standard of care or buyer beware." *J Soc Gynecol Investig* 1997;4:267–273.

369. **Stovall DW, Van Voorhis BJ.** Immunologic tests and treatments in patients with unexplained infertility, IVF-ET, and recurrent pregnancy loss. *Clin Obstet Gynecol* 1999;42:979–1000.

370. **Stephenson M, Kutteh W.** Evaluation and management of recurrent early pregnancy loss. *Clin Obstet Gynecol* 2007;50:132–145.

371. **Agrawal S, Pandey MK, Pandey A.** Prevalence of MLR blocking antibodies before and after immunotherapy. *J Hematother Stem Cell Res* 2000;9:257–262.

372. **Clark DA, Gorczynski RM, Blajchman MA.** Transfusion-related immunomodulation due to peripheral blood dendritic cells expressing the CD200 tolerance signaling molecule and alloantigen. *Transfusion* 2008;48:814–821.

373. **Gafter U, Sredni B, Segal J, et al.** Suppressed cell-mediated immunity and monocyte and natural killer cell activity following allogeneic immunization of women with spontaneous recurrent abortion. *J Clin Immunol* 1997;17:408–419.

374. **Ito K, Tanaka T, Tsutsumi N, et al.** Possible mechanisms of immunotherapy for maintaining pregnancy in recurrent spontaneous aborters: analysis of anti-idiotypic antibodies directed against autologous T-cell receptors. *Hum Reprod* 1999;14:650–655.

375. **Prigoshin N, Tambutti ML, Redal MA, et al.** Microchimerism and blocking activity in women with recurrent spontaneous abortion (RSA) after alloimmunization with the partner's lymphocytes. *J Reprod Immunol* 1999;44:41–54.

376. **Adachi H, Takakuwa K, Mitsui T, et al.** Results of immunotherapy for patients with unexplained secondary recurrent abortions. *Clin Immunol* 2003;106:175–180.

377. **Daya S, Gunby J.** The effectiveness of allogeneic leukocyte immunization in unexplained primary recurrent spontaneous abortion. Recurrent Miscarriage Immunotherapy Trialists Group. *Am J Reprod Immunol* 1994;32:294–302.

378. **Fraser EJ, Grimes DA, Schulz KF.** Immunization as therapy for recurrent spontaneous abortion: a review and meta-analysis. *Obstet Gynecol* 1993;82:854–859.

379. **Mowbray JF, Gibbings C, Liddell H, et al.** Controlled trial of treatment of recurrent spontaneous abortion by immunisation with paternal cells. *Lancet* 1985;1:941–943.

380. **Ober C, Karrison T, Odem RR, et al.** Mononuclear-cell immunisation in prevention of recurrent miscarriages: a randomised trial. *Lancet* 1999;354:365–369.

381. **Porter FT, LaCoursiere Y, Scott RT Jr.** Immunotherapy for recurrent miscarriage. *Cochrane Database Syst Rev* 2010;4:CD00.

382. **Kling C, Steinmann J, Westphal E, et al.** Adverse effects of intradermal allogeneic lymphocyte immunotherapy: acute reactions and role of autoimmunity. *Hum Reprod* 2006;21:429–435.

383. **Christiansen OB.** Intravenous immunoglobulin in the prevention of recurrent spontaneous abortion: the European experience. *Am J Reprod Immunol* 1998;39:77–81.

384. **Hill JA, Anderson DJ.** Blood transfusions for recurrent abortion: is the treatment worse than the disease? *Fertil Steril* 1986;46:152–154.

385. **Hofmeyr GJ, Joffe MI, Bezwoda WR, et al.** Immunologic investigation of recurrent pregnancy loss and consequences of immunization with husbands' leukocytes. *Fertil Steril* 1987;48:681–684.

386. **Katz I, Fisch B, Amit S, et al.** Cutaneous graft-versus-host-like reaction after paternal lymphocyte immunization for prevention of recurrent abortion. *Fertil Steril* 1992;57:927–929.

387. **Johnson PM, Ramsden GH.** Recurrent miscarriage. *Ballieres Clin Immunol Allergy* 1992;2:607–624.

388. **Porter TF, LaCoursiere Y, Scott JR.** Immunotherapy for recurrent miscarriage. *Cochrane Database Syst Rev* 2006;2:CD000112.

389. **Coulam CB, Stern JJ.** Seminal plasma treatment of recurrent spontaneous abortion. In: **Dondero F, Johnson PM, eds.** Reproductive immunology. Serono Symposia 97. New York: Raven Press, 1993:205–216.

390. **Thaler CJ.** Immunological role for seminal plasma in insemination and pregnancy. *Am J Reprod Immunol* 1989;21:147–150.

391. **Jerzak M, Rechberger T, Gorski A.** Intravenous immunoglobulin therapy influences T cell adhesion to extracellular matrix in women with a history of recurrent spontaneous abortions. *Am J Reprod Immunol* 2000;44:336–341.

392. **Dwyer JM.** Manipulating the immune system with immune globulin. *N Engl J Med* 1992;326:107–116.

393. **Samuelsson A, Towers TL, Ravetch JV.** Anti-inflammatory activity of IVIG mediated through the inhibitory Fc receptor. *Science* 2001;291:484–486.

394. **Mollnes TE, Hogasen K, De Carolis C, et al.** High-dose intravenous immunoglobulin treatment activates complement in vivo. *Scand J Immunol* 1998;48:312–317.

395. **Stephenson MD, Kutteh WH, Purkiss S, et al.** Intravenous immunoglobulin and idiopathic secondary recurrent miscarriage: a multicentered randomized placebo-controlled trial. *Hum Reprod* 2010;25:2203–2209.

396. **Jablonowska B, Selbing A, Palfi M, et al.** Prevention of recurrent spontaneous abortion by intravenous immunoglobulin: a double-blind placebo-controlled study. *Hum Reprod* 1999;14:838–841.

397. **Mueller-Eckhardt G, Heine O, Polten B.** IVIG to prevent recurrent spontaneous abortion. *Lancet* 1991;337:424–425.

398. **Perino A, Vassiliadis A, Vucetich A, et al.** Short-term therapy for recurrent abortion using intravenous immunoglobulins: results of a double-blind placebo-controlled Italian study. *Hum Reprod* 1997;12:2388–2392.

399. **Stephenson MD, Dreher K, Houlihan E, et al.** Prevention of unexplained recurrent spontaneous abortion using intravenous immunoglobulin: a prospective, randomized, double-blinded, placebo-controlled trial. *Am J Reprod Immunol* 1998;39:82–88.

400. **Harris EN, Pierangeli SS.** Utilization of intravenous immunoglobulin therapy to treat recurrent pregnancy loss in the antiphospholipid syndrome: a review. *Scand J Rheumatol Suppl* 1998;107:97–102.

401. **Vaquero E, Lazzarin N, Valensise H, et al.** Pregnancy outcome in recurrent spontaneous abortion associated with antiphospholipid antibodies: a comparative study of intravenous immunoglobulin versus prednisone plus low-dose aspirin. *Am J Reprod Immunol* 2001;45:174–179.

402. **Practice Committee of the American Society for Reproductive Medicine.** Intravenous immunoglobulin (IVIG) and recurrent spontaneous pregnancy loss. *Fertil Steril* 2006;86(Suppl 4):S226–S227.

403. **Thornton CA, Ballow M.** Safety of intravenous immunoglobulin. *Arch Neurol* 1993;50:135–136.

404. **Choi BC, Polgar K, Xiao L, et al.** Progesterone inhibits *in-vitro* embryotoxic Th1 cytokine production to trophoblast in women with recurrent pregnancy loss. *Hum Reprod* 2000;15(Suppl 1):46–59.

405. **Haas DM, Ramsey PS.** Progestogen for preventing miscarriage. *Cochrane Database Syst Rev* 2008;2:CD003511.

406. **Oates-Whitehead RM, Haas DM, Carrier JA.** Progestogen for preventing miscarriage. *Cochrane Database Syst Rev* 2003;4: CD003511.

407. **Battistella FD, Widergren JT, Anderson JT, et al.** A prospective, randomized trial of intravenous fat emulsion administration in trauma victims requiring total parenteral nutrition. *J Trauma* 1997;43:52–60.

408. **Mayer K, Meyer S, Reinholz-Muhly M, et al.** Short-time infusion of fish oil-based lipid emulsions, approved for parenteral nutrition, reduces monocyte proinflammatory cytokine generation and adhesive interaction with endothelium in humans. *J Immunol* 2003;171:4837–4843.

409. **Sedman PC, Somers SS, Ramsden CW, et al.** Effects of different lipid emulsions on lymphocyte function during total parenteral nutrition. *Br J Surg* 1991;78:1396–1399.

410. **Clark DA.** Intralipid as treatment for recurrent unexplained abortion? *Am J Reprod Immunol* 1994;32:290–293.

411. **Roussev RG, Acacio B, Ng SC, et al.** Duration of intralipid's suppressive effect on NK cell's functional activity. *Am J Reprod Immunol* 2008;60:258–263.

412. **Roussev RG, Ng SC, Coulam CB.** Natural killer cell functional activity suppression by intravenous immunoglobulin, intralipid and soluble human leukocyte antigen-G. *Am J Reprod Immunol* 2007;57:262–269.

413. **Arslan E, Colakolu M, Celik C, et al.** Serum TNF-alpha, IL-6, lupus anticoagulant and anticardiolipin antibody in women with and without a past history of recurrent miscarriage. *Arch Gynecol Obstet* 2004;270:227–229.

414. **Palmirotta R, La Farina F, Ferroni P, et al.** TNFA gene promoter polymorphisms and susceptibility to recurrent pregnancy loss in Italian women. *Reprod Sci* 2010;17:659–666.

415. **Zammiti W, Mtiraoui N, Finan RR, et al.** Tumor necrosis factor alpha and lymphotoxin alpha haplotypes in idiopathic recurrent pregnancy loss. *Fertil Steril* 2009;91:1903–1908.

416. **Robinson WH, Genovese MC, Moreland LW.** Demyelinating and neurologic events reported in association with tumor necrosis factor alpha antagonism: by what mechanisms could tumor necrosis factor alpha antagonists improve rheumatoid arthritis but exacerbate multiple sclerosis? *Arthritis Rheum* 2001;44:1977–1983.

417. **Mossner R, Schon MP, Reich K.** Tumor necrosis factor antagonists in the therapy of psoriasis. *Clin Dermatol* 2008;26:486–502.

418. **Winger EE, Reed JL.** Treatment with tumor necrosis factor inhibitors and intravenous immunoglobulin improves live birth rates in women with recurrent spontaneous abortion. *Am J Reprod Immunol* 2008;60:8–16.

419. **Carter JD, Ladhani A, Ricca LR, et al.** A safety assessment of tumor necrosis factor antagonists during pregnancy: a review of the Food and Drug Administration database. *J Rheumatol* 2009;36:635–641.

420. **Ferro D, Quintarelli C, Russo G, et al.** Successful removal of antiphospholipid antibodies using repeated plasma exchanges and prednisone. *Clin Exp Rheumatol* 1989;7:103–104.

421. **Doss BJ, Greene MF, Hill J, et al.** Massive chronic intervillositis associated with recurrent abortions. *Hum Pathol* 1995;26:1245–1251.

422. **Lubbe WF, Butler WS, Palmer SJ, et al.** Fetal survival after prednisone suppression of maternal lupus-anticoagulant. *Lancet* 1983;1:1361–1363.

423. **Quenby S, Farquharson R, Young M, et al.** Successful pregnancy outcome following 19 consecutive miscarriages: case report. *Hum Reprod* 2003;18:2562–2564.

424. **Quenby S, Kalumbi C, Bates M, et al.** Prednisolone reduces preconceptual endometrial natural killer cells in women with recurrent miscarriage. *Fertil Steril* 2005;84:980–984.

425. **Tang AW, Alfirevic Z, Turner MA, et al.** Prednisolone Trial: Study protocol for a randomised controlled trial of prednisolone for women with idiopathic recurrent miscarriage and raised levels of uterine natural killer (uNK) cells in the endometrium. *Trials* 2009;10:102.

426. **Laskin CA, Bombardier C, Hannah ME, et al.** Prednisone and aspirin in women with autoantibodies and unexplained recurrent fetal loss. *N Engl J Med* 1997;337:148–153.

427. **Ermel LD, Marshburn PB, Kutteh WH.** Interaction of heparin with antiphospholipid antibodies (APA) from the sera of women with recurrent pregnancy loss (RPL). *Am J Reprod Immunol* 1995;33:14–20.

428. **Górski A, Makula J, Morzycka-Michalik M, et al.** Low-dose heparin: a novel approach in immunosuppression. *Transpl Int* 1994;7(Suppl 1):S567–S569.

429. **Kutteh WH.** Antiphospholipid antibody-associated recurrent pregnancy loss: treatment with heparin and low-dose aspirin is superior to low-dose aspirin alone. *Am J Obstet Gynecol* 1996;174:1584–1589.

430. **Lima F, Khamashta MA, Buchanan NM, et al.** A study of sixty pregnancies in patients with the antiphospholipid syndrome. *Clin Exp Rheumatol* 1996;14:131–136.

431. **Mak A, Cheung MW, Cheak AA, et al.** Combination of heparin and aspirin is superior to aspirin alone in enhancing live births in patients with recurrent pregnancy loss and positive anti-phospholipid antibodies: a meta-analysis of randomized controlled trials and meta-regression. *Rheumatology (Oxford)* 2010;49:281–288.

432. **Rai R, Cohen H, Dave M, et al.** Randomised controlled trial of aspirin and aspirin plus heparin in pregnant women with recurrent miscarriage associated with phospholipid antibodies (or antiphospholipid antibodies). *BMJ* 1997;314:253–257.

433. **Ziakas PD, Pavlou M, Voulgarelis M.** Heparin treatment in antiphospholipid syndrome with recurrent pregnancy loss: a systematic review and meta-analysis. *Obstet Gynecol* 2010;115:1256–1262.

434. **Bates SM, Ginsberg JS.** Anticoagulation in pregnancy. *Pharm Pract Manag Q* 1999;19:51–60.

435. **Bates SM, Greer IA, Pabinger I, et al.** Venous thromboembolism, thrombophilia, antithrombotic therapy, and pregnancy: American College of Chest Physicians Evidence-Based Clinical Practice Guidelines (8th edition). *Chest* 2008;133(6 Suppl):844S–886S.

436. **Bijsterveld NR, Hettiarachchi R, Peters R, et al.** Low-molecular weight heparins in venous and arterial thrombotic disease. *Thromb Haemost* 1999;82(Suppl 1):139–147.

437. **Deruelle P, Coulon C.** The use of low-molecular-weight heparins in pregnancy—how safe are they? *Curr Opin Obstet Gynecol* 2007;19:573–577.

438. **Stephenson MD, Ballem PJ, Tsang P, et al.** Treatment of antiphospholipid antibody syndrome (APS) in pregnancy: a randomized pilot trial comparing low molecular weight heparin to unfractionated heparin. *J Obstet Gynaecol Can* 2004;26:729–734.

439. **Bar J, Cohen-Sacher B, Hod M, et al.** Low-molecular-weight heparin for thrombophilia in pregnant women. *Int J Gynaecol Obstet* 2000;69:209–213.

440. **Carp H, Dolitzky M, Inbal A.** Thromboprophylaxis improves the live birth rate in women with consecutive recurrent miscarriages and hereditary thrombophilia. *J Thromb Haemost* 2003;1:433–438.

441. **Younis JS, Ohel G, Brenner B, et al.** The effect of thrombophylaxis on pregnancy outcome in patients with recurrent pregnancy loss associated with factor V Leiden mutation. *Bjog* 2000;107:415–419.

442. **Lepercq J, Conard J, Borel-Derlon A, et al.** Venous thromboembolism during pregnancy: a retrospective study of enoxaparin safety in 624 pregnancies. *BJOG* 2001;108:1134–1140.

443. **Sanson BJ, Lensing AW, Prins MH, et al.** Safety of low-molecular-weight heparin in pregnancy: a systematic review. *Thromb Haemost* 1999;81:668–672.

444. **Pattison NS, Chamley LW, Birdsall M, et al.** Does aspirin have a role in improving pregnancy outcome for women with the antiphospholipid syndrome? A randomized controlled trial. *Am J Obstet Gynecol* 2000;183:1008–1012.

445. **Rai R, Regan L.** Thrombophilia and adverse pregnancy outcome. *Semin Reprod Med* 2000;18:369–377.

446. **James AH, Brancazio LR, Price T.** Aspirin and reproductive outcomes. *Obstet Gynecol Surv* 2008;63:49–57.

447. **Richards EM, Makris M, Preston FE.** The successful use of protein C concentrate during pregnancy in a patient with type 1 protein C deficiency, previous thrombosis and recurrent fetal loss. *Br J Haematol* 1997;98:660–661.

448. **Brouwer IA, van Dusseldorp M, Thomas CM, et al.** Low-dose folic acid supplementation decreases plasma homocysteine concentrations: a randomized trial. *Am J Clin Nutr* 1999;69:99–104.

449. **Carlsson CM, Pharo LM, Aeschlimann SE, et al.** Effects of multivitamins and low-dose folic acid supplements on flow-mediated vasodilation and plasma homocysteine levels in older adults. *Am Heart J* 2004;148: E11.

450. **de la Calle M, Usandizaga R, Sancha M, et al.** Homocysteine, folic acid and B-group vitamins in obstetrics and gynaecology. *Eur J Obstet Gynecol Reprod Biol* 2003;107:125–134.

451. **O'Donnell J, Perry DJ.** Pharmacotherapy of hyperhomocysteinaemia in patients with thrombophilia. *Expert Opin Pharmacother* 2002;3:1591–1598.

452. **Neugebauer R, Kline J, Shrout P, et al.** Major depressive disorder in the 6 months after miscarriage. *JAMA* 1997;277:383–388.

453. **Harger JH, Archer DF, Marchese SG, et al.** Etiology of recurrent pregnancy losses and outcome of subsequent pregnancies. *Obstet Gynecol* 1983;62:574–581.

454. **Phung Thi T, Byrd JR, McDonough PG.** Etiologies and subsequent reproductive performance of 100 couples with recurrent abortion. *Fertil Steril* 1979;32:389–395.

455. **Vlaanderen W, Treffers PE.** Prognosis of subsequent pregnancies after recurrent spontaneous abortion in first trimester. *Br Med J (Clin Res Ed)* 1987;295:92–93.

456. **DeCherney AH, Russell JB, Graebe RA, et al.** Resectoscopic management of mullerian fusion defects. *Fertil Steril* 1986;45:726–728.

457. **March CM, Israel R.** Hysteroscopic management of recurrent abortion caused by septate uterus. *Am J Obstet Gynecol* 1987;156:834–842.

458. **Colacurci N, De Franciscis P, Mollo A, et al.** Small-diameter hysteroscopy with Versapoint versus resectoscopy with a unipolar knife for the treatment of septate uterus: a prospective randomized study. *J Minim Invasive Gynecol* 2007;14:622–627.

459. **Hollett-Caines J, Vilos GA, Abu-Rafea B, et al.** Fertility and pregnancy outcomes following hysteroscopic septum division. *J Obstet Gynaecol Can* 2006;28:156–159.

460. **Branch DW, Silver RM, Blackwell JL, et al.** Outcome of treated pregnancies in women with antiphospholipid syndrome: an update of the Utah experience. *Obstet Gynecol* 1992;80:614–620.

461. **Lubbe WF, Liggins GC.** Role of lupus anticoagulant and autoimmunity in recurrent pregnancy loss. *Semin Reprod Endocrinol* 1988;6:161–190.

462. **Prakash A, Laird S, Tuckerman E, et al.** Inhibin A and activin A may be used to predict pregnancy outcome in women with recurrent miscarriage. *Fertil Steril* 2005;83:1758–1763.

463. **Pratt DE, Kaberlein G, Dudkiewicz A, et al.** The association of antithyroid antibodies in euthyroid nonpregnant women with recurrent first trimester abortions in the next pregnancy. *Fertil Steril* 1993;60:1001–1005.

464. **Laufer MR, Ecker JL, Hill JA.** Pregnancy outcome following ultrasound-detected fetal cardiac activity in women with a history of multiple spontaneous abortions. *J Soc Gynecol Investig* 1994;1:138–142.

465. **Rai RS, Clifford K, Cohen H, et al.** High prospective fetal loss rate in untreated pregnancies of women with recurrent miscarriage and antiphospholipid antibodies. *Hum Reprod* 1995;10:3301–3304.

466. **Brigham SA, Conlon C, Farquharson RG.** A longitudinal study of pregnancy outcome following idiopathic recurrent miscarriage. *Hum Reprod* 1999;14:2868–2871.

34

Menopause

Jan L. Shifren
Isaac Schiff

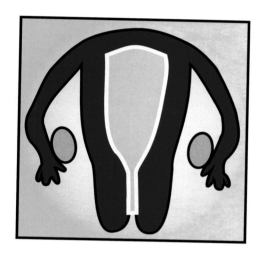

- Vasomotor symptoms affect up to 75% of perimenopausal women. Symptoms last for 1 to 2 years after menopause in most women but may continue for 10 years or longer in others.

- Topical vaginal application of low doses of *estrogen* is an effective and safe treatment of vaginal dryness, dyspareunia, and some urinary symptoms.

- Counseling women to alter modifiable risk factors is important for the prevention and treatment of osteoporosis. Many women have diets deficient in calcium and vitamin D and will benefit from dietary changes and supplementation. Women should receive 1,000 to 1,500 mg of *calcium* and 400 to 800 IU of *vitamin D* daily.

- Contraindications to hormone therapy use include known or suspected breast or endometrial cancer, undiagnosed abnormal genital bleeding, cardiovascular disease (including coronary heart disease, cerebrovascular disease, and thromboembolic disorders), and active liver or gallbladder disease. Relative contraindications include high-risk states for the above disorders.

Menopause, the permanent cessation of menstruation, occurs at a mean age of 51 years. Despite a great increase in the life expectancy of women, the age at menopause remains remarkably constant. A woman in the United States today will live approximately 30 years, or greater than a third of her life, beyond the menopause. The age at menopause appears to be genetically determined and is unaffected by race, socioeconomic status, age at menarche, or number of prior ovulations. Factors that are toxic to the ovary often result in an earlier age of menopause; women who smoke experience an earlier menopause, as do many women exposed to chemotherapy or pelvic radiation (1). Women who had surgery on their ovaries or had a hysterectomy, despite retention of their ovaries, may experience early menopause (2). ***Premature ovarian insufficiency,* defined as menopause before the age of 40 years, occurs in approximately 1% of women.** It may be idiopathic or associated with a toxic exposure, chromosomal abnormality, or an autoimmune disorder.

Although menopause is associated with changes in the hypothalamic and pituitary hormones that regulate the menstrual cycle, menopause is not a central event, but rather primary ovarian failure. At the level of the ovary, there is a depletion of ovarian follicles, most likely secondary to apoptosis or programmed cell death. The ovary, therefore, is no longer able to respond to the pituitary hormones, follicle-stimulating hormone (FSH), and luteinizing hormone (LH), and ovarian estrogen and progesterone production ceases. **The ovarian–hypothalamic–pituitary axis remains intact during the menopausal transition; thus, FSH levels rise in response to ovarian failure and the absence of negative feedback from the ovary.** Atresia of the follicular apparatus, in particular the granulosa cells, leads to decreased production of estrogen and inhibin, resulting in elevated FSH levels, a cardinal sign of menopause. Antimüllerian hormone (AMH) is produced by small ovarian follicles, so levels decrease with declining ovarian reserve (3). Although still considered experimental, AMH may one day be used as a reliable marker of the menopause transition.

Androgen production from the ovary continues beyond the menopausal transition because of sparing of the stromal compartment. Androgen concentrations are lower in menopausal women than in women of reproductive age. This finding appears to be associated with aging and decreased functioning of the ovary and adrenal glands over time rather than with menopause *per se*. Menopausal women continue to have low levels of circulating estrogens, principally from peripheral aromatization of ovarian and adrenal androgens. Adipose tissue is a major site of aromatization, so obesity affects many of the sequelae of menopause.

Several staging systems were developed to describe the many changes that encompass the transition from reproductive life to postmenopause. **The late reproductive years are characterized by regular menses associated with elevated FSH levels** (4).

- *Menopausal transition* is characterized by elevated FSH levels associated with variable cycle lengths and missed menses, whereas the postmenopausal period is marked by amenorrhea. The menopausal transition begins with variability in menstrual cycle length accompanied by rising FSH levels and ends with the final menstrual period.

- *Menopause* is defined retrospectively as the time of the final menstrual period followed by 12 months of amenorrhea

- *Postmenopause* describes the period following the final menses (4).

The pathophysiologic consequences of menopause may be best understood by considering that the ovary is a women's only source of oocytes, her primary source of estrogen and progesterone, and a major source of androgens. Menopause results in infertility secondary to oocyte depletion. Ovarian cessation of progesterone production appears to have no clinical consequences except for the increased risk of endometrial proliferation, hyperplasia, and cancer associated with continued endogenous estrogen production or administration of unopposed estrogen therapy in menopausal women. The possible effects of declining androgen concentrations that occur with aging are an area of controversy and active investigation.

The major consequences of menopause are related primarily to estrogen deficiency. It is very difficult to distinguish the consequences of estrogen deficiency from those of aging, as aging and menopause are inextricably linked. Studying the effects of estrogen deficiency and replacement in young women with ovarian failure or of drugs that suppress estrogen synthesis (such as gonadotropin-releasing hormone antagonists) helps to distinguish between the effects of aging and estrogen deficiency. These models are imperfect, though, and differ from natural menopause in many ways.

Principal health concerns of menopausal women include vasomotor symptoms, urogenital atrophy, osteoporosis, cardiovascular disease, cancer, cognitive decline, and sexual problems. Options for caring for menopausal women have increased greatly since hormone therapy was first introduced in the 1960s. With respect to hormone use, there are many choices of hormone type, dose, and method of administration. In addition to hormones, estrogen agonist-antagonists, centrally acting agents, and bisphosphonates are available to treat menopausal health concerns. Women are requesting more information on complementary and alternative therapies, which are being studied more carefully. The many options now available make caring for the postmenopausal woman more challenging and more rewarding.

Health Concerns After Menopause

Vasomotor Symptoms

Vasomotor symptoms affect up to 75% of perimenopausal women. Symptoms last for 1 to 2 years after menopause in most women, but may continue for up to 10 years or longer in others. Hot flashes are the primary reason women seek care at menopause. Hot flashes disturb women at work, interrupt daily activities and disrupt sleep (5). Many women report difficulty concentrating and emotional lability during the menopausal transition. **Treatment of vasomotor symptoms should improve these cognitive and mood symptoms if they are secondary to sleep disruption and its resulting daytime fatigue. The incidence of thyroid disease increases as women age; therefore, thyroid function tests should be performed if vasomotor symptoms are atypical or resistant to therapy.**

The physiologic mechanisms underlying hot flashes are incompletely understood. A central event, probably initiated in the hypothalamus, drives an increased core body temperature, metabolic rate, and skin temperature; this reaction results in peripheral vasodilation and sweating in some women. The central event may be triggered by noradrenergic, serotoninergic, and/or dopaminergic activation. Although an LH surge often occurs at the time of a hot flash, it is not causative, because vasomotor symptoms occur in women who had their pituitary glands removed. In symptomatic postmenopausal women, hot flashes likely are triggered by small elevations in core body temperature acting within a narrow thermoneutral zone (6). Exactly how estrogen and alternative therapies play a role in modulating these events is unknown. Vasomotor symptoms are a consequence of estrogen withdrawal, not simply estrogen deficiency. For example, a young woman with primary ovarian insufficiency resulting from Turner syndrome will have a very high FSH level and low estrogen levels, but she will not experience hot flashes until she is treated with estrogens and then therapy is withdrawn.

Lifestyle interventions may safely decrease vasomotor symptoms. Being in a cool environment is associated with fewer subjective and objective hot flashes, so women experiencing symptoms should be advised to keep the room temperature low and wear light, layered clothing (7). **Overweight women and those who smoke have more severe vasomotor symptoms than women of normal weight and nonsmokers.** These findings provide additional reasons to encourage women to lose weight and stop smoking (8,9).

Many menopausal women are interested in trying complementary and alternative (CAM) therapies for relief of hot flashes. These are diverse medical and health care products and practices generally not considered part of conventional medicine. Vasomotor symptoms are particularly sensitive to placebo treatments, and numerous nutritional supplements and other interventions claim to relieve hot flashes but are rarely studied in controlled trials (10). *Phytoestrogens* are plant-derived substances that may act as estrogen agonists-antagonists, with their effects modulated through interactions with the estrogen receptor. Although they decrease hot flash severity and frequency, symptom improvement is similar to that seen with placebo treatment (11). *Black cohosh* is another popular alternative treatment, with efficacy likely similar to that of placebo (12). Although often recommended, *vitamin E* (800 IU per day) only minimally reduced hot flashes in a placebo-controlled, randomized, crossover trial (13).

Acupuncture reduced vasomotor symptoms in several studies, although a traditional Chinese medicine approach may be no more effective than shallow or "sham" needling techniques (14). Exercise and paced respiration demonstrated an improvement in hot flashes in several uncontrolled studies, with additional health benefits, including stress reduction. Women may choose to use alternative and complementary therapies for relief of symptoms, but they should be aware that the safety and efficacy of these approaches often are unproven.

Systemic *estrogen* therapy is the most effective treatment for vasomotor symptoms and the only therapy currently approved by the U.S. Food and Drug Administration (FDA) for this indication (see Table 34.1 for available hormone therapy formulations). **Although standard doses are usually effective, younger women and those with recent oophorectomy may require higher doses. Healthy, nonsmoking women in the perimenopausal transition who are experiencing bothersome hot flashes but still menstruating may benefit from oral contraceptives. The supraphysiologic doses of estrogens and progestins in oral contraceptives effectively treat vasomotor symptoms and provide cycle control.** Low-dose *estrogen* therapy

Table 34.1 Hormone Therapy Options

Oral Estrogen Products

Composition	Product Name	Dose (mg/day)
Conjugated estrogens	Premarin	0.3, 0.45, 0.625, 0.9, 1.25
Synthetic conjugated estrogens	Cenestin, Enjuvia	0.3. 0.45, 0.625, 0.9, 1.25
Esterified estrogens	Menest	0.3, 0.625, 1.25, 2.5
17β-estradiol	Estrace, generics	0.5, 1.0, 2.0
Estropipate (Estrone)	Ortho-Est, Ogen, generics	0.625, 1.25

Transdermal/Topical Estrogen Products

Composition	Product Name	Delivery Rate (mg/day)	Dosing
17β-estradiol matrix patch	Alora	0.025, 0.05, 0.075, 0.1	Twice weekly
	Climara	0.025, 0.0375, 0.05, 0.075, 0.1	Once weekly
	Esclim	0.025, 0.0375, 0.05, 0.075, 0.1	Twice weekly
	FemPatch	0.025	Once weekly
	Menostar	0.014	Once weekly
	Vivelle, Vivelle-Dot	0.025, 0.0375, 0.05, 0.075, 0.1	Twice weekly
	Various generics	0.05, 0.1	Once or twice weekly
17β-estradiol reservoir patch	Estraderm	0.05, 0.1	Twice weekly
17β-estradiol transdermal gel	EstroGel	0.035	Daily application via metered-dose pump
	Elestrin	0.0125	Daily application via metered-dose pump
	Divigel	0.003, 0.009, 0.027	Daily application of 1 packet
17β-estradiol topical emulsion	Estrasorb	0.05	Daily application of 2 packets
17β-estradiol transdermal spray	Evamist	0.021 (per spray)	Daily application via metered-dose pump (1–3 sprays daily)

Vaginal Estrogen Products

Composition	Product Name	Recommended Dose
Vaginal Creams		
17β-estradiol	Estrace vaginal cream	0.5–1 g, 2–3 times weekly
Conjugated estrogens	Premarin vaginal cream	0.5–1 g, 2–3 times weekly
Vaginal Rings		
17β-estradiol	Estring	Device releases 7.5 μg/day for 90 days
Estradiol acetate	Femring	Device releases 0.05 or 0.1 mg/day for 90 days (systemic estradiol levels achieved)
Vaginal Tablet		
Estradiol hemihydrate	Vagifem	1 tablet (10 μg) twice weekly

(Continued)

Table 34.1 *Continued*

Progestogens

Composition	Product Name	Dose
Progestin: Oral Tablet		
Medroxyprogesterone acetate	Provera, generics	2.5, 5, 10 mg
Norethindrone	Micronor, Nor-QD, generics	0.35 mg
Norethindrone acetate	Aygestin, generics	5 mg
Megestrol acetate	Megace	20, 40 mg
Progesterone: Oral Capsule		
Micronized progesterone	Prometrium	100, 200 mg
Progestin: Intrauterine System		
Levonorgestrel IUS	Mirena	20 µg/day release rate (5-year use)
Progesterone: Vaginal Gel		
Progesterone	Prochieve 4%, 8% Crinone 4%, 8%	45 or 90 mg/applicator

Combination Estrogen-Progestogen Products

Composition	Product Name	Dose (per day)
Oral Continuous-Cyclic Regimen		
Conjugated estrogens (E) + medroxyprogesterone acetate (P)	Premphase	0.625 mg E + 5.0 mg P (E alone days 1–14, E + P days 15–28)
Oral Continuous-Combined Regimen		
Conjugated estrogens (E) + medroxyprogesterone acetate (P)	Prempro	0.625 mg E + 2.5 or 5.0 mg P 0.3 or 0.45 mg E + 1.5 mg P
Ethinyl estradiol (E) + norethindrone acetate (P)	Femhrt	2.5 µg E + 0.5 mg P 5 µg E + 1 mg P
17β-estradiol (E) + norethindrone acetate (P)	Activella	0.5 mg E + 0.1 mg P 1 mg E + 0.5 mg P
17β-estradiol (E) + drosperinone (P)	Angeliq	1 mg E + 0.5 mg P
Oral Intermittent-Combined Regimen		
17β-estradiol (E) + norgestimate (P)	Prefest	1 mg E + 0.09 mg P (E alone for 3 days, followed by E + P for 3 days)
Transdermal Continuous-Combined Regimen		
17β-estradiol (E) + norethindrone acetate (P)	CombiPatch	0.05 mg E + 0.14 P twice weekly
17β-estradiol (E) + levonorgestrel (P)	Climara Pro	0.045 mg E + 0.0015 mg P once weekly

E, estrogen; P, progestin.
Products available in the United States.
Table modified and used with permission; North American Menopause Society; www.menopause.org.

also effectively treats hot flashes for many women. Low-dose oral *esterified and conjugated estrogens (CE)* (0.3 mg daily), oral *estradiol* (0.5 mg daily), and transdermal *estradiol* (0.025 and 0.014 mg weekly) often are effective and associated with minimal side effects and endometrial stimulation (15–17). **Progestin therapy must be given concurrently if a woman has not had a hysterectomy, although with low-dose estrogen therapy, intermittent progestin treatment may be an option.**

Given the known risks, described in detail later in this chapter, hormone therapy should be used at the lowest effective dose for the shortest amount of time that meets treatment goals. The majority of healthy women with very bothersome hot flashes at the time of the menopausal transition will benefit from short-term therapy and be able to wean off hormones after several years of use.

Because vasomotor symptoms appear to be the result of estrogen withdrawal, rather than simply low estrogen levels, if cessation of *estrogen* therapy is desired, the dose should be reduced slowly over time. Abruptly stopping treatment may result in a return of disruptive vasomotor symptoms. This recommendation is based on clinical experience, as no controlled trials have been performed to examine the optimal way to cease hormone therapy use. One possible approach to stopping therapy is to reduce the dose and dosing interval slowly (e.g., every 2 or 3 months) and let the patient's symptoms guide the pace at which she discontinues therapy.

When a woman chooses not to take estrogen or when it is contraindicated, other options are available (Table 34.2) (18). *Progestin* therapy alone is an option for some women. *Medroxy-progesterone acetate (MPA; Provera)* (20 mg per day) and *megestrol acetate (Megace)* (20 mg per day) effectively treat vasomotor symptoms (19,20). Several drugs that alter central neurotransmitter pathways are effective. Agents that decrease central noradrenergic tone, such as *clonidine (Catapres)*, decrease hot flashes, although the effect size is not great. Potential side effects include orthostatic hypotension and drowsiness.

Selective serotonin or serotonin norepinephrine reuptake inhibitors (SSRIs/SNRIs) are effective and are the mainstay of nonhormonal treatment of hot flashes, although none are FDA approved for this purpose. In a double-blind, randomized, placebo-controlled trial of *paroxetine CR (Paxil)* (12.5 and 25 mg per day), menopausal women with hot flashes experienced a significant reduction in both hot flash frequency and severity (21). Actual hot flash frequency decreased by 3.3 hot flashes per day on *paroxetine* versus 1.8 on placebo, and the improvement in

Table 34.2 Options for the Treatment of Vasomotor Symptoms
Hormone therapy
• *Estrogen* therapy
• *Progestin* therapy[a]
• Combination *estrogen/progestin* therapy
Nonhormonal prescription medications[a]
• *Clonidine*
• Selective serotonin and norepinephrine reuptake inhibitors
Paroxetine
Venlafaxine
• *Gabapentin*
Nonprescription medications
• Isoflavone supplements
• Soy products
• *Black cohosh*
• *Vitamin E*
Lifestyle changes
• Reducing body temperature
• Maintaining a healthy weight
• Smoking cessation
• Relaxation response techniques
• Acupuncture

[a]Not U.S. Food and Drug Administration–approved for treatment of vasomotor symptoms.

vasomotor symptoms was independent of any significant change in mood or anxiety symptoms. The most common side effects were headache, nausea, and insomnia. *Paroxetine* is a potent inhibitor of the cytochrome P450 system (CYP2D6) required to convert *tamoxifen* to its active form. It should not be used in women with breast cancer who are receiving *tamoxifen,* as concurrent use may result in a higher rate of breast cancer recurrence. *Venlafaxine (Effexor)* (75 mg per day), an SNRI, significantly reduced hot flashes in a controlled trial, though the active treatment group experienced significantly more side effects, including dry mouth, nausea, and anorexia (22). Most studies of SSRI or SNRI use for vasomotor symptoms are only short term and not all show an improvement in symptoms. In a double-blind, parallel-group trial of 9 months' duration, there was no significant improvement in hot flashes with either *fluoxetine (Prozac)* or *citalopram (Celexa)* (10 to 30 mg per day) compared to placebo (23).

Gabapentin (Neurontin) is a γ-aminobutyric acid analogue approved for the treatment of seizures that reduced hot flash frequency and severity significantly more than placebo in several randomized, double-blind trials (24). Hot flash scores decreased 54% in the women treated with *gabapentin* (900 mg per day) compared with a 31% reduction in placebo-treated women. Side effects include disorientation, dizziness, and drowsiness. Women who are principally bothered by night sweats and disrupted sleep may benefit from sleeping medication. In a double-blind, placebo-controlled study of peri- and postmenopausal women, the prescription insomnia treatment, *eszopiclone,* significantly improved sleep and menopause-related symptoms, with a positive impact on next-day functioning, mood, and quality of life (25). The antihistamine *diphenhydramine hydrochloride* is an inexpensive, over-the-counter sleep aid.

Urogenital Atrophy

Urogenital atrophy results in vaginal dryness and pruritus, dyspareunia, dysuria, and urinary urgency. These common problems in menopausal women respond well to therapy (26). **Systemic** *estrogen* **therapy is a very effective treatment for vaginal dryness, dyspareunia, and associated symptoms. Low doses of** *estrogen* **applied vaginally are preferred to systemic** *estrogen* **therapy when vasomotor symptoms are not present, given minimal systemic absorption and increased safety.** Low doses of *estrogen cream (Premarin, Estrace)* (0.5 g) are effective when used only once or twice a week (27). An *estradiol vaginal* tablet *(Vagifem)* (10 μg) inserted twice weekly may be less messy and easier to use than *estrogen* cream. An *estrogen*-containing vaginal ring *(Estring)* (7.5 μg per day) is another convenient formulation, which is placed in the vagina every 3 months and slowly releases a low dose of estradiol (28). Studies of the low-dose *estrogen* vaginal ring and tablet confirm a small increase in serum estradiol and estrone levels, but these levels remain within the normal range for postmenopausal women (29).

Studies of the vaginal tablets and ring of up to 1 years' duration confirmed endometrial safety, but long-term studies on the effects of low-dose vaginal *estrogen* **therapy on the endometrium are not available. Women using vaginal** *estrogen* **therapy should be reminded to report any vaginal bleeding, and a thorough evaluation should be performed.** Typically, concurrent *progestin* therapy is not prescribed with low-dose vaginal *estrogen* preparations. Long-acting vaginal moisturizers, available without a prescription, are an effective nonhormonal alternative for treating symptoms of urogenital atrophy when used two to three times weekly (e.g., *Replens, KY-Long Acting*). Nonhormonal vaginal lubricants (e.g., *Astroglide, KY-Silk*) increase comfort with intercourse.

Vaginal *estrogen* **therapy appears to reduce urinary symptoms, such as frequency and urgency, and reduces the likelihood of recurrent urinary tract infections in postmenopausal women** (30). The effect of *estrogen* therapy on urinary incontinence is unclear. Whereas the results of some studies suggest improvement in incontinence with *estrogen* therapy, others show a worsening of symptoms (31).

Osteoporosis

Low bone mass and osteoporosis affect an estimated 30 million US women, or approximately 55% of women older than age 50 years (32). Because therapy is most likely to benefit those at highest risk, it is important to review a woman's risk factors for osteoporosis when making treatment decisions. **Bone mineral density screening should be considered for high-risk women** (Table 34.3). **Nonmodifiable risk factors include age, family history, Asian or Caucasian race, history of a prior fracture, small body frame, early menopause, and prior oophorectomy. Modifiable risk factors include smoking, decreased intake of calcium and vitamin D, and a sedentary lifestyle.** Medical conditions associated with an increased risk of

Table 34.3 Risk Factors for Osteoporosis
Nonmodifiable
• Age
• Race (white, Asian)
• Small body frame
• Early menopause
• Prior fracture
• Family history of osteoporosis
Modifiable
• Inadequate intake of *calcium* and *vitamin D*
• Smoking
• Low body weight
• Excess alcohol use
• Sedentary lifestyle
Associated Medical Conditions
• Hyperthyroidism
• Hyperparathyroidism
• Chronic renal disease
• Conditions requiring systemic corticosteroid use

osteoporosis include anovulation during the reproductive years (e.g., secondary to excess exercise or an eating disorder), chronic renal disease, hyperparathyroidism, hyperthyroidism, and diseases requiring systemic *corticosteroid* use.

Assessment

Bone mineral density (BMD) measurements may be used to determine fracture risk, diagnose osteoporosis, and identify women who would benefit from therapeutic interventions. Dual x-ray absorptiometry (DXA) of the hip and spine is the primary technique for BMD assessment. BMD is expressed as a T score, which is the number of standard deviations from the mean for a young, healthy woman. A T score above −1 is considered normal, a score between −1 and −2.5 indicates low bone mass, and a score below −2.5 denotes osteoporosis. Although there is a strong association between BMD and fracture risk, a woman's age, risk for falls, and overall health status significantly influence fracture risk. **Evaluation of BMD by DXA is recommended for all women aged 65 and older, regardless of risk factors, and for younger postmenopausal women with one or more risk factors, other than being white and menopausal (33).**

Modifiable Risk

Women should be counseled to alter modifiable risk factors as an important step in the prevention and treatment of osteoporosis. Women with diets deficient in calcium and vitamin D will benefit from dietary modification and supplementation. Daily intake of *calcium* 1,000 to 1,500 mg and *vitamin D* 400 to 800 IU is recommended. This may be achieved through a combination of diet and vitamin and mineral supplementation. Treatment with *calcium* and *vitamin D* may reduce fracture risk, especially in older women, according to some but not all studies (34–36). Reducing the risk of osteoporosis is another of the many health benefits of regular exercise and smoking cessation. Treatment is indicated for all women with osteoporosis and for those at high fracture risk. **FRAX, an online fracture risk assessment tool, provides the 10-year probability of a major osteoporotic fracture for an individual woman (37,38).**

Treatment

Drugs used in the prevention and treatment of osteoporosis are principally antiresorptive agents that reduce bone loss and anabolic drugs that stimulate new bone formation (Table 34.4). **Hormone therapy effectively prevents and treats osteoporosis.** In observational studies, estrogen therapy started soon after menopause and continued long term reduces

Table 34.4 Options for Osteoporosis Prevention and Treatment

Bisphosphonates

Alendronate (Fosamax) (35 or 70 mg/week orally)

Risedronate (Actonel) (35 mg/week or 150 mg/month orally)

Ibandronate (Boniva) (150 mg/month orally or 3 mg/every 3 months intravenous)

Zoledronic Acid (Zometa) (5 mg/year intravenous)

- Additional potential benefits: none

- Potential risks: esophageal ulcers, osteonecrosis of jaw (rare), atypical femoral fractures (rare)
  Zoledronic acid: hypocalcemia, atrial fibrillation, renal impairment

- Side effects: gastrointestinal distress, arthralgias/myalgias

Hormone Therapy

Estrogen or Estrogen/Progestin Therapy

- Additional potential benefits: treatment of vasomotor symptoms and urogenital atrophy

- Potential risks: breast cancer, gallbladder disease, venous thromboembolic events, coronary heart disease, stroke

- Side effects: vaginal bleeding, breast tenderness

Estrogen Agonists-Antagonists

Raloxifene (Evista) (60 mg/day orally)

- Additional potential benefits: reduced risk of breast cancer

- Potential risks: venous thromboembolic events

- Side effects: vasomotor symptoms, leg cramps

Other

Calcitonin (Miacalcin) (200 IU/day intranasally or 100 IU/day subcutaneously or intramuscularly)

- Additional potential benefits: none

- Potential risks: none

- Side effects: rhinitis, back pain

Forteo (Teriparatide) (20 μg/day subcutaneously)

- Additional potential benefits: none

- Potential risks: osteosarcoma (after long-term use in rodents), hypercalcemia

- Side effects: musculoskeletal pain

Prolia (Denosumab) (60 mg subcutaneously every 6 months)

- Additional potential benefits: none

- Potential risks: rash, serious infection, hypocalcemia

- Side effects: musculoskeletal pain

osteoporosis-related fractures by approximately 50% (39). **The Women's Health Initiative (WHI) trial confirmed a significant (34%) reduction in hip fractures in healthy women randomized to hormone therapy** (*conjugated estrogen* 0.625 mg per day) after a mean follow-up of 5.6 years (40). Combined with *calcium* and *vitamin D*, even very low-dose *estrogen* therapy (*conjugated estrogen* 0.3 mg per day; *transdermal estradiol* 0.014 mg per day) produces significant increases in bone mineral density compared with placebo (41).

Bisphosphonates, including *alendronate* (*Fosamax,* 35 or 70 mg orally weekly), *risedronate* (*Actonel,* 35 mg weekly or 150 mg orally monthly), *ibandronate* (*Boniva,* 150 mg orally monthly or 3 mg every 3 months intravenous), and *zoledronic acid* (*Zometa,* 5 mg intravenous yearly) specifically inhibit bone resorption and are very effective for both the

prevention and treatment of osteoporosis (42–44). Patients should take oral bisphosphonates on an empty stomach with a large glass of water and remain upright for at least 30 minutes. The major side effect is gastrointestinal distress; esophageal ulceration, osteonecrosis of the jaw, and atypical femoral fractures are very rare occurrences.

The estrogen agonist-antagonist *raloxifene (Evista,* 60 mg per day orally) prevents vertebral fractures in women with low bone mass and osteoporosis, though does not appear to reduce the risk of nonvertebral fractures (45). *Raloxifene* exercises estrogen-like actions on bone and lipids without stimulating the breast or endometrium. *Calcitonin* nasal spray (*Miacalcin,* 200 IU per day intranasal) is another approved treatment for established osteoporosis. Unlike most treatments for osteoporosis that inhibit bone resorption, parathyroid hormone (human recombinant PTH 1–34) (*teriparatide, Forteo,* 20 μg per day subcutaneously) stimulates new bone formation, resulting in significant reductions in vertebral and nonvertebral fractures (46). Recently approved for the treatment of postmenopausal osteoporosis, *denosumab (Prolia)* 60 mg, a monoclonal antibody to the receptor activator of nuclear factor-κB ligand, decreases the risk of vertebral and hip fractures in postmenopausal osteoporotic women when given subcutaneously twice yearly for 36 months' duration (47).

Cardiovascular Disease

Cardiovascular disease (CVD) is the leading cause of death for women, accounting for approximately 45% of mortality. Nonmodifiable risk factors include family history and age. Modifiable risk factors include a sedentary lifestyle, obesity, and smoking. Medical conditions associated with an increased risk of heart disease include diabetes, hypertension, and hyperlipidemia. Advising women to alter modifiable risk factors for CVD and adequately treating diabetes, hypertension, and hyperlipidemia are important parts of the comprehensive care of midlife women.

As epidemiologic studies identify an approximately 50% decrease in coronary heart disease (CHD) in woman who use hormone therapy, prevention of heart disease was considered a potential benefit of postmenopausal hormones (48). This observed reduction in CHD was considered secondary to beneficial effects of hormone therapy on the vascular wall and lipid levels (49). Observational studies are prone to bias, and women who used hormone therapy were generally healthier and at lower risk for CHD than nonusers (50).

The WHI randomized controlled trial of combination hormone therapy versus placebo showed that hormone therapy did not prevent heart disease in healthy women, but instead, it increased the risk of cardiovascular events in older women (51). The WHI was a 15-year study sponsored by the National Institutes of Health that examined ways to prevent heart disease, osteoporosis, and breast and colorectal cancer in women. There were several different studies in WHI, involving more than 160,000 healthy postmenopausal women. The WHI randomized controlled trial enrolled approximately 16,000 women nationwide between the ages of 50 and 79 years. The average age of women in the study was 63 years. The major goal of the WHI clinical trial was to determine whether combined *estrogen* and *progestin* hormone therapy prevented heart disease and to evaluate associated benefits and risks. **After an average of 5 years of follow-up,** risks (hazard ratio) were increased for CHD (1.3), breast cancer (1.3), stroke (1.4), and pulmonary embolism (PE) (2.1), and decreased for hip fracture (0.7) and colorectal cancer (0.6) (51). The absolute excess risk per 10,000 woman-years attributable to hormone therapy was small, with seven more CHD events, eight breast cancers, eight strokes, and eight pulmonary embolisms, with six fewer colorectal cancers and five fewer hip fractures.

Approximately 11,000 women without a uterus participated in a separate WHI study and were randomized either to *estrogen* alone or placebo. After an average follow-up of 7 years, there was no increased risk of heart disease or breast cancer in *estrogen* users. Outcomes were similar to those seen in the *estrogen* plus *progestin* arm of WHI with respect to venous thromboembolism, stroke, and osteoporotic fractures; there was no effect on colorectal cancer (52) (see Table 34.5 for a summary of WHI findings).

Studies confirmed that the increased risk of CHD in WHI occurs principally in older women and those who are a number of years beyond menopause (Table 34.6). In a secondary analysis of data from the combined WHI trials, no increased risk of CHD was seen in women between the ages 50 to 59 or in those within 10 years of menopause (53). Although stroke was increased with hormone therapy, regardless of age or years since menopause, the absolute excess risk of stroke in the younger women was minimal. **These data do not support a**

Table 34.5 Summary of Women's Health Initiative Study Results

Risks per 10,000 Woman-Years Attributable to Estrogen Plus Progestin [a]

Excess Risk	Additional Cases
Coronary heart disease	7
Stroke	8
Pulmonary embolism	8
Invasive breast cancer	8
Dementia (WHIMS) (subset older than age 65)	23
Reduced Risk	**Fewer Cases**
Hip fracture	5
Colorectal cancer	6

Risks per 10,000 Woman-Years Attributable to Estrogen Alone (Hysterectomized Women) [b]

Excess Risk	Additional Cases
Stroke	12
Deep venous thrombosis	6
Reduced Risk	**Fewer Cases**
Hip fracture	6
No Difference	
Coronary heart disease	
Invasive breast cancer	
Colorectal cancer	

WHIMS, Women's Health Initiative Memory Study.
[a]From **Writing Group for the Women's Health Initiative Investigators.** Risks and benefits of estrogen plus progestin in healthy postmenopausal women: principal results from the Women's Health Initiative randomized controlled trial. *JAMA* 2002;288:321–333; and **Shumaker S, Legault C, Rapp S, et al.** Estrogen plus progestin and the incidence of dementia and mild cognitive impairment in postmenopausal women. *JAMA* 2003;289:2651–2662.
[b]From **Women's Health Initiative Steering Committee.** Effects of conjugated equine estrogen in postmenopausal women with hysterectomy. *JAMA* 2004;291:1701–1712.

Table 34.6 Absolute Excess Risk of Coronary Heart Disease and Mortality

	Age (yr)			Years Since Menopause		
Outcome	50–59	60–69	70–79	<10	10–19	>20
Coronary heart disease	−2	−1	+19[a]	−6	+4	+17[a]
Total mortality	−10	−4	+16[a]	−7	−1	+14
Global index[b]	−4	+15	+43	+5	+20	+23

Absolute excess risk of coronary heart disease and mortality (cases per 10,000 woman-years) by age and years since menopause in the combined trials (*estrogen + progestin* and *estrogen* alone) of the WHI.
(**Rossouw J, Prentice R, Manson J, et al.** Postmenopausal hormone therapy and risk of cardiovascular disease by age and years since menopause. *JAMA* 2007;297:1465–1477).
[a]$P = .03$ compared with age 50–59 years or less than 10 years since menopause.
[b]Global index is a composite of coronary heart disease, stroke, pulmonary embolism, breast cancer, colorectal cancer, endometrial cancer, hip fracture, and mortality.
From **Martin K, Manson J.** Approach to the patient with menopausal symptoms. *J Clin Endocrinol Metab* 2008;93:4567–4575. Copyright 2008, The Endocrine Society.

role for hormone therapy in the prevention of heart disease, but they do provide reassurance regarding the safety of hormone therapy use for bothersome hot flashes and night sweats in otherwise healthy women at the time of the menopausal transition.

The WHI trials examined treatment only with conjugated equine *estrogens* and *medroxyprogesterone acetate*. The effects of other oral *estrogen* agents, transdermal *estradiol*, therapy with other *progestins*, or cyclic hormone therapy may be different. In observational studies, transdermal *estrogen* therapy is not associated with an increased risk of venous thromboembolic disease (54). The average age of women participating in these trials was more than 15 years beyond the age at which women typically initiate hormone therapy for the treatment of vasomotor symptoms. It is possible that early initiation of hormone therapy may result in a more favorable risk–benefit profile.

The effects of the estrogen agonist-antagonist *raloxifene* on CHD was studied in a multicenter, randomized trial of approximately 10,000 older postmenopausal women with heart disease or multiple risk factors. **Compared with placebo, *raloxifene* had no significant effect on death from any cause, coronary events, or total stroke, though risk of fatal stroke and venous thromboembolic disease was increased** (55). The risks of clinical vertebral fractures and invasive breast cancer were significantly reduced.

Breast Cancer

Breast cancer is a major health concern for menopausal women, as it is the most common cancer in women and the second leading cause of cancer death (56). The lifetime risk of invasive breast cancer for US women is 12%; therefore, any therapies that increase or reduce this risk will have a major impact on women's health. Risk factors for breast cancer include age, family history, early menarche, late menopause, and prior breast disease, including epithelial atypia and cancer. Risk is reduced in women who had bilateral oophorectomy or a term pregnancy before the age of 30. **Many of these risk factors are consistent with the hypothesis that prolonged *estrogen* exposure increases breast cancer risk.**

Long-term use of hormone therapy, generally defined as greater than 5 years, is associated with an increased risk of breast cancer (relative risk [RR] = 1.3) in observational studies (57). There is no increased risk of breast cancer in past users of hormone therapy. The results of several studies suggest that the risk of breast cancer associated with the use of *estrogen* alone may be lower, with a higher risk in users of *estrogen* plus *progestin* (58). **The WHI randomized controlled trial demonstrated a significant (26%) increase in the risk of invasive breast cancer after approximately 5 years of use of hormone therapy** (51). In women with a prior hysterectomy, there was no increased risk of breast cancer after an average of 7 years of use of *estrogen* alone (52).

Hormone therapy should not be prescribed to women with a history of breast cancer and should be used by women at high risk only after a very careful assessment of potential benefits and risks. A randomized trial of hormone therapy use in women with a history of breast cancer and bothersome hot flashes was stopped after only 2 years, as more new breast cancers were diagnosed in woman randomized to hormone therapy (59).

The *estrogen* agonist-antagonist *tamoxifen* (*Nolvadex*, 20 mg per day orally) is used in the treatment of estrogen-receptor positive breast cancer. Both *tamoxifen* and *raloxifene* reduce the risk of breast cancer in high-risk women by approximately 50% and are approved for this indication (60). **The risk of venous thromboembolism is increased approximately threefold with the use of *tamoxifen* and *raloxifene*, similar to the increase seen with hormone therapy.** *Tamoxifen* acts as an estrogen agonist in the endometrium, increasing the risk of endometrial polyps, hyperplasia, and cancer, whereas no endometrial stimulation is seen with *raloxifene*. **Performing a screening mammography examination annually for women older than age 50 years reduces breast cancer mortality.** Monthly breast self-examination is advised.

Alzheimer's Disease

Alzheimer's disease is the most common form of dementia. Women are at greater risk for developing the disease than men, and the number of affected individuals in the United States is estimated to be more than 5 million with an annual cost of 183 billion dollars. Although several small studies suggest that hormone therapy may decrease the risk of Alzheimer's disease, a randomized controlled study in women with mild to moderate Alzheimer's disease showed that

1 year of *estrogen* therapy neither slowed disease progression nor improved cognition (61). The WHI Memory Study (WHIMS) was a randomized placebo-controlled study of women aged 65 years or older enrolled in WHI, which assessed the effect of hormone therapy on cognitive function. In contrast to observational studies, **women in WHIMS randomized to hormone therapy experienced a significant twofold increased risk of dementia, most commonly Alzheimer's disease** (62). Hormone therapy use was associated with an adverse effect on cognition, as women randomized to hormone therapy scored significantly lower on the Modified Mini-Mental State Examination compared with placebo-treated women (63). Given the increased incidence of stroke identified in hormone therapy users in the WHI trial, it is possible that small, undetected cerebrovascular events were more likely to occur in the hormone therapy group, increasing the risk of dementia.

Hormone Therapy Use

For a healthy woman with bothersome hot flashes, hormone therapy remains a very reasonable option, especially if she is within 10 years of menopause or less than age 60. **Hormone therapy should be used at the lowest effective dose for the shortest duration consistent with treatment goals (64–66). The need for continued hormone therapy use should be assessed at least annually.**

The use of unopposed *estrogen* is associated with an increased risk of endometrial hyperplasia and cancer. Therefore, combination *estrogen-progestin* therapy is recommended for all women with a uterus. Treatment may be provided in a sequential manner, with *estrogen* daily and *progestin* for 12 to 14 days of each month, or in a continuous-combined fashion with *estrogen* and a lower dose of *progestin* daily. Sequential regimens result in regular, predictable vaginal bleeding. The majority of women using continuous-combined regimens will experience amenorrhea by the end of 1 year of therapy, but the bleeding that does occur is irregular and unpredictable. Low-dose combination hormone therapy products (e.g., *Prempro* 0.45/1.5 and 0.3/1.5 mg per day) generally result in a lower incidence of breakthrough bleeding and breast tenderness (67).

Women using low doses of oral or transdermal *estrogens* may elect intermittent *progestin* use (e.g., 14 days every 3 to 4 months) (68), although these are not approved regimens. **A *progestin*-containing intrauterine device approved for contraception in premenopausal women provides endometrial protection in *estrogen*-treated menopausal women, although it is not approved for this indication** (69). Increased endometrial surveillance is advised with these alternative regimens.

Transdermal administration of *estradiol* with a patch, spray, or gel may be preferred by some women. Avoiding the "first pass hepatic effect" of oral *estrogens* on lipids, binding globulins and clotting factors may have benefits for women on thyroid replacement or those with low libido (70). In contrast to oral administration, transdermal *estradiol* does not appear to increase the risk of venous thromboembolic events or gallbladder disease, though it remains contraindicated in women at high risk for venous thromboembolic disease or those with active liver or gallbladder disease.

Popularized by the media, many women are interested in using "bioidentical hormones" for treatment of menopausal symptoms. Bioidentical generally refers to hormones structurally identical to "natural" hormones made by the ovary, including estradiol and progesterone. FDA-approved oral and transdermal *estradiol* products are available in a wide range of doses, as is an oral form of micronized *progesterone* (*Prometrium*, 100 to 200 mg per day). *Progesterone* should be taken at bedtime, as it may cause drowsiness. **There is potentially significant increased risk and no known benefit to the use of custom-compounded bioidentical hormone therapy formulations, preparations that are "custom" mixed and packaged by a compounding pharmacist for an individual patient** (see Table 34.1 for approved hormone therapy formulations).

Contraindications to hormone therapy use include known or suspected breast or endometrial cancer, undiagnosed abnormal genital bleeding, cardiovascular disease (including coronary heart disease, cerebrovascular disease, and thromboembolic disorders), and active liver or gallbladder disease. Relative contraindications include high-risk states for the above disorders. These situations require a thoughtful assessment of potential risks and benefits and documentation of informed patient consent before treatment.

Sexual Dysfunction

Sexual problems are highly prevalent, reported in approximately 40% of US women, with 12% reporting a sexual problem associated with personal distress (71). Although sexual problems generally increase with aging, distressing sexual problems peak in midlife women (aged 45 to 64) and are lowest in women 65 years or older. The etiology of female sexual dysfunction is often multifactorial, including depression or anxiety, relationship conflict, stress, fatigue, prior abuse, medications, or physical problems that make sexual activity uncomfortable, such as endometriosis or atrophic vaginitis. The impact of the menopausal transition on sexual function was examined in a prospective, longitudinal cohort study of approximately 3,000 women who were pre- or perimenopausal at baseline and followed for 6 years. Pain during sexual intercourse increased and sexual desire decreased over the menopausal transition, but other factors were unaffected, including sexual arousal, frequency, and pleasure (72). In contrast to menopausal factors, which were unrelated to most aspects of sexual functioning, age, social, health, and psychological factors were strongly linked.

Treatment Options

Hormone Therapy

Estrogen therapy is very effective in treating vaginal dryness and dyspareunia; however, a significant effect of *estrogen* therapy on sexual interest, arousal, and orgasmic response, independent from its role in treating menopausal symptoms, is not supported by evidence. A woman with distressing low libido concurrent with the onset of bothersome night sweats, sleep disruption, and fatigue likely will experience increased sexual interest with effective treatment of her menopausal symptoms, but this is probably secondary to improved well-being, rather than a direct effect of *estrogen* therapy on libido. **A double-blind, randomized trial of combined oral and vaginal *estrogen* therapy in 285 sexually active postmenopausal women demonstrated decreased dyspareunia and significant improvements in pleasure of orgasm and sexual interest in women treated with *estrogen* therapy compared to placebo** (73). As this trial used a combination of systemic and vaginal *estrogens,* it is not possible to determine the relative impact of systemic versus local effects.

In contrast to *estrogen* therapy, *androgen* therapy is consistently shown to improve sexual function in selected populations of postmenopausal women (74–76). Potential risks of *androgen* therapy include hirsutism, acne, irreversible deepening of the voice, and adverse changes in liver function and lipids. As most *androgens* are aromatized to *estrogens,* there is potential for an increased risk of cardiovascular events or breast cancer. A transdermal *testosterone* patch is approved in Europe for the treatment of hypoactive sexual desire disorder in surgically post-menopausal women using concomitant *estrogen* therapy. An advisory panel of the FDA did not recommend approval in the United States pending additional data on long-term safety.

Alternatives to Hormone Therapy

Although vaginal atrophy and dyspareunia respond very well to *estrogen* therapy, most other sexual problems may be effectively treated without hormones. Relationship quality and conflict, stress, and fatigue predict sexual satisfaction, so couples often benefit from counseling, lifestyle changes, and prescribed "date nights." Women and their partners should be referred to sex therapists who provide education, materials, counseling, and instruction in specific exercises (77). In one study, 65% of 365 couples undergoing sex therapy for a range of sexual dysfunctions described their treatment as successful (78). Underlying depression and anxiety should be treated, and antidepressant medication may need adjustment. *Bupropion* may be an alternative to SSRIs, and one small, double-blind study reported increased sexual pleasure, arousal, and orgasm in nondepressed women with distressing low desire treated with *bupropion* (79). *Sildenafil citrate* may benefit women who develop problems with arousal and orgasmic response on SSRIs but generally is no more effective than placebo for most female sexual problems (80,81).

Despite the fact that sexual problems are common, the majority of women with distressing sexual problems do not seek formal care, but when they do, it is typically the woman, rather than the physician, who initiates the conversation (82,83). Clinicians should routinely ask their menopausal patients whether vaginal dryness, dyspareunia, or another bothersome sexual problem is present, as many effective interventions are available.

Summary

There are many options available to address the health and quality of life concerns of menopausal women. **The primary indication for hormone therapy is the alleviation of hot flashes and associated symptoms. Women must be informed of the potential risks and benefits of all therapeutic options. Care should be individualized based on a woman's medical history, needs, and preferences.**

References

1. **Adena M, Gallagher H.** Cigarette smoking and the age at menopause. *Ann Hum Biol* 1982;9:121–130.
2. **Siddle N, Sarrel P, Whitehead M.** The effect of hysterectomy on the age at ovarian failure: identification of a subgroup of women with premature loss of ovarian function and literature review. *Fertil Steril* 1987;47:94–100.
3. **de Vet A, Laven J, de Jong F, et al.** Antimullerian hormone serum levels: a putative marker for ovarian aging. *Fertil Steril* 2002;77:357–362.
4. **Soules M, Sherman S, Parrott E, et al.** Executive summary: stages of reproductive aging workshop (STRAW). *Fertil Steril* 2001;76:874–878.
5. **Schiff I, Regestein Q, Tulchinsky D, et al.** Effects of estrogens on sleep and psychological state of the hypogonadal woman. *JAMA* 1979;242:2405–2407.
6. **Freedman R, Subramanian M.** Effects of symptomatic status and the menstrual cycle on hot flash-related thermoregulatory parameters. *Menopause* 2005;12:156–159.
7. **Kronenberg F, Barnard RM.** Modulation of menopausal hot flashes by ambient temperature. *J Therm Biol* 1992;17:43–49.
8. **Gold E, Sternfeld B, Kelsey J, et al.** Relation of demographic and lifestyle factors to symptoms in a multi-racial/ethnic population of women 40–55 years of age. *Am J Epidemiol* 2000;152:463–473.
9. **Whiteman M, Staropoli C, Langenberg P, et al.** Smoking, body mass, and hot flashes in midlife women. *Obstet Gynecol* 2003;101:264–272.
10. **Kronenberg F, Fugh-Berman A.** Complementary and alternative medicine for menopausal symptoms: a review of randomized, controlled trials. *Ann Intern Med* 2002;137:805–813.
11. **Krebs E, Ensrud K, MacDonald R, et al.** Phytoestrogens for treatment of menopausal symptoms: a systematic review. *Obstet Gynecol* 2004;104:824–836.
12. **Newton K, Reed S, LaCroix A, et al.** Treatment of vasomotor symptoms of menopause with black cohosh, multibotanicals, soy, hormone therapy, or placebo. *Ann Intern Med* 2006;145:869–879.
13. **Barton D, Loprinzi C, Quella S, et al.** Prospective evaluation of vitamin E for hot flashes in breast cancer survivors. *J Clin Oncol* 1998;16:495–500.
14. **Avis N, Legault C, Coeytaux R, et al.** A randomized, controlled pilot study of acupuncture treatment for menopausal hot flashes. *Menopause* 2008;15:1070–1078.
15. **Utian WH, Shoupe D, Bachmann G, et al.** Relief of vasomotor symptoms and vaginal atrophy with lower doses of conjugated equine estrogens and medroxyprogesterone acetate. *Fertil Steril* 2001;75:1065–1078.
16. **Notelovitz M, Lenihan J, McDermott M, et al.** Initial 17B-estradiol dose for treating vasomotor symptoms. *Obstet Gynecol* 2000;95:726–731.
17. **Bachmann G, Schaefers M, Uddin A, et al.** Lowest effective transdermal 17b-estradiol dose for relief of hot flushes in postmenopausal women. *Obstet Gynecol* 2007;110:771–779.
18. **North American Menopause Society.** Treatment of menopause-associated vasomotor symptoms: position statement of the North American Menopause Society. *Menopause* 2004;11:11–33.
19. **Schiff I, Tulchinsky D, Cramer D, et al.** Oral medroxyprogesterone in the treatment of postmenopausal symptoms. *JAMA* 1980;244:1443–1445.
20. **Goodwin J, Green S, Moinpour C, et al.** Phase III randomized placebo-controlled trial of two doses of megestrol acetate as treatment for menopausal symptoms in women with breast cancer: Southwest Oncology Group Study 9626. *J Clin Oncol* 2008;26:1650–1656.
21. **Stearns V, Beebe K, Iyengar M, et al.** Paroxetine controlled release in the treatment of menopausal hot flashes. *JAMA* 2003:2827–2834.
22. **Loprinzi C, Kugler J, Sloan J, et al.** Venlafaxine in management of hot flashes in survivors of breast cancer: a randomised controlled trial. *Lancet* 2000;356:2059–2063.
23. **Suvanto-Luukkonen E, Koivunen R, Sundstrom H, et al.** Citalopram and fluoxetine in the treatment of postmenopausal symptoms: a prospective, randomized, 9-month, placebo-controlled, double-blind study. *Menopause* 2005;12:18–26.
24. **Guttuso T, Kurlan R, McDermott M, et al.** Gabapentin's effects on hot flashes in postmenopausal women: a randomized controlled trial. *Obstet Gynecol* 2003;101:337–345.
25. **Soares C, Joffe H, Rubens R, et al.** Eszopiclone in patients with insomnia during perimenopause and early postmenopause. *Obstet Gynecol* 2006;108:1402–1410.
26. **North American Menopause Society.** The role of local vaginal estrogen for treatment of vaginal atrophy in postmenopausal women: 2007 position statement of the North American Menopause Society. *Menopause* 2007;14:357–369.
27. **Handa VL, Bachus KE, Johnston WW, et al.** Vaginal administration of low-dose conjugated estrogens: systemic absorption and effects on the endometrium. *Obstet Gynecol* 1994;84:215–218.
28. **Henriksson L, Stjernquist M, Boquist L, et al.** A one-year multicenter study of efficacy and safety of a continuous, low-dose, estradiol-releasing vaginal ring (Estring) in postmenopausal women with symptoms and signs of urogenital aging. *Am J Obstet Gynecol* 1996;174:85–92.
29. **Weisberg E, Ayton R, Darling G, et al.** Endometrial and vaginal effects of low-dose estradiol delivered by vaginal ring or vaginal tablet. *Climacteric* 2005;8:83–92.
30. **Eriksen BC.** A randomized, open, parallel-group study on the preventive effect of an estradiol-releasing vaginal ring (Estring) on recurrent urinary tract infections in postmenopausal women. *Am J Obstet Gynecol* 1999;180:1072–1079.
31. **Hendrix S, Cochrane B, Nygaard I, et al.** Effects of estrogen with and without progestin on urinary incontinence. *JAMA* 2005;293:935–948.
32. **National Osteoporosis Foundation.** Fast facts on osteoporosis. www.nof.org.2010.
33. **National Osteoporosis Foundation.** Clinician's guide to prevention and treatment of osteoporosis. Washington, DC: National Osteoporosis Foundation, 2008.
34. **Chapuy MC, Arlot ME, Duboeuf F, et al.** Vitamin D_3 and calcium to prevent hip fractures in elderly women. *N Engl J Med* 1992;327:1637–1642.
35. **Bischoff-Ferrari H, Willett W, Wong J, et al.** Prevention of non-vertebral fractures with oral vitamin D and dose dependency: a meta-analysis of randomized controlled trials. *Arch Intern Med* 2009;169:551–561.
36. **Jackson R, LaCroix A, Gass M, et al.** Calcium plus vitamin D supplementation and the risk of fractures. *N Engl J Med* 2006;354:669–683.
37. World Health Organization Collaborating Centre for Metabolic Bone Diseases, University of Sheffield, UK. *Welcome to FRAX.* Available at http://www.sheffield.ac.uk/FRAX/. Accessed September 15, 2011.
38. **Watts N, Ettinger B, LeBoff M.** Perspective: FRAX facts. *J Bone Min Res* 2009;24:975–979.

39. **Cauley J, Zmuda J, Ensrud K, et al.** Timing of estrogen replacement therapy for optimal osteoporosis prevention. *J Clin Endocrinol Metab* 2001;86:5700–5705.

40. **Cauley J, Robbins J, Chen Z, et al.** Effects of estrogen plus progestin on risk of fracture and bone mineral density. *JAMA* 2003;290:1729.

41. **Ettinger B, Ensrud K, Wallace R, et al.** Effects of ultralow-dose transdermal estradiol on bone mineral density: a randomized clinical trial. *Obset Gynecol* 2004;104:443–451.

42. **Cummings S, Black D, Thompson D, et al.** Effect of alendronate on risk of fracture in women with low bone density but without vertebral fractures. *JAMA* 1998;280:2077–2082.

43. **Harris ST, Watts NB, Genant HK, et al.** Effects of risedronate treatment on vertebral and nonvertebral fractures in women with postmenopausal osteoporosis. *JAMA* 1999;282:1344–1352.

44. **Black D, Delmas P, Eastell R, et al.** Once-yearly zoledronic acid for treatment of postmenopausal osteoporosis. *N Engl J Med* 2007;356:1809–1822.

45. **MORE Investigators.** Reduction of vertebral fracture risk in postmenopausal women with osteoporosis treated with raloxifene. *JAMA* 1999;282:637–645.

46. **Neer R, Arnaud C, Zanchetta J, et al.** Effect of parathyroid hormone on fractures and bone mineral density in postmenopausal women with osteoporosis. *N Engl J Med* 2001;344:1434–1441.

47. **Cummings S, San Martin J, McClung M, et al.** Denosumab for prevention of fractures in postmenopausal women with osteoporosis. *N Engl J Med* 2009;361:756–765.

48. **Stampfer M, Colditz G, Willet W, et al.** Postmenopausal estrogen therapy and cardiovascular disease: ten-year follow-up from the Nurses' Health Study. *N Engl J Med* 1991;325:756–762.

49. **Writing Group for the PEPI Trial.** Effects of estrogen or estrogen/progestin regimens on heart disease risk factors in postmenopausal women. *JAMA* 1995;273:199–208.

50. **Barrett-Connor I.** Postmenopausal estrogen and prevention bias. *Ann Intern Med* 1991;115:455–456.

51. **Writing Group for the Women's Health Initiative Investigators.** Risks and benefits of estrogen plus progestin in healthy postmenopausal women: principal results from the Women's Health Initiative randomized controlled trial. *JAMA* 2002;288:321–333.

52. **Women's Health Initiative Steering Committee.** Effects of conjugated equine estrogen in postmenopausal women with hysterectomy. *JAMA* 2004;291:1701–1712.

53. **Rossouw J, Prentice R, Manson J, et al.** Postmenopausal hormone therapy and risk of cardiovascular disease by age and years since menopause. *JAMA* 2007;297:1465–1477.

54. **Canonico M, Oger E, Plu-Bureau G, et al.** Hormone therapy and venous thromboembolism among postmenopausal women: Impact of the route of estrogen administration and progestins. *Circulation* 2007;115:840–845.

55. **Barrett-Connor E, Mosca L, Collins P, et al.** Effects of raloxifene on cardiovascular events and breast cancer in postmenopausal women. *N Engl J Med* 2006;355:125–137.

56. **Parkin D, Pisani P, Ferlay J.** Global cancer statistics. *CA Cancer J Clin* 1999;49:33–64.

57. **Collaborative Group on Hormonal Factors in Breast Cancer.** Breast cancer and hormone replacement therapy. *Lancet* 1997;350:1047–1059.

58. **Schairer C, Lubin J, Troisi R, et al.** Menopausal estrogen and estrogen-progestin replacement therapy and breast cancer risk. *JAMA* 2000;283:485–491.

59. **Holmberg L, Anderson H.** HABITS, a randomised comparison: trial stopped. *Lancet* 2003;363:453–455.

60. **Vogel V, Costantino JP, Wickerham DL, et al.** Effects of tamoxifen vs. raloxifene on the risk of developing invasive breast cancer and other disease outcomes. *JAMA* 2006;295:2727–2741.

61. **Mulnard RA, Cotman CW, Kawas C, et al.** Estrogen replacement therapy for treatment of mild to moderate Alzheimer disease. *JAMA* 2000;283:1007–1015.

62. **Shumaker S, Legault C, Rapp S, et al.** Estrogen plus progestin and the incidence of dementia and mild cognitive impairment in postmenopausal women. *JAMA* 2003;289:2651–2662.

63. **Espeland MA, Rapp S, Shumaker S, et al.** Conjugated equine estrogens and global cognitive function in postmenopausal women: Women's Health Initiative Memory Study. *JAMA* 2004;291:2959–2968.

64. **North American Menopause Society.** Estrogen and progestogen use in postmenopausal women: 2010 position statement of the North American Menopause Society. *Menopause* 2010;17:242–255.

65. **American College of Obstetricians and Gynecologists.** Hormone therapy. *Obstet Gynecol* 2004;104(Suppl 4):S1–S129.

66. **Shifren J, Schiff I.** Role of hormone therapy in the management of menopause. *Obstet Gynecol* 2010;115:839–855.

67. **Archer D, Dorin M, Lewis V, et al.** Effects of lower doses of conjugated equine estrogens and medroxyprogesterone acetate on endometrial bleeding. *Fertil Steril* 2001;75:1080.

68. **Ettinger B, Selby J, Citron JT, et al.** Cyclic hormone replacement therapy using quarterly progestin. *Obstet Gynecol* 1994;83:693–700.

69. **Varila E, Wahlstrom T, Raura I.** A 5-year follow-up study on the use of a levonorgestrel intrauterine system in women receiving hormone replacement therapy. *Fertil Steril* 2001;76:969–973.

70. **Shifren J, Desindes S, McIlwain M, et al.** A randomized, open label, crossover study comparing the effects of transdermal vs. oral estrogen therapy on serum androgens, thyroid hormones, and adrenal hormones in naturally menopausal women. *Menopause* 2007;14:985–994.

71. **Shifren J, Monz B, Russo P, et al.** Sexual problems and distress in United States women: prevalence and correlates. *Obstet Gynecol* 2008;112:970–978.

72. **Avis N, Brockwell S, Randolph J, et al.** Longitudinal changes in sexual functioning as women transition through menopause: results from the Study of Women's Health Across the Nation. *Menopause* 2009;16:442–452.

73. **Gast M, Freedman M, Vieweg A, et al.** A randomized study of low-dose conjugated estrogens on sexual function and quality of life in postmenopausal women. *Menopause* 2009;16:247–526.

74. **Shifren J, Braunstein G, Simon J, et al.** Transdermal testosterone treatment in women with impaired sexual function after oophorectomy. *N Engl J Med* 2000;343:682–688.

75. **Shifren J, Davis S, Moreau M, et al.** Testosterone patch for the treatment of hypoactive sexual desire disorder in naturally menopausal women: results from the INTIMATE NM1 study. *Menopause* 2006;13:770–779.

76. **Davis S, Moreau M, Kroll R, et al.** Testosterone for low libido in postmenopausal women not taking estrogen. *N Engl J Med* 2008;359:2005–2017.

77. **Sarwer D, Durlak J.** A field trial of the effectiveness of behavioral treatment for sexual dysfunctions. *J Sex Marital Ther* 1997;23:87–97.

78. **American Association of Sexuality Educators, Counselors, and Therapists (AASECT).** *Homepage.* Available at http://www.aasect.org. Accessed September 15, 2011.

79. **Seagraves R, Clayton A, Croft H, et al.** Bupropion sustained release for the treatment of hypoactive sexual desire disorder in premenopausal women. *J Clin Psychopharmacol* 2004;24:339–342.

80. **Nurnberg H, Hensley P, Heiman J, et al.** Sildenafil treatment of women with antidepressant-associated sexual dysfunction: a randomized controlled trial. *JAMA* 2008;300:395–404.

81. **Basson R, McInnes R, Smith M, et al.** Efficacy and safety of sildenafil citrate in women with sexual dysfunction associated with female sexual arousal disorder. *J Womens Health Gend Based Med* 2002;11:367–377.

82. **Shifren J, Johannes C, Monz B, et al.** Help-seeking behavior of women with self-reported distressing sexual problems. *J Womens Health* 2009;18:461–468.

83. **Martin K, Manson J.** Approach to the patient with menopausal symptoms. *J Clin Endocrinol Metab* 2008;93:4567–4575.

GYNECOLOGIC ONCOLOGY

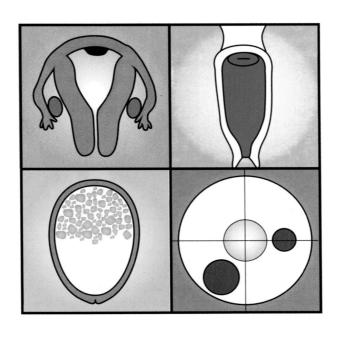

35

Uterine Cancer

Sean C. Dowdy
Andrea Mariani
John R. Lurain

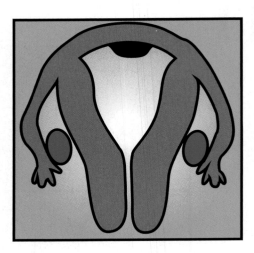

- Most risk factors for the development of endometrial carcinoma are related to prolonged, unopposed estrogen stimulation.

- Office endometrial aspiration biopsy is the accepted first step in evaluating a woman with abnormal uterine bleeding or suspected endometrial pathology.

- Serous and clear cell endometrial carcinomas make up less than 10% of endometrial cancers, yet account for more than one-half of all endometrial cancer deaths.

- Most patients with endometrial cancer should undergo surgical staging, including hysterectomy, bilateral salpingo-oophorectomy, pelvic and para-aortic lymphadenectomy, and peritoneal cytology. Lymphadenectomy may be omitted in patients with negligible risk of lymphatic spread.

- The most important adverse prognostic variables in endometrial cancer are advancing patient age, nonendometrioid or grade 3 histology, deep myometrial invasion, lymphovascular space invasion, large tumor size, cervical extension, lymph node metastasis, and intraperitoneal spread.

- Postoperative adjuvant radiotherapy in selected patients with endometrial cancer decreases the risk of local vaginal/pelvic recurrence and improves disease-free survival.

- Overall 5-year survival rate in endometrial cancer is approximately 75%.

- Uterine sarcomas are, in general, the most malignant group of uterine tumors and differ from endometrial cancers with regard to risk factors, diagnosis, clinical behavior, pattern of spread, and management.

Endometrial carcinoma is the most common malignancy of the female genital tract, accounting for almost one-half of all gynecologic cancers in the United States. In 2011, an estimated 46,470 new cases and 8,120 cancer-related deaths are anticipated. Endometrial carcinoma is the fourth most common cancer, ranking behind breast, lung, and colorectal cancers, and the eighth leading cause of death from malignancy in women. Overall, about 2% to 3% of women develop endometrial cancer during their lifetimes (1). Certain factors are increasing awareness of and emphasis on diagnosis and treatment of endometrial cancer. These factors include the declining incidence of cervical cancer-related deaths in the United States, prolonged life expectancy, postmenopausal use of hormone therapy, and earlier diagnosis. The availability of easily applied diagnostic tools and a clearer understanding of premalignant lesions of the endometrium led to an increase in the number of women diagnosed with endometrial cancer. Although endometrial carcinoma usually presents as early-stage disease and often is managed without radical surgery or radiotherapy, deaths from endometrial carcinoma now exceed those from cervical carcinoma in the United States. **Endometrial cancer is a disease that occurs primarily in postmenopausal women and is increasingly virulent with advancing age. The definite role of estrogen in the development of most endometrial cancers is established. Any factor that increases exposure to unopposed estrogen increases the risk for endometrial cancer.**

The histopathology, spread patterns, and clinicopathologic factors that affect the prognosis of endometrial cancers have become better defined. Management of endometrial cancer evolved from a program of preoperative intrauterine or external pelvic radiation followed by hysterectomy based on clinical staging, to an individualized approach using hysterectomy as primary therapy and employing additional postoperative treatment depending on surgical and pathologic findings. Further analysis and investigation are needed to determine whether this initial operative approach to treatment and staging, followed by targeted postoperative therapy, will translate into improved survival rates and lower morbidity.

Epidemiology and Risk Factors

There appear to be two pathogenetic types of endometrial cancer (2). Type I, accounting for about 75% to 85% of cases, occurs in younger, perimenopausal women with a history of exposure to unopposed estrogen, either endogenous or exogenous. In these women, tumors begin as hyperplastic endometrium and progress to carcinoma. These "estrogen-dependent" tumors tend to be better differentiated and have a more favorable prognosis than tumors that are not associated with hyperestrogenism. **Type II endometrial carcinoma occurs in women without estrogenic stimulation of the endometrium.** These spontaneously occurring cancers are not associated pathologically with endometrial hyperplasia, but may arise in a background of atrophic endometrium. They are less differentiated and associated with a poorer prognosis than estrogen-dependent tumors. These "estrogen-independent" tumors tend to occur in older, postmenopausal, thin women and are present disproportionately in AfricanAmerican and Asian women. Over the past decade, molecular genetic studies showed that these two tumor types evolve via distinct pathogenetic pathways (3) (see Type I and II Endometrial Carcinoma: Molecular Aberrations, below).

Several risk factors for the development of endometrial cancer are identified (4–9) (Table 35.1). **Most of these risk factors are related to prolonged, unopposed estrogen stimulation of the endometrium.** Nulliparous women have twoto threetimes the risk of parous women. Infertility and a history of irregular menses as a result of anovulatory cycles (prolonged exposure to estrogen

Table 35.1 Risk Factors for Endometrial Cancer	
Characteristic	*Relative Risk*
Nulliparity	2–3
Late menopause	2.4
Obesity	
21–50 lb overweight	3
>50 lb overweight	10
Diabetes mellitus	2.8
Unopposed *estrogen* therapy	4–8
Tamoxifen therapy	2–3
Atypical endometrial hyperplasia	8–29
Lynch II syndrome	20

without sufficient progesterone) increase risk. Natural menopause occurring after age 52 years increases the risk for endometrial cancer 2.4-fold compared with women who experienced menopause before 49 years of age, probably as a result of prolonged exposure of the uterus to progesterone-deficient menstrual cycles. **The risk of endometrial cancer is increased 3 times in women who are 21 to 50 pounds overweight and 10 times in those more than 50 pounds overweight** (resulting from excess estrone as a result of peripheral conversion of adrenallyderived androstenedione by aromatization in fat). The obesity epidemic in Western countries, together with growing rates of insulin resistance and "metabolic syndrome," can be expected to increase the incidence of endometrial cancer in coming years.

Other factors leading to long-term estrogen exposure, such as polycystic ovary syndrome and functioning ovarian tumors, also are associated with an increased risk for endometrial cancer. Menopausal *estrogen* therapy without *progestins* increases the risk of endometrial cancer fourto eighttimes. This risk increases with higher doses and with more prolonged use and can be reduced to essentially baseline levels by the addition of *progestin* (8). The use of the antiestrogen *tamoxifen* for treatment of breast cancer is associated with a two- to threefold increased risk for the development of endometrial cancer, although this finding is confounded by the apparent greater risk of endometrial cancer in women who have breast cancer, with or without treatment with *tamoxifen* (9,10). Diabetes mellitus increases a women's risk for endometrial cancer by 1.3 to 2.8 times. **Women with Lynch II syndrome (previously referred to as hereditary nonpolyposis colorectal cancer syndrome, or HNPCC), a cancer susceptibility syndrome with germline mutations in mismatch repair genes *MLH1, MSH2,* and *MSH6,* have a 40% to 60% lifetime risk for endometrial and colon cancer** (11). Other medical conditions, such as hypertension and hypothyroidism, are associated with endometrial cancer, but a causal relationship is not confirmed.

Endometrial Hyperplasia

Endometrial hyperplasia represents a spectrum of morphologic and biologic alterations of the endometrial glands and stroma, ranging from an exaggerated physiologic state to carcinoma *in situ.* **Clinically significant hyperplasias usually evolve within a background of proliferative endometrium as a result of protracted estrogen stimulation in the absence of progestin influence.** Endometrial hyperplasias are important clinically because they may cause abnormal bleeding, be associated with estrogen-producing ovarian tumors, result from hormonal therapy, and precede or occur simultaneously with endometrial cancer.

The classification scheme endorsed by the International Society of Gynecological Pathologists is based on architectural and cytologic features and long-term studies that reflect the natural history of the lesions (12) (Table 35.2). Architecturally, hyperplasias are either simple or complex; the major differing features are complexity and crowding of the glandular elements. **Simple hyperplasia** is characterized by dilated or cystic glands with round to slightly irregular shapes, an increased glandular-to-stromal ratio without glandular crowding, and no cytologic atypia. **Complex hyperplasia** has architecturally complex (budding and infolding) crowded glands, with less intervening stroma without atypia. **Atypical hyperplasia refers to cytologic atypia and can be categorized as simple or complex, depending on the corresponding glandular architecture.** Criteria for cytologic atypia include large nuclei of variable size and shape that have lost polarity, increased nuclear-to-cytoplasmic ratios, prominent nucleoli, and irregularly clumped chromatin with parachromatin clearing (Fig. 35.1).

Table 35.2 Classification of Endometrial Hyperplasias	
Type of Hyperplasia	*Progression to Cancer (%)*
Simple (cystic without atypia)	1
Complex (adenomatous without atypia)	3
Atypical	
Simple (cystic with atypia)	8
Complex (adenomatous with atypia)	29

From **Kurman RJ, Kaminski PF, Norris HJ.** The behavior of endometrial hyperplasia: a long term study of "untreated" hyperplasia in 170 patients. *Cancer* 1985;56:403–412, with permission.

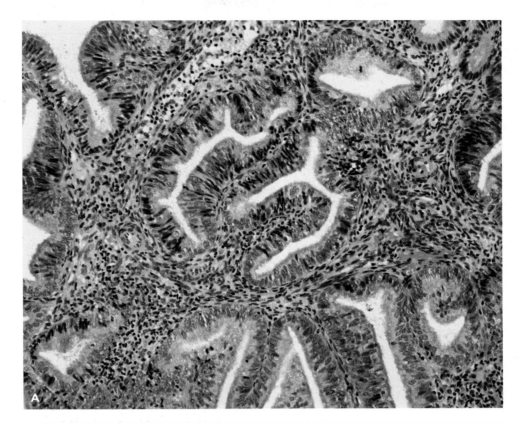

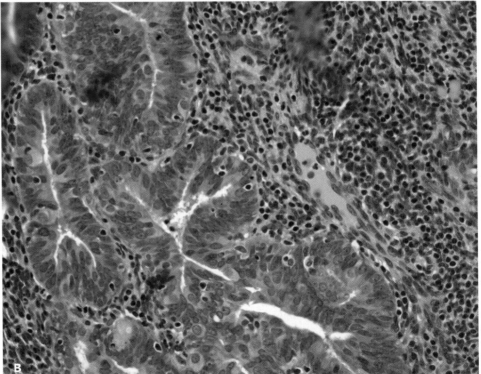

Figure 35.1 **Atypical hyperplasia (complex hyperplasia with severe nuclear atypia) of endometrium.** **A:** The proliferative endometrial glands reveal considerable crowding and papillary infoldings. The endometrial stroma, although markedly diminished, can still be recognized between the glands. **B:** Higher magnification demonstrates disorderly nuclear arrangement and nuclear enlargement and irregularity. Some contain small nucleoli. (Provided by Gordana Stevanovic, MD, and Jianyu Rao, MD, Department of Pathology, UCLA.)

The risk of endometrial hyperplasia progressing to carcinoma is related to the presence and severity of cytologic atypia. Kurman et al. retrospectively studied endometrial curettings from 170 patients with untreated endometrial hyperplasia followed a mean of 13.4 years (13). They found that **progression to carcinoma occurred in 1% of patients with simple hyperplasia, 3% of patients with complex hyperplasia, 8% of patients with atypical simple hyperplasia, and 29% of patients with atypical complex hyperplasia.** Most of the hyperplasias seemed to remain stable (18%) or regress (74%). The premalignant potential of hyperplasia is influenced by age, underlying ovarian disease, endocrinopathy, obesity, and exogenous hormone exposure (14,15).

As many as 25% to 43% of patients with atypical hyperplasia detected in an endometrial biopsy or curettage specimen will have an associated, usually well-differentiated, endometrial carcinoma detected during hysterectomy (16). Marked cytologic atypia, a high mitotic rate, and marked cellular stratification are features of atypical endometrial hyperplasia most often associated with the finding of an undiagnosed carcinoma at hysterectomy.

Fertility Sparing Treatment of Endometrial Hyperplasia and Cancer

Younger patients with endometrial cancer tend to have disorders such as polycystic ovarian syndrome, chronic anovulation, and infertility, indicative of exposure to intrinsic estrogen excess (17). Lesions in this age group are usually welldifferentiated and of endometrioid subtype with the potential to regress with progestational therapy (18). Althoughstandard treatment for all endometrial cancer is hysterectomy and staging, nonsurgical treatment with hormonal therapy may be an option for appropriately selected women desiring to preserve fertility. Surrogate staging techniques, such as magnetic resonance imaging (MRI), may be employed to evaluate the depth of myometrial invasion or identify extrauterine disease (19,20). The sensitivity of MRI to evaluate these factors is limited and has the potential for underdiagnosis (21).

High regression rates for both endometrial cancer and atypical hyperplasia following treatment with *progestin* therapy are extensively documented (18,22–28). However, relatively small cohorts of patients and reports of hormone failure suggest caution when counseling patients for conservative management (27,29). In a 2004 meta-analysis, Ramirez et al. reported a comprehensive review of hormonal treatment of grade 1endometrial cancer, including 27 articles with a combined total of 81 patients. A variety of progestational agents were utilized with an overall response rate of 76% (62/81) and the median time to regression was 12 weeks (30). The recurrence rate was 24% among responders; nearly all recurrences occurred within 1year of diagnosis. Only 1month of progestational treatment was required to achieve a response in the 76% of patients without recurrence. Twenty patients achieved pregnancy following treatment. It is important to note that 24% (19/81) of the original cohort never responded to treatment, and only 68% had any documented follow-up endometrial sampling. Progestational therapy can successfully treat disease while preserving fertility for patients with atypical hyperplasia and well-differentiated presumed stage I endometrial cancer. Appropriate patient selection and exclusion criteria remain undefined. Patients must be counseled that failure to identify recurrence or extension of disease during progestational treatment may lead to a delay in definitive surgery and ultimately a compromised prognosis (27).

Continuous *progestin* therapy with *megestrol acetate* (40–160 mg per day) is probably the most reliable treatment for reversing complex or atypical hyperplasia. No clear consensus exists for an optimal follow-up interval. Therapy should be continued for at least 2 to 3 months, and endometrial biopsy should be performed 3 to 4 weeks after completion of therapy to assess response. **Periodic endometrial biopsy or transvaginal ultrasonography is advisable in patients being monitored after progestin therapy for atypical hyperplasia because of the presence of undiagnosed cancer in 25% of cases, the 29% progression rate to cancer, and the high recurrence rate after treatment with progestins.** In this setting the use of progesterone should be considered a temporary, rather than long-term, treatment. **For women with atypical complex hyperplasia who no longer desire fertility, hysterectomy is recommended.**

Endometrial Cancer Screening in the General Population

Screening for endometrial cancer should not be undertaken because of the lack of an appropriate, cost-effective, and acceptable test that reduces mortality (31–33). **Routine Papanicolaou (Pap)** testing is inadequate, and endometrial cytologic assessment is too insensitive and nonspecific to be useful in screening for endometrial cancer, even in a high-risk population. A progesterone challenge test reveals whether the endometrium is primed by estrogen, but it does not identify abnormal endometrial pathology. Transvaginal ultrasonographic examination of the uterus and endometrial biopsy are too expensive to be employed as screening tests.

Although many risk factors for endometrial cancer have been identified, screening of high-risk individuals using current technologies could, at best, detect only one-half of all cases of endometrial cancer. Furthermore, no controlled trials were carried out to evaluate the effectiveness of screening for endometrial cancer. Screening for endometrial cancer or its precursors may be justified for certain high-risk women, such as those receiving postmenopausal *estrogen* therapy without *progestins* and members of families with hereditary nonpolyposis colorectal cancer (34). Women taking *tamoxifen* receive no benefit from routine screening with transvaginal ultrasonography or endometrial biopsy (35,36).

Most patients who have endometrial cancer present with abnormal perimenopausal or postmenopausal uterine bleeding early in the development of the disease, when the tumor is still confined to the uterus. Application of an appropriate and accurate diagnostic test in this situation usually results in early diagnosis, timely treatment, and a high cure rate. It is important to recognize that the workup of abnormal uterine bleeding should include endometrial biopsy even in premenopausal patients as 5% are in women under the age of 40.

Surveillance and Prevention in Patients at High Risk

Most endometrial carcinomas are sporadic, but about 10% of cases have a hereditary basis (37–41). Two genetic models were described in the development of familial endometrial cancer: HNPCC or Lynch II syndrome and a predisposition for endometrial cancer alone; both are inherited in an autosomal dominant fashion (42). The majority of studies focused on the increased incidence of endometrial cancer associated with Lynch II syndrome, a highly penetrant disorder (80% to 85%) (43). HNPCC or Lynch II syndrome is caused by an inherited mutation in one of the following mismatch repair genes: *hMSH2, hMLH1, PMS1, PMS2,* or *hMSH6* (44–47). The disorder is characterized by early age (average age younger than 45 years) at onset of neoplastic lesions in a variety of tissues, including the colon, uterus, stomach, ureters, ovaries, and skin (43,48,49). The lifetime risk of endometrial cancer in women with Lynch II syndrome is 32% to 60% and the lifetime risk of ovarian cancer is 10% to 12% (50,51). Interestingly, colorectal cancer is less prevalent in women with HNPCC or Lynch II syndrome than in men, whose risk approaches 100%. In a study of 1,763 patients from 50 HNPCC or Lynch II syndrome families in the Finnish Cancer Registry, the cumulative incidence of colorectal cancer in women was 54% by age 70, while the cumulative incidence of endometrial cancer was 60% (11). Although these data appear to support the use of endometrial cancer surveillance strategies for women with Lynch syndrome, a specific algorithm is not defined (50,52). No effective screening method exists for patients at increased risk for ovarian cancer.

In 2006, a European workshop of 21 experts in the treatment of hereditary gastrointestinal cancers from ninecountries (the Mallorca group) recommended the following endometrial cancer surveillance strategy for patients with HNPCC or Lynch II syndrome: annual pelvic examination, transvaginal ultrasound, and endometrial biopsy beginning at 30 to 35 years of age (53). These recommendations are by expert opinion only, and it is unknown whether these interventions are cost-effective or will impact mortality from endometrial or ovarian cancer in patients with Lynch II syndrome. An attractive alternative to early detection is prophylactic surgery after completion of childbearing (54,55). In 2006 a multi-institutional, matched case-control study found that prophylactic hysterectomy withbilateral salpingo-oophorectomy is an effective primary prevention strategy in women with Lynch II syndrome (51). No woman with hysterectomy and bilateral salpingo-oophorectomy developed endometrial, ovarian, or primary peritoneal carcinoma during the period of follow-up. In contrast, endometrial cancer developed in 33% and ovarian cancer in 5% of women who did not undergo prophylactic surgery (51).

There are rare reports of pedigrees in which family members are affected by endometrial cancer alone, and genetic studies have not found a germline mutation associated with site-specific endometrial cancer (42,56,57). A population-based study of endometrial cancer and familial risk in younger women (Cancer and Steroid Hormone, or CASH, Study Group) reported that a history of endometrial cancer in a first-degree relative increased the risk of endometrial cancer by nearly threefold (odds ratio of 2.8; 95% confidence interval [CI], 1.9–4.2) (58). A significant association was found with colorectal cancers, with an observed odds ratio of 1.9 (95% CI, 1.1–3.3). The presence of Lynch II syndrome families within the cohort may explain the latter association, but a family history of endometrial caner was an independent risk factor for endometrial cancer, after adjusting for age, obesity, and number of relatives (58).

Endometrial cancer and breast cancer share some of the same reproductive and hormonal risk factors such as nulliparity and exposure to unopposed estrogen (4,8,59–63). However, the familial association between breast and endometrial cancer is still uncertain and studies report conflicting results (63–67). For example, in the past it was thought that patients with *BRCA* mutations were at elevated risk for endometrial cancer, in addition to breast and ovarian cancer. A study suggests that this increase in risk is seen only in those patients with a personal history of breast cancer who are taking *tamoxifen* (68).

Endometrial Cancer

Clinical Features

Symptoms

Endometrial carcinoma most often occurs in women in the sixth and seventh decades of life, at an average age of 60 years; 75% of cases occur in women older than 50 years of age. **About 90% of women with endometrial carcinoma have vaginal bleeding or discharge as their only presenting symptom.** Most women recognize the importance of this symptom and seek medical consultation within 3 months. Some women experience pelvic pressure or discomfort indicative of uterine enlargement or extrauterine disease spread. Bleeding may not have occurred because of cervical stenosis, especially in older patients, and may be associated with hematometra or pyometra, causing a purulent vaginal discharge. This finding is often associated with a poor prognosis (69). **Less than 5% of women diagnosed with endometrial cancer are asymptomatic.** In the absence of symptoms, endometrial cancer usually is detected as the result of investigation of abnormal Pap test results, discovery of cancer in a uterus removed for some other reason, or evaluation of an abnormal finding on a pelvic ultrasonography examination or computed tomography (CT) scan obtained for an unrelated reason. Women who are found to have malignant cells on Pap test are more likely to have a more advanced stage of disease (70).

Abnormal perimenopausal and postmenopausal bleeding should always be taken seriously and be properly investigated, no matter how minimal or nonpersistent. Causes may be nongenital, genital extrauterine, or uterine (71). Nongenital tract sites should be considered based on the history or examination, including testing for blood in the urine and stool.

Invasive tumors of the cervix, vagina, and vulva are usually evident on examination, and any tumors discovered should be biopsied. Traumatic bleeding from an atrophic vagina may account for up to 15% of all causes of postmenopausal vaginal bleeding. This diagnosis can be considered if inspection reveals a thin, friable vaginal wall, but the possibility of a uterine source of bleeding must first be eliminated.

Possible uterine causes of perimenopausal or postmenopausal bleeding include endometrial atrophy, endometrial polyps, *estrogen* therapy, hyperplasia, and cancer or sarcoma (72–75) (Table 35.3). Uterine leiomyomas should never be accepted as a cause of postmenopausal bleeding. **Endometrial atrophy is the most common endometrial finding in women with postmenopausal bleeding, accounting for 60% to 80% of such bleeding.** Women with endometrial

Table 35.3 Causes of Postmenopausal Uterine Bleeding	
Cause of Bleeding	*Percentage*
Endometrial atrophy	60–80
Estrogen replacement therapy	15–25
Endometrial polyps	2–12
Endometrial hyperplasia	5–10
Endometrial cancer	10

atrophy usually were menopausal for about 10 years. **Endometrial biopsy often yields insufficient tissue or only blood and mucus, and usually bleeding ceases after biopsy.** Endometrial polyps account for 2% to 12% of postmenopausal bleeding. Polyps are often difficult to identify with office endometrial biopsy or curettage. Hysteroscopy, transvaginal ultrasonography, or both may be useful adjuncts in identifying endometrial polyps. Unrecognized and untreated polyps may be a source of continued or recurrent bleeding, leading eventually to unnecessary hysterectomy.

Estrogen therapy is an established risk factor for endometrial hyperplasia and cancer. **The risk for endometrial cancer is fourto eighttimes greater in postmenopausal women receiving unopposed *estrogen* therapy, and the risk increases with time and higher *estrogen* doses.** This risk can be decreased by the addition of a *progestin* to the *estrogen,* either cyclically or continuously. Endometrial biopsy should be performed as indicated to assess unscheduled bleeding or annually in women not taking a *progestin.* **Endometrial hyperplasia occurs in 5% to 10% of patients with postmenopausal uterine bleeding.** The sources of excess estrogen should be considered, including obesity, exogenous estrogen, or an estrogen-secreting ovarian tumor. **Only about 10% of patients with postmenopausal bleeding have endometrial cancer.**

Premenopausal women with endometrial cancer invariably have abnormal uterine bleeding, which is often characterized as menometrorrhagia or oligomenorrhea, or cyclical bleeding that continues past the usual age of menopause. The diagnosis of endometrial cancer must be considered in premenopausal women if abnormal bleeding is persistent or recurrent or if obesity or chronic anovulation is present.

Signs

Physical examination seldom reveals any evidence of endometrial carcinoma, although **obesity and hypertension are commonly associated constitutional factors.** Special attention should be given to the more common sites of metastasis. Peripheral lymph nodes and breasts should be assessed carefully. Abdominal examination is usually unremarkable, except in advanced cases in which ascites or hepatic or omental metastases may be palpable. On gynecologic examination, the vaginal introitus and suburethral area, and the entire vagina and cervix, should be carefully inspected and palpated. Bimanual rectovaginal examination should be performed specifically to evaluate the uterus for size and mobility, the adnexa for masses, the parametria for induration, and the cul-de-sac for nodularity.

Diagnosis

Office endometrial aspiration biopsy is the accepted first step in evaluating a patient with abnormal uterine bleeding or suspected endometrial pathology (76). The diagnostic accuracy of office-based endometrial biopsy is 90% to 98% when compared with subsequent findings at dilation and curettage (D&C) or hysterectomy (77–79).

The narrow plastic cannulas are relatively inexpensive, often can be used without a tenaculum, cause less uterine cramping (resulting in increased patient acceptance), and are successful in obtaining adequate tissue samples in more than 95% of cases. If cervical stenosis is encountered, a paracervical block can be performed, and the cervix can be dilated. Premedication with an antiprostaglandin agent can reduce uterine cramping. Complications following endometrial biopsy are exceedingly rare; uterine perforation occurs in only 1 to 2 cases per 1,000. Endocervical curettage may be performed at the time of endometrial biopsy if cervical pathology is suspected. **A Pap test is an unreliable diagnostic test because only 30% to 50% of patients with endometrial cancer have abnormal Pap test results** (80).

Hysteroscopy and D&C should be reserved for situations in which cervical stenosis or patient tolerance does not permit adequate evaluation by aspiration biopsy, bleeding recurs after a negative endometrial biopsy, or the specimen obtained is inadequate to explain the abnormal bleeding. Hysteroscopy is more accurate in identifying polyps and submucous myomas than endometrial biopsy or D&C alone (81–83).

Transvaginal ultrasonography may be a useful adjunct to endometrial biopsy for evaluating abnormal uterine bleeding and selecting patients for additional testing (84–87). Transvaginal ultrasonography, with or without endometrial fluid instillation (sonohysterography), may be helpful in distinguishing between patients with minimal endometrial tissue whose bleeding is related to perimenopausal anovulation or postmenopausal atrophy and patients with significant amounts of endometrial tissue or polyps who are in need of further evaluation. The finding of an endometrial thickness greater than 4 mm, a polypoid endometrial mass, or a collection of fluid

Table 35.4 Classification of Endometrial Carcinomas

Endometrioid adenocarcinoma
    Variants
    Villoglandular or papillary
    Secretory
    With squamous differentiation

Mucinous carcinoma
Papillary serous carcinoma
Clear cell carcinoma
Squamous carcinoma
Undifferentiated carcinoma
Mixed carcinoma

within the uterus requires further evaluation. Although most studies agree that an endometrial thickness of 5 mm or less in a postmenopausal woman is consistent with atrophy, more data are needed before ultrasonography findings can be considered to eliminate the need for endometrial biopsy in a patient with symptoms (88).

Pathology

The histologic classification of carcinoma arising in the endometrium is shown in Table 35.4 (12,89).

Endometrioid Adenocarcinoma

The endometrioid type of adenocarcinoma accounts for about 80% of endometrial carcinomas. These tumors are composed of glands that resemble normal endometrial glands; they have columnar cells with basally oriented nuclei, little or no intracytoplasmic mucin, and smooth intraluminal surfaces (Fig. 35.2). As tumors become less differentiated, they contain more solid areas, less glandular formation, and more cytologic atypia. The well-differentiated lesions may be difficult to separate from atypical hyperplasia.

Criteria that indicate the presence of invasion and are used to diagnose carcinoma are desmoplastic stroma, back-to-back glands without intervening stoma, extensive papillary pattern, and squamous epithelial differentiation. These changes, with the exception of the infiltrating pattern with desmoplastic reaction, require an area of involvement equal to or exceeding one-half of a low-power microscopic field (LPF) (>1 LPF; 4.2 mm in diameter) (90,91).

The differentiation of a carcinoma, expressed as its grade, is determined by architectural growth pattern and nuclear features (Table 35.5). **In the International Federation of Gynecology and Obstetrics (FIGO) grading system proposed in 1989, tumors are grouped into three grades:** *grade 1*, **5% or less of the tumor shows a solid growth pattern;** *grade 2*, **6% to 50% of the tumor shows a solid growth pattern; and** *grade 3*, **more than 50% of the tumor shows a solid growth pattern. The presence of notable nuclear atypia that is inappropriate for the architectural grade increases the tumor grade by one.**

Adenocarcinomas with squamous differentiation are graded according to the nuclear grade of the glandular component. This FIGO system is applicable to all endometrioid carcinomas, including its variants, and to mucinous carcinomas. In serous and clear cell carcinomas, nuclear grading takes precedence; however, most investigators believe that these two carcinomas should always be considered high-grade lesions, making grading unnecessary.

About 15% to 25% of endometrioid carcinomas have areas of squamous differentiation (Fig. 35.3). In the past, tumors with benign-appearing squamous areas were called *adenoacanthomas,* and tumors with malignant-looking squamous elements were called *adenosquamous carcinomas.* It is recommended that the term *endometrial carcinoma with squamous differentiation* be used to replace these two designations because the degree of differentiation of the squamous component parallels that of the glandular component, and the behavior of the tumor is largely dependent on the grade of the glandular component (92,93).

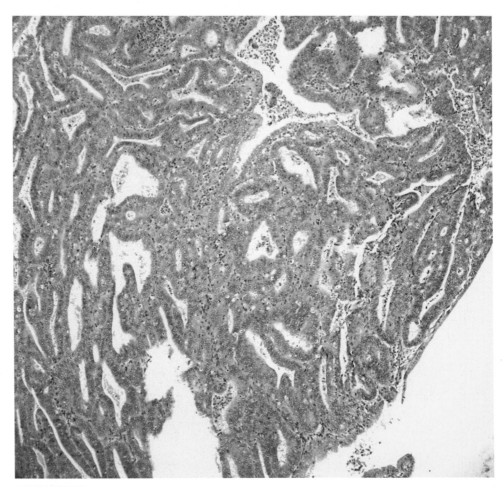

Figure 35.2 **Well-differentiated adenocarcinoma of endometrium.** The glands and complex papillae are in direct contact with no intervening endometrial stroma, the so-called back-to-back pattern. (Provided by Gordana Stevanovic, MD, and Jianyu Rao, MD, Department of Pathology, UCLA.)

Table 35.5 FIGO Definition for Grading of Endometrial Carcinoma

Histopathologic degree of differentiation:

G1 <5% nonsquamous or nonmorular growth pattern

G2   6%–50% nonsquamous or nonmorular growth pattern

G3 >50% nonsquamous or nonmorular growth pattern

Notes on pathologic grading:

Notable nuclear atypia, inappropriate for the architectural grade, raises a grade 1 (G1) or grade 2 (G2) tumor by one grade.

In serous adenocarcinoma, clear cell adenocarcinoma, and squamous cell carcinoma, nuclear grading takes precedence.

Adenocarcinomas with squamous differentiation are graded according to the nuclear grade of the glandular component.

FIGO Committee on Gynecologic Oncology. Revised FIGO staging for carcinoma of the vulva, cervix, and endometrium. *Int J Gynecol Obst* 2009;105:103–104.

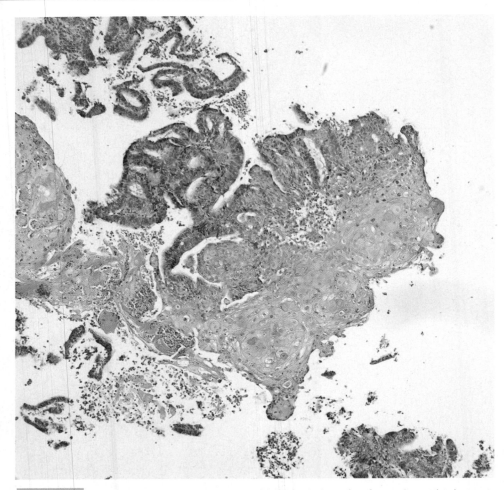

Figure 35.3 **Adenocarcinoma with squamous differentiation of endometrium.** This lesion is also classified as adenoacanthoma. Squamous cells with eosinophilic cytoplasm and distinct cell borders form solid clusters in the lumina of neoplastic glands. (Provided by Gordana Stevanovic, MD, and Jianyu Rao, MD, Department of Pathology, UCLA.)

A*villoglandular* **configuration is present in about 2% of endometrioid carcinomas** (94,95). In these tumors, the cells are arranged along fibrovascular stalks, giving a papillary appearance but maintaining the characteristics of endometrioid cells. The villoglandular variants of endometrioid carcinomas are always well-differentiated lesions that behave like the regular endometrioid carcinomas, and they should be distinguished from serous carcinomas. ***Secretory carcinoma* is a rare variant of endometrioid carcinoma that accounts for about 1% of cases** (96,97). It occurs mostly in women in their early postmenopausal years. The tumors are composed of well-differentiated glands with intracytoplasmic vacuoles similar to early secretory endometrium. These tumors behave as regular well-differentiated endometrioid carcinomas and have an excellent prognosis. Secretory carcinoma may be an endometrioid carcinoma that exhibits progestational changes, but a history of progestational therapy is rarely elicited. Secretory carcinoma must be differentiated from clear cell carcinoma because both tumors have predominately clear cells. These two tumors can be distinguished by their structure: secretory carcinomas have uniform glandular architecture, uniform cytology, and low nuclear grade, whereas clear cell carcinomas have more than one architectural pattern and a high nuclear grade.

Mucinous Carcinoma	**About 5% of endometrial carcinomas have a predominant mucinous pattern in which more than one-half of the tumor is composed of cells with intracytoplasmic mucin** (98,99). Most of these tumors have a well-differentiated glandular architecture; their behavior is similar to that of common endometrioid carcinomas, and the prognosis is good. It is important to recognize mucinous carcinoma of the endometrium as an entity and to differentiate it from endocervical

adenocarcinoma. Features that favor a primary endometrial carcinoma are the merging of the tumor with areas of normal endometrial tissue, presence of foamy endometrial stromal cells, presence of squamous metaplasia, or presence of areas of typical endometrioid carcinoma. Positive perinuclear immunohistochemical staining with vimentin suggests an endometrial origin (100).

Serous Carcinoma

About 3% to 4% of endometrial carcinomas resemble serous carcinoma of the ovary and fallopian tube (101–104). Most often, these tumors are composed of fibrovascular stalks lined by highly atypical cells with tufted stratification (Fig. 35.4). Psammoma bodies frequently are observed.

Serous carcinomas, **also referred to as** *uterine papillary serous carcinomas*, **are considered high-risk lesions.** The first description in 1982, noted that this entity usually occurred in elderly, hypoestrogenic women who presented with advanced-stage disease and accounted for up to one-half of deaths from endometrial carcinoma (101). Since then, several reports documented the aggressive nature and poor prognosis of serous carcinomas.

They are commonly admixed with other histologic patterns, but mixed tumors behave as aggressively as pure serous carcinomas. Even patients with a very small proportion of serous features (5%) remain at high risk of recurrence (105). Serous carcinomas are often associated with lymph–vascular space and deep myometrial invasion. The presence of lymph node metastases, positive

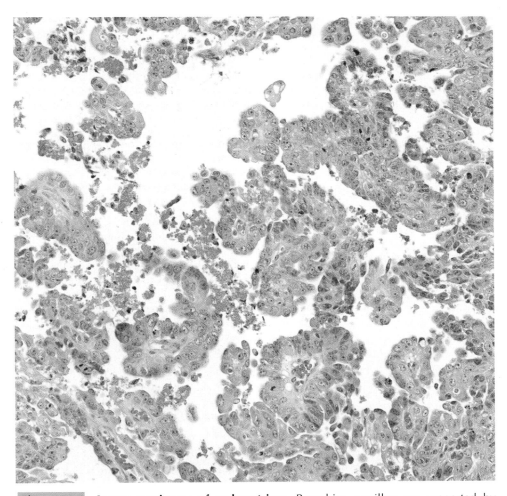

Figure 35.4   Serous carcinoma of endometrium. Branching papillae are supported by delicate fibrovascular cores and lined with columnar cells with moderate nuclear atypism, multiple nucleoli, and mitotic figures. (Provided by Gordana Stevanovic, MD, and Jianyu Rao, MD, Department of Pathology, UCLA.)

peritoneal cytology, and intraperitoneal tumor does not necessarily correlate with increasing myometrial invasion (104). **Even when these tumors appear to be confined to the endometrium or endometrial polyps without myometrial or vascular invasion, they behave more aggressively than endometrioid carcinomas and have a propensity to spread intraabdominally, simulating the behavior of ovarian carcinoma.** In one series, 37% of patients with serous carcinomas of the endometrium confined to a polyp demonstrated extrauterine disease when subjected to exploration and surgical staging (106).

A multi-institutional review of 206 patients with surgical stage I and II serous carcinomas demonstrated recurrence in 21% (105). Substage and treatment with platinum-based chemotherapy were associated with improved overall survival. Survival of surgically staged patients without myometrial invasion or extrauterine disease is between 89% and 100%, suggesting that observation may be appropriate in select patients, particularly in elderly patients with comorbidities (107). However, stage I patients, particularly those with myometrial invasion, remain at high risk of both peritoneal and vaginal recurrence. Therefore, platinum-based chemotherapy and vaginal brachytherapy should be considered in these patients (107–109).

Surgical treatment of advanced disease is no different from the endometrioid subtype, consisting of complete extirpation of visible disease (108). In one investigation from the Mayo Clinic, cytoreduction to microscopic residual was associated with a median overall survival of 51 versus 12 months for those patients with any residual (110). Postoperative treatment of advanced disease in the United States consists of chemotherapy and pelvic radiation, with or without para-aortic radiation. The Gynecologic Oncology Group study GOG184 included serous carcinomas and randomized patients to *carboplatin* and *paclitaxel* versus *cisplatin, doxorubicin (Adriamycin)*, and *paclitaxel* together with tumor volume–directed radiation (111). The former regimen demonstrated similar outcomes with less toxicity. Limited data suggest that delivering radiation "sandwiched" with chemotherapy improves progression-free and overall 3-year survival rates (112). Ongoing studies are evaluating the role of chemotherapy alone for these tumors, especially because of the high rate of peritoneal dissemination and recurrences. It remains unknown whether radiation improves survival in addition to chemotherapy alone. For elderly patients with multiple comorbidities who cannot tolerate multimodal therapy, chemotherapy alone.

Clear Cell Carcinoma

Clear cell carcinoma accounts for less than 5% of all endometrial carcinomas (96,113,114). Clear cell carcinoma usually has a mixed histologic pattern, including papillary, tubulocystic, glandular, and solid types. The cells have highly atypical nuclei and abundant clear or eosinophilic cytoplasm. Often, the cells have a hobnail configuration arranged in papillae with hyalinized stalks (Fig. 35.5).

Clear cell carcinoma characteristically occurs in older women and like serous carcinoma is considered a poor prognosticator. Traditionally clear cell carcinoma was associated with very poor outcomes with overall survival rates varying from 33% to 64%. A multi-institutional review of 99 patients with uterine clear cell carcinoma documented only 1 recurrence (vaginal) in the 22 patients without extrauterine disease subjected to thorough surgical staging (115). Considering all 49 patients with stage I or II disease (regardless of the extent of staging), only 1 hematologic failure was noted. These data argue against the use of systemic therapy in patients with clear cell carcinoma limited to the pelvis, while the 10% vaginal cuff failure suggests that vaginal brachytherapy alone may be sufficient treatment. In contrast, others argued for systemic treatment of patients with stage I disease (116).

Complete surgical staging is important because 52% of patients with clinical stage I clear cell carcinoma have metastatic disease. Patients who undergo a complete cytoreduction appear to have improved progression-free and overall survivals compared to women left with residual disease following surgery (115). Postoperative therapy for patients with advanced disease is platinum-based (116).

Squamous Carcinoma

Squamous carcinoma of the endometrium is rare. Some tumors are pure, but most have a few glands. To establish primary origin within the endometrium, there must be no connection with or spread from cervical squamous epithelium. Squamous carcinoma often is associated with cervical stenosis, chronic inflammation, and pyometra at the time of diagnosis. This tumor has a poor prognosis, with an estimated 36% survival rate in patients with clinical stage I disease (117).

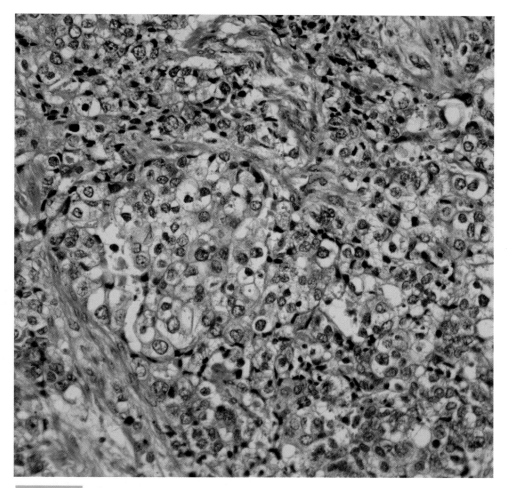

Figure 35.5   **Clear cell adenocarcinoma of the endometrium.** Back-to-back glands lined by polygonal to columnar cells with distinct cell membrane, abundant granular to clear cytoplasm, and variably sized nuclei (including binucleated and multinucleated forms) with prominent nucleoli (magnification X400). (Provided by Gordana Stevanovic, MD, and Jianyu Rao, MD, Department of Pathology, UCLA.)

Simultaneous Tumors of the Endometrium and Ovary

Synchronous endometrial and ovarian cancers are the most frequent simultaneously occurring genital malignancies, with a reported incidence of 1.4% to 3.8% (118–122). Most commonly, both the ovarian and endometrial tumor are well-differentiated endometrioid adenocarcinomas of low stage, resulting in an excellent prognosis. Patients often are premenopausal and present with abnormal uterine bleeding. The ovarian cancer usually is discovered as an incidental finding and is diagnosed at an earlier stage because of the symptomatic endometrial tumor, leading to a more favorable outcome. Up to 29% of patients with endometrioid ovarian adenocarcinomas have associated endometrial cancer. If more poorly differentiated, nonendometrioid histologic subtypes are present or if the uterine and ovarian tumors are histologically dissimilar, the prognosis is less favorable. Immunohistochemical studies, flow cytometry, and assessment of molecular DNA patterns to detect loss of heterozygosity may be helpful in distinguishing between metastatic and independent tumors, but the differential diagnosis can usually be determined by conventional clinical and pathologic criteria.

Pretreatment Evaluation

After establishing the diagnosis of endometrial carcinoma, the next step is to evaluate the patient thoroughly to determine the best and safest approach to management of the disease. A complete history and physical examination areof utmost importance. Patients with endometrial carcinoma are often elderly and obese with a variety of medical problems, such as diabetes mellitus and hypertension, which complicate surgical management. Any abnormal symptoms, such as bladder or intestinal symptoms, should be evaluated.

On physical examination, attention should be directed to enlarged or suspicious lymph nodes, including the inguinal area, abdominal masses, and possible areas of cancer spread within the pelvis. Evidence of distant metastasis or locally advanced disease in the pelvis, such as gross cervical involvement or parametrial spread, may alter the treatment approach.

Chest radiography should be performed to exclude pulmonary metastasis and to evaluate the cardiorespiratory status of the patient. Other routine preoperative studies should include electrocardiography, complete blood and platelet counts, serum chemistries (including renal and liver function tests), and blood type and screen. Other preoperative or staging studies are neither required nor necessary for most patients with endometrial cancer. Studies such as cystoscopy, colonoscopy, intravenous pyelography, and barium enema are not indicated unless dictated by patient symptoms, physical findings, or other laboratory tests (123). CT scanning of the abdomen and pelvis may be considered in patients with type II uterine cancer to determine if minimally invasive surgery is appropriate. Stage IV disease is usually clinically evident based on patient symptomatology and clinical examination. Ultrasonography and MRI can be used to assess myometrial invasion preoperatively with a fairly high degree of accuracy (124). This information may be of use in planning the surgical procedure with regard to whether lymph node sampling should be undertaken.

Serum CA125, an antigenic determinant that is elevated in 80% of patients with advanced epithelial ovarian cancers, is elevated in most patients with advanced or metastatic endometrial cancer (125). In one study, 23 of 81 patients with apparently localized disease preoperatively had elevated CA125 levels. At surgery, 20 (87%) of these 23 patients with an elevated CA125 were found to have extrauterine disease, whereas only 1 of 58 patients with a normal CA125 had disease spread outside the uterus (126). Another study found that 78% of endometrial cancer patients with lymph node metastases had an elevated preoperative CA125 level (127). Preoperative measurement of serum CA125 may help determine the extent of surgical staging and, if elevated, may be useful as a tumor marker in assessing response to subsequent therapy (128,129).

Clinical Staging

Clinical staging, according to the 1971 FIGO system, should be performed only in patients who are deemed not to be surgical candidates because of their poor medical condition or the degree of disease spread (130). The current FIGO staging is surgical, as discussed below, which has supplanted the old clinical system. With improvements in preoperative and postoperative care, anesthesia administration, and surgical techniques, almost all patients are medically suitable for operative therapy. One study reported an operability rate of 87% in a series of 595 consecutive patients with clinical early-stage endometrial cancer (131). A small percentage of patients will not be candidates for surgical staging because of gross cervical involvement, parametrial spread, invasion of the bladder or rectum, or distant metastasis.

Surgical Staging

Widely accepted management of endometrial cancer consists of hysterectomy, removal of remaining adnexal structures, and appropriate surgical staging in patients considered at risk for extrauterine disease (132–134). Surgical staging was recommended for patients with endometrial cancer since 1988 (134). In spite of this general recommendation, the incorporation of a systematic pelvic and para-aortic lymphadenectomy in all patients is not universally accepted (135–137). This recommendation became more controversial after the publication of two large prospective randomized trials that failed to demonstrate improved outcomes for patients who underwent pelvic lymphadenectomy (138,139). These two studies show differences in their design: in the ASTEC trial all women with clinical stage I were included without exclusion criteria, whereas the Italian study excluded women with stage IA and IB grade 1 tumors, and nonendometrioid malignancies. In the Italian study, systematic nodal dissection was performed, as opposed to pelvic node sampling in the ASTEC trial (median number of lymph nodes harvested 30 vs. 12, respectively). The studies share characteristics that could lead to misinterpretation of their results. The percentage of nodal positivity is low in both studies (13% and 9%), suggesting that regardless of differences in exclusion criteria, low-risk cases were included in both studies, thus diluting possible (if any) therapeutic benefit of lymphadenectomy. Another important limitation is that nodal dissection was limited to the pelvis without any recommendation for para-aortic lymphadenectomy. It was demonstrated previously that radiotherapy limited to the pelvis does not improve survival (136). It is not surprising that pelvic lymphadenectomy alone has no therapeutic impact, considering that 67% of patients with nodal involvement have para-aortic lymph node metastases and 16% of patients with documented lymphatic dissemination have isolated para-aortic metastases (140). Neither study used the information derived from lymphadenectomy to target postoperative treatment (i.e., to spare patients with negative nodes from radiotherapy or to target postoperative treatment to the metastatic areas), thus eliminating one of the potential benefits of this surgical procedure.

Systematic pelvic and para-aortic lymphadenectomy remains one of the most important steps to assess the presence of extrauterine disease and to guide targeted postoperative treatment. GOG33 demonstrated that patients with absent or superficial myometrial invasion have a low probability of lymphatic metastases (141). Furthermore, Mariani et al. demonstrated that no patient with endometrioid grade 1 or 2 disease and superficial myometrial invasion harbored a lymphatic metastasis when the tumor diameter was 2 cm or less (137). The importance of tumor size as a predictor for lymphatic spread was reported by Schink et al. (142). It is possible to identify a group of patients in whom lymphadenectomy is likely to increase the risk of surgical complications without producing any concrete benefits. Tumor diameter, along with myometrial invasion and histologic grade and subtype, can be utilized to determine whether or not lymphadenectomy is appropriate.

An observational study reported a significant survival benefit of para-aortic lymphadenectomy in patients at intermediate or high risk of recurrence (based on presence of histologic grade 3 or deep myometrial invasion, or lymphovascular invasion, or evidence of spread outside of the uterine corpus), compared to patients who had hysterectomy with pelvic lymphadenectomy but without para-aortic dissection. This benefit was not observed in patients with low-risk endometrial cancer (143). In addition, the Postoperative Radiation Therapy in Endometrial Carcinoma (PORTEC) studies identified patients with stage IC, grade 3 endometrial carcinoma as being at high risk of early distant spread and death when treated with hysterectomy only (no staging), followed by pelvic external-beam radiation therapy. These patients had a 31% risk of distant recurrence (136). From the literature, it seems that the patients who have the potential to benefit from surgical staging are those with risk factors such as histologic grade 3, deep myometrial invasion, or lymphovascular invasion.

In summary, surgical staging should (i) identify patients with disseminated disease who are at high risk of recurrence; (ii) target postoperative treatment; (iii) reduce the number of patients potentially requiring postoperative treatment when the provided information is used appropriately (avoiding the risk of morbidity without reasonable benefit); and (iv) possibly eradicate lymphatic disease. In spite of these potential benefits in high-risk patients, prospective randomized data demonstrating a survival advantage or reduction in overall morbidity resulting from a potential reduction of adjuvant treatment still are not available.

The FIGO published the updated surgical staging system for endometrial cancer (Table 35.6) (144). In comparison with recommendations from 1988, the new system introduces the following

Table 35.6 Carcinoma of the Endometrium (2008)	
Stage I*	Tumor confined to the corpus uteri
IA	No or less than half myometrial invasion
IB	Invasion equal to or more than half of the myometrium
Stage II*	Tumor invades cervical stroma, but does not extend beyond the uterus**
Stage III*	Local and/or regional spread of the tumor
IIIA	Tumor invades the serosa of the corpus uteri and/or adnexae#
IIIB	Vaginal and/or parametrial involvement#
IIIC	Metastases to pelvic and/or para-aortic lymph nodes#
IIIC1	Positive pelvic nodes
IIIC2	Positive para-aortic lymph nodes with or without positive pelvic lymph nodes
Stage IV*	Tumor invades bladder and/or bowel mucosa, and/or distant metastases
IVA	Tumor invasion of bladder and/or bowel mucosa
IVB	Distant metastases, including intra-abdominal metastases and/or inguinal lymph nodes

FIGO Committee on Gynecologic Oncology. Revised FIGO staging for carcinoma of the vulva, cervix, and endometrium. *Int J Gynecol Obst* 2009;105:103–104.
*Either G_1, G_2, or G_3.
**Endocervical glandular involvement only should be considered as Stage I and no longer as Stage II.
#Positive cytology has to be reported separately without changing the stage.

changes: (i) former stages IA and IB are combined; (ii) former stage IIA was eliminated so that only the presence of cervical stroma involvement is considered stage II disease; (iii) alone, peritoneal cytologic findings positive for endometrial cancer are no longer a criterion for disease upstaging (although FIGO still recommends the collection of peritoneal washing, recognizing the predictive value of positive cytologic findings when combined with other poor-prognosis factors); and (iv) stage IIIC was divided into IIIC1 and IIIC2 in accordance with the absence or presence of positive para-aortic nodes. The presence of parametrial disease is now formally recognized as stage IIIB disease.

Prognostic Variables

Although disease stage is the most significant variable affecting survival, a number of other individual prognostic factors for disease recurrence or survival are known, including tumor grade, histopathology, depth of myometrial invasion, patient age, and surgical–pathologic evidence of extrauterine disease spread (Tables 35.7 and 35.8). Other factors, such as **tumor size, peritoneal cytology, hormone receptor status, flow cytometric analysis, and oncogene perturbations, are implicated as having prognostic importance.**

Age

In general, younger women with endometrial cancer have a better prognosis than older women. Two reports observed no deaths related to disease in patients with endometrial cancer diagnosed before 50 years of age (145,146). Another series demonstrated a 60.9% 5-year survival rate for patients older than 70 years of age, compared with 92.1% survival rate for patients younger than 50 years of age (147). Decreased survival was associated with an increased risk for extrauterine spread (38% vs. 21%) and deep myometrial invasion (57% vs. 24%) for these two groups. The GOG reported 5-year survival rates of 96.3% for patients 50 years of age or younger, 87.3% for patients 51 to 60 years, 78% for patients 61 to 70 years, 70.7% for patients 71 to 80 years, and 53.6% for patients older than 80 years (148).

Increased risk for recurrence in older patients was related to a higher incidence of grade 3 tumors or unfavorable histologic subtypes; however, age appears to be an independent

Table 35.7 Surgical-Pathologic Findings in Clinical Stage I Endometrial Cancer

Surgical-Pathologic Finding	Percentage of Patients
Histology	
Adenocarcinoma	80
Adenosquamous	16
Other (papillary serous, clear cell)	4
Grade	
1	29
2	46
3	25
Myometrial invasion	
None	14
Inner third	45
Middle third	19
Outer third	22
Lymph–vascular space invasion	15
Isthmic tumor	16
Adnexal involvement	5
Positive peritoneal cytology	12
Pelvic lymph node metastasis	9
Aortic lymph node metastasis	6
Other extrauterine metastasis	6

Modified from **Creasman WT, Morrow CP, Bundy BN, et al.** Surgical pathologic spread patterns of endometrial cancer. *Cancer* 1987;60:2035–2041, with permission.

Table 35.8 Prognostic Variables in Endometrial Carcinoma
Age
Histologic type
Histologic grade
Myometrial invasion
Lymph–vascular space invasion
Isthmus–cervix extension
Adnexal involvement
Lymph node metastasis
Intraperitoneal tumor
Tumor size
Peritoneal cytology
Hormone receptor status
DNA ploidy/proliferative index
Genetic/molecular tumor markers

prognostic variable. Increasing patient age appears to be independently associated with disease recurrence in endometrial cancer. In one study, the mean age at diagnosis of patients who had recurrence or died of disease was 68.6 years, compared with 60.3 years for patients without recurrence. For every 1 year increase in age, the estimated rate of recurrence increased 7%. None of the patients younger than 50 years of age developed recurrent cancer, compared with 12% of patients aged 50 to 75 years and 33% of patients older than 75 years (149).

Histologic Type

Nonendometrioid histologic subtypes account for about 10% of endometrial cancers and carry an increased risk for recurrence and distant spread (150,151). In a retrospective review of 388 patients treated at the Mayo Clinic for endometrial cancer, 52 (13%) had an uncommon histologic subtype, including 20 adenosquamous, 14 serous, 11 clear cell, and 7 undifferentiated carcinomas. In contrast to the 92% survival rate among patients with endometrioid tumors, the overall survival for patients with one of these more aggressive subtypes was only 33%. At the time of surgical staging, 62% of the patients with an unfavorable histologic subtype had extrauterine spread of disease (150).

Histologic Grade

Histologic grade of the endometrial tumor is strongly associated with prognosis (132,141,149,152–156). In one study, recurrences developed in 7.7% of grade 1 tumors, 10.5% of grade 2 tumors, and 36.1% of grade 3 tumors. Patients with grade 3 tumors were in excess of fivetimes more likely to have a recurrence than were patients with grades 1 and 2 tumors. The 5-year disease-free survival rates for patients with grades 1 and 2 tumors were 92% and 86%, respectively, compared with 64% for patients with grade 3 tumors (149). Another study reported similar results, noting recurrences in 9% of patients with grades 1 and 2 tumors compared with 39% of patients with grade 3 lesions (153). Increasing tumor anaplasia is associated with deep myometrial invasion, cervical extension, lymph node metastasis, and both local recurrence and distant metastasis.

Tumor Size

Tumor size is a significant prognostic factor for lymph node metastasis and survival in patients with endometrial cancer (142,157). One report determined tumor size in 142 patients with clinical stage I endometrial cancer and found lymph node metastasis in 4% of patients with tumors 2 cm or smaller, in 15% of patients with tumors larger than 2 cm, and in 35% of patients with tumors involving the entire uterine cavity (156). Tumor size better defined an intermediate-risk group for lymph nodes metastasis (i.e., patients with grade 2 tumors with less than 50% myometrial invasion). Overall, these patients had a 10% risk for lymph node metastasis, but there was no nodal metastasis associated with tumors 2 cm or smaller, compared with 18% when tumors were larger than 2 cm. Five-year survival rates were 98% for patients with tumors 2 cm or smaller, 84% for patients with tumors larger than 2 cm, and 64% for patients with tumors involving the whole uterine cavity (137,157).

Hormone Receptor Status

Estrogen receptor and progesterone receptor levels are prognostic indicators for endometrial cancer independent of grade in several studies (158–164). Patients whose tumors are positive for one or both receptors have longer survival times than patients whose carcinomas lack the corresponding receptors. Even patients with metastasis have an improved prognosis with receptor-positive tumors (161). Progesterone receptor levels appear to be stronger predictors of survival than estrogen receptor levels, and the higher the absolute level of the receptors, the better the prognosis.

DNA Ploidy and Proliferative Index

About two-thirds of endometrial adenocarcinomas have a diploid DNA content as determined by flow cytometric analysis (162,165–174). **The proportion of nondiploid tumors increases with stage, lack of tumor differentiation, and depth of myometrial invasion.** In several studies, DNA content was related to clinical course of the disease, with death rates reported to be higher in women whose tumors contained aneuploid populations of cells. The proliferative index is related to prognosis.

Myometrial Invasion

Because access to the lymphatic system increases as cancer invades into the outer one-half of the myometrium, increasing depth of invasion is associated with increasing likelihood of extrauterine spread and recurrence (153,155,175). The association of depth of myometrial invasion with extrauterine disease and lymph node metastases was reported (175). Of patients without demonstrable myometrial invasion, only 1% had pelvic lymph node metastasis, compared with patients with outer one-third myometrial invasion who had 25% pelvic and 17% aortic lymph node metastases. Deep myometrial invasion (>50% for all stages; ≥66% for stage I) is the strongest predictor of hematogenous recurrence (176). Survival decreases with increasing depth of myometrial invasion. In general, patients with noninvasive or superficially invasive tumors have an 80% to 90% 5-year survival rate, whereas those with deeply invasive tumors have a 60% survival rate. The most sensitive indicator of the effect of myometrial invasion on survival is distance from the tumor–myometrial junction to the uterine serosa. Patients with tumors that are less than 5 mm from the serosal surface are at much higher risk for recurrence and death than those with tumors greater than 5 mm from the serosal surface (177,178).

Lymph–Vascular Space Invasion

Lymph–vascular space invasion (LVSI) appears to be an independent risk factor for recurrence and death from all types of endometrial cancer (178–181). The overall incidence of LVSI in early endometrial cancer is about 15%, although it increases with increasing tumor grade and depth of myometrial invasion. One study reported LVSI in 2% of grade 1 tumors and 5% of superficially invasive tumors, compared with 42% of grade 3 tumors and 70% of deeply invasive tumors (180). LVSI was demonstrated to be a strong predictor of lymphatic dissemination and lymphatic recurrence (182). Another study reported deaths in 26.7% of patients with clinical stage I disease who had LVSI, compared with 9.1% of those without LVSI (183). Likewise, an 83% 5-year survival rate was reported for patients without demonstrable LVSI, compared with a 64.5% survival rate for those in whom LVSI was present (181). Using multivariate analysis, only depth of myometrial invasion, DNA ploidy, and vascular invasion–associated changes correlated significantly with survival of patients with stage I endometrial adenocarcinomas in another report (165).

Isthmus and Cervix Extension

The location of the tumor within the uterus is important. Involvement of the uterine isthmus, cervix, or both is associated with an increased risk for extrauterine disease, lymph node metastasis, and recurrence. Cervical stromal invasion was a strong predictor of lymphatic dissemination and lymphatic recurrence, especially for pelvic lymph nodes (182). One study reported that if the fundus of the uterus alone was involved with tumor, there was a 13% recurrence rate, whereas if the lower uterine segment or cervix was involved with occult tumor, there was a 44% recurrence rate (151). A subsequent GOG study found that tumor involvement of the isthmus or cervix without evidence of extrauterine disease was associated with a 16% recurrence rate and a relative risk of 1.6 (132). Patients with cervical involvement tended to have higher-grade, larger, and more deeply invasive tumors, undoubtedly contributing to the increased risk for recurrence.

Peritoneal Cytology

Several reports noted increased recurrence rates and decreased survival rates and, on this basis, recommended treatment for positive cytology (184–186). Most of the studies included patients with other evidence of extrauterine disease spread and were performed without appropriate multivariate analysis and with patients who were incompletely staged. The GOG studycritically analyzed 1,180 clinical stagesI and II endometrial cancer patients in whom appropriate surgical and pathologic staging was performed (132). Considering only the 697 patients for whom peritoneal cytology status and adequate follow-up were available, 25 (29%) of 86 patients with positive cytology developed recurrence, compared with 64 (10.5%) of 611 patients with negative cytology. They noted that 17 of the 25 recurrences in the positive cytology group were outside the peritoneal cavity.

In contrast to these reports, an equal number of studies found no significant relationship between malignant peritoneal cytology and an increased incidence of disease recurrence in the absence of other risk factors such as extrauterine disease (186–189). Patients with positive peritoneal cytology as the only site of extrauterine disease (i.e., no adnexal or uterine serosal invasion) and without poor prognosticators (i.e., myometrial invasion more than50%, nonendometrioid histologic subtype, grade 3, lymphovascular space invasion, cervical invasion) have a very favorable outcome with an absence of extra-abdominal recurrences (190). These patients have an associated 5-year survival of 98% to 100% even when not treated with adjuvant therapy (148,191,192). On the other hand, patients with positive cytology in addition to poor prognostic factors demonstrate a high rate (47%) of distant extra-abdominal failure and may potentially benefit from systemic chemotherapy. **Positive peritoneal cytology seems to have an adverse effect on survival only if the endometrial cancer has spread to the adnexa, peritoneum, or lymph nodes, not if the disease is otherwise confined to the uterus** (188,189,191). These considerations led to the omission of cytology as a factor impacting stage in the FIGO 2009 staging criteria.

The following conclusions may be reached regarding the prognostic implications of positive peritoneal cytology:

1. **Positive peritoneal cytology is associated with other known poor prognostic factors.**
2. **Positive peritoneal cytology in the absence of other evidence of extrauterine disease or poor prognostic factors has no significant effect on recurrence and survival.**
3. **Positive peritoneal cytology, when associated with other poor prognostic factors or extrauterine disease, increases the likelihood for distant as well as intra-abdominal disease recurrence and has a significant adverse effect on survival.**
4. **Use of several different therapeutic modalities has not resulted in any proven benefit to patients with endometrial cancer and positive peritoneal cytology.**

Stage IIIA: Adnexal or Uterine Serosal Involvement

Most patients with stage IIIA disease have other poor prognostic factors that place them at high risk for recurrence. One series described treatment of all patients with serosal or adnexal invasion (or both) with whole-abdomen radiotherapy. Failures were observed outside the abdomen in 100% of patients with full thickness myometrial invasion or uterine serosal invasion, and in 20% to 25% of cases in the presence of isolated adnexal invasion (132,193). These patients may benefit from postoperative systemic chemotherapy.

Lymph Node Metastasis

Lymph node metastasis is the most important prognostic factor in clinical early-stage endometrial cancer. Of patients with clinical stage I disease, about 10% will have pelvic and 6% will have para-aortic lymph node metastases. Patients with lymph node metastases have almost a sixfold higher likelihood of developing recurrent cancer than patients without lymph node metastases. One study reported a recurrence rate of 48% with positive lymph nodes, including 45% with positive pelvic nodes and 64% with positive aortic nodes, compared with 8% with negative nodes. **The 5-year disease-free survival rate for patients with lymph node metastases was 54%, compared with 90% for patients without lymph node metastases** (148). The GOG found that the presence or absence of para-aortic lymph node metastases was of paramount importance in determining prognosis. Of 48 para-aortic node–positive patients, 28 (58%) developed progressive or recurrent cancer, and only 36% of these patients were alive at 5 years, compared with 85% of patients without para-aortic node involvement (194). One series examined patients with lymph nodes metastases in addition to other extrauterine sites of disease (vagina, uterine serosa, positive peritoneal cytology, adnexal invasion). The recurrence rateswere67% (41% extranodal) for those with lymphatic dissemination versus. 32% (5% extranodal) for those with other sites of extrauterine disease spread (190).

Intraperitoneal Metastases

Extrauterine metastasis, excluding peritoneal cytology and lymph node metastasis, occurs in about 4% to 6% of patients with clinical stage I endometrial cancer. Gross intraperitoneal spread is highly correlated with lymph node metastases; one study noted that 51% of patients with intraperitoneal tumor had positive lymph nodes, whereas only 7% of patients without gross peritoneal spread had positive nodes (141). Extrauterine spread other than lymph node metastasis issignificantly associated with tumor recurrence. Another study found that 50% of patients with extrauterine disease developed recurrence, compared with 11% of patients without extrauterine disease, making recurrence almost fivetimes more likely in patients with extrauterine disease spread. The 5-year disease-free survival rate for patients with nonlymphatic extrauterine disease was 50%, compared with 88% in other patients (148). Predictors of peritoneal relapse include stage IV disease or stage II or III disease with two or more of the following risk factors: cervical invasion, positive peritoneal cytology, positive lymph nodes, and nonendometrioid histology (195).

Types I and II Endometrial Carcinoma: Molecular Aberrations

Based on their etiological and pathological features, sporadic endometrial cancer is classified into two subtypes (2,134). Type I (endometrioid histology) represents the majority of lesions (approximately 80%), whichare mostly low grade, estrogen receptor positive, associated with hyperestrogenism, and arise from atypical complex hyperplasia (196,197). Hyperestrogenism may be attributed to obesity with peripheral conversion of androgens to estrogens, anovulation, or exposure to excessive exogenous estrogen (134,198–202). Obesity, polycystic ovarian syndrome, *tamoxifen* use, and unopposed *estrogen* use are all associated with increased risk of endometrial cancer. Other associated findings include late onset of menopause, nulliparity, diabetes mellitus, and hypertension. The molecular basis for the progression from hyperplasia to invasive endometrial carcinoma as a result of hyperestrogenism remains unknown because the involvement of only a minority of factors is reproducible (203). In contrast, type II endometrial cancer (serous, clear cell carcinoma) appears to be unrelated to high estrogen levels and often develops in nonobese women. Type II cancers arise from its precursor, endometrial intraepithelial carcinoma (EIC) adjacent to an atrophic endometrium background in relatively older women (204). Distinct molecular changes are associated with these two subtypes. Common genetic changes in endometrioid endometrial cancer include mutations in *PTEN* (205–212), or β-catenin genes (213–215). In contrast, type II cancers frequently demonstrate alterations in HER2/*neu*, p53, p16, e-cadherin, and loss of heterozygosity (LOH) (216–218). These distinct molecular alterations underscore prognostic differences. Type I endometrial cancer is limited to the uterus in 70% of cases with a 5-year survival greater than 85%. Type II endometrial cancer displays a more aggressive clinical course and a poor prognosis; even in tumors with little or no myometrial invasion, more than one in three patients will have extensive extrauterine spread with complete surgical staging, resulting in an overall survival of 20% (106,110,114,219).

Inactivation of the *PTEN* tumor-suppressor gene is one of the earliest aberrations observed in endometrial cancer precursors and is the most common genetic defect in type I cancers, observed in up to 83% of tumors (206). Tumors with *PTEN* mutations tend to be well differentiated and minimally invasive (220–222). Approximately 20% of sporadic endometrioid cancers demonstrate a molecular phenotype referred to as microsatellite instability (MSI) (223–225). Microsatellites are short segments of repetitive DNA bases scattered throughout the genome. MSI describes the accumulation of sequence changes in these DNA segments that occur because of the inactivation of intranuclear proteins that comprise the mismatch repair system (226). Inactivation of MLH1, a component of the mismatch repair system, is a common event in type I endometrial cancer. This alteration occurs through hypermethylation of CpG islands in the gene promoter, a process known as epigenetic silencing (227). This is in contrast to colon cancer, in which MSI and inactivation of the mismatch repair genes occurs through mutations in mismatch repair genes, including *hMSH2, hMLH1, PMS1, PMS2,* or *hMSH6* (44–46). MSI and abnormal methylation of MLH1 are early events in endometrial carcinogenesis and are described in precancerous lesions (196,224). Mutations in codons 12 or 13 of the K-ras oncogene are reported in 10% to 20% of endometrial adenocarcinomas (228). The presence of mutations of K-ras appears to be an independent unfavorable prognostic factor (229,230).

Chromosomal instability with extensive genomic derangements is commonly found in type II endometrial cancers (231). The most frequent genetic alteration is TP53 mutation, present in about 90% of serous carcinomas (205,227,232,233). In contrast to endometrioid carcinoma, MSI is rare (<5%), as are K-ras and *PTEN* mutations (210,234,235). Other genetic alterations that occur more frequently in serous compared to endometrioid carcinomas are inactivation of

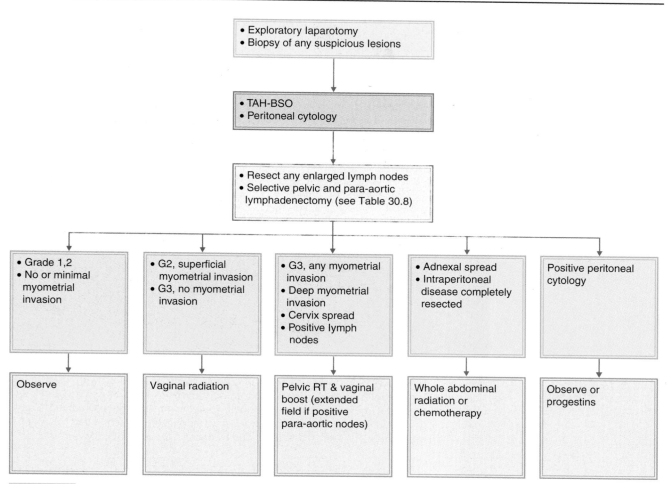

Figure 35.6   Surgical management of patients with stage I–II endometrial carcinoma.

p16 (45%) and overexpression and gene amplification of HER2/*neu* oncogene (45% and 70%, respectively) (232,236,237). HER-2/*neu* overexpression is related to diminished, progression-free survival (238–240). E-cadherin, an oncogene responsible for cell-to-cell adhesion that seems to play a critical role in initiation and progression of endometrial neoplasia, is absent or reduced in 62% to 87% of cases. Loss of E-cadherin is often associated with advanced stage and LOH in both serous and clear cell carcinomas (214,241,242).

Surgical Treatment

An algorithm for the management of patients with clinical stage I and II endometrial cancer is presented in Figure 35.6. The most common current protocol for surgical management of endometrial cancer includes peritoneal cytology, hysterectomy and bilateral salpingo-oophorectomy, and surgical staging. In patients with nonendometrioid cancer, omentectomy along with appendectomy and peritoneal biopsies may be performed. The need to perform lymphadenectomy is based on the type of endometrial cancer, the grade of the tumor, the tumor size and extent of myometrial invasion determined during the surgery, and the presence of extrauterine disease. Bilateral pelvic and para-aortic lymphadenectomy is performed if the patient has any of the following factors: evidence of extrauterine disease, tumor that is FIGO grade 3, nonendometrioid type endometrial cancer, or evidence of tumor invasion more than 50% of the thickness of the myometrium. In the absence of these risk factors only bilateral pelvic lymphadenectomy is performed, if the tumor size is greater than 2 cm; para-aortic lymphadenectomy would be performed only if pelvic lymph nodes were positive (Fig. 35.7). Lymphadenectomy is omitted altogether for patients without the above risk factors, absence of cervical involvement, and tumor size less than 2 cm. The decision to administer postoperative radiation, chemotherapy, or both is predicated on the final results of pathological examination of the surgical specimen and cytology, according to previously described criteria (243).

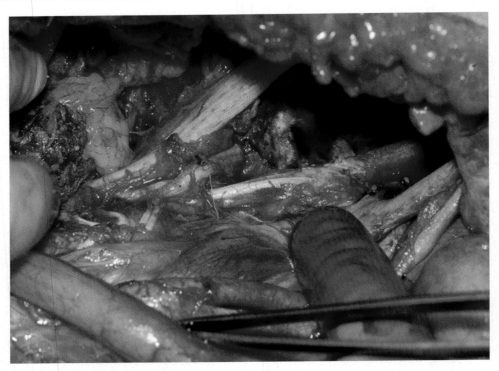

Figure 35.7   Radical pelvic sidewall resection. Photo taken of a patient with a left pelvic sidewall recurrence following resection of psoas muscle and bony ilium. Structures from lower to upper aspect of the photo (medial to lateral) include ureter, internal and external iliac artery, common iliac vein, lumbosacral trunk, obturator nerve (sacrificed), and femoral nerve. The cut edge of the psoas muscle is seen at left. (Provided by Sean C. Dowdy, MD, Mayo Clinic.)

Hysterectomy with bilateral salpingo-oophorectomy represents the first step in the treatment of endometrial cancer. The most debated issue in endometrial cancer management concerns the utility of lymph node dissection. This topic is extensively discussed in the "Surgical Staging" section of this chapter.

Vaginal Hysterectomy

Vaginal hysterectomy may be considered for selected patients who are extremely obese and have a poor medical status or for patients with extensive uterovaginal prolapse. Vaginal hysterectomy with bilateral salpingo-oophorectomy may be considered adequate treatment for patients with low risk tumors (endometrioid, grade 1 or 2, <50% myometrial invasion, and tumor diameter <2 cm; Fig. 35.7. **Vaginal hysterectomy is particularly suitable for patients who are at lowrisk for extrauterine spread of disease (i.e., those with clinical stage I, well-differentiated tumors). In one report, a 94% survival rate was found in 56 patients with clinical stage I endometrial carcinoma treated by vaginal hysterectomy, with or without postoperative radiotherapy (mostly brachytherapy).** Three-fourths of these patients had grade 1 lesions (244). Others reported similar good results (245–247). Vaginal hysterectomy is preferable to radiation therapy alone, but should be reserved for specific patients.

Laparoscopic Management

Advances in endoscopic technologies and power sources allowed application of a laparoscopic approach to the management of endometrial cancer. Since 1992, **there were multiple reports documenting the feasibility of laparoscopicallyassisted vaginal hysterectomy with bilateral salpingo-oophorectomy and laparoscopic lymphadenectomy for staging and treatment of patients with endometrial cancer** (248–256). These early studies demonstrated no differences in lymph node counts, estimated blood loss, and recurrence or survival rates with laparoscopy versus laparotomy, whereas decreased perioperative morbidity, longer operating times, shorter hospital stays, and earlier return to work were associated with laparoscopy.

Although the literature has isolated case reports of port site metastases, there are few data documenting the incidence. Martinez et al. analyzed 1,216 patients with endometrial and cervical cancer and showed that the port site metastasis rate was less than 0.5%; no port site metastases occurred after excluding patients with peritoneal disease (257).

A large prospective study by GOG randomized patients to laparoscopy versus laparotomy for the primary treatment of patients with endometrial cancer (258). Over 2,500 patients were enrolled, 1,696 to laparoscopy and 920 to laparotomy. Consistent with early reports, patients randomized to laparoscopy had shorter hospital stay (52% more than 2 days vs. 94% in the laparotomy group), less blood loss, and fewer postoperative complications (14% vs. 21%). The rate of intra-operative complications was similar, and the operative time was longer in the laparoscopy cohort. There was no difference in lymph node counts, and stage distribution was identical between groups. A follow-up quality-of-life investigation of the same cohorts revealed improved Functional Assessment of Cancer Therapy–General (FACT-G) scores, better physical functioning, better body image, less pain and its interference with quality of life, and an earlier resumption of normal activities and return to work over the 6-week recovery period in the laparoscopic group (259). Although the differences were modest and negligible by 6 months, the analysis was performed as per intention to treat. Of concern is the 24% rate of conversions in the laparoscopic cohort; only 4% were converted because of advanced disease. Furthermore, the conversion rate increased dramatically with body mass index (BMI). This is problematic recognizing that the vast majority of patients with endometrial cancer are obese. The conversion rate for patients with a BMI of 40 was 57%. This implies a limitation of the surgical technique in obese patients.

The use of extraperitoneal laparoscopic staging for para-aortic lymphadenectomy was reported in a prospective investigation of 293 patients with endometrial cancer (260). The extraperitoneal approach greatly improved exposure by circumventing handling of the small bowel and was successful in over 90% of unselected patients up to a BMI of 51. There was no difference in lymph node counts, all dissections were performed to the level of the renal veins, and significant improvements in blood loss, postoperative complications, and length of stay were noted compared to the laparotomy group. The ability to gain access to the renal veins is important, given that 60% of patients with nodal involvement above the inferior mesenteric artery have negative ipsilateral inframesenteric para-aortic nodes (140). Thus, 38% to 46% of patients with para-aortic metastases will be missed if the dissection is limited to the region below the inframesenteric artery. Althoughinfrarenal lymphadenectomy has yet to be proven necessary, the extraperitoneal approach offers the most reliable method to consistently perform a thorough dissection.

Robotic-assisted surgery gained popularity for endometrial cancer treatment (see Chapter 25). Improved instrumentation and visualization allow minimally invasive surgery to be performed by surgeons with less laparoscopic experience, and in patients, particularly obese patients, who otherwise might not be candidates for minimally invasive surgery. In one report limited to obese patients with endometrial carcinoma, the robotic approach offered reduced operating times, less blood loss, higher lymph node yields, and shorter hospital stays compared to laparoscopy (261). The extent of para-aortic dissection was not described in this report, and infrarenal para-aortic lymphadenectomy remains challenging, even with robotic assistance.

When not limited to obese patients, robotic-assisted surgery appears to offer the same benefits as laparoscopy in regards to postoperative morbidity and convalescence compared to laparotomy, but with shorter operative times (262). Althoughoncologic outcomes have yet to be proven in patients with endometrial cancer, robotic surgery is simply an advanced laparoscopic tool, and it can be expected to find equal outcomes. Given the great costs associated with robotic instruments and the absence of differential reimbursement, it is still undetermined which group of patients will benefit most from this approach from a clinical and financial perspective.

Radical Hysterectomy

Radical hysterectomy, with removal of the parametria and upper vagina, and bilateral pelvic lymphadenectomy, does not improve survival of patients with clinical stage I disease compared with extrafascial hysterectomy and bilateral salpingo-oophorectomy alone (263–266). Radical hysterectomy increases both intraoperative and postoperative morbidity and should not be performed for treatment of apparent early endometrial cancer. In the presence of demonstrable invasion of the cervix, a modified extrafascial hysterectomy may be performed. This may improve outcomes and decrease the risk of local recurrences, especially if postoperative local radiation is not planned in younger patients (267).

Table 35.9 Review of Recent Series of Endometrial Carcinoma Treated with Radiation Alone

Author (Ref.)	Year	Stage	No. of Patients	Local Recurrence Rate (%)	Disease-specific Survival Rate (%)	Major Complication Rate (%) [a]
Landgren et al. (268)	1976	I–II	124	22	68	7
		III–IV	26	42	22	
Abayomi et al. (269)	1982	I–II	50	26	78	15
		III–IV	16	—	10	
Patanaphan et al. (270)	1985	I–II	42	14	64	2
		III–IV	10	60	20	
Jones and Stout (271)	1986	I–II	146	22	61	4
		III–IV	14	79	14	
Varia et al. (272)	1987	I–II	73	21	43	10
Wang et al. (273)	1987	I–II	41	22	76	5
Grigsby et al. (274)	1987	I	69	9	88	16
Taghian et al. (275)	1988	I–II	94	6	70	17
		III–IV	10	10	27	
Lehoczky et al. (276)	1991	I	171	20	75	0
Kupelian et al. (277)	1993	I–II	137	14	85	3
		III–IV	15	32	49	

[a]For all stages combined.
From **Kupelian PA, Eifel PJ, Tornos C, et al.** Treatment of endometrial carcinoma with radiation therapy alone. *Int J Radiat Oncol Biol Phys* 1993;27:817–824, with permission.

Radiation Therapy as Primary Treatment

Primary surgery followed by individualized radiation therapy is the most widely accepted treatment for early-stage endometrial cancers. However, about 5% to 15% of endometrial cancer patients have severe medical conditions that render them unsuitable for surgery (131). These patients tend to be elderly and obese with multiple chronic or acute medical illnesses, such as hypertension, cardiac disease, diabetes mellitus, and pulmonary, renal, and neurologic diseases.

Several series show that radiotherapy is effective treatment for patients with inoperable endometrial cancer (268–277) (Table 35.9). One reported on the treatment of 120 patients with clinical stage I and 17 patients with clinical stage II endometrial cancer with radiation alone, 85% of whom received only intracavitary radiation. Because of the high incidence of death caused by intercurrent illness in this group of patients, the 5- and 10-year overall survival rates were only 55% and 28%, respectively, compared with disease-specific survival rates of 87% and 85%, respectively. There was no difference in disease-specific survival rates between patients with stage I and II disease. Intrauterine cancer recurred in 14% of patients, and extrauterine pelvic disease recurred in 3%. The authors treated 15 patients with stage III and IV disease, usually with a combination of external-beam and intracavitary radiation therapy, yielding a 5-year disease-specific survival rate of 49%. Five patients (3%) had serious late complications of radiation therapy (277).

Although it is generally agreed that intracavitary radiation is necessary to achieve adequate local control, the indications for external-beam radiation therapy in the primary treatment of endometrial cancer are less well defined. Patients with cervical involvement and known or suspected extrauterine pelvic spread undoubtedly would benefit from external-beam radiation therapy. Theoretically, external-beam radiation could sterilize microscopic nodal disease and possibly increase the radiation dose to deep myometrial or subserosal uterine disease, which may receive an insufficient dose from intracavitary radiation alone. A correlation between tumor grade and recurrence was noted in several reports. One found that the 5-year progression-free survival rate for medically inoperable patients with clinical stage I disease treated with radiotherapy alone was 94% for grade 1, 92% for grade 2, and 78% for grade 3 tumors (274). Therefore, **patients with grade 3 tumors and a known propensity for deep myometrial invasion and lymph node metastasis may benefit from external-beam therapy.**

The decision to treat a patient who has endometrial cancer with radiation alone must involve a careful analysis of the relative risks and benefits of surgery. Although radiation alone can produce excellent survival and local control, it should be considered for definitive treatment only if the operative risk is estimated to exceed the 10% to 15% risk for uterine recurrence that is expected with radiation treatment alone.

Patterns of Metastatic Dissemination: Implications for Postoperative and Disease-Based Adjuvant Treatment

Endometrial cancer is commonly diagnosed early in its natural history with approximately 80% of patients presenting with stage I disease. Nevertheless, approximately one of every three women who die of endometrial cancer was considered to have early locoregional disease at primary diagnosis. The majority of treatment failures and the accompanying compromised longevity probably result from the failure to recognize sites of occult extrauterine dissemination at primary diagnosis. Traditional postoperative therapy (modality-based) for high-risk endometrial cancer is external-beam radiotherapy that is frequently supplemented with vaginal brachytherapy (278). This approach improves local control but not survival in early stage disease (135,155,279).

Understanding the different pathways of metastatic dissemination of endometrial cancer and their predictive factors allows the development of an individualized model for target-based therapeutic approaches to the predicted site(s) of failure. The natural history of epithelial corpus cancer includes four potential routes of metastasis: (i) contiguous extension (mainly to the vagina), (ii) hematogenous dissemination, (iii) lymphatic embolization, and (iv) exfoliation with intraperitoneal spread. On the basis of regression analysis, independent pathologic risk factors predictive of the four routes of metastatic spread were identified:

1. **Contiguous extension: histologic grade 3 and lymphovascular space invasion are proven predictors of vaginal relapse in stage I endometrial cancer** (280).
2. **Hematogenous: deep myometrial invasion is the strongest predictor of hematogenous recurrence (>50% for all stages and ≥66% for stage I)** (176,281).
3. **Lymphatic: lymphatic failure is more likely to occur when cervical stroma involvement or positive lymph nodes are present** (182).
4. **Peritoneal: predictors of peritoneal relapse are: (i) stage IV disease or (ii) stage II or III disease with two or more of the following risk factors: cervical invasion, peritoneal cytologic results positive for endometrial cancer, positive lymph nodes, and nonendometrioid histologic findings** (195).

Patients with the risk factors summarized in Table 35.10 account for 35% of the overall population with endometrial cancer, but 89% of the observed hematogenous, lymphatic, and peritoneal relapses. Importantly, 46% of the patients considered at risk subsequently experienced a recurrence in one or more of the three sites, compared with only 2% of patients not judged to be at risk based on these criteria ($p < 0.001$). The identification of subgroups of patients at risk for the different patterns of recurrence would allow postoperative treatment targeted to the predicted areas of tumor dissemination. The recurrence sites predicted by risk factors would presuppose different adjuvant treatment strategies. Patients at risk for hematogenous or peritoneal recurrence would potentially benefit from systemic cytotoxic treatment, while patients at risk for lymphatic or vaginal recurrence would potentially benefit from radiation treatment directed at areas at risk.

Modalities of Postoperative Treatment

Observation

Patients with grades 1 and 2 lesions without myometrial invasion or any of the above risk factors (Table 35.10) **have an excellent prognosis and require no postoperative therapy.** In a GOG study, there were no recurrences and a 100% disease-free 5-year survival rate in the 91 patients in this category, 72 of whom received no additional treatment after hysterectomy (132). Other investigators reported equally favorable results with only surgical therapy in similar patients (282,283).

Vaginal Vault Radiation

Vaginal brachytherapy is an attractive alternative to external radiation therapy (ERT). High-dose rate (HDR) brachytherapy is well tolerated with low rates of severe or chronic complications.

Table 35.10 Rates of Recurrence at 5 Years According to the Different Risk Categories for 915 Patients	
Risk Category	**Recurrence at 5 Years (%)**
Hematogenous	
All stages	
Myometrial invasion ≤50%	4
Myometrial invasion >50%	28
Stage I (negative lymph nodes)	
Myometrial invasion <66%	2
Myometrial invasion ≥66%	34
Lymphatic	
No risk factors	2
CSI and/or positive lymph nodes	31
Peritoneal	
Stage IV disease	63
Stage II–III disease and ≥2 risk factors[a]	21
Stage I–III disease and ≤1 risk factor[a]	1
Overall[b]	
Not at risk[c]	2
At risk[c]	46

CSI, cervical stromal invasion.
[a]CSI, nonendometrioid histologic subtype, positive lymph nodes, or positive result on peritoneal cytologic evaluation.
[b]Excluding vaginal recurrences.
[c]*For at least one of the three categories of recurrence (i.e. hematogenous, lymphatic, or peritoneal).*
From **Mariani A, Dowdy SC, Keeney GL, et al.** High-risk endometrial cancer subgroups: candidates for target-based adjuvant therapy. *Gynecol Oncol* 2004;95:120–126.

Vaginal control rates with the more convenient, better-tolerated HDR brachytherapy are comparable to control rates with the lengthier low-dose rate (LDR) brachytherapy. Pearcey and Petereit established the HDR dosing of 21 Gy to 5-mm depth in threefractions as the standard brachytherapy dose, providing local control rates of 98% to 100% (284). Additional retrospective data demonstrate 98% to 100% vaginal control rates with HDR in high risk early-stage endometrial cancer (285,286). Retrospective data suggestthat the vaginal relapse rate after brachytherapy averages 4% to 5% (Table 35.11) and this is similar to the 5-year vaginal failure rate of 3.5% reported among the highest-risk patients who received ERT in PORTEC-1 (135,282,285,287–291).

PORTEC-2 randomized patients with apparent uterine-confined endometrial cancer at high risk for recurrence (>60 years of age with grade 1 or 2, stage IB and grade 3, stage IA; or any age, any grade IIA with <50% myometrial invasion), to pelvic ERT (46 Gy, in 23 fractions) versus vaginal brachytherapy (21 Gy in three HDR fractions or 30 Gy LDR, to a depth of 0.5 cm). At 3 years, there was no difference in vaginal failure rates (0.9% for vaginal brachytherapy, 2% for pelvic ERT; $p = .97$).There was a higher rate of nonvaginal pelvic relapse in the brachytherapy group (3.6 %) compared to the ERT group (0.7%; $p = .03$), however, the absolute difference was small and there was no difference in overall survival (292). The difference between nonvaginal pelvic recurrences may be a reflection of unrecognized lymph node metastases at the time of initial surgery treated with ERT. One concern regarding PORTEC-2 is that there was not a surgery-only control in the study. However, the highest risk endometrial cancer subgroup in PORTEC-1 (patients >60 years of age with grade 3 or deeply invasive grade 1 or 2, all stage I) was similar to the cohort included in PORTEC-2 and the locoregional recurrence rate in patients who did not receive adjuvant ERT in PORTEC-1 was 18% (135).

Table 35.11 Recurrence in High-Risk, Comprehensively Staged, Early-Stage Endometrial Cancer after Adjuvant Vaginal Brachytherapy Alone (No Pelvic ERT)

Author (Ref.)	No. of Patients	Lymphadenectomy Performed	Postoperative Vaginal Brachytherapy	No. of Recurrences N (%)
Orr et al. (282)	115	+	+	6 (5.2)
Mohan et al. (287)	28	+	+	2 (7)
Chadha et al. (288)	38	+	+	3 (7.9)
Fanning (289)	66	+	+	2 (3)
Horowitz et al. (285)	102	+	+	10 (9.8)
Straughn et al. (290)	56	+	+	0 (0)
Solhjem et al. (291)	100	+	+	0 (0)
Total	505			23 (4.6)[a]

ERT, external radiation therapy.

[a] Includes 18 distant (78% of all recurrences), 3 vaginal (13%), 1 isolated pelvic sidewall (4.3%), 1 unknown site (4.3%).

Grade 3 histology and lymphovascular space invasion are proven predictors of vaginal relapse in stage I endometrial cancer. Patients with these risk factors are the most likely group to benefit from vaginal vault brachytherapy (280). Although vaginal recurrences can be successfully treated and controlled in up to 81% of cases, the addition of vaginal brachytherapy to the initial surgical intervention can significantly reduce the risk of such recurrences (293).

External Pelvic Radiation

Radiation therapy traditionally was suggested to patients who were deemed to have intermediate or high risk of recurrence, according to grade and depth of myometrial invasion. Several retrospective studies and large, randomized trials did not show an overall survival benefit for intermediate- and high-risk patients with stage I endometrial cancer (or occult IIA endometrial cancer according to the 1988 FIGO staging) who received adjuvant pelvic radiotherapy.

The PORTEC trial tested the role of postoperative pelvic radiation therapy for presumed stage I endometrial cancer in 714 patients. Eligibility criteria were stage IB, grades 1 to 2, and stage IA, grades 2 to 3; patients with stage IA, grade 3, were only 10% of the study population, and lymph node biopsies and peritoneal cytology were not required. Local-regional recurrences developed in 14% of the surgery group, compared with 4% of the postoperative pelvic radiation group. Overall, the 5-year survival rate was no different between the two groups (85% vs. 81%, respectively) (135). These results were confirmed by GOG99, a prospective, randomized investigation of surgery alone (including lymphadenectomy to the level of the inferior mesentery artery in some patients) versus surgery plus adjuvant pelvic radiation in intermediate-risk endometrial cancer (stages IA to IIb occult). Of 392 patients accrued to the study, more than 80% were actually low-risk patients (90.6% stage I, 81.6% grades 1 to 2, 82% <50% myometrial invasion). Disease recurrence was reduced by 58% ($p = 0.007$) with the use of postoperative pelvic radiation. After 2 years, the cumulative recurrence rate was 12% in the group with no postoperative treatment compared with 3% in the group that received pelvic radiation. The pelvic failure rate was 8.9% in the surgery-alone group compared with 1.6% in the postoperative pelvic radiation group. **Overall survival rates were not significantly improved in patients receiving postoperative pelvic radiation compared with those treated only with surgery (92% vs. 86%, respectively) (279). Recently, the intergroup ASTEC/EN.5 trial provided further confirmation that external-beam radiation therapy in patients at intermediate to high risk of recurrence has no significant effect on overall survival (294).**

Postoperative whole-pelvis external-beam radiation usually involves the delivery of 4,500 to 5,040 cGy in 180 cGy daily fractions over 5 to 6 weeks to a field encompassing the upper one-half of the vagina inferiorly, the lower border of the L4 vertebral body superiorly, and 1 cm lateral to the margins of the bony pelvis. The dose of radiation at the surface of the vaginal apex usually is boosted to 6,000 to 7,000 cGy by a variety of techniques. The most frequently reported side effects are gastrointestinal, usually abdominal cramps and diarrhea, although more serious complications such as bleeding, proctitis, bowel obstruction, and fistula can occur and may require surgical correction. The urinary system may be affected in the form of hematuria, cystitis, or fistula. The overall complication rate ranges from 25% to 40%; and the rate of serious complications requiring surgical intervention is about 1.5% to 3%.

External-beam pelvic radiation does not appear to impact survival in patients with high-risk stage I endometrial cancer. Patients with extrauterine pelvic disease, including adnexal spread, parametrial involvement, and pelvic lymph node metastases, in the absence of extrapelvic disease, are likely to benefit from postoperative pelvic radiation.

Extended-Field Radiation

Patients with histologically proven para-aortic node metastases and no other evidence of disease spread outside the pelvis should be treated with extended-field radiation. The entire pelvis, common iliac lymph nodes, and para-aortic lymph nodes are included within the radiation field. The para-aortic radiation dose is limited to 4,500 to 5,000 cGy. **Extended-field radiotherapy appears to improve survival in patients with endometrial cancer who have positive para-aortic lymph nodes** (132,295–298).

Five-year survival rates of 47% and 43% were reported for patients with surgically confirmed isolated para-aortic lymph node metastases and for those with para-aortic and pelvic lymph node metastases, respectively, using postoperative extended-field radiation. In one report, only one case of severe enteric morbidity occurred in 48 patients, a complication rate of 2% (295). In a GOG study, 37 of 48 patients with positive para-aortic nodes received postoperative para-aortic radiation, 36% of whom remained tumor free at 5 years (132). A comparison of patients with positive para-aortic nodes treated with *megestrol acetate* alone versus *megestrol acetate* and extended-field radiation showed that the survival rate in the patients receiving extended-field radiation was significantly better: 53% versus 12.5%, respectively (296). In another study of 18 patients with positive para-aortic nodes, 5-year survival rates were 67% for microscopic nodal disease and 17% for gross nodal disease (297).

Whole-Abdomen Radiation

Whole-abdomen radiation therapy is usually reserved for patients with stages III and IV endometrial cancer. It may be considered for patients who have serous or carcinosarcomas, which have a propensity for upper-abdominal recurrence (299–304). The recommended dose to the whole abdomen is 3,000 cGy in 20 daily fractions of 150 cGy, with kidney shielding at 1,500 to 2,000 cGy, along with an additional 1,500 cGy to the para-aortic lymph nodes and 2,000 cGy to the pelvis. Gastrointestinal side effects, including nausea, vomiting, and diarrhea, sometimes make it necessary to interrupt therapy, but it is rare for patients to discontinue treatment because of these symptoms. Hematologic toxicity can be expected to occur during whole-abdomen radiation, but it is usually mild. The incidence of late complications, mainly chronic diarrhea and small bowel obstruction, is low (5% to 10%).

In a series of 27 patients treated with surgical stage III endometrial cancer with whole-abdomen radiation, patients with spread to the adnexa, positive peritoneal cytology, or both had a 5-year, relapse-free survival of 90%, whereas all patients with macroscopic disease beyond the adnexa had recurrence (298). Similar results were reported by others (300,301). Some advocated the use of adjuvant whole-abdomen radiotherapy for patients with high-risk stages I and II endometrial carcinoma, including those with deep myometrial invasion, high-grade tumors, and serous histology, because of the high proportion of recurrences in the upper abdomen. A 5-year recurrence-free survival rate of 85% was reported (302,303). With whole-abdomen radiation in patients at increased risk for intra-abdominal metastatic disease, such as those with nonnodal extrauterine disease and serous histology, an actuarial 5-year relapse-free survival rate of 70% was reported, with no significant toxicity (304). Similarly, others noted a 3-year disease-free survival rate of 79% in patients with stages III and IV endometrial adenocarcinoma treated with whole-abdomen radiation (305). Other reports of using adjuvant postoperative whole-abdomen radiation in early-stage uterine serous carcinoma suggest a reduction in recurrence rates (304–306). Most recurrences are in the upper abdomen in all of these patients, despite use of this type of radiotherapy. **After the publication of GOG122, demonstrating the superiority of chemotherapy over whole-abdominal radiotherapy in advanced endometrial cancer, the utilization of whole-abdominal radiotherapy is not common** (see section on "Chemotherapy") (307).

Progestins

Because most endometrial cancers have both estrogen and progesterone receptors and *progestins* were used successfully to treat metastatic endometrial cancer, postoperative adjuvant *progestin* therapy attempted to reduce the risk of recurrence. This therapy is attractive because it provides systemic treatment and has few side effects. Unfortunately, **several large randomized, placebo-controlled studies failed to identify a benefit for adjuvant *progestin* therapy** (308–313).

Chemotherapy

Adjuvant cytotoxic chemotherapy was studied in a few trials. The GOG treated 181 patients who had poor prognostic factors with postoperative radiation and then randomly assigned patients to receive no further therapy or *doxorubicin* chemotherapy. After 5 years of observation, there was no difference in recurrence rates between the two groups (314).

In cases of advanced disease, chemotherapy is now standard treatment. The GOG122 trial compared whole-abdominal radiotherapy versus systemic chemotherapy (eightcycles of *doxorubicin* and *cisplatin*) in 388 patients with stage III or IV disease who underwent maximal surgical resection of disease to less than 2 cm. Its results showed a significant advantage of chemotherapy on 5-year survival (307). Patients who received chemotherapy had a 13% improvement in 2-year progression-free survival (50% vs. 46%) and an 11% improvement in overall 2-year survival (70% vs. 59%) compared with patients treated with whole-abdomen radiation. Although this study was the first to suggest an improvement in outcome for use of adjuvant chemotherapy compared with radiation, toxicity was more prevalent with chemotherapy; patients with gross residual disease were assigned to the radiation arm, almost guaranteeing failure; and overall, 55% of patients experienced a recurrence or progression during the study period (315). GOG184 randomized 552 patients with advanced disease to sixcycles of *cisplatin* and *doxorubicin* with or without *paclitaxel* following surgical debulking and radiotherapy. Side effects were more pronounced with the three-drug regimen, and recurrence-free survival at 36 months was no different between arms (62% vs. 64% for the three-drug regimen). The investigation was closed to patients with stage IV disease during the trial, but subgroup analysis suggested a 50% reduction in recurrence or death in the 57 patients with gross residual disease who received *cisplatin, doxorubicin,* and *paclitaxel* (111).

Other GOG studies and the PORTEC-3 trial are investigating the combination of chemotherapy and radiotherapy in advanced or high-risk endometrial cancer. Results of these trials await maturation. GOG258 is comparing chemoradiation followed by chemotherapy versus chemotherapy alone in advanced endometrial cancer. PORTEC-3 is investigating overall survival and failure-free survival of patients with high-risk and advanced stage endometrial carcinoma treated after surgery with chemoradiation followed by chemotherapy versus pelvic radiation alone.

Regarding the use of chemotherapy in high-risk populations with early stage endometrial cancer, the European Organisation for Research and Treatment of Cancer, along with the Nordic Society of Gynecologic Oncology, presented the results of a collaborative trial comparing external radiotherapy versus chemoradiotherapy in patients with stages I or II or IIIC1 (positive pelvic nodes only) and one of the following characteristics: grade 3 or myometrial invasion greater than 50%, DNA aneuploidy, or clearcell or serous histologic type. Performance of a systematic lymphadenectomy was optional. A total of 375 patients were enrolled over a 10-year period and the study was closed early because of slow recruitment. The hazard ratio for progression-free survival was 0.58 (95% CI, 0.34–0.99) in favor of chemoradiation after a median follow-up of 3.5 years (316).

The Japanese GOG randomized patients to pelvic radiotherapy versus platinum-based chemotherapy in patients with stage IB to IIIC endometrial cancer and myometrial invasion greater than 50%. Assessment of para-aortic nodal status was performed in only 29% of cases. The investigators found no differences between the twoexperimental arms in terms of progression-free survival and overall survival. A subgroup analysis of 120 patients with either (i) stage IB tumor and age greater than 70 years or grade 3 endometrioid adenocarcinoma or (ii) stage II or IIIA tumor (positive cytologic findings) showed that chemotherapy was associated with significantly improved disease-free and overall survival rates (317). **The benefits achieved with combined chemoradiation, identification of the best chemotherapeutic regimen, and the identification of subgroups of patients who may benefit from these treatments deserves further investigation.**

Clinical Stage II

Endometrial cancer involving the cervix either contiguously or by lymphatic spread has a poorer prognosis than disease confined to the corpus (267,278,318–334). Preoperative assessment of cervical involvement is difficult. **Endocervical curettage has relatively high false-positive (50% to 80%) and false-negative rates.** Histologic proof of cancer infiltration of the cervix or presence of obvious tumor on the cervix is the only reliable means of diagnosing cervical involvement, although ultrasonography, hysteroscopy, or MRI may show cervical invasion.

The relatively small number of true stage II cases in reported series and the lack of randomized, prospective studies preclude formulation of a definitive treatment plan. **Three areas must be addressed in any treatment plan:**

1. **For optimal results, the uterus should be removed in all patients.**
2. **Because the incidence of pelvic lymph node metastases is about 36% in stage II endometrial cancer, any treatment protocol should include treatment of these lymph nodes.**
3. **Because the incidence of disease spread outside the pelvis to the para-aortic lymph nodes, adnexal structures, and upper abdomen is higher than in stage I disease, attention should be directed to evaluating and treating extrapelvic disease.**

Two approaches usually were used in the treatment of clinical stage II disease:

1. **Radical hysterectomy, bilateral salpingo-oophorectomy, and pelvic and para-aortic lymphadenectomy**
2. **Combined radiation and surgery (external pelvic radiation and intracavitary radium or cesium followed in 6 weeks by total abdominal hysterectomy and bilateral salpingo-oophorectomy)**

An initial radical surgical approach to treatment of clinical stage II endometrial cancer has the advantage of collecting accurate surgical–pathologic information. Conversely, many patients with endometrial cancer are elderly and obese and have medical problems that make this approach unsuitable. Reported results are no better than those with combined radiation and less radical surgical therapy (267). The use of radical hysterectomy may be limited to patients with anatomic problems that prevent optimum dosimetry or other conditions that conflict with the use of radiation therapy.

The most common, **traditional approach to the management of clinical stage II endometrial cancer is to use external and intracavitary radiation followed by extrafascial hysterectomy.** This combined approach resulted in 5-year survival rates of 60% to 80%, with severe gastrointestinal or urologic complications occurring in about 10% of patients (319–327). Patients who have medically inoperable disease are usually treated with external-beam radiation and one or two intracavitary insertions. Compared with combined radiation and surgery, the results with radiation alone are diminished, but about 50% of patients are long-term survivors (279) (Table 35.9).

Another method of management of clinical stage II endometrial cancer that is gaining favor is an initial surgical approach followed by radiation. This method is based on the difficulty in establishing the preoperative diagnosis of cervical involvement in the absence of a gross cervical tumor, the evidence that radiation is equally effective when given after hysterectomy, and the high incidence of extrapelvic disease when the cervix is involved. Exploratory laparotomy with an extrafascial or modified radical hysterectomy, bilateral salpingo-oophorectomy, peritoneal washings for cytology, and resection of grossly enlarged lymph nodes are performed. These procedures are followed by appropriate pelvic or extended-field external and intravaginal radiation, depending on the results of surgical staging. Excellent results were reported using this treatment scheme (329–331).

Clinical Stages III and IV

Clinical stage III disease accounts for about 7% to 10% of all endometrial carcinomas (335–340). Patients usually have clinical evidence of disease spread to the parametria, pelvic sidewall, or adnexal structures; less frequently, there is spread to the vagina or pelvic peritoneum. **Treatment for stage III endometrial carcinoma must be individualized, but initial operative evaluation and treatment should be considered because of the high risk for occult lymph node metastases and intraperitoneal spread when disease is known to extend outside of the uterus into the pelvis.** In the presence of an adnexal mass, the initial impetus for surgery is to determine the nature of the mass. Surgery is performed to determine the extent of disease and to remove the bulk of the disease if possible. This procedure should include peritoneal washings for cytologic examination, para-aortic and pelvic lymphadenectomy, biopsy or excision of any suspicious areas within the peritoneal cavity, and omentectomy and peritoneal biopsies. Except in patients with bulky parametrial disease, total abdominal hysterectomy and bilateral salpingo-oophorectomy should be performed. **The goal of surgery is eradication of all macroscopic disease because this finding is of major prognostic importance in the management of patients with clinical stage III disease.** Postoperative therapy can be tailored to the extent of disease.

Results of therapy depend on the extent and nature of disease. A 5-year survival rate of 54% was reported for all patients with stage III disease; however, the survival was 80% when only adnexal metastases were present, compared with 15% when other extrauterine pelvic structures were involved (335). Patients with surgical–pathologic stage III disease have a much better survival rate (40%) than those with clinical stage III disease (16%) (326). Patients who are treated with combined surgery and radiation fare better than patients who receive radiation therapy alone (340).

Stage IV endometrial adenocarcinoma, in which tumor invades the bladder or rectum or extends outside the pelvis, makes up about 3% of cases (340–344). **Treatment of stage IV disease is patient dependent but usually involves a combination of surgery, radiation therapy, and systemic hormonal therapy or chemotherapy.** One objective of surgery and radiation therapy is to achieve local disease control in the pelvis to provide palliative relief of bleeding, discharge, and complications involving the bladder and rectum. In one report, control of pelvic disease was achieved in 28% of 72 patients with stage IV disease treated with radiation alone or in combination with surgery, *progestins,* or both (342). **Several reports noted a positive impact of cytoreductive surgery on survival, the median survival being about threetimes greater with optimal cytoreduction (18 to 34 months vs. 8 to 11 months, respectively)** (342–344). Pelvic exenteration may be considered in the very rare patient in whom disease is limited to the bladder, rectum, or both (345,346).

Recurrent Disease

About one-fourth of patients treated for early endometrial cancer develop recurrent disease. More than one-half of the recurrences develop within 2 years, and about three-fourths occurs within 3 years of initial treatment. The distribution of recurrences is dependent in large part on the type of primary therapy: surgery alone versus surgery plus local or regional radiotherapy. In a GOG study of 390 patients with surgical stage I disease, vaginal and pelvic recurrences were noted to comprise 53% of all recurrences in the group treated with surgery alone, whereas only 30% of recurrences were vaginal or pelvic in the group treated with combined surgery and radiotherapy (132). Therefore, after combined surgery and radiotherapy (vaginal or external beam), 70% or more of patients with treatment failures have distant metastases, and most of these patients do not have evidence of local or pelvic recurrence. The most common sites of extrapelvic metastases are the lung, abdomen, lymph nodes (aortic, supraclavicular, inguinal), liver, brain, and bone. Patients with isolated vaginal recurrences fare better than those with pelvic recurrences, who in turn have a better chance of cure than those with distant metastases. Patients who initially have well-differentiated tumors or who develop recurrent cancer more than 3 years after the primary therapy also tend to have an improved prognosis.

In a 1984 report on 379 patients with recurrent endometrial cancer seen at the Norwegian Radium Hospital from 1960 to 1976, site of recurrence was local or regional in 190 patients (50%), distant in 108 patients (28%), and local and distant in 81 patients (21%) (347). The median time of recurrence was 14 months for patients with local recurrences and 19 months for patients with distant metastases. Of all recurrences, 34% were detected within 1 year, and 76% were detected within 3 years of primary treatment. At the time of diagnosis of recurrence, 32% of patients had no symptoms. **Vaginal bleeding was the most common symptom associated with local recurrence, and pelvic pain was most often present with pelvic recurrence.** Hemoptysis was the initial symptom in 32% of patients with lung metastases, but 45% of cases of lung metastases were asymptomatic and picked up on routine chest x-ray. Only 9% of patients with metastases at other sites did not have symptoms; most had pain (37%) or other symptoms such as anorexia, nausea and vomiting, or ascites related to intra-abdominal carcinomatosis, neurologic symptoms such as seizures from brain metastases, or jaundice caused by liver metastases. Overall, only 29 (7.7%) of the 379 patients were alive without evidence of disease from 3 to 19 years. This included 22 patients (12%) with local or pelvic recurrence, 5 patients (5%) with distant metastases, and 2 patients (2%) with both local and distant recurrences. The best results were obtained in the 42 patients with vaginal vault recurrences who were treated with radiotherapy, resulting in a 24% survival rate. None of the 78 patients with pelvic soft tissue recurrence survived. Three patients (7%) with only lung metastases treated with *progestins,* two patients with lymph node metastases treated with combined radiotherapy and *progestins,* and two patients with local recurrence and lung metastases treated with radiotherapy, surgery, and *progestins* survived.

Surgery

A small subset of patients with isolated recurrent endometrial cancer may benefit from surgical intervention. A search for distant recurrences prior to treatment is obligatory as such patients are best treated with chemotherapy. In one small series, upper-abdominal disease was found at laparotomy in three(37.5%) of eightpatients with presumed localized pelvic recurrence. Presence of subclinical extrapelvic metastases was associated with larger pelvic tumor size (>2 cm) and elevated serum CA125 levels (348). As discussed in the next section, isolated vaginal recurrence in patients who have not received prior pelvic radiation is best treated with external radiation plus some type of brachytherapy.

Treatment of patients with pelvic recurrence (generally located on the pelvic sidewall secondary to lymphatic failure) is more complex. Althoughthe study by Aalders et al. reviewed above showed no survivors in patients with pelvic recurrences, there is evidence that a multimodality approach consisting of radiotherapy followed by radical surgical resection and intraoperative radiotherapy (IORT) will cure some patients (347). A retrospective investigation at Mayo Clinic of 25 heavily pretreated patients with recurrent endometrial cancer demonstrated a survival of 71% in patients with complete surgical resection (349). Over 50% of these patients underwent radiation as primary therapy and one-half of those treated with radiationalso received chemotherapy or an attempt at surgical resection at the time of recurrence. Radical procedures performed at the time of IORT included resection of the pelvic sidewall *en bloc* with the obturator nerve, external iliac vein, psoas, iliacus, or obturator internus muscles, ureter, or boney ileum (Fig. 35.7). Seven patients required exenteration in combination with resection of the pelvic sidewall. Two patients with isolated para-aortic recurrences were alive and diseasefree at 54 and 71 months. Althoughsurvival in this cohort was impressive, the complication rate was similarly impressive at 64%. The most common complication was neuropathy; other complications included functional ureteral obstruction and fourpatients developed fistulas. Until more active agents are developed, radical multimodality treatment remains the only viable alternative for patients with pelvic recurrences. Memorial Sloan-Kettering Cancer Center reported on 36 patients with isolated central pelvic recurrence who underwent pelvic exenteration for recurrent endometrial carcinoma. Seventy-five percent died of their cancer within 1 year of operation, and 14% were alive after 5 years (349).

Radiation Therapy

Radiotherapy is the best treatment option for patients with isolated local or regional recurrences who are unable or unwilling to undergo radical pelvic resection (350–356). The best local control and subsequent cure are usually achieved by a combination of ERT followed by a brachytherapy boost to deliver a total tumor dose of at least 6,000 cGy. Women with low-volume disease limited to the pelvis have the best outcome. For patients with isolated vaginal recurrence treated with radiation, reported 5-year survival rates range from 24% to 45%. The reclamation rate was 81% in one multi-institutional series that was limited to stage I patients with isolated vaginal failures (357). Conversely, for those patients who undergo radiation for the pelvic extension of their disease, lower survival rates (0% to 26%) are reported. Factors associated with improved survival and control of pelvic disease in patients with locally recurrent endometrial cancer include initial endometrial cancer grade 1, younger age at recurrence, recurrent tumor size 2 cm or less, time from initial treatment to recurrence of more than 1 year, vaginal versus pelvic disease, and use of vaginal brachytherapy.

Hormonal Therapy

The use of progestational agents for treatment of metastatic endometrial cancer was first described in 1961 when researchers observed an objective response rate of 29% in 21 patients (358). In a report from 1974, a beneficial response was observed in 35% of 308 patients (359). Subsequent reports noted somewhat less optimistic response rates, probably as a result of more strictly applied criteria for objective responses (359–362) (Table 35.12). Reports from Roswell Park Cancer Center and the Mayo Clinic observed objective response rates of 16% and 11%, respectively, with an additional 15% to 40% of patients exhibiting stable disease for at least 3 months (358,363). In 1986, the **GOG reported on the use of oral *medroxyprogesterone acetate* for treatment of patients with advanced or recurrent endometrial cancer** (361). **Of 219 patients with measurable disease, 8% had a complete response, 6% had a partial response, 52% had stable disease, and 34% developed progressive disease within 1 month.** The mean survival time for the entire group was 10.4 months. In a follow-up study comparing

Table 35.12 Response to Progestin Therapy in Advanced or Recurrent Endometrial Cancer

Author (Ref.)		Progestin	No. of Patients	Response Rate (%)
Piver et al. (365)	HPC	1,000 mg/week IM	51	14
	MPA	1,000 mg/week IM	37	19
Podratz et al. (366)	HPC	1–3 g/week IM	33	9
	MA	320 mg/day PO	81	11
Thigpen et al. (367,368)	MPA	150 mg/day PO	219	14
		200 mg/day PO	138	26
		1,000 mg/day PO	140	18

HPC, hydroxyprogesterone caproate (Delalutin); MPA, medroxyprogesterone acetate (Provera, Depo-Provera); MA, megestrol acetate (Megace); IM, intramuscular; PO, oral.

two different doses of oral *medroxyprogesterone acetate,* similar response rates were achieved (26% for 200 mg per day and 18% for 1,000 mg per day) (362). The type, dosage, and route of administration of the *progestin* seemed to have no effect on response in these studies.

The response of metastatic endometrial carcinoma to *progestin* therapy is related to several clinical and pathologic factors. **Higher response rates are observed in well-differentiated tumors.** A 20.5% response in low-grade tumors and only 1.4% response in high-grade tumors are noted (360). Likewise, the probability of an objective response to *progestin* therapy is about 70% for tumors that are estrogen- and progesterone-receptor positive, compared with about 5% to 15% for tumors that are negative for both receptors. A longer disease-free interval is associated with higher response rates to *progestins.* The response rate to *progestins* ranged from 6% in patients with an interval from primary treatment to recurrence of less than 6 months to 65% in patients in whom disease recurred more than 5 years after initial treatment (359). Other observed but less well-documented factors that may have an adverse effect on response to *progestins* are disease recurrence within a prior radiation field, large tumor burden, and advanced primary versus recurrent disease (360, 363).

A phase II investigation of the aromatase inhibitor *anastrozole* showed minimal activity in an unselected subset of patients with advanced or recurrent endometrial cancer (364).

Tamoxifen, a nonsteroidal antiestrogen with some estrogenic properties, was evaluated for treatment of metastatic endometrial carcinoma based on experience in using this agent in breast cancer treatment. Its use as either a single agent or in combination with a *progestin* is related to its ability to inhibit the binding of *estradiol* to the estrogen receptor and to increase progesterone-receptor expression. **In a review of eight studies using *tamoxifen,* 20 to 40 mg per day, in patients with metastatic endometrial carcinoma, the overall response rate was 22%, with a range of 0% to 53% (365). Responses to *tamoxifen* were more likely to be observed in patients with low-grade, hormone receptor–positive tumors who had a prior response to *progestin* therapy.** In an attempt to reverse the hormone receptor down-regulation seen with *progestin* therapy, *tamoxifen* was given along with *progestins,* but the overall responses to combined *tamoxifen* and *progestin* therapy were similar to those noted for single-agent *progestin* therapy.

***Progestins* are recommended as initial treatment for all patients with recurrent endometrioid tumors with hormone receptor–positive tumors.** Radiation therapy, surgery, or both should be used whenever feasible for treatment of localized recurrent cancer such as vaginal, pelvic, bone, and peripheral lymph node disease; however, these patients should also be given long-term *progestin* therapy unless they are known to have a progesterone-receptor–negative tumor. Patients with nonlocalized recurrent tumors, especially if progesterone receptors are known to be positive, are candidates for *progestin* therapy, either *megestrol acetate,* 80 mg twice daily, or *medroxyprogesterone acetate,* 50 to 100 mg three times daily. *Progestin* therapy should be continued for at least 2 to 3 months before assessing response. **If a response is obtained, the *progestin* should be continued for as long as the disease is static or in remission. In the presence of a relative contraindication to high-dose *progestin* therapy (e.g., prior or current thromboembolic disease, severe heart disease, or inability of the patient to tolerate progestin therapy), *tamoxifen,* **20 mg twice daily, is recommended.** Failure to respond to hormonal therapy is an indication for initiating chemotherapy.

Chemotherapy

Several chemotherapeutic agents or combinations of agents are capable of inducing objective responses and even remissions in patients with metastatic endometrial carcinoma, but all cytotoxic therapy should be considered palliative because response and survival times are short (365–368). The most active chemotherapeutic agents are *doxorubicin,* the *platinum* compounds *cisplatin* and *carboplatin,* and *paclitaxel* (Taxol). *Doxorubicin,* 50 to 60 mg/m^2 every 3 weeks (366–368); *cisplatin,* 60 to 75 mg/m^2 every 3 weeks; and *carboplatin,* 350 to 400 mg/m^2 every 4 weeks are associated with response rates of 21% to 29%. *Paclitaxel,* 250 mg/m^2 as a 24-hour infusion with granulocyte colony-stimulating factor support, or 175 mg/m^2 as a 3-hour infusion every 3 weeks, produced response rates of about 36% (369–371). Alkylating agents such as *cyclophosphamide* and *melphalan, 5-fluorouracil, altretamine* (*hexamethylmelamine*), *liposomal doxorubicin,* and *topotecan* show activity against endometrial cancer (371–374). Most responses obtained with use of these agents were partial, averaging only 3 to 6 months, with the median survival time ranging from 4 to 8 months.

Combination chemotherapy regimens employing *doxorubicin* and *cisplatin*; *cyclophosphamide, doxorubicin,* and *cisplatin*; *paclitaxel* and *cisplatin* with or without *doxorubicin*; and *carboplatin* and *paclitaxel* resulted in response rates ranging from 38% to 76% (375–390). Despite these fairly impressive response rates, most responses are partial, with durations of 4 to 8 months, and the median survival time is less than 12 months.

Response to chemotherapy in patients with metastatic endometrial cancer does not appear to be affected by prior or concurrent *progestin* therapy. Metastatic site, age, disease-free interval, histology, and tumor grade appear to have no effect on chemotherapy response. Patients with long disease-free intervals and better performance status may live longer.

Treatment Results

Comprehensive survival data for endometrial cancer are provided by the FIGO (391). Survival in relation to the old clinical and surgical stage is shown in Table 35.13 and in relation to surgical stage and grade in Table 35.14. **The overall 5-year survival rate was 76%. Patients who underwent surgical staging had much better 5-year survival rates than those staged clinically across all stages** (respectively): stage I, 87% versus 54%; stage II, 76% versus 41%; stage III, 57% versus 23%; stage IV, 18% versus 12%. Survival in surgical stage I disease ranged from more than 90% for patients with grade 1 and 2 tumors without myometrial invasion to 63% for stage IB grade 3.

Table 35.13 Carcinoma of the Endometrium: Stage Distribution and Actuarial Survival by Stage (Surgical and Clinical)

Stage	Patients Treated		Survival	
	N	Percent	3-Year	5-Year
Surgical				
I	3,996	70	92	87
II	709	12	82	76
III	758	13	66	59
IV	231	4	23	18
Clinical				
I	232	61	63	54
II	64	16	53	41
III	54	14	30	23
IV	33	8	12	12
Total	6,260	100	82	76

Adapted from **Creasman WT, Odicino F, Maisonneuve P, et al.** Carcinoma of the corpus uteri. FIGO Annual Report on the results of treatment in gynecological cancer. *J Epidemiol Biostat* 2001;6:45–86, with permission.

Table 35.14 Surgically Staged Endometrial Cancer: Actuarial 5-Year Survival Rate (%) by Histologic Grade and Stage (1988 staging criteria)

Stage	Grade		
	1	2	3
Ia	93	90	69
Ib	90	93	84
Ic	89	81	63
IIa	91	78	57
IIb	78	75	58
IIIa	79	69	44
IIIb	77	40	21
IIIc	61	61	44
IVa	—	—	19
IVb	35	27	7

Adapted from **Creasman WT, Odicino F, Maisonneuve P, et al.** Carcinoma of the corpus uteri. FIGO Annual Report on the results of treatment in gynecological cancer. *J Epidemiol Biostat* 2001;6:45–86, with permission.

Follow-Up after Treatment

History and physical examination remain the most effective methods of follow-up in patients treated for endometrial cancer (392–394). Patients should be examined every 3 to 4 months during the first 2 years and every 6 months thereafter. About one-half of patients discovered to have recurrent cancer have symptoms, and 75% to 80% of recurrences are detected initially on physical examination. Particular attention should be given to peripheral lymph nodes, the abdomen, and the pelvis. Very few asymptomatic recurrences are detected by vaginal cytology.

Chest x-ray every 12 months is an important method of posttreatment surveillance. **Almost one-half of all asymptomatic recurrences are detected by chest x-ray.** Other radiologic studies, such as CT scans, are not indicated for routine follow-up of patients who do not have symptoms.

Serum CA125 measurement was suggested for posttreatment surveillance of endometrial cancer (392–394). Elevated CA125 levels were documented in patients with recurrent tumor, and these levels correlated with the clinical course of disease. However, CA125 levels may be normal in the presence of small recurrences, making the utility of CA125 measurements for follow-up of patients after treatment of early-stage disease suspect. Determinations of CA125 should be obtained in patients with elevated levels at the time of diagnosis or with known extrauterine disease.

Ovarian Preservation and Estrogen Replacement

Twenty-five percent of women with endometrial cancer are premenopausal and 5% are under the age of 40, indicating that interest in ovarian preservation or postoperative *estrogen* replacement is not uncommon (395). Isolated investigations suggest that premenopausal women have a much higher likelihood (23%) of a synchronous ovarian cancer (396). If both ovaries appear grossly normal, the risk of adnexal malignancy decreases to less than 1% (397).Careful inspection of the adnexa is imperative when ovarian preservation is considered (23,396–398).

Most endometrial cancers are associated with excess estrogen exposure, calling into question the appropriateness of *estrogen* therapy for premenopausal patients with endometrial cancer following hysterectomy and bilateral salpingo-oophorectomy. In 1986, Creasman et al. and others reported that *estrogen* therapy appeared safe with no documented increase in the risk of recurrence following surgical treatment for endometrial carcinoma (397,399,400). Some investigations reported higher intercurrent death rates, such as from myocardial infarction, in the group in which *estrogen* was withheld (397,401). A randomized, double-blind, placebo-controlled study was designed to determine whether *estrogen* replacement increased rates of disease recurrence in women with stage I or II endometrial cancer. This investigation closed early because of a fall off in accrual after the findings of the Women's Health Initiative were made public in 2002. At the time of closure, the enrollment of over 1,200 patients in the study was insufficient, given the exceptionally low recurrence rate is this low-risk group (399). Although the safety of *estrogen* therapy in patients with endometrial cancer was not verified with level 1evidence, this investigation provided sufficient reassurance to justify the practice of offering *estrogen* therapy to patients with low-grade, FIGO 2009 stage IA disease in the absence of other contraindications. The American College of Obstetricians and Gynecologists issued a committee opinion recommending that providers should take into consideration prognostic indicators such as depth of invasion, grade, and stage when deciding to administer *estrogen* therapy to these patients (402).

For women who decline systemic *estrogen* replacement, symptoms of vaginal dryness and dyspareunia may be judiciously treated with **topical *estrogen* alone. Symptomatic relief of hot flashes can be achieved by prescribing *progestins* such a *medroxyprogesterone acetate*, 10 mg orally daily or 150 mg intramuscularly every 3 months, or nonhormonal agents such as *Bellergal, clonidine,* and *venlafaxine.***

Uterine Sarcoma

Uterine sarcomas are relatively rare tumors of mesodermal origin. They constitute 2% to 6% of uterine malignancies (403–405). There is an increased incidence of uterine sarcomas after radiation therapy to the pelvis for either carcinoma of the cervix or a benign condition. The relative risk of uterine sarcoma after pelvic radiotherapy is estimated to be 5.38, with an interval of 10 to 20 years (405). Uterine sarcomas are, in general, the most malignant group of uterine tumors and differ from endometrial cancers with regard to diagnosis, clinical behavior, pattern of spread, and management.

Classification and Staging

The three most common histologic variants of uterine sarcoma are endometrial stromal sarcoma (ESS), leiomyosarcoma, and carcinosarcoma (malignant mixed müllerian tumor, or MMMT) of both homologous and heterologous type (406) (Table 35.15). Variations in the relative incidences of uterine sarcomas occur in published series, probably related to the strictness of criteria used to classify smooth muscle and endometrial stromal tumors as sarcomas. Leiomyosarcoma and carcinosarcoma each constitute approximately 40% of tumors, with carcinosarcoma predominating in more recent reports, followed by ESS (15%) and other sarcomas (5%).

Staging

Staging of uterine sarcomas is based on the FIGO system (Table 35.16).

Endometrial Stromal Tumors

Stromal tumors occur primarily in perimenopausal women between ages 45 and 50 years; about one-third occurs in postmenopausal women. There is no relationship to parity, associated diseases, or prior pelvic radiotherapy. These tumors are rare in African-American women. The most frequent symptom is abnormal uterine bleeding; abdominal pain and pressure caused by an enlarging pelvic mass occur less often, and some patients do not have symptoms. Pelvic examination usually reveals regular or irregular uterine enlargement, sometimes associated with rubbery parametrial induration. The diagnosis may be determined by endometrial biopsy, but the usual preoperative diagnosis is uterine leiomyoma. At surgery, the diagnosis is suggested by the presence of an enlarged uterus filled with soft, gray-white to yellow necrotic and hemorrhagic tumors with bulging surfaces associated with wormlike elastic extensions into the pelvic veins.

Endometrial stromal tumors are composed purely of cells resembling normal endometrial stroma. They are divided into three types on the basis of mitotic activity, vascular invasion, and observed differences in prognosis: (i) endometrial stromal nodule, (ii) endometrial stromal sarcoma, and (iii) high-grade or undifferentiated sarcoma.

Endometrial stromal nodule **is an expansive, noninfiltrating, solitary lesion confined to the uterus with pushing margins, no lymphatic or vascular invasion, and usually less than 5 mitotic figures per 10 high-power microscopic fields (5 MF/10 HPF).** These tumors should be considered benign because there are no recurrences or tumor-associated deaths reported after surgery (406,407).

Table 35.15 Classifications of Uterine Sarcomas

I. Pure nonepithelial tumors

  A. Homologous

    1. Endometrial stromal tumors

      a. Low-grade stromal sarcoma

      b. High-grade or undifferentiated stromal sarcoma

    2. Smooth muscle tumors

      a. Leiomyosarcoma

      b. Leiomyoma variants

        1. Cellular leiomyoma

        2. Leiomyoblastoma (epithelioid leiomyoma)

      c. Benign metastasizing tumors

        1. Intravenous leiomyomatosis

        2. Benign metastasizing leiomyoma

        3. Disseminated peritoneal leiomyomatosis

  B. Heterologous

    1. Rhabdomyosarcoma

    2. Chondrosarcoma

    3. Osteosarcoma

    4. Liposarcoma

II. Mixed epithelial–nonepithelial tumors

  A. Malignant mixed müllerian tumor

    1. Homologous (carcinosarcoma)

    2. Heterologous

  B. Adenosarcoma

Modified from **Clement P, Scully RE.** Pathology of uterine sarcomas. In: **Coppleson M, ed.** *Gynecologic oncology: principles and practice.* New York: Churchill-Livingston, 1981, with permission.

Endometrial stromal sarcoma **(formerly termed low-grade ESS or endolymphatic stromal myosis) is distinguished from high-grade ESS or undifferentiated endometrial sarcoma microscopically by a mitotic rate of less than 10 MF/10 HPF and a more protracted clinical course.** Recurrences typically occur late, and local recurrence is more common than distant metastases (408–412). Although endometrial stromal sarcoma often behaves in a histologically aggressive fashion, it lacks the aneuploid DNA content and high proliferative index associated with high-grade stromal sarcoma. Flow cytometric analysis can be used to differentiate the two conditions and predict response to therapy.

Endometrial stromal sarcoma extends beyond the uterus in 40% of cases at the time of diagnosis, but the extrauterine spread is confined to the pelvis in two-thirds of the cases. Upper-abdominal, pulmonary, and lymph node metastases are uncommon. Recurrence occurs in almost one-half of cases at an average interval of 5 years after initial therapy. Prolonged survival and cure are common even after the development of recurrent or metastatic disease.

Optimum initial therapy for patients with endometrial stromal sarcoma consists of surgical excision of all grossly detectable tumor. Total abdominal hysterectomy and bilateral salpingo-oophorectomy should be performed. The adnexa should always be removed because of the propensity for tumor extension into the parametria, broad ligaments, and adnexal structures, and the possible estrogen-stimulating effect on the tumor cells if ovaries are retained. A beneficial effect of radiation therapy is reported, and pelvic radiation is recommended for

Table 35.16 Staging for Uterine Sarcomas (Leiomyosarcomas, Endometrial Stromal Sarcomas, Adenosarcomas, and Carcinosarcomas) (2008)

(1) Leiomyosarcomas

Stage	Definition
Stage I	Tumor limited to uterus
IA	<5 cm
IB	>5 cm
Stage II	Tumor extends to the pelvis
IIA	Adnexal involvement
IIB	Tumor extends to extrauterine pelvic tissue
Stage III	Tumor invades abdominal tissues (not just protruding into the abdomen).
IIIA	One site
IIIB	> one site
IIIC	Metastasis to pelvic and/or para-aortic lymph nodes
Stage IV	
IVA	Tumor invades bladder and/or rectum
IVB	Distant metastasis

(2) Endometrial stromal sarcomas (ESS) and adenosarcomas*

Stage	Definition
Stage I	Tumor limited to uterus
IA	Tumor limited to endometrium/endocervix with no myometrial invasion
IB	Less than or equal to half myometrial invasion
IC	More than half myometrial invasion
Stage II	Tumor extends to the pelvis
IIA	Adnexal involvement
IIB	Tumor extends to extrauterine pelvic tissue
Stage III	Tumor invades abdominal tissues (not just protruding into the abdomen).
IIIA	One site
IIIB	> one site
IIIC	Metastasis to pelvic and/or para-aortic lymph nodes
Stage IV	
IVA	Tumor invades bladder and/or rectum
IVB	Distant metastasis

(3) Carcinosarcomas

Carcinosarcomas should be staged as carcinomas of the endometrium.

FIGO Committee on Gynecologic Oncology. FIGO staging for uterine sarcomas. *Int J Gynecol Obst* 2009;104:179.
*Note: Simultaneous tumors of the uterine corpus and ovary/pelvis in association with ovarian/pelvic endometriosis should be classified as independent primary tumors.

inadequately excised or locally recurrent pelvic disease (408). There is evidence that endometrial stromal sarcoma is hormone dependent or responsive. Objective responses to *progestin* therapy were reported in 48% of patients in one series (410). Recurrent or metastatic lesions may be amenable to surgical excision. Long-term survival and apparent cures were noted in patients with pulmonary metastases (413).

***High-grade ESS or undifferentiated endometrial sarcoma* is a highly malignant neoplasm. Histologically, it exhibits greater than 10 MF/10 HPF and often completely lacks recognizable stromal differentiation.** This tumor has a much more aggressive clinical course and poorer prognosis than endometrial stromal sarcoma (406,408,413–416). The 5-year disease-free survival is about 25%. Treatment of undifferentiated endometrial sarcoma should consist of total abdominal hysterectomy and bilateral salpingo-oophorectomy. The poor therapeutic results suggest that radiation therapy, chemotherapy, or both should be used in combination with surgery. These tumors, unlike endometrial stromal sarcoma, are not responsive to *progestin* therapy.

Uterine tumor resembling ovarian sex-cord tumor **(UTROSCT) is a rare variant of endometrial stromal sarcoma in which benign glands and epithelial cells are found.** Immunohistochemically, these tumors express cytokeratin, epithelial membrane antigen, vimentin, and smooth muscle actin. Although some of these tumors have infiltrative margins, almost all of them behave benignly. The so-called mixed UTROSCT have a significant endometrial stromal sarcoma component and tend to behave more aggressively (417,418).

Leiomyosarcoma

The median age for women with leiomyosarcoma (43 to 53 years) is somewhat lower than for other uterine sarcomas, and premenopausal patients have a better chance of survival. This malignancy has no relationship with parity, and the incidence of associated diseases is not as high as in carcinosarcoma or endometrial adenocarcinoma. AfricanAmerican women have a higher incidence and a poorer prognosis than women of other races. A history of prior pelvic radiation therapy can be elicited in about 4% of patients with leiomyosarcoma. The incidence of sarcomatous change in benign uterine leiomyomas is reported to be between 0.13% and 0.81% (419–429).

Presenting symptoms, which are of short duration (mean, 6 months) and not specific to the disease, include vaginal bleeding, pelvic pain or pressure, and awareness of an abdominopelvic mass. The principal physical finding is the presence of a pelvic mass. The diagnosis should be suspected if severe pelvic pain accompanies a pelvic tumor, especially in a postmenopausal woman. Endometrial biopsy, although not as useful as in other sarcomas, may establish the diagnosis in as many as one-third of cases when the lesion is submucosal.

Survival rates for patients with uterine leiomyosarcoma range from 20% to 63% (mean, 47%). The pattern of tumor spread is to the myometrium, pelvic blood vessels and lymphatics, contiguous pelvic structures, abdomen, and then distantly, most often to the lungs. The number of mitoses in the tumor traditionally was the most reliable microscopic indicator of malignant behavior (Fig. 35.8).

Tumors with less than 5 MF/10 HPF behave in a benign fashion, and tumors with more than 10 MF/10 HPF are frankly malignant with a poor prognosis. Tumors with 5 to 10 MF/10 HPF, termed *cellular leiomyomas* **or** *smooth muscle tumors of uncertain malignant potential,* **are less predictable. In addition to mitotic index greater than 10, other histologic indicators used to classify uterine smooth muscle tumors as malignant are severe cytologic atypia and coagulative tumor cell necrosis** (430). Uterine smooth muscle tumors with any two of these three features are associated with a poor prognosis. Gross presentation of the tumor at the time of surgery is an important prognostic indicator. Tumors with infiltrating tumor margins or extension beyond the uterus are associated with poor prognosis, whereas tumors less than 5 cm, originating within myomas, or with pushing margins are associated with prolonged survival.

Five other clinical pathologic variants of uterine smooth muscle tumors deserve special comment: (i) myxoid leiomyosarcoma, (ii) leiomyoblastoma, (iii) intravenous leiomyomatosis, (iv) benign metastasizing uterine leiomyoma, and (v) disseminated peritoneal leiomyomatosis.

Myxoid leiomyosarcoma **is characterized grossly by a gelatinous appearance and apparent circumscribed border.** Microscopically, the tumors have a myxomatous stroma and extensively invade adjacent tissue and blood vessels (431). The mitotic rate is low (0 to 2 MF/10 HPF), which belies their aggressive behavior and poor prognosis. Surgical excision by hysterectomy is the mainstay of treatment. The low mitotic rate and abundance of intracellular myxomatous tissue suggest that these tumors would not be responsive to radiation therapy or chemotherapy.

Leiomyoblastoma **includes smooth muscle tumors designated as epithelioid leiomyomas, clear cell leiomyomas, and plexiform tumorlets** (432,433). This group of atypical smooth muscle tumors is distinguished by the predominance of rounded rather than spindle-shaped cells and by a clustered or cordlike pattern. These lesions should be regarded as specialized low-grade leiomyosarcomas with fewer than 5 MF/10 HPF. Leiomyoblastoma is treated with hysterectomy, and the prognosis is excellent.

Intravenous leiomyomatosis **is characterized by the growth of histologically benign smooth muscle into venous channels within the broad ligament and then into uterine and iliac veins** (434-437). The intravascular growth takes the form of visible, wormlike projections that extend

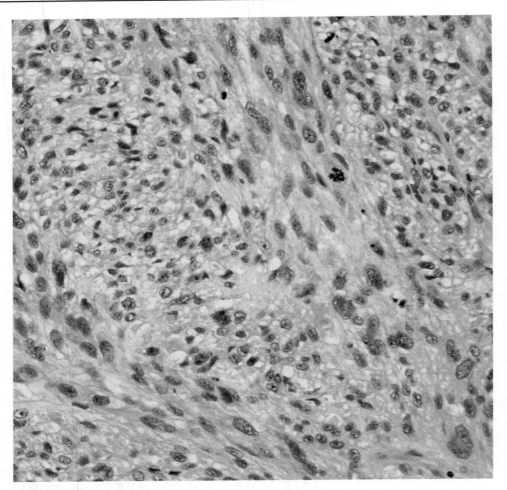

Figure 35.8   **Leiomyosarcoma of the uterus.** Interlacing bundles of spindle cells have fibrillar cytoplasm, irregular and hyperchromatic nuclei, and multiple mitotic figures. (Provided by Gordana Stevanovic, MD, and Jianyu Rao, MD, Department of Pathology, UCLA.)

out from a myomatous uterus into the parametria toward the pelvic sidewalls. It may be confused with low-grade stromal sarcoma. Symptoms are related to the associated uterine myomas. Most patients are in the late fifth and early sixth decades of life. The prognosis is excellent, even when tumor is left in pelvic vessels. Late local recurrences can occur, and deaths from extension into the inferior vena cava or metastases to the heart were reported. Estrogen may stimulate the proliferation of these intravascular tumors. Treatment should be total abdominal hysterectomy and bilateral salpingo-oophorectomy with removal of as much of the tumor as possible.

***Benign metastasizing uterine leiomyoma* is a rare condition in which a histologically benign uterine smooth muscle tumor acts in a somewhat malignant fashion and produces benign metastases, usually to the lungs or lymph nodes** (438). In most instances, intravenous leiomyomatosis is not apparent. The metastasizing myomas are capable of growth at distant sites, whereas the intravenous tumors spread only by direct extension within blood vessels. Both experimental and clinical evidence suggests that these tumors are stimulated by estrogen. Removing the source of estrogen, by castration or withdrawal of exogenous *estrogen,* or by treatment with *progestins, tamoxifen,* or a gonadotropin agonist, has an ameliorating effect (439). Surgical treatment should consist of total abdominal hysterectomy and bilateral salpingo-oophorectomy and resection of pulmonary metastases, if possible.

***Disseminated peritoneal leiomyomatosis* is a rare clinical entity characterized by benign smooth muscle nodules scattered throughout the peritoneal cavity** (440). This condition probably arises as a result of metaplasia of subperitoneal mesenchymal stem cells to smooth muscle, fibroblasts, myofibroblasts, and decidual cells under the influence of estrogen and progesterone. Most reported cases occurred in 30- to 40-year-old women who are or who recently were pregnant or who have a long history of oral contraceptive use. Intriguing features of this disease are its grossly malignant appearance, benign histology, and favorable clinical outcome. Intraoperative diagnosis requires frozen-section examination. Extirpative surgery, including total abdominal hysterectomy, bilateral salpingo-oophorectomy, omentectomy, and excision of as much gross disease as possible, may be indicated in menopausal women. Removal of the source of excess estrogen, treatment with *progestins,* or both resulted in regression of unresected tumor masses. Almost all patients have a good prognosis.

Carcinosarcoma

Carcinosarcoma is composed histologically of a mixture of sarcoma and carcinoma. The carcinomatous element is usually glandular, whereas the sarcomatous element may resemble the normal endometrial stroma (homologous or the so-called carcinosarcoma), or it may be composed of tissues foreign to the uterus, such as cartilage, bone, or striated muscle (heterologous). These tumors are most likely derived from totipotential endometrial stromal cells (441–444).

Almost all of these tumors occur after menopause, at a median age of 62 years. The incidence is higher in AfricanAmerican women. These tumors are often found in association with other medical conditions, such as obesity, diabetes mellitus, and hypertension. A history of previous pelvic radiation can be obtained in 7% to 37% of patients.

The most frequent presenting symptom is postmenopausal bleeding, which occurs in 80% to 90% of cases. Other less common symptoms are vaginal discharge, abdominal or pelvic pain, weight loss, and passage of tissue from the vagina. The duration of symptoms usually is only a few months. On physical examination, uterine enlargement is present in 50% to 95% of patients, and a polypoid mass may be seen within or protruding from the endocervical canal in up to 50% of patients. Diagnosis can usually be determined by biopsy of an endocervical mass or endometrial curettage.

The tumor grows as a large, soft, polypoid mass, filling and distending the uterine cavity; necrosis and hemorrhage are prominent features. The myometrium is invaded to various degrees in almost all cases. The most frequent areas of spread are the pelvis, lymph nodes, peritoneal cavity, lungs, and liver. This metastatic pattern suggests that these neoplasms spread by local extension and regional lymph node metastasis in a manner similar to that of endometrial adenocarcinoma, although they behave more aggressively.

The most important single factor affecting prognosis in patients with carcinosarcoma is the extent of tumor at the time of treatment. One study noted that in patients with tumor apparently confined to the uterine corpus (stage I), the 2-year survival rate was 53%, whereas the survival rate dropped to 8.5% when disease had extended to the cervix, vagina, or parametria (stage II and III); no patients with disease outside the pelvis (stage IV) survived (445). In another study, 5-year survival for patients with disease confined to the corpus (74%) was significantly greater than for those with more advanced disease (24%) (446).

Disease extends outside the uterus in 40% to 60% of cases at the time of diagnosis, indicating the highly malignant nature of this lesion. Even when disease is believed to be confined to the uterus preoperatively, surgical and pathologic staging identifies extrauterine spread of disease in a significant number of cases. In one study, 55% of women with clinical stage I carcinosarcoma had a higher surgical–pathologic stage. Only 28% of tumors were actually confined to the uterine corpus, 16% had extension to the cervix, and 56% showed extrauterine spread (447). In a significant number of patients, lymph node metastases and positive peritoneal cytology werefound with early-stage carcinosarcoma (446,448,449). Deep myometrial invasion, which is present in about one-half of stage I cases, is associated with poor prognosis. Almost all patients in whom tumor involves the outer one-half of the myometrium die from the disease. Patients who die from carcinosarcoma tend to have larger tumors and a higher incidence of LVSI. Patients with a history of prior pelvic radiation have a poorer prognosis. Overall, the 5-year survival rate for patients with carcinosarcoma is about 20% to 30%.

Adenosarcoma **is an uncommon variant of carcinosarcoma** (450,451). It consists of an admixture of benign-appearing neoplastic glands and a sarcomatous stroma. Most patients present with postmenopausal vaginal bleeding, and the disease is diagnosed or suspected based on endometrial curettage. Most adenosarcomas are well circumscribed and limited to the endometrium or superficial myometrium. The treatment is hysterectomy and bilateral salpingo-oophorectomy, with or without adjuvant radiotherapy. Because recurrences, mostly in the form of local pelvic or vaginal disease, are reported in 40% to 50% of cases, adjuvant postoperative intravaginal or pelvic radiation is recommended.

Treatment

Recurrences develop in more than one-half of cases of uterine sarcoma, even when disease is apparently localized at the time of treatment (452–454). At least one-half of recurrences occur outside the pelvis, with isolated pelvic failures accounting for less than 10% of recurrences. The most common sites of recurrence are the abdomen and lungs. These data emphasize that the major limitation to cure of uterine sarcomas is distant spread.

Based on this evidence, treatment of most stage I and II uterine sarcomas should include hysterectomy, bilateral salpingo-oophorectomy, and treatment of the pelvic lymphatics by radiation or surgery. Strong consideration should be given to the use of adjuvant chemotherapy to decrease the incidence of distant metastases. Stage III uterine sarcomas are probably best treated by an aggressive combined approach of surgery, radiation therapy, and chemotherapy, while patients with stage IV disease are candidates for combination chemotherapy.

Surgery

The first step in the treatment of early uterine sarcoma should be exploration. Because extirpative survey is the most important aspect of treatment, and knowledge of the extent and spread of the disease is important for further management, one should not forgo or delay surgery by using radiation therapy or chemotherapy first. At the time of surgery, the peritoneal cavity should be carefully explored and peritoneal washings obtained. Special attention should be given to the pelvic and para-aortic lymph nodes; lymphadenectomy should be performed with ESS and carcinosarcoma, but may be omitted in leiomyosarcoma, in which the risk of lymph node metastases is low and the therapeutic and diagnostic value is questionable (428). **Total abdominal hysterectomy is the standard procedure, and bilateral salpingo-oophorectomy should be performed in all patients except premenopausal women with leiomyosarcoma.** Based on the surgical and pathologic findings, additional therapy with radiation therapy or chemotherapy can be planned. Rarely, a patient may be cured by excision of an isolated pulmonary metastasis (455,456).

Radiation Therapy

Several studies showed that adjuvant preoperative or postoperative radiation therapy is beneficial in decreasing pelvic recurrences and increasing quality of life in patients with localized ESS and carcinosarcoma, but not with leiomyosarcoma (457–465). Radiation was not demonstrated to improve survival. One trial randomized patients with uterine sarcomas to pelvic radiotherapy versus observation. Althoughthe risk of local relapse significantly decreased from 24% to 14%, there was no difference in survival between groups (466). The GOG randomized patients to whole abdomen radiation versus three cycles of *cisplatin, ifosfamide,* and *mesna* in patients with less than 1 cm of residual disease (467). Whole-abdomen radiation was associated with significant toxicity and the chemotherapy regimen appeared to confer a nonsignificant survival advantage.

Chemotherapy

Several chemotherapeutic agents have activity in sarcomas, including *vincristine, actinomycin D, cyclophosphamide, doxorubicin, dimethyl triazeno imidazole carboxamide (dacarbazine, DTIC), cisplatin, ifosfamide paclitaxel, gemcitabine,* and *liposomal doxorubicin* (468). *Doxorubicin* appears to be the most active single agent in the treatment of leiomyosarcoma, producing a 25% response rate (469). *Ifosfamide* has a lesser degree of activity (470). *Cisplatin* and *ifosfamide* demonstrated clear activity in carcinosarcoma, with response rates of 18% to 42% and 32%, respectively (471–473). *Doxorubicin* demonstrated less than a 10% response rate in carcinosarcoma (469). *Paclitaxel* yielded an 18% response rate with carcinosarcoma, but had limited activity in leiomyosarcomas (474,475). *Gemcitabine* and *liposomaldoxorubicin* showed activity in leiomyosarcomas (476,477).

Combination chemotherapy with *doxorubicin* and *DTIC,* or these two drugs plus *vincristine* and *cyclophosphamide,* was yielded somewhat higher response rates (478–480). Similarly, *ifosfamide* was combined with *mesnauroprotection, doxorubicin,* and *DTIC* to treat metastatic pure sarcomas (481). ***Gemcitabine* combined with *docetaxel* for treatment of metastatic leiomyosarcoma yielded an overall response rate of 53%, including patients previously treated with *doxorubicin*** (482). Median time to progression was 5.6 months. Several retrospective investigations concluded that neither chemotherapy nor radiation impacts survival for patients with ESS or leiomyosarcoma (428,483,484).

Combined *ifosfamide* and *cisplatin* chemotherapy resulted in a higher response rate (54% versus 36%) and a longer progression-free survival than *ifosfamide* chemotherapy alone for treatment of advanced carcinosarcoma (485). Overall survival was unchanged (8 versus 9 months), and the combined regimen was significantly more toxic. A 3-day regimen of *ifosfamide* with or without *paclitaxel* in patients with advanced and recurrent carcinosarcoma demonstrated improved response rates (29% versus 45%) and median overall survival (8 versus 13 months) in the combination chemotherapy arm (486). This regimen appears to be the most efficacious for patients with advanced or recurrent carcinosarcoma. **A combination of *paclitaxel* and *carboplatin* for treatment of advanced uterine carcinosarcoma resulted in a complete response rate of 80% and a median progression-free interval of 18 months** (487). The GOG completed a phase II evaluation of *paclitaxel* and *carboplatin* with the results awaiting maturation. A randomized phase III evaluation of *paclitaxel* plus *carboplatin* versus *ifosfamide* plus *paclitaxel* in chemotherapy naive patients with carcinosarcoma is accruing.

Adjuvant Treatment

Because of the relatively low survival rate in localized uterine sarcomas and the high incidence of failure resulting from subsequent distant metastasis, adjuvant treatment programs employing chemotherapy were tested (487–490). **Most reports were unable to show a clear improvement in survival by the addition of postoperative adjuvant chemotherapy in early uterine sarcoma.** The GOG conducted a trial of postoperative adjuvant *doxorubicin* in stage I and II uterine sarcoma patients. Of the 75 patients randomized to receive *doxorubicin*, 41% developed a recurrence, compared with 53% of 81 patients receiving no adjuvant chemotherapy, but these differences were not significant (487). Other smaller, nonrandomized adjuvant chemotherapy studies employing *cyclophosphamide*, *cisplatin* plus *doxorubicin*, and *ifosfamide* plus *cisplatin* reported recurrence rates of 33%, 24%, and 31%, respectively (488–490).

References

1. **Siegel R, Ward E, Brawley O, et al.** Cancer statistics, 2011. *CA Cancer J Clin* 2011;61:212–236. http://cacancerjournal.org
2. **Bokhman JV.** Two pathogenetic types of endometrial carcinoma. *Gynecol Oncol* 1983;15:10–17.
3. **Lax SF.** Molecular genetic pathways in various types of endometrial carcinoma: from a phenotypical to a molecular-based classification. *Virchows Arch* 2004;444:213–223.
4. **MacMahon B.** Risk factors for endometrial cancer. *Gynecol Oncol* 1974;2:122–129.
5. **Parazzini F, LaVecchia C, Bocciolone L, et al.** The epidemiology of endometrial cancer. *Gynecol Oncol* 1991;41:1–16.
6. **Parazzini F, LaVecchia C, Negri E, et al.** Reproductive factors and risk of endometrial cancer. *Am J Obstet Gynecol* 1991;64:522–527.
7. **Brinton LA, Berman ML, Mortel R, et al.** Reproductive, menstrual and medical risk factors for endometrial cancer: results from a case control study. *Am J Obstet Gynecol* 1993;81:265–271.
8. **Grady D, Gebretsadik T, Kerlikowske K, et al.** Hormone replacement therapy and endometrial cancer risk: a meta-analysis. *Obstet Gynecol* 1995;85:304–313.
9. **Fisher B, Constantino JP, Redmond CK, et al.** Endometrial cancer in tamoxifen-treated breast cancer patients: findings from the National Surgical Adjuvant Breast and Bowel Project B-14. *J Natl Cancer Inst* 1994;86:527–537.
10. **Assikis VJ, Jordan VC.** Gynecologic effects of tamoxifen and the association with endometrial carcinoma. *Int J Gynaecol Obstet* 1995;49:241–257.
11. **Aarnio M, Sankila R, Pukkala E, et al.** Cancer risk in mutation carriers of DNA-mismatch-repair genes. *Int J Cancer* 1999;81:214–218.
12. **Gordon MD, Ireland K.** Pathology of hyperplasia and carcinoma of the endometrium. *Semin Oncol* 1994;21:64–70.
13. **Kurman RJ, Kaminski PF, Norris HJ.** The behavior of endometrial hyperplasia: a long term study of "untreated" hyperplasia in 170 patients. *Cancer* 1985;56:403–412.
14. **Tavassoli F, Kraus FT.** Endometrial lesions in uteri resected for atypical endometrial hyperplasia. *Am J Clin Pathol* 1978;70:770–779.
15. **Hunter JE, Tritz DE, Howell MG, et al.** The prognostic and therapeutic implications of cytologic atypia in patients with endometrial hyperplasia. *Gynecol Oncol* 1994;55:66–71.
16. **Trimble C, Kauderer J, Silverberg S, et al.** Concurrent endometrial carcinoma in women with biopsy diagnosis of atypical endometrial hyperplasia: a Gynecologic Oncology Group study. *Gynecol Oncol* 2004;92:393(abst).
17. **Ota T, Yoshida M, Kimura M, et al.** Clinicopathologic study of uterine endometrial carcinoma in young women aged 40 years and younger. *Int J Gynecol Cancer* 2005;15:657–662.
18. **Randall TC, Kurman RJ.** Progestin treatment of atypical hyperplasia and well-differentiated carcinoma of the endometrium in women under age 40. *Obstet Gynecol* 1997;90:434–440.
19. **Ben-Shachar I, Vitellas KM, Cohn DE.** The role of MRI in the conservative management of endometrial cancer. *Gynecol Oncol* 2004;93:233–237.
20. **Minderhoud-Bassie W, Treurniet FE, Koops W, et al.** Magnetic resonance imaging (MRI) in endometrial carcinoma; preoperative estimation of depth of myometrial invasion. *Acta Obstet Gynecol Scand* 1995;74:827–831.
21. **Nakao Y, Yokoyama M, Hara K, et al.** MR imaging in endometrial carcinoma as a diagnostic tool for the absence of myometrial invasion. *Gynecol Oncol* 2006;102:343–347.
22. **Lai CH, Huang HJ.** The role of hormones for the treatment of endometrial hyperplasia and endometrial cancer. *Curr Opin Obstet Gynecol* 2006;18:29–34.
23. **Shamshirsaz AA, Withiam-Leitch M, Odunsi K, et al.** Young patients with endometrial carcinoma selected for conservative treatment: a need for vigilance for synchronous ovarian carcinomas, case report and literature review. *Gynecol Oncol* 2007;104:757–760.
24. **Wildemeersch D, Dhont M.** Treatment of nonatypical and atypical endometrial hyperplasia with a levonorgestrel-releasing intrauterine system. *Am J Obstet Gynecol* 2003;188:1297–1298.
25. **Montz FJ, Bristow RE, Bovicelli A, et al.** Intrauterine progesterone treatment of early endometrial cancer. *Am J Obstet Gynecol* 2002;186:651–657.
26. **Giannopoulos T, Butler-Manuel S, Tailor A.** Levonorgestrel-releasing intrauterine system (LNG-IUS) as a therapy for endometrial carcinoma. *Gynecol Oncol* 2004;95:762–764.
27. **Huang S-Y, Jung S-M, Ng K-K, et al.** Ovarian metastasis in a nulliparous woman with endometrial adenocarcinoma failing conservative hormonal treatment. *Gynecol Oncol* 2005;97:652–655.

28. **Kaku T, Yoshikawa H, Tsuda H, et al.** Conservative therapy for adenocarcinoma and atypical endometrial hyperplasia of the endometrium in young women: central pathologic review and treatment outcome. *Cancer Lett* 2001;167:39–48.

29. **Dhar KK, Needhi-Rajan T, Koslowski M, et al.** Is levonorgestrel intrauterine system effective for treatment of early endometrial cancer? Report of four cases and review of the literature. *Gynecol Oncol* 2005;97:924–927.

30. **Ramirez PT, Frumovitz M, Bodurka DC, et al.** Hormonal therapy for the management of grade 1 endometrial adenocarcinoma: a literature review. *Gynecol Oncol* 2004;95:133–138.

31. **Koss LG, Schreiber K, Oberlander SG, et al.** Detection of endometrial carcinoma and hyperplasia in asymptomatic women. *Obstet Gynecol* 1984;64:1–11.

32. **Abayomi O, Dritschilo A, Emami B, et al.** The value of "routine tests" in the staging evaluation of gynecologic malignancies: a cost effective analysis. *Int J Radiat Oncol Biol Phys* 1982;8:241–244.

33. **Mettlin C, Jones G, Averette H, et al.** Defining and updating the American Cancer Society guidelines for the cancer-related checkup: prostate and endometrial cancers. *CA Cancer J Clin* 1993;43:42–46.

34. **Smith RA, Cokkinides V, von Eschenbach AC, et al.** American Cancer Society guidelines for the early detection of cancer. *CA Cancer J Clin* 2002;52:8–22.

35. **Gerber B, Krause A, Heiner M, et al.** Effects of adjuvant tamoxifen in postmenopausal women with breast cancer: a prospective long-term study using transvaginal ultrasound. *J Clin Oncol* 2000;18:3464–3470.

36. **Barakat RR, Gilewski TA, Almadrones L, et al.** Effect of adjuvant tamoxifen on the endometrium in women with breast cancer: a prospective study using office endometrial biopsy. *J Clin Oncol* 2000;18:3459–3463.

37. **Ollikainen M, Abdel-Rahman WM, Moisio A-L, et al.** Molecular analysis of familial endometrial carcinoma: a manifestation of hereditary nonpolyposis colorectal cancer or a separate syndrome? *J Clin Oncol* 2005;23:4609–4616.

38. **Parc YR, Halling KC, Burgart LJ, et al.** Microsatellite instability and hMLH1/hMSH2 expression in young endometrial carcinoma patients: associations with family history and histopathology. *Int J Cancer* 2000;86:60–66.

39. **Dunlop M, Farrington S, Carothers A, et al.** Cancer risk associated with germline DNA mismatch repair gene mutations. *Hum Mol Genet* 1997;6:105–110.

40. **Kunkel TA, Erie DA.** DNA mismatch repair. *Annu Rev Biochem* 2005;74:681–710.

41. **Marti TM, Kunz C, Fleck O.** DNA mismatch repair and mutation avoidance pathways. *J Cell Physiol* 2002;191:28–41.

42. **Boltenberg A, Furgyik S, Kullander S.** Familial cancer aggregation in cases of adenocarcinoma corporis uteri. *Acta Obstet Gynecol Scand* 1990;69:249–258.

43. **Vasen HFA, Watson P, Mecklin J-P, et al.** New clinical criteria for hereditary nonpolyposis colorectal cancer (HNPCC, Lynch syndrome) proposed by the International Collaborative Group on HNPCC. *Gastroenterology* 1999;116:1453–1456.

44. **Peltomaki P, Vasen HF.** The International Collaborative Group on Hereditary Nonpolyposis Colorectal Cancer. Mutations predisposing to hereditary nonpolyposis colorectal cancer: database and results of a collaborative study. *Gastroenterology* 1997;113:1146–1158.

45. **Miyaki M, Konishi M, Tanaka K, et al.** Germline mutation of MSH6 as the cause of hereditary nonpolyposis colorectal cancer. *Nat Genet* 1997;17:271–272.

46. **Akiyama Y, Sato H, Yamada T, et al.** Germ-line mutation of the hmSH6/GTPB gene in an atypical hereditary nonpolyposis colorectal cancer kindred. *Cancer Res* 1997;57:3920–3923.

47. **Hendriks YMC, Jagmohan-Changur S, van der Klift HM, et al.** Heterozygous mutations in PMS2 cause hereditary nonpolyposis colorectal carcinoma (Lynch syndrome). *Gastroenterology* 2006;130:312–322.

48. **Umar A, Boland CR, Terdiman JP, et al.** Revised Bethesda guidelines for hereditary nonpolyposis colorectal cancer (Lynch Syndrome) and microsatellite instability. *J Natl Cancer Inst* 2004;96:261–268.

49. **Lynch HT, Lynch JF.** The Lynch syndrome: melding natural history and molecular genetics to genetic counseling and cancer control. *Cancer Control* 1996;3:13–19.

50. **Renkonen-Sinisalo L, Bützow R, Leminen A, et al.** Surveillance for endometrial cancer in hereditary nonpolyposis colorectal cancer syndrome. *Int J Cancer* 2007;120:821–824.

51. **Schmeler KM, Lynch HT, Chen LM, et al.** Prophylactic surgery to reduce the risk of gynecologic cancers in the Lynch syndrome. *N Engl J Med* 2006;354:261–269.

52. **Lindor NM, Petersen GM, Hadley DW, et al.** Recommendations for the care of individuals with an inherited predisposition to Lynch syndrome: a systematic review. *JAMA* 2006;296:1507–1517.

53. **Vasen HFA, Moslein G, Alonso A, et al.** Guidelines for the clinical management of Lynch syndrome (HNPCC). *J Med Genet* 2007;44:353–362.

54. **Bertagnolli, Monica M.** Surgical prevention of cancer. *J Clin Oncol* 2005;23:324–332.

55. **Lynch HT, Watson P, Shaw TG, et al.** Clinical impact of molecular genetic diagnosis, genetic counseling, and management of hereditary cancer. *Cancer* 1999;86:2457–2463.

56. **Lynch HT, Krush AJ, Larsen AL, et al.** Endometrial carcinoma: multiple primary malignancies, constitutional factors, and heredity. *Am J Med Sci* 1966;252:381–390.

57. **Sandles LG, Shulman LP, Elias S, et al.** Endometrial adenocarcinoma: genetic analysis suggesting heritable site-specific uterine cancer. *Gynecol Oncol* 1992;47:167–171.

58. **Gruber S, Thompson W.** Cancer and Steroid Hormone Study Group. A population-based study of endometrial cancer and familial risk in younger women. *Cancer Epidemiol Biomarkers Prev* 1996;5:411–417.

59. **Sasco AJ.** Epidemiology of breast cancer: an environmental disease? *APMIS* 2001;109:321–332.

60. **MacMahon B, Cole P, Lin TM, et al.** Age at first birth and breast cancer risk. *Bull World Health Organ* 1970;43:209–221.

61. **Brinton LA, Berman ML, Mortel R, et al.** Reproductive, menstrual, and medical risk factors for endometrial cancer: results from a case-control study. *Am J Obstet Gynecol* 1992;167:1317–1325.

62. **Henderson BE, Casagrande JT, Pike MC, et al.** The epidemiology of endometrial cancer in young women. *Br J Cancer* 1983;47:749–756.

63. **Kazerouni N, Schairer C, Friedman HB, et al.** Family history of breast cancer as a determinant of the risk of developing endometrial cancer: a nationwide cohort study. *J Med Genet* 2002;39:826–832.

64. **Kelsey JL, LiVolsi VA, Holford TR, et al.** A case-control study of cancer of the endometrium. *Am J Epidemiol* 1982;116:333–342.

65. **Anderson DE, Badzioch MD.** Familial breast cancer risks. Effects of prostate and other cancers. *Cancer* 1993;72:114–119.

66. **Parazzini F, La Vecchia C, Negri E, et al.** Family history of breast, ovarian and endometrial cancer and risk of breast cancer. *Int J Epidemiol* 1993;22:614–618.

67. **Lynch HT, Krush AJ, Lemon HM, et al.** Tumor variation in families with breast cancer. *JAMA* 1972;222:1631–1635.

68. **Beiner ME, Finch A, Rosen B, et al.** The risk of endometrial cancer in women with BRCA1 and BRCA2 mutations: a prospective study. *Gynecol Oncol* 2007;104:7–10.

69. **Smith M, McCartney AJ.** Occult, high-risk endometrial carcinoma. *Gynecol Oncol* 1985;22:154–161.

70. **Dubeshter B, Warshal DP, Angel C, et al.** Endometrial carcinoma: the relevance of cervical cytology. *Obstet Gynecol* 1991;77:458–462.

71. **Choo YC, Mak KC, Hsu C, et al.** Postmenopausal uterine bleeding of nonorganic cause. *Obstet Gynecol* 1985;66:225–228.

72. **Pacheco JC, Kempers RD.** Etiology of postmenopausal bleeding. *Obstet Gynecol* 1968;32:40–46.

73. **Hawwa ZM, Nahhas WA, Copenhaver EH.** Postmenopausal bleeding. *Lahey Clin Found Bull* 1970;19:61–70.

74. **Lidor A, Ismajovich B, Confino E, et al.** Histopathological findings in 226 women with postmenopausal uterine bleeding. *Acta Obstet Gynecol Scand* 1986;65:41–43.

75. **Fortier KJ.** Postmenopausal bleeding and the endometrium. *Clin Obstet Gynecol* 1986;29:440–445.

76. **Chambers JT, Chambers SK.** Endometrial sampling: When? Where? Why? With what? *Clin Obstet Gynecol* 1992;35:28–39.

77. **Grimes DA.** Diagnostic dilation and curettage: a reappraisal. *Am J Obstet Gynecol* 1982;142:1–6.

78. **Kaunitz AM, Masciello A, Ostrowski M, et al.** Comparison of endometrial biopsy with the endometrial Pipelle and Vabra aspirator. *J Reprod Med* 1988;33:427–431.

79. **Dijkuizen FPHLJ, Mol BWJ, Brolmann HAM, et al.** The accuracy of endometrial sampling in the diagnosis of patients with endometrial carcinoma and hyperplasia: a meta-analysis. *Cancer* 2000;89:1765–1772.

80. **Zucker PK, Kasdon EJ, Feldstein ML.** The validity of Pap smear parameters as predictors of endometrial pathology in menopausal women. *Cancer* 1985;56:2256–2263.

81. **Stelmachow J.** The role of hysteroscopy in gynecologic oncology. *Gynecol Oncol* 1982;14:392–395.

82. **Gimpleson RJ, Rappold HO.** A comparative study between panoramic hysteroscopy with directed biopsies and dilation and curettage: a review of 276 cases. *Am J Obstet Gynecol* 1988;158:489–492.

83. **Clark TJ, Bakour SH, Gupta JK, et al.** Evaluation of outpatient hysteroscopy and ultrasonography in the diagnosis of endometrial disease. *Obstet Gynecol* 2002;99:1001–1007.

84. **Bourne TH, Campbell S, Steer CV, et al.** Detection of endometrial cancer by transvaginal sonography with color flow imaging and blood flow analysis: a preliminary report. *Gynecol Oncol* 1991;40:253–259.

85. **Granberg S, Wikland M, Karlsson B, et al.** Endometrial thickness as measured by endovaginal ultrasonography for identifying endometrial abnormality. *Am J Obstet Gynecol* 1991;164:47–52.

86. **Varner RE, Sparks JM, Cameron CD, et al.** Transvaginal sonography of the endometrium in postmenopausal women. *Obstet Gynecol* 1991;78:195–199.

87. **Karlsson B, Granberg S, Wikland M, et al.** Transvaginal ultrasonography of the endometrium in women with postmenopausal bleeding: a Nordic multicenter study. *Am J Obstet Gynecol* 1995;172:1488–1494.

88. **Tabor A, Watt HC, Wald NJ.** Endometrial thickness as a test for endometrial cancer in women with postmenopausal vaginal bleeding. *Obstet Gynecol* 1995;172:1488–1494.

89. **Silverberg SG, Kurman RJ.** Tumors of the uterine corpus and gestational trophoblastic disease (3rd series). Washington, DC: Armed Forces Institute of Pathology, 1992.

90. **Hendrickson MR, Ross JC, Kempson RL.** Toward the development of morphologic criteria for well differentiated adenocarcinoma of the endometrium. *Am J Surg Pathol* 1983;7:819–838.

91. **Norris HJ, Tavassoli FA, Kurman RJ.** Endometrial hyperplasia and carcinoma: diagnostic considerations. *Am J Surg Pathol* 1983;7:839–847.

92. **Zaino RJ, Kurman RJ.** Squamous differentiation in carcinoma of the endometrium: a critical appraisal of adenoacanthoma and adenosquamous carcinoma. *Semin Diagn Pathol* 1988;5:154–171.

93. **Zaino RJ, Kurman R, Herbold D, et al.** The significance of squamous differentiation in endometrial carcinoma. *Cancer* 1991;68:2293–2302.

94. **Chen JL, Trost DC, Wilkinson EJ.** Endometrial papillary adenocarcinomas: two clinicopathologic types. *Int J Gynecol Pathol* 1985;4:279–288.

95. **Sutton GP, Brill L, Michael H, et al.** Malignant papillary lesions of the endometrium. *Gynecol Oncol* 1987;27:294–304.

96. **Christophenson WM, Alberhasky RC, Connelly PJ.** Carcinoma of the endometrium: a clinicopathologic study of clear cell carcinoma and secretory carcinoma. *Cancer* 1982;49:1511–1523.

97. **Tobon H, Watkins GJ.** Secretory adenocarcinoma of the endometrium. *Int J Gynecol Pathol* 1985;4:328–335.

98. **Ross JC, Eifel PJ, Cox RS, et al.** Primary mucinous adenocarcinoma of the endometrium: a clinicopathologic and histochemical study. *Am J Surg Pathol* 1983;7:715–729.

99. **Melhern MF, Tobon H.** Mucinous adenocarcinoma of the endometrium: a clinico-pathologic review of 18 cases. *Int J Gynecol Pathol* 1987;6:347–355.

100. **Dabbs DJ, Geisinger KR, Norris HT.** Intermediate filaments in endometrial and endocervical carcinomas. *Am J Surg Pathol* 1986;10:568–576.

101. **Hendrickson M, Ross J, Eifel P, et al.** Uterine papillary serous carcinoma: a highly malignant form of endometrial adenocarcinoma. *Am J Surg Pathol* 1982;6:93–108.

102. **Silva EG, Jenkins R.** Serous carcinoma in endometrial polyps. *Mod Pathol* 1990;3:120–128.

103. **Sherman ME, Bitterman P, Rosenshein NB, et al.** Uterine serous carcinoma. *Am J Surg Pathol* 1992;16:600–610.

104. **Goff BA, Kato D, Schmidt RA, et al.** Uterine papillary serous carcinoma: patterns of metastatic spread. *Gynecol Oncol* 1994;54:264–268.

105. **Fader AN, Starks D, Gehrig PA, et al.** UPSC Consortium. An updated clinicopathologic study of early-stage uterine papillary serous carcinoma (UPSC). *Gynecol Oncol* 2009;115:244–248.

106. **Slomovitz BM, Burke TW, Eifel PJ, et al.** Uterine papillary serous carcinoma (UPSC): a single institution review of 129 cases. *Gynecol Oncol* 2003;91:463–469.

107. **Thomas MB, Mariani A, Cliby WA, et al.** Role of systematic lymphadenectomy and adjuvant therapy in stage I uterine papillary serous carcinoma. *Gynecol Oncol* 2007;107:186–189.

108. **Boruta DM 2nd, Gehrig PA, Fader AN, et al.** Management of women with uterine papillary serous cancer: a Society of Gynecologic Oncology (SGO) review. *Gynecol Oncol* 2009;115:142–153.

109. **Fakiris AJ, Moore DH, Reddy SR, et al.** Intraperitoneal radioactive phosphorus (32P) and vaginal brachytherapy as adjuvant treatment for uterine papillary serous carcinoma and clear cell carcinoma: a phase II Hoosier Oncology Group (HOG 97-01) study. *Gynecol Oncol* 2005;96:818–823.

110. **Thomas MB, Mariani A, Cliby WA, et al.** Role of cytoreduction in stage III and IV uterine papillary serous carcinoma. *Gynecol Oncol* 2007;107:190–193.

111. **Homesley HD, Filiaci V, Gibbons SK, et al.** A randomized phase III trial in advanced endometrial carcinoma of surgery and volume directed radiation followed by cisplatin and doxorubicin with or without paclitaxel: a Gynecologic Oncology Group study. *Gynecol Oncol* 2009;112:543–552.

112. **Secord AA, Havrilesky LJ, O Malley DM, et al.** A multicenter evaluation of sequential multimodality therapy and clinical outcome for the treatment of advanced endometrial cancer. *Gynecol Oncol* 2009;112:S12.

113. **Abeler VM, Kjorstad KE.** Clear cell carcinoma of the endometrium: a histopathologic and clinical study of 97 cases. *Gynecol Oncol* 1991;40:207–217.

114. **Abeler VM, Vergote IB, Kjorstad KE, et al.** Clear cell carcinoma of the endometrium: prognosis and metastatic pattern. *Cancer* 1996;78:1740–1747.

115. **Thomas MB, Wright JD, Leiser AL, et al.** Clear cell carcinoma of the cervix: a multi-institutional review in the post-DES era. *Gynecol Oncol* 2008;109:335–339.

116. **Olawaiye AB, Boruta DM 2nd.** Management of women with clear cell endometrial cancer: a Society of Gynecologic Oncology (SGO) review. *Gynecol Oncol* 2009;113:277–283.

117. **Abeler VM, Kjorstad KE.** Endometrial squamous cell carcinoma: report of three cases and review of the literature. *Gynecol Oncol* 1990;36:321–326.

118. **Eifel P, Hendrickson M, Ross J, et al.** Simultaneous presentation of carcinoma involving the ovary and the uterine corpus. *Cancer* 1982;50:163–170.

119. **Zaino RJ, Unger ER, Whitney C.** Synchronous carcinomas of the uterine corpus and ovary. *Gynecol Oncol* 1984;19:329–335.

120. **Eisner RF, Nieberg RK, Berek JS.** Synchronous primary neoplasms of the female reproductive tract. *Gynecol Oncol* 1989;33:335–339.

121. **Kline RC, Wharton JT, Atkinson EN, et al.** Endometrioid carcinoma of the ovary: retrospective review of 145 cases. *Gynecol Oncol* 1990;39:337–346.

122. **Prat J, Matias-Guiu X, Barreto J.** Simultaneous carcinoma involving the endometrium and the ovary. *Cancer* 1991;68:2455–2459.

123. **Zerbe MJ, Bristow R, Crumbine FC, et al.** Inability of preoperative computed tomography scans to accurately predict the extent of myometrial invasion and extracorporeal spread in endometrial cancer. *Gynecol Oncol* 2000;78:67–70.

124. **Gordon AN, Fleischer AC, Dudley BS, et al.** Preoperative assessment of myometrial invasion of endometrial adenocarcinoma by sonography (US) and magnetic resonance imaging (MRI). *Gynecol Oncol* 1989;34:175–179.

125. **Niloff JM, Klug TL, Schaetzl E, et al.** Elevation of serum CA125 in carcinoma of the fallopian tube, endometrium, and endocervix. *Am J Obstet Gynecol* 1984;148:1057–1058.

126. **Patsner B, Mann WJ, Cohen H, et al.** Predictive value of preoperative serum CA 125 levels in clinically localized and advanced endometrial carcinoma. *Am J Obstet Gynecol* 1988;158:399–402.

127. **Hsieh CH, Chang Chien CC, Lin H, et al.** Can a preoperative CA-125 level be a criterion for full pelvic lymphadenectomy in surgical staging of endometrial cancer? *Gynecol Oncol* 2002;86:28–33.

128. **Dotters DJ.** Preoperative CA125 in endometrial cancer: is it useful? *Am J Obstet Gynecol* 2000;182:1328–1334.

129. **Jhang H, Chuang L, Visintainer P, et al.** CA125 levels in the preoperative assessment of advanced-stage uterine cancer. *Am J Obstet Gynecol* 2003;188:1195–1197.

130. **Inter Federation of Obstetrics and Gynecolo7y (FIGO).** Classification and staging of malignant tumors in the female pelvis. *Int J Gynecol Obstet* 1971;9:172–180.

131. **Marziale P, Atlante G, Pozzi M, et al.** 426 Cases of stage I endometrial carcinoma: a clinicopathologic analysis. *Gynecol Oncol* 1989;32:278–281.

132. **Morrow CP, Bundy BN, Kurman RJ, et al.** Relationship between surgical-pathological risk factors and outcome in clinical stage I and II carcinoma of the endometrium: a Gynecologic Oncology Group study. *Gynecol Oncol* 1991;40:55–65.

133. **Rotman M, Aziz H, Halpern J, et al.** Endometrial carcinoma. Influence of prognostic factors on radiation management. *Cancer* 1993;71:1471–1479.

134. **Amant F, Moerman P, Neven P, et al.** Endometrial cancer. *Lancet* 2005;366:491–505.

135. **Creutzberg CL, van Putten WL, Koper PC, et al.** PORTEC Study Group. Postoperative radiation therapy in endometrial carcinoma. Surgery and postoperative radiotherapy versus surgery alone for patients with stage-1 endometrial carcinoma: multicentre randomised trial. *Lancet* 2000;355:1404–1411.

136. **Creutzberg CL, van Putten WL, Wárlám-Rodenhuis CC, et al.** Outcome of high-risk stage IC, grade 3, compared with stage I endometrial carcinoma patients: the Postoperative Radiation Therapy in Endometrial Carcinoma Trial. *J Clin Oncol* 2004;22:1234–1241.

137. **Mariani A, Webb MJ, Keeney GL, et al.** Low-risk corpus cancer: is lymphadenectomy or radiotherapy necessary? *Am J Obstet Gynecol* 2000;182:1506–1519.

138. **Benedetti Panici P, Basile S, Maneschi F, et al.** Systematic pelvic lymphadenectomy vs no lymphadenectomy in early-stage endometrial carcinoma: randomized clinical trial. *J Natl Cancer Inst* 2008;100:1707–1716.

139. **Kitchener H, Swart AM, Qian Q, et al.** ASTEC Study Group. Efficacy of systematic pelvic lymphadenectomy in endometrial cancer (MRC ASTEC trial): a randomised study. *Lancet* 2009;373:125–136.

140. **Mariani A, Dowdy SC, Cliby WA, et al.** Prospective assessment of lymphatic dissemination in endometrial cancer: a paradigm shift in surgical staging. *Gynecol Oncol* 2008;109:11–18.

141. **Creasman WT, Morrow CP, Bundy BN, et al.** Surgical pathologic spread patterns of endometrial cancer: a Gynecologic Oncology Group Study. *Cancer* 1987;60:2035–2041.

142. **Schink JC, Lurain JR, Wallemark CB, et al.** Tumor size in endometrial cancer: a prognostic factor for lymph node metastasis. *Obstet Gynecol* 1987;70:216–219.

143. **Todo Y, Kato H, Kaneuchi M, et al.** Survival effect of para-aortic lymphadenectomy in endometrial cancer (SEPAL study): a retrospective cohort analysis. *Lancet* 2010;375:1165–1172.

144. **Pecorelli S.** Revised FIGO staging for carcinoma of the vulva, cervix, and endometrium. *Int J Gynecol Obstet* 2009;105:103–104.

145. **Christopherson WM, Connelly PJ, Aberhasky RC.** Carcinoma of the endometrium: an analysis of prognosticators in patients with favorable subtypes and stage II disease. *Cancer* 1983;51:1705–1709.

146. **Crissman JD, Azoury RS, Banner AE, et al.** Endometrial carcinoma in women 40 years of age or younger. *Obstet Gynecol* 1981;57:699–704.

147. **Nilson PA, Koller O.** Carcinoma of the endometrium in Norway 1957–1960 with special reference to treatment results. *Am J Obstet Gynecol* 1969;105:1099–1109.

148. **Zaino RJ, Kurman RJ, Diana KL, et al.** Pathologic models to predict outcome for women with endometrial adenocarcinoma. *Cancer* 1996;77:1115–1121.

149. **Lurain JR, Rice BL, Rademaker AW, et al.** Prognostic factors associated with recurrence in clinical stage I adenocarcinoma of the endometrium. *Obstet Gynecol* 1991;78:63–69.

150. **Wilson TO, Podratz KC, Gaffey TA, et al.** Evaluation of unfavorable histologic subtypes in endometrial adenocarcinoma. *Am J Obstet Gynecol* 1990;162:418–426.

151. **Fanning J, Evans MC, Peters AJ, et al.** Endometrial adenocarcinoma histologic subtypes: clinical and pathologic profile. *Gynecol Oncol* 1989;32:288–291.

152. **DiSaia PJ, Creasman WT, Boronow RC, et al.** Risk factors and recurrent patterns in stage I endometrial cancer. *Am J Obstet Gynecol* 1985;151:1009–1015.

153. **Sutton GP, Geisler HE, Stehman FB, et al.** Features associated with survival and disease-free survival in early endometrial cancer. *Am J Obstet Gynecol* 1989;160:1385–1393.

154. **Bucy GS, Mendenhall WM, Morgan LS, et al.** Clinical stage I and II endometrial carcinoma treated with surgery and/or radiation therapy: analysis of prognostic and treatment related factors. *Gynecol Oncol* 1989;33:290–295.

155. **Kadar N, Malfetano JH, Homesley HD.** Determinants of survival of surgically staged patients with endometrial carcinoma histologically confined to the uterus: implications for therapy. *Obstet Gynecol* 1992;80:655–659.

156. **Aalders J, Abeler V, Kolstad P, et al.** Postoperative external irradiation and prognostic parameters in stage I endometrial carcinoma: clinical and histopathologic study of 540 patients. *Obstet Gynecol* 1980;56:419–427.

157. **Schink JC, Rademaker AW, Miller DS, et al.** Tumor size in endometrial cancer. *Cancer* 1991;67:2791–2794.

158. **Martin JD, Hahnel R, McCartney AJ, et al.** The effect of estrogen receptor status on survival in patients with endometrial cancer. *Am J Obstet Gynecol* 1983:147;322–324.

159. **Zaino RJ, Satyaswaroop PG, Mortel R.** The relationship of histologic and histochemical parameters to progesterone receptor status in endometrial adenocarcinomas. *Gynecol Oncol* 1983;16:196–208.

160. **Creasman WT, Soper JT, McCarty KS, et al.** Influence of cytoplasmic steroid receptor content on prognosis of early stage endometrial carcinoma. *Am J Obstet Gynecol* 1985;151:922–932.

161. **Liao BS, Twiggs LB, Leung BS, et al.** Cytoplasmic estrogen and progesterone receptors as prognostic parameters in primary endometrial carcinoma. *Obstet Gynecol* 1986;67:463–467.

162. **Geisinger KR, Homesley HD, Morgan TM, et al.** Endometrial adenocarcinoma: a multiparameter clinicopathologic analysis including the DNA profile and sex hormone receptors. *Cancer* 1986;58:1518–1525.

163. **Palmer DC, Muir IM, Alexander AI, et al.** The prognostic importance of steroid receptors in endometrial carcinoma.*Obstet Gynecol* 1988;72:388–393.

164. **Chambers JT, MacLusky N, Eisenfeld A, et al.** Estrogen and progestin receptor levels as prognosticators for survival in endometrial cancer. *Gynecol Oncol* 1988;31:65–81.

165. **Ambros RA, Kurman RJ.** Identification of patients with stage I uterine endometrioid adenocarcinoma at high risk of recurrence by DNA ploidy, myometrial invasion, and vascular invasion. *Gynecol Oncol* 1992;45:235–239.

166. **Iverson OE.** Flow cytometric deoxyribonucleic acid index: a prognostic factor in endometrial carcinoma. *Am J Obstet Gynecol* 1986;155:770–776.

167. **Newbury R, Schuerch C, Goodspeed N, et al.** DNA content as a prognostic factor in endometrial carcinoma. *Obstet Gynecol* 1990;76:251–257.

168. **Stendahl U, Strang P, Wegenius G, et al.** Prognostic significance of proliferation in endometrial adenocarcinomas: a multivariate analysis of clinical and flow cytometric variables. *Int J Gynecol Pathol* 1991;10:271–284.

169. **Ikeda M, Watanabe Y, Nanjoh T, et al.** Evaluation of DNA ploidy in endometrial cancer. *Gynecol Oncol* 1993;50:25–29.

170. **Podratz KC, Wilson TO, Gaffey TA, et al.** Deoxyribonucleic acid analysis facilitates the pretreatment identification of high-risk endometrial cancer patients. *Am J Obstet Gynecol* 1993;168:1206–1213.

171. **Friberg LG, Noren H, Delle U.** Prognostic value of DNA ploidy and S-phase fraction in endometrial cancer stage I and II: a prospective 5-year survival study. *Gynecol Oncol* 1994;53:64–69.

172. **Susini T, Rapi S, Savino L, et al.** Prognostic value of flow cytometric deoxyribonucleic acid index in endometrial carcinoma: comparison with other clinical-pathologic parameters. *Am J Obstet Gynecol* 1994;170:527–534.

173. Pisani AL, Barbuto DA, Chen D, et al. HER-2/neu, p53, and DNA analysis as prognosticators for survival in endometrial carcinoma. *Obstet Gynecol* 1995;85:729–734.

174. Zaino RJ, Davis ATL, Ohlsson-Wilhelm BM, et al. DNA content is an independent prognostic indicator in endometrial adenocarcinoma. *Int J Gynecol Pathol* 1998;17:312–319.

175. Boronow RC, Morrow CP, Creasman WT, et al. Surgical staging in endometrial cancer: clinical-pathologic findings of a prospective study. *Obstet Gynecol* 1984;63:825–883.

176. Mariani A, Webb MJ, Keeney GL, et al. Hematogenous dissemination in corpus cancer. *Gynecol Oncol* 2001;80:233–238.

177. Lutz MH, Underwood PB, Kreutner A Jr, et al. Endometrial carcinoma: a new method of classification of therapeutic and prognostic significance. *Gynecol Oncol* 1978;6:83–94.

178. Kaku T, Tsuruchi N, Tsukamoto N, et al. Reassessment of myometrial invasion in endometrial carcinoma. *Obstet Gynecol* 1994;84:979–982.

179. Cowles TA, Magrina JF, Materson BJ, et al. Comparison of clinical and surgical staging in patients with endometrial carcinoma. *Obstet Gynecol* 1985;66:413–416.

180. Hanson MB, Van Nagell JR, Powell DE, et al. The prognostic significance of lymph-vascular space invasion in stage I endometrial cancer. *Cancer* 1985;55:1753–1757.

181. Abeler VM, Kjorstad KE, Berle E. Carcinoma of the endometrium in Norway: a histopathological and prognostic survey of a total population. *Int J Gynecol Pathol* 1992;2:9–32.

182. Mariani A, Webb MJ, Keeney GL, et al. Predictors of lymphatic failure in endometrial cancer. *Gynecol Oncol* 2002;84:437–442.

183. Mariani A, Webb MJ, Galli L, et al. Potential therapeutic role of para-aortic lymphadenectomy in node-positive endometrial cancer. *Gynecol Oncol* 2000;76:348–356.

184. Creasman WT, DiSaia PJ, Blessing J, et al. Prognostic significance of peritoneal cytology in patients with endometrial cancer and preliminary data concerning therapy with intraperitoneal radiopharmaceuticals. *Am J Obstet Gynecol* 1981;141:921–929.

185. Harouny VR, Sutton EP, Clark SA, et al. The importance of peritoneal cytology in endometrial carcinoma. *Obstet Gynecol* 1988;72:394–398.

186. Turner DA, Gershenson DM, Atkinson N, et al. The prognostic significance of peritoneal cytology for stage I endometrial cancer. *Obstet Gynecol* 1989;74:775–780.

187. Lurain JR, Rumsey NK, Schink JC, et al. Prognostic significance of positive peritoneal cytology in clinical stage I adenocarcinoma of the endometrium. *Obstet Gynecol* 1989;74:175–179.

188. Kadar N, Homesley HD, Malfetano JH. Positive peritoneal cytology is an adverse factor in endometrial carcinoma only if there is other evidence of extrauterine disease. *Gynecol Oncol* 1992;46:145–149.

189. Milosevic MF, Dembo AJ, Thomas GM. The clinical significance of malignant peritoneal cytology in stage I endometrial carcinoma. *Int J Gynecol Cancer* 1992;2:225–235.

190. Mariani A, Webb MJ, Keeney GL, et al. Stage IIIC endometrioid corpus cancer includes distinct subgroups. *Gynecol Oncol* 2002;87:112–117.

191. Takeshima N, Nishida H, Tabata T, et al. Positive peritoneal cytology in endometrial cancer: enhancement of other prognostic indicators. *Gynecol Oncol* 2001;82:470–473.

192. Ebina Y, Hareyama H, Sakuragh N, et al. Peritoneal cytology and its prognostic value in endometrial carcinoma. *Int Surg* 1997;82:244–248.

193. Mariani A, Webb MJ, Keeney GL, et al. Assessment of prognostic factors in stage IIIA endometrial cancer. *Gynecol Oncol* 2002;86:38–44.

194. Moore DH, Fowler WC, Walton LA, et al. Morbidity of lymph node sampling in cancers of the uterine corpus and cervix. *Obstet Gynecol* 1989;74:180–184.

195. Mariani A, Webb MJ, Keeney GL, et al. Endometrial cancer: predictors of peritoneal failure. *Gynecol Oncol* 2003;89:236–242.

196. Levine RL, Cargile CB, Blazes MS, et al. PTEN mutations and microsatellite instability in complex atypical hyperplasia, a precursor lesion to uterine endometrioid carcinoma. *Cancer Res* 1998;58:3254–3258.

197. Emons G, Fleckenstein G, Hinney B, et al. Hormonal interactions in endometrial cancer. *Endocr Relat Cancer* 2000;7:227–242.

198. Kaaks R, Lukanova A, Kurzer MS. Obesity, endogenous hormones, and endometrial cancer risk: a synthetic review. *Cancer Epidemiol Biomarkers Prev* 2002;11:1531–1543.

199. Parslov M, Lidegaard O, Klintorp S, et al. Risk factors among young women with endometrial cancer: a Danish case-control study. *Am J Obstet Gynecol* 2000;182:23–29.

200. Potischman N, Hoover RN, Brinton LA, et al. Case-control study of endogenous steroid hormones and endometrial cancer. *J Natl Cancer Inst* 1996;88:1127–1135.

201. Zeleniuch-Jacquotte A, Akhmedkhanov A, Kato I, et al. Postmenopausal endogenous oestrogens and risk of endometrial cancer: results of a prospective study. *Br J Cancer* 2001;84:975–981.

202. Calle EE, Rodriguez C, Walker-Thurmond K, et al. Overweight, obesity, and mortality from cancer in a prospectively studied cohort of U.S. adults. *N Engl J Med* 2003;348:1625–1638.

203. Clement PB, Young RH. Endometrioid carcinoma of the uterine corpus: a review of its pathology with emphasis on recent advances and problematic aspects. *Adv Anat Pathol* 2002;9:145–184.

204. Ambros RA, Sherman ME, Zahn CM, et al. Endometrial intraepithelial carcinoma: a distinctive lesion specifically associated with tumors displaying serous differentiation. *Human Pathol* 1995;26:1260–1267.

205. Zheng W, Cao P, Zheng M, et al. p53 Overexpression and bcl-2 persistence in endometrial carcinoma: comparison of papillary serous and endometrioid subtypes. *Gynecol Oncol* 1996;61:167–174.

206. Mutter GL, Lin M-C, Fitzgerald JT, et al. Altered PTEN expression as a diagnostic marker for the earliest endometrial precancers. *J Natl Cancer Inst* 2000;92:924–930.

207. Mutter GL, Lin M-C, Fitzgerald JT, et al. Changes in endometrial PTEN expression throughout the human menstrual cycle. *J Clin Endocrinol Metab* 2000;85:2334–2338.

208. Mutter GL, Baak JPA, Fitzgerald JT, et al. Global expression changes of constitutive and hormonally regulated genes during endometrial neoplastic transformation. *Gynecol Oncol* 2001;83:177–185.

209. Risinger JI, Hayes AK, Berchuck A, et al. PTEN/MMAC1 mutations in endometrial cancers. *Cancer Res* 1997;57:4736–4738.

210. Lax SF, Kendall B, Tashiro H, et al. The frequency of p53, K-ras mutations, and microsatellite instability differs in uterine endometrioid and serous carcinoma: evidence of distinct molecular genetic pathways. *Cancer* 2000;88:814–824.

211. Lagarda H, Catasus L, Arguelles R, et al. K-ras mutations in endometrial carcinomas with microsatellite instability. *J Pathol* 2001;193:193–199.

212. Enomoto T, Inoue M, Perantoni AO, et al. K-ras activation in premalignant and malignant epithelial lesions of the human uterus. *Cancer Res* 1991;51:5308–5314.

213. Scholten AN, Creutzberg CL, van den Broek L, et al. Nuclear beta-catenin is a molecular feature of type 1 endometrial carcinoma. *J Pathol* 2003;201:460–465.

214. Moreno-Bueno G, Hardisson D, Sanchez C, et al. Abnormalities of the APC/beta-catenin pathway in endometrial cancer. *Oncogene* 2002;21:7981–7990.

215. Mirabelli-Primdahl L, Gryfe R, Kim H, et al. β-Catenin mutations are specific for colorectal carcinomas with microsatellite instability but occur in endometrial carcinomas irrespective of mutator pathway. *Cancer Res* 1999;59:3346–3351.

216. Mariani A, Sebo TJ, Webb MJ, et al. Molecular and histopathologic predictors of distant failure in endometrial cancer. *Cancer Detect Prev* 2003;27:434–441.

217. Lax SF. Molecular genetic pathways in various types of endometrial carcinoma: from a phenotypical to a molecular-based classification. *Virchows Arch* 2004;444:213–223.

218. Lax SF, Pizer ES, Ronnett BM, et al. Clear cell carcinoma of the endometrium is characterized by a distinctive profile of p53, Ki-67, estrogen, and progesterone receptor expression. *Hum Pathol* 1998;29:551–558.

219. Wheeler DT, Bell KA, Kurman RJ, et al. Minimal uterine serous carcinoma: diagnosis and clinicopathologic correlation. *Am J Surg Pathol* 2000;24:797–806.

220. Risinger JI, Hayes AK, Berchuck A, et al. PTEN/MMAC1 mutations in endometrial cancers. *Cancer Res* 1997;57:4736–4738.

221. Risinger JI, Hayes K, Maxwell GL, et al. PTEN mutation in endometrial cancers is associated with favorable clinical and pathological characteristics. *Clin Cancer Res* 1998;4:3005–3010.

222. **Inaba F, Kawamata H, Teramoto T, et al.** PTEN and p53 abnormalities are indicative and predictive factors for endometrial carcinoma. *Oncol Rep* 2005;13:17–24.

223. **Duggan BD, Felix JC, Mudersbach Ll, et al.** Microsatellite instability in sporadic endometrial carcinoma. *J Natl Cancer Inst* 1994;86:1216–1221.

224. **Mutter GL, Boynton KA, Faquin WC, et al.** Allelotype mapping of unstable microsatellites establishes direct lineage continuity between endometrial precancers and cancer. *Cancer Res* 1996;56:4483–4486.

225. **Risinger JI, Berchuck A, Kohler MF, et al.** Genetic instability of microsatellites in endometrial carcinoma. *Cancer Res* 1993;53:5100–5103.

226. **Gryfe R, Kim H, Hsieh ETK, et al.** Tumor microsatellite instability and clinical outcome in young patients with colorectal cancer. *N Engl J Med* 2000;342:69–77.

227. **Sherman ME, Bur ME, Kurman RJ.** p53 in endometrial cancer and its putative precursors: evidence for diverse pathways of tumorigenesis. *Hum Pathol* 1995;26:1268–1274.

228. **Mizuuchi H, Nasim S, Kudo R, et al.** Clinical implications of K-ras mutations in malignant epithelial tumors of the endometrium. *Cancer Res* 1992;52:2777–2781.

229. **Fujimoto I, Shimizu Y, Hirai Y, et al.** Studies on ras oncogene activation in endometrial carcinoma. *Gynecol Oncol* 1993;48:196–202.

230. **Semczuk A, Berbec H, Kostuch M, et al.** K-ras gene point mutations in human endometrial carcinomas: correlation with clinicopathological features and patients' outcome. *J Cancer Res Clin Oncol* 1998;124:695–700.

231. **Sonoda G, du Manoir S, Godwin AK, et al.** Detection of DNA gains and losses in primary endometrial carcinomas by comparative genomic hybridization. *Genes Chromosomes Cancer* 1997;18:115–125.

232. **Niederacher D, An H-X, Cho Y-J, et al.** Mutations and amplification of oncogenes in endometrial cancer. *Oncology* 1999;56:59–65.

233. **Tashiro H, Isacson C, Levine R, et al.** p53 gene mutations are common in uterine serous carcinoma and occur early in their pathogenesis. *Am J Pathol* 1997;150:177–185.

234. **Goodfellow PJ, Buttin BM, Herzog TJ, et al.** Prevalence of defective DNA mismatch repair and MSH6 mutation in an unselected series of endometrial cancers. *PNAS* 2003;100:5908–5913.

235. **Tashiro H, Lax SF, Gaudin PB, et al.** Microsatellite instability is uncommon in uterine serous carcinoma. *Am J Pathol* 1997;150:75–79.

236. **Saffari B, Jones LA, Elnaggar A, et al.** Amplification and overexpression of Her-2/Neu (C-Erbb2) in endometrial cancers: correlation with overall survival. *Cancer Res* 1995;55:5693–5698.

237. **Halperin R, Zehavi S, Habler L, et al.** Comparative immunohistochemical study of endometrioid and serous papillary carcinoma of endometrium. *Eur J Gynaecol Oncol* 2001;22:122–126.

238. **Berchuck A, Rodriguez G, Kinney RB, et al.** Overexpression of HER-2/neu in endometrial cancer is associated with advanced stage disease. *Am J Obstet Gynecol* 1991;164:15–21.

239. **Hetzel DJ, Wilson TO, Keeney GL, et al.** HER-2/neu expression: a major prognostic factor in endometrial cancer. *Gynecol Oncol* 1992;47:179–185.

240. **Cianciulli AM, Guadagni F, Marzano R, et al.** HER-2/neu oncogene amplification and chromosome 17 aneusomy in endometrial carcinoma: correlation with oncoprotein expression and conventional pathological parameters. *J Exp Clin Cancer Res* 2003;22:265–271.

241. **Holcomb K, Delatorre R, Pedemonte B, et al.** E-cadherin expression in endometrioid, papillary serous, and clear cell carcinoma of the endometrium. *Obstet Gynecol* 2002;100:1290–1295.

242. **Moreno-Bueno G, Hardisson D, Sanchez C, et al.** Abnormalities of E- and P-cadherin and catenin (beta-gamma-catenin, and p120 ctn) expression in endometrial cancer and endometrioid cancer and endometrial atypical hyperplasia. *J Pathol* 2003;199:471–478.

243. **Mariani A, Dowdy SC, Keeney GL, et al.** High-risk endometrial cancer subgroups: candidates for target-based adjuvant therapy. *Gynecol Oncol* 2004;95:120–126.

244. **Peters WA III, Anderson WA, Thornton N Jr, et al.** The selective use of vaginal hysterectomy in the management of adenocarcinoma of the endometrium. *Am J Obstet Gynecol* 1983;146:285–289.

245. **Malkasian GD, Annegers JF, Fountain KS.** Carcinoma of the endometrium: stage. *Am J Obstet Gynecol* 1980;136:872–883.

246. **Bloss JD, Berman ML, Bloss LP, et al.** Use of vaginal hysterectomy for the management of stage I endometrial cancer in the medically compromised patient. *Gynecol Oncol* 1991;40:74–77.

247. **Chan JK, Lin YG, Monk BJ, et al.** Vaginal hysterectomy as primary treatment of endometrial cancer in medically compromised women. *Obstet Gynecol* 2001;97:707–711.

248. **Childers JM, Brzechffa PR, Hatch K, et al.** Laparoscopically-assisted surgical staging (LASS) of endometrial cancer. *Gynecol Oncol* 1993;51:33–38.

249. **Boike G, Lurain J, Burke J.** A comparison of laparoscopic management of endometrial cancer with traditional laparotomy. *Gynecol Oncol* 1994;52:105(abst).

250. **Gemignani M, Curtin JP, Zelmanovich J, et al.** Laparoscopic-assisted vaginal hysterectomy for endometrial cancer: clinical outcomes and hospital charges. *Gynecol Oncol* 1999;73:5–11.

251. **Spirtos NM, Schlaerth JB, Grous GM, et al.** Cost and quality-of-life analyses of surgery for early endometrial cancer: laparotomy versus laparoscopy. *Am J Obstet Gynecol* 1996;174:1795–1799.

252. **Schribner DR, Mannel RS, Walker JL, et al.** Cost analysis of laparoscopy versus laparotomy for early endometrial cancer. *Gynecol Oncol* 1999;75:460–463.

253. **Magrina JF, Mutone NF, Weaver Al, et al.** Laparoscopic lymphadenectomy and vaginal or laparoscopic hysterectomy with bilateral salpingo-oophorectomy for endometrial cancer. *Am J Obstet Gynecol* 1999;181:376–381.

254. **Eltabbakh GH, Shamonki MJ, Moody JM, et al.** Laparoscopy as the primary modality for the treatment of women with endometrial carcinoma. *Cancer* 2001;91:378–387.

255. **Obermair A, Manolitsas TP, Leung Y, et al.** Total laparoscopic hysterectomy for endometrial cancer: patterns of recurrence and survival. *Gynecol Oncol* 2004;92:789–793.

256. **Malur S, Possover M, Wolfgang M, et al.** Laparoscopic-assisted vaginal versus abdominal surgery in patients with endometrial cancer: a prospective randomized trial. *Gynecol Oncol* 2001;80:239–244.

257. **Martínez A, Querleu D, Leblanc E, et al.** Low incidence of port-site metastases after laparoscopic staging of uterine cancer. *Gynecol Oncol* 2010;118:145–150.

258. **Walker JL, Piedmonte MR, Spirtos NM, et al.** Laparoscopy compared with laparotomy for comprehensive surgical staging of uterine cancer: Gynecologic Oncology Group Study LAP2. *J Clin Oncol* 2009;27:5331–5336.

259. **Kornblith AB, Huang HQ, Walker JL, et al.** Quality of life of patients with endometrial cancer undergoing laparoscopic international federation of gynecology and obstetrics staging compared with laparotomy: a Gynecologic Oncology Group study. *J Clin Oncol* 2009;27:5337–5342.

260. **Dowdy SC, Aletti G, Cliby WA, et al.** Extra-peritoneal laparoscopic para-aortic lymphadenectomy: a prospective cohort study of 293 patients with endometrial cancer. *Gynecol Oncol* 2008;111:418–424.

261. **Gehrig PA, Cantrell LA, Shafer A, et al.** What is the optimal minimally invasive surgical procedure for endometrial cancer staging in the obese and morbidly obese woman? *Gynecol Oncol* 2008;111:41–45.

262. **Boggess JF, Gehrig PA, Cantrell L, et al.** A comparative study of 3 surgical methods for hysterectomy with staging for endometrial cancer: robotic assistance, laparoscopy, laparotomy. *Am J Obstet Gynecol* 2008;199:360.e1–e9.

263. **Lewis BV, Stallworthy JA, Cowdell R.** Adenocarcinoma of the body of the uterus. *J Obstet Gynecol Br Commonw* 1970;77:343–348.

264. **DeMuelenaere GFGO.** The case against Wertheim's hysterectomy in endometrial carcinoma. *J Obstet Gynaecol Br Commonw* 1973;80:728–734.

265. **Rutledge F.** The role of radical hysterectomy in adenocarcinoma of the endometrium. *Gynecol Oncol* 1974;2:331–347.

266. **Jones HW III.** Treatment of adenocarcinoma of the endometrium. *Obstet Gynecol Surv* 1975;30:147–169.

267. **Mariani A, Webb MJ, Keeney GL, et al.** Role of wide/radical hysterectomy and pelvic lymph node dissection in endometrial cancer with cervical involvement. *Gynecol Oncol* 2001;83:72–80.

268. **Landgren R, Fletcher G, Delclos L, et al.** Irradiation of endometrial cancer in patients with medical contraindication to surgery or with unresectable lesions. *AJR Am J Roentgenol* 1976;126:148–154.

269. **Abayomi O, Tak W, Emami B, et al.** Treatment of endometrial carcinoma with radiation therapy alone. *Cancer* 1982;49:2466–2469.

270. **Patanaphan V, Salazar O, Chougule P.** What can be expected when radiation therapy becomes the only curative alternative for endometrial cancer? *Cancer* 1985;55:1462–1467.

271. **Jones D, Stout R.** Results of intracavitary radium treatment for adenocarcinoma of the body of the uterus. *Clin Radiol* 1986;37:169–171.

272. **Varia M, Rosenman, Halle J, et al.** Primary radiation therapy for medically inoperable patients with endometrial carcinoma-stages I–II. *Int J Radiat Oncol Biol Phys* 1987;13:11–15.

273. **Wang M, Hussey D, Vigliotti A, et al.** Inoperable adenocarcinoma of the endometrium: radiation therapy. *Radiology* 1987;165:561–565.

274. **Grigsby P, Kuske R, Perez C, et al.** Medically inoperable stage I adenocarcinoma of the endometrium treated with radiotherapy alone. *Int J Radiat Oncol Biol Phys* 1987;13:483–488.

275. **Taghian A, Pernot M, Hoffstetter S, et al.** Radiation therapy alone for medically inoperable patients with adenocarcinoma of the endometrium. *Int J Radiat Oncol Biol Phys* 1988;15:1135–1140.

276. **Lehoczky O, Busze P, Ungar L, et al.** Stage I endometrial carcinoma: treatment of nonoperable patients with intracavitary radiation therapy alone. *Gynecol Oncol* 1991;43:211–216.

277. **Kupelian PA, Eifel PJ, Tornos C, et al.** Treatment of endometrial carcinoma with radiation therapy alone. *Int J Radiat Oncol Biol Phys* 1993;27:817–824.

278. **Podczaski ES, Kaminski P, Manetta A, et al.** Stage II endometrial carcinoma treated with external-beam radiotherapy, intracavitary application of cesium, and surgery. *Gynecol Oncol* 1989;35:251–254.

279. **Keys HM, Roberts JA, Brunetto VL, et al.** Gynecologic Oncology Group. A phase III trial of surgery with or without adjunctive external pelvic radiation therapy in intermediate risk endometrial adenocarcinoma. *Gynecol Oncol* 2004;92:744–751.

280. **Mariani A, Dowdy SC, Keeney GL, et al.** Predictors of vaginal relapse in stage I endometrial cancer. *Gynecol Oncol* 2005;97:820–827.

281. **Mariani A, Webb MJ, Keeney GL, et al.** Surgical stage I endometrial cancer: predictors of distant failure and death. *Gynecol Oncol* 2002;87:274–280.

282. **Orr JW Jr, Holman JL, Orr PF.** Stage I corpus cancer: Is teletherapy necessary? *Am J Obstet Gynecol* 1997;176:777–789.

283. **Straughn JM Jr, Huh WK, Kelly FJ, et al.** Conservative management of stage I endometrioid carcinoma after surgical staging. *Gynecol Oncol* 2002;84:194–200.

284. **Pearcey RG, Petereit DG.** Post-operative high dose rate brachytherapy in patients with low to intermediate risk endometrial cancer. *Radiother Oncol* 2000;56:17–22.

285. **Horowitz NS, Peters WA 3rd, Smith MR, et al.** Adjuvant high dose rate vaginal brachytherapy as treatment of stage I and II endometrial carcinoma. *Obstet Gynecol* 2002;99:235–240.

286. **Weiss E, Hirnle P, Arnold-Bofinger H, et al.** Adjuvant vaginal high-dose-rate afterloading alone in endometrial carcinoma: patterns of relapse and side effects following low-dose therapy. *Gynecol Oncol* 1998;71:72–76.

287. **Mohan DS, Samuels MA, Selim MA, et al.** Long-term outcomes of therapeutic pelvic lymphadenectomy for stage I endometrial adenocarcinoma. *Gynecol Oncol* 1998;70:165–171.

288. **Chadha M, Nanavati PJ, Liu P, et al.** Patterns of failure in endometrial carcinoma stage IB grade 3 and IC patients treated with postoperative vaginal vault brachytherapy. *Gynecol Oncol* 1999;75:103–107.

289. **Fanning J.** Long-term survival of intermediate risk endometrial cancer (stage IG3, IC, II) treated with full lymphadenectomy and brachytherapy without teletherapy. *Gynecol Oncol* 2001;82:371–374.

290. **Straughn JM, Huh WK, Orr JW, et al.** Stage IC adenocarcinoma of the endometrium: survival comparisons of surgically staged patients with and without adjuvant radiation therapy. *Gynecol Oncol* 2003;89:295–300.

291. **Solhjem MC, Petersen IA, Haddock MG.** Vaginal brachytherapy alone is sufficient adjuvant treatment of surgical stage I endometrial cancer. *Int J Rad Oncol Biol Phys* 2005;62:1379–1384.

292. **Nout RA, Smit VT, Putter H, et al.** PORTEC Study Group. Vaginal brachytherapy versus pelvic external beam radiotherapy for patients with endometrial cancer of high-intermediate risk (PORTEC-2): an open-label, non-inferiority, randomised trial. *Lancet* 2010;375:816–823.

293. **Huh WK.** Salvage of isolated vaginal recurrences in women with

294. **Blake P, Swart AM, Orton J, et al.** ASTEC/EN.5 Study Group. Adjuvant external beam radiotherapy in the treatment of endometrial cancer (MRC ASTEC and NCIC CTG EN.5 randomised trials): pooled trial results, systematic review, and meta-analysis. *Lancet* 2009;373:137–146.

295. **Potish RA, Twiggs LB, Adcock LL, et al.** Para-aortic lymph node radiotherapy in cancer of the uterine corpus. *Obstet Gynecol* 1985;65:251–256.

296. **Rose PG, Cha SD, Tak WK, et al.** Radiation therapy for surgically proven para-aortic node metastasis in endometrial carcinoma. *Int J Radiat Oncol Biol Phys* 1992;24:229–233.

297. **Feuer GA, Calanog A.** Endometrial carcinoma: treatment of positive para-aortic nodes. *Gynecol Oncol* 1987;27:104–109.

298. **Corn BW, Lanciano RM, Greven KM, et al.** Endometrial cancer with para-aortic adenopathy: patterns of failure and opportunities for cure. *Int J Radiat Oncol Biol Phys* 1992;24:223–227.

299. **Potish RA, Twiggs LB, Adcock LL, et al.** Role of whole abdominal radiation therapy in the management of endometrial cancer; prognostic importance of factors indicating peritoneal metastases. *Gynecol Oncol* 1985;21:80–86.

300. **Greer BE, Hamberger AD.** Treatment of intraperitoneal metastatic adenocarcinoma of the endometrium by the whole-abdomen moving-strip technique and pelvic boost irradiation. *Gynecol Oncol* 1983;16:365–373.

301. **Loeffler JS, Rosen EM, Niloff JM, et al.** Whole abdominal irradiation for tumors of the uterine corpus. *Cancer* 1988;61:1322–1335.

302. **Martinez A, Schray M, Podratz K, et al.** Postoperative whole abdomino-pelvic irradiation for patients with high-risk endometrial cancer. *Int J Radiat Oncol Biol Phys* 1989;17:371–377.

303. **Gibbons S, Martinez A, Schray M, et al.** Adjuvant whole abdominopelvic irradiation for high-risk endometrial carcinoma. *Int J Radiat Oncol Biol Phys* 1991;21:1019–1025.

304. **Small W, Mahadevan A, Roland P, et al.** Whole abdominal radiation in endometrial carcinoma: an analysis of toxicity, patterns of recurrence, and survival. *J Cancer* 2000;6:394–400.

305. **Smith RS, Kapp DS, Chen Q, et al.** Treatment of high-risk uterine cancer with whole abdominopelvic radiation therapy. *Int J Radiat Oncol Biol Phys* 2000;48:767–778.

306. **Frank AH, Tseng PC, Haffty BG, et al.** Adjuvant whole abdominal radiation in uterine papillary serous carcinoma. *Cancer* 1991;68:1516–1519.

307. **Randall ME, Filiaci VL, Muss H, et al.** Gynecologic Oncology Group Study. Randomized phase III trial of whole-abdominal irradiation versus doxorubicin and cisplatin chemotherapy in advanced endometrial carcinoma. *J Clin Oncol* 2006;24:36–44.

308. **Lewis GC Jr, Slack NH, Mortel R, et al.** Adjuvant progestogen therapy in the primary definitive treatment of endometrial cancer. *Gynecol Oncol* 1974;2:368–376.

309. **DePalo G, Merson M, Del Vecchio M, et al.** A controlled clinical study of adjuvant medroxyprogesterone acetate (MPA) therapy in pathologic stage I endometrial carcinoma with myometrial invasion. *Proc Am Soc Clin Oncol* 1985;4:121(abst).

310. **Vergote I, Kjorstad J, Abeler V, et al.** A randomized trail of adjuvant progestogen in early endometrial cancer. *Cancer* 1989;64:1011–1016.

311. **MacDonald RR, Thorogood J, Mason MK.** A randomized trial of progestogens in the primary treatment of endometrial carcinoma. *BJOG* 1988;95:166–174.

312. **COSA-NZ-UK Endometrial Cancer Study Groups.** Adjuvant medroxyprogesterone acetate in high-risk endometrial cancer. *Int J Gynecol Cancer* 1998;8:387–391.

313. **von Minckwitz G, Loibl S, Brunnert K, et al.** Adjuvant endocrine treatment with medroxyprogesterone acetate or tamoxifen in stage I and II endometrial cancer—a multicentre, open, controlled, prospectively randomized trial. *Eur J Cancer* 2002;38:2265–2271.

314. **Morrow CP, Bundy B, Homesley H, et al.** Doxorubicin as an adjuvant following surgery and radiation therapy in patients with high-risk endometrial carcinoma, stage I and occult stage II. *Gynecol Oncol* 1990;36:166–171.

315. **Randall ME, Brunetto G, Muss H, et al.** Whole abdominal radiotherapy versus combination doxorubicin-cisplatin chemotherapy in advanced endometrial carcinoma: a randomized phase III

trial of the Gynecologic Oncology Group. *Proc Am Soc Clin Oncol* 2003;22:abstr 3.

316. **Hogberg T, Signorelli M, de Oliveira CF, et al.** Sequential adjuvant chemotherapy and radiotherapy in endometrial cancer: results from two randomised studies. *Eur J Cancer* 2010;46:2422–2431.

317. **Susumu N, Sagae S, Udagawa Y, et al.** Japanese Gynecologic Oncology Group. Randomized phase III trial of pelvic radiotherapy versus cisplatin-based combined chemotherapy in patients with intermediate- and high-risk endometrial cancer. *Gynecol Oncol* 2008;108:226–233.

318. **Homesley HD, Boronow RC, Lewis JL Jr.** Stage II endometrial adenocarcinoma: Memorial Hospital for Cancer, 1949–1965. *Obstet Gynecol* 1977;49:604–608.

319. **Surwit EA, Fowler WC Jr, Rogoff EE, et al.** Stage II carcinoma of the endometrium. *Int J Radiat Oncol Biol Phys* 1979;5:323–326.

320. **Kinsella TJ, Bloomer WD, Lavin PT, et al.** Stage II endometrial carcinoma: a 10-year follow-up of combined radiation and surgical treatment. *Gynecol Oncol* 1980;10:290–297.

321. **Nahhas WA, Whitney CW, Stryker JA, et al.** Stage II endometrial carcinoma. *Gynecol Oncol* 1980;10:303–311.

322. **Onsrud M, Aalders J, Abeler V, et al.** Endometrial carcinoma with cervical involvement (stage II): prognostic factors and value of combined radiological-surgical treatment. *Gynecol Oncol* 1982;13:76–86.

323. **Berman ML, Afridi MA, Kanbour AI, et al.** Risk factors and prognosis in stage II endometrial cancer. *Gynecol Oncol* 1982;14:49–61.

324. **Nori D, Hilaris BS, Tome M, et al.** Combined surgery and radiation in endometrial carcinoma: an analysis of prognostic factors. *Int J Radiat Oncol Biol Phys* 1987;13:489–496.

325. **Larson DM, Copeland LJ, Gallager HS, et al.** Prognostic factors in stage II endometrial carcinoma. *Cancer* 1987;60:1358–1361.

326. **Larson DM, Copeland LJ, Gallager HS, et al.** Stage II endometrial carcinoma: results and complications of a combined radiotherapeutic-surgical approach. *Cancer* 1988;61:1528–1534.

327. **Boothby RA, Carlson JA, Neiman W, et al.** Treatment of stage II endometrial carcinoma. *Gynecol Oncol* 1989;33:204–208.

328. **Pitson G, Colgan T, Levin W, et al.** Stage II endometrial carcinoma: prognostic factors and risk classification in 170 patients. *Int J Radiat Oncol Biol Phys* 2002;53:862–867.

329. **Mannel RS, Berman ML, Walker JL, et al.** Management of endometrial cancer with suspected cervical involvement. *Obstet Gynecol* 1990;75:1016–1022.

330. **Andersen ES.** Stage II endometrial carcinoma: prognostic factors and the results of treatment. *Gynecol Oncol* 1990;38:220–223.

331. **Lanciano RM, Curran WJ Jr, Greven KM, et al.** Influence of grade, histologic subtype, and timing of radiotherapy on outcome among patients with stage II carcinoma of the endometrium. *Gynecol Oncol* 1990;39:368–373.

332. **Sartori E, Gadducci A, Landoni F, et al.** Clinical behavior of 203 stage II endometrial cancer cases: the impact of primary surgical approach and of adjunct radiation therapy. *Int J Gynecol Cancer* 2001;11:430–437.

333. **Higgins RV, van Nagell JR Jr, Horn EJ, et al.** Preoperative radiation therapy followed by extrafascial hysterectomy in patients with stage II endometrial cancer. *Cancer* 1991;68:1261–1264.

334. **Rubin SC, Hoskins WJ, Saigo PE, et al.** Management of endometrial adenocarcinoma with cervical involvement. *Gynecol Oncol* 1992;45:294–298.

335. **Aalders JG, Abeler V, Kolstad P.** Clinical (stage III) as compared with subclinical intrapelvic extrauterine tumor spread in endometrial carcinoma: a clinical and histopathological study of 175 patients. *Gynecol Oncol* 1984;17:64–74.

336. **Genest P, Drouin P, Girard A, et al.** Stage III carcinoma of the endometrium: a review of 41 cases. *Gynecol Oncol* 1987;26:77–86.

337. **Grigsby PW, Perez CA, Kuske RR, et al.** Results of therapy, analysis of failures and prognostic factors for clinical and pathologic stage III adenocarcinoma of the endometrium. *Gynecol Oncol* 1987;27:44–57.

338. **Greven K, Curran W, Whittington R, et al.** Analysis of failure patterns in stage III endometrial carcinoma and therapeutic implications. *Int J Radiat Biol Phys* 1989;17:35–39.

339. **Pliskow S, Penalver M, Averette HE.** Stage III and IV endometrial carcinoma: a review of 41 cases. *Gynecol Oncol* 1990;38:210–215.

340. **Aalders JG, Abeler V, Kolstad P.** Stage IV endometrial carcinoma: a clinical and histopathological study of 83 patients. *Gynecol Oncol* 1984;17:75–84.

341. **Bristow RE, Zerbe MJ, Rosenshein NB, et al.** Stage IV endometrial carcinoma: the role of cytoreductive surgery and determinants of survival. *Gynecol Oncol* 2000;78:85–91.

342. **Goff BA, Goodman A, Muntz HG, et al.** Surgical stage IV endometrial carcinoma: a study of 47 cases. *Gynecol Oncol* 1994;52:237–240.

343. **Chi DS, Welshinger M, Venkatraman ES, et al.** The role of surgical cytoreduction in stage IV endometrial carcinoma. *Gynecol Oncol* 1997;67:56–60.

344. **Rutledge F, Smith JP, Wharton JT, et al.** Pelvic exenteration: analysis of 296 patients. *Am J Obstet Gynecol* 1977;129:881–890.

345. **Barber HRK, Brunschwig A.** Treatment and results of recurrent cancer of corpus uteri in patients receiving anterior and total exoneration 1947–1963. *Cancer* 1968; 22:949–955.

346. **Aalders JG, Abeler V, Kolstad P.** Recurrent adenocarcinoma of the endometrium: a clinical and histopathological study of 379 patients. *Gynecol Oncol* 1984;17:85–103.

347. **Angel C, DuBeshter B, Dawson AE, et al.** Recurrent stage I endometrial adenocarcinoma in the nonirradiated patient: preliminary results of surgical "staging." *Gynecol Oncol* 1993;48:221–226.

348. **Dowdy SC, Mariani A.** Lymphadenectomy in endometrial cancer: when, not if. *Lancet* 2010;375:1138–1140.

349. Insert IORT publication

350. **Jhingran A, Burke TW, Eifel PJ.** Definitive radiotherapy for patients with isolated vaginal recurrence of endometrial carcinoma after hysterectomy. *Int J Radiat Oncol Biol Phys* 2003;56:1366–1372.

351. **Phillips GL, Prem KA, Adcock LL, et al.** Vaginal recurrence of adenocarcinoma of the endometrium. *Gynecol Oncol* 1982;13:323–328.

352. **Greven K, Olds W.** Isolated vaginal recurrences of endometrial adenocarcinoma and their management. *Cancer* 1987;60:419–421.

353. **Curran WJ, Whittington R, Peters AJ, et al.** Vaginal recurrences of endometrial carcinoma: the prognostic value of staging by a primary vaginal carcinoma system. *Int J Radiat Oncol Biol Phys* 1988;15:803–808.

354. **Poulsen MG, Roberts SJ.** The salvage of recurrent endometrial carcinoma in the vagina and pelvis. *Int J Radiat Oncol Biol Phys* 1988;15:809–813.

355. **Kuten A, Grigsby PW, Perez CA, et al.** Results of radiotherapy in recurrent endometrial carcinoma: a retrospective analysis. *Int J Radiat Oncol Biol Phys* 1989;17:29–34.

356. **Sears JD, Greven KM, Hoen HM, et al.** Prognostic factors and treatment outcome for patients with locally recurrent endometrial cancer. *Cancer* 1994;74:1303–1308.

357. **Wylie J, Irwin C, Pintilie M, et al.** Results of radical radiotherapy for recurrent endometrial cancer. *Gynecol Oncol* 2000;77:66–72.

358. **Kelley RM, Baker WH.** Progestational agents in the treatment of carcinoma of the endometrium. *N Engl J Med* 1961;264:216–222.

359. **Piver MS, Barlow JJ, Lurain JR, et al.** Medroxyprogesterone acetate (Depo-Provera) versus hydroxyprogesterone caproate (Delalutin) in women with metastatic endometrial adenocarcinoma. *Cancer* 1980;45:268–272.

360. **Podratz KC, O'Brien PC, Malkasian GD Jr, et al.** Effects of progestational agents in treatment of endometrial carcinoma. *Obstet Gynecol* 1985;66:106–110.

361. **Thigpen T, Blessing J, DiSaia P, et al.** Oral medroxyprogesterone acetate in advanced or recurrent endometrial carcinoma: results of therapy and correlation with estrogen and progesterone receptor levels. The Gynecologic Oncology Group experience. In: Baulier EE, Iacobelli S, McGuire WL,eds. Endocrinology of malignancy. Park Ridge, NJ: Parthenon, 1986:446–454.

362. **Thigpen T, Blessing J, Hatch K, et al.** A randomized trial of medroxyprogesterone acetate (MPA) 200 mg versus 1000 mg daily in advanced or recurrent endometrial carcinoma: a Gynecologic Oncology Group study. *Proc ASCO* 1991;10:185.

363. **Reifenstein EC Jr.** The treatment of advanced endometrial cancer with hydroxyprogesterone caproate. *Gynecol Oncol* 1974;2:377–414.

364. **Rose PG, Brunetto VL, VanLe L, et al.** A phase II trial of anastrozole in advanced recurrent or persistent endometrial carcinoma: a

Gynecologic Oncology Group study. *Gynecol Oncol* 2000;78:212–216.

365. **Elit L, Hirte H.** Current status and future innovations of hormonal agents, chemotherapy and investigational agents in endometrial cancer. *Curr Opin Obstet Gynecol* 2002;14:67–73.

366. **Levin DA, Hoskins WJ.** Update in the management of endometrial cancer. *Cancer J* 2002;8S:31–40.

367. **Sonoda Y.** Optimal therapy and management of endometrial cancer. *Expert Rev Anticancer Ther* 2003;3:37–47.

368. **Thigpen JT, Buchsbaum HJ, Mangan C, et al.** Phase II trial of adriamycin in the treatment of advanced or recurrent endometrial carcinoma: a Gynecologic Oncology Group study. *Cancer Treat Rep* 1979;63:21–27.

369. **Burke TW, Munkarah A, Kavanagh JJ, et al.** Treatment of advanced or recurrent endometrial carcinoma with single-agent carboplatin. *Gynecol Oncol* 1993;51:397–400.

370. **Ball HG, Blessing J, Leuntz S, et al.** A phase II trial of taxol in advanced and recurrent adenocarcinoma of the endometrium: a Gynecologic Oncology Group study. *Gynecol Oncol* 1996;62:278–281.

371. **Woo HL, Swenerton KD, Hoskins PJ.** Taxol is active in platinum-resistant endometrial adenocarcinoma. *Am J Clin Oncol* 1996;19:290–291.

372. **Lissoini A, Zanetta G, Losa G, et al.** Phase II study of paclitaxel as salvage treatment in advanced endometrial cancer. *Ann Oncol* 1996;7:861–865.

373. **Thigpen JT, Blessing JA, Ball H, et al.** Hexamethylmelanine in first-line therapy in the treatment of advanced or recurrent carcinoma of the endometrium: a phase II trial of the Gynecologic Oncology Group. *Gynecol Oncol* 1988;31:435–438.

374. **Muggia FM, Blessing JA, Sorosky J, et al.** Phase II trial of the pegylated liposomal doxorubicin in previously treated metastatic endometrial cancer: a Gynecologic Oncology Group study. *J Clin Oncol* 2002;20:2360–2364.

375. **Thigpen JT, Brady MF, Homesley HD, et al.** Phase III trial of doxorubicin with or without cisplatin in advanced endometrial carcinoma: a Gynecologic Oncology Group study. *J Clin Oncol* 2004;22:3902–3907.

376. **Deppe G, Cohen CJ, Bruckner HW.** Treatment of advanced endometrial adenocarcinoma with cis-dichlorodiamine platinum (II) after intensive prior therapy. *Gynecol Oncol* 1980;10:51–54.

377. **Thigpen JT, Blessing JA, Homesley H, et al.** Phase II trial of cisplatin as first-line chemotherapy in patients with advanced or recurrent endometrial carcinoma: a Gynecologic Oncology Group study. *Gynecol Oncol* 1989;33:68–70.

378. **Long HJ, Pfeifle DM, Wieand HS, et al.** Phase II evaluation of carboplatin in advanced endometrial carcinoma. *J Natl Cancer Inst* 1988;80:276–278.

385. **Miller DS, Blessing JA, Lentz SS, et al.** A phase II trial of topotecan in patients with advanced, persistent, or recurrent endometrial carcinoma: a Gynecologic Oncology Group study. *Gyneocol Oncol* 2002;87:247–251.

386. **Wadler S, Levy DE, Lincoln ST, et al.** Topotecan is an active agent in first line treatment of metastatic or recurrent endometrial carcinoma. Eastern Oncology Cooperative Group Study E3E93. *J Clin Oncol* 2003;21:2110–2114.

387. **Aapro MS, van Wijk FH, Bolis G, et al.** Doxorubicin versus doxorubicin and cisplatin in endometrial carcinoma: definitive results of a randomized study by the EORTC Gynecologic Cancer Group. *Ann Oncol* 2003;14:441–448.

388. **Edmonson JH, Krook JE, Hilton JF, et al.** Randomized phase II studies of cisplatin and a combination of a cyclophosphamide-doxorubicin-cisplatin (CAP) in patients with progestin-refractory advanced endometrial carcinoma. *Gynecol Oncol* 1987;28:20–24.

389. **Burke TW, Stringer CA, Morris M, et al.** Prospective treatment of advanced or recurrent endometrioid carcinoma with cisplatin, doxorubicin, and cyclophosphamide. *Gynecol Oncol* 1991;40:264–267.

390. **Dimopoulos MP, Papadimitriou CA, Georgoulias V, et al.** Paclitaxel and cisplatin in advanced or recurrent carcinoma of the endometrium: long-term results of a phase II multicenter study. *Gynecol Oncol* 2000;78:52–57.

391. **Creasman WT, Odicino F, Maisonneuve P, et al.** Carcinoma of the corpus uteri. FIGO annual report on the results of treatment in gynecological cancer. *J Epidemiol Biostat* 2001;6:45–86.

392. **Shumsky AG, Stuart GE, Brasher PM, et al.** An evaluation of routine follow up of patients treated for endometrial carcinoma. *Gynecol Oncol* 1994;55:229–233.

393. **Berchuck A, Auspach C, Evans AC, et al.** Postsurgical surveillance of patients with FIGO stage I/II endometrial adenocarcinoma. *Gynecol Oncol* 1995;59:20–24.

394. **Reddoch JM, Burke TW, Morris M, et al.** Surveillance for recurrent endometrial carcinoma: development of a follow-up scheme. *Gynecol Oncol* 1995;59:221–225.

395. **Gallup DG, Stock RJ.** Adenocarcinoma of the endometrium in women 40 years of age or younger. *Obstet Gynecol* 1984;64:417–420.

396. **Walsh C, Holschneider C, Hoang Y, et al.** Coexisting ovarian malignancy in young women with endometrial cancer. *Obstet Gynecol* 2005;106:693–699.

397. **Lee TS, Jung JY, Kim JW, et al.** Feasibility of ovarian preservation in patients with early stage endometrial carcinoma. *Gynecol Oncol* 2007;104:52–57.

398. **Morice P, Fourchotte V, Sideris L, et al.** A need for laparoscopic evaluation of patients with endometrial carcinoma selected for conservative treatment. *Gynecol Oncol* 2005;96:245–248.

399. **Creasman WT, Henderson D, Hinshaw W, et al.** Estrogen replacement therapy in the patient treated for endometrial cancer. *Obstet Gynecol* 1986;67:326–330.

400. **Suriano KA, McHale M, McLaren CE, et al.** Estrogen replacement therapy in endometrial cancer patients: a matched control study. *Obstet Gynecol* 2001;97:555–560.

401. **Levenback C, Rubin SC, McCormack PM, et al.** Resection of pulmonary metastases from uterine sarcomas. *Gynecol Oncol* 1992;45:202–205.

402. **Committee on Gynecologic Practice.** ACOG committee opinion. Hormone replacement therapy in women treated for endometrial cancer. *Int J Gynecol Obstet* 2001;73:283–284.

403. **Harlow BL, Weiss NS, Lofton S.** The epidemiology of sarcomas of the uterus. *J Natl Cancer Inst* 1986;76:399–402.

404. **Clement PB, Young RH.** Mesenchymal and mixed epithelial-mesenchymal tumors of the uterine corpus and cervix. In: **Clement PB, Young RH, eds.** Atlas of gynecologic surgical pathology. Philadelphia, PA: Saunders, 2000:177–210.

405. **Brooks SE, Zhan M, Cote T, Baquet CR.** Surveillance, epidemiology, and end results analysis of 2677 cases of uterine sarcoma 1989–1999. *Gynecol Oncol* 2004;93:204–208.

406. **Kempson RL, Bari W.** Uterine sarcomas: classification, diagnosis and prognosis. *Hum Pathol* 1970;1:331–349.

407. **Dionigi A, Oliva E, Clement PB, et al.** Endometrial stromal nodules and endometrial stromal tumors with limited infiltration: a clinicopathologic study of 50 cases. *Am J Surg Pathol* 2002;26:567–581.

408. **Norris HJ, Taylor HB.** Mesenchymal tumors of the uterus. I. A clinical and pathologic study of 53 endometrial stromal tumors. *Cancer* 1966;19:755–766.

409. **Hart WR, Yoonessi M.** Endometrial stromatosis of the uterus. *Obstet Gynecol* 1977;49:393–403.

410. **Krieger PD, Gusberg SB.** Endolymphatic stromal myosis: a grade 1 endometrial sarcoma. *Gynecol Oncol* 1973;1:299–313.

411. **Thatcher SS, Woodruff JD.** Uterine stromatosis: a report of 33 cases. *Obstet Gynecol* 1982;59:428–434.

412. **Piver MS, Rutledge FN, Copeland L, et al.** Uterine endolymphatic stromal myosis: a collaborative study. *Obstet Gynecol* 1984;64:173–178.

413. **Aubrey MC, Myers JL, Colby TV, et al.** Endometrial stromal sarcoma metastatic to the lung: a detailed analysis of 16 patients. *Am J Surg Pathol* 2002;26:440–449.

414. **Yoonessi M, Hart WR.** Endometrial stromal sarcomas. *Cancer* 1977;40:898–906.

415. **Evans HL.** Endometrial stromal sarcoma and poorly differentiated endometrial sarcoma. *Cancer* 1982;52:2170–2182.

416. **Chang KL, Crabtree GS, Lim Tan SK, et al.** Primary uterine endometrial stromal neoplasms: a clinicopathologic study of 117 cases. *Am J Surg Pathol* 1990;14:415–438.

417. **Clement PB, Scully RE.** Uterine tumors resembling ovarian sex-cord tumors: a clinicopathologic study of fourteen cases. *Am J Clin Pathol* 1976;66:512–525.

418. **Hauptman S, Nadjari B, Kraus J, et al.** Uterine tumor resembling ovarian sex-cord tumor: a case report and review of the literature. *Virchows Arch* 2001;439:97–101.

419. **Taylor HB, Norris HJ.** Mesenchymal tumors of the uterus. IV. Diagnosis and prognosis of leiomyosarcoma. *Arch Pathol* 1966;82:40–44.

420. **Gudgeon DH.** Leiomyosarcoma of the uterus. *Obstet Gynecol* 1968;32:96–100.

421. **Silverberg SG.** Leiomyosarcoma of the uterus: a clinicopathologic study. *ObstetGynecol* 1971;38:613–628.

422. **Christopherson WM, Williamson EO, Gray LA.** Leiomyosarcoma of the uterus. *Cancer* 1972;29:1512–1517.

423. **Gallup DG, Cordray DR.** Leiomyosarcoma of the uterus: case reports and a review. *Obstet Gynecol Surv* 1979;34:300–312.

424. **Vardi JR, Tovell HMM.** Leiomyosarcoma of the uterus: clinico-pathologic study. *Obstet Gynecol* 1980;56:428–434.

425. **Van Dinh T, Woodruff JD.** Leiomyosarcoma of the uterus. *Am J Obstet Gynecol* 1982;144:817–823.

426. **Berchuck A, Rubin SC, Hoskins WJ, et al.** Treatment of uterine leiomyosarcoma. *Obstet Gynecol* 1988;71:845–850.

427. **Leibsohn S, d'Ablaing G, Mishell DR, et al.** Leiomyosarcoma in a series of hysterectomies performed for presumed uterine leiomyomas. *Am J Obstet Gynecol* 1990;162:968–976.

428. **Giuntoli RL 2nd, Metzinger DS, DiMarco CS, et al.** Retrospective review of 208 patients with leiomyosarcoma of the uterus: prognostic indicators, surgical management, and adjuvant therapy. *Gynecol Oncol* 2003;89:460–469.

429. **Dinh TA, Oliva EA, Fuller AF Jr, et al.** The treatment of uterine leiomyosarcoma: results from a 10-year experience (1990–1999) at the Massachusetts General Hospital. *Gynecol Oncol* 2004;92:648–652.

430. **Bell SW, Kempson RL, Hendrickson MR.** Problematic uterine smooth muscle neoplasms: a clinicopathologic study of 213 cases. *Am J Surg Pathol* 1994;18:535–558.

431. **King ME, Dickersin GR, Scully RE.** Myxoid leiomyosarcoma of the uterus: a report of six cases. *Am J Surg Pathol* 1982;6:589–598.

432. **Kurman RJ, Norris HJ.** Mesenchymal tumors of the uterus. VI. Epithelioid smooth muscle tumors including leiomyoblastoma and clear cell leiomyoma: a clinical and pathologic analysis of 26 cases. *Cancer* 1976;37:1853–1865.

433. **Prayson RA, Goldblum JR, Hart WR.** Epithelioid smooth muscle tumors of the uterus: a clinicopathologic study of 18 patients. *Am J Surg Pathol* 1997;21:383–391.

434. **Norris HJ, Parmley T.** Mesenchymal tumors of the uterus. V. Intravenous leiomyomatosis: a clinical and pathologic study. *Cancer* 1975;36:2164–2178.

435. **Scharfenberg JC, Geary WL.** Intravenous leiomyomatosis. *Obstet Gynecol* 1974;43:909–914.

436. **Evans AT III, Symmonds RE, Gaffey TA.** Recurrent pelvic intravenous leiomyomatosis. *Obstet Gynecol* 1981;57:260–264.

437. **Clement PB, Young RH, Scully RE.** Intravenous leiomyomatosis of the uterus: a clinicopathologic analysis of 16 cases with unusual histologic features. *Am J Surg Pathol* 1988;12:932–945.

438. **Abell MR, Littler ER.** Benign metastasizing uterine leiomyoma: multiple lymph node metastases. *Cancer* 1975;36:2206–2213.

439. **Banner AS, Carrington CB, Emory WB, et al.** Efficacy of oophorectomy in lymph-angioleiomyomatosis and benign metastasizing leiomyoma. *N Engl J Med* 1981;305:204–209.

440. **Tavassoli FA, Norris HJ.** Peritoneal leiomyomatosis (leiomyomatosis peritonealis disseminata): a clinicopathologic study of 20 cases with ultrastructural observations. *Int J Gynecol Pathol* 1982;1:59–74.

441. **Norris HJ, Roth E, Taylor HB.** Mesenchymal tumors of the uterus. II. A clinical and pathologic study of 31 mixed mesodermal tumors. *Obstet Gynecol* 1966;28:57–63.

442. **Norris HJ, Taylor HB.** Mesenchymal tumors of the uterus. III. A clinical pathologic study of 31 carcinosarcomas. *Cancer* 1966;19:1459–1465.

443. **Silverberg SG, Major FJ, Blessing JA, et al.** Carcinosarcoma (malignant mixed mesodermal tumor) of the uterus: a Gynecologic Oncology Group pathologic study of 203 cases. *Int J Gynecol Pathol* 1990;9:1–19.

444. **Inthasorn P, Carter J, Valmadre S, et al.** Analysis of clinicopathologic factors in malignant mixed mullerian tumors of the uterine corpus. *Int J Gynecol Cancer* 2002;12:348–353.

445. **DiSaia PJ, Castro JR, Rutledge FN.** Mixed mesodermal sarcoma of the uterus. *AJR Am J Roentgenol* 1973;117:632–636.

446. **Yamada SD, Burger RA, Brewster WR, et al.** Pathologic variables and adjuvant therapy as predictors of recurrence and survival for patients with surgically evaluated carcinoma of the uterus. *Cancer* 2000;88:2782–2786.

447. **Macasaet MA, Waxman M. Fruchter RG, et al.** Prognostic factors in malignant mesodermal (mullerian) mixed tumors of the uterus. *Gynecol Oncol* 1985;20:32–42.

448. **DiSaia PJ, Morrow CP, Boronow R, et al.** Endometrial sarcoma: lymphatic spread pattern. *Am J Obstet Gynecol* 1978;130:104–105.

449. **Geszler G, Szpak CA, Harris RE, et al.** Prognostic value of peritoneal washings in patients with malignant mixed mullerian tumors of the uterus. *Am J Obstet Gynecol* 1986;155:83–89.

450. **Clement PB, Scully RE.** Mullerian adenosarcoma of the uterus: a clinico-pathologic analysis of 100 cases with a review of the literature. *Hum Pathol* 1990;21:363–381.

451. **Kaku T, Silverberg SG, Major FJ.** Adenosarcoma of the uterus: a Gynecologic Oncology Group study of 31 cases. *Int J Gynecol Pathol* 1992;11:75–88.

452. **Salazar OM, Bonfiglio TA, Patten SF, et al.** Uterine sarcomas: analysis of failures with special emphasis on the use of adjuvant radiation therapy. *Cancer* 1978;42:1161–1170.

453. **Spanos WJ, Peters LJ, Oswald MJ.** Patterns of recurrence in malignant mixed mullerian tumors of the uterus. *Cancer* 1986;57:155–159.

454. **Vongtama V, Karlen JR, Piver MS, et al.** Treatment results and prognostic factors in stage I and II sarcomas of the corpus uteri. *AJR Am J Roentgenol* 1976;126:139–147.

455. **Leitao MM, Brennan MF, Hensley M, et al.** Surgical resection of pulmonary and extrapulmonary recurrences of uterine leiomyosarcoma. *Gynecol Oncol* 2002;87:287–294.

456. **Belgrad R, Elbadawi N, Rubin P.** Uterine sarcomas. *Radiology* 1975;114:181–188.

457. **Salazar OM, Bonfiglio TA, Patten SF, et al.** Uterine sarcomas: natural history, treatment, and prognosis. *Cancer* 1978;42:1152–1160.

458. **Perez CA, Askin F, Baglan RJ, et al.** Effects of irradiation on mixed mullerian tumors of the uterus. *Cancer* 1979;43:1274–1284.

459. **Hornback NB, Omura G, Major FJ.** Observations on the use of adjuvant radiation therapy in patients with stage I and II uterine sarcoma. *Int J Radiat Oncol Biol Phys* 1986;12:2127–2130.

460. **Knocke TH, Kucera H, Dotfler D, et al.** Results of postoperative radiotherapy in the treatment of sarcoma of the corpus uteri. *Cancer* 1998;83:1972–1979.

461. **Molpus KL, Redlin-Frazier S, Reed G, et al.** Postoperative pelvic irradiation in early stage uterine mixed mullerian tumors. *Eur J Gynecol Oncol* 1998;19:541–546.

462. **Le T.** Adjuvant pelvic radiotherapy for uterine carcinosarcoma in a high-risk population. *Eur J Surg Oncol* 2001;27:282–285.

463. **Livi L, Paiar F, Shah N, et al.** Uterine sarcoma: twenty-seven years experience. *Int J Radiat Oncol Biol Phys* 2003;57:1366–1373.

464. **Menczer J, Levy T, Piuva B, et al.** A comparison between different postoperative treatment modalities of uterine carcinosarcoma. *Gynecol Oncol* 2005;97:166–170.

465. **Reed NS, Mangioni C, Malmstrom H, et al.** Phase III randomized study to evaluate the role of adjuvant pelvic radiotherapy in the treatment of uterine sarcomas stages I and II: an EORTC Gynaecological Cancer Group study (protocol 55874). *Int J Gynecol Cancer* 2003;13:4.

466. **Wolfson AH, Brady MF, Rocereto TF, et al.** Gynecologic Oncology Group randomized trial of whole abdominal irradiation (WAI) vs cisplatin-ifosfamide+mesna (CIM) in optimally debulked stage I-IV carcinosarcoma (CS) of the uterus. *J Clin Oncol* 2006;24:5001.

467. **Kanjeekal S, Chambers A, Fung MF, et al.** Systemic therapy for advanced uterine sarcoma: a systemic review of the literature. *Gynecol Oncol* 2005;97:624–637.

468. **Omura GA, Blessing JA, Major F, et al.** A randomized study of adriamycin with and without triazenoimidazole carboxamide in advanced uterine sarcomas. *Cancer* 1983;52:626–632.

469. **Sutton G, Blessing J, Barrett R, et al.** Phase II trial of ifosfamide and mesna in leiomyosarcoma of the uterus: a Gynecology Oncology Group study. *Am J Obstet Gynecol* 1992;166:556–559.

470. **Thigpen JT, Blessing JA, Beecham J, et al.** Phase II trial of cisplatin as first-line chemotherapy in patients with advanced or recurrent

uterine sarcomas: a Gynecologic Oncology Group study. *J Clin Oncol* 1991;9:1962.

471. **Gershenson DM, Kavanagh JJ, Copeland LJ, et al.** Cisplatin therapy for a disseminated mixed mesodermal sarcoma of the uterus. *J Clin Oncol* 1987;5:618–621.

472. **Sutton GP, Blessing JA, Rosenshein N, et al.** Phase II trial of ifosfamide and mesna in mixed mesodermal tumors of the uterus: a Gynecologic Oncology Group Study. *Am J Obstet Gynecol* 1989;161:309–312.

473. **Curtin JP, Blessing JA, Soper JT, et al.** Paclitaxel in the treatment of carcinosarcoma of the uterus: a Gynecologic Oncology Group Study. *Gynecol Oncol* 2001;83:268–270.

474. **Sutton G, Blessing JA, Ball H.** Phase II trial of paclitaxel in leiomyosarcoma of the uterus: a Gynecologic Oncology Group study. *Gynecol Oncol* 1999;74:346–349.

475. **Look KY, Sandler A, Blessing JA, et al.** Phase II trial of gemcitabine as second-line chemotherapy of uterine leiomyosarcoma: a Gynecologic Oncology Group study. *Gynecol Oncol* 2004;92:644–647.

476. **Sutton G, Blessing J, Hanjani P, et al.** Phase II evaluation of liposomal doxorubicin (Doxil) in recurrent or advanced leiomyosarcoma of the uterus: a Gynecologic Oncology Group study. *Gynecol Oncol* 2005;96:749–752.

477. **Gottlieb JA, Baker LH, O'Bryan RM, et al.** Adriamycin used alone and in combination for soft tissue and bony sarcomas. *Cancer Chemother Rep (Part 3)* 1975;6:271–282.

478. **Blum RH, Corson JM, Wilson RE, et al.** Successful treatment of metastatic sarcomas with cyclophosphamide, Adriamycin, and DTIC (CAD). *Cancer* 1980;46:1722–1726.

479. **Piver MS, DeEulis TG, Lele SB, et al.** Cyclophosphamide, vincristine, adriamycin, and dimethyltriazenoimidazole carboxamide (CYVADIC) for sarcomas of the female genital tract. *Gynecol Oncol* 1981;14:319–323.

480. **Pearl ML, Inagami M, McCauley DL, et al.** Mesna, doxorubicin, ifosfamide, and dacarbazine (MAID) chemotherapy for gynecologic sarcomas. *Int J Gynecol Cancer* 2002;12:745–748.

481. **Hensley ML, Maki R, Venkatraman E, et al.** Gemcitabine and docetaxel in patients with unresectable leiomyosarcoma. *J Clin Oncol* 2002;20:2824–2831.

482. **Nordal RN, Kjørstad KE, Stenwig AE, et al.** Leiomyosarcoma (LMS) and endometrial stromal sarcoma (ESS) of the uterus: a survey of patients treated in the Norwegian Radium Hospital 1976–1985. *Int J Gynecol Cancer* 1993;3:110–115.

483. **Berchuck A, Rubin SC, Hoskins WJ, et al.** Treatment of endometrial stromal tumors. *Gynecol Oncol* 1990;36:60–65.

484. **Sutton G, Brunetto VL, Kilgore L, et al.** A phase III trial of ifosfamide with or without cisplatin in carcinosarcoma of the uterus: a Gynecologic Oncology Group study. *Gynecol Oncol* 2000;79:47–53.

485. **Homesley HD, Filiaci V, Markman M, et al.** Gynecologic Oncology Group. Phase III trial of ifosfamide versus ifosfamide plus paclitaxel as first-line treatment of advanced or recurrent uterine carcinosarcoma (mixed mesodermal tumors): a Gynecologic Oncology Group study. *J Clin Oncol* 2007;25:526–531.

486. **Toyoshima M, Akahira J, Matsunaga G, et al.** Clinical experiences with combination paclitaxel and carboplatin therapy for advanced or recurrent carcinosarcoma for the uterus. *Gynecol Oncol* 2004;94:774–778.

487. **Omura GA, Blessing JA, Major F, et al.** A randomized clinical trial of adjuvant adriamycin in uterine sarcomas: a Gynecologic Oncology Group study. *J Clin Oncol* 1985;3:1240–1245.

36

Cervical and Vaginal Cancer

Caela Miller

John C. Elkas

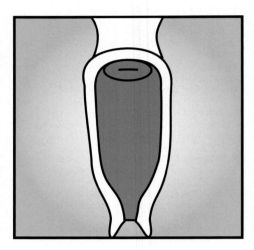

- **Human papillomavirus (HPV) infection is the causal agent of cervical cancer.**

- **Screening programs are effective at decreasing the incidence of cervical cancer. Vaccines also help decrease the incidence of cervical cancer.**

- **The most common histologic type of cervical cancer is squamous, and the relative and absolute incidence of adenocarcinoma is increasing; both histologies are caused by HPV infection.**

- **Cervical cancer is clinically staged, although modern radiographic modalities such as computed tomography, magnetic resonance imaging, ultrasound, or positron emission tomography may be beneficial for individual treatment planning.**

- **Treatment of cervical cancer is based on stage of disease. Early stage disease (stages I to IIA) can be treated with either radical surgery or radiation therapy. Advanced stage disease (stages IIB to IV) is best treated with chemoradiation.**

- **Vaginal cancer is a rare disease with many similarities to cervical cancer. Radiation therapy is the mainstay of treatment for most patients; however, select patients may be treated with radical surgery.**

Cervical cancer ranks as the third most common gynecologic neoplasm in the United States, behind cancer of the corpus and ovary, mainly as a result of the effectiveness of screening programs. **Worldwide, cervical carcinoma continues to be a significant health care problem. In developing countries, where health care resources are limited, cervical carcinoma is the second most frequent cause of cancer death in women.** Because cervical cancer is preventable, it is imperative that gynecologists and other primary health care providers to women be familiar with vaccination programs, screening techniques, diagnostic procedures, and risk factors for cervical cancer and management of preinvasive disease. Vaginal cancer is a rare tumor that shares an epidemiology and risk factor profile that is similar to cervical cancer.

Cervical Cancer

Epidemiology and Risk Factors

Invasive cancer of the cervix is considered a preventable disease because it has a long preinvasive state, cervical cytology screening programs are currently available, and the treatment of preinvasive lesions is effective. In spite of the preventable nature of this disease, 12,710 new cases of invasive cervical cancer resulting in 4290 deaths were anticipated in the United States in 2011 (1). Nationally, the lifetime probability of developing cervical cancer is 1:128. Although screening programs in the United States are well established, it is estimated that 30% of cervical cancer cases will occur in women who have never had a Papanicolaou (Pap) test. In developing countries, this percentage approaches 60% (2). Nevertheless, the worldwide incidence of invasive disease is decreasing, and cervical cancer is being diagnosed earlier, leading to better survival rates (1,3). The mean age for cervical cancer in the United States is 47 years, and the distribution of cases is bimodal, with peaks at 35 to 39 years and 60 to 64 years of age (1).

There are numerous risk factors for cervical cancer: young age at first intercourse (younger than 16 years), multiple sexual partners, cigarette smoking, race, high parity, low socioeconomic status, and chronic immune suppression. The relationship to oral contraceptive use was debated. Some investigators proposed that use of oral contraceptives might increase the incidence of cervical glandular abnormalities; however, this hypothesis was not consistently supported (4,5). Many of these risk factors are linked to sexual activity and exposure to sexually transmitted diseases. Infection with the herpes virus was thought to be the initiating event in cervical cancer; however, infection with human papillomavirus (HPV) was determined to be the causal agent in the development of cervical cancer, with herpes virus and *Chlamydia trachomatis* likely acting as cofactors. The role of human immunodeficiency virus (HIV) in cervical cancer is mediated through immune suppression (4). The Centers for Disease Control and Prevention described cervical cancer as an acquired immune deficiency syndrome (AIDS)–defining illness in patients infected with HIV (6).

The initiating event in cervical dysplasia and carcinogenesis is infection with HPV. HPV infection was detected in up to 99% of women with squamous cervical carcinoma. HPV is the causative agent in both squamous and adenocarcinoma of the cervix, but the respective tumors may have different carcinogenic pathways (7). There are more than 100 different types of HPV, more than 30 of which can affect the lower genital tract. There are 14 high-risk HPV subtypes; two of the high-risk subtypes, 16 and 18, are found in up to 62% of cervical carcinomas. The mechanism by which HPV affects cellular growth and differentiation is through the interaction of viral E6 and E7 proteins with tumor suppressor genes p53 and Rb, respectively. Inhibition of p53 prevents cell cycle arrest and cellular apoptosis, which normally occurs when damaged DNA is present, whereas inhibition of Rb disrupts transcription factor E2F, resulting in unregulated cellular proliferation (8). Both steps are essential for the malignant transformation of cervical epithelial cells. Two HPV vaccines, the quadrivalent *Gardasil* and the bivalent *Cervarix,* are approved by the U.S. Food and Drug Administration (FDA) and protect against subtypes 16 and 18. After 3 years, the efficacy of *Gardasil* was 99% for preventing cervical intraepithelial neoplasia grades 2 and 3 caused by HPV 16 or 18 in females who were not previously infected with either HPV 16 or 18 before vaccination; however, efficacy was only 44% in those who were infected prior to vaccination (9). Because the quadrivalent and bivalent HPV vaccines both protect only against certain types of HPV, vaccinated women need to continue to receive Pap test screening according to guidelines.

Evaluation

Vaginal bleeding is the most common symptom occurring in patients with cancer of the cervix. Most often, this is postcoital bleeding, but it may occur as irregular or postmenopausal bleeding. Patients with advanced disease may present with a malodorous vaginal discharge, weight loss, or obstructive uropathy. In asymptomatic women, cervical cancer is most commonly identified through evaluation of abnormal cytologic screening tests. The false-negative rate for Pap tests in the presence of invasive cancer is up to 50%, so a negative Pap test should never be relied on in a symptomatic patient (10).

Initially, all women suspected of having cervical cancer should have a general physical examination performed to include evaluation of the supraclavicular, axillary, and inguinofemoral lymph

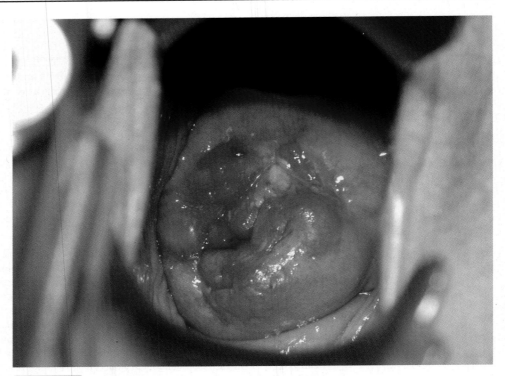

Figure 36.1   Gross appearance of cervical cancer on examination.

nodes to exclude the presence of metastatic disease. On pelvic examination, a speculum is inserted into the vagina, and the cervix is inspected for suspicious areas (Fig. 36.1). The vaginal fornices also should be closely inspected. With invasive cancer, the cervix is usually firm and expanded, and these features should be confirmed by digital examination. Rectal examination is important to help establish cervical consistency and size, particularly in patients with endocervical carcinomas. Rectal examination is the only way to determine cervical size if the vaginal fornices have been obliterated by menopausal changes or by the extension of disease. Parametrial extension of disease is best determined by the finding of nodularity beyond the cervix on rectal examination.

When obvious tumor growth is present, a cervical biopsy is usually sufficient for diagnosis. If gross disease is not present, a colposcopic examination with cervical biopsies and endocervical curettage is warranted. If the diagnosis cannot be established conclusively with colposcopy and directed biopsies, which may be the case with adenocarcinoma, cervical conization may be necessary.

Colposcopic Findings of Invasion	**Colposcopic examination is mandatory for patients with suspected early invasive cancer based on cervical cytology and a grossly normal-appearing cervix. Colposcopic findings that suggest invasion are (i) abnormal blood vessels, (ii) irregular surface contour with loss of surface epithelium, and (iii) color tone change. Colposcopically directed biopsies may permit the diagnosis of frank invasion and thus avoid the need for diagnostic cone biopsy, allowing treatment to be administered without delay.** If there is debate about the depth of invasion based on the cervical biopsies, and if the clinical stage may be upstaged to stage IA2 or IB1, the patient should undergo a conization. In the presence of a large cervical biopsy specimen showing invasion greater than 3 mm, or two biopsy specimens separated by 7 mm showing invasive cervical carcinoma, therapy should proceed without delay, and the patient could undergo radical surgery or radiation therapy.

Abnormal Blood Vessels   Abnormal vessels may be looped, branched, or reticular. **Abnormal looped vessels are the most common colposcopic finding and arise from the punctated and mosaic vessels present in cervical intraepithelial neoplasia (CIN).** As the neoplastic growth process proceeds and the need for oxygen and nutrition increases, angiogenesis occurs as a result of tumor and local tissue production of vascular endothelial growth factor (VEGF), platelet-derived growth factor (PDGF), epidermal growth factor (EGF), and other cytokines, resulting in the proliferation of blood vessels and neovascularization. Punctate vessels push out over the surface of the epithelium in an erratic fashion, producing the looped, corkscrew, or J-shaped pattern of abnormal vessels characteristic of invasive disease. Abnormal blood vessels arise from the cervical stroma and are pushed to the surface as the underlying cancer invades. The normally branching cervical stromal vessels are best observed over nabothian cysts. In this area, the branches are generally at acute angles, with the caliber of vessels becoming smaller after branching, much like the arborization of a tree. The abnormal branching blood vessels seen with cancer tend to form obtuse or right angles, with the caliber sometimes enlarging after branching. Sharp turns, dilations, and luminal narrowing also characterize these vessels. The surface epithelium may be lost in these areas, leading to irregular surface contour and friability.

Abnormal reticular vessels represent the terminal capillaries of the cervical epithelium. Normal capillaries are best seen in postmenopausal women with atrophic epithelium. When cancer involves this epithelium, the surface is eroded, and the capillary network is exposed. These vessels are very fine and short and appear as small comma-shaped vessels without an organized pattern. They are not specific to invasive cancer; atrophic cervicitis may also have this appearance.

Irregular Surface Contour Abnormal surface patterns are observed as tumor growth proceeds. The surface epithelium ulcerates as the cells lose intercellular cohesiveness secondary to loss of desmosomes. Irregular contour may occur as a result of papillary characteristics of the lesion. **This finding can be confused with a benign HPV papillary growth on the cervix. For that reason, biopsies should be performed on all papillary cervical growths to avoid missing invasive disease.**

Color Tone Color tone may change as a result of increasing vascularity, surface epithelial necrosis, and in some cases, production of keratin. The color tone is yellow-orange rather than the expected pink of intact squamous epithelium or the red of the endocervical epithelium.

Adenocarcinoma **Adenocarcinoma of the cervix does not have a specific colposcopic appearance.** All of the aforementioned blood vessels may be seen in these lesions. Because adenocarcinomas tend to develop within the endocervix, endocervical curettage is required as part of the colposcopic examination, and traditional screening methods are less reliable (10).

Histologic Appearance of Invasion	**Cervical conization is required to assess correctly the depth and the linear extent of involvement when microinvasion is suspected.** Early invasion is characterized by a protrusion of malignant cells from the stromal–epithelial junction. This focus consists of cells that appear better differentiated than the adjacent noninvasive cells and have abundant pink-staining cytoplasm, hyperchromatic nuclei, and small- to medium-sized nucleoli (11). **These early invasive lesions form tonguelike processes without measurable volume and are classified as International Federation of Gynecology and Obstetrics (FIGO) stage IA1.** With further progression, more tonguelike processes and isolated malignant cells appear in the stroma, followed by a proliferation of fibroblasts (desmoplasia) and a bandlike infiltration of chronic inflammatory cells (Fig. 36.2). **With increasing depth of invasion, lesions occur at multiple sites, and the growth becomes measurable by depth and linear extent. Lesions that are less than 3 mm in depth are classified as FIGO stage IA1. Lesions that are 3 to 5 mm or more in depth and up to 7 mm in linear extent are classified as FIGO stage IA2** (12). As the depth of stromal invasion increases, so does the risk of capillary lymphatic space involvement. Dilated capillaries, lymphatic spaces, and foreign-body multinucleated giant cells containing keratin debris are often seen in the stroma.

The depth of invasion should be measured with a micrometer from the base of the epithelium to the deepest point of invasion. **Depth of invasion is a significant predictor for the development of pelvic lymph node metastasis and tumor recurrence. Although lesions that have invaded 3 mm or less rarely metastasize, patients in whom lesions invade between 3 to 5 mm have positive pelvic lymph nodes in 3% to 8% of cases** (13). The significance of the cutoff at 3 mm is not identified completely; it was postulated that small capillary–lymphatic spaces at this level are incapable of facilitating the transport of malignant cells. Uneven shrinkage of tissue by fixative often creates space between the tumor nests and the surrounding fibrous stroma, simulating vascular lymphatic invasion (Fig. 36.2). Therefore, suspected vascular–lymphatic involvement

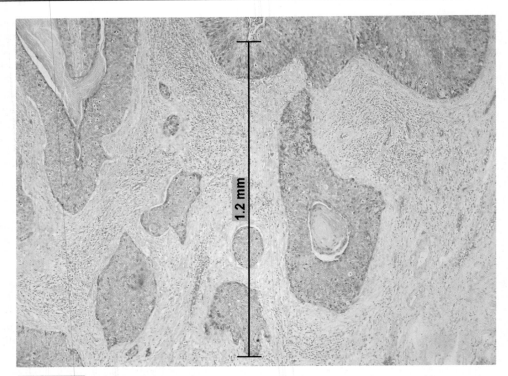

Figure 36.2   **Microinvasive squamous carcinoma.** Multiple irregular tonguelike processes and isolated nests of malignant cells are seen, some surrounded by clear spaces, simulating capillary lymphatic invasion. This is an artifact caused by tissue shrinkage. The depth of stromal invasion is measured from the basement membrane of the overlying cervical intraepithelial neoplasia (CIN). In this case, it is 1.2 mm.

with invasion of less than 3 mm should be interpreted with care. A lack of endothelial lining indicates that the space is a fixation artifact rather than true vascular invasion.

Staging

Cervical cancer is a clinically staged disease. The FIGO staging system is the standard and is applicable to all histologic types of cervical cancer. The FIGO staging system is presented in Table 36.1 and Figure 36.3. The staging procedures allowed by FIGO are listed in Table 36.2. **When there is doubt concerning the stage to which a cancer should be allocated, the earlier stage should be selected. After a clinical stage is assigned and treatment is initiated, the stage must not be changed because of subsequent findings by either extended clinical staging or surgical staging.** The upstaging of patients during treatment will produce an erroneous perception of improvement in the results of treatment of low-stage disease. Following is a breakdown of the incidence of cervical cancer by stage at diagnosis: 38%, stage I; 32%, stage II; 26%, stage III; and 4%, stage IV (3,13,14).

Additional Staging Modalities

Various investigators used lymphangiography, computed tomography (CT), ultrasonography, magnetic resonance imaging (MRI), and positron emission tomography (PET) in an attempt to improve the accuracy of clinical staging (15–25). These modalities suffer from poor sensitivity and high false-negative rates. Evaluation of the para-aortic lymph nodes with lymphangiography is associated with a false-positive rate of 20% to 40% and a false-negative rate of 10% to 20% (15–17). Overall, lymphangiography has a sensitivity of 79% and specificity of 73% (20). CT has poor sensitivity (34%) but excellent specificity (97%) (21). The accuracy of CT scanning is 80% to 85%; the false-negative rate is 10% to 15%, and the false-positive rate is 20% to 25% (16–18). Ultrasound has a high false-negative rate (30%), low sensitivity (19%), but high specificity (99%) (19). Early data showed that MRI results were comparable to those of CT scanning, a finding confirmed on meta-analysis (21,22). However, **a systematic review comparing CT scan with MRI showed that MRI is significantly more sensitive with**

Table 36.1 FIGO Staging of Carcinoma of the Cervix Uteri (2008)

Stage I	The carcinoma is strictly confined to the cervix (extension to the corpus would be disregarded)
IA	Invasive carcinoma which can be diagnosed only by microscopy, with deepest invasion ≤5 mm and largest extension ≤7 mm
IA1	Measured stromal invasion of ≤3.0 mm in depth and extension of ≤7.0 mm
IA2	Measured stromal invasion of >3.0 mm and not >5.0 mm with an extension of not >7.0 mm
IB	Clinically visible lesions limited to the cervix uteri or pre-clinical cancers greater than stage IA[a]
IB1	Clinically visible lesion ≤4.0 cm in greatest dimension
IB2	Clinically visible lesion >4.0 cm in greatest dimension
Stage II	Cervical carcinoma invades beyond the uterus, but not to the pelvic wall or to the lower third of the vagina
IIA	Without parametrial invasion
IIA1	Clinically visible lesion ≤4.0 cm in greatest dimension
IIA2	Clinically visible lesion >4 cm in greatest dimension
IIB	With obvious parametrial invasion
Stage III	The tumor extends to the pelvic wall and/or involves lower third of the vagina and/or causes hydronephrosis or non-functioning kidney[b]
IIIA	Tumor involves lower third of the vagina, with no extension to the pelvic wall
IIIB	Extension to the pelvic wall and/or hydronephrosis or non-functioning kidney
Stage IV	The carcinoma has extended beyond the true pelvis or has involved (biopsy proven) the mucosa of the bladder or rectum. A bullous edema, as such, does not permit a case to be allotted to Stage IV
IVA	Spread of the growth to adjacent organs
IVB	Spread to distant organs

FIGO Committee on Gynecologic Oncology. Revised FIGO staging for carcinoma of the vulva, cervix, and endometrium. *Int Cynecol Obst* 2009;105:103–104.

[a]All macroscopically visible lesions, even those with superficial invasion, are allotted to stage IB carcinomas. Invasion is limited to a measured stroma invasion with a maximal depth of 5.0 mm and a horizontal extension greater than 7.0 mm. Dept of invasion should not be greater than 5 mm taken from the base of the epithelium of the original tissue squamous or glandular. The depth of invasion should always be reported in millimeters, even those cases with "early minimal stromal invasion" (~1 mm). The involvement of vascular/lymphatic spaces should not change stage allotment.

[b]On rectal examination, there is no cancer-free space between the tumor and the pelvic wall. All cases with hydronephrosis or non-functioning kidney are included, unless they are known to be due to another cause.

equivalent specificity. Additionally, MRI has excellent sensitivity on T2-weighted images for the detection of parametrial disease (23). As a result, MRI is the preferred study to evaluate tumor size, lymph node metastasis, and local tumor extension.

PET scans are increasingly being utilized either alone or in conjunction with CT or MRI to detect metastatic disease; however, large prospective data series are limited. Early studies suggest that PET may be more useful than other techniques for the detection of abdominal and extrapelvic disease, with comparable or better sensitivity (76% to 100%) and specificity (94%) (24,25). In addition, PET scans may be better predictors of treatment outcome. Although early studies show promise for the use of PET scans in evaluating cervical cancer, the sensitivity for detecting metastatic disease less than 1 cm in size appears to be limited (26).

When abnormalities are noted on CT, MRI, or PET, radiographic-guided fine-needle aspirations (FNA) can be performed to confirm metastatic disease and individualize treatment planning. Because these tests are not available equally throughout the world and the interpretation of results can be variable, these studies are not used for staging. They may be useful in individual treatment planning.

The clinical staging system developed by FIGO is based on the belief that cervical cancer is a local disease until rather late in its course. **The accuracy of clinical staging is limited, and surgical evaluation, although not practical or feasible in all patients, can more accurately identify metastatic disease.** Surgical staging is advocated by providers who believe that surgical information details the extent of disease, allowing the treatment to be tailored to the individual (27). However, other providers believe that surgical staging should be limited to patients who are enrolled in clinical trials. These beliefs are based on the lack of randomized controlled studies demonstrating a survival benefit in patients who had surgical staging.

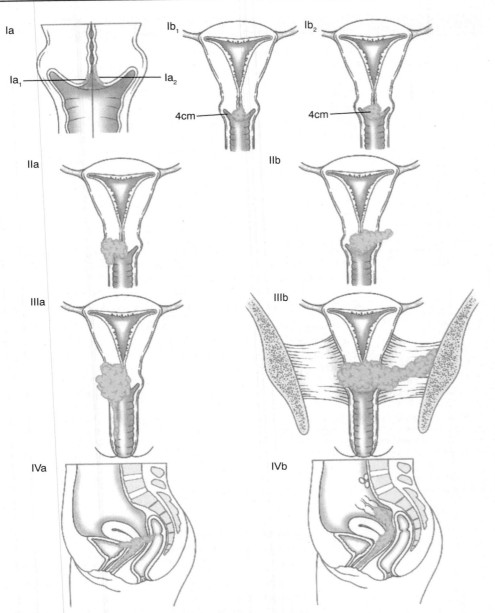

Figure 36.3 **Carcinoma of the cervix uteri: staging cervical cancer (primary tumor and metastases).** (From **Benedet JL, Odicino F, Maisonneuve P, et al.** Carcinoma of the cervix. *J Epidemiol Biostat* 2001;6:5–44, with permission.)

Pathology

Squamous Cell Carcinoma **Invasive squamous cell carcinoma is the most common variety of invasive cancer in the cervix.** Histologically, variants of squamous cell carcinoma include **large cell keratinizing, large cell nonkeratinizing, and small cell types** (28). Large cell keratinizing tumors consist of tumor cells forming irregular infiltrative nests with laminated keratin pearls in the center. Large cell nonkeratinizing carcinomas reveal individual cell keratinization but do not form keratin pearls (Fig. 36.4). The category of small cell carcinoma includes poorly differentiated squamous cell carcinoma and small cell anaplastic carcinoma. If possible, these two tumors should be differentiated. The former contains cells that have small- to medium-sized nuclei and more abundant cytoplasm than those of the latter. The designation of small cell anaplastic

Table 36.2 Staging Procedures	
Physical examination[a]	Palpate lymph nodes
	Examine vagina
	Bimanual rectovaginal examination (under anesthesia recommended)
Radiologic studies[a]	Intravenous pyelogram
	Barium enema
	Chest x-ray
	Skeletal x-ray
Procedures[a]	Biopsy
	Conization
	Hysteroscopy
	Colposcopy
	Endocervical curettage
	Cystoscopy
	Proctoscopy
Optional studies[b]	Computerized axial tomography
	Lymphangiography
	Ultrasonography
	Magnetic resonance imaging
	Positron emission tomography
	Radionucleotide scanning
	Laparoscopy

[a]Allowed by the International Federation of Gynecology and Obstetrics (FIGO).
[b]Information that is not allowed by FIGO to change the clinical stage.

carcinoma should be reserved for lesions resembling oat cell carcinoma of the lung. Small cell anaplastic carcinoma infiltrates diffusely and consists of tumor cells that have scanty cytoplasm, round to oval small nuclei, coarsely granular chromatin, and high mitotic activity. The nucleoli are absent or small. **Immunohistochemistry or electron microscopy can differentiate the small cell neuroendocrine tumors.** Patients with the large cell type of carcinoma, with or without keratinization, have a better prognosis than those with the small cell variant. Small cell anaplastic carcinomas behave more aggressively than poorly differentiated squamous carcinomas that contain small cells. Infiltration of parametrial tissue and pelvic lymph node metastasis affect the prognosis.

Other less common variants of squamous carcinoma include **verrucous carcinoma** and **papillary (transitional) carcinoma.** Verrucous carcinomas may resemble giant condyloma acuminatum, are locally invasive, and rarely metastasize. Papillary carcinomas histologically resemble transitional cells of the bladder and may have more typical squamous cell invasion at the base of the lesion. Papillary carcinomas behave and are treated in a manner similar to traditional squamous cell cancers, except that late recurrences were noted.

Adenocarcinoma

There is an increasing number of cervical adenocarcinomas reported in women in their 20s and 30s. Although the total number of cases of adenocarcinoma is relatively stable, this disease is appearing more frequently in young women, especially as the number of cases of invasive squamous cell carcinoma decreases. Older reports indicated that 5% of all cervical cancers were adenocarcinomas, whereas newer reports show a proportion as high as 18.5% to 27% (29–31). Much of this proportional increase is related to a decreasing incidence

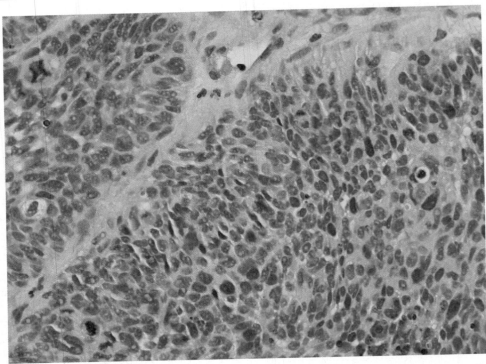

Figure 36.4 **Invasive squamous cell carcinoma, large cell nonkeratinizing type.** Tumor cells form irregular nests and have abundant eosinophilic cytoplasm and distinct cell borders indicative of squamous differentiation.

of squamous carcinoma secondary to screening programs (which are less accurate at identifying preinvasion adenocarcinoma), greater exposure to oral contraceptives, and a greater exposure to HPV (4,5).

Adenocarcinoma *in situ* (AIS) is believed to be the precursor of invasive adenocarcinoma, and it is not surprising that the two often coexist (32). In addition to AIS, intraepithelial or invasive squamous neoplasia occurs in 30% to 50% of cervical adenocarcinomas (33). A squamous intraepithelial lesion may be observed colposcopically on the ectocervix, and the coexistent adenocarcinoma often is higher in the cervical canal.

Patients with AIS who are treated with conization should undergo close clinical follow-up. Endocervical curettage, often used in surveillance, may miss residual or invasive disease, and false-negative rates as high as 50% were reported (34). In addition, skip lesions not resected at the time of conization may be present. For these reasons, hysterectomy should be considered the standard therapy for patients who have completed their childbearing. In two reports, patients with negative cone biopsy margins were followed conservatively, with few requiring repeat surgical procedures (35,36). Because cervical AIS tends to affect women during their reproductive years, a thorough discussion of risks and benefits should take place, and treatment should be individualized.

Adenocarcinoma of the cervix is managed in the same manner used for squamous cell carcinoma. Adenocarcinoma was believed to be associated with a worse prognosis and outcome when compared with squamous cell carcinoma. A study of 203 women with adenocarcinoma and 756 women with squamous carcinoma supported this assertion (30). This study showed 5-year survival rates of 90% versus 60%, 62% versus 47%, and 36% versus 8% for stages I, II, and III, respectively. Although some attributed these rates to a relative resistance to radiation, they are more likely a reflection of the tendency of adenocarcinomas to grow endophytically and to be undetected until a large volume of tumor is present. When adjusted for tumor size, it appears that there is no difference in prognosis between the two histologic subtypes. Adenocarcinoma may be detected by cervical sampling, but less reliably so than squamous carcinomas. A definitive diagnosis may require cervical conization.

The clinical features of stage I adenocarcinomas are well studied (30,37–39). These studies identified size of tumor, depth of invasion, grade of tumor, and age of the patient as significant correlates of lymph node metastasis and survival. When matched with squamous carcinomas for lesion size, age, and depth of invasion, the incidence of lymph node metastases and the survival rate appear to be the same (38,39). **Patients with stage I adenocarcinomas can be selected for treatment according to the same criteria as for those with squamous cancers** (39).

The choice of treatment for bulky stage I and II tumors is controversial. Some advocated treatment with radiation alone, whereas others support radiation plus extrafascial hysterectomy (40–42). In 1975, Rutledge et al. reported an 85.2% 5-year survival rate for all patients with stage I disease treated with radiation alone and an 83.8% survival rate for those who had radiation plus surgery (41). The central persistent disease rate was 8.3%, compared with 4% for those who had radiation plus surgery. In stage II disease, the 5-year survival rate was 41.9% for radiation alone and 53.7% for radiation plus surgery. **A subsequent report revealed no significant difference in survival among patients treated with radiation alone or radiation plus extrafascial hysterectomy** (43).

Invasive adenocarcinoma may be pure (Fig. 36.5A, B) or mixed with squamous cell carcinoma. Within the category of pure adenocarcinoma, the tumors are quite heterogeneous, with a wide range of cell types, growth patterns, and differentiation (30). **About 80% of cervical adenocarcinomas consist predominantly of the endocervical type cells with mucin production. The remaining tumors are populated by endometrioid cells, clear cells, intestinal cells, or a mixture of more than one cell type. By histologic examination alone, some of these tumors are indistinguishable from those arising elsewhere in the endometrium or ovary.** Within each cell type, the growth patterns and nuclear abnormalities vary according to the degree of differentiation. In well-differentiated tumors, tall columnar cells line the well-formed branching glands and papillary structures, whereas pleomorphic cells tend to form irregular nests and solid sheets in poorly differentiated neoplasms. The latter may require mucicarmine and periodic acid–Schiff (PAS) staining to confirm their glandular differentiation.

There are several special variants of adenocarcinoma. **Minimal deviation adenocarcinoma (adenoma malignum)** is an extremely well-differentiated form of adenocarcinoma in which the branching glandular pattern strongly simulates that of the normal endocervical glands. The lining cells have abundant mucinous cytoplasm and uniform nuclei (44,45). Because of this, the tumor may not be recognized as malignant in small biopsy specimens, thereby causing considerable delay in diagnosis. Special immunohistochemical staining may be required to establish the diagnosis. Earlier studies reported a dismal outcome for women with this tumor, but more recent studies found a favorable prognosis if the disease is detected early (46). Although rare, similar tumors were reported in association with endometrioid, clear, and mesonephric cell types (47).

An entity described as **villoglandular papillary adenocarcinoma** deserves special attention (48). It primarily affects young women, some of whom are pregnant or users of oral contraceptives. Histologically, the tumors have smooth, well-defined borders, are well differentiated, and are either *in situ* or superficially invasive. Follow-up information is encouraging. None of these tumors recurred after cervical conization or hysterectomy, and no metastasis was detected among women undergoing pelvic lymphadenectomy. This tumor appears to have limited risk for spread beyond the uterus.

Adenosquamous Carcinoma

Carcinomas with a mixture of malignant glandular and squamous components are known as **adenosquamous carcinomas.** Patients with adenosquamous carcinoma of the cervix were reported to have a poorer prognosis than those with pure adenocarcinoma or squamous carcinoma (49). Whether this is true when corrected for size of lesion is controversial (38,39).

In mature adenosquamous carcinomas, the glandular and squamous carcinomas are readily identified on routine histologic evaluation and do not cause diagnostic problems. **In poorly differentiated or immature adenosquamous carcinomas, however, glandular differentiation can be appreciated only with special stains, such as mucicarmine and PAS.** In one study, 30% of squamous cell carcinomas demonstrated mucin secretion when stained with mucicarmine (47). These squamous cell carcinomas with mucin secretion have a higher incidence of pelvic lymph node metastases than do squamous cell carcinomas without mucin secretion, and they are similar to the signet-ring variant of adenosquamous carcinoma (47,50).

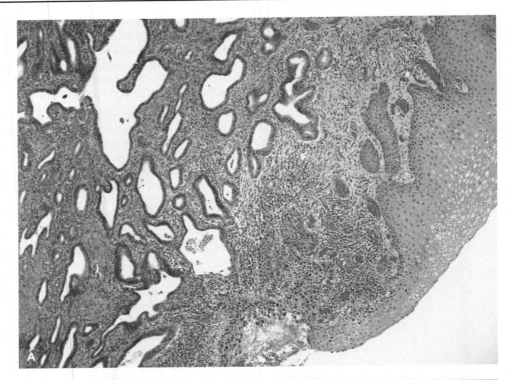

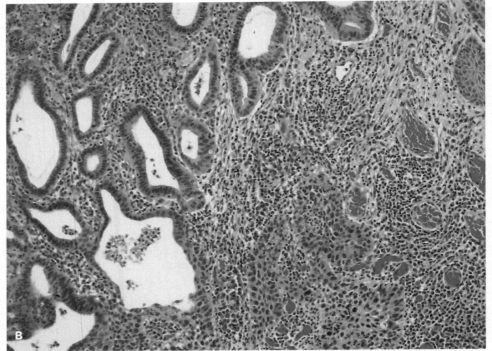

Figure 36.5   Invasive adenocarcinoma of the cervix, well-differentiated. A. Irregular glands are lined with tall columnar cells with vacuolated mucinous cytoplasm resembling endocervical cells. B. Nuclear stratification, mild nuclear atypism, and mitotic figures are evident in higher power.

Glassy cell carcinoma is recognized as a poorly differentiated form of adenosquamous carcinoma (51). Individual cells have abundant eosinophilic, granular, ground-glass cytoplasm, large round to oval nuclei, and prominent nucleoli. The stroma is infiltrated by numerous lymphocytes, plasma cells, and eosinophils. Approximately half of these tumors contain glandular structures or stain positive for mucin. The poor diagnosis of this tumor is linked to understaging and resistance to radiotherapy.

Other variants of adenosquamous carcinoma include **adenoid basal carcinoma** and **adenoid cystic carcinoma.** Adenoid basal carcinoma simulates the basal cell carcinoma of the skin (51). Nests of basaloid cells extend from the surface epithelium deep into the underlying tissue. Cells at the periphery of tumor nests form a distinct parallel nuclear arrangement, so-called peripheral palisading. An "adenoid" pattern occasionally develops, with "hollowed-out" nests of cells. Mitoses are rare, and the tumor often extends deep into the cervical stroma.

Adenoid cystic carcinoma of the cervix behaves much like such lesions elsewhere in the body. The tumors tend to invade into the adjacent tissues and metastasize late, often 8 to 10 years after the primary tumor was removed. Like other adenoid cystic tumors, they may metastasize directly to the lung. The pattern simulates that of the adenoid basal tumor, but there is a cystic component, and the glands of the cervix are involved (51). Mitoses may be seen but are not numerous.

Sarcoma

The most important sarcoma of the cervix is **embryonal rhabdomyosarcoma,** which occurs in children and young adults. The tumor has grapelike polypoid nodules, known as botryoid sarcoma, and the diagnosis depends on the recognition of rhabdomyoblasts. **Leiomyosarcomas** and **mixed mesodermal tumors** involving the cervix may be primary but are more likely to be secondary to uterine tumors. **Cervical adenosarcoma** is described as a low-grade tumor with a good prognosis (52). If recurrence develops, it is generally a central recurrence that may be treated with resection and hormonal therapy.

Malignant Melanoma

On rare occasions, melanosis is seen in the cervix. **Malignant melanoma** may arise *de novo* in this area. Histopathologically, it simulates melanoma elsewhere, and the prognosis depends on the depth of invasion into the cervical stroma.

Neuroendocrine Carcinoma

The classification of neuroendocrine cervical carcinoma includes four histologic subtypes: **(i) small cell, (ii) large cell, (iii) classical carcinoid,** and **(iv) atypical carcinoid** (53). Neuroendocrine tumors of the cervix are rare, and treatment regimens are based on small case series of patients.

Small cell (neuroendocrine type) carcinoma of the cervix is aggressive in nature and is similar to cancer arising from the bronchus (54). The hallmark of neuroendocrine tumors is their aggressive malignant behavior with the propensity to metastasize. At the time of diagnosis, it is usually disseminated, with bone, brain, liver, and bone marrow being the most common sites of metastases. In one study of 11 patients with disease apparently confined to the cervix, a high rate of lymph node metastasis was noted (55). Pathologically, the diagnosis is aided by the finding of neuroendocrine granules on electron microscopy and by immunoperoxidase studies that are positive for a variety of neuroendocrine proteins such as calcitonin, insulin, glucagon, somatostatin, gastrin, and adrenocorticotropic hormone (ACTH). In addition to the traditional staging for cancer of the cervix, these patients should undergo bone, liver and brain scanning and bone marrow aspiration and biopsy to evaluate the possibility of metastatic disease. Therapy consists of surgery, chemotherapy, and radiation. Because patients with early-stage disease have distant metastases, multimodal therapy is recommended. The main active chemotherapeutic agent is *etoposide.*

Local therapy alone gives almost no chance of cure of small cell carcinoma. Regimens of combination chemotherapy improved the median survival rates in small cell bronchogenic carcinoma, and these regimens are used for treatment of small cell carcinoma of the cervix. Combination chemotherapy may consist of *vincristine, doxorubicin,* and *cyclophosphamide (VAC)* or *VP-16 (etoposide)* and *cisplatin (EP)* (56). Patients must be monitored carefully because they are at high risk for developing recurrent metastatic disease (57).

Table 36.3 Incidence of Pelvic and Para-aortic Lymph Node Metastasis by Stage			
Stage	*No. of Patients*	*Positive Pelvic Nodes (%)*	*Positive Para-aortic Nodes (%)*
IA1 (≤3 mm)	179[a]	0.5	0
IA2 (>3–5 mm)	84[a]	4.8	<1
IB	1,926[b]	15.9	2.2
IIA	110[c]	24.5	11
IIB	324[c]	31.4	19
III	125[c]	44.8	30
IVA	23[c]	55	40

[a]References 74, 103, 110, 113, 114, 156.
[b]References 14, 74, 76, 86, 87, 90–94, 157.
[c]References 14, 15, 87, 90, 91, 95, 123.

Patterns of Spread

Cancer of the cervix spreads by (i) direct invasion into the cervical stroma, corpus, vagina, and parametrium; (ii) lymphatic metastasis; (iii) blood-borne metastasis; and (iv) intraperitoneal implantation. The incidence of pelvic and para-aortic nodal metastasis is shown in Table 36.3.

The cervix is commonly involved in cancer of the endometrium and vagina. The latter is rare, and most lesions that involve the cervix and vagina are designated cervical primaries. Consequently, the clinical classification is that of cervical neoplasia extending to the vagina, rather than vice versa. Endometrial cancer may extend into the cervix by three modes: direct extension from the endometrium, submucosal involvement by lymph vascular extension, and multifocal disease. The latter is most unusual, but occasionally a focus of adenocarcinoma may be seen in the cervix, separate from the endometrium. This lesion should not be diagnosed as metastasis but rather as multifocal disease. Malignancies involving the peritoneal cavity (e.g., ovarian cancer) may be found in the cul-de-sac and extend directly into the vagina and cervix. Carcinomas of the urinary bladder and colon occasionally extend into the cervix. Cervical involvement by lymphoma, leukemia, and carcinoma of the breast, stomach, and kidney is usually part of the systemic pattern of spread for these malignancies. Isolated metastasis to the cervix in such cases may be the first sign of a primary tumor elsewhere in the body.

Treatment Options

The treatment of cervical cancer is similar to the treatment of any other type of malignancy in that both the primary lesion and potential sites of spread should be evaluated and treated. The therapeutic modalities for achieving this goal include primary treatment with surgery, radiotherapy, chemotherapy, or chemoradiation. **Whereas radiation therapy can be used in all stages of disease, surgery is limited to patients with stage I to IIa disease. The 5-year survival rate for stage I cancer of the cervix is approximately 85% with either radiation therapy or radical hysterectomy.** A study using the National Cancer Institute's Surveillance Epidemiology and End Results data by an intent-to-treat analysis showed that patients in the surgery arm had an improved survival when compared with patients in the radiation arm (58). Optimal therapy consists of radiation, or surgery alone, to limit the increased morbidity that occurs when the two treatment modalities are combined. Recent improvements in the treatment of cervical carcinoma include adjuvant chemoradiation in patients discovered to have high-risk cervical carcinoma after radical hysterectomy and in patients with locally advanced cervical carcinoma.

Surgery

There are advantages to the use of surgery instead of radiotherapy, particularly in younger women for whom conservation of the ovaries is important. Chronic bladder and bowel problems that require medical or surgical intervention occur in up to 8% of patients undergoing radiation therapy (59). Such problems are difficult to treat because they result from fibrosis and decreased vascularity. This is in contrast to surgical injuries, which usually can be repaired without long-term complications. Sexual dysfunction is less likely to occur after surgical therapy

Table 36.4 Management of Invasive Cancer of the Cervix		
Stage IA1	≤3 mm invasion, no LVSI	Conization or type I hysterectomy
	≤3 mm invasion, w/LVSI	Radical trachelectomy or type II radical hysterectomy with pelvic lymphadenectomy
IA2	>3–5 mm invasion	Radical trachelectomy or type II radical hysterectomy with pelvic lymphadenectomy
IB1	>5 mm invasion, <2 cm	Radical trachelectomy or type III radical hysterectomy with pelvic lymphadenectomy
	>5 mm invasion, >2 cm	Type III radical hysterectomy with pelvic lymphadenectomy
IB2		Type III radical hysterectomy with pelvic and para-aortic lymphadenectomy or primary chemoradiation
Stage IIA1, IIA2		Type III radical hysterectomy with pelvic and para-aortic lymphadenectomy or primary chemoradiation
IIB, IIIA, IIIB		Primary chemoradiation
Stage IVA		Primary chemoradiation or primary exenteration
IVB		Primary chemotherapy ± radiation

LVSI, lymphovascular space invasion.

than radiation, because of vaginal shortening, fibrosis, and atrophy of the epithelium associated with radiation. Surgical therapy shortens the vagina, but gradual lengthening can be brought about by sexual activity. The epithelium does not become atrophic because it responds either to endogenous estrogen or to exogenous estrogens if the patient is postmenopausal.

Radical hysterectomy is reserved for women who are in good physical condition. Advanced chronologic age should not be a deterrent. With improvements in anesthesia, elderly patients withstand radical surgery almost as well as their younger counterparts (60). **It is prudent not to operate on lesions that are larger than 4 cm in diameter because these patients will require postoperative radiation therapy.** When selected in this manner, the urinary fistula rate is less than 2%, and the operative mortality rate is less than 1% (61,62). A summary of the management of cervical cancer is presented in Table 36.4.

If radiation therapy is needed, transposing the ovaries out of the planned radiation field may preserve ovarian function. Although transposition provides some protection, studies suggest that normal ovarian function is preserved in fewer than 50% of patients (63,64). Metastasis to the ovaries occurs in 0.9% of cases of early stage cervical cancer, so preservation of the ovaries, particularly with adenocarcinoma, may confer a small recurrence risk (65).

Cone Biopsy of the Cervix

Cone biopsy of the cervix serves both a diagnostic and therapeutic role in cervical cancer. The procedure is indicated to confirm the diagnosis of cancer, and to definitively treat stage Ia1 disease when preservation of fertility is desired. For effective treatment, there must be no evidence of lymph–vascular space invasion, and both endocervical margins and curettage findings must be negative for cancer or dysplasia. Because stage Ia1 cancers have less than a 1% risk of lymph node metastasis, lymphadenectomy is not necessary. If the endocervical margin or curettage is positive for dysplasia or malignancy, further treatment is necessary because these findings are strong predictors of residual disease. For squamous cell carcinoma, the risk of residual disease is 4% if both the endocervical margin and curettage are negative for dysplasia or malignancy, 22% if the endocervical margin alone is positive, and 33% if both are positive (66). In cases of AIS, the status of the cone margins is particularly important, with residual preinvasive and invasive disease noted in up to 25% and 3%, respectively, of cases with negative margins, and up to 80% and 7%, respectively, in cases with positive margins (67,68).

Simple (Extrafascial) Hysterectomy

Type I hysterectomy is an appropriate therapy for patients with stage Ia1 tumors without lymph–vascular space invasion who are not desirous of future fertility. In such cases,

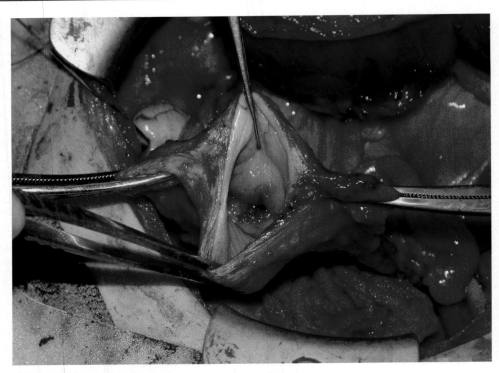

Figure 36.6   Abdominal radical trachelectomy.

lymphadenectomy is not recommended. If lymph–vascular space invasion is found, a modified radical hysterectomy with pelvic lymphadenectomy is appropriate and effective therapy.

Radical Trachelectomy

Radical trachelectomy is a procedure that is gaining popularity as a surgical management option for women with stage 1A2 and IB1 disease who desire uterine preservation and fertility. This procedure may be performed vaginally, abdominally, laparoscopically, or robotically (Fig. 36.6), and it usually is accompanied by pelvic lymphadenectomy and cervical cerclage placement. The risk of positive pelvic lymph nodes with stage Ia2 cancer may be as high as 8%, indicating the need for lymphadenectomy. Lymphadenectomy may be performed laparoscopically, robotically, or by the open laparotomy technique. Experience with this therapeutic modality is limited, although early results are promising, and it is uncertain whether the long-term outcome is similar to that of traditional therapy. Patients who are ideal candidates for this procedure have tumors less than 2 cm in diameter and have negative lymph nodes. Lymphadenectomy can be performed at the beginning of the procedure, and depending on those results, the procedure can be continued or abandoned. A retrospective trial comparing patients who had tumors with these attributes and were treated with either laparoscopic radical hysterectomy or laparoscopic radical trachelectomy showed similar outcomes and recurrence (69). There are limited data on subsequent pregnancy outcomes after radical trachelectomy; however, successful outcomes were reported. A study found that for women attempting to conceive after radical trachelectomy, the 5-year cumulative pregnancy rate was 52.8%, with an increased risk of miscarriage (70). Although radical trachelectomy and lymphadenectomy are performed with curative intent, it should be remembered that if a recurrence develops, definitive therapy with surgery or radiation is necessary.

Radical Hysterectomy

The **radical hysterectomy** (Fig. 36.7A, B) performed most often in the United States is that described by Meigs in 1944 (71). **The operation includes pelvic lymphadenectomy along with removal of most of the uterosacral and cardinal ligaments and the upper one-third of the vagina. This operation is referred to as the type III radical hysterectomy (72).**

The **hysterectomy described by Wertheim is less extensive than a radical hysterectomy and removes the medial half of the cardinal and uterosacral ligaments (62). This procedure**

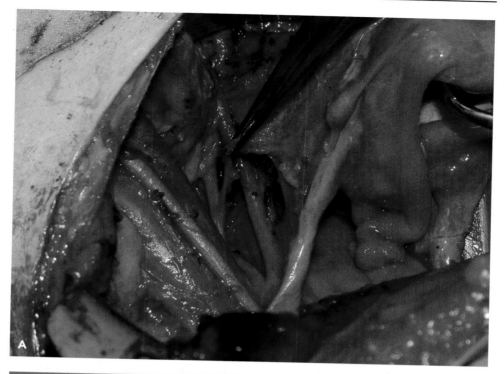

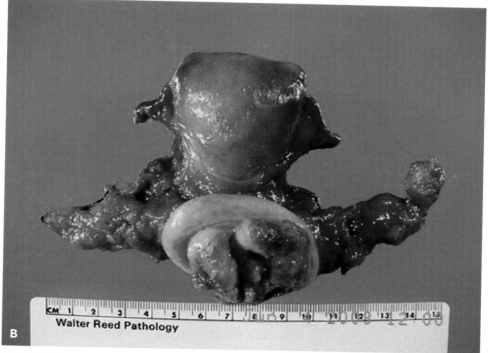

Figure 36.7   A: **Radical hysterectomy.** An intraoperative photograph showing the lateral dissection during a radical hysterectomy. Note the ureter running beneath the uterine artery (tissue in the clamp). B: **Radical hysterectomy specimen.**

is often referred to as the modified radical or type II hysterectomy. Wertheim's original operation did not include pelvic lymphadenectomy but instead included selective removal of enlarged lymph nodes. **The modified radical hysterectomy (type II) differs from the radical hysterectomy (type III) in the following ways:**

1. **The uterine artery is transected at the level of the ureter, thus preserving the ureteral branch to the ureter.**
2. **The cardinal ligament is not divided near the sidewall but instead is divided close to its midportion near the ureteral dissection.**
3. **The anterior vesicouterine ligament is divided, but the posterior vesicouterine ligament is conserved.**
4. **A smaller margin of vagina is removed.**

Radical hysterectomies can be further classified as extended radical hysterectomy (type IV and type V). In the type IV operation, the periureteral tissue, superior vesicle artery, and as much as three-fourths of the vagina are removed. In the type V operation, portions of the distal ureter and bladder are resected. This procedure is rarely performed because radiotherapy should be used when such extensive disease is encountered (72).

The abdomen is opened through either a midline incision or a low transverse incision after the methods of Maylard or Cherney. The low transverse incision requires division of the rectus muscles and provides excellent exposure of the lateral pelvis. It allows adequate pelvic lymphadenectomy and wide resection of the primary tumor. After the abdomen is entered, the peritoneal cavity is explored to exclude metastatic disease. The stomach is palpated to ensure that it has been decompressed to facilitate packing of the intestines. The liver is palpated, and the omentum is inspected for metastases. Both kidneys are palpated to ensure their proper placement and lack of congenital and other abnormalities. The para-aortic nodes are palpated transperitoneally.

During exploration of the pelvis, the fallopian tubes and ovaries are inspected for any abnormalities. **In premenopausal patients, the ovaries can be conserved.** The peritoneum of the vesicouterine fold and the rectouterine pouch should be inspected for signs of tumor extension or implantation. The cervix is palpated between the thumb anteriorly and the fingers posteriorly to determine its extent, and the cardinal ligaments are palpated for evidence of lateral tumor extension or nodularity.

Lymphadenectomy   **After inspection of the abdomen and pelvis, the pelvic and para-aortic lymph nodes should be inspected and palpated. Lymph nodes suspicious for gross disease should be excised and evaluated by frozen section.** If metastatic disease is identified, consideration should be given to abandoning radical surgery in favor of primary chemoradiation therapy. If the patient has no gross evidence of metastatic disease, the pelvic lymphadenectomy is begun.

Pelvic Lymphadenectomy   The pelvic lymphadenectomy is begun by opening the round ligaments at the pelvic sidewall and developing the paravesical and pararectal spaces. The ureter is elevated on the medial flap by a Deaver retractor to expose the common iliac artery. The common iliac and external iliac nodes are dissected, with care taken to avoid injuring the genitofemoral nerve, which lies laterally on the psoas muscle. At the bifurcation of the common iliac artery, the external iliac node chain is divided into lateral and medial portions.

The lateral chain is stripped free from the artery to the circumflex iliac vein distally. A hemoclip is placed across the distal portion of the lymph node chain to reduce the incidence of lymphocyst formation. The medial chain is dissected. The obturator lymph nodes are dissected; for this procedure, the lymph nodes are grasped just under the external iliac vein, and traction is applied medially. In most patients the obturator artery and vein are dorsal to the obturator nerve; however, 10% have an aberrant vein arising from the external iliac vein. The node chain is separated from the nerve and vessels and clipped caudally. Dissection continues cephalad to the hypogastric artery. The cephalad portion of the obturator space should be entered lateral to the external iliac artery and medial to the psoas muscle, where the remainder of the obturator node tissue can be dissected as far cephalad as the common iliac artery. Drainage of the pelvic and para-aortic lymph node beds is not performed because of the increase in complications in patients in whom drains were used (73).

Patients who have bulky cervical tumors or grossly positive pelvic nodes, or for whom frozen section evaluation will be performed, should undergo para-aortic lymph node evaluation to determine the full extent of disease and to guide adjuvant therapy.

Para-aortic Lymph Node Evaluation   The bowel is packed to expose the peritoneum overlying the bifurcation of the aorta. The peritoneum is incised medial to the ureter and over the right common iliac artery. A retractor is placed retroperitoneally to expose the aorta and the vena cava. Any enlarged para-aortic lymph nodes are removed, hemoclips are applied for hemostasis, and specimens are sent for analysis by frozen section. If the lymph nodes are positive for metastatic cancer, an option is to discontinue the operation and treat the patient with radiation therapy (71). If the lymph nodes are negative for disease, the left side of the aorta is palpated through the peritoneal incision with a finger passed under the inferior mesenteric artery. The lymph nodes on this side of the aorta are more lateral and nearly behind the aorta and the common iliac artery. If the left para-aortic lymph nodes appear healthy and the cervical tumor is small with no suspicious pelvic lymph nodes, these additional lymph nodes are not submitted for frozen-section analysis. If they are removed, they may be dissected through the incision made for the right para-aortic nodes, or they may be dissected after reflection of the sigmoid colon medially.

Development of Pelvic Spaces   The pelvic spaces are developed by sharp and blunt dissection (Fig. 36.8).

The paravesical space is bordered by the following structures:

1. The obliterated umbilical artery running along the bladder medially.
2. The obturator internus muscle along the pelvic sidewall laterally.
3. The cardinal ligament posteriorly.
4. The pubic symphysis anteriorly.

The attachments of the vagina to the tendinous arch form the floor of the paravesical space.

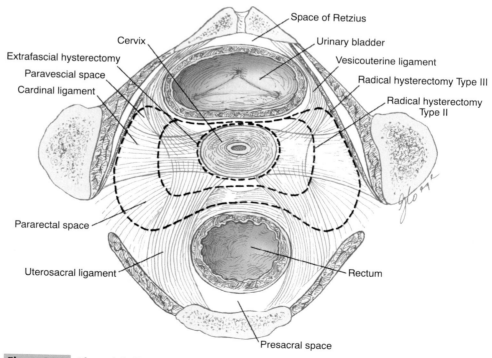

Figure 36.8   The pelvic ligaments and spaces. (From **Berek JS, Hacker NF.** *Berek & Hacker's Gynecologic Oncology.* 5th ed. Philadelphia, PA: Lippincott Williams & Wilkins, 2010:360, with permission.)

The pararectal space is bordered by the following structures:

1. Rectum medially
2. Cardinal ligament anteriorly
3. Hypogastric artery laterally
4. Sacrum posteriorly

The coccygeus (levator ani) muscle forms the floor of the pararectal space.

The development of these spaces before pelvic lymphadenectomy will aid in identification and dissection of the pelvic lymph nodes and dissection of the ureter as it passes into the vesicouterine ligament tunnel.

Dissection of the Bladder   **The dissection of the bladder from the anterior part of the cervix and vagina is a critical step. Occasionally, tumor extension into the base of the bladder (which cannot be detected with cystoscopy) precludes adequate mobilization of the bladder flap, leading to the abandonment of the operation. Therefore, this portion of the operation should be undertaken early in the procedure.** The bladder should be mobilized off of the upper third of the vagina to remove the tumor safely and with adequate margins.

Dissection of the Uterine Artery   The superior vesicle artery is dissected away from the cardinal ligament at a point near the uterine artery. **The uterine artery, which usually arises from the superior vesicle artery, is thus isolated and divided, preserving the superior vesicle arteries.** The uterine vessels are brought over the ureter by application of gentle traction. Occasionally, the uterine vein passes under the ureter.

Dissection of the Ureter   **The ureter is dissected free from the medial peritoneal flap at the level of the uterosacral ligament.** As the ureter passes near the uterine artery, there is a consistent arterial branch from the uterine artery to the ureter. This branch is sacrificed in the standard radical (type III) hysterectomy but preserved in the modified radical (type II) hysterectomy. Dissection of the ureter from the vesicouterine ligament (ureteral tunnel) may now be accomplished. If the patient has a deep pelvis, ligation of the uterosacral and cardinal ligaments may be undertaken first to bring the ureteral tunnel dissection closer to the operator. The roof of the ureteral tunnel is the anterior vesicouterine ligament. It should be ligated and divided to expose the posterior ligament. **The posterior ligament is divided in the radical (type III) hysterectomy but conserved in the modified radical (type II) hysterectomy.**

Posterior Dissection   The peritoneum across the cul-de-sac is incised, exposing the uterosacral ligaments. **The rectum is rolled free from the uterosacral ligaments, which are divided midway to the sacrum in a radical (type III) hysterectomy and near the rectum in the modified radical (type II) operation. This allows the operator to isolate and separate the cardinal ligament from the rectum.** A surgical clamp is placed on the cardinal ligament at the lateral pelvic sidewall in a radical hysterectomy and at the level of the ureteral bed in the modified radical procedure. A clamp is placed on the specimen side to maintain traction and to ensure that the full cardinal ligament is excised with the specimen. A right-angled clamp is placed caudad to this clamp across the paravaginal tissues. A second paravaginal clamp is usually needed to reach the vagina.

The vagina is entered anteriorly, and a suitable margin of proximal vagina is removed with the specimen. More vaginal epithelium can be excised if necessary, depending on the previous colposcopic findings. The vaginal edge may be sutured in a hemostatic fashion and left open with a drain from the pelvic space or closed with a suction drain placed percutaneously. The ureteral fistula and pelvic lymphocyst rates from these two techniques are similar.

Complications of Radical Hysterectomy

Acute Complications   The acute complications of radical hysterectomy include (74):

- Blood loss (average, 0.8 L)
- Ureterovaginal fistula (1% to 2%)
- Vesicovaginal fistula (1%)
- Pulmonary embolus (1% to 2%)

- Small bowel obstruction (1%)

- Febrile morbidity (25% to 50%)

Febrile morbidity is most often caused by pulmonary infection (10%) and is seen frequently with pelvic cellulitis (7%) and urinary tract infection (6%). Wound infection, pelvic abscess, and phlebitis all occur in fewer than 5% of patients (75).

Subacute Complications   **The subacute effects of radical hysterectomy are postoperative bladder dysfunction and lymphocyst formation.** For the first few days after radical hysterectomy, bladder volume is decreased, and filling pressure is increased. The sensitivity to filling is diminished, and the patient is unable to initiate voiding. The cause of this dysfunction is unclear. It is important to maintain adequate bladder drainage during this time to prevent overdistention. Bladder drainage is usually accomplished with a suprapubic catheter. It is more comfortable for the patient and allows the physician to perform cystometrography and determine residual urine volume without the need for frequent catheterization. In addition, the patient is able to accomplish voiding trials at home by clamping the catheter, voiding, and releasing to check the residual urine level. Cystometrography may be performed 3 to 4 weeks after surgery. For the catheter to be discontinued, the patient must be able to sense the fullness of the bladder, initiate voiding, and void with a residual urine level of less than 75 to 100 mL. Otherwise, voiding trials should continue at home until these criteria can be fulfilled.

Lymphocyst formation occurs in fewer than 5% of patients, and the cause is uncertain (75). Adequate drainage of the pelvis after radical hysterectomy may be an important step in prevention. However, routine placement of retroperitoneal drains did not reduce this morbidity (73). Ureteral obstruction, partial venous obstruction, and thrombosis may occur from lymphocyst formation. Simple aspiration of the lymphocyst is generally not curative, but percutaneous catheters with chronic drainage may allow healing. If this treatment is unsuccessful, operative intervention with excision of a portion of the lymphocyst wall and placement of either large bowel or omentum into the lymphocyst should be performed.

Chronic Complications   **The most common chronic effect of radical hysterectomy is bladder hypotonia or, in extreme instances, atony.** This condition occurs in about 3% of patients, regardless of the method of bladder drainage used (76,77). It may be a result of bladder denervation and not simply a problem associated with bladder overdistention (78). Voiding every 4 to 6 hours, increasing intra-abdominal pressure with Credé's maneuver, and intermittent self-catheterization may be used to manage bladder hypotonia.

Ureteral strictures are uncommon in the absence of postoperative radiation therapy, recurrent cancer, or lymphocyst formation (78). If the stricture is associated with lymphocyst formation, treatment of the lymphocyst usually alleviates the problem. Strictures that occur after radiation therapy should be managed with ureteral stenting. If a ureteral stricture is noted in the absence of radiotherapy or lymphocyst formation, recurrent carcinoma is the most common cause. A CT scan of the area of obstruction should be obtained and cytologic assessment by FNA should be performed if there is a target lesion to exclude carcinoma. If the results of these tests are negative, a ureteral stent may be placed to relieve the stricture. Close observation for recurrent carcinoma is necessary, and the diagnosis of recurrence may ultimately require laparotomy.

Nerve-Sparing Radical Hysterectomy

Nerve-sparing radical hysterectomies were described in recent years in an attempt to diminish the bladder dysfunction, sexual dysfunction, and colorectal motility disorders commonly encountered after traditional radical hysterectomy. Multiple techniques were described involving the identification of the pelvic autonomic nerves at the sacral promontory followed by various surgical methods of nerve preservation as the nerves transit the cardinal ligaments. These techniques are promising and in small series did reduce postoperative bladder dysfunction (79,80).

Laparoscopic Radical Hysterectomy

Laparoscopic-assisted radical vaginal hysterectomy is being performed with increasing frequency in highly selected patients. In one large series of 200 women with stages IA1 to IIB cervical cancer treated with laparoscopic lymphadenectomy followed by radical vaginal hysterectomy, the authors found a 5-year survival rate comparable to patients treated with a similar abdominal approach and a comparable rate of intraoperative complications (81).

The use of laparoscopy in cervical cancer patients is appealing because it may lead to less blood loss, improved cosmetic results, shorter duration of hospitalization, and faster recovery.

Robotic Laparoscopic Radical Hysterectomy

Robotic laparoscopic radial hysterectomy is a relatively new technique. Proponents argue that in highly selected patients it can decrease hospital admission time and decrease the surgical morbidity in obese patients. One study reports comparable body mass index, operative times, parametrial margin, and number of lymph nodes collected when compared to open cases. Robotic cases had significantly shorter hospital stays and blood loss, while having significantly larger incidence of postoperative bladder dysfunction. The technique is still too new to tabulate cancer outcome data (82,83).

Sentinel Lymph Node Evaluation

Sentinel lymph node detection has become an integral part of the management strategy for breast cancer and melanoma and is being investigated as a diagnostic tool in multiple human malignancies, including carcinoma of the cervix. The sentinel node is a specific lymph node (or nodes) that is the first to receive drainage from a malignancy and is a primary site of nodal metastasis. In theory, the presence or absence of metastatic disease in the sentinel node should reflect the status of the nodal basin as a whole. Thus, a negative sentinel lymph node would allow omission of lymphadenectomy of the involved nodal basin. Sentinel lymph nodes are detected through perilesional injection of radiolabeled technicium-99 or blue dye followed by intraoperative identification of the sentinel lymph nodes utilizing handheld gamma probes or visual identification of blue-stained nodes. These techniques are primarily applicable in patients with early-stage disease and clinically negative lymph nodes, in whom lymph node status may influence the extent of the procedure or the use of adjuvant treatment.

Although data utilizing sentinel lymph node detection techniques in cervical cancer are limited, several interesting conclusions can be drawn from completed studies. Sentinel nodes can be detected in 80% to 100% of cervical cancer patients, and these rates were confirmed by both laparotomy and laparoscopy. A combination of dye and radiolabeled techniques appears to be superior for the detection of sentinel lymph nodes over either technique used alone. Test sensitivity of 65% to 87% can be expected with a 90% to 97% negative predictive value. The likelihood of detecting sentinel nodes may depend on the tumor volume, the time from injection to retrieval of the sentinel nodes, and the volume of dye or radiolabeled tracer injected. Sentinel node detection rates do not appear to be influenced by prior cold knife cone biopsy. False-negative results were reported. **The role of sentinel node detection in cervix cancer is investigational; although the technique is promising, complete lymphadenectomy, when indicated, remains the standard of care** (84).

Postoperative Management

Prognostic Variables for Early-Stage Cervical Cancer (Ia2–IIa)

The survival of patients with early-stage cervical cancer after radical hysterectomy and pelvic lymphadenectomy depends on the presence or absence of several intermediate and high-risk pathologic factors (76,85–99).

Intermediate risk factors for recurrent disease are:

1. Large tumor size
2. Cervical stromal invasion to the middle or deep one-third
3. Lymph–vascular space invasion

High risk factors for recurrent disease are:

1. Positive or close margins
2. Positive lymph nodes
3. Microscopic parametrial involvement

Patients treated with radical hysterectomy who have intermediate or high risk factors have a 30% and 40% risk, respectively, of recurrence within 3 years (100–102).

Lesion Size   Lesion size is an independent predictor of survival. Patients with lesions smaller than 2 cm have a survival rate of approximately 90%, and patients with lesions larger than 2 cm have a 60% survival rate (89). When the primary tumor is larger than 4 cm, the survival rate drops to 40% (87,97). An analysis of a Gynecologic Oncology Group (GOG) prospective study of 645 patients showed a 94.6% 3-year disease-free survival rate for patients with occult lesions, 85.5% for those with tumors smaller than 3 cm, and 68.4% for patients with tumors larger than 3 cm (98).

Depth of Invasion   Patients in whom depth of invasion is less than 1 cm have a 5-year survival rate of approximately 90%, but the survival rate falls to 63% to 78% if the depth of invasion is more than 1 cm (76,98,102–105).

Parametrial Spread   Patients with spread to the parametrium have a 5-year survival rate of 69%, compared with 95% when the parametrium is negative. When the parametrium is involved and pelvic lymph nodes are positive, the 5-year survival rate falls to 39% to 42% (90,106).

Lymph–Vascular Space Involvement   The significance of finding lymph–vascular space involvement is somewhat controversial. Several reports show a 50% to 70% 5-year survival rate when lymph–vascular space invasion is present and a 90% 5-year survival rate when invasion is absent (76,89,93,107,108). Others found no significant difference in survival if the study is controlled for other risk factors (98,99,109–112). Lymph–vascular space involvement may be a predictor of lymph node metastasis and not an independent predictor of survival.

Lymph Nodes   The variable that is most independently predictive of survival is the status of the lymph nodes. Patients with negative nodes have an 85% to 90% 5-year survival rate, whereas the survival rate for those with positive nodes ranges from 20% to 74%, depending on the number of nodes involved and the location and size of the metastases (94–96,99,102,105,111–113).

Data on lymph node status is summarized as follows:

1. When the common iliac lymph nodes are positive, the 5-year survival rate is about 25%, compared with about 65% when only the pelvic lymph nodes are involved (106,114,115).

2. Bilateral positive pelvic lymph nodes portend a less favorable prognosis (22% to 40% survival rate) than unilateral positive pelvic nodes (59% to 70%) (114,115).

3. The presence of more than three positive pelvic lymph nodes is accompanied by a 68% recurrence rate, compared with 30% to 50% when three or fewer lymph nodes are positive (94,112).

4. Patients in whom tumor emboli are the only findings in the pelvic lymph node have an 82.5% 5-year survival rate, whereas the survival rate is 62.1% and 54% with microscopic invasion and macroscopic disease, respectively (84).

Given the high risk of recurrent disease in surgically treated patients with early-stage cervical cancer who exhibit intermediate- or high-risk pathologic factors, adjuvant radiation or chemoradiation therapy should be considered.

Primary Radiation Therapy

Radiotherapy can be used to treat all stages of cervical cancer, with cure rates of about 70% for stage I, 60% for stage II, 45% for stage III, and 18% for stage IV (3). A comparison of surgery and radiation for treatment of low-stage disease is shown in Table 36.5. Primary radiation treatment plans consist of a combination of external teletherapy to treat the regional lymph nodes and to decrease the tumor volume, and brachytherapy delivered by intracavitary applicators or interstitial implants to provide a treatment boost to the central tumor. Intracavitary therapy alone may be used in patients with early disease when the incidence of lymph node metastasis is negligible.

The treatment sequence depends on tumor volume. Stage IB lesions smaller than 2 cm may be treated first with an intracavitary source to treat the primary lesion, followed by external therapy

	Table 36.5 Comparison of Surgery versus Radiation for Stage IB/IIA Cancer of the Cervix	
	Surgery	*Radiation*
Survival	85%	85%
Serious complications	Urologic fistulas 1%–2%	Intestinal and urinary strictures and fistulas 1.4%–5.3%
Vagina	Initially shortened, but may lengthen with regular intercourse	Fibrosis and possible stenosis, particularly in postmenopausal patients
Ovaries	Can be conserved	Destroyed
Chronic effects	Bladder atony in 3%	Radiation fibrosis of bowel and bladder in 6%–8%
Applicability	Best candidates are younger than 65 years of age, <200 lb, and in good health	All patients are potential candidates
Surgical mortality	1%	1% (from pulmonary embolism during intracavitary therapy)

to treat the pelvic lymph nodes. Larger lesions require external radiotherapy first to shrink the tumor and to reduce the anatomic distortion caused by the cancer. Such a treatment strategy enables the therapist to achieve intracavitary dosimetry. **The usual doses delivered are 7,000 to 8,000 cGy to point A (defined as 2 cm superior to the external cervical os and 2 cm lateral to the internal uterine canal) and 6,000 cGy to point B (defined as 3 cm lateral to point A),** limiting the bladder and rectal dosage to less than 6,000 cGy. To achieve this level, it is necessary to adequately pack the bladder and bowel away from the intracavitary source. Localization films and careful calculation of dosimetry are mandatory to optimize the dose of radiation and to reduce the incidence of bowel and bladder complications. Local control depends on delivering an adequate dose to the tumor from the intracavitary source.

Although brachytherapy was traditionally prescribed using a low-dose rate technique, high-dose rate techniques are becoming more popular, and controversy exists over which technique is superior. Low-dose rates use caesium-137 as the source, whereas high-dose rates use iridium-192. Proponents of high-dose rate techniques argue that the exposure of radiation to medical personnel is less, ambulatory therapy is possible, and total treatment time is less. Advocates of low-dose rate techniques cite literature suggesting that complication rates are higher with higher-dose rate therapy. **Several published trials show that there may be slight stage-related differences in survival between patients treated with low- and high-dose rate regimens, but the techniques have comparable survival and complication rates** (116–118).

As noted, clinical staging is imprecise and fails to accurately predict disease extension to the para-aortic nodes in 7% of patients with stage IB, 18% with stage IIB, and 28% with stage III disease (119). Such patients will have "geographic" treatment failures if standard pelvic radiotherapy ports are used. As a result, treatment plans for these patients are individualized based on CT scans, PET scans, and biopsies of the para-aortic lymph nodes for consideration of extended-field radiotherapy. The routine use of extended-field radiation for prophylactic para-aortic radiation without documentation of distant metastasis to the para-aortic nodes was evaluated and is not practiced because of the increased enteric morbidity associated with this treatment modality.

Intensity Modulated Radiation Therapy

A method of providing external beam therapy, known as intensity modulated radiation therapy (IMRT), may be a significant therapeutic development. This technique uses computer-generated algorithms that accurately distinguish between target treatment volumes and normal tissue. The radiation beam intensity is modulated to optimize the delivery of radiation to the specified treatment volume while sparing adjacent normal tissue. The result appears to be much more accurate treatment of the tumor with minimal toxicity. Emphasizing this point is a study in 40 gynecologic cancer patients in which IMRT was used. Excellent coverage of the planned treatment volume was obtained, with no patient suffering grade 3 toxicity, and only 60% of patients suffering grade 2 toxicity, compared with a historical rate of 90% toxicity with conventional techniques (120). This technique is especially promising for treating cervical cancer because it allows higher doses to be delivered much more precisely, allowing patients who are unable to undergo brachytherapy because of pelvic anatomy and tumor geometry a chance for curative therapy. Studies utilizing IMRT in treating patients with cervical cancer are limited, but experience with this technique is increasing. Initial papers comparing the two techniques report decreased toxicity with comparable locoregional control, but they do not have long-term data on 5-year survival rates, so this technique is yet to be validated (121).

Adjuvant Radiation

In an effort to improve survival rates, postoperative radiotherapy was recommended for patients with high and intermediate risk factors such as metastasis to pelvic lymph nodes, invasion of paracervical tissue, deep cervical invasion, or positive surgical margins (76,86,89,90,106,111,112,122). Although most authors agree that postoperative radiotherapy is necessary in the presence of positive surgical margins, the use of radiation in patients with other high risk factors is controversial. Increasing evidence supports the use of adjuvant radiation. Particularly controversial, but best studied, is the use of radiation in the presence of positive pelvic lymph nodes. The rationale for treatment is the knowledge that pelvic lymphadenectomy does not remove all of the nodal and lymphatic tissue and subsequent radiotherapy can eradicate microscopic disease. The hesitancy to recommend postoperative radiotherapy derives from the significant rate of postradiation bowel and urinary tract complications (123). Most of the available data are retrospective. However, a randomized study by the GOG comparing radiation with no further treatment for patients at high risk for recurrence with negative pelvic nodes revealed a 30% serious complication rate, 16% reoperation rate, and a 2% mortality rate as a result of treatment-related complications (124).

Based on retrospective studies, it appears that postoperative radiation therapy for positive pelvic nodes can decrease pelvic recurrence but does not improve 5-year actuarial survival rates. One multi-institutional study showed no difference in survival in patients with three or fewer positive pelvic nodes (59% versus 60%) (112). However, there seemed to be a benefit when radiotherapy was given to those with more than three positive nodes.

In a study of 60 pairs of irradiated and nonirradiated women matched for age, lesion size, number, and location of positive nodes after radical hysterectomy, no significant difference was found in projected 5-year survival rates (72% for surgery alone, 64% for surgery plus radiation) (125). The proportion of recurrences confined to the pelvis was 67% in patients treated with surgery only and 27% in patients treated with postoperative radiation ($p = 0.03$). In a Cox regression analysis of 320 women who underwent radical hysterectomy, for the 72 who received postoperative radiation, there was a significant decrease in pelvic recurrence but no survival benefit (95). A multi-institutional retrospective study was performed on 185 women with positive pelvic nodes after radical hysterectomy, including 103 who received postoperative radiotherapy (97). Multivariate analysis disclosed that radiotherapy was not an independent predictor of survival, whereas age, lesion diameter, and number of positive nodes did influence survival. These authors concluded that additional treatment is needed to improve survival rates. Because survival is limited by distant recurrence, the addition of chemotherapy to postoperative radiotherapy was proposed. A 75% disease-free survival rate was reported at 3 years in 40 high-risk patients given *cisplatin*, *vinblastine*, and *bleomycin* after radical hysterectomy, and a 46% disease-free survival rate was found in 79 comparable patients who refused treatment (126). Only 4 (11.8%) of 34 patients with positive pelvic nodes had recurrences, whereas disease recurred in 8 (33%) of 24 untreated patients with positive nodes. An 82% rate of disease-free survival was reported at 2 years among 32 patients who were treated postoperatively with radiation therapy plus *cisplatin* and *bleomycin* (127).

The location of lymph node metastases apparently is relevant to postirradiation recurrence rates. When common iliac lymph nodes are involved, the survival rate drops to 20%. As the number of positive pelvic nodes increases, the percentage of positive common iliac and low para-aortic nodes increases (i.e., 0.6% when pelvic lymph nodes are negative, 6.3% with one positive pelvic node, 21.4% with two or three positive nodes, and 73.3% with four or more positive nodes). This information was used to recommend extended-field radiotherapy to patients with positive pelvic lymph nodes in an attempt to treat undetected extrapelvic nodal disease (107). A 3-year disease-free survival rate of 85% occurred in patients with positive pelvic nodes, and a survival rate of 51% occurred in patients with positive common iliac nodes; these rates are better than the survival rates of 50% and 23%, respectively, for historical control groups receiving radiotherapy to the pelvis alone.

The GOG reported the results of a randomized controlled trial on patients with cervical cancer treated by radical hysterectomy and found to have at least two of the following risk factors: capillary lymphatic space invasion, more than one-third stromal invasion, and large tumor burden (101). A total of 277 patients were entered into the study, with 140 patients randomized to no further therapy and 137 patients randomized to adjuvant pelvic radiotherapy. Patients with these risk factors who were treated postoperatively with radiation therapy had a statistically significant (47%) decrease in recurrent disease. After extensive follow-up, there is no statistically significant difference in mortality rates (128). The morbidity with combination therapy was acceptable, with a low rate of enteric and urinary complications. A second GOG study of patients with high-risk cervical cancer randomized patients to concurrent chemoradiation therapy or radiation therapy alone, as discussed below (100).

Concurrent Chemoradiation

Radiation therapy fails to achieve tumor control in 20% to 65% of patients with advanced cervical cancer. Chemotherapy, despite its relative lack of success in treating patients with cervical cancer, was evaluated as neoadjuvant treatment in combination with surgery. Concomitant use of chemotherapy and radiation was studied extensively by the GOG and results of five randomized studies were reported. The concept of chemoradiation encompasses the benefits of systemic chemotherapy with the benefits of regional radiation therapy. The use of chemotherapy to sensitize cells to radiation therapy improved local–regional control. These new results changed the way cervical cancer is treated in many medical centers.

An Intergroup trial involving the GOG, the Southwestern Oncology Group, and the Radiation Therapy Oncology Group evaluated postoperative chemoradiation therapy in patients with stage IA2, IB, or IIA cervical cancer who had positive pelvic lymph nodes, positive parametrial extension, or positive vaginal margins at the completion of radical hysterectomy (127). A total of 243 patients were assessed in this trial, with 127 receiving chemoradiation (*cisplatin, 5-fluorouracil [5-FU], radiation therapy*) and 116 receiving radiation. The results of this trial showed a statistically significant improvement in progression-free survival and overall survival at 43 months for the patients receiving concurrent chemoradiation. The 4-year survival rates for the patients receiving chemoradiation versus radiation alone were 81% and 71%, respectively. The toxicity levels in the two groups were acceptable, with a higher rate of hematologic toxicity in the concurrent chemoradiation arm. This study showed that in patients with these high-risk factors after radical hysterectomy for stage IA2, IB, and IIA disease, chemoradiation is the postoperative treatment of choice.

Concurrent chemoradiation was evaluated in patients with advanced cervical carcinoma. GOG protocol 85 was a prospective study that enrolled patients with stage IIb to IVA cervical cancer and compared concurrent chemoradiation (129). There were 177 patients treated with *cisplatin, 5-FU,* and radiation. These patients were compared with 191 patients treated with *hydroxyurea* and radiation. The median follow-up of patients who were alive at the time of the analysis was 8.7 years. Patients who received concurrent chemoradiation and were treated with *cisplatin* and *5-FU* had a statistically significant improvement in progression-free interval and overall survival (129). Hematologic toxicity levels in the two groups were similar. This study showed that *cisplatin*-based concurrent chemoradiation was a superior treatment when compared with *hydroxyurea* and concurrent radiation.

GOG Protocol 120 was initiated to evaluate patients with negative para-aortic nodes and cervical carcinoma stage IIB to IVA treated with concurrent chemoradiation. The treatment arms in this study consisted of radiation plus weekly *cisplatin;* or *cisplatin, 5-FU,* and *hydroxyurea;* or *hydroxyurea.* There were 176 patients in the weekly *cisplatin* arm; 173 patients in the *cisplatin, 5-FU,* and *hydroxyurea* arm; and 177 patients in the *hydroxyurea* arm (130). The two treatment arms with *cisplatin*-based chemotherapy and radiation showed an improvement in progression-free interval and overall survival at a median follow-up of 35 months. The relative risks for progression of disease or death were 0.55 and 0.57, respectively, for patients treated with *cisplatin*-based chemotherapy and radiation, compared with the patients treated with *hydroxyurea* and radiation (130). This study confirmed the findings of GOG Protocol 85 and reaffirmed the finding that *cisplatin*-based concurrent chemoradiation is the treatment of choice for patients with advanced-stage cervical cancer.

A third GOG trial evaluated patients with stage IB to IVA cervical cancer. Of the patients enrolled in this study, 70% had stage IB or IIA disease (131). A total of 403 patients were enrolled and evaluated. The 5-year survival rates were 73% in patients treated with chemoradiation and 58% in patients treated with radiation therapy alone. The cumulative rates of disease-free survival at 5 years were 67% in patients treated with concurrent chemoradiation and 40% in patients treated with radiation therapy alone. Survival and progression-free intervals for patients receiving concurrent chemoradiation were significantly improved (131). **The results of this study suggested that chemoradiation is the treatment of choice for stage IIB to IVA disease and that those patients with stage IB2 and IIA disease may benefit from chemoradiation.**

A GOG study of chemoradiation comparing concurrent *cisplatin* and radiation with radiation alone in patients with bulky IB cervical cancer included adjuvant hysterectomy after completion of the radiation (132). There were 183 patients assigned to the concurrent chemotherapy and radiation arm and 186 patients treated with radiation alone. The median duration of follow-up was 36 months, with disease recurrence detected in 37% of the patients treated with radiation alone, compared with 21% who were treated with concurrent chemoradiation (132). The 3-year survival rates were 83% in the group who received concurrent chemoradiation and 74% in the group who received radiation alone (132). The study also included adjuvant hysterectomy after completion of radiation treatment. Because the results did not show an improvement in survival by using adjuvant hysterectomy, the authors concluded that adjuvant hysterectomy would not be part of their recommendations. **This study supports the results of previous studies and shows that patients with bulky stage IB and IIA cervical cancer treated with concurrent chemoradiation have survival rates superior to those treated with radiation alone. These two studies indicate that patients with bulky stage IB and IIA disease should have primary treatment consisting of chemoradiation, with the chemotherapy agent being weekly *cisplatin*.**

Surgical Staging before Radiation

Surgical staging procedures designed to discover positive lymph nodes may be forgone with use of PET/CT imaging studies. The use of transperitoneal exploration was associated with a 16% to 33% mortality rate from radiotherapy-induced bowel complications and a 5-year survival rate of only 9% to 12% (133,134). **To avoid these complications, extraperitoneal dissection of the para-aortic nodes is recommended, and the radiation dose should be reduced to 5,000 cGy or less** (135,136). **When this approach is used, postradiotherapy bowel complications occur in fewer than 5% of patients, and the 5-year survival rate is 15% to 26% in patients with positive para-aortic nodes** (19,137,138). Survival appears to be related to the amount of disease in the para-aortic nodes and to the size of the primary tumor. In patients whose metastases to the para-aortic lymph nodes are microscopic and whose central tumor has not extended to the pelvic sidewall, the 5-year survival rate improves to 20% to 50% (139,140). Surgical staging techniques have improved to include laparoscopic assessment of the para-aortic and pelvic lymph nodes. Studies demonstrated benefit from surgical staging with improved survival and changes in treatment plans in 40% of patients (136,137). When PET/CT is compared with surgicopathological staging of para-aortic lymph nodes, some patients with histologically positive para-aortic lymph nodes are missed with surgicopathological staging (141).

Management of Grossly Positive Para-aortic Lymph Nodes

The management of patients with macroscopic or grossly positive para-aortic lymph nodes discovered at the time of surgery or by imaging studies is controversial. It is likely that grossly positive nodes are beyond the ability of radiation therapy alone to sterilize. Therefore, to improve survival, additional therapy is required. In a representative study of the multiple reports in the literature, lymph node metastases were noted in 133 of 266 patients. Pelvic and para-aortic nodes were positive in 44 patients and positive para-aortic nodes were noted in only 2 patients. Five- and 10-year survival rates were similar for patients with macroscopically positive resectable nodes and microscopically positive nodes. Patients with unresectable nodal disease had a worse survival rate than those with resectable disease. All patients underwent extraperitoneal lymph node resections and subsequent radiotherapy. There was a 10% incidence of severe morbidity related to radiation use. Consistent with other reports in the literature, this study showed that **extraperitoneal debulking lymphadenectomy confers a survival advantage similar to that enjoyed by patients with micrometastatic disease without additional morbidity** (27).

Prophylactic Para-aortic Radiation Therapy

Prophylactic extended-field radiation therapy is an alternative to surgical staging of the para-aortic lymph node chain in women with advanced cervical cancer judged to be at high risk but without radiological or clinical evidence of para-aortic lymph node involvement. This treatment strategy was evaluated in 441 patients with stages I to III disease (142). High rates of gastrointestinal toxicity were noted in the treatment group. There was no difference in disease-free survival or overall survival between the control and treated groups, although treated patients had fewer para-aortic failures. A lack of difference in survival rates in this study may be related to high local and regional failure rates, suggesting that ideal patients for prophylactic radiotherapy would be those in whom there is a high likelihood of achieving pelvic control. A survival benefit was noted in a study by the Radiation Therapy Oncology Group, in which 367 patients with stages IB to IIB disease were randomized to pelvic radiotherapy versus pelvic and extended field radiotherapy (143). The extended field treatment arm suffered more grade 4 and 5 toxicity, confirming previous studies. Complicating the issue is another study from the Radiation Therapy Oncology Group that revealed that in locally advanced cervical cancer, pelvic radiation therapy with concurrent *cisplatin* chemotherapy was superior to extended-field radiation therapy (131). **The appropriate role of prophylactic para-aortic radiation therapy is still under investigation.**

Supraclavicular Lymph Node Biopsy

Although not standard practice, the performance of a supraclavicular lymph node biopsy was advocated in patients with positive para-aortic lymph nodes before the initiation of extended-field irradiation and in patients with a central recurrence before exploration for possible exenteration. The incidence of metastatic disease in the supraclavicular lymph nodes in patients with positive para-aortic lymph nodes is 5% to 30% (144). Node enlargement and increased metabolic activity can be assessed with chest PET/CT scanning. Cytologic assessment by FNA can obviate the need for an excisional biopsy and should be performed if any enlarged nodes are present. If the scalene lymph nodes are positive, chemotherapy should be considered.

Complications of Radiation Therapy

Perforation of the uterus may occur with the insertion of the uterine tandem. This is particularly a problem for elderly patients and those who had a previous diagnostic conization procedure. When perforation is recognized, the tandem should be removed, and the patient should be observed for bleeding or signs of peritonitis. Survival may be decreased in patients who have uterine perforation, possibly because these patients have more extensive uterine disease (145). Fever may occur after insertion of the uterine tandem and ovoids. Fever most often results from infection of the necrotic tumor and occurs 2 to 6 hours after insertion of the intracavitary system. If uterine perforation was excluded by ultrasonography, intravenous broad-spectrum antibiotic coverage, usually with a *cephalosporin*, should be administered. If the fever does not decrease promptly or if the temperature is higher than 38.5°C, an aminoglycoside and a *bacteroides* species–specific antibiotic should administered. If fever persists or if the patient shows signs of septic shock or peritonitis, the intracavitary system must be removed. Antibiotics are continued until the patient recovers, and the intracavitary application is delayed for 1 to 2 weeks.

Acute Morbidity   **The acute effects of radiotherapy are caused by ionizing radiation on the epithelium of the intestine and bladder and occur after administration of 2,000 to 3,000 cGy.** Symptoms include diarrhea, abdominal cramps, nausea, frequent urination, and occasionally bleeding from the bladder or bowel mucosa. Bowel symptoms can be treated with a low-gluten, low-lactose, and low-protein diet. Antidiarrheal and antispasmodic agents may help. Bladder symptoms may be treated with antispasmodic medication. Severe symptoms may require a week of rest from radiotherapy.

Chronic Morbidity   **The chronic effects of radiotherapy result from radiation-induced vasculitis and fibrosis and are more serious than the acute effects. These complications occur several months to years after radiotherapy is completed. The bowel and bladder fistula rate after pelvic radiation therapy for cervical cancer is 1.4% to 5.3%, respectively** (59,61). Other serious toxicity (e.g., bowel bleeding, stricture, stenosis, or obstruction) occurs in 6.4% to 8.1% of patients (59,61).

Proctosigmoiditis   **Bleeding from proctosigmoiditis should be treated with a low-residue diet, antidiarrheal medications, and steroid enemas.** In extreme cases, a colostomy may be required to rest the bowel completely. Occasionally resection of the rectosigmoid must be performed.

Rectovaginal Fistula   **Rectovaginal fistulas or rectal strictures occur in fewer than 2% of patients.** The successful closure of fistulas with bulbocavernosus flaps or sigmoid colon transposition was reported (146,147). Occasionally, resection with anastomosis is feasible. Diversion resulting in colostomy may be the optimal therapy in patients who have poor vascular supply to the pelvis and a history of an anastomotic leak or breakdown from prior repairs.

Small Bowel Complications   **Patients with previous abdominal surgery are more likely to have pelvic adhesions and thus sustain more radiotherapy complications in the small bowel. The terminal ileum may be particularly susceptible to chronic damage because of its relatively fixed position at the cecum.** Patients with small bowel complications have a long history of crampy abdominal pain, intestinal rushes, and distention characteristic of partial small bowel obstruction. Often, low-grade fever and anemia accompany the symptoms. **Patients who have no evidence of disease should be treated aggressively with total parenteral nutrition, nasogastric suction, and early surgical intervention after the anemia resolves and good nutritional status is attained.** The type of procedure performed depends on individual circumstances (148). Small bowel fistulas that occur after radiotherapy rarely close spontaneously while total parenteral nutrition is maintained. Recurrent cancer should be excluded; aggressive fluid replacement, nasogastric suction, and wound care should be instituted. Fistulography and a barium enema should be performed to exclude a combined large and small bowel fistula. The fistula-containing loop of bowel may be either resected or isolated and left *in situ*. In the latter case, the fistula will act as its own mucous fistula.

Urinary Tract   **Chronic urinary tract complications occur in 1% to 5% of patients and depend on the dose of radiation to the base of the bladder. Vesicovaginal fistulas are the most common complication and usually require supravesicular urinary diversion.** Occasionally, a small fistula can be repaired with either a bulbocavernosus flap or an omental pedicle. Ureteral strictures are usually a sign of recurrent cancer, and a cytologic sample should be obtained at the site of the obstruction using FNA guided by a CT scan. If the findings are negative, the patient should undergo exploratory surgery to evaluate the presence of recurrent disease. If radiation fibrosis is the cause, ureterolysis may be possible or indwelling ureteral stents may be passed through the open urinary bladder to relieve obstruction.

Chemotherapy

Neoadjuvant Chemotherapy   Randomized trials were initiated by the GOG and other large centers to determine the efficacy of neoadjuvant chemotherapy. **In the era of effective chemoradiation therapy, there is no evidence that neoadjuvant chemotherapy offers superior results or a survival advantage over standard therapy.**

Chemotherapy for Advanced Disease   **Chemotherapy was studied in advanced cervical cancer with mixed results.** Single-agent chemotherapy was the standard for advanced or recurrent disease. Active agents include *cisplatin, carboplatin, paclitaxel,* and *ifosfamide,* but response rates are only 10% to 20% with a median duration of only 4 to 6 months. A number of trials were performed to determine whether multiagent chemotherapy is superior. The GOG Protocol 149 studied patients with histologically confirmed, advanced stage (IVb), recurrent or persistent squamous cell cancer of the cervix and randomized these patients to one of two combination chemotherapy treatment arms. Of the 287 patients, 146 patients were randomized to the *cisplatin* and *ifosfamide* arm, and 141 patients received *cisplatin, ifosfamide,* and *bleomycin.* There were no differences in overall survival, progression-free survival, response rates, or overall toxicity between the two combination chemotherapy regimens (149). In another trial sponsored by the GOG, single-agent *cisplatin* was compared to *cisplatin* plus either *dibromodulcitol* or *ifosfamide* plus *mesna.* In this trial, the combination of *cisplatin* plus *ifosfamide* had a better response rate (31% vs. 18%) and median time to progression (4.6 months vs. 3.2 months) compared with single agent *cisplatin.* Toxicity was notably higher in the combination regimen, and there was no overall survival advantage demonstrated (150). The GOG published the results of a study comparing single-agent *cisplatin* to *cisplatin* plus *paclitaxel* in women with stage IVb squamous cell cancer of the cervix. Although the response rate (36% vs. 19%) and progression-free survival (4.8 months vs. 2.8 months) were greater for the combination regimen, there was only a 1-month increase in overall survival (151). Finally, the regimen of *methotrexate, vinblastine, doxorubicin,* and *cisplatin* (*MVAC*), which received considerable attention because of preliminary studies suggesting high response rates, was evaluated in **POG Protocol 179.** In this study,

MVAC was compared to *cisplatin* alone, and *cisplatin* combined with *topotecan*. The *MVAC* arm was prematurely closed because of excessive toxicity, and the remaining *cisplatin* arms were compared. **Although the combination of *cisplatin* and *topotecan* was superior to *cisplatin* alone, the improvement in overall survival was only 3 months.** The combination arm had a higher complete response rate, overall response rate, progression-free survival, and overall survival (152). Doublet therapy with *cisplatin* and *paclitaxel* is considered standard therapy based on GOG 204, which analyzed four *cisplatin*-containing doublets (*topotecan, paclitaxel, vinorelbine*, and *gemcitabine*) for the best efficacy; although no major differences existed in overall survival for the four doublets, the *cisplatin* and *paclitaxel* doublet trended toward the best results (153). Overall, it appears that multiagent regimens offer an improved response rate and slightly higher overall survival but with increased toxicity. Other studies showed comparable survival and less toxicity with *carboplatin* and *paclitaxel* (154).

Treatment of Cervical Cancer by Stage

Stage IA   Until 1985, no FIGO recommendation existed concerning the size of lesion or the depth of invasion that should be considered microinvasive (stage Ia). This led to considerable confusion and controversy in the literature. Over the years, as many as 18 different definitions were used to describe microinvasion. In 1974, the Society of Gynecologic Oncologists recommended a definition that is accepted by FIGO: **A microinvasive lesion is one in which neoplastic epithelium invades the stroma to a depth of less than 3 mm beneath the basement membrane and in which lymphatic or blood vascular involvement is not demonstrated.** The purpose of defining microinvasion is to identify a group of patients who are not at risk for lymph node metastases or recurrence and who therefore may be treated with less than radical therapy.

Diagnosis must be determined on the basis of a cone biopsy of the cervix. The treatment decision rests with the gynecologist and should based on a review of the conization specimen with the pathologist. It is important that the pathologic condition be described in terms of (i) depth of invasion, (ii) width and breadth of the invasive area, (iii) presence or absence of lymph–vascular space invasion, and (iv) margin status. These variables are used to determine the degree of radicality of the operation and whether the regional lymph nodes should be treated (12).

Stage IA1 ≤3 mm Invasion   **Lesions with invasion less than or equal to 3 mm have less than 1% incidence of pelvic node metastases.** Within this group, it appears that the patients most at risk for nodal metastases or central pelvic recurrence are those with definitive evidence of tumor emboli in lymph vascular spaces (74,155). Therefore, patients with less than 3 mm invasion and no lymph–vascular space invasion may be treated with extrafascial hysterectomy without lymphadenectomy. Therapeutic conization appears to be adequate therapy for these patients if preservation of childbearing capability is desired. Surgical margins and postconization endocervical curettage must be free of disease. If there is lymph–vascular space invasion, a type I (extrafascial) or II (modified radical) hysterectomy with pelvic lymphadenectomy should be considered.

Treatment of microinvasive cervical adenocarcinoma is complicated by a lack of agreement on approaches. Recent reports show that patients with stage Ia1 cervical adenocarcinoma may be treated in a fashion similar to patients with this stage and a squamous lesion (103–105). Some experts disagree with this interpretation because of the difficulty in establishing a pathologic diagnosis of microinvasion from a frankly invasive adenocarcinoma. **Patients diagnosed with microinvasive cervical adenocarcinoma should have expert pathologic assessment before considering treatment with extrafascial hysterectomy or conization.**

Stage IA2 >3–5 mm Invasion   **Lesions with invasion of greater than 3 to 5 mm have a 3% to 8% incidence of pelvic node metastases;** thus, pelvic lymphadenectomy is necessary for these lesions (155,156). The primary tumor may be treated with a modified radical hysterectomy (type II) or a radical trachelectomy if preservation of fertility is desired. If intermediate- or high-risk pathologic factors are identified in the surgical specimen, adjuvant radiation or chemoradiation therapy is recommended.

Stages IB1, IB2, and IIA1 Invasive Cancer   **Stage Ib lesions are subdivided into stage IB1, which denotes lesions that are 4 cm or smaller in maximum diameter, and stage IB2, which denotes lesions that are greater than 4 cm. Stage IIA1 disease involves the upper two-thirds of the vagina, but total lesion size is 4 cm or less. These patients may be managed with either radical trachelectomy or a type III radical hysterectomy, with pelvic lymphadenectomy.**

Radical trachelectomy should be restricted to candidates with low-risk disease and a tumor size less than 2 cm. The para-aortic lymph node chain must be evaluated, especially if pelvic nodal disease is encountered. Adjuvant radiation therapy is recommended if intermediate risk factors are identified postoperatively. Adjuvant chemoradiation is indicated if high risk features are found.

Alternatively, primary chemoradiation therapy with curative intent is appropriate. A comparison of radical hysterectomy with radiation resulted in similar survival rates for the two treatment modalities. Several studies comparing patients treated by either radical hysterectomy or radiation therapy showed similar survival rates and outcomes for both groups (85,157). However, patients treated with type III radical hysterectomy who subsequently received postoperative radiation had a higher rate of intestinal and urinary morbidity compared with patients treated with either modality alone. Therefore, some clinicians advocate using radiation and avoiding surgery in these patients because many will require adjuvant postoperative radiation.

Bulky Stages IB2 and IIA2 Invasive Cancer   Patients with bulky IB2 and IIA2 disease may be treated with either primary chemoradiation or radical surgery. Because many of these patients will have intermediate or high risk factors postoperatively, strong consideration should be given to primary chemoradiation. If surgical therapy is desired, a type III radical hysterectomy with pelvic and para-aortic lymphadenectomy, followed by adjuvant chemoradiation if intermediate or high risk factors are present, is appropriate therapy. This option has benefits of complete surgical staging and ovarian preservation, if desired. Disadvantages of primary surgery include increased morbidity if multimodality therapy is utilized (157).

Stages IIB to IIIB Invasive Cancer   Therapy for patients with stage IIB or greater cervical cancer traditionally was radiation therapy. Primary pelvic radiation fails to control disease progression in 30% to 82% of patients with advanced cervical carcinoma (3). Two-thirds of these failures occur in the pelvis (158). A variety of agents were used in an attempt to increase the effectiveness of radiation therapy in patients with large primary tumors. Because chemoradiation was superior to radiation therapy alone, chemoradiation is the preferred treatment strategy for these patients, with *cisplatin* the chemotherapy agent of choice. Nodal involvement, particularly the para-aortic lymph nodes, is the most important factor related to survival (see section above on Concurrent Chemoradiation).

Stages IVA and IVB Cancer   Primary exenteration may be considered for patients with direct extension to the rectum or bladder, but it is rarely performed. For patients with extension to the bladder, the survival rate with radiation therapy is as high as 30%, with a urinary fistula rate of only 3.8% (159). The presence of tumor in the bladder may prohibit cure with radiation therapy alone; thus, consideration must be given to removal of the bladder on completion of external beam radiation treatment. This is particularly true if the disease persists at that time and the geometry is not conducive to brachytherapy. Rectal extension is less commonly observed but may require diversion of the fecal stream before chemoradiation to avoid septic episodes from fecal contamination. In certain clinical situations, such as with patients who have stage IVA disease and present with vesicovaginal or rectovaginal fistula, urinary or rectal diversion may be performed, followed by chemoradiation.

Patients with stage IVB cervical carcinoma are candidates for chemotherapy and palliative pelvic radiation therapy. Control of symptoms with the least morbidity is of primary concern in this patient population.

Patient Evaluation and Follow-up after Therapy

Patients who receive radiotherapy should be monitored closely to assess treatment response. Tumors may be expected to regress for up to 3 months after radiotherapy. During the pelvic examination, progressive shrinkage of the cervix and possible stenosis of the cervical os and surrounding upper vagina is expected and should be noted. During rectovaginal examination, careful palpation of the uterosacral and cardinal ligaments for nodularity is important. Cytologic assessment by FNA of suspicious areas should be performed to allow early diagnosis of persistent disease. In addition to the pelvic examination, the supraclavicular and inguinal lymph nodes should be carefully examined, and cervical or vaginal assessment should be performed every 3 months for 2 years and then every 6 months for the next 3 years. Endocervical curettage may be performed in patients with large central tumors.

Radiography of the chest may be performed yearly in patients who have advanced disease. Metastasis to the lung was reported in 1.5% of cases. Solitary nodules are present in 25% of cases with metastasis. Resection of a solitary nodule in the absence of other persistent disease may yield some long-term survivors (160). Although intravenous pyelography (IVP) is not a part of routine postradiotherapy surveillance, it should be performed if a pelvic mass is detected or if urinary symptoms warrant evaluation. The finding of ureteral obstruction after radiotherapy in the absence of a palpable mass may indicate unresectable pelvic sidewall disease, but this finding should be confirmed, usually by FNA cytologic assessment (161).

Patients who had radical hysterectomy and who are at high risk for recurrence may benefit from early recognition of recurrence because they might be saved with radiation therapy. In these patients, a routine CT urogram 6 to 12 months after surgery may be beneficial. After radical hysterectomy, about 80% of recurrences are detected within 2 years (162). The larger the primary lesion, the shorter the median time is to recurrence (163).

Special Considerations

Cervical Cancer during Pregnancy

The incidence of invasive cervical cancer associated with pregnancy is 1.2 in 10,000 (164). A Pap test should be performed on all pregnant patients at the initial prenatal visit, and any grossly suspicious lesions should be biopsied. Diagnosis is often delayed during pregnancy because bleeding is attributed to pregnancy-related complications. **If the result of the Pap test is positive for malignant cells, and invasive cancer cannot be diagnosed using colposcopy and biopsy, a diagnostic conization procedure may be necessary. Conization in the first trimester of pregnancy is associated with hemorrhagic and infectious complications, and an abortion rate as high as 33%** (165,166). **Because conization subjects the mother and fetus to complications, it should not be performed before the second trimester and only in patients with colposcopy findings consistent with cancer, biopsy-proven microinvasive cervical cancer, or strong cytologic evidence of invasive cancer.** Inadequate colposcopic examination may be encountered during pregnancy in patients who had prior ablative therapy. Close follow-up throughout pregnancy may allow the cervix to evert and develop an ectropion, allowing satisfactory colposcopy in the second or third trimester. Patients with obvious cervical carcinoma may undergo cervical biopsy and clinical staging similar to that of nonpregnant patients.

After conization, there appears to be no harm in delaying definitive treatment until fetal maturity is achieved in patients with stage Ia cervical cancer (165,167,168). Patients with less than 3 mm of invasion and no lymphatic or vascular space involvement may be followed to term. Historically, these patients were allowed to deliver vaginally, and a hysterectomy was performed 6 weeks postpartum if further childbearing was not desired. However, in a multivariate analysis of 56 women with cervical cancer diagnosed during pregnancy and 27 women with cervical cancer diagnosed within 6 months of delivery, vaginal delivery was the most significant predictor of recurrence. In addition, most recurrences after vaginal delivery involved distant sites. The ideal delivery method for these patients is not known definitively; however, strong consideration should be given to performing a cesarean birth in women with cervical cancer of any stage (169). If vaginal delivery is chosen, close inspection of the episiotomy site is required during follow-up because of rare reports of metastatic cervical cancer at these locations (170).

Patients with 3 to 5 mm of invasion and those with lymph–vascular space invasion may be followed to term or delivered early after establishment of fetal pulmonary maturity (165,168). They may have cesarean delivery, immediately followed by modified radical hysterectomy and pelvic lymphadenectomy. **Patients with more than 5 mm invasion should be treated as having frankly invasive carcinoma of the cervix.** Treatment depends on the gestational age of the pregnancy and the wishes of the patient. Modern neonatal care affords a 75% survival rate for infants delivered at 28 weeks of gestation and 90% for those delivered at 32 weeks of gestation. Fetal pulmonary maturity can be determined by amniocentesis, and prompt treatment can be instituted when pulmonary maturity is documented. Although timing is controversial, it is probably unwise to delay therapy for longer than 4 weeks (167,168). The recommended treatment is classic cesarean delivery followed by radical hysterectomy with pelvic lymphadenectomy. There should be a thorough discussion of the risks and options with both parents before any treatment is undertaken.

Patients with stages II to IV cervical cancer should be treated with radiotherapy. If the fetus is viable, it is delivered by classic cesarean birth, and therapy is begun postoperatively. If the pregnancy is in the first trimester, external radiation therapy can be started with the expectation that spontaneous abortion will occur before the delivery of 4,000 cGy. In the second trimester, a delay of therapy may be entertained to improve the chances of fetal survival. If the patient wishes to delay therapy, it is important to ensure fetal pulmonary maturity before delivery is undertaken. Neoadjuvant chemotherapy has been administered to women during pregnancy with cervical cancer after 13 weeks gestation, without clear short-term harm to the fetus, although longer clinical follow-up is necessary (171).

The clinical stage is the most important prognostic factor for cervical cancer during pregnancy. Overall survival for these patients is slightly better because an increased proportion of these patients have stage I disease. For patients with advanced disease, there is evidence that pregnancy impairs the prognosis (165,168). The diagnosis of cancer in the postpartum period is associated with a more advanced clinical stage and a corresponding decrease in survival (169).

Cancer of the Cervical Stump

Cancer of the cervical stump was more common many decades ago when supracervical hysterectomy was popular; because this operation is being performed more frequently, this situation may become increasingly familiar. Early-stage disease is treated surgically, with very little change in technique from that used when the uterus is intact (172). **Radical parametrectomy with upper vaginectomy and pelvic lymphadenectomy is the standard procedure.** Advanced-stage disease may present a therapeutic problem for the radiotherapist if the length of the cervical canal is less than 2 cm. This length is necessary to allow satisfactory placement of the uterine tandem. If the uterine tandem cannot be placed, radiation therapy can be completed with vaginal ovoids or with an external treatment plan in which lateral ports are used to augment the standard anterior and posterior ports. Such a technique will reduce the dosage to the bowel and bladder and thus reduce the incidence of complications.

Pelvic Mass

The origin of a pelvic mass must be clarified before treatment is initiated. A CT urogram can exclude a pelvic kidney, and a barium enema helps to identify diverticular disease or carcinoma of the colon. An abdominal x-ray film may show calcifications typically associated with benign ovarian teratomas or uterine leiomyomas. Pelvic ultrasonography differentiates between solid and cystic masses and indicates uterine or adnexal origin. Solid masses of uterine origin are most often leiomyomas and do not need further investigation.

Pyometra and Hematometra

An enlarged fluid-filled uterine cavity may be a pyometra or a hematometra. The hematometra can be drained by dilation of the cervical canal and will not interfere with treatment. The pyometra also should be drained, and the patient should be given antibiotics to cover *bacteroides* species, anaerobic *staphylococcus* and *streptococcus* species, and aerobic coliform bacterial infection. Placement of a large mushroom catheter through the cervix was advocated, but the catheter itself may become obstructed, leading to further occlusion of the drainage. Repeated dilation of the cervix with aspiration of pus every 2 to 3 days is more effective.

If the disease is stage I, a radical hysterectomy and pelvic lymphadenectomy may be performed. However, a pyometra is usually found in patients with advanced disease, and thus radiotherapy is required. External-beam therapy can begin after the pyometra is healed. Patients often have a significant amount of pus in the uterus or a tubo-ovarian abscess without signs of infection; therefore, a normal temperature and a normal white blood cell count do not necessarily exclude infection. Repeat physical examination or pelvic ultrasonography is necessary to ensure adequate drainage.

Cervical Carcinoma after Extrafascial Hysterectomy

When invasive cervical cancer is found after simple hysterectomy, further treatment is predicated on the extent of disease. Microinvasive disease in patients at low risk for lymph node metastasis does not require further treatment. Invasive disease may be treated with radiotherapy or reoperation involving a pelvic lymphadenectomy and radical excision of parametrial tissue, cardinal ligaments, and the vaginal stump (173).

Reoperation   **Reoperation is indicated for a young patient who has a small lesion and in whom preservation of ovarian function is desirable.** It is not indicated for patients who have positive margins or obvious residual disease (173). Survival rates after radical reoperation are similar to those after radical hysterectomy for stage I disease.

Concurrent *cisplatin*-based chemoradiation is recommended for gross residual disease, positive imaging, disease in the lymph nodes or parametrium, or a positive surgical margin; individualized brachytherapy is clearly indicated for a positive vaginal margin (174).

Radiation Therapy **Survival after radiotherapy depends on the volume of disease, the status of the surgical margins, and the length of delay from surgery to radiotherapy. Patients with microscopic disease have a 95% to 100% 5-year survival rate; the 5-year survival rate is 82% to 84% in those with macroscopic disease and free margins, 38% to 87% in those with microscopically positive margins, and 20% to 47% in those with obvious residual cancer** (175–177). A delay in treatment of more than 6 months is associated with a 20% survival rate (177).

Acute Hemorrhage

Occasionally, a large lesion can produce life-threatening hemorrhage. A biopsy of the lesion should be performed to verify neoplasia, and a vaginal pack soaked in Monsel's solution (*ferric subsulfate*) should be packed tightly against the cervix. After proper evaluation, **external radiation therapy can be started with the expectation that control of bleeding may require 8 to 10 daily treatments at 180 to 200 cGy per day.** Broad-spectrum antibiotics should be used to reduce the incidence of infection. If the patient becomes febrile, the pack should be removed. Rapid replacement of the pack may be necessary, and a fresh pack should be immediately available. This approach to management of hemorrhage in patients previously untreated is preferable to exploration and vascular ligation. **Vascular embolization under fluoroscopic control may be required in severe cases, and this procedure may obviate a laparotomy.** However, vascular occlusion ultimately may lead to decreased blood flow and oxygenation of the tumor, compromising the effectiveness of subsequent radiotherapy.

Ureteral Obstruction

Treatment of bilateral ureteral obstruction and uremia in previously untreated patients should be determined on an individual basis. Transvesical or percutaneous ureteral catheters should be placed in patients with no evidence of distant disease, and radiotherapy with curative intent should be instituted. Patients with metastatic disease beyond curative treatment fields should be presented with the options of ureteral stenting, palliative radiotherapy, and chemotherapy. With aggressive management, a median survival rate of 17 months may be achieved for these patients (178).

Barrel-Shaped Cervix

The expansion of the upper endocervix and lower uterine segment by tumor is referred to as a **barrel-shaped cervix. Patients with tumors larger than 6 cm in diameter have a 17.5% central failure rate when treated with radiotherapy alone because the tumor at the periphery of the lower uterine segment is too far from the standard intracavitary source to receive an adequate tumoricidal dose** (179). Attempts were made to overcome this problem radiotherapeutically by means of interstitial implants into the tumor with a perineal template, but high central failure rates were reported with this technique (180).

One approach is to use a combination of radiotherapy and surgery for treatment of patients with a barrel-shaped cervix. An extrafascial hysterectomy is performed 2 to 3 months after the completion of radiation therapy in an effort to resect a small, centrally persistent tumor. The dose of external radiotherapy is reduced to 4,000 cGy, and a single intracavitary treatment is given, which is followed by an extrafascial hysterectomy (181,182). This method appears to result in a lower rate of central failure (2%), although it is not clear that the overall survival rate is improved. **There is disagreement concerning the need for extrafascial hysterectomy**, and the GOG is undertaking a randomized study to compare adjuvant hysterectomy with radiotherapy alone in patients who have no evidence of occult metastases in the para-aortic nodes (see stages IB and IIA discussion).

The narrow upper vagina of older patients may preclude the use of an intracavitary source of radiation. These patients must receive their entire course of therapy from external sources, leading to a higher central failure rate and more significant bowel and bladder morbidity. If stage I disease is present in such a patient, a radical hysterectomy with pelvic lymphadenectomy is preferable, if the patient's medical condition allows this approach. There may be a role for IMRT in the management of such tumors.

Recurrent Cervical Cancer

Treatment of recurrent cervical cancer depends on the mode of primary therapy and the site of recurrence. Patients who were treated initially with surgery should be considered for radiation therapy, and those who had radiation therapy should be considered for surgical treatment. Chemotherapy is palliative only and is reserved for patients who are not considered curable by either surgery or radiation therapy.

Radiotherapy for recurrence after surgery consists primarily of external treatment. Vaginal ovoids may be placed in patients with isolated vaginal cuff recurrences. Patients with a regional recurrence may require interstitial implantation with a Syed type of template in addition to external therapy. A 25% survival rate can be expected in patients treated with radiation for a postsurgical recurrence (162).

Radiation Retreatment

Retreatment of recurrent pelvic disease by means of radiotherapy with curative intent is confined to patients who had suboptimal or incomplete primary therapy. This may allow the radiotherapist to deliver curative doses of radiation to the tumor. The proximity of the bladder and rectum to the cancer and the relative sensitivity of these organs to radiation injury are the major deterrents to retreatment with radiation. The insertion of multiple interstitial radiation sources into locally recurrent cancer through a perineal template may help overcome these dosimetric considerations (173,183). The fistula rates are high, and those consequences must be considered before interstitial therapy is initiated. For patients considered curable with interstitial implant therapy, pelvic exenteration is a better treatment choice. Palliative radiotherapy can be given to patients with localized metastatic lesions that are deemed incurable. Painful bony metastases, central nervous system lesions, and severe urologic or vena caval obstructions are specific indications.

Surgical Therapy

Surgical therapy for postirradiation recurrence is limited to patients with central pelvic disease. A few carefully selected patients with small-volume disease limited to the cervix may be treated with an extrafascial or radical hysterectomy. However, the difficulty of assessing tumor volume and the 30% to 50% rate of serious urinary complications in these previously irradiated patients have led most gynecologic oncologists to recommend pelvic exenteration as a last chance for cure (184,185).

Exenteration

There are three types of exenterative procedures: (i) an anterior exenteration (removal of the bladder, vagina, cervix, and uterus), (ii) a posterior exenteration (removal of the rectum, vagina, cervix, and uterus), and (iii) a total exenteration (removal of both bladder and rectum with the vagina, cervix, and uterus (Fig. 36.9). A total exenteration that includes a large perineal phase includes the entire rectum and leaves the patient with a permanent colostomy and a urinary conduit (infralevator). In selected patients, a total exenteration may take place above the levator muscle (supralevator), leaving a rectal stump that may be anastomosed to the sigmoid, thus avoiding a permanent colostomy.

Preoperative Evaluation and Patient Selection   **It is imperative to search for metastatic disease before undergoing an exenteration. The presence of metastatic disease in this setting is considered a contraindication to exenterative procedures.** Physical examination includes careful palpation of the peripheral lymph nodes with FNA cytologic sampling of any nodes that appear suspicious. A random biopsy of nonsuspicious supraclavicular lymph nodes is advocated by some clinicians but is not routinely practiced (145,186). A PET/CT scan of the chest and abdomen and pelvis CT helps in the detection of liver metastases and enlarged nodes. Cytologic study of any abnormality should be undertaken with CT-guided FNA. If a positive cytologic diagnosis is obtained, it will obviate the need for exploratory laparotomy.

Extension of the tumor to the pelvic sidewall is a contraindication to exenteration; however, this may be difficult for even the most experienced examiner to determine because of radiation fibrosis. If any question of resectability arises, exploratory laparotomy and parametrial biopsies should be offered (187–190). **The clinical triad of unilateral leg edema, sciatic pain, and ureteral obstruction is nearly always pathognomonic of unresectable disease on the pelvic sidewall.** Preoperatively, the patient should be prepared for a major operation. Total parenteral nutrition may be necessary to place the patient in an anabolic state for optimal healing. A bowel preparation, preoperative antibiotic administration, and prophylaxis for deep venous thrombosis with low-dose *heparin* or pneumatic calf compression should be undertaken (191).

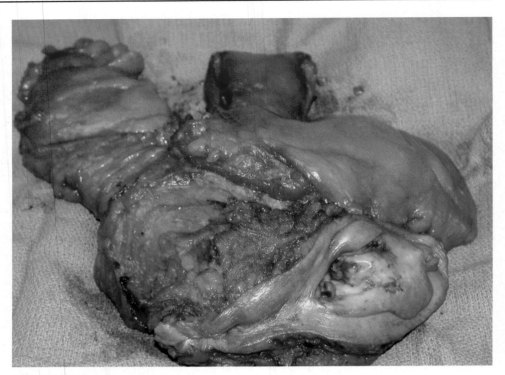

Figure 36.9   **Pelvic exenteration specimen.**

Surgical mortality increases with age, and the operation should rarely be considered in a patient who is older than 70 years. Other medical illnesses should be taken into account. When life expectancy is limited, exenterative surgery is unwise.

Anterior Exenteration   **Candidates for anterior exenteration are those in whom the disease is limited to the cervix and anterior portion of the upper vagina.** Proctoscopic examination should be performed because a positive finding would mandate a total exenteration. However, a negative proctoscopic examination finding does not exclude disease in the rectal muscularis, and findings at laparotomy still must be considered. The presence of disease in the posterior vaginal mucosa directly over the rectum mandates removal of the underlying rectum.

Posterior Exenteration   **A posterior exenteration is rarely performed for recurrent cervical cancer.** It is indicated, however, for the patient with an isolated posterior vaginal recurrence in which dissection of the ureters through the cardinal ligaments will not be necessary.

Total Exenteration   **Total exenteration with a large perineal phase is indicated when the disease extends to the lower part of the vagina** (Fig. 36.9). Because distal vaginal lymphatics may empty into the nodal basins of the inguinal region, these nodes should be carefully evaluated preoperatively. A supralevator total exenteration with low rectal anastomosis is indicated in the patient whose disease is confined to the upper vagina and cervix (192,193). Samples from margins of the rectal edge should be obtained for frozen-section evaluation because occult metastases to the muscularis may occur.

The development of techniques to establish continent urinary diversion help improve a woman's physical appearance after exenteration (194–196). When both a rectal anastomosis and a continent diversion are performed, the patient will not have a permanent external appliance. Associated psychological trauma in such cases may be avoided. **Every effort should be made to create a neovagina simultaneously with the exenteration** (197). This procedure helps in the reconstruction of the pelvic floor after extirpation of the pelvic viscera. Regardless of whether a neovagina is constructed, it is desirable to mobilize the omentum on the left gastroepiploic artery to create a new pelvic floor.

Surgical mortality from exenterative procedures has steadily decreased to less than 10%. Common causes of postoperative death are sepsis, pulmonary thromboembolism, and hemorrhage.

Fistulas of the gastrointestinal and genitourinary tract are serious surgical complications, with a 30% to 40% mortality rate despite attempts at surgical repair. The risk for fistula formation is decreased if nonirradiated segments of bowel are used for formation of the urinary conduit (191). **The 5-year survival rate is 33% to 60% for patients undergoing anterior exenteration and 20% to 46% for those undergoing total exenteration** (187–197). Survival rates are worse for patients with recurrent disease (larger than 3 cm), invasion into the bladder, positive pelvic lymph nodes, and recurrence diagnosed within 1 year after radiotherapy (190). The 5-year survival rate of patients with positive pelvic lymph nodes is less than 5%; thus, the performance of an extensive lymphadenectomy in the irradiated field is not warranted. Discontinuation of the procedure is advisable if any nodes are positive for metastatic cancer. Patients who have any disease in the peritoneal cavity have no chance of survival.

Laterally Extended Endopelvic Resection

Locally recurrent cervical cancer in a previously irradiated field is associated with a dismal prognosis. Exenterative therapy traditionally was reserved for the highly select patient with centrally recurrent disease, a selection criteria that excludes most patients with recurrence. A technique called the **laterally extended endopelvic resection (LEER)** procedure was described, which offers a surgical treatment option for patients with recurrent disease involving the pelvic sidewall. The LEER procedure involves extending the lateral resection plane of the traditional pelvic exenteration to include resection of the internal iliac vessels; the endopelvic portion of the obturator internus muscle; and the coccygeus, iliococcygeus, and pubococcygeus muscles. Extension of the surgical plane allows for resection of lateral tumors with a negative margin. Experience with it is limited to one center, which reports as high as a 62% recurrence-free survival, but as high as 70% moderate to severe morbidity (198).

Chemotherapy for Recurrent Cervical Cancer

Recurrent cervical cancer is not considered curable with chemotherapy. The delivery of chemotherapy to recurrent tumor in a prior radiated field may be compromised because of altered blood supply caused by radiation. *Topotecan* and *cisplatin* **had response rates of 15% to 20%, with a median duration of 6 to 9 months** (199). Many other agents showed activity against cervical cancer and may be used in attempt to help control symptoms. **Several clinical trials with various drugs (e.g.,** *paclitaxel, topotecan, cisplatin,* **and** *carboplatin*) **showed response rates of up to 45%. Most responses are partial; complete responses are unusual and limited to patients with chest metastases** in whom the dose of drug delivered to the disease is stronger than that delivered to the fibrotic postirradiated pelvis (200,201). Doublet therapy with *cisplatin* and *paclitaxel* is considered standard therapy based on GOG 204, which analyzed four *cisplatin*-containing doublets for the best efficacy; although no major differences existed in overall survival for the four doublets, the *cisplatin* and *paclitaxel* doublet trended toward the best results (153). Other studies showed comparable survival and less toxicity with *carboplatin* and *paclitaxel* (154).

Palliative Therapy

Palliative therapy for patients with incurable disease consists of radiation or chemotherapy or both. **Palliative radiation therapy is intended to relieve symptoms of pain or bleeding associated with advanced disease and may be administered as either external beam therapy (teletherapy) or brachytherapy.** Special care should be given to previously irradiated sites because additional radiation therapy may be associated with unacceptable morbidity. Single or multiagent palliative chemotherapy may be used with variable response rates. Symptomatic recurrent disease within previously irradiated fields may not respond well to palliative chemotherapy.

Vaginal Carcinoma

Primary vaginal cancer is a relatively uncommon tumor, representing only 2% to 3% of malignant neoplasms of the female genital tract. In the United States it is estimated that there were 2,160 new cases in 2009, and 770 deaths from the disease (1). Squamous histology accounts for 80% (202). **Primary vaginal cancer should be differentiated from cancers metastatic to the vagina, which constitute the majority of cancers found in the vagina (84%)** (203).

Staging

The FIGO staging of vaginal cancer dictates that a tumor extending to the vagina from the cervix be regarded as a cancer of the cervix, whereas a tumor involving both the vulva and the vagina should be classified as a cancer of the vulva.

Table 36.6 FIGO Staging of Vaginal Cancer	
Stage I	The carcinoma is limited to the vaginal wall.
Stage II	The carcinoma has involved the subvaginal tissue but has not extended to the pelvic wall.
Stage III	The carcinoma has extended to the pelvic wall.
Stage IV	The carcinoma has extended beyond the true pelvis or has involved the mucosa of the bladder or rectum; bullous edema as such does not permit a case to be allotted to Stage IV
IVA	Tumor invades bladder and/or rectal mucosa and/or direct extension beyond the true pelvis
IVB	Spread to distant organs.

FIGO, International Federation of Gynecology and Obstetrics.
From **FIGO Annual Report.** *Int J Gynecol Obstet* 2006;95:S29 and *Int J Gynecol Obstet* 2009;105:3–4.

The FIGO staging for vaginal carcinoma is shown in Table 36.6. **Staging is performed by clinical examination** and, if indicated, cystoscopy, proctoscopy, and chest and skeletal radiography. Information derived from lymphangiography, CT, MRI, or PET cannot be used to change the FIGO stage; however, it can be used for planning treatment. Less than 30% of vaginal cancers present at stage I (204–206).

Surgical staging and resection of enlarged lymph nodes may be indicated in selected patients. FIGO staging does not include a category for microinvasive disease. Because vaginal cancer is rare and treatment is by radiotherapy, there is very little information concerning the spread of disease in relation to depth of invasion, lymph–vascular space invasion, and size of the lesion.

Etiology

The association of cervical cancer with HPV suggests that vaginal cancer may have a similar association (207). A study of 341 cases revealed that in younger patients the disease seemed to be related to HPV infection, while in older patients there was no association (206). **In addition, as many as 30% of women with vaginal cancer have a history of cervical cancer treated within the previous 5 years** (208–210). As with cervical cancer, there appears to be a premalignant phase called **vaginal intraepithelial neoplasia (VAIN)** (see Chapter 19). **The exact incidence of progression to invasive vaginal cancer from VAIN is not known;** however, there are documented cases of invasive disease occurring despite adequate treatment of VAIN (211,212).

By convention, any new vaginal carcinoma developing at least 5 years after cervical cancer is considered a new primary lesion. There are three possible mechanisms for the occurrence of vaginal cancer after cervical neoplasia:

1. Residual disease in the vaginal epithelium after treatment of the cervical neoplasia

2. New primary disease arising in a patient with increased susceptibility to lower genital tract carcinogenesis (the role of HPV in this setting is suspected)

3. Increased susceptibility to carcinogenesis caused by radiation therapy

Screening

Routine screening of all patients for vaginal cancer is inappropriate. For women who had a cervical or vulvar neoplasm, the Pap test is an important part of routine follow-up with each physician visit, because these patients are at an increased lifetime risk for developing vaginal cancer. It is recommended that Pap test surveillance for vaginal cancer be performed yearly after the patient has completed surveillance for cancer of the cervix or vulva. **For women who had a hysterectomy for benign disease and have no antecedent history of CIN 2–3, performance of Pap testing is unnecessary. If the patient has a history of cervical dysplasia or cervical cancer, yearly screening is recommended.** When adjusted for age and prior cervical disease, the incidence of vaginal cancer is not increased in women who had hysterectomy for benign disease (213). Because primary vaginal tumors tend to be multicentric, the entire vaginal mucosa should

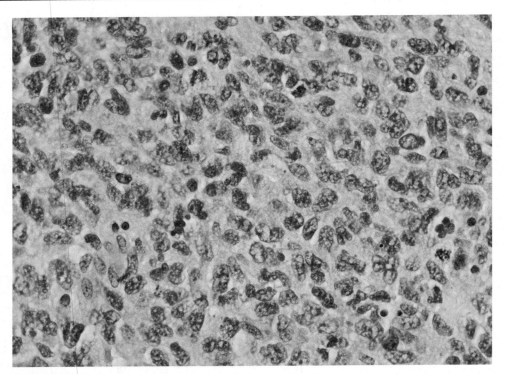

Figure 36.11 **Embryonal rhabdomyosarcoma of the vagina (botryoid sarcoma).** This lesion consists of primitive mesenchymal cells and rhabdomyoblasts, which have abundant eosinophilic cytoplasm. With further differentiation, cross striations may become evident.

uteri during postmenopausal years. Preoperative chemotherapy with *vincristine, actinomycin D,* and *cyclophosphamide,* followed by conservative surgery or radiation, has improved survival.

Treatment

Treatment selection is based on the clinical examination, CT scan results, chest radiography results, age, and condition of the patient. PET scans may give more accurate information about disease spread than MRI or CT scan alone (230). Most tumors are treated by radiation therapy. Surgery is limited to selected cases. These are as follows:

1. **Women with stage I disease involving the upper posterior vagina may be treated by radical vaginectomy and pelvic lymphadenectomy.** If the uterus is *in situ*, it is removed as a radical hysterectomy specimen. When margins are clear and lymph nodes are negative, no additional therapy is necessary.

2. **Patients with stage IV disease with either rectovaginal or vesicovaginal fistula** may be candidates for primary pelvic exenteration with pelvic and para-aortic lymphadenectomy (225). Low rectal anastomosis, continent urinary diversion, and vaginal reconstruction are indicated and are more successful in these nonirradiated patients than in patients who received prior radiation therapy.

3. **Women with central pelvic recurrence after radiation therapy are candidates for pelvic exenteration similar to that used for cervical cancer.**

4. **Surgical staging with resection of enlarged lymph nodes followed by radiation therapy may improve the control of pelvic disease.**

Radiation therapy is the treatment of choice for all patients except those described previously. Small superficial lesions may be treated with intracavitary radiation alone (225). Larger, thicker lesions should be treated first with external teletherapy to decrease tumor volume and to treat the regional pelvic nodes, followed by intracavitary and interstitial therapy to deliver a high dose to the primary tumor (218,226). If the uterus is intact and the lesion involves the upper vagina, an intrauterine tandem and ovoids can be used. If the uterus was previously removed, a vaginal cylinder may be used for superficial irradiation. When brachytherapy

Table 36.7 Primary Vaginal Carcinoma: 5-Year Survival			
Stage	*No. of Patients*	*No. Surviving 5 Years*	*Percentage*
I	509	378	74.3
II	622	333	53.5
III	377	128	34.0
IV	163	24	15.3
Total	**1,671**	**864**	**51.7**

Data compiled from **Pride et al.**, 1979 (233); **Houghton and Iversen**, 1982 (229); **Benedet et al.**, 1983 (205); **Rubin et al.**, 1985 (207); **Kucera et al.**, 1985 (228); **Eddy et al.**, 1991 (232); **Kirkbride et al.**, 1995 (234); **Perez et al.**, 1999 (235); **Tewari et al.**, 2001 (236); **Otton et al.**, 2004 (237); **Frank et al.**, 2005 (238); **Hellman et al.**, 2006 (204); **Tran et al.**, 2007 (239).

is used, high- and low-dose rate techniques were described. If the lesion is more than 0.5 cm thick, interstitial radiation techniques can improve the dose distribution to the primary tumor. Surgical exploration or laparoscopy at the time of insertion of Syed interstitial implants defines more precisely the placement of the needles and ensures that needles do not pass into adherent loops of bowel. Extended-field radiation may be used for vaginal cancer in a manner similar to its use for cervical carcinoma, although there is no experience reported with the use of this technique in the treatment of vaginal cancer. Likewise, there is little reported experience with combination chemoradiation treatment (231). Although there will never be enough patients for a proper randomized control trial, concurrent use of *5-FU* and *cisplatin* was highly successful in anal and cervical cancer and thus should be considered for treatment of vaginal cancer.

Sequelae

The proximity of the rectum, bladder, and urethra leads to a major complication rate of 10% to 15% for both surgery and radiation treatment. For large tumors, the risk of bladder or bowel fistula is significant. Radiation cystitis and proctitis are common, as are rectal strictures or ulcerations. Radiation necrosis of the vagina occasionally occurs, requiring debridement, and often leads to fistula formation. Vaginal fibrosis, stenosis, and stricture are common after radiation therapy. **Use of vaginal dilators and resumption of regular sexual relations should be encouraged, along with the use of topical *estrogen* to maintain adequate vaginal function.**

Survival

The overall 5-year survival rate for patients with vaginal cancer is 52% (Table 36.7). This reflects the difficulties of treatment and the fact the disease presents at late stage. **For patients with stage I disease, the 5-year survival rate is 74%.** Most recurrences are in the pelvis, either from enlarged regional nodes or from large central tumors. Radiation techniques, including interstitial implants with Syed applicator and combination chemoradiation, are the mainstay of therapy. Careful evaluation of patients who receive radiation therapy to detect central recurrence may allow some patients to be saved by pelvic exenteration. Because of the rarity of vaginal cancer, these patients should be treated in a center that is familiar with the complexity of treatment and modalities of therapy.

References

1. **Siegel R, Ward E, Brawley O, et al.** Cancer statistics, 2011. *CA Cancer J Clin* 2011;61:212–236. http://cacancerjournal.org
2. **Womack C, Warren AY.** *Achievable laboratory standards: a review of cytology of 99 women with cervical cancer.* Cytopathology 1998; 9:171.
3. **Pettersson F.** Annual report on the results of treatment in gynecological cancer. Radiumhemmet, Stockholm, Sweden: International Federation of Gynecology and Obstetrics (FIGO), 1994:132–168.[MB6]
4. **International Collaboration of Epidemiological Studies of Cervical Cancer.** Comparison of risk factors for invasive squamous cell carcinoma and adenocarcinoma of the cervix: collaborative reanalysis of individual data on 8,097 women with squamous cell carcinoma and 1,374 women with adenocarcinoma from 12 epidemiological studies. *Int J Cancer* 2007;120:885–891.
5. **Ursin G, Peters RK, Henderson BE, et al.** Oral contraceptive use and adenocarcinoma of the cervix. *Lancet* 1994;344:1390–1393.
6. **Centers for Disease Control and Prevention.** Sexually transmitted disease guidelines. *MMWR Morb Mortal Wkly Rep* 1993;42:90–100.
7. **Reimers LL, Anderson WF, Rosenberg PS, et al.** Etiologic heterogeneity for cervical carcinoma by histopathologic type, using comparative age-period-cohort models. *Cancer Epidemiol Biomarkers Prev* 2009;18:792–800.
8. **Munger K, Scheffner M, Huibregtse JM, et al.** Interactions of HPV E6 and E7 oncoproteins with tumor suppressor gene products. *Cancer Surv* 1992;12:197–217.
9. **Ault KA.** Effect of prophylactic human papillomavirus L1 virus-like- particle vaccine on risk of cervical intraepithelial neoplasia grade 2, grade 3, and adenocarcinoma *in situ:* a combined

analysis of four randomised clinical trials. *Lancet* 2007;369:1861–1868.

10. **Sasieni P, Castanon A, Cuzick J.** Screening and adenocarcinoma of the cervix. *Int J Cancer* 2009;125:525–529.

11. **Fu YS, Berek JS.** Minimal cervical cancer: definition and histology. In: **Grundmann E, Beck L, eds.** *Minimal neoplasia—diagnosis and therapy.* Recent results in cancer research, Vol. 106. Berlin: Springer-Verlag, 1988:47–56.

12. **Creasman W.** New gynecologic cancer staging. *Gynecol Oncol* 1995;58:157–158.

13. **Fu YS, Reagan JW.** *Pathology of the uterine cervix, vagina and vulva.* Philadelphia, PA: Saunders, 1989.

14. **Averette HE, Ford JH Jr, Dudan RC, et al.** Staging of cervical cancer. *Clin Obstet Gynecol* 1975;18:215–232.

15. **Lagasse LD, Ballon SC, Berman ML, et al.** Pretreatment lymphangiography and operative evaluation in carcinoma of the cervix. *Am J Obstet Gynecol* 1979;134:219–224.

16. **Koehler PR.** Current status of lymphangiography in patients with cancer. *Cancer* 1976;37:503–516.

17. **King LA, Talledo OE, Gallup DG, et al.** Computed tomography in evaluation of gynecologic malignancies: a retrospective analysis. *Am J Obstet Gynecol* 1986;155:960–964.

18. **Bandy LC, Clarke-Pearson DL, Silverman PM, et al.** Computed tomography in evaluation of extrapelvic lymphadenopathy in carcinoma of the cervix. *Obstet Gynecol* 1986;65:73–76.

19. **Hacker NF, Berek JS.** Surgical staging. In: **Surwit E, Alberts D, eds.** *Cervix cancer.* Boston, MA: Martinus Nijhoff, 1987:43–57.

20. **Heller PB, Malfetano JH, Bundy BN.** Clinical pathologic study of stages IIB, III, and IVA carcinoma of the cervix: extended diagnostic study for paraaortic metastasis (a GOG study). *Gynecol Oncol* 1990;38:425.

21. **Worthington JL, Balfe DM, Lee JK, et al.** Uterine neoplasms: MR imaging. *Radiology* 1986;159:725–730.

22. **Scheidler J, Hricak H, Yu KK, et al.** Radiological evaluation of lymph node metastases in patients with cervical cancer: a meta-analysis. *JAMA* 1997;278:1096.

23. **Bipat S, Glas AS, Velden J, et al.** Computed tomography and magnetic resonance imaging in staging of uterine cervical carcinoma: a systematic review. *Gynecol Oncol* 2003;91:59.

24. **Rose RG.** Stage IIB-IVA cancer of the cervix. *Cancer J* 2003;9:404.

25. **Lin WC, Hung YC, YEH LS, et al.** Usefulness of (18)F-fluorodeoxyglucose positron emission tomography to detect paraaortic lymph node metastasis in advanced cervical cancer with negative computed tomography findings. *Gynecol Oncol* 2003;89:73.

26. **Park SY, Roh JW, Park YJ, et al.** Positron emission tomography (PET) for evaluating para-aortic and pelvic lymph node metastasis in cervical cancer before surgical staging: a surgico-pathologic study. *Proc Am Soc Clin Oncol* 2003;22:456.

27. **Cosin JA, Fowler JM, Chen MD, et al.** Pretreatment surgical staging of patients with cervical carcinoma: the case for lymph node debulking. *Cancer* 1998;82:2241–2248.

28. **Robert ME, Fu YS.** Squamous cell carcinoma of the uterine cervix: a review with emphasis on prognostic factors and unusual variants. *Semin Diagn Pathol* 1990;7:173–189.

29. **Kjorstad KE.** Adenocarcinoma of the uterine cervix. *Gynecol Oncol* 1977;5:219–223.

30. **Berek JS, Hacker NF, Fu YS, et al.** Adenocarcinoma of the uterine cervix: histologic variables associated with lymph node metastasis and survival. *Obstet Gynecol* 1985;65:46–52.

31. **Hopkins MP, Morley GW.** A comparison of adenocarcinoma and squamous cell carcinoma of the cervix. *Obstet Gynecol* 1991;77:912–917.

32. **Fu YS, Berek JS, Hilborne LH.** Diagnostic problems of cervical *in situ* and invasive adenocarcinoma. *Appl Pathol* 1987;5:47–56.

33. **Maier RC, Norris HJ.** Coexistence of cervical intraepithelial neoplasia with primary adenocarcinoma of the endocervix. *Obstet Gynecol* 1980;56:361–364.

34. **Denehy TR, Gregori CA, Breen JL.** Endocervical curettage, cone margins, and residual adenocarcinoma *in situ* of the cervix. *Obstet Gynecol* 1997;90:1–6.

35. **Shin CH, Schorge JO, Lee KR, et al.** Conservative management of adenocarcinoma *in situ* of the cervix. *Gynecol Oncol* 2000;69:6–10.

36. **Ostor AG, Duncan A, Quinn M, et al.** Adenocarcinoma *in situ* of the uterine cervix: an experience with 100 cases. *Gynecol Oncol* 2000;79:207–210.

37. **Shingleton HM, Gore H, Bradley DH, et al.** Adenocarcinoma of the cervix. I. Clinical evaluation and pathologic features. *Am J Obstet Gynecol* 1981;139:799–814.

38. **Kilgore LC, Soong S-J, Gore H, et al.** Analysis of prognostic features in adenocarcinoma of the cervix. *Gynecol Oncol* 1988;31:137–153.

39. **Berek JS, Castaldo TW, Hacker NF, et al.** Adenocarcinoma of the uterine cervix. *Cancer* 1981;48: 2734–2741.

40. **Mayer EG, Galindo J, Davis J, et al.** Adenocarcinoma of the uterine cervix: incidence and the role of radiation therapy. *Radiology* 1976;121:725–729.

41. **Rutledge FN, Galakatos AE, Wharton JT, et al.** Adenocarcinoma of the uterine cervix. *Am J Obstet Gynecol* 1975;122:236–245.

42. **Gallup DG, Abell MR.** Invasive adenocarcinoma of the uterine cervix. *Obstet Gynecol* 1977;49:596–603.

43. **Eifel PJ, Morris M, Oswald MJ, et al.** Adenocarcinoma of the uterine cervix: prognosis and patterns of failure in 367 cases. *Cancer* 1990;65:2507–2514.

44. **Kaku T, Enjoji M.** Extremely well-differentiated adenocarcinoma ("adenoma malignum"). *Int J Gynecol Pathol* 1983;2:28–41.

45. **Gilks CB, Young R, Aguirre P, et al.** Adenoma malignum (minimal deviation adenocarcinoma) of the uterine cervix. *Am J Surg Pathol* 1989;13:717–729.

46. **Kaminski PF, Norris HJ.** Minimal deviation carcinoma (adenoma malignum) of the cervix. *Int J Gynecol Pathol* 1983;2:141–152.

47. **Benda JA, Platz CE, Buchsbaum H, et al.** Mucin production in defining mixed carcinoma of the uterine cervix: a clinicopathologic study. *Int J Gynecol Pathol* 1985;4:314–327.

48. **Young RH, Scully RE.** Villoglandular papillary adenocarcinoma of the uterine cervix: a clinicopathologic analysis of 13 cases. *Cancer* 1989;63:1773–1779.

49. **Gallup DG, Harper RH, Stock RJ.** Poor prognosis in patients with adenosquamous cell carcinoma of the cervix. *Obstet Gynecol* 1985;65:416–422.

50. **Glucksmann A, Cherry CP.** Incidence, histology and response to radiation of mixed carcinomas (adenoacanthomas) of the uterine cervix. *Cancer* 1956;9:971–979.

51. **Ferry JA, Scully RE.** "Adenoid cystic" carcinoma and adenoid basal carcinoma of the uterine cervix: a study of 28 cases. *Am J Surg Pathol* 1988;12:134–144.

52. **Rotmensch J, Rosenshein NB, Woodruff JD.** Cervical sarcoma: a review. *Obstet Gynecol Surv* 1983;38:456–461.

53. **Albores-Saavedra J, Gersell D, Gilks CB, et al.** Terminology of endocrine tumors of the uterine cervix: results of a workshop sponsored by the College of American Pathologists and National Cancer Institute. *Arch Pathol Lab Med* 1997;121:34–39.

54. **Van Nagell JR Jr, Donaldson ES, Wood EC, et al.** Small cell carcinoma of the cervix. *Cancer* 1979;40:2243–2249.

55. **Sheets EE, Berman ML, Hrountas CE, et al.** Surgically treated, early stage neuroendocrine small-cell cervical carcinoma. *Obstet Gynecol* 1988;7:10–14.

56. **Oldham RK, Greco FA.** Small cell lung cancer, a curable disease. *Cancer Chemother Pharmacol* 1980;4:173–177.

57. **Groben P, Reddick R, Askin F.** The pathologic spectrum of small cell carcinoma of the cervix. *Int J Gynecol Pathol* 1985;4:42–57.

58. **Brewster WR, Monk BJ, Ziogas A, et al.** Intent-to-treat analysis of stage IB and IIA cervical cancer in the United States: radiotherapy or surgery 1988–1995. *Obstet Gynecol* 2001;97:245–254.

59. **Van Nagell JR Jr, Parker JC Jr, Maruyama Y, et al.** Bladder or rectal injury following radiation therapy for cervical cancer. *Am J Obstet Gynecol* 1974;119:727–732.

60. **Lawton FG, Hacker NF.** Surgery for invasive gynecologic cancer in the elderly female population. *Obstet Gynecol* 1990;76:287–289.

61. **Hatch KD, Parham G, Shingleton HM, et al.** Ureteral strictures and fistulae following radical hysterectomy. *Gynecol Oncol* 1984;19:17–23.

62. **Webb M, Symmonds R.** Wertheim hysterectomy: a reappraisal. *Obstet Gynecol* 1979;54:140–145.

63. **Feeny DD, Moore DH, Look KY, et al.** The fate of the ovaries after radical hysterectomy and ovarian transposition. *Gynecol Oncol* 1995;56:3.

64. **Anderson B, LaPolla J, Turner D, et al.** Ovarian transposition in cervical cancer. *Gynecol Oncol* 1993;49:206.

65. **Landoni F, Zanagnolo V, Lovato-Diaz L, et al.** Ovarian metastases in early-stage cervical cancer (IA2–IIA): a multicenter retrospective study of 1965 patients (a Cooperative Task Force study). *Int J Gynecol Cancer* 2007;17:623–628.

66. **Roman LD, Felix JC, Muderspach LI, et al.** Risk of residual invasive disease in women with microinvasive squamous cancer in a conization specimen. *Obstet Gynecol* 1997;90:759.

67. **Wolf JK, Levenback C, Maslpica A, et al.** Adenocarcinoma *in situ* of the cervix: significance of cone biopsy margins. *Obstet Gynecol* 1996;88:82–86.

68. **Hopkins MP.** Adenocarcinoma *in situ* of the cervix: the margins must be clear. *Gynecol Oncol* 2000;79:4–5.

69. **Shepherd JH, Spencer C, Herod J, et al.** Radical vaginal trachelectomy as a fertility-sparing procedure in women with early-stage cervical cancer-cumulative pregnancy rate in a series of 123 women. *BJOG* 2006;113:719–724.

70. **Marchiole P, Benchaib M, Buenerd A, et al.** Oncological safety of laparoscopic-assisted vaginal radical trachelectomy (LARVT or Dargent's operation): a comparative study with laparoscopic-assisted vaginal radical hysterectomy (LARVH). *Gynecol Oncol* 2007;106:132–141.

71. **Meigs J.** Radical hysterectomy with bilateral pelvic node dissections: a report of 100 patients operated five or more years ago. *Am J Obstet Gynecol* 1951;62:854–870.

72. **Piver M, Rutledge F, Smith J.** Five classes of extended hysterectomy for women with cervical cancer. *Obstet Gynecol* 1974;44:265–272.

73. **Morice P, Lassau N, Pautier P, et al.** Retroperitoneal drainage after complete para-aortic lymphadenectomy for gynecologic cancer: a randomized trial. *Obstet Gynecol* 2001;97:243–247.

74. **Boyce J, Fruchter R, Nicastri A.** Prognostic factors in stage I carcinoma of the cervix. *Gynecol Oncol* 1981;12:154–165.

75. **Orr JW Jr, Shingleton HM, Hatch KD.** Correlation of perioperative morbidity and conization to radical hysterectomy interval. *Obstet Gynecol* 1982;59:726–731.

76. **Potter ME, Alvarez RD, Shingleton HM, et al.** Early invasive cervical cancer with pelvic lymph node involvement: to complete or not to complete radical hysterectomy? *Gynecol Oncol* 1990;37:78–81.

77. **Mann WJ Jr, Orr JW Jr, Shingleton HM, et al.** Perioperative influences on infectious morbidity in radical hysterectomy. *Gynecol Oncol* 1981;11:207–212.

78. **Green T.** Ureteral suspension for prevention of ureteral complications following radical Wertheim hysterectomy. *Obstet Gynecol* 1966;28:1–11.

79. **Raspagliesi F, Ditto A, Fontanelli R, et al.** Nerve-sparing radical hysterectomy: a surgical technique for preserving the autonomic hypogastric nerve. *Gynecol Oncol* 2004;93:307–314.

80. **Sakuragi N, Todo Y, Kudo M, et al.** A systematic nerve-sparing radical hysterectomy technique in invasive cervical cancer for preserving postsurgical bladder function. *Int J Gynecol Cancer* 2005;15:389–397.

81. **Hertel H, Kohler C, Michels W, et al.** Laparoscopic-assisted radical vaginal hysterectomy (LARVH): prospective evaluation of 200 patients with cervical cancer. *Gynecol Oncol* 2003;90:505.

82. **Geisler JP, Orr CJ, Khurshid N, et al.** Robotically assisted laparoscopic radical hysterectomy compared with open radical hysterectomy. *Int J Gynecol Cancer* 2010;20:438–442.

83. **Lowe MP, Chamberlain DH, Kamelle SA, et al.** A multi-institutional experience with robotic assisted radical hysterectomy for early stage cervical cancer. *Gynecol Oncol* 2009;113:191–194.

84. **Bidus MA, O'Boyle JD, Elkas JC.** Sentinel lymph node detection in gynecologic malignancies. *Postgrad Obstet Gynecol* 2004;24:1–5.

85. **Morley GW, Seski JC.** Radial pelvic surgery versus radiation therapy for stage I carcinoma of the cervix (exclusive of microinvasion). *Am J Obstet Gynecol* 1976;126:785–798.

86. **Baltzer J, Lohe K, Kopke W, et al.** Histologic criteria for the prognosis of patients with operated squamous cell carcinoma of the cervix. *Gynecol Oncol* 1982;13:184–194.

87. **Chung C, Nahhas W, Stryker J, et al.** Analysis of factors contributing to treatment failures in stage IB and IIA carcinoma of the cervix. *Am J Obstet Gynecol* 1980;138:550–556.

88. **Creasman W, Soper J, Clarke-Pearson D.** Radical hysterectomy as therapy for early carcinoma of the cervix. *Am J Obstet Gynecol* 1986;155:964–969.

89. **Van Nagell J, Donaldson E, Parker J.** The prognostic significance of cell type and lesion size in patients with cervical cancer treated by radical surgery. *Gynecol Oncol* 1977;5:142–151.

90. **Inoue T, Okumura M.** Prognostic significance of parametrial extension in patients with cervical carcinoma stage IB, IIA, and IIIB. *Cancer* 1984;54:1714–1719.

91. **Bleker O, Ketting B, Wayjean-eecen B, et al.** The significance of microscopic involvement of the parametrium and/or pelvic lymph nodes in cervical cancer stages IB and IIA. *Gynecol Oncol* 1983;16:56–62.

92. **Gauthier P, Gore I, Shingleton HM.** Identification of histopathologic risk groups in stage IB squamous cell carcinoma of the cervix. *Obstet Gynecol* 1985;66:569–574.

93. **Van Nagell J, Donaldson E, Wood E, et al.** The significance of vascular invasion and lymphocytic infiltration in invasive cervical cancer. *Cancer* 1978;41:228–234.

94. **Nahhas W, Sharkey F, Whitney C, et al.** The prognostic significance of vascular channel involvement in deep stromal penetration in early cervical carcinoma. *Am J Clin Oncol* 1983;6:259–264.

95. **Soisson AP, Soper JT, Clarke-Pearson DL, et al.** Adjuvant radiotherapy following radical hysterectomy for patients with stage IB and IIA cervical cancer. *Gynecol Oncol* 1990;37:390–395.

96. **Tinga DJ, Timmer PR, Bouma J, et al.** Prognostic significance of single versus multiple lymph node metastases in cervical carcinoma stage IB. *Gynecol Oncol* 1990;39:175–180.

97. **Alvarez RD, Soong SJ, Kinney WK, et al.** Identification of prognostic factors and risk groups in patients found to have nodal metastasis at the time of radical hysterectomy for early stage squamous carcinoma of the cervix. *Gynecol Oncol* 1989;35:130–135.

98. **Fuller AF, Elliott N, Kosloff C, et al.** Determinants of increased risk for recurrence in patients undergoing radical hysterectomy for stage IB and IIA carcinoma of the cervix. *Gynecol Oncol* 1989;33:34–39.

99. **Delgado G, Bundy B, Zaino R, et al.** Prospective surgical-pathological study of disease free interval in patients with stage IB squamous cell carcinoma of the cervix: a Gynecologic Oncology Group study. *Gynecol Oncol* 1990;38:352–357.

100. **Peters WA, Liu PY, Barrett RJ, et al.** Concurrent chemotherapy and pelvic radiation therapy compared with pelvic radiation therapy alone as adjuvant therapy after radical surgery in high-risk early-stage cancer of the cervix. *J Clin Oncol* 2000:18;1606–1613.

101. **Sedlis A, Bundy BN, Rotman MZ, et al.** A randomized trial of pelvic radiation therapy versus no further therapy in selected patients with stage IB carcinoma of the cervix after radical hysterectomy and pelvic lymphadenectomy: a Gynecologic Oncology Group study. *Gynecol Oncol* 1999;73:177.

102. **Morrow P.** Panel report: is pelvic irradiation beneficial in the postoperative management of stage Ib squamous cell carcinoma of the cervix with pelvic node metastases treated by radical hysterectomy and pelvic lymphadenectomy? *Gynecol Oncol* 1980;10:105–110.

103. **Lohe KJ, Burghardt E, Hillemanns HG, et al.** Early squamous cell carcinoma of the uterine cervix. II. Clinical results of a cooperative study in the management of 419 patients with early stromal invasion and microcarcinoma. *Gynecol Oncol* 1978;6:31–50.

104. **Burghardt E, Holzer E.** Diagnosis and treatment of microinvasive carcinoma of the cervix uteri. *Obstet Gynecol* 1977;49:641–653.

105. **Van Nagell J Jr, Greenwell N, Powell D, et al.** Microinvasive carcinoma of the cervix. *Am J Obstet Gynecol* 1983;145:981–991.

106. **Pilleron J, Durand J, Hamelin J.** Prognostic value of node metastasis in cancer of the uterine cervix. *Am J Obstet Gynecol* 1974;119:458–462.

107. **Inoue T, Chihara T, Morita K.** Postoperative extended field irradiation in patients with pelvic and/or common iliac node metastasis from cervical carcinoma stages IB to IIB. *Gynecol Oncol* 1986;25:234–243.

108. **Larsson G, Alm P, Gullberg B, et al.** Prognostic factors in early invasive carcinoma of the uterine cervix. *Am J Obstet Gynecol* 1983;146:145–153.

109. **Leman M, Benson W, Kurman R, et al.** Microinvasive carcinoma of the cervix. *Obstet Gynecol* 1976;48:571–578.

110. **Seski JC, Abell MR, Morley GW.** Microinvasive squamous cell carcinoma of the cervix: definition, histologic analysis, late results of treatment. *Obstet Gynecol* 1977;50:410–414.

111. **Gonzalez DG, Ketting BW, Van Bunningen B, et al.** Carcinoma of the uterine cervix stage IB and IIA: results of postoperative irradiation in patients with microscopic infiltration in the parametrium and/or lymph node metastasis. *Int J Radiat Oncol Biol Phys* 1989;16:389–395.

112. **Martinbeau P, Kjorstad K, Iversen T.** Stage IB carcinoma of the cervix: the Norwegian Radium Hospital. II. Results when pelvic nodes are involved. *Obstet Gynecol* 1982;60:215–218.

113. **Inoue T.** Prognostic significance of the depth of invasion relating to nodal metastases, parametrial extension, and cell types. *Cancer* 1984;54:3035–3042.

114. **Piver M, Chung W.** Prognostic significance of cervical lesion size and pelvic node metastases in cervical carcinoma. *Obstet Gynecol* 1975;46:507–510.

115. **Hsu CT, Cheng YS, Su SC.** Prognosis of uterine cervical cancer with extensive lymph node metastasis. *Am J Obstet Gynecol* 1972;114:954–962.

116. **Hareyama M, Sakata K, Oouchi A, et al.** High dose rate versus low dose rate intracavitary therapy for carcinoma of the uterine cervix: a randomized trial. *Cancer* 2002;94:117.

117. **Teshima T, Inoue T, Ikeda H, et al.** High dose rate and low dose rate intracavitary therapy for carcinoma of the uterine cervix. *Cancer* 1993;72:2409.

118. **Shigematsu Y, Nishiyama K, Masaki N, et al.** Treatment of carcinoma of the uterine cervix by remotely controlled afterloading radiotherapy with high dose rate: a comparative study with a low dose rate system. *Int J Radiat Oncol Biol Phys* 1983;9:351.

119. **Berman M, Keys N, Creasman W, et al.** Survival and patterns of recurrence in cervical cancer metastatic to para-aortic lymph nodes. *Gynecol Oncol* 1984;19:8–16.

120. **Mundt AJ, Lujan AE, Rotmensch J, et al.** Intensity modulated whole radiotherapy in women with gynecologic malignancies. *Int J Radiat Oncol Biol Phys* 2002;52:1330.

121. **Chen MF, Tseng CJ, Tseng CC, et al.** Clinical outcome in posthysterectomy cervical cancer patients treated with concurrent cisplatin and intensity-modulated pelvic radiotherapy: comparison with conventional radiotherapy. *Int J Radiat Oncol Biol Phys* 2007;67:1438–1444.

122. **Roche WO, Norris HC.** Microinvasive carcinoma of the cervix. *Cancer* 1975;36:180–186.

123. **Shingleton HM, Orr JW Jr.** Primary surgical and combined treatment. In: **Singer A, Jordan J, eds.** *Cancer of the cervix.* New York: Churchill Livingstone, 1983:76–100.

124. **Barter JF, Soong SJ, Shingleton HM, et al.** Complications of combined radical hysterectomy: postoperative radiation therapy in women with early stage cervical cancer. *Gynecol Oncol* 1989;32:292–296.

125. **Kinney WK, Alvarez RD, Reid GC, et al.** Value of adjuvant whole-pelvic irradiation after Wertheim hysterectomy for early-stage squamous carcinoma of the cervix with pelvic nodal metastasis: a matched-control study. *Gynecol Oncol* 1989;34:258–262.

126. **Lai CH, Lin TS, Soong YK, et al.** Adjuvant chemotherapy after radical hysterectomy for cervical carcinoma. *Gynecol Oncol* 1989;35:193–198.

127. **Wertheim MS, Hakes TB, Daghestani AN, et al.** A pilot study of adjuvant therapy in patients with cervical cancer at high risk of recurrence after radical hysterectomy and pelvic lymphadenectomy. *J Clin Oncol* 1985;3:912–916.

128. **Rotman M, Sedlis A, Piedmonte MR, et al.** A phase III randomized trial of postoperative pelvic irradiation in stage IB cervical carcinoma with poor prognostic features: follow-up of a gynecologic oncology group study. *Int J Radiat Oncol Biol Phys* 2006;65:169–176.

129. **Whitney CW, Sause W, Bundy BN, et al.** Randomized comparison of fluorouracil plus cisplatin versus hydroxyurea as an adjunct to radiation therapy in stage IIB–IVA carcinoma of the cervix with negative para-aortic lymph nodes: a Gynecologic Oncology Group and Southwest Oncology Group study. *J Clin Oncol* 1999;17:1339–1348.

130. **Rose PG, Bundy BN, Watkins EB, et al.** Concurrent cisplatin-based radiotherapy and chemotherapy for locally advanced cervical cancer. *N Engl J Med* 1999;340:1144–1153.

131. **Morris M, Eifel PJ, Lu J, et al.** Pelvic radiation with concurrent chemotherapy compared with pelvic and para-aortic radiation for high risk cervical cancer. *N Engl J Med* 1999;340:1137–1143.

132. **Keys HM, Bundy BN, Stehman FB, et al.** Cisplatin, radiation, and adjuvant hysterectomy compared with radiation and adjuvant hysterectomy for bulky stage IB cervical carcinoma. *N Engl J Med* 1999;340:1154–1161.

133. **Piver MS, Barlow JJ, Krishnamsetty R.** Five-year survival (with no evidence of disease) in patients with biopsy-confirmed aortic node metastasis from cervical carcinoma. *Am J Obstet Gynecol* 1981;193:575–578.

134. **Wharton JT, Jones HW 3rd, Day TG, et al.** Preirradiation celiotomy and extended field irradiation for invasive carcinoma of the cervix. *Obstet Gynecol* 1977;49:333–338.

135. **Ballon SC, Berman ML, Lagasse LD, et al.** Survival after extraperitoneal pelvic and paraaortic lymphadenectomy and radiation therapy in cervical carcinoma. *Obstet Gynecol* 1981;57:90–95.

136. **Twiggs LB, Potish RA, George RJ, et al.** Pretreatment extraperitoneal surgical staging in primary carcinoma of the cervix uteri. *Surg Gynecol Obstet* 1984;158:243–250.

137. **Weiser EB, Bundy BN, Hoskins WJ, et al.** Extraperitoneal versus transperitoneal selective paraaortic lymphadenectomy in the pretreatment surgical staging of advanced cervical carcinoma (a Gynecologic Oncology Group study). *Gynecol Oncol* 1989;33:283–289.

138. **Stehman FB, Bundy BN, DiSaia PJ, et al.** Carcinoma of the cervix treated with radiation therapy. I. A multi-variate analysis of prognostic variables in the Gynecologic Oncology Group. *Cancer* 1991;67:2776–2785.

139. **Lovecchio JL, Averette HE, Donato D, et al.** 5-Year survival of patients with periaortic nodal metastases in clinical stage IB and IIA cervical carcinoma. *Gynecol Oncol* 1990;38:446.

140. **Rubin SC, Brookland R, Mikuta JJ, et al.** Paraaortic nodal metastases in early cervical carcinoma: long-term survival following extended-field radiotherapy. *Gynecol Oncol* 1984;18:213–217.

141. **Boughanim M, Leboulleux S, Rey A, et al.** Histologic results of para-aortic lymphadenectomy in patients treated for stage IB2/II cervical cancer with negative [18F]fluorodeoxyglucose positron emission tomography scans in the para-aortic area. *J Clin Oncol* 2008;26:2558–2561.

142. **Haie C, Pejovic MH, Gerbaulet A, et al.** Is prophylactic paraaortic irradiation worthwhile in the treatment of advanced cervical carcinoma? Results of a controlled clinical trial of the EORTC radiotherapy group. *Radiother Oncol* 1998;11:101.

143. **Rotman M, Pajak TF, Choi K, et al.** Prophylactic extended-field irradiation of paraaortic lymph nodes in stages IIB and bulky IB and IIA cervical carcinomas. Ten-year treatment results of RTOG 79-20. *JAMA* 1995;274:387.

144. **Stehman FB, Bundy BN, Hanjani P, et al.** Biopsy of the scalene fat pad in carcinoma of the cervix uteri metastatic to the periaortic lymph nodes. *Surg Gynecol Obstet* 1987;165:503–506.

145. **Kim RY, Levy DS, Brascho DJ, et al.** Uterine perforation during intracavitary application: prognostic significance in carcinoma of the cervix. *Radiology* 1983;147:249–251.

146. **White AJ, Buchsbaum HJ, Blythe JG, et al.** Use of the bulbocavernosus muscle (Martius procedure) for repair of radiation-induced rectovaginal fistulas. *Obstet Gynecol* 1982;60:114–118.

147. **Bricker EM, Johnston WD.** Repair of postirradiation rectovaginal fistula and stricture. *Surg Gynecol Obstet* 1979;148:499–506.

148. **Smith ST, Seski JC, Copeland LJ, et al.** Surgical management of irradiation-induced small bowel damage. *Obstet Gynecol* 1985;65:563–567.

149. **Bloss JD, Blessing JA, Behrens BC, et al.** Randomized trial of cisplatin and ifosfamide with and without bleomycin in squamous cell carcinoma of the cervix: a Gynecologic Oncology Group study. *J Clin Oncol* 2002;20:1832–1837.

150. **Omura GA, Blessing JA, Vaccarello L, et al.** Randomized trial of cisplatin versus cisplatin plus mitolactol versus cisplatin plus ifosfamide in advanced squamous carcinoma of the cervix: a Gynecologic Oncology Group study. *J Clin Oncol* 1997;15:165.

151. **Moore DH, Blessing JA, McQuellon RP, et al.** Phase III study of *cisplatin* with or without *paclitaxel* in stage IVB, recurrent, or persistent squamous cell carcinoma of the cervix: a Gynecologic Oncology Group study. *J Clin Oncol* 2004;22:3113.

152. **Long HJ, Monk BJ, Huang HQ, et al.** Clinical results and quality of life analysis of the MVAC combination in carcinoma of the cervix: a Gynecologic Oncology Group study. *Gynecol Oncol* 2006;100:537–543.

153. **Monk BJ, Sill MW, McMeekin DS, et al.** Phase III trial of four cisplatin-containing doublet combinations in stage IVb, recurrent, or persistent cervical carcinoma: a Gynecologic Oncology Group study. *J Clin Oncol* 2009;27:4649–4655.

154. **Pectasides D, Fountzilas G, Papaxoinis G, et al.** Carboplatin and paclitaxel in metastatic or recurrent cervical cancer. *Int J Gynecol Cancer* 2009;19:777–781.

155. **Simon NL, Gore H, Shingleton HM, et al.** Study of superficially invasive carcinoma of the cervix. *Obstet Gynecol* 1986;68:19–24.

156. **Delgado G, Bundy BN, Fowler WC, et al.** A prospective surgical pathological study of stage I squamous carcinoma of the cervix: a Gynecologic Oncology Group study. *Gynecol Oncol* 1989;35:314–320.

157. **Landoni F, Maneo A, Columbo A, et al.** Randomised study of radical surgery versus radiotherapy for stage IB–IIA cervical cancer. *Lancet* 1997;350:535–540.

158. **Jampolis S, Andras J, Fletcher GH.** Analysis of sites and causes of failure of irradiation in invasive squamous cell carcinoma of the intact uterine cervix. *Radiology* 1975;115:681–685.

159. **Million RR, Rutledge F, Fletcher GH.** Stage IV carcinoma of the cervix with bladder invasion. *Am J Obstet Gynecol* 1972;113:239–246.

160. **Gallousis S.** Isolated lung metastases from pelvic malignancies. *Gynecol Oncol* 1979;7:206–214.

161. **Nordqvist SR, Sevin BU, Nadji M, et al.** Fine-needle aspiration cytology in gynecologic oncology. I. Diagnostic accuracy. *Obstet Gynecol* 1979;54:719–724.

162. **Krebs HB, Helmkamp BF, Sevin B-U, et al.** Recurrent cancer of the cervix following radical hysterectomy and pelvic node dissection. *Obstet Gynecol* 1982;59:422–427.

163. **Shingleton HM, Orr JW Jr.** Posttreatment surveillance. In: **Singer A, Jordan J, eds.** *Cancer of the cervix.* New York: Churchill Livingstone, 1983:135–122.

164. **Duggan B, Muderspach LI, Roman LD, et al.** Cervical cancer in pregnancy: reporting on planned delay in therapy. *Obstet Gynecol* 1993;82:598.

165. **Hacker NF, Berek JS, Lagasse LD, et al.** Carcinoma of the cervix associated with pregnancy. *Obstet Gynecol* 1982;59:735–746.

166. **Averette HE, Nasser N, Yankow SL, et al.** Cervical conization in pregnancy. *Am J Obstet Gynecol* 1970;106:543–549.

167. **Lee RB, Neglia W, Park RC.** Cervical carcinoma in pregnancy. *Obstet Gynecol* 1981;58:584–589.

168. **Shingleton HM, Orr JW Jr.** Cancer complicating pregnancy. In: **Singer A, Jordan J, eds.** *Cancer of the cervix.* New York: Churchill Livingstone, 1983:193–209.

169. **Sood AK, Sorosky JI, Mayr N, et al.** Cervical cancer diagnosed shortly after pregnancy: prognostic variables and delivery routes. *Obstet Gynecol* 2000;95:832–838.

170. **Committee on Practice Bulletins–Gynecology.** Diagnosis and treatment of cervical carcinoma. *Obstet Gynecol* 2002;99:855.

171. **Bader AA, Petru E, Winter R.** Long-term follow-up after neoadjuvant chemotherapy for high-risk cervical cancer during pregnancy. *Gynecol Oncol* 2007;105:269–272.

172. **Green TH, Morse WJ Jr.** Management of invasive cervical cancer following inadvertent simple hysterectomy. *Obstet Gynecol* 1969;33:763–769.

173. **Orr JW Jr, Ball GC, Soong SJ, et al.** Surgical treatment of women found to have invasive cervix cancer at the time of total hysterectomy. *Obstet Gynecol* 1986;68:353–356.

174. **Journal of the National Comprehensive Cancer Network.** JNCCN consensus guidelines for cervical carcinoma. *JNCCN* December 2010.

175. **Durrance FY.** Radiotherapy following simple hysterectomy in patients with stage I and II carcinoma of the cervix. *AJR Am J Roentgenol* 1968;102:165–169.

176. **Andras EJ, Fletcher GH, Rutledge F.** Radiotherapy of carcinoma of the cervix following simple hysterectomy. *Am J Obstet Gynecol* 1973;115:647–655.

177. **Heller PB, Barnhill DR, Mayer AR, et al.** Cervical carcinoma found incidentally in a uterus removed for benign indications. *Obstet Gynecol* 1986;67:187–190.

178. **Taylor PT, Andersen WA.** Untreated cervical cancer complicated by obstructive uropathy and renal failure. *Gynecol Oncol* 1981;11:162–174.

179. **Fletcher GH, Wharton JT.** Principles of irradiation therapy for gynecologic malignancy. *Curr Probl Obstet Gynecol* 1978;2:2–44.

180. **Gaddis O** Jr, **Morrow CP, Klement V, et al.** Treatment of cervical carcinoma employing a template for transperineal interstitial iridium brachytherapy. *Int J Radiat Oncol Biol Phys* 1983;9:819–827.

181. **O'Quinn AG, Fletcher GH, Wharton JT.** Guidelines for conservative hysterectomy after irradiation. *Gynecol Oncol* 1980;9:68–79.

182. **Homesley HD, Raben M, Blake DD, et al.** Relationship of lesion size to survival in patients with stage IB squamous cell carcinoma of the cervix uteri treated by radiation therapy. *Surg Gynecol Obstet* 1980;150:529–531.

183. **Feder BH, Syed AMN, Neblett D.** Treatment of extensive carcinoma of the cervix with the "transperineal parametrial butterfly"—a preliminary report on the revival of Waterman's approach. *Int J Radiat Oncol Biol Phys* 1978;4:735–742.

184. **Mikuta JJ, Giuntoli RL, Rubin EL, et al.** The radical hysterectomy. *Am J Obstet Gynecol* 1977;128:119–127.

185. **Symmonds RE, Pratt JH, Welch JS.** Extended Wertheim operation for primary, recurrent, or suspected recurrent carcinoma of the cervix. *Obstet Gynecol* 1964;24:15–27.

186. **Ketcham AS, Chretien PB, Hoye RC, et al.** Occult metastases to the scalene lymph nodes in patients with clinically operable carcinoma of the cervix. *Cancer* 1973;31:180–183.

187. **Fleisch MC, Pantke P, Beckmann MW, et al.** Predictors for long-term survival after interdisciplinary salvage surgery for advanced or recurrent gynecologic cancers. *J Surg Oncol* 2007;95:476–484.

188. **Rutledge FN, Smith JP, Wharton JT, et al.** Pelvic exenteration: an analysis of 296 patients. *Am J Obstet Gynecol* 1977;129:881–892.

189. **Maggioni A, Roviglione G, Landoni F, et al.** Pelvic exenteration: ten-year experience at the European Institute of Oncology in Milan. *Gynecol Oncol* 2009;114:64–68.

190. **Hatch KD, Shingleton HM, Soong SJ, et al.** Anterior pelvic exenteration. *Gynecol Oncol* 1988;31:205–216.

191. **Orr JW Jr, Shingleton HM, Hatch KD, et al.** Gastrointestinal complications associated with pelvic exenteration. *Am J Obstet Gynecol* 1983;145:325–332.

192. **Berek JS, Hacker NF, Lagasse LD.** Rectosigmoid colectomy and reanastomosis to facilitate resection of primary and recurrent gynecologic cancer. *Obstet Gynecol* 1984;64:715–720.

193. **Hatch KD, Shingleton HM, Potter ME, et al.** Low rectal resection and anastomosis at the time of pelvic exenteration. *Gynecol Oncol* 1988;31:262–267.

194. **Kock NG, Nilson AE, Nilsson LO, et al.** Urinary diversion via a continent ileal reservoir: clinical results in 12 patients. *J Urol* 1982;128:469–475.

195. **Penalver MA, Bejany DE, Averette HE, et al.** Continent urinary diversion in gynecologic oncology. *Gynecol Oncol* 1989;34:274–288.

196. **Mannel RS, Braly PS, Buller RE.** Indiana pouch continent urinary reservoir in patients with previous pelvic irradiation. *Obstet Gynecol* 1990;75:891–893.

197. **Berek JS, Hacker NF, Lagasse LD.** Vaginal reconstruction performed simultaneously with pelvic exenteration. *Obstet Gynecol* 1984;63:318–323.

198. **Hockel M.** Laterally extended endopelvic resection: principles and practices. *Gynecol Oncology* 2008;111:S13–S17.

199. **Abu-Rusteem NR, Lee S, Massad LS.** Topotecan for recurrent cervical cancer after platinum based therapy. *Int J Gynecol Cancer* 2000;10:285–288.

200. **Thigpen JT.** Single agent chemotherapy in carcinoma of the cervix. In: Surwit EA, Alberts DS, eds. Cervix cancer. Boston, MA: Martinus Nijhoff, 1987:119–136.

201. **Barter JF, Soong SJ, Hatch KD, et al.** Diagnosis and treatment of pulmonary metastases from cervical carcinoma. *Gynecol Oncol* 1990;38:347–351.

202. **Beller U, Benedet JL, Creasman WT, et al.** Carcinoma of the vagina: 26th annual report on the results of treatment in gynecological cancer. *Int J Gynecol Obstet* 2006;95:S29–S42.

203. **Fu YS.** Intraepithelial, invasive and metastatic neoplasms of the vagina. In: *Pathology of the uterine cervix vagina and vulva.* 2nd ed. Philadelphia: Saunders, 2002:531.

204. **Hellman K, Lundell M, Silfversward C, et al.** Clinical and histopathological factors related to prognosis in primary squamous cell carcinoma of the vagina. *Int J Gynecol Cancer* 2006:16;1201–1211.

205. **Benedet JL, Murphy KJ, Fairey RN, et al.** Primary invasive carcinoma of the vagina. *Obstet Gynecol* 1983;62:715–719.

206. **Hellman K, Silfversward C, Nilsson B, et al.** Primary cancer of the vagina factors influencing the age at diagnosis: the Radiumhemmet Series 1956–1996. *Int J Gynecol Oncol Cancer* 2004;14:491–501.

207. **Rubin SC, Young J, Mikuta JJ.** Squamous carcinoma of the vagina: treatment, complications, and long-term follow up. *Gynecol Oncol* 1985;20:346–353.

208. **Benedet JL, Saunders BH.** Carcinoma *in situ* of the vagina. *Am J Obstet Gynecol* 1984;148:695–700.

209. **Lenehan PM, Meffe F, Lickrish GM.** Vaginal intraepithelial neoplasia: biologic aspects and management. *Obstet Gynecol* 1986;68:333–337.

210. **Herman JM, Homesley HD, Dignan MB.** Is hysterectomy a risk factor for vaginal cancer? *JAMA* 1986;256:601–603.

211. **Frick HC, Jacox HW, Taylor HC.** Primary carcinoma of the vagina. *Am J Obstet Gynecol* 1986;101:695.

212. **Hoffman MS, DeCesare SL, Roberts WS, et al.** Upper vaginectomy for *in situ* and occult superficially invasive carcinoma of the vagina. *Am J Obstet Gynecol* 1992;166:30–33.

213. **Al-Kurdi M, Monaghan JM.** Thirty-two years experience in management of primary tumors of the vagina. *BJOG* 1981;88:1145–1150.

214. **Rutledge F.** Cancer of the vagina. *Am J Obstet Gynecol* 1967;97:635–655.

215. **Perez CA, Arneson AN, Dehner LP, et al.** Radiation therapy in carcinoma of the vagina. *Obstet Gynecol* 1974;44:862–872.

216. **Chung AF, Casey MJ, Flannery JT, et al.** Malignant melanoma of the vagina—report of 19 cases. *Obstet Gynecol* 1980;55:720–727.

217. **Iversen K, Robins RE.** Mucosal malignant melanomas. *Am J Surg* 1980;139:660.

218. **Norris HJ, Taylor HB.** Melanomas of the vagina. *Am J Clin Pathol* 1966;46:420.

219. **Ballon SC, Lagasse LD, Chang NH, et al.** Primary adenocarcinoma of the vagina. *Surg Gynecol Obstet* 1979;149:233–237.

220. **Herbst AL, Scully RE.** Adenocarcinoma of the vagina in adolescence. *Cancer* 1970;25:745–757.

221. **Herbst AL, Ulfelder H, Poskanzer DC.** Adenocarcinoma of the vagina: association of maternal stilbestrol therapy with tumor appearance in young women. *N Engl J Med* 1971;284:878–881.

222. **Herbst AL, Cole P, Norusis MJ, et al.** Epidemiologic aspects of factors related to survival in 384 registry cases of clear cell adenocarcinoma of the vagina and cervix. *Am J Obstet Gynecol* 1979;135:876–886.

223. **Reid GC, Schmidt RW, Roberts JA, et al.** Primary melanoma of the vagina: a clinicopathologic analysis. *Obstet Gynecol* 1989;74:190–199.

224. **Morrow CP, DiSaia PJ.** Malignant melanoma of the female genitalia: a clinical analysis. *Obstet Gynecol Surv* 1976;31:233.

225. **Cramer DW, Cutler SJ.** Incidence and histopathology of malignancies of the female genital organs in the United States. *Am J Obstet Gynecol* 1974;118:443–460.

226. **Eddy GL, Singh KP, Gansler TS.** Superficially invasive carcinoma of the vagina following treatment for cervical cancer: a report of six cases. *Gynecol Oncol* 1990;36:376–379.

227. **Reddy S, Lee MS, Graham JE, et al.** Radiation therapy in primary carcinoma of the vagina. *Gynecol Oncol* 1987;26:19–24.

228. **Kucera H, Langer M, Smekal G, et al.** Radiotherapy of primary carcinoma of the vagina: management and results of different therapy schemes. *Gynecol Oncol* 1985;21:87–93.

229. **Houghton CRS, Iversen T.** Squamous cell carcinoma of the vagina: a clinical study of the location of the tumor. *Gynecol Oncol* 1982;13:365–372.

230. **Lamoreaux WT, Grigsby PW, Dehdashti F, et al.** FDG-PET evaluation of vaginal carcinoma. *Int J Radiat Oncol Biol Phys* 2005;62:733–737.

231. **Dalrymple JL, Russell AH, Lee SW, et al.** Chemoradiation for primary invasive squamous carcinoma of the vagina. *Int J Gynecol Cancer* 2004;14:110–117.

232. **Eddy GL, Marks RD, Miller MC 3rd, et al.** Primary invasive vaginal carcinoma. *Am J Obstet Gynecol* 1991;165:292–296.

233. **Pride GL, Schultz AE, Chuprevich TW, et al.** Primary invasive squamous carcinoma of the vagina. *Obstet Gynecol* 1979;53:218–225.

234. **Kirkbride P, Fyles A, Rawlings GA, et al.** Carcinoma of the vagina: experience at the Princess Margaret Hospital (1974–1989). *Gynecol Oncol* 1995;56:435–443.

235. **Perez CA, Grigsby PW, Garipagaoglu M, et al.** Factors affecting long-term outcome of irradiation in carcinoma of the vagina. *Int J Radiat Oncol Biol Phys* 1999;44:37–45.

236. **Tewari KS, Cappuccini F, Puthawala AA, et al.** Primary invasive carcinoma of the vagina: treatment with interstitial brachytherapy. *Cancer* 2001;91:758–770.

237. **Otton GR, Nicklin JL, Dickie GJ, et al.** Early-stage vaginal carcinoma—an analysis of 70 patients. *Int J Gynecol Cancer* 2004;14:304–310.

238. **Frank SJ, Thingran A, Levenbach C, et al.** Definitive radiation therapy for squamous cell carcinoma of the vagina. *Int J Radiat Oncol Biol Phys* 2005;62:138–147.

239. **Tran PT, Su Z, Lee P, et al.** Prognostic factors for outcomes and complications for primary squamous cell carcinoma of the vagina treated with radiation. *Gynecol Oncol* 2007;105:641–649.

37

Ovarian, Fallopian Tube, and Peritoneal Cancer

Jonathan S. Berek
Teri A. Longacre
Michael Friedlander

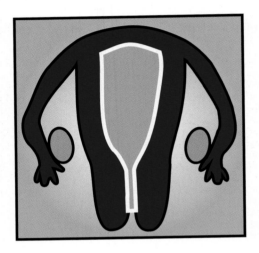

- The peak incidence of invasive epithelial ovarian cancer is at about 60 years of age. About 30% of ovarian neoplasms in postmenopausal women are malignant, whereas only about 7% of ovarian epithelial tumors in premenopausal patients are frankly malignant. The average age of patients with borderline tumors is approximately 46 years.

- Ovarian cancer is associated with low parity and infertility. Because parity is inversely related to the risk of ovarian cancer, having at least one child is protective for the disease, with a risk reduction of 0.3 to 0.4.

- Oral contraceptive use reduces the risk of epithelial ovarian cancer. Women who use oral contraceptives for 5 or more years reduce their relative risk to 0.5 (i.e., there is a 50% reduction in the likelihood of development of ovarian cancer).

- Given the false-positive results for both CA125 and transvaginal ultrasonography, particularly in premenopausal women, and the absence of evidence from randomized trials that these tests reduce the mortality of ovarian cancer, these tests should not be used routinely to screen women at risk for ovarian cancer.

- Most epithelial ovarian cancers are sporadic, but at least 5% to 10% result from inherited susceptibility and are hereditary. Hereditary ovarian cancers, particularly those caused by *BRCA1* mutations, occur in women approximately 10 years younger than those with nonhereditary tumors.

- Most hereditary ovarian cancers result from germline mutations in the *BRCA1* and *BRCA2* genes. The mutations are inherited in an autosomal dominant fashion, and therefore a full pedigree analysis (i.e., both maternal and paternal sides of the family history for both breast and ovarian cancer) must be carefully evaluated in all patients with epithelial ovarian cancer, and those with fallopian tube cancer and peritoneal cancer. The value of prophylactic salpingo-oophorectomy in these patients is well documented and is the most effective way to reduce risk of these cancers.

- The importance of thorough surgical staging cannot be overemphasized, because subsequent treatment and prognosis will be determined by the stage of disease. Patients with advanced-stage disease should undergo *debulking* or cytoreductive surgery to remove as much of the tumor and its metastases as possible, if the patient is medically fit for major surgery. The performance of a debulking operation as early as possible in the course of the patient's treatment is considered the standard of care for most patients. Most patients have a primary debulking surgery, while a smaller proportion of patients not suitable for initial surgery receive two to three cycles of primary chemotherapy followed by interval debulking surgery.

- Combination chemotherapy with *carboplatin* and *paclitaxel* is recommended for patients with high-risk, low-stage disease. For advanced-stage epithelial ovarian cancer, the choice of intravenous versus intraperitoneal *platinum* and *taxane* chemotherapy should be individualized.

- In the first two decades of life, almost 70% of ovarian tumors are of germ cell origin, and one-third of these are malignant. In contrast to the relatively slow-growing epithelial ovarian tumors, germ cell malignancies grow rapidly.

- The most common types of malignant germ cell tumors are dysgerminomas, immature teratomas, and endodermal sinus tumors. Preservation of fertility should be standard in most patients. The most effective chemotherapy is *bleomycin, etoposide,* and *cisplatin* (BEP).

- Stromal tumors include granulosa cell tumors, which are low-grade malignancies. In premenopausal women, they can be treated conservatively. Adjuvant chemotherapy is of unproven value.

- Metastatic tumors to the ovaries are most frequently from the breast and gastrointestinal tract.

- Fallopian tube carcinomas and peritoneal cancers are treated the same as ovarian cancer, with staging and cytoreductive surgery followed by *platinum* and *taxane* chemotherapy.

Of all the gynecologic cancers, ovarian malignancies represent the greatest clinical challenge because they have a high mortality. Epithelial cancers are the most common ovarian malignancy, and over two-thirds of patients have advanced disease at diagnosis. Ovarian cancer represents a major surgical challenge, and optimal therapy includes surgical debulking followed by *platinum*-based combination chemotherapy. It has the highest fatality-to-case ratio of all the gynecologic malignancies. There are nearly 22,000 new cases annually in the United States, and 15,460 women can be expected to succumb to their illness (1). Ovarian cancer is the seventh most common cancer in women in the United States, accounting for 3% of all malignancies and 6% of deaths from cancer in women and almost one-third of invasive malignancies of the female genital organs. Ovarian cancer is the fifth most common cause of death from malignancy in women. **A woman's risk at birth of having ovarian cancer at some point in her lifetime is 1% to 1.5% and that of dying from ovarian cancer is almost 0.5%** (2).

Epithelial Ovarian Cancer

Approximately 90% of ovarian cancers are derived from the coelomic epithelium or mesothelium (2). The cells are a product of the primitive mesoderm, which can undergo metaplasia. A classification of the histologic types of epithelial tumors of the ovary is presented in Table 37.1. Neoplastic transformation can occur when the cells are genetically predisposed to oncogenesis or exposed to an oncogenic agent or both (3).

Pathology

Invasive Cancer

Seventy-five percent to 80% of epithelial cancers are of the serous histologic type. Less common types are endometrioid (10%), clear cell (5%), mucinous (5%), transitional (Brenner), and undifferentiated carcinomas, with each of the last two types representing less than 1% of epithelial lesions (2). Each of the major tumor types is named on the basis of a histologic

Table 37.1 Epithelial Ovarian Tumors	
Histologic Type	*Cellular Type*
I. Serous	*Endosalpingeal*
A. Benign	
B. Borderline	
C. Malignant	
II. Mucinous	*Intestinal, Endocervical*
A. Benign	
B. Borderline	
C. Malignant	
III. Endometrioid	*Endometrial*
A. Benign	
B. Borderline	
C. Malignant	
IV. Clear-cell	*Müllerian*
A. Benign	
B. Borderline	
C. Malignant	
V. Brenner	*Transitional*
A. Benign	
B. Borderline (proliferating)	
C. Malignant	
VI. Mixed epithelial	*Mixed*
A. Benign	
B. Borderline	
C. Malignant	
VII. Undifferentiated	*May be anaplastic*
VIII. Unclassified	

From **Seroy SF, Scully RE, Sobin LH.** *International histological classification of tumours no. 9. Histological typing of ovarian tumors.* Geneva, Switzerland: World Health Organization, 1973, with permission.

pattern that resembles epithelium in the lower genital tract (3). For example, serous tumors have an appearance similar to that of the glandular epithelial lining of the fallopian tube, endometrioid tumors resemble proliferative endometrium, and clear cell tumors resemble secretory or gestational endometrium. Mucinous tumors may contain cells that resemble endocervical glands, but more commonly these cells resemble the gastrointestinal epithelium. Transitional (Brenner) tumors are so named because of a resemblance to the epithelium in Walthard rests and bladder urothelium.

Although it was believed that epithelial ovarian cancers arise from either the surface epithelium of the ovary or from inclusion cysts within the ovary, there is growing evidence to suggest that many, if not most, high-grade serous carcinomas of the ovary arise from the fimbrial end of the fallopian tube rather than from the ovary (4,5). It is suggested that **serous epithelial ovarian cancers be separated into two distinct groups—type I and type II serous tumors—as they differ considerably in the cell of origin, molecular pathogenesis, and their biological behavior** (6). **Type I tumors include serous borderline tumors and low-grade serous carcinoma; they are** genetically stable and are characterized by mutations in *KRAS* and *BRAF.* Type II serous tumors are rapidly growing, highly aggressive neoplasms that lack well-defined precursor lesions; most are advanced stage at, or soon after, their inception and many appear to arise in the fimbrial end of the fallopian tube (7). The type II tumors are genetically unstable and harbor p53 mutations.

Borderline Tumors

An important group of tumors to distinguish is the *tumor of low malignant potential*, also called the *borderline tumor.* Borderline tumors are lesions that tend to remain confined to the ovary for long periods, occur predominantly in premenopausal women, and are associated with a very good prognosis (2,3,8–12). They are encountered most frequently in women between the ages of 30 and 50 years, whereas invasive carcinomas occur more often in women between the ages of 50 and 70 years (2).

Although uncommon, implants may occur with serous borderline tumors. Such implants are divided into *noninvasive* and *invasive* forms. The latter group has a higher likelihood of developing into progressive, proliferative disease in the peritoneal cavity, which can lead to intestinal obstruction and death (2,6).

Classification of Epithelial Ovarian Tumors

Serous Tumors

Serous tumors are so classified because they resemble tubal secretory cells. *Psammoma bodies* are frequently found in these neoplasms, and they are made up of concentric rings of calcification. Several hypotheses pertaining to the origin and development of psammoma bodies are proposed, including apoptosis of tumor cells and osteoinductive cytokines produced by macrophages (6). In the wall of the mesothelial invaginations, papillary ingrowths are common, representing the early stages of development of a papillary serous cystadenoma. There are many variations in the proliferation of these mesothelial inclusions. Several foci may be lined with flattened inactive epithelium; in adjacent cavities, papillary excrescences are present, often resulting from local irritants (2).

Borderline Serous Tumors Approximately 10% of all ovarian serous tumors fall into the category of a tumor of low malignant potential or borderline tumor (Fig. 37.1), and 50% occur before the age of 40 years. The criteria for the diagnosis of serous borderline tumors are as follows (11):

1. Epithelial hyperplasia in the form of pseudostratification, tufting, cribriform, and micropapillary architecture
2. Mild nuclear atypia and mild increased mitotic activity
3. Detached cell clusters
4. Absence of destructive stromal invasion (i.e., without tissue destruction)

Serous borderline tumors that are composed of an exuberant micropapillary architecture are designated as serous borderline tumors with micropapillary features (Fig. 37.2); these tumors are more frequently bilateral, exophytic, and high-stage than the usual serous borderline tumor.

It should be emphasized that up to 40% of serous borderline tumors are associated with spread beyond the ovary, but high-stage disease does not necessarily warrant a diagnosis of carcinoma. The diagnosis of a serous borderline tumor versus serous carcinoma is based on the histologic features of the primary tumor (11). Up to 10% of women with ovarian serous borderline tumors and extraovarian implants may have invasive implants, and these can behave more aggressively (13). The 5-year overall survival for women with invasive implants is about 50% if stringent criteria are applied (10,13–15). Most implants are noninvasive (10,16). In the noninvasive implants, papillary proliferations of atypical cells involve the peritoneal surface and form smooth invaginations (10). In contrast, the invasive implants resemble well-differentiated serous carcinoma and are characterized by atypical cells forming irregular glands with sharp borders. Implants are usually confined to the abdominal cavity and may be seen in the pelvis, omentum, and adjacent tissues, including lymph nodes, but spread outside the abdominal cavity is rare. Death can occur as the result of intestinal obstruction (16–19).

Borderline serous tumors may harbor foci of stromal microinvasion (18). Most patients are young and International Federation of Gynecology and Obstetrics (FIGO) stage I. Stromal microinvasion is increased about ninefold in pregnant women with serous borderline tumors.

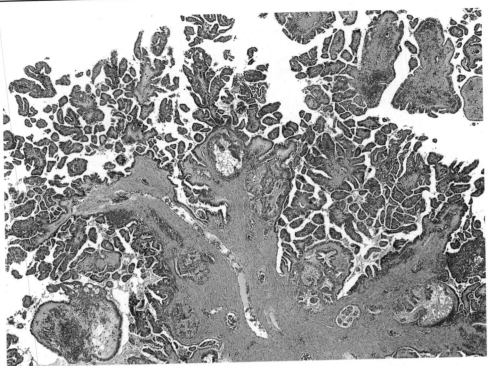

Figure 37.1   **Serous borderline tumor of the ovary.** Complex papillary fronds with hierarchical branching are lined with pseudostratified columnar cells. The epithelium and the stroma are clearly separated by a basement membrane, indicating no stromal invasion.

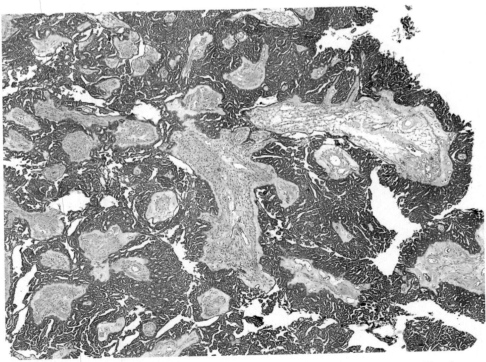

Figure 37.2   **Serous borderline tumor with micropapillary features.** The papillae have a non-hierarchical branching pattern and are lined by a monomorphous population of cells.

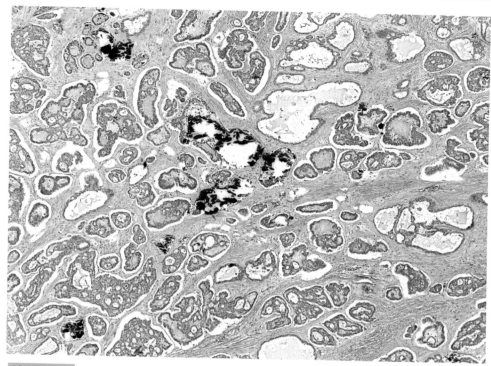

Figure 37.3 **Low-grade serous adenocarcinoma of the ovary.** Clusters and papillae of malignant cells are in direct contact with fibrous stroma indicative of stromal invasion.

The presence of stromal microinvasion is associated with lymphovascular space invasion in the primary ovarian tumor (and likely represents a form of true stromal invasion), but it is not associated with an aggressive clinical course, and patients with this finding should be managed in the same way as patients without stromal microinvasion.

Serous Carcinomas   **In malignant serous tumors, stromal invasion is present** (2). The grade of tumor is important and needs to be documented. In low-grade serous adenocarcinomas, papillary and glandular structures predominate (Fig. 37.3); high-grade neoplasms are characterized by solid sheets of cells, nuclear pleomorphism, and high mitotic activity (Fig. 37.4). Laminated, calcified psammoma bodies are found in 80% of serous carcinomas. ***Serous psammocarcinoma is a rare variant of serous carcinoma characterized by massive psammoma body formation and low-grade cytological features.*** At least 75% of the epithelial nests are associated with psammoma body formation. Patients with serous psammocarcinoma have a protracted clinical course and a relatively favorable prognosis; their clinical course more closely resembles that of high-stage, progressive serous borderline tumor than serous carcinoma.

Mucinous Tumors

These cystic ovarian tumors have loculi lined with mucin-secreting epithelium. The lining epithelial cells contain intracytoplasmic mucin and resemble those of endocervix, gastric pylorus, or intestine. **They represent about 8% to 10% of epithelial ovarian tumors.** They may reach enormous size, filling the entire abdominal cavity (2).

Borderline Mucinous Tumors   The mucinous tumor of low malignant potential is often difficult to diagnose. Although it is common to find a rather uniform pattern from section to section in the serous borderline tumor, this is not true in the mucinous tumors. **Well-differentiated mucinous epithelium may be seen immediately adjacent to a poorly differentiated focus. It is important to take multiple sections from many areas in the mucinous tumor to identify the most malignant alteration** (2).

Mucinous Carcinomas   **Bilateral tumors occur in 8% to 10% of cases.** The mucinous lesions are confined to the ovary in 95% to 98% of cases (Fig. 37.5). **Because most ovarian mucinous carcinomas contain intestinal-type cells, they cannot be distinguished from**

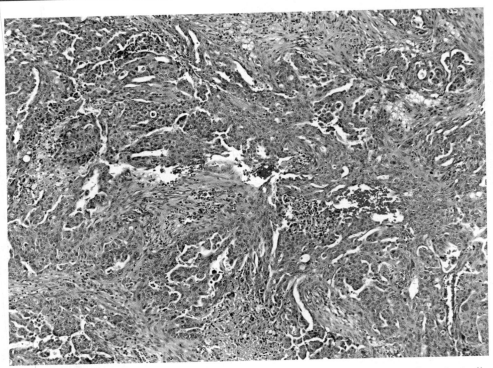

Figure 37.4   **High-grade serous adenocarcinoma.** Papillae lined by sheets of cytologically malignant cells invade stroma, often with associated necrosis.

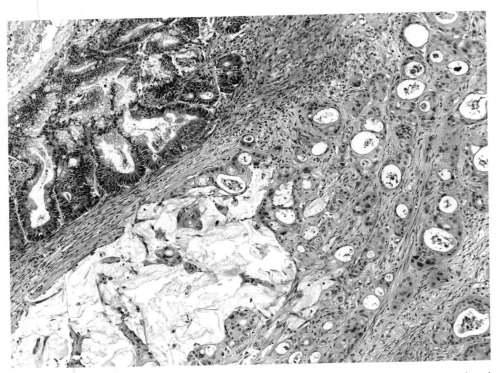

Figure 37.5   **Mucinous adenocarcinoma of the ovary.** Irregular glandular spaces are lined with a layer of tall columnar cells with abundant mucinous cytoplasm, resembling intestinal epithelium at the left. At the right, there is destructive invasion into the ovarian stroma.

metastatic carcinoma of the gastrointestinal tract on the basis of histology alone (2,6). Primary ovarian neoplasms rarely metastasize to the mucosa of the bowel, although they commonly involve the serosa, whereas gastrointestinal lesions frequently involve the ovary by direct extension or lymphatic spread (2).

Pseudomyxoma Peritonei ***Pseudomyxoma peritonei*** is a clinical term used to describe the finding of abundant mucoid or gelatinous material in the pelvis and abdominal cavity surrounded by fibrous tissue. It is **most commonly secondary to a well-differentiated appendiceal mucinous neoplasm** or other gastrointestinal primary; rarely, mucinous tumors arising in an ovarian mature teratoma are associated with pseudomyxoma peritonei.

Endometrioid Tumors

Endometrioid lesions constitute 6% to 8% of epithelial tumors. Endometrioid neoplasia includes all the benign demonstrations of endometriosis. In 1925, Sampson suggested that certain cases of adenocarcinoma of the ovary probably arose in areas of endometriosis (19). The adenocarcinomas are similar to those seen in the uterine corpus. The malignant potential of endometriosis is very low, although a transition from benign to malignant epithelium may be demonstrated.

Borderline Endometrioid Tumors **The endometrioid tumor of low malignant potential has a wide morphologic spectrum.** Tumors may resemble an endometrial polyp or complex endometrial hyperplasia with glandular crowding. When there are back-to-back, architecturally complex glands with no intervening stroma, the tumor is classified as a well-differentiated endometrioid carcinoma. Some borderline endometrioid tumors have a prominent fibromatous component. In such cases, the term *adenofibroma* is used to describe them (2).

Endometrioid Carcinomas Endometrioid tumors are characterized by a markedly complex glandular pattern with all the potential variations of epithelia found in the uterus (Fig. 37.6).

Multifocal Disease The endometrioid tumors afford the greatest opportunity to evaluate multifocal disease. **Endometrioid carcinoma of the ovary is associated in 15% to 20% of the**

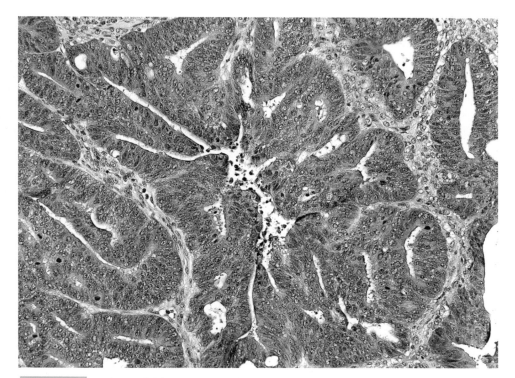

Figure 37.6 Endometrioid cancer. Round to tubular glands lined by stratified columnar cells with confluent growth pattern.

cases with carcinoma of the endometrium. Identification of multifocal disease is important because patients with disease metastatic from the uterus to the ovaries have a 30% to 40% 5-year survival, whereas those with synchronous multifocal disease have a 75% to 80% 5-year survival (20). When the histologic appearance of endometrial and ovarian tumors is different, the two tumors most likely represent two separate primary lesions. When they appear similar, the endometrial tumor can be considered a separate primary tumor if it is well differentiated and only superficially invasive.

Clear Cell Carcinomas

Several basic histologic patterns are present in the clear cell adenocarcinoma (i.e., tubulocystic, papillary, reticular, and solid). The tumors are made up of clear and hobnail cells that project their nuclei into the apical cytoplasm. The clear cells have abundant clear or vacuolated cytoplasm, hyperchromatic irregular nuclei, and nucleoli of various sizes (Fig. 37.7). **Focal areas of endometriosis are common and mixed clear cell and endometrioid carcinoma may occur** (20). The clear cell carcinoma seen in the ovary is histologically identical to that seen in the uterus or vagina of the young patient who has been exposed to *diethylstilbestrol* (DES) *in utero*. Nuclei of clear cell carcinoma range from grade 1 to grade 3, but pure grade 1 tumors are extremely rare. **Almost invariably high-grade (grade 3) nuclei are identified. Hence, clear cell carcinoma is not graded.**

Transitional (Brenner) Tumors

Borderline Brenner Tumors   In the past, proliferative Brenner tumors were subclassified as proliferating tumors (those tumors that resemble low-grade papillary urothelial carcinoma of the urinary bladder) and borderline tumors (those tumors that resemble high-grade papillary urothelial carcinoma), but both groups of tumors are now classified as borderline Brenner tumors (21). Complete surgical removal usually results in cure.

Malignant Brenner Tumors   **These rare tumors are defined as benign or borderline Brenner tumors coexisting with invasive transitional cell carcinoma.**

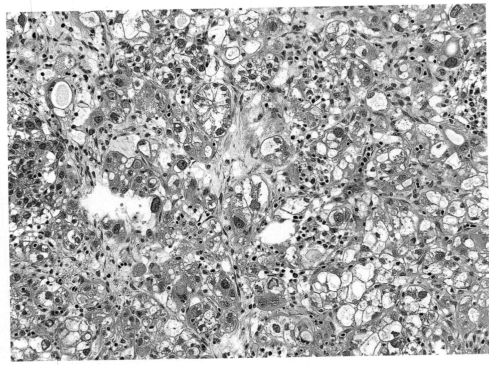

Figure 37.7   **Clear cell carcinoma of the ovary.** Note the solid variant of clear cell carcinoma with sheets of cells that have clear cytoplasm ("hobnail" cells).

Transitional Cell Carcinoma

The designation *transitional cell carcinoma* refers to a primary ovarian carcinoma resembling transitional cell carcinoma of the urinary bladder without a recognizable Brenner tumor. It is reported that those ovarian carcinomas that contain more than 50% of transitional cell carcinoma are more sensitive to chemotherapy and have a more favorable prognosis than other poorly differentiated ovarian carcinomas of comparable stage (22,23). Transitional cell tumors differ from malignant Brenner tumors in that they are more frequently diagnosed in an advanced stage and are associated with a poorer survival rate (24).

Peritoneal Carcinomas

Peritoneal tumors are histologically indistinguishable from ovarian serous tumors. In the case of *borderline serous peritoneal tumors* and *serous peritoneal carcinomas*, the ovaries are normal or minimally involved, and the tumors affect predominantly the uterosacral ligaments, pelvic peritoneum, or omentum. The overall prognosis for borderline serous peritoneal tumors is excellent and comparable to that of ovarian borderline serous tumors (25–27). In the review of 38 cases of peritoneal borderline serous tumors from the literature, 32 women had no persistent disease, 4 were well after resection of recurrence, 1 developed an invasive serous carcinoma, and 1 died from the effects of the tumor (25).

Carcinoma that appears predominantly as peritoneal carcinomatosis without appreciable ovarian or fallopian tube enlargement is called *peritoneal carcinoma* or müllerian carcinoma when tumors spread from the breast, gastrointestinal tract, and other organs of nonmüllerian origin are excluded. Most are *peritoneal serous carcinomas*, which have the appearance of a moderately to poorly differentiated serous ovarian carcinoma. Peritoneal endometrioid carcinoma is less common.

Peritoneal carcinoma should be considered clinically the same as ovarian and fallopian tube cancers. In patients for whom exploratory surgery is performed, there may be microscopic or small macroscopic cancer on the surface of the ovary and extensive disease in the upper abdomen, particularly in the omentum (28).

Mesotheliomas

Peritoneal malignant mesotheliomas may be epithelial, sarcomatous, or biphasic (2,29). Deciduoid peritoneal mesothelioma is an unusual variant that resembles exuberant, ectopic decidual reaction of the peritoneum. Asbestos exposure is not correlated with peritoneal mesotheliomas in women. These lesions typically appear as multiple intraperitoneal masses, often coating the entire peritoneum and can develop after hysterectomy and bilateral salpingo-oophorectomy for benign disease. Malignant mesotheliomas should be distinguished from benign multicystic peritoneal mesothelioma (multilocular peritoneal inclusion cyst), and ovarian tumor implants and primary peritoneal müllerian neoplasms.

Clinical Features

More than 80% of epithelial ovarian cancers are found in postmenopausal women (Fig. 37.8). **The peak incidence of invasive epithelial ovarian cancer is at 56 to 60 years of age** (2,3,30). The age-specific incidence of ovarian epithelial cancer rises precipitously from 20 to 80 years of age and subsequently declines (30). These cancers are relatively uncommon in women younger than age 45. Fewer than 1% of epithelial ovarian cancers occur before the age of 21 years, two-thirds of ovarian malignancies in such patients being germ cell tumors (2,30,31). **About 30% of ovarian neoplasms in postmenopausal women are malignant, whereas only about 7% of ovarian epithelial tumors in premenopausal patients are frankly malignant** (2,3).

The average age of patients with borderline tumors is approximately 46 years (2,3,9). Eighty percent to 90% of ovarian cancers, including borderline forms, occur after the age of 40 years, whereas 30% to 40% of malignancies occur after the age of 65 years. The chance that a primary epithelial tumor will be of borderline or invasive malignancy in a patient younger than 40 years is approximately 1 in 10, but after that age it rises to 1 in 3 (2,3). Less than 1% of epithelial ovarian cancers occur before the age of 20 years, with two-thirds of ovarian malignancies in such patients being germ cell tumors (31).

Etiology

Ovarian cancer is associated with low parity and infertility (32). Although there are a variety of epidemiologic variables correlated with ovarian cancer, such as talc use, galactose consumption, and tubal ligation (see Chapter 4), none is so strongly correlated as prior reproductive history

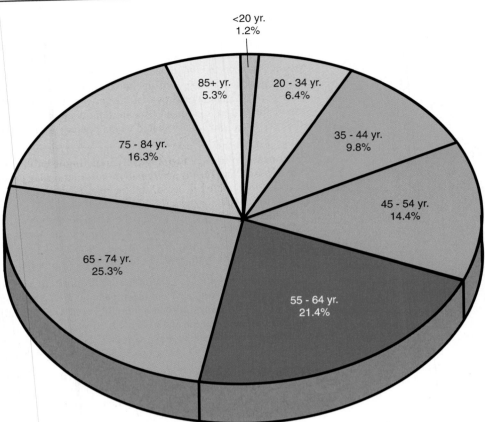

Figure 37.8 **Ovarian cancer incidence: distribution by age.** (From **Nagy K.** The side effects of managed care on the drug industry. *J Natl Cancer Inst* 1995;87:1280, with permission.)

and duration of the reproductive career (32,33). Early menarche and late menopause increase the risk of ovarian cancer (33). These factors and the relationship of parity and infertility to the risk of ovarian cancer led to the hypothesis that suppression of ovulation may be an important factor. **Theoretically, the surface epithelium undergoes repetitive disruption and repair. It is thought that this process might lead to a higher probability of spontaneous mutations that can unmask germline mutations or otherwise lead to the oncogenic phenotype** (see Chapter 6).

Prevention

Because parity is inversely related to the risk of ovarian cancer, having at least one child is protective for the disease, with a risk reduction of 0.3 to 0.4. Oral contraceptive use reduces the risk of epithelial ovarian cancer (32). **Women who use oral contraceptives for 5 or more years reduce their relative risk to 0.5 (i.e., there is a 50% reduction in the likelihood of development of ovarian cancer).** Women who had two children and used oral contraceptives for 5 or more years have a relative risk of ovarian cancer as low as 0.3, or a 70% reduction (34). **The oral contraceptive pill is the only documented method of chemoprevention for ovarian cancer, and it should be recommended to women for this purpose. When counseling patients regarding birth control options, this important benefit of oral contraceptive use should be emphasized. This is important for women with a strong family history of ovarian cancer.**

The performance of a prophylactic salpingo-oophorectomy significantly reduces, but does not totally eliminate, the risk of nonuterine pelvic cancers; because the entire peritoneum is at risk, peritoneal carcinomas can occur in 2% to 3% of women even after prophylactic bilateral salpingo-oophorectomy (25,28).

A thorough discussion of the risks and benefits of oophorectomy should be undertaken in premenopausal women who are undergoing a hysterectomy for benign disease, who do not

carry germline mutations, and do not have a family history that suggests that they are at higher than average risk for ovarian cancer (35). The ovaries may provide protection from cardiovascular disease and osteoporosis, and long-term mortality may not be decreased by the performance of prophylactic oophorectomy in women at population risk of ovarian cancer (36).

Screening

The value of tumor markers and ultrasonography to screen for epithelial ovarian cancer is not established by prospective studies. Screening results with transabdominal ultrasonography are encouraging in postmenopausal women, but specificity is limited (37–39). Advances in transvaginal ultrasonography showed a very high (>95%) sensitivity for the detection of early-stage ovarian cancer, although this test alone might require performance of as many as 10 to 15 laparotomy procedures for each case of ovarian cancer detected (37,38). Routine annual pelvic examinations have disappointing results in the early detection of ovarian cancer (40). Transvaginal color flow Doppler to assess the vascularity of the ovarian vessels is a useful adjunct to ultrasonography, but it is not useful in screening (41,42).

CA125 is useful for monitoring epithelial ovarian cancer patients during their chemotherapy, but the role of CA125 is still being defined in a screening setting (43–49). **Regarding the sensitivity of the test, elevated CA125 levels are seen in 50% of patients with stage I disease** (43,48). **Data suggest that the specificity of CA125 is improved when the test is combined with transvaginal ultrasonography or when the CA125 levels are followed over time** (49,50). These data encouraged the development of prospective screening studies in Sweden and the United Kingdom (45,47). In these studies, patients with elevated CA125 levels (>30 U/mL) underwent abdominal ultrasonography, and 14 ovarian cancers were discovered among 27,000 women screened. About four laparotomies were performed for each case of cancer detected (47).

A randomized trial of nearly 22,000 women aged 45 years or older was performed in the United Kingdom (50). The patients were assigned to either a control group of routine pelvic examination (n = 0,977) or to a screening group (n = 10,958). The screening consisted of three annual screens that involved measurement of serum CA125 levels, pelvic ultrasonography if the CA125 was 30 U/mL or higher, and referral for gynecologic examination if the ovarian volume was 8.8 mL or greater on the ultrasonography. Of the 468 women in the screened group with an elevated CA125, 29 were referred for surgery, 6 cancers were discovered, and 23 had false-positive screening results, yielding a positive predictive value of 20.7%. During a 7-year follow-up period, cancer developed in 10 additional women in the screened group, as it did in 20 women in the control group. Although the median survival of women in whom cancer developed in the screened group was 72.9 months, compared with 41.8 months in the control group ($p = .0112$), the number of deaths did not differ significantly between the control and screened groups (18/10,977 vs. 9/10,958; relative risk 2.0 [0.78 to 5.13]). These data show that a multimodal approach to ovarian cancer screening is feasible, but a larger trial is necessary to determine whether this approach affects mortality. Such a three-arm randomized trial is ongoing in the United Kingdom, and the anticipated accrual is approximately 50,000 women per study arm and 100,000 women in the control arm. Based on the risk of ovarian cancer (ROC) algorithm for CA125 levels, patients in the third group will be referred for transvaginal ultrasonography and/or surgery (51). Women will be screened for 3 years and studied for 7 years. **The aims of this trial are to determine the feasibility of screening for ovarian cancer and whether ovarian cancers can be diagnosed at an earlier stage and the impact of early detection on survival.**

Another approach is the use of *proteomic patterns* to identify ovarian cancer using surface-enhanced laser desorption ionization time-of-flight (SELDI-TOF) technology (52). In a study using this technology, the sensitivity for predicting ovarian cancer was 100%, with a specificity of 95% and a positive predictive value of 94%. The assay correctly identified all 18 women with stage I tumors. This technology is in the early phases of development and validation, and its efficacy has yet to be demonstrated in large population-based studies (53).

Given the false-positive and false-negative results for both CA125 and transvaginal ultrasonography and the absence of good data to show that screening detects ovarian cancers at an earlier stage, these tests are not recommended and should not be used routinely to screen women with a population risk or high risk for ovarian cancer (54–56). In the future, new markers or technologies may improve the specificity of ovarian cancer screening, but proof of this will require a large, prospective study (47,48). Screening in women who have a familial risk may have a better yield, but to date there is no evidence to demonstrate a benefit of screening even in high-risk women, and this is being actively investigated (55,57). The findings of two prospective studies of annual transvaginal ultrasound and CA125 screening in 888 *BRCA1* and *BRCA2* mutation carriers in the Netherlands and 279 mutation carriers in the United Kingdom are not encouraging and suggest a very limited benefit of screening in high-risk women (55,56). Despite annual gynecologic screening Hermsen et al. reported that a high proportion of ovarian cancers in *BRCA1-2* carriers were interval cancers and the large majority of all cancers diagnosed were at advanced stages; similar results were reported by Woodward et al. (55,56).

Genetic Risk for Epithelial Ovarian Cancer

The lifetime risk of ovarian carcinoma for women in the United States is about 1.4% (1–3). The risk of ovarian cancer is higher than that in the general population in women with certain family histories (51–60). **Most epithelial ovarian cancer is sporadic, with familial or hereditary causes accounting for 5% to 10% of invasive epithelial ovarian cancer** (59).

Hereditary Ovarian Cancer

BRCA1 and *BRCA2*

Most hereditary ovarian cancer is associated with mutations in the *BRCA1* gene, located on chromosome 17 (58–69). **A small proportion of inherited disease is associated with germline mutations in another gene, *BRCA2*, located on chromosome 13** (60). Discovered through linkage analyses, these two high-penetrance genes are associated with the genetic predisposition to both ovarian and breast cancers. There are almost certainly other low- to moderate-penetrance genes that predispose to ovarian and breast cancer, and this is an area of intense research interest (1).

It was thought that there were two distinct syndromes associated with a genetic risk, *site-specific hereditary ovarian cancer* and *hereditary breast-ovarian cancer syndrome*. It is now believed that these groups represent a continuum of mutations with different degrees of penetrance within a given family (62,70). There is a higher-than-expected risk of ovarian and endometrial cancer in *Lynch syndrome*, known as the ***hereditary nonpolyposis colorectal cancer syndrome* (HNPCC syndrome)** (71).

The mutations are inherited in an autosomal dominant fashion, and therefore a full pedigree analysis (i.e., both maternal and paternal sides of the family) must be carefully evaluated (62). There are numerous distinct mutations that were identified on each of these genes, and the mutations have different degrees of penetrance that may account for the preponderance of either breast cancer, ovarian cancer, or both, in any given family. Based on analysis of women who have a mutation in the *BRCA1* gene and are from high-risk families, the lifetime risk of ovarian cancer may be as high as 28% to 44%, and the risk was calculated to be as high as 27% for those women with a *BRCA2* mutation (59,60,66–69). The risk of breast cancer in women with a *BRCA1* or *BRCA2* mutation may be as high as 56% to 87%.

Hereditary ovarian cancers occur in women approximately 10 years younger than those with nonhereditary tumors (i.e., closer to age 50 compared to age 60 for those with sporadic cancer) (59). A woman with a first- or second-degree relative who had premenopausal ovarian cancer may have a higher probability of carrying an affected gene. Breast and ovarian cancer may exist in a family in which there is a combination of epithelial ovarian and breast cancers, affecting a mixture of first- and second-degree relatives. Women with this syndrome tend to have these tumors at a young age, and the breast cancers may be bilateral. If two first-degree relatives are affected, this pedigree is consistent with an autosomal dominant mode of inheritance (50,58). Most *BRCA1* ovarian cancers are high-grade serous carcinomas (Fig. 37.9).

Founder Effect

There is a higher carrier rate of *BRCA1* and *BRCA2* mutations in women of Ashkenazi Jewish descent, in Icelandic women, and in many other ethnic groups (64,65,67–69). There are three specific founder mutations carried by the Ashkenazi population, 185delAG and 5382insC on *BRCA1*, and 6174delT on *BRCA2*. **Individuals of Ashkenazi Jewish descent have a 1 in 40, or 2.5%**, chance of having a mutation in *BRCA1* or *BRCA2*, and thus there is a greater risk in this population. The increased risk is a result of the *founder effect*, in which a higher rate of specific mutations occurs in an ethnic group from a defined geographic area. These founder mutations

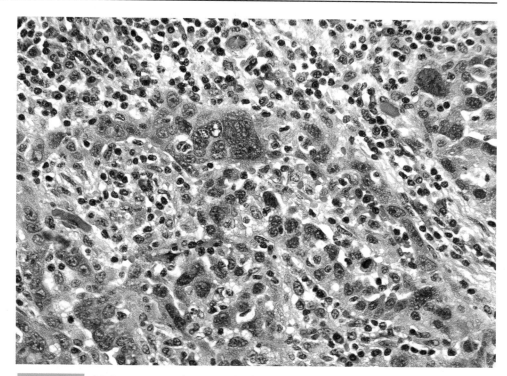

Figure 37.9 *BRCA1*-associated ovarian carcinoma is typically a high-grade serous adenocarcinoma with numerous mitotic figures and marked nuclear pleomorphism. A brisk lymphocytic infiltrate with tumor infiltrating lymphocytes is not uncommon in these tumors.

generated considerable interest, because they facilitate studies of prevalence and penetrance and can be used to quantify the degree of homogeneity within a population.

Pedigree Analysis

The risk of carrying a germline mutation that predisposes to ovarian cancer depends on the number of first- or second-degree relatives (or both) with a history of epithelial ovarian carcinoma or breast cancer (or both) and on the number of malignancies that occurs at an earlier age. The degree of risk is difficult to determine precisely unless a full pedigree analysis is performed.

1. In families with two first-degree relatives (i.e., mother, sister, or daughter) with documented premenopausal epithelial ovarian cancer, the risk that a female first-degree relative has an affected gene could be as high as 35% to 40% (60).

2. In families with a single first-degree relative and a single second-degree relative (i.e., grandmother, aunt, first cousin, or granddaughter) with epithelial ovarian cancer, the risk that a woman has an affected gene may be increased. The risk may be two- to 10-fold higher than in those without a familial history of the disease (60).

3. In families with a single postmenopausal first-degree relative with epithelial ovarian carcinoma, a woman may not have an increased risk of having an affected gene because the case is most likely to be sporadic. If the ovarian cancer occurs in a premenopausal relative, this could be significant, and a full pedigree analysis should be undertaken.

4. Women with a primary history of breast cancer have twice the expected incidence of subsequent ovarian cancer (59).

Lynch Syndrome or Hereditary Nonpolyposis Colon Cancer

Lynch syndrome (HNPCC), which includes multiple adenocarcinomas, involves a combination of colon cancer and endometrial or ovarian cancer and other malignancies of the gastrointestinal and genitourinary systems (71). The mutations that are associated with this syndrome are *MSH2, MLH1, PMS1,* and *PMS2*. The risk that a woman who is a member of one of these families will develop epithelial ovarian cancer depends on the frequency of this disease in first- and second-degree relatives, although these women appear to have at least three times the relative risk of the general population. A full pedigree analysis of such families should be performed by a geneticist to more accurately determine the risk.

Management of Women at High Risk for Ovarian Cancer

The management of a woman with a strong family history of epithelial ovarian cancer must be individualized and depends on her age, her reproductive plans, and the extent of risk. In all of these syndromes, women at risk benefit from a thorough pedigree analysis. A geneticist should evaluate the family pedigree for at least three generations. Decisions about management are best made after careful study and, whenever possible, verification of the histologic diagnosis of the family members' ovarian cancer.

The value of testing for *BRCA1* and *BRCA2* is established, and there are guidelines for testing (62,70,72). The importance of genetic counseling cannot be overemphasized because the decision is complex. The American Society of Clinical Oncology offered guidelines that emphasize careful evaluation by geneticists, careful maintenance of medical records, and an understanding in a genetic screening clinic of how to effectively counsel and manage these patients. Concerns remain over the use of the information, the impact on insurability, the interpretation of the results, and how the information will be used within a specific family (e.g., to counsel children).

Although there are some conflicting data, the behavior of breast cancers arising in women with germline mutations in *BRCA1* or *BRCA2* is comparable to the behavior of sporadic tumors (61,73). **Women with breast cancer who carry these mutations are at a greatly increased risk of ovarian cancer and a second breast cancer: the lifetime risk of ovarian cancer is 54% for women who have a *BRCA1* mutation and 23% for those with a *BRCA2* mutation, and for the two groups together, there is an 82% lifetime risk of breast cancer** (73).

Despite recommendation by the National Institutes of Health Consensus Conference on Ovarian Cancer, the value of screening with transvaginal ultrasonography, CA125 levels, or other procedures is not established in women at high risk (74). Bourne and coworkers showed that, using this approach, tumors can be detected approximately 10 times more often than in the general population, and they recommend screening in high-risk women, but other groups have not confirmed these findings, and bilateral salpingo-oophorectomy remains the most effective way to reduce risk (57,75).

Data derived from a multicenter consortium of genetic screening centers indicate that the use of the oral contraceptive pill is associated with a lower risk for development of ovarian cancer in women who have a mutation in either *BRCA1* or *BRCA2* (76). The risk reduction is significant: in women who take oral contraceptives for 5 or more years, the relative risk of ovarian cancer is 0.4, or a 60% reduction in the incidence of the disease.

Prophylactic Salpingo-oophorectomy in High-Risk Women

The value of prophylactic salpingo-oophorectomy in these patients is documented (77–83). Women at high risk for ovarian cancer who undergo prophylactic salpingo-oophorectomy have a risk of harboring occult neoplasia: in one series of 98 such operations, 3 (3.1%) patients had a low-stage ovarian malignancy (80). **The protection against ovarian cancer is excellent: the performance of a prophylactic salpingo-oophorectomy reduced the risk of *BRCA*-related gynecologic cancer by 96%** (80). In a series of 42 such operations, 4 patients (9.5%) had a malignancy, 1 of which was noted at surgery and 3 that were microscopic; all were smaller than 5 mm (78). Although the risk of ovarian cancer is significantly diminished, there remains the small risk of peritoneal carcinoma, a tumor for which women who have mutations in *BRCA1* and *BRCA2* may have a higher predisposition. In these series, the subsequent development of peritoneal carcinoma was 0.8% and 1%, respectively (78,79). **The risk of developing subsequent breast cancer was reduced by 50% to 80%.**

The role of hysterectomy is more controversial. Most studies show no increase in the rate of uterine and cervical tumors, but there are rare reports of an increase of papillary serous tumors of the endometrium (83). Women on *tamoxifen* are at higher risk for benign endometrial lesions (e.g., polyps) and endometrial cancer. **It is reasonable to consider the performance of a prophylactic hysterectomy in conjunction with salpingo-oophorectomy,** but this decision should be individualized.

The survival of women who have a *BRCA1* or *BRCA2* mutation and develop ovarian cancer is longer than that for those who do not have a mutation. In one study, the median survival for mutation carriers was 53.4 months compared with 37.8 months for those with sporadic ovarian cancer from the same institution (84).

Recommendations

Current recommendations for management of women at high risk for ovarian cancer are summarized as follows (72,82):

1. **Women who appear to be at high risk for ovarian or breast cancer should undergo genetic counseling and, if the risk appears to be substantial (i.e., a calculated risk of at least 10% in having a mutation in *BRCA1* or *BRCA2*), may be offered genetic testing for *BRCA1* and *BRCA2*.**

2. **Women who wish to preserve their reproductive capacity can undergo screening by transvaginal ultrasonography every 6 months**, although the efficacy of this approach is not established.

3. **Oral contraceptives should be recommended** to young women before they embark on an attempt to have a family.

4. **Women who do not wish to maintain their fertility or who have completed their families should be recommended to undergo prophylactic bilateral salpingo-oophorectomy after the age of 35**, but by age 40 years. The risk of ovarian cancers under the age of 40 is very low but the decision regarding the age of surgery should be based on the age of onset of ovarian cancers in the family. Most *BRCA2*-related ovarian cancers tend to occur after the age of 50, whereas *BRCA1*-related cancers occur at an earlier age. The risk should be clearly documented, preferably established by *BRCA1* and *BRCA2* testing, before salpingo-oophorectomy is performed. These women should be counseled that this operation does not offer absolute protection, because peritoneal carcinomas can occur after bilateral salpingo-oophorectomy (25,28,83).

5. **In women who have a strong family history of breast or ovarian cancer, annual breast screening should be performed beginning at age 30 years using a combination of magnetic resonance imaging (MRI), mammograms, and ultrasound. Ideally, these women should be followed in clinics that manage women at high risk for cancer.**

6. **Women with a documented HNPCC syndrome should be treated as mentioned above, and they should undergo periodic colonoscopy, endometrial biopsy, or prophylactic hysterectomy after the completion of childbearing (71).**

Symptoms

The majority of women with epithelial ovarian cancer have vague and nonspecific symptoms (3,85–87). In early-stage disease, if the patient is premenopausal, she may experience irregular menses. If a pelvic mass is compressing the bladder or rectum, she may report urinary frequency or constipation (85–87). Occasionally, she may perceive lower abdominal distention, pressure, or pain, such as dyspareunia. Acute symptoms, such as pain secondary to rupture or torsion, are unusual.

In advanced-stage disease, patients have symptoms related to the presence of ascites, omental metastases, or bowel metastases. The symptoms include abdominal distention, bloating, constipation, nausea, anorexia, or early satiety. Premenopausal women may report irregular or heavy menses, whereas vaginal bleeding may occur in postmenopausal women (86).

Traditionally, ovarian cancer was considered a "silent killer" that did not produce symptoms until far advanced. Some patients with ovarian cancers confined to the ovary are asymptomatic, but the majority will have nonspecific symptoms that do not necessarily suggest an origin in the ovary (86,88–90). In one survey of 1,725 with ovarian cancer, 95% recalled symptoms before diagnosis, including 89% with stage I and II disease and 97% with stages III and IV disease (86). Some 70% had abdominal or gastrointestinal symptoms, 58% pain, 34% urinary symptoms, and 26% pelvic discomfort. At least some of these symptoms could have reflected pressure on the pelvic viscera from the enlarging ovary. Goff et al. developed an ovarian cancer symptom index and reported that symptoms associated with ovarian cancer, when present for less than 1 year and occurring longer than 12 days a month, were pelvic/abdominal pain, urinary frequency/urgency, increased abdominal size or bloating, and difficulty eating or feeing full (88). The index had a sensitivity of 56.7% for early ovarian cancer and 79.5% for advanced stage disease. A population-based study from Australia found that there did not appear to be a significant difference in the duration of symptoms or the nature of symptoms in patients with early as opposed to advanced stage ovarian cancer, reinforcing the concept that they are biologically different entities and arguing against the widely held misconception that early stage ovarian cancers are at an early stage because they were diagnosed earlier than patients with more advanced stage cancers (89).

Signs

The most important sign of epithelial ovarian cancer is the presence of a pelvic mass on physical examination. A solid, irregular, fixed pelvic mass is highly suggestive of an ovarian malignancy. If an upper abdominal mass or ascites is present, the diagnosis of ovarian cancer is almost certain. Because the patient usually reports abdominal symptoms, she may not have a pelvic examination, and a tumor may be missed.

In patients who are at least 1 year past menopause, the ovaries should be atrophic and not palpable. It was proposed that any palpable pelvic mass in these patients should be considered potentially malignant, a situation that was referred to as the postmenopausal palpable ovary syndrome (91). This concept was challenged, because subsequent authors reported that only about 3% of palpable masses measuring less than 5 cm in postmenopausal women are malignant (57).

Diagnosis

Ovarian epithelial cancers must be differentiated from benign neoplasms and functional cysts of the ovaries. A variety of benign conditions of the reproductive tract, such as pelvic inflammatory disease, endometriosis, and pedunculated uterine leiomyomas, can simulate ovarian cancer. Nongynecologic causes of a pelvic tumor, such as an inflammatory (e.g., diverticular) disease or neoplastic colonic mass, must be excluded (3). A pelvic kidney can simulate ovarian cancer.

Serum CA125 levels are useful in distinguishing malignant from benign pelvic masses (92). For a postmenopausal patient with an adnexal mass and a very high serum CA125 level (>200 U/mL), there is a 96% positive predictive value for malignancy. For premenopausal patients, the specificity of the test is low because the CA125 level tends to be elevated in common benign conditions.

For the premenopausal patient, a period of observation is reasonable provided the adnexal mass does not have characteristics that suggest malignancy (i.e., it is mobile, mostly cystic, unilateral, and of regular contour). An interval of no more than 2 months is allowed, during which hormonal suppression with an oral contraceptive may be used. If the lesion is not neoplastic, it should regress, as measured by pelvic examination and pelvic ultrasonography. If the mass does not regress or if it increases in size, it must be presumed to be neoplastic and must be removed surgically.

The size of the lesion is important. If a cystic mass is greater than 8 cm in diameter, the probability is high that the lesion is neoplastic, unless the patient is taking *clomiphene citrate* or other agents to induce ovulation (37–40). **Premenopausal patients whose lesions are clinically suspicious (i.e., large, predominantly solid, relatively fixed, or irregularly shaped) should undergo laparotomy, as should postmenopausal patients with complex adnexal masses of any size.**

Ultrasonographic signs of malignancy include an adnexal pelvic mass with areas of complexity, such as irregular borders, multiple echogenic patterns within the mass, and dense multiple irregular septae. Bilateral tumors are more likely to be malignant, although the individual characteristics of the lesions are of greater significance. Transvaginal ultrasonography may have a somewhat better resolution than transabdominal ultrasonography for adnexal neoplasms (93–96). Doppler color flow imaging may enhance the specificity of ultrasonography for demonstrating findings consistent with malignancy (97–99).

In postmenopausal women with unilocular cysts measuring 8 to 10 cm or less and normal serial CA125 levels, expectant management is acceptable, and this approach may decrease the number of surgical interventions (100–102).

The diagnosis of an ovarian cancer requires an exploratory laparotomy. The preoperative evaluation of the patient with an adnexal mass is outlined in Figure 14.19 (see Chapter 14).

Before the planned exploration, the patient should undergo routine hematologic and biochemical assessments. A preoperative evaluation in a patient undergoing laparotomy should include a radiograph of the chest. Abdominal and pelvic computed tomography (CT) or MRI are of limited value for a patient with a definite pelvic mass (103–105). A CT or MRI should be performed for patients with ascites and no pelvic mass to look for liver or pancreatic tumors. The findings only rarely preclude laparotomy (103). The value of PET scanning is still being evaluated (105–107). If the hepatic enzyme values are normal, the likelihood of liver disease is low. Liver-spleen scans, bone scans, and brain scans are unnecessary unless symptoms or signs suggest metastases to these sites.

The preoperative evaluation should exclude other primary cancers metastatic to the ovary. A barium enema or colonoscopy is indicated in selected patients with symptoms and signs suspicious for colon cancer. This study should be performed for any patient who has evidence of occult blood in the stool or of intestinal obstruction. An upper gastrointestinal radiographic series or gastroscopy is indicated if there are upper gastrointestinal symptoms such as nausea, vomiting, or hematemesis (3,108). Bilateral mammography is indicated if there is any breast mass, because breast cancer metastatic to the ovaries can simulate primary ovarian cancer.

A Papanicolaou (Pap) test should be performed, although its value for the detection of ovarian cancer is very limited. Patients who have irregular menses or postmenopausal vaginal bleeding should have endometrial biopsy and endocervical curettage to exclude the presence of uterine or endocervical cancer metastatic to the ovary.

Differential Diagnosis

Ovarian epithelial cancers must be differentiated from benign neoplasms and functional cysts of the ovaries (100–102). **A variety of benign conditions of the reproductive tract, such as pelvic inflammatory disease, endometriosis, and pedunculated uterine leiomyomata, can simulate ovarian cancer.** Nongynecologic causes of a pelvic tumor, such as an inflammatory or neoplastic colonic mass, must be excluded. A pelvic kidney can simulate ovarian cancer.

Patterns of Spread

Ovarian epithelial cancers spread primarily by exfoliation of cells into the peritoneal cavity, by lymphatic dissemination, and by hematogenous spread.

Transcoelomic **The most common and earliest mode of dissemination of ovarian epithelial cancer is by exfoliation of cells that implant along the surfaces of the peritoneal cavity.** The cells tend to follow the circulatory path of the peritoneal fluid. The fluid moves with the forces of respiration from the pelvis, up the paracolic gutters, especially on the right, along the intestinal mesenteries, to the right hemidiaphragm. Metastases are typically seen on the posterior cul-de-sac, paracolic gutters, right hemidiaphragm, liver capsule, the peritoneal surfaces of the intestines and their mesenteries, and the omentum. The disease seldom invades the intestinal lumen but progressively agglutinates loops of bowel, leading to a functional intestinal obstruction. This condition is known as carcinomatous ileus (3).

Lymphatic **Lymphatic dissemination to the pelvic and para-aortic lymph nodes is common, particularly in advanced-stage disease** (109–111). Spread through the lymphatic channels of the diaphragm and through the retroperitoneal lymph nodes can lead to dissemination above the diaphragm, especially to the supraclavicular lymph nodes (109). Burghardt et al. reported that 78% of patients with stage III disease have metastases to the pelvic lymph nodes (111). In another series, the rate of para-aortic lymph nodes positive for metastasis was 18% in stage I, 20% in stage II, 42% in stage III, and 67% in stage IV (109).

Hematogenous **Hematogenous dissemination at the time of diagnosis is uncommon.** Spread to vital organ parenchyma, such as the lungs and liver, occurs in only about 2% to 3% of patients. Most patients with disease above the diaphragm when diagnosed have a right pleural effusion (3). Systemic metastases appear more frequently in patients who survived for some years. Dauplat et al. reported that distant metastasis consistent with stage IV disease ultimately occurred in 38% of the patients whose disease was originally intraperitoneal (112).

Prognostic Factors

The outcome of treatment can be evaluated in the context of prognostic factors, which can be grouped into pathologic, biologic, and clinical factors (113).

Pathologic Factors

The morphology and histologic pattern, including the architecture and grade of the lesion, are important prognostic variables (3). Histologic type was not believed to have prognostic significance, but several papers contained suggestions that clear cell carcinomas are associated with a prognosis worse than that of other histologic types (113,114).

Histologic grade, as determined either by the pattern of differentiation or by the extent of cellular anaplasia and the proportion of undifferentiated cells, seems to be of prognostic significance (115–118). Studies of the reproducibility of grading ovarian cancers show a high degree of intraobserver and interobserver variation (119,120). **Because there is significant heterogeneity of tumors and observational bias, the value of histologic grade as an independent prognostic factor is not established.** Baak et al. have presented a standard grading system based on morphometric analysis, and the system seems to correlate with prognosis, especially in its ability to distinguish low-grade or borderline patterns from other tumors (121).

Clinical Factors

In addition to stage, the extent of residual disease after primary surgery, the volume of ascites, patient age, and performance status are all independent prognostic variables (122–131). Among patients with stage I disease, Dembo et al. showed, in a multivariate analysis, that tumor grade and dense adherence to the pelvic peritoneum had a significant adverse impact on prognosis, whereas intraoperative tumor spillage or rupture did not (128). Sjövall et al. confirmed that **ovarian cancers that undergo intraoperative rupture or spillage do not worsen prognosis, whereas tumors that are ruptured preoperatively do have a poorer prognosis** (129). A multivariate analysis of these and several other studies was performed by Vergote et al., who found that for **early-stage disease, poor prognostic variables were tumor grade, capsular penetration, surface excrescences, and malignant ascites, but not iatrogenic rupture** (131).

Initial Surgery for Ovarian Cancer

Staging

Ovarian epithelial malignancies are staged according to the FIGO system listed in Table 37.2 (30). The FIGO staging is based on findings at surgical exploration. A preoperative evaluation should exclude the presence of extraperitoneal metastases.

The importance of thorough surgical staging cannot be overemphasized, because subsequent treatment will be determined by the stage of disease. For patients in whom exploratory laparotomy does not reveal any macroscopic evidence of disease on inspection and palpation of the entire intra-abdominal space, a careful search for microscopic spread must be undertaken. In earlier series in which patients did not undergo careful surgical staging, the overall 5-year survival for patients with apparent stage I epithelial ovarian cancer was only about 60% (132). Since then, survival rates of 90% to 100% are reported for patients who were properly staged and were found to have stage IA or IB disease (133,134).

Technique for Surgical Staging

In patients whose preoperative evaluation suggests a probable malignancy, a midline or paramedian abdominal incision is recommended to allow adequate access to the upper abdomen (3,132). When a malignancy is unexpectedly discovered in a patient who has a lower transverse incision, the rectus muscles can be either divided or detached from the symphysis pubis to allow better access to the upper abdomen. If this is not sufficient, the incision can be extended on one side to create a "J" incision (3).

The ovarian tumor should be removed intact, if possible, and a frozen histologic section should be obtained. If ovarian malignancy is present and the tumor is apparently confined to the ovaries or the pelvis, thorough surgical staging should be performed. Staging involves the following steps (3,132):

1. **Any free fluid, especially in the pelvic cul-de-sac, should be submitted for cytologic evaluation.**

Table 37.2 FIGO Staging for Primary Carcinoma of the Ovary	
Stage I	**Growth limited to the ovaries.**
IA	Growth limited to one ovary; no ascites containing malignant cells.
	No tumor on the external surface; capsule intact.
IB	Growth limited to both ovaries; no ascites containing malignant cells.
	No tumor on the external surfaces; capsules intact.
IC[a]	Tumor either stage IA or IB but with tumor on the surface of one or both ovaries; or with capsule ruptured; or with ascites present containing malignant cells or with positive peritoneal washings.
Stage II	**Growth involving one or both ovaries with pelvic extension.**
IIA	Extension and/or metastases to the uterus and/or fallopian tubes.
IIB	Extension to other pelvic tissues.
IIC[a]	Tumor either stage IIA or IIB but with tumor on the surface of one or both ovaries; or with capsule(s) ruptured; or with ascites present containing malignant cells or with positive peritoneal washings.
Stage III	**Tumor involving one or both ovaries with peritoneal implants outside the pelvis and/or positive retroperitoneal or inguinal nodes. Superficial liver metastasis equals stage III. Tumor is limited to the true pelvis, but with histologically proven malignant extension to small bowel or omentum.**
IIIA	Tumor grossly limited to the true pelvis with negative nodes but with histologically confirmed microscopic seeding of abdominal peritoneal surfaces.
IIIB	Tumor of one or both ovaries with histologically confirmed implants of abdominal peritoneal surfaces, none exceeding 2 cm in diameter. Nodes negative.
IIIC	Abdominal implants >2 cm in diameter or positive retroperitoneal or inguinal nodes or both.
Stage IV	**Growth involving one or both ovaries with distant metastasis. If pleural effusion is present, there must be positive cytologic test results to allot a case to stage IV. Parenchymal liver metastasis equals stage IV.**

These categories are based on findings at clinical examination or surgical exploration or both. The histologic characteristics are to be considered in the staging, as are results of cytologic testing as far as effusions are concerned. It is desirable that a biopsy be performed on suspicious areas outside the pelvis.

FIGO, International Federation of Obstetrics and Gynecology.

[a]To evaluate the impact on prognosis of the different criteria for allotting cases to stage IC or IIC, it would be of value to know if rupture of the capsule was (i) spontaneous or (ii) caused by the surgeon and if the source of malignant cells detected was (i) peritoneal washings or (ii) ascites.

Reproduced from **Berek JS, Hacker NF**, *Berek & Hacker's Gynecologic Oncology*. 5th ed. Lippincott Williams & Wilkins. 2010:455, adapted from FIGO Annual Report, Vol 26, *Int J Gynecol Obstet* 2006;105:3–4.

2. **If no free fluid is present, peritoneal washings should be performed by instilling and recovering 50 to 100 mL of saline from the pelvic cul-de-sac, each paracolic gutter, and beneath each hemidiaphragm.** Obtaining the specimens from under the diaphragms can be facilitated with the use of a rubber catheter attached to the end of a bulb syringe.

3. **A systematic exploration of all the intra-abdominal surfaces and viscera is performed**, proceeding in a clockwise fashion from the cecum cephalad along the paracolic gutter and the ascending colon to the right kidney, the liver and gallbladder, the right hemidiaphragm, the entrance to the lesser sac at the para-aortic area, across the transverse colon to the left hemidiaphragm, down the left gutter and the descending colon to the rectosigmoid colon. The small intestine and its mesentery from the Treitz ligament to the cecum should be inspected.

4. **Any suspicious areas or adhesions on the peritoneal surfaces should be biopsied.** If there is no evidence of disease, multiple intraperitoneal biopsies should be performed. Tissue from the peritoneum of the pelvic cul-de-sac, both paracolic gutters, the peritoneum over the bladder, and the intestinal mesenteries should be taken for biopsy.

5. **The diaphragm should be sampled, either by biopsy or by scraping with a tongue depressor, and a sample obtained for cytologic assessment.** Biopsies of any irregularities on the surface of the diaphragm can be facilitated by use of the laparoscope and the associated biopsy instrument.

6. **The omentum should be resected from the transverse colon, a procedure called an *infracolic omentectomy.*** The procedure is initiated on the underside of the greater omentum, where the peritoneum is incised just a few millimeters away from the transverse colon. The branches of the gastroepiploic vessels are clamped, ligated, and divided, along with all the small branching vessels that feed the infracolic omentum. If the gastrocolic ligament is palpably normal, it does not need to be resected.

7. **The retroperitoneal spaces should be explored to evaluate the pelvic and para-aortic lymph nodes.** The retroperitoneal dissection is performed by incision of the peritoneum over the psoas muscles. This may be performed on the ipsilateral side only for unilateral tumors. Any enlarged lymph nodes should be resected and submitted for frozen section. If no metastases are present, a formal pelvic lymphadenectomy should be performed. The para-aortic area should be explored.

Results

Metastases in apparent stage I and II epithelial ovarian cancer occur in as many as 3 in 10 patients whose tumors appear to be confined to the pelvis but who have occult metastatic disease in the upper abdomen or the retroperitoneal lymph nodes (110,133–140). In a literature review, occult metastases in such patients were found in biopsies of the diaphragm in 7.3%, biopsies of the omentum in 8.6%, the pelvic lymph nodes in 5.9%, the aortic lymph nodes in 18.1%, and in 26.4% of peritoneal washings (132).

The importance of careful initial surgical staging is emphasized by the findings of a cooperative national study in which 100 patients with apparent stage I and II disease were referred for subsequent therapy and underwent additional surgical staging (133). In this series, 28% of the patients initially believed to have stage I disease were upstaged and 43% of those believed to have stage II disease had more advanced lesions. **A total of 31% of the patients were upstaged as a result of additional surgery, and 77% were reclassified as having actual stage III disease. Histologic grade was a significant predictor of occult metastasis.** Sixteen percent of the patients with grade 1 lesions were upstaged, compared with 34% with grade 2 disease and 46% with grade 3 disease.

Borderline Tumors

The principal treatment of borderline (low malignant potential) ovarian tumors is surgical resection of the primary tumor. There is no evidence that either subsequent chemotherapy or radiation therapy improves survival. When a **frozen section determines that the histology is borderline, premenopausal patients who desire preservation of ovarian function may undergo a conservative operation, a unilateral oophorectomy** (3,141). In a study of patients who underwent unilateral ovarian cystectomy only for apparent stage I borderline serous tumors, Lim-Tan et al. found that this conservative operation was safe, with only 8% of the patients developing recurrences 2 to 18 years later, all with curable disease confined to the ovaries (141). Recurrence was associated with positive margins of the removed ovarian cyst. Thus, hormonal function and fertility can be maintained (3,141). For patients who had an oophorectomy or cystectomy and a borderline tumor is documented later in the permanent pathology, no additional immediate surgery is necessary.

Stage I

After a comprehensive staging laparotomy, only a minority of women will have local disease (FIGO stage I). There are over 20,000 women diagnosed yearly with epithelial ovarian cancer in the United States, and nearly 4,000 of these have disease confined to the ovaries (1,142). The prognosis for these patients depends on the clinical–pathologic features, as outlined below. Because of this emphasis on the importance of surgical staging, the rate of lymph node sampling increased in the United States, with a study showing that for women with stages I and II disease, the percentage having lymph nodes sampled increased from 38% to 59% from 1991 to 1996 (143).

The primary surgical treatment for stage I epithelial ovarian cancer is surgical, and patients should undergo total abdominal hysterectomy, bilateral salpingo-oophorectomy, and surgical staging (132,133). **In certain circumstances, a unilateral salpingo-oophorectomy may be performed.** Based on the findings at surgery and the pathologic evaluation, patients with stage I ovarian cancer can be grouped into low-risk and high-risk categories (Table 37.3).

Table 37.3 Prognostic Variables in Early-Stage Epithelial Ovarian Cancer	
Low Risk	*High Risk*
Low grade	High grade
Intact capsule	Tumor growth through capsule
No surface excrescences	Surface excrescences
No ascites	Ascites
Negative peritoneal cytologic findings	Malignant cells in fluid
Unruptured or intraoperative rupture	Preoperative rupture
No dense adherence	Dense adherence
Diploid tumor	Aneuploid tumor

Modified from **Berek JS, Hacker NF**. *Berek & Hacker's Gynecologic Oncology.* 5th ed. Philadelphia, PA: Lippincott Williams & Wilkins, 2010:458, with permission.

Stage I Low Risk

Fertility Preservation in Early-Stage Ovarian Cancer   **For patients who underwent a thorough staging laparotomy and who have no evidence of spread beyond the ovary, abdominal hysterectomy and bilateral salpingo-oophorectomy are appropriate therapy. The uterus and the contralateral ovary can be preserved in women with stage IA, grade 1 to 2 disease who desire to preserve fertility.** The conditions of the women should be monitored carefully with routine periodic pelvic examinations and determinations of serum CA125 levels. Generally, the other ovary and the uterus are removed at the completion of childbearing.

Guthrie et al. studied the outcome of 656 patients with early-stage epithelial ovarian cancer (140). No untreated patients who had stage IA, grade 1 cancer died of their disease; thus, adjuvant radiation and chemotherapy are unnecessary. Furthermore, the Gynecologic Oncology Group (GOG) carried out a prospective, randomized trial of observation versus *melphalan* for patients with stage IA and IB, grade 1 or 2 disease (114). Five-year survival for each group was 94% and 96%, respectively, confirming that no further treatment is needed for such patients.

Stage I High Risk

Patients who have more poorly differentiated disease or who have malignant cells, either in ascites fluid or in peritoneal washings, must undergo complete surgical staging (3). The surgery should include the performance of a hysterectomy and bilateral salpingo-oophorectomy in addition to the staging laparotomy. Although the optimal supportive therapy for these patients is not known, most patients are treated with chemotherapy, as outlined below.

Advanced-Stage Ovarian Cancer

The surgical management of all patients with advanced-stage disease is approached in a similar manner, with modifications made in response to the overall status and general health of the patient and the extent of residual disease present at the time treatment is initiated. A treatment scheme is outlined in Figure 37.10. **Most patients subsequently receive combination chemotherapy for an empiric number of cycles.**

Cytoreductive Surgery for Advanced-Stage Disease

If the patient is medically stable, she should undergo cytoreductive surgery to remove as much of the tumor and its metastases as possible (144–171). The operation to remove the primary tumor and the associated metastatic disease is referred to as *debulking* or cytoreductive surgery. The operation typically includes the performance of a total abdominal hysterectomy and bilateral salpingo-oophorectomy, along with a complete omentectomy and resection of any metastatic lesions from the peritoneal surfaces or from the intestines. The pelvic tumor often directly involves the rectosigmoid colon, the terminal ileum, and the cecum

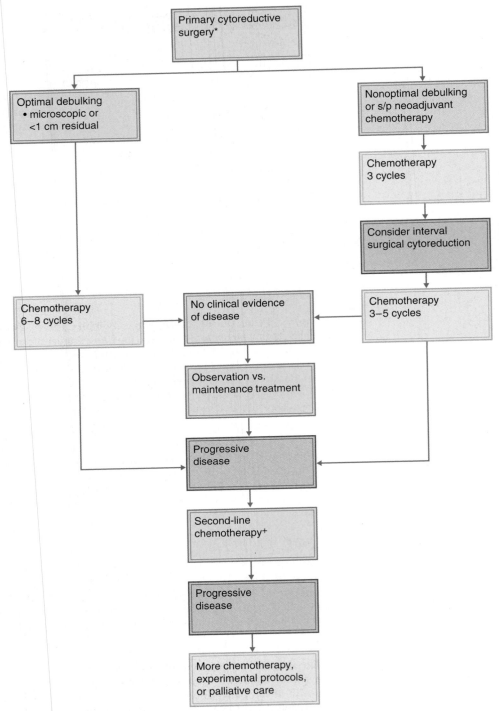

Figure 37.10 **Treatment scheme for patients with advanced-stage ovarian cancer.**
*In selected cases of Stage IIIc/IV disease, neoadjuvant chemotherapy may be given, and then an interval cytoreductive surgery is performed after 3 cycles.
+Chemotherapy depends on whether platinum-sensitive or platinum-resistant. (Modified from **Berek JS, Hacker NF.** *Berek & Hacker's Gynecologic Oncology.* 5th ed. Philadelphia, PA: Lippincott Williams & Wilkins, 2010:460, with permission.)

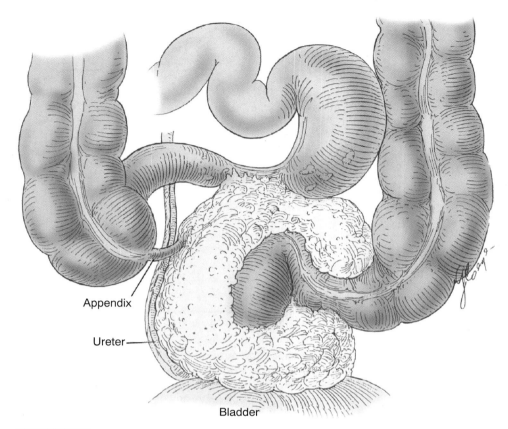

Figure 37.11 Extensive ovarian carcinoma involving the bladder, rectosigmoid, and ileocecal area. (Redrawn from **Heintz APM, Berek JS.** Cytoreductive surgery for ovarian carcinoma. In: **Piver MS, ed.** *Ovarian malignancies.* Edinburgh, UK: Churchill Livingstone, 1987:134, with permission.)

(Fig. 37.11). In a minority of patients, most or all of the disease is confined to the pelvic viscera and the omentum, so that removal of these organs will result in extirpation of all gross tumor, a situation that is associated with a reasonable chance of prolonged progression-free survival.

The removal of bulky tumor masses may reduce the volume of ascites present. Often, ascites will disappear after removal of the primary tumor and a large omental "cake." Removal of the omental cake may alleviate the nausea and early satiety that many patients experience. Removal of intestinal metastases may restore adequate intestinal function and improve the overall nutritional status of the patient, thereby facilitating the patient's ability to tolerate subsequent chemotherapy.

A large, bulky tumor may contain areas that are poorly vascularized, and these areas will be exposed to suboptimal concentrations of chemotherapeutic agents. Similarly, these areas are poorly oxygenated, so that radiation therapy, which requires adequate oxygenation to achieve maximal cell kill, will be less effective. Surgical removal of these bulky tumors may eliminate areas that could be relatively resistant to radiation and chemotherapeutic treatment.

Larger tumor masses tend to be composed of a higher proportion of cells that are either nondividing or in the "resting" phase (i.e., G_0 cells, which are essentially resistant to the therapy). A low growth fraction is characteristic of bulky tumor masses, and cytoreductive surgery can result in smaller residual masses with a relatively higher growth fraction.

Goals of Cytoreductive Surgery **The principal goal of cytoreductive surgery is removal of all of the primary cancer and, if possible, all metastatic disease.** If resection of all metastases is not feasible, the goal is to reduce the tumor burden by resection of all individual tumors to an optimal status. Griffiths initially proposed that all metastatic nodules should be reduced to less

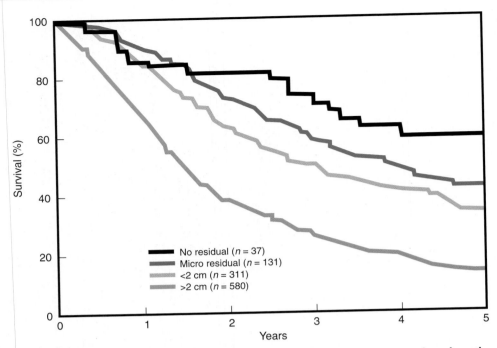

Figure 37.12 **Survival of patients with stage IIIC epithelial ovarian cancer based on the maximal size of residual tumor after exploratory laparotomy and tumor resection.** (From **Heintz APM, Odicino F, Maisonneuve P, et al.** Carcinoma of the ovary. Twenty-sixth annual report of the results of treatment of gynaecological cancer. Int *J Gynecol Oncol 2006;95(suppl 1):S161–S192*, with permission.)

than 1.5 cm in maximal diameter and showed that survival was significantly longer in patients for whom this was achieved (144).

Hacker and Berek demonstrated that patients whose largest residual lesions were less than 5 mm had a superior survival rate, which was substantiated by Van Lindert et al. (145–148). The median survival of patients in this category was 40 months, compared with 18 months for patients whose lesions were less than 1.5 cm and 6 months for patients with nodules greater than 1.5 cm. **Patients whose disease is completely resected to no macroscopic (microscopic only) residual disease have the best overall survival** (149) (Fig. 37.12). **Approximately 30% to 40% of patients in this category will be free of disease at 5 years.**

The resectability of the metastatic tumor is usually determined by the location of the disease. Optimal cytoreduction is difficult to achieve in the presence of extensive disease on the diaphragm, in the parenchyma of the liver, along the base of the small bowel mesentery, in the lesser omentum, or in the porta hepatis.

The ability of cytoreductive surgery to influence survival is limited by the extent of metastases before cytoreduction, presumably because of the presence of phenotypically resistant clones of cells in large metastatic masses. A patient whose metastatic tumor is very large (i.e., >10 cm before cytoreductive surgery) has a shorter survival than those with smaller areas of disease (147,149). Extensive carcinomatosis, the presence of ascites, and poor tumor grade, even with lesions that measure less than 5 mm, may shorten the survival (150–153).

Exploration   The supine position on the operating table may be sufficient for surgical exploration of most patients. For patients with extensive pelvic disease and for whom a low resection of the colon may be necessary, the low lithotomy position should be used. Debulking operations should be performed through a vertical incision to gain adequate access to the upper abdomen and to the pelvis.

After the peritoneal cavity is opened, ascites fluid, if present, should be evacuated. In some centers, fluid is submitted for *in vitro* research studies, such as molecular analyses. In cases of massive ascites, careful attention must be given to hemodynamic monitoring, especially for patients with borderline cardiovascular function.

The peritoneal cavity and retroperitoneum are thoroughly inspected and palpated to assess the extent of the primary tumor and the metastatic disease. All abdominal viscera must be palpated to exclude the possibility that the ovarian disease is metastatic, particularly from the stomach, colon, or pancreas. If optimal status is not considered achievable, extensive bowel and urologic resections are not indicated, except to overcome a bowel obstruction. Removal of the primary tumor and omental cake is usually both feasible and desirable.

Pelvic Tumor Resection **The essential principle of pelvic tumor removal is the retroperitoneal approach.** To accomplish this, the retroperitoneum is entered laterally, along the surface of the psoas muscles, which avoids the iliac vessels and the ureters. If the uterus is present, the procedure is initiated by bilateral division of the round ligaments. The peritoneal incision is extended cephalad, lateral to the ovarian vessels within the infundibulopelvic ligament, and caudally toward the bladder. With careful dissection, the retroperitoneal space is explored, and the ureter and pelvic vessels are identified. The pararectal and paravesicular spaces are identified and developed, as described in Chapter 36.

The peritoneum overlying the bladder is dissected to connect the peritoneal incisions anteriorly. The vesicouterine plane is identified, and with careful sharp dissection the bladder is mobilized from the anterior surface of the cervix. The ovarian vessels are isolated, doubly ligated, and divided.

Hysterectomy is then performed. The ureters must be carefully displayed to avoid injury. During this procedure, the uterine vessels can be identified. Ligation of the uterine vessels

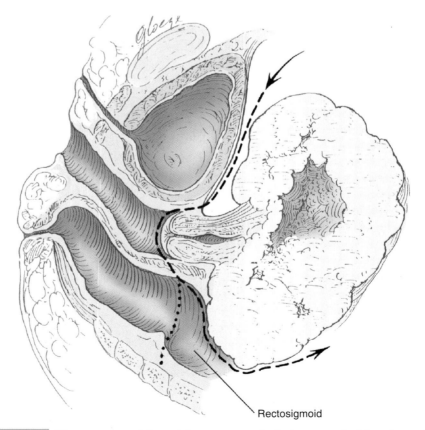

Rectosigmoid

Figure 37.13 **The resection of the pelvic tumor may include removal of the uterus, tubes, and ovaries, as well as portions of the lower intestinal tract.** The *arrows* represent the plane of resection. (From **Berek JS, Hacker NF.** *Berek & Hacker's Gynecologic Oncology.* 5th ed. Philadelphia, PA: Lippincott Williams & Wilkins, 2010:465, with permission.)

and the remainder of the tissues within the cardinal ligaments completes the hysterectomy and resection of the contiguous tumor.

Because epithelial ovarian cancers tend not to invade the lumina of the colon or bladder, it is usually feasible to resect pelvic tumors without having to resect portions of the lower colon or the urinary tract (154,155). Resection of a small portion of the bladder may be required and, if so, a cystotomy should be performed to assist in resection of the disease (155).

Intestinal Resection   **Resection of focal areas of disease involving the small or large intestine should be performed if that would permit the removal of all or most of the abdominal metastases and leave the patient with optimal disease at the end of the cytoreduction.** Apart from the rectosigmoid colon, the most frequent sites of intestinal metastasis are the terminal ileum, the cecum, and the transverse colon. Resection of one or more of these segments of bowel may be necessary (154,156).

If the disease surrounds the rectosigmoid colon and its mesentery, that portion of the colon may have to be removed in order to clear the pelvic disease (Fig. 37.13) (154). When the pararectal space is identified in such patients, the proximal site of colonic involvement is identified, the colon and its mesentery are divided, and the rectosigmoid is removed along with the uterus *en bloc.* A reanastomosis of the colon is performed.

Omentectomy   **Advanced epithelial ovarian cancer often completely replaces the omentum, forming an "omental cake."** This disease may be adherent to the parietal peritoneum of the anterior abdominal wall, making entry into the abdominal cavity difficult. After freeing the omentum from any adhesions to parietal peritoneum, adherent loops of small intestine are freed by sharp dissection. The omentum is lifted and pulled gently in the cranial direction, exposing the attachment of the infracolic omentum to the transverse colon. The peritoneum is incised to open the appropriate plane, which is developed by sharp dissection along the serosa of the transverse colon. Small vessels are ligated with hemoclips. The omentum is separated from the greater curvature of the stomach by ligation of the right and left gastroepiploic arteries and ligation of the short gastric arteries (Fig. 37.14).

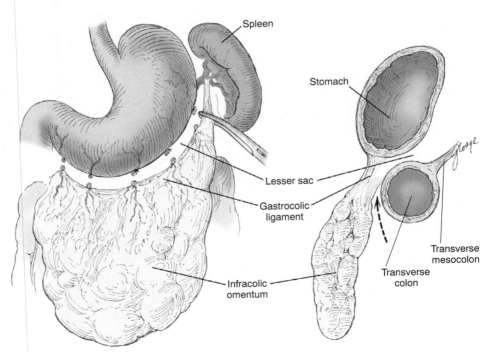

Figure 37.14   **Separation of the omentum from stomach and transverse colon.** *Arrow,* the direction of the initial surgical approach. (From **Heintz APM, Berek JS.** Cytoreductive surgery for ovarian carcinoma. In: **Piver MS, ed.** *Ovarian malignancies.* Edinburgh, UK: Churchill Livingstone, 1987:134, with permission.)

The disease in the gastrocolic ligament can extend to the hilus of the spleen and splenic flexure of the colon on the left and to the capsule of the liver and the hepatic flexure of the colon on the right. Usually, the disease does not invade the parenchyma of the liver or spleen, and a plane can be found between the tumor and these organs. It will occasionally be necessary to perform splenectomy to remove all the omental disease (157).

Resection of Other Metastases   **Other large masses of tumor located on the parietal peritoneum should be removed, particularly if they are isolated masses and their removal will permit optimal cytoreduction.** Resection of extensive disease from the surfaces of the diaphragm is neither practical nor feasible, although solitary metastases may be resected, the diaphragm sutured, and a chest tube placed for a few days (157,158). The use of the Cavitron Ultrasonic Surgical Aspirator (CUSA) and the argon beam coagulator may facilitate resection of small tumor nodules, especially those on flat surfaces (159,160).

Feasibility and Outcome

There was no randomized prospective study performed to define the value of primary cytoreductive surgery, but all retrospective studies indicate that the diameter of the largest residual tumor nodule before the initiation of chemotherapy is significantly related to progression-free survival in patients with advanced ovarian cancer (163). Quality of life may be significantly enhanced by removal of bulky tumor masses from the pelvis and upper abdomen (166).

An analysis of the retrospective data indicates that, when performed by gynecologic oncologists, successful operations are feasible in 70% to 90% of patients (152,153). Major morbidity is approximately 5% and operative mortality is 1% (156,161,162). Intestinal resection in these patients does not appear to increase the overall morbidity caused by the operation (156).

In a meta-analysis of 81 studies of women who underwent cytoreductive surgery for advanced ovarian cancer, Bristow et al. documented that the extent of debulking correlated with incremental benefits in survival (i.e., the greater the percentage of tumor reduction, the longer the survival). Each 10% increase in cytoreduction equaled a 5.5% increase in median survival (163). Women whose cytoreduction was greater than 75% of their tumor burden had a median survival of 33.9 months compared with 22.7 months for women whose tumors were cytoreduced less than 75% ($p < 0.001$). The performance of a pelvic and para-aortic lymphadenectomy in patients with stage III disease does not prolong survival, based on the results of a large prospective, randomized trial (164).

A prospective randomized study of "interval" cytoreductive surgery was carried out by the European Organisation for the Research and Treatment of Cancer (EORTC). Interval surgery was performed after three cycles of *platinum*-combination chemotherapy in patients whose primary attempt at cytoreduction was suboptimal. The initial surgery for most of these patients was not an aggressive attempt to debulk their tumors. Patients in the surgical arm of the study demonstrated a survival benefit when compared with those who did not undergo interval debulking (165). The risk of mortality was reduced by more than 40% in the group that was randomized to the debulking arm of the study. Based on these data, the performance of a debulking operation as early as possible in the course of the patient's treatment should be considered the standard of care (166).

A prospective phase III study of interval cytoreductive surgery was conducted by the GOG; the patients entered on the trial had a maximal attempt at tumor resection at their initial surgery (167). The randomized findings showed no difference between the patients who had an additional attempt at debulking after three cycles of chemotherapy compared with those who did not. The median survival of the 216 women who underwent interval cytoreduction was 32 months compared with 33 months for the 209 women who did not undergo surgical cytoreduction.

There is evidence that the survival of women with advanced ovarian cancer is improved when the surgeon is specifically trained to perform cytoreductive surgery and when there is centralization of care (168–171). **Whenever feasible, patients with advanced ovarian malignancy should be referred to a subspecialty unit for primary surgery, and every effort should be made to attain as complete a cytoreduction as possible.**

Chemotherapy

Stage I Epithelial Ovarian Cancer

Early Stage, Low Risk

Guthrie et al. studied the outcome of 656 patients with early-stage epithelial ovarian cancer (140). Patients who had stage IA, grade 1 cancer and did not receive radiation or chemotherapy did not die of their disease; indicating that adjuvant therapy is unnecessary. The GOG carried out a prospective, randomized trial of observation versus *melphalan* for patients with stage IA and IB, grades 1 and 2 disease (114). **Five-year survival for each group was 94% and 96%, respectively, confirming that adjuvant treatment did not improve survival. Therefore, no adjuvant chemotherapy is recommended for these patients.**

Early Stage, High Risk

In patients whose disease is high risk (e.g., more poorly differentiated or in whom there are malignant cells either in ascites fluid or in peritoneal washings), additional therapy is indicated. Most investigators recommend chemotherapy for these patients (172–185). Chemotherapy for patients with early-stage high-risk epithelial ovarian cancer can be either single agent or multiagent. Some researchers question the wisdom of overly aggressive chemotherapy in women with early-stage disease, suggesting that the evidence for a durable impact on survival is marginal (174,175,181). The risk of leukemia with alkylating agents and *platinum* make the administration of adjuvant therapy hazardous unless there is a significant benefit (186,187).

Because *cisplatin, carboplatin, cyclophosphamide*, and *paclitaxel* (*Taxol*) are active single agents against epithelial ovarian cancer, these drugs are administered in various combinations. There are some series in which *cisplatin* or *cyclophosphamide* (*PC*) or both have been used to treat patients with stage I disease (176–181). In a GOG trial of three cycles of *cisplatin* and *cyclophosphamide* versus intraperitoneal chromic phosphate (^{32}P) in patients with stage IB and IC disease, the progression-free survival of women receiving the *platinum*-based chemotherapy was 31% higher than those receiving the radiocolloid (178). Similar results were reported by a multicenter trial performed in Italy by the Gruppo Italiano Collaborativo Oncologica Ginecologica (GICOG) for progression-free survival, although there was no overall survival advantage (179).

Two large parallel randomized phase III clinical trials were conducted on women with early-stage disease: the **International Collaborative Ovarian Neoplasm Trial 1 (ICON1)** and the **Adjuvant Chemotherapy Trial in Ovarian Neoplasia (ACTION)** (188,189).

In the ICON1 trial, 477 patients from 84 centers in Europe were entered. Patients of all stages were eligible for the trial if, in the opinion of the investigator, it was unclear whether adjuvant therapy would be of benefit. Most patients were considered to have stage I and IIA disease, but optimal **surgical staging was not required**, and it is likely that a significant number of these women had stage III disease. Adjuvant *platinum*-based chemotherapy was given to 241 patients, and no adjuvant chemotherapy was given to 236 patients. **The 5-year survival was 73% in the group who received adjuvant chemotherapy compared with 62% in the control group** (hazard ratio [HR] = 0.65, $p = 0.01$) (189).

In the ACTION trial, 440 patients from 40 European centers were randomized; 224 patients received adjuvant *platinum*-based chemotherapy, and 224 patients did not (188). **Patients with As I and IIa, grades 2 and 3 were eligible.** Only about one-third of the total group was optimally staged (151 patients). **In the observation arm, optimal staging was associated with a better survival (HR = 2.31, $p = 0.03$), and in the suboptimally staged patients, adjuvant chemotherapy was associated with an improvement in survival (HR = 1.78, $p = 0.009$).** In optimally staged patients, no benefit of adjuvant chemotherapy was seen. **In the ACTION trial, the benefit from adjuvant chemotherapy was limited to the patients with suboptimal staging, suggesting that patients benefit only if they had a likelihood of occult microscopic dissemination.**

When the data from the two trials were combined and analyzed, a total of 465 patients were randomized to receive *platinum*-based adjuvant chemotherapy and 460 to observation until disease progression (190). After a median follow-up of more than 4 years, the overall survival was 82% in the chemotherapy arm and 74% in the observation arm (HR = 0.67, $p = 0.001$).

Recurrence-free survival was better in the chemotherapy arm: 76% versus 65% (HR = 0.64, $p = 0.001$). The results of this analysis must be interpreted with caution, because most of the patients did not undergo thorough surgical staging, but the **findings suggest that** *platinum*-**based chemotherapy should be given to patients who were not optimally staged.**

Carboplatin is widely used instead of *cisplatin,* as it is equivalent in efficacy and much better tolerated with significantly fewer side effects (191). A randomized phase III trial of three versus six cycles of adjuvant *carboplatin* and *paclitaxel* in 457 patients with early stage epithelial ovarian carcinoma was conducted by the GOG (192). An unexpectedly large number of patients (126 patients, 29%) had incomplete or inadequately documented surgical staging in this study. The recurrence rate for six cycles was 24% lower (HR = 0.76; confidence interval [CI], 0.5–1.13; $p = 0.18$) versus three cycles, but this was not statistically significant. The estimates of probability of recurrence at 5 years were 20.1% for six cycles and 25.4% for three cycles. The authors concluded that three cycles of adjuvant *carboplatin* and *paclitaxel* was a reasonable option for women with high-risk early stage ovarian cancer. The current GOG trial includes patients with high-risk stage I and stage II disease, and offers three cycles of *carboplatin* and *paclitaxel* followed by a randomization to either observation versus 26 weeks of weekly low-dose (40 mg/m^2) *paclitaxel.* High-risk stage I is defined as stage IA or IB, grade 3, stage IC, or clear cell carcinomas.

The recommendations for therapy follow:

- Patients with high-grade, high-risk stage I epithelial ovarian cancer should be given adjuvant chemotherapy. The type depends on the patient's overall health and medical comorbidities

- Treatment with *carboplatin* and *paclitaxel* chemotherapy for three to six cycles is used in these patients, whereas single agent *carboplatin* may be preferable for older women and patients with other medical comorbidities.

Advanced-Stage Epithelial Ovarian Cancer

Systemic multiagent chemotherapy is the standard treatment for metastatic epithelial ovarian cancer (193–217). After the introduction of *cisplatin* in the latter half of the 1970s, *platinum*-based combination chemotherapy became the most frequently used treatment regimen in the United States. *Paclitaxel* became available in the 1980s, and this drug was incorporated into the combination chemotherapy in the 1990s (192–196). Comparative trials of *paclitaxel, cisplatin,* and *carboplatin* are summarized below.

In a meta-analysis performed on studies of patients with advanced-stage disease, those patients given *cisplatin*-containing combination chemotherapy were compared with those treated with regimens that did not include *cisplatin* (197). Survival differences between the groups were seen from 2 to 5 years, with the *cisplatin* group having a slight survival advantage, but this difference disappeared by 8 years.

A major advance in the treatment of advanced-stage disease was the incorporation of *paclitaxel* **into the chemotherapeutic regimens in the late 1990s. A series of randomized, prospective clinical trials with** *paclitaxel*-**containing arms defined** *carboplatin* **and** *paclitaxel* **as the standard treatment protocol in advanced epithelial ovarian cancer,** although there are data to support intraperitoneal chemotherapy in selected patients (194,195,201,202).

Reporting the GOG data (Protocol 111), McGuire et al. showed that the combination of *cisplatin* (75 mg/m^2) and *paclitaxel* (135 mg/m^2) was superior to *cisplatin* (75 mg/m^2) and *cyclophosphamide* (600 mg/m^2), each given for six cycles (194). In suboptimally resected patients, the *paclitaxel*-containing arm produced a 36% reduction in mortality. These data were verified in a trial conducted jointly by the EORTC, the Nordic Ovarian Cancer Study Group (NOCOVA), and the National Cancer Institute of Canada (NCIC), in which patients with both optimal and suboptimal disease were treated (195). In this study, the *paclitaxel*-containing arm produced a significant improvement in both progression-free interval and overall survival in both optimal and suboptimal groups. **Based on these two studies,** *paclitaxel* **is included in the primary treatment of all women with advanced-stage epithelial ovarian cancer, unless there are contraindications to** *paclitaxel,* **such as preexisting peripheral neuropathy.**

A three-arm comparison of *paclitaxel* (T) versus *cisplatin* (P) versus PT in suboptimal stage III and IV patients (Protocol 132) showed equivalency in the three groups, but crossover from one drug to the other was permitted (196). The study showed that the combination regimen was better tolerated than the sequential administration of the agents in suboptimally resected patients.

The second-generation *platinum* analogue, *carboplatin*, was developed to have less toxicity than its parent compound, *cisplatin*. In early trials, *carboplatin* had lower overall toxicity (204). Fewer gastrointestinal side effects, especially nausea and vomiting, were observed than with *cisplatin*, and there was less nephrotoxicity, neurotoxicity, and ototoxicity. *Carboplatin* is associated with a higher degree of myelosuppression (206).

The dose of carboplatin is calculated by using the area under the curve (AUC) and the glomerular filtration rate (GFR) according to the *Calvert formula* (207). The target AUC is 5 to 6 for previously untreated patients with ovarian cancer.

Carboplatin and Paclitaxel

Two randomized, prospective clinical studies compared the combination of *paclitaxel* and *carboplatin* to *paclitaxel* and *cisplatin* (201,202). In both studies, the efficacy and survivals were similar, but the toxicity was more acceptable with the *carboplatin*-containing regimen. In the first trial, GOG Protocol 158, the randomization was *carboplatin* AUC = 7.5 and *paclitaxel* 175 mg/m^2 over 3 hours versus *cisplatin* 75 mg/m^2 and *paclitaxel* 135 mg/m^2 over 24 hours (Fig. 37.15). The disease progression-free survival of the *carboplatin*-containing arm was 22 months versus 21.7 months for the control arm (201). The gastrointestinal and neurotoxicity of the *carboplatin* arm were appreciably lower than that of the *cisplatin* arm. A similar result was obtained in a large randomized trial in Germany, in which the dose of *carboplatin* was AUC = 6 and *paclitaxel* was 185 mg/m^2 over 3 hours compared with the same dose of *paclitaxel* and *cisplatin* 75 mg/m^2 (202). Based on these data, **the preferred regimen in patients with advanced-stage disease is the *paclitaxel* plus *carboplatin* combination** (203).

The ICON3 trial was a study of 2,074 women with all stages of ovarian cancer, including 20% who had stage I or II disease (208). *Carboplatin* plus *paclitaxel* **was compared with two non-*paclitaxel* regimens, *carboplatin* (70%), or *cyclophosphamide*, *Adriamycin*, and *cisplatin* (CAP) (30%). The regimens were chosen before randomization and based on the clinical preference of the treating physician.** One-third of patients who received *carboplatin* or *CAP* subsequently received second-line *paclitaxel*, and this additional chemotherapy was often given before clinical progression. With a median follow-up of 51 months, the *carboplatin* plus *paclitaxel* and the control groups had a similar progression-free survival (0.93) and overall survival (0.98). **The median survival for the *paclitaxel* plus *carboplatin* and control groups was 36.1 and 35.4 months, respectively.** The median duration of progression-free survival was 17.3 and 16.1 months, respectively. **The researchers concluded that single agent *carboplatin* and *CAP* were as effective as *paclitaxel* and *carboplatin* for first-line chemotherapy.** Because *carboplatin* as a single agent had a lower toxicity than the other regimens and the median survival (33 months) was similar in the prior trial (ICON2) that compared *carboplatin* and *CAP* as first-line treatment, the researchers suggested that *carboplatin* alone was the preferred therapy (209). **The design of the study limited the interpretation of the results and was criticized, because patients with FIGO stages I to IV disease were included, the extent of primary surgery was variable, and the majority (85%) of patients who relapsed after single-agent *carboplatin* or *CAP* received *paclitaxel*. The results of this study did not change the practice in the United Kingdom where the study was predominantly carried out.**

Carboplatin and Docetaxel

***Docetaxel* has a different toxicity profile from *paclitaxel*.** The SCOT-ROC (Scottish Gynaecological Cancer Trials Group) study randomly assigned 1,077 women with stages Ic to IV epithelial ovarian cancer to *carboplatin* with either *paclitaxel* or *docetaxel* (210). **The efficacy of *docetaxel* appeared to be similar to *paclitaxel*:** The median progression-free survival was 15.1 months versus 15.4 months, and the ***docetaxel* group had fewer neurologic effects, arthralgias, myalgias, and extremity weakness than the *paclitaxel* group.** The *docetaxel* plus *carboplatin* regimen was associated with significantly more myelosuppression and its consequences (i.e., serious infections and prolonged grade 3 to 4 neutropenia). Additional study is necessary to determine whether *docetaxel* should supplant *paclitaxel* in the primary treatment of epithelial ovarian cancer.

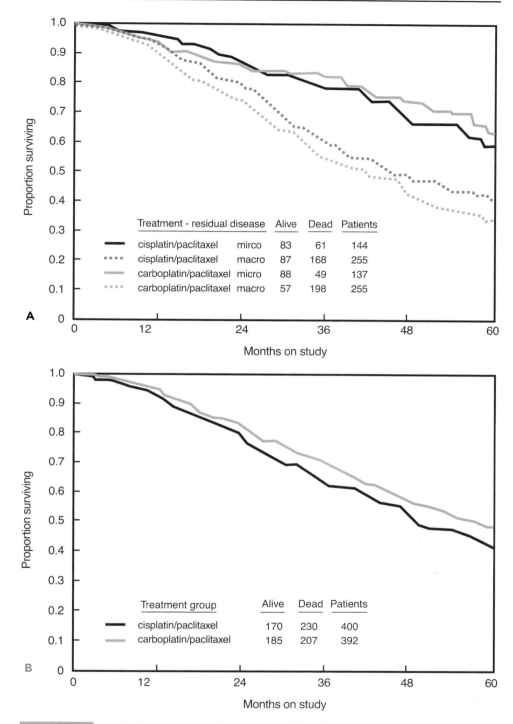

Figure 37.15 Survival of patients with stage III epithelial ovarian cancer treated with *carboplatin* and *paclitaxel* versus *cisplatin* and *paclitaxel:* a Gynecologic Oncology Group study. **A:** Survival by treatment. **B:** Survival by treatment group (micro vs. macro). (From **Ozols RF, Bundy BN, Greer BE, et al.** Phase III trial of carboplatin and paclitaxel compared with cisplatin and paclitaxel in patients with optimally resected stage III ovarian cancer: a Gynecologic Oncology Group Study. *J Clin Oncol* 2003;21:3194–3200, with permission; **Berek JS, Hacker NF.** *Berek & Hacker's Gynecologic Oncology.* 4th ed. Philadelphia, PA: Lippincott Williams & Wilkins, 2010:475, with permission.)

Five-Arm Trial

An Intergroup, international trial—GOG 182/Southwest Oncology Group (SWOG) 182/ICON5—compared the standard combination of *carboplatin* and *paclitaxel* with these drugs in combination with *gemcitabine, topotecan,* or *liposomal doxorubicin* in sequential doublets or triplets (211). The study showed that the addition of any these three drugs to the standard chemotherapy with *carboplatin* and *paclitaxel* did not improve progression-free survival or overall survival.

Intraperitoneal Chemotherapy

A randomized, prospective GOG study (Protocol 104) of intraperitoneal *cisplatin* versus intravenous *cisplatin* (100 mg/m^2), each given with 750 mg/m^2 *cyclophosphamide*, was performed jointly by the SWOG and the GOG in patients with minimal residual disease (212). **The intraperitoneal *cisplatin* arm had a somewhat longer overall median survival than the intravenous arm, 49 versus 41 months** ($p = 0.03$). In the patients with minimal residual disease (<0.5 cm maximal residual), paradoxically, there was no difference between the two treatments, 51 versus 46 months ($p = 0.08$).

In a follow-up GOG study (Protocol 114), the dose-intense arm was initiated by giving a moderately high dose of *carboplatin* (dose AUC = 9) for two induction cycles, followed by intraperitoneal *cisplatin* 100 mg/m^2 and intravenous *paclitaxel* 135 mg/m^2 over 24 hours, versus intravenous *cisplatin* 75 mg/m^2 and intravenous *paclitaxel* 135 mg/m^2 (213). The dose-intense arm results were slightly better—the disease progression-free median survival was 27.6 months compared with 22.5 months for the control arm ($p = 0.02$). There was no difference in overall survival (52.9 months versus 47.6 months, $p = 0.056$). Based on this study, it was unclear whether dose intensification with intraperitoneal *cisplatin* has a sustained long-term impact on the survival of these patients.

A third randomized prospective GOG study (Protocol 172) compared intraperitoneal *cisplatin* and *paclitaxel* versus intravenous *cisplatin* and *paclitaxel* (214). The combination of *cisplatin* 75 mg/m^2 and *paclitaxel* 135 mg/m^2 given intravenously every 3 weeks was compared with *paclitaxel* 135 mg/m^2 intravenous day 1, followed by *cisplatin* 100 mg/m^2 intraperitoneal day 2, and *paclitaxel* 60 mg/m^2 intraperitoneal day 8 every 3 weeks, each given for six cycles. **Although 83% of the patients randomized to intravenous chemotherapy completed all six cycles of therapy, only 42% of those treated with intraperitoneal chemotherapy completed the six cycles, principally because of catheter-related complications. For patients in either group who could not complete the therapy because of *cisplatin*-related toxicity, the chemotherapy was switched to intravenous *carboplatin*.** Comparing the intravenous and intraperitoneal arms, the median duration of progression-free survival was 18.3 and 23.8 months, respectively ($p = 0.05$). **The median duration of overall survival in the intravenous-therapy and intraperitoneal-therapy groups was 49.7 and 65.6 months, respectively** ($p = 0.03$) (214). Quality of life was significantly worse in the intraperitoneal-therapy group before cycle four and 3 to 6 weeks after treatment but not 1 year after treatment. A summary of the intraperitoneal catheter-related issues in this trial was presented (215).

Based on these randomized trials, the intraperitoneal route of administration for *cisplatin* and *paclitaxel* chemotherapy in the primary treatment of optimally resected stage III ovarian cancer is an acceptable therapeutic alternative to intravenous chemotherapy with *carboplatin* and *paclitaxel* (216). There are no reports of randomized direct comparisons of this intraperitoneal regimen to intravenous *carboplatin* and *paclitaxel* or to intraperitoneal *carboplatin* and *paclitaxel*. Intraperitoneal therapy can be used in patients with optimally resected tumors who have a good performance status and are in overall good health. Because intraperitoneal chemotherapy is more cumbersome and has a higher morbidity than intravenous therapy, the use of this technique of drug delivery should be individualized after thorough discussion with the patient.

Dose-Dense Intravenous Chemotherapy

The Japanese GOG randomized 637 patients with ovarian cancer to receive *carboplatin* AUC 6 and *paclitaxel* 180 mg/m^2 every 3 weeks or the same dose of *carboplatin* and 80 mg/m^2 *paclitaxel* every week for at least six cycles (217). The median progression-free survival was 28 months in the dose-dense arm and 17 months in the control group, and they reported relatively little difference in toxicity between the two arms and that grade 3 to 4 neurotoxicity in particular was very low. In the 417 patients who had stage III disease, about half had less than 1 cm maximum residual disease, similar to the patients in GOG 172. There is no subgroup analysis to determine whether these optimally debulked patients fared better with dose-dense *paclitaxel*, but the hazard ratio for recurrence was 0.69 for stage III as a group. These findings are very encouraging but need to be validated in another study. **There is good evidence that weekly *paclitaxel* is more effective than *paclitaxel* every 3 weeks in breast cancer and the Japanese GOG study suggests that the same may apply to ovarian cancer.** This important question is being studied in GOG and other studies comparing intravenous dose-dense treatment with intraperitoneal chemotherapy.

Neoadjuvant Chemotherapy

Some authors suggested that selected patients with suboptimal stage III and stage IV disease and those with large volume ascites and pleural effusions should have chemotherapy prior to debulking surgery. A series performed by Schwartz et al. suggested that these patients treated with neoadjuvant or cytoreductive chemotherapy had survival that was comparable to those patients treated in the same institution with debulking surgery followed by conventional chemotherapy (218). It is accepted that two or three cycles of chemotherapy before cytoreductive surgery may be helpful in patients with massive ascites and large pleural effusions. The chemotherapy may "dry up" the effusions, improve the patient's performance status, and decrease postoperative morbidity, particularly chest morbidity (219,220).

The EORTC completed a large randomized trial in 718 patients with advanced ovarian cancer comparing initial surgery followed by six cycles of *carboplatin* and *paclitaxel* with three cycles of neoadjuvant chemotherapy followed by surgical debulking and another three cycles of chemotherapy. The study found that the progression-free survival was identical in both arms (12 months) and similarly the overall survival (30 months) was the same in both arms (221). The morbidity of surgery was significantly less in patients receiving neoadjuvant chemotherapy, suggesting that in selected patients with very advanced (stages IIIC and IV) ovarian cancer two to three cycles of neoadjuvant chemotherapy prior to surgical debulking is a reasonable option.

Chemotherapy and Bevacizumab

Inhibition of angiogenesis with drugs such as *bevacizumab* demonstrated activity and benefit in women with recurrent ovarian cancer. There is evidence in other tumor types such as breast cancer and colon cancer that the addition of *bevacizumab* to chemotherapy increases response rates, progression-free survival, and survival in some studies (222–224). Two large randomized trials (GOG 218 and ICON7) investigating the impact of the addition of *bevacizumab* to standard *carboplatin* and *paclitaxel* in patients with advanced ovarian cancer were completed (225,226). GOG 218 is a phase III three-arm randomized double-blind placebo-controlled trial. Patients in arm one received six cycles of *carboplatin* and *paclitaxel* and placebo starting with the second cycle and continuing for 16 additional cycles after the completion of chemotherapy. Patients in arm two received six cycles of chemotherapy with *bevacizumab* starting with cycle two and administered with chemotherapy followed by 16 cycles of placebo, and in arm three patients received *bevacizumab* starting with cycle two of chemotherapy and then received 16 additional cycles after the completion of chemotherapy. This study was designed to investigate the benefit of *bevacizumab* in combination with chemotherapy and as a maintenance therapy. The *bevacizumab* was administered at a does of 15 mg/kg, starting with the second cycle of chemotherapy, to decrease the risk of gastrointestinal perforation, which is a rare complication of this agent in the setting of its use in colorectal cancer. The results of GOG 218 reported a modest improvement of 3.8 months in progression-free survival in patients randomized to receive *bevacizumab* in combination with *carboplatin* and *paclitaxel* every 3 weeks and then as a maintenance therapy every 3 weeks for an additional 16 cycles for a total of 15 months' treatment (225). The toxicity of *bevacizumab* was acceptable and the risk of bowel perforation very low (below 2%). The study did not find any improvement in overall survival, but follow-up is required. The ICON7 study is similar to the GOG study, although it is a two-arm study of *carboplatin* and *paclitaxel* plus or minus *bevacizumab* 7.5 mg/kg administered every 3 weeks with chemotherapy for six cycles and then as maintenance therapy for 12 additional cycles. The ICON7 results were presented and reported a statistically significant, yet modest, 1.7-month improvement in median progression-free survival in the experimental arm (226). The results of these studies support a role of *bevacizumab* in combination with chemotherapy in patients with advanced ovarian cancer. However, the cost of *bevacizumab* is very high and the improvement in progressive-free survival is short.

Chemotherapeutic Recommendation in Advanced Epithelial Ovarian Cancer

For the treatment of advanced-stage epithelial ovarian cancer, the following is recommended (Table 37.4):

- Combination chemotherapy or intravenous *carboplatin* and *paclitaxel* or intraperitoneal *cisplatin* and *paclitaxel* (using the GOG 172 protocol) are the treatments of choice for patients with advanced disease. The advantages and disadvantages of the intravenous versus intraperitoneal routes of administration of these drugs should be discussed with the patient.

- The recommended doses and schedule for intravenous chemotherapy are: *carboplatin* (starting dose AUC = 5–6), and *paclitaxel* (175 mg/m^2), every 3 weeks for six to eight cycles, or the dose-dense regimen of *carboplatin* AUC 6 every 3 weeks for six cycles and weekly *paclitaxel* 80 mg/m^2 (217).

- The recommended doses and schedule for intraperitoneal chemotherapy are *paclitaxel* 135 mg/m^2 intravenous on day 1, followed by *cisplatin* 75 to 100 mg/m^2 intraperitoneal on day 2, followed by *paclitaxel* 60 mg/m^2 intraperitoneal on day 8, every 3 weeks for

Table 37.4 Combination Chemotherapy for Advanced Epithelial Ovarian Cancer: Recommended Regimens

Drugs*	Dose (mg/m^2)[a]	Route	Interval (weeks)	Treatments (cycles)
Standard regimens				
Intraperitoneal chemotherapy				
Paclitaxel	135	IV	3, day 1	6
Cisplatin	50–100	IP	day 2	
Paclitaxel	60	IP	day 8	
Intravenous chemotherapy				
Paclitaxel	175	IV	3	6–8
Carboplatin	AUC = 5–6[a]	IV		
Paclitaxel	135	IV	3	6–8
Cisplatin	75	IV		
Alternative drugs[b]				
Docetaxel	75	IV	3	
Doxorubicin, liposomal	35–50	IV	3–4	
Topotecan	1.0–1.25	IV	1	
	4.0	IV	3 (daily × 3–5 days)	
Etoposide	50	PO	3, days 14–21	

*Bevacizumab 7.5–15 mg/kg can be added to any of these regimens.
[a]Except for *carboplatin* dosing, where AUC—area under the curve—dose calculated by using Calvert formula (**Calvert AH, Newell DR, Gumbrell LA, et al.** Carboplatin dosage: prospective evaluation of a simple formula based on renal function. *J Clin Oncol* 1989;7:1748–1756).
[b]Drugs that can be substituted for *paclitaxel* if hypersensitivity to that drug occurs; the number of treatments administered as tolerated.

six cycles, as tolerated. (Many centers modified the dose of *cisplatin* to 75 mg/m^2 rather than 100 mg/m^2 to reduce toxicity. Others substitute *carboplatin* (AUC 6) for *cisplatin* in the regimen.) The impact on outcome of these pragmatic modifications is unknown.

- *Bevacizumab* 7.5–15 mg/kg can be added to any of these intravenous or intraperitoneal chemotherapy regimens.

- In patients who cannot tolerate combination chemotherapy, single-agent, intravenously administered *carboplatin* (AUC 5–6) can be given.

- In patients who have a hypersensitivity to *paclitaxel* or *carboplatin*, an alternative active drug can be substituted (e.g., *docetaxel*, nanoparticle *paclitaxel*, cisplatin). In the case of *carboplatin* hypersensitivity, desensitization could be attempted.

The treatment of all patients with advanced-stage disease is approached in a similar manner, with modifications based on the overall status and general health of the patient and the extent of residual disease present at the time treatment is initiated.

Maintenance of Complete Clinical Response to First-Line Chemotherapy

Because as many as 80% of women with advanced-stage disease who completely respond to their first-line chemotherapy will ultimately relapse, several trials were conducted that administer a drug to these patients immediately following their primary treatment in an effort to decrease the relapse rate.

Paclitaxel   In a study conducted by the GOG and SWOG, 277 women with advanced ovarian cancer who had a complete clinical remission to first-line chemotherapy were randomized to receive 3 or 12 cycles of additional single-agent *paclitaxel* (175 or 135 mg/m^2 every 28 days) (227). Patients were excluded if they developed grade 2 or 3 neurotoxicity during their initial chemotherapy. Because of cumulative toxicity, the mean number of actual cycles of *paclitaxel* received by the group assigned to receive 12 cycles was 9. The treatment-related grade 2 to 3 neuropathy was more common with longer treatment, 24% versus 14% of patients, respectively. **The study closed after a median follow-up of only 8.5 months, and an interim analysis showed a significant 7-month prolongation in median progression-free survival (28 versus 21 months) with 9 versus 3 months of consolidation *paclitaxel*. There was no difference in median overall survival and this study has not changed practice.** The rate of disease progression increased significantly after maintenance therapy was discontinued, which suggested that long-term survival was not likely to be improved. It is improbable that a survival benefit will appear with longer follow-up, because patients assigned to three cycles were given the option of receiving an additional nine courses of *paclitaxel* after the study was discontinued (228). Another placebo-controlled, randomized trial using two formulations of *paclitaxel* is being conducted by the GOG.

Topotecan   Four additional treatment courses of *topotecan* were administered to patients following six cycles of *carboplatin* and *paclitaxel* in two randomized trials, one conducted in Italy and the other in Germany (229,230). In the larger trial conducted in Germany, 1,059 evaluable patients were randomly assigned to six cycles of *paclitaxel* (175 mg/m^2 over 3 hours) and *carboplatin* (AUC 5) with (537 patients) or without (522 patients) four additional cycles of *topotecan* (1.25 mg/m^2 intravenous days 1 to 5 every 3 weeks) (230). In the Italian trial, 273 women were randomly assigned to receive four additional cycles (137 patients) of *topotecan* at a dose of 1 mg/m^2 on days 1 to 5 every 3 weeks or no further chemotherapy (136 patients) (229). **Preliminary reports suggest no significant differences in either progression-free or overall survival in patients who received four to six cycles of consolidation *topotecan*.**

Cisplatin   **In a randomized clinical trial of intraperitoneal *cisplatin* for consolidation versus observation, there was no difference in survival between the treatment arms** (231).

Biologic Therapies   As noted above, the use of the monoclonal antibody (MonAb) *bevacizumab* with first-line *carboplatin* and *paclitaxel* chemotherapy followed by maintenance *bevacizumab* for a year was associated with a modest improvement in progression-free survival, (225,226). Patients and their physicians may consider maintenance therapy with *bevacizumab* as delivered in GOG 218 and ICON7. There are a number of ongoing trials addressing the role of oral angiogenesis inhibitors as maintenance therapy after completion of first-line therapy in women with advanced ovarian cancer.

Studies MonAbs directed toward CA125 (OvaRex) and toward the HMFG (human milk fat globulin) tumor–associated antigens were conducted (232–234). In a randomized, placebo-controlled trial of intravenous *oregovomab* (anti-CA125 MonAb) as maintenance therapy, Berek et al. reported that *oregovomab* did not demonstrate a survival advantage as a maintenance therapy (233). A randomized trial of an intraperitoneally administered yttrium-labeled antimucin (HMFG) MonAb versus placebo was not associated with an improved overall survival after a negative second-look laparoscopy (234).

Treatment Assessment

Many patients who undergo optimal cytoreductive surgery and subsequent chemotherapy for epithelial ovarian cancer have no evidence of disease at the completion of treatment. Tumor markers and radiologic assessments are too insensitive to exclude the presence of subclinical disease. **Historically, a second-look surgery was performed to evaluate these patients, but was abandoned, as there is no evidence of a meaningful benefit to patients** (132,235–244).

Tumor Markers

The level of CA125, a surface glycoprotein associated with müllerian epithelial tissues, is elevated in about 80% of patients with epithelial ovarian cancers, particularly those with nonmucinous tumors (245–247). The levels frequently become undetectable after the initial surgical resection and one or two cycles of chemotherapy. Carcinoembryonic antigen (CEA) levels are often elevated in patients with ovarian cancer, and the test is too nonspecific and insensitive to be used in the management of these patients, apart from patients with a mucinous cancer of the ovary (48).

Levels of CA125 were correlated with findings at second-look operations. Elevated levels are useful in predicting the presence of disease, but negative levels are an insensitive determinant of the absence of disease. In a prospective study, the predictive value of a positive test was 100%; if the level of CA125 was elevated (>35 U/mL), disease was always detectable in patients at the second-look procedure (245). The predictive value of a negative test was only 56%; if the level was less than 35 U/mL, disease was present in 44% of the patients at the time of the second-look surgery. **A literature review suggests that an elevated CA125 level predicts persistent disease at second-look surgery in 97% of the cases, but the CA125 level is not sensitive enough to exclude subclinical disease in many patients** (246).

Serum CA125 levels can be used during chemotherapy to follow those patients whose levels were positive at the initiation of therapy (245). The change in level correlates with response. Those patients with persistently elevated levels after three cycles of treatment probably have persistent disease. When levels rise after treatment, almost invariably treatment has failed, and continuation of the current regimen is futile. A retrospective study determined that a doubling of the CA125 level from its nadir in those patients with a persistently elevated level accurately predicts disease progression (247).

Radiologic Assessment

Radiologic tests assess response in patients with measurable lesions at the start of therapy. In patients who have no or minimal residual disease following cytoreductive surgery, the value of these tests is limited, but they may be useful in follow-up, especially to document the site of recurrence. Ascites can be readily detected, but quite large omental metastases can be missed on CT scan in patients with recurrent disease (248). If liver enzyme levels are abnormal, the liver can be evaluated with a CT scan or ultrasonography. A positive CT scan and fine-needle aspiration (FNA) cytology indicating tumor persistence could document persistent or recurrent disease, but the false-negative rate of a CT scan is about 45% (249). **Positron-emission tomography (PET) alone, or with CT imaging, may help detect relapse, although the relative value of adding PET is not established. There appears to be a higher false-positive rate with PET compared with CT** (106,107). MRI can be used as an alternative to CT in patients with allergies to the contrast medium (105).

Second-Line Therapy

Secondary Cytoreductive Surgery

Secondary cytoreduction may be defined as an attempt at cytoreductive surgery at some stage following completion of first-line chemotherapy (250–253). Patients with progressive disease on chemotherapy are not suitable candidates for secondary cytoreduction, but patients with recurrent disease are occasionally candidates for surgical excision of their disease. **Tumor resection under these circumstances should be restricted to those who have a disease-free interval of at least 12, but preferably 24, months or those in whom it is expected that all macroscopic disease can be resected,** regardless of the disease-free interval (250–258). Complete resection is possible when there are only one or two isolated recurrences in patients without diffuse carcinomatosis (258).

Chemotherapy for Persistent-Recurrent Ovarian Cancer

The majority of women who relapse will be offered more chemotherapy with the likelihood of benefit related to the initial response and the duration of response. **The goals of treatment include improving control of disease-related symptoms, maintaining or improving quality of life, delaying time to progression, and possibly prolonging survival, particularly in women with *platinum*-sensitive recurrences.** Many active chemotherapy agents (*platinum, paclitaxel, topotecan, liposomal doxorubicin, docetaxel, gemcitabine,* and *etoposide*) and targeted agents (*bevacizumab*) are available, and the choice of treatment is based on many factors including likelihood of benefit, potential toxicity, and patient convenience.

Women who relapse later than 6 months after primary chemotherapy are classified as *platinum*-sensitive and usually receive further *platinum*-based chemotherapy with response rates ranging from 27% to 65% and a median survival of 12 to 24 months (259–263). **Patients who relapse within 6 months of completing first-line chemotherapy are classified as *platinum*-resistant and have a median survival of 6 to 9 months and a 10% to 30% likelihood of responding to chemotherapy. Patients who progress while on treatment are classified as having *platinum*-refractory disease.** Objective response rates to chemotherapy in patients with *platinum*-refractory ovarian cancer are low—less than 20% (264).

The potential adverse effects associated with chemotherapy in trials in women with recurrent ovarian cancer are well documented and should not be underestimated. The three most commonly used drugs are *paclitaxel, topotecan,* and *liposomal doxorubicin* (265–291). The reported adverse effects associated with *paclitaxel* were alopecia in 62% to 100%, neurotoxicity (any grade) in 5% to 42% of patients, and severe leukopenia in 4% to 24% of patients. *Topotecan* is associated with significantly greater myelosuppression than *liposomal doxorubicin* or *paclitaxel* and is observed in 49% to 76% of patients. *Liposomal doxorubicin* is associated with palmer-planter erythrodysesthesia (PPE) of any grade in over 50% of patients and is severe in 23%. Severe stomatitis is reported in up to 10% of patients (265–268).

Platinum-Sensitive Disease   The use of combination *platinum* plus *paclitaxel* chemotherapy versus a single-agent *platinum* was tested in two multinational randomized phase III trials and a randomized phase II study (292,293). In a report of the ICON4 and AGO-OVAR-2.2 (AGO Studiengruppe Ovarialkarzinom) trials, 802 women with *platinum*-sensitive ovarian cancer, who relapsed after being treatment free for at least 6 to 12 months were randomized to *platinum*-based chemotherapy (72% *carboplatin* or *cisplatin* alone; 17% *CAP*; 4% *carboplatin* plus *cisplatin*; and 3% *cisplatin* plus *doxorubicin*) or *paclitaxel* plus *platinum*-based chemotherapy (80% *paclitaxel* plus *carboplatin*; 10% *paclitaxel* plus *cisplatin*; 5% *paclitaxel* plus both *carboplatin* and *cisplatin*; and 4% *paclitaxel* alone) (292). The AGO-OVAR-2.2 trial did not accrue its planned number of patients. **In both trials, a significant proportion of the patients did not receive *paclitaxel* as part of their initial chemotherapeutic regimen. Combining the trials for analysis, there was a significant survival advantage for the *paclitaxel*-containing therapy** (HR = 0.82) with a median follow-up of 42 months. **The absolute 2-year survival advantage was 7% (57% versus 50%), and there was a 5-month improvement in median survival (29 versus 24 months).** Progression-free survival was better with the *paclitaxel* regimen (HR = 0.76); there was a 10% difference in 1-year progression-free survival (50% versus 40%) and a 3-month prolongation in median progression-free survival (13 versus 10 months). The toxicities were comparable, except for a significantly higher incidence of neurologic toxicity and alopecia in the *paclitaxel* group, while myelosuppression was significantly greater with the *non-paclitaxel*-containing regimens. **These data support the slight advantage of a second-line regimen containing both** *paclitaxel* and a *platinum* agent compared with *platinum*-based therapy alone in patients who have not received *paclitaxel* in their primary chemotherapeutic regimen.

There were two randomized trials comparing *carboplatin alone to carboplatin and gemcitabine or liposomal doxorubicin* (294,295). There was a higher response rate with the combination therapy and a longer progression-free survival, but the studies were not powered to look at overall survival. In the Gynecologic Oncology Intergroup (GCIG) study comparing *carboplatin* and *gemcitabine* with *carboplatin* alone, the response rate was 47.2% for the combination and 30.9% for *carboplatin*, with the progression-free survival being 8.6 months and 5.8 months, respectively (294). A large GCIG study (CALYPSO) compared *carboplatin and liposomal doxorubicin* (CD) with *carboplatin* and *paclitaxel* (*CP*) in 976 patients (296). The progression-free survival for the CD arm was statistically superior to *CP* arm with a median progression-free survival of 11.3 months versus 9.4 months, respectively. Overall survival data are not yet available. The CD arm was better tolerated with less severe toxicities, and this combination is now widely used (296).

Platinum-Resistant and Refractory Disease   Patients with *platinum*-refractory and resistant ovarian cancer are treated with chemotherapy and may have a number of lines of therapy depending on response and performance status. In *platinum*-refractory patients (i.e., those progressing on treatment), response rates to second-line chemotherapy are less than 10% and the median survival is short, around 3 to 5 months (260–264). The management of women who are *platinum*-resistant (i.e., progressing within 6 months of completion of chemotherapy) is difficult and "non-cross-resistant agents" are selected, but there does not appear to be one best treatment. Single-agent therapy is typically used because combination regimens are associated with more toxicity without any apparent additional benefit. High response rates of 48% to 64% were reported with dose-dense weekly *carboplatin* (AUC4) plus *paclitaxel* (90 mg/m^2), and this deserves more study (297). There are a variety of potentially active drugs: *paclitaxel, docetaxel, topotecan, liposomal doxorubicin, gemcitabine, oral etoposide, tamoxifen,* and *bevacizumab* are the most frequently used. Other agents include *vinorelbine* and newer drugs such as *trabectedin.*

The results of a study comparing *topotecan* with *liposomal doxorubicin* demonstrate the low response rates and poor prognosis among women with *platinum*-resistant ovarian cancer (265). There were two randomized trials comparing *liposomal doxorubicin* with either *topotecan* or *paclitaxel*. In a study of 237 women who relapsed after receiving one *platinum*-containing regimen, 117 of whom (49.4%) had *platinum*-refractory disease, *liposomal doxorubicin* 50 mg/m^2 over 1 hour every 4 weeks was compared with *topotecan* 1.5 mg/m^2/day for 5 days every 3 weeks (265). The two treatments had a similar overall response rate (20% versus 17%), time to progression (22 versus 20 weeks), and median overall survival (66 versus 56 weeks). The myelotoxicity was significantly lower in the *liposomal doxorubicin*-treated patients than with those receiving *topotecan*. In a second study comparing *liposomal doxorubicin* with single-agent *paclitaxel* in 214 *platinum*-treated patients who had not received prior *taxanes*, the overall response rates for *liposomal doxorubicin* and *paclitaxel* were 18% versus 22%, respectively, and median survival durations were 46 and 56 weeks, respectively, and these were not significantly different (266). In practice, most patients are treated with a starting dose of 40 mg/m^2 of *liposomal doxorubicin* every 4 weeks, because of the toxicity associated with the higher dose and the need to dose reduce when 50 mg/m^2 is used. In a subset analysis of *platinum*-resistant patients, the median time to progression ranged from 9.1 to 13.6 weeks for *topotecan* and *liposomal doxorubicin*, respectively. The median survival ($p = 0.455$) was 35.6 weeks for pegylated *liposomal doxorubicin* and 41.3 weeks for *topotecan*. Objective response rates were recorded in 6.5% of patients who received *topotecan* and in 12.3% of those who received pegylated *liposomal doxorubicin* ($p = 0.118$). It is not known whether the treatment improved symptoms control or quality of life because this was not specifically addressed.

In another randomized trial in 195 patients with *platinum*-resistant ovarian cancer, patients were randomized to receive either liposomal doxorubicin (PLD) or *gemcitabine* (298). In the *gemcitabine* and PLD groups, median progression-free survival was 3.6 versus 3.1 months; median overall survival was 12.7 versus 13.5 months; overall response rate was 6.1% versus 8.3%; and in the subset of patients with measurable disease, overall response rate was 9.2% versus 11.7%, respectively. None of the efficacy end points showed a statistically significant difference between treatment groups. The PLD group experienced significantly more hand-foot syndrome and mucositis; the gemcitabine group experienced significantly more constipation, nausea or vomiting, fatigue, and neutropenia.

Some researchers attempted to treat patients with non-*platinum* drugs to prolong the *platinum*-free interval, hoping that would allow the tumor to become *platinum*-sensitive during the interval use of non-cross-resistant agents. The rationale for this approach is the belief that the *platinum*-free interval is equivalent to the treatment-free interval, and before the availability of other active drugs, these two terms were synonymous. **There are no data to support the hypothesis that the interposition of another drug can produce an increased *platinum* sensitivity as a result of a longer interval since the last *platinum* treatment.**

Taxanes

Single-agent *paclitaxel* shows objective responses in 20% to 30% in phase II trials of women with *platinum*-resistant ovarian cancer (269–274). The main toxicities are fatigue and peripheral neuropathy. **Weekly *paclitaxel* is active, and the toxicity, especially myelosuppression, is less than with the every 3-week regimens.** In a study of 53 women with *platinum*-resistant ovarian cancer, weekly *paclitaxel* (80 mg/m^2 over 1 hour) had an objective response of 25% in patients with measurable disease, and 27% of patients without measurable disease had a 75% decline in serum CA125 levels (269).

Docetaxel has some activity in these patients (299–301). The GOG studied 60 women with *platinum*-resistant ovarian or primary peritoneal cancer (301). Although there was a 22% objective response rate, the median response duration was only 2.5 months, and therapy was complicated by severe neutropenia in three-quarters of the patients.

Topotecan   *Topotecan* is an active second-line treatment for patients with *platinum*-sensitive and *platinum*-resistant disease (277–291). In a study of 139 women receiving *topotecan* 1.5 mg/m^2 daily for 5 days, response rates were 19% and 13% in patients with *platinum*-sensitive and *platinum*-resistant disease, respectively (287). **The predominant toxicity of *topotecan* is hematologic, especially neutropenia.** With the 5-day dosing schedule, approximately 70% to 80% of patients have severe neutropenia, and 25% have febrile neutropenia with or without infection. In some studies, regimens of 5 days produce better response rates than regimens of shorter duration, but in others, reducing the dose to 1.0 mg/m^2 per day for 3 days is associated with similar response rates but lower toxicity (280,290). In a study of 31 patients, one-half of whom were *platinum* refractory, *topotecan* 2 mg/m^2 per day for 3 days every 21 days had a 32% response rate (285). Continuous infusion *topotecan* (0.4 mg/m^2 per day for 14 to 21 days) had a 27% to 35% objective response rate in *platinum*-refractory patients (284). **Weekly *topotecan* administered at a dose of 4 mg/m^2 per week for 3 weeks with a week off every month produced a response rate similar to the 5-day regimen with considerably less toxicity, and this is the preferred dose schedule in the recurrent setting** (290).

Oral *topotecan*, not available in the United States, **results in similar response rates with less hematologic toxicity** (286). The intravenous and oral formulations of *topotecan* were compared in a randomized trial of 266 women as a third-line regimen after an initial *platinum*-based regimen (291). Compared with intravenous *topotecan* (1.5 mg/m^2 daily for 5 days every 3 weeks), oral *topotecan* (2.3 mg/m^2 per day for 5 days every 3 weeks) produced a similar response rate (13% versus 20%), less severe myelosuppression, and only a slightly shorter median survival (51 versus 58 weeks).

Liposomal Doxorubicin   Liposomal doxorubicin (*Doxil* in the United States and *Caelyx* in Europe), as noted above, has activity in *platinum*- and *taxane*-refractory disease (265–268,295). One of the **most important side effects of *liposomal doxorubicin* is the hand-foot syndrome, also known as palmar-plantar erythrodysesthesia or acral erythema, which occurs in 20% of patients who receive 50 mg/m^2 every 4 weeks** (266). Most oncologists administer 40 mg/m^2 and escalate only if there are no side effects. *Liposomal doxorubicin* has a low rate of alopecia. In a study of 89 patients with *platinum*-refractory disease, including 82 *paclitaxel*-resistant patients, *liposomal doxorubicin* (50 mg/m^2 every 3 weeks) produced a response in 17% (1 complete and 14 partial responses) (268). In another study, an objective response of 26% was reported, although there were no responses in women who progressed during first-line therapy (265).

Gemcitabine   *Gemcitabine* is associated with response rates of 20% to 50%, with 15% to 30% in patients who are *platinum*-resistant (302–306). **The principal toxicities are myelosuppression and gastrointestinal.** The drug is used in doublet combinations with *cisplatin* or *carboplatin* with acceptable responses and toxicities, and in the triplet combination with *carboplatin* and *paclitaxel* (304).

Oral Etoposide **The most common toxicities with oral *etoposide* are myelosuppression and gastrointestinal:** grade 4 neutropenia is observed in about one-fourth of patients, and 10% to 15% have severe nausea and vomiting (307,308). A study of oral *etoposide* given for a prolonged treatment (50 mg/m^2 daily for 21 days every 4 weeks) had a 27% response rate in 41 women with *platinum*-resistant disease, 3 of whom had durable complete responses (308). In 25 patients with *platinum* and *taxane*-resistant disease, 8 objective responses (32%) were reported.

Hormonal Therapy

***Tamoxifen* is associated with CA125 response rates of 15% to 20% in small studies of patients with recurrent ovarian cancer** (309–315). Aromatase inhibitors (e.g., *letrozole, anastrozole*, and *exemestane*), which have activity in metastatic breast cancer, are being studied in relapsed ovarian cancer (316). One of the principal advantages of this class of agents is its very low toxicity (317).

Targeted Therapies

Knowledge of molecular pathways within normal and malignant cells is leading to the development of cancer treatment agents with specific molecular targets. There is great potential in targeting angiogenesis, in particular vascular endothelial growth factor (VEGF), which plays a major role in the biology of epithelial ovarian cancer (318). There are three main approaches to target angiogenesis: the first is to target VEGF itself, the second to target the VEGF receptor, and the third is to inhibit tyrosine kinase activation and downstream signaling with small molecules that work at the intracellular level.

Bevacizumab is the first targeted agent to show significant single agent activity in ovarian cancer. It is a humanized monoclonal antibody that targets angiogenesis by binding to VEGF-A, thereby blocking the interaction of VEGF with its receptor. There are a number of phase II studies reported using *bevacizumab* in patients with *platinum*-sensitive and *platinum*-resistant ovarian cancer with response rates ranging from 16% to 22% in both *platinum*-sensitive and -refractory patients (319). Up to 40% of patients had stabilization of disease for at least 6 months. A study of low-dose metronomic chemotherapy with 50 mg of cyclophosphamide daily and bevacizumab 10 mg/kg intravenously every 2 weeks showed significant activity in a study of 70 patients with recurrent ovarian cancer (320). The primary end point was progression-free survival at 6 months. The probability of being alive and progression free at 6 months was 56%. A partial response was achieved in 17 patients (24%). Median time to progression and survival were 7.2 and 16.9 months, respectively. This comes with toxicity. The side effects of *bevacizumab* are well recognized and include hypertension, fatigue, proteinuria, gastrointestinal perforation or fistula, and uncommonly, vascular thrombosis and central nervous system ischemia, pulmonary hypertension, and bleeding and wound healing complications. The most common side effects are hypertension that is grade 3 in 7% of patients and is usually treatable. The most concerning side effect is bowel perforation and the study by Cannistra et al. was stopped after recruiting 44 patients because of an 11% incidence of perforation of the bowel (321).

It was suggested that the bowel perforation complication could be avoided by carefully screening patients. Simpkins et al. limited *bevacizumab* treatment to patients without clinical symptoms of bowel obstruction or evidence of rectosigmoid involvement on pelvic examination or bowel involvement on CT scan (322). Their study included 25 patients with *platinum*-resistant ovarian cancer who were heavily pretreated, and they observed a response rate of 28% and no bowel perforations or any other grade 3 or 4 toxicities were reported. This highlights the importance of patient selection and suggests that increased experience with these agents will result in less toxicity.

VEGF Trap functions as a soluble decoy receptor soaking up ligand before it can interact with its receptor and is being evaluated in phase II trials in patients with recurrent ovarian cancer. There are other oral agents that target angiogenesis through tyrosine kinase inhibition that are in clinical trial (323).

Radiation Therapy

Whole-abdominal radiation therapy given as a treatment for recurrent or persistent disease is associated with a high morbidity and is not used. The principal problem associated with this approach is the development of acute and chronic intestinal morbidity. As many as 30% of patients treated with this approach develop intestinal obstruction, which necessitated exploratory surgery with potential morbidity (324).

Intestinal Obstruction

Patients with epithelial ovarian cancer often develop intestinal obstruction, either at the time of initial diagnosis or in association with recurrent disease (325–340). Obstruction may be related to a mechanical blockage or to carcinomatous ileus.

The intestinal blockage can be corrected in most patients whose obstruction appears at initial diagnosis. The decision to perform an exploratory procedure to ease intestinal obstruction in patients with recurrent disease is more difficult. For patients whose life expectancy is very short (e.g., less than 2 months), surgical relief of the obstruction is not indicated (325–330). **In those patients with a longer projected lifespan, features predicting a reasonable likelihood of correcting the obstruction include young age, good nutritional status, and the absence of rapidly accumulating ascites** (326).

For most patients with recurrent ovarian cancer and intestinal obstruction, initial management should include proper radiographic documentation of the obstruction, hydration, correction of any electrolyte disturbances, parenteral alimentation, and intestinal intubation. For some patients, the obstruction may be alleviated by this conservative approach. A preoperative upper gastrointestinal radiographic series and a barium enema will define possible sites of obstruction.

If exploratory surgery is deemed appropriate, the type of operation to be performed will depend on the site and the number of obstructions. **Multiple sites of obstruction are not uncommon in patients with recurrent epithelial ovarian cancer.** More than one-half of the patients have small bowel obstruction, one-third have colonic obstruction, and one-sixth have both (327–331). If the obstruction is principally contained in one area of the bowel (e.g., the terminal ileum), this area can be either resected or bypassed, depending on what is easier to accomplish safely. Intestinal bypass is less morbid than resection, and in patients with progressive cancer, the survival time after these two operations is the same (332–337).

If multiple obstructions are present, resection of several segments of intestine is usually not indicated, and intestinal bypass and/or colostomy should be performed. A gastrostomy may be useful in this circumstance, and this can usually be placed percutaneously (336,339).

Surgery for bowel obstruction in patients with ovarian cancer carries an operative mortality of about 10% and a major complications rate of about 30% (325–337). The need for multiple reanastomoses and prior radiation therapy increase the morbidity, which consists primarily of sepsis and enterocutaneous fistulae. The median survival ranges from 3 to 12 months, although about 20% of such patients survive longer than 12 months (337–340).

Survival

The prognosis for patients with epithelial ovarian cancer is related to several clinical variables. Survival analyses based on prognostic variables are presented (1,3,30,123–127). Including patients at all stages, patients younger than 50 years of age have a 5-year survival rate of about 40%, compared with about 15% for patients older than 50 years.

The 5-year survival rate for carefully and properly staged patients with stage I disease is as high as 94%, for stage II is 73%, for stage III or IV 28% (1). The 5-year survival rate for stage IIIA is 41%, for stage IIIB about 25%, for stage IIIC 23%, and for stage IV disease 11% (Fig. 37.16). An analysis of the National Cancer Institute's Surveillance, Epidemiology, and End Results (SEER) database reveals a trend toward improved survival for ovarian cancer in the United States. In this cohort, the survival for stage I was 93%, for stage II 70%, for stage III 37%, and for stage IV 25% (341).

Survival of patients with borderline tumors is excellent, with stage I lesions having a 98% 15-year survival (30). When all stages of borderline tumors are included, the 5-year survival rate is about 86% to 90%.

Patients with stage III disease with microscopic residual disease at the start of treatment have a 5-year survival rate of about 40% to 75%, compared with about 30% to 40% for those with optimal disease and only 5% for those with suboptimal disease (126,127,149). Patients whose Karnofsky index (KI) is low (<70) have a significantly shorter survival than those with a KI greater than 70 (30).

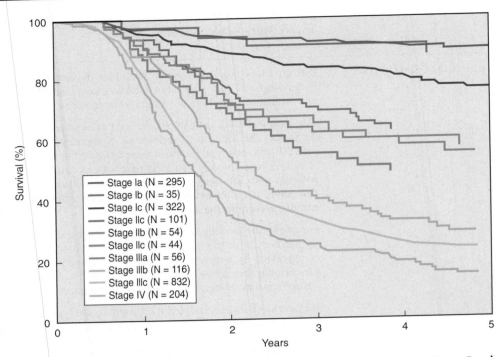

Figure 37.16 Survival of patients with epithelial ovarian cancer by substage. (From **Berek JS, Hacker NF.** *Berek & Hacker's Gynecologic Oncology.* 5th ed. Philadelphia, PA: Lippincott Williams & Wilkins, 2010:491, adapted with permission from **Heintz APM, Odicino F, Maisonneuve P, et al.** Carcinoma of the ovary. In Twenty-sixth annual report of the results of treatment of gynaecological cancer. *Int J Gynecol Oncol* 2006;95(suppl 1):S161–S192.

Nonepithelial Ovarian Cancers

Compared with epithelial ovarian cancers, other malignant tumors of the ovary are uncommon. **Nonepithelial malignancies of the ovary account for about 10% of all ovarian cancers** (2,3,342). Nonepithelial ovarian cancers include malignancies of germ cell origin, sex cord–stromal cell origin, metastatic carcinomas to the ovary, and a variety of extremely rare ovarian cancers (e.g., sarcomas). Although there are similarities in the presentation, evaluation, and management of these patients, the tumors have unique qualities that require a special approach (2,342–345).

Germ Cell Malignancies

Germ cell tumors are derived from the primordial germ cells of the ovary. Their incidence is about one-tenth the incidence of malignant germ cell tumors of the testis, so most of the advances in the management of these tumors are extrapolations from experience with the corresponding testicular tumors. Although malignant germ cell tumors can arise in extragonadal sites such as the mediastinum and the retroperitoneum, most germ cell tumors arise in the gonad from undifferentiated germ cells. The variation in the site of these cancers is explained by the embryonic migration of the germ cells from the caudal part of the yolk sac to the dorsal mesentery before their incorporation into the sex cords of the developing gonads (2,3,342).

Classification

A histologic classification of ovarian germ cell tumors is presented in Table 37.5 (3,342). **Both α-fetoprotein (AFP) and human chorionic gonadotropin (hCG) are secreted by some germ cell malignancies; therefore, the presence of circulating hormones can be clinically useful in the diagnosis of a pelvic mass and in monitoring the course of a patient after surgery. Placental alkaline phosphatase (PLAP) and lactate dehydrogenase (LDH) are produced by up to 95% of dysgerminomas, and serial measurements of LDH may be useful for monitoring the disease.** When the histologic and immunohistologic identification of these

Table 37.5 Histologic Typing of Ovarian Germ Cell Tumors

1. Primitive germ cell tumors	3. Monodermal teratoma and somatic-type tumors associated with dermoid cysts
A. Dysgerminoma	
B. Yolk sac tumor	A. Thyroid tumor
C. Embryonal carcinoma	1. Struma ovarii
D. Polyembryoma	a. Benign
E. Non-gestational choriocarcinoma	b. Malignant
F. Mixed germ cell tumor	B. Carcinoid
2. Biphasic or triphasic teratoma	C. Neuroectodermal tumor
A. Immature teratoma	D. Carcinoma
B. Mature teratoma	E. Melanocytic
1. Solid	F. Sarcoma
2. Cystic	G. Sebaceous tumor
a. Dermoid cyst	H. Pituitary-type tumor
b. Fetiform teratoma (homunculus)	I. Others

Adapted from Tavassoll FA, Devllee P, eds. World Health Organization classification of tumours. *Pathology and genetics of tumors of the breast and female organs.* Lyon: IARC Press, 2003.

substances in tumors is correlated, a classification of germ cell tumors emerges (Fig. 37.17) (346).

In this scheme, **embryonal carcinoma (a cancer composed of undifferentiated cells) synthesizes both hCG and AFP**, and this lesion is the progenitor of several other germ cell tumors (346–348). More differentiated germ cell tumors, such as the endodermal sinus tumor, which secretes AFP, and the choriocarcinoma, which secretes hCG, are derived from the extraembryonic tissues; the immature teratomas derived from the embryonic cells have lost the ability to secrete these substances. Pure germinomas do not secrete these markers.

Epidemiology

Although 20% to 25% of all benign and malignant ovarian neoplasms are of germ cell origin, only about 3% of these tumors are malignant (2,3). Germ cell malignancies account for fewer than 5% of all ovarian cancers in Western countries. Germ cell malignancies represent up to 15% of ovarian cancers in Asian and African American societies, where epithelial ovarian cancers are much less common.

In the first two decades of life, almost 70% of ovarian tumors are of germ cell origin, and one-third of these are malignant (2,3,342). Germ cell cancers are seen in the third decade, but thereafter they become quite rare.

Clinical Features

Symptoms

In contrast to the slower-growing epithelial ovarian tumors, germ cell malignancies grow rapidly and are characterized by subacute pelvic pain related to capsular distention, hemorrhage, or necrosis. The rapidly enlarging pelvic mass may produce pressure symptoms on the bladder or rectum, and menstrual irregularities may occur in menarcheal patients. Some young patients misinterpret the early symptoms of a neoplasm as those of pregnancy, which can lead to a delay in the diagnosis. Acute symptoms associated with torsion or rupture of the adnexa can develop. These symptoms may be confused with acute appendicitis. In more advanced cases, ascites may develop, and the patient can have abdominal distention (336).

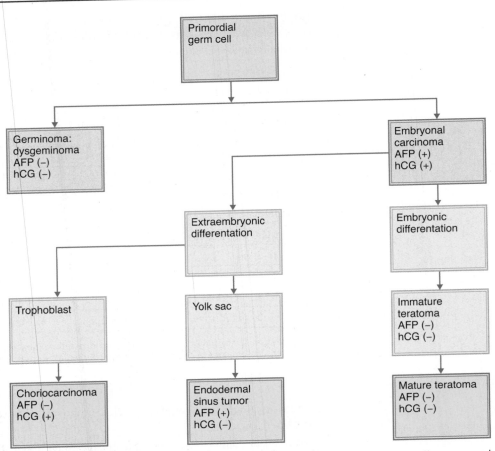

Figure 37.17 **Relationship between types of pure malignant tumors.** Germ cell tumors and their secreted marker substances. (From **Berek JS, Hacker NF.** *Berek & Hacker's Gynecologic Oncology.* 5th ed. Philadelphia: Lippincott Williams & Wilkins, 2010:511, with permission.

Signs

For a patient with a palpable adnexal mass, the evaluation can proceed as outlined. Some patients with germ cell tumors will be premenarcheal and may require examination under anesthesia. **If the lesions are principally solid or a combination of solid and cystic, as might be noted on an ultrasonographic evaluation, a neoplasm is probable and a malignancy is possible** (see Fig. 14.8 and Chapter 14). During the remainder of the physical examination, effort should be directed to searching for signs of ascites, pleural effusion, and organomegaly.

Diagnosis

Adnexal masses measuring 2 cm or larger in premenarcheal girls or 8 cm or larger in other premenopausal patients will usually require surgical exploration. For young patients, blood tests should include serum hCG and AFP and LDH. A CT scan of the chest is important because germ cell tumors can metastasize to the lungs or mediastinum. **A karyotype should be obtained preoperatively for all premenarcheal girls, particularly those with dysgerminomas, because of the propensity of these tumors to arise in dysgenetic gonads** (343,349). A preoperative CT scan or MRI may document the presence and extent of retroperitoneal lymphadenopathy or liver metastases; however, because these patients require surgical exploration, preoperative imaging is not usually required. If postmenarcheal patients have predominantly cystic lesions up to 8 cm in diameter, they may be observed or given oral contraceptives for two menstrual cycles (350).

Dysgerminoma	**Dysgerminoma is the most common malignant germ cell tumor, accounting for about 30% to 40% of all ovarian cancers of germ cell origin** (2,3,346). The tumors represent only 1%

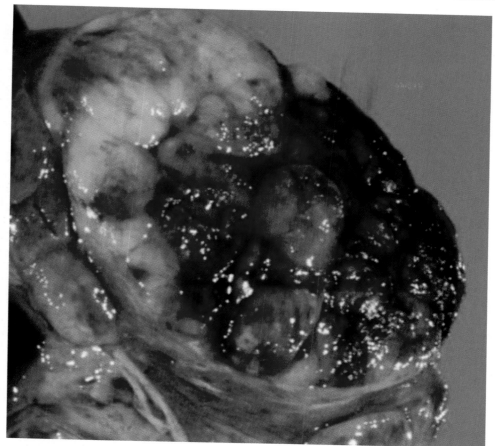

Figure 37.18 **Dysgerminoma of the ovary.** Note that the lesion is principally solid with some cystic areas and necrosis.

to 3% of all ovarian cancers, but they represent as many as 5% to 10% of ovarian cancers in patients younger than 20 years. Seventy-five percent of dysgerminomas occur between the ages of 10 and 30 years, 5% occur before the age of 10 years, and they rarely occur after 50 years of age (2,3,336). Because these malignancies occur in young women, 20% to 30% of ovarian malignancies associated with pregnancy are dysgerminomas.

Germinomas are found in both sexes and may arise in gonadal or extragonadal sites. The latter include the midline structures from the pineal gland to the mediastinum and the retroperitoneum. Histologically, they represent abnormal proliferations of the basic germ cell. In the ovary, the germ cells are encapsulated at birth (the primordial follicle), and the unencapsulated or free cells die. If either of the latter processes fails, it is possible that the germ cell could free itself of its normal control and multiply indiscriminately.

The size of dysgerminomas varies widely, but they are usually 5 to 15 cm in diameter (2,3). The capsule is slightly bosselated, and the consistency of the cut surface is fleshy and pale tan to gray-brown in color (Fig. 37.18).

The histologic characteristics of the dysgerminoma are very distinctive. The large round, ovoid, or polygonal cells have abundant, clear, very-pale–staining cytoplasm, large and irregular nuclei, and prominent nucleoli (Fig. 37.19). Mitotic figures are seen in varying numbers, although they are usually numerous. Another characteristic feature is the arrangement of the elements in lobules and nests separated by fibrous septa, which are often extensively infiltrated with lymphocytes, plasma cells, and granulomas with epithelioid cells and multinucleated giant cells. When necrosis is extensive, the lesion may be confused with tuberculosis. Dysgerminomas may contain syncytiotrophoblastic giant cells and may be associated with precocious puberty or virilization. The presence of these cells does not seem to alter the behavior of the

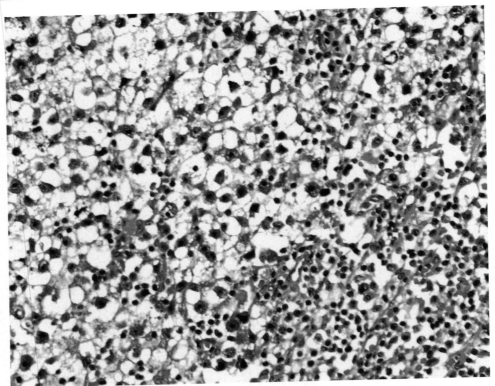

Figure 37.19   **Dysgerminoma of ovary.** Primitive germ cells are divided into clusters and lobules by fibrous septa rich in lymphocytes.

tumor (2,3). The presence of calcifications should prompt a search for a possible underlying gonadoblastoma.

Because the dysgerminoma is a germ cell tumor and parthenogenesis (stimulation of the basic germ cell to atypical division) is the accepted genesis for the more immature teratomas, it is logical that these two tumors may coexist. Choriocarcinoma, endodermal sinus tumor, and other extraembryonal lesions may be associated with the dysgerminoma.

Approximately 5% of dysgerminomas are discovered in phenotypic women with abnormal gonads (2,349,351). This malignancy can be associated with patients who have pure gonadal dysgenesis (46,XY, bilateral streak gonads), mixed gonadal dysgenesis (45,X/46,XY, unilateral streak gonad, contralateral testis), and the androgen insensitivity syndrome (46,XY, testicular feminization). For premenarcheal patients with a pelvic mass, the karyotype should be determined (see Chapter 29).

For most patients with gonadal dysgenesis, dysgerminomas arise in gonadoblastomas, which are benign ovarian tumors that are composed of germ cells and sex cord stroma. If gonadoblastomas are left *in situ* in patients with gonadal dysgenesis, more than 50% will develop into ovarian malignancies (351).

About 65% of dysgerminomas are stage I (i.e., confined to one or both ovaries) at diagnosis (2,3,352–356). About 85% to 90% of stage I tumors are confined to one ovary; 10% to 15% are bilateral. Dysgerminoma is the only germ cell malignancy that has this significant rate of bilaterality. Other germ cell tumors are rarely bilateral.

For patients whose contralateral ovary is preserved, disease can develop in 5% to 10% of the retained gonads over the next 2 years (2). This figure includes those not given additional therapy and patients with gonadal dysgenesis.

In the 25% of patients who are diagnosed initially with metastatic disease, the tumor commonly spreads via the lymphatic system. It can spread hematogenously or by direct extension through the capsule of the ovary with exfoliation and dissemination of cells throughout the peritoneal surfaces. Metastases to the contralateral ovary may be present when there is no other evidence of spread. An uncommon site of metastatic disease is bone; when metastasis to this site occurs, the lesions are principally in the lower vertebrae. Metastases to the lungs, liver, and brain are often in patients with longstanding or recurrent disease. Metastasis to the mediastinum and supraclavicular lymph nodes is usually a late manifestation of disease (352,353).

Treatment

The treatment of patients with early dysgerminoma is primarily surgical, including resection of the primary lesion and proper surgical staging. Chemotherapy is administered to patients with metastatic disease. Because the disease principally affects girls and young women, special consideration must be given to the preservation of fertility and use of chemotherapy whenever possible. An algorithm for the management of ovarian dysgerminoma is presented in Figure 37.20.

Surgery   **The minimal surgical operation for ovarian dysgerminoma is a unilateral oophorectomy (354). If there is a desire to preserve fertility, as there almost always is, the contralateral ovary, fallopian tube, and uterus should be left *in situ*, even in the presence of metastatic disease, because of the sensitivity of the tumor to chemotherapy.** If fertility need not be preserved, it may be appropriate to perform a total abdominal hysterectomy and bilateral salpingo-oophorectomy for patients with advanced disease (356). For patients whose karyotype analysis reveals a Y chromosome, both ovaries should be removed, although the uterus may be left *in situ* for possible future embryo transfer (351). Whereas cytoreductive surgery is of unproved value, bulky disease that can be readily resected (e.g., an omental cake) should be removed during the initial operation.

In patients in whom the neoplasm appears on inspection to be confined to the ovary, a careful staging operation should be undertaken to determine the presence of any occult metastatic disease. All peritoneal surfaces should be inspected and palpated, and any suspicious lesions should be sampled for biopsy. Unilateral pelvic lymphadenectomy and careful palpation and biopsy of enlarged para-aortic nodes are particularly important parts of the staging. These tumors often metastasize to the para-aortic nodes around the renal vessels. Dysgerminoma is the only germ cell tumor that tends to be bilateral, excisional biopsy of any suspicious masses is desirable (354–356). If a small contralateral tumor is found, it may be possible to resect it and preserve some normal ovary.

Many patients with a dysgerminoma will have a tumor that is apparently confined to one ovary and will be referred after unilateral salpingo-oophorectomy without surgical staging. The options for such patients are (i) repeat laparotomy for surgical staging, (ii) regular pelvic and abdominal CT scans, or (iii) adjuvant chemotherapy. Because these are rapidly growing tumors, the preference is to perform regular surveillance. Tumor markers (LDH, AFP, and β-hCG) should be monitored in case occult mixed germ cell elements are present.

Radiation Therapy   Dysgerminomas are very sensitive to radiation therapy, and doses of 2,500 to 3,500 cGy may be curative, even for gross metastatic disease. Loss of fertility is a problem with radiation therapy, and radiation is rarely used as first-line treatment ().

Chemotherapy   **There is very good evidence to demonstrate the effectiveness of *platinum*-based chemotherapy, which is regarded as the treatment of choice (356–367). The obvious advantage is the preservation of fertility** (368).

The most frequently used chemotherapeutic regimen for germ cell tumors is *BEP* (*bleomycin, etoposide*, and *cisplatin*), EP or EC (*etoposide and carboplatin*) (356–373) (Table 37.6).

The GOG studied three cycles of the EC regimen, consisting of *etoposide* (120 mg/m^2 intravenously on days 1, 2, and 3 every 4 weeks) and *carboplatin* (400 mg/m^2 intravenously on day 1 every 4 weeks) for patients with completely resected ovarian dysgerminoma, stage IB, IC, II, or III (364). The results showed a sustained disease-free remission rate of 100%.

For patients with advanced, incompletely resected germ cell tumors, the GOG studied *cisplatin*-based chemotherapy in two consecutive protocols (357,358). In the first study, patients received four cycles of *vinblastine* (12 mg/m^2 every 3 weeks), *bleomycin* (20 units/m^2 intravenously every week for 12 weeks), and *cisplatin* (20 mg/m^2 per day intravenously for 5 days every 3 weeks). Patients with persistent or progressive disease at second-look laparotomy were treated

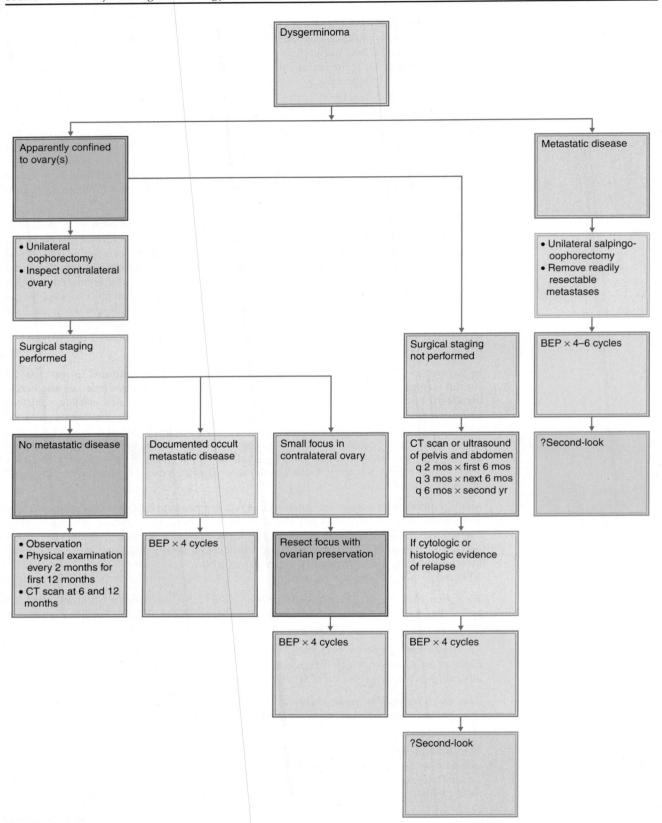

Figure 37.20   **Management of dysgerminoma of the ovary.** BEP = *bleomycin, etoposide,* and *cisplatin;* CT = computed tomogram. (From **Berek JS, Hacker NF.** *Berek & Hacker's Gynecologic Oncology.* 5th ed. Philadelphia, PA: Lippincott Williams & Wilkins, 2010:515, with permission.

Table 37.6 Combination Chemotherapy for Germ Cell Tumors of the Ovary	
Regimen and Drugs	*Dose and Schedule* [a]
BEP	
Bleomycin	15 units/m²/week × 5; then on day 1 of course 4
Etoposide	100 mg/m²/day × 5 days every 3 weeks
Cisplatin	20 mg/m²/day × 5 days, or 100 mg/m²/day × 1 day every 3 weeks
VBP	
Vinblastine	0.15 mg/kg days 1 and 2 every 3 weeks
Bleomycin	15 units/m²/week × 5; then on day 1 of course 4
Cisplatin	100 mg/m² on day 1 every 3 weeks
VAC	
Vincristine	1–1.5 mg/m² on day 1 every 4 weeks
Actinomycin D	0.5 mg/day × 5 days every 4 weeks
Cyclophosphamide	150 mg/m²/day × 5 days every 4 weeks

[a] All doses given intravenously.

with six cycles of VAC (*vincristine, actinomycin D*, and *cyclophosphamide*). In the second trial, patients received three cycles of *BEP* initially, followed by consolidation with VAC, which was later discontinued in patients with dysgerminomas (358). The VAC consolidation after *BEP* is no longer used. A total of 20 evaluable patients with stages III and IV dysgerminoma were treated in these two protocols, and 19 were alive and free of disease after 6 to 68 months (median = 26 months). Fourteen of these patients had a second-look laparotomy, and all findings were negative. Another study at M. D. Anderson Cancer Center used *BEP* in 14 patients with residual disease, and all patients were free of disease during long-term follow-up (361). **These results demonstrate that patients with advanced-stage, incompletely resected dysgerminoma have an excellent prognosis when treated with *cisplatin*-based combination chemotherapy. The standard regimen is three to four cycles of *BEP*, depending on assigned risk based on the data from testicular cancers** (372,373).

Recurrent Disease

About 75% of recurrences occur within the first year after initial treatment, the most common sites being the peritoneal cavity and the retroperitoneal lymph nodes (2,335,336). These patients should be treated with chemotherapy, although radiation may be appropriate in selected patients. Patients with recurrent disease who had no therapy other than surgery should be treated with chemotherapy. If prior chemotherapy with *BEP* was given, there are a number of second-line options including *TIP* (*paclitaxel, iphosphamide, cisplatin*) or VIP (*vinblastine, iphosphamide, cisplatin*) (Table 35.7), and consideration should be given to the use of high-dose chemotherapy in selected patients. Patients with recurrent disease should be managed in specialized centers. Radiation therapy is effective for this disease, with the major disadvantage being loss of fertility if pelvic and abdominal irradiation is required.

Pregnancy

Because dysgerminomas tend to occur in young patients, they may coexist with pregnancy. When a stage IA cancer is found, the tumor can be removed intact and the pregnancy continued. For patients with more advanced disease, continuation of the pregnancy depends on the gestational age of the fetus. Chemotherapy can be given in the second and third trimesters in the same dosages as given for the nonpregnant patient without apparent detriment to the fetus (368).

Prognosis

For patients whose initial disease is stage Ia (i.e., a unilateral encapsulated dysgerminoma), unilateral oophorectomy alone results in a 5-year disease-free survival rate of greater than 95% (355). The features associated with a higher tendency to recur, include lesions larger than

Table 37.7 POMB-ACE Chemotherapy for Germ Cell Tumors of the Ovary

POMB

Day 1	*Vincristine* 1 mg/m² IV; *methotrexate* 300 mg/m² as a 12-hr infusion
Day 2	*Bleomycin* 15 mg as a 24-hr infusion: *folinic acid* rescue started at 24 hr after the start of *methotrexate* in a dose of 15 mg every 12 hr for 4 doses
Day 3	*Bleomycin* infusion 15 mg by 24-hr infusion
Day 4	*Cisplatin* 120 mg/m² as a 12-hr infusion, given with hydration and 3 g magnesium sulfate supplementation

ACE

Days 1–5	*Etoposide* (VP16–213) 100 mg/m², days 1–5
Days 3, 4, 5	*Actinomycin D* 0.5 mg IV, days 3, 4, and 5
Day 5	*Cyclophosphamide* 500 mg/m² IV, day 5

OMB

Day 1	*Vincristine* 1 mg/m² IV; *methotrexate* 300 mg/m² as a 12-hr infusion
Day 2	*Bleomycin* 15 mg by 24-hr infusion; *folinic acid* rescue started at 24 hrs after start of *methotrexate* in a dose of 15 mg every 12 hr for 4 doses
Day 3	*Bleomycin* 15 mg by 24-hr infusion

IV, intravenous.

The sequence of treatment schedules is two courses of POMB followed by ACE. POMB is then alternated with ACE until patients are in biochemical remission as measured by human chorionic gonadotropin (hCG) and α-fetoprotein (AFP), placental alkaline phosphatase (PLAP), and lactate dehydrogenase (LDH). The usual number of courses of POMB is three to five. Following biochemical remission, patients alternate ACE with OMB until remission has been maintained for approximately 12 weeks. The interval between courses of treatment is kept to the minimum (usually 9 to 11 days). If delays are caused by myelosuppression after courses of ACE, the first 2 days of etoposide are omitted from subsequent courses of ACE.

From **Newlands ES, Southall PJ, Paradinas FJ, et al.** Management of ovarian germ cell tumours. In: **Williams CJ, Kaikorian JG, Green MR, et al., eds.** *Textbook of uncommon cancer.* New York: John Wiley and Sons, 1988:47, with permission.

10 to 15 cm in diameter, age younger than 20 years, and a microscopic pattern that includes numerous mitoses, anaplasia, and a medullary pattern (2,346).

Surgery for advanced disease followed by pelvic and abdominal radiation resulted in a 5-year survival rate of 63% to 83%, for this same group of patients cure rates of 85% to 90% are reported with the use of *VBP* (*vinblastine, bleomycin, cisplatin*), *BEP*, or *EC* combination chemotherapy and radiation is infrequently indicated (356–376).

Immature Teratomas

Immature teratomas contain elements that resemble tissues derived from the embryo. Immature teratomatous elements may occur in combination with other germ cell tumors as mixed germ cell tumors. The pure immature teratoma accounts for fewer than 1% of all ovarian cancers, but it is the second most common germ cell malignancy and accounts for 10% to 20% of all ovarian malignancies seen in women younger than 20 years (2). About 50% of pure immature teratomas of the ovary occur in women between the ages of 10 and 20 years, and they rarely occur in postmenopausal women.

Pathology and Grading

Of fundamental importance in the understanding of the teratoma is recognition of the maturation of the various elements. If maturation continues along normal lines, the mature or adult teratoma results, and the prognosis is excellent. Conversely, abnormal maturation of these elements can result in an immature teratoma that has metastatic potential.

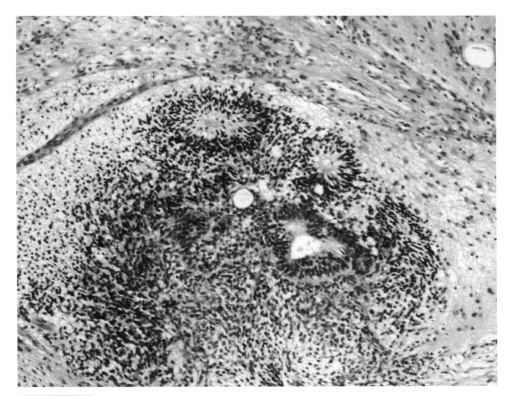

Figure 37.21 **Ovarian teratoma.** This tumor contains both mature and immature neural elements with a neural tube-like structure near its center.

Teratomas containing immature elements, although relatively rare, were recognized more often as pathologists became more alert to their presence (Fig. 37.21). Among the tumors with embryonal elements, those containing neural tissues demonstrate the ability to mature.

Semiquantification of immature neuroepithelium correlates with survival in ovarian immature teratoma and is the basis for grading of these tumors (377–379). **Those with less than one low power field (X 4) of immature neuroepithelium on the slide with the greatest amount of such tissue (grade 1) have a survival of at least 95%, whereas greater amounts of immature neuroepithelium (grades 2 and 3) appear to have a lower overall survival (approximately 85%)** (379). This may not apply to immature teratomas of the ovary in children because they have a good outcome with surgery alone, regardless of the degree of immaturity (380,381). The significant inter- and intraobserver difficulty with a three-tier system led some authorities to recommend the two-tier grading system in use, with immature teratomas categorized as either low grade or high grade (377). Immature ovarian teratomas may be associated with gliomatosis peritonei, a favorable prognostic finding if composed of completely mature tissues; reports using molecular methods indicate these glial implants are not tumor derived but represent teratoma-induced metaplasia of pluripotent müllerian stem cells in the peritoneum (382,383).

Somatic malignant change in benign cystic teratomas was recorded as occurring in 0.5% to 2% of cases, usually in patients older than 40 years of age (377). The most common malignancy developing in the initially benign teratoma is squamous cell carcinoma. Other neoplasms were reported (e.g., adenocarcinomas, melanomas, which may arise from the skin or retinal anlage, and sarcomas, including leiomyosarcomas and mixed mesodermal tumors) (2). Carcinomas may arise from any of the epithelial elements.

Diagnosis

The preoperative evaluation and differential diagnosis of immature teratomas are the same as for other germ cell tumors. Some of these lesions will contain calcifications similar to those of mature teratomas, which can be detected by a radiograph of the abdomen or by ultrasonography. Rarely they are associated with the production of steroid hormones and can be accompanied by sexual pseudoprecocity (342). Tumor markers are negative unless a mixed germ cell tumor is present.

Treatment

Surgery   **In a premenopausal patient whose lesion appears to be confined to a single ovary, unilateral oophorectomy and surgical staging should be performed. For a postmenopausal patient, a total abdominal hysterectomy and bilateral salpingo-oophorectomy may be performed. Contralateral involvement is rare, and routine resection or wedge biopsy of the contralateral ovary is unnecessary** (3,378,379). Any lesions on the peritoneal surfaces should be sampled and submitted for histologic evaluation. The most frequent site of dissemination is the peritoneum and, much less commonly, the retroperitoneal lymph nodes. Blood-borne metastases to organ parenchyma, such as the lungs, liver, or brain, are uncommon. When present, they are usually seen in patients with late or recurrent disease and most often in tumors that are poorly differentiated (i.e., grade 3).

It is unclear whether debulking of metastatic implants enhances the response to combination chemotherapy (384–390). Unlike epithelial lesions, immature teratomas are chemosensitive. Because cure depends on the prompt delivery of chemotherapy, any surgical resection that is potentially morbid and could delay chemotherapy should be resisted.

Chemotherapy   **Patients with IA, grade 1 tumors have an excellent prognosis, and no adjuvant therapy is required. For patients whose tumors are stage IA, grade 2 or 3, adjuvant chemotherapy should be used** (359–361,374,375–378). Chemotherapy is indicated for patients who have ascites, regardless of tumor grade. The standard approach is *BEP*. The most frequently used combination chemotherapeutic regimen was *VAC*, but this regimen is no longer used (359,360,391–397).

The GOG is prospectively studying three courses of *BEP* therapy for patients with completely resected stages I, II, and III ovarian germ cell tumors (359,360,397). Overall, the toxicity is acceptable, and 91 of 93 patients whose nondysgerminomatous tumors were treated are clinically free of disease. **The *BEP* regimen, which is standard of care for testicular cancer, is also the most appropriate chemotherapy regimen for nondysgerminomatous germ cells tumors of the ovary.** As these tumors can progress rapidly, treatment should be initiated as soon as possible after surgery, preferably within 7 to 10 days (398).

The switch from *VBP* to *BEP* was prompted by the experience in patients with testicular cancer, in which the replacement of *vinblastine* with *etoposide* was associated with a better therapeutic index (i.e., equivalent efficacy and lower morbidity), especially less neurologic and gastrointestinal toxicity. The use of *bleomycin* seems to be important for this group of patients. In a randomized study of three cycles of *etoposide* plus *cisplatin* with or without *bleomycin* (*EP* versus *BEP*) in 166 patients with germ cell tumors of the testes, the *BEP* regimen had a relapse-free survival rate of 84% compared with 69% for the *EP* regimen ($p = 0.03$) (372). *Cisplatin* may be slightly better than *carboplatin* in the setting of metastatic germ cell tumors. One hundred ninety-two patients with germ cell tumors of the testes were entered into a study of four cycles of *etoposide* plus *cisplatin* (*EP*) versus four cycles of *etoposide* plus *carboplatin* (EC). There were three relapses with the *EP* regimen versus seven with the EC regimen, although the overall survival of the two groups is identical thus far (373). In view of these results, ***BEP* is the preferred treatment regimen for patients with gross residual disease and has replaced the VAC regimen for patients with completely resected disease.**

It is unclear whether adjuvant chemotherapy is indicated or required for all patients with resected immature teratomas. Several reports support the successful management of these patients with surgery alone and close surveillance (390,399). In the largest series, an Intergroup study from the Pediatric Oncology Group and the Children's Cancer Group, 73 children with immature teratoma (44 of ovarian origin) underwent surgery followed by surveillance. With a median follow-up of 35 months, the overall 3-year event-free survival rates for all patients and those with ovarian teratomas were 93% and 100%, respectively. Thirteen of the 44 girls with an immature ovarian teratoma had microscopic foci of yolk sac tumor in the teratoma; one developed recurrent disease and was successfully treated with *cisplatin*-based chemotherapy. Of note, 82% of the tumors were grade 1 or 2; however, 92% of those with foci of yolk sac tumor were grade 2 or 3.

Second-Look Laparotomy

The need for a second-look operation was questioned (375,376). It seems not to be justified in patients who received chemotherapy in an adjuvant setting, because chemotherapy in these patients is effective. Second-look laparotomy in patients with macroscopic residual disease at the start of chemotherapy may be of value in selected patients, as some patients may have residual mature teratoma and are at risk of growing teratoma syndrome, a rare complication of immature teratomas (400,401). Cancers can arise at a later date in residual mature teratoma. It is important to resect any residual mass and exclude persistent disease because further chemotherapy may be indicated. The principles of surgery are based on the much larger experience of surgery in males with residual masses following chemotherapy for germ cell tumors with a component of immature teratoma (402). Mathew et al. reported their experience of laparotomy in assessing the nature of postchemotherapy residue in ovarian germ cell tumors. Sixty-eight patients completed combination chemotherapy with *cisplatin* regimes, and 35 had radiological residual masses. Twenty-nine of these 35 patients underwent laparotomy and 3 patients had viable tumor, 7 immature teratomas, 3 mature teratoma, and 16 only necrosis or fibrosis. None of the patients with dysgerminoma, embryonal carcinoma, absence of teratoma element in the primary tumor, and radiological residual mass of less than 5 cm had viable tumor, whereas all patients with tumors containing the teratoma component initially had residual tumor, strengthening the case for surgery in patients with immature teratoma and any residual mass (403,404).

Prognosis

The most important prognostic feature of the immature teratoma is the grade of the lesion (2,370). The stage of disease and the extent of tumor at the initiation of treatment have an impact on the curability of the lesion. Overall, the 5-year survival rate for patients with all stages of pure immature teratomas is 70% to 80%, and it is 90% to 95% for patients with surgically staged, stage I lesions (374,377,386).

Endodermal Sinus Tumors

Endodermal sinus tumors (EST) are referred to as *yolk sac carcinomas* because they are derived from the primitive yolk sac (2, 3). These lesions are the third most frequent malignant germ cell tumors of the ovary. ESTs occur in patients with a median age of 16 to 18 years (2,3,405). About one-third of the patients are premenarcheal at the time of diagnosis. Abdominal or pelvic pain is the most frequent initial symptom, occurring in about 75% of patients, whereas an asymptomatic pelvic mass is documented in 10% of patients (343).

Pathology

The gross appearance of an EST is soft grayish-brown. Cystic areas caused by degeneration or necrosis are present in these rapidly growing lesions. The capsule is intact in most cases.

The EST is unilateral in 100% of cases; thus, biopsy of the opposite ovary is contraindicated. The association of such lesions with gonadal dysgenesis must be appreciated, and chromosomal analysis should be performed preoperatively in premenarcheal patients (3).

Microscopically, the characteristic feature is the endodermal sinus, or *Schiller-Duval body* (Fig. 37.22). The cystic space is lined with a layer of flattened or irregular endothelium into which projects a glomerulus-like tuft with a central vascular core. These structures vary throughout the tumor, and the reticular, myxoid elements simulate undifferentiated mesoblast. The lining of the papillary infolding and the cavity is irregular, with an occasional cell containing clear, glassy cytoplasm, simulating the hobnail appearance of the epithelium in clear cell tumors. The association of EST with dysgerminoma must be emphasized if diagnosis and therapy are to be optimal (2,3).

Most EST lesions secrete AFP and, rarely, they may elaborate detectable alpha-1 antitrypsin (AAT). AFP can be demonstrated in the tumor by means of the immunoperoxidase technique. There is a good correlation between the extent of disease and the level of AFP, although discordance is observed. The serum level of these markers, particularly AFP, is useful in monitoring the patient's response to treatment (405–409).

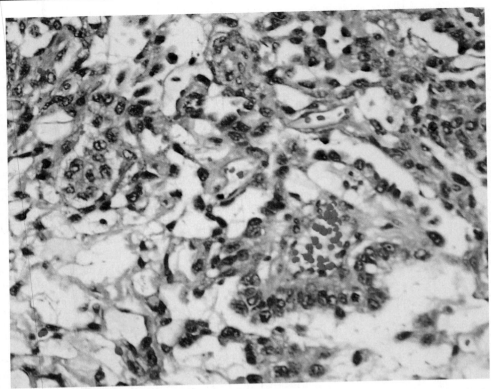

Figure 37.22   **Endodermal sinus tumor of the ovary.** Note the classic Schiller-Duval body with its central vessel and mantle of endoderm.

Treatment

Surgery   **The treatment of the EST consists of surgical exploration, unilateral salpingo-oophorectomy, and a frozen section for diagnosis. The addition of a hysterectomy and contralateral salpingo-oophorectomy does not alter outcome** (407). Any gross metastases should be removed, if possible, but thorough surgical staging is not indicated because all patients need chemotherapy. At surgery, the tumors tend to be solid and large, ranging in size from 7 to 28 cm (median, 15 cm) in the GOG series (397). Bilaterality does not occur, and the other ovary is involved with metastatic disease only when there are other metastases in the peritoneal cavity. Most patients have early-stage disease: 71%, stage I; 6%, stage II; and 23%, stage III (409).

Chemotherapy   **All patients with ESTs are treated with either adjuvant or therapeutic chemotherapy.** Before the routine use of combination chemotherapy for this disease, the 2-year survival rate was only about 25%. After the introduction of the VAC regimen, this rate improved to 60% to 70%, indicating the chemosensitivity of most of these tumors (392,393). With conservative surgery and adjuvant chemotherapy, fertility can be preserved as with other germ cell tumors.

Cisplatin-**containing combination chemotherapy with three to four cycles of** *BEP* **should be used as primary chemotherapy for EST.** The GOG protocols used three to four treatment cycles given every 3 weeks (397,410).

Rare Germ Cell Tumors of the Ovary

Embryonal Carcinoma

Embryonal carcinoma of the ovary is an extremely rare tumor that is distinguished from a choriocarcinoma of the ovary by the absence of syncytiotrophoblastic and cytotrophoblastic cells. The patients are very young; ages ranged between 4 and 28 years (median, 14 years) in two series (411). Older patients were reported (412). Embryonal carcinomas may secrete estrogen, with the patient exhibiting symptoms and signs of precocious pseudopuberty or irregular bleeding (2). The clinical picture is otherwise similar to that of the EST. The primary lesions tend to be large, and about two-thirds are confined to one ovary at the time of diagnosis. These lesions frequently secrete AFP and hCG, which are useful for following the response to subsequent therapy (408). **The treatment of embryonal carcinomas is the same as for the EST (i.e., a unilateral oophorectomy followed by combination chemotherapy with *BEP*)** (360,397).

Choriocarcinoma of the Ovary

Pure nongestational choriocarcinoma of the ovary is an extremely rare tumor. Histologically, it has the same appearance as gestational choriocarcinoma metastatic to the ovaries (413). Most patients with this cancer are younger than 20 years. The presence of hCG can be useful in monitoring the patient's response to treatment. **In the presence of high hCG levels, isosexual precocity occurs in about 50% of patients whose lesions appear before menarche** (413,414).

There are only a few limited reports on the use of chemotherapy for nongestational choriocarcinomas, but complete responses were reported with the MAC (*methotrexate, actinomycin D*, and *cyclophosphamide*) regimen used in a manner described for gestational trophoblastic disease (379) (see Chapter 39). Alternatively, the *BEP* regimen can be used. The prognosis of ovarian choriocarcinomas is poor, with most patients having metastases to organ parenchyma at the time of diagnosis.

Polyembryoma

Polyembryoma of the ovary is another extremely rare tumor, which is composed of embryoid bodies. This tumor replicates the structures of early embryonic differentiation (i.e., the three somatic layers: endoderm, mesoderm, and ectoderm) (2,346). The lesion tends to occur in very young, premenarcheal girls with signs of pseudopuberty and elevated AFP and hCG levels. Anecdotally, the VAC chemotherapeutic regimen is reported to be effective (346,415).

Mixed Germ Cell Tumors

Mixed germ cell malignancies of the ovary contain two or more elements of the lesions described above. In one series, the most common component of a mixed malignancy was dysgerminoma, which occurred in 80%, followed by EST in 70%, immature teratoma in 53%, choriocarcinoma in 20%, and embryonal carcinoma in 16% (415). **The most frequent combination was a dysgerminoma and an EST. The mixed lesions may secrete either AFP, hCG, or both or neither of these markers, depending on the components.**

These lesions should be managed with combination chemotherapy, preferably *BEP*. The serum marker, if positive initially, may become negative during chemotherapy, but this finding may reflect regression of only a particular component of the mixed lesion. Therefore, for these patients, a second-look laparotomy may be indicated to determine the precise response to therapy if macroscopic disease was present at initiation of chemotherapy.

The most important prognostic features are the size of the primary tumor and the relative size of its most malignant component (416). For stage IA lesions smaller than 10 cm, survival is 100%. Tumors composed of less than one-third EST, choriocarcinoma, or grade 3, immature teratoma have an excellent prognosis, but it is less favorable when these components constitute most of the mixed lesions.

Late Effects of Treatment of Malignant Germ Cell Tumors of the Ovary

Although there are substantial data regarding late effects of *cisplatin*-based therapy in men with testicular cancer, sparse information is available for women with ovarian germ cell tumors. Among the adverse events from chemotherapy reported in men are renal and gonadal dysfunction, neurotoxicity, cardiovascular toxicity, and secondary malignancies.

Gonadal Function

An important cause of infertility in patients with ovarian germ cell tumors is unnecessary bilateral salpingo-oophorectomy and hysterectomy. **Although temporary ovarian dysfunction or failure is common with *platinum*-based chemotherapy, most women will resume normal ovarian function, and childbearing is usually preserved** (349,355). In one representative series of 47 patients treated with combination chemotherapy for germ cell malignancies, 91.5% resumed normal menstrual function, and there were 14 healthy live births and no birth defects (370). Factors such as older age at initiation of chemotherapy, greater cumulative drug dose, and longer duration of therapy all have an adverse effect on future gonadal function.

Secondary Malignancies

An important cause of late morbidity and mortality in patients receiving chemotherapy for germ cell tumors is the development of secondary tumors. ***Etoposide* in particular was implicated in the development of treatment-related leukemias** (417,418).

The chance of developing treatment-related leukemia following *etoposide* is dose related. **The incidence of leukemia is approximately 0.4% to 0.5%** (representing a 30-fold increased likelihood) in patients receiving a cumulative *etoposide* dose of less than 2,000 mg/m^2, compared with as much as 5% (representing a 336-fold increased likelihood) in those receiving more than 2,000 mg/m^2 (417). In a typical three- or four-cycle course of *BEP*, patients receive a cumulative *etoposide* dose of 1,500 or 2,000 mg/m^2, respectively.

Despite the risk of secondary leukemia, risk-benefit analyses concluded that *etoposide*-containing chemotherapy regimens are beneficial in advanced germ cell tumors; one case of treatment-induced leukemia would be expected for every 20 additionally cured patients who receive *BEP* as compared with *platinum, vincristine, bleomycin (PVB)*. The risk–benefit balance for low-risk disease, or for high-dose *etoposide* in the salvage setting, is less clear (418).

Sex Cord–Stromal Tumors

Sex cord–stromal tumors of the ovary account for about 5% to 8% of all ovarian malignancies (2,3,342,343,419–425). This group of ovarian neoplasms is derived from the sex cords and the ovarian stroma or mesenchyme. The tumors usually are composed of various combinations of elements, including the "female" cells (i.e., granulosa and theca cells) and "male" cells (i.e., Sertoli and Leydig cells), and morphologically indifferent cells. A classification of this group of tumors is presented in Table 37.8.

Table 37.8 Sex Cord–Stromal and Steroid Cell Tumors
1.
A. Granulosa cell tumor
B. Tumors in thecoma-fibroma group
1. Thecoma
2. Fibroma
3. Unclassified
2. ***Androblastomas; Sertoli-Leydig cell tumors***
A. Well-differentiated
1. Sertoli cell tumor
2. Sertoli-Leydig cell tumor
3. Leydig cell tumor; hilus cell tumor
B. Moderately differentiated
C. Poorly differentiated (sarcomatoid)
D. With heterologous elements
3. ***Gynandroblastoma***
4. ***Sex cord tumor with annular tubules***
5. ***Sex cord-stromal tumors, unclassified***
6. ***Steroid cell tumors***
A. Stromal luteoma
B. Leydig cell tumor
C. Steroid cell tumor, not otherwise classified

Granulosa-Stromal Cell Tumors

Granulosa-stromal cell tumors include granulosa cell tumors, thecomas, and fibromas. The granulosa cell tumor is a low-grade malignancy; rarely, thecomas and fibromas have morphologic features of malignancy and may be referred to as fibrosarcomas.

Granulosa cell tumors, which secrete estrogen, are seen in women of all ages. They are found in prepubertal girls in 5% of cases; the remainder are found in women throughout their reproductive and postmenopausal years (422). Granulosa cell tumors are bilateral in only 2% of patients.

Pathology

Granulosa cell tumors range from a few millimeters to 20 cm or more in diameter. **The tumors are rarely bilateral** and have a smooth, lobulated surface. The solid portions of the tumor are granular, frequently trabeculated, and yellow or gray-yellow in color. After clear cell carcinoma, the granulosa-theca cell tumor is probably the most inaccurately diagnosed tumor of the female gonad. Of 477 ovarian tumors from the Emil Novak Ovarian Tumor Registry diagnosed initially as granulosa-theca cell tumors, almost 15% were reclassified after histologic review. Lesions misdiagnosed as granulosa cell tumors included primary or metastatic carcinomas, teratoid tumors, and poorly differentiated mesothelial tumors (419).

The classic adult granulosa cell is round or ovoid with scant cytoplasm. The nucleus contains compact, finely granular chromatin and is either euchromatic or hypochromatic (3). "Coffee bean" grooved nuclei are characteristic; mitotic figures may be present, but numerous mitotic figures should prompt consideration for poorly differentiated or undifferentiated carcinoma. **In the most common variety, the adult granulosa cells show a tendency to arrange themselves in small clusters or rosettes around a central cavity, so there is a resemblance to primordial follicles (i.e., *Call-Exner bodies*)** (Fig. 37.23). The stroma is similar to the theca and may be luteinized. In children and adolescents, the granular cell tumors are often cystic, contain luteinized cells, and can be associated with precocious puberty. Juvenile granulosa cell tumors, so named because of their tendency to occur in younger patients, feature rounder, more

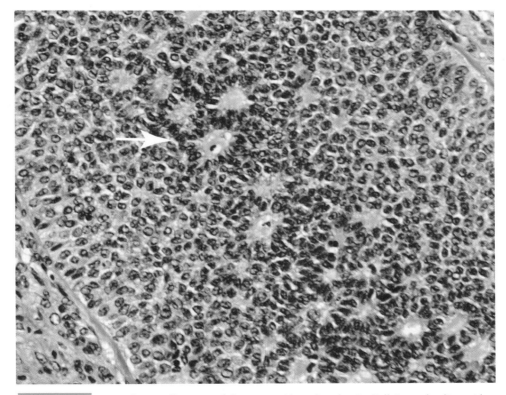

Figure 37.23 **Granulosa cell tumor of the ovary.** Note the classic Call-Exner bodies with a minimal stromal component in this tumor of folliculoid pattern. (*Arrow* points to an example.)

hyperchromatic nuclei and may contain numerous mitotic figures. The presence of large, irregular follicle spaces is an additional distinguishing feature of the juvenile granulosa cell tumor. The adult granulosa cell tumor tends to occur in older women and the juvenile tumor in children and young women, but the diagnosis is not based on age of presentation, but on histology. Adult granulosa cell tumors, but not juvenile granulose cell tumors, harbor a somatic mutation in the *FOXL2* gene (426).

Diagnosis

Granulosa cell tumors, which secrete estrogen, are seen in women of all ages. They are found in prepubertal girls in 5% of cases (typically the juvenile form); the remainder are distributed throughout the reproductive and postmenopausal years (422– 425). **They are bilateral in only 2% of patients.**

Of the rare prepubertal lesions, 75% are associated with sexual pseudoprecocity because of the estrogen secretion (422). Most reproductive-age patients have menstrual irregularities or secondary amenorrhea, and, frequently, cystic hyperplasia of the endometrium. Abnormal uterine bleeding is often the initial symptom for postmenopausal women. The estrogen secretion in these patients can be sufficient to stimulate the development of endometrial cancer. **Low-grade endometrial cancer occurs in association with granulosa cell tumors in at least 5% of cases, and 25% to 50% are associated with endometrial hyperplasia** (2,413,419–422,426).

The other symptoms and signs of granulosa cell tumors are nonspecific and the same as most ovarian malignancies. Ascites is present in about 10% of cases, and, rarely, a pleural effusion is present (419–422). Granulosa tumors tend to be hemorrhagic; occasionally, they rupture and produce a hemoperitoneum.

Adult granulosa cell tumors are usually stage I at diagnosis, but may recur 5 to 30 years after initial diagnosis (421). Most juvenile granulosa cell tumors are clinically benign; only about 10% recur and when they do so, it is generally within 5 years of the initial diagnosis. The tumors may spread hematogenously, and metastases can develop in the lungs, liver, and brain years after initial diagnosis. When adult granulosa cell tumors do recur, they can progress rapidly. Malignant thecomas are extremely rare, and their signs and symptoms, management, and outcome are similar to those of the granulosa cell tumors (419). **Inhibin is secreted by some granulosa cell tumors and is a useful marker for the disease** (427–431). An elevated serum inhibin level in a premenopausal woman presenting with amenorrhea and infertility is suggestive of a granulosa cell tumor (432).

Treatment

The treatment of granulosa cell tumors depends on the age of the patient and the extent of disease. For most patients, surgery alone is sufficient primary therapy; radiation and chemotherapy are reserved for the treatment of recurrent or metastatic disease (422–429,433–436).

Surgery   Because granulosa cell tumors are bilateral in only about 2% of patients, a unilateral salpingo-oophorectomy is appropriate therapy for stage IA tumors in children or in women of reproductive age (420). At the time of laparotomy, if a granulosa cell tumor is identified by frozen section, a staging operation is performed, including an assessment of the contralateral ovary. If the opposite ovary appears enlarged, it should be sampled for biopsy. For perimenopausal and postmenopausal women for whom ovarian preservation is not important, a hysterectomy and bilateral salpingo-oophorectomy should be performed. **For premenopausal patients in whom the uterus is left *in situ*, an endometrial biopsy should be performed because of the possibility of a coexistent adenocarcinoma of the endometrium** (422).

Radiation Therapy   There is no evidence to support the use of adjuvant radiation therapy for granulosa cell tumors, although pelvic irradiation may help to palliate isolated pelvic recurrences (422,434).

Chemotherapy   There is no evidence that adjuvant chemotherapy will prevent recurrence of disease (436–439). Metastatic lesions and recurrences were treated with a variety of antineoplastic drugs. Although the data are inconclusive, *BEP* or *carboplatin* and *paclitaxel* are used in selected patients with stage III or IV tumors or recurrent disease (433). In a GOG study, 37% (14 of 30) patients treated with *BEP* had a negative second-look laparotomy, and these patients had a median time to progression of 24.4 months (440). Granulosa cell tumors are potentially hormonally responsive, with about 30% of granulosa tumors expressing estrogen receptors and almost 100% expressing progesterone receptors. Hormonal agents such as progestins or luteinizing hormone-releasing hormone agonists are used to treat these patients because they are often elderly (441–445). There are case reports of durable response to aromatase inhibitors in patients with metastatic granulosa cell tumors who received multiple prior treatment (443). Small clinical series and case reports indicated that luteinizing hormone-releasing hormone agonists had a 50% response rate in 13 patients, while 4 of 5 patients in the literature responded to a progestational agent. Two case series reported durable responses in a total of six patients receiving aromatase inhibitors among those who progressed on or were intolerant of chemotherapy (442–445).

Prognosis

Adult granulosa cell tumors have a prolonged natural history and a tendency toward late relapse, reflecting their low-grade biology. Ten-year survival rates of about 90% are reported, with 20-year survival rates dropping to 75% (420–422,432,433). Most histologic types have the same prognosis, but patients with the more poorly differentiated diffuse or sarcomatoid type tend to do worse (419).

The DNA ploidy of the tumors is correlated with survival. Holland et al. reported DNA aneuploidy in 13 of 37 patients (35%) with primary adult granulosa cell tumors (437). The presence of residual disease is the most important predictor of progression-free survival, but DNA ploidy is an independent prognostic factor. **Patients with residual-negative DNA diploid tumors had a 10-year progression-free survival of 96%.**

Juvenile granulosa cell tumors of the ovary are rare and constitute less than 5% of ovarian tumors in childhood and adolescence (446). About 90% are diagnosed in stage I, and they have a favorable prognosis. The juvenile subtype behaves less aggressively than the adult type. Only about 10% of juvenile granulosa cell tumors are malignant and late relapse is unusual. Advanced-stage tumors are successfully treated with *platinum*-based combination chemotherapy (e.g., *BEP*) (433,440).

Sertoli-Leydig Tumors

Sertoli-Leydig tumors occur most frequently in the third and fourth decades of life; 75% of these tumors are seen in women younger than 40 years. These neoplasms are extremely rare and account for less than 0.2% of ovarian cancers (2,447,448). Sertoli-Leydig cell tumors are most frequently low-grade malignancies; a poorly differentiated variety may behave more aggressively (Fig. 37.24) (447–449).

The tumors typically produce androgens, and clinical virilization is noted in 70% to 85% of patients (449). Signs of virilization include oligomenorrhea followed by amenorrhea, breast atrophy, acne, hirsutism, clitoromegaly, deepening of the voice, and a receding hairline. Measurement of plasma androgens may reveal elevated testosterone and androstenedione, with normal or slightly elevated dehydroepiandrosterone sulphate (2,450). Rarely, the Sertoli-Leydig tumor is associated with manifestations of estrogenization (i.e., isosexual precocity, irregular or post-menopausal bleeding).

Treatment

Because these low-grade lesions are only rarely bilateral (<1%), the usual treatment is unilateral salpingo-oophorectomy and evaluation of the contralateral ovary for patients who are in their reproductive years (3,422). For older patients, hysterectomy and bilateral salpingo-oophorectomy are appropriate (447,448).

There are insufficient data to document the utility of radiation or chemotherapy for patients with persistent disease, but some responses in patients with measurable disease were reported with pelvic irradiation and the VAC chemotherapy regimen (3,451–455).

Prognosis

The 5-year survival rate is 70% to 90%, and recurrences thereafter are uncommon (3,450–455). Most fatalities occur in the presence of poorly differentiated tumors.

Uncommon Ovarian Cancers

There are several varieties of malignant ovarian tumors that together constitute only 0.1% of ovarian malignancies (2). Two of these lesions are the lipoid (or lipid) cell tumors and the primary ovarian sarcomas.

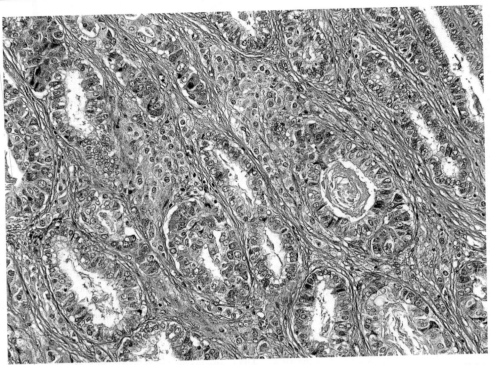

Figure 37.24 **Sertoli-Leydig cell tumor of the ovary.** Note the aggregates of eosinophilic Leydig cells in the stroma adjacent to Sertoli cell tubules.

Lipoid Cell Tumors

Lipoid cell tumors are believed to arise in adrenal cortical rests that reside in the vicinity of the ovary. More than 100 cases were reported, and bilateral disease was noted in only a few (2). Most are associated with virilization and, occasionally, with obesity, hypertension, and glucose intolerance, reflecting corticosteroid secretion. Rare cases of estrogen secretion and isosexual precocity were reported.

Most of these tumors have benign or low-grade behavior, but about 20%, most of which are initially larger than 8 cm in diameter, are associated with metastatic lesions. Metastases are usually in the peritoneal cavity but can occur at distant sites. The primary treatment is surgical extirpation of the primary lesion. There are no data regarding the effectiveness of radiation or chemotherapy for this disease.

Sarcomas

Malignant mixed mesodermal tumors (MMMT) of the ovary or carcinosarcomas are uncommon. Clinical, morphologic and molecular data suggest that MMMTs are monoclonal and are metaplastic carcinomas in which the mesenchymal part reflects dedifferentiation. Most tumors are heterologous, and 80% occur in postmenopausal women. The signs and symptoms are similar to those of most ovarian malignancies. These tumors are biologically aggressive, and most patients have evidence of metastases at presentation. They are treated either with *carboplatin* and *paclitaxel* or *iphosphamide* and *cisplatin*, but in general have a poor prognosis.

Small Cell Carcinoma, Hypercalcemic Type

This rare tumor occurs at an average age of 24 years (range 2 to 46 years) (456). The tumors are typically unilateral. Approximately two-thirds of the tumors are accompanied by paraendocrine hypercalcemia. This tumor accounts for one-half of all of the cases of hypercalcemia associated with ovarian tumors. About 50% of the tumors have spread beyond the ovaries when they are diagnosed (456). Immunohistochemical stains are helpful to differentiate this tumor from a lymphoma, leukemia, or sarcoma.

The management of these malignancies consists of surgery followed by *platinum*-based chemotherapy or radiation therapy or both. In addition to the primary treatment of the disease, control of the hypercalcemia may require aggressive hydration, loop diuretics, and the use of bisphosphonates or *calcitonin*. The prognosis tends to be poor, with most patients dying within 2 years of diagnosis in spite of treatment.

Metastatic Tumors

About 5% to 6% of ovarian tumors are metastatic from other organs, most frequently from the female genital tract, the breast, or the gastrointestinal tract (457–473). The metastases may occur from direct extension of another pelvic neoplasm, by hematogenous or lymphatic spread, or by transcoelomic dissemination, with surface implantation of tumors that spread in the peritoneal cavity.

Gynecologic

Nonovarian cancers of the genital tract can spread by direct extension or metastasize to the ovaries. Tubal carcinoma involves the ovaries secondarily in 13% of cases, usually by direct extension (2,3). Under some circumstances, it is difficult to know whether the tumor originated in the tube or in the ovary when both are involved. Cervical cancer spreads to the ovary only in rare cases (<1%), and most of these are of an advanced clinical stage or are adenocarcinomas. Adenocarcinoma of the endometrium can spread and implant directly onto the surface of the ovaries in about 5% of cases, but two synchronous primary tumors probably occur with greater frequency (472). In these cases, an endometrioid carcinoma of the ovary is usually associated with the adenocarcinoma of the endometrium.

Nongynecologic

The frequency of metastatic breast carcinoma to the ovaries varies according to the method of determination, but the phenomenon is common (Fig. 37.25). In autopsy data of women who died of metastatic breast cancer, the ovaries were involved in 24% of cases, and 80% of the involvement was bilateral (457–462). Similarly, when ovaries are removed to palliate

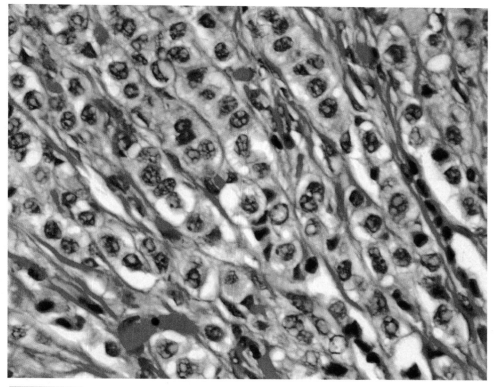

Figure 37.25   **Metastatic carcinoma in the ovary.** Note the linear, single cell pattern found in this metastatic breast carcinoma.

advanced breast cancer, about 20% to 30% of the cases reveal ovarian involvement, 60% of those bilaterally. The involvement of ovaries in early-stage breast cancer seems to be considerably lower, but precise figures are not available. In almost all cases, either ovarian involvement is occult or a pelvic mass is discovered after other metastatic disease becomes apparent.

Krukenberg Tumor

The Krukenberg tumor, which can account for 30% to 40% of metastatic cancers to the ovaries, arises in the ovarian stroma and has characteristic mucin-filled, signet-ring cells (463–465) (Fig. 37.26). The primary tumor is frequently located in the stomach and less commonly in the colon, appendix (so-called goblet cell carcinoid), breast, or biliary tract. Rarely, the cervix or the bladder may be the primary site. Krukenberg tumors can account for about 2% of ovarian cancers at some institutions, and they are usually bilateral. The lesions are usually not discovered until the primary disease is advanced, and, therefore, most patients die of their disease within 1 year. In some cases, a primary tumor is never found.

Other Gastrointestinal Tumors

In other cases of metastasis from the gastrointestinal tract to the ovary, the tumor does not have the classic histologic appearance of a Krukenberg tumor; most of these are from the colon and, less commonly, the pancreato-biliary tract, appendix, and small intestine (Fig. 37.27). **As many as 1% to 2% of women with intestinal carcinomas will develop metastases to the ovaries during the course of their disease** (459). Before exploration for an adnexal tumor in a woman older than 40 years, a barium enema is indicated to exclude a primary gastrointestinal carcinoma with metastases to the ovaries, particularly if there are any gastrointestinal symptoms. Metastatic colon cancer can mimic a mucinous cystadenocarcinoma of the ovary histologically, and the histological distinction between the two can be difficult (458,459,466–470). Lesions that arise in the appendix may be associated with ovarian metastasis and confused with primary ovarian malignancies, especially when associated with pseudomyxoma peritonei (466,470). It is reasonable to consider the performance of prophylactic bilateral salpingo-oophorectomy at the time of surgery for women with colon cancer (471).

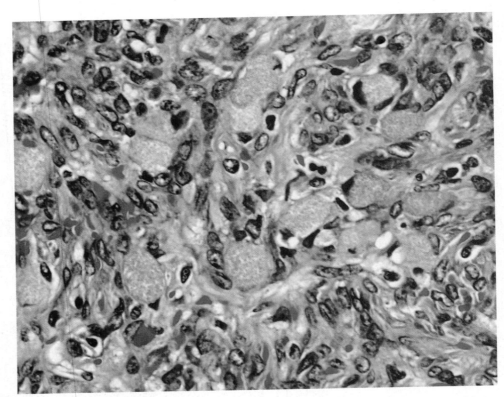

Figure 37.26   Krukenberg tumor of the ovary metastatic from a gastric carcinoma. Malignant cells have discrete vacuoles that push nuclei eccentrically, giving a signet-ring appearance. Mucicarmine stain demonstrates the cytoplasmic vacuoles to be mucin.

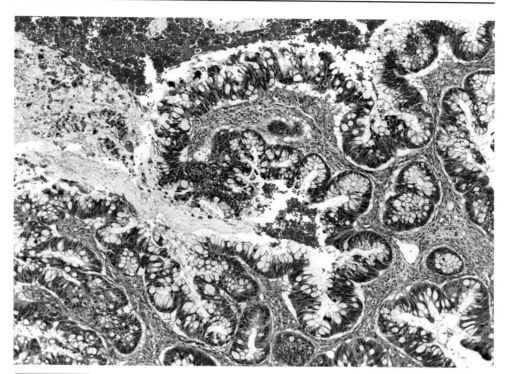

Figure 37.27 Metastatic colorectal carcinoma in the ovary often has areas of necrotic debris (so-called dirty necrosis) adjacent to partial gland structures showing a cribriform pattern.

Melanoma

Rare cases of malignant melanoma metastatic to the ovaries were reported (473). In these circumstances, the melanomas are usually widely disseminated. Removal would be warranted for palliation of abdominal or pelvic pain, bleeding, or torsion. Malignant melanoma can arise, rarely, in a mature cystic teratoma (474).

Carcinoid Tumors

Metastatic carcinoid tumors represent fewer than 2% of metastatic lesions to the ovaries (475). Only about 2% of patients with primary carcinoids have evidence of ovarian metastasis, and only 40% of them have the carcinoid syndrome at the discovery of the metastatic carcinoid. In perimenopausal and postmenopausal women explored for an intestinal carcinoid, it is reasonable to remove the ovaries to prevent subsequent ovarian metastasis. The discovery of an ovarian carcinoid should prompt a careful search for a primary intestinal lesion (476).

Lymphoma and Leukemia

Lymphomas and leukemia can involve the ovary. When they do, the involvement is usually bilateral (477–479). About 5% of patients with Hodgkin's lymphoma will have lymphomatous involvement of the ovaries, but this involvement occurs typically with advanced-stage disease. **With Burkitt's lymphoma, ovarian involvement is very common. Other types of lymphoma involve the ovaries less frequently, and leukemic infiltration of the ovaries is uncommon** (479). Sometimes the ovaries can be the only apparent sites of involvement of the abdominal or pelvic viscera with a lymphoma; if this circumstance is found, a careful surgical exploration may be necessary. Intraoperatively, a hematologist-oncologist should be consulted to determine the need for these procedures if frozen section of a solid ovarian mass reveals a lymphoma. Most lymphomas no longer require extensive surgical staging; biopsy of enlarged lymph nodes should be performed. In some cases of Hodgkin's lymphoma, a more extensive evaluation may be necessary. Treatment involves that of the lymphoma or leukemia. Removal of a large ovarian mass may improve patient comfort and facilitate a response to subsequent radiation or chemotherapy.

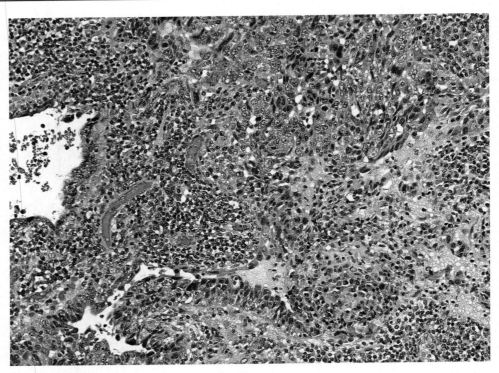

Figure 37.28 **Carcinoma of the fallopian tube.** This is a high-grade serous carcinoma that has invaded the lamina propria of the tubal mucosa. Most primary fallopian tube carcinomas arise in the distal (fimbria) portion of the fallopian tube.

Fallopian Tube Cancer

Historically, carcinoma of the fallopian tube accounted for 0.3% of all cancers of the female genital tract (2,3,480–486). Data suggest primary fallopian tube carcinoma may be more common. **In histologic features and behavior, fallopian tube carcinoma is similar to ovarian cancer; thus, the evaluation and treatment are essentially the same** (Fig 37.28). The fallopian tubes frequently are involved secondarily from other primary sites, most often the ovaries, endometrium, gastrointestinal tract, or breast. They may be involved in primary peritoneal carcinomatosis. Almost all cancers are of epithelial origin, frequently of serous histology. Rarely, sarcomas are reported.

As noted above, there is growing evidence to suggest that many high-grade serous carcinomas of the ovary may prove to arise from the fimbrial end of the fallopian tube (5,7). The true incidence of fallopian tube cancer may be historically underestimated because of the convention of assigning many of these as ovarian cancer when the site of origin is unclear. Despite the uncertainty concerning site of origin, all evidence suggests that our evaluation and treatment of these high-grade serous carcinomas should be the same. In recognition of this, many pathologists resorted to diagnosing these tumors as (nonuterine) high-grade serous carcinomas without definite assignment to primary site.

Clinical Features

Tubal cancers are seen most frequently in the fifth and sixth decades, with a mean age of 55 to 60 years (480). **Women who have germline mutations in *BRCA1* and *BRCA2* are at substantially higher risk for developing fallopian tube carcinoma; therefore, prophylactic surgery in these women should include a complete removal of both tubes along with the ovaries** (78,487).

Symptoms and Signs

The classic triad of symptoms and signs associated with fallopian tube cancer is (i) a prominent watery vaginal discharge (i.e., hydrops tubae profluens), (ii) pelvic pain, and

(iii) a pelvic mass. This triad is noted in fewer than 15% of patients, and may be less common based on the histopathologic origins of fallopian tube cancers (3).

Vaginal discharge or bleeding is the most common symptom reported by patients with tubal carcinoma and is documented in more than 50% of patients (3,481). Lower abdominal or pelvic pressure and pain are noted in many patients. The symptoms may be rather vague and nonspecific. For perimenopausal and postmenopausal women with unusual, unexplained, or persistent vaginal discharge, in the absence of bleeding, the clinician should be concerned about the possibility of occult tubal cancer. Fallopian tube cancer may be found incidentally in asymptomatic women at the time of abdominal hysterectomy and bilateral salpingo-oophorectomy.

On examination, a pelvic mass is present in about 60% of patients, and ascites may be present if advanced disease exists. For patients with tubal carcinoma, the results of dilation and curettage will be negative, although abnormal or adenocarcinomatous cells may be seen in cytologic specimens obtained from the cervix in 10% of patients (483).

Spread Pattern

Tubal cancers spread in the same manner as epithelial ovarian malignancies, principally by the transcoelomic exfoliation of cells that implant throughout the peritoneal cavity. In about 80% of the patients with advanced disease, metastases are confined to the peritoneal cavity at the time of diagnosis (482).

The fallopian tubes are richly permeated with lymphatic channels, as are the ovaries, and spread to the para-aortic and pelvic lymph nodes is common. Metastases to the para-aortic lymph nodes are documented in at least 33% of the patients with all stages of disease (486).

Staging

Fallopian tube cancer is staged according to FIGO (480,485). The staging is based on the surgical findings at laparotomy (Table 37.9). According to this system, about 20% to 25% of patients have stage I disease, 20% to 25% have stage II disease, 40% to 50% have stage III disease, and 5% to 10% have stage IV disease (480). A somewhat lower incidence of advanced disease is seen in these patients than in patients with epithelial ovarian carcinomas, presumably because of the earlier occurrence of symptoms, particularly vaginal bleeding or unusual vaginal discharge. Findings on transvaginal ultrasonography and CT scan may be suspicious for tubal carcinomas (488).

Treatment

The treatment of this disease is the same as that of epithelial ovarian cancer (480,483,489–495). Exploratory laparotomy is necessary to remove the primary tumor, to stage the disease, and to resect metastases. After surgery, the chemotherapy is the same as with epithelial ovarian cancer (i.e., *carboplatin* and *paclitaxel*).

Surgery

Patients with tubal carcinoma should undergo total abdominal hysterectomy and bilateral salpingo-oophorectomy (3). If there is no evidence of gross tumor spread, a staging operation is performed. The retroperitoneal lymph nodes should be adequately evaluated, and peritoneal cytologic studies and biopsies should be performed, along with an infracolic omentectomy.

In patients with metastatic disease, an effort should be made to remove as much tumor bulk as possible. The role of cytoreductive surgery in this disease is unclear, but extrapolation from the experience with epithelial ovarian cancer indicates that significant benefit might be expected, particularly if all macroscopic disease can be resected (490).

Chemotherapy

As with epithelial ovarian cancer, the most active agents are *platinum* and the *taxanes* (489,490). **The recommended treatment for fallopian tube cancer is the same as that for epithelial ovarian cancer (i.e., *platinum* and *taxane*-based chemotherapy).** A variety of other chemotherapeutic agents that are effective against recurrent ovarian cancer appear to be active in recurrent or persistent fallopian tube carcinomas. These agents include *docetaxel*, *etoposide*, *topotecan*, *gemcitabine*, and liposomally encapsulated *doxorubicin* (491–495). As data on well-staged lesions are scarce, it is unclear whether patients with disease confined to the fallopian tube (i.e., a stage IA, grade 1 or 2 carcinoma) benefit from additional therapy.

Table 37.9 FIGO Staging for Carcinoma of the Fallopian Tube

Stage 0	**Carcinoma *in situ* (limited to tubal mucosa).**
Stage I	**Growth is limited to the fallopian tubes.**
IA	Growth is limited to one tube with extension into the submucosa[c] and/or muscularis but not penetrating the serosal surface; no ascites.
IB	Growth is limited to both tubes with extension into the submucosa[c] and/or muscularis but not penetrating the serosal surface; no ascites.
IB	Tumor either stage IA or IB but with tumor extension through or onto the tubal serosa; or with ascites present containing malignant cells or with positive peritoneal washings.
Stage II	**Growth involving one or both fallopian tubes with pelvic extension.**
IIA	Extension and/or metastasis to the uterus and/or ovaries.
IIB	Extension to other pelvic tissues.
IIC	Tumor either stage IIA or IIB but with tumor extension through or onto the tubal serosa; or with ascites present containing malignant cells or with positive peritoneal washings.
Stage III	**Tumor involves one or both fallopian tubes with peritoneal implants outside of the pelvis and/or positive retroperitoneal or inguinal nodes. Superficial liver metastases equals stage III. Tumor appears limited to the true pelvis but with histologically proven malignant extension to the small bowel or omentum.**
IIIA	Tumor is grossly limited to the true pelvis with negative nodes but with histologically confirmed microscopic seeding of abdominal peritoneal surfaces.
IIIB	Tumor involving one or both tubes with histologically confirmed implants of abdominal peritoneal surfaces, none exceeding 2 cm in diameter. Lymph nodes are negative.
IIIC	Abdominal implants greater than 2 cm in diameter and/or positive retroperitoneal or inguinal nodes.
Stage IV	**Growth involving one or both fallopian tubes with distant metastases. If pleural effusion is present, there must be positive cytology to be stage IV. Parenchymal liver metastases equals stage IV.**

FIGO, International Federation of Gynecology and Obstetrics.
From **Berek JS, Hacker NF.** *Berek and Hacker's Gynecologic Oncology.* 5th ed. Philadelphia, PA: Lippincott Williams & Wilkins, 2010:494; adapted from FIGO Annual Report. Vol 26, *Int J Gynecol Obstet* 2006;105:3–4.

Prognosis

The overall 5-year survival for patients with epithelial tubal carcinomas is about 40%. This number is higher than for patients with ovarian cancer and reflects the somewhat higher proportion of patients diagnosed with early-stage disease. These data may reflect the fact that some advanced stage tubal cancers were classified as ovarian cancers. The reported 5-year survival rate for patients with stage I disease is only about 65%. The 5-year survival rate for patients with stage II disease is 50% to 60%, but it is only 10% to 20% for patients with stages III and IV disease (480,485).

Tubal Sarcomas

Tubal sarcomas, particularly malignant mixed mesodermal tumors, are described, but rare. They occur mainly in the sixth decade and typically are advanced at the time of diagnosis. If all gross disease can be resected, *platinum*-based combination chemotherapy should be tried. Survival is poor, and most patients die of their disease within 2 years (2,450).

References

1. **Siegel R, Ward E, Brawley O, et al.** Cancer statistics, 2011. *CA Cancer J Clin* 2011;61:212–236. http://cacancerjournal.org
2. **Scully RE, Young RH, Clement PB.** Tumors of the ovary, maldeveloped gonads, fallopian tube, and broad ligament. In: *Atlas of tumor pathology*. Washington, DC: Armed Forces Institute of Pathology, 1998:Fascicle 23, 3rd series.
3. **Berek JS, Friedlander M, Hacker NF.** Epithelial ovarian, fallopian tube and peritoneal cancer. In: *Berek and Hacker's gynecologic oncology*. 5th ed. Philadelphia, PA: Lippincott Williams & Wilkins, 2009:443–508.
4. **Kindelberger DW, Lee Y, Miron A, et al.** Intraepithelial carcinoma of the fimbria and pelvic serous carcinoma: evidence for a causal relationship. *Am J Surg Pathol* 2007;31:161–169.
5. **Callahan MJ, Crum CP, Medeiros F, et al.** Primary fallopian tube malignancies in *BRCA*-positive women undergoing surgery for ovarian cancer risk reduction. *J Clin Oncol* 2007;25:3985–3990.

6. **Kurman RJ, Shih IeM.** Pathogenesis of ovarian cancer: lessons from morphology and molecular biology and their clinical implications [review]. *Int J Gynecol Pathol* 2008;27:151–160.

7. **Crum CP, Drapkin R, Miron A, et al.** The distal fallopian tube: a new model for pelvic serous carcinogenesis [review]. *Curr Opin Obstet Gynecol* 2007;19:3–9.

8. **Barnhill DR, Kurman RJ, Brady MF, et al.** Preliminary analysis of the behavior of stage I ovarian serous tumors of low malignant potential: a Gynecologic Oncology Group study. *J Clin Oncol* 1995;13:2752–2756.

9. **Seidman JD, Kurman RJ.** Subclassification of serous borderline tumors of the ovary into benign and malignant types: a clinicopathologic study of 65 advanced stage cases. *Am J Surg Pathol* 1996;20:1331–1345.

10. **Bell DA, Weinstock MA, Scully RE.** Peritoneal implants of ovarian serous borderline tumors: histologic features and prognosis. *Cancer* 1988;62:2212–2222.

11. **Bell DA.** Ovarian surface epithelial-stromal tumors. *Hum Pathol* 1991;22:750–762.

12. **Bell DA, Scully RE.** Clinical perspectives on borderline tumors of the ovary. In: **Greer BE, Berek JS, eds.** *Gynecologic oncology: treatment rationale and techniques.* New York: Elsevier Science, 1991;119–134.

13. **McCaughey WT, Kirk ME, Lester W, et al.** Peritoneal epithelial lesions associated with proliferative serous tumours of the ovary. *Histopathology* 1984;8:195–208.

14. **Longacre TA, McKenney JK, Tazelaar HD, et al.** Ovarian serous tumors of low malignant potential (borderline tumors): outcome-based study of 276 patients with long term (>5 year) follow-up. *Am J Surg Pathol* 2005;29:707–723.

15. **Seidman JD, Kurman RJ.** Ovarian serous borderline tumors: a critical review of the literature with emphasis on prognostic indicators. *Hum Pathol* 2000;31:539–557.

16. **Michael H, Roth LM.** Invasive and noninvasive implants in ovarian serous tumors of low malignant potential. *Cancer* 1986;57:1240–1247.

17. **Gershenson DM, Silva EG.** Serous ovarian tumors of low malignant potential with peritoneal implants. *Cancer* 1990;65:578–585.

18. **Bell DA, Scully RE.** Ovarian serous borderline tumors with stromal microinvasion: a report of 21 cases. *Hum Pathol* 1990;21:397–403.

19. **Sampson JA.** Endometrial carcinoma of the ovary. *Arch Surg* 1925;10:1.

20. **Kurman RJ, Craig JM.** Endometrioid and clear cell carcinomas of the ovary. *Cancer* 1972;29:1653–1664.

21. **Roth LM, Dallenbach-Hellweg G, Czernobilsky B.** Ovarian Brenner tumors. I. Metaplastic proliferating and of low grade potential. *Cancer* 1985;56:582–591.

22. **Robey SS, Silva EG, Gershenson DM, et al.** Transitional cell carcinoma in high-grade stage ovarian carcinoma: an indicator of favorable response to chemotherapy. *Cancer* 1989;63:839–847.

23. **Silva EG, Robey-Cafferty SS, Smith TL, et al.** Ovarian carcinomas with transitional cell carcinoma pattern. *Am J Clin Pathol* 1990;93:457–462.

24. **Austin RM, Norris HJ.** Malignant Brenner tumor and transitional cell carcinoma of the ovary: a comparison. *Int J Gynecol Pathol* 1987;6:29–34.

25. **Piver MS, Jishi MF, Tsukada Y, et al.** Primary peritoneal carcinoma after prophylactic oophorectomy in women with a family history of ovarian cancer: a report of the Gilda Radner Familial Ovarian Cancer Registry. *Cancer* 1993;71:2751–2755.

26. **Fowler JM, Nieberg RK, Schooler TA, et al.** Peritoneal adenocarcinoma (serous) of müllerian type: a subgroup of women presenting with peritoneal carcinomatosis. *Int J Gynecol Cancer* 1994;4:43–51.

27. **Truong LD, Maccato ML, Awalt H, et al.** Serous surface carcinoma of the peritoneum: a clinicopathology study of 22 cases. *Hum Pathol* 1990;21:99–110.

28. **Tobachman JK, Greene MH, Tucker MA, et al.** Intraabdominal carcinomatosis after prophylactic oophorectomy in ovarian cancer-prone families. *Lancet* 1982;2:795–797.

29. **Thor AD, Young RH, Clement PB.** Pathology of the fallopian tube, broad ligament, peritoneum, and pelvic soft tissue. *Hum Pathol* 1991;22:856–867.

30. **Pecorelli S, Odicino F, Maisonneuve P, et al.** Carcinoma of the ovary. Annual report on the results of treatment of gynaecological

cancer, vol. 23. International Federation of Gynecology and Obstetrics. *J Epidemiol Biostat* 1998;3:75–102.

31. **Norris HJ, Jensen RD.** Relative frequency of ovarian neoplasms in children and adolescents. *Cancer* 1972;30:713–719.

32. **Negri E, Franceschi S, Tzonou A, et al.** Pooled analysis of three European case-control studies of epithelial ovarian cancer: I. Reproductive factors and risk of epithelial ovarian cancer. *Int J Cancer* 1991;49:50–56.

33. **Franceschi S, La Vecchia C, Booth M, et al.** Pooled analysis of three European case-control studies of epithelial ovarian cancer: II. Age at menarche and menopause. *Int J Cancer* 1991;49:57–60.

34. **Franceschi S, Parazzini F, Negri E, et al.** Pooled analysis of three European case-control studies of epithelial ovarian cancer: III. Oral contraceptive use. *Int J Cancer* 1991;49:61–65.

35. **Berek JS, Chalas E, Edelson M, et al.** Prophylactic and risk-reducing bilateral salpingo-oophorectomy: recommendations based on risk of ovarian cancer. *Obstet Gynecol* 2010;116:733–743.

36. **Parker WH, Broder MS, Chang E, et al.** Ovarian conservation at the time of hysterectomy and long-term health outcomes in the nurses' health study. *Obstet Gynecol* 2009;113:1027–1037.

37. **Campbell S, Bhan V, Royston P, et al.** Transabdominal ultrasound screening for early ovarian cancer. *BMJ* 1989;299:1363–1367.

38. **Higgins RV, van Nagell JR Jr, Donaldson ES, et al.** Transvaginal sonography as a screening method for ovarian cancer. *Gynecol Oncol* 1989;34:402–406.

39. **van Nagell JR Jr, DePriest PD, Puls LE, et al.** Ovarian cancer screening in asymptomatic postmenopausal women by transvaginal sonography. *Cancer* 1991;68:458–462.

40. **Rulin MC, Preston AL.** Adnexal masses in postmenopausal women. *Obstet Gynecol* 1987;70:578–581.

41. **Kurjak A, Zalud I, Jurkovic D, et al.** Transvaginal color flow Doppler for the assessment of pelvic circulation. *Acta Obstet Gynecol Scand* 1989;68:131–135.

42. **Kurjak A, Zalud I, Alfirevic Z.** Evaluation of adnexal masses with transvaginal color ultrasound. *J Ultrasound Med* 1991;10:295–297.

43. **Rustin GJS, van der Burg MEL, Berek JS.** Tumor markers. *Ann Oncol* 1993;4:S71–S77.

44. **Jacobs I, Davies AP, Bridges J, et al.** Prevalence screening for ovarian cancer in postmenopausal women by CA 125 measurements and ultrasonography. *BMJ* 1993;306:1030–1034.

45. **Jacobs IJ, Skates S, Davies AP, et al.** Risk of diagnosis of ovarian cancer after raised serum CA 125 concentration: a prospective cohort study. *BMJ* 1996;313:1355–1358.

46. **Einhorn N, Sjovall K, Knapp RC, et al.** A prospective evaluation of serum CA 125 levels for early detection of ovarian cancer. *Obstet Gynecol* 1992;80:14–18.

47. **Jacobs IJ, Oram DH, Bast RC Jr.** Strategies for improving the specificity of screening for ovarian cancer with tumor-associated antigens CA125, CA15-3, and TAG 72.3. *Obstet Gynecol* 1992;80:396–399.

48. **Berek JS, Bast RC Jr.** Ovarian cancer screening: the use of serial complementary tumor markers to improve sensitivity and specificity for early detection. *Cancer* 1995;76:2092–2096.

49. **Skates SJ, Xu FJ, Yu YH, et al.** Towards an optimal algorithm for ovarian cancer screening with longitudinal tumour markers. *Cancer* 1995;76:2004–2010.

50. **Jacobs IJ, Skates SJ, MacDonald N, et al.** Screening for ovarian cancer: a pilot randomised controlled trial. *Lancet* 1999;353:1207–1210.

51. **Skates SJ, Menon U, MacDonald N, et al.** Calculation of the risk of ovarian cancer from serial CA-125 values for preclinical detection in postmenopausal women. *J Clin Oncol* 2003;21(Suppl):206–210.

52. **Petricoin EF, Ardekani AM, Hitt BA, et al.** Use of proteomic patterns in serum to identify ovarian cancer. *Lancet* 2002;359:572–577.

53. **Zhang Z, Bast RC Jr, Fung E, et al.** A panel of serum biomarkers identified through proteomic profiling for the detection of early stage ovarian cancer. *Cancer Res* 2004;64:5882–5890.

54. **American College of Obstetricians and Gynecologists.** Genetic risk and screening techniques for epithelial ovarian cancer. ACOG Committee Opinion 117. Washington, DC: ACOG, 1992.

55. **Woodward ER, Sleightholme HV, Considine AM, et al.** Annual surveillance by CA125 and transvaginal ultrasound for ovarian cancer in both high-risk and population risk women is ineffective. *BJOG* 2007;114:1500–1509.

56. **Hermsen BB, Olivier RI, Verheijen RH, et al.** No efficacy of annual gynaecological screening in *BRCA1/2* mutation carriers; an observational follow-up study. *Br J Cancer* 2007;96:1335–1342.

57. **Bourne TH, Campbell S, Reynolds KM, et al.** Screening for early familial ovarian cancer with transvaginal ultrasonography and colour blood flow imaging. *BMJ* 1993;306:1025–1029.

58. **Easton DF, Ford D, Bishop DT.** Breast Cancer Linkage Consortium: breast and ovarian cancer incidence in *BRCA1*-mutation carriers. *Am J Hum Genet* 1995;56:265–271.

59. **Whittemore AS, Gong G, Itnyre J.** Prevalence and contribution of *BRCA1* mutations in breast cancer and ovarian cancer: results from three U.S. population-based case-control studies of ovarian cancer. *Am J Hum Genet* 1997;60:496–504.

60. **Frank TS, Manley SA, Olopade OI, et al.** Sequence analysis of *BRCA1* and *BRCA2:* correlation of mutations with family history and ovarian cancer risk. *J Clin Oncol* 1998;16:2417–2425.

61. **Johannsson OT, Ranstam J, Borg A, et al.** Survival of *BRCA1* breast and ovarian cancer patients: a population-based study from southern Sweden. *J Clin Oncol* 1998;16:397–404.

62. **Burke W, Daly M, Garber J, et al.** Recommendations for follow-up care of individuals with an inherited predisposition to cancer. II. *BRCA1* and *BRCA2*. Cancer Genetics Studies Consortium. *JAMA* 1997;277:997–1003.

63. **Berchuck A, Cirisano F, Lancaster JM, et al.** Role of *BRCA1* mutation screening in the management of familial ovarian cancer. *Am J Obstet Gynecol* 1996;175:738–746.

64. **Struewing JP, Hartge P, Wacholder S, et al.** The risk of cancer associated with specific mutations of *BRCA1* and *BRCA2* among Ashkenazi Jews. *N Engl J Med* 1997;336:1401–1408.

65. **Beller U, Halle D, Catane R, et al.** High frequency of *BRCA1* and *BRCA2* germline mutations in Ashkenazi Jewish ovarian cancer patients, regardless of family history. *Gynecol Oncol* 1997;67:123–126.

66. **Lerman C, Narod S, Schulman K, et al.** *BRCA1* testing in families with hereditary breast-ovarian cancer: a prospective study of patient decision making and outcomes. *JAMA* 1996;275:1885–1892.

67. **Risch HA, McLaughlin JR, Cole DE, et al.** Population *BRCA1* and *BRCA2* mutation frequencies and cancer penetrances: a kin-cohort study in Ontario, Canada. *J Natl Cancer Inst.* 2006;98:1694–1706.

68. **Brozek I, Ochman K, Debniak J, et al.** High frequency of *BRCA1/2* germline mutations in consecutive ovarian cancer patients in Poland. *Gynecol Oncol* 2008;108:433–437.

69. **Chetrit A, Hirsh-Yechezkel G, Ben-David Y, et al.** Effect of *BRCA1/2* mutations on long-term survival of patients with invasive ovarian cancer: the national Israeli study of ovarian cancer. *J Clin Oncol* 2008;26:20–25.

70. **Ponder B.** Genetic testing for cancer risk. *Science* 1997;278:1050–1058.

71. **Lynch HT, Cavalieri RJ, Lynch JF, et al.** Gynecologic cancer clues to Lynch syndrome II diagnosis: a family report. *Gynecol Oncol* 1992;44:198–203.

72. **American Society of Clinical Oncology.** Genetic testing for cancer susceptibility. *J Clin Oncol* 1996;14:1730–1736.

73. **King MC, Marks JH, Mandell JB, et al.** Breast and ovarian cancer risks due to inherited mutations in *BRCA1* and *BRCA2*. *Science* 2003;302:643–646.

74. **NIH Consensus Development Panel on Ovarian Cancer.** Ovarian cancer: screening, treatment and follow-up. *JAMA* 1995;273:491–497.

75. **Greene MH, Piedmonte M, Alberts D, et al.** Prospective study of risk-reducing salpingo-oophorectomy and longitudinal CA-125 screening among women at increased genetic risk of ovarian cancer: design and baseline characteristics: a Gynecologic Oncology Group Study. *Cancer Epidemiol Biomarkers Prev* 2008;17:594–604.

76. **Narod SA, Risch H, Moslehi R, et al.** Oral contraceptives and the risk of hereditary ovarian cancer. *N Engl J Med* 1998;339:424–428.

77. **Averette HE, Nguyen HN.** The role of prophylactic oophorectomy in cancer prevention. *Gynecol Oncol* 1994;55:S38–S41.

78. **Kauff ND, Satagopan JM, Robson ME, et al.** Risk-reducing salpingo-oophorectomy in women with a *BRCA1* or *BRCA2* mutation. *N Engl J Med* 2002;346:1609–1615.

79. **Rebbeck TR, Lynch HT, Neuhausen SL, et al.** Prevention and Observation of Surgical End Points Study Group. Prophylactic oophorectomy in carriers of *BRCA1* or *BRCA2* mutations. *N Engl J Med* 2002;346:1616–1622.

80. **Haber D.** Prophylactic oophorectomy to reduce the risk of ovarian and breast cancer in carriers of *BRCA* mutations. *N Engl J Med* 2002;346:1660–1661.

81. **Rebbeck TR, Levin AM, Eisen A, et al.** Breast cancer risk after bilateral prophylactic oophorectomy in *BRCA1* mutation carriers. *J Natl Cancer Inst* 1999;91:1475–1479.

82. **Schrag D, Kuntz KM, Garber JE, et al.** Decision analysis—effects of prophylactic mastectomy and oophorectomy on life expectancy among women with *BRCA1* and *BRCA2* mutations. *N Engl J Med* 1997;336:1465–1471 [erratum, *N Engl J Med* 1997;337:434].

83. **Li AJ, Karlan BY.** Surgical advances in the treatment of ovarian cancer. *Hematol Oncol Clin North Am* 2003;17:945–956.

84. **Ben David Y, Chetrit A, Hirsh-Yechezkel G, et al.** Effect of *BRCA* mutations on the length of survival in epithelial ovarian tumors. *J Clin Oncol* 2002;20:463–466.

85. **Smith EM, Anderson B.** The effects of symptoms and delay in seeking diagnosis on stage of disease at diagnosis among women with cancers of the ovary. *Cancer* 1985;56:2727–2732.

86. **Goff BA, Mandel LS, Muntz HG, et al.** Ovarian cancer diagnosis: results of a national ovarian cancer survey. *Cancer* 2000;89:2068–2075.

87. **Olson SSH, Mignone L, Nakraseive C, et al.** Symptoms of ovarian cancer. *Obstet Gynecol* 2001;98:212–217.

88. **Goff BA, Mandel LS, Drescher CW, et al.** Development of an ovarian cancer symptom index: possibilities for earlier detection. *Cancer* 2007;109:221–227.

89. **Olsen CM, Cnossen J, Green AC, et al.** Comparison of symptoms and presentation of women with benign, low malignant potential and invasive ovarian tumors. *Eur J Gynaecol Oncol* 2007;28:376–380.

90. **Hogg R, Friedlander M.** Biology of epithelial ovarian cancer: implications for screening women at high genetic risk. *J Clin Oncol* 2004;22:1315–1327.

91. **Barber HK, Grober EA.** The PMPO syndrome (postmenopausal palpable ovary syndrome). *Obstet Gynecol* 1971;138:921–923.

92. **Malkasian GD, Knapp RC, Lavin PT, et al.** Preoperative evaluation of serum CA 125 levels in premenopausal and postmenopausal patients with pelvic masses: discrimination of benign from malignant disease. *Am J Obstet Gynecol* 1988;159:341–346.

93. **Campbell S, Royston P, Bhan V, et al.** Novel screening strategies for early ovarian cancer by transabdominal ultrasonography. *BJOG* 1990;97:304–311.

94. **van Nagell JR Jr, Higgins RV, Donaldson ES, et al.** Transvaginal sonography as a screening method for ovarian cancer: a report of the first 1000 cases screened. *Cancer* 1990;65:573–577.

95. **van Nagell JR Jr, Gallion HH, Pavlik EJ, et al.** Ovarian cancer screening. *Cancer* 1995;76:2086–2091.

96. **van Nagell JR Jr, DePriest PD, Reedy MB, et al.** The efficacy of transvaginal sonographic screening in asymptomatic women at risk for ovarian cancer. *Gynecol Oncol* 2000;77:350–356.

97. **Ueland FR, DePriest PD, Pavlik EJ, et al.** Preoperative differentiation of malignant from benign ovarian tumors: the efficacy of morphology indexing and Doppler flow sonography. *Gynecol Oncol* 2003;91:46–50.

98. **Cohen LS, Escobar PF, Scharm C, et al.** Three-dimensional power Doppler ultrasound improves the diagnostic accuracy for ovarian cancer prediction. *Gynecol Oncol* 2001;82:40–48.

99. **Kurjak A, Kupesic S, Sparac V, et al.** The detection of stage I ovarian cancer by three-dimensional sonography and power Doppler. *Gynecol Oncol* 2003;90:258–264.

100. **Nardo LG, Kroon ND, Reginald PW.** Persistent unilocular ovarian cysts in a general population of postmenopausal women: is there a place for expectant management? *Obstet Gynecol* 2003;102:589–593.

101. **Modesitt SC, Pavlik EJ, Ueland FR, et al.** Risk of malignancy in unilocular ovarian cystic tumors less than 10 centimeters in diameter. *Obstet Gynecol* 2003;102:594–599.

102. **Roman LD.** Small cystic pelvic masses in older women: is surgical removal necessary? *Gynecol Oncol* 1998;69:1–2.

103. **Bristow RE, Duska LR, Lambrou NC, et al.** A model for predicting surgical outcome in patients with advanced ovarian carcinoma using computed tomography. *Cancer* 2000;89:1532–1540.

104. **Togashi K.** Ovarian cancer: the clinical role of US, CT, and MRI. *Eur Radiol* 2003;13(Suppl 4):L87–L104.

105. **Jung SE, Lee JM, Rha SE, et al.** CT and MR imaging of ovarian tumors with emphasis on differential diagnosis. *Radiographics* 2002;22:1305–1325.

106. **Makhija S, Howden N, Edwards R, et al.** Positron emission tomography/computed tomography imaging for the detection of recurrent ovarian and fallopian tube carcinoma: a retrospective review. *Gynecol Oncol* 2002;85:53–58.

107. **Kurokawa T, Yoshida Y, Kawahara K, et al.** Whole-body PET with FDG is useful for following up an ovarian cancer patient with only rising CA-125 levels within the normal range. *Ann Nucl Med* 2002;16:491–493.

108. **Hacker NF, Berek JS, Lagasse LD.** Gastrointestinal operations in gynecologic oncology. In: **Knapp RE, Berkowitz RS, eds.** *Gynecologic oncology.* 2nd ed. New York: McGraw-Hill, 1993:361–375.

109. **Plentl AM, Friedman EA.** *Lymphatic system of the female genitalia.* Philadelphia, PA: WB Saunders, 1971.

110. **Chen SS, Lee L.** Incidence of para-aortic and pelvic lymph node metastasis in epithelial ovarian cancer. *Gynecol Oncol* 1983;16:95–100.

111. **Burghardt E, Pickel H, Lahousen M, et al.** Pelvic lymphadenectomy in operative treatment of ovarian cancer. *Am J Obstet Gynecol* 1986;155:315–319.

112. **Dauplat J, Hacker NF, Neiberg RK, et al.** Distant metastasis in epithelial ovarian carcinoma. *Cancer* 1987;60:1561–1566.

113. **Krag KJ, Canellos GP, Griffiths CT, et al.** Predictive factors for long term survival in patients with advanced ovarian cancer. *Gynecol Oncol* 1989;34:88–93.

114. **Young RC, Walton LA, Ellenberg SS, et al.** Adjuvant therapy in stage I and stage II epithelial ovarian cancer: results of two prospective randomized trials. *N Engl J Med* 1990;322:1021–1027.

115. **Bjorkholm E, Pettersson F, Einhorn N, et al.** Long term follow-up and prognostic factors in ovarian carcinoma: the Radiumhemmet series 1958 to 1973. *Acta Radiol Oncol* 1982;21:413–419.

116. **Malkasian GD, Decker DG, Webb MJ.** Histology of epithelial tumours of the ovary: clinical usefulness and prognostic significance of histologic classification and grading. *Semin Oncol* 1975;2:191–201.

117. **Silverberg SG.** Prognostic significance of pathologic features of ovarian carcinoma. *Curr Top Pathol* 1989;78:85–109.

118. **Jacobs AJ, Deligdisch L, Deppe G, et al.** Histologic correlations of virulence in ovarian adenocarcinoma. 1. Effects of differentiation. *Am J Obstet Gynecol* 1982;143:574–580.

119. **Baak JP, Langley FA, Talerman A, et al.** Interpathologist and intra-pathologist disagreement in ovarian tumor grading and typing. *Anal Quant Cytol Histol* 1986;8:354–357.

120. **Hernandez E, Bhagavan BS, Parmley TH, et al.** Interobserver variability in the interpretation of epithelial ovarian cancer. *Gynecol Oncol* 1984;17:117–123.

121. **Baak JP, Chan KK, Stolk JG, et al.** Prognostic factors in borderline and invasive ovarian tumours of the common epithelial type. *Pathol Res Pract* 1987;182:755–774.

122. **Berek JS, Martínez-Maza O, Hamilton T, et al.** Molecular and biological factors in the pathogenesis of ovarian cancer. *Ann Oncol* 1993;4:S3–S16.

123. **Omura GA, Brady MF, Homesley HD, et al.** Long-term follow-up and prognostic factor analysis in advanced ovarian carcinoma: the Gynecologic Oncology Group experience. *J Clin Oncol* 1991;9:1138–1150.

124. **Voest EE, van Houwelingen JC, Neijt JP.** A meta-analysis of prognostic factors in advanced ovarian cancer with median survival and overall survival measured with log (relative risk) as main objectives. *Eur J Cancer Clin Oncol* 1989;25:711–720.

125. **van Houwelingen JC, ten Bokkel Huinink WW, van der Burg ATM, et al.** Predictability of the survival of patients with ovarian cancer. *J Clin Oncol* 1989;7:769–773.

126. **Berek JS, Bertlesen K, du Bois A, et al.** Advanced epithelial ovarian cancer: 1998 consensus statement. *Ann Oncol* 1999;10(Suppl 1):87–92.

127. **Sharp F, Blackett AD, Berek JS, et al.** Conclusions and recommendations from the Helene Harris Memorial Trust sixth biennial international forum on ovarian cancer. *Int J Gynecol Cancer* 1997;7:416–424.

128. **Dembo AJ, Davy M, Stenwig AE, et al.** Prognostic factors in patients with stage I epithelial ovarian cancer. *Obstet Gynecol* 1990;75:263–273.

129. **Sjövall K, Nilsson B, Einhorn N.** Different types of rupture of the tumor capsule and the impact on survival in early ovarian cancer. *Int J Gynecol Cancer* 1994;4:333–336.

130. **Sevelda P, Dittich C, Salzer H.** Prognostic value of the rupture of the capsule in stage I epithelial ovarian carcinoma. *Gynecol Oncol* 1989;35:321–322.

131. **Vergote I, De Branbanter J, Fyles A, et al.** Prognostic importance of degree of differentiation and cyst rupture in stage I epithelial ovarian carcinoma. *Lancet* 2001;357:176–182.

132. **Berek JS, Hacker NF.** Staging and second-look operations in ovarian cancer. In: **Alberts DS, Surwit EA, eds.** *Ovarian cancer.* Boston, MA: Martinus Nijhoff, 1985:109–127.

133. **Young RC, Decker DG, Wharton JT, et al.** Staging laparotomy in early ovarian cancer. *JAMA* 1983;250:3072–3076.

134. **Buchsbaum HJ, Lifshitz S.** Staging and surgical evaluation of ovarian cancer. *Semin Oncol* 1984;11:227–237.

135. **Yoshimuna S, Scully RE, Bell DA, et al.** Correlation of ascitic fluid cytology with histologic findings before and after treatment of ovarian cancer. *Am J Obstet Gynecol* 1984;148:716–721.

136. **Piver MS, Barlow JJ, Lele SB.** Incidence of subclinical metastasis in stage I and II ovarian carcinoma. *Obstet Gynecol* 1978;52:100–104.

137. **Delgado G, Chun B, Caglar H.** Para-aortic lymphadenectomy in gynecologic malignancies confined to the pelvis. *Obstet Gynecol* 1977;50:418–423.

138. **Rosenoff SH, Young RC, Anderson T, et al.** Peritoneoscopy: a valuable staging tool in ovarian carcinoma. *Ann Intern Med* 1975;83:37–41.

139. **Knapp RC, Friedman EA.** Aortic lymph node metastases in early ovarian cancer. *Am J Obstet Gynecol* 1974;119:1013–1017.

140. **Guthrie D, Davy MLJ, Phillips PR.** Study of 656 patients with "early" ovarian cancer. *Gynecol Oncol* 1984;17:363–369.

141. **Lim-Tan SK, Cajigas HE, Scully RE.** Ovarian cystectomy for serous borderline tumors: a follow-up study of 35 cases. *Obstet Gynecol* 1988;72:775–781.

142. **Green JA.** Early ovarian cancer—time for a rethink on stage? *Gynecol Oncol* 2003;90:235–237.

143. **Harlan LC, Clegg LX, Trimble EL.** Trends in surgery and chemotherapy for women diagnosed with ovarian cancer in the United States. *J Clin Oncol* 2003;21:3488–3494.

144. **Griffiths CT.** Surgical resection of tumor bulk in the primary treatment of ovarian carcinoma. *Natl Cancer Inst Monogr* 1975;42:101–104.

145. **Hacker NF, Berek JS.** Cytoreductive surgery in ovarian cancer. In: **Albert PS, Surwit EA, eds.** *Ovarian cancer.* Boston, MA: Martinus Nijhoff, 1986:53–67.

146. **Heintz APM, Berek JS.** Cytoreductive surgery in ovarian cancer. In: **Piver MS, eds.** *Ovarian cancer.* Edinburgh, UK: Churchill Livingstone, 1987:129–143.

147. **Hacker NF, Berek JS, Lagasse LD, et al.** Primary cytoreductive surgery for epithelial ovarian cancer. *Obstet Gynecol* 1983;61:413–420.

148. **Van Lindert AM, Alsbach GJ, Barents JW, et al.** The role of the abdominal radical tumor reduction procedure (ARTR) in the treatment of ovarian cancer. In: **Heintz APM, Griffiths CT, Trimbos JB, eds.** *Surgery in gynecologic oncology.* The Hague, Netherlands: Martinus Nijhoff, 1984:275–287.

149. **Hoskins WJ, Bundy BN, Thigpen TJ, et al.** The influence of cytoreductive surgery on recurrence-free interval and survival in small volume stage III epithelial ovarian cancer: a Gynecologic Oncology Group study. *Gynecol Oncol* 1992;47:159–166.

150. **Farias-Eisner R, Teng F, Oliveira M, et al.** The influence of tumor grade, distribution and extent of carcinomatosis in minimal residual stage III epithelial ovarian cancer after optimal primary cytoreductive surgery. *Gynecol Oncol* 1995;5:108–110.

151. **Hunter RW, Alexander NDE, Soutter WP.** Meta-analysis of surgery in advanced ovarian carcinoma: is maximum cytoreductive surgery an independent determinant of prognosis? *Am J Obstet Gynecol* 1992;166:504–511.

152. **Berek JS.** Complete debulking of advanced ovarian cancer. *Cancer J* 1996;2:134–135.

153. **Hacker NF.** Cytoreduction for advanced ovarian cancer in perspective. *Int J Gynecol Cancer* 1996;6:159–160.

154. **Berek JS, Hacker NF, Lagasse LD.** Rectosigmoid colectomy and reanastomosis to facilitate resection of primary and recurrent gynecologic cancer. *Obstet Gynecol* 1984;64:715–720.

155. **Berek JS, Hacker NF, Lagasse LD, et al.** Lower urinary tract resection as part of cytoreductive surgery for ovarian cancer. *Gynecol Oncol* 1982;13:87–92.

156. **Heintz AM, Hacker NF, Berek JS, et al.** Cytoreductive surgery in ovarian carcinoma: feasibility and morbidity. *Obstet Gynecol* 1986;67:783–788.

157. **Deppe G, Malviya VK, Boike G, et al.** Surgical approach to diaphragmatic metastases from ovarian cancer. *Gynecol Oncol* 1986;24:258–260.

158. **Montz FJ, Schlaerth J, Berek JS.** Resection of diaphragmatic peritoneum and muscle: role in cytoreductive surgery for ovarian carcinoma. *Gynecol Oncol* 1989;35:338–340.

159. **Brand E, Pearlman N.** Electrosurgical debulking of ovarian cancer: a new technique using the argon beam coagulator. *Gynecol Oncol* 1990;39:115–118.

160. **Deppe G, Malviya VK, Boike G, et al.** Use of Cavitron surgical aspirator for debulking of diaphragmatic metastases in patients with advanced carcinoma of the ovaries. *Surg Gynecol Obstet* 1989;168:455–456.

161. **Chen SS, Bochner R.** Assessment of morbidity and mortality in primary cytoreductive surgery for advanced ovarian cancer. *Gynecol Oncol* 1985;20:190–195.

162. **Venesmaa P, Ylikorkala O.** Morbidity and mortality associated with primary and repeat operations for ovarian cancer. *Obstet Gynecol* 1992;79:168–172.

163. **Bristow RE, Tomacruz RS, Armstrong DK, et al.** Survival effect of maximal cytoreductive surgery for advanced ovarian carcinoma during the *platinum* era: a meta-analysis. *J Clin Oncol* 2002;20:1248–1259.

164. **Panici PB, Maggioni A, Hacker N, et al.** Systematic aortic and pelvic lymphadenectomy versus resection of bulky nodes only in optimally debulked advanced ovarian cancer: a randomized clinical trial. *J Natl Cancer Inst* 2005;20;97:560–566.

165. **van der Burg MEL, van Lent M, Buyse M, et al.** The effect of debulking surgery after induction chemotherapy on the prognosis in advanced epithelial ovarian cancer. *N Engl J Med* 1995;332:629–634.

166. **Berek JS.** Interval debulking of epithelial ovarian cancer: an interim measure. *N Engl J Med* 1995;332:675–677.

167. **Rose PG, Nerenstone S, Brady MF, et al.** Secondary surgical cytoreduction for advanced ovarian carcinoma. *N Engl J Med* 2004;351:2489–2497.

168. **Junor EJ, Hole DJ, McNulty L, et al.** Specialist gynecologists and survival outcome in ovarian cancer: a Scottish National Study of 1966 patients. *Br J Obstet Gyn* 1999;106:1130–1136.

169. **Tingulstad S, Skjeldestad FE, Hagen B.** The effect of centralization of primary surgery on survival in ovarian cancer patients. *Obstet Gynecol* 2003;102:499–505.

170. **Paulson T, Kjaerheim K, Kaern J, et al.** Improved short-term survival for advanced ovarian, tubal, and peritoneal cancer patients operated at teaching hospitals. *Int J Gynecol Cancer* 2006;16:11–17.

171. **Engelen MJA, Kos HE, Willemse PHB, et al.** Surgery by consultant gynecologic oncologists improves survival in patients with ovarian carcinoma. *Cancer* 2006;106:589–598.

172. **Hreshchyshyn MM, Park RC, Blessing JA, et al.** The role of adjuvant therapy in stage I ovarian cancer. *Am J Obstet Gynecol* 1980;138:139–145.

173. **Berek JS.** Adjuvant therapy for early-stage ovarian cancer. *N Engl J Med* 1990;322:1076–1078.

174. **Ahmed FY, Wiltshaw E, Hern RP, et al.** Natural history and prognosis of untreated stage I epithelial ovarian carcinoma. *J Clin Oncol* 1996;14:2968–2975.

175. **Finn CB, Luesley DM, Buxton EJ, et al.** Is stage I epithelial ovarian cancer overtreated both surgically and systemically? Results of a five-year cancer registry review. *Br J Obstet Gyn* 1992;99:54–58.

176. **Vergote I, Vergote S, De Vos LN, et al.** Randomized trial comparing cisplatin with radioactive phosphorus or whole abdominal irradiation as adjuvant treatment of ovarian cancer. *Cancer* 1992;69:741–749.

177. **Rubin SC, Wong GY, Curtin JP, et al.** Platinum based chemotherapy of high risk stage I epithelial ovarian cancer following comprehensive surgical staging. *Obstet Gynecol* 1993;82:143–147.

178. **Young RC, Brady MF, Nieberg RM, et al.** Adjuvant treatment for ovarian cancer: a randomized phase III trial of intraperitoneal ^{32}P or intravenous cyclophosphamide and cisplatin: a Gynecologic Oncology Group study. *J Clin Oncol* 2003;21:4350–4355.

179. **Bolis G, Colombo N, Pecorelli S, et al.** Adjuvant treatment for early epithelial ovarian cancer: results of two randomized clinical trials comparing cisplatin to no further treatment or chromic phosphate (^{32}P). *Ann Oncol* 1995;6:887–893.

180. **Young RC, Pecorelli S.** Management of early ovarian cancer. *Semin Oncol* 1998;25:335–339.

181. **Colombo N, Chiari S, Maggioni A, et al.** Controversial issues in the management of early epithelial ovarian cancer: conservative surgery and the role of adjuvant therapy. *Gynecol Oncol* 1994;55:S47–S51.

182. **Colombo N, Maggioni A, Bocciolone L, et al.** Multimodality therapy of early-stage (FIGO I-II) ovarian cancer: review of surgical management and postoperative adjuvant treatment. *Int J Gynecol Cancer* 1996;6:13–17.

183. **Vermorken JB, Pecorelli S.** Clinical trials in patients with epithelial ovarian cancer: past, present and future. *Eur J Surg Oncol* 1996;22:455–466.

184. **Tropé C, Kaern J, Hogberg T, et al.** Randomized study on adjuvant chemotherapy in stage I high-risk ovarian cancer with evaluation of DNA-ploidy as prognostic instrument. *Ann Oncol* 2000;11:259–261.

185. **Gadducci A, Sartori E, Maggino T, et al.** Analysis of failure in patients with stage I ovarian cancer: an Italian multicenter study. *Int J Gynecol Cancer* 1997;7:445–450.

186. **Greene MH, Boice JD, Greer BE, et al.** Acute nonlymphocytic leukemia after therapy with alkylating agents for ovarian cancer. *N Engl J Med* 1982;307:1416–1421.

187. **Travis LB, Holowaty EJ, Bergfeldt K, et al.** Risk of leukemia after platinum-based chemotherapy for ovarian cancer. *N Engl J Med* 1999;340:351–357.

188. **Trimbos JB, Vergote I, Bolis G, et al.** Impact of adjuvant chemotherapy and surgical staging in early-stage ovarian carcinoma: European Organisation for Research and Treatment of Cancer-Adjuvant Chemotherapy in Ovarian Neoplasm Trial. *J Natl Cancer Inst* 2003;95:113–125.

189. **International Collaborative Ovarian Neoplasm (ICON1) Collaborators.** International collaborative ovarian neoplasm trial 1: a randomized trial of adjuvant chemotherapy in women with early-stage ovarian cancer. *J Natl Cancer Inst* 2003;95:125–132.

190. **Trimbos JB, Parmar M, Vergote I, et al.** International Collaborative Ovarian Neoplasm Trial 1 and Adjuvant Chemotherapy in Ovarian Neoplasm Trial: two parallel randomized phase III trials of adjuvant chemotherapy in patients with early-stage ovarian carcinoma. *J Natl Cancer Inst* 2003;95:105–112.

191. **Bell J, Brady MF, Young RC, et al.** Randomized phase III trial of three versus six cycles of adjuvant carboplatin and paclitaxel in early stage epithelial ovarian carcinoma: a Gynecologic Oncology Group study. *Gynecol Oncol* 2006;102:432–439.

192. **Bookman MA, McGuire WP, Kilpatrick D, et al.** Carboplatin and paclitaxel in ovarian carcinoma: a phase I study of the Gynecologic Oncology Group. *J Clin Oncol* 1996;14:1895–1902.

193. **Eisenhauer EA, ten Bokkel Huinink WW, Swenerton KD, et al.** European-Canadian randomized trial of paclitaxel in relapsed ovarian cancer: high-dose versus low-dose and long versus short infusion. *J Clin Oncol* 1994;12:2654–2666.

194. **McGuire WP, Hoskins WJ, Brady MF, et al.** Cyclophosphamide and cisplatin compared with paclitaxel and cisplatin in patients with stage III and stage IV ovarian cancer. *N Engl J Med* 1996;334:1–6.

195. **Piccart MJ, Bertelsen K, Stuart G, et al.** Long-term follow-up confirms a survival advantage of the paclitaxel-cisplatin regimen over the cyclophosphamide-cisplatin combination in advanced ovarian cancer. *Int J Gynecol Cancer* 2003;13:144–148.

196. **Muggia FM, Braly PS, Brady MF, et al.** Phase III randomized study of cisplatin versus paclitaxel versus cisplatin and paclitaxel in patients with suboptimal stage III or IV ovarian cancer: a Gynecologic Oncology Group study. *J Clin Oncol* 2000;18:106–115.

197. **Advanced Ovarian Cancer Trialists Group.** Chemotherapy in advanced ovarian cancer: an overview of randomized clinical trials. *BMJ* 1991;303:884–891.

198. **Omura G, Bundy B, Berek JS, et al.** Randomized trial of cyclophosphamide plus cisplatin with or without doxorubicin in ovarian carcinoma: a Gynecologic Oncology Group study. *J Clin Oncol* 1989;7:457–465.

199. **Ovarian Cancer Meta-analysis Project.** Cyclophosphamide plus cisplatin versus cyclophosphamide, doxorubicin, and cisplatin chemotherapy of ovarian carcinoma: a meta-analysis. *J Clin Oncol* 1991;9:1668–1674.

200. **Swenerton K, Jeffrey J, Stuart G, et al.** Cisplatin-cyclophosphamide versus carboplatin-cyclophosphamide in advanced ovarian cancer: a randomized phase III study of the National Cancer Institute of Canada Clinical Trials Group. *J Clin Oncol* 1992;10:718–726.

201. **Ozols RF, Bundy BN, Greer B, et al.** Phase III trial of carboplatin and paclitaxel versus cisplatin and paclitaxel in patients with optimally resected stage III ovarian cancer: a Gynecologic Oncology Group study. *J Clin Oncol* 2003;21:3194–3200.

202. **Du Bois A, Luck HJ, Meier W, et al.** A randomized clinical trial of cisplatin/paclitaxel versus carboplatin/paclitaxel as first-line treatment of ovarian cancer. *J Natl Cancer Inst* 2003;95:1320–1330.

203. **Polverino G, Parazzini F, Stellato G, et al.** Survival and prognostic factors of women with advanced ovarian cancer and complete response after a carboplatin-paclitaxel chemotherapy. *Gynecol Oncol* 2005;99:343–347.

204. **Alberts DS, Green S, Hannigan EV, et al.** Improved therapeutic index of carboplatin plus cyclophosphamide versus cisplatin plus cyclophosphamide: final report by the Southwest Oncology Group of a phase III randomized trial in stages III (suboptimal) and IV ovarian cancer. *J Clin Oncol* 1992;10:706–717.

205. **McGuire WP, Hoskins WJ, Brady MS, et al.** An assessment of dose-intensive therapy in suboptimally debulked ovarian cancer: a Gynecologic Oncology Group study. *J Clin Oncol* 1995;13:1589–1599.

206. **Ozols RF, Ostchega Y, Curt G, et al.** High-dose carboplatin in refractory ovarian cancer patients. *J Clin Oncol* 1987;5:197–201.

207. **Calvert AH, Newell DR, Gumbrell LA, et al.** Carboplatin dosage: prospective evaluation of a simple formula based on renal function. *J Clin Oncol* 1989;7:1748–1756.

208. **The International Collaborative Ovarian Neoplasm (ICON) Group.** Paclitaxel plus carboplatin versus standard chemotherapy with either single agent carboplatin or cyclophosphamide, doxorubicin, and cisplatin in women with ovarian cancer: the ICON3 randomised trial. *Lancet* 2002;360:505–515.

209. **The ICON Collaborators.** International Collaborative Ovarian Neoplasm Study 2 (ICON2): randomised trial of single-agent carboplatin against three-drug combination of CAP (cyclophosphamide, doxorubicin, and cisplatin) in women with ovarian cancer. *Lancet* 1998;352:1571–1576.

210. **Vasey PA, Paul J, Birt A, et al.** Docetaxel and cisplatin in combination as first-line chemotherapy for advanced epithelial ovarian cancer. Scottish Gynaecological Cancer Trials Group. *J Clin Oncol* 1999;17:2069–2080.

211. **Bookman MA, Brady MF, McGuire WP, et al.** Evaluation of new platinum-based treatment regimens in advanced-stage ovarian cancer: A phase III tiral of the Gynecologic Cancer InterGroup. *J Clin Oncol* 2009;27:1419–1425.

212. **Alberts DS, Liu PY, Hannigan EV, et al.** Intraperitoneal cisplatin plus intravenous cyclophosphamide versus intravenous cisplatin plus intravenous cyclophosphamide for stage III ovarian cancer. *N Engl J Med* 1996;335:1950–1955.

213. **Markman M, Bundy BN, Alberts DS, et al.** Phase III trial of standard-dose intravenous cisplatin plus paclitaxel versus moderately high-dose intravenous carboplatin followed by intraperitoneal paclitaxel and intraperitoneal cisplatin in small-volume stage III ovarian cancer: an intergroup study of the Gynecologic Oncology Group, Southwestern Oncology Group, and the Eastern Cooperative Oncology Group. *J Clin Oncol* 2001;19:1001–1007.

214. **Armstrong DK, Bundy B, Wenzel L, et al.** Intraperitoneal cisplatin and paclitaxel in ovarian cancer. *N Engl J Medl* 2006;354:34–43.

215. **Walker JL, Armstrong DK, Huang HQ, et al.** Intraperitoneal catheter outcomes in a phase III trial of intravenous versus intraperitoneal chemotherapy in optimal stage III ovarian and primary peritoneal cancer: a Gynecologic Oncology Group study. *Gynecol Oncol* 2006;100:27–32.

216. **Jaaback K, Johnson N.** Intraperitoneal chemotherapy for the initial management of primary epithelial ovarian cancer. *Cocharane Database Syst Rev* 2006;1:CD005340

217. **Katsumata N, Yasuda M, Takahashi F, et al.** Dose-dense *paclitaxel* once a week in combination with carboplatin every 3 weeks for advanced ovarian cancer: a phase 3, open-label, randomised controlled trial. *Lancet* 2009;374:1331–1338.

218. **Schwartz PE, Rutherford TJ, Chambers JT, et al.** Neoadjuvant chemotherapy for advanced ovarian cancer: long-term survival. *Gynecol Oncol* 1999;72:93–99.

219. **Shibata K, Kikkawa F, Mika M, et al.** Neoadjuvant chemotherapy for FIGO stage III or IV ovarian cancer: survival benefit and prognostic factors. *Int J Gynecol Cancer* 2003;13:587–592.

220. **Chan YM, Ng TY, Ngan HY, et al.** Quality of life in women treated with neoadjuvant chemotherapy for advanced ovarian cancer: a prospective longitudinal study. *Gynecol Oncol* 2003;88:9–16.

221. **Vergote I, Tropé CG, Amant F, et al.** Neoadjuvant chemotherapy or primary surgery in stage IIIC or IV ovarian cancer. *N Engl J Med* 2010;363:943–953.

222. **Cohen MH, Gootenberg J, Keegan P, et al.** FDA drug approval summary: bevacizumab (Avastin) plus carboplatin and paclitaxel as first-line treatment of advanced/metastatic recurrent nonsquamous non-small cell lung cancer. *Oncologist* 2007;12:713–718.

223. **Miller K, Wang M, Gralow J, et al.** Paclitaxel plus bevacizumab versus paclitaxel alone for metastatic breast cancer. *N Engl J Med* 2007;357:2666–2676.

224. **Hurwitz H, Fehrenbacher L, Novotny W, et al.** Bevacizumab plus irinotecan, fluorouracil, and leucovorin for metastatic colorectal cancer. *N Engl J Med* 2004;350:2335–2342.

225. **Burger RA, Brady MF, Fleming GF, et al.** Phase III trial of bevacizumab in the primary treatment of advanced ovarian, primary peritoneal or fallopian tube cancer: a GOG study. *Int J Gynecol Cancer* 2010;28(Suppl):LBA1.

226. **Pfisterer J, Perren T, Swart AM, et al.** ICON7: A randomised controlled trial of bevacizumab in women with newly diagnosed epithelial ovarian, primary peritoneal or fallopian tube cancer. *Int J Gynecol Cancer* 2010;20(Suppl 2).

227. **Markman M, Liu PY, Wilczynski S, et al.** Phase III randomized trial of 12 versus 3 months of maintenance paclitaxel in patients with advanced ovarian cancer after complete response to platinum and paclitaxel-based chemotherapy: a Southwest Oncology Group and Gynecologic Oncology Group trial. *J Clin Oncol* 2003;21:2460–2465.

228. **Ozols RF.** Maintenance therapy in advanced ovarian cancer: progression-free survival and clinical benefit. *J Clin Oncol* 2003;21:2451–2453.

229. **De Placido S, Scambia G, Di Vagno G, et al.** Topotecan compared with no therapy after response to surgery and carboplatin/paclitaxel in patients with ovarian cancer: Multicenter Italian Trials in Ovarian Cancer (MITO-1) randomized study. *J Clin Oncol* 2004;22:2635–2642.

230. **Pfisterer J, Weber B, Reuss A, et al.** Randomized phase III trial of topotecan following carboplatin and paclitaxel in first-line treatment of advanced ovarian cancer: a Gynecologic Cancer Intergroup Trial of the AGO-OVAR and GINECO. *J Natl Cancer Inst* 2006;98:1036–1045.

231. **Piccart MJ, Floquet A, Scarfone G, et al.** Intraperitoneal cisplatin versus no further treatment: 8-year results of EORTC 55875, a randomized phase III study in ovarian cancer patients with a pathologically complete remission after platinum-based intravenous chemotherapy. *Int J Gynecol Cancer* 2003;13(Suppl 2):196–203.

232. **Berek JS, Taylor PT, Gordon A, et al.** Randomized placebo-controlled study of oregovomab for consolidation of clinical remission in patients with advanced ovarian cancer. *J Clin Oncol* 2004;22:3507–3516.

233. **Berek H, Taylor P, McGuire W, et al.** Oregovomab maintenance monoimmunotherapy does not improve outcomes in advanced ovarian cancer. *J Clin Oncol* 2009;27:418–425.

234. **Verheijen RH, Massuger LF, Benigno BB, et al.** Phase III trial of intraperitoneal therapy with yttrium-90-labeled HMFG1 murine monoclonal antibody in patients with epithelial ovarian cancer after a surgically defined complete remission. *J Clin Oncol* 2004;22:2635–2642.

235. Berek JS, Hacker NF, Lagasse LD, et al. Second-look laparotomy in stage III epithelial ovarian cancer: clinical variables associated with disease status. *Obstet Gynecol* 1984;64:207–212.

236. Copeland LJ, Gershenson DM, Wharton JT, et al. Microscopic disease at second-look laparotomy in advanced ovarian cancer. *Cancer* 1985;55:472–478.

237. Gershenson DM, Copeland LJ, Wharton JT, et al. Prognosis of surgically determined complete responders in advanced ovarian cancer. *Cancer* 1985;55:1129–1135.

238. Smira LR, Stehman FB, Ulbright TM, et al. Second-look laparotomy after chemotherapy in the management of ovarian malignancy. *Am J Obstet Gynecol* 1985;152:661–668.

239. Freidman JB, Weiss NS. Second thoughts about second-look laparotomy in advanced ovarian cancer. *N Engl J Med* 1990;322:1079–1082.

240. Berek JS. Second-look versus second-nature. *Gynecol Oncol* 1992;44:1–2.

241. Rubin SC, Hoskins WJ, Hakes TB, et al. Recurrence after negative second-look laparotomy for ovarian cancer: analysis of risk factors. *Am J Obstet Gynecol* 1988;159:1094–1098.

242. Berek JS, Griffith CT, Leventhal JM. Laparoscopy for second-look evaluation in ovarian cancer. *Obstet Gynecol* 1981;58:192–198.

243. Berek JS, Hacker NF. Laparoscopy in the management of patients with ovarian carcinoma. In: DiSaia P, ed. The treatment of ovarian cancer. Philadelphia, PA: WB Saunders, 1983:213–222.

244. Lele S, Piver MS. Interval laparoscopy prior to second-look laparotomy in ovarian cancer. *Obstet Gynecol* 1986;68:345–347.

245. Berek JS, Knapp RC, Malkasian GD, et al. CA125 serum levels correlated with second-look operations among ovarian cancer patients. *Obstet Gynecol* 1986;67:685–689.

246. Lavin PT, Knapp RC, Malkasian GD, et al. CA125 for the monitoring of ovarian carcinoma during primary therapy. *Obstet Gynecol* 1987;69:223–227.

247. Rustin GJ, Bast RC, Kelloff GJ, et al. Use of CA125 in clinical trial evaluation of new therapeutic drugs for ovarian cancer. *Clin Cancer Res* 2004;10:3919–3926.

248. De Rosa V, Mangioni di Stefano ML, et al. Computed tomography and second-look surgery in ovarian cancer patients: correlation, actual role and limitations of CT scan. *Eur J Gynaecol Oncol* 1995;16:123–129.

249. Lund B, Jacobson K, Rasch L, et al. Correlation of abdominal ultrasound and computed tomography scans with second- or third-look laparotomy in patients with ovarian carcinoma. *Gynecol Oncol* 1990;37:279–283.

250. Berek JS, Hacker NF, Lagasse LD, et al. Survival of patients following secondary cytoreductive surgery in ovarian cancer. *Obstet Gynecol* 1983;61:189–193.

251. Hoskins WJ, Rubin SC, Dulaney E, et al. Influence of secondary cytoreduction at the time of second-look laparotomy on the survival of patients with epithelial ovarian carcinoma. *Gynecol Oncol* 1989;34: 365–371.

252. Bristow RE, Lagasse LD, Karlan BY. Secondary surgical cytoreduction in advanced epithelial ovarian cancer: patient selection and review of the literature. *Cancer* 1996;78:2049–2062.

253. Berek JS, Tropé C, Vergote I. Surgery during chemotherapy and at relapse of ovarian cancer. *Ann Oncol* 1999;10:S3–7.

254. Eisenkop SM, Friedman RL, Spirtos NM. The role of secondary cytoreductive surgery in the treatment of patients with recurrent epithelial ovarian carcinoma. *Cancer* 2000;88:144–153.

255. Gadducci A, Iacconi P, Cosio S, et al. Complete salvage surgical cytoreduction improves further survival of patients with late recurrent ovarian cancer. *Gynecol Oncol* 2000;79:344–349.

256. Munkarah A, Levenback C, Wolf JK, et al. Secondary cytoreductive surgery for localized intra-abdominal recurrences in epithelial ovarian cancer. *Gynecol Oncol* 2001;81:237–241.

257. Tay EH, Grant PT, Gebski V, et al. Secondary cytoreductive surgery for recurrent epithelial ovarian cancer. *Obstet Gynecol* 2002;100:1359–1360.

258. Chi DS, McCaughty K, Diaz JP, et al. Guidelines and selection criteria for secondary cytoreductive surgery in patients with recurrent, platinum-sensitive epithelial ovarian carcinoma. *Cancer* 2006;106:1933–1939.

259. Markman M, Rothman R, Hakes T, et al. Second-line platinum therapy in patients with ovarian cancer previously treated with cisplatin. *J Clin Oncol* 1991;9:389–393.

260. Gore ME, Fryatt I, Wiltshaw E, et al. Treatment of relapsed carcinoma of the ovary with cisplatin or carboplatin following initial treatment with these compounds. *Gynecol Oncol* 1990;36:207–211.

261. Markman M, Markman J, Webster K, et al. Duration of response to second-line, platinum-based chemotherapy for ovarian cancer: implications for patient management and clinical trial design. *J Clin Oncol* 2004;22:3120–3125.

262. Markman M. Second-line therapy for potentially platinum-sensitive recurrent ovarian cancer: what is optimal treatment? *Gynecol Oncol* 2001;81:1–2.

263. Cannistra SA. Is there a "best" choice of second-line agent in the treatment of recurrent, potentially platinum-sensitive ovarian cancer? *J Clin Oncol* 2002;20:1158–1160.

264. Eisenhauer EA, Vermorken JB, van Glabbeke M. Predictors of response to subsequent chemotherapy in platinum pretreated ovarian cancer: a multivariate analysis of 704 patients. *Ann Oncol* 1997;8:963–968.

265. Gordon AN, Fleagle JT, Guthrie D, et al. Recurrent epithelial ovarian carcinoma: a randomized phase III study of pegylated liposomal doxorubicin versus topotecan. *J Clin Oncol* 2001;19:3312–3322.

266. Gordon AN, Tonda M, Sun S, et al. Doxil Study 30–49 Investigators. Long-term survival advantage for women treated with pegylated liposomal doxorubicin compared with topotecan in a phase 3 randomized study of recurrent and refractory epithelial ovarian cancer. *Gynecol Oncol* 2004;95:1–8.

267. Gordon AN, Granai CO, Rose PG, et al. Phase II study of liposomal doxorubicin in platinum- and paclitaxel-refractory epithelial ovarian cancer. *J Clin Oncol* 2000;18:3093–3100.

268. Muggia F, Hainsworth J, Jeffers S, et al. Phase II study of liposomal doxorubicin in refractory ovarian cancer: antitumor activity and toxicity modification by liposomal encapsulation. *J Clin Oncol* 1997;15:987–993.

269. Greco FA, Hainsworth JD. One-hour paclitaxel infusion schedules: a phase I/II comparative trial. *Semin Oncol* 1995;22:118–123.

270. Chang AY, Boros L, Garrow G, et al. Paclitaxel by 3-hour infusion followed by 96-hour infusion on failure in patients with refractory malignant disease. *Semin Oncol* 1995;22:124–127.

271. Kohn EC, Sarosy G, Bicher A, et al. Dose-intense taxol: high response rate in patients with platinum-resistant recurrent ovarian cancer. *J Natl Cancer Inst* 1994;86:1748–1753.

272. Omura GA, Brady MF, Look KY, et al. Phase III trial of paclitaxel at two dose levels, the higher dose accompanied by filgrastim at two dose levels in platinum-pretreated epithelial ovarian cancer: an Intergroup study. *J Clin Oncol* 2003;21:2843–2848.

273. Markman M, Hall J, Spitz D, et al. Phase II trial of weekly single-agent paclitaxel in platinum/paclitaxel-refractory ovarian cancer. *J Clin Oncol* 2002;20:2365–2369.

274. Ghamande S, Lele S, Marchetti D, et al. Weekly paclitaxel in patients with recurrent or persistent advanced ovarian cancer. *Int J Gynecol Cancer* 2003;13:142–147.

275. Thigpen JT, Blessing JA, Ball H, et al. Phase II trial of paclitaxel in patients with progressive ovarian carcinoma after platinum-based chemotherapy: a Gynecologic Oncology Group study. *J Clin Oncol* 1994;12:1748–1753.

276. Trimble EL, Adams JD, Vena D, et al. Paclitaxel for platinum-refractory ovarian cancer: results from the first 1000 patients registered to National Cancer Institute Treatment Referral Center 9103. *J Clin Oncol* 1993;11:2405–2410.

277. Bookman MA, Malstrom H, Bolis G, et al. Topotecan for the treatment of advanced epithelial ovarian cancer: an open-label phase II study in patients treated after prior chemotherapy that contained cisplatin or carboplatin and paclitaxel. *J Clin Oncol* 1998;16:3345–3352.

278. ten Bokkel Huinink W, Gore M, Carmichael J, et al. Topotecan versus paclitaxel for the treatment of recurrent epithelial ovarian cancer. *J Clin Oncol* 1997;15:2183–2193.

279. ten Bokkel Huinink W, Lane SR, Ross GA; International Topotecan Study Group. Long-term survival in a phase III, randomised study of topotecan versus paclitaxel in advanced epithelial ovarian carcinoma. *Ann Oncol* 2004;15:100–103.

280. **Hoskins P, Eisenhauer E, Beare S, et al.** Randomized phase II study of two schedules of topotecan in previously treated patients with ovarian cancer: a National Cancer Institute of Canada Clinical Trials Group study. *J Clin Oncol* 1998;16:2233–2237.

281. **Markman M, Blessing JA, Alvarez RD, et al.** Phase II evaluation of 24-h continuous infusion topotecan in recurrent, potentially platinum-sensitive ovarian cancer: a Gynecologic Oncology Group study. *Gynecol Oncol* 2000;77:112–115.

282. **Kudelka AP, Tresukosol D, Edwards CL, et al.** Phase II study of intravenous topotecan as a 5-day infusion for refractory epithelial ovarian cancer. *J Clin Oncol* 1996;14:1552–1557.

283. **Hochster H, Wadler S, Runowicz C, et al.** Activity and pharmacodynamics of 21-day topotecan infusion in patients with ovarian cancer previously treated with platinum-based chemotherapy. New York Gynecologic Oncology Group. *J Clin Oncol* 1999;17:2553–2561.

284. **Elkas JC, Holschneider CH, Katz B, et al.** The use of continuous infusion topotecan in persistent and recurrent ovarian cancer. *Int J Gynecol Cancer* 2003;13:138–141.

285. **Markman M, Kennedy A, Webster K, et al.** Phase 2 evaluation of topotecan administered on a 3-day schedule in the treatment of platinum- and paclitaxel-refractory ovarian cancer. *Gynecol Oncol* 2000;79:116–119.

286. **Clarke-Pearson DL, Van Le L, Iveson T, et al.** Oral topotecan as single-agent second-line chemotherapy in patients with advanced ovarian cancer. *J Clin Oncol* 2001;19:3967–3975.

287. **McGuire WP, Blessing JA, Bookman MA, et al.** Topotecan has substantial antitumor activity as first-line salvage therapy in platinum-sensitive epithelial ovarian carcinoma: a Gynecologic Oncology Group Study. *J Clin Oncol* 2000;18:1062–1067.

288. **Gronlund B, Hansen HH, Hogdall C, et al.** Efficacy of low-dose topotecan in second-line treatment for patients with epithelial ovarian carcinoma. *Cancer* 2002;95:1656–1662.

289. **Brown JV III, Peters WA III, Rettenmaier MA, et al.** Three-consecutive-day topotecan is an active regimen for recurrent epithelial ovarian cancer. *Gynecol Oncol* 2003;88:136–140.

290. **Gore M, Oza A, Rustin G, et al.** A randomised trial of oral versus intravenous topotecan in patients with relapsed epithelial ovarian cancer. *Eur J Cancer* 2002;38:57–63.

291. **Homesley HD, Hall DJ, Martin DA, et al.** A dose-escalating study of weekly bolus topotecan in previously treated ovarian cancer patients. *Gynecol Oncol* 2001;83:394–399.

292. **Parmar MK, Ledermann JA, Colombo N, et al.** Paclitaxel plus platinum-based chemotherapy versus conventional platinum-based chemotherapy in women with relapsed ovarian cancer: the ICON4/AGO-OVAR-2.2 trial. *Lancet* 2003;361:2099–2106.

293. **Gonzalez-Martin AA, Calvo E, Bover I, et al.** Randomized phase II trial of carboplatin versus paclitaxel and carboplatin in platinum-sensitive recurrent advanced ovarian carcinoma: a GEICO (Grupo Espanol de Investigacion en Cancer de Ovario) study. *Ann Oncol* 2005;16:749–755.

294. **Pfisterer J, Plante M, Vergote I, et al.** Gemcitabine plus carboplatin compared with carboplatin in patients with platinum-sensitive recurrent ovarian cancer: an intergroup trial of the AGO-OVAR, the NCIC CTG, and the EORTC GCG. *J Clin Oncol* 2006;24:4699–4707.

295. **Alberts DS, Liu PY, Wilczynski SP, et al.** Randomized trial of pegylated liposomal doxorubicin (PLD) plus carboplatin versus carboplatin in platinum-sensitive (PS) patients with recurrent epithelial ovarian or peritoneal carcinoma after failure of initial platinum-based chemotherapy (Southwest Oncology Group Protocol S0200). *Gynecol Oncol* 2008;108:90–94.

296. **Pujade-Lauraine E, Wagner U, Aavall-Lundqvist E, et al.** Pegylated liposomal doxorubicin and carboplatin compared with paclitaxel and carboplatin for patients with platinum-sensitive ovarian cancer in late relapse. *J Clin Oncol* 2010;28:3323–3329.

297. **Havrilesky LJ, Alvarez AA, Sayer RA, et al.** Weekly low-dose carboplatin and paclitaxel in the treatment of recurrent ovarian and peritoneal cancer. *Gynecol Oncol* 2003;88:51–57.

298. **Mutch DG, Orlando M, Goss T, et al.** Randomized phase III trial of gemcitabine compared with pegylated liposomal doxorubicin in patients with platinum-resistant ovarian cancer. *J Clin Oncol* 2007;25:2811–2818.

299. **Piccart MJ, Gore M, ten Bokkel Huinink W, et al.** Docetaxel: an active new drug for treatment of advanced epithelial ovarian cancer. *J Natl Cancer Inst* 1995;87:676–681.

300. **Francis P, Schneider J, Hann L, et al.** Phase II trial of docetaxel in patients with platinum-refractory advanced ovarian cancer. *J Clin Oncol* 1994;12:2301–2308.

301. **Rose PG, Blessing JA, Ball HG, et al.** A phase II study of docetaxel in paclitaxel-resistant ovarian and peritoneal carcinoma: a Gynecologic Oncology Group study. *Gynecol Oncol* 2003;88:130–135.

302. **Shapiro JD, Millward MJ, Rischin D, et al.** Activity of gemcitabine in patients with advanced ovarian cancer: responses seen following platinum and paclitaxel. *Gynecol Oncol* 1996;63:89–93.

303. **Papadimitriou CA, Fountzilas G, Aravantinos G, et al.** Second-line chemotherapy with gemcitabine and carboplatin in paclitaxel-pretreated, platinum-sensitive ovarian cancer patients. A Hellenic Cooperative Oncology Group Study. *Gynecol Oncol* 2004;92:152–159.

304. **Look KY, Bookman MA, Schol J, et al.** Phase I feasibility trial of carboplatin, paclitaxel, and gemcitabine in patients with previously untreated epithelial ovarian or primary peritoneal cancer: a Gynecologic Oncology Group study. *Gynecol Oncol* 2004;92:93–100.

305. **Belpomme D, Krakowski I, Beauduin M, et al.** Gemcitabine combined with cisplatin as first-line treatment in patients with epithelial ovarian cancer: a phase II study. *Gynecol Oncol* 2003;91:32–38.

306. **Markman M, Webster K, Zanotti K, et al.** Phase 2 trial of single-agent gemcitabine in platinum-paclitaxel refractory ovarian cancer. *Gynecol Oncol* 2003;90:593–596.

307. **Hoskins PJ, Swenerton KD.** Oral etoposide is active against platinum-resistant epithelial ovarian cancer. *J Clin Oncol* 1994;12:60–63.

308. **Rose PG, Blessing JA, Mayer AR, et al.** Prolonged oral etoposide as second-line therapy for platinum-resistant and platinum-sensitive ovarian carcinoma: a Gynecologic Oncology Group study. *J Clin Oncol* 1998;16:405–410.

309. **Perez-Gracia JL, Carrasco EM.** Tamoxifen therapy for ovarian cancer in the adjuvant and advanced settings: systematic review of the literature and implications for future research. *Gynecol Oncol* 2002;84:201–209.

310. **Ansink AC, Williams CJ.** The role of tamoxifen in the management of ovarian cancer. *Gynecol Oncol* 2002;86:390–391.

311. **Williams CJ.** Tamoxifen for relapse of ovarian cancer. *Cochrane Database Syst Rev* 2001;1:CD001034.

312. **Hatch KD, Beecham JB, Blessing JA, et al.** Responsiveness of patients with advanced ovarian carcinoma to tamoxifen: a Gynecologic Oncology Group study of second-line therapy in 105 patients. *Cancer* 1991;68:269–271.

313. **Van der Velden J, Gitsch G, Wain GV, et al.** Tamoxifen in patients with advanced epithelial ovarian cancer. *Int J Gynecol Cancer* 1995;5:301–305.

314. **Miller DS, Brady MF, Barrett RJ.** A phase II trial of leuprolide acetate in patients with advanced epithelial ovarian cancer. *J Clin Oncol* 1992;15:125–128.

315. **Lopez A, Tessadrelli A, Kudelka AP, et al.** Combination therapy with leuprolide acetate and tamoxifen in refractory ovarian cancer. *Int J Gynecol Cancer* 1996;6:15–19.

316. **Smith IE, Dowsett M.** Aromatase inhibitors in breast cancer. *N Engl J Med* 2003;348:2431–2442.

317. **Le T, Leis A, Pahwa P, et al.** Quality of life evaluations in patients with ovarian cancer during chemotherapy treatment. *Gynecol Oncol* 2004;92:839–844.

318. **Alvarez AA, Krigman HR, Whitaker RS, et al.** The prognostic significance of angiogenesis in epithelial ovarian carcinoma. *Clin Cancer Res* 1999;5:587–591.

319. **Burger RA, Sill MW, Monk BJ, et al.** Phase II trial of bevacizumab in persistent or recurrent epithelial ovarian cancer or primary peritoneal cancer: a Gynecologic Oncology Group Study. *J Clin Oncol* 2007;25:5165–5171.

320. **Garcia AA, Hirte H, Fleming G, et al.** Phase II clinical trial of bevacizumab and low-dose metronomic oral cyclophosphamide in recurrent ovarian cancer: a trial of the California, Chicago, and Princess Margaret Hospital phase II consortia. *J Clin Oncol* 2008;26:76–82.

321. **Cannistra SA, Matulonis UA, Penson RT, et al.** Phase II study of bevacizumab in patients with platinum-resistant ovarian cancer or

peritoneal serous cancer. *J Clin Oncol* 2007;25:5180–5186 [Erratum in: *J Clin Oncol* 2008;26:1773].

322. **Simpkins F, Belinson JL, Rose PG.** Avoiding bevacizumab related gastrointestinal toxicity for recurrent ovarian cancer by careful patient screening. *Gynecol Oncol* 2007;107:118–123.

323. **Moroney JW, Sood AK, Coleman RL.** Aflibercept in epithelial ovarian carcinoma [review]. *Future Oncol* 2009;5:591–600.

324. **Hacker NF, Berek JS, Burnison CM, et al.** Whole abdominal radiation as salvage therapy for epithelial ovarian cancer. *Obstet Gynecol* 1985;65:60–66.

325. **Castaldo TW, Petrilli ES, Ballon SC, et al.** Intestinal operations in patients with ovarian carcinoma. *Am J Obstet Gynecol* 1981;139:80–84.

326. **Krebs HB, Goplerud DR.** Surgical management of bowel obstruction in advanced ovarian cancer. *Obstet Gynecol* 1983;61:327–330.

327. **Tunca JC, Buchler DA, Mack EA, et al.** The management of ovarian cancer caused bowel obstruction. *Gynecol Oncol* 1981;12:186–192.

328. **Piver MS, Barlow JJ, Lele SB, et al.** Survival after ovarian cancer induced intestinal obstruction. *Gynecol Oncol* 1982;13:44–49.

329. **Clarke-Pearson DL, DeLong ER, Chin N, et al.** Intestinal obstruction in patients with ovarian cancer: variables associated with surgical complications and survival. *Arch Surg* 1988;123:42–45.

330. **Fernandes JR, Seymour RJ, Suissa S.** Bowel obstruction in patients with ovarian cancer: a search for prognostic factors. *Am J Obstet Gynecol* 1988;158:244–249.

331. **Rubin SC, Hoskins WJ, Benjamin I, et al.** Palliative surgery for intestinal obstruction in advanced ovarian cancer. *Gynecol Oncol* 1989;34:16–19.

332. **Coukos G, Rubin SC.** Surgical management of epithelial ovarian cancer. *Oncol Spect* 2001;2:350–361.

333. **Pothuri B, Vaidya A, Aghajanian C, et al.** Palliative surgery for bowel obstruction in recurrent ovarian cancer: an updated series. *Gynecol Oncol* 2003;89:306–313.

334. **Tamussino KF, Lim PC, Webb MJ, et al.** Gastrointestinal surgery in patients with ovarian cancer. *Gynecol Oncol* 2001;80:79–84.

335. **Jong P, Sturgeon J, Jamieson CG.** Benefit of palliative surgery for bowel obstruction in advanced ovarian cancer. *Can J Surg* 1995;38:454–457.

336. **Winter WE, McBroom JW, Carlson JW, et al.** The utility of gastrojejunostomy in secondary cytoreduction and palliation of proximal intestinal obstruction in recurrent ovarian cancer. *Gynecol Oncol* 2003;91:261–264.

337. **Bryan DN, Radbod R, Berek JS.** An analysis of surgical versus chemotherapeutic intervention for the management of intestinal obstruction in advanced ovarian cancer. *Int J Gynecol Cancer* 2006;16:125–134.

338. **Feuer DJ, Broadley KE, Shepherd JH, et al.** Surgery for the resolution of symptoms in malignant bowel obstruction in advanced gynaecological and gastrointestinal cancer. *Cochrane Database Syst Rev* 2000;4:CD002764.

339. **Malone JM Jr, Koonce T, Larson DM, et al.** Palliation of small bowel obstruction by percutaneous gastrostomy in patients with progressive ovarian carcinoma. *Obstet Gynecol* 1986;68:431–433.

340. **Campagnutta E, Cannizzaro R, Gallo A, et al.** Palliative treatment of upper intestinal obstruction by gynecologic malignancy: the usefulness of percutaneous endoscopic gastrostomy. *Gynecol Oncol* 1996;62:103–105.

341. **Kosary CL.** Cancer of the ovary. Surveillance Survival and End Results (SEER) survival monograph. *J Natl Cancer Inst* 2007;16:133–144.

342. **Berek JS, Friedlander M, Hacker NF.** Germ cell and other nonepithelial ovarian cancers. In: *Berek and Hacker's gynecologic oncology*. 5th ed. Philadelphia, PA: Lippincott Williams & Wilkins, 2009:509–535.

343. **Imai A, Furui T, Tamaya T.** Gynecologic tumors and symptoms in childhood and adolescence: 10-years' experience. *Int J Gynaecol Obstet* 1994;45:227–234.

344. **Gershenson DM.** Management of early ovarian cancer: germ cell and sex-cord stromal tumors. *Gynecol Oncol* 1994;55:S62–S72.

345. **Gershenson DM.** Update on malignant ovarian germ cell tumors. *Cancer* 1993;71:1581–1590.

346. **Kurman RJ, Scardino PT, Waldmann TA, et al.** Malignant germ cell tumors of the ovary and testis: an immunohistologic study of 69 cases. *Ann Clin Lab Sci* 1979;9:462–466.

347. **Koulouris CR, Penson RT.** Ovarian stromal and germ cell tumors. *Semin Oncol* 2009;36:126–136.

348. **Pectasides D, Pectasides E, Kassanos D.** Germ cell tumors of the ovary. *Cancer Treat Rev* 2008;34:427–441.

349. **Obata NH, Nakashima N, Kawai M, et al.** Gonadoblastoma with dysgerminoma in one ovary and gonadoblastoma with dysgerminoma and yolk sac tumor in the contralateral ovary in a girl with 46XX karyotype. *Gynecol Oncol* 1995;58:124–128.

350. **Spanos WJ.** Preoperative hormonal therapy of cystic adnexal masses. *Am J Obstet Gynecol* 1973;116:551–556.

351. **Bremer GL, Land JA, Tiebosch A, et al.** Five different histologic subtypes of germ cell malignancies in an XY female. *Gynecol Oncol* 1993;50:247–248.

352. **Mayordomo JI, Paz-Ares L, Rivera F, et al.** Ovarian and extragonadal malignant germ-cell tumors in females: a single-institution experience with 43 patients. *Ann Oncol* 1994;5:225–231.

353. **Piura B, Dgani R, Zalel Y, et al.** Malignant germ cell tumors of the ovary: a study of 20 cases. *J Surg Oncol* 1995;59:155–161.

354. **Gordon A, Lipton D, Woodruff JD.** Dysgerminoma: a review of 158 cases from the Emil Novak Ovarian Tumor Registry. *Obstet Gynecol* 1981;58:497–504.

355. **Thomas GM, Dembo AJ, Hacker NF, et al.** Current therapy for dysgerminoma of the ovary. *Obstet Gynecol* 1987;70:268–275.

356. **Low JJ, Perrin LC, Crandon AJ, et al.** Conservative surgery to preserve ovarian function in patients with malignant ovarian germ cell tumors: a review of 74 cases. *Cancer* 2000;89:391–398.

357. **Williams SD, Birch R, Einhorn LH, et al.** Treatment of disseminated germ cell tumors with cisplatin, bleomycin and either vinblastine or etoposide. *N Engl J Med* 1987;316:1435–1440.

358. **Williams SD, Blessing JA, Hatch K, et al.** Chemotherapy of advanced ovarian dysgerminoma: trials of the Gynecologic Oncology Group. *J Clin Oncol* 1991;9:1950–1955.

359. **Williams SD, Blessing JA, Moore DH, et al.** Cisplatin, vinblastine, and bleomycin in advanced and recurrent ovarian germ-cell tumors. *Ann Intern Med* 1989;111:22–27.

360. **Williams S, Blessing JA, Liao S, et al.** Adjuvant therapy of ovarian germ cell tumors with cisplatin, etoposide, and bleomycin: a trial of the Gynecologic Oncology Group. *J Clin Oncol* 1994;12:701–706.

361. **Gershenson DM, Morris M, Cangir A, et al.** Treatment of malignant germ cell tumors of the ovary with bleomycin, etoposide, and cisplatin. *J Clin Oncol* 1990;8:715–720.

362. **Bekaii-Saab T, Einhorn LH, Williams SD.** Late relapse of ovarian dysgerminoma: case report and literature review. *Gynecol Oncol* 1999;72:111–112.

363. **Kurtz JE, Jaeck D, Maloisel F, et al.** Combined modality treatment for malignant transformation of a benign ovarian teratoma. *Gynecol Oncol* 1999;73:319–321.

364. **Williams SD, Kauderer J, Burnett A, et al.** Adjuvant therapy of completely resected dysgerminoma with carboplatin and etoposide: a trial of the Gynecologic Oncology Group. *Gynecol Oncol* 2004;95:496–499.

365. **Pawinski A, Favalli G, Ploch E, et al.** PVB chemotherapy in patients with recurrent or advanced dysgerminoma: a phase II study of the EORTC Gynaecological Cancer Cooperative Group. *Clin Oncol (R Coll Radiol)* 1998;10:301–305.

366. **Culine S, Lhomme C, Kattan J, et al.** Cisplatin-based chemotherapy in dysgerminoma of the ovary: thirteen-year experience at the Institut Gustave Roussy. *Gynecol Oncol* 1995;58:344–348.

367. **Brewer M, Gershenson DM, Herzog CE, et al.** Outcome and reproductive function after chemotherapy for ovarian dysgerminoma. *J Clin Oncol* 1999;17:2670–2675.

368. **Gershenson DM.** Menstrual and reproductive function after treatment with combination chemotherapy for malignant ovarian germ cell tumors. *J Clin Oncol* 1988;6:270–275.

369. **Kanazawa K, Suzuki T, Sakumoto K.** Treatment of malignant ovarian germ cell tumors with preservation of fertility: reproductive performance after persistent remission. *Am J Clin Oncol* 2000;23:244–248.

370. **El-Lamie IK, Shehata NA, Abou-Loz SK, et al.** Conservative surgical management of malignant ovarian germ cell tumors: the experience of the Gynecologic Oncology Unit at Ain Shams University. *Eur J Gynaecol Oncol* 2000;21:605–609.

371. **Tangir J, Zelterman D, Ma W, et al.** Reproductive function after conservative surgery and chemotherapy for malignant germ cell tumors of the ovary. *Obstet Gynecol* 2003;101:251–257.

372. **Loehrer PJ, Johnson D, Elson P, et al.** Importance of bleomycin in favorable-prognosis disseminated germ cell tumors: an Eastern Cooperative Oncology Group trial. *J Clin Oncol* 1995;13:470–476.

373. **Bajorin DF, Sarosdy MF, Pfister GD, et al.** Randomized trial of etoposide and cisplatin versus etoposide and carboplatin in patients with good-risk germ cell tumors: a multi-institutional study. *J Clin Oncol* 1993;11:598–606.

374. **Schwartz PE, Chambers SK, Chambers JT, et al.** Ovarian germ cell malignancies: the Yale University experience. *Gynecol Oncol* 1992;45:26–31.

375. **Williams SD, Blessing JA, DiSaia PJ, et al.** Second-look laparotomy in ovarian germ cell tumors. *Gynecol Oncol* 1994;52:287–291.

376. **Culine S, Lhomme C, Michel G, et al.** Is there a role for second-look laparotomy in the management of malignant germ cell tumors of the ovary? Experience at Institute Gustave Roussy. *J Surg Oncol* 1996;62:40–45.

377. **O'Conner DM, Norris HJ.** The influence of grade on the outcome of stage I ovarian immature (malignant) teratomas and the reproducibility of grading. *Int J Gynecol Pathol* 1994;13:283–289.

378. **Ulbright TM.** Gonadal teratomas: a review and speculation. *Adv Anat Pathol* 2004;11:10–23.

379. **Norris HJ, Zirkin HJ, Benson WL.** Immature (malignant) teratoma of the ovary: a clinical and pathologic study of 58 cases. *Cancer* 1976;37:2359–2372.

380. **Heifetz SA, Cushing B, Giller R, et al.** Immature teratomas in children: pathologic considerations: a report from the combined Pediatric Oncology Group/Children's Cancer Group. *Am J Surg Pathol* 1998;22:1115–1124.

381. **Marina NM, Cushing B, Giller R, et al.** Complete surgical excision is effective treatment for children with immature teratomas with or without malignant elements: a Pediatric Oncology Group/Children's Cancer Group Intergroup Study. *J Clin Oncol* 1999;17:2137–2143.

382. **Ferguson AW, Katabuchi H, Ronnett BM, et al.** Glial implants in gliomatosis peritonei arise from normal tissue, not from the associated teratoma. *Am J Pathol* 2001;159:51–55.

383. **Best DH, Butz GM, Moller K, et al.** Molecular analysis of an immature ovarian teratoma with gliomatosis peritonei and recurrence suggests genetic independence of multiple tumors. *Int J Oncol* 2004;25:17–25.

384. **Dimopoulos MA, Papadopoulou M, Andreopoulou E, et al.** Favorable outcome of ovarian germ cell malignancies treated with cisplatin or carboplatin-based chemotherapy: a Hellenic Cooperative Oncology Group study. *Gynecol Oncol* 1998;70:70–74.

385. **Bafna UD, Umadevi K, Kumaran C, et al.** Germ cell tumors of the ovary: is there a role for aggressive cytoreductive surgery for nondysgerminomatous tumors? *Int J Gynecol Cancer* 2001;11:300–304.

386. **De Palo G, Zambetti M, Pilotti S, et al.** Non-dysgerminomatous tumors of the ovary treated with cisplatin, vinblastine, and bleomycin: long-term results. *Gynecol Oncol* 1992;47:239–246.

387. **Culine S, Kattan J, Lhomme C, et al.** A phase II study of high-dose cisplatin, vinblastine, bleomycin, and etoposide (PVeBV regimen) in malignant non-dysgerminomatous germ-cell tumors of the ovary. *Gynecol Oncol* 1994;54:47–53.

388. **Mann JR, Raafat F, Robinson K, et al.** The United Kingdom Children's Cancer Study Group's second germ cell tumor study: carboplatin, etoposide, and bleomycin are effective treatment for children with malignant extracranial germ cell tumors, with acceptable toxicity. *J Clin Oncol* 2000;18:3809–3818.

389. **Segelov E, Campbell J, Ng M, et al.** Cisplatin-based chemotherapy for ovarian germ cell malignancies: the Australian experience. *J Clin Oncol* 1994;12:378–384.

390. **Bonazzi C, Peccatori F, Colombo N, et al.** Pure ovarian immature teratoma, a unique and curable disease: 10 years' experience of 32 prospectively treated patients. *Obstet Gynecol* 1994;84:598–604.

391. **Cangir A, Smith J, van Eys J.** Improved prognosis in children with ovarian cancers following modified VAC (vincristine sulfate, dactinomycin, and cyclophosphamide) chemotherapy. *Cancer* 1978;42:1234–1238.

392. **Wong LC, Ngan HYS, Ma HK.** Primary treatment with vincristine, dactinomycin, and cyclophosphamide in non-dysgerminomatous germ cell tumour of the ovary. *Gynecol Oncol* 1989;34:155–158.

393. **Slayton RE, Park RC, Silverberg SC, et al.** Vincristine, dactinomycin, and cyclophosphamide in the treatment of malignant germ cell tumors of the ovary: a Gynecologic Oncology Group study (a final report). *Cancer* 1985;56:243–248.

394. **Creasman WJ, Soper JT.** Assessment of the contemporary management of germ cell malignancies of the ovary. *Am J Obstet Gynecol* 1985;153:828–834.

395. **Taylor MH, DePetrillo AD, Turner AR.** Vinblastine, bleomycin and cisplatin in malignant germ cell tumors of the ovary. *Cancer* 1985;56:1341–1349.

396. **Culine S, Lhomme C, Kattan J, et al.** Cisplatin-based chemotherapy in the management of germ cell tumors of the ovary: the Institute Gustave Roussy experience. *Gynecol Oncol* 1997;64:160–165.

397. **Williams SD, Wong LC, Ngan HYS.** Management of ovarian germ cell tumors. In: **Gershenson DM, McGuire WP, eds.** *Ovarian cancer.* New York: Churchill Livingston, 1998:399–415.

398. **Tay SK, Tan LK.** Experience of a 2-day BEP regimen in postsurgical adjuvant chemotherapy of ovarian germ cell tumors. *Int J Gynecol Cancer* 2000;10:13–18.

399. **Dark GG, Bower M, Newlands ES, et al.** Surveillance policy for stage I ovarian germ cell tumors. *J Clin Oncol* 1997;15:620–624.

400. **Hariprasad R, Kumar L, Janga D, et al.** Growing teratoma syndrome of ovary. *Int J Clin Oncol* 2008;13:83–87.

401. **Tangjitgamol S, Manusirivithaya S, Leelahakorn S, et al.** The growing teratoma syndrome: a case report and a review of the literature. *Int J Gynecol Cancer* 2006;16(Suppl 1):384–390.

402. **Carver BS, Bianco FJ Jr, Shayegan B, et al.** Predicting teratoma in the retroperitoneum in men undergoing post-chemotherapy retroperitoneal lymph node dissection. *J Urol* 2006;176:100–103.

403. **Mathew GK, Singh SS, Swaminathan RG, et al.** Laparotomy for post chemotherapy residue in ovarian germ cell tumors. *J Postgrad Med* 2006;52:262–265.

404. **Geisler JP, Goulet R, Foster RS, et al.** Growing teratoma syndrome after chemotherapy for germ cell tumors of the ovary. *Obstet Gynecol* 1994;84:719–721.

405. **Talerman A.** Germ cell tumors of the ovary. *Curr Opin Obstet Gynecol* 1997;9:44–47.

406. **Sasaki H, Furusata M, Teshima S, et al.** Prognostic significance of histopathological subtypes in stage I pure yolk sac tumour of the ovary. *Br J Cancer* 1994;69:529–536.

407. **Fujita M, Inoue M, Tanizawa O, et al.** Retrospective review of 41 patients with endodermal sinus tumor of the ovary. *Int J Gynecol Cancer* 1993;3:329–335.

408. **Kawai M, Kano T, Kikkawa F, et al.** Seven tumor markers in benign and malignant germ cell tumors of the ovary. *Gynecol Oncol* 1992;45:248–253.

409. **Abu-Rustum NR, Aghajanian C.** Management of malignant germ cell tumors of the ovary. *Semin Oncol* 1998;25:235–242.

410. **Newlands ES, Southall PJ, Paradinas FJ, et al.** Management of ovarian germ cell tumours. In: **Williams CJ, Krikorian JG, Green MR, et al., eds.** *Textbook of uncommon cancer.* New York: John Wiley and Sons, 1988:37–53.

411. **Ueda G, Abe Y, Yoshida M, et al.** Embryonal carcinoma of the ovary: a six-year survival. *Gynecol Oncol* 1990;31:287–292.

412. **Kammerer-Doak D, Baurick K, Black W, et al.** Endodermal sinus tumor and embryonal carcinoma of the ovary in a 53-year-old woman. *Gynecol Oncol* 1996;63:133–137.

413. **Simosek T, Trak B, Tunoc M, et al.** Primary pure choriocarcinoma of the ovary in reproductive ages: a case report. *Eur J Gynaecol Oncol* 1998;19:284–286.

414. **Oliva E, Andrada E, Pezzica E, et al.** Ovarian carcinomas with choriocarcinomatous differentiation. *Cancer* 1993;72:2441–2446.

415. **Chapman DC, Grover R, Schwartz PE.** Conservative management of an ovarian polyembryoma. *Obstet Gynecol* 1994;83:879–882.

416. **Gershenson DM, Del Junco G, Copeland LJ, et al.** Mixed germ cell tumors of the ovary. *Obstet Gynecol* 1984;64:200–206.

417. **Nichols CR, Breeden ES, Lloehrer PJ, et al.** Secondary leukemia associated with a conventional dose of etoposide: review of serial germ cell tumor protocols. *J Natl Cancer Inst* 1993;85:36–40.

418. **Pedersen-Bjergaard J, Daugaard G, Hansen SW, et al.** Increased risk of myelodysplasia and leukaemia after etoposide, cisplatin, and bleomycin for germ-cell tumours. *Lancet* 1991;338:359–363.

419. **Young RE, Scully RE.** Ovarian sex cord-stromal tumors: problems in differential diagnosis. *Pathol Annu* 1988;23:237–296.

420. **Miller BE, Barron BA, Wan JY, et al.** Prognostic factors in adult granulosa cell tumor of the ovary. *Cancer* 1997;79:1951–1955.

421. **Malmstrom H, Hogberg T, Bjorn R, et al.** Granulosa cell tumors of the ovary: prognostic factors and outcome. *Gynecol Oncol* 1994;52:50–55.

422. **Segal R, DePetrillo AD, Thomas G.** Clinical review of adult granulosa cell tumors of the ovary. *Gynecol Oncol* 1995;56:338–344.

423. **Cronje HS, Niemand I, Bam RH, et al.** Review of the granulosa-theca cell tumors from the Emil Novak ovarian tumor registry. *Am J Obstet Gynecol* 1999;180:323–328.

424. **Aboud E.** A review of granulosa cell tumours and thecomas of the ovary. *Arch Gynecol Obstet* 1997;259:161–165.

425. **Young R, Clement PB, Scully RE.** The ovary. In: Sternberg SS, ed. Diagnostic surgical pathology. New York: Raven Press, 1989:1687.

426. **Shah SP, Köbel M,, Senz J, et al.** Mutation of *FOXL2* in granulosa-cell Tumors of the ovary. *N Engl J Med* 2009;360:2719–2729.

427. **Lappohn RE, Burger HG, Bouma J, et al.** Inhibin as a marker for granulosa-cell tumors. *N Engl J Med* 1989;321:790–793.

428. **Hildebrandt RH, Rouse RV, Longacre TA.** Value of inhibin in the identification of granulosa cell tumors of the ovary. *Hum Pathol* 1997;28:1387–1395.

429. **Richi M, Howard LN, Bratthauae GL, et al.** Use of monoclonal antibody against human inhibin as a marker for sex-cord-stromal tumors of the ovary. *Am J Surg Pathol* 1997;21:583–589.

430. **Matias-Guiu X, Pons C, Prat J.** Mullerian inhibiting substance, alpha-inhibin, and CD99 expression in sex cord-stromal tumors and endometrioid ovarian carcinomas resembling sex cord-stromal tumors. *Hum Pathol* 1998;29:840–845.

431. **McCluggage WG.** Recent advances in immunohistochemistry in the diagnosis of ovarian neoplasms. *J Clin Pathol* 2000;53:327–334.

432. **Rey RA, Lhomme C, Marcillac I, et al.** Antimullerian hormone as a serum marker of granulosa cell tumors of the ovary: comparative study with serum alpha-inhibin and estradiol. *Am J Obstet Gynecol* 1996;174:958–965.

433. **Schumer ST, Cannistra SA.** Granulosa cell tumor of the ovary. *J Clin Oncol* 2003;21:1180–1189.

434. **Wolf JK, Mullen J, Eifel PJ, et al.** Radiation treatment of advanced or recurrent granulosa cell tumor of the ovary. *Gynecol Oncol* 1999;73:35–41.

435. **Savage P, Constenla D, Fisher C, et al.** Granulosa cell tumours of the ovary: demographics, survival and the management of advanced disease. *Clin Oncol (R Coll Radiol)* 1998;10:242–245.

436. **Gershenson DM, Copeland LJ, Kavanauh JJ, et al.** Treatment of metastatic stromal tumors of the ovary with cisplatin, doxorubicin, and cyclophosphamide. *Obstet Gynecol* 1987;5:765–769.

437. **Holland DR, Le Riche J, Swenerton KD, et al.** Flow cytometric assessment of DNA ploidy is a useful prognostic factor for patients with granulosa cell ovarian tumors. *Int J Gynecol Cancer* 1991;1:227–232.

438. **Uygun K, Aydiner A, Saip P, et al.** Clinical parameters and treatment results in recurrent granulosa cell tumor of the ovary. *Gynecol Oncol* 2003;88:400–403.

439. **Al-Badawi IA, Brasher PM, Ghatage P, et al.** Postoperative chemotherapy in advanced ovarian granulosa cell tumors. *Int J Gynecol Cancer* 2002;12:119–123.

440. **Homesley HD, Bundy BN, Hurteau JA, et al.** Bleomycin, etoposide, and cisplatin combination therapy of ovarian granulosa cell tumors and other stromal malignancies: a Gynecologic Oncology Group study. *Gynecol Oncol* 1999;72:131–137.

441. **Freeman SA, Modesitt SC.** Anastrozole therapy in recurrent ovarian adult granulosa cell tumors: a report of 2 cases. *Gynecol Oncol* 2006;103:755–758.

442. **Fishman A, Kudelka AP, Tresukosol D, et al.** Leuprolide acetate for treating refractory or persistent ovarian granulosa cell tumor. *J Reprod Med* 1996;41:393–396.

443. **Korach J, Perri T, Beiner M, et al.** Promising effect of aromatase inhibitors on recurrent granulosa cell tumors. *Int J Gynecol Cancer* 2009;19:830–833.

444. **Hardy RD, Bell JG, Nicely CJ, et al.** Hormonal treatment of a recurrent granulosa cell tumor of the ovary: case report and review of the literature. *Gynecol Oncol* 2005;96:865–869.

445. **Martikainen H, Penttinen J, Huhtaniemi I, et al.** Gonadotropin-releasing hormone agonist analog therapy effective in ovarian granulosa cell malignancy. *Gynecol Oncol* 1989;35:406–408.

446. **Powell JL, Otis CN.** Management of advanced juvenile granulosa cell tumor of the ovary. *Gynecol Oncol* 1997;64:282–284.

447. **Tomlinson MW, Treadwell MC, Deppe G.** Platinum based chemotherapy to treat recurrent Sertoli-Leydig cell ovarian carcinoma during pregnancy. *Eur J Gynaecol Oncol* 1997;18:44–46.

448. **Le T, Krepart GV, Lotocki RJ, et al.** Malignant mixed mesodermal ovarian tumor treatment and prognosis: a 20-year experience. *Gynecol Oncol* 1997;65:237–240.

449. **Roth LM, Anderson MC, Govan AD, et al.** Sertoli-Leydig cell tumors: a clinicopathologic study of 34 cases. *Cancer* 1981;48:187–197.

450. **Berek JS, Hacker NF.** Sarcomas of the female genital tract. In: Eilber FR, Morton DL, Sondak VK, et al., eds. *The soft tissue sarcomas.* Orlando, FL: Grune & Stratton, 1987:229–238.

451. **Piura B, Rabinovich A, Yanai-Inbar I, et al.** Primary sarcoma of the ovary: report of five cases and review of the literature. *Eur J Gynaecol Oncol* 1998;19:257–261.

452. **Topuz E, Eralp Y, Aydiner A, et al.** The role of chemotherapy in malignant mixed mullerian tumors of the female genital tract. *Eur J Gynaecol Oncol* 2001;22:469–472.

453. **van Rijswijk RE, Tognon G, Burger CW, et al.** The effect of chemotherapy on the different components of advanced carcinosarcomas (malignant mixed mesodermal tumors) of the female genital tract. *Int J Gynecol Cancer* 1994;4:52–60.

454. **Barakat RR, Rubin SC, Wong G, et al.** Mixed mesodermal tumor of the ovary: analysis of prognostic factors in 31 cases. *Obstet Gynecol* 1992;80:660–664.

455. **Fowler JM, Nathan L, Nieberg RK, et al.** Mixed mesodermal sarcoma of the ovary in a young patient. *Eur J Obstet Gynecol Reprod Biol* 1996;65:249–253.

456. **Young RH, Oliva E, Scully RE.** Small cell sarcoma of the ovary, hypercalcemic type: a clinicopathological analysis of 150 cases. *Am J Surg Pathol* 1994;18:1102–1116.

457. **Petru E, Pickel H, Heydarfadai M, et al.** Non-genital cancers metastatic to the ovary. *Gynecol Oncol* 1992;44:83–86.

458. **Demopoulos RI, Touger L, Dubin N.** Secondary ovarian carcinoma: a clinical and pathological evaluation. *Int J Gynecol Pathol* 1987;6:166–175.

459. **Young RH, Scully RE.** Metastatic tumors in the ovary: a problem-oriented approach and review of the recent literature. *Semin Diagn Pathol* 1991;8:250–276.

460. **Yada-Hashimoto N, Yamamoto T, Kamiura S, et al.** Metastatic ovarian tumors: a review of 64 cases. *Gynecol Oncol* 2003;89:314–317.

461. **Ayhan A, Tuncer ZS, Bukulmez O.** Malignant tumors metastatic to the ovaries. *J Surg Oncol* 1995;60:268–276.

462. **Curtin JP, Barakat RR, Hoskins WJ.** Ovarian disease in women with breast cancer. *Obstet Gynecol* 1994;84:449–452.

463. **Yakushiji M, Tazaki T, Nishimura H, et al.** Krukenberg tumors of the ovary: a clinicopathologic analysis of 112 cases. *Acta Obstet Gynaecol Jpn* 1987;39:479–485.

464. **Kim HK, Heo DS, Bang YJ, et al.** Prognostic factors of Krukenberg's tumor. *Gynecol Oncol* 2001;82:105–109.

465. **Yakushiji M, Tazaki T, Nishimura H, et al.** Krukenberg tumors of the ovary: a clinicopathologic analysis of 112 cases. *Acta Obstet Gynaecol Jpn* 1987;39:479–485.

466. **Misdraji J, Yantiss RK, Graeme-Cook FM, et al.** Appendiceal mucinous neoplasms: a clinicopathologic analysis of 107 cases. *Am J Surg Pathol* 2003;27:1089–1103.

467. **Chou YY, Jeng YM, Kao HL, et al.** Differentiation of ovarian mucinous carcinoma and metastatic colorectal adenocarcinoma by immunostaining with beta-catenin. *Histopathology* 2003;43:151–156.

468. **Seidman JD, Kurman RJ, Ronnett BM.** Primary and metastatic mucinous adenocarcinomas in the ovaries: incidence in routine practice with a new approach to improve intraoperative diagnosis. *Am J Surg Pathol* 2003;27:985–993.

469. **Lee KR, Young RH.** The distinction between primary and metastatic mucinous carcinomas of the ovary: gross and histologic findings in 50 cases. *Am J Surg Pathol* 2003;27:281–292.

470. **McBroom JW, Parker MF, Krivak TC, et al.** Primary appendiceal malignancy mimicking advanced stage ovarian carcinoma: a case series. *Gynecol Oncol* 2000;78:388–390.

471. Schofield A, Pitt J, Biring G, et al. Oophorectomy in primary colorectal cancer. *Ann R Coll Surg Engl* 2001;83:81–84.

472. Ayhan A, Guvenal T, Coskun F, et al. Survival and prognostic factors in patients with synchronous ovarian and endometrial cancers and endometrial cancers metastatic to the ovaries. *Eur J Gynaecol Oncol* 2003;24:171–174.

473. Young RH, Scully RE. Malignant melanoma metastatic to the ovary: a clinicopathologic analysis of 20 cases. *Am J Surg Pathol* 1991;15:849–860.

474. Davis GL. Malignant melanoma arising in mature ovarian cystic teratoma (dermoid cyst). Report of two cases and literature analysis. *Int J Gynecol Pathol* 1996;15:356–362.

475. Motoyama T, Katayama Y, Watanabe H, et al. Functioning ovarian carcinoids induce severe constipation. *Cancer* 1991;70:513–518.

476. Robbins ML, Sunshine TJ. Metastatic carcinoid diagnosed at laparoscopic excision of pelvic endometriosis. *J Am Assoc Gynecol Laparosc* 2000;7:251–253.

477. Fox H, Langley FA, Govan AD, et al. Malignant lymphoma presenting as an ovarian tumour: a clinicopathological analysis of 34 cases. *BJOG* 1988;95:386–390.

478. Monterroso V, Jaffe ES, Merino MJ, et al. Malignant lymphomas involving the ovary: a clinicopathologic analysis of 39 cases. *Am J Surg Pathol* 1993;17:154–170.

479. Azizoglu C, Altinok G, Uner A, et al. Ovarian lymphomas: a clinicopathological analysis of 10 cases. *Arch Gynecol Obstet* 2001;265:91–93.

480. Pecorelli S, Odicino F, Maisonneuve P, et al. Carcinoma of the fallopian tube. FIGO annual report on the results of treatment in gynaecological cancer. *J Epidemiol Biostat* 1998;3:363–374.

481. Cormio G, Maneo A, Gabriele A, et al. Primary carcinoma of the fallopian tube: a retrospective analysis of 47 patients. *Ann Oncol* 1996;7:271–275.

482. Alvarado-Cabrero I, Young RH, Vamvakas EC, et al. Carcinoma of the fallopian tube: a clinicopathological study of 105 cases with observations on staging and prognostic factors. *Gynecol Oncol* 1999;72:367–379.

483. Podratz KC, Podczaski ES, Gaffey TA, et al. Primary carcinoma of the fallopian tube. *Am J Obstet Gynecol* 1986;154:1319–1326.

484. Romagosa C, Torne A, Iglesias X, et al. Carcinoma of the fallopian tube presenting as acute pelvic inflammatory disease. *Gynecol Oncol* 2003;89:181–184.

485. Kosary C, Trimble EL. Treatment and survival for women with fallopian tube carcinoma: a population-based study. *Gynecol Oncol* 2002;86:190–191.

486. Hellstrom AC, Silfversward C, Nilsson B, et al. Carcinoma of the fallopian tube: a clinical and histopathologic review. The Radiumhemmet series. *Int J Gynecol Cancer* 1994;4:395–407.

487. Levine DA, Argenta PA, Yee CJ, et al. Fallopian tube and primary peritoneal carcinomas associated with *BRCA* mutations. *Clin Oncol* 2003;21:4222–4227.

488. Mikami M, Tei C, Kurahashi T, et al. Preoperative diagnosis of fallopian tube cancer by imaging. *Abdom Imaging* 2003;28:743–747.

489. Barakat RR, Rubin SC, Saigo PE, et al. Cisplatin-based combination chemotherapy in carcinoma of the fallopian tube. *Gynecol Oncol* 1991;42:156–160.

490. Cormio G. Experience at the Memorial Sloan-Kettering Cancer Center with paclitaxel-based combination chemotherapy following primary cytoreductive surgery in carcinoma of the fallopian tube. *Gynecol Oncol* 2002;84:185–186.

491. Markman M, Zanotti K, Webster K, et al. Phase 2 trial of single agent docetaxel in platinum and paclitaxel-refractory ovarian cancer, fallopian tube cancer, and primary carcinoma of the peritoneum. *Gynecol Oncol* 2003;91:573–576.

492. Kuscu E, Oktem M, Haberal A, et al. Management of advanced-stage primary carcinoma of the fallopian tube: case report and literature review. *Eur J Gynaecol Oncol* 2003;24:557–560.

493. Matulonis U, Campos S, Duska L, et al. A phase II trial of three sequential doublets for the treatment of advanced mullerian malignancies. *Gynecol Oncol* 2003;91:293–298.

494. Markman M, Glass T, Smith HO, et al. Phase II trial of single agent carboplatin followed by dose-intense paclitaxel, followed by maintenance paclitaxel therapy in stage IV ovarian, fallopian tube, and peritoneal cancers: a Southwest Oncology Group trial. *Gynecol Oncol* 2003;88:282–288.

495. Rose PG, Rodriguez M, Walker J, et al. A phase I trial of prolonged oral etoposide and liposomal doxorubicin in ovarian, peritoneal, and tubal carcinoma: a Gynecologic Oncology Group Study. *Gynecol Oncol* 2002;85:136–139.

38 Vulvar Cancer

Christine H. Holschneider
Jonathan S. Berek

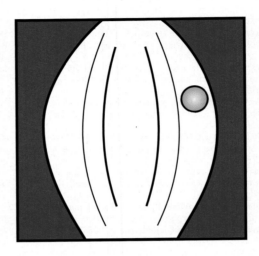

- Vulvar lesions require biopsy to avoid delay in diagnosis.

- The modern approach to patients with vulvar cancer is multidisciplinary and individualized.

- Management of the primary lesion and groin nodes is determined separately.

- Most T_1, T_2, and early T_3 lesions can be managed with radical local excision.

- Large T_3 and T_4 primary tumors are best treated with chemoradiation followed by more limited surgical resection.

- When groin dissection is indicated, it should be a thorough inguinofemoral lymphadenectomy.

- The potential role of the sentinel lymph node procedure to eliminate the need of a complete inguinofemoral lymphadenectomy is being investigated.

- The single most important prognostic factor is lymph node status: 5-year survival without groin node metastases is greater than 90%; with groin node metastases 5-year survival is 50%.

- Postoperative radiation decreases the risk of groin recurrence in patients with multiple positive inguinofemoral lymph nodes.

- Recurrence in the groin is almost universally fatal.

With 4,340 new cases and 940 deaths annually in the United States, vulvar cancer is uncommon, representing about 4% of malignancies of the female genital tract and 0.6% of all cancers in women (1,2). Squamous cell carcinomas account for about 90% of all primary vulvar malignancies, whereas melanomas, adenocarcinomas, basal cell carcinomas, and sarcomas are less common. **The incidence of *in situ* vulvar cancer is increasing worldwide, primarily because of the increasing occurrence in young women, who account for 75% of the cases. The overall rate of invasive vulvar carcinoma is increasing, but at a much lower rate** (3,4). In women younger than 50 years, there is a striking increase in the incidence of *in situ* and invasive squamous cell carcinoma of the vulva (5).

Following the reports of Taussig in the United States and Way in Great Britain, radical vulvectomy and *en bloc* groin dissection, with or without pelvic lymphadenectomy, was standard treatment for all patients with operable disease (6,7). Postoperative morbidity was high and prolonged hospitalization common. **During the past 25 years, there were significant advances in the management of vulvar cancer, reflecting a paradigm shift toward a more conservative surgical approach without compromised survival and with markedly decreased physical and psychological morbidity:**

1. **Individualization of treatment for all patients with invasive disease.**

2. **Vulvar conservation for patients with unifocal tumors and an otherwise normal vulva.**

3. **Omission of the groin dissection for patients with microinvasive tumors (T1a, ≤ 2 cm diameter and ≤ 1 mm of stromal invasion).**

4. **Elimination of routine pelvic lymphadenectomy.**

5. **Investigation of the role of the sentinel lymph node procedure to eliminate requirement for complete inguinofemoral lymphadenectomy.**

6. **The use of separate incisions for the groin dissection to improve wound healing.**

7. **Omission of the contralateral groin dissection in patients with lateral T_1 lesions and negative ipsilateral nodes.**

8. **The use of preoperative radiation therapy to obviate the need for exenteration in patients with advanced disease.**

9. **The use of postoperative radiation therapy to decrease the incidence of groin recurrence in patients with multiple positive groin nodes.**

Etiology

The etiology of vulvar cancer is only partially elucidated and likely to be multifactorial. Reported risk factors for vulvar cancer include human papillomavirus (HPV) infection, vulvar intraepithelial neoplasia (VIN), cervical intraepithelial neoplasia (CIN), lichen sclerosus, squamous hyperplasia, cigarette smoking, alcohol consumption, immunosuppression, a prior history of cervical cancer, and northern European ancestry (8,9). **Based on histopathologic and environmental factors, there appear to be at least two distinct etiologic entities of squamous cell carcinoma of the vulva:**

1. *Basaloid or warty types*, **which tend to be multifocal, occur generally in younger patients and are related to HPV infection, VIN, and cigarette smoking.**

2. *Keratinizing, differentiated, or simplex types*, **which tend to be unifocal, occur predominantly in older patients, are not related to HPV, and often are found in areas adjacent to lichen sclerosus and squamous hyperplasia.**

High-grade vulvar intraepithelial neoplasia (VIN 3) was closely studied as a potential precancerous lesion. The direct progression of VIN to cancer is difficult to document, but a review of 3,322 published patients with VIN 3 reports a 9% progression rate to cancer for untreated cases (10). VIN is found adjacent to basaloid or warty vulvar squamous cell carcinomas in more than 80% of cases and 10% to 20% of vulvar carcinoma *in situ* lesions harbor an occult invasive component (11,12). HPV DNA is documented in 89% of patients with VIN 3, in 60% of vulvar cancers overall, and in up to 86% of warty or basaloid type carcinomas of the vulva; but it occurs in less than 10% of the keratinizing type of carcinomas of the vulva (13). HPV 16 and 33 are the prevalent subtypes, accounting for 55.5% of all HPV-related vulvar cancers (14). **Epidemiologic risk factors for the basaloid or warty type squamous cell carcinoma of the vulva are similar to those for cervical cancer and include a history of multiple lower genital tract neoplasias, immunosuppression, and smoking (13,15).**

Frequently implied as an etiologic variable for the keratinizing carcinoma is the itch–scratch cycle associated with lichen sclerosus and squamous hyperplasia, with atypical changes occurring in the repaired epithelium. Differentiated (or simplex) VIN is a precursor to squamous cell carcinoma and is associated with lichen sclerosus. **In keratinizing carcinoma, associated lichen sclerosus or squamous hyperplasia is found in more than 80% of patients (16,17).** Women with vulvar lichen sclerosus are at increased risk of developing invasive squamous cell

Table 38.1 Types of Vulvar Cancer	
Type	*Percent*
Squamous	92
Melanoma	2–4
Basal cell	2–3
Bartholin gland (adenocarcinoma, squamous cell, transitional cell, adenoid cystic)	1
Metastatic	1
Verrucous	<1
Sarcoma	<1
Appendage (e.g., hidradenocarcinoma)	Rare

cancer of the vulva, reported at 2.5% to 7.2% with a median follow-up of 4.7 to 6.2 years (18–20). Supportive evidence that some of these lesions could be precancerous comes from molecular studies that demonstrate aneuploid DNA content, *p53* overexpression, high Ki67 expression, indicating high proliferation indices and monoclonal expansion of keratinocytes in lichen sclerosus and associated squamous hyperplasia (21–23). An area of active research explores whether treatment of lichen sclerosus with superpotent topical steroids can impact the malignancy risk (18–20). Some studies reported vulvar cancer to be more common in patients who are obese, have hypertension and diabetes mellitus, or are nulliparous, but a case-control study of vulvar cancer did not confirm any of these as risk factors (15,24,25).

Types of Invasive Vulvar Cancer

The histologic subtypes of invasive vulvar cancer are shown in Table 38.1.

Squamous Cell Carcinoma

Approximately 90% to 92% of all invasive vulvar cancers are of the squamous cell type. Squamous carcinomas of the vulva can be divided into distinct histologic subtypes designated as *basaloid carcinoma*, *warty carcinoma*, and *keratinizing squamous carcinoma* (16). Mitoses are noted in these malignancies, but atypical keratinization is the histologic hallmark of invasive vulvar cancer (26). Most vulvar squamous carcinomas reveal keratinization (Fig. 38.1). Histologic features that correlate with the occurrence of inguinal lymph node metastasis are lymph–vascular space invasion, tumor thickness, depth of stromal invasion, histologic pattern of invasion (spray and stellate versus broad and pushing), and increased amount of keratin (27–30).

Microinvasive carcinoma of the vulva (T_{1a}) is defined as a lesion 2 cm or less in diameter with 1 mm or less stromal invasion (31). Depth of stromal invasion is measured vertically from the epithelial–stromal junction (basement membrane) of the adjacent most superficial dermal papilla to the deepest point of tumor invasion (Fig. 38.2). **When the tumor invades 1 mm or less, metastasis to the inguinal lymph nodes is extremely rare among reported series. When invasion is greater than 1 mm, there is a significant risk of inguinal lymph node metastasis.**

Clinical Features

Squamous cell carcinoma of the vulva is predominantly a disease of postmenopausal women. The mean age at diagnosis is about 65 years and 15% of patients who develop vulvar cancer do so before age 40. There may be a longstanding history of an associated vulvar intraepithelial disorder, such as lichen sclerosus, squamous hyperplasia, or VIN. As many as 27% of patients with vulvar cancer have a second primary malignancy (32–34). Based on data from the National Cancer Institute's Surveillance Epidemiology and End Results (SEER) program, patients with invasive vulvar cancer have an increased risk of 1.3% for developing a subsequent cancer. **Most of the excess second cancers were smoking related** (e.g., cancers of the lung, buccal cavity and pharynx, esophagus, nasal cavity, and larynx) **or related to infection with human papillomavirus** (e.g., cervix, vulva, vagina, and anus) (35).

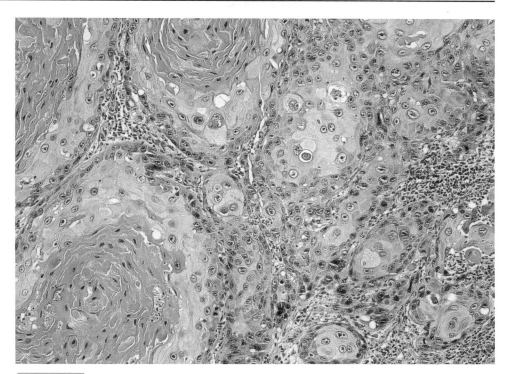

Figure 38.1 **Squamous cell carcinoma of the vulva, keratinizing type.** The multiple pearl formations consist of laminated keratin.

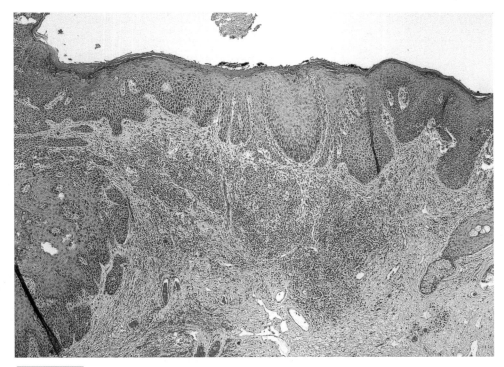

Figure 38.2 **Early invasive carcinoma of vulva originating from vulvar intraepithelial neoplasia.** An irregular nest of malignant cells extend from the base of rete pegs. Desmoplastic stromal reaction and chronic inflammation are useful diagnostic signs of stromal invasion. The depth of stromal invasion is measured from the base of the most superficial dermal papilla vertically to the deepest tumor cells.

Most patients are asymptomatic at the time of diagnosis. If symptoms exist, vulvar pruritus, a lump, or a mass are the most common findings. Less frequent symptoms include a bleeding or ulcerative lesion, discharge, pain, or dysuria. Occasionally, a large metastatic mass in the groin is the initial symptom.

A careful inspection of the vulva should be part of every gynecologic examination. On physical examination, vulvar carcinoma is usually raised and may be fleshy, ulcerated, plaquelike or warty in appearance. It may be pigmented, red or white, and tender or painless. The lesion may be clinically indistinct, especially in the presence of VIN or vulvar dystrophies (12). Any lesion of the vulva warrants a biopsy.

Most squamous carcinomas of the vulva occur on the labia majora and minora (60%), but the clitoris (15%) and perineum (10%) may be primary sites. Approximately 10% of the cases are too extensive to determine a site of origin, and about 5% of the cases are multifocal.

As part of the clinical evaluation, a careful assessment of the extent of the lesion, including whether it is unifocal or multifocal, should be performed. The groin lymph nodes should be evaluated carefully, and a complete pelvic examination should be performed. A cytologic sample should be taken from the cervix, and **colposcopy of the cervix and vagina should be performed because of the common association with other squamous intraepithelial or invasive neoplasms of the lower genital tract.**

Diagnosis

Diagnosis requires a Keys punch biopsy or wedge biopsy, which can be obtained in the office using local anesthesia. The biopsy must include sufficient underlying dermis to assess for microinvasion.

Physician delay is a common problem in the diagnosis of vulvar cancer, particularly if the lesion has a warty appearance. Any large or confluent warty lesion requires biopsy before medical or ablative therapy is initiated.

Routes of Spread

Vulvar cancer spreads by the following routes:

1. **Direct extension**, to involve adjacent structures such as the vagina, urethra, and anus.
2. **Lymphatic embolization** to the regional inguinal and femoral lymph nodes.
3. **Hematogenous spread** to distant sites, including the lungs, liver, and bone.

Lymphatic metastases may occur early in the disease. Twelve percent of tumors 2 cm in diameter or smaller have regional metastases (32,36). Initially, spread is usually to the inguinal lymph nodes, which are located between Camper's fascia and the fascia lata (37). From these superficial groin nodes, the disease spreads to the deep femoral nodes, which are located medial to the femoral vessels (Fig. 38.3). *Cloquet's* or *Rosenmüller's node*, situated beneath the inguinal ligament, is the most cephalad of the femoral node group. **Metastases to the femoral nodes without involvement of the inguinal nodes is reported** (38–41). A study from the M. D. Anderson Cancer Center reported a 9% groin recurrence rate in 104 patients with vulvar cancer who had negative nodes on superficial inguinal lymphadenectomy at initial surgery, and intraoperative lymphatic mapping studies found the sentinel node deep to the cribriform fascia in 5% to 16% of these cases (42–44).

From the inguinal-femoral nodes, the cancer spreads to the pelvic nodes, particularly the external iliac group. Although direct lymphatic pathways from the clitoris and Bartholin gland to the pelvic nodes were described, these channels seem to be of minimal clinical significance (45–47). The lymphatics from either side of the vulva form a rich network of anastomoses along the midline. Lymphatic drainage from the clitoris, anterior labia minora, and perineum is bilateral. Metastases to contralateral lymph nodes in the absence of ipsilateral nodal involvement is very rare (0% to 0.4%) for lateral vulvar tumors that are either 2 cm or less in diameter or with 5 mm or less invasion (36,48).

The overall incidence of inguinal-femoral lymph node metastases is reported to be about 32% (41,43,46–56) (Table 38.2). **Metastases to pelvic nodes occur in about 12% of cases.** Pelvic nodal metastases are rare (0.6%) in the absence of groin node involvement, but they occur in about 16% of cases with positive groin nodes (Table 38.2). The risk increases to 33% in the presence of clinically suspicious groin nodes and to 40% to 50% if there are three or more pathologically positive inguinal-femoral nodes (33,48,57–60). The incidence of lymph node

Table 38.2 Incidence of Lymph Node Metastases in Squamous Cell Carcinoma of the Vulva

Author	Positive Inguinal-femoral Nodes	Positive Pelvic Nodes/Patients s/p Lymphadenectomy	Positive Pelvic Nodes/Patients with Negative Inguinal-femoral Nodes	Positive Pelvic Nodes/Patients with Positive Inguinal-femoral Nodes
Rutledge et al., 1970 (32)	33/86 (38%)	12/72 (17%)	0/53 (0%)	12/33 (36%)
Collins et al., 1971 (51)	27/98 (28%)	11/98 (11%)	4/71 (6%)	7/27 (26%)
Morley, 1976 (52)	67/180 (37%)	6/23 (26%)	0/113 (0%)	6/67 (9%)
Krupp and Bohm, 1978 (53)	40/195 (21%)	10/195 (5%)	1/155 (0.6%)	9/40 (23%)
Benedet et al., 1979 (55)	34/120 (28%)	4/51 (8%)	N/A	N/A
Curry et al., 1980 (45)	57/191 (30%)	9/52 (17%)	0/134 (0%)	9/57 (16%)
Iversen et al., 1980 (56)	90/262 (34%)	7/100 (7%)	1/172 (0.6%)	6/90 (7%)
Hacker et al., 1983 (57)	31/113 (27%)	6/18 (33%)	0/82 (0%)	6/31 (19%)
Podratz et al., 1983 (33)	59/175 (34%)	7/114 (6%)	0/116 (0%)	7/59 (12%)
Monaghan and Hammond, 1984 (58)	37/134 (28%)	3/80 (4%)	N/A	N/A
Hopkins et al., 1991 (59)	61/145 (42%)	13/38 (34%)	0/84 (0%)	13/61 (21%)
Keys, 1993 (54)	203/588 (35%)	15/53 (28%)	N/A	N/A
Gonzales Bosquet, 2007 (48)	108/320 (34%)	NA	NA	14/108 (13%)
Total	847/2,607 (32%)	103/894 (12%)	6/980 (0.6%)	89/573 (16%)

N/A, data not available.

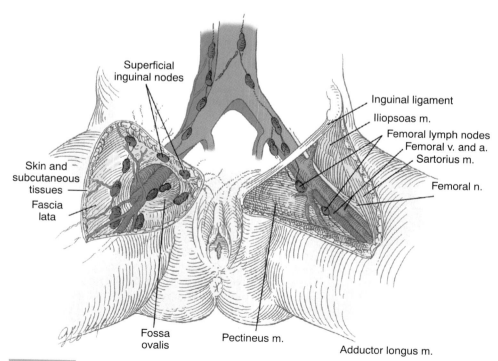

Figure 38.3 Inguinal-femoral lymph nodes. (From **Berek JS, Hacker NF.** *Berek & Hacker's Gynecologic Oncology.* 5th ed. Philadelphia, PA: Lippincott Williams & Wilkins, 2010:541, with permission.)

Table 38.3 Nodal Status in T_1 Squamous Cell Carcinoma of the Vulva versus Depth of Stromal Invasion

Depth of Invasion	No. of Patients	Positive Nodes	Nodes
1 mm	163	0	0
1.1–2 mm	145	11	7.7
2.1–3 mm	131	11	8.3
3.1–5 mm	101	27	26.7
>5	38	13	34.2
Total	578	62	10.7

From **Berek JS, Hacker NF.** *Berek & Hacker's Gynecologic Oncology.* 5th ed. Philadelphia, PA: Lippincott Williams & Wilkins 2010:543, with permission.

metastases correlates positively with depth of invasion, as shown in Table 38.3. Hematogenous spread usually occurs late in the course of vulvar cancer and is rare in the absence of lymph node metastases.

Staging

Initially, vulvar carcinoma was staged clinically based on tumor size and location, palpable regional lymph node status, and a limited search for distant metastases. The prognostic importance of the lymph node status is significant, but clinical assessment of the lymph nodes has limited accuracy. This led the Cancer Committee of FIGO to introduce a surgical staging system for vulvar cancer in 1988, which underwent several revisions, most recently in 2009, to provide better prognostic discrimination between stages and less heterogeneity within stages (31,61,62) (Table 38.4). The main changes are:

1. While stage Ia remains unchanged as the only group of patients with a negligible risk of lymph node metastases, former stages I and II have been combined into stage Ib.
2. The new stage II segregates patients whose tumors involve the lower adjacent perineal structures from those with positive lymph nodes.
3. For stages III and IV, the number and morphology of the involved nodes are taken into account and the bilaterality of lymph nodes is discounted.

The new FIGO staging system was validated in 269 patients, 42% of whom were restaged (63). The number of positive nodes negatively correlated with survival, as did the presence of extracapsular growth. This study confirmed Gynecologic Oncology Group (GOG) and SEER data indicating that in patients with negative nodes, tumor size was not predictive of survival (62). This study confirmed reports demonstrating that, when corrected for the number of positive nodes, bilaterality of nodal metastases was not predictive of survival (64–67).

Paralleling the changes to the FIGO staging, the American Joint Committee on Cancer (AJCC) significantly modified the vulvar cancer tumor-node-metastasis (TNM) classification with the release of the 2009 edition of the AJCC Cancer Staging Manual (Table 38.4) (68).

Prognosis and Survival

Survival of patients with vulvar cancer correlates with FIGO stage (69). The prognosis for patients with early-stage disease is generally good (Table 38.5). **The single most important prognostic factor is lymph node status** (54–56,59,70,71). A report from the Mayo Clinic on 330 patients with primary squamous cell carcinoma of the vulva demonstrated a significant correlation between lymph node status and risk of treatment failure, especially in the first 2 years following initial therapy: 44.2% overall recurrence rate with positive versus 17.5% with negative lymph nodes. **More than one-third of relapses presented 5 years or more after initial therapy** (72). There is a strong negative correlation between the number of positive lymph nodes and survival (Table 38.6). **Patients with negative lymph nodes have a 5-year survival rate of over 80%; for patients with positive nodes 5-year survival falls below 50%.** The number of positive nodes is of critical importance: **Patients with one microscopically positive lymph node have a prognosis similar to those with all negative lymph nodes, whereas patients with three or more positive nodes have a poor prognosis and a 2-year survival rate of 20%** (73). The survival rate for patients with positive pelvic nodes is about 11% (74). In addition

Table 38.4 FIGO Staging and TNM classification for Vulvar Cancer (2008)

FIGO Stage	TNM Classification	Clinical/Pathologic Findings
Stage IA	$T_{1a}N_0M_0$	Lesions ≤2 cm in size, confined to the vulva or perineum and with stromal invasion ≤1 mm,* no nodal metastasis
Stage IB	$T_{1b}N_0M_0$	Lesions >2 cm in size or with stromal invasion >1 mm, confined to the vulva or perineum, with negative nodes
Stage II	$T_2N_0M_0$	Tumor of any size with extension to adjacent perineal structures (1/3 lower urethra, 1/3 lower vagina, anus) with negative nodes
Stage III		Tumor of any size with or without extension to adjacent perineal structures (1/3 lower urethra, 1/3 lower vagina, anus) with positive inguino-femoral lymph nodes
IIIA	$T_{1or2}\ N_{1b}\ M_0$ $T_{1or2}\ N_{1a}\ M_0$	(i) with 1 lymph node metastasis (≥5 mm) or (ii) 1–2 lymph node metastasis(es) (<5 mm)
IIIB	$T_{1or2}\ N_{2b}\ M_0$ $T_{1or2}\ N_{2a}\ M_0$	(i) with 2 or more lymph node metastasis (≥5 mm) or (ii) 3 or more lymph node metastases (<5 mm)
IIIC	$T_{1or2}\ N_{2c}\ M_0$	with positive nodes with extracapsular spread
Stage IV		Tumor invades other regional (2/3 upper urethra, 2/3 upper vagina), or distant structures
IVA	$T_3N_{any}\ M_0$ $T_{any}N_3$	Tumor invades any of the following: (i) upper urethral and/or vaginal mucosa, bladder mucosa, rectal musosa, or fixed to pelvic bone or (ii) fixed or ulcerated inguino-femoral lymph nodes
IVB	$T_{any}N_{any}M_1$	Any distant metastasis including pelvic lymph nodes

FIGO, International Federation of Gynecology and Obstetrics; TNM, tumor node metastasis.

FIGO Committee on Gynecologic Oncology. Revised FIGO staging for carcinoma of the vulva, cervix, and endometrium. *Int J Gynecol Obstet* 2009;105:103–104 (31).

American Joint Committee on Cancer. *AJCC Cancer Staging Manual.* 7th ed. Chicago, Illinois: Springer New York, Inc., 2010.

*The depth of stromal invasion is measured from the epithelial–stromal junction of the adjacent most superficial dermal papilla to the deepest point of invasion.

[a]**TNM Classification:**

T: Primary tumor
T_x: Primary tumor cannot be assessed
T_0: No evidence of primary tumor
T_{is}: Carcinoma *in situ* (preinvasive carcinoma)
T_{1a}: Lesions ≤2 cm in size, confined to the vulva or perineum and with stromal invasion ≤1 mm
T_{1b}: Lesions >2 cm in size or any size with stromal invasion >1 mm, confined to the vulva or perineum
T_2: Tumor of any size with extension to adjacent perineal structures (lower 1/3 of urethra, lower of 1/3 vagina, anal involvement)
T_3: Tumor of any size with extension to any of the following: upper 2/3 of urethra, upper 2/3 of vagina, bladder mucosa, rectal mucosa, or fixed to pelvic bone

N: Regional lymph nodes (femoral and inguinal nodes)
N_x: Regional lymph nodes cannot be assessed
N_0: No regional lymph node metastases
N_1: One or two regional lymph node metastases with the following features:
N_{1a}: One or two lymph node metastases each <5 mm
N_{1b}: One lymph node metastasis ≥5 mm
N_2: Regional lymph node metastases with the following features
N_{2a}: ≥3 lymph node metastases, each <5 mm in diameter
N_{2b}: ≥2 lymph node metastases ≥5 mm
N_{2c}: Lymph node metastases with extracapsular spread
N_3: Fixed or ulcerated regional lymph node metastasis
M: Distant metastasis
M_0: No distant metastasis
M_1: Distant metastasis (including pelvic lymph node metastasis)

to the number of nodes involved, the morphology of the positive groin nodes is of prognostic significance. As demonstrated in several studies, significant negative predictors of survival are the size of the nodal metastasis, the proportion of the node replaced by tumor cells, and the presence of any extracapsular spread (62,70,75,76). Histologic grade, tumor thickness, depth of stromal invasion, and lymph–vascular space involvement contribute to the risk of lymph node involvement but are not independent predictors of survival (73).

Treatment

After the pioneering work of Taussig and Way, *en bloc* radical vulvectomy and bilateral dissection of the groin and pelvic nodes were the standard treatment for most patients with operable vulvar cancer (6,7). When the disease involved the anus, rectovaginal septum, or proximal urethra, some type of pelvic exenteration was combined with the dissection.

Table 38.5 Five-Year Survival for Patients with Vulvar Carcinoma		
FIGO Stage	**No. of Patients**	**5-Year Survival (%)**
I	286 (34%)	79
II	266 (32%)	59
III	216 (26%)	43
IV	71 (8%)	13

FIGO, International Federation of Gynecology and Obstetrics.
Modified from the FIGO Annual Report on the Results of Treatment in Gynecological Cancer using 1994 FIGO staging classification (31).

Although the survival rate improved markedly with this aggressive surgical approach, several factors led to modifications of this treatment plan. These factors are summarized as follows:

1. An increasing proportion of patients present with early-stage disease—up to 50% of patients in many centers have tumors 2 cm in diameter or smaller.
2. Concerns about the postoperative morbidity and associated long-term hospitalization common with the *en bloc* radical dissection.
3. Increasing awareness of the psychosexual consequences of radical vulvectomy.

To individualize the patient's care and determine the appropriate therapy, it is necessary to independently manage the primary lesion and groin lymph nodes. Before initiation of therapy, all patients should undergo colposcopy of the cervix, vagina, and vulva. Preinvasive (and rarely invasive) lesions may be present at other sites along the lower genital tract.

Management of the Primary Lesion

Microinvasive Vulvar Cancer (T_{1a})   **Tumors 2 cm or less in diameter with 1 mm or less invasion are appropriately treated with a wide local excision, which is as effective as radical surgery for the prevention of vulvar recurrences for these tumors** (77). The excision should go sufficiently deep into the dermis that depth of invasion is fully assessed.

Early Vulvar Cancer (T_{1b})   **The modern approach to the management of patients with T_{1b} carcinoma of the vulva should be individualized.** There is no standard approach applicable to every patient, and emphasis is on performing the most conservative operation that is consistent with cure of the disease. Radical vulvectomy was considered the standard treatment for primary vulvar lesions, but this operation is associated with significant surgical morbidity and disturbances of sexual function and body image. Psychosexual sequelae are a major long-term morbidity associated with the treatment of vulvar cancer (37). One study reported that sexual arousal was reduced to the eighth percentile and body image was reduced to the fourth percentile for women who had undergone vulvectomy when compared with healthy adult women (66). Traditionally, the concern was that without an *en bloc* resection of vulva and groin nodes, intervening tissue left between the primary tumor and the regional lymph nodes contained

Table 38.6 Five-year Survival for Patients with Vulvar Squamous Cell Carcinoma by Number of Lymph Node Metastases		
No. of Lymph Node Metastases	**No. of Patients**	**5-Year Survival (%)**
0	302 (61%)	81
1	66 (13%)	63
2	43 (9%)	30
3	24 (5%)	19
4 or more	62 (12%)	13

FIGO, International Federation of Gynecology and Obstetrics.
Modified from the FIGO Annual Report on the Results of Treatment in Gynecological Cancer (31).

microscopic tumor foci in draining lymphatics. **Experience with a separate incision technique for node dissection confirmed that metastases rarely occur in the skin bridge in patients without clinically suspicious nodes in the groin** (78).

During the past 20 years, several investigators advocated a radical local excision rather than a radical vulvectomy for the primary lesion for patients with T_{1b} tumors (37,49,79,80). Regardless of whether a radical vulvectomy or a radical local excision is performed, the surgical margins adjacent to the tumor are the same. An analysis of the literature indicates that the incidence of local invasive recurrence after radical local excision or radical hemivulvectomy is not higher than that after radical vulvectomy (36,49,74,81–83). This finding suggests that in the presence of an otherwise normal-appearing vulva, **radical local excision is a safe surgical option, regardless of the size of the tumor or the depth of invasion.** Based on cumulative data of 413 patients reported in four studies, an 8 mm or greater histopathological resection margin results in a high rate of local disease control (81,84–86). Of the 252 patients whose tumors were resected with margins of 8 mm or greater, 2.4% experienced a local recurrence, compared to 30.3% of the 161 patients whose margins were less than 8 mm. Neither clinical tumor size nor the presence of coexisting benign vulvar pathology correlated with local recurrence. It is important to bear in mind that paraffin-embedded tissue shrinks by about 25%. **At the time of radical local excision, at least a 1-cm grossly negative margin, without putting the skin under tension, should be obtained and extended down to the level of the inferior fascia of the urogenital diaphragm.**

When vulvar cancer arises in the presence of VIN, vulvar dystrophy, or some nonneoplastic epithelial disorder, treatment is influenced by the patient's age. Elderly patients who often had many years of chronic itching may not be disturbed by the prospect of a vulvectomy. In younger women, it is desirable to conserve as much of the vulva as possible. Radical local excision should be performed for the invasive disease, and the associated intraepithelial disease should be treated in the manner most appropriate to the patient. For example, topical steroids may be required for lichen sclerosus or squamous hyperplasia, whereas VIN may require superficial local excision with primary closure or laser ablation.

Radical local excision is most appropriate for lesions on the lateral or posterior aspects of the vulva (Fig. 38.4). Midline lesions pose special challenges because of their proximity to clitoris, urethra, or anus. For anterior lesions, conservative clitoris-sparing surgery allows for excellent local control as long as pathological margins are at least 8 mm (87). For tumors that involve the clitoris or that are in close proximity to it, any type of surgical excision will have psychosexual consequences. In addition, marked edema of the posterior vulva may occur. For young patients with periclitoral lesions, the primary lesion can be treated with a small field of radiation therapy, possibly with concomitant sensitizing chemotherapy. Small vulvar lesions should respond very well to about 5,000 cGy external radiation, and biopsy can be performed after therapy to confirm the absence of any residual disease (61).

Early T_2 Vulvar Cancer **The indications for vulvar conservation can be extended to selected patients with early T_2 tumors. The tumor-free margin should be the same, whether or not a radical vulvectomy or a radical local excision is performed. It seems both feasible and desirable to extend the indications for vulvar conservation, particularly for younger patients. Tumors that are suitable for a conservative resection are those involving the posterior vulva and lower vagina, where preservation of the anus, clitoris, and urethra is feasible.**

For patients with more advanced T_2 lesions, management consists of radical vulvectomy and/or chemoradiation therapy, as discussed below. When the disease involves the distal urethra or anus, partial resection of these organs is required. Alternatively, it is often preferable to give preoperative radiation therapy with chemosensitization to allow for a less radical resection (see below).

Closure of Large Defects

After radical local excision, primary closure without tension can be accomplished for smaller defects. If an extensive dissection is required to treat a large primary lesion, a number of options are available to repair the defect:

1. An area may be left open to granulate, which it will usually do over a period of 6 to 8 weeks (88).

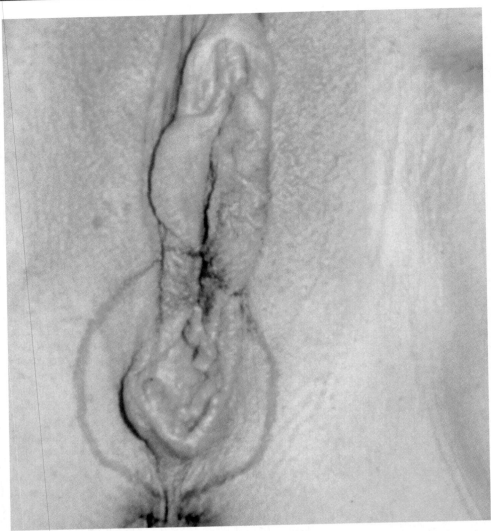

Figure 38.4   **Small (T1) vulvar carcinoma at the posterior fourchette.** (From **Berek JS, Hacker NF.** *Berek & Hacker's Gynecologic Oncology.* 5th ed. Philadelphia, PA: Lippincott Williams & Wilkins, 2010:547, with permission.)

2. Full-thickness skin flaps may be devised (89–92). The rhomboid flap is best suited to covering large defects of the posterior vulva, whereas for lateral defects, a mons pubis pedicle flap is advocated (89,92).

3. Myocutaneous flaps may be developed to cover the defect. Unilateral or bilateral gracilis myocutaneous grafts are useful when an extensive area from the mons pubis to the perianal area was resected. Because the graft brings a new blood supply to the area, it is particularly applicable if the vulva is poorly vascularized from prior surgical resection or radiation (93).

4. If extensive defects exist in the groin and vulva, the tensor fascia lata myocutaneous graft may be the most applicable (94).

Advanced Disease: Large T_2 and T_3 Primary Tumors

To achieve primary surgical clearance for tumors involving the upper urethra, anus, rectum, or rectovaginal septum, pelvic exenteration is needed in addition to radical vulvectomy and inguinal-femoral lymphadenectomy, which carries an extremely high physical and psychological morbidity (95,96). Reported 5-year survival rates with this approach are about 50% (97–100). For many of these patients, a combined approach of surgery and radiation therapy offers improved survival and reduced morbidity and is the preferred treatment approach. Numerous small prospective and retrospective series report on the use of external beam radiation, often with concomitant chemotherapy to shrink the primary tumor. Reported initial response rates to chemoradiation are 80% to 90%, and operability is achieved in 63% to 92% of cases (101–108). **It is important that this chemoradiation is followed by a more limited resection of the tumor bed on an individualized basis.** About one-half of the specimens will contain residual tumor, and local relapse rates are as high as 50% to 79% with external radiation alone (with or without concomitant chemotherapy), emphasizing the need for a combined approach that involves radiation and surgery (109–112).

As experience with this combination therapy evolved, it appeared that **external beam therapy is appropriate for most cases, with more selective use of brachytherapy. The extensiveness of the surgery is significantly modified. A limited vulvar resection is advocated, and bulky N2 and N3 nodes are resected without full groin lymphadenectomy to avoid the leg edema associated with groin lymphadenectomy and radiation. With this combined radiation-surgical approach, 5-year survival rates as high as 76% are reported** (110). With the experience accrued, preoperative radiation, with or without concurrent chemotherapy, is regarded as the first treatment of choice for patients with advanced vulvar cancer who would otherwise require some type of pelvic exenteration or stoma. Neoadjuvant therapy is not justified in patients with tumors that can be adequately treated with primary radical vulvectomy and bilateral groin node dissection.

Management of the Lymph Nodes

Appropriate groin dissection is the single most important factor in decreasing the mortality from early vulvar cancer.

When assessing a patient for groin dissection, the following facts should to be kept in mind:

1. The only patients with virtually no risk of lymph node metastases are those whose tumor is small and invades the stroma to 1 mm or less (T_{1a}).
2. Patients who develop recurrent disease in an undissected groin have a greater than 90% mortality (113).
3. Based on the laterality of the vulvar lesions and the status of the ipsilateral groin, an ipsilateral or bilateral lymphadenectomy becomes necessary.

Groin dissection is associated with postoperative wound infection and breakdown. Although the incidence of wound breakdown is reduced significantly when separate incisions are used for the groin dissection, lymphocyst formation and chronic leg edema remain a major problem (Fig. 38.5) (78).

All patients whose tumors demonstrate more than 1 mm of stromal invasion or whose tumors are larger than 2 cm (T_{1b} and above) require inguinal-femoral lymphadenectomy. If there is any question regarding the need for inguinofemoral lymphadenectomy, a Keys biopsy or wedge biopsy of the primary tumor should be obtained, and the depth of invasion should be determined. If it is smaller than 1 mm on the wedge biopsy specimen, the entire lesion should be locally excised and analyzed histologically to determine the depth of invasion. If the lesion is 2 cm in diameter or smaller and there is no invasive focus larger than 1 mm, groin dissection may be omitted, provided there is no lymph–vascular space invasion and there are no clinically suspicious groin lymph nodes. An occasional patient with less than 1 mm of stromal invasion has documented groin node metastases, but the incidence is so low that it is of no practical significance (114,115).

Inguinal-Femoral Lymphadenectomy   **If groin dissection is indicated in patients with vulvar cancer, it should be a thorough inguinal-femoral lymphadenectomy.** The GOG reported six groin recurrences among 121 patients with tumors 2 cm or less after a superficial (inguinal) dissection, although the removed inguinal nodes were negative, and a study from the M. D. Anderson Cancer Center reported a 9% groin recurrence rate in 104 patients with vulvar cancer and negative nodes on superficial inguinal lymphadenectomy (41,42). Whether all of these recurrences were in the femoral nodes is unclear, but both studies indicate that an incomplete groin dissection will increase the number of groin recurrences and mortality. GOG data indicate that radiation therapy cannot substitute for groin dissection followed by selective radiation as indicated, even in patients with clinically nonsuspicious lymph nodes (116). This GOG study was closed early because a significantly higher incidence of recurrences occurred in women who were receiving groin radiation therapy only (19% versus 0%). The dose of radiation was 5,000

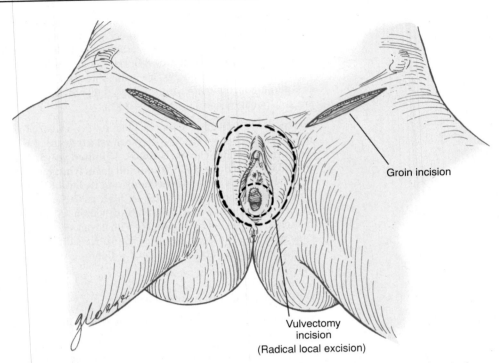

Figure 38.5 **Skin incision for groin dissection through a separate incision.** A line is drawn 1 cm above and parallel to the groin crease, and a narrow ellipse of skin is removed. (Revised from **Berek JS, Hacker NF.** *Practical Gynecologic Oncology.* 2nd ed. Baltimore, MD: Williams & Wilkins, 1994:418, with permission.)

cGy given in daily 200-cGy fractions to a depth of 3 cm below the anterior skin surface. Although the radiation regimen prescribed was criticized extensively, other uncontrolled studies give no evidence for better groin control with radiotherapy (117,118). Surgery remains the treatment of choice for the groin for women with vulvar cancer.

Unilateral versus Bilateral Groin Dissection **It is not necessary to perform a bilateral groin dissection if the primary lesion is unilateral and the ipsilateral lymph nodes are negative.** In a patient with a unilateral lesion and negative ipsilateral groin nodes, the risk of contralateral lymph node metastasis is very low (36,48). In a study from the Mayo Clinic, 8 of 163 patients with unilateral vulvar cancers (4.8%) had bilateral lymph node metastases and only 3 (1.8%) had isolated contralateral lymph node metastases. None of the patients with unilateral vulvar lesions that were either 2 cm or less or had 5 mm or less depth of invasion had bilateral groin node involvement at diagnosis (48). There is an increase in the risk of contralateral nodal involvement proportional to the number of positive ipsilateral inguinal nodes (60,48). **It is recommended that patients with any bulky or multiple microscopically positive ipsilateral groin lymph nodes undergo contralateral inguinal-femoral lymphadenectomy. Bilateral inguinal-femoral lymphadenectomy should be performed for midline lesions (clitoris, anterior labia minora, posterior fourchette) or those within 2 cm of the midline because of the more frequent contralateral lymph flow from these regions** (119).

Management of Bulky Groin Nodes All clinically or radiologically suspicious groin nodes should be resected. If nodal metastasis is confirmed by frozen section, the question arises whether a full inguinofemoral lymphadenectomy may be safely omitted to decrease morbidity without compromising survival. One small, retrospective, multi-institutional study suggests that targeted nodal debulking compared with full lymphadenectomy does not jeopardize survival when both are followed by groin and pelvic radiation (120). Patients with fixed, unresectable groin nodes should be treated with primary chemoradiation. If there is no other evidence of metastatic disease following chemoradiation, GOG data suggest that it may be appropriate to resect the residual nodes (121).

Management of Pelvic Lymph Nodes In the past, pelvic lymphadenectomy was part of the routine surgery for invasive vulvar cancer. The incidence of pelvic lymph node metastasis is rare in the absence of groin node involvement, and a more selective approach is preferred (Table 38.2). Patients most prone to pelvic lymph node metastasis are those with three or more pathologically positive groin nodes (33,45,57,122). In addition to the number of nodes involved, the morphology of the positive groin nodes is of prognostic significance. As demonstrated in several studies, significant negative predictors of survival are the number of positive nodes, the size of the nodal metastasis, the proportion of the node replaced by tumor cells, and the presence of any extracapsular spread (65,70,75,76). In these patients, the pelvis requires treatment by radiation (discussed below). **If a preoperative pelvic imaging study reveals bulky pelvic lymph nodes, resection of these nodes should be performed via an extraperitoneal approach prior to radiation because of the limited ability of external beam radiation therapy to sterilize bulky positive pelvic nodes.**

Sentinel Lymph Node Studies **Considerable investigation was conducted regarding the use of intraoperative lymphatic mapping using lymphoscintigraphy with technetium-99m-labeled nanocolloid or isosulfan blue dye to identify a sentinel node that would predict the presence or absence of regional nodal metastases** (43,123–125). A systematic review of 29 small studies of 961 groins found lymphoscintigraphy to be the most accurate technique, with a pooled sensitivity and negative likelihood ratio of 97% and 0.12, respectively (126). Studies suggested that a sentinel node could be identified in most patients (127–129). A GOG study of 403 evaluable patients in whom 697 groins were assessed demonstrated that a sentinel node was successfully identified in 78.8% (67 of 85) of patients using blue dye only and in 96.2% (306 of 318) using combination of radiolocalization and blue dye, demonstrating the superiority of the combination of blue dye and radiocolloid over blue dye alone for sentinel node identification (130). The sensitivity of the sentinel node assessment is enhanced by ultrastaging using serial sectioning or immunohistochemistry to detect micrometastases (129,131–133).

The strong interest in the sentinel node concept lies in the desire to reduce the significant life-long morbidity of lymphedema associated with a thorough inguinofemoral lymphadenectomy. Reliable identification of the sentinel node and forgoing full lymphadenectomy in patients with clinically nonsuspicious groin lymph nodes and a negative sentinel node may significantly reduce the number of patients who undergo unnecessary, extensive lymphadenectomy in the absence of disease. This is contingent upon a negative sentinel lymph node reliably predicting the absence of any other nodal metastases given the greater than 90% mortality associated with a groin recurrence.

The largest study published to date on the safety of the sentinel node procedure in vulvar cancer, GROINSS-V, included 403 assessable patients with a sentinel node procedure performed in 623 groins (Table 38.2) (129). Metastatic sentinel nodes were found in 26% of patients. In eight of 276 patients (3%) groin recurrences were diagnosed at a median follow-up time of 35 months. At the time of groin recurrence these patients all underwent bilateral inguinofemoral lymphadenectomy followed by chemoradiotherapy; six of the eight patients died of disease.

False-negative sentinel nodes were reported by others, but were thought to occur with low incidence in patients with clinically nonsuspicious nodes (44,134,135). Two recent studies of sentinel nodes in vulvar cancer, one single institution study of 56 patients and one multi-institution study of 127 patients with inclusion criteria similar to those in GROINSS-V, showed an unexpectedly high false-negative rate (27% and 7.7%, respectively), some of which may be attributable to insufficient experience of low-volume providers (128,136). This highlights one of the key concerns that any wide implantation of the sentinel node procedure beyond select expert centers might carry with it an unjustifiable rise in the frequency of groin recurrences.

The 2008 International Sentinel Node Society's expert panel statement stresses the importance of a well-informed patient treated by a skilled multidisciplinary team of a gynecologic oncologist, a nuclear medicine specialist, and a pathologist with expertise in the sentinel lymph node technique (137). They recommended the following eligibility criteria for the performance of the sentinel node procedure: unifocal primary tumor of 4 cm or less in diameter with greater than 1 mm invasion; and absence of any obvious metastatic disease on physical examination or imaging studies, including the absence of suspicious groin nodes. Until data from prospective randomized controlled trials document comparable survival for patients undergoing the sentinel node procedure compared to full inguinofemoral lymphadenectomy, complete inguinofemoral lymphadenectomy remains indicated in all but stage Ia disease, given the high mortality of recurrence in an undissected groin. The sentinel node technique should be limited to carefully selected patients in expert centers, ideally on research protocols.

Postoperative Management

Despite the age and general medical condition of many elderly patients with vulvar cancer, surgery is usually remarkably well tolerated. Patients should be able to commence eating a low-residue diet on the first postoperative day. In the past, bed rest was advised for 3 to 5 days postoperatively to allow for immobilization of the wounds and to foster healing. **Because radical local excisions are being performed with increasing frequency and groin lymphadenectomy is done through separate incisions, patients begin ambulation on postoperative day 1 or 2.** Pneumatic calf compression or subcutaneous *heparin* should be given to help prevent deep venous thrombosis, and active leg movements are to be encouraged. Frequent dressing changes are performed to keep the vulvar wound dry. Meticulous perineal hygiene is maintained. Suction drainage of each side of the groin is continued until output is minimal to help decrease the incidence of groin seromas. It is not uncommon for suction drainage to continue for 10 or more days. The Foley catheter is removed when the patient is ambulatory. If there is significant periurethral swelling, prolonged bladder drainage may be advisable. If there is breakdown of the vulvar wound, sitz baths or whirlpool therapy is helpful, followed by drying of the perineum with a hair dryer.

Early Postoperative Complications

The major immediate morbidity is related to groin wound infection, necrosis, and breakdown. This complication is reported in as many as 53% to 85% of patients having an *en bloc* operation (32,33). **With the separate-incision approach,** the incidence of wound breakdown can be reduced to about 44%; **major breakdown occurs in about 14% of patients** (34,78,138,139). With appropriate antibiotics, debridement, and wound dressings, the area will granulate and re-epithelialize over several weeks and may be managed with home nursing. Whirlpool therapy is effective for areas of extensive breakdown. The most common complications with the separate incision approach continues to be wound infection requiring antibiotic therapy and lymphocyst formation, both reported in about 40% of cases (139). Symptomatic lymphocysts should be managed by periodic sterile aspiration.

Other early postoperative complications include urinary tract infection, seromas in the femoral triangle, deep venous thrombosis, pulmonary embolism, myocardial infarction, hemorrhage, and, rarely, osteitis pubis. Anesthesia of the anterior thigh resulting from femoral nerve injury is common and usually resolves slowly.

Late Complications

One major late complication is chronic lymphedema, which occurs in about 30% of patients (32–34,138–140). Recurrent lymphangitis or cellulitis of the leg develops in about 10% of patients and usually responds to oral antibiotics. Urinary stress incontinence, with or without genital prolapse, occurs in about 10% of patients after radical vulvectomy and may require corrective surgery. Introital stenosis can lead to dyspareunia and may require a vertical relaxing incision, which is sutured transversely. An uncommon late complication is femoral hernia, which can be prevented intraoperatively by closure of the femoral canal with a suture from the inguinal ligament to Cooper's ligament. Pubic osteomyelitis and rectovaginal or rectoperineal fistulas are rare late complications.

Other major long-term treatment complications associated with the extent of vulvar surgery include depression, altered body image, and sexual dysfunction (96,97). Modifications in the radical extent of the surgical approach and appropriate preoperative and postoperative counseling may help lessen some of the psychological trauma.

Role of Radiation Therapy

Radiation therapy traditionally had a limited role in the management of patients with vulvar cancer. In the orthovoltage era, local tissue tolerance was poor and vulvar necrosis was common, but with megavoltage therapy, tolerance improved significantly. Radiation therapy, frequently with concurrent chemotherapy, has an increasingly important role in the management of patients with vulvar cancer. It is important to remember that, with a rare exception, radiation therapy alone has little place in the primary management of vulvar cancer. It is indicated in conjunction with surgery.

The indications for radiation therapy for patients with primary vulvar cancer are evolving. **Radiation seems to be indicated in the following situations:**

1. Preoperatively, in patients with advanced disease who would otherwise require pelvic exenteration or suffer loss of anal or urethral sphincteric function.
2. Preoperatively, in patients with fixed, unresectable groin nodes (141).
3. Postoperatively, to treat the pelvic lymph nodes and groins of patients with multiple microscopically positive groin nodes, one or more macrometastasis (10 mm or larger), or any evidence of extracapsular spread.

Possible roles for radiation therapy include the following:

1. Postoperatively, to help prevent local recurrences in patients with involved or close surgical margins (141–143).
2. As primary therapy for patients with small primary tumors, particularly clitoral or periclitoral lesions in young and middle-aged women, for whom surgical resection would have significant psychological consequences (80).

No additional treatment is recommended if one microscopically positive groin node (5 mm or less tumor deposit) is found in a fully dissected groin. The prognosis for this group of patients is excellent, and only careful observation is required (57). If unilateral groin dissection was performed for a lateral lesion, there seems to be no indication for dissection of the other side, because contralateral lymph node involvement is likely only if there are multiple microscopic or any gross ipsilateral inguinal node metastases (57,60). For patients with a single groin node metastasis, a recent retrospective SEER database review suggests that adjuvant radiation may provide a therapeutic benefit, especially if the groin dissection was limited (144).

If clinically evident groin metastases, any extracapsular spread or two or more microscopically positive groin nodes are found, the patient is at increased risk of groin and pelvic recurrence and should receive postoperative groin and pelvic irradiation. In 1977, the GOG initiated a prospective trial in which patients with positive groin nodes were randomized to either ipsilateral pelvic node dissection or bilateral pelvic plus groin irradiation (60). The survival rate for the radiation group (68% at 2 years) was significantly better than the survival rate for the pelvic lymphadenectomy group (54% at 2 years) ($p = 0.03$). The survival advantage was limited to patients with clinically evident groin nodes or more than one microscopically positive groin node. Groin recurrence occurred in 3 of 59 patients (5%) treated with radiation, compared with 13 of 55 (23.6%) patients treated with lymphadenectomy ($p = 0.02$). Four patients who received radiation had a pelvic recurrence, compared with one who had lymphadenectomy. These data indicate no benefit from pelvic irradiation compared with pelvic lymphadenectomy for the prevention of pelvic recurrence, but they do highlight the value of groin irradiation in preventing groin recurrence in patients with multiple positive groin nodes.

Recurrent Vulvar Cancer

Recurrence of vulvar cancer correlates closely with the number of positive groin nodes (57). Patients with fewer than three positive nodes, particularly if the nodes are only microscopically involved, have a low incidence of recurrence at any site, whereas patients with three or more positive nodes have a high incidence of local, regional, and systemic recurrences (57,60).

Most recurrences of vulvar cancer occur within the first 2 years from initial therapy, with groin recurrences occurring sooner (median time to recurrence 6 to 7 months) than vulvar recurrences (median time to recurrence 3 years) (72,145–147). **About one-third of vulvar cancer relapses present 5 or more years after initial therapy** (72). In a long-term follow-up study at the Mayo Clinic, nearly 1 in 10 patients with vulvar cancer had a late (longer than 5 years) reoccurrence of disease (72). Over 95% of those late relapses had local reoccurrences (same site recurrence or second primary vulvar site). Because of this propensity for late local reoccurrence, regular and long-term careful examinations of the vulva and groin constitute the cornerstone of posttreatment surveillance for these patients.

The published literature on the management and outcome of recurrent disease is limited. The timing and primary site of recurrence is critical to the prognosis postrecurrence. Although groin recurrences tend to occur early and are nearly always fatal, 5-year overall survival rates of 50%

Table 38.7 Microstaging of Vulvar Melanoma		
Clark Level (168)	**Chung Depth of Invasion (167)**	**Breslow Tumor Thickness (169)**
I Intraepithelial	Intraepithelial	<0.76 mm
II Into papillary dermis	≤1 mm from granular layer	0.76–1.5 mm Superficial invasion
III Filling dermal papillae	1.1–2.0 mm from granular layer	1.51–2.25 mm Intermediate invasion
IV Into reticular dermis	>2 mm from granular layer	2.26–3.0 Intermediate invasion
V Into subcutaneous fat	Into subcutaneous fat	>3 mm Deep invasion

2. The *superficial spreading melanoma* tends to remain relatively superficial early in its development.

3. The *nodular melanoma*, which is the most aggressive, is characterized by a raised lesion that penetrates deeply and may metastasize widely.

In one of the largest reported series, more than one-fourth of the cases of melanomas were macroscopically amelanotic (158). Vulvar melanoma tends to spread early, not only lymphatically but also hematogenously.

Staging

The FIGO staging used for squamous lesions is not applicable to melanomas because the lesions are usually much smaller and the prognosis is related to the depth of tumor invasion rather than to the diameter of the lesion (162,165,166). The leveling system established by Clark et al. for cutaneous melanomas is less readily applicable to vulvar lesions because of the different skin morphology (166). The vulvar skin lacks a well-defined papillary dermis. Breslow measured the thickest portion of the melanoma from the surface of intact epithelium to the deepest point of invasion (167). This system is more adequate for the vulva. Chung et al. proposed a modified system that retained Clark's definitions for levels I and V but arbitrarily defined levels II, III, and IV, using measurements in millimeters (165). A comparison of these systems is shown in Table 38.7.

The revised 2009 AJCC staging for cutaneous melanoma indicates that tumor thickness remains the primary determinant of the T staging, but mitotic rate was integrated to subcategorize T_1 tumors in addition to the presence of ulcerations. Specific immunohistochemistry criteria for the detection of micrometastases were included. The number and volume of metastatic nodes, site(s) of distant metastatic disease, serum lactate dehydrogenase level, and sentinel node results remained part of the staging (168).

Treatment

With better understanding of the prognostic significance of the microstage, some individualization of treatment developed. Treatment of vulvar melanoma continues to be controversial, in part because of the lack of large prospective studies, which makes it difficult to draw conclusions regarding its behavior and best treatment. Treatments are guided by experience from cutaneous melanoma and squamous cell carcinomas of the vulva. Paralleling the trend toward more conservative surgical management of cutaneous melanoma, there is a shift toward more conservative management of vulvar melanoma (163,164,169–171).

It is accepted that lesions with less than 1 mm of invasion may be treated with radical local excision alone (165,172). With more invasive lesions, *en bloc* resection of the primary tumor and regional groin nodes was traditionally recommended. In the past 15 years, **radical vulvectomy was performed less frequently and survival did not seem to be compromised** (173). One study reported on 32 patients with vulvar melanoma who underwent local excision (n = 14), simple vulvectomy (n = 7), or radical resection (n = 11) (174). No group had a superior survival rate, although the overall survival rate at 5 years was only 25%. Another study reported on 59 patients who underwent radical vulvectomy and 19 who underwent more conservative resections (163). Survival was not improved by the more radical approach, and they recommended radical local excision for the primary tumor, with groin dissection for tumors with a thickness of more than 1 mm. A recent SEER data analysis of 644 patients with vulvar melanoma did not find a survival difference in patients with localized disease treated with more conservative versus radical surgery. Five-year disease specific survival rates for patients undergoing conservative surgery for localized disease were 75% versus 79% for those undergoing radical surgery (174). Literature on cutaneous melanoma suggests that a 1-cm margin of skin and subcutaneous tissue is sufficient for the treatment of superficial localized melanoma (Breslow tumor thickness <0.76 mm), whereas a 2-cm margin suffices for intermediate-thickness lesions (1 to 4 mm) (175,176). At least a 1-cm tumor-free deep surgical margin is recommended, irrespective of tumor thickness. Because melanomas commonly involve the clitoris and labia minora, the vaginourethral margin of resection is a common site of failure, and care should be taken to obtain an adequate "inner" resection margin (177). A 10-year survival rate of 61% was shown for lateral lesions, compared with 37% for medial lesions ($p = 0.027$) (149).

Controversy exists as to which patients may benefit from inguinal-femoral lymphadenectomy. A prospective study by the GOG demonstrated that the risk of inguinal-femoral lymph node metastasis correlated with the Breslow microstage (165). As with cutaneous melanoma, it appears that for superficial lesions (Breslow tumor thickness <0.76 mm), the risk for nodal spread is so low that routine lymphadenectomy is not indicated as long as the nodes appear clinically free of disease. **For intermediate-thickness (1 to 4 mm) cutaneous melanoma, a randomized controlled trial of elective lymph node dissection versus observation showed a 5-year survival advantage for patients who underwent elective lymph node dissection, who were younger than 60 years, and whose tumors were characterized by 1- to 2-mm thickness and no ulcerations (178). Patients with deeply invasive cutaneous melanomas (>4-mm tumor thickness) have a high risk of regional and systemic metastases and are unlikely to benefit from regional lymphadenectomy** (179). Given some of the epidemiologic, histologic, and prognostic differences between vulvar and cutaneous melanoma, extrapolation of these data to the vulva should be done with caution (180). Specific to patients with vulvar melanoma, there is a small body of literature to suggest that there may be a clinical benefit in elective groin lymphadenectomy and the resection of clinically positive nodes (162,163). The role of the sentinel lymph node procedure in vulvar melanoma is under investigation. In cutaneous melanoma, sentinel lymph node biopsy replaced elective lymph node dissection in patients with clinically negative nodes, as it provides the same prognostic information with reduced morbidity. Only patients with metastatic disease undergo completion lymphadenectomy. Results from an interim analysis of the Multicenter Selective Lymphadenectomy Trial confirmed the prognostic value of the sentinel node procedure. These data suggest that an immediate completion lymphadenectomy following detection of a positive sentinel lymph node improves survival in patients with regional nodal metastases (181). Studies on the sentinel lymph node procedure for vulvar melanoma are limited. A review of the literature estimates a false-negative rate of about 15% (182). Although the sentinel node procedure appears appropriate for select patients with vulvar melanoma, the importance of an expert team familiar with the procedure and consisting of a gynecologic oncologist, a nuclear medicine specialist, and a pathologist with expertise in microstaging cannot be overemphasized.

Pelvic node metastases do not occur in the absence of groin node metastases (177,183,184). The prognosis for patients with positive pelvic nodes is so poor that there seems to be no value in performing pelvic lymphadenectomy for this disease. Immunotherapy and chemotherapy have demonstrated modest results in cutaneous melanoma. Several randomized cooperative and Intergroup trials of high-risk melanoma patients demonstrated a small but significant improvement in disease-free and overall survival with adjuvant *interferon alpha* (185–187). *Dacarbazine (DTIC)* is considered the most active single-agent chemotherapy, with a response rate of 16%, and randomized controlled trials failed to demonstrate superiority of any multiagent regimen (188). Targeted therapy is an area of promising development as single agents, in combination, and combined with chemotherapy. A vaccine stimulating both antibody and T-cell responses against melanoma is a promising but experimental treatment that is under investigation (189). Estrogen receptors were demonstrated in human melanomas, and an occasional response to *tamoxifen* was reported (190,191). Traditionally, melanomas were thought to be radiation resistant. There is a growing body of literature for advanced, high-risk, lymph node–metastatic cutaneous melanoma, demonstrating improved locoregional disease control compared to surgery with therapeutic lymphadenectomy alone (192,193).

Table 38.8 Prognosis for Patients with Vulvar Melanoma Stratified by Breslow Microstaging		
Breslow Tumor Thickness	*No. of Patients*	*% DOD*
<0.76 mm	31	7 (23%) [1 (5%)][a]
0.76–1.5 mm	35	6 (17%)
1.51–3.0 mm	42	23 (55%)
>3.0 mm	195	131 (67%)

DOD, died of disease.
[a]All but one of these seven deaths were reported in one study with an unusually low 5-year survival of 48% for 12 patients with superficial melanomas of Breslow thickness <0.76 mm. If these 12 cases were excluded, 5% of patients with superficial melanoma of the vulva died of disease.
From references 160, 165, 174, 185, 186, 196–199.

Prognosis

The behavior of melanomas can be unpredictable, but the prognosis is poor. The reported 5-year overall survival rate for vulvar melanoma is in the range of 50% to 60% (158,159,171). A SEER database analysis showed disease-specific survival rates for patients with localized, regional, and distant disease of 76%, 39%, and 22%, respectively (171). Localized disease, negative lymph nodes, and younger age were significant independent prognostic factors for improved survival. Because vulvar melanoma has a propensity for late recurrences, 5-year survival may not reflect cure. Prognosis is best predicted by microstaging. Patients with lesions invading to 1 mm or less have a good prognosis, but as depth of invasion increases, the prognosis worsens (Table 38.8). Tumor volume is reported to correlate with prognosis; patients whose lesions have a volume less than 100 mm^3 have an excellent prognosis (184). Additional prognostic factors are the patient's age, AJCC stage, presence of multifocal or satellite lesions, tumor ulceration, central tumor location, histologic growth pattern, lymph–vascular space involvement, and aneuploidy (158,162–164,194–197).

Bartholin Gland Carcinoma

Epidemiology

Primary carcinoma of the Bartholin gland is a rare form of vulvar cancer, which accounts for about 2% to 7% of vulvar malignancies (198). Because of its rarity, individual experience with the tumor is limited, and recommendations for management must be based on the review of small published series. Only about 300 cases are reported (46,198,199). Bartholin gland carcinoma is five times more common in postmenopausal than in premenopausal women (200).

Histopathology

The bilateral Bartholin glands are greater vestibular glands situated posterolaterally in the vulva. Their main duct is lined with stratified squamous epithelium, which changes to transitional epithelium as the terminal ducts are reached. Because tumors may arise from the gland or the duct, a variety of histologic types occur, including adenocarcinomas, squamous carcinomas, and, rarely, transitional cell, adenosquamous, and adenoid cystic carcinomas.

Classification of a vulvar tumor as a Bartholin gland carcinoma typically required that it fulfill Honan's criteria, which are as follows:

1. The tumor is in the correct anatomic position.
2. The tumor is located deep in the labium majus.
3. The overlying skin is intact.
4. There is some recognizable normal gland present.

Strict adherence to these criteria results in underdiagnosis of some cases. Large tumors may ulcerate through the overlying skin and obliterate the residual normal gland. Although transition between normal and malignant tissue is the best criterion, some cases will be diagnosed on the basis of their histologic characteristics and anatomic location.

		Table 38.9 Survival of Patients with Bartholin Gland Carcinoma	
FIGO Stage	*No. of Patients*	*No. of Patients with Recurrent Disease*	*No. of Patients NED at Last F/U* [a]
I	15 (21%)	3 (20%)	14 (93%)
II	16 (23%)	2 (13%)	15 (94%)
III	30 (42%)	11 (37%)	22 (73%)
IV	10 (14%)	5 (50%)	5 (50%)
Total	71 (100%)	21 (30%) [b]	56 (79%) [b]

FIGO, International Federation of Gynecology and Obstetrics; NED, no evidence of disease; F/U, follow-up.
[a] Median follow-up in each study was at least 5 years.
[b] Total >100% because some patients with recurrence remained NED.
From references 46, 200, 201, 205.

Signs and Symptoms

The most common initial symptom of Bartholin gland carcinoma is a vulvar mass or perineal pain. About 10% of patients have a history of inflammation of the Bartholin gland, and malignancies may be mistaken for benign cysts or abscesses. Delay of diagnosis is common, particularly for premenopausal patients. The differential diagnosis of any pararectovaginal neoplasm should include cloacogenic carcinoma and secondary neoplasm (199).

Treatment

Traditionally, treatment was radical vulvectomy with bilateral groin and pelvic node dissection (201). There seems to be no indication for dissection of the pelvic nodes in the absence of positive groin nodes, and good results were reported with hemivulvectomy or radical local excision for the primary tumor (199). Because these lesions are deep in the vulva, extensive dissection is required in the ischiorectal fossa; surgical margins are often close. Postoperative radiation to the vulva decreased the likelihood of local recurrence from 27% (6 of 22 patients) to 7% (1 of 14 patients) (199). If the ipsilateral groin nodes are positive, bilateral groin and pelvic irradiation may decrease regional recurrence. If the tumor is fixed to the inferior pubic ramus or involves adjacent structures, such as the anal sphincter or rectum, preoperative radiation and chemotherapy is preferable to avoid ultraradical surgery. A recent report of 10 consecutive patients with primary Bartholin gland carcinoma suggests that treatment with radiation or chemoradiation using teletherapy combined with a boost to the primary site or regional nodes and/or interstitial brachytherapy may offer an effective alternative to surgery with 3- and 5-year survival rates of 72% and 66%, respectively (202).

Prognosis

Because of the deep location of the gland, disease tends to be more advanced than squamous carcinomas at the time of diagnosis but, stage for stage, the prognosis is similar. Five-year disease-free survival rates by stage are summarized in Table 38.9.

Adenoid Cystic Carcinoma of the Bartholin Gland

The adenoid cystic variety accounts for 15% of Bartholin gland carcinomas. A review of 62 cases reported in the literature demonstrates that adenoid cystic carcinoma of the Bartholin gland is a slow growing tumor characterized by perineural infiltration and a marked propensity for local relapse preceding distant recurrences by years. It is less likely to metastasize to lymph nodes and carries a somewhat better prognosis (Fig. 38.8) (203–205). The slowly progressive nature of these tumors and the tendency for late recurrences is reflected in the disparity between progression-free interval and overall survival (204).

Other Adenocarcinomas

Adenocarcinomas of the vulva usually arise in a Bartholin gland or occur in association with Paget disease. They may arise rarely from the skin appendages, paraurethral glands, minor vestibular glands, aberrant breast tissue, endometriosis, or a misplaced cloacal remnant (206).

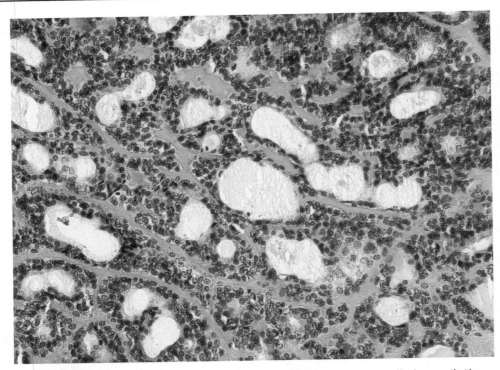

Figure 38.8 **Adenoid cystic tumor of the Bartholin gland.** Basaloid cells form cribriform, sievelike spaces containing mucinous material. The hyaline stroma is another distinct feature of this tumor.

Adenosquamous Carcinoma

A particularly aggressive type of carcinoma is the adenosquamous carcinoma. This tumor has a number of synonyms, including cylindroma, pseudoglandular squamous cell carcinoma, adenoid squamous cell carcinoma, and adenoacanthoma of the sweat gland of Lever. The tumor has a propensity for perineural invasion, early lymph node metastasis, and local recurrence. One study noted a crude 5-year survival rate of 5.5% (1 of 18) for adenosquamous carcinoma of the vulva, compared with 62.3% (48 of 77) for patients with squamous cell carcinoma (207). Treatment should be radical vulvectomy and bilateral groin dissection. Postoperative radiation therapy may be appropriate.

Basal Cell Carcinoma

Basal cell carcinomas represent about 2% of vulvar cancers. As with other basal cell carcinomas, vulvar lesions commonly appear as a "rodent ulcer" with rolled edges, although nodules and macules are other morphologic varieties that occur. Most lesions are smaller than 2 cm in diameter and are usually situated on the anterior labia majora. Giant lesions occasionally occur (208). Basal cell carcinoma usually affects postmenopausal white women and is locally aggressive. Symptoms are frequently present for a prolonged period and most often include pruritus, soreness, and irritation (209). It is diagnosed by biopsy, and **radical local excision is adequate treatment** (210). **Metastasis to regional lymph nodes is reported but is rare** (211–213). The local recurrence rate is about 10% to 20% (209,214). Basal cell carcinoma of the vulva is associated with a high incidence of antecedent or concomitant malignancies elsewhere (209). In a series of 28 women with vulvar basal cell carcinoma, 10 patients had other basal cell carcinomas, and 10 patients suffered from other primary malignancies (209).

About 3% to 5% of basal cell carcinomas contain a malignant squamous component, the so-called *basosquamous carcinoma*. These lesions are more aggressive and should be treated as squamous carcinomas (213). Another subtype of basal cell carcinoma is the adenoid basal cell carcinoma, which must be differentiated from the more aggressive adenoid cystic carcinoma arising in a Bartholin gland or the skin (213).

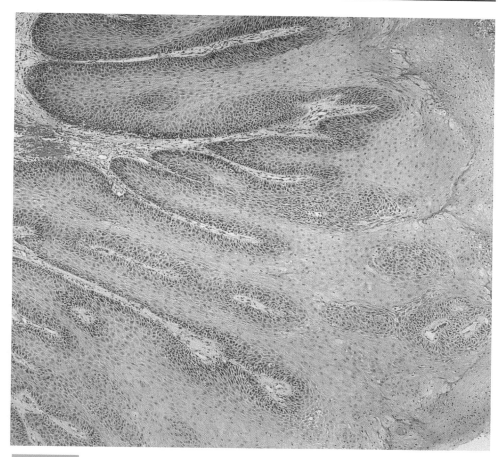

Figure 38.9   Verrucous carcinoma of the vulva. Note the exophytic hyperkeratotic papillary fronds and endophytic bulky rete pegs with smooth borders.

Verrucous Carcinoma

Verrucous carcinoma is a variant of squamous cell carcinoma and has distinctive clinical and pathologic characteristics (215). Although most commonly found in the oral cavity, verrucous lesions may be found on any moist membrane composed of squamous epithelium (216). In the female genital tract, these lesions may develop on the cervix, vulva, and vagina. The cause of the lesion in the female genital tract is not fully understood, but associated HPV-6 and HPV-11 were found in some studies, whereas others find it to have no association with HPV infection (217,218). Some studies found as many as one-third of the cases to have coexisting squamous carcinoma of the vulva, underscoring the importance of careful histopathologic assessment of these tumors (219).

Grossly, the tumors have a cauliflowerlike appearance; microscopically, they contain multiple papillary fronds that lack the central connective tissue core that characterizes condylomata acuminata (Fig. 38.9). The gross and microscopic features of a verrucous carcinoma are very similar to those of the **giant condyloma of Buschke-Loewenstein**, and they probably represent the same disease entity (206). Adequate biopsy from the base of the lesion is required to differentiate a verrucous carcinoma from a benign condyloma acuminatum or a squamous cell carcinoma with a verrucous growth pattern.

Verrucous carcinomas usually occur in postmenopausal women, and they are slow-growing but locally destructive lesions. Even bone may be invaded. Metastasis to regional lymph nodes is rare but was reported (220). Radical local excision is the basic treatment, although any palpably suspicious groin nodes should be evaluated with fine-needle aspiration cytology or excisional biopsy. Usually, enlarged nodes will be caused by inflammatory hypertrophy (221). If the nodes contain metastases, radical vulvectomy and bilateral inguinal-femoral lymphadenectomy are indicated.

Several small studies failed to document any therapeutic advantage with radiation therapy (221). There is concern that radiation may induce anaplastic transformation with subsequent regional and distant metastasis (222). One study reported a corrected 5-year survival rate of 94% for 17 patients treated with surgery alone, compared with 42% for 7 patients treated with surgery and radiation (221). The latter patients had more advanced disease. If there is a recurrence, further surgical excision is the treatment of choice, which occasionally may necessitate some type of exenteration.

Vulvar Sarcoma

Sarcomas represent 1.5% of vulvar malignancies and constitute a heterogenous group of tumors (223). Leiomyosarcomas are the most common, and other histologic types include fibrosarcomas, neurofibrosarcomas, liposarcomas, rhabdomyosarcomas, angiosarcomas, epithelioid sarcomas, and malignant schwannomas.

Leiomyosarcomas **usually appear as enlarging, often painful masses, usually in the labium majus.** Smooth muscle tumors of the vulva that show at least three of the following four criteria should be regarded as sarcomas: (i) diameter greater than 5 cm, (ii) infiltrating margins, (iii) 5 or more mitotic figures per 10 high-power fields, (iv) moderate-to-severe cytological atypia (224). The absence of one, or even all, of these features does not guarantee against recurrence (225). Lymphatic metastases are uncommon, and radical local excision is the usual treatment.

Epithelioid sarcomas **characteristically develop in the soft tissues of the extremities of young adults but rarely may occur on the vulva.** In a description of two cases and review of three other reports, the authors concluded that these tumors might mimic a Bartholin cyst, leading to inadequate initial treatment (226). They believed that vulvar epithelioid sarcomas behave more aggressively than their extragenital counterparts, with four of the five patients dying of metastatic disease. They suggested that early recognition and wide excision should improve the prognosis.

Rhabdomyosarcomas **are the most common soft tissue sarcomas in childhood, and 20% involve the pelvis or genitourinary tract** (227). Dramatic gains were made in the treatment of these tumors during the past 20 years. Previously, radical pelvic surgery was the standard approach, but results were poor. A multimodal approach evolved, and survival rates improved significantly, with a corresponding decrease in morbidity. In a report of the experience of the Intergroup Rhabdomyosarcoma Study I and II (1972 to 1984) with primary tumors of the female genital tract, nine patients aged 1 to 19 years had primary vulvar tumors, and these tumors were often regarded as a form of Bartholin gland infection before biopsy (228). They were all managed with chemotherapy (*vincristine*, or *actinomycin D* and *cyclophosphamide* and *doxorubicin*), with or without radiotherapy. Wide local excision of the tumor, with or without inguinal-femoral lymphadenectomy, was carried out before or after the chemotherapy. Seven of the nine patients were free of disease 4 or more years from diagnosis, one patient was free of disease when lost to follow-up at 5 years, and one patient was alive with disease.

Rare Vulvar Malignancies

In addition to the previously mentioned tumors, a number of malignancies more commonly seen in other areas of the body may rarely occur as isolated vulvar tumors.

Lymphomas

The genital tract may be involved primarily by malignant lymphomas but, more commonly, involvement is a manifestation of systemic disease. In the lower genital tract, the cervix is most often involved, followed by the vulva and the vagina (229). Most patients are in their third to sixth decades of life, and about three-fourths of the cases involve diffuse large cell or histiocytic non-Hodgkin's lymphomas. The remainder are nodular or Burkitt's lymphomas. Treatment is by surgical excision followed by chemotherapy and radiation or both, and the overall 5-year survival rate is about 70% (229).

Endodermal Sinus Tumor

There were four case reports of endodermal sinus tumor of the vulva, and three of the four patients died of distant metastases (230). All patients were in their third decade of life, but none was treated with modern chemotherapy.

Merkel Cell Carcinoma

Merkel cell carcinomas are primary small cell carcinomas of the skin that resemble oat cell carcinomas of the lung. They metastasize widely and have a very poor prognosis (231–233). They should be locally excised and treated with *cisplatin*-based chemotherapy.

Dermatofibrosarcoma Protuberans

This rare, low-grade cutaneous malignancy occasionally involves the vulva. It has a marked tendency for local recurrence but a low risk of systemic spread (234). Radical local excision should be sufficient treatment.

Metastatic Tumors of the Vulva

Eight percent of vulvar tumors are metastatic. The most common primary site is the cervix, followed by the endometrium, kidney, and urethra. Most patients in whom vulvar metastases develop have advanced primary tumors when diagnosed, and in about one-fourth of the patients, the primary lesion and the vulvar metastasis are diagnosed simultaneously (235).

References

1. **Siegel R, Ward E, Brawley O, et al.** Cancer statistics, 2011. *CA Cancer J Clin* 2011;61:212–236. http://cacancerjournal.org
2. **US Cancer Statistics Working Group.** *United States cancer statistics.* Available online at: http://apps.nccd.cdc.gov/uscs/
3. **Judson PL, Habermann EB, Baxter NN, et al.** Trends in the incidence of invasive and *in situ* vulvar carcinoma. *Obstet Gynecol* 2006;107:1018–1022.
4. **Joura EA, Losch A, Haider-Angeler MG, et al.** Trends in vulvar neoplasia. Increasing incidence of vulvar intraepithelial neoplasia and squamous cell carcinoma of the vulva in young women. *J Reprod Med* 2000;45:613–615.
5. **Jones RW, Baranyai J, Stables S.** Trends in squamous cell carcinoma of the vulva: the influence of vulvar intraepithelial neoplasia. *Obstet Gynecol* 1997;90:448–452.
6. **Taussig FJ.** Cancer of the vulva: an analysis of 155 cases. *Am J Obstet Gynecol* 1940;40:764–778.
7. **Way S.** Carcinoma of the vulva. *Am J Obstet Gynecol* 1960;79:692–697.
8. **Madsen BS, Jensen HL, van den Brule AJ, et al.** Risk factors for invasive squamous cell carcinoma of the vulva and vagina—population-based case-control study in Denmark. *Int J Cancer* 2008;122:2827—2834.
9. **Ansink A.** Vulvar squamous cell carcinoma. *Semin Dermatol* 1996;15:51–59.
10. **van Seters M, van Beurden M, de Craen AJ.** Is the assumed natural history of vulvar intraepithelial neoplasia III based on enough evidence? A systematic review of 3322 published patients. *Gynecol Oncol* 2005;97:645–651.
11. **Hording U, Junge J, Poulsen H, et al.** Vulvar intraepithelial neoplasia III: a viral disease of undetermined progressive potential. *Gynecol Oncol* 1995;56:276–279.
12. **Modesitt SC, Waters AB, Walton L, et al.** Vulvar intraepithelial neoplasia III: occult cancer and the impact of margin status on recurrence. *Obstet Gynecol* 1998;92:962–966.
13. **Trimble CL, Hildesheim A, Brinton LA, et al.** Heterogeneous etiology of squamous carcinoma of the vulva. *Obstet Gynecol* 1996;87:59–64.
14. **Insinga RP, Liaw KL, Johnson LG, et al.** A systematic review of the prevalence and attribution of human papillomavirus types among cervical, vaginal, and vulvar precancers and cancers in the United States. *Cancer Epidemiol Biomarkers Prev* 2008;17:1611–1622.
15. **Brinton LA, Nasco PC, Mallin K, et al.** Case-control study of cancer of the vulva. *Obstet Gynecol* 1990;75:859–866.
16. **Kurman RJ, Toki T, Schiffman MH.** Basaloid and warty carcinomas of the vulva: distinctive types of squamous cell carcinoma frequently associated with human papillomaviruses. *Am J Surg Pathol* 1993;17:133–145.
17. **Vilmer C, Cavelier-Balloy B, Nogues C, et al.** Analysis of alterations adjacent to invasive vulvar carcinoma and their relationship with the associated carcinoma: a study of 67 cases. *Eur J Gynaecol Oncol* 1998;19:25–31.
18. **Cooper SM, Gao XH, Powell JJ, et al.** Does treatment of vulvar lichen sclerosus influence its prognosis? *Arch Dermatol* 2004;140:702–706.
19. **Renaud-Vilmer C, Cavelier-Balloy B, Porcher R, et al.** Vulvar lichen sclerosus: effect of long-term topical application of a potent steroid on the course of the disease. *Arch Dermatol* 2004;140:709–712.
20. **Bradford J, Fischer G.** Long-term management of vulval lichen sclerosus in adult women. *Aust N Z J Obstet Gynaecol* 2010;50:148–152.
21. **Carlson JA, Ambros R, Malfetano J, et al.** Vulvar lichen sclerosus and squamous cell carcinoma: a cohort, case control, and investigational study with historical perspective; implications for chronic inflammation and sclerosis in the development of neoplasia. *Hum Pathol* 1998;29:932–948.
22. **Tate JE, Mutter GL, Boynton KA, et al.** Monoclonal origin of vulvar intraepithelial neoplasia and some vulvar hyperplasias. *Am J Pathol* 1997;150:315–322.
23. **Raspollini MR, Asirelli G, Moncini D, et al.** A comparative analysis of lichen sclerosus of the vulva and lichen sclerosus that evolves to vulvar squamous cell carcinoma. *Am J Obstet Gynecol* 2007;197:592.e1–e5.
24. **Franklin EW, Rutledge FD.** Epidemiology of epidermoid carcinoma of the vulva. *Obstet Gynecol* 1972;39:165–172.
25. **Green TH Jr, Ulfelder H, Meigs JV.** Epidermoid carcinoma of the vulva: an analysis of 238 cases. Parts I and II. *Am J Obstet Gynecol* 1958;73:834–864.
26. **Woodruff JD.** Early invasive carcinoma of the vulva. *Clin Oncol* 1982;1:349.
27. **Binder SW, Huang I, Fu YS, et al.** Risk factors for the development of lymph node metastasis in vulvar squamous cell carcinoma. *Gynecol Oncol* 1990;37:9–16.
28. **Boyce J, Fruchter RG, Kasambilides E, et al.** Prognostic factors in carcinoma of the vulva. *Gynecol Oncol* 1985;20:364–377.
29. **Donaldson ES, Powell DE, Hanson MB, et al.** Prognostic parameters in invasive vulvar cancer. *Gynecol Oncol* 1981;11:184–190.
30. **Buscema J, Woodruff JD.** Progressive histobiologic alterations in the development of vulvar cancer. *Am J Obstet Gynecol* 1980;138:146–150.
31. **Pecorelli S.** Revised FIGO staging for carcinoma of the vulva, cervix, and endometrium. *Int J Gynaecol Obstet* 2009;105:103–104.
32. **Rutledge F, Smith JP, Franklin EW.** Carcinoma of the vulva. *Am J Obstet Gynecol* 1970;106:1117–1130.
33. **Podratz KC, Symmonds RE, Taylor WF, et al.** Carcinoma of the vulva: analysis of treatment and survival. *Obstet Gynecol* 1983;61:63–74.

34. **Cavanagh D, Fiorica JV, Hoffman MS, et al.** Invasive carcinoma of the vulva: changing trends in surgical management. *Am J Obstet Gynecol* 1990;163:1007–1115.

35. **Sturgeon SR, Curtis RE, Johnson K, et al.** Second primary cancers after vulvar and vaginal cancers. *Am J Obstet Gynecol* 1996;174:929–933.

36. **Hacker NF, Van der Velden J.** Conservative management of early vulvar cancer. *Cancer* 1993;71:1673–1677.

37. **DiSaia PJ, Creasman WT, Rich WM.** An alternative approach to early cancer of the vulva. *Am J Obstet Gynecol* 1979;133:825–832.

38. **Hacker NF, Nieberg RK, Berek JS, et al.** Superficially invasive vulvar cancer with nodal metastases. *Gynecol Oncol* 1983;15:65–77.

39. **Chu J, Tamimi HK, Figge DC.** Femoral node metastases with negative superficial inguinal nodes in early vulvar cancer. *Am J Obstet Gynecol* 1981;140:337–339.

40. **Podczaski E, Sexton M, Kaminski P, et al.** Recurrent carcinoma of the vulva after conservative treatment for "microinvasive" disease. *Gynecol Oncol* 1990;39:65–68.

41. **Stehman FB, Bundy BN, Dvoretsky PM, et al.** Early stage I carcinoma of the vulva treated with ipsilateral superficial inguinal lymphadenectomy and modified radical hemivulvectomy: a prospective study of the Gynecologic Oncology Group. *Obstet Gynecol* 1992;79:490–497.

42. **Gordinier ME, Malpica A, Burke TW, et al.** Groin recurrence in patients with vulvar cancer with negative nodes on superficial inguinal lymphadenectomy. *Gynecol Oncol* 2003;90:625–628.

43. **Levenback C, Burke TW, Morris M, et al.** Potential applications of intraoperative lymphatic mapping in vulvar cancer. *Gynecol Oncol* 1995;59:216–220.

44. **Rob L, Robova H, Pluta M, et al.** Further data on sentinel lymph node mapping in vulvar cancer by blue dye and radiocolloid Tc99. *Int J Gynecol Cancer* 2007;17:147–153.

45. **Curry SL, Wharton JT, Rutledge F.** Positive lymph nodes in vulvar squamous carcinoma. *Gynecol Oncol* 1980;9:63–67.

46. **Leuchter RS, Hacker NF, Voet RL, et al.** Primary carcinoma of the Bartholin gland: a report of 14 cases and a review of the literature. *Obstet Gynecol* 1982;60:361–368.

47. **Piver MS, Xynos FP.** Pelvic lymphadenectomy in women with carcinoma of the clitoris. *Obstet Gynecol* 1977;49:592–595.

48. **Gonzalez Bosquet J, Magrina JF, Magtibay PM, et al.** Patterns of inguinal groin metastases in squamous cell carcinoma of the vulva. *Gynecol Oncol* 2007;105:742–746.

49. **Burke TW, Levenback C, Coleman RL, et al.** Surgical therapy of T1 and T2 vulvar carcinoma: further experience with radical wide excision and selective inguinal lymphadenectomy. *Gynecol Oncol* 1995;57:215–220.

50. **Burrell MO, Franklin EW III, Campion MJ, et al.** The modified radical vulvectomy with groin dissection: an eight-year experience. *Am J Obstet Gynecol* 1988;159:715–722.

51. **Collins CG, Lee FY, Roman-Lopez JJ.** Invasive carcinoma of the vulva with lymph node metastases. *Am J Obstet Gynecol* 1971;109:446–452.

52. **Morley GW.** Infiltrative carcinoma of the vulva: results of surgical treatment. *Am J Obstet Gynecol* 1976;124:874–888.

53. **Krupp PJ, Bohm JW.** Lymph gland metastases in invasive squamous cell cancer of the vulva. *Am J Obstet Gynecol* 1978;130:943–952.

54. **Keys H.** Gynecologic Oncology Group randomized trials of combined technique therapy of vulvar cancer. *Cancer* 1993;71:1691–1696.

55. **Benedet JL, Turko M, Fairey RN, et al.** Squamous carcinoma of the vulva: results of treatment, 1938 to 1976. *Am J Obstet Gynecol* 1979;134:201–207.

56. **Iversen T, Aalders JG, Christensen A, et al.** Squamous cell carcinoma of the vulva: a review of 424 patients, 1956–1974. *Gynecol Oncol* 1980;9:271–279.

57. **Hacker NF, Berek JS, Lagasse LD, et al.** Management of regional lymph nodes and their prognostic influence in vulvar cancer. *Obstet Gynecol* 1983;61:408–412.

58. **Monaghan JM, Hammond IG.** Pelvic node dissection in the treatment of vulvar carcinoma—is it necessary? *BJOG* 1984;91:270–274.

59. **Hopkins MP, Reid CG, Vettrano I, et al.** Squamous cell carcinoma of the vulva: prognostic factors influencing survival. *Gynecol Oncol* 1991;43:113–117.

60. **Homesley HD, Bundy BN, Sedlis A, et al.** Radiation therapy versus pelvic node resection for carcinoma of the vulva with positive groin nodes. *Obstet Gynecol* 1986;68:733–740.

61. **Hacker NF.** Vulvar cancer. In: **Berek JS, Hacker NF, eds.** *Berek & Hacker's Gynecologic Oncology.* 5th ed. Philadelphia, PA: Lippincott Williams & Wilkins, 2010:536–575.

62. **Hacker NF.** Revised FIGO staging for carcinoma of the vulva. *Int J Gynaecol Obstet* 2009;105:105–106.

63. **van der Steen S, de Nieuwenhof HP, Massuger L, et al.** New FIGO staging system of vulvar cancer indeed provides a better reflection of prognosis. *Gynecol Oncol* 2010;119:520–525.

64. **Hopkins MP, Reid GC, Johnston CM, et al.** A comparison of staging systems for squamous cell carcinoma of the vulva. *Gynecol Oncol* 1992;47:34–37.

65. **Raspagliesi F, Hanozet F, Ditto A, et al.** Clinical and pathological prognostic factors in squamous cell carcinoma of the vulva. *Gynecol Oncol* 2006;102:333–337.

66. **Lataifeh I, Nascimento MC, Nicklin JL, et al.** Patterns of recurrence and disease-free survival in advanced squamous cell carcinoma of the vulva. *Gynecol Oncol* 2004;95:701–705.

67. **Fons G, Hyde SE, Buist MR, et al.** Prognostic value of bilateral positive nodes in squamous cell cancer of the vulva. *Int J Gynecol Cancer* 2009;19:1276–1280.

68. **College of American Pathologists.** Protocol for the examination of specimens from patients with carcinoma of the vulva. October 2009. Available online at: http://www.cap.org/apps/docs/committees/cancer/cancer protocols/2009/Vulva 09protocol.pdf

69. **Beller U, Quinn MA, Benedet JL, et al.** 26th annual report on the results of treatment in gynecological cancer: carcinoma of the vulva. *Int J Gynecol Obstet* 2006;95:S7–S27.

70. **Paladini D, Cross P, Lopes A, et al.** Prognostic significance of lymph node variables in squamous cell carcinoma of the vulva. *Cancer* 1994;74:2491–2496.

71. **Homesley HD, Bundy BN, Sedlis A, et al.** Assessment of current International Federation of Gynecology and Obstetrics staging of vulvar carcinoma relative to prognostic factors for survival (a Gynecologic Oncology Group study). *Am J Obstet Gynecol* 1991;164:997–1003.

72. **Gonzalez Bosquet J, Magrina JF, Gaffey TA, et al.** Long-term survival and disease recurrence in patients with primary squamous cell carcinoma of the vulva. *Gynecol Oncol* 2005;97:828–833.

73. **Homesley HD, Bundy BN, Sedlis A, et al.** Prognostic factors for groin node metastasis in squamous cell carcinoma of the vulva (a Gynecologic Oncology Group Study). *Gynecol Oncol* 1993;49:279–283.

74. **van der Velden J, Hacker NF.** Update on vulvar carcinoma. In: **Rothenberg ML, ed.** *Gynecologic oncology: controversies and new developments.* Boston, MA: Kluwer Academic Publishers, 1994:101–119.

75. **Van der Velden J, van Lindert AC, Lammes FB, et al.** Extracapsular growth of lymph node metastases in squamous cell carcinoma of the vulva. The impact on recurrence and survival. *Cancer* 1995;75:2885–2890.

76. **Origoni M, Sideri M, Garsia S, et al.** Prognostic value of pathological patterns of lymph node positivity in squamous cell carcinoma of the vulva stage III and IVA FIGO. *Gynecol Oncol* 1992;45:313–316.

77. **Magrina JF, Gonzalez Bosquet J, Weaver AL, et al.** Squamous cell carcinoma of the vulva stage IA: long-term results. *Gynecol Oncol* 2000;76:24–27.

78. **Hacker NF, Leuchter RS, Berek JS, et al.** Radical vulvectomy and bilateral inguinal lymphadenectomy through separate groin incisions. *Obstet Gynecol* 1981;58:574–579.

79. **Iversen T, Abeler V, Aalders J.** Individualized treatment of stage I carcinoma of the vulva. *Obstet Gynecol* 1981;57:85–89.

80. **Hacker NF, Berek JS, Lagasse LD, et al.** Individualization of treatment for stage I squamous cell vulvar carcinoma. *Obstet Gynecol* 1984;63:155–162.

81. **Tantipalakorn C, Robertson G, Marsden DE, et al.** Outcome and patterns of recurrence for International Federation of Gynecology and Obstetrics (FIGO) stages I and II squamous cell vulvar cancer. *Obstet Gynecol* 2009;113:895–901.

82. **DeSimone CP, Van Ness JS, Cooper AL, et al.** The treatment of lateral T1 and T2 squamous cell carcinomas of the vulva confined to the labium majus or minus. *Gynecol Oncol* 2007;104:390–395.

83. **Farias-Eisner R, Cirisano FD, Grouse D, et al.** Conservative and individualized surgery for early squamous carcinoma of the vulva: the treatment of choice for stages I and II (T1–2, N0–1, M0) disease. *Gynecol Oncol* 1994;53:33–38.

84. **Heaps JM, Fu YS, Montz FJ, et al.** Surgical-pathologic variables predictive of local recurrence in squamous cell carcinoma of the vulva. *Gynecol Oncol* 1990;38:309–314.

85. **De Hullu JA, Hollema H, Lolkema S, et al.** Vulvar carcinoma. The price of less radical surgery. *Cancer* 2002;95:2331–2338.

86. **Chan JK, Sugiyama V, Pham H, et al.** Margin distance and other clinico-pathologic prognostic factors in vulvar carcinoma: a multivariate analysis. *Gynecol Oncol* 2007;104:636–641.

87. **Chan JK, Sugiyama V, Tajalli TR, et al.** Conservative, clitoral preservation surgery in the treatment of vulvar squamous cell carcinoma. *Gynecol Oncol* 2004;95:152–156.

88. **Simonsen E, Johnsson JE, Tropé C.** Radical vulvectomy with warm-knife and open-wound techniques in vulvar malignancies. *Gynecol Oncol* 1984;17:22–31.

89. **Potkul RK, Barnes WA, Barter JF, et al.** Vulvar reconstruction using a mons pubis pedicle flap. *Gynecol Oncol* 1994;55:21–24.

90. **Trelford JD, Deer DA, Ordorica E, et al.** Ten-year prospective study in a management change of vulvar carcinoma. *Am J Obstet Gynecol* 1984;150:288–296.

91. **Julian CG, Callison J, Woodruff JD.** Plastic management of extensive vulvar defects. *Obstet Gynecol* 1971;38:193–198.

92. **Barnhill DR, Hoskins WJ, Metz P.** Use of the rhomboid flap after partial vulvectomy. *Obstet Gynecol* 1983;62:444–447.

93. **Ballon SC, Donaldson RC, Roberts JA.** Reconstruction of the vulva using a myocutaneous graft. *Gynecol Oncol* 1979;7:123–127.

94. **Chafe W, Fowler WC, Walton LA, et al.** Radical vulvectomy with use of tensor fascia lata myocutaneous flap. *Am J Obstet Gynecol* 1983;145:207–213.

95. **Andersen BL, Hacker NF.** Psychological adjustment after vulvar surgery. *Obstet Gynecol* 1983;62:457–462.

96. **Andersen BL, Hacker NF.** Psychosexual adjustment following pelvic exenteration. *Obstet Gynecol* 1983;61:457–462.

97. **Kaplan AL, Kaufman RH.** Management of advanced carcinoma of the vulva. *Gynecol Oncol* 1975;3:220–232.

98. **Phillips B, Buchsbaum HJ, Lifshitz S.** Pelvic exenteration for vulvovaginal carcinoma. *Am J Obstet Gynecol* 1981;141:1038–1044.

99. **Cavanagh D, Shepherd JH.** The place of pelvic exenteration in the primary management of advanced carcinoma of the vulva. *Gynecol Oncol* 1982;13:318–322.

100. **Grimshaw RN, Aswad SG, Monaghan JM.** The role of anovulvectomy in locally advanced carcinoma of the vulva. *Int J Gynecol Cancer* 1991;1:15.

101. **Moore DH, Thomas GM, Montana GS, et al.** Preoperative chemoradiation for advanced vulvar cancer: a phase II study of the GOG. *Int J Radiat Oncol Biol Phys* 1998;42:79–85.

102. **Cunningham MJ, Goyer RP, Gibbons SK, et al.** Primary radiation, cisplatin, and 5-fluorouracil for advanced squamous carcinoma of the vulva. *Gynecol Oncol* 1997;66:258–261.

103. **Eifel PJ, Morris M, Burke TW, et al.** Prolonged continuous infusion cisplatin and 5-fluorouracil for advanced squamous carcinoma of the vulva. *Gynecol Oncol* 1995;59:51–56.

104. **Gerszten K, Selvaraj RN, Kelley J, et al.** Preoperative chemoradiation for locally advanced carcinoma of the vulva. *Gynecol Oncol* 2005;99:640–644.

105. **Lupi G, Raspagliesi F, Zucali R, et al.** Combined preoperative chemoradiotherapy followed by radical surgery in locally advanced vulvar carcinoma. A pilot study. *Cancer* 1996;77:1472–1478.

106. **Landoni F, Maneo A, Zanetta G, et al.** Concurrent preoperative chemotherapy with 5-fluorouracil and mitomycin C and radiotherapy (FUMIR) followed by limited surgery in locally advanced and recurrent vulvar carcinoma. *Gynecol Oncol* 1996;61:321–327.

107. **Beriwal S, Coon D, Heron DE, et al.** Preoperative intensity-modulated radiotherapy and chemotherapy for locally advanced vulvar carcinoma. *Gynecol Oncol* 2008;109:291–295.

108. **van Doorn HC, Ansink A, Verhaar-Langereis M, et al.** Neoadjuvant chemoradiation for advanced primary vulvar cancer. *Cochrane Database Syst Rev* 2006;3:CD003752.

109. **Hacker NF, Berek JS, Juillard GJF, et al.** Preoperative radiation therapy for locally advanced vulvar cancer. *Cancer* 1984;54:2056–2061.

110. **Boronow RC, Hickman BT, Reagan MT, et al.** Combined therapy as an alternative for exenteration for locally advanced vulvovaginal cancer. II. Results, complications and dosimetric and surgical considerations. *Am J Clin Oncol* 1987;10:171–181.

111. **Backstrom A, Edsmyr F, Wicklund H.** Radiotherapy of carcinoma of the vulva. *Acta Obstet Gynecol* 1972;51:109–115.

112. **Thomas G, Dembo A, DePetrillo A, et al.** Concurrent radiation and chemotherapy in vulvar carcinoma. *Gynecol Oncol* 1989;34:263–267.

113. **Marsden DE, Hacker NF.** Contemporary management of primary carcinoma of the vulva. *Surg Clin North Am* 2001;81:799–813.

114. **Atamdede F, Hoogerland D.** Regional lymph node recurrence following local excision for microinvasive vulvar carcinoma. *Gynecol Oncol* 1989;34:125–128.

115. **Vernooij F, Sie-Go DM, Heintz AP.** Lymph node recurrence following stage IA vulvar carcinoma: two cases and a short overview of literature. *Int J Gynecol Cancer* 2007;17:517–520.

116. **Stehman FB, Bundy BN, Thomas G, et al.** Groin dissection versus groin radiation in carcinoma of the vulva: a Gynecologic Oncology Group study. *Int J Radiat Oncol Biol Phys* 1992;24:389–396.

117. **van der Velden K, Ansink A.** Primary groin irradiation vs primary groin surgery for early vulvar cancer. *Cochrane Database Syst Rev* 2001;4:CD002224.

118. **Hallak S, Ladi L, Sorbe B.** Prophylactic inguinal-femoral irradiation as an alternative to primary lymphadenectomy in treatment of vulvar carcinoma. *Int J Oncol* 2003;31:1077–1085.

119. **Iversen T, Aas M.** Lymph drainage from the vulva. *Gynecol Oncol* 1983;16:179–189.

120. **Hyde SE, Valmadre S, Hacker NF, et al.** Squamous cell carcinoma of the vulva with bulky positive groin nodes-nodal debulking versus full groin dissection prior to radiation therapy. *Int J Gynecol Cancer* 2007;17:154–158.

121. **Montana GS, Thomas GM, Moore DH, et al.** Preoperative chemoradiation for carcinoma of the vulva with N2/N3 nodes: a gynecologic oncology group study. *Int J Radiat Oncol Biol Phys* 2000;48:1007–1013.

122. **Hoffman JS, Kumar NB, Morley GW.** Prognostic significance of groin lymph node metastases in squamous carcinoma of the vulva. *Obstet Gynecol* 1985;66:402–405.

123. **Terada K, Shimizu D, Wong J.** Sentinel node dissection and ultrastaging in squamous cell carcinoma of the vulva. *Gynecol Oncol* 2000;76:40–44.

124. **Ansink AC, Sie-Go DM, van der Velden J, et al.** Identification of sentinel lymph nodes in vulvar carcinoma patients with the aid of a patent blue V injection: a multicenter study. *Cancer* 1999;86:652–656.

125. **De Cicco C, Sideri M, Bartolomei M, et al.** Sentinel node biopsy in early vulvar cancer. *Br J Cancer* 2000;82:295–299.

126. **Selman TJ, Luesley DM, Acheson N, et al.** A systematic review of the accuracy of diagnostic tests for inguinal lymph node status in vulvar cancer. *Gynecol Oncol* 2005;99:206–214.

127. **Plante M, Renaud MC, Roy M.** Sentinel node evaluation in gynecologic cancer. *Oncology (Williston Park)* 2004;18:75–87.

128. **Hampl M, Hantschmann P, Michels W, et al.** Validation of the accuracy of the sentinel lymph node procedure in patients with vulvar cancer: results of a multicenter study in Germany. *Gynecol Oncol* 2008;111:282–288.

129. **Van der Zee AG, Oonk MH, de Hullu JA, et al.** Sentinel node dissection is safe in the treatment of early-stage vulvar cancer. *J Clin Oncol* 2008;26:884–889.

130. **Levenback CF, Tian C, Coleman RL, et al.** Sentinel node (SN) biopsy in patients with vulvar cancer: a Gynecologic Oncology Group (GOG) study. *J Clin Oncol* 2009;27(Suppl):abstr 5505.

131. **Moore RG, Granai CO, Gajewski W, et al.** Pathologic evaluation of inguinal sentinel lymph nodes in vulvar cancer patients: a comparison of immunohistochemical staining versus ultrastaging with hematoxylin and eosin staining. *Gynecol Oncol* 2003;91:378–382.

132. **Hakam A, Nasir A, Raghuwanshi R, et al.** Value of multilevel sectioning for improved detection of micrometastases in sentinel lymph nodes in invasive squamous cell carcinoma of the vulva. *Anticancer Res* 2004;24:1281–1286.

133. **Narayansingh GV, Miller ID, Sharma M, et al.** The prognostic significance of micrometastases in node-negative squamous cell carcinoma of the vulva. *Br J Cancer* 2005;92:222–224.

134. **Merisio C, Berretta R, Gualdi M, et al.** Radioguided sentinel lymph node detection in vulvar cancer. *Int J Gynecol Cancer* 2005;15:493–497.

135. **Raspagliesi F, Ditto A, Fontanelli R, et al.** False-negative sentinel node in patients with vulvar cancer: a case study. *Int J Gynecol Cancer* 2003;13:361–363.

136. **Kowalewska M, Szkoda MT, Radziszewski J, et al.** The frequency of human papillomavirus infection in polish patients with vulvar squamous cell carcinoma. *Int J Gynecol Cancer* 2010;20:434–437.

137. **Levenback CF, van der Zee AG, Rob L, et al.** Sentinel lymph node biopsy in patients with gynecologic cancers expert panel statement from the International Sentinel Node Society Meeting, February 21, 2008. *Gynecol Oncol* 2009;114:151–156.

138. **Hopkins MP, Reid GC, Morley GW.** Radical vulvectomy: the decision for the incision. *Cancer* 1993;72:799–803.

139. **Gaarenstroom KN, Kenter GG, Trimbos JB, et al.** Postoperative complications after vulvectomy and inguinofemoral lymphadenectomy using separate groin incisions. *Int J Gynecol Cancer* 2003;13:522–527.

140. **Gould N, Kamelle S, Tillmanns T, et al.** Predictors of complications after inguinal lymphadenectomy. *Gynecol Oncol* 2001;82:329–332.

141. **Podratz KC, Symmonds RE, Taylor WF.** Carcinoma of the vulva: analysis of treatment failures. *Am J Obstet Gynecol* 1982;143:340–351.

142. **Malfetano J, Piver MS, Tsukada Y.** Stage III and IV squamous cell carcinoma of the vulva. *Gynecol Oncol* 1986;23:192–198.

143. **Faul CM, Mirmow D, Huang Q, et al.** Adjuvant radiation for vulvar carcinoma: improved local control. *Int J Radiat Oncol Biol Phys* 1997;38:381–389.

144. **Parthasarathy A, Cheung MK, Osann K, et al.** The benefit of adjuvant radiation therapy in single-node-positive squamous cell vulvar carcinoma. *Gynecol Oncol* 2006;103:1095–1099.

145. **Oonk MHM, de Hullu JA, Hollema H, et al.** The value of routine follow-up in patients treated for carcinoma of the vulva. *Cancer* 2003;98:2624–2629.

146. **Stehman FB, Bundy BN, Ball H, et al.** Sites of failure and time to failure in carcinoma of the vulva treated conservatively: a GOG study. *Am J Obstet Gynecol* 1996;174:1128–1133.

147. **Cormio G, Loizzi V, Carriero C, et al.** Groin recurrence in carcinoma of the vulva: management and outcome. *Eur J Cancer Care* 2010;19:302–307.

148. **Crosbie EJ, Slade RJ, Ahmed AS.** The management of vulval cancer. *Cancer Treat Rev* 2009;35:533–539.

149. **Homesley HD.** Management of vulvar cancer. *Cancer* 1995; 76(Suppl 1):2159–2170.

150. **Rouzier R, Haddad B, Plantier F, et al.** Local relapse in patients treated for squamous cell vulvar carcinoma: incidence and prognostic values. *Obstet Gynecol* 2002;100:1159–1167.

151. **Hopkins MP, Reid GC, Morley GW.** The surgical management of recurrent squamous cell carcinoma of the vulva. *Obstet Gynecol* 1990;75:1001–1005.

152. **Hruby G, MacLeod C, Firth I.** Radiation treatment in recurrent squamous cell cancer of the vulva. *Int J Radiat Oncol Biol Phys* 2000;46:1193–1197.

153. **Wagenaar HC, Colombo N, Vergote I, et al.** Bleomycin, methotrexate, and CCNU in locally advanced or recurrent, inoperable, squamous-cell carcinoma of the vulva: an EORTC Gynaecological Cancer Cooperative Group Study. *Gynecol Oncol* 2001;81:348–354.

154. **Durrant KR, Mangioni C, Lacave AJ, et al.** Bleomycin, methotrexate, and CCNU in advanced inoperable squamous cell carcinoma of the vulva: a phase II study of the EORTC Gynaecological Cancer Cooperative Group (GCCG). *Gynecol Oncol* 1990;37:359–362.

155. **Tropé C, Johnsson JE, Larsson G, et al.** Bleomycin alone or combined with mitomycin C in treatment of advanced or recurrent squamous cell carcinoma of the vulva. *Cancer Treat Rev* 1980;64:639–642.

156. **Cormio G, Loizzi V, Gissi F, et al.** Cisplatin and vinorelbine chemotherapy in recurrent vulvar carcinoma. *Oncology* 2009; 77:281–284.

157. **Witteveen PO, van der Velden J, Vergote I, et al.** Phase II study on paclitaxel in patients with recurrent, metastatic or locally advanced vulvar cancer not amenable to surgery or radiotherapy: a study of the EORTC-GCG (European Organisation for Research and Treatment of Cancer—Gynaecological Cancer Group). *Ann Oncol* 2009;20:1511–1516.

158. **Ragnarsson-Olding BK, Nilsson BR, Kanter-Lewensohn LR, et al.** Malignant melanoma of the vulva in a nationwide, 25-year study of 219 Swedish females: clinical observations and histopathologic features. Predictors of survival. *Cancer* 1999;86:1273–1293.

159. **Weinstock MA.** Malignant melanoma of the vulva and vagina in the United States: patterns of incidence and population-based estimates of survival. *Am J Obstet Gynecol* 1994;171:1225–1230.

160. **Dunton CJ, Kautzky M, Hanau C.** Malignant melanoma of the vulva: a review. *Obstet Gynecol Surv* 1995;50:739–746.

161. **Hu DN, Yu GP, McCormick SA.** Population-based incidence of vulvar and vaginal melanoma in various races and ethnic groups with comparisons to other site-specific melanomas. *Melanoma Res* 2010;20:153–158.

162. **Podratz KC, Gaffey TA, Symmonds RE, et al.** Melanoma of the vulva: an update. *Gynecol Oncol* 1983;16:153–168.

163. **Trimble EL, Lewis JL Jr, Williams LL, et al.** Management of vulvar melanoma. *Gynecol Oncol* 1992;45:254–258.

164. **Phillips GL, Bundy BN, Okagaki T, et al.** Malignant melanoma of the vulva treated by radical hemivulvectomy: a prospective study by the Gynecologic Oncology Group. *Cancer* 1994;73:2626–2632.

165. **Chung AF, Woodruff JM, Lewis JL Jr.** Malignant melanoma of the vulva: a report of 44 cases. *Obstet Gynecol* 1975;45:638–646.

166. **Clark WH, From L, Bernardino EA, et al.** The histogenesis and biologic behavior of primary human malignant melanomas of the skin. *Cancer Res* 1969;29:705–727.

167. **Breslow A.** Thickness, cross-sectional area and depth of invasion in the prognosis of cutaneous melanoma. *Ann Surg* 1970;172:902–908.

168. **Balch CM, Gershenwald JE, Soong SJ, et al.** Final version of 2009 AJCC melanoma staging and classification. *J Clin Oncol* 2009;27:6199–6206.

169. **Aitken DR, Clausen K, Klein JP, et al.** The extent of primary melanoma excision—a re-evaluation. How wide is wide? *Ann Surg* 1983;198:634–641.

170. **Day CL, Mihm MC Jr, Sober AJ, et al.** Narrower margins for clinical stage I malignant melanoma. *N Engl J Med* 1982;306:479–482.

171. **Sugiyama VE, Chan JK, Shin JY, et al.** Vulvar melanoma: a multivariable analysis of 644 patients. *Obstet Gynecol* 2007;110:296–301.

172. **Phillips GL, Twiggs LB, Okagaki T.** Vulvar melanoma: a microstaging study. *Gynecol Oncol* 1982;14:80–88.

173. **Rose PG, Piver MS, Tsukada Y, et al.** Conservative therapy for melanoma of the vulva. *Am J Obstet Gynecol* 1988;159:52–55.

174. **Davidson T, Kissin M, Wesbury G.** Vulvovaginal melanoma—should radical surgery be abandoned? *Br J Obstet Gynaecol* 1987;94:473–476.

175. **Veronesi U, Cascinelli N.** Narrow excision (1-cm margin): a safe procedure for thin cutaneous melanoma. *Arch Surg* 1991;126:438–441.

176. **Balch CM, Urist MM, Karakousis CP, et al.** Efficacy of 2-cm surgical margins for intermediate-thickness melanoma (1–4 mm): results of a multi-institutional randomized surgical trial. *Ann Surg* 1993;218:262–269.

177. **Morrow CP, Rutledge FN.** Melanoma of the vulva. *Obstet Gynecol* 1972;39:745–752.

178. **Balch CM, Soong SJ, Bartolucci AA, et al.** Efficacy of an elective regional lymph node dissection of 1–4 mm thick melanomas for patients 60 years of age or younger. *Ann Surg* 1996;224:255–263.

179. **Balch CM, Soong SJ, Milton GW, et al.** A comparison of prognostic factors and surgical results in 1,786 patients with localized (stage I) melanoma treated in Alabama, USA, and New South Wales, Australia. *Ann Surg* 1982;196:677–684.

180. **Dunton JD, Berd D.** Vulvar melanoma, biologically different from other cutaneous melanomas. *Lancet* 1999;354:2013–2014.

181. **Morton DL, Thompson JF, Cochran AJ, et al.** Sentinel-node biopsy or nodal observation in melanoma. *N Engl J Med* 2006;355:1307–1317.

182. **Dhar KK, DAS N, Brinkman DA, et al.** Utility of sentinel node biopsy in vulvar and vaginal melanoma: report of two cases and review of the literature. *Int J Gynecol Cancer* 2007;17:720–723.

183. **Jaramillo BA, Ganjei P, Averette HE, et al.** Malignant melanoma of the vulva. *Obstet Gynecol* 1985;66:398–401.

184. **Beller U, Demopoulos RI, Beckman EM.** Vulvovaginal melanoma: a clinicopathologic study. *J Reprod Med* 1986;31:315–319.

185. **Kirkwood JM, Strawderman MH, Ernstoff MS, et al.** Interferon alfa-2b adjuvant therapy of high-risk resected cutaneous melanoma: the Eastern Cooperative Oncology Group Trial EST 1684. *J Clin Oncol* 1996;14:7–17.

186. **Kirkwood JM, Ibrahim JG, Sondak VK, et al.** High- and low-dose interferon alpha-2b in high-risk melanoma: first analysis of intergroup trial E1690/S9111/C9190. *J Clin Oncol* 2000;18:2444–2458.

187. **Kirkwood JM, Ibrahim J, Sosman JA, et al.** High-dose interferon alpha-2b significantly prolongs relapse-free and overall compared with the GM2-KLH/QS-21 vaccine in patients with resected stage IIB–III melanoma: results of Intergroup trial E1694/S9512/C509801. *J Clin Oncol* 2001;19:2370–2380.

188. **Atallah E, Flaherty L.** Treatment of metastatic malignant melanoma. *Curr Treat Options Oncol* 2005;6:185–193.

189. **Bystryn JC, Reynolds SR.** Melanoma vaccines: what we know so far. *Oncology (Williston Park)* 2005;19:97–108.

190. **Masiel A, Buttrick P, Bitran J.** Tamoxifen in the treatment of malignant melanoma. *Cancer Treat Rep* 1981;65:531–532.

191. **Nesbit RA, Woods RL, Tattersall MH, et al.** Tamoxifen in malignant melanoma. *N Engl J Med* 1979;301:1241–1242.

192. **Agrawal S, Kane JM 3rd, Guadagnolo BA, et al.** The benefits of adjuvant radiation therapy after therapeutic lymphadenectomy for clinically advanced, high-risk, lymph node-metastatic melanoma. *Cancer* 2009;115:5836–5844.

193. **Mendenhall WM, Amdur RJ, Grobmyer SR, et al.** Adjuvant radiotherapy for cutaneous melanoma. *Cancer* 2008;112:1189–1196.

194. **Scheistroen M, Tropé C, Kaern J, et al.** Malignant melanoma of the vulva: evaluation of prognostic factors with emphasis on DNA ploidy in 75 patients. *Cancer* 1995;75:72–80.

195. **Woolcott RJ, Henry RJW, Houghton CRS.** Malignant melanoma of the vulva: Australian experience. *J Reprod Med* 1988;33:699–702.

196. **Piura B, Egan M, Lopes A, et al.** Malignant melanoma of the vulva: a clinicopathologic study of 18 cases. *J Surg Oncol* 1992;50:234–240.

197. **Look KY, Roth LM, Sutton GP.** Vulvar melanoma reconsidered. *Cancer* 1993;72:143–146.

198. **Cardosi RJ, Speights A, Fiorica JV, et al.** Bartholin's gland carcinoma: a 15-year experience. *Gynecol Oncol* 2001;82:247–251.

199. **Copeland LJ, Sneige N, Gershenson DM, et al.** Bartholin gland carcinoma. *Obstet Gynecol* 1986;67:794–801.

200. **Visco AG, Del Priore G.** Postmenopausal Bartholin gland enlargement: a hospital-based cancer risk assessment. *Obstet Gynecol* 1996;87:286–290.

201. **Barclay DL, Collins CG, Macey HB.** Cancer of the Bartholin gland: a review and report of 8 cases. *Obstet Gynecol* 1964;24:329–336.

202. **López-Varela E, Oliva E, McIntyre JF, et al.** Primary treatment of Bartholin's gland carcinoma with radiation and chemoradiation: a report on ten consecutive cases. *Int J Gynecol Cancer* 2007;17:661–667.

203. **Wheelock JB, Goplerud DR, Dunn LJ, et al.** Primary carcinoma of the Bartholin gland: a report of 10 cases. *Obstet Gynecol* 1984;63:820–824.

204. **Copeland LJ, Sneige N, Gershenson DM, et al.** Adenoid cystic carcinoma of Bartholin gland. *Obstet Gynecol* 1986;67:115–120.

205. **Yang SY, Lee JW, Kim WS, Jung et al.** Adenoid cystic carcinoma of the Bartholin's gland: report of two cases and review of the literature. *Gynecol Oncol* 2006;100:422–425.

206. **Fu YS, Reagan JW.** Benign and malignant epithelial tumors of the vulva. In: **Fu YS, Reagan JW, eds.** *Pathology of the uterine cervix, vagina, and vulva.* Philadelphia, PA: WB Saunders, 1989:138–192.

207. **Underwood JW, Adcock LL, Okagaki T.** Adenosquamous carcinoma of skin appendages (adenoid squamous cell carcinoma, pseudoglandular squamous cell carcinoma, adenoacanthoma of sweat gland of Lever) of the vulva: a clinical and ultrastructural study. *Cancer* 1978;42:1851–1858.

208. **Dudzinski MR, Askin FB, Fowler WC.** Giant basal cell carcinoma of the vulva. *Obstet Gynecol* 1984;63:57S–60S.

209. **Benedet JL, Miller DM, Ehlen TG, et al.** Basal cell carcinoma of the vulva: clinical features and treatment results in 28 patients. *Obstet Gynecol* 1997;90:765–768.

210. **de Giorgi V, Salvini C, Massi D, et al.** Vulvar basal cell carcinoma: retrospective study and review of literature. *Gynecol Oncol* 2005;97:192–194.

211. **Jimenez HT, Fenoglio CM, Richart RM.** Vulvar basal cell carcinoma with metastasis: a case report. *Am J Obstet Gynecol* 1975;121:285–286.

212. **Sworn MJ, Hammond GT, Buchanan R.** Metastatic basal cell carcinoma of the vulva: a case report. *Br J Obstet Gynaecol* 1979;86:332–334.

213. **Hoffman MS, Roberts WS, Ruffolo EH.** Basal cell carcinoma of the vulva with inguinal lymph node metastases. *Gynecol Oncol* 1988;29:113–119.

214. **Palladino VS, Duffy JL, Bures GJ.** Basal cell carcinoma of the vulva. *Cancer* 1969;24:460–470.

215. **Isaacs JH.** Verrucous carcinoma of the female genital tract. *Gynecol Oncol* 1976;4:259–269.

216. **Partridge EE, Murad R, Shingleton HM, et al.** Verrucous lesions of the female genitalia. II. Verrucous carcinoma. *Am J Obstet Gynecol* 1980;137:419–424.

217. **Kondi-Paphitis A, Deligeorgi-Politi H, Liapis A, et al.** Human papillomavirus in verrucous carcinoma of the vulva: an immunopathological study of three cases. *Eur J Gynecol Obstet* 1998;19:319–320.

218. **Gualco M, Bonin S, Foglia G, et al.** Morphologic and biologic studies on ten cases of verrucous carcinoma of the vulva supporting the theory of a discrete clinicopathologic entity. *Int J Gynecol Cancer* 2003;13:317–324.

219. **Haidopoulos D, Diakomanolis E, Rodolakis A, et al.** Coexistence of verrucous and squamous carcinoma of the vulva. *Aust N Z J Obstet Gynaecol* 2005;45:60–63.

220. **Gallousis S.** Verrucous carcinoma: report of three vulvar cases and a review of the literature. *Obstet Gynecol* 1972;40:502–507.

221. **Japaze H, Van Dinh TV, Woodruff JD.** Verrucous carcinoma of the vulva: study of 24 cases. *Obstet Gynecol* 1982;60:462–466.

222. **Demian SDE, Bushkin FL, Echevarria RA.** Perineural invasion and anaplastic transformation of verrucous carcinoma. *Cancer* 1973;32:395–401.

223. **Ulutin HC, Zellars RC, Frassica D.** Soft tissue sarcoma of the vulva: a clinical study. *Int J Gynecol Cancer* 2003;13:528–531.

224. **Nielsen GP, Rosenberg AE, Koerner FC, et al.** Smooth-muscle tumors of the vulva: a clinicopathological study of 25 cases and review of the literature. *Am J Surg Pathol* 1996;20:779–793.

225. **Tavassoli FA, Norris HJ.** Smooth muscle tumors of the vulva. *Obstet Gynecol* 1979;53:213–217.

226. **Ulbright TM, Brokaw SA, Stehman FB, et al.** Epithelioid sarcoma of the vulva. *Cancer* 1983;52:1462–1469.

227. **Bell J, Averette H, Davis J, et al.** Genital rhabdomyosarcoma: current management and review of the literature. *Obstet Gynecol Surv* 1986;41:257–263.

228. **Hays DM, Shimada H, Raney RB Jr, et al.** Clinical staging and treatment results in rhabdomyosarcoma of the female genital tract among children and adolescents. *Cancer* 1988;61:1893–1903.

229. **Harris NL, Scully RE.** Malignant lymphoma and granulocytic sarcoma of the uterus and vagina. *Cancer* 1984;53:2530–2545.

230. **Dudley AG, Young RH, Lawrence WD, et al.** Endodermal sinus tumor of the vulva in an infant. *Obstet Gynecol* 1983;61:76S–79S.

231. **Bottles K, Lacy CG, Goldberg J, et al.** Merkel cell carcinoma of the vulva. *Obstet Gynecol* 1984;63:61S–65S.

232. **Husseinzadeh N, Wesseler T, Newman N, et al.** Neuroendocrine (Merkel cell) carcinoma of the vulva. *Gynecol Oncol* 1988;29:105–112.

233. **Khoury-Collado F, Elliott KS, Lee YC, et al.** Merkel cell carcinoma of the Bartholin's gland. *Gynecol Oncol* 2005;97:928–931.

234. **Bock JE, Andreasson B, Thorn A, et al.** Dermatofibromasarcoma protuberans of the vulva. *Gynecol Oncol* 1985;20:129–135.

235. **Dehner LP.** Metastatic and secondary tumors of the vulva. *Obstet Gynecol* 1973;42:47–57.

39 Gestational Trophoblastic Disease

Ross S. Berkowitz
Donald P. Goldstein

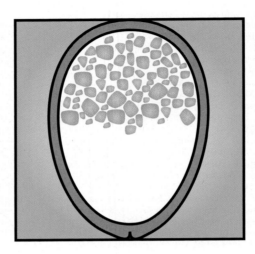

- Complete molar pregnancies are generally diploid and all chromosomes are of paternal origin.

- Partial molar pregnancies are triploid and the extra set of chromosomes is paternal.

- Complete moles are diagnosed earlier in pregnancy and less frequently present with the classic signs and symptoms.

- Single-agent chemotherapy achieves a high remission rate in nonmetastatic and low-risk metastatic gestational trophoblastic neoplasia.

- After achieving remission with chemotherapy, patients with gestational trophoblastic neoplasia can anticipate normal reproduction in the future.

Gestational trophoblastic disease (GTD) is the term used to describe the heterogeneous group of interrelated lesions that arise from abnormal proliferation of placental trophoblasts. GTD lesions are histologically distinct and can be benign or malignant. Benign lesions consist of hydatidiform moles, complete and partial, whereas malignant lesions consist of invasive mole, placental-site trophoblastic tumor (PSTT), and choriocarcinoma. This subset of malignant lesions that have varying propensities for local invasion and metastasis is referred to as gestational trophoblastic neoplasia (GTN). GTNs are among the rare human tumors that can be cured even in the presence of widespread dissemination (1,2). Although GTNs commonly follow a molar pregnancy, they can occur after any gestational event, including induced or spontaneous abortion, ectopic pregnancy, or term pregnancy.

Hydatidiform Mole

Epidemiology

Estimates of the incidence of molar pregnancy vary dramatically in different regions of the world. For example, the incidence of molar pregnancy in Japan (2:1,000 pregnancies) is reported to be about threefold higher than the incidence in Europe or North America (about 0.6 to 1.1 per 1,000 pregnancies) (3). In Taiwan, 1 in 125 pregnancies are molar, while in the

Table 39.1 Features of Complete and Partial Hydatidiform Moles

Features	*Complete Mole*	*Partial Mole*
Fetal or embryonic tissue	Absent	Present
Hydatidiform swelling of chorionic villi	Diffuse	Focal
Trophoblastic hyperplasia	Diffuse	Focal
Scalloping of chorionic villi	Absent	Present
Trophoblastic stromal inclusions	Absent	Present
Karyotype	46,XX (90%); 46,XY	Triploid

United States the incidence is 1 in 1,500 live births. The incidences of complete and partial hydatidiform mole in Ireland were investigated by reviewing all products of conception from first- and second-trimester abortions (4). **Based on a thorough pathologic review, the incidence of complete and partial hydatidiform mole was 1:1,945 and 1:695 pregnancies, respectively.**

While variations in the worldwide incidence of molar pregnancy may result in part from reporting population-based versus hospital-based data, a number of studies suggest that the high incidence in some populations can be attributed to socioeconomic and nutritional factors. The decreasing incidence of molar pregnancy in South Korea is attributed to a more Western diet and improved standard of living (5). Case-control studies from Italy and the United States show that the rate of complete mole increases with decreasing consumption of dietary carotene (vitamin A precursor) and animal fat (6,7). Maternal age and reproductive history influence the rate of molar pregnancy. Women older than 40 years have a 5- to 10-fold greater risk of having a complete mole, while one in three pregnancies in women older than 50 years results in a molar gestation (8,9). **These findings suggest that ova from older women may be more susceptible to abnormal fertilization, resulting in a complete hydatidiform mole.**

Limited information is available concerning risk factors for partial molar pregnancy. The epidemiologic characteristics of complete and partial mole appear to differ significantly (8–11). The risk for partial mole is associated with the use of oral contraceptives and a history of irregular menstruation, but not with dietary factors (10). Nor does there appear to be an association between maternal age and the risk for partial mole.

Pathology and Cytogenetics

Hydatidiform moles may be categorized as either complete or partial moles on the basis of gross morphology, histopathology, and karyotype (Table 39.1).

Complete Hydatidiform Mole

Complete hydatidiform moles exhibit characteristic swelling and trophoblastic hyperplasia (Fig. 39.1). **They usually have a 46,XX karyotype, but about 10% have a 46,XY karyotype** (12,13). **The molar chromosomes are entirely of paternal origin,** with mitochondrial DNA of maternal origin (Fig. 39.2) (14). Complete moles usually arise from an ovum fertilized by a haploid sperm, which duplicates its own chromosomes. The ovum nucleus may be absent or inactivated (15).

Partial Hydatidiform Mole

Partial hydatidiform mole is characterized by the following pathologic features (16) (Fig. 39.3):

1. Chorionic villi of varying size with focal hydatidiform swelling, cavitation, and trophoblastic hyperplasia
2. Marked villous scalloping
3. Prominent stromal trophoblastic inclusions
4. Identifiable embryonic or fetal tissues

Partial moles have a triploid karyotype (69 chromosomes); the extra haploid set of chromosomes usually is derived from the father (Fig. 39.4) (17). It is possible that nontriploid partial moles do not exist (18). When a fetus is present in conjunction with a partial mole, it

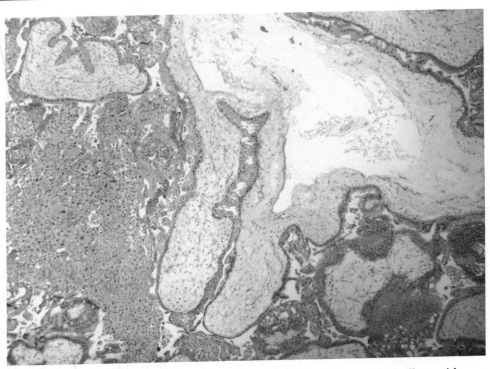

Figure 39.1   Photomicrograph of complete mole demonstrating enlarged villous with central cavitation and surrounding trophoblastic hyperplasia.

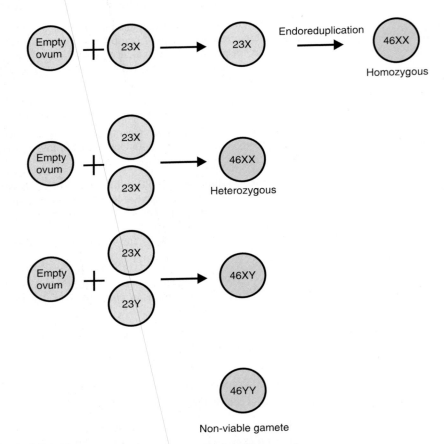

Figure 39.2   The karyotype of complete hydatidiform mole.

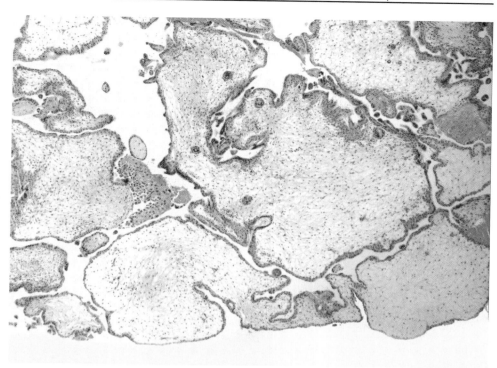

Figure 39.3 Photomicrograph of partial mole showing marked disparity in villous size, trophoblastic inclusions (*center*), and mild trophoblastic hyperplasia. (From Berkowitz RS, Goldstein OP. Gestational trophoblastic diseases. In: Ryan KJ, BerkowitzR, Barbieri R, eds. *Kistner's gynecology principles and practice,* 5th ed. Chicago: Year Book Medical Publishers, 1990:433, with permission.)

generally exhibits the stigmata of triploidy, including growth retardation and multiple congenital malformations such as syndactyly and hydrocephaly (Fig. 39.5).

Advances in Pathologic Diagnosis

When molar pregnancy is diagnosed early in the first trimester, the pathologist can have difficulty distinguishing complete hydatidiform mole from partial hydatidiform mole or hydropic abortions because of smaller villi, less trophoblastic hyperplasia, more primitive villous stroma, and less global necrosis (19,20). Accurate diagnosis can be facilitated through the use of flow cytometry to determine ploidy (i.e., diploid vs. triploid moles) (21) and through assessment of biomarkers of paternally imprinted and maternally expressed gene products (22). Biomarkers that take advantage of imprinted genes to distinguish complete mole and hydropic abortions from other gestations are identified. Because complete moles generally have no maternal chromosomes, paternally imprinted gene products normally expressed only by maternal chromosomes, should be absent. In complete moles, the nuclei of the villous stroma and cytotrophoblastic cells do not express p57, whereas all other gestations, including partial moles, are characterized by nuclear immunostaining in these cells. Thus, a complete mole is diploid and negative for p57, a hydropic abortion is diploid (sometimes triploid) and positive for p57, and a partial mole is triploid and positive for p57.

Familial Recurrent Molar Pregnancy

Evaluation of families with recurrent molar pregnancy suggests that dysregulation of normal parental imprinting of genes, with loss of maternally transcribed genes, is likely to contribute to the pathogenesis of molar pregnancy. Familial recurrent hydatidiform mole, is a rare occurrence, characterized by recurrent complete hydatidiform mole of biparental origin, rather than the more usual androgenetic origin (23). Genetic mapping shows that in most families the gene responsible is located in a 1.1 Mb region on chromosome 19q13.4. Mutations in the gene result in dysregulation of imprinting in the female germ line with abnormal development of both embryonic and extraembryonic tissue.

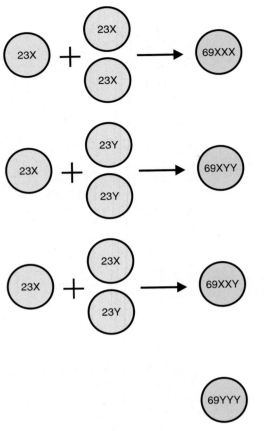

Figure 39.4   **The karyotype of partial hydatidiform mole.**

Clinical Features

Patients with complete molar pregnancy are diagnosed increasingly earlier in pregnancy and treated before they develop the classic clinical signs and symptoms. This is the result of many changes in clinical practice, such as the frequent use of human chorionic gonadotropin (hCG) measurement and transvaginal ultrasonography in early pregnancy for women with vaginal staining and for determining the gestational dates in asymptomatic women. The following is a description of the classic and current clinical features of complete molar pregnancy (24,25).

Complete Hydatidiform Mole

Vaginal Bleeding   **Vaginal bleeding is the most common symptom causing patients to seek treatment for complete molar pregnancy.** It had been reported to occur in 97% of cases, whereas currently it is reported to occur in 84% of patients. Molar tissues may separate from the decidua and disrupt maternal vessels, and large volumes of retained blood may distend the endometrial cavity. Because vaginal bleeding may be considerable and prolonged, one-half of these patients had anemia (hemoglobin <10 g/100 mL). Anemia is present in only 5% of patients.

Excessive Uterine Size   **Excessive uterine enlargement relative to gestational age is one of the classic signs of a complete mole, although it was present in only about half of patients.** Currently, excessive uterine size occurs in only 28% of patients. The endometrial cavity may be expanded by both chorionic tissue and retained blood. Excessive uterine size is generally associated with markedly elevated levels of hCG, because uterine enlargement results in part from trophoblastic overgrowth.

Preeclampsia   **Preeclampsia was observed in 27% of patients with a complete hydatidiform mole.** Preeclampsia is now reported in only 1 of 74 patients with complete mole at the initial visit. Although preeclampsia is associated with hypertension, proteinuria, and hyperreflexia,

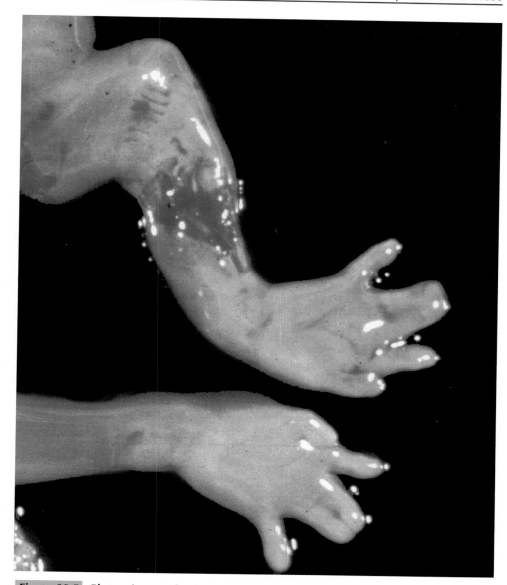

Figure 39.5 **Photomicrograph of a fetal hand demonstrating syndactyly.** The fetus had a triploid karyotype, and the chorionic tissues were a partial mole.

eclamptic convulsions rarely occur. Preeclampsia develops almost exclusively in patients with excessive uterine size and markedly elevated hCG levels. Hydatidiform mole should be considered whenever preeclampsia develops early in pregnancy.

Hyperemesis Gravidarum **Hyperemesis requiring antiemetic or intravenous replacement therapy occurred in one-fourth of women with a complete mole, particularly those with excessive uterine size and markedly elevated hCG levels.** Severe electrolyte disturbances may develop and require treatment with parenteral fluids. Currently, only 8% of patients have hyperemesis.

Hyperthyroidism **Clinically evident hyperthyroidism was observed in 7% of patients with a complete molar gestation.** These women may have tachycardia, warm skin, and tremor, and the diagnosis can be confirmed by detection of elevated serum levels of free thyroxine (T_4) and tri-iodothyronine (T_3). Clinical evidence of hyperthyroidism with complete mole is rare.

Anesthesia or surgery may precipitate thyroid storm. Thus, if hyperthyroidism is suspected before the induction of anesthesia for molar evacuation, β-adrenergic blocking agents should be administered. Thyroid storm may be manifested by hyperthermia, delirium, convulsions, tachycardia, high-output heart failure, or cardiovascular collapse. Administration of β-adrenergic blocking agents prevents or rapidly reverses many of the metabolic and cardiovascular complications of thyroid storm. After molar evacuation, thyroid function test results rapidly return to normal.

Hyperthyroidism develops almost exclusively in patients with very high hCG levels. Some investigators suggest that hCG is the thyroid stimulator in women with molar pregnancy because positive correlations between serum hCG levels and total T_4 or T_3 concentrations were observed. However, in one study in which thyroid function was measured in 47 patients with a complete mole, no significant correlation was found between serum hCG levels and serum values of free T_4 index or free T_3 index (26). Although some investigators speculated about a separate chorionic thyrotropin, this substance is not yet isolated.

Trophoblastic Embolization   **Respiratory distress rarely occurs in patients with a complete mole.** It is usually diagnosed in patients with excessive uterine size and markedly elevated hCG levels. These patients may have chest pain, dyspnea, tachypnea, and tachycardia and may experience severe respiratory distress during and after molar evacuation. Auscultation of the chest usually reveals diffuse rales, and chest radiographic evaluation may show bilateral pulmonary infiltrates. Respiratory distress usually resolves within 72 hours with cardiopulmonary support. In some circumstances, patients may require mechanical ventilation. Respiratory insufficiency may result from trophoblastic embolization and the cardiopulmonary complications of thyroid storm, preeclampsia, and massive fluid replacement.

Theca Lutein Ovarian Cysts   **Prominent theca lutein ovarian cysts (6 cm in diameter) develop in about one-half of patients with a complete mole** (27). Theca lutein ovarian cysts result from high serum hCG levels, which cause ovarian hyperstimulation (28). Because the uterus may be excessively enlarged, theca lutein cysts can be difficult to palpate during physical examination; however, ultrasonography can accurately document their presence and size. **After molar evacuation, theca lutein cysts normally regress spontaneously within 2 to 4 months.**

Prominent theca lutein cysts may cause symptoms of marked pelvic pressure, and they can be decompressed by laparoscopic or ultrasonographically directed aspiration. If acute pelvic pain develops, laparoscopy should be performed to assess possible cystic torsion or rupture.

Partial Hydatidiform Mole

Patients with partial hydatidiform mole usually do not have the dramatic clinical features characteristic of complete molar pregnancy. **These patients have the signs and symptoms of incomplete or missed abortion, and partial mole is diagnosed after histologic review of the tissue obtained by curettage** (29).

In a survey of 81 patients with a partial mole, the main initial sign was vaginal bleeding, which occurred in 59 patients (72.8%) (30). Excessive uterine enlargement and preeclampsia were present in three patients (3.7%) and two patients (2.5%), respectively. No patient had theca lutein ovarian cysts, hyperemesis, or hyperthyroidism. The initial clinical diagnosis was an incomplete or missed abortion in 74 patients (91.3%) and hydatidiform mole in five patients (6.2%). Pre-evacuation hCG levels were measured in 30 patients and were higher than 100,000 mIU/mL in two patients (6.6%).

Natural History

Complete Hydatidiform Mole

Complete moles have a potential for local invasion and dissemination. **After molar evacuation, local uterine invasion occurs in 15% of patients, and metastasis occurs in 4%** (27).

A review of 858 patients with complete hydatidiform mole at the New England Trophoblastic Disease Center (NETDC) revealed that two-fifths of the patients had the following signs of marked trophoblastic proliferation at the time they sought treatment:

1. **hCG level greater than 100,000 mIU/mL**
2. **Excessive uterine enlargement**
3. **Theca lutein cysts 6 cm in diameter or larger**

In this review, patients with any one of these signs were considered at high risk for developing postmolar tumor. After molar evacuation, local uterine invasion occurred in 31%, and metastases developed in 8.8% of the 352 high-risk patients. For the 506 low-risk patients, local invasion was found in only 3.4%, and metastases developed in 0.6%.

Older patients are at increased risk of developing postmolar GTN. One study reported that persistent tumor developed after a complete molar pregnancy in 37% of women older than 40 years (27), whereas in another study this finding occurred in 60% of women older than 50 years (31).

Partial Hydatidiform Mole

Persistent tumor, usually nonmetastatic, develops in approximately 2% to 4% of patients with a partial mole, and chemotherapy is required to achieve remission (32). Patients who develop persistent disease have no distinguishing clinical or pathologic characteristics (33).

Diagnosis

Ultrasonography is a reliable and sensitive technique for the diagnosis of complete molar pregnancy. Because the chorionic villi exhibit diffuse hydropic swelling, complete moles produce a characteristic vesicular ultrasonographic pattern as soon as in the first trimester (Fig. 39.6).

Ultrasonography may contribute to the diagnosis of partial molar pregnancy by demonstrating focal cystic spaces in the placental tissues and an increase in the transverse diameter of the gestational sac (34). When these criteria are present, the positive predictive value for partial mole is 90%.

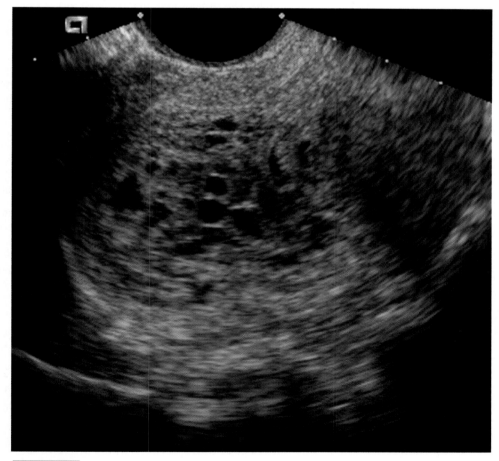

Figure 39.6 Ultrasonogram of a uterus showing a typical pattern of a complete hydatidiform mole. Note the characteristic vesicular ultrasonographic pattern.

Treatment

When molar pregnancy is diagnosed, the patient should be evaluated for the presence of associated medical complications, including preeclampsia, hyperthyroidism, electrolyte imbalance, and anemia. After the patient's condition is stabilized, a decision must be made concerning the most appropriate method of evacuation.

Suction Curettage

Suction curettage is the preferred method of evacuation, regardless of uterine size, for patients who desire to preserve fertility (32). It involves the following steps:

1. **Oxytocin infusion**—This procedure is begun before the induction of anesthesia.
2. **Cervical dilation**—As the cervix is being dilated, uterine bleeding often increases. Retained blood in the endometrial cavity may be expelled during cervical dilation. Active uterine bleeding should not deter the prompt completion of cervical dilation.
3. **Suction curettage**—Within a few minutes of commencing suction curettage, uterine size may decrease dramatically, and the bleeding will be well controlled. The use of a 12-mm cannula is strongly advised to facilitate evacuation. If the uterus is larger than 14 weeks of gestation, one hand should be placed on top of the fundus, and the uterus should be massaged to stimulate uterine contraction and reduce the risk of perforation.
4. **Sharp curettage**—When suction evacuation is believed to be complete, gentle sharp curettage is performed to remove any residual molar tissue.

Because trophoblast cells express RhD factor, patients who are Rh negative should receive Rh immune globulin at the time of evacuation.

Hysterectomy

If the patient desires surgical sterilization, a hysterectomy may be performed with the mole in situ. The ovaries may be preserved at the time of surgery, even in the presence of prominent theca lutein cysts. Large ovarian cysts may be decompressed by aspiration. Hysterectomy does not prevent metastasis; patients still require follow-up with assessment of hCG levels.

Prophylactic Chemotherapy

The use of prophylactic chemotherapy at the time of molar evacuation is controversial. The debate concerns the wisdom of exposing all patients to potentially toxic treatment when only about 20% are at risk of developing persistent tumor.

In a study of 247 patients with complete molar pregnancy who prophylactically received a single course of *actinomycin D (ActD)* at the time of evacuation, local uterine invasion developed in 10 patients (4%), and no patients experienced metastasis (35). All 10 patients with local invasion achieved remission after one additional course of chemotherapy. **Prophylactic chemotherapy, prevented metastasis and reduced the incidence and morbidity of local uterine invasion.**

In two prospective randomized studies of prophylactic chemotherapy in patients with a complete mole, a significant decrease in persistent tumor was detected in patients with high-risk mole who received prophylactic chemotherapy (47% and 50% vs. 14%) (36–38). **Prophylaxis may be particularly useful in the management of high-risk complete molar pregnancy, especially when hCG assessments for follow-up are unavailable or unreliable.**

Follow-Up

Human Chorionic Gonadotropin

After molar evacuation, patients should be monitored with weekly determinations of β-subunit hCG levels until these levels are normal for 3 consecutive weeks, followed by monthly determinations until the levels are normal for 6 consecutive months (39). The average time to achieve the first normal hCG level after evacuation is about 9 weeks (40). After achieving nondetectable serum hCG levels, the risk of developing GTN approaches zero (41–43). If these findings are confirmed, it is possible that postmolar hCG surveillance could be safely abbreviated.

Contraception

Patients are encouraged to use effective contraception during the entire interval of hCG follow-up. Because of the potential risk of uterine perforation, bleeding, and infection, intrauterine devices should not be inserted until the patient achieves a normal hCG level. If the patient does not desire surgical sterilization, either oral contraceptives or barrier methods should be used.

Increased incidence of postmolar persistent tumor was reported among patients who used oral contraceptives before gonadotropin remission (44). However, data from a prospective trial and other centers indicate that oral contraceptive use does not increase the risk of postmolar trophoblastic disease (45–47). **It appears that oral contraceptives may be used safely after molar evacuation during the entire interval of hormonal follow-up.**

Gestational Trophoblastic Neoplasia

Nonmetastatic Disease

Locally invasive GTN develops in about 15% of patients after evacuation of a complete mole and infrequently after other gestations (1). These patients usually present with the following symptoms:

1. Irregular vaginal bleeding
2. Theca lutein cysts
3. Uterine subinvolution or asymmetric enlargement
4. Persistently elevated serum hCG levels.

The trophoblastic tumor may perforate the myometrium, causing intraperitoneal bleeding, or erode into uterine vessels, causing vaginal hemorrhage. Bulky, necrotic tumor may involve the uterine wall and serve as a nidus for infection. Patients with uterine sepsis may have a purulent vaginal discharge and acute pelvic pain.

After molar evacuation, persistent GTN may exhibit the histologic features of either hydatidiform mole or choriocarcinoma. After a nonmolar pregnancy, persistent GTN always has the histologic pattern of choriocarcinoma. Histologic characterization of choriocarcinoma depends on sheets of anaplastic syncytiotrophoblast and cytotrophoblast without chorionic villi.

Placental-Site Trophoblastic Tumor

Placental-site trophoblastic tumor is an uncommon but important variant of choriocarcinoma that consists predominantly of intermediate trophoblast (48). Relative to their mass, these tumors produce small amounts of hCG and human placental lactogen (hPL), and they tend to remain confined to the uterus, metastasizing late in their course. **In contrast to other trophoblastic tumors, placental-site tumors are relatively insensitive to chemotherapy.**

Metastatic Disease

Metastatic GTN occurs in about 4% of patients after evacuation of a complete mole, but it is seen more often when GTN develops after nonmolar pregnancies (1). GTN usually metastasizes as choriocarcinoma because of its tendency for early vascular invasion with widespread dissemination. Trophoblastic tumors often are perfused by fragile vessels and are frequently hemorrhagic. Symptoms of metastases may result from spontaneous bleeding at metastatic foci. The most common sites of metastases are lung (80%), vagina (30%), pelvis (20%), liver (10%), and brain (10%).

Pulmonary

At the time of diagnosis, lung involvement is visible by chest radiography in 80% of patients with metastatic GTN. Patients with pulmonary metastasis may have chest pain, cough, hemoptysis, dyspnea, or an asymptomatic lesion visible by chest radiography. Respiratory symptoms may be acute or chronic, persisting over many months.

GTN may produce four principal pulmonary patterns:

1. An alveolar or "snowstorm" pattern
2. Discrete rounded densities
3. Pleural effusion
4. An embolic pattern caused by pulmonary arterial occlusion.

Table 39.2 Staging of Gestational Trophoblastic Tumors[b]	
Stage I	Disease confined to uterus
Stage II	GTN extending outside uterus but limited to genital structures (adnexa, vagina, broad ligament)
Stage III	GTN extending to lungs with or without known genital tract involvement
Stage IV	All other metastatic sites

Because respiratory symptoms and radiographic findings may be dramatic, the patient may be thought to have a primary pulmonary disease. Some patients with extensive pulmonary involvement have minimal, if any, gynecologic symptoms because the reproductive organs may be free of trophoblastic tumor. The diagnosis of GTN may be confirmed only after thoracotomy is performed, particularly in patients with a nonmolar antecedent pregnancy.

Pulmonary hypertension may develop in patients with GTN secondary to pulmonary arterial occlusion by trophoblastic emboli. The development of early respiratory failure requiring intubation is associated with a poor clinical outcome (49).

Vaginal

Vaginal metastases occur in 30% of the patients with metastatic tumor. These lesions are highly vascular and may bleed vigorously when biopsied. Metastases to the vagina may occur in the fornices or suburethrally and may produce irregular bleeding or a purulent discharge.

Hepatic

Liver metastases occur in 10% of patients with disseminated trophoblastic tumor. Hepatic involvement is encountered when there is a protracted delay in diagnosis and the patient has an extensive tumor burden. Epigastric or right upper quadrant pain may develop if metastases stretch the hepatic capsule. Hepatic lesions may be hemorrhagic, causing hepatic rupture and exsanguinating intraperitoneal bleeding.

Central Nervous System

Metastatic trophoblastic disease involves the brain in 10% of patients. Cerebral involvement is seen in patients with advanced disease; virtually all patients with brain metastasis have concurrent pulmonary or vaginal involvement or both. Because cerebral lesions frequently hemorrhage spontaneously, most patients develop acute focal neurologic deficits (50,51).

Staging and Prognostic Score

Staging

An anatomic staging system for GTN was adopted by the International Federation of Gynecology and Obstetrics (FIGO) (Table 39.2). It is hoped that this staging system will encourage the objective comparison of data from various centers (52).

Stage I: **Patients have persistently elevated hCG levels and tumor confined to the uterine corpus.**
Stage II: **Patients have metastases to the genital tract.**
Stage III: **Patients have pulmonary metastases with or without uterine, vaginal, or pelvic involvement.** The diagnosis is based on a rising hCG level in the presence of pulmonary lesions viewed by chest radiography.
Stage IV: **Patients have advanced disease and involvement of the brain, liver, kidneys, or gastrointestinal tract.** These patients are in the highest risk category because they are most likely to be resistant to chemotherapy. Choriocarcinoma is usually present, and the disease commonly follows a nonmolar pregnancy.

Prognostic Scoring System

In addition to anatomic staging, it is important to consider other variables to predict the likelihood of drug resistance and to assist in selecting appropriate chemotherapy (53). **A prognostic scoring system proposed by the World Health Organization reliably predicts the potential for resistance to chemotherapy** (Table 39.3).

Table 39.3 Scoring System Based on Prognostic Factors[a]

	0	1	2	4
Age (years)	≤39	>39		
Antecedent pregnancy	Hydatidiform mole	Abortion	Term	
Interval between end of antecedent pregnancy and start of chemotherapy (months)	<4	4–6	7–12	>12
Human chorionic gonadotropin (IU/L)	$<10^3$	10^3–10^4	10^4–10^5	$>10^5$
ABO groups		O or A	B or AB	
Largest tumor, including uterine (cm)	<3	3–5	>5	
Site of metastases		Spleen, kidney	GI tract	Brain, Liver
Number of metastases		1–3	4–8	>8
Prior chemotherapy			1 drug	≥2 drugs

[a]The total score for a patient is obtained by adding the individual scores for each prognostic factor. Total score: <7, low risk; ≥7, high risk.

When the prognostic score is higher than 6, the patient is categorized as high risk and requires multimodal therapy, which includes intensive combination chemotherapy, and may also include surgery and radiation to achieve remission. Patients with stage I disease usually have a low-risk score, and those with stage IV disease have a high-risk score. The distinction between low and high risk applies mainly to patients with stage II or III disease.

Diagnostic Evaluation

Optimal management of persistent GTN requires a thorough assessment of the extent of the disease before the initiation of treatment. **All patients with persistent GTN should undergo a careful pretreatment evaluation, including the following:**

1. Complete history and physical examination
2. Measurement of the serum hCG level
3. Hepatic, thyroid, and renal function tests
4. Determination of baseline peripheral white blood cell and platelet counts

The metastatic workup should include the following:

1. Chest radiograph or computed tomography (CT) scan
2. Ultrasonography or CT scan of the abdomen and pelvis
3. CT or magnetic resonance imaging (MRI) scan of the head

When the pelvic examination and chest radiographic findings are negative, metastatic involvement of other sites is uncommon.

Liver ultrasonography and CT or MRI scanning will disclose most hepatic metastases in patients with abnormal liver function tests. CT or MRI scan of the head facilitates the early diagnosis of asymptomatic cerebral lesions. Chest CT scans may detect micrometastases not visible on chest radiography. Chest CT will demonstrate pulmonary micrometastases in about 40% of patients with presumed nonmetastatic disease (54).

In patients with choriocarcinoma or metastatic disease, hCG levels may be measured in the cerebrospinal fluid (CSF) to exclude cerebral involvement if the results of CT scanning of the brain are normal. The ratio of plasma-to-CSF hCG tends to be lower than 60 in the presence of cerebral metastases (55). A single plasma-to-CSF hCG ratio may be misleading, because rapid changes in plasma hCG levels may not be reflected promptly in the CSF (56).

Table 39.4 Protocol for Treatment of GTN	
Stage I	
Initial	Single-agent chemotherapy or hysterectomy with adjunctive chemotherapy
Resistant	Combination chemotherapy
	Hysterectomy with adjunctive chemotherapy
	Local resection
	Pelvic infusion
Stage II and III	
Low risk[a]	
Initial	Single-agent chemotherapy
Resistant	Combination chemotherapy
High risk[a]	
Initial	Combination chemotherapy
Resistant	Second-line combination chemotherapy
Stage IV	
Initial	Combination chemotherapy
Brain	Whole-head radiation (3,000 cGy)
	Craniotomy to manage complications
Liver	Resection or embolization to manage complications
Resistant[a]	Second-line combination chemotherapy
	Hepatic arterial infusion

[a]Local resection optional.

Pelvic ultrasonography appears to be useful in detecting extensive trophoblastic uterine involvement and may aid in identifying sites of resistant uterine tumor (57). Because ultrasonography can accurately and noninvasively detect extensive uterine tumor, it may help identify patients who would benefit from hysterectomy.

Management of GTN

A protocol for the management of GTN is presented in Table 39.4.

Low-Risk Disease

Low-risk GTN includes patients with both nonmetastatic (stage I) and metastatic GTN whose prognostic score is less than 7. In patients with stage I disease, the selection of treatment is based primarily on whether the patient desires to retain fertility.

Hysterectomy Plus Chemotherapy

If the patient does not wish to preserve fertility, hysterectomy with adjuvant single-agent chemotherapy may be performed as primary treatment. Adjuvant chemotherapy is administered for three reasons:

1. To reduce the likelihood of disseminating viable tumor cells at surgery.
2. To maintain a cytotoxic level of chemotherapy in the bloodstream and tissues in case viable tumor cells are disseminated at surgery.
3. To treat any occult metastases that may be present at the time of surgery.

Chemotherapy can be administered safely at the time of hysterectomy without increasing the risk of bleeding or sepsis. In a series of 31 patients treated with primary hysterectomy and a single course of adjuvant chemotherapy, all achieved complete remission with no additional therapy (58).

Hysterectomy is performed in all patients with stage I placental-site trophoblastic tumor. Because placental-site tumors are resistant to chemotherapy, hysterectomy for presumed nonmetastatic disease is the only curative treatment. Patients with metastatic placental site trophoblastic tumor may still achieve remission, but their tumors are less responsive to chemotherapy (59).

Chemotherapy Alone

Single-agent chemotherapy is the preferred treatment in patients with stage I disease who desire to retain fertility (60). At the NETDC from July 1965 through June 2008, primary single-agent chemotherapy was administered to 561 patients with stage I GTN and 434 patients (77.4%) attained complete remission. The remaining 127 patients with resistant disease subsequently achieved remission after combination chemotherapy or surgical intervention.

When a patient's disease is resistant to single-agent chemotherapy and she desires to preserve fertility, combination chemotherapy should be administered. If the patient's disease is resistant to single-agent and combination chemotherapy and she wants to retain fertility, local uterine resection may be considered. When local resection is planned, a preoperative ultrasonography, MRI, or arteriography may help to define the site of the resistant tumor.

Low-Risk Metastatic GTN (Stages II and III)

Vaginal and Pelvic Metastasis

Low-risk disease treated with primary single-agent chemotherapy has a high (approximately 80%) rate of remission in contrast to high-risk disease that usually does not achieve remission with single-agent treatment and requires treatment with primary intensive combination chemotherapy.

Vaginal metastases may bleed profusely because they are highly vascular and friable. When bleeding is substantial, it may be controlled by packing the vagina or by wide local excision. Infrequently, arteriographic embolization of the hypogastric arteries may be required to control hemorrhage from vaginal metastases (61).

Pulmonary Metastasis

At the NETDC from July 1965 through June 2008, of the 139 patients with low-risk stages II or III disease, 114 (82%) attained complete remission with single-agent chemotherapy. The remaining 25 (18%) patients who had disease resistant to single-agent treatment subsequently achieved remission with combination chemotherapy.

Thoracotomy   Thoracotomy has a limited but important role in the management of pulmonary metastases. **If a patient has a persistent viable pulmonary metastasis following intensive chemotherapy, thoracotomy may be indicated to excise the resistant focus.** A thorough metastatic workup should be performed before surgery is undertaken to exclude other sites of persistent disease. It is important to realize that fibrotic pulmonary nodules may persist indefinitely on chest radiography, even after complete gonadotropin remission is attained. In patients undergoing thoracotomy for resistant disease, chemotherapy should be administered postoperatively to treat potential occult sites of micrometastasis.

Hysterectomy

Hysterectomy may be required in patients with metastatic disease to control uterine hemorrhage or sepsis. In patients with extensive uterine tumor, hysterectomy may substantially reduce the trophoblastic tumor burden and limit the need for multiple courses of chemotherapy (62).

Follow-Up

All patients with low-risk GTN (stages I through III) should undergo follow-up with:

1. **Weekly measurement of hCG levels until they are normal for 3 consecutive weeks.**

2. **Monthly measurement of hCG values until levels are normal for 12 consecutive months.**

3. **Effective contraception during the entire interval of hormonal follow-up.**

<table>
<tr><td>

High-Risk Metastatic GTN (Stages II–IV)

</td><td>

All patients with high-risk GTN (stages II–IV) should be treated with primary intensive combination chemotherapy and the selective use of radiation therapy and surgery. Between July 1965 and June 2008, of the 103 patients with high-risk GTN stages II–IV treated at the NETDC, 83 (80.5%) achieved complete remission. Before 1975, when single agent therapy was used primarily to treat patients with stage IV GTN, only 6 of 20 patients (30%) attained complete remission. Since 1975, 17 of 21 patients (80.9%) achieved remission. This improvement in survival resulted from the use of multimodal therapy, including primary combination chemotherapy in conjunction with radiation and surgical treatment. Patients with stage IV disease are at the greatest risk of developing rapidly progressive and unresponsive tumors despite intensive multimodal therapy. They should be referred to centers with special expertise in the management of trophoblastic disease.

Hepatic Metastasis

The management of resistant hepatic metastasis is particularly difficult (63). If a patient becomes resistant to systemic chemotherapy, hepatic arterial infusion of chemotherapy may induce complete remission in selected cases. Hepatic resection may be required to control acute bleeding or to excise a focus of resistant tumor. New techniques of arterial embolization may reduce the need for surgical intervention.

Cerebral Metastasis

At the NETDC, cerebral metastases are treated with either whole-brain radiation (3,000 cGy in 10 fractions) or stereotactic radiosurgery in conjunction with combination chemotherapy. **Because irradiation may be hemostatic and tumoricidal, the risk of spontaneous cerebral hemorrhage may be lessened by the concurrent use of combination chemotherapy and brain irradiation.** Excellent remission rates (86%) were reported in patients with cranial metastases treated with intensive intravenous combination chemotherapy and intrathecal *methotrexate (MTX)* (64).

Craniotomy   **Craniotomy may be required to provide acute decompression or to control bleeding.** It should be performed to manage life-threatening complications so that the patient ultimately will be cured with chemotherapy. In a study of six patients (65), the use of craniotomy to control bleeding resulted in complete remission in three patients. Infrequently, cerebral metastases that are resistant to chemotherapy may be amenable to local resection (66). Patients with cerebral metastases who achieve sustained remission generally have no residual neurologic deficits.

Follow-Up

Patients with stage IV disease should receive follow-up with:

1. **Weekly determination of hCG levels until they are normal for 3 consecutive weeks.**
2. **Monthly determination of hCG levels until they are normal for 24 consecutive months.**

These patients require prolonged gonadotropin follow-up because they are at increased risk of late recurrence.

An algorithm for the management of persistent GTN is presented in Figure 39.7.

</td></tr>
</table>

Chemotherapy

<table>
<tr><td>

Single-Agent Treatment

</td><td>

Single-agent chemotherapy with either *actinomycin D (ActD)* or *MTX* achieved comparable and excellent remission rates in both nonmetastatic and low-risk metastatic GTN (67). Several protocols using these agents are available. *ActD* can be given every other week as a 5-day regimen or in a pulsatile fashion; similarly, *MTX* can be given either in a 5-day regimen or pulsatile weekly (68,69). No study compared all of these protocols with regard to success. An optimal regimen should maximize the response rate while minimizing morbidity and cost.

An important phase III randomized trial examining *MTX* and *ActD* in the treatment of low-risk GTN was published by the Gynecologic Oncology Group (GOG) (70). Two hundred sixteen

</td></tr>
</table>

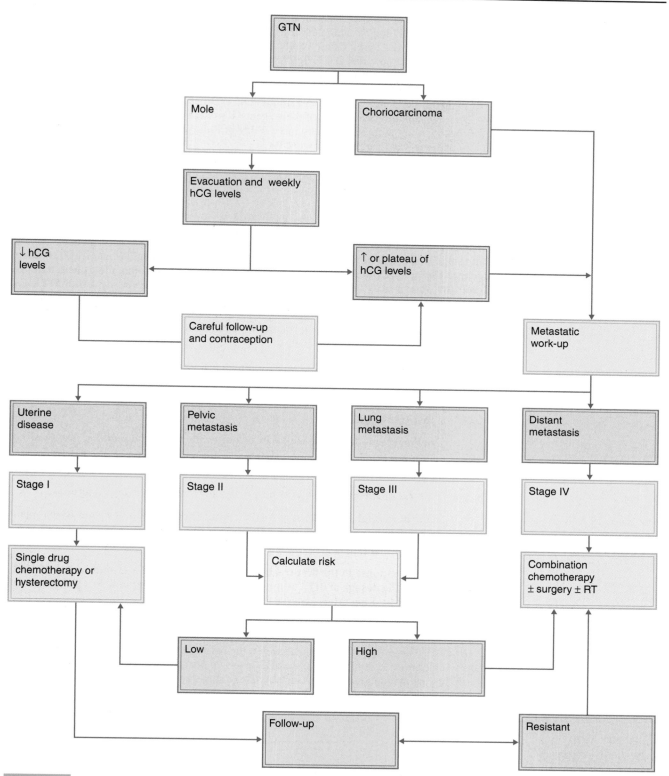

Figure 39.7   Management of gestational trophoblastic tumor. GTN, gestational trophoblastic neoplasia; hCG, human chorionic gonadotropin; RT, radiotherapy. (From **Berkowitz RS, Goldstein DP.** Gestational trophoblastic neoplasia. In: **Berek JS, Hacker NF.** *Berek and Hacker's Gynecologic Oncology,* 5th ed. Philadelphia, PA: Lippincott Williams & Wilkins, 2010;607, with permission.)

patients were randomized to receive either biweekly *ActD* 1.25mg/m^2 intravenous (IV) bolus or weekly *MTX* 30 mg/m^2 intramuscular (IM). The remission rate was 58% in the *MTX* arm and 73% in the *ActD* arm. These results suggest that *ActD* is superior to the weekly *MTX* regimen in treating low-risk GTN. Before recommending pulse *ActD* as the primary modality in the treatment of patients with low-risk GTN, it is important to be aware of the potential for significant toxicity of this regimen compared to those receiving *MTX*. All patients with low-risk disease in this study ultimately achieved remission, regardless of their initial response. Regarding the true comparative effectiveness of these agents, it would be prudent to compare the biweekly *ActD* regimen to the more commonly used 5-day or 8-day *MTX* regimens, which offer a high initial remission rate with minimal toxicity.

The administration of *methotrexate* with folinic acid (*MTX*-FA) in GTN to limit systemic toxicity was first reported in 1964 (71).Subsequently, it has been confirmed that *MTX*-FA is both effective and safe in the management of GTN.

An evaluation of 185 patients treated with *MTX*-FA revealed that complete remission was achieved in 162 patients (87.6%); of these patients, 132 (81.5%) required only one course of *MTX*-FA to attain remission (72). *MTX*-FA induced remission in 147 of 163 patients (90.2%) with stage I GTN and in 15 of 22 patients (68.2%) with low-risk stages II and III GTN. **Resistance to therapy was more common in patients with choriocarcinoma, metastasis, and pretreatment serum hCG levels higher than 50,000 mIU/mL.** After treatment with **MTX-FA**, thrombocytopenia, granulocytopenia, and hepatotoxicity developed in 3 (1.6%), 11 (5.9%), and 26 (14.1%) patients, respectively. **Thus, *MTX*-FA achieved an excellent therapeutic outcome with minimal toxicity and attained this goal with limited exposure to chemotherapy.**

Technique of Single-Agent Treatment

The serum hCG level is measured weekly after each course of chemotherapy. The hCG regression curve serves as the primary basis for determining the need for additional treatment.

After the first treatment:

1. **Further chemotherapy is withheld as long as the hCG level is falling progressively.**
2. **Additional single-agent chemotherapy is not administered at any predetermined or fixed interval.**

A second course of chemotherapy is administered under the following conditions:

1. **If the hCG level plateaus for more than 3 consecutive weeks or begins to rise again.**
2. **If the hCG level does not decline by 1 log within 18 days after completion of the first treatment.**

If the patient's response to the first treatment was adequate and a second course of *MTX*-FA is required, the dosage of *MTX* is unaltered. An adequate response is defined as a fall in the hCG level by 1 log after a course of chemotherapy.

If the response to the first treatment is inadequate, the dosage of *MTX* is increased from 1.0 mg/kg/day to 1.5 mg/kg/day for each of the 4 treatment days. If the response to two consecutive courses of *MTX*-FA is inadequate, the patient is considered to be resistant to *MTX*, and *ActD* is promptly substituted. If the hCG levels do not decline by 1 log after treatment with *ActD*, the patient is considered resistant to *ActD* as a single agent. She must be treated intensively with combination chemotherapy to achieve remission.

Combination Chemotherapy

Triple Therapy

Prior to the introduction of *etoposide* in combination with *MTX, ActD, cyclophosphamide,* and *vincristine* (*EMA-CO*), triple therapy with *MTX, ActD,* and *cyclophosphamide* was the treatment of choice as initial therapy for patients with low-risk disease resistant to single-agent therapy and as primary therapy for high-risk patients. Collectively, data from three centers indicate that triple therapy induced remission in 21 (49%) of 43 patients with metastasis and a high-risk score (score >6) (73–75). **Triple therapy is no longer indicated in patients with high-risk disease. It maybe useful in selected patients with low-risk scores resistant to single agents.**

EMA-CO

Etoposide induces complete remission in 56 (95%) of 60 patients with nonmetastatic and low-risk metastatic GTN (76). **The use of *EMA-CO* induced an 83% remission rate in patients with metastasis and a high-risk score** (77). Another study confirmed that primary *EMA-CO* induced complete remission in 76% of the patients with metastatic GTN and a high-risk score (78). Another study reported that *EMA-CO* induced complete sustained remission in 87 (90.6%) of 96 patients with high-risk (score >6) GTN (79). Remission occurred with *EMA-CO* in 30 (86%) of 35 patients with brain metastasis (65).

The *EMA-CO* regimen is well tolerated, and treatment seldom has to be suspended because of toxicity. The *EMA-CO* regimen is the preferred primary treatment in patients with metastasis and a high-risk prognostic score (score >6).

EMA-EP

Patients resistant to *EMA-CO* can be treated successfully by substituting *etoposide* and *cisplatin* on day 8 (*EMA-EP*). *EMA-EP* induced remission alone or with surgery in 16 (76%) of 21 patients who were resistant to *EMA-CO* (80). The optimal combination drug protocol will most likely include *etoposide, MTX,* and *ActD* and perhaps other agents administered in the most dose-intensive manner.

Management of Refractory GTN

Efforts continue to identify new agents and regimens effective in treating patients who prove resistant to all standard chemotherapy regimens. A combination of *cisplatin, vinblastine,* and *bleomycin* (*PVB*) was used effectively in patients with drug-resistant tumor (74,75,81). Although *ifosfamide* and *paclitaxel* were used successfully, further studies are needed to define their potential role in either primary or second-line therapy (82,83). Osborne et al. reported that a novel three-drug doublet regimen consisting of *paclitaxel, etoposide,* and *cisplatin* (*TE/TP*) induced complete remission in two patients with relapsed high-risk GTN (84). Wan et al. demonstrated that *floxuridine* (*FUDR*)-containing regimens induced complete remission in all of 21 patients with drug-resistant GTN (85). Matsui et al. found that 5-*fluorouracil* (5-*FU*) in combination with *ActD* induced remission in 9 of 11 (82%) patients with drug resistance (86). The potential role for autologous bone marrow transplantation or stem cell rescue in conjunction with ultra-high-dose chemotherapy has yet to be defined, although complete remissions was reported in patients with refractory GTN (87,88).

Duration of Therapy

Patients who require combination chemotherapy must be treated intensively to attain remission. Combination chemotherapy should be given as often as toxicity permits until the patient achieves three consecutive normal hCG levels. After normal hCG levels are attained, at least two additional courses of chemotherapy are administered to reduce the risk of relapse.

False-Positive hCG Tests

The concept of false-positive hCG tests caused by heterophile antibodies is critical to remember when following patients with molar gestation or GTN. Some assay systems used by commercial laboratories are particularly vulnerable to false-positive tests resulting from the presence of heterophilic antibodies in the test kits they were using (89). For the most part this problem was corrected by adding blocking antibodies to the test systems. Since the hCG molecules in GTN are significantly more degraded or heterogeneous than in normal pregnancy, with higher proportions of free *B*-hCG, nicked hCG, and *B*-core fragments, it is important to use an assay that detects both intact hCG and its metabolites and fragments in order to accurately assess the tumor burden (90–92). Additionally, cross-reactivity with luteinizing hormone (LH) can cause confusion when dealing with women in the perimenopausal age group whose hCG level may plateau above assay even when there is no longer active tumor. The use of hormone suppression will suppress LH and prevent unnecessary treatment. False-positive hCG tests caused by heterophile agglutinins or LH release may cause confusion in the diagnosis of early pregnancy, ectopic pregnancy, and so-called phantom choriocarcinoma. When there is concern about the possibility of a false-positive serum hCG test, a urine sample should be tested, because patients with phantom hCG generally have no measurable hCG in a parallel urine sample.

Persistent Low-Level "Real" hCG

Some patients with molar pregnancy and GTN have persistent (weeks to months) very low levels of real hCG (usually <500 mIU/mL). In these women, extensive radiologic and clinical evaluations fail to reveal any lesions, and chemotherapy is usually not effective. This condition of "real" low-level hCG, where hCG is not hyperglycosylated, is called "quiescent GTN." These patients should be managed with careful follow-up, because 6% to 10% ultimately will relapse into active disease and rising hCG levels. The risk of relapse to active disease is correlated with the amount of hyperglycosylated hCG. If relapse does occur, chemotherapy usually proves effective (93).

Subsequent Pregnancies

Pregnancies After Uncomplicated Hydatidiform Mole

Patients with hydatidiform moles can anticipate normal reproduction in the future (94). At the NETDC from 1965 until 2007, patients with uncomplicated complete mole had 1,337 subsequent pregnancies that resulted in 912 term live births (68.1%), 101 premature deliveries (7.5%), 11 ectopic pregnancies (0.9%), 7 stillbirths (0.5%), and 20 repeat molar pregnancies (1.5%). First- and second-trimester spontaneous abortions occurred in 245 (18.3%) pregnancies. Major and minor congenital malformations were detected in 40 infants (3.9%), and primary cesarean delivery was performed in 81 of 414 (19.6%) term or preterm births from 1979 to 2007.

Although data regarding pregnancies after partial mole are limited (296 subsequent pregnancies), the information is reassuring (94). **Patients with both complete and partial mole should be reassured that they are generally at no increased risk of complications in later gestations.**

When a patient has had a molar pregnancy, either partial or complete, she should be informed of the increased risk of having a molar gestation in subsequent conceptions. After one molar pregnancy, the risk of having molar disease in a future gestation is about 1% to 1.5%. Of 35 patients with at least two documented molar pregnancies, every possible combination of repeat molar pregnancy was observed. After two molar gestations, these 35 patients had 39 later conceptions resulting in 24 (61.5%) term deliveries, 7 (17.9%) moles (6 complete, 1 partial), 3 spontaneous abortions, 3 therapeutic abortions, 1 intrauterine fetal death, and 1 ectopic pregnancy. In six patients, the medical records indicated that the patient had a different partner at the time of different molar pregnancies (95).

For any subsequent pregnancy, it seems prudent to undertake the following approach:

1. **Perform pelvic ultrasonographic examination during the first trimester to confirm normal gestational development.**
2. **Obtain an hCG measurement 6 weeks after completion of the pregnancy to exclude occult trophoblastic neoplasia.**

Pregnancies After GTN

Patients with GTN who are treated successfully with chemotherapy can expect normal reproduction in the future. Patients who were treated with chemotherapy at the NETDC from 1965 to 2007 had 631 subsequent pregnancies that resulted in 422 term live births (66.9%), 42 preterm deliveries (6.7%), 7 ectopic pregnancies (1.1%), 9 stillbirths (1.4%), and 9 repeat molar pregnancies (1.7%) (94). First- and second-trimester spontaneous abortions occurred in 114 (18.1%) pregnancies. Major and minor congenital malformations were detected in 10 infants (2.1%). Primary cesarean delivery was performed in 81 (21.8%) of 371 subsequent term and preterm births from 1979 to 2007. The frequency of congenital anomalies is not increased, although chemotherapeutic agents have teratogenic and mutagenic potential.

References

1. **Berkowitz RS, Goldstein DP.** The management of molar pregnancy and gestational trophoblastic tumors. In: Knapp RC, Berkowitz RS, eds. *Gynecologic oncology.* 2nd ed. New York: McGraw-Hill, 1993:328–338.
2. **Bagshawe KD.** Risks and prognostic factors in trophoblastic neoplasia. *Cancer* 1976;38:1373–1385.
3. **Palmer JR.** Advances in the epidemiology of gestational trophoblastic disease. *J Reprod Med* 1994;39:155–162.
4. **Jeffers MD, O'Dwyer P, Curran B, et al.** Partial hydatidiform mole: a common but underdiagnosed condition. *Int J Gynecol Pathol* 1993;12:315–323.
5. **Martin BH, Kim JM.** Changes in gestational trophoblastic tumors over four decades: a Korean experience. *J Reprod Med* 1998;43:60–68.
6. **Parazzini F, La Vecchia C, Mangili G, et al.** Dietary factors and risk of trophoblastic disease. *Am J Obstet Gynecol* 1988;158:93–99.

7. **Berkowitz RS, Cramer DW, Bernstein MR, et al.** Risk factors for complete molar pregnancy from a case-control study. *Am J Obstet Gynecol* 1985;52:1016–1020.

8. **Parazzini F, La Vecchia C, Pampallona S.** Parental age and risk of complete and partial hydatidiform mole. *Br J Obstet Gynaecol* 1986;93:582–585.

9. **Sebire NJ, Foskett M, Fisher RA, et al.** Risk of partial and complete molar pregnancy in relation to maternal age. *Br J Obstet Gynecol* 2002;109:99–102.

10. **Berkowitz RS, Bernstein MR, Harlow BL, et al.** Case-control study of risk factors for partial molar pregnancy. *Am J Obstet Gynecol* 1995;173:788–794.

11. **Acaia B, Parazzini F, La Vecchia C, et al.** Increased frequency of complete hydatidiform mole in women with repeated abortion. *Gynecol Oncol* 1988;31:310–314.

12. **Kajii T, Ohama K.** Androgenetic origin of hydatidiform mole. *Nature* 1977;268:633–634.

13. **Pattillo RA, Sasaki S, Katayama KP, et al.** Genesis of 46XY hydatidiform mole. *Am J Obstet Gynecol* 1981;141:104–110.

14. **Azuma C, Saji F, Tokugawa Y, et al.** Application of gene amplification by polymerase chain reaction to genetic analysis of molar mitochondrial DNA: the detection of anuclear empty ovum as the cause of complete mole. *Gynecol Oncol* 1991;40:29–33.

15. **Yamashita K, Wake N, Araki T, et al.** Human lymphocyte antigen expression in hydatidiform mole: androgenesis following fertilization by a haploid sperm. *Am J Obstet Gynecol* 1979;135:597–600.

16. **Szulman AE, Surti U.** The syndromes of hydatidiform mole. I. Cytogenetic and morphologic correlations. *Am J Obstet Gynecol* 1978;131:665–671.

17. **Lawler SD, Fisher RA, Dent J.** A prospective genetic study of complete and partial hydatidiform moles. *Am J Obstet Gynecol* 1991;164:1270–1277.

18. **Genest DR, Ruiz RE, Weremowicz S, et al.** Do non-triploid partial hydatidiform moles exist?: a histologic and flow cytometric reevaluation of non-triploid specimens. *J Reprod Med* 2002;47:363–368.

19. **Mosher R, Goldstein DP, Berkowitz RS.** Complete hydatidiform mole—comparison of clinicopathologic features, current and past. *J Reprod Med* 1998;43:21–27.

20. **Keep D, Zaragoza MV, Hasold T, et al.** Very early complete hydatidiform mole. *Hum Pathol* 1996;27:708–713.

21. **Lage JM, Berkowitz RS, Rice LW, et al.** Flow cytometric analysis of DNA content in partial hydatidiform moles with persistent gestational trophoblastic tumors. *Obstet Gynecol* 1991;77:111.

22. **Berkowitz RS, Goldstein DP.** Molar pregnancy. *N Engl J Med* 2009;360:1639–1645.

23. **Fisher RA, Hodges MD, Rees HC, et al.** The maternally transcribed gene p57 (KIP2) (CDNK1C) is abnormally expressed in both androgenetic and biparental complete hydatidiform moles. *Hum Mol Genet* 2002;11:3267.

24. **Soto-Wright V, Bernstein MR, Goldstein DP, et al.** The changing clinical presentation of complete molar pregnancy. *Obstet Gynecol* 1995;86:775–779.

25. **Goldstein DP, Berkowitz RS.** Current management of complete and partial molar pregnancy. *J Reprod Med* 1994;39:139–146.

26. **Amir SM, Osathanondh R, Berkowitz RS, et al.** Human chorionic gonadotropin and thyroid function in patients with hydatidiform mole. *Am J Obstet Gynecol* 1984;150:723–728.

27. **Berkowitz RS, Goldstein DP.** Presentation and management of molar pregnancy. In: **Hancock BW, Newlands ES, Berkowitz RS, eds.** Gestational trophoblastic disease. London: Chapman and Hall, 1997:127–142.

28. **Osathanondh R, Berkowitz RS, de Cholnoky C, et al.** Hormonal measurements in patients with theca lutein cysts and gestational trophoblastic disease. *J Reprod Med* 1986;31:179–183.

29. **Szulman AE, Surti U.** The clinicopathologic profile of the partial hydatidiform mole. *Obstet Gynecol* 1982;59:597–602.

30. **Berkowitz RS, Goldstein DP, Bernstein MR.** Natural history of partial molar pregnancy. *Obstet Gynecol* 1985;66:677–681.

31. **Elias K, Goldstein DP, Berkowitz RS.** Complete hydatidiform mole in women over than age 50. *J Reprod Med* 2010;55:208–212.

32. **Berkowitz RS, Goldstein DP.** Current management of gestational trophoblastic disease. *Gynecol Oncol* 2009;112:654–662.

33. **Rice LW, Berkowitz RS, Lage JM, et al.** Persistent gestational trophoblastic tumor after partial hydatidiform mole. *Gynecol Oncol* 1990;36:358–362.

34. **Fine C, Bundy AL, Berkowitz RS, et al.** Sonographic diagnosis of partial hydatidiform mole. *Obstet Gynecol* 1989;73:414–418.

35. **Goldstein DP, Berkowitz RS.** Prophylactic chemotherapy of complete molar pregnancy. *Semin Oncol* 1995;22:157–160.

36. **Kim DS, Moon H, Kim KT, et al.** Effects of prophylactic chemotherapy for persistent trophoblastic disease in patients with complete hydatidiform mole. *Obstet Gynecol* 1986;67:690–694.

37. **Limpongsanurak S.** Prophylactic *actinomycin D* for high-risk complete hydatidiform mole. *J Reprod Med* 2001;46:110–116.

38. **Uberti EMH, Fajardo Mde C, da Cunha AGV, et al.** Prevention of postmolar gestational trophoblastic neoplasia using prophylactic single bolus dose of *actinomycin D* in high-risk hydatidiform mole: a simple, effective, secure and low cost approach without adverse effects on compliance to general follow-up or subsequent treatment. *Gynecol Oncol* 2009;114:299–305.

39. **Committee on Practice Bulletins-Gynecology.** American College of Obstetricians and Gynecologists. ACOG Practice Bulletin 53. Diagnosis and treatment of gestational trophoblastic neoplasms. *Obstet Gynecol* 2004;103:1365–1373.

40. **Genest DR, LaBorde O, Berkowitz RS, et al.** A clinicopathologic study of 153 cases of complete hydatidiform mole (1980–1990): histologic grade lacks prognostic significance. *Obstet Gynecol* 1991;78:402–409.

41. **Wolfberg A, Feltmate C, Goldstein DP, et al.** Low risk of relapse after achieving undetectable hCG levels in women with complete molar pregnancy. *Obstet Gynecol* 2004;104:551–554.

42. **Lavie I, Rao G, Castrillon DH, et al.** Duration of human chorionic gonadotropin surveillance or partial hydatidiform moles. *Am J Obstet Gynecol* 2005;192:1362–1364.

43. **Sebire NJ, Foskett M, Short D, et al.** Shortened duration of human chorionic gonadotropin surveillance following complete or partial hydatidiform mole: evidence for a revised protocol of a regional UK trophoblastic disease unit. *Br J Obstet Gynaecol* 2007;114:760–762.

44. **Stone M, Dent J, Kardana A, et al.** Relationship of oral contraception to development of trophoblastic tumour after evacuation of a hydatidiform mole. *BJOG* 1976;83:913–916.

45. **Berkowitz RS, Goldstein DP, Marean AR, et al.** Oral contraceptives and postmolar trophoblastic disease. *Obstet Gynecol* 1981;58:474–477.

46. **Curry SL, Schlaerth JB, Kohorn EI, et al.** Hormonal contraception and trophoblastic sequelae after hydatidiform mole (a Gynecologic Oncology Group study). *Am J Obstet Gynecol* 1989;160:805–809.

47. **Parrazzini F, Cipriani S, Mangili G, et al.** Oral contraceptives and risk of gestational trophoblastic disease. *Contraception* 2002;65:425-7.

48. **Feltmate CM, Genest DR, Goldsein DP, et al.** Advances in the understanding of placental site trophoblastic tumor. *J Reprod Med* 2002;47:337–341.

49. **Bakri YN, Berkowitz RS, Khan J, et al.** Pulmonary metastases of gestational trophoblastic tumor—risk factors for early respiratory failure. *J Reprod Med* 1994;39:175–178.

50. **Bakri YN, Berkowitz RS, Goldstein DP, et al.** Brain metastases of gestational trophoblastic tumor. *J Reprod Med* 1994;39:179–184.

51. **Athanassiou A, Begent RHJ, Newlands ES, et al.** Central nervous system metastases of choriocarcinoma: 23 years' experience at Charing Cross Hospital. *Cancer* 1983;52:1728–1735.

52. **Kohorn EI.** Negotiating a staging and risk factor scoring system for gestational trophoblastic neoplasia: a progress report. *J Reprod Med* 2002;47:445–450.

53. **Goldstein DP, Vzanten-Przybysz I, Bernstein MR, et al.** Revised FIGO staging system for gestational trophoblastic tumors: recommendations regarding therapy. *J Reprod Med* 1998;43:37–43.

54. **Garner EIO, Garrett A, Goldstein DP, et al.** Significance of chest computed tomography findings in the evaluation and treatment of persistent gestational trophoblastic neoplasia. *J Reprod Med* 2004;49:411–414.

55. **Bagshawe KD, Harland S.** Immunodiagnosis and monitoring of gonadotropin-producing metastases in the central nervous system. *Cancer* 1976;38:112–118.

56. **Bakri Y, Al-Hawashim N, Berkowitz RS.** Cerebrospinal fluid/serum β-subunit human gonadotropin ratio in patients with brain

metastases of gestational trophoblastic tumor. *J Reprod Med* 2000;45:94–96.

57. **Berkowitz RS, Birnholz J, Goldstein DP, et al.** Pelvic ultrasonography and the management of gestational trophoblastic disease. *Gynecol Oncol* 1983;15:403–412.

58. **Lurain JR, Singh DK, Schink JC.** Role of surgery in the management of high-risk gestational trophoblastic neoplasia. *J Reprod Med* 2006;51:773–776.

59. **Papadopoulos AJ, Foskett M, Seckl MJ, et al.** Twenty-five years' clinical experience with placental site trophoblastic tumors. *J Reprod Med* 2002;47:460–464.

60. **Kohorn EI.** Single-agent chemotherapy for nonmetastatic gestational trophoblastic neoplasia. *J Reprod Med* 1992;36:49.

61. **Tse KY, Chan KKI, Tam KF, Ngan HYS.** 20-year experience of managing profuse bleeding in gestational trophoblastic disease. *J Reprod Med* 2007;52:397–401.

62. **Soper JT.** Role of surgery and radiation therapy in the management of gestational trophoblastic disease. *Clin Obstet Gynecol* 2003;17:943–957.

63. **Crawford RAS, Newlands ES, Rustin GJR, et al.** Gestational trophoblastic disease with liver metastases: the Charing Cross experience. *Br J Obstet Gyaecol* 1997;104:105–109.

64. **Newlands ES, Holden L, Seckl MJ, et al.** Management of brain metastases in patients with high risk gestational trophoblastic tumors. *J Reprod Med* 2002;47:465–469.

65. **Weed JC Jr, Hammond CB.** Cerebral metastatic choriocarcinoma: intensive therapy and prognosis. *Obstet Gynecol* 1980;55:89–94.

66. **Soper JT, Spillman M, Sampson JH, et al.** High-risk gestational trophoblastic neoplasia with brain metastases: individualized multidisciplinary therapy in the management of four patients. *Gynecol Oncol* 2007;104:691–694.

67. **Osborne R, Gerulath A.** What is the best regimen for low-risk gestational trophoblastic neoplasia? A review. *J Reprod Med* 2004;49:602–616.

68. **Osborne R, Filiaci V, Schink J, et al.** A randomized phase III trial comparing weekly parental methotrexate and pulsed dactinomycin as primary management of low-risk gestational trophoblastic neoplasia: a Gynecologic Oncology Group study. *Gynecol Oncol* 2008;108:S2.

69. **Yerandi F, Eftekhar Z, Shojaei H, et al.** Pulse methotrexate versus pulse actinomycin D in the treatment of low-risk gestational trophoblastic neoplasia. *Int J Gynecol Obstet* 2008;103:33–39.

70. **Osborne R, Filiaci VL, Schink JC, et al.** Phase III trial of weekly methotrexate or pulsed dactinomycin for low-risk gestational trophoblastic neoplasia: a Gynecologic Oncology Group study. *J Clin Oncol* 2011;29:825–831.

71. **Bagshawe KD, Wilde CE.** Infusion therapy for pelvic trophoblastic tumors. *J Obstet Gynaecol Br Commonw* 1964;71:565–570.

72. **Berkowitz RS, Goldstein DP, Bernstein MR.** Ten years' experience with methotrexate and folinic acid as primary therapy for gestational trophoblastic disease. *Gynecol Oncol* 1986;23:111–118.

73. **Curry SL, Blessing JA, DiSaia PJ, et al.** A prospective randomized comparison of methotrexate, dactinomycin and chlorambucil versus methotrexate, dactinomycin, cyclophosphamide, doxorubicin, melphalan, hydroxyurea and vincristine in "poor prognosis" metastatic gestational trophoblastic disease: a Gynecologic Oncology Group study. *Obstet Gynecol* 1989;73:357–362.

74. **Gordon AN, Gershenson DM, Copeland LJ, et al.** High-risk metastatic gestational trophoblastic disease: further stratification into clinical entities. *Gynecol Oncol* 1989;34:54–56.

75. **DuBeshter B, Berkowitz RS, Goldstein DP, et al.** Metastatic gestational trophoblastic disease: experience at the New England Trophoblastic Disease Center, 1965–1985. *Obstet Gynecol* 1987;69:390–395.

76. **Wong LC, Choo YC, Ma HK.** Primary oral etoposide therapy in gestational trophoblastic disease: an update. *Cancer* 1986;58:14–17.

77. **Bagshawe KD.** Treatment of high-risk choriocarcinoma. *J Reprod Med* 1984;29:813–820.

78. **Bolis G, Bonazzi C, Landoni F, et al.** EMA-CO regimen in high-risk gestational trophoblastic tumor (GTT). *Gynecol Oncol* 1988;31:439–444.

79. **Kim SJ, Bae SN, Kim JH, et al.** Risk factors for the prediction of treatment failure in gestational trophoblastic tumors treated with EMA/CO regimen. *Gynecol Oncol* 1998;71:247–251.

80. **Bower M, Newlands ES, Holden L, et al.** EMA-CO for high-risk gestational trophoblastic tumors: results from a cohort of 272 patients. *J Clin Oncol* 1997;15:2636–2643.

81. **Azab M, Droz JP, Theodore C, et al.** Cisplatin, vincristine and bleomycin combination in the treatment of resistant high-risk gestational trophoblastic tumors. *Cancer* 1989;64:1829–1832.

82. **Sutton GP, Soper JT, Blessing JA, et al.** Ifosfamide alone and in combination in the treatment of refractory malignant gestational trophoblastic disease. *Am J Obstet Gynecol* 1992;167:489–495.

83. **Jones WB, Schneider J, Shapiro F, et al.** Treatment of resistant gestational choriocarcinoma with Taxol: a report of two cases. *Gynecol Oncol* 1996;61:126–130.

84. **Osborne R, Covens A, Merchandani DE, et al.** Successful salvage of relapsed high-risk gestational trophoblastic neoplasia patients using a novel paclitaxel-containing doublet. *J Reprod Med* 2004;49:655–661.

85. **Wan X, Yang Y, Wu Y, et al.** Floxuridine-containing regimens in the treatment of gestational trophoblastic tumor. *J Reprod Med* 2004;49:453–456.

86. **Matsui H, Iitsuka Y, Suzuka K, et al.** Salvage chemotherapy for high-risk gestational trophoblastic tumor. *J Reprod Med* 2004;49:438–442.

87. **Giacalone PL, Benos P, Donnadio D, et al.** High dose chemotherapy with autologous bone marrow transplantation for refractory metastatic gestational trophoblastic disease. *Gynecol Oncol* 1999;5:38–45.

88. **VanBesien K, Verschraegen C, Mehta R, et al.** Complete remission of refractory gestational trophoblastic disease with brain metastases treated with multicycle *ifosfamide, carboplatin,* and *etoposide* (ICE) and stem cell rescue. *Gynecol Oncol* 1997;65:366–369.

89. **Khanlian SA, Cole LA.** Management of gestational trophoblastic disease and other cases with low serum levels of human chorionic gonadotropin. *J Reprod Med* 2006;51:812–818.

90. **Hancock BW.** hCG measurement in gestational trophoblastic neoplasia: a critical appraisal. *J Reprod Med* 2006;51:859–860.

91. **Mitchell H, Bagshawe KD, Newlands ES, et al.** Importance of accurate human chorionic gonadotropin measurement in the treatment of gestational trophoblastic disease and testicular cancer. *J Reprod Med* 2006;51:868–870.

92. **Cole LA, Kohorn EI.** The need for an hCG assay that appropriately detects trophoblastic disease and other hCG-producing tumors. *J Reprod Med* 2006;51:793–811.

93. **Kohorn EI.** What we know about low-level hCG: definition, classification and management. *J Reprod Med* 2004;49:433–437.

94. **Garrett LA, Garner EO, Feltmate CM, et al.** Subsequent pregnancy outcomes in patients with molar pregnancy and persistent gestational trophoblastic neoplasia. *J Reprod Med* 2008;53:481–486.

95. **Tuncer ZS, Bernstein MR, Wang J, et al.** Repetitive hydatidiform mole with different male partners. *Gynecol Oncol* 1999;75:224–226.

40 Breast Cancer

Junko Ozao-Choy
Armando E. Giuliano

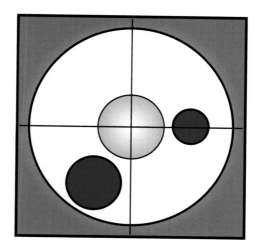

- **Breast cancer accounts for one-third of cancers in women. The risk of breast cancer increases with a positive family history and the use of hormone therapy. Breast cancer may be either** *in situ* **(ductal carcinoma** *in situ* **or lobular carcinoma** *in situ***) or invasive (infiltrating ductal carcinoma, infiltrating lobular carcinoma).**

- **The standard screening modalities for detection of breast cancer include yearly mammography and physical examination.**

- **Tissue diagnosis is achieved using fine-needle aspiration cytology (FNAC) or core needle biopsy (CNB). Open biopsy is performed if FNAC or CNB results are equivocal or discordant with the clinical findings.**

- **The combination of segmental mastectomy (with negative surgical margins), axillary lymph node dissection, and postoperative radiation therapy has the same overall survival compared to modified radical mastectomy for the management of patients with stages I and II breast cancer.**

- **Axillary lymph node status and the number of involved nodes are the most important prognostic indicators in primary breast cancer.**

- **Sentinel lymph node dissection alone can replace axillary lymph node dissection if the sentinel lymph node is found to be negative on pathology.**

- **Adjuvant systemic therapy prolongs survival and is recommended for women with a greater than 10% chance of relapse within 10 years.**

Breast cancer accounts for approximately one-third of all cancers in women and is second only to lung cancer as the leading cause of cancer deaths among women. Breast cancer has the highest incidence rate of all cancers. According to statistics from the American Cancer Society (ACS), over 230,000 new cases of invasive breast cancer will be diagnosed in women during 2011 in the United States as well as over 55,000 patients of *in situ* cancers, with almost 40,000 women succumbing to the disease during the same period (1). Over the past 50 years, the incidence of breast cancer in the United States increased significantly; one in every seven women will develop the disease during her lifetime. Fortunately, the mortality rate has declined since 1990.

Predisposing Factors

Less than 1% of breast cancers occur in women younger than 25 years of age. After age 30, there is a sharp increase in the incidence of breast cancer. Except for a short plateau between the ages of 45 and 50 years, the incidence increases steadily with age (2).

Family History

Of women who develop breast cancer, 20% to 30% have a family history of the disease. Although any family history of breast cancer increases the overall relative risk, this risk is not significantly increased if the disease was diagnosed postmenopausally in a first-degree or more distant relative (3). **If a woman's mother or sister had unilateral breast cancer premenopausally, her lifetime risk of developing the disease approaches 30%, whereas a woman whose mother or sister had bilateral breast cancers premenopausally has at least a 40% to 50% lifetime risk. The increased incidence in these women is probably the result of inherited oncogenes.**

Approximately 5% to 10% of breast cancers have an inherited basis. All inherited genes are autosomal dominant but have variable penetrance. Men carry the gene 50% of the time. The most common mutations are the **BRCA1** (chromosome 17q21) and **BRCA2** (chromosome 13q12-13) gene deletions. **Carriers of these germline mutations have up to a 4% per year risk of developing breast cancer and a lifetime risk that ranges from 35% to 85%** (4). These individuals have up to a 65% risk of developing a contralateral breast cancer. The *BRCA1* mutation is associated with an increased risk of ovarian and prostate cancer, whereas *BRCA2* carriers, although less common, demonstrate increased risks of male breast and prostate cancers. Both mutations are rare in the general public (0.1%) but are more commonly identified in Jews of Ashkenazi descent (1% to 2.3%) (5). **Genetic testing is available and should be considered if there is a high likelihood that results will be positive and will be used to influence decisions regarding the clinical management of the care of the patient and her family. Patients with three of more relatives with breast or ovarian cancer with one of the relatives being diagnosed before the age of 50, two first- or second-degree relatives with breast or ovarian cancer, any relative with male breast cancer, patients whose cancer has been diagnosed before the age of 50, and any patients with both breast and ovarian cancer in their family should undergo genetic counseling for BRCA testing. Ashkenazi Jewish patients should undergo genetic counseling if any first-degree relative, or two second-degree relatives on the same side have breast or ovarian cancer** (6). **Genetic testing is increasingly important given the evidence that prophylactic surgery may prevent new cancers from occurring, as well as prolong survival, in some cases. A prospective multicenter cohort study of 2,482 women with BRCA1 and BRCA2 mutations between 1974 and 2008 showed risk-reducing mastectomy was associated with a decreased risk of breast cancer. Risk-reducing salpingo-oophorectomy was associated with decreased risk of ovarian cancer, first diagnosis of breast cancer, all-cause mortality, breast cancer–specific mortality, and ovarian cancer–specific mortality** (7).

Diet, Obesity, and Alcohol

There are marked geographic differences in the incidence of breast cancer that may be related to diet. A meta-analysis demonstrated an association between a healthy diet and lower risk of breast cancer (8). Although a definitive relationship between total alcohol consumption and increased risk of breast cancer has yet to be determined, high wine intake was associated with elevated risk (8,9).

Reproductive and Hormonal Factors

The risk of breast cancer increases with the length of a woman's reproductive phase (10). **Although early menarche was reported among breast cancer patients, early menopause appears to protect against the development of the disease, with artificial menopause from oophorectomy lowering the risk more than early natural menopause** (11). There is no clear association between the risk of breast cancer and menstrual irregularity or the duration of menses. **Although lactation does not affect the incidence of breast cancer, women who were never pregnant have a higher risk of breast cancer than those who are multiparous.** Women who give birth to their first child later in life have a higher incidence of breast cancer than do younger primigravida women (12).

A historic well-controlled study from the Centers for Disease Control and Prevention showed that oral contraceptive use does not increase the risk of breast cancer, regardless of duration of use, family history, or coexistence of benign breast disease (13). A pooled analysis from 54 epidemiologic studies showed current users of oral contraceptives had a small but significant increased risk when compared with nonusers. Ten years after discontinuation, the risk of past users declined to that of the normal population (14).

It was reported that short-term *estrogen* treatment for menopausal symptoms did not increase the risk of breast cancer, but this belief was refuted by the results of the Women's Health Initiative randomized trial. This prospective trial, involving 16,000 postmenopausal women randomly assigned to receive *estrogen* plus *progesterone* or placebo, revealed an association between hormone therapy use and the development of breast cancer. When invasive breast cancer developed, it was diagnosed at a more advanced stage compared with tumors that developed among placebo users. Based on interim analysis, the trial was stopped early and the **investigators concluded that even relatively short-term use of combined *estrogen–progesterone* therapy increases the development of invasive breast cancer** (15). The risk demonstrated by this study must be considered when postmenopausal hormone therapy is used to treat conditions such as hot flashes and osteoporosis.

History of Cancer

Women with a history of breast cancer have a 50% risk of developing microscopic cancer and a 20% to 25% risk of developing clinically apparent cancer in the contralateral breast, which occurs at a rate of 1% to 2% per year (16). Lobular carcinoma has a higher incidence of bilaterality than does ductal carcinoma. A history of endometrial, ovarian, or colon cancer is associated with an increased risk of subsequent breast cancer, as is a history of radiation therapy for Hodgkin's lymphoma, even if the patient is *BRCA1* and *BRCA2* negative.

Diagnosis

Breast cancer commonly arises in the upper outer quadrant, where there is proportionally more breast tissue. Masses are often discovered by the patient and less frequently by the physician during routine breast examination. The increasing use of screening mammography has enhanced the ability to detect nonpalpable breast abnormalities. Metastatic breast cancer is found as an axillary mass without obvious malignancy in less the 1% of cases.

The standard screening modalities of mammography and physical examination are complementary. Approximately **10% to 50% of cancers detected mammographically are not palpable, whereas physical examination detects 10% to 20% of cancers not seen radiographically** (17). The purpose of screening is to detect tumors when they are small (<1 cm) and have the highest potential for surgical cure. Most trials show a 20% to 30% reduction in breast cancer mortality for women age 50 and older who undergo annual screening mammography. Data on screening women younger than 40 years are more controversial. **Results from the Gothenburg screening trial showed a 45% reduction in mortality for women screened between the ages of 40 and 49** (18). **Because of these findings, it is recommended that all women undergo yearly screening mammography starting at age 40, along with clinical breast examination at least every 3 years** (19). Monthly breast self-examination (BSE) is no longer recommended because there is little evidence to show that BSE is superior to heightened breast awareness such that any new symptoms related to the breast in daily activities would be reported promptly when noticed. BSE was not shown to improve survival. Women should be informed about the benefits and limitations of monthly BSE, mainly the risk of a false-positive result. Women who would still prefer to perform BSE should be instructed in the technique and occasionally have their technique reviewed. No other tests, including ultrasonography, computed tomography (CT) scans, sestamibi scans, positron emission tomography (PET) scans, or serum blood markers, have been shown to be effective screening modalities. Screening guidelines recommended by the American College of Radiology and the American Cancer Society are presented in Table 40.1. In 2010, the ACS recommended annual screening mammography and magnetic resonance imaging (MRI) starting at age 30 for women with a known *BRCA* mutation and other high-risk genetic syndromes, women who are untested with a first-degree relative with the *BRCA* mutation and women with an approximately 20% to 25% or greater lifetime risk of breast cancer, or women who have been treated with radiation for Hodgkin's lymphoma (19). Although breast MRI may prove to be advantageous for other women with an elevated risk of breast cancer, there

Table 40.1 Screening Recommendations
Bilateral mammograms
Beginning at age 40 yearly mammograms, which should continue as long as the patient is in good health.
Self-examination
Is an option for women starting in their 20s. Women should be counseled on the benefits and limitation of breast self-examination and should be told to report any changes in their breasts to their health professional right away.
Clinical breast examination
Age 20–40 examination by physician every 3 years, annually if positive history
(May do annually if there is a positive family history)
Age ≥ 40 examination by physician every year
Breast magnetic resonance imaging (MRI)
High risk women (greater than 20% lifetime risk) should undergo MRI and mammography every year
Medium risk women (15%–20% lifetime risk) should talk to their health care professional about the benefits and limitations of adding MRI to their yearly mammographic screening.
Low risk women (less than 15% lifetime risk) are not recommended to undergo additional MRI screening.

From American Cancer Society Screening Guidelines. **Smith RA, Cokkinides V, Brooks D, et al.** Cancer screening in the United States, 2010: a review of current American Cancer Society Guidelines and Issues in Cancer Screening. *CA Cancer J Clin* 2010;60:99–119.

is currently insufficient evidence to make recommendations for women with lower than a 20% lifetime risk of breast cancer (19).

Masses are easier to palpate in older women with fatty breasts than in younger women with dense, nodular breasts. An area of thickening amid normal nodularity may be the only clue to an underlying malignancy. Skin dimpling, nipple retraction, or skin erosion, while obvious, are later-stage disease signs. Algorithms for the evaluation of breast masses in premenopausal and postmenopausal women are presented in Chapter 21.

When a dominant breast mass is identified, the presence of a carcinoma must be considered, and biopsy should be performed to establish a tissue diagnosis. About 30% to 40% of lesions clinically believed to be malignant will be benign on histologic examination (20). Conversely, 25% of clinically benign-appearing lesions will be malignant when biopsied (21).

Biopsy Techniques

It is preferable for the patient to be involved in planning her therapy. In most instances, initial biopsy can be followed by definitive treatment at a later date. This approach allows the physician to discuss alternative forms of surgical therapy with the patient who has a malignancy. It gives the patient an opportunity to obtain a second opinion before undergoing definitive treatment.

Fine-Needle Aspiration Cytology

Fine-needle aspiration cytology (FNAC) is usually performed on palpable lesions or under ultrasound guidance using a 20- or 22-gauge needle. The technique has a high level of diagnostic accuracy, with low false-negative rates and rare, but persistent, false-positive results (20,22). In most reported series, **false-negative rates range from 10% to 15%, and false-positive rates are generally less than 1%, whereas insufficient specimens account for about 15% of samples** (23). If a mass appears malignant on physical examination, mammography, or both, FNAC cytology results can be used for definitive diagnosis, although in these circumstances a core biopsy is usually the biopsy of choice. Negative FNAC results do not exclude malignancy and should be evaluated by either a core needle or traditional excisional biopsy for suspicious lesions. In younger women, it is prudent to monitor a benign-appearing mass for one or two menstrual cycles. Confirmation of a clinically apparent fibroadenoma with FNAC can serve as the basis for observational follow-up without excision. FNAC may be used in cystic lesions to aspirate fluid, especially in benign-appearing cystic lesions. For benign cysts, cytologic examination is not necessary if the fluid is nonbloody and the cyst resolves after aspiration.

Core Needle Biopsy

Core needle biopsy (CNB) can be performed on both palpable and nonpalpable breast masses. **Performing a core biopsy instead of FNAC on a palpable lesion has the advantage of obtaining more tissue for diagnostic purposes, including tests for estrogen and progesterone receptors and Her-2/*neu*, and has generally replaced FNAC unless aspiration of a cystic mass is being performed. Core biopsy of nonpalpable breast lesions usually is performed using mammographic or ultrasonographic guidance.** MRI-detected lesions that cannot be seen with mammography or ultrasonography may be biopsied under MRI guidance. Mammographic units with computerized stereotactic modifications can be used to localize abnormalities and perform CNB without surgery. **Under imaging guidance, a biopsy needle is inserted into the lesion and a core of tissue is removed for histologic examination.** Devices with suction assistance often are used to increase the volume of tissue removed for evaluation. A titanium clip often is used to mark the biopsy site and serve as a guide should further excision be required. Ultrasonography may be used to perform core biopsy on a nonpalpable lesion. Because it is less invasive and less expensive than open mammographic localization biopsy, CNB is preferred for accessible lesions. If a definitive diagnosis is not established, these procedures must be followed by open biopsy.

Open Biopsy

Open biopsy may be performed if the lesion cannot be successfully biopsied with a needle, or if FNAC or CNB has shown a lesion that may be associated with malignancy, such as atypical ductal hyperplasia (ADH) or lobular carcinoma *in situ* (LCIS). Excision must be performed if the results with needle biopsy are equivocal or discordant with the clinical findings. **An unequivocal histologic diagnosis of cancer should be obtained before treatment of breast cancer is undertaken.** Cytologic diagnosis may be relied on if the mass clinically or mammographically appears to be malignant.

Open biopsy can be performed in the outpatient setting with local anesthesia in the following manner (although this technique largely is replaced by core biopsy and usually is not necessary):

1. The patient is positioned and the location of the mass confirmed.
2. Local anesthesia is used to infiltrate the skin and subcutaneous tissue surrounding the palpable mass.
3. The skin in incised directly over the mass. Placement of this incision is critical. It should be situated in such a way that it can be excised with an ellipse of skin should the patient require a subsequent mastectomy, or placed cosmetically so that partial mastectomy can be performed successfully through it. Para-areolar incisions are appropriate only for lesions in proximity to the nipple–areolar complex.
4. The mass is gently grasped with Allis forceps or with a stay suture and moved into the operative field.
5. The mass should be excised completely whenever possible. Larger lesions that are difficult to totally excise can be incised for diagnostic purposes only. When an incisional biopsy is performed, a frozen section should be obtained to confirm that appropriate tissue for diagnosis is present. Such masses are preferably sampled with FNAC or CNB, with incisional biopsy rarely, if ever, indicated.
6. Once the mass is removed, hemostasis is achieved and the incision is closed. A cosmetically superior result will be achieved if the deep breast parenchyma is not reapproximated. The most superficial subcutaneous fat can be reapproximated with fine absorbable sutures, and the skin can be closed with a subcuticular suture and adhesive strips.

Image-Guided Localization Biopsy

Biopsy of nonpalpable lesions is a potentially difficult procedure that requires close cooperation between the surgeon and radiologist. Using ultrasonographic, mammographic, or MRI guidance, a needle or specialized wire is placed into the breast parenchyma at or near

the site of the suspected abnormality. Some mammographers will inject a biologic dye into the breast parenchyma to assist localization. The surgeon reviews the films and localizes the abnormality with respect to the tip of the wire or needle. Alternatively, the surgeon will perform ultrasonography intraoperatively to directly localize the lesion. An incision is made directly over the abnormality, and a small portion of the breast tissue suspected of containing the abnormality is excised. For mammographically detected lesions, a specimen radiograph is obtained to ensure that the abnormality has been recovered. Often, the radiologist can place a needle in the specimen at the site of the abnormality to facilitate histologic evaluation and ensure that the pathologist examines the site of the abnormality. Image-guided biopsy should be performed only for lesions inaccessible to needle biopsy or those lesions that may be associated with malignancy such as ADH.

Pathology and Natural History

Breast cancer may arise in the intermediate-size ducts, terminal ducts, or lobules. In most cases, the diagnosis of lobular and intraductal carcinoma is based more on histologic appearance than site of origin. The cancer may be either *in situ* (ductal carcinoma *in situ* or lobular carcinoma *in situ*) or invasive (infiltrating ductal carcinoma, infiltrating lobular carcinoma). Morphologic subtypes of infiltrating ductal carcinoma include scirrhous, tubular, medullary, and mucinous carcinoma.

True invasive ductal carcinoma accounts for 80% of all invasive tumors, with the final 20% split evenly between lobular carcinoma and special variants of infiltrating ductal carcinoma (24). Mammographically, invasive ductal cancers are characterized by a stellate density or microcalcifications. Macroscopically, gritty, chalky streaks are present within the tumor that most likely represent a desmoplastic response. Invasion of the surrounding stroma and fat, with a fibrotic, desmoplastic reaction surrounding the invasive carcinoma, generally is present.

Special types of infiltrating ductal carcinoma are uncommon and typically account for nearly 10% of all invasive cancers. Medullary carcinoma, which accounts for 5% to 8% of breast carcinomas, arises from larger ducts within the breast and has a dense lymphocytic infiltrate. The tumor appears to be a slower growing and less-aggressive malignancy than other forms of carcinoma. Even when axillary disease is present, the prognosis with medullary carcinoma is better than that of other variants of invasive ductal carcinoma. **Mucinous (colloid) carcinoma accounts for 5% of all breast cancers.** Grossly, areas of the tumor may appear mucinous or gelatinous, whereas microscopically they are relatively acellular. Infiltrating comedo carcinoma accounts for less than 1% of all breast malignancies and is an invasive cancer characterized by foci of necrosis that exude a comedonecrosis-like substance when biopsied. Usually, comedo-carcinomas are *in situ* malignancies. Papillary carcinoma is predominantly a noninvasive ductal carcinoma; when invasive components are present, it should be specified as invasive papillary carcinoma. **Tubular carcinoma, a well-differentiated breast cancer that accounts for 1% to 2% of all malignant breast neoplasms,** rarely metastasizes to axillary lymph nodes and tends to have a better prognosis than infiltrating ductal carcinoma. **Adenoid cystic carcinomas are extremely rare breast tumors that histologically are similar to those seen in the salivary glands.** They are well-differentiated cancers that are slow to metastasize.

Growth Patterns

The growth potential of breast cancer and the patient's resistance to malignancy vary widely with the individual and the stage of disease. **The doubling time of breast cancer ranges from several weeks for rapidly growing tumors to months or years for slowly growing lesions.** If the doubling time of a breast tumor were constant and a tumor originated from one cell, a doubling time of 100 days would result in a 1-cm tumor in about 8 years (Fig. 40.1) (25). During the preclinical phase, tumor cells may be circulating throughout the body. Because of the long preclinical tumor growth phase and the tendency of infiltrating lesions to metastasize early, many clinicians view breast cancer as a systemic disease at the time of diagnosis. Although cancer cells may be released from the tumor before diagnosis, variations in the tumor's ability to grow in other organs and the host's response to tumor cells may inhibit dissemination of the disease. Many women with breast cancer can be treated successfully with surgery alone, and some patients have been cured even in the presence of palpable axillary disease. A pessimistic attitude that breast cancer is systemic and incurable at diagnosis is unwarranted.

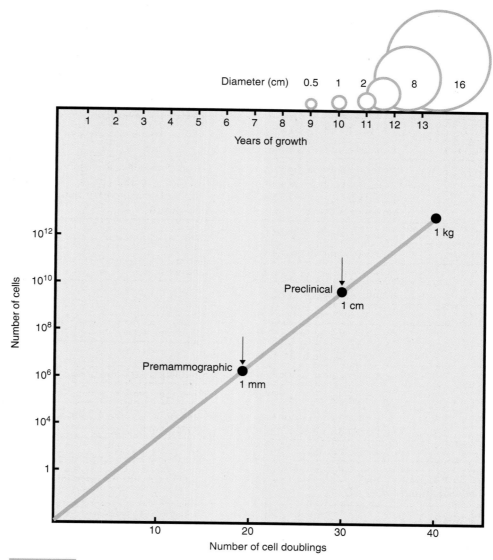

Figure 40.1   Growth rate of breast cancer indicating long preclinical phase. (From **Gullino PM.** Natural history of breast cancer: progression from hyperplasia to neoplasia as predicted by angiogenesis. *Cancer* 1977;39:2699.)

A more realistic approach may be to view breast cancer as a two-component disease involving the breast and the body as a whole. Although the primary breast tumor and issues of local control must be managed, the possibility of systemic metastases with their life-threatening consequences should not be overlooked.

Breast cancer can metastasize to any organ, and involvement of bone, lungs, or liver occurs in up to 85% of women who develop distant disease (26,27). In addition to these sites, invasive lobular carcinoma is known to disseminate to the abdominal viscera, uterus, ovaries, and peritoneal surfaces.

Staging

After the diagnosis of breast cancer is definitively established, the clinical stage of the disease should be determined. The Columbia Clinical Staging System was used historically but is replaced by the tumor-node-metastases (TNM) system of the American Joint Committee on Cancer (28,29). The TNM system allows both preoperative clinical staging and postoperative pathologic staging to be determined (Tables 40.2 and 40.3).

Table 40.2 Tumor-Node-Metastasis (TNM) System for Staging of Breast Cancer

Primary Tumor (T)

TX	Primary tumor cannot be assessed
T_0	No evidence of primary tumor
Tis	Carcinoma *in situ*
Tis (DCIS)	Ductal carcinoma *in situ*
Tis (LCIS)	Lobular carcinoma *in situ*
Tis (Paget's)	Paget's disease of the nipple NOT associated with invasive carcinoma and/or carcinoma *in situ* (DCIS and/or LCIS) in the underlying breast parenchyma. Carcinomas in the breast parenchyma associated with Paget's disease are categorized based on the size and characteristics of the parenchymal disease, although the presence of Paget's disease should still be noted.
T_1	Tumor ≤20 mm in greatest dimension
T_{1mi}	Tumor ≤1 mm in greatest dimension
T_{1a}	Tumor >1 mm but ≤5 mm in greatest dimension
T_{1b}	Tumor >5 mm but ≤10 mm in greatest dimension
T_{1c}	Tumor >10 mm but ≤20 mm in greatest dimension
T_2	Tumor >20 mm but ≤50 mm in greatest dimension
T_3	Tumor >50 mm in greatest dimension
T_4	Tumor of any size with direct extension to chest wall and/or skin (ulceration or skin nodules)
T_{4a}	Extension to chest wall, not including only pectoralis muscle adherence/invasion
T_{4b}	Ulceration and/or ipsilateral satellite nodules and/or edema (including peau d'orange) of the skin which do not meet the criteria for inflammatory carcinoma
T_{4c}	Both T_{4a} and T_{4b}
T_{4d}	Inflammatory carcinoma

Regional Lymph Nodes (N)

Clinical

N X	Regional lymph nodes cannot be assessed (e.g., previously removed)
N_0	No regional lymph node metastasis
N_1	Metastases to movable ipsilateral level I, II axillary lymph node(s)
N_2	Metastases in ipsilateral level I, II axillary lymph node(s) that are clinically fixed or matted, or in clinically detected ipsilateral internal mammary nodes in the absence of clinically evident axillary lymph node metastases
N_{2a}	Metastases in ipsilateral level I, II axillary lymph nodes fixed to one another (matted) or to other structures
N_{2b}	Metastases only in clinically detected ipsilateral internal mammary nodes and in the absence of clinically evident level I, II axillary lymph node metastases
N_3	Metastases in ipsilateral infraclavicular (level III axillary) lymph node(s) with or without level I, II axillary lymph node involvement; or in clinically detected ipsilateral internal mammary lymph nodes and with clinically evident level I, II axillary lymph node metastases; or metastases in ipsilateral supraclavicular lymph node(s) with or without axillary or internal mammary lymph node involvement
N_{3a}	Metastases in ipsilateral infraclavicular lymph node(s)
N_{3b}	Metastases in ipsilateral internal mammary lymph node(s) and axillary lymph node(s)
N_{3c}	Metastases in ipsilateral supraclavicular lymph node(s)

(Continued)

Table 40.2 *Continued*

Pathologic classification (pN)

pN$_X$	Regional lymph nodes cannot be assessed (e.g., previously removed or not removed for pathologic study)
pN$_0$	No regional lymph node metastasis identified histologically
pN$_{0(i-)}$	No regional lymph node metastases histologically, negative IHC
pN$_{0(i+)}$	Malignant cells in regional lymph node(s) no greater than 0.2 mm (detected by H&E or IHC including ITC)
pN$_{0(mol-)}$	No regional lymph node metastases histologically, negative molecular findings (RT-PCR)
pN$_{0(mol+)}$	Positive molecular findings (RT-PCR), but no regional lymph node metastases detected by histology or IHC
pN$_1$	Micrometastases; or metastases in 1 to 3 axillary lymph nodes; and/or in internal mammary nodes with metastases detected by sentinel lymph node biopsy but not clinically detected
pN$_{1mi}$	Micrometastasis (>0.2 mm and/or more than 200 cells, but none >2.0 mm)
pN$_{1a}$	Metastases in 1 to 3 axillary lymph nodes, at least one metastasis >2.0 mm
pN$_{1b}$	Metastases in internal mammary nodes with micrometastases or macrometastases detected by sentinel lymph node biopsy but not clinically apparent
pN$_{1c}$	Metastases in 1 to 3 axillary lymph nodes, and in internal mammary lymph nodes with micrometastases or macrometastases detected by sentinel lymph node biopsy but not clinically detected
pN$_2$	Metastases in 4 to 9 axillary lymph nodes; or in clinically detected internal mammary lymph nodes in the absence of axillary lymph node metastases
pN$_{2a}$	Metastases in 4 to 9 axillary lymph nodes (at least one tumor deposit >2.0 mm)
pN$_{2b}$	Metastases in clinically detected internal mammary lymph nodes in the absence of axillary lymph node metastases
pN$_3$	Metastases in ten or more axillary lymph nodes; or in infraclavicular (level III axillary) lymph nodes; or in clinically detected ipsilateral internal mammary lymph nodes in the presence of one or more positive level I, II axillary lymph nodes; or in more than three axillary lymph nodes and in internal mammary lymph nodes with micrometastases or macrometastases detected by sentinel lymph node biopsy but not clinically detected; or in ipsilateral supraclavicular lymph nodes
pN$_{3a}$	Metastases in ten or more axillary lymph nodes (at least one tumor deposit greater than 2.0 mm); or metastasis to the infraclavicular (level III axillary lymph) nodes
pN$_{3b}$	Metastases in clinically detected ipsilateral internal mammary nodes in the presence of one or more positive axillary lymph nodes; or in more than three axillary lymph nodes and in internal mammary lymph nodes with micrometastases or macrometastases detected by sentinel lymph node biopsy but not clinically detected
pN$_{3c}$	Metastases in ipsilateral supraclavicular node(s)

Distant metastasis (M)

M$_0$	No clinical or radiologic evidence of distant metastasis
cM$_{0(i+)}$	No clinical or radiographic evidence of distant metastases, but deposits of molecularly or microscopically detected tumor cells in circulating blood, bone marrow, or other nonregional nodal tissue that are no larger than 0.2 mm in a patient without symptoms or signs of metastases
M$_1$	Distant detectable metastases as determined by classic clinical and radiographic means and/or histologically proven larger than 0.2 mm

From **Edge SB, Byrd DB, Compton CC, et al., eds.** Breast. In *AJCC cancer staging manual.* 7th ed. New York: Springer, 2010:419–460, with permission.

Table 40.3 Staging of Breast Carcinoma Anatomic Stage/Prognostic Groups			
	TNM Classification		
	Tumor	*Node*	*Metastasis*
Stage 0	Tis	N_0	M_0
Stage IA	T_1*	N_0	M_0
Stage IB	T_0	N_{1mi}	M_0
	T_1*	N_{1mi}	M_0
Stage IIA	T_0	N_1**	M_0
	T_1*	N_1**	M_0
	T_2	N_0	M_0
IIB	T_2	N_1	M_0
	T_3	N_0	M_0
Stage IIIA	T_0	N_2	M_0
	T_1*	N_2	M_0
	T_2	N_2	M_0
	T_3	N_1	M_0
	T_3	N_2	M_0
IIIB	T_4	N_0	M_0
	T_4	N_1	M_0
	T_4	N_2	M_0
IIIC	Any T	N_3	M_0
Stage IV	Any T	Any N	M_1

*T_1 includes T_{1mi}
**T_0 and T_1 tumors with nodal micrometastases only are excluded from stage IIA and are classified stage IB.
From **Edge SB, Byrd DB, Compton CC, et al., eds.** Breast. In *AJCC cancer staging manual*. 7th ed. New York: Springer, 2010:419–460, with permission.

Treatment

Preoperative Evaluation

The extent of the preoperative workup varies with the initial stage of the disease (30). For most patients with small tumors, clinically negative lymph nodes, and no evidence of metastasis (TNM stage I), the preoperative evaluation should consist of bilateral mammography, chest radiography, complete blood count, and screening blood chemistry tests. Bone, CT, and MRI scanning are unnecessary unless there are symptoms or abnormal blood chemistry levels to suggest the existence of bone or intra-abdominal involvement. For patients with clinical stage II, node-positive disease, a bone scan is recommended, but CT scan of the abdomen is not necessary unless symptoms or laboratory results suggest liver disease. Patients with clinical stage III or stage IV disease should undergo both bone and liver scanning. PET scanning is becoming a popular means of total body scanning for breast cancer, but there have been concerns that this modality may miss some bony metastasis. A study found that PET scan is highly concordant (81%) with bone scan in a study of 132 paired studies of breast cancer patients (31). Of 31 (19%) discordant pairs, 12 patients had pathology proven metastatic disease. Nine of these 12 patients had a positive PET scan but negative bone scan, supporting the use of PET scan in detecting osseous metastasis in breast cancer, although further studies are needed to ascertain whether this modality should supplant the use of bone scan in this setting.

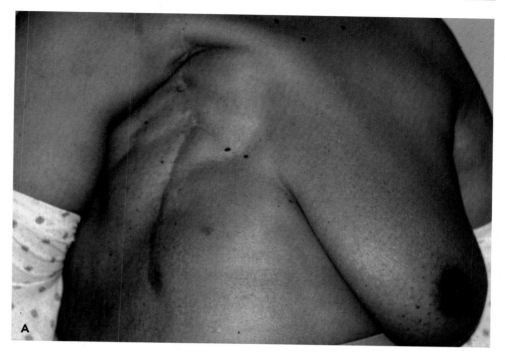

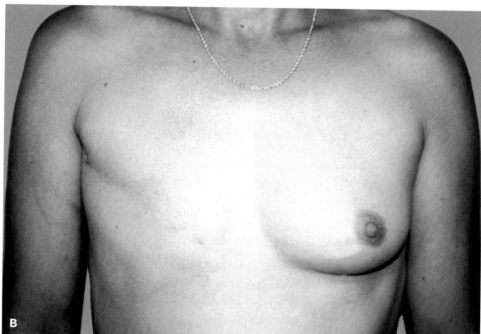

Figure 40.2   Appearance of breast after radical mastectomy (A) versus modified mastectomy (B). (From **Kruper L, Giuliano AE.** Breast disease. In: **Berek JS, Hacker NF.** *Berek & Hacker's Gynecologic Oncology.* 5th ed. Philadelphia, PA: Lippincott Williams & Wilkins, 2010:636.)

Radical Mastectomy

Traditionally, the treatment of breast cancer has been surgical, but the type of procedure has remained a controversial and highly emotional issue. During the 19th century, surgical treatment of breast cancer was haphazard, varying from local excision alone to total mastectomy. The radical mastectomy was based on the principle that breast carcinoma was a locally infiltrative process that spread in a stepwise fashion from breast, to nodes, to distant sites (32). Thus, **radical mastectomy removes the entire breast, the underlying pectoral muscles, and the contiguous axillary lymph nodes in continuity** (33) (Fig. 40.2A). A report of 51 years of experience with radical mastectomy, which included 1,036 patients with a follow-up of 47 years, is unequaled in evaluating any single method of treating breast cancer (34).

During the 20th century, extensions and modifications of the radical mastectomy were devised that involved removal of more local and regional tissue. At one time, supraclavicular lymph node dissections were considered a routine component of surgical treatment (35). Supraclavicular, mediastinal, and internal mammary lymph node dissections were performed (36).

An *en bloc* internal mammary lymph node dissection was added to the standard radical mastectomy in the 1960s (37). This technique became popular and is the operation commonly referred to as the *extended radical mastectomy*. Extended radical mastectomy did not enhance overall survival rates, because only 3% to 5% of patients with negative axillary nodes will have involvement of internal mammary nodes (38). Locally destructive surgery is not justified, based on current understanding of the biologic behavior of breast cancer. Radical mastectomy is no longer an indicated procedure, except in the most unusual circumstances, with extensive pectoralis involvement by direct tumor extension.

Modified Radical Mastectomy

In contrast to radical mastectomy, modified radical mastectomy preserves the pectoralis major muscle (39,40) (Fig. 40.2B). The breast is removed in a manner similar to that of radical mastectomy, but neither the axillary lymph node dissection nor the skin excision is as extensive. Consequently, there is no need for skin grafting. There are no differences in survival rates between radical and modified radical mastectomy, but the latter procedure has a better functional outcome and a superior cosmetic result (41). Modified radical mastectomy has replaced radical mastectomy in the United States and is an alternative to breast conserving surgery and axillary dissection for some patients.

Total Mastectomy

Total mastectomy involves removal of the entire breast, nipple, and areolar complex without resection of the underlying muscles or intentional excision of axillary lymph nodes. Low-lying lymph nodes in the upper outer portion of the breast and low axilla often are excised. Total mastectomy has local control rates comparable with those of radical or modified radical mastectomy but has a higher risk of axillary recurrence. In the past, regional recurrence would occur in at least 15% to 20% of patients treated with total mastectomy alone. With the addition of sentinel lymph node biopsy, which selects patients who are lymph node negative, local recurrence rates should be lowered in patients with total mastectomy and node negative disease compared to those in the past with unknown axillary status.

Skin-Sparing and Nipple-Sparing Mastectomy

More patients have early small cancers and others are undergoing prophylactic mastectomy for genetic mutations and for other high-risk lesions. Patients may elect to undergo a skin-sparing mastectomy (SSM) with nipple–areolar complex (NAC) removal that leaves a skin envelope to accommodate the breast reconstruction, as well as providing a nipple-sparing mastectomy (NSM) with preservation of the NAC. Both of these procedures are being studied for their potential utility and safety in various clinical situations. Retrospective series show that performing NSM does not impact survival, although a prospective randomized trial has not been performed (42).

Postmastectomy Radiation Therapy

McWhirter developed the combination of total mastectomy followed by radiation (43). Many advocated adjuvant radiation therapy used in combination with various operative procedures. Studies claiming improvements in overall survival usually are flawed by the use of historical controls and inaccurate preoperative staging. Classic trials, both prospective randomized and historical control studies, showed that adjuvant radiation therapy improves local control but not overall survival rates (44–47). In a prospective randomized trial performed by the National Surgical Adjuvant Breast Project (NSABP), the roles of postoperative radiation therapy and axillary treatment were examined. Patients were randomly assigned to either total mastectomy, radical mastectomy, or total mastectomy with radiation therapy. This trial showed no difference in survival among the three treatment arms, whereas radiation therapy and axillary treatment improved local and regional control. Twenty-five-year follow-up data continue to support these conclusions (48).

Three randomized control studies from the 1990s showed that postmastectomy radiation therapy reduced the risk of local–regional failure by 20% and produced an absolute sur-

vival benefit of 10% at 10 years among women with stage II to III breast cancer, regardless of menopausal status (49–51). Additional trials challenged the need for postmastectomy radiation among women with only one to three involved axillary nodes and T_1 or T_2 primary tumors. These studies showed adequate local–regional control rates with mastectomy and chemotherapy alone (52–54). In a large meta-analysis, an absolute risk reduction in local recurrence was found in women with radiation therapy after both breast conservation and mastectomy. One breast cancer death is avoided for every four local recurrences, reducing the 15-year mortality among patients with a greater than 10% risk of local recurrence (55). **Guidelines from the American Society of Clinical Oncology recommend postmastectomy radiation therapy for women with T_3 (>5 cm) primary tumors and four or more positive axillary lymph nodes** (56).

Breast Conservation Therapy with or without Radiation Therapy

Radiation therapy alone, without excision of the tumor, is associated with a high local failure rate, as is local excision without radiation (57–60). Throughout the last quarter of the 20th century, a paradigm shift occurred in the surgical management of breast cancer. Data from the NSABP B-04 trial, for which 25-year follow-up exists, established the equivalency of radical versus total mastectomy with regard to overall survival. Shortly after initiation of the B-04 trial, a number of studies were designed to evaluate the efficacy of breast preservation among women with early-stage breast cancers. **The Milan trial, a major prospective randomized trial that began accruing patients in 1973, compared treatment with either radical mastectomy or a combination of quadrantectomy, axillary lymph node dissection, and postoperative radiation therapy.** In total, 701 clinically node-negative patients with noncentrally located, small tumors (<2 cm) ($T_1 N_0 M_0$) were enrolled. **After 25 years of follow-up, there continues to be no statistically significant difference between the two groups in either local control or overall survival rates** (61).

At nearly the same time, in the **NSABP B-06 trial, patients with early breast cancer (stage I or stage II, T_1 or T_2, and N_0 or N_1) were randomized to modified radical mastectomy, segmental mastectomy (lumpectomy) and axillary lymph node dissection, or segmental mastectomy, axillary lymph node dissection and postoperative radiation therapy.** Unlike the quadrantectomy performed in the Milan study, segmental mastectomy consists of removing only the tumor and a small rim of normal surrounding tissue, yielding cosmetically superior results (Fig. 40.3). A total of 1,843 women were enrolled, with the lowest local recurrence rate

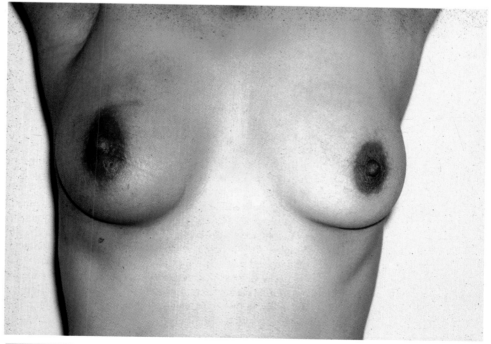

Figure 40.3 **Appearance of breast after lumpectomy, axillary dissection, and radiation therapy.** (From **Kruper L, Giuliano AE.** Breast disease. In: **Berek JS, Hacker NF.** *Berek & Hacker's Gynecologic Oncology.* 5th ed. Philadelphia, PA: Williams & Wilkins, 2010:638.)

seen among patients treated with segmental mastectomy and postoperative radiation therapy. The addition of radiation improved the local control rate, but no significant differences in overall survival or disease-free survival rates were detected among the three treatment arms; there was a trend, however, in favor of patients who had received radiation. **This NSABP study established, now with 25-year follow-up, that the combination of segmental mastectomy (with negative surgical margins), axillary lymph node dissection, and postoperative radiation therapy is as effective as modified radical mastectomy for the management of patients with stages I and II breast cancer** (62). A number of additional prospective randomized studies also demonstrated no decrease in overall survival among women being treated with breast preservation therapy (63–65).

Axillary lymph node status and the number of involved nodes are the most important prognostic indicators for patients with primary breast cancer (66). Axillary lymphadenectomy traditionally was used to detect and quantify the extent of nodal metastasis (67). Before the introduction of sentinel lymph node dissection in the 1990s, axillary lymph node dissection was performed routinely on all patients with early breast cancer. Although axillary dissection is associated with a very low risk of regional recurrence (1% to 3%), the rate of acute complications is as high as 30% (68). Similarly, the risk of chronic lymphedema ranges from 6% to as high 30% (69). Limiting the dissection to level I nodes or random sampling is associated with unacceptably high false-negative rates and should not be done (70). Only one-third of patients with a clinically negative axilla will have nodal metastasis after histopathologic examination of all harvested lymph nodes (71). This means that two-thirds of patients will be exposed to the morbidity of axillary lymph node dissection without proven benefit when performed routinely in the presence of invasive breast cancer.

In 1991 intraoperative lymphatic mapping and sentinel lymph node dissection were introduced to address these problems (72). The concept behind sentinel lymph node dissection is best described by the definition of a sentinel node. The sentinel node is the lymph node that has the greatest potential to harbor metastasis if axillary disease is present. Examination of the sentinel lymph node dissection can accurately predict the status of the entire nodal basin. Removing only one or two lymph nodes can accurately stage the axilla with minimal morbidity. Numerous investigators have demonstrated that, with proper training, sentinel lymph node dissection identification rates range from 90% to 99%, with false-negative rates of less than 5% found in most large studies (73). **In one study of 107 patients with T$_1$ and T$_2$ breast cancer who underwent sentinel lymph node dissection followed by axillary lymph node dissection, the sentinel node was successfully identified in 100 patients (93.5%)** (73). **There were no false-negative results, and the sentinel node accurately predicted axillary status in all 100 patients.**

The technique of sentinel lymph node dissection is validated by a number of authors using a variety of techniques (74,75). The information obtained from sentinel lymph node dissection appears to be equivalent to that of axillary lymph node dissection. One prospective study demonstrated that in node-negative patients undergoing only sentinel lymph node dissection, the recurrence rate in the axilla was zero at a median follow-up of 39 months (76). Overall survival for patients who undergo sentinel lymph node dissection without axillary dissection appears to be excellent. In a randomized controlled trial, Veronesi et al. showed that the long-term breast cancer–related event-free survival among patients in the sentinel node biopsy arm (89.9%) was similar to that in the axillary lymph node dissection arm (88.8%), affirming not only that sentinel lymph node biopsy is as good as complete axillary dissection at staging the axilla, but that it is as safe as the once standard method of complete axillary dissection (77). Sentinel node biopsy alone without complete axillary lymph node dissection may have value in patients with micrometastatic and macrometastatic disease given low recurrence rates after sentinel lymph node biopsy. In a randomized controlled trial, in patients with hematoxylin and eosin (H&E) positive sentinel lymph nodes, there was no statistically significant difference in overall survival between patients randomized to complete axillary lymph node dissection and sentinel lymph node biopsy alone (78). **The degree of accuracy in predicting axillary metastasis, combined with its very low morbidity rate, makes sentinel lymph node dissection the preferred procedure for staging the axilla in breast cancer.**

Adjuvant Systemic Therapy

For many patients, local and regional control of breast cancer is achieved with a combination of surgery and radiation therapy. About 90% of patients will never experience an in-breast recurrence; these patients may develop metastatic disease. The goal of adjuvant systemic therapy is to eliminate occult metastases during the early postoperative period and thus reduce the risk of local and distant recurrence (79).

Adjuvant systemic therapy will prolong survival in selected breast cancer patients. In patients with favorable tumors and a low risk of recurrence and subsequent death, such as those with node-negative cancers smaller than 1 cm and favorable biology, this benefit is small and may not justify the risks of systemic therapy. **Adjuvant systemic therapy reduces the odds of death by 25% per year in both node-negative and node-positive patients** (80). Because this risk reduction is relatively constant, patients with favorable, node-negative disease have a much smaller absolute benefit compared with patients who have higher-risk, node-positive disease and/or patients with unfavorable biologic markers such as patients with triple negative disease or Her-2/*neu* positive disease. For patients with node-negative disease, the absolute benefit may be minimal versus 10% to 20% for those with nodal involvement.

Cytotoxic chemotherapy and hormonal therapy have inherent risks that must be considered when treatment decisions are made. There are many known acute side effects with standard regimens, and there is growing evidence that patients who undergo chemotherapy report more frequent chronic neurocognitive deficits than do untreated controls (81). The impact of these deficits remains undefined. Systemic therapy with *tamoxifen* is associated with an increased incidence of uterine cancer, vaginal dryness, and hot flashes, whereas aromatase inhibitors are linked to osteoporosis and musculoskeletal symptoms. Choosing those patients who should receive adjuvant therapy can be a difficult decision that often entails analyzing a variety of prognostic and predictive factors, identifying patients at risk for recurrence, and quantifying that risk. **Based on available data, adjuvant chemotherapy is recommended for women with greater than a 10% chance of relapse within 10 years.** The choice of therapy depends on an evaluation of specific risk factors. Two multigene assays such as the Oncotype DX and the Mammaprint have been introduced to help identify those estrogen receptor–positive, lymph node–negative patients who will benefit most from systemic chemotherapy. These tests, which calculate a recurrence risk score for each individual based on a 21-gene assay and 70-gene signature, respectively, allow the treating physician to determine the average rate of distant disease at 10 years and make treatment recommendations based on this risk (82).

Prognostic Indicators

Factors that determine each patient's risk of recurrence include nodal involvement, tumor size, estrogen and progesterone receptor status, nuclear grade, histologic type, proliferative rate, and biologic markers such as Her-2/*neu* status. These prognostic factors and their effects on recurrence are summarized in Table 40.4. Patients with high-risk prognostic factors are more likely to benefit from adjuvant cytotoxic or hormonal therapy and usually are offered such treatment.

Table 40.4 Prognostic Factors in Node-Negative Breast Carcinoma

Factor	Increased Risk of Recurrence	Decreased Risk of Recurrence
Size	T_3, T_2	T_1, T_0
Hormone receptors	Negative	Positive
DNA flow cytometry	Aneuploid tumors	Diploid
Histologic grade	High	Low
Tumor labeling index	<3%	>3%
S phase fraction	>5%	<5%
Lymphatic or vascular invasion	Present	Absent
Cathepsin D	High	Low
HER-2/*neu* oncogene	High	Low
Epidermal growth factor receptor	High	Low

From **Giuliano AE, Hurvitz SA.** Breast Disorders. In: **McPhee SJ, Papadakis MA, eds.** 2011 *current medical diagnosis and treatment.* New York: McGraw Hill, 2011;710, with permission.

Table 40.5 Year Survival According to Stage of Breast Cancer		
AJCC Stage	*5-Year Survival (%)*	*10-Year Survival (%)*
Stage 0	95	90
Stage I	85	70
Stage IIA	70	50
IIB	60	40
Stage IIIA	55	30
IIIB	30	20
Stage IV	5—10	2
All	65	30

AJCC, American Joint Committee on Cancer.
From **Giuliano AE, Hurvitz SA.** Breast disorders. In: **McPhee SJ, Papadakis MA, eds.** 2011 *current medical diagnosis and treatment.* New York: McGraw Hill, 2011;716, with permission.

Patients with lymph node metastasis have a higher risk of recurrence than patients with node-negative disease. The 10-year survival rate for women with palpable metastatic axillary lymph nodes who fail to receive systemic therapy is about 50% to 60%. The number of lymph nodes involved and the presence of extracapsular invasion are important indicators of poor prognosis.

Another prognostic indicator of relapse is primary tumor size. In an evaluation of 767 patients with node-negative disease who underwent radical or modified radical mastectomy without adjuvant chemotherapy, the relapse rate in patients with tumors larger than 1 cm or special tumor types larger than 3 cm (tubular, mucinous, or papillary) was 27% at 10 years, compared with 9% for tumors smaller than 1 cm (83).

Hormone receptor status is an important predictor not only of long-term prognosis but also of response to endocrine therapy. Several studies demonstrated that patients with positive estrogen and progesterone receptor status have **improved overall survival** (84,85). Receptor status should be known when determining the need for and choice of adjuvant therapy. Histologic grade appears to predict overall survival. Patients with well-differentiated tumors tend to have more favorable outcomes than those with poorly differentiated ones (Table 40.5). In a British study of 1,168 women, histologic grade, along with tumor size and lymph node status, was an independent predictor of overall survival at 10 years (86).

Two multigene assays were rapidly developed and are commercially available including the 21-gene assay (Oncotype DX) and the 70-gene signature (Mammaprint). Oncotype DX was developed for identifying patients who have a high risk of recurrence distantly and for patients with node negative ER+ breast cancer. Large-scale phase III trials are under way in the United States and in Europe to test the clinical utility of these multigene assays, which will assist in determining the use of adjuvant systemic therapy.

The possible roles of specific tumor markers in predicting which patients will respond to chemotherapy regimens were investigated. The most thoroughly researched of these markers is HER-2/*neu*. In an NSABP study, patients with HER-2/*neu* overexpression who were not treated with *anthracycline*-based regimens fared worse (87). Another study showed that the addition of *trastuzumab* (*Herceptin*), an antibody directed against the HER-2/*neu* receptor, significantly increased the response rate to therapy over standard chemotherapy alone in the presence of metastatic disease (88). **Reports from trials investigating the adjuvant use of *trastuzumab* for women with early-stage Her-2/*neu* breast cancers show significant improvements in disease-free survival for women receiving *trastuzumab; trastuzumab* is used as systemic adjuvant therapy for patients with Her-2/*neu* positive breast cancer, and the standard length of treatment is one full year (89–91).**

Systemic Regimens

Based on the results of more than 100 prospective, randomized trials examining the role of adjuvant chemotherapy in breast cancer, a variety of systemic regimens emerged. Systemic therapy includes cytotoxic agents and hormonal agents, used alone or in combination. Following is a brief description of the more commonly used regimens. Initially, trials involved a single perioperative course of chemotherapy aimed at eradicating circulating tumor cells. The Nissen-Meyer study from Norway showed that a single course of *cyclophosphamide* improved overall survival rates (92). Numerous trials demonstrated the benefit of adjuvant chemotherapy for certain subgroups of patients (93). In the initial NSABP adjuvant trial, a 2-year course of *melphalan* was superior to no treatment, and further trials demonstrated enhanced beneficial effect with the use of multiple drugs as well as with the combination of hormonal manipulation with chemotherapy (94,95).

Historically, the most frequently used adjuvant combination chemotherapy was *CMF: cyclophosphamide (C), methotrexate (M),* and *5-fluorouracil (5-FU)*. In the original study by Bonadonna et al., patients with positive axillary lymph nodes were randomized to receive either 12 monthly cycles of *CMF* or no therapy after radical mastectomy (96). A statistically significant benefit was found with *CMF* treatment for premenopausal patients, especially those with one to three positive nodes. A subsequent study showed six cycles of *CMF* to be as effective as 12 cycles (97). No significant effect was seen for postmenopausal women, which may result from the fact that these women were less likely to tolerate the full course of therapy (98). **After 20 years of follow-up, this trial demonstrated a persistent survival advantage for premenopausal women receiving *CMF* adjuvant therapy (99). In a later study involving node-negative, estrogen receptor–negative breast cancer patients, after 12 years of follow-up, 71% of patients treated with adjuvant *CMF* remained disease free compared with 48% in the control group, regardless of menopausal status (100).**

Anthracylines (A) were more commonly used in the adjuvant and metastatic treatment of breast cancer than any other agents. A large randomized NSABP study compared *CMF* with *AC* regimens in node-positive patients and found similar treatment outcomes among both groups. The *AC* regimen was preferred because of its shorter duration (four cycles for 3 months vs. six cycles for 6 months) and better tolerance (101).

Several landmark trials showed that taxanes such as *paclitaxel* and *docetaxel* in combination with *anthracyclines* have significant efficacy and are the new standard adjuvant therapy for node-positive breast cancer. **The Cancer and Leukemia Group B was the first to show a 17% improvement in the rate of recurrence and 18% reduction in the rate of death with the addition of *paclitaxel* to *cyclophosphamide* (102).** Given concerns over the cardiotoxicity of anthracyclines as well as the 0.21% risk of leukemia after the *AC* regimen at 5 years, a US oncology trial randomized stage I, II, and III patients to *AC* or *docetaxel* and *cyclophosphamide (TC)* every 3 weeks for four cycles and found that after 7 years' follow-up disease-free survival and overall survival statistically favored the *TC* group (103). This was the first trial to compare a *taxane*-based regimen to an *anthracycline*-based regimen. Concerns remain because multiple trials demonstrate that the duration of therapy is significant and the *TC* regimen used was a short-duration treatment of four cycles (104). Until results of an ongoing US oncology trial designed to assess whether an incremental benefit exists for adding an *anthracycline* to *TC*-based therapy for six cycles on a 3-week dosing schedule for Her-2/*neu* negative patients, oncologists will need to decide whether to add *anthracycline* to *taxane*-based chemotherapy guided by their clinical judgment.

Neoadjuvant Systemic Therapy

The use of neoadjuvant chemotherapy traditionally was limited to those individuals with either inoperable locally advanced or inflammatory breast cancers. The goal of preoperative systemic therapy was to convert inoperable patients into resectable candidates on the basis of pathologic and clinical responses (105). Indications for neoadjuvant chemotherapy were broadened to include individuals presenting with large operable tumors and wanting to undergo breast preservation instead of mastectomy. Reports indicate that breast conservation therapy is possible and that low rates of in-breast or local–regional recurrences occur when neoadjuvant chemotherapy results in clinical and pathological tumor downstaging (106). In addition to large, operable tumors, neoadjuvant therapy continues to have a role in the treatment of inflammatory breast cancers and those presenting in a locally advanced state.

Hormonal Therapy

Hormonal manipulation with *tamoxifen* or an aromatase inhibitor, used alone or in combination with a cytotoxic regimen, is beneficial in select groups of women. *Tamoxifen*, an estrogen analogue, offers substantial benefits in both premenopausal and postmenopausal women. Taken at a dose of 20 mg per day for 5 years, *tamoxifen* reduces the annual risk of recurrence by about 50% and the annual risk of death by about 25%. These benefits occur

in women with estrogen receptor–positive disease regardless of chemotherapy treatment (107).

Tamoxifen, **when used in combination with cytotoxic chemotherapy, improves survival in women with positive axillary lymph nodes and tumor estrogen receptor expression** (108). In patients with node-negative, estrogen receptor–positive disease, the addition of *tamoxifen* to chemotherapy improved disease-free survival rates after 5 years of follow-up (109). In NSABP study B-14, 2,644 patients with estrogen receptor–positive tumors and no axillary metastases were randomized to either *tamoxifen* (10 mg orally twice daily for 5 years) or a placebo control. After a 4-year median follow-up, the disease-free survival rate for the 1,318 patients treated with *tamoxifen* was 82% compared with 77% for the 1,326 patients treated with placebo ($p = .00001$), again regardless of menopausal status.

The Early Breast Cancer Trialists' Collaborative Group (EBCTCG) performed a meta-analysis of adjuvant systemic therapy for breast cancer. They analyzed randomized trials involving adjuvant systemic hormonal, cytotoxic, or immune therapy administered to more than 75,000 women with stage I or II carcinoma. **The investigators concluded that for postmenopausal women with estrogen receptor–positive tumors, *tamoxifen* daily for at least 2 years had a significant beneficial effect on disease-free survival rates, with these effects lasting up to 10 years. The incidence of both carcinoma in the contralateral breast and death rate from heart disease decreased.**

In addition to *tamoxifen,* **aromatase inhibitors have been approved for use in the adjuvant treatment of patients with estrogen receptor–positive cancers.** Aromatase inhibitors act by inhibiting the aromatase enzyme, thus blocking the conversion of androgens into estrogens. These drugs should be used only in postmenopausal patients or premenopausal women who have undergone chemical ovarian suppression or oophorectomy. Although aromatase inhibitors cause fewer episodes of thrombotic events, hot flashes, and endometrial cancers, musculoskeletal symptoms and osteoporosis are more commonly encountered among aromatase inhibitor users than those taking *tamoxifen.* Results from the *anastrozole (Arimidex), tamoxifen,* Alone or in Combination (ATAC) trial showed overall lower recurrence rates, as well as fewer contralateral tumors, among women treated with *anastrozole* alone after 68 months of follow-up (110). A meta-analysis confirmed that aromatase inhibitor therapy alone conferred a 2.9% absolute decrease in recurrence; aromatase inhibitor therapy after 2 to 3 years of *tamoxifen* conferred a 3.1% reduction in recurrence, as well as a 0.7% decrease in mortality at 5-year follow-up, although additional long-term follow-up is needed (111). Based on these results, **aromatase inhibitors are now often offered as a first-line treatment option for adjuvant therapy. Research suggests that conversion of patients from** *tamoxifen* **to an aromatase inhibitor, such as** *letrozole (Femara),* **after 2.5 or 5 years may improve survival, although concurrent use of the two agents offers no benefit** (110,112).

General Recommendations

Adjuvant systemic therapy lowers the incidence of recurrence by 25% to 30%. It is important to understand that the proportional reduction in risk of relapse is relatively constant regardless of absolute risk (113). The EBCTCG meta-analysis showed that the risk reduction of recurrence and breast cancer–specific mortality from polychemotherapy occurs in all women, but the most benefit occurs in women under the age of 50 (Table 40.6). A meta-analysis from the EBCTCG assessing the effect of polychemotherapy and *tamoxifen* on estrogen receptor–poor breast cancer found that women under the age of 50 or between the ages of 50 and 69 had statistically significant decreases in 10-year risks of recurrence and mortality, with more benefit in women under the age of 50, confirming the results of the earlier study in patients with estrogen receptor–poor breast cancer (114). Tamoxifen did not add any benefit in patients with estrogen receptor–poor tumors. Adjuvant cytotoxic chemotherapy appears to affect the natural history of patients with either axillary node–negative or node–positive breast cancer. All high-risk patients with node-negative disease are considered candidates for adjuvant cytotoxic therapy.

In postmenopausal, estrogen receptor–positive women, chemotherapy is about one-half as effective as *tamoxifen* **in the adjuvant setting** (115). For most postmenopausal women with hormone-responsive disease (estrogen- and progesterone-responsive positivity), including node-positive patients, hormonal therapy alone may be adequate treatment. High-risk patients with hormone-resistant disease benefit from cytotoxic systemic therapy. Caution should be exercised when using chemotherapeutic agents. Patients in whom the risk of recurrence is low are likely to derive little overall benefit from the use of adjuvant systemic therapy, whereas those with a

Table 40.6 Effect of Systemic Therapy on Recurrence and Survival from Breast Cancer

Age	Therapy	Reduction in Annual Odds of Recurrence	Reduction in Annual Odds of Death
<50	Tamoxifen × 5 yrs	45 ± 8	32 ± 10
50–59	Tamoxifen × 5 yrs	37 ± 6	11 ± 8
60–69	Tamoxifen × 5 yrs	54 ± 5	33 ± 6
<40	Polychemotherapy	37 ± 7	27 ± 8
40–49	Polychemotherapy	34 ± 5	27 ± 5
50–59	Polychemotherapy	22 ± 4	14 ± 4
60–69	Polychemotherapy	18 ± 4	8 ± 4

From **Early Breast Cancer Trialists' Collaborative Group.** Polychemotherapy for early breast cancer: an overview of the randomized trials. *Lancet* 1998;352:930, with permission.

high risk of recurrence are likely to receive the greatest benefit. Comorbidities must always be considered on an individual basis.

The current recommendations for adjuvant systemic therapy in breast cancer are summarized as follows:

1. Premenopausal women with lymph node involvement should be treated with adjuvant combination chemotherapy. *Tamoxifen* should be added for patients with estrogen receptor–positive tumors following cytotoxic therapy.

2. Premenopausal women without evidence of lymph node involvement but with large (>1 cm) size, aneuploid, or estrogen receptor–negative tumors should be treated with combination chemotherapy. *Tamoxifen* should be given to patients with estrogen receptor–positive tumors.

3. Postmenopausal patients with negative lymph nodes who are hormone receptor–positive should receive adjuvant aromatase inhibitor therapy as primary therapy. Those with positive lymph nodes should receive multidrug cytotoxic therapy, or a combination thereof if there are no medical contraindications.

4. Postmenopausal women with lymph node metastases who are hormone receptor–negative may be treated with adjuvant chemotherapy.

5. Adjuvant systemic therapy is not recommended for patients with favorable tumors smaller than 1 cm. Hormonal therapy may be considered if the patient's tumor is estrogen receptor–positive.

6. Trastuzumab is recommended as adjuvant treatment in addition to chemotherapy for patients with Her-2/*neu* positive breast cancer, especially those with positive nodes, young women, and women with large tumors.

Prognosis

The treatment of advanced, metastatic breast cancer is largely palliative. For most physicians, quality-of-life issues are paramount when choosing which type of therapy is offered. In patients with locally advanced disease in conjunction with distant metastasis, palliative radiotherapy may be advised to control pain or avoid pathologic fractures. This approach is best exemplified in the treatment of isolated bone metastases, chest wall recurrences, brain metastases, and spinal cord compression.

Systemic disease may be controlled by hormonal or cytotoxic therapy. Because the quality of life during an endocrine-induced remission is usually superior to one following cytotoxic chemotherapy, it is preferable to try endocrine manipulation first. As many as one-third of patients with disseminated disease respond favorably to either functional end-organ ablation (ovary, pituitary, adrenal glands) or administration of drugs that block hormonal function. For patients with estrogen receptor–positive tumors, this response rate may be as high as 60%.

Because only 5% to 10% of women with estrogen receptor–negative cancers respond to endocrine treatment, they should not routinely receive hormonal therapy except in unusual cases, such as elderly women who are intolerant of cytotoxic therapy (116).

Cytotoxic chemotherapy should be considered for the treatment of metastatic breast cancer if organ involvement is potentially life-threatening (brain, lung, or liver), if hormonal treatment is unsuccessful, if the disease has progressed after an initial response to endocrine manipulation, or if the tumor is estrogen receptor–negative. The most useful single chemotherapeutic agent is an *anthracycline* such as *doxorubicin,* which has an estimated response rate of 40% to 50%. Combination therapy using multiple agents has response rates as high as 60% to 80% (117). Clinical trials, including those investigating the use of *trastuzumab* for Her-2/*neu*-positive women with metastases, are underway to examine a variety of combinations for stage IV disease. In Her-2/*neu*-positive women, the *trastuzumab* and *vinorelbine* or *taxane* (TRAVIOTA) study showed that both regimens were active as first-line treatments for metastatic breast cancer (118). The historically prominent side effects of debilitating nausea and vomiting are well controlled with central-acting antiemetics. The importance of controlling these potentially devastating symptoms cannot be overemphasized.

Bisphosphonates have played an increasing role in the treatment of breast cancer that has metastasized to bone. *Zoledronic acid* (*Zometa*) was found to be superior to *pamidronate* (Aredia) in patients with breast cancer, with a relative risk reduction of skeletal-related events, defined as pathological fracture, spinal cord compression, radiation therapy, or surgery to bone, by an additional 16% (119). A review that compared all oral and intravenous bisphosphonates that were approved for breast cancer treatment in 2005 demonstrated a 41% risk reduction in skeletal related events with *zoledronic acid* versus placebo, compared with a 14% to 23% risk reduction for *ibandronate* (*Boniva*), *clodronate*, and *pamidronate* (120). Bisphosphonates may be important in preventing bone loss during hormone-based therapies for breast cancer. Bisphosphonates garnered interest as a possible adjuvant treatment for breast cancer, with early trials showing a decrease in breast cancer recurrence. Further investigations in randomized, controlled trials, including a trial by the Southwest Oncology Group, are comparing stages I through III breast cancer patients randomized to three different bisphosphonates prescribed after adjuvant systemic antitumor treatment.

Special Breast Cancers

Paget's Disease

In the 1870s, Sir James Paget described a nipple lesion similar to eczema and recognized that this nipple change was associated with an underlying breast malignancy (121). The erosion results from invasion of the nipple and surrounding areola by characteristic large cells with irregular nuclei, now called Paget cells. Although the origin of these cells is much debated by pathologists, they are probably extensions of an underlying carcinoma into the major ducts of the nipple–areolar complex. There may be no visible changes associated with the initial invasion of the nipple. Often, the patient's presenting symptom will be nipple discharge, which is actually a combination of serum and blood from the involved ducts. The patient may have a delay in the diagnosis because the presenting symptoms are overlooked. The diagnosis is established by incisional or punch biopsy of the area of the skin changes.

The overall prognosis for patients with this rare form of breast cancer depends on the stage of the underlying malignancy. When an intraductal carcinoma alone is identified, the prognosis remains favorable, whereas patients with infiltrating ductal carcinoma metastatic to the regional lymph nodes have worse outcomes. Traditional treatment was total mastectomy and lymph node dissection, although breast conservation therapy with resection of the tumor and nipple–areolar complex, followed by whole breast radiation, is being performed in appropriately identified patients (122).

Inflammatory Carcinoma

Patients presenting with inflammatory carcinoma initially appear to have acute inflammation of the breast with corresponding redness and edema. Additional clinical findings are variable and range from complete absence of a dominant mass to the presence of either satellite skin nodules or a large palpable abnormality.

Inflammatory cancer, rather than infiltrating ductal carcinoma, should be diagnosed when more than one-third of the breast is involved with erythema and edema and when biopsy of the involved area, including the skin, demonstrates metastatic cancer in the subdermal lymphatics. Most of these tumors are poorly differentiated. Mammographically, the breast shows skin thickening with an infiltrative process and may or may not show a mass or calcifications.

Except for biopsy of the lesion to establish the diagnosis, surgery is not part of the initial management of inflammatory carcinoma. Mastectomy usually fails locally within 2 years of the initial diagnosis and does not improve overall or disease-free survival rates. Better results are achieved with a combination of chemotherapy and radiation therapy. Mastectomy may be indicated for patients who remain free of distant metastatic disease after initial chemotherapy and radiation (123).

In Situ Carcinomas

Both lobular and ductal carcinoma may be confined by the basement membrane of the ducts. These carcinomas do not invade the surrounding tissue and, theoretically, lack the ability to spread.

Lobular Carcinoma *In Situ*

Lobular carcinoma *in situ* should not be considered a true malignancy but rather a risk factor for the subsequent development of invasive ductal or lobular carcinoma in either breast (124). A more appropriate nomenclature for lobular carcinoma *in situ* may be lobular neoplasia. Most women with lobular carcinoma *in situ* are premenopausal and have neither clinical nor mammographic signs of an abnormality. The lesion typically is not a discrete mass, but rather a multifocal entity within one or both breasts incidentally discovered by the pathologist during the evaluation of a completely unrelated issue. Lobular carcinoma *in situ* usually is managed with an excisional biopsy followed by careful surveillance with clinical breast examinations and mammography. Occasionally, a patient may request either bilateral prophylactic mastectomy or *tamoxifen* for chemoprevention. Women with lobular carcinoma *in situ* have a 1% per year and up to a 30% lifetime risk of developing an invasive cancer.

An increasingly diagnosed subtype of LCIS that has more of a pleomorphic and florid appearance appears to act in a more aggressive manner similar to ductal carcinoma *in situ* (DCIS). In this instance, the lesions should be managed as DCIS with wide segmental mastectomy and radiation treatment (125).

Ductal Carcinoma *In Situ*

DCIS is more common in postmenopausal women. It may manifest as a palpable mass but usually is detected mammographically as a cluster of branched or Y-shaped pleomorphic microcalcifications. By definition, intraductal disease does not invade beyond the basement membrane. Unlike patients with LCIS, 30% to 50% of patients with DCIS will develop an invasive ductal cancer within the same breast if treated by excisional biopsy alone (126).

Although modified radical mastectomy was previously the standard treatment for intraductal carcinoma, more conservative surgery, with or without radiation therapy, yielded good results. In NSABP trial B17, 818 patients were randomly assigned to excision alone or excision followed by radiation therapy. The mean extent of DCIS lesions was 13 mm, and 88% were larger than 20 mm. All lesions were completely resected with negative margins. After a median follow-up of 43 months, the actuarial 5-year local recurrence rate was 10.4% without radiation versus 7.5% with radiation ($p = .055$) for noninvasive cancers, and 10.5% without radiation versus 2.9% with radiation ($p > .001$) for invasive cancers. Of 83 recurrences, only 9 (11%) were not in the index quadrant. A reanalysis with a mean follow-up of 90 months confirmed these results (127). These data suggest that segmental mastectomy offers excellent local control.

Axillary metastases occur in fewer than 5% of patients diagnosed with DCIS, making routine axillary dissection unnecessary. When axillary disease is identified, further evaluation of the breast or surgical specimen or both is warranted because nodal metastases indicate that an invasive ductal component was missed. Sentinel node biopsy may be offered to certain individuals with DCIS, especially if the lesion is high grade, contains comedonecrosis, or was diagnosed on core biopsy and has clinical or radiographic features suggesting invasive disease. About 5% of patients whose initial biopsy results show intraductal carcinoma will have infiltrating ductal carcinoma when treated with mastectomy, whereas core biopsy may underestimate the invasiveness of the disease in up to 20% of patients. The incidence of contralateral breast cancer in women with intraductal carcinoma is the same as in those with invasive ductal carcinoma (5% to 8%) (128).

Breast Cancer in Pregnancy

Breast cancer complicates 1 in 3,000 pregnancies (129,130). It is the second most common malignancy seen in association with pregnancy, surpassed only by cervical cancer. Initial studies suggested a significantly worse prognosis for patients first diagnosed during pregnancy, but data indicate that the hormonal changes associated with pregnancy seem to have little, if any, influence on prognosis. **When pregnant patients are matched stage for stage with nonpregnant patients, survival rates seem equivalent** (131). Patients typically present with a painless mass. Up to 60% will have concurrent lymph node involvement. The evaluation includes imaging with ultrasonography and mammography, which, although controversial, expose the fetus to less than 0.02 cGy of radiation when used with proper abdominal shielding (132). If biopsy is warranted, the procedure can be performed safely and should not be delayed until after delivery. Needle biopsy is safe and easily accomplished in the office setting.

The treatment of breast cancer in pregnant women must be highly individualized. Considerations include the patient's age and desire to continue the pregnancy. The overall prognosis should be considered, especially when axillary lymph nodes are involved, because adjuvant chemotherapy can be teratogenic or lethal to the fetus during the first trimester, but may be given later in the pregnancy. It is believed that interruption of pregnancy does not alter the prognosis for patients with potentially curable breast cancer.

Following are generalized recommendations for treatment of pregnant women with breast cancer:

1. **Traditionally, cancers diagnosed during the first or second trimester of pregnancy were treated with modified radical mastectomy.** Sentinel node biopsy remains a controversial procedure in pregnancy; the use of blue dye is contraindicated as it is classified as a pregnancy category C drug, and there are serious concerns about the risk of fetal irradiation with the use of radiocolloid despite some literature supporting its safety (133). Most centers do not offer breast conservation therapy based on the theory that radiation therapy should not be given to the gravid patient. In a patient diagnosed before the third trimester, waiting until after delivery may result in an unacceptable delay in the initiation of therapy and should not be encouraged. Adjuvant chemotherapy can be given after the first trimester, although many oncologists prefer not to give it to pregnant women outside of clinical trials. A classic study reported the risk of fetal malformations to be 20% during the first trimester, a rate that dropped to 1.5% during the second and third trimesters (134). *Tamoxifen*, however, is a class D drug and should not be given to pregnant or lactating patients with breast cancer.

2. **Localized tumors found during the third trimester of pregnancy can be managed with breast conservation therapy, with radiation delayed until after delivery, or with modified radical mastectomy.** Tumors should be excised early in the third trimester using local anesthesia. If delivery is imminent, standard therapy can be performed immediately postpartum. In the patient with a viable fetus, it may be preferable to induce early labor to avoid delaying definitive cancer therapy.

3. **If the breast cancer is diagnosed during lactation, lactation should be suppressed and the cancer should be treated definitively.**

4. **Advanced, incurable cancer should be treated with palliative therapy.** Decisions regarding continuation of the pregnancy should be based on the therapy necessary and the desires of the mother.

Counseling regarding future childbearing is important for women who have had carcinoma of the breast. It was assumed that subsequent pregnancies would be detrimental because of the high levels of circulating estrogens, but **there is no clear difference in survival for women who become pregnant after the diagnosis of breast cancer.** One study evaluated the effect of subsequent pregnancy on overall survival after the diagnosis of early-stage breast cancer. Approximately 40% of the women in the study had node-positive disease. The 5- and 10-year survival rates were better in women who became pregnant than in matched pair controls who did not. This study suggests that subsequent pregnancy does not adversely affect the prognosis of early-stage breast cancer (135). A subsequent investigation demonstrated no increase in the relative risk of death for patients who gave birth more than 10 months after their initial diagnosis of cancer (136). Theoretically, it may be that only women with estrogen receptor–positive or progesterone-positive tumors would be affected deleteriously by subsequent pregnancy, but this possibility has not been studied. Because recurrences are most frequent within the first 2 to 3 years after diagnosis, patients with receptor-positive tumors and advanced-stage disease probably should wait until after that time before becoming pregnant again.

References

1. **Siegel R, Ward E, Brawley O, et al.** Cancer statistics, 2011. *CA Cancer J Clin* 2011;61:212–236. http://cacancerjournal.org
2. **Anderson WF, Chu KC, Devesa SS.** Distinct incidence patterns among *in situ* and invasive breast carcinomas, with possible etiologic implications. *Breast Cancer Res Treat* 2004;88:149–159.
3. **American Cancer Society.** Breast cancer facts and figures 2010. Atlanta: American Cancer Society.
4. **Greene MH.** Genetics of breast cancer. *Mayo Clin Proc* 1997;72:54–65.
5. **FitzGerald MG, MacDonald DJ, Krainer M, et al.** Germ-line *BRCA1* mutations in Jewish and non-Jewish women with early-onset breast cancer. *N Engl J Med* 1996;334:143–149.
6. **US Preventative Services Task Force.** Genetic risk assessment and *BRCA* mutation testing for breast and ovarian cancer susceptibility: recommendation statement. *Ann Int Med* 2005;143:355–361.
7. **Domchek SM, Friebel TM, Singer CF, et al.** Association of risk-reducing surgery in *BRCA1* or *BRCA2* mutation carriers with cancer risk and mortality. *JAMA* 2010;304:967–975.
8. **Brennan SF, Cantwell MM, Cardwell CR, et al.** Dietary patterns and breast cancer risk: a systematic review and meta-analysis. *Am J Clin Nutr* 2010;91:1294–1302.
9. **Mattisson I, Wirfalt E, Wallstrom, et al.** High fat and alcohol intakes are risk factors of postmenopausal breast cancer: a prospective study from the Malmo diet and cancer cohort. *Int J Cancer* 2004;110:589–597.
10. **Chavez-MacGregor M, Elias SG, Onland-Moret NC, et al.** Postmenopausal breast cancer risk and cumulative number of menstrual cycles. *Cancer Epidemiol Biomarkers Prev* 2005;14:799–804.
11. **Eisen A, Rebbeck TR, Wood WC, et al.** Prophylactic surgery in women with a hereditary predisposition to breast and ovarian cancer. *J Clin Oncol* 2000;18:1980–1995.
12. **Russo J, Moral R, Balogh GA.** The protective role of pregnancy in breast cancer. *Breast Cancer Res* 2005;7:131–142.
13. **The Cancer and Steroid Hormone Study of the Centers for Disease Control and the National Institute of Child Health and Human Development.** Oral-contraceptive use and the risk of breast cancer. *N Engl J Med* 1986;315:405–411.
14. **Collaborative Group on Hormonal Factors in Breast Cancer.** Breast cancer and hormonal contraceptives: collaborative reanalysis of individual data on 53,297 women with breast cancer and 100,239 women without breast cancer from 54 epidemiological studies. *Lancet* 1996;347:1713–1727.
15. **Chlebowski RT, Hendrix SL, Langer RD, et al.** Influence of estrogen plus progestin on breast cancer and mammography in healthy postmenopausal women: the Women's Health Initiative Randomized Trial. *JAMA* 2003;289:3243–3253.
16. **Gao X, Fisher SG, Enami B.** Risk of second primary cancer in the contralateral breast in women treated for early-stage breast cancer: a population-based study. *Int J Radiat Oncol Biol Phys* 2003;56:1038–1045.
17. **Majid AS, de Paredes ES, Doherty RD, et al.** Missed breast carcinoma: pitfalls and pearls. *Radiographics* 2003;23:881–895.
18. **Bjurstam N, Bjorneld L, Duffy SW, et al.** The Gothenburg Breast Cancer Screening Trial: preliminary results on breast cancer mortality for women aged 39–49. *J Natl Cancer Inst Monogr* 1997;22:53–55.
19. **Smith RA, Cokkinides V, Brooks D, et al.** Cancer screening in the United States, 2010: a review of current American Cancer Society Guidelines and Issues in Cancer Screening. *CA Cancer J Clin* 2010;60:99–119.

20. **Bassett LW, Liu TH, Giuliano AE, et al.** The prevalence of carcinoma in palpable vs nonpalpable mammographically detected lesions. *Am J Roentgenol* 1991;157:21–24.
21. **Elmore JG, Armstrong K, Lehman CD, et al.** Screening for breast cancer. *JAMA* 2005;293:1245–1256.
22. **Collaco LM, de Lima RS, Werner B, et al.** Value of fine needle aspiration in the diagnosis of breast lesions. *Acta Cytol* 1999;43:587–592.
23. **Morrow M.** Breast. In: **Greenfield LJ, Mulholland MW, Oldham KT, et al., eds.** *Surgery: scientific principles and practice*. 3rd ed. Philadelphia, PA: Lippincott Williams & Wilkins, 2001:1334–1372.
24. **Arpino G, Bardou VJ, Clark GM, et al.** Infiltrating lobular carcinoma of the breast: tumor characteristics and clinical outcome. *Breast Cancer Res* 2004;6:R149–R156.
25. **Tubiana M, Pejovic JM, Renaud A, et al.** Kinetic parameters and the course of the disease in breast cancer. *Cancer* 1981;47:937–943.
26. **Perrone MA, Musolino A, Michiara M, et al.** Early detection of recurrences in the follow-up of primary breast cancer in an asymptomatic or symptomatic phase. *Tumori* 2004;90:276–279.
27. **Giuliano A.** The pattern of recurrence of early stage breast cancer. *J Surg Oncol* 1989;31:152–158.
28. **Haagensen CD.** *Diseases of the breast*. 3rd ed. Philadelphia, PA: WB Saunders, 1986.
29. **American Joint Committee on Cancer.** Breast. In: **Edge SB, Byrd DR, Compton CC, et al., eds.** *AJCC cancer staging manual*. 7th ed. New York: Springer, 2010:419–460.
30. **Barry MC, Thornton F, Murphy M, et al.** The value of metastatic screening in early primary breast cancer. *Ir J Med Sci* 1999;168:248–250.
31. **Morris PG, Lynch C, Feeney JN, et al.** Integrated positron emission tomography/computed tomography may render bone scintigraphy unnecessary to investigate suspected metastatic breast cancer. *J Clin Oncol* 2010;28:3154–3159.
32. **Halsted WS.** The results of radical operation for cure of carcinoma of the breast. *Ann Surg* 1907;46:1–19.
33. **Meyer W.** Carcinoma of the breast; ten years experience with my method of radical operation. *JAMA* 1905;45:297–313.
34. **Haagensen CD, Bodian C.** A personal experience with Halsted's radical mastectomy. *Ann Surg* 1984;199:143–150.
35. **Dahl-Iversen E, Tobiassen T.** Radical mastectomy with parasternal and supraclavicular dissection for mammary carcinoma. *Ann Surg* 1963;157:170–173.
36. **Lewis FJ.** Extended or super radical mastectomy for cancer of the breast. *Minn Med* 1953;36:763–766.
37. **Urban JA.** Extended radical mastectomy for breast cancer. *Ann Surg* 1963;106:399–404.
38. **Veronesi U, Valagussa P.** Inefficacy of internal mammary node dissection in breast cancer surgery. *Cancer* 1981;47:170–173.
39. **Handley RS.** The conservative radical mastectomy of Patey: 10-year results in 425 patients. *Breast* 1976;2:16–19.
40. **Maier WP, Leber D, Rosemond GP, et al.** The technique of modified radical mastectomy. *Surg Gynecol Obstet* 1977;145:68–74.
41. **Cody HS III, Laughlin EH, Trillo C, et al.** Have changing treatment patterns affected outcome of operable breast cancer? Ten year follow-up in 1288 patients, 1965 to 1978. *Ann Surg* 1991;213:297–307.
42. **Sacchini V, Pinotti JA, Barros AC.** Nipple-sparing mastectomy for breast cancer and risk reduction: oncologic or technical problem? *J Am Coll Surg* 2006;203:704–714.
43. **McWhirter R.** Should more radical treatment be attempted in breast cancer? *AJR Am J Roentgenol* 1964;92:3–13.

44. **Montague ED.** Radiation therapy and breast cancer: past, present and future. *Am J Clin Oncol* 1985;8:455–462.

45. **Montague ED, Fletcher GH.** The curative value of irradiation in the treatment of nondisseminated breast cancer. *Cancer* 1980;46:995–998.

46. **Wallgren A, Arner O, Bergstrom J, et al.** The value of preoperative radiotherapy in operable mammary carcinoma. *Int J Radiat Oncol Biol Phys* 1980;6:287–290.

47. **Nevin JE, Baggerly JT, Laird TK.** Radiotherapy as an adjuvant in the treatment of cancer of the breast. *Cancer* 1982;49:1194–1200.

48. **Fisher B, Jeong JH, Anderson S, et al.** Twenty-five-year follow-up of a randomized trial comparing radical mastectomy, total mastectomy, and total mastectomy followed by irradiation. *N Engl J Med* 2002;347:567–575.

49. **Overgaard M, Hansen P, Overgaard J, et al.** Postoperative radiotherapy in high-risk premenopausal women with breast cancer who receive adjuvant chemotherapy. *N Engl J Med* 1997;337:949–955.

50. **Ragaz J, Jackson SM, Le N, et al.** Adjuvant radiotherapy and chemotherapy in node-positive premenopausal women with breast cancer. *N Engl J Med* 1997;337:956–962.

51. **Overgaard M, Jensen MB, Overgaard J, et al.** Postoperative radiotherapy in high-risk postmenopausal breast cancer patients given adjuvant tamoxifen: Danish Breast Cancer Cooperative Group DBCG 82c randomised trial. *Lancet* 1999;353:1641–1648.

52. **Katz A, Strom EA, Buchholz TA, et al.** Locoregional recurrence patterns after mastectomy and doxorubicin-based chemotherapy: implications for postoperative irradiation. *J Clin Oncol* 2000;18:2817–2827.

53. **Woodward WA, Strom EA, Tucker SL, et al.** Locoregional recurrence after doxorubicin-based chemotherapy and postmastectomy: implications for breast cancer patients with early stage disease and predictors for recurrence after postmastectomy radiation. *Int J Radiat Oncol Biol Phys* 2003;57:336–344.

54. **Sharma R, Bedrosian I, Lucci A, et al.** Present-day locoregional control in patients with T1 or T2 breast cancer with 0 and 1 to 3 positive lymph nodes after mastectomy without radiotherapy. *Ann Surg* 2010;17:2899–2908.

55. **Clarke M, Collins R, Darby S, et al.** Effect of radiotherapy and of difference in the extent of surgery for early breast cancer on local recurrence and the 15 years survival: an overview of the randomised trials. *Lancet* 2005;9503:2087–2106.

56. **Recht A, Edge SB, Solin LJ, et al.** Postmastectomy radiotherapy: clinical practice guidelines of the American Society of Clinical Oncology. *J Clin Oncol* 2001;19:1539–1569.

57. **Keynes G.** Conservative treatment of cancer of the breast. *BMJ* 1937;2:643–647.

58. **Calle R, Pilleron JP, Schlienger P, et al.** Conservative management of operable breast cancer: ten years' experience at the Foundation Curie. *Cancer* 1978;42:2045–2053.

59. **Prosnitz LR, Goldenberg IS, Packard RA, et al.** Radiation therapy as initial treatment for early stage cancer of the breast without mastectomy. *Cancer* 1977;39:917–923.

60. **Harris JR, Hellman S, Silen W.** *Conservative management of breast cancer.* Philadelphia, PA: JB Lippincott, 1983.

61. **Veronesi U, Cascinelli N, Mariani L, et al.** Twenty-year follow-up of a randomized study comparing breast-conserving surgery with radical mastectomy for early breast cancer. *N Engl J Med* 2002;347:1227–1232.

62. **Fisher B, Anderson S, Bryant J, et al.** Twenty-year follow-up of a randomized trial comparing total mastectomy, lumpectomy, and lumpectomy plus irradiation for the treatment of invasive breast cancer. *N Engl J Med* 2002;347:1233–1241.

63. **Sarrazin D, Le MG, Arrigada R, et al.** Ten-year results of a randomized trial comparing a conservative treatment to mastectomy in early breast cancer. *Radiother Oncol* 1989;14:177–184.

64. **Jacobson JA, Danforth DN, Cowan KH, et al.** Ten-year results of a comparison of conservation with mastectomy in the treatment of stage I and II breast cancer. *N Engl J Med* 1995;332:907–911.

65. **van Dongen JA, Voogd AC, Fentiman IS, et al.** Long-term results of a randomized trial comparing breast-conserving therapy with mastectomy: European Organization for Research and Treatment of Cancer 10801 trial. *J Natl Cancer Inst* 2000;92:1143–1150.

66. **Truong PT, Berthelet E, Lee J, et al.** The prognostic significance of the percentage of positive/dissected axillary lymph nodes in breast cancer recurrence and survival in patients with one to three positive axillary lymph nodes. *Cancer* 2005;103:2006–2014.

67. **National Institutes of Health.** NIH consensus conference on the treatment of early-stage breast cancer. *JAMA* 1991;265:391–395.

68. **Ivens D, Hoe AL, Podd TJ, et al.** Assessment of morbidity from complete axillary dissection. *Br J Cancer* 1992;66:136–138.

69. **Goffman TE, Laronga C, Wilson L, et al.** Lymphedema of the arm and breast in irradiated breast cancer patients: risks in an era of dramatically changing axillary surgery. *Breast J* 2004;10:405–411.

70. **Gui GP, Joubert DJ, Reichert R, et al.** Continued axillary sampling is unnecessary and provides no further information to sentinel node biopsy in staging breast cancer. *Eur J Surg Oncol* 2005;31:707–714.

71. **Changsri C, Prakash S, Sandweiss L, et al.** Prediction of additional axillary metastasis of breast cancer following sentinel lymph node surgery. *Breast J* 2004;10:392–397.

72. **Giuliano AE, Kirgan DM, Guenther JM, et al.** Lymphatic mapping and sentinel lymphadenectomy for breast cancer. *Ann Surg* 1994;220:391–401.

73. **Wilson L, Giuliano A.** Sentinel lymph node mapping for primary breast cancer. *Curr Oncol Rep* 2005;7:12–17.

74. **Krag DN, Weaver DL, Alex JC, et al.** Surgical resection and radiolocalization of the sentinel lymph node in breast cancer using a gamma probe. *Surg Oncol* 1993;2:335–339.

75. **Veronesi U, Paganelli G, Galimberti V, et al.** Sentinel-node biopsy to avoid axillary dissection in breast cancer with clinically negative lymph-nodes. *Lancet* 1997;349:1864–1867.

76. **Giuliano AE, Haigh PI, Brennan MB, et al.** Prospective observational study of sentinel lymphadenectomy without further axillary dissection in patients with sentinel node-negative breast cancer. *J Clin Oncol* 2000;13:2553–2559.

77. **Veronesi U, Viale G, Paganelli G.** Sentinel lymph node biopsy in breast cancer: ten year results of a randomized controlled study. *Ann Surg* 2010;251:595–600.

78. **Giuliano AE, Hunt KK, Ballman KV, et al.** Axillary dissection vs. no axillary dissection in women with invasive breast cancer and sentinel node metastasis: a randomized clinical trial. *JAMA* 2011;305:569–575.

79. **Green MC, Hortobagyi GN.** Adjuvant chemotherapy for breast cancer. *Langenbecks Arch Surg* 2002;387:109–116.

80. **Murphy GP, Lawrence W, Lenhard RE, eds.** *American Cancer Society textbook of clinical oncology.* Atlanta, GA: American Cancer Society, 1995:213.

81. **Brezden C, Phillips KA, Abdolell M, et al.** Cognitive function in breast cancer patients receiving adjuvant chemotherapy. *J Clin Oncol* 2000;18:2695–2701.

82. **Paik S, Shak S, Tang G, et al.** A multigene assay to predict recurrence of tamoxifen-treated, node-negative breast cancer. *N Engl J Med* 2004;351:2817–2826.

83. **Rosen PP, Groshen S, Kinne DW, et al.** Factors influencing prognosis in node-negative breast carcinoma: analysis of 767 T1N0M0/T2N0M0 patients with long-term follow-up. *J Clin Oncol* 1993;11:2090–2100.

84. **Rapiti E, Fioretta G, Verkooigen HM, et al.** Survival of young and older breast cancer patients in Geneva from 1990 to 2001. *Eur J Cancer* 2005;41:1446–1452.

85. **Trudeau ME, Pritchard KI, Chapman JA, et al.** Prognostic factors affecting the natural history of node-negative breast cancer. *Breast Cancer Res Treat* 2005;89:35–45.

86. **Kollias J, Elston CW, Ellis IO, et al.** Early-onset breast cancer—histopathological and prognostic considerations. *Br J Cancer* 1997;75:1318–1323.

87. **Paik S, Bryant J, Park C, et al.** ErbB-2 and response to doxorubicin in patients with node-positive breast cancer. *J Natl Cancer Inst* 1998;90:1361–1370.

88. **Slamon DJ, Leyland-Jones B, Shak S, et al.** Use of chemotherapy plus a monoclonal antibody against *HER2* for metastatic breast cancer that overexpresses HER2. *N Engl J Med* 2001;344:783–792.

89. **Romond E, Perez E, Bryant J, et al.** Trastuzumab plus adjuvant chemotherapy for operable HER2-positive breast cancer. *N Engl J Med* 2005;353:1673–1684.

90. **Smith I, Procter M, Gelber RD, et al.** HERA study team. 2-year follow-up of trastuzumab after adjuvant chemotherapy in

HER2-positive breast cancer: a randomised controlled trial. *Lancet* 2007;369:29–36.

91. **Piccart-Gebhart MJ, Procter M, Leyland-Jones B.** Trastuzumab after adjuvant chemotherapy in *HER2*-positive breast cancer. *N Engl J Med* 2005;353:1659–1672.

92. **Nissen-Meyer R.** The Scandinavian clinical trials. *Experientia Suppl* 1982;41:571–579.

93. **Bonadonna G, Valagussa P.** Adjuvant systemic therapy for resectable breast cancer. *J Clin Oncol* 1985;3:259–275.

94. **Fisher B, Carbone P, Economou SG, et al.** L-phenylalanine mustard in the management of primary breast cancer: a report of early findings. *N Engl J Med* 1975;292:117–122.

95. **Mueller CB, Lesperance ML.** NSABP trials of adjuvant chemotherapy for breast cancer: a further look at the evidence. *Ann Surg* 1991;214:206–211.

96. **Bonadonna G, Rossi A, Valagussa P.** Adjuvant CMF chemotherapy in operable breast cancer: ten years later. *World J Surg* 1985;9:707–713.

97. **Tancine G, Bonadonna G, Valagussa P, et al.** Adjuvant CMF in breast cancer: comparative 5-year results of 12 versus 6 cycles. *J Clin Oncol* 1983;1:2–10.

98. **Bonadonna G, Valagussa P.** Dose-response effect of adjuvant chemotherapy in breast cancer. *N Engl J Med* 1981;304:10–15.

99. **Bonadonna G, Valagussa P, Moliterni A, et al.** Adjuvant cyclophosphamide, methotrexate, and fluorouracil in node-positive breast cancer: the results of 20 years of follow-up. *N Engl J Med* 1995;332:901–906.

100. **Zambetti M, Valagussa P, Bonadonna G.** Adjuvant CMF in node-negative and estrogen receptor negative breast cancer: updated results. *Ann Oncol* 1996;7:481–485.

101. **Fisher B, Brown AM, Dimitrov NV, et al.** Two months of doxorubicin-cyclophosphamide with and without interval reinduction therapy compared with 6 months of cyclophosphamide, methotrexate, and fluorouracil in positive-node breast cancer patients with tamoxifen-nonresponsive tumors: results from the National Surgical Adjuvant Breast and Bowel Project B-15. *J Clin Oncol* 1990;8:1483–1496.

102. **Henderson IC, Berry DA, Demetri GD, et al.** Improved outcomes from adding sequential paclitaxel but not from escalating doxorubicin dose in an adjuvant chemotherapy regimen for patients with node positive primary breast cancer. *J Clin Oncol* 2003;21:976–983.

103. **Jones S, Holmes FA, O'Shaughnessy J, et al.** Docetaxel with cyclophosphamide is associated with an overall survival benefit compared with doxorubicin and cyclophosphamide:7 year follow-up of US Oncology Research Trial 9735. *J Clin Oncol* 2009;27:1177–1183.

104. **Saurel CA, Patel TA, Perez EA.** Changes to adjuvant systemic therapy in breast cancer: a decade in review. *Clin Breast Cancer* 2010;10:196–208.

105. **Trudeau M, Sinclair SE, Clemons M, et al.** Neoadjuvant taxanes in the treatment of non-metastatic breast cancer: a systemic review. *Cancer Treat Rev* 2005;31:283–302.

106. **Chen AM, Meric-Berstam F, Hunt KK, et al.** Breast conservation after neoadjuvant chemotherapy. *Cancer* 2005;103:689–695.

107. **Early Breast Cancer Trialists' Collaborative Group.** Polychemotherapy for early breast cancer: an overview of the randomised trials. *Lancet* 1998;352:930–942.

108. **Albain K, Green S, Ravdin P, et al.** Overall survival after cyclophosphamide, adriamycin, 5-FU, and tamoxifen is superior to tamoxifen alone in post-menopausal, receptor(+), node(+) breast cancer: new findings from phase III Southwest Oncology Group Intergroup Trial S8814 (INT-0100). *Proc Am Soc Clin Oncol* 2001;20:94(abst).

109. **Fisher B, Digman J, Wolmark N, et al.** Tamoxifen and chemotherapy for lymph node-negative, estrogen receptor–positive breast cancer. *J Natl Cancer Inst* 1997;89:1673–1682.

110. **Howell A, Cuzick J, Baum M, et al.** Results of the ATAC (Arimidex, tamoxifen, alone or in combination) trial after completion of 5 years' adjuvant treatment for breast cancer. *Lancet* 2005;365:60–62.

111. **Dowsett M, Cuzick J, Ingle J, et al.** Meta-analysis of breast cancer outcomes in adjuvant trials of aromatase inhibitors versus tamoxifen. *J Clin Oncol* 2010;28:509–518.

112. **Goss PE, Ingle JN, Martino S, et al.** A randomized trial of letrozole in postmenopausal women after five years of tamoxifen therapy for early-stage breast cancer. *N Engl J Med* 2003;349:1793–1802.

113. **Winer EP, Morrow M, Osborne CK, et al.** Malignant tumors of the breast. In: **Devita VT, Hellman S, Rosenberg S, eds. Cancer principles and practice of oncology.** 6th ed. Philadelphia, PA: Lippincott Williams & Wilkins, 2001:1651–1717.

114. **Early Breast Cancer Trialists' Collaborative Group.** Effects of chemotherapy and hormonal therapy for early breast cancer on recurrence and 15-year survival: an overview of the randomised trials. *Lancet* 2005;365:1687–1717.

115. **Early Breast Cancer Trialists' Collaborative Group.** Adjuvant chemotherapy in oestrogen-receptor-poor breast cancer: patient-level meta-analysis of randomised trials. *Lancet* 2008;371:29–40.

116. **Dhodapkar MV, Ingle JN, Cha SS, et al.** Prognostic factors in elderly women with metastatic breast cancer treated with tamoxifen: an analysis of patients entered on four prospective clinical trials. *Cancer* 1996;77:683–690.

117. **Valero V.** Combination docetaxel/cyclophosphamide in patients with advanced solid tumors. *Oncology* 1997;11:34–36.

118. **Burstein HJ, Keshaviah A, Baron AD.** Trastuzumab plus vinorelbine or taxane chemotherapy for HER2-overexpressing metastatic breast cancer: the trastuzumab and vinorelbine or taxane study. *Cancer* 2007;110:965–972.

119. **Rosen LS, Gordon D, Kaminski M, et al.** Long-term efficacy and safety of zoledronic acid compared with pamidronate disodium in the treatment of skeletal complications in patients with advanced multiple myeloma or breast carcinoma: a randomized, double-blind, multicenter, comparative trial. *Cancer* 2003;98:1735–1744.

120. **Pavlakis B, Scmidt RL, Stockier M.** Bisphosphonates for breast cancer. *Cochrane Database Syst Rev* 2005;3:CD003474.

121. **Paget J.** Disease of the mammary areola preceding cancer of the mammary gland. *St Barts Hosp Rep* 1874;10:89.

122. **Pezzi CM, Kukora JS, Audet IM, et al.** Breast conservation surgery using nipple-areolar resection for central breast cancers. *Arch Surg* 2004;139:32–37.

123. **Barnes DM, Newman L.** Pregnancy-associated breast cancer: a literature review. *Surg Clin North Am* 2007;87:417–430.

124. **Simpson PT, Gale T, Fulford LG, et al.** The diagnosis and management of pre-invasive breast disease: pathology of atypical lobular hyperplasia and lobular carcinoma *in situ*. *Breast Cancer Res* 2003;5:258–262.

125. **Barth A, Brenner RJ, Giuliano AE.** Current management of ductal carcinoma *in situ*. *West J Med* 1995;163:360–366.

126. **Sneige N, Wang J, Baker BA, et al.** Clinical, histopathologic, and biologic features of pleomorphic lobular (ductal-lobular) carcinoma *in situ* of the breast: a report of 24 cases. *Mod Pathol* 2002;15:1044–1050.

127. **Fisher B, Dignam J, Wolmark N, et al.** Lumpectomy and radiation therapy for the treatment of intraductal breast cancer: findings from the National Surgical Adjuvant Breast and Bowel Project B-17. *J Clin Oncol* 1998;16:441–452.

128. **Claus EB, Stowe M, Carter D, et al.** The risk of contralateral breast cancer among women diagnosed with ductal and lobular breast carcinoma *in situ*: data from the Connecticut Tumor Registry. *Breast* 2003;12:451–456.

129. **Psyrri A, Burtness B.** Pregnancy-associated breast cancer. *Cancer J* 2005;11:83–95.

130. **Partridge A, Schapira L.** Pregnancy and breast cancer: epidemiology, treatment, and safety issues. *Oncology* 2005;19:693–697.

131. **Petrek JA.** Breast cancer and pregnancy. *J Natl Cancer Inst Monogr* 1994;16:113–121.

132. **Rosene-Montella K, Larson L.** Diagnostic imaging. In: **Lee RV, Rosene-Montella K, Barbour A, et al. eds.,** *Medical care of the pregnant patient.* Philadelphia, PA: American College of Physicians Press, 2000:103–115.

133. **Bodner-Adler B, Bodner K, Zeisler H.** Breast cancer diagnosed during pregnancy. *Anticancer Res* 2007;27:1705–1707.

134. **Gentilini O, Cremonesi M, Toesca A, et al.** Sentinel lymph node biopsy in pregnant patients with breast cancer. *Eur J Nucl Med Mol Imaging* 2010;37:78–83.

135. **Gelber S, Coates A, Goldhirsch A, et al.** Effect of pregnancy on overall survival after the diagnosis of early stage breast cancer. *J Clin Oncol* 2001;19:1671–1675.

136. **Mueller BA, Simon MS, Deapen D, et al.** Childbearing and survival after breast carcinoma in young women. *Cancer* 2003;98:1131–1140.

Index

Note: Page number followed by f and t indicates figure and table respectively.

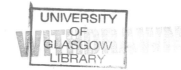